BENUMOF'S AIRWAY MANAGEMENT

BENUMOF'S AIRWAY MANAGEMENT

PRINCIPLES AND PRACTICE

SECOND EDITION

Edited by

Carin A. Hagberg, MD

Professor of Anesthesiology
University of Texas Medical School at Houston
Director, Neuroanesthesia and Advanced Airway Management
Memorial Hermann Hospital
Houston, Texas

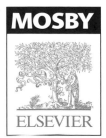

MOSBY

ELSEVIER

1600 John F. Kennedy Blvd.
Ste 1800
Philadelphia, PA 19103-2899

Benumof's Airway Management: Principles and Practice

ISBN-13: 978-0-323-02233-0
ISBN-10: 0-323-02233-2

Library of Congress Cataloging-in-Publication Data

Benumof's airway management : principles and practice / [edited by] Carin A. Hagberg.
--2nd ed.
    p. cm.
Rev. ed. of Airway management. 1996.
ISBN 0-323-02233-2
  1. Airway (Medicine). 2. Respiratory therapy. 3. Anesthesia. 4. Trachea--Intubation.
I. Benumof, Jonathan. II. Hagberg, Carin A.
RC735.I5A396 2006
616.2--dc22

2006044890

Acquisitions Editor: Natasha Andjelkovic
Publishing Services Manager: Tina Rebane
Project Manager: Norm Stellander
Design Direction: Gene Harris

Printed in the United States

Last digit is the print number: 9 8 7 6 5 4 3 2 1

DEDICATION

Dedicated to my family in gratitude for their enthusiastic support and to the readers who will greatly benefit from the contents of this book.

CONTRIBUTORS

Felice E. Agro, MD
Professor and Chairman,
Department of Anesthesiology and Intensive Care,
University School of Medicine,
Campus BioMedico, Rome, Italy

Anis Baraka, MD, FRCA (Hon)
Professor and Chairman,
Department of Anesthesiology,
American University of Beirut School of Medicine,
American University of Beirut Medical Center,
Beirut, Lebanon

Robert F. Bedford, MD
Professor, Department of Anesthesiology,
University of Virginia School of Medicine;
Attending Anesthesiologist,
University of Virginia Health System,
Charlottesville, Virginia

Elizabeth C. Behringer, MD
Clinical Professor of Anesthesiology and Surgery,
Director of Fellowship in Critical Care Medicine,
Department of Anesthesiology,
University of California, Irvine,
Orange, California

Jacqueline A. Bello, MD
Clinical Professor and Director,
Division of Neuroradiology, Department of Radiology;
Clinical Professor,
The Leo M. Davidoff
Department of Neurological Surgery,
Albert Einstein College of Medicine of Yeshiva University,
Montefiore Medical Center,
Bronx, New York

Jonathan L. Benumof, MD
Professor, Department of Anesthesiology,
University of California, San Diego,
San Diego, California

James M. Berry, MD
Professor of Anesthesiology,
Director of Multispecialty Anesthesia,
Department of Anesthesiology,
Vanderbilt University;
Medical Director of Operating Rooms,
Vanderbilt University Hospital,
Nashville, Tennessee

Nasir I. Bhatti, MD
Assistant Professor of Head and Neck Surgery,
Department of Otolaryngology,
Johns Hopkins University School of Medicine;
Director, Percutaneous Tracheostomy Service,
Johns Hopkins Hospital,
Baltimore, Maryland

Michael J. Bishop, MD
Professor and Director, Department of Anesthesiology,
Adjunct Professor of Medicine,
University of Washington;
Attending Physician,
University of Washington Medical Center,
Veteran Affairs Puget Sound Health System,
Seattle, Washington

Archie I. J. Brain, MD, LMSSA, FFARCS
Honorary Research Fellow,
Institute of Laryngology, University of London;
Honorary Consultant, Department of Anaesthesia,
Royal Berkshire Hospital,
Reading, Berkshire, United Kingdom

Roy D. Cane, MB, BCh, FCCM

Professor Emeritus,
Department of Anesthesiology,
Northwestern University Medical School,
Chicago, Illinois

Robert A. Caplan, MD

Clinical Professor, Department of Anesthesiology,
University of Washington School of Medicine;
Director of Quality, Department of Anesthesiology,
Virginia Mason Medical Center,
Seattle, Washington

Jacques E. Chelly, MD, PhD, MBA

Professor and Vice Chair for Clinical Research,
Department of Anesthesiology, and
Professor of Orthpedic Surgery,
University of Pittsburgh School of Medicine;
Director of Orthopedic Anesthesia Acute Interventional
Postoperative Pain, Shadyside Hospital,
University of Pittsburgh Medical Center,
Pittsburgh, Pennsylvania

T. Linda Chi, MD

Associate Professor, Diagnostic Radiology,
The University of Texas MD Anderson Cancer Center;
Neuroradiologist,
Southwest Radiology Associates,
Houston, Texas

Chris C. Christodoulou, MD

Assistant Professor of Anesthesia,
University of Manitoba;
Anesthetist, Department of Anesthesia and
Perioperative Medicine,
St. Boniface General Hospital,
Winnipeg, Manitoba, Canada

Neal H. Cohen, MD, MPH, MS

Professor of Anesthesia and Medicine,
Vice Dean, Academic Affairs,
University of California, San Francisco, Medical School,
San Francisco, California

Tim M. Cook, MD

Consultant Anaesthetist,
Department of Anaesthesia,
Royal United Hospital,
Combe Park, Bath, United Kingdom

Richard M. Cooper, MD, BSc, MSc, FRCPC

Professor of Anesthesiology,
University of Toronto;
Anesthesiologist, Toronto General Hospital,
Toronto, Ontario, Canada

Edward T. Crosby, MD, BSc, FRCPC

Professor, Department of Anesthesiology,
University of Ottawa,
Ottawa Hospital,
Ottawa, Ontario, Canada

Steven A. Deem, MD

Associate Professor of Anesthesiology and Medicine,
Pulmonary and Critical Care,
University of Washington;
Co-Director, Neurosurgical Intensive Care Unit,
Associate Medical Director, Respiratory Care,
Harborview Medical Center,
Seattle, Washington

Stephen F. Dierdorf, MD

Professor of Anesthesiology and
Perioperative Medicine,
Medical University of South Carolina,
Charleston, South Carolina

D. John Doyle, MD, PhD, FRCPC

Staff Anesthesiologist,
Department of General Anesthesiology,
Cleveland Clinic Foundation,
Cleveland, Ohio

Tiberiu Ezri, MD

Senior Lecturer,
Tel Aviv University;
Director, Department of Anesthesia,
Wolfson Medical Center,
Sackler School of Medicine,
Tel Aviv, Israel

David Z. Ferson, MD

Professor and Director of Neuroanesthesia,
Department of Anesthesiology and Pain Medicine,
The University of Texas MD Anderson Cancer Center,
Houston, Texas

Lorraine J. Foley, MD

Clinical Assistant Professor of Anesthesia,
Tufts School of Medicine,
Boston, Massachusetts;
Anesthesiologist, Winchester Hospital,
Winchester, Massachusetts

Michael Frass, MD

Professor of Medicine,
Department of Internal Medicine,
Head of Intensive Care Unit,
Medical University of Vienna,
Vienna, Austria

Rainer Georgi, MD

Department of Anesthesia and
Operative Intensive Care,
Katharinen Hospital,
Stuttgart, Germany

Michael A. Gibbs, MD

Chief,
Department of Emergency Medicine,
Maine Medical Center,
Portland, Maine

David Goldenberg, MD

Associate Professor,
Head and Neck Surgery,
Department of Otolaryngology,
Milton S. Hershey Medical Center,
Penn State College of Medicine,
Hershey, Pennsylvania

Carin A. Hagberg, MD

Professor, Department of Anesthesiology,
University of Texas Medical School at Houston;
Director of Neuroanesthesia and
Advanced Airway Management,
Memorial Hermann Hospital,
Houston, Texas

Gregory B. Hammer, MD

Professor of Anesthesiology and Pediatrics,
Stanford University School of Medicine,
Stanford, California;
Associate Director, Pediatric Intensive Care Unit,
Lucile Packard Children's Hospital,
Palo Alto, California

Amy C. Hessel, MD

Assistant Professor of Head and Neck Surgery,
Associate Director of Head and Neck Fellowship,
University of Texas MD Anderson Cancer Center,
Houston, Texas

Orlando R. Hung, MD, BSc, FRCP

Professor, Departments of Anesthesia,
Surgery, and Pharmacology,
Queen Elizabeth II Health Sciences Centre,
Dalhousie University,
Halifax, Nova Scotia, Canada

Raj R. Iyer, MD, RPh

Head, Division of Cardiac Anesthesia,
Department of Anesthesiology,
Rush-Copley Medical Center,
Aurora, Illinois

Robert M. Kacmarek, PhD, RRT

Professor of Anesthesiology,
Harvard Medical School;
Director, Department of Respiratory Care,
Massachusetts General Hospital,
Boston, Massachusetts

P. Allan Klock, Jr., MD

Associate Professor and
Associate Chair for Clinical Affairs,
Department of Anesthesia and Critical Care,
University of Chicago,
Chicago, Illinois

Stephen M. Koch, MD

Associate Professor,
Department of Anesthesiology,
University of Texas Medical School at Houston,
Houston, Texas

Karen M. Kost, MDCM, FRCSC

Associate Professor of Head and Neck Surgery,
Department of Otolaryngology, and
Director of Voice Laboratory,
McGill University;
Director of Otolaryngology,
Montreal General Hospital,
Montreal, Quebec, Canada

Peter Krafft, MD, PhD

Professor,
Department of Anesthesiology and
Intensive Care Medicine,
Medical University of Vienna,
Vienna, Austria

David C. Kramer, MD

Assistant Professor of Anesthesiology,
Associate Director of Neuroanesthesia,
Mount Sinai School of Medicine,
New York, New York

Claude Krier, MD

Professor of Anesthesiology and
Medical Director,
Katharinen Hospital,
Stuttgart, Germany

Robert G. Krohner, DO

Associate Professor, Department of Anesthesiology,
University of Pittsburgh School of Medicine;
Staff Anesthesiologist, Residency Director,
Magee-Women's Hospital,
University of Pittsburgh Medical Center,
Pittsburgh, Pennsylvania

J. Adam Law, MD, BSc, FRCPC

Associate Professor,
Departments of Anesthesia and Surgery,
Dalhousie University;
Attending Anesthesiologist,
Queen Elizabeth II Health Sciences Centre,
Halifax, Nova Scotia, Canada

Stephen R. Luney, MB, BCh, BAO

Consultant Neuroanaesthetist,
Department of Clinical Anaesthesia,
Royal Victoria Hospital,
Belfast, United Kingdom

Atul Malhotra, MD, FRCPC

Assistant Professor of Medicine,
Harvard Medical School;
Attending Physician, Brigham and Women's Hospital,
Beth Israel Deaconess Medical Center,
Boston, Massachusetts

Lynette Mark, MD

Associate Professor,
Department of Anesthesiology and
Critical Care Medicine,
Johns Hopkins Medical Institutions,
Baltimore, Maryland

John P. McGee II, MD, MS

Assistant Professor of Clinical Anesthesia,
Feinberg School of Medicine, Northwestern University,
Chicago, Illinios;
Senior Attending Anesthesiologist,
Evanston Northwestern Healthcare,
Evanston, Illinois

Richard J. Melker, MD, PhD, MS

Professor of Anesthesiology,
Pediatrics and Biomedical Engineering,
University of Florida College of Medicine,
Gainesville, Florida

James Michelson, MD

Professor, Department of Orthopedic Surgery,
Director of Clinical Informatics,
The George Washington University School of
Medicine and Health Sciences,
Washington, DC

David Mirsky, MD

Division of Neuroradiology,
Department of Radiology,
Albert Einstein College of Medicine of Yeshiva University,
Montefiore Medical Center,
Bronx, New York

Ian R. Morris, MD, FRCPC, FACEP

Professor, Department of Anesthesia,
Dalhousie University;
Chief, Thoracic Anesthesia
and Liver Transplantation Anesthesia,
Department of Anesthesia,
Queen Elizabeth II Health Sciences Centre,
Halifax, Nova Scotia, Canada

Debra E. Morrison, MD

Director of Preoperative Services,
Department of Anesthesiology,
University of California, Irvine,
Orange, California

Uma Munnur, MD

Assistant Professor,
Department of Anesthesiology,
Baylor College of Medicine,
Houston, Texas

Michael F. Murphy, MD

Professor and Chair,
Department of Anesthesia,
Professor of Emergency Medicine,
Dalhousie University,
Halifax, Nova Scotia, Canada

Kevin F. O'Grady, MD, BASc, MHSc, FRCSC

Staff Plastic Surgeon,
York Central Hospital,
Richmond Hill, Ontario, Canada

Irene P. Osborn, MD

Associate Professor,
Department of Anesthesiology,
Director of Neuroanesthesia,
Mount Sinai School of Medicine,
New York, New York

Andranik Ovassapian, MD

Professor,
Department of Anesthesiology and Critical Care,
University of Chicago,
Chicago, Illinois

Donald H. Parks, MD, FRCSC, FACS

Professor and Director,
Department of Plastic and Reconstructive Surgery,
University of Texas Medical School at Houston;
Medical Director, John S. Dunn Sr. Burn Center, and
Chief of Plastic and Reconstructive Surgery,
Memorial Hermann Hospital,
Houston, Texas

C. Lee Parmley, MD, JD

Professor and Director,
Department of Anesthesiology,
Division of Critical Care Medicine,
Vanderbilt University Medical Center,
Nashville, Tennessee

Kevin D. Pereira, MD, MS

Professor and Vice Chairman
Department of Otolaryngology,
The University of Texas Medical School at Houston;
Chief of Pediatric Otolaryngology,
Memorial Hermann Children's Hospital,
Houston, Texas

Karen L. Posner, PhD

Research Professor,
Department of Anesthesiology,
University of Washington,
Seattle, Washington

Robert M. Pousman, DO

Associate Professor,
Department of Anesthesiology,
David Geffen School of Medicine,
University of California, Los Angeles;
Director of Surgical Intensive Care Unit,
West Los Angeles Veteran Affairs,
Los Angeles, California

Mary F. Rabb, MD

Associate Professor and Residency Director,
Department of Anesthesiology,
The University of Texas School of Medicine;
Director of Pediatric Anesthesia,
Memorial Hermann Hospital,
Houston, Texas

Sivam Ramanathan, MD

Professor Emeritus,
University of Pittsburgh School of Medicine,
Pittsburgh, Pennsylvania; Attending Physician,
Cedars-Sinai Medical Center,
Los Angeles, California

Allan P. Reed, MD

Associate Professor,
Department of Anesthesiology,
Mount Sinai School of Medicine,
New York, New York

William H. Rosenblatt, MD

Professor,
Department of Anesthesiology,
Yale University School of Medicine,
New Haven, Connecticut

M. Ramez Salem, MD

Clinical Professor of Anesthesiology,
University of Illinois College of Medicine;
Chairman, Department of Anesthesiology,
Advocate Illinois Masonic Medical Center,
Chicago, Illinois

Antonio Sanchez, MD

Associate Clinical Professor,
Department of Anesthesiology,
University of California, Irvine,
Orange, California;
Staff Anesthesiologist,
Kaiser Permanente Baldwin Park Medical Center,
Baldwin Park, California

John J. Schaefer III, MD

Professor of Anesthesiology and Preoperative Medicine,
Medical University of South Carolina,
Charleston, South Carolina

Bettina U. Schmitz, MD, PhD

Assistant Professor of Anesthesiology,
Texas Tech University Medical School;
Director of Regional Pain Service,
University Medical Center,
Lubbock, Texas

David E. Schwartz, MD, FCCM

Professor of Anesthesiology,
Director of Critical Care Medicine,
University of Illinois College of Medicine,
Chicago, Illinois

Roy Sheinbaum, MD

Associate Professor,
Department of Anesthesiology,
University of Texas Medical School at Houston;
Director of Cardiovascular Anesthesia,
Memorial Hermann Hospital,
Houston, Texas

George J. Sheplock, MD

Associate Professor,
Department of Anesthesia and Critical Care,
Indiana University School of Medicine,
Riley Hospital for Children,
Indianapolis, Indiana

Ronald D. Stewart, MD, OC, FACEP

Professor,
Department of Community Health and Epidemiology,
Dalhousie University,
Halifax, Nova Scotia, Canada

Robert K. Stoelting, MD

Professor, Department of Anesthesiology,
Indiana University School of Medicine;
President, Anesthesia Patient Safety Foundation,
Indianapolis, Indiana

Maya S. Suresh, MB, BS

Professor, Department of Anesthesiology;
Chief, Obstetric and Gynecological Anesthesia,
Baylor College of Medicine,
Houston, Texas

Peter Szmuk, MD

Associate Professor,
Department of Anesthesiology,
University of Texas Southwestern Medical School;
Attending Anesthesiologist,
Children's Medical Center of Dallas,
Dallas, Texas

Joseph W. Szokol, MD

Associate Professor, Department of Anesthesiology,
Feinberg School of Medicine, Northwestern University,
Chicago, Illinois;
Vice Chairman, Department of Anesthesiology,
Evanston Northwestern Healthcare,
Evanston, Illinios

Mark D. Tasch, MD

Associate Professor, Department of Anesthesiology,
Indiana University School of Medicine,
Indianapolis, Indiana

Andreas R. Thierbach, MD

Senior Lecturer and Director,
Department of Anesthesiology and
Intensive Care Medicine,
Johannes Gutenberg University of Mainz,
Mainz, Germany

Ricardo M. Urtubia, MD

Anesthesiologist,
Intensive Care and Anesthesia Unit,
Mutual de Seguridad Hospital CCHC,
Santiago, Chile

Jeffrey S. Vender, MD, FCCM

Professor and Associate Chairman,
Department of Anesthesiology,
Feinberg School of Medicine, Northwestern University,
Chicago, Illinois;
Chairman, Department of Anesthesiology,
Director, Medical-Surgical ICU,
Evanston Northwestern Healthcare,
Evanston, Illinois

Robert J. Vissers, MD, FACEP, FRCPC

Adjunct Associate Professor of Medicine,
Oregon Health and Sciences University;
Medical Director, Emergency Department,
Legacy Emanuel Hospital;
Director of Education,
Northwest Acute Care Specialists,
Portland, Oregon

Ashutosh Wali, MD, FFARCSI

Associate Professor,
Department of Anesthesiology,
Baylor College of Medicine,
Houston, Texas

Ron M. Walls, MD, FRCPC, FACEP

Professor of Medicine,
Division of Emergency Medicine,
Harvard Medical School;
Chairman, Department of Emergency Medicine,
Brigham and Women's Hospital,
Boston, Massachusetts

David O. Warner, MD

Professor of Anesthesiology,
Mayo Clinic College of Medicine,
Rochester, Minnesota

R. David Warters, MD

Professor,
Department of Anesthesia and Perioperative Medicine,
Medical University of South Carolina;
Chief of Anesthesiology,
Ralph H. Johnson Medical Center,
Charleston, South Carolina

Melissa Wheeler, MD

Chief of Anesthesiology,
Shriners Hospitals for Children,
Chicago, Illinois

William C. Wilson, MD

Clinical Professor,
Anesthesiology and Critical Care Medicine,
University of California, San Diego;
Associate Director, Surgical Intensive Care Unit,
and Director, Anesthesiology and Critical Care,
University of California, San Diego, Medical Center,
San Diego, California

PREFACE

This second edition of *Benumof's Airway Management* is published 10 years after the first edition appeared in 1996. Since publication of the first edition, the practice of airway management has experienced many new innovations. As a reflection of these changes, several chapters have been added and many new authors have been recruited whose experience and expertise in certain areas have emerged in the past decade. Although several chapters have been removed, all the material retained from the first edition was updated to reflect the state of anesthesia practice in the new millennium. There is liberal use of illustrations, lists, and tables to reinforce written materials. As with the first edition, the goal and purpose of this book is to encompass and clearly present the knowledge and forethought that will allow the clinician to avoid airway complications and solve airway problems.

This in-depth, highly referenced textbook is intended to be a resource that is divided into seven parts. The first section (Chapters 1-6) provides basic clinical science considerations of airway management. The second section (Chapters 7-9) presents difficult airway terminology and recognition, as well as the latest version of the American Society of Anesthesiologists' Difficult Airway Algorithm. The third section (Chapters 10-12) emphasizes patient preparation and preintubation ventilation procedures. The fourth section (Chapters 13-30) covers specific methods and problems in securing an airway.

New airway devices and techniques are reviewed. It also provides the indications for and confirmation of tracheal intubation. The fifth section (31-43) covers management of difficult airway situations, such as the difficult airway in conventional head and neck surgery, as well as neurosurgery. The sixth section (Chapters 44-48) emphasizes postintubation procedures and discusses issues such as endotracheal tube and respiratory care and complications of managing the airway. Lastly, the seventh section (Chapters 49-53) presents societal considerations of airway management, including instruction and learning of airway management skills, both in and out of the operating room, as well as effective dissemination of critical airway information and medical-legal considerations.

Management of the difficult airway remains one of the most relevant and challenging tasks for all those involved in airway management. The diversity of this textbook should provide greater insight into airway problems and strengthen the clinician's understanding of the airway by contributing to the general knowledge and safe practice of airway management, both in and out of the hospital setting. Future research will uncover even different options and cause new attitudes to emerge, as the practice of airway management is evolving and we, as practitioners, must evolve with it.

Carin A. Hagberg, MD

ACKNOWLEDGMENTS

I would like to sincerely acknowledge the scholarly efforts of the individual contributors, consisting of expert anesthesiologists, emergency room specialists, surgeons, radiologists and basic scientists, each examining the airway from a different perspective. The success of any multiauthored text is dependent on the expertise and dedication of the contributors. It is both an honor and privilege to have worked with all of the authors and present this book to the medical community at large.

I would also like to recognize the invaluable efforts of Dawn Iannucci, my research assistant, who went well beyond the call of duty with her organizational and secretarial contributions. In addition, I am very appreciative and want to recognize the support of Elsevier in the preparation of this second edition of *Benumof's Airway Management*. In particular, I am grateful to Natasha Andjelkovic.

I am especially indebted to three wonderful mentors whom I admire and respect: Jon Benumof, M.D., who launched my interest in this area of clinical practice and gave me the opportunity to edit this book, Andranik Ovassapian, M.D., a great teacher, for his enthusiastic encouragement, guidance and wisdom, and Jacques Chelly, M.D., Ph.D., M.B.A., a close friend, for his endless willingness to listen and for believing so passionately that I will succeed in my endeavors. Finally, I am grateful to my father, John Hagberg, whose integrity, humility, and love has made an incredible impression in my life, and to my wonderful husband, Steven Roberts, for his patience and support through the many hours that went into editing this book.

CONTENTS

Section V
DIFFICULT AIRWAY SITUATIONS

BASIC CLINICAL SCIENCE CONSIDERATIONS

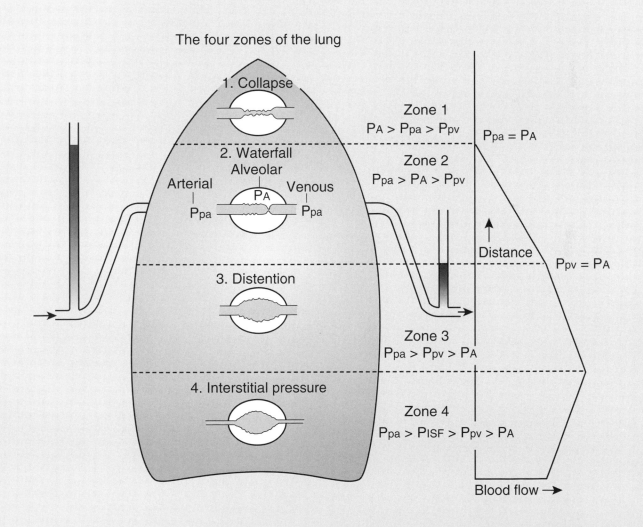

The four zones of the lung

1

FUNCTIONAL ANATOMY OF THE AIRWAY

Robert G. Krohner
Sivam Ramanathan

I. INTRODUCTION

The air passages starting from the nose and ending at the bronchioles are vital to the delivery of respiratory gas to and from the alveoli. During clinical anesthesia, the anesthesiologist uses these air passages to deliver the anesthetic gases to the alveoli while, at the same time, maintaining vital respiratory gas transport. To accomplish proper airway management, anesthesiologists often gain access to the airways by means of an endotracheal tube (ET) or other devices that are directly introduced into the patient's upper or lower air passages. In addition, anesthesiologists are called upon to establish access to the airways in certain cases of dire emergencies. For the purpose of description, the airway is divided into the upper airway, which extends from the nose to the glottis, and the lower airway, which includes the trachea, the bronchi, and the subdivisions of the bronchi. The airways also serve other important functions such as olfaction, deglutition, and phonation. A detailed anatomic description of these structures is beyond the scope of this chapter. Structural details as they relate to function in health and disease are described.

II. UPPER AIRWAY

A. NOSE

The airway functionally begins at the nares and the mouth, where air first enters the body. Phylogenetically, breathing was intended to occur through the nose. This arrangement not only enables the animal to smell danger but also permits uninterrupted conditioning of the inspired air while feeding. Resistance to airflow through the nasal passages is twice the resistance that occurs through the mouth. Therefore, during exercise or respiratory distress, mouth breathing occurs to facilitate a reduction in airway resistance and increased airflow.

The nose serves a number of functions: respiratory, olfaction, humidification, filtration, and phonation. In the adult human, the two nasal fossae extend 10 to 14 cm from the nostrils to the nasopharynx. The two fossae are divided mainly by a midline quadrilateral cartilaginous septum together with the two extreme medial portions of the lateral cartilages. The nasal septum is composed mainly of the perpendicular plate of the ethmoid bone descending from the cribriform plate, septal cartilage, and the vomer. Disruption of the cribriform plate secondary to facial trauma or head injury may allow direct communication with the anterior fossa. The use of positive-pressure mask ventilation in this scenario may lead to the entry of bacteria or foreign material leading to meningitis or sepsis. In addition, nasal airways, nasotracheal tubes, and nasogastric tubes may be inadvertently introduced into the subarachnoid space.

Each nasal fossa is convoluted and provides approximately 60 cm² surface area per side for warming and humidifying the inspired air.[49] The nasal fossa is bounded laterally by inferior, middle, and superior turbinate bones (conchae),[52] which divide the fossa into scroll-like spaces called the inferior, middle, and superior meatuses (Fig. 1-1).[49,66,67] The inferior turbinate usually limits the size of the nasotracheal tube that can be passed through the nose. Thus, damage to the lateral walls may occur as a result of vigorous attempts during nasotracheal intubation. The arterial supply to the nasal cavity is mainly from the ethmoid branches of the ophthalmic artery,

sphenopalatine and greater palatine branches of the maxillary artery, and superior labial and lateral nasal branches of the facial artery. Kiesselbach's plexus, where these vessels anastomose, is situated in Little's area on the anterior-inferior portion of the nasal septum. This is a common source of clinically significant epistaxis. The vascular mucous membrane overlying the turbinates can be damaged easily, leading to profuse hemorrhage. The paranasal sinuses, named for the bone in which they are located, are the sphenoid, ethmoid, maxillary, and frontal. They drain through apertures into the lateral wall of the nose. Prolonged nasotracheal intubation has most often been associated with infection of the maxillary sinus as its drainage is hindered by the location of the ostia superiorly in the sinus promoting a chronic infectious process.[9]

The olfactory area is located in the upper third of the nasal fossa and consists of the middle and upper septum and the superior turbinate bone. The respiratory portion is located in the lower third of the nasal fossa.[67] The respiratory mucous membrane consists of ciliated columnar cells containing goblet cells and nonciliated columnar cells with microvilli and basal cells. The olfactory cells have specialized hairlike processes, called the olfactory hair, innervated by the olfactory nerve.[67] The nonolfactory sensory nerve supply to the nasal mucosa is derived from the first two divisions of the trigeminal nerve. The parasympathetic autonomic nerves reach the mucosa from the facial nerve after relay through the sphenopalatine ganglion, and sympathetic fibers are derived from the plexus surrounding the internal carotid artery through the vidian nerve.[35]

Approximately 10,000 L of ambient air passes through the nasal airway per day, and 1 L of moisture is added to this air in the process.[19] The moisture is derived partly from transudation of fluid through the mucosal epithelium and from secretions produced by glands and goblet cells. These secretions have significant bacteriocidal properties. Foreign body invasion is further minimized by the stiff hairs (vibrissae), the ciliated epithelium, and the extensive lymphatic drainage of the area.

A series of complex autonomic reflexes controls the blood supply to the nasal mucosa and allows it to shrink and swell quickly. Reflex arcs also connect this area with other parts of the body. For example, the Kratschmer reflex leads to bronchiolar constriction upon stimulation of the anterior nasal septum in animals. A demonstration of this reflex may be seen in the postoperative period when a patient becomes agitated when the nasal passage is packed.[35]

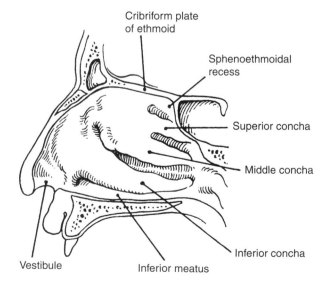

Figure 1-1 Lateral wall of right nasal cavity. Conchae are also known as turbinate bones. Sphenoid sinus opens into the sphenoethmoidal recess. Frontal, maxillary, and ethmoidal sinuses open into meatuses of the nose. (From Ellis H, Feldman S: Anatomy for Anaesthetists, 6th ed. Oxford, Blackwell Scientific, 1993.)

B. PHARYNX

The pharynx, 12 to 15 cm long, extends from the base of the skull to the level of the cricoid cartilage anteriorly and the inferior border of the sixth cervical vertebrae posteriorly.[4] It is widest at the level of the hyoid bone

(5 cm) and narrowest at the level of the esophagus (1.5 cm), which is the most common site for obstruction after foreign body aspiration. It is further subdivided into the nasopharynx, oropharynx, and laryngopharynx. The nasopharynx, which primarily has a respiratory function, lies posterior to the termination of the turbinates and nasal septum and extends to the soft palate. The oropharynx has primarily a digestive function, starts below the soft palate, and extends to the superior edge of the epiglottis. The laryngopharynx (hypopharynx) lies between the fourth and sixth cervical vertebrae, starts at the superior border of the epiglottis, and extends to the inferior border of the cricoid cartilage, where it narrows and becomes continuous with the esophagus (Fig. 1-2). The eustachian tubes open into the lateral walls of the nasopharynx. In the lateral walls of the oropharynx are situated the tonsillar pillars of the fauces. The anterior pillar contains the glossopharyngeus muscle and the posterior pillar the palatoglossus muscle.[51] The wall of the pharynx consists of two layers of muscles, an external circular and an internal longitudinal. Each layer is composed of three paired muscles. The stylopharyngeus, the salpingopharyngeus, and the palatopharyngeus form the internal layer. They elevate the pharynx and shorten the larynx during deglutition. The superior, middle, and inferior constrictors form the external layer, and they advance the food in a coordinated fashion from the oropharynx into the esophagus.

The constrictors are innervated by filaments arising out of the pharyngeal plexus (formed by motor and sensory branches from the vagus, the glossopharyngeal, and the external branch of the superior laryngeal nerves). The inferior constrictor is additionally innervated by branches from recurrent laryngeal and external laryngeal nerves. The internal layer is innervated by the glossopharyngeal nerve.

1. Defense against Pathogens

Inhaled particles of size greater than 10 µm are removed by inertial impaction upon the posterior nasopharynx. In addition, the inhaled airstream changes direction sharply at 90 degrees at the nasopharynx, thus causing some loss of momentum of the suspended particles. Being unable to remain suspended, the particles are trapped by the pharyngeal walls. The impacted particles are trapped by the circularly arrayed lymphoid tissue located at the entrance to the respiratory and alimentary tracts known as the ring of Waldeyer (Fig. 1-3). The ring includes masses of lymphoid tissue or tonsils, including the two large palatine, lingual, tubal, and the nasopharyngeal tonsils (adenoids, see Fig. 1-3).[20,43] These structures occasionally impede the passage of ETs, especially if they are infected and enlarged. Specifically, enlarged adenoid tissue may impede passage of a nasotracheal tube or nasal airway or simply obstruct the nasal airway passages. The lingual tonsils are located between the base of the tongue and the epiglottis. During routine anesthetic evaluation of the oropharynx, the lingual tonsils are typically not visible. Lingual tonsillar hypertrophy, which is usually asymptomatic, has been reported as a cause of unanticipated difficult intubation and fatal upper airway obstruction.[45] In addition, sepsis originating from one of the numerous lymphoid aggregates may lead to a retropharyngeal or peritonsillar abscess, which indeed poses anesthetic challenges.[9]

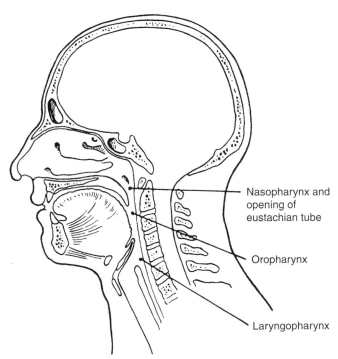

Figure 1-2 Diagrammatic representation of a sagittal section through head and neck to show divisions of the pharynx. Laryngopharynx is also known as the hypopharynx. (From Ellis H, Feldman S: Anatomy for Anaesthetists, 6th ed. Oxford, Blackwell Scientific, 1993.)

Nasopharynx and opening of eustachian tube

Oropharynx

Laryngopharynx

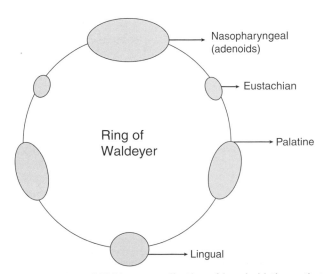

Nasopharyngeal (adenoids)

Eustachian

Palatine

Ring of Waldeyer

Lingual

Figure 1-3 Ring of Waldeyer, a collection of lymphoid tissue that guards against pathogen invasion. (From Hodder Headline PLC, London.)

2. Upper Airway Obstruction

a. Sedation and Anesthesia

The pharynx is the common pathway for food and the respiratory gases. Patency of the pharynx is vital to the patency of the airway and proper gas exchange. Proper placement of an ET relies upon an understanding of the distance relationships from the oropharynx to the vocal cords and carina. Complications such as a cuff leak at the level of the vocal cords and endobronchial intubation may thus be avoided (Fig. 1-4). Traditionally, it has been taught that upper airway obstruction in patients who are sedated or anesthetized (without an ET), or have altered levels of consciousness for other reasons, occurs as a result of the tongue falling back onto the posterior pharyngeal wall. Specifically, it is thought that a reduction in genioglossus muscle activity leads to posterior displacement of the tongue with subsequent obstruction.[41] However, a number of publications offer a different explanation. Nandi and colleagues, using lateral radiographs in patients under general inhalational anesthesia, showed that obstructive changes in the airway occurred at the level of the soft palate and epiglottis.[42] Shorten and coworkers, using magnetic resonance imaging (MRI), found that patients receiving intravenous sedation for anxiolysis with midazolam had anterior-posterior dimensional changes in the upper airway also at the level of the soft palate and epiglottis while sparing the tongue[58] (Fig. 1-5). In addition, Mathru and coauthors, using MRI to evaluate volunteers receiving propofol anesthesia, found that obstruction occurs at the level of the soft palate and not the tongue.[39] Thus, it appears that the soft palate and epiglottis may play a more significant role than the tongue in pharyngeal upper airway obstruction.

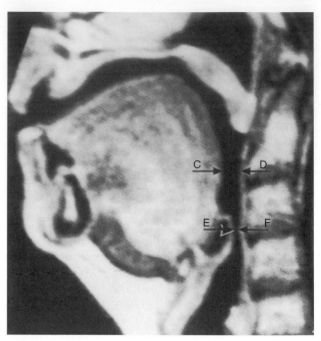

Figure 1-5 Medial sagittal view of upper airway showing site of airway obstruction in sedated patients. Soft palate is in contact with the posterior pharyngeal wall. CD, Minimum anteroposterior diameter at level of tongue; EF, minimum anteroposterior diameter at level of epiglottis. (From Shorten GD, Opie NJ, Graziotti P, et al: Assessment of upper airway anatomy in awake, sedated and anaesthetized patients using magnetic resonance imaging. Anaesth Intensive Care 22:165, 1994.)

b. Obstructive Sleep Apnea

The reduction in the size of the pharynx is also a factor in the development of respiratory obstruction in patients with obstructive sleep apnea (OSA).[25] This problem has been studied utilizing several imaging techniques including computed tomography (CT) and MRI, nasopharyngoscopy, fluoroscopy, and acoustic reflection.[2] In awake male patients with OSA, CT has shown a reduced airway caliber at all levels of the pharynx when compared with normal patients, with the narrowest portion posterior to the soft palate.[23] The subatmospheric intra-airway pressure created by contraction of the diaphragm against the resistance of the nose can lead to a reduction in size of the pharyngeal airway. These collapsible segments of the pharynx are divided into three areas, retropalatal, retroglossal, and retroepiglottic. Patency is dependent upon the contractile function of pharyngeal dilator muscles of these segments. The muscles involved are the tensor palatini retracting the soft palate away from the posterior pharyngeal wall, the genioglossus moving the tongue anteriorly, and the muscles moving the hyoid bone forward including the geniohyoid, sternohyoid, and thyrohyoid.[6] Studies show that the configuration of the airway may differ in patients with OSA.[53] Normally, the longer axis of the pharyngeal airway is transverse; however, in OSA patients the anterior-posterior axis is predominant. It is believed that this orientation is less efficient and may affect upper

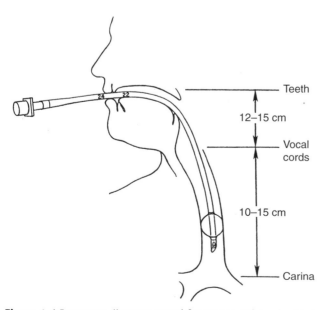

Figure 1-4 Important distances noted for proper endotracheal tube placement. (From Stone DJ, Bogdonoff DL: Airway considerations in the management of patients requiring long-term endotracheal intubation. Anesth Analg 74:276, 1992.)

airway muscle function. This alteration in shape is attributed to an increased thickness of the lateral pharyngeal walls for reasons not clearly understood.[34] Continuous positive airway pressure (CPAP) has been found to be effective in treating airway obstruction in these patients. The application of CPAP appears to increase the volume and cross-sectional area of the oropharynx, especially in the lateral axis.[56]

C. LARYNX

The larynx, which lies in the adult neck opposite the third through sixth cervical vertebrae,[51] is situated at the crossroads between the food and air passages (or conduits). It is made up of cartilages forming the skeletal framework, ligaments, membranes, and muscles. Its primary function is to serve as the "watchdog" of the respiratory tract, allowing passage only to air and preventing secretions, food, or foreign bodies from entering the trachea. In addition, it functions as the organ of phonation. The larynx may be somewhat higher in females and children. Until puberty, no differences in the laryngeal sizes exist between males and females. At puberty, the larynx develops more rapidly in males than females, nearly doubling in the anteroposterior diameter. The female larynx is smaller and more cephalad.[51] The measurements of the adult male and female larynx length, transverse diameter, and sagittal diameter are 44 and 36 mm, 43 and 41 mm, and 36 and 26 mm, respectively.[3] Most larynxes develop somewhat asymmetrically.[24] The inlet to the larynx is bounded anteriorly by the upper edge of the epiglottis, posteriorly by a fold of mucous membrane stretched between the two arytenoid cartilages, and laterally by the aryepiglottic folds.[35]

1. Bones of the Larynx

The hyoid bone suspends and anchors the larynx during respiratory and phonatory movement. It is U shaped, as its name is derived from the Greek word *hyoeides*, meaning shaped like the letter upsilon. It has a body, which is 2.5 cm wide by 1 cm thick, and greater and lesser horns (cornu). This bone does not articulate with any other bone. It is attached to the styloid processes of the temporal bones by the stylohyoid ligament and to the thyroid cartilage by the thyrohyoid membrane and muscle. Intrinsic tongue muscles originate on the hyoid, and the pharyngeal constrictors are attached here as well.[50-52]

2. Cartilages of the Larynx

Nine cartilages provide the framework of the larynx (Figs. 1-6 and 1-7). These are the unpaired thyroid, cricoid, and epiglottis and the paired arytenoids, corniculates, and cuneiforms. They are connected and supported by membranes, synovial joints, and ligaments.

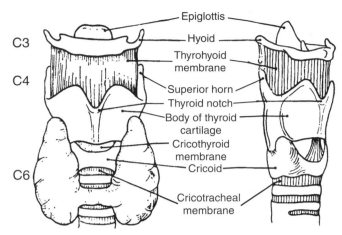

Figure 1-6 External frontal *(left)* and anterolateral *(right)* views of the larynx. Note location of cricothyroid membrane and thyroid gland in relation to thyroid and cricoid cartilage in the frontal view. Horn of the thyroid cartilage is also known as the cornu. In the anterolateral lateral view, the shape of the cricoid cartilage and its relation to thyroid cartilage are shown. (From Ellis H, Feldman S: Anatomy for Anaesthetists, 6th ed. Oxford, Blackwell Scientific, 1993.)

The ligaments, when covered by mucous membranes, are called folds.

a. Thyroid Cartilage

The thyroid cartilage, the longest laryngeal cartilage and largest structure in the larynx, acquires its shieldlike shape from the embryologic midline fusion of the two

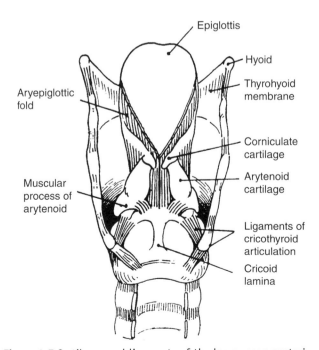

Figure 1-7 Cartilages and ligaments of the larynx seen posteriorly. Note location of the corniculate cartilage within the aryepiglottic fold. (From Ellis H, Feldman S: Anatomy for Anaesthetists, 6th ed. Oxford, Blackwell Scientific, 1993.)

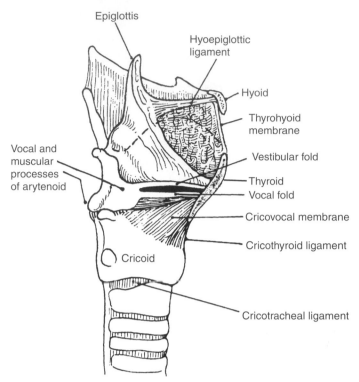

Figure 1-8 Sagittal (lateral) view of the larynx. Vocal and vestibular folds and thyroepiglottic ligament attach to midline of inner surface of the thyroid cartilage. Also note relationship between cricovocal membrane and vocal folds. (Modified from Ellis H, Feldman S: Anatomy for Anaesthetists, 6th ed. Oxford, Blackwell Scientific, 1993.)

distinct quadrilateral laminae.[22] In females, the sides join at approximately 120 degrees, and in males at closer to 90 degrees. This smaller thyroid angle explains the greater laryngeal prominence in males (the "Adam's apple"), the longer vocal cords, and the lower pitched voice.[15] The thyroid notch lies in the midline at the top of the fusion site of the two laminae.[62] On the inner side of this fusion line are attached the vestibular ligaments and, below them, the vocal ligaments (Fig. 1-8). The superior (greater) and inferior (lesser) cornu of the thyroid are the slender posteriorly directed extensions of the edges of the lamina. The lateral thyrohyoid ligament attaches the superior cornu to the hyoid bone, and the cricoid cartilage articulates with the inferior cornu at the cricothyroid joint. The movements of this joint are rotatory and gliding, which leads to changes in the length of the vocal folds.

b. Cricoid Cartilage

The cricoid cartilage represents the anatomic lower limit of the larynx and helps support it.[22] It is thicker and stronger than the thyroid cartilage and represents the only complete cartilaginous ring in the airway. Thus, cautious downward pressure on the cricoid cartilage to prevent passive regurgitation is possible without subsequent airway obstruction. The name cricoid is derived from the Greek words *krikos* and *eidos*, meaning shaped like a ring, hence its frequent reference to a signet ring shape. The bulky

portion or laminae are located posteriorly. The tracheal rings connect to the cricoid by ligaments and muscles. The cricoid lamina has ball and socket synovial articulations with the arytenoids posterosuperiorly and the thyroid cartilage more inferolaterally and anteriorly.[22] It also attaches to the thyroid cartilage by the cricothyroid membrane, a relatively avascular and easily palpated landmark in most adults.

Attempts have been made to measure the inner diameters of the cricoid cartilage in cadaveric specimens, with great variability noted.[11,47] Randestad and colleagues reported that the smallest diameter is in the frontal plane in females, ranging from 8.9 to 17.0 mm (mean 11.6), and that in males ranged from 11.0 to 21.5 mm (mean 15.0 mm). They further noted that placement of a standard size ET (7 mm inner diameter for females and 8 mm inner diameter for males) through the cricoid cartilage while preventing mucosal necrosis may be difficult in certain individuals.[47] The cricothyroid membrane represents an important identifiable landmark, providing access to the airway by percutaneous or surgical cricothyroidotomy. The various dimensions of the cricothyroid membrane have been identified in cadaveric specimens.[5,8,10] However the actual methodology of obtaining the anatomic measurements varies, making comparisons difficult to interpret. Caparosa and Zavatsky described the cricothyroid membrane as a trapezoid with a width ranging from 27 to 32 mm, representing the actual anatomic limit of the membrane, and a height of 5 to 12 mm.[8] Bennett and coauthors reported the dimensions as a width of 9 to 19 mm and a height of 8 to 19 mm, and Dover and coworkers reported a width of 6.0 to 11.0 mm and a height of 7.5 to 13.0 mm, using the distance between the cricothyroid muscles as their horizontal limit.[5,10] In females it was reported that the width and height of the membrane are smaller than in males.[10] Anteriorly vascular structures overlie the membrane and pose a risk of hemorrhage.[10,18,36] Cadaveric studies have noted the presence of a transverse cricothyroid artery, a branch of the superior thyroid artery, traversing the upper half of the membrane. Thus, a transverse incision in the lower third of the membrane is recommended. The superior thyroid artery was noted to course along the lateral edge of the membrane as well. Also, various branches of the superior and inferior thyroid veins and the jugular veins were reported to traverse the membrane.[10]

c. Arytenoids

The two light arytenoid cartilages are shaped like three-sided pyramids, and they lie in the posterior aspect of the larynx.[16] The arytenoid's medial surface is flat and covered with only a firm, tight layer of mucoperichondrium.[63] The base of the arytenoid is concave and articulates by a true diarthrodial joint with the superior lateral aspect of the posterior lamina of the cricoid cartilage. It is described as a ball and socket with three movements, rocking or rotating, gliding, and pivoting, controlling adduction and abduction of the vocal cords. All such synovial joints can be affected by rheumatoid arthritis. Cricoarytenoid arthritis, noted to be present in a majority of these patients, has been identified as a cause of life-threatening upper airway obstruction.[32] Cricoarytenoid arthropathy has also been reported as a rare but potentially fatal cause of acute upper airway obstruction in patients with systemic lupus erythematosus.[28]

The lateral extension of the arytenoid base is called the muscular process. Important intrinsic laryngeal muscles, lateral and posterior cricoarytenoids, originate here. The medial extension of the arytenoid base is called the vocal process. Vocal ligaments, the bases of the true vocal folds, extend from the vocal process to the midline of the inner surface of the thyroid lamina (see Fig. 1-8). The fibrous membrane that connects the vocal ligament to the thyroid cartilage actually penetrates the body of the thyroid. This membrane is called Broyles' ligament. This ligament contains lymphatics and blood vessels and therefore can act as an avenue for extension of laryngeal cancer outside the larynx.[7,22] The relationship between the anterior commissure of the larynx and the inner aspect of the thyroid cartilage is important to otolaryngologists, who perform thyroplasties and supraglottic laryngectomies on the basis of its location. A study of cadavers reported that the anterior commissure of the larynx can usually be found above the midpoint of the vertical midline fusion of the thyroid cartilage ala.[40,63]

d. Epiglottis

The epiglottis is considered to be vestigial by many authorities.[68] Composed primarily of fibroelastic cartilage, the epiglottis does not ossify and maintains some flexibility throughout life.[16,22,46] It is shaped like a leaf or a tear and is found between the larynx and the base of the tongue (see Fig. 1-7).[50,63] In approximately 1% of the population, the tip and posterior aspect of the epiglottis are visible during a pharyngoscopic view with the mouth opened and tongue protruded.[38] Contrary to reports, this does not always predict ease of intubation.[21] The upper border of the epiglottis is attached by its narrow tip or petiole to the midline of the thyroid cartilage by the thyroepiglottic ligament (Fig. 1-9; see Fig. 1-8). The hyoepiglottic ligament connects the epiglottis to the back of the body of the hyoid bone.[13,15] The mucous membrane that covers the anterior aspect of the epiglottis sweeps forward to the tongue as the median glossoepiglottic fold and to the pharynx as the paired lateral pharyngoepiglottic folds.[22] The pouchlike areas found between the median and lateral folds are the valleculae. The tip of a properly placed Macintosh laryngoscope blade rests in this area. The vallecula is a common site of impaction of foreign bodies, such as fish bones, in the upper airway.

e. Cuneiform and Corniculate Cartilages

The epiglottis is connected to the arytenoid cartilages by the laterally placed aryepiglottic ligaments and folds (see Fig. 1-7). Two sets of paired fibroelastic cartilages are

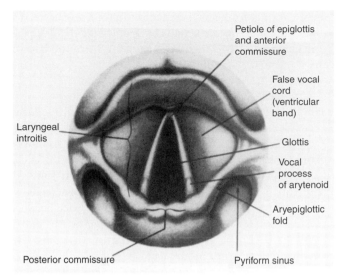

Figure 1-9 Larynx viewed from above with a laryngeal mirror. Note location of the anterior and posterior commissures of the larynx and the aryepiglottic fold. Elevations in the aryepiglottic folds are the cuneiform cartilages. (From Tucker HM, Harvey M: Anatomy of the larynx. In Tucker HM [ed]: The Larynx, 2nd ed. New York, Thieme Medical, 1993, p 9.)

embedded in each aryepiglottic fold.[16] The sesamoid cuneiform cartilage is roughly cylindrical and lies antero-superior to the corniculate in the fold. The cuneiform may be seen laryngoscopically as a whitish elevation through the mucosa (see Fig. 1-9). The corniculate is a small triangular object visible directly over the arytenoid cartilage. The cuneiform and corniculate cartilages reinforce and support the aryepiglottic folds[22,63] and may help the arytenoids move.[46,51]

f. False and True Vocal Cords

The thyrohyoid membrane (see Figs. 1-7 to 1-9), attaching the superior edge of the thyroid cartilage to the hyoid bone, provides cranial support and suspension.[51] It is separated from the hyoid body by a bursa that facilitates movement of the larynx during deglutition.[63] The thicker median section of the thyrohyoid membrane is the thyrohyoid ligament and its thinner lateral edges are pierced by the internal branches of the superior laryngeal nerves.

Beneath the laryngeal mucosa is a fibrous sheet containing many elastic fibers, the fibroelastic membrane of the larynx. Its upper area, the quadrangular membrane, extends in the aryepiglottic fold between the arytenoids and the epiglottis. The lower free border of the membrane is called the vestibular ligament and forms the vestibular folds, or false cords (see Figs. 1-8 and 1-9).[15,32,50]

The cricothyroid membrane joins the cricoid and thyroid cartilages. The thickened median area of this fibrous tissue, the "conus elasticus," extends up inside the thyroid lamina to the anterior commissure and continues and blends with the vocal ligament. The cricothyroid ligament thus connects the cricoid, thyroid, and arytenoid cartilages.[15,32] The thickened inner edges of the cricothyroid ligament, called the vocal ligament, form the basis of the vocal folds (see Fig. 1-8).[51,63]

g. Laryngeal Cavity

The laryngeal cavity (Fig. 1-10) extends from the laryngeal inlet to the lower border of the cricoid cartilage. Viewed laryngoscopically from above, two paired inward projections of tissue are visible in the laryngeal cavity (see Fig. 1-9): the superiorly placed vestibular folds, or false cords, and the more inferiorly placed vocal folds, or true vocal cords (see Figs. 1-8 to 1-10). The space between the true cords is called the rima glottidis, or the glottis (see Fig. 1-9). The glottis is divided into two parts. The anterior intermembranous section is situated between the two vocal folds. The two vocal folds meet at the anterior commissure of the larynx (see Fig. 1-9). The posterior intercartilaginous part passes between the two arytenoid cartilages and the mucosa, stretching between them in the midline posteriorly, forming the posterior commissure of the larynx (see Fig. 1-9).[15] At rest the vocal processes are approximately 8 mm apart.[65] The area extending from the laryngeal inlet to the vestibular folds is known as the vestibule or supraglottic larynx (see Fig. 1-10). The laryngeal space from the free border of the cords to the cricoid cartilage is called the subglottic or infraglottic larynx. On the basis of cadaver studies, the measurements of the subglottis have been identified.[8,27,31] Understanding the anatomic relationships between the cricothyroid space and the vocal folds is important to minimize complications after cricothyrotomy (Fig. 1-11).[37] Bennett and colleagues reported this distance as 9.78 mm.

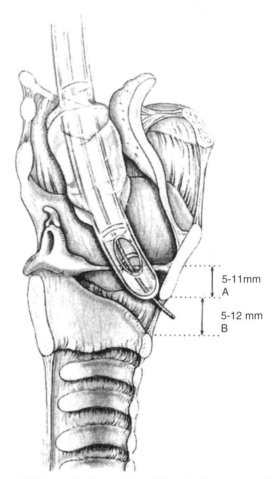

Figure 1-11 Schematic illustration noting the distance relationships (ranges) of the larynx, thyroid, and cricoid cartilages. **A,** Distance from the vocal cords to the anteroinferior edge of the thyroid cartilage. **B,** Distance from the anteroinferior edge of the thyroid cartilage to the anterosuperior edge of the cricoid cartilage. (From Kuriloff DB, Setzen M, Portnoy W: Laryngotracheal injury following cricothyroidotomy. Laryngoscope 99:125, 1989.)

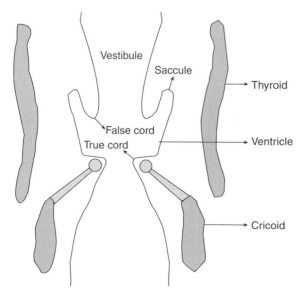

Figure 1-10 Diagrammatic representation of the laryngeal cavity. Note location of false and true cords and laryngeal saccule. (Modified from Pectu LP, Sasaki CT: Laryngeal anatomy and physiology. Clin Chest Med 12:415, 1991.)

The region between the vestibular folds and the glottis is termed the ventricle or the sinus. The ventricle may expand anterolaterally to a pouchlike area with many lubricating mucous glands called the laryngeal saccule (see Fig. 1-10).[22] The saccule is believed to help in voice resonance in apes.[63,68] The pyriform sinus lies laterally to the aryepiglottic fold within the inner surface of the thyroid cartilage (see Fig. 1-9).[63]

The epithelium of the vestibular folds is the ciliated-pseudostratified variety (respiratory), whereas the epithelium of the vocal folds is the nonkeratinized squamous type.[62] Thus, the entire interior of the larynx is covered with respiratory epithelium except the vocal folds.[35]

Airway protection is enhanced by the orientation of the cords. The false cords are directed inferiorly at their free border. This position can help to stop egress of air during a Valsalva maneuver. The true cords are oriented slightly superiorly. This prevents air or matter from entering the lungs. Great pressure is needed to separate adducted true cords.[46] Air trapped in the ventricle during closure pushes each false cord and true cord more tightly together.[62]

3. Muscles of the Larynx

The complex and delicate functions of the larynx are made possible by an intricate group of small muscles. These muscles can be divided into the extrinsic and the intrinsic groups.[13,68] The extrinsic group connects the larynx with its anatomic neighbors, such as the hyoid bone, and modifies the position and movement of the larynx. The intrinsic group facilitates the movements of the laryngeal cartilages against one another and directly affects glottic movement.[46,63]

a. Extrinsic Muscles of the Larynx

The suprahyoid muscles attach the larynx to the hyoid bone and elevate the larynx. These muscles are the stylohyoid, geniohyoid, mylohyoid, thyrohyoid, digastric, and stylopharyngeus muscles. In the infrahyoid muscle group are the omohyoid, sternothyroid, thyrohyoid, and sternohyoid muscles. These "strap" muscles, in addition to lowering the larynx, can modify the internal relationship of laryngeal cartilages and folds to one another. The inferior constrictor of the pharynx primarily assists in deglutition (Table 1-1).[15,22,51,62]

b. Intrinsic Muscles of the Larynx

The function of the intrinsic musculature is threefold: (1) open the vocal cords during inspiration, (2) close the cords and the laryngeal inlet during deglutition, and (3) alter the tension of the cords during phonation.[22,51,63] The larynx can close at three levels: the aryepiglottic folds close by the contraction of the aryepiglottic and oblique arytenoid muscles, the false

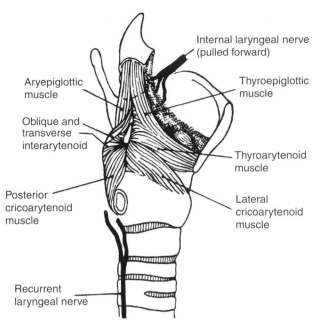

Figure 1-12 Intrinsic muscles of the larynx and their nerve supply. (Modified from Ellis H, Feldman S: Anatomy for Anaesthetists, 6th ed. Oxford, Blackwell Scientific, 1993.)

vocal cords close by the action of the lateral thyroarytenoids, and the true vocal cords close by the contraction of interarytenoids, lateral cricoarytenoids, and the cricothyroid.[51] The intrinsic muscles include the aryepiglottic and thyroepiglottic, thyroarytenoid and vocalis, oblique and transverse arytenoids, lateral and posterior cricoarytenoids, and cricothyroids (Fig. 1-12). All but the transverse arytenoids are paired.

Some authors consider the cricothyroid muscle to be both an extrinsic and intrinsic muscle of the larynx because its actions affect both laryngeal movements and the glottic structures.[63] It is the only intrinsic muscle found external to the larynx itself. The paired cricothyroid

Table 1-1 **Extrinsic Muscles of the Larynx**

Muscle	Function	Innervation
Sternohyoid	Indirect depressor of the larynx	Cervical plexus Ansa hypoglossi C1, C2, C3
Sternothyroid	Depresses the larynx Modifies the thyrohyoid and aryepiglottic folds	Same as above
Thyrohyoid	Same as above	Cervical plexus Hypoglossal nerve C1, C2
Thyroepiglottic	Mucosal inversion of aryepiglottic fold	Recurrent laryngeal nerve
Stylopharyngeus	Assists folding of thyroid cartilage	Glossopharyngeal
Inferior pharyngeal constrictor	Assists in swallowing	Vagus, pharyngeal plexus

From Benumof JL: Airway Management: Principles and Practice. St. Louis, Mosby, 1996.

muscles join the cricoid cartilage and the thyroid cartilage (Fig. 1-13). The muscle has two parts. A larger, ventral section runs vertically between the cricoid and the inferior thyroid border. The smaller oblique segment attaches to the posterior inner thyroid border and the lesser cornu of the thyroid. During swallowing, the muscle contracts and the ventral head draws the anterior part of the cricoid cartilage toward the relatively fixed lower border of the thyroid cartilage. The oblique head of the muscle rocks the cricoid lamina posteriorly. Because the arytenoids do not move, the vocal ligaments are tensed and the glottic length is increased 30%.[1,63]

The thick posterior cricoarytenoid muscle originates near the entire posterior midline of the cricoid cartilage. Muscle fibers run superiorly and laterally to the posterior area of the muscular process of the arytenoid cartilage.[39] Upon contraction, the posterior cricoarytenoid rotates the arytenoids and moves the vocal folds laterally. The posterior cricoarytenoid is the only true abductor of the vocal folds.[15,16,46,63]

The lateral cricoarytenoid muscle joins the superior border of the lateral cricoid cartilage and the muscular process of the arytenoid. This muscle rotates the arytenoids medially, adducting the true vocal folds.[22] The unpaired transverse arytenoid muscle joins the posterolateral aspects of the arytenoids. The muscle, covered anteriorly by a mucous membrane, forms the posterior commissure of the larynx. Contraction of this muscle brings the arytenoids together and ensures posterior adduction of the glottis.[15,16,22]

The oblique arytenoids (see Fig. 1-12) ascend diagonally from the muscular processes posteriorly across the cartilage to the opposite superior arytenoid and help close the glottis. Fibers of the oblique arytenoid may

continue from the apex through the aryepiglottic fold as the aryepiglottic muscle, which attaches itself to the lateral aspect of the epiglottis. The aryepiglottic muscle and the oblique arytenoid act as a "purse-string" sphincter during deglutition.[63]

The thyroarytenoid muscle (see Fig. 1-12) is broad and sometimes divided into three parts. It is among the fastest contracting striated muscles.[46] The muscle arises along the entire lower border of the thyroid cartilage. It passes posteriorly, superiorly, and laterally to attach to the anterolateral surface and the vocal process of the arytenoid.

The segment of thyroarytenoid muscle that lies adjacent to the vocal ligament (and frequently surrounds it) is called the vocalis muscle. The vocalis is the major tensor of vocal fold and can "thin" the fold to achieve a high pitch. Beneath the mucosa of the fold, extending from the anterior commissure back to the vocal process, is a potential space called Reinke's space. This area can become edematous if traumatized. The more laterally attached fibers of the thyroarytenoid function as the prime adductor of the vocal folds.[63]

The most lateral section of the muscle, sometimes called the thyroepiglottic muscle, attaches to the lateral aspects of arytenoids, the aryepiglottic fold, and even the epiglottis. When it contracts, the arytenoids are pulled medially, down, and forward.[22,63] This shortens and relaxes the vocal ligament. The function and innervation of the extrinsic muscles are summarized in Table 1-1. Table 1-2 describes the intrinsic musculature of the larynx.

c. Innervation of the Larynx

The main nerves of the larynx are the recurrent laryngeal nerves and the internal and external branches of the superior laryngeal nerves. The external branch of the superior laryngeal nerve supplies motor innervation to the cricothyroid muscle. All other motor supply to the laryngeal musculature is provided by the recurrent laryngeal nerve (see Fig. 1-12). Both the superior and recurrent laryngeal nerves are derivatives of the vagus nerve.

The superior laryngeal nerve generally separates from the main trunk, off the inferior vagal ganglion, just outside the jugular foramen. At approximately the level of the hyoid bone, it divides into the smaller external and larger internal branches. The external branch travels below the superior thyroid artery to the cricothyroid muscle, giving off a branch to the inferior constrictor of the pharynx along the way. The internal branch travels along with the superior laryngeal artery and passes through the thyrohyoid membrane laterally between the greater cornu of the thyroid and hyoid. The nerve and artery together pass through the pyriform recess, where the nerve may be anesthetized intraorally. The nerve divides almost immediately into a series of sensory branches and provides sensory innervation from the posterior aspect of the tongue base to as far down as the vocal cords.[22,63] Sensory innervation of the epiglottis is dense, and the

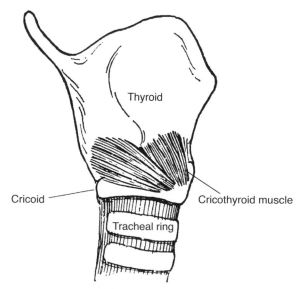

Figure 1-13 Cricothyroid muscle and its attachments. (Modified from Ellis H, Feldman S: Anatomy for Anaesthetists, 6th ed. Oxford, Blackwell Scientific, 1993.)

Table 1-2 **Intrinsic Musculature of the Larynx**

Muscle	Function	Innervation
Posterior cricoarytenoid	Abductor of vocal cords	Recurrent laryngeal
Lateral cricoarytenoid	Adducts arytenoids closing glottis	Recurrent laryngeal
Transverse arytenoid	Adducts arytenoids	Recurrent laryngeal
Oblique arytenoid	Closes glottis	Recurrent laryngeal
Aryepiglottic	Closes glottis	Recurrent laryngeal
Vocalis	Relaxes the cords	Recurrent laryngeal
Thyroarytenoid	Relaxes tension cords	Recurrent laryngeal
Cricothyroid	Tensor of the cords	Superior laryngeal (external branch)

From Benumof JL: Airway Management: Principles and Practice. St. Louis, Mosby, 1996.

true vocal folds are more heavily innervated posteriorly than anteriorly.[46]

The left recurrent laryngeal nerve branches from the vagus in the thorax and courses cephalad after hooking around the arch of the aorta in close relation to the ligamentum arteriosum, at approximately the level of the fourth and fifth thoracic vertebrae. On the right, the nerve loops posteriorly beneath the subclavian artery, at approximately the first and second thoracic vertebrae, before following a cephalad course to the larynx. Both nerves ascend the neck in the tracheoesophageal groove before they reach the larynx. The nerves enter the larynx just posterior to, or sometimes anterior to, the cricothyroid articulation. The recurrent laryngeal nerve supplies all the intrinsic muscles of the larynx except the cricothyroid. The recurrent laryngeal nerve also provides sensory innervation to the larynx below the vocal cords. Parasympathetic fibers to the larynx travel along the laryngeal nerves, and the sympathetics from the superior cervical ganglion travel to the larynx with blood vessels. Tables 1-1 and 1-2 summarize the innervation of the laryngeal musculature.

i. Glottic Closure and Laryngeal Spasm Stimulation of the superior laryngeal nerve endings in the supraglottic region can induce protective closure of the glottis. This short-lived phenomenon is a polysynaptic involuntary reflex.[46] Triggering of other nerves, notably cranial nerves such as the trigeminal and glossopharyngeal, can, to a lesser degree, also produce reflex glottic closure.[30,60] The nerve endings in the mammalian supraglottic area are highly sensitive to touch, heat, and chemical stimuli.[48] This sensitivity is especially intense in the posterior commissure of the larynx, close to where the pyriform recesses blend with the hypopharynx.[61] Complex sensory receptors, similar in structure to lingual taste buds, have been demonstrated here.[26] Instillation of water, saline, bases, and acids has been demonstrated to cause glottic closure in vitro and in vivo.[59] Infants also respond to stimulation with prolonged apnea, although this response disappears later in life.[52]

The term episodic paroxysmal laryngospasm has been coined to describe laryngeal dysfunction, which may or may not arise as true episodes of respiratory distress.[17] However, postoperative laryngeal nerve injury has been reported to cause paroxysmal laryngospasm arising with stridor and acute airway obstruction. Superior laryngeal nerve blockade may be temporarily effective in some patients.[64]

Laryngospasm occurs when glottic closure persists long after the removal of the stimulus.[60,61] This has led to speculation that laryngospasm represents a focal seizure of the adductors subtended by the recurrent laryngeal nerve.[55] This state is initiated by repeated superior laryngeal nerve stimulation.[60] It was reported that the recurrent laryngeal nerve may also be responsible for laryngospasm.[57] Symptoms abate, perhaps through a central mechanism, as hypoxia and hypercarbia worsen.[44]

ii. Vocal Cord Palsies The recurrent laryngeal nerve may be traumatized during surgery on the thyroid and parathyroid glands.[14] Malignancy or benign processes of the neck, trauma, pressure from an ET or a laryngeal mask airway, and stretching the neck may also affect the nerve.[13,35,37,54] The left recurrent laryngeal nerve may be compressed by neoplasms in the thorax, aneurysm of the aortic arch, or an enlarged left atrium (mitral stenosis).[50] It may be occasionally injured during ligation of a patent ductus arteriosus. The left nerve is likely to be paralyzed twice as frequently as the right one because of its close relationship to many intrathoracic structures. Damage to the superior laryngeal nerve (external branch) during thyroidectomy is the commonest cause of voice change.[29]

Under normal circumstances, the vocal cords meet in the midline during phonation (Fig. 1-14). On inspiration they move away from each other. They return toward the midline on expiration, leaving a small opening between them. When laryngeal spasm occurs, both true and false vocal cords lie tightly in the midline opposite each other. To arrive at a clinical diagnosis, the position of the cords

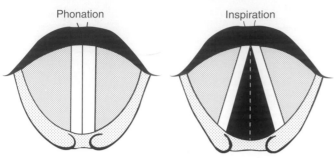

Figure 1-14 Position of vocal cords during phonation and inspiration. (From Hodder Headline PLC, London.)

must be examined laryngoscopically during phonation and inspiration (Fig. 1-15; see Fig. 1-14).

The recurrent laryngeal nerve carries both abductor and adductor fibers to the vocal cords. The abductor fibers are more vulnerable, and moderate trauma causes a pure abductor paralysis (Selmon's law).[12] Severe trauma causes both abductor and adductor fibers to be affected.[35] Pure adductor paralysis does not occur as a clinical entity. In the case of pure unilateral abductor palsy, both cords meet in the midline on phonation (because adduction is still possible on the affected side) (see Fig. 1-15). However, only the normal cord abducts during inspiration (see Fig. 1-15). In the case of complete unilateral palsy of the recurrent laryngeal nerve, both abductors and adductors are affected. On phonation, the unaffected cord crosses the midline to meet its paralyzed counterpart, appearing to lie in front of the affected cord (see Fig. 1-15).[35] On inspiration, the unaffected cord

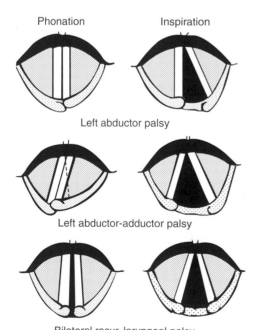

Figure 1-15 Diagrammatic representation of different types of vocal cord palsies. Note that in complete bilateral recurrent laryngeal palsy *(bottom)*, vocal cords remain in the abducted position and the glottic opening is preserved. recur., recurrent. For details see text. (From Hodder Headline PLC, London.)

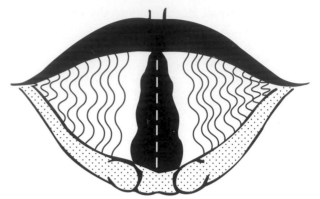

Figure 1-16 Cadaveric position of vocal cords. For details see text. (From Hodder Headline PLC, London.)

moves to full abduction. When abductor fibers are damaged bilaterally (incomplete bilateral damage to the recurrent laryngeal nerve), the adductor fibers draw the cords toward each other and the glottic opening is reduced to a slit, resulting in severe respiratory distress (see Fig. 1-15).[13,68] However, with a complete palsy, each vocal cord lies midway between abduction and adduction and a reasonable glottic opening exists. Thus, bilateral incomplete palsy is more dangerous than the complete variety (see Fig. 1-15).

Damage to the external branch of the superior laryngeal nerve or to the superior laryngeal nerve trunk causes paralysis of the cricothyroid muscle (the tuning fork of the larynx) and causes hoarseness that improves with time because of increased compensatory action of the opposite muscle. The glottic chink appears oblique during phonation. The aryepiglottic fold on the affected side appears shortened and the one on the normal side is lengthened. The cords may appear wavy. The symptoms include frequent throat clearing and difficulty in raising the vocal pitch.[1] A total bilateral paralysis of vagus nerves affects the recurrent laryngeal nerves and the superior laryngeal nerves. In this condition, the cords assume the abducted, cadaveric position.[35] The vocal cords are relaxed and appear wavy (Fig. 1-16).[1,35] A similar picture may be seen following the use of muscle relaxants.

Topical anesthesia of the larynx may affect the fibers of the external branch of the superior laryngeal nerve and paralyze the cricothyroid muscle, signified by a "gruff" voice. Similarly, a superior laryngeal nerve block may affect the cricothyroid muscle in the same manner as surgical trauma does. These factors must be taken into consideration when evaluating post-thyroidectomy vocal cord dysfunction after surgery.

d. Blood Supply of the Larynx

Blood supply to the larynx is derived from the external carotid and the subclavian arteries. The external carotid gives rise to the superior thyroid artery, which bifurcates, forming the superior laryngeal artery. This artery courses with the superior laryngeal nerve through the thyrohyoid membrane to supply the supraglottic region. The inferior thyroid artery, derived from the thyrocervical trunk, terminates as the inferior laryngeal artery. This vessel travels in the tracheoesophageal groove with the recurrent laryngeal nerve and supplies the infraglottic larynx. There are extensive connections with the ipsilateral superior laryngeal artery and across the midline. A small cricothyroid artery may branch from the superior thyroid and cross the cricothyroid membrane. It most commonly travels near the inferior border of the thyroid cartilage.[63]

III. LOWER AIRWAY

A. GROSS STRUCTURE OF THE TRACHEA AND BRONCHI

The adult trachea begins at the cricoid cartilage, opposite the sixth cervical vertebra (see Figs. 1-10 and 1-11). It is 10 to 20 cm long and 12 mm in diameter. It is flattened posteriorly and contains 16 to 20 horseshoe-shaped cartilaginous rings. At the sixth ring, the trachea becomes intrathoracic. The first and last rings are broader than the rest. The lower borders of the last ring split and curve interiorly between the two bronchi to form the carina at the T5 level (angle of Louis, second intercostal space). The posterior part of the trachea, void of cartilage, consists of a membrane of smooth muscle and fibroelastic tissue joining the ends of the cartilages. The muscle of the trachea is stratified in an inner circular and an outer longitudinal layer. The longitudinal bundles predominate in children but are virtually absent in adults.[16,18]

In the adult, the right main bronchus is wider and shorter and takes off at a steeper angle than the left main stem bronchus. Thus, ETs, suction catheters, or foreign bodies more readily enter the right bronchial lumen. However, the angulations of the two bronchi are nearly equal in children younger than 3 years. The right main stem bronchus gives rise to three lobar bronchi and the left, two. Both main bronchi and the lower lobe bronchi are situated outside the lung substance (large bronchi, 7 to 12 mm in diameter). Main bronchi divide into 20 bronchopulmonary divisions supplying each respective lobule's medium bronchi (4 to 7 mm) that lead into small bronchi (0.8 to 4 mm). Bronchioles are bronchi that are less than 0.8 mm in size. Bronchioles do not have any cartilage in their walls.[63]

Bronchioles are of two types, terminal and respiratory. The terminal bronchioles do not bear any alveoli and lead into the alveoli-bearing respiratory bronchioles. Each terminal bronchiole leads to three respiratory bronchioles, and each respiratory bronchiole leads to four generations of alveolar ducts (Fig. 1-17).[63]

Although the diameter of each new generation of airway decreases progressively, the aggregate cross-sectional area increases. This is especially true beyond airways 2 mm in diameter or smaller, where further

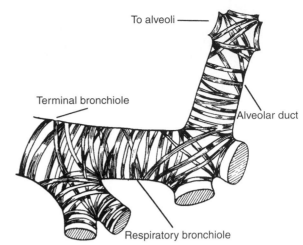

Figure 1-17 Bronchiolar division and geodesic network of muscle layer surrounding the airway. (From Hodder Headline PLC, London.)

branching is not accompanied by concomitant decreases in caliber. The failure of the airway diameter to decrease with subsequent divisions produces the inverted thumbtack appearance on a graph depicting increasing surface area as a function of distance from the mouth (Fig. 1-18).[9]

The bronchi are surrounded by irregular, cartilaginous rings similar in structure to the trachea except that the attachment of the posterior membrane is more anterior (Fig. 1-19).[32] Rings give way to discrete, cartilaginous plates as the bronchi become intrapulmonary at the lung

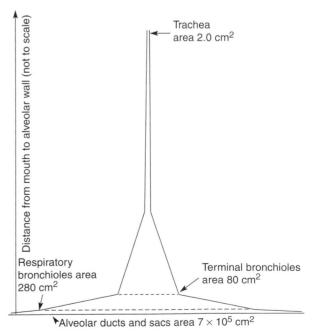

Figure 1-18 Relationship between cross-sectional area and generation of the airway. Note abrupt increase in cross section when the respiratory bronchiole is reached (inverted thumbtack arrangement). For details see text. (From Hodder Headline PLC, London.)

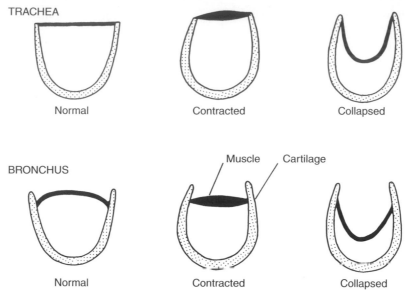

Figure 1-19 Cross-sectional view of trachea and bronchus. Note different sites of attachment of posterior membrane in the tracheal and bronchial sections. Also note invagination of posterior membrane into the lumen in the collapsed state. (From Horsfield K: The relation between structure and function of the airways of the lung. Br J Dis Chest 68:145, 1974.)

roots (Fig. 1-20). Eventually, even these plates disappear, usually at airway diameters of about 0.6 mm.[32]

The rings or the plates of the bronchi are interconnected by a strong fibroelastic sheath within which a myoelastic layer consisting of smooth muscle and elastic tissue is arrayed.[9] The myoelastic band is arranged in a special pattern called the geodesic network, representing the shortest distance between two points on a curved surface (see Fig. 1-17). This architectural design serves as the strongest and most effective mechanism for withstanding or generating pressures within a tube without fiber slippage along the length of the outer surface of the tube. The primary function of the muscular component is to change the size of the airway according to the respiratory phase. The smooth muscle tone (bronchomotor tone) is predominantly under the influence of the vagus nerve. The elastic layer runs longitudinally but encircles the bronchus at the points of division.[9]

The muscular layer becomes progressively thinner distally, but its thickness relative to the bronchial wall increases. Therefore, the terminal bronchiole with the narrowest lumen has perhaps the thickest muscle, nearly 20% of the total thickness of the wall that lacks cartilaginous support.[32,63] Thus, smaller bronchioles may be readily closed off by action of the musculature during prolonged bronchial spasm. Such an arrangement may facilitate closure of unperfused portions of the lung when a ventilation-perfusion mismatch occurs (pulmonary embolism). The smooth muscles and the glands of the cartilaginous airways are innervated by the autonomic nervous system. They are stimulated by the vagus and inhibited by sympathetic impulses derived from the upper thoracic ganglia.

B. AIRWAY EPITHELIUM AND AIRWAY DEFENSE MECHANISMS

The cartilaginous airways are lined by a tall, columnar, pseudostratified epithelium containing at least 13 cell types.[3] An important function of this lining is the production of

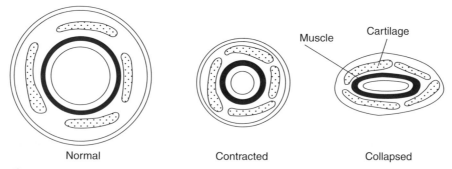

Figure 1-20 Cross-sectional views of medium bronchi (4 to 8 mm diameter) with peribronchial space. (From Horsfield K: The relation between structure and function of the airways of the lung. Br J Dis Chest 68:145, 1974.)

mucus, a part of the respiratory defense mechanism. The mucus is steadily propelled to the outside by a conveyer belt mechanism. The large airways have a mucous secretory apparatus that consists of serous and goblet cells and submucous glands. The submucous glands empty into secretory tubules, which, in turn, connect with the larger connecting ducts. Several connecting ducts unite and form the ciliated duct that opens into the airway lumen. No mucous glands are seen in the bronchioles.[28,35]

The most populous cell of the large airways is the ciliated epithelial cell, bearing 250 cilia per cell.[3,35] The length of the cilia decreases progressively in the smaller airways. On the surface of the cell are found small claws and microvilli. The microvilli probably regulate the volume of secretions through resorption, a function that may be shared with the brush cells scattered along the airways. The basal cell, more numerous in the large airways, imparts the epithelium's pseudostratified appearance. The other cell types, except the K cell, develop from the basal cell through the intermediate cell. This cell lies in the layer above the basal cell and differentiates into cells with secretory or ciliary function.[3,28,35] The K cell, or Kulchitsky-like cell, resembles the Kulchitsky cells of the gastrointestinal tract. These cells take up, decarboxylate, and store amine precursors, such as levodopa (L-dopa), and are thus known as amine precursor uptake and decarboxylation (APUD) cells. The functions of the K cells are not definitely known, but proposed roles include mechanoreception or chemoreception (stretch, carbon dioxide [CO_2]). Globule leukocytes are derived from subepithelial mast cells and interact with them to transfer immunoglobulin E to the secretions and to alter membrane permeability to locally produced or circulating antibodies. The ubiquitous lymphocytes and plasma cells defend against pathogens. Table 1-3 lists important cell types that constitute the airway epithelium.

The nonciliated bronchiolar epithelial cell, or Clara cell, largely composes the cuboidal epithelium of the bronchioles. The Clara cells assume the role of basal cells as a stem cell in the bronchiole. Only six cell types have been recorded in the human bronchiole: the ciliated, brush, basal, K, Clara, and globular leukocyte. These cells form a single-layered simple cuboidal epithelium.

C. BLOOD SUPPLY

Bronchial arteries supply the bronchi and the bronchioles. Arterial supply extends into the respiratory bronchiole. Arterial anastomoses occur in the adventitia of the bronchiole. The branches enter the submucosa after piercing the muscle layer to form the submucosal capillary plexus. The venous radices arising from the capillary plexus reach the venous plexus in the adventitia by penetrating the muscle layer. When the muscle layer contracts, the arteries can maintain forward flow to the capillary plexus. However, the capillaries cannot force the blood back into the venous plexus. Thus, prolonged bronchial

Table 1-3 Types of Tracheobronchial Cell

Cell	Probable Function
Epithelial	
Goblet	Mucous secretion
Serous	Mucous secretion
Ciliated	Mucous propulsion-resorption, supportive
Brush	Mucous resorption
Basal	Supportive, parent
Intermediate	Parent
Clara	Supportive, parent
Kulchitsky	Neuroendocrine possible mechanoreceptor, chemoreceptor
Mesenchymal	
"Globule" leukocyte	Immunologic defense
Lymphocyte	Defense

Modified from Jeffrey PK, Reid L: New features of the rat airway epithelium: A quantitative and electron microscopic study. J Anat 120:295, 1975.

spasm can lead to mucous membrane swelling in the small airways.[9] The venous drainage of the bronchi occurs through the bronchial, azygous, hemiazygos, and intercostal veins. There is some communication between the pulmonary artery and the bronchiolar capillary plexus leading to normally occurring "anatomic shunting."

D. FUNCTION OF THE LOWER AIRWAY

1. Forces Acting on the Airway

Different forces act upon the airway to alter its morphology continuously. These forces are modified by (1) the location of a given airway segment (intrathoracic or extrathoracic), (2) the phases of respiration, (3) lung volume, (4) gravity, (5) age, and (6) disease.[28,32]

Intrathoracic, intrapulmonary airways such as the distal bronchi and bronchioles are surrounded by a potential space, the peribronchial space (Fig. 1-21). The bronchi are untethered and, therefore, move longitudinally within this sheath. However, the bronchiolar adventitia is attached by an elastic tissue matrix to the adjoining elastic framework of the surrounding alveoli and parenchyma. Consequently, the bronchioles are subject to transmitted tissue forces.[18,35]

Many forces act in concert to modify the airway lumen (Fig. 1-22). The forces that tend to expand the lumen include pressure of the gas in the bronchi-bronchioles and the elastic tissue forces of the alveoli. Forces that tend to close the airway include the elasticity of the bronchial wall, which increases as the lumen expands; the

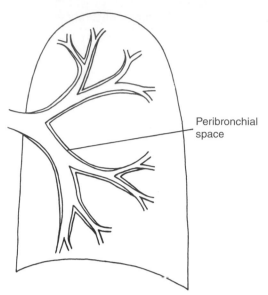

Figure 1-21 Diagram showing formation of peribronchial space by invagination of the visceral pleura. (From Horsfield K: The relation between structure and function of the airways of the lung. Br J Dis Chest 68:145, 1974.)

forces related to bronchial muscle contraction; and the pressure of the gas in the surrounding alveoli. The algebraic sum of these forces at any given time determines the diameter of the airway.[32,63]

The lower part of the trachea and proximal bronchi are intrathoracic but extrapulmonary. Consequently, they are subject to the regular intrathoracic pressures (intrapleural pressure) but not to the tissue elastic recoil forces.

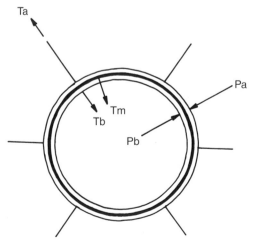

Figure 1-22 Vector diagram showing transmural forces influencing airway caliber. Ta, alveolar elastic forces; Tb, bronchial elastic forces; Tm, bronchial muscular forces; Pb, barometric pressure; Pa, alveolar gas pressure. Arrow direction indicates direction of the force. Algebraic sum of these forces determines size of airway lumen at any given time. (From Horsfield K: The relation between structure and function of the airways of the lung. Br J Dis Chest 68:145, 1974.)

The upper trachea is both extrathoracic and extrapulmonary. Although it is unaffected by the elastic recoil of the lung, it is subject to the effects of ambient pressure and cervical tissue forces.[18,32]

During spontaneous inspiration, the lung expands, lowering the alveolar pressure more than it does the bronchial pressure, to create a pressure gradient that induces airflow. This increases the elastic retractive forces of the connective tissue and opens the intrathoracic airways. However, extrathoracic intraluminal pressure decreases relative to atmospheric pressure, with the result that the diameter of the upper trachea decreases. During expiration, alveolar pressure rises and exceeds the tissue retractive forces, thus decreasing intrathoracic airway diameter. In this case, the extrathoracic intraluminal pressure rises above the atmospheric pressure, and the upper trachea expands. On forced expiration alveolar pressure is greatly elevated, further reducing the diameter of the smaller airways.

The dynamic forces are altered by gravity such that the forces tending to expand the lung are greater at the top than at the bottom whether the patient is prone, supine, or erect.[7] The diameter and length of the airways of all sizes vary directly as the cube root of the lung volume varies when the lung expands.[40] On expiration below functional residual capacity, the retractive forces gradually decrease the airway size toward the point of closing volume. Because of the effect of gravity, the basal airways close first. The retractive forces of the elastic tissues decrease with aging, which explains why closing volume increases with age. This effect is exaggerated in diseases with elastic tissue damage (pulmonary emphysema).

2. Relationship between Structure and Function

The extent to which the retractive forces affect the airway morphology is related to the specific structure of the airway segment in question. When the fibromuscular membrane of the trachea contracts, the ends of the cartilages are approximated, and the lumen narrows in both the intrathoracic and extrathoracic trachea. When the radial forces decrease airway diameter, the posterior membrane invaginates into the lumen (see Fig. 1-19). However, the rigid cartilaginous hoops prevent luminal occlusion. Extrapulmonary bronchi behave in a similar fashion.

The medium intrapulmonary bronchi within the peribronchial sheath are surrounded by cartilaginous plates. Although these plates add some rigidity to the wall, they do not prevent collapse, and so these airways are dependent on the elastic retractive forces of the surrounding tissue (see Fig. 1-22).[32] Therefore, forced expiration can collapse many bronchioles in emphysema.

The miniature carinas at small airway bifurcations maintain airway lumens. Intrinsic bronchial muscles reduce the lumen and increase the mean velocity of the

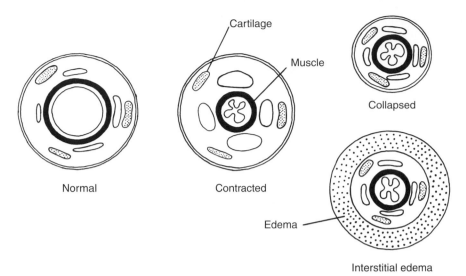

Figure 1-23 Structure of small bronchi (0.8 to 4 mm in diameter). Note that the mucous membrane is thrown into folds in contracted and collapsed states, reducing the airway lumen. (From Horsfield K: The relation between structure and function of the airways of the lung. Br J Dis Chest 68:145, 1974.)

airflow during forced expiratory maneuvers, particularly in the peripheral airways with small flow rates. Here, two additional anatomic adaptations contribute to increasing flow rates: (1) as the muscular ring contracts, the mucous lining is thrown into accordion-type folds that project into the lumen, further narrowing the lumen (Fig. 1-23)[32]; (2) the venous plexus situated between the muscle and the cartilage fills and invaginates into the lumen during muscle contraction. These mechanisms permit bronchoconstriction without distorting the surrounding tissues and minimize the muscular effort required to reduce airway lumen. The drawback of such an arrangement is that even a small amount of fluid or sputum can result in complete occlusion of the small airways.[32] Thus, it is not surprising that the airway resistance is increased tremendously during an asthmatic attack that is characterized by both bronchospasm and increased secretions.[38,46,68] The small airways can also be affected by interstitial pulmonary edema, a condition in which the peribronchial space can accumulate fluid and isolate the bronchus from the surrounding retractive forces (see Fig. 1-23).

IV. CONCLUSION

In this chapter we described certain salient features of the human respiratory passages as they relate to their functional anatomy in health and disease from the anesthesiologist's point of view. It is necessary for students of anesthesia to possess some knowledge of the structures that they will most frequently use as a passageway to care of patients in their professional career.

REFERENCES

1. Abelson TI, Tucker HM: Laryngeal findings in superior laryngeal nerve paralysis: A controversy. Otolaryngol Head Neck Surg 89:463, 1981.
2. Ayappa I, Rapoport DM: The upper airway in sleep: Physiology of the pharynx. Sleep Med Rev 7:9, 2003.
3. Bannister LH, Berry MM, Collins P, et al: Gray's Anatomy, 38th ed. New York, Churchill Livingstone, 1995, p 1637.
4. Beasley P: Anatomy of the pharynx and oesophagus. In Kerr AG (ed): Scott Brown's Otolaryngology. Oxford, Butterworth-Heinemann, 1997, p 8.
5. Bennett JDC, Guha SC, Sankar AB: Cricothyrotomy: The anatomical basis. J R Coll Surg Edinb 41:57, 1996.
6. Benumof JL: Obstructive sleep apnea in the adult obese patient: Implications for airway management. J Clin Anesth 13:144, 2001.
7. Broyles EN: The anterior commissure tendon. Ann Otol Rhinol Laryngol 52:341, 1943.
8. Caparosa RJ, Zavatsky AR: Practical aspects of the cricothyroid space. Laryngoscope 67:577, 1957.
9. Deutschman CS, Wilton P, Sinow J, et al: Paranasal sinusitis associated with nasotracheal intubation: A frequently unrecognized and treatable source of sepsis. Crit Care Med 14:111, 1986.
10. Dover K, Howdieshell TR, Colborn GL: The dimensions and vascular anatomy of the cricothyroid membrane: Relevance to emergent surgical airway access. Clin Anat 9:291, 1995.
11. Eckel HE, Sittel C: Morphometry of the larynx in horizontal sections. Am J Otol 16:40, 1995.
12. Ellis H: Clinical Anatomy, 10th ed. Oxford, Blackwell Scientific, 2002, p 310.

13. Ellis H, Feldman S: Anatomy for Anaesthetists, 6th ed. Oxford, Blackwell Scientific, 1993.
14. Fewins J, Simpson CB, Miller FR: Complications of thyroid and parathyroid surgery. Otolaryngol Clin North Am 36:189, 2003.
15. Fink RF: Anatomy of the larynx. In The Human Larynx: A Functional Study. New York, Raven Press, 1975.
16. Fried MP, Meller SM: Adult laryngeal anatomy. In Fried MP (ed): The Larynx: A Multidisciplinary Approach. Boston, Little, Brown, 1988, p 41.
17. Gallivan GJ, Hoffman L, Gallivan KH: Episodic paroxysmal laryngospasm: Voice and pulmonary function assessment and management. J Voice 10:93, 1996.
18. Goumas P, Kokkinis K, Petrochelios J, et al: Cricothyroidotomy and the anatomy of the cricothyroid space: An autopsy study. J Laryngol Otol 111:354, 1997.
19. Grande CM, Ramanathan S, Turndorf H: The structural correlates of airway function. Probl Anesth 2:175, 1988.
20. Green GM: Lung defense mechanisms. Symposium on chronic respiratory disease. Med Clin North Am 57:547, 1973.
21. Grover VK, Mahajan R, Tomar M: Class zero airway and laryngoscopy. Anesth Analg 96:911, 2003.
22. Hanafee WN, Ward PH: Anatomy and physiology. In Hanafee WN, Ward PH (eds): The Larynx: Radiology, Surgery, Pathology. New York, Thieme Medical, 1990, p 3.
23. Haponik EF, Smith PL, Bohlman ME, et al: Computerized tomography in obstructive sleep apnea: Correlation of airway size with physiology during sleep and wakefulness. Am Rev Respir Dis 127:221, 1983.
24. Hirano M, Kurita S, Yukizane K, et al: Asymmetry of the laryngeal framework: A morphologic study of cadaver larynges. Ann Otol Rhinol Laryngol 98:135, 1989.
25. Hudgel DW: The role of upper airway anatomy and physiology in obstructive sleep apnea. Clin Chest Med 13:383, 1992.
26. Ide C: The cytologic composition of laryngeal chemosensory corpuscles. Am J Anat 158:193, 1980.
27. Isshiki N: Phonosurgery. In Lawrence VL, Gould WJ (eds): Disorders of Human Communication. New York, Springer-Verlag, 1984, p 61.
28. Karim A, Ahmed S, Siddiqui R, et al: Severe upper airway obstruction from cricoarytenoiditis as the sole presenting manifestation of a systemic lupus erythematosus flare. Chest 121:990, 2002.
29. Kark AE, Kissin MW, Auerback R, et al: Voice changes after thyroidectomy: Role of the external laryngeal nerve. Br Med J 289:1412, 1984.
30. Kirchner J: Laryngeal reflex system. In Baer T, Sasaki C (eds): Laryngeal Function in Phonation and Respiration. Boston, Little, Brown, 1987, p 65.
31. Kirchner JA: Cricothyroidotomy and subglottic stenosis. Plast Reconstr Surg 68:828, 1981.
32. Kolman J, Morris I: Cricoarytenoid arthritis: A cause of acute upper airway obstruction in rheumatoid arthritis. Can J Anesth 49:729, 2002.
33. Kuriloff DB, Setzen M, Portnoy W, et al: Laryngotracheal injury following cricothyroidotomy. Laryngoscope 99:125, 1989.
34. Leiter JC: Upper airway shape: Is it important in the pathogenesis of obstructive sleep apnea? Am J Respir Crit Care Med 153:894, 1996.
35. Linton RF: Structure and function of the respiratory tract in relation to anaesthesia. In Churchill-Davidson HC (ed): A Practice of Anaesthesia, 5th ed. Chicago, Year Book Medical, 1984, p12.
36. Little CM, Parker MG, Tarnopolsky R: The incidence of vasculature at risk during cricothyroidostomy. Ann Emerg Med 15:805, 1986.
37. Lowinger D, Benjamin B, Gadd L: Recurrent laryngeal nerve injury caused by a laryngeal mask airway. Anaesth Intensive Care 27:202, 1999.
38. Maleck WH, Koetter KK, Less SD: Pharyngoscopic views. Anesth Analg 89:256, 1999.
39. Mathru M, Esch O, Lang J, et al: Magnetic resonance imaging of the upper airway: Effects of propofol anesthesia and nasal continuous positive airway pressure in humans. Anesthesiology 84:273, 1996.
40. Meitelles LZ, Lin P, Wenk EJ: An anatomic study of the external laryngeal framework with surgical implications. Otolaryngol Head Neck Surg 106:235, 1992.
41. Morikawa S, Safar P, DeCarlo J: Influence of head-jaw position on airway patency. Anesthesiology 22:265, 1961.
42. Nandi PR, Charlesworth CR, Taylor SJ, et al: Effects of general anesthesia on the pharynx. Br J Anaesth 66:157, 1991.
43. Newhouse M, Sanchis J, Bienstock J, et al: Lung defense mechanisms, part I. N Engl J Med 295:990, 1976.
44. Nishino T, Yonezawa T, Honda Y: Modification of laryngospasm in response to changes in Pa_{CO_2} and Pa_{O_2} in the cat. Anesthesiology 55:286, 1981.
45. Ovassapian A, Glassenber R, Randel GI, et al: The unexpected difficult airway and lingual tonsil hyperplasia: A case series and a review of the literature. Anesthesiology 97:124, 2002.
46. Pectu LP, Sasaki CT: Laryngeal anatomy and physiology. Clin Chest Med 12:415, 1991.
47. Randestad A, Lindholm CE, Fabian P: Dimensions of the cricoid cartilage and the trachea. Laryngoscope 110:1957, 2000.
48. Rex MAE: The production of laryngospasm in the cat by volatile anesthetic agents. Br J Anaesth 42:941, 1970.
49. Reznik GK: Comparative anatomy, physiology and function of the upper respiratory tract. Environ Health Perspect 85:171, 1990.
50. Roberts J: Functional anatomy of the larynx. Int Anesthesiol Clin 28:101, 1990.
51. Roberts J: Fundamentals of Tracheal Intubation. New York, Grune & Stratton, 1983.
52. Roberts JT, Pino R: Functional anatomy of the upper airway. In Roberts JT (ed): Clinical Management of the Airway. Philadelphia, WB Saunders, 1994, p 2.
53. Rodenstein DO, Dooms G, Thomas Y, et al: Pharyngeal shape and dimensions in healthy subjects, snorers, and patients with obstructive sleep apnoea. Thorax 45:722, 1990.
54. Salem MR, Wond AY, Barangan VC, et al: Postoperative vocal cord paralysis in pediatric patients. Br J Anaesth 43:696, 1971.
55. Sasaki CT: Physiology of the larynx. In English GM (ed): Otolaryngology. Philadelphia, Harper & Row, 1984, p 10.
56. Schwab RJ, Gefter WB, Pack AL, et al: Dynamic imaging of the upper airway in normal subjects. J Appl Physiol 74:1504, 1993.

57. Sercarz JA, Nasri S, Gerratt BR, et al: Recurrent laryngeal nerve afferents and their role in laryngospasm. Am J Otolaryngol 16:49, 1995.

58. Shorten GD, Opie NJ, Graziotti P, et al: Assessment of upper airway anatomy in awake, sedated and anaesthetized patients using magnetic resonance imaging. Anaesth Intensive Care 22:165, 1994.

59. Storey AT, Johnson P: Laryngeal water receptors initiating apnea in the lamb. Exp Neurol 47:42, 1975.

60. Suzuki M, Sasaki CT: Laryngeal spasm: A neuroradiologic redefinition. Ann Otol Rhinol Laryngol 86:150, 1977.

61. Thach BT: Neuromuscular control of upper airway patency. Clin Perinatol 19:773, 1992.

62. Tucker HM: Physiology of the larynx. In Tucker HM (ed): The Larynx, 2nd ed. New York, Thieme Medical, 1993, p 23.

63. Tucker HM, Harvey M: Anatomy of the larynx. In Tucker HM (ed): The Larynx, 2nd ed. New York, Thieme Medical, 1993, p 1.

64. Wani MK, Woodson GE: Paroxysmal laryngospasm after laryngeal nerve injury. Laryngoscope 109:694, 1999.

65. Weir N: Anatomy of the larynx and tracheobronchial tree. In Kerr AG (ed): Scott Brown's Otolaryngology. Oxford, Butterworth-Heinemann, 1997, p 8.

66. Williams P, Warwick R, Dyson M, et al: Gray's Anatomy, 37th ed. New York, Churchill Livingstone, 1989, p 365.

67. Williams P, Warwick R, Dyson M, et al: Gray's Anatomy, 37th ed. New York, Churchill Livingstone, 1989, p 1171.

68. Williams P, Warwick R, Dyson M, et al: Gray's Anatomy, 37th ed. New York, Churchill Livingstone, 1989, pp 1248-1286.

2

RADIOLOGY OF THE AIRWAY

T. Linda Chi
David Mirsky
Jacqueline A. Bello
David Z. Ferson

I. INTRODUCTION

Ordering and interpreting radiologic studies are not in the usual domain of anesthesiologists. However, imaging studies provide a wealth of information regarding the airway, which could be useful for formulating an anesthetic plan, especially if the anesthesiologist has a good basic knowledge of radiology. Currently, radiology is not part of the curriculum of any anesthesia residency training program; thus, the majority of anesthesiologists have only rudimentary skills in interpreting radiologic studies. With the rapid pace of technological advances in the field of radiology and especially with the introduction of several new imaging techniques such as magnetic resonance imaging (MRI), computed tomography (CT), and helical CT, it is harder than ever to stay current. The main goal of this chapter is to introduce anesthesiologists to images of normal airway anatomy by conventional radiography (plain film or x-ray), CT, and MRI and to illustrate the anatomic variants and pathologic processes that can compromise the airway. The technology behind the different imaging modalities, as well as their technical differences, is briefly reviewed, with the main emphasis placed on evaluation of the airway using available radiologic studies, which most patients already have as part of their often extensive medical work-up. Familiarity with the normal anatomy and its variants is sometimes more useful than an exhaustive list of esoteric diagnoses. Therefore, our clinical examples focus on the pathologic processes involving the airway that are most relevant to anesthesiologists and include a short discussion of some common abnormalities.

The macroscopic airway is a tubular conduit for air inhaled from the nares to the tracheobronchial tree. Imaging of this airspace as a unique entity is gaining popularity. The soft tissue structures bordering the airway have warranted more of the radiologist's attention. The integrity of the airway with its natural contrast is usually referenced with respect to extrinsic impression, compression, encroachment, or displacement. Segmentation of the airway into the head and neck, and chest compartments is usually done for the ease of discussion. Different imaging modalities (x-ray, CT, and MRI) evaluate the airway structures and surrounding tissues with different levels of accuracy and spatial resolution. Any clinician attempting to analyze imaging studies needs to be familiar with the advantages and disadvantages of different imaging techniques. This is especially important when selecting a study that will best depict the anatomic structures and pathologic processes of the airway that are of clinical interest.

II. IMAGING MODALITIES

A brief history and description of the different imaging modalities are presented here in chronologic order, starting with plain x-ray films. This will enable the reader to develop a good foundation for understanding how different imaging modalities are used in modern diagnostic imaging.

A. PLAIN FILM (X-RAY)

Wilhelm Conrad Roentgen, a German physicist, discovered x-rays on November 8, 1895, while studying the behavior of cathode rays (electrons) in high-energy cathode ray tubes. When a high-tension discharge was passed through the tube, which was shrouded by black cardboard, a mysterious ray escaped the tube and serendipitously struck a small piece of paper coated with fluorescent barium platinocyanide on a workbench 3 feet away, causing a faint fluorescent glow. Different objects placed between the cathode ray tube and the fluorescent screen changed the brightness of the fluorescence, indicating that the mysterious ray penetrated objects differently. When Roentgen held his hand between the tube and the screen and saw the outline of the bony skeleton of his hand, he quickly realized the significance of his discovery. Less than 2 months later, he had prepared a manuscript describing his experiments. For his work, he was awarded the first Nobel Prize for Physics in 1901.[13]

X-rays are a type of electromagnetic radiation, which, as its name implies, transports energy through space as a combination of electric and magnetic fields. Other types of electromagnetic radiation include radio waves, radiant heat, and visible light. In diagnostic radiology, the predominant energy source used for imaging is ionizing radiation such as alpha, beta, gamma, and x-rays. The science of electromagnetic waves and x-ray generation is very complex and exceeds the scope of this text. In principle, x-rays are produced by energy conversion as a fast stream of electrons is suddenly decelerated in an x-ray tube.[12] The localized x-ray beam produced passes through the part of the body being studied. The final image is dependent on the degree of attenuation of the beam by matter. Attenuation, the reduction in the intensity of the beam as it traverses matter of different constituents, is caused by the absorption or deflection of photons from the beam. The transmitted beam determines the final image, which is represented in shades of gray.[7,8,11] The lightest or brightest area on the film or image represents the greatest attenuation of the beam by tissue and the least amount of beam transmitted to film. An example would be bone, a high-density material that attenuates much of the x-ray beam; images of bone on x-rays are very bright or white. Plain film is a two-dimensional collapsed or compressed view of the body part being imaged. This information can now also be presented in a digital format without the use of traditional x-ray films.

As compared to other more sophisticated imaging modalities, conventional plain film radiography is limited in displaying pathologic processes. Its advantage, however, is the anatomic presentation in a larger field of view. The head, chest, abdomen, or extremity can be visualized on a single film or digitized image. Thus, the image on the x-ray appears more familiar to nonradiologists. The plain x-ray is inexpensive and can be obtained quickly at the patient's bedside in any location in the hospital. Also, combining x-rays with cine mode allows radiologists to obtain dynamic images, which are used to evaluate organ function (e.g., barium swallow to evaluate deglutition and intravenous pyelogram to assess renal function).

B. COMPUTED TOMOGRAPHY

After the discovery of x-rays, it became apparent that images of the internal structures of the human body could yield important diagnostic information. However, the usefulness of the x-rays is limited by the projection of a three-dimensional object onto a two-dimensional display. With x-rays, the details of internal objects are masked by the shadows of overlying and underlying structures. Thus, the goal of diagnostic imaging is to bring forth the organ or area of interest in detail and eliminate the unwanted information. Various film-based traditional tomographic techniques were developed, culminating in the creation of computed tomography or computerized axial tomography (CAT).[9] The first clinically viable CT scanner was developed by Hounsfield[22] and commercially marketed by EMI (EMI Limited, Middlesex, England) for brain imaging in the early 1970s. Since then, several generations of CT scanners have been developed.

As with conventional plain film radiography, CT technology requires x-rays as the energy source. Whereas conventional radiography employs a single beam of x-rays from a single direction and yields a static image, CT images are obtained using multiple collimated x-ray beams from multiple angles and the transmitted radiation is counted by a row or rows of detectors. The patient is enclosed in a gantry, and a fan-shaped x-ray source rotates around him or her. The radiation counted by the detectors is analyzed using mathematical equations to localize and characterize, by density and attenuation measurements, and a single cross-sectional image is produced with one rotation of the gantry.[9] The gantry must then "unwind" to prepare for the next slice while the table with the patient moves forward or backward a distance predetermined by slice thickness. An intrinsic limitation of this technique is the time necessary for moving the mechanical parts.

The introduction of slip-ring technology in the 1990s and the development of faster computers, high-energy x-ray tubes, and multidetectors enabled continuous activation of the x-ray source without having to unwind the gantry and, at the same time, allows continuous movement of the tabletop. This process, known as helical CT, is used in the latest generation of CT scanners. Because the information acquired using helical CT is volumetric, as compared with the single slice obtained with conventional CT, the entire thorax or abdomen can be scanned in a single breath-hold. Volumetric information also makes it possible to identify small lesions more accurately and allows better three-dimensional reformation. Because of the higher speed of data acquisition, misregistration and image degradation caused by the patient's motion are no longer significant concerns. This is especially important when scanning uncooperative patients and trauma victims. The absorbed radiation dose used in multidetector helical CT as compared with conventional single-detector row CT is dependent on scanning protocol and varies with the desired high-speed or high-quality study.[20]

Practically speaking, CT examinations have become routine. The spatial resolution of CT is the best of all the imaging modalities currently available. The advantage of CT technology is that it can depict accurately any pathology involving bones. Data acquisition by using CT is very quick and CT can be used to produce images in all three planes as well as provide information for surface rendering and three-dimensional reformation, which allows the display of different organs in an anatomic format that can be easily recognized by clinicians.

C. MAGNETIC RESONANCE IMAGING

MRI has become one of the most widely used imaging modalities in diagnostic radiology. In contrast to conventional radiography and CT, MRI uses no ionizing radiation. Instead, imaging is based on the resonance of the atomic nuclei of certain elements such as sodium, phosphorus, and hydrogen in response to radio waves of the same frequency produced in a static magnetic field environment. Current clinical MRI units use protons from the nuclei of hydrogen atoms to generate images. Hydrogen is the most abundant element in the body. Every water molecule contains two hydrogen atoms, and larger molecules, such as lipids and proteins, contain many hydrogen atoms. MRI data are acquired by utilizing powerful electromagnets to create a magnetic field, which influences the alignment of protons in hydrogen atoms in the body. When radio waves are applied, protons are knocked out of natural alignment, and when the radio wave is stopped, the protons return to their original state of equilibrium, realigning to the steady magnetic field and emitting energy, which is translated into weak radio signals. The time it takes for the protons to realign is referred to as a relaxation time[10] and is dependent on the tissue composition and cellular environment. The different relaxation times and signal strength of the protons are processed by a computer, generating diagnostic images. With MRI, the chemical and physical properties of matter are examined at the molecular level. The relaxation times, T1 and T2, for each tissue type are expressed as constants at a given magnetic field strength. Imaging that optimizes T1 or T2 characteristics is referred to as T1-weighted or T2-weighted imaging. Tissue response to pathologic processes usually includes an increase in bound water, or edema, which lengthens the T2 relaxation time and appears as a bright focus on T2-weighted images.[10]

MRI is more sensitive, but not necessarily more specific, in detecting pathology than CT, which depicts anatomy with unparalleled clarity. The advantage of MRI technology is that it provides metabolic information at the cellular level, allowing one to link organ function and physiology to anatomic information. MRI and CT technologies also have other differences: (1) MRI shows no bone detail, whereas CT provides excellent images of bone structures; (2) acute hemorrhage is clearly visible on CT scans but may be difficult to diagnose with MRI because MRI blood signal characteristics depend on the breakdown products of hemoglobin; and (3) MRI is very susceptible to all types of motion artifacts, ranging from patient's movement, breathing, swallowing, and phonation to vascular and cerebral spinal fluid pulsation and flow.

It is important to mention that MRI scanners operate in a strong magnetic field environment, and strict precautions must be observed. Because any item containing ferromagnetic substances introduced into the magnetic field environment can become a projectile and result in deleterious consequences for patients, personnel, and the MRI scanner itself. No metal objects should be brought into the MRI suite if one is not absolutely certain about their composition. Only specially designed nonferromagnetic equipment is used in the MRI suite, including anesthesia machines, monitoring equipment, oxygen tanks, intravenous poles, infusion pumps, and stretchers. One must also remove pagers, telephones, hand-held organizers and computers, credit cards, and analog watches because the strong magnetic field can cause malfunction or permanent damage to them. Patients must be carefully screened for implantable pacemakers, intracranial aneurysm clips, cochlear implants, and other metallic foreign objects prior to entering the MRI environment.

III. BASICS OF PLAIN FILM (X-RAY) INTERPRETATION

To illustrate the usefulness of conventional radiography in evaluating the airway, we focus our discussion on the interpretation of plain films of the cervical spine, chest, and neck. These are probably the most frequently ordered x-ray studies in the hospital setting and are ubiquitous in patients' film jackets. They are also the most relevant to anesthesiologists, as a composite of these studies gives a picture of the entire airway. Although these radiologic studies are usually obtained for reasons other than airway evaluation, it is actually in this group of patients who are "normal" or "cleared for surgery" that one may glean important observations about the airway. The anatomy and pathology displayed by plain film radiographs may alert the anesthesiologist to potential difficulties in securing the patient's airway and help him or her to develop an alternative anesthetic plan. In this sense, the information about the airway that is inherent to these x-ray examinations is gratuitous. The following sections address the basics of plain film interpretation with respect to imaging of the airway anatomy and pathology.

A. CERVICAL SPINE X-RAY

1. Radiologic Anatomy

The cervical spine connects the skull to the trunk, articulating with the occiput above and the thoracic vertebrae below. The bony elements, muscles, ligaments, and intervertebral discs support and provide protection to the spinal cord. On plain film x-ray, one can appreciate the bony morphology of the vertebrae and the disc spaces and assess the alignment of the vertebral column, which indirectly provides information regarding the integrity of the ligaments, which are crucial in maintaining alignment of the cervical spine. Individual ligaments and muscle groups, however, all have the same attenuation and cannot be soft tissue differentiated from one another on plain film.

There are seven cervical vertebrae (C1 through C7). C1 and C2 are different from the other cervical vertebrae and are considered more a part of the cervicocranium. The atlas (C1) is a ringlike vertebra characterized by the absence of a vertebral body. It does not contain pedicles or laminae, as do other vertebrae, and has no true spinous process. It consists of an anterior arch, the anterior tubercle, a lateral mass on each side, and a posterior arch. The anterior and posterior arches are relatively thin and the lateral masses are heavy and thick structures. A rudimentary transverse process extends laterally and contains the transverse foramen, through which passes the vertebral artery.[6]

Ossification of the atlas begins with the lateral masses during intrauterine life. At birth, neither the anterior nor the posterior arches are fused. Fusion of the anterior arch is complete between the 7th and 10th years. During the second year, the center of the posterior tubercle appears, and by the end of the fourth year, the posterior arch becomes complete.[21] Nonfusion of the anterior and/or the posterior arch exists as a normal variant in adults and should not be mistaken as fractures (Fig. 2-1).

The second cervical vertebra, the axis (C2), is the largest and heaviest cervical segment. The odontoid process (dens) serves as the conceptual body of C1, around which the atlas rotates and bends laterally. In contrast to the other cervical vertebrae, C2 does not have a discrete pedicle.

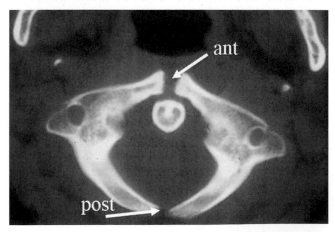

Figure 2-1 Nonfused anterior and posterior arches of C1, normal variant. Axial computed tomography, bone algorithm.

The dens is situated between the lateral masses of the atlas and is maintained in its normal sagittal relationship to the anterior arch of C1 by several ligaments, most important of which is the transverse atlantal ligament. Superiorly, the dentate (apical) ligament extends from the tip of the clivus to the tip of the dens. Alar ligaments secure the tip of the dens to the occipital condyles and to the lateral masses of the atlas. They are the second line of defense in maintaining the proper position of the dens. The tectorial membrane is a continuum of the posterior longitudinal ligament from the body of C2 to the upper surface of the occipital bone anterior to the foramen magnum.

The C2 vertebra arises from five or six separate ossification centers, depending upon whether the centrum has one or two centers. The vertebral body is ossified at birth, and the posterior arch is partially ossified. They fuse posteriorly by the second or third year and unite with the body of the vertebrae by the seventh year. The dens ossifies from two vertically oriented centers that fuse by the seventh fetal month. Cranially, a central cleft separates the tips of these ossification centers (Fig. 2-2), which can mimic a fracture when ossification is incomplete. The ossiculum terminale, the ossification center for the tip of the dens, may be visible on plain film, conventional tomograms, or CT scans and unites with the body by age 11 or 12 years. Failure of the ossiculum terminale to either develop or unite with the dens may result in a bulbous cleft dens tip. A nonunited terminal dental ossification center is called the *os terminale* and may be mistaken for a fracture of the odontoid tip.

From C3 to C7, the cervical vertebrae are uniform in shape but increase in size, with the seventh vertebra being the largest and heaviest. All the vertebrae have transverse processes containing the foramen transversarium through which the vertebral artery passes. The articular masses are dense, heavy, rhomboid-shaped structures bounded by articulating superior and inferior facets. The pedicles are short and are posterolaterally oblique in orientation.[4,21]

2. Film Interpretation and Pathology

To answer a specific clinical question, different views of the cervical spine are frequently needed. The most common views are the lateral, anteroposterior (AP), open-mouth odontoid, oblique, and pillar views (Fig. 2-3). A systematic approach is recommended to assess the integrity of the cervical spine. Examination of the cervical spine should include visualization of all seven cervical vertebrae. This is especially important for trauma victims because 7% to 14% of fractures are known to occur at the C7 or C7-T1 level.[26] One must evaluate the spine for bone integrity, alignment, cartilage, joint space, and soft tissue abnormalities. The disadvantages of cervical spine x-rays are the limited range of tissue attenuation and the loss of spatial resolution caused by overlapping bone structures. In brief, a normal lateral cervical radiograph should demonstrate intact vertebrae and normal alignment of the anterior and posterior aspects of the vertebral bodies. The posterior vertebral body line, which is more reliable (the anterior vertebral body line is often encumbered by the presence of anterior osteophytes), must be intact. The facet joints overlap in an orderly fashion, similar to shingles on a rooftop. The spinolaminar line is uninterrupted, and the interlaminar, or interspinous, distances are uniform. The spinolaminar line is the dense cortical line representing the junction of the posterior laminae with the posterior spinous process, as seen on lateral radiographs. The posterior spinal line is an imaginary line extending from the spinolaminar line of the atlas to C3 (Fig. 2-4*A* and *B*).[21]

The anatomy and integrity of the craniocervical junction are crucial to the anesthesiologist. To achieve successful and safe endotracheal intubation, the anterior atlantodental interval (AADI), the vertical and anterior-posterior position of the dens, and the degree of extension of the head on the neck must be considered. The anterior arch of C1 bears a constant relationship to the dens called the AADI, or the predental space. It is defined as the space between the posterior surface of the anterior arch of C1 and the anterior surface of the dens. In flexion, because of the physiologic laxity of the cervicocranial ligaments, the anterior tubercle of the atlas assumes a more normal-appearing relationship to the dens, and the AADI increases in width, greater rostrally than caudally. In children and in flexion, the AADI is normally about 5 mm. In adults, it is generally accepted that the AADI is less than or equal to 3 mm (Fig. 2-5).[21]

The bone structures of the atlantoaxial joint provide mobility, such as rotational movement, rather than stability.

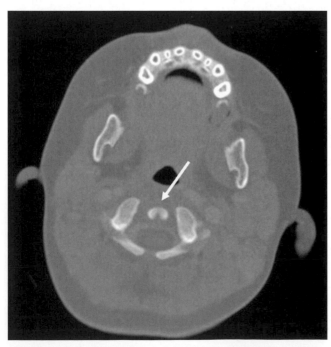

Figure 2-2 Cleft dens, normal variant. Axial computed tomography, bone algorithm.

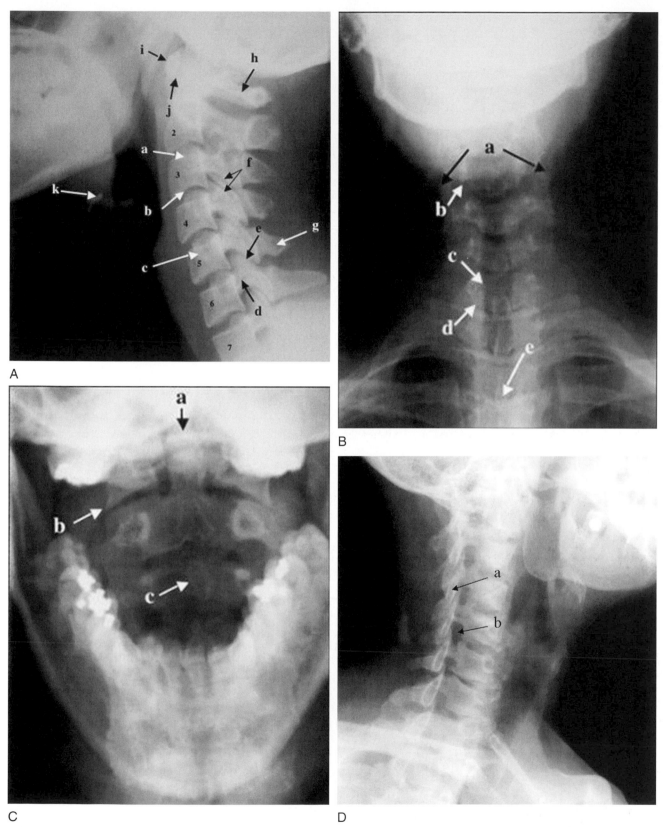

Figure 2-3 Normal cervical spine series. Lateral **(A)**, anteroposterior **(B)**, open-mouth odontoid **(C)**, and oblique **(D)** views of the cervical spine. **A,** Upper and lower end plates of C3 cervical vertebra, a and b; transverse process, c; pedicle, d; facet joint, e; articulating facets, f; posterior spinous process, g; posterior arch of C1, h; anterior arch of C1, i; atlantoaxial distance, j; hyoid bone, k. **B,** Smoothly undulating cortical margins of the lateral masses, a; joint of Luschka, b; superior and inferior end plates, c and d; midline posterior spinous process, e. **C,** Odontoid tip, a, centered between the lateral masses of the axis; symmetrical lateral margins of the lateral atlantoaxial joints, b; spinous process, c. **D,** Laminae of the articular masses, a, reflecting shingling effect of the articular masses; intervertebral (neural) foramen, b.

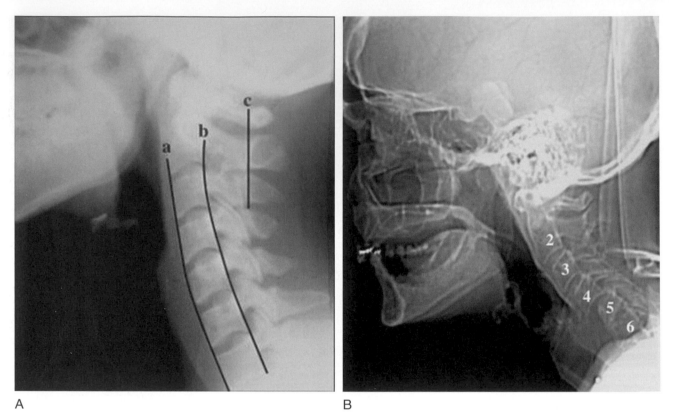

A   B

Figure 2-4 Normal lateral cervical spine x-ray **(A)** demonstrates normal alignment. Anterior spinal line, a; posterior vertebral line, b; posterior spinal line, c. Lateral scout view of a computed tomography examination **(B)** demonstrates anterior subluxation of C4 on C5.

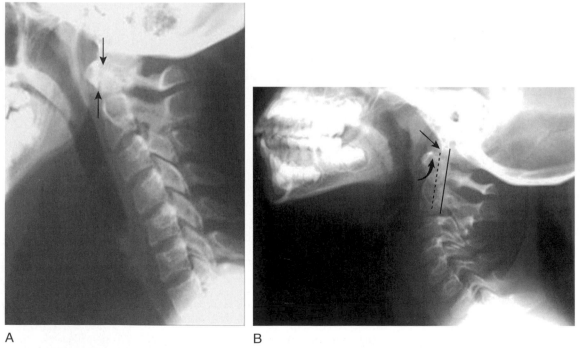

A   B

Figure 2-5 Anterior atlantodental interval (AADI). Lateral radiograph of the cervical spine in an adult patient **(A)**. AADI *(arrows)* or predental space is normally less than 3 mm. Lateral radiograph of the cervical spine in a pediatric patient **(B)**. The AADI can be normal up to 5 mm in a pediatric patient. Basion *(short arrow)*; posterior axial line *(solid line)*; distance between the dotted line and the solid line is the basion-axial interval (BAI) and should be 12 mm or less for a normal occipitovertebral relationship in a child.

Thus, the ligaments play a significant role in stability. The most important ligaments in the upper cervical spine are the transverse ligament, alar ligaments, and tectorial membrane. If the transverse ligament is disrupted and the alar and apical ligaments remain intact, up to 5 mm of movement at the atlantoaxial joint can be seen.[6] If all the ligaments have been disrupted, AADI can measure 10 mm or more. In atlantoaxial subluxation, the dens is invariably displaced posteriorly, which causes narrowing of the spinal canal and potential impingement of the spinal cord. The space available for the spinal cord is defined as the diameter of the spinal canal as measured in the AP plane, at the C1 level, that is not occupied by the odontoid process. In the normal spine, this space is approximately 20 mm.[6]

Important to rigid laryngoscopy and endotracheal intubation is the distance between the occiput and the posterior tubercle of C1, the atlanto-occipital distance (Fig. 2-6*A* and 6*B*), which is quite variable from individual to individual. Head extension is limited by the abutment of the occiput to the posterior tubercle of C1. It has been proposed that a shorter atlanto-occipital distance decreases the effectiveness of head extension and contributes to difficult intubation.[6,31] Occipitalization of C1 with the occiput not only limits head extension but also adds stress to the atlantoaxial joint.

Although the majority of head extension occurs at the atlanto-occipital joint, some extension can also occur at C1-C2.[31] Of note is the distinction made between the maneuver of general hyperextension of the head and neck and flexing the neck, then extending the head and neck, at the atlanto-occipital joint to improve the alignment of the airway structures and thus ease of intubation. It was observed by Nichol and Zuck[31] that in patients with limited or no extension possible at the atlanto-occipital joint, general extension of the head actually brings the larynx "anterior," thus limiting the visibility of the larynx on laryngoscopy.

The position and anatomy of the dens with respect to the anterior arch of C1 and the foramen magnum are worthy of attention. Congenital anomalies of the odontoid process, such as hypoplasia, can result in a loss of the buttressing action of the dens during extension and subsequent compression of neural elements. Conditions that are associated with odontoid hypoplasia are Morquio, Klippel-Feil, and Down syndromes; neurofibromatosis; dwarfism; spondyloepiphyseal dysplasia; osteogenesis imperfecta; and congenital scoliosis.[6,25] These patients are predisposed to atlantoaxial subluxation and craniocervical instability, and hyperextension of the head for intubation should be avoided. In addition, congenital fusion of C2 and C3 (Fig. 2-7*A* to *C*), whether occurring as an isolated

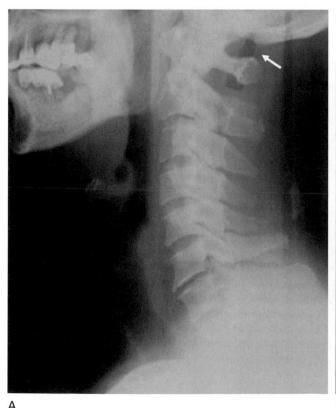

A

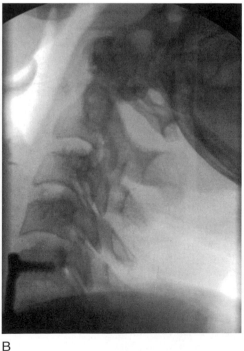

B

Figure 2-6 Atlanto-occipital distance. Lateral cervical spine in neutral position **(A)** with the atlanto-occipital distance demarcated *(arrow)*. Lateral cervical spine in hyperextension **(B).** Head extension is limited by the abutment of the occiput to the posterior tubercle of C1.

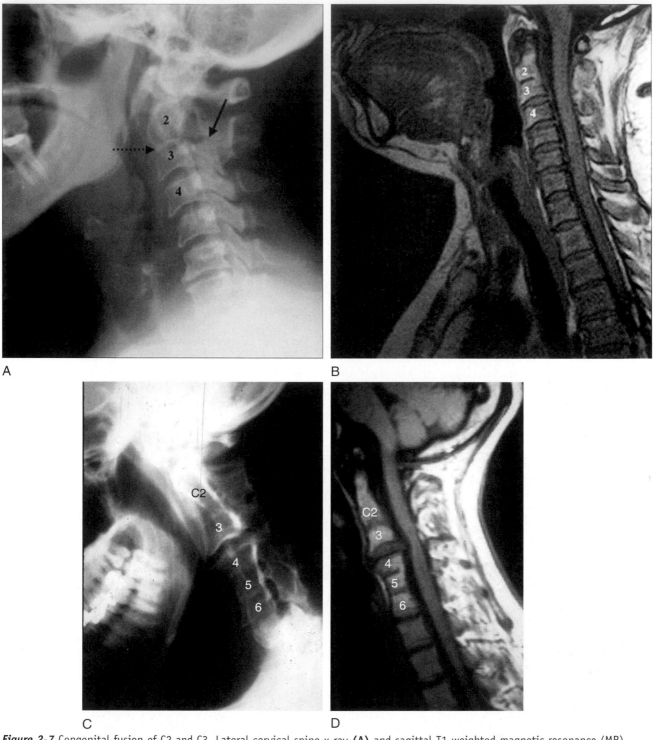

Figure 2-7 Congenital fusion of C2 and C3. Lateral cervical spine x-ray **(A)** and sagittal T1-weighted magnetic resonance (MR) study **(B)** demonstrating fusion of C2 and C3 vertebral bodies and lateral and posterior elements. A lateral radiograph **(C)** and T1-weighted MR cervical spine **(D)** of a patient with Klippel-Feil syndrome. There is fusion of C2 to C3 and fusion of C4 to C6. Not surprisingly, a disc herniation is present at the point of greatest mobility at C3-C4.

anomaly or as part of Klippel-Feil syndrome, places added stress at the C1-C2 junction.

Inflammatory arthropathies involving the atlantoaxial joint with subluxation are classically illustrated in rheumatoid arthritis and ankylosing spondylitis. The underlying cause of atlantoaxial subluxation is quite different in these two entities. Ankylosing spondylitis is characterized by progressive fibrosis and ossification of ligaments and joint capsules. In rheumatoid arthritis, there are bone erosion, synovial overgrowth, and destruction of the ligaments. Patients with rheumatoid arthritis are not only susceptible to AP subluxation at the C1-C2 junction but also at risk for vertical subluxation of the dens. Whether this condition is referred to as "cranial settling,"[21] superior migration of the odontoid process, or basilar invagination, the end result is the same. The odontoid process protrudes above the foramen magnum, narrowing the available space for the spinal cord and potentially leading to cord compression with the slightest head extension (Fig. 2-8*A* to *C*).

In response to the effective foreshortening of the spine secondary to the superior migration of the odontoid process, there is acquired rotational malalignment between the spine and larynx.[23] The larynx and the trachea, because they are semirigid structures and as a result of the tethering effect of the arch of aorta as it passes posteriorly over the left main bronchus, are predictably displaced caudally, deviated laterally to the left, rotated to the right, and anteriorly angulated. The effective neck length can be affected by superior migration of the dens, severe spondylosis with loss of disc space, or iatrogenic causes secondary to surgery. The soft tissues of the pharynx

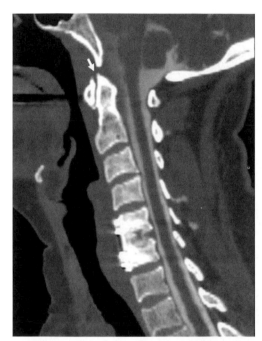

Figure 2-8 Position of the dens. Normal **(A);** rheumatoid patient **(B);** basilar invagination and platybasia in nonrheumatoid patient **(C).** Postmyelogram computed tomography with sagittal reformation **(A)** demonstrates normal relationship of the dens with respect to the foramen magnum, brain stem, and anterior arch of C1. Normal atlantoaxial distance (AADI) is seen *(arrow)*. **B,** T1-weighted sagittal magnetic resonance (MR) study of the cervical spine in a rheumatoid patient with erosion and pannus formation at the atlantoaxial joint resulting in increased AADI *(arrow)*, posterior subluxation of the dens, and brain stem compression. Sagittal MR study of the brain in a nonrheumatoid patient **(C)** with normal AADI, but basilar invagination and platybasia result in vertical subluxation of the dens and brain stem compression. The line drawn from the hard palate to the posterior lip of the foramen magnum is Chamberlain's line *(dotted line)*, which defines basilar invagination when the odontoid tip extends 5 mm or above this line. Also, note fusion of C2 and C3 vertebrae. The small linear dark line at the level of mid-C2 is the subdental synchondrosis *(white arrow)*.

A

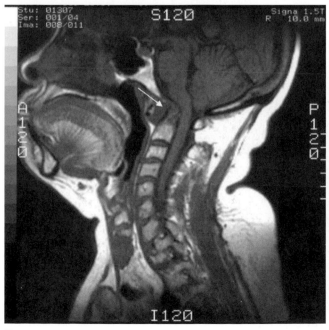

B

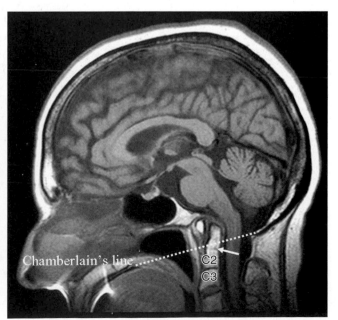

C

become more redundant owing to the relative shortening of the neck, which further obscures the view of the larynx. On laryngoscopy, the vocal cords are rotated clockwise. The presence of a rotated airway is suspected when the frontal view of the cervical spine demonstrates a deviated tracheal air column.

Historically, bone landmarks other than the spine, appreciated on a lateral cervical spine x-ray study, have been used in the anesthesia arena to predict preoperatively difficult laryngoscopy and endotracheal intubation on the basis of anatomic factors. Mandibular size and the ratios of the various measurements and their relationship to the hyoid bone have been proposed as predictors of difficult laryngoscopy (Fig. 2-9).[45] These measurements are meant to reflect the oral capacity, degree of mouth opening, and the level of larynx.[5,17] It is apparent that the causes of difficult laryngoscopy and endotracheal intubation are multifactorial. Combined with the clinical examination, anatomic measurements and findings assessed by x-ray study can help to alert the anesthesiologist to a potentially difficult airway. Thus, difficult laryngoscopy and endotracheal intubation can be anticipated and not unexpected.

Pseudosubluxation and pseudodislocation are terms applied to the physiologic anterior displacement of C2 on C3 that is frequently seen in infants and young children (Fig. 2-10). Physiologic anterior displacement of C2 on C3 and of C3 on C4 occurs in 24% and 14%, respectively, of children up to the age of 8 years.[4] In pediatric trauma cases, if C2 is noted to be anteriorly displaced and there are no other signs of trauma such as posterior arch fracture or prevertebral soft tissue hematoma, the spinolaminar lines of C1 through C3 should have a normal anatomic relationship. In a neutral position, the spinolaminar line of C2 lies upon, or up to 1 mm anterior or posterior to, the imaginary posterior spinal line. If the C2 vertebra is intact, in flexion, as the C2 body glides forward with respect to C3, the spinolaminar line of C2 moves 1 to 2 mm anterior to the posterior spinal line. Similarly, in extension, the posterior translation of the C2 body is mirrored by similar posterior displacement of the spinolaminar line of C2 with respect to the posterior spinal line. In traumatic spondylolisthesis, which is rare in children but more common in adults, the C2 body would translate anteriorly in flexion and posteriorly in extension, and the posterior spinal line would be maintained because of intact ligaments. However, flexion and extension films are not advisable when traumatic spondylolisthesis is suspected.

Acute cervical spine injury is often the indication for ordering a cervical spine examination. Although CT and MRI are exceptional in detailing bone and soft tissue abnormalities, plain film of the cervical spine remains a good initial screening study. It is useful to tailor and

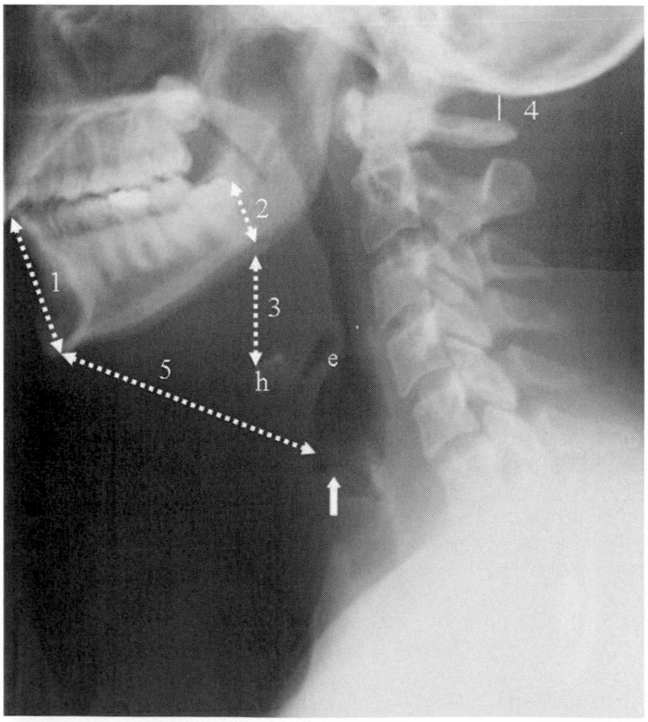

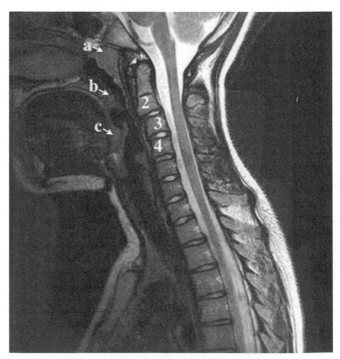

Figure 2-9 Mandibular and hyoid measurements proposed as predictors of difficult laryngoscopy. Anterior depth of mandible, 1; posterior depth of mandible, 2; mandibulohyoid distance, 3; atlanto-occipital distance, 4; thyromental distance, 5; epiglottis, e; hyoid bone, h; laryngeal ventricle *(solid arrow)* demarcating the level of the larynx. The true vocal cords are just below the level of the laryngeal ventricle.

Figure 2-10 Pseudosubluxation at C2-C3. T2-weighted sagittal magnetic resonance cervical spine study demonstrates physiologic anterior displacement of C2 on C3 in a child. Also seen are normal soft tissue masses encroaching on the airway from adenoids, a; palatine tonsils, b; lingual tonsils at the base of the tongue, c.

focus further imaging of the spine. For evaluation of trauma, cross-table lateral, AP, and open-mouth odontoid views are recommended. A lateral view reveals the majority of injuries (Fig. 2-11); however, patients who are rendered quadriplegic by severe ligamentous injuries may demonstrate a normal lateral cervical spine x-ray. By adding the AP and open-mouth odontoid views to the cross-table lateral view of the cervical spine, the sensitivity of detecting significant injury is increased from 74% to 82% to 93%.[41] In reality, cross-sectional imaging (i.e., CT of the spine) has become a mainstay in the evaluation of the cervical spine, especially in the setting of acute trauma.

Cervical spine x-rays are also ordered for the evaluation of cervical spondylosis (Fig. 2-12). The hypertrophic bone changes associated with this condition are well depicted on x-ray studies. Large anterior osteophytes that project forward may cause dysphagia and difficult intubation. The bone canal and neural foramina are assessed for stenosis, and, when present, precautions can be taken when hyperextending the neck and positioning the patient to avoid exacerbation of baseline neurologic symptomatology. Calcification and ossification are well depicted on x-ray examination. Ossification of the anterior longitudinal ligament and diffuse idiopathic skeletal hyperostosis have been reported as causes of difficult intubation.[2] This can be readily appreciated on plain films. Another condition, which also may signal difficult intubation, is calcification of the stylohyoid ligament (Fig. 2-13).[35]

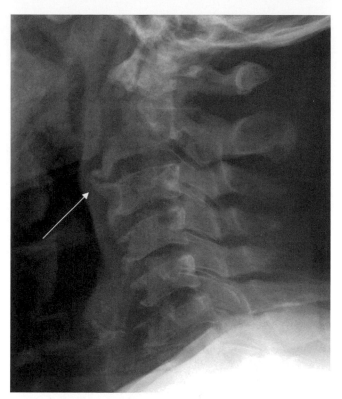

Figure 2-12 Cervical spondylosis. Lateral cervical spine x-ray film. Large anterior osteophytes indent the airway and oropharynx.

3. Cervical Spine X-Ray and the Airway

The lateral cervical spine x-ray, obtained to evaluate the integrity and alignment of the bony cervical spine, allows an incidental view of the aerodigestive tract and a gross assessment of the overall patency of the airway. Useful bone landmarks of the pharynx and larynx, which can be appreciated on the lateral neck x-ray, are the hard palate, hyoid bone, thyroid, and cricoid cartilages (Fig. 2-14). The hard palate separates the nasopharynx from the oropharynx. The larynx can be thought of as being suspended from the hyoid bone. Muscles acting on the hyoid bone elevate the larynx and provide the primary protection from aspiration. The largest cartilage in the neck is the thyroid cartilage, which along with the cricoid cartilage acts as a protective shield for the inner larynx. The cricoid cartilage is the only complete cartilaginous ring in the respiratory system. It is located at the level where the larynx ends and the trachea begins.

Normal air-filled structures seen on lateral plain film are the nasopharynx, oropharynx, and hypopharynx. Air in the pharynx outlines the soft palate, uvula, base of the tongue, and nasopharyngeal airway (Fig. 2-15). Any sizable soft tissue pathology results in deviation or effacement of the airway. The tongue constitutes the bulk of the soft tissues at the level of the oropharynx. In children, and sometimes in adults, prominent lymphatic tissues, such as adenoids, and palatine tonsils may encroach on the nasopharyngeal and oral airways. Lingual tonsils are located at the base of the tongue above the

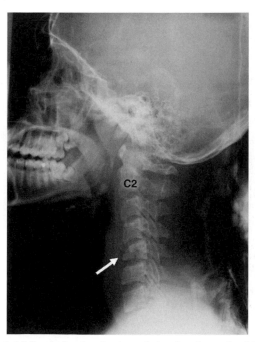

Figure 2-11 Cervical spine fracture. Lateral radiograph of the cervical spine demonstrates a compression fracture of the C5 vertebra (block arrow). A retropulsed fragment impinges on the spinal canal.

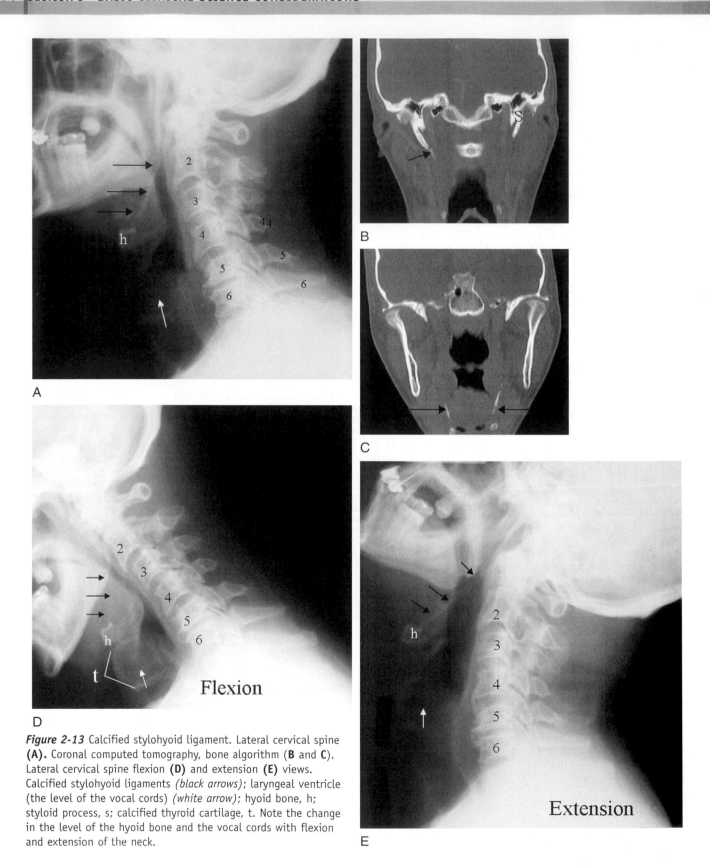

Figure 2-13 Calcified stylohyoid ligament. Lateral cervical spine **(A)**. Coronal computed tomography, bone algorithm (**B** and **C**). Lateral cervical spine flexion **(D)** and extension **(E)** views. Calcified stylohyoid ligaments *(black arrows)*; laryngeal ventricle (the level of the vocal cords) *(white arrow)*; hyoid bone, h; styloid process, s; calcified thyroid cartilage, t. Note the change in the level of the hyoid bone and the vocal cords with flexion and extension of the neck.

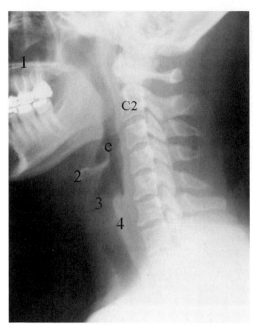

Figure 2-14 Normal bone landmarks. Lateral cervical spine. Hard palate, 1; hyoid bone, 2; calcified thyroid cartilage, 3; calcified cricoid cartilage, 4; epiglottis, e.

valleculae, which are air-filled pouches between the tongue base and the free margin of the epiglottis.

The epiglottis is an elastic fibrocartilage in the shape of a flattened teardrop or leaf that tapers inferiorly and attaches to the thyroid cartilage. The epiglottis tends to be more angular in infants than in adults. During the first several years of life, the larynx changes its position in the neck.[32,47] The free edge of the epiglottis in neonates is

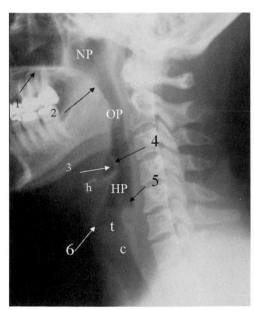

Figure 2-15 Normal airway structures. Lateral cervical spine x-ray film. Hard palate, 1; soft palate and uvula, 2; air-filled vallecula, 3; epiglottis, 4; air-filled pyriform sinus, 5; air-filled stripe laryngeal ventricle, 6; nasopharynx, NP; oropharynx, OP; hypopharynx, HP; hyoid bone, h; thyroid cartilage, t; noncalcified cricoid cartilage, c.

found at or near the C1 level, and the cricoid cartilage, representing the most caudal portion of the larynx, is at the C4-C5 level. By adolescence, the epiglottis is found at the C2-C3 level, and the cricoid is at the C6 level. The adult epiglottis is usually seen at the C3 level, with the cricoid at C6-C7. However, the position of these structures in the normal population varies by at least one vertebral body level. Sometimes visualized by a cervical spine x-ray study, soft tissue neck technique, and on the CT scout view or the MR sagittal view of the neck is a transversely oriented air-containing lucent stripe, just below the base of the aryepiglottic folds, which indicates the position of the air-filled laryngeal ventricle (Fig. 2-16). This marks the position of the true vocal cords, which are just below this lucent stripe. Lateral to the aryepiglottic fold is the pyriform sinus of the pharynx. This anterior mucosal recess is between the posterior third of the thyroid cartilage and the aryepiglottic fold. The extreme lower aspect of the pyriform sinus is situated between the mucosa-covered arytenoids and the mucosa-covered thyroid cartilage. This is at the level of the true vocal cords. The air column caudally represents the cervical trachea. On the AP view, the false and true vocal cords above and below the laryngeal ventricles may be identified, as well as the subglottic region and the trachea. Calcified thyroid cartilage can also sometimes be visualized.

The landmarks dorsal to the airway are shadows representing the normal soft tissue structures of the posterior wall of the nasopharynx, which is closely adherent to the anterior surface of the atlas and the axis and extends superiorly to the clivus and inferiorly to become continuous with the soft tissues of the posterior wall of the hypopharynx. The ligaments of the cervicocranium critical to maintaining stability throughout this region are directly involved in the range of motion of the cervicocranium and anteriorly contribute to the prevertebral soft tissue shadow. Superimposed upon these deep structures are the constrictor muscles and the mucosa of the posterior pharyngeal wall. The cervicocranial prevertebral soft tissue contour should normally be slightly posteriorly concave rostral to the anterior tubercle of C1, anteriorly convex in front of the anterior tubercle, and posteriorly concave caudal to the anterior tubercle, depending on the amount of adenoidal tissue and on the amount of air in the pharynx. Adenoidal tissue appears as a homogeneous, smoothly lobulated mass of varying size and configuration. The anterior surface of the adenoid is demarcated by air anteriorly and inferiorly. The air inferior to the adenoids allows differentiation between adenoids and the presence of a nasopharyngeal hematoma commonly associated with major midface fractures. In infants and young children, the soft tissues of the cervicocranium are lax and redundant. Depending on the phase of respiration and position, the thickness of the prevertebral soft tissues may appear to increase and simulate a retropharyngeal hematoma. This finding may extend to the lower cervical spine. This anomaly becomes normal if imaging is repeated with the neck extended and

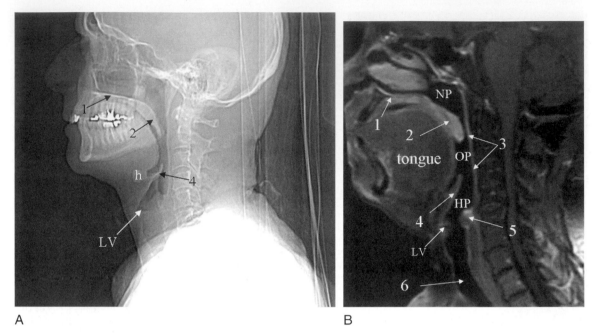

Figure 2-16 Normal airway structures. Computed tomography lateral scout view **(A).** T1-weighted, fat-suppressed postcontrast sagittal magnetic resonance cervical spine study **(B).** Hard palate, 1; soft palate and uvula, 2; retropharyngeal or prevertebral soft tissue, 3; epiglottis, 4; arytenoid prominence, 5; trachea air column, 6; hyoid bone, h; laryngeal ventricle, LV; nasopharynx, NP; oropharynx, OP; hypopharynx, HP.

during inspiration. By 8 years of age, the contour of the soft tissues should resemble that seen in adults. Of note, in pediatric patients, sedation may result in a decrease in the AP diameter of the pharynx at the level of the palatine tonsils, in the soft palate, and at the level of the epiglottis.

In the lower neck, from C3 to C7, the prevertebral soft tissue shadow differs from that in the cervicocranium by virtue of the beginning of the esophagus and the prevertebral fascial space, which are recognized on the lateral radiograph as a fat stripe. By standard anatomic description, the esophagus begins at the level of C4; however, in vivo, the esophageal ostium may normally be found as high as C3 and as low as C6 and varies with the phase of swallowing and the flexion and extension of the

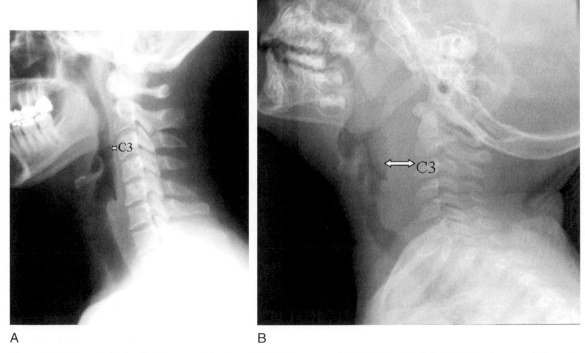

Figure 2-17 Prevertebral soft tissues on lateral cervical spine x-ray study. **A,** Normal adult. **B,** Retropharyngeal abscess in a child. The airway is displaced anteriorly. (Courtesy of Dr. Alan Schlesinger, Texas Children's Hospital, Houston.)

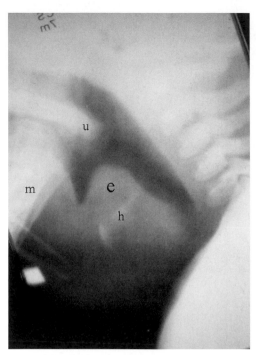

Figure 2-18 Epiglottitis. Lateral soft tissue neck examination in flexion of a child demonstrating an enlarged and swollen epiglottis, the "thumb" sign. Epiglottis, e; mandible, m; uvula, u; hyoid, h. (Courtesy of Dr. Alan Schlesinger, Texas Children's Hospital, Houston.)

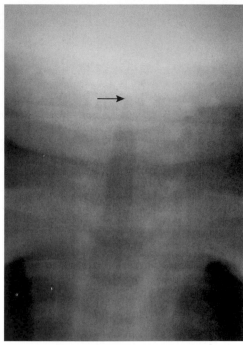

Figure 2-19 Croup. Anteroposterior soft tissue neck x-ray in an infant. Long segment narrowing of the subglottic airway is present with loss of the normal angle between the vocal cords and the subglottic airway, the "steeple" sign. (Courtesy of Dr. Alan Schlesinger, Texas Children Hospital, Houston.)

cervical spine.[46] The prevertebral soft tissue thickness, the distance between the posterior pharyngeal air column and the anterior portion of the third or fourth vertebra, should not exceed one half to three quarters of the diameter of the vertebral body. In the opinion of Harris and Mirvis, only the measurement at C3 is valid, and it should not exceed 4 mm (Fig. 2-17).[21] More caudally, at the cervicothoracic junction, assessment of the prevertebral soft tissues is based on contour rather than actual measurement. This contour should parallel the arch formed by the anterior cortices of the lower cervical and upper thoracic vertebral bodies.

In truth, plain film diagnosis of upper airway diseases has been supplanted by cross-sectional imaging, except in a few situations, in which plain x-ray findings are pathognomonic of the disease. Two classical examples of plain film radiologic diagnosis are acute epiglottitis and croup. In acute epiglottitis, or supraglottitis, a more encompassing term, there is edema and swelling of the epiglottis, with or without involvement of the aryepiglottic folds and arytenoids. The offending organism is usually *Haemophilus influenzae*. Airway compromise with a rapidly progressive course requiring emergency tracheostomy is a possibility if the entity goes unrecognized and untreated. In general, the infection is milder in adults than in children. This entity, usually a more indolent form, is making a comeback in patients with acquired immunodeficiency syndrome (AIDS).

The plain x-ray findings are swelling or enlargement of the epiglottis. On the conventional lateral radiograph of the neck, thickening of the free edge of the epiglottis can be appreciated and is referred to as the "thumb" sign (Fig. 2-18). The width of the adult epiglottis should be less than one third of the AP width of the C4 body. Cross-sectional imaging is superfluous. However, theoretically the degree of airway compromise can be quantified by three-dimensional reformation.

In laryngotracheobronchitis or croup, the subglottic larynx is involved. It affects younger children and has a less fulminant course than acute epiglottitis. The swelling of the soft tissues in subglottic neck can be appreciated on an AP view of the neck (Fig. 2-19). There is usually a long segment narrowing of the glottis and subglottic airway with loss of the normal angle between the vocal cords and the subglottic airway. This has been referred to as the "steeple" sign. The hypopharynx is usually dilated because of the airway obstruction distally.

Cervical spine examination using soft tissue technique is also useful for the evaluation for the presence of radiopaque foreign bodies such as a fish bone. Ingested foreign bodies most often lodge at the level of the pyriform sinus (Fig. 2-20).

B. CHEST X-RAY

Prior to the advent of CT, chest x-ray (CXR) was routinely ordered to assess pulmonary and cardiovascular status, and CXR is still a cost-efficient examination that yields a great deal of general information. The most common views of the chest are the posteroanterior (PA), AP, and

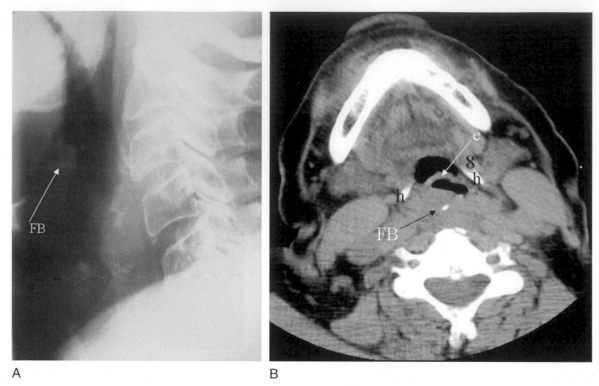

A   B

Figure 2-20 Foreign body, fishbone. **A,** Lateral cervical spine. **B,** Axial computed tomography of the neck in a different patient. Tip of the epiglottis, e; hyoid, h; fishbone, FB.

lateral projections (Fig. 2-21). The PA chest view is obtained with the patient's anterior chest closest to the film cassette and the x-ray beam directed from a posterior to anterior direction. Alternatively, the AP chest view is done with the patient's back closest to the film cassette and the x-ray beam directed in the anterior to posterior direction. The part of the chest closest to the film cassette is the least magnified; therefore, the cardiac silhouette is larger on the AP projection. The lateral projection is most often performed with the patient's left chest closest to the film cassette for better delineation of the structures in the left hemithorax, which is more obscured by the heart on a PA projection. Other common projections obtained include oblique, decubitus, and lordotic views. The oblique view is useful for assessing a lesion with respect to other structures in the chest. The decubitus view is helpful to assess whether an apparent elevated hemidiaphragm is due to a large subpulmonic pleural effusion. The lordotic view is helpful to look for suspected small apical pneumothorax, which can also be accentuated on an expiratory phase view.

1. Chest X-Ray Interpretation and Pathology

It is useful to train one's eyes to analyze the CXR systematically to cover the details of the chest wall, including the ribs, lungs (field and expansion), and mediastinal structures that include the heart and the outline of the tracheal-bronchial tree. On an adequate inspiratory film, the hemidiaphragms are below the anterior end of the sixth rib, or at least below the 10th posterior rib, and the

lung expansion should be symmetrical. The right hemidiaphragm is usually half an interspace higher than the left, which is depressed by the heart (see Fig. 2-21). A high hemidiaphragm implies reduced lung volume, which can be caused by phrenic nerve paralysis, thoracic conditions causing chest pain resulting in splinting, and extrapulmonic processes such as an enlarged spleen or liver, pancreatitis, and subphrenic abscess. The presumed level of the hemidiaphragm is seen as an edge or transition between aerated lungs and the opacity of the organs in the abdomen. If the thin leaves of the hemidiaphragm are outlined by air, a pneumoperitoneum should be considered (Fig. 2-22).

A well-expanded lung should appear radiographically lucent but be traversed by "lung markings," thin threads of interstitium consisting of septa and arterial, venous, and lymphatic vessels. In the majority of normal individuals, the lungs appear more lucent at the top owing to the distribution of the pulmonary vasculature, the effect of gravity, and overlying soft tissues such as breast tissues. In congestive heart failure or pulmonary venous hypertension, this pattern is reversed, with "cephalization" and engorgement of the pulmonary veins in the upper lung zones (Fig. 2-23; see Fig. 2-21). In general, any process such as fluid, pus, or cells that replaces the airspaces of the lungs causes the x-ray beam to be more attenuated, allowing less of the beam to be transmitted through the patient to the film. This would make this area or areas on the film less dark or more opaque (white). A whole host of diseases could be responsible, depending on the clinical picture, including pleural effusion, pulmonary edema,

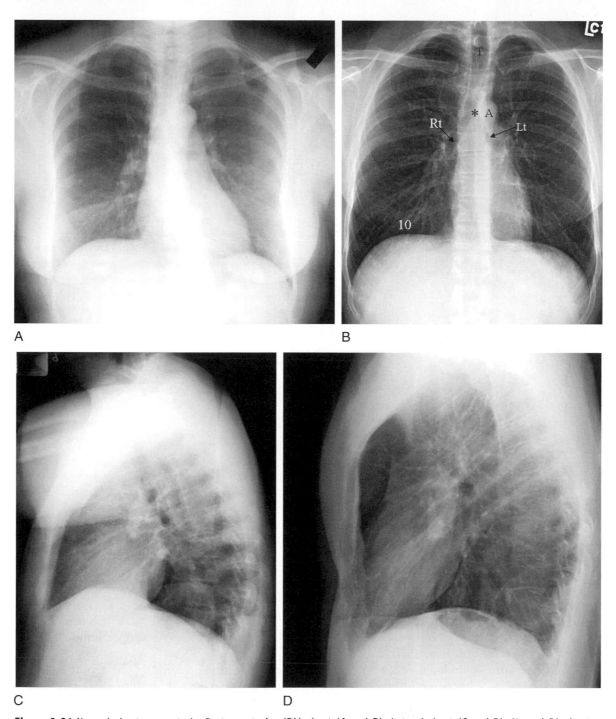

A

B

C

D

Figure 2-21 Normal chest x-ray study. Posteroanterior (PA) chest (**A** and **B**). Lateral chest (**C** and **D**). Normal PA chest of a female with increased density at the lung bases related to overlying breast tissues **(A).** PA chest of a male with lucent lungs **(B).** Normal lateral chest view **(C)** and lateral chest of a patient with chronic obstructive pulmonary disease **(D)** showing barrel-shaped chest with increase in the retrosternal air. Note that on the lateral examination the lung base appears progressively more lucent overlying the dorsal spine. Trachea, T; aorta, A; carina, asterisk; right and left bronchi, Rt and Lt; 10th posterior rib, 10.

pneumonia, lung mass, lung collapse or atelectasis, lung infarct or contusion, and metastatic disease (Fig. 2-24). The key, from an anesthesiologist's point of view, is not to make the correct pathologic diagnosis but to note the abnormality, which may affect ventilation, and adjust the anesthetic practice accordingly.

In contrast to the increased opacity of the lung caused by the preceding conditions is a hemithorax, which appears too lucent and devoid of the expected lung markings. Two entities should be considered. Foremost is a pneumothorax (Fig. 2-25); if large, the collapsed lung is medially applied against the mediastinum. If the mediastinum is shifted away from the midline, a tension pneumothorax may be present, and emergent management is required. More often than not, the cause is the presence of large emphysematous blebs in patients with chronic obstructive

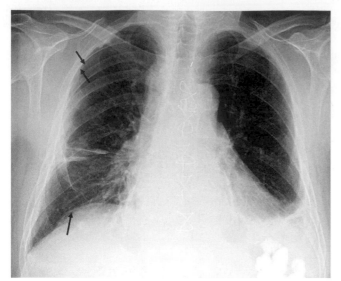

Figure 2-22 Pneumoperitoneum. Postoperative anteroposterior chest in a patient after thoracotomy. Arrows in right upper chest outline thin pleural line defining a tiny pneumothorax. Arrow in right lower chest demarcates the right hemidiaphragm outlined by a small pneumoperitoneum. This patient also has cardiomegaly, right midlung and left basilar atelectasis.

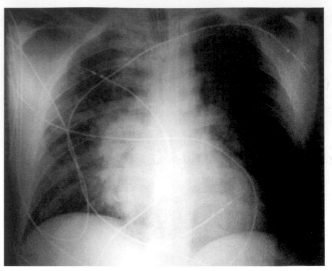

Figure 2-23 Congestive heart failure. Anteroposterior chest demonstrates engorgement of the perihilar vasculature. Endotracheal tube and nasogastric tube are in place.

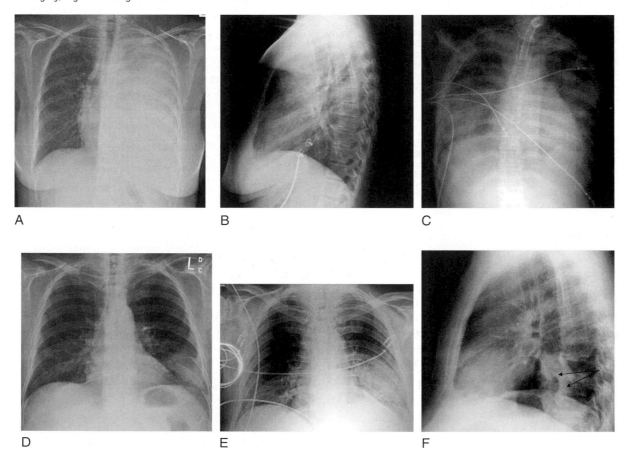

A

B

C

D

E

F

Figure 2-24 Left pleural effusion—posteroanterior (PA) **(A)** and lateral **(B)** chest x-ray films. PA chest shows almost complete "white-out" of the left hemithorax and minimal residual aerated left upper lung zone. There is a mass effect with deviation of the trachea to the right. On the lateral view **(B)**, the pleural effusion is less apparent. The tipoff is the lack of the expected lucency overlying the spine at the base; see Figure 2-21*C* and *D*. Pulmonary edema—anteroposterior (AP) view of the chest **(C)** demonstrates bilateral hazy lung fields with air bronchogram. Tracheostomy tube is noted. Left lower lung mass—PA **(D)** and AP **(E)** radiographs of the chest. Note that although the inspiratory effort is the same on both the PA and AP views (hemidiaphragm below ninth posterior rib), the cardiac silhouette and the left lower lobe mass appear larger on the AP view by virtue of the film geometry and magnification factor. The lateral view **(F)** helps to localize the disease process to the lateral segment of the left lower lobe. A mass is noted with postobstructive atelectasis.

Continued

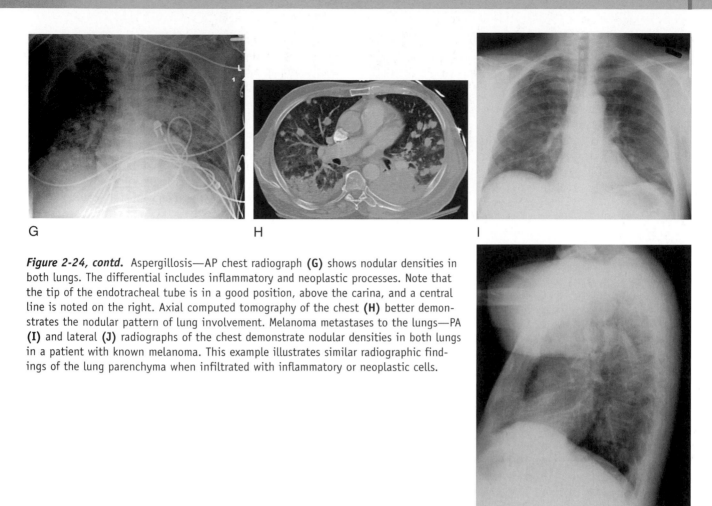

G   H   I

Figure 2-24, contd. Aspergillosis—AP chest radiograph **(G)** shows nodular densities in both lungs. The differential includes inflammatory and neoplastic processes. Note that the tip of the endotracheal tube is in a good position, above the carina, and a central line is noted on the right. Axial computed tomography of the chest **(H)** better demonstrates the nodular pattern of lung involvement. Melanoma metastases to the lungs—PA **(I)** and lateral **(J)** radiographs of the chest demonstrate nodular densities in both lungs in a patient with known melanoma. This example illustrates similar radiographic findings of the lung parenchyma when infiltrated with inflammatory or neoplastic cells.

J

pulmonary disease, which are sometimes difficult to differentiate from a moderate to large pneumothorax. More rare causes of a unilateral lucent lung are pulmonary oligemia, with decreased pulmonary flow from a thromboembolism of the right or left pulmonary artery, pulmonary neoplasm, and obstructive hyperinflation. Bilateral lucent lungs are harder to appreciate. These are usually seen in patients with pulmonary stenosis secondary to cyanotic heart disease and right-to-left shunts. A discussion of the pediatric chest and congenital heart and lung diseases is beyond the scope of this chapter.

Moving centrally in the chest, one encounters the mediastinum, containing the hila, tracheobronchial tree, heart and great vessels, lymph nodes, esophagus, and thymus. The mediastinum is extrapleural and outlined by air in the adjacent lungs. Except for the air within the trachea and the main stem bronchi, the remainder of the mediastinal structures are soft tissues or water density, including the fat, on conventional chest radiographs. Therefore, it is extremely difficult to localize a mediastinal lesion. There are traditional pleural reflections or vertical lines described for a frontal CXR that, if deviated, would suggest the presence of mediastinal pathology.

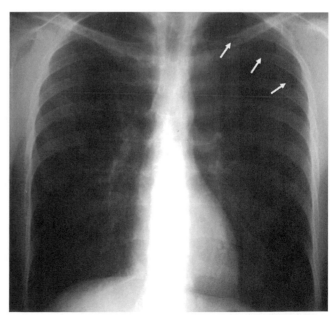

Figure 2-25 Pneumothorax. Posteroanterior chest x-ray in a young male with spontaneous pneumothorax. (Courtesy of Dr. John Pagani, IRPA, Houston.)

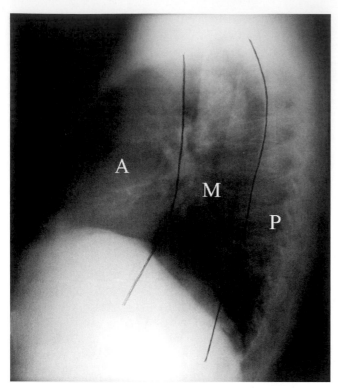

Figure 2-26 Mediastinal compartments. Lateral chest x-ray with imaginary lines drawn on the film to demonstrate the three mediastinal compartments. The anterior (A) and middle (M) mediastinal compartments are divided by the line extending along the back of the heart and front of the trachea. A line drawn connecting each thoracic vertebra about a centimeter behind its anterior margin separates the middle from the posterior compartment (P).

Felson[16] has proposed a radiologic approach to subdividing the mediastinum on a lateral radiograph into three compartments: anterior, middle, and posterior. The anterior and middle mediastinum are divided by the line extending along the back of the heart and front of the trachea. The middle and posterior mediastinal compartments are separated by the line connecting a point on each thoracic vertebra about a centimeter behind its anterior margin (Fig. 2-26).[16] Conditions that can be found in each of the compartments of the mediastinum are logically based on the anatomic structures found within the compartments. For example, tracheal, esophageal, and thyroid lesions would lie in the middle mediastinum. Neurogenic tumors and spinal problems would be in the posterior mediastinum. Cardiac and thymic lesions would occupy the anterior mediastinum. Certain diseases such as lymph node disorders, lymphoma, and aortic aneurysms may arise in any or all three compartments.[16] Many modifications to the divisions of the mediastinum have been proposed.[19]

The great vessels and the heart should be centrally located on the AP view of the mediastinum. The aortic knob is usually on the left, and the cardiothoracic ratio on the AP view is roughly less than 50%. The hila are composed of the pulmonary arteries and their main branches, the upper lobe pulmonary veins, the major bronchi, and the lymph glands (Fig. 2-27). This is an excellent opportunity to visualize the position of the trachea, carina, and main stem bronchi, which are outlined by air. The carinal bifurcation angle is typically 60 to 75 degrees.[19] The right main stem bronchus has a steeper angle than the left (see Fig. 2-21); it usually branches off

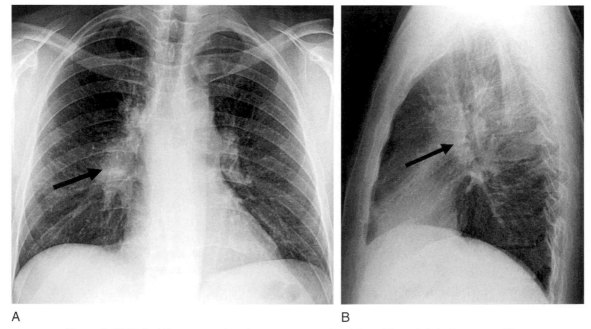

A   B

Figure 2-27 Right hilar mass and nodes. Posteroanterior **(A)** and lateral **(B)** chest x-ray films.

the trachea at 25- to 30-degrees, whereas the left main stem bronchus leaves the trachea at a 45- to 50-degree angle. The trachea is a tubular structure extending from the cricoid cartilage to the carina, which is located approximately at the T5 level. C-shaped hyaline cartilage rings, which can calcify with age, outline the trachea anteriorly. The posterior trachea is membranous. The mean transverse diameter of the trachea is approximately 15 mm for women and 18 mm for men.[19] The trachea in the cervical region is midline, but it is deviated to the right in the thorax.

Adequate positioning of an endotracheal tube (ET) in an intubated patient can be documented. The tip should be intrathoracic and at a distance above the carina that ensures equal ventilation to both lungs. After translaryngeal intubation, CXR is frequently obtained to assess the position of the ET. One should evaluate the ET position with the patient's head and neck in a neutral position; however, in an intensive care unit setting, this may not be possible. The tip of the ET may move, up or down, by 1 to 2 cm with either flexion or extension of the head. Rotation of the head and neck usually results in ascent of the tip.[19] The optimum position of the tip of the ET should be approximately 3 to 5 cm above the carina, to allow enough latitude in movement of the tube with turning of patient's head, and the inflated cuff position below the vocal cords (Fig. 2-28).[18] Malpositioning of the cuff at the level of the vocal cords or pharynx increases the risk of aspiration. Overinflation of the cuff at the level of

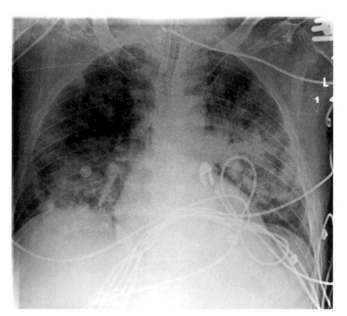

Figure 2-28 Anteroposterior (AP) portable chest x-ray. Most chest examinations in the intensive care unit are done with a portable x-ray machine in the AP projection. Note the acceptable position of the endotracheal tube above the carina. A right subclavian central venous line is present with the tip in the superior vena cava. Multiple cables attached to monitors are noted crossing the chest.

the vocal cords may lead to necrosis.[1] The inflated cuff of the ET should fill the tracheal air column without changing its contour. Overall, the ET size should be about two thirds the diameter of the tracheal lumen. At times, the tip of the ET extends beyond the carina, resulting in intubation of the right main bronchus, which can be detected by asymmetric breath sounds or on CXR. If unrecognized, atelectasis in the underaerated lung may result.

If a nasogastric or orogastric tube is in place, it should more or less course inferiorly and to the left, toward the fundus of the stomach in the left upper quadrant, except for the unusual case of situs inversus. Inadvertently the gastric tube may achieve bronchial intubation; the errant course of the tube would be evident. Without doubt, the art of CXR interpretation has been supplanted by the advent of CT, which demonstrates chest pathology with unparalleled clarity. However, CXR can still afford a composite survey of the chest at one quick glance. One can easily compare the lung volumes, position of the mediastinum, presence or absence of major airspace disease, and gross assessment of the cardiac status.

IV. CROSS-SECTIONAL ANATOMY AND PATHOLOGY: COMPUTED TOMOGRAPHY AND MAGNETIC RESONANCE IMAGING

The anatomy of the airway from the nasal cavity, pharynx, and larynx to the lungs is exceptionally well depicted by CT, but MRI can be a useful complement in the evaluation of these regions. It is superior to CT in evaluating tumor infiltration of soft tissues but lacks the ability to depict bone erosions secondary to tumor because cortical bone gives no MRI signal. MRI is susceptible to motion artifacts, including breathing artifacts, whereas spiral CT technology allows the entire neck or thorax to be scanned in a single breath-hold. Both techniques allow either direct scanning or reformation in all three planes.

A. NOSE AND NASAL CAVITY

The nose, which refers to both the external apparatus and the nasal cavity or internal architecture, is one of the two gateways to the aerodigestive tract. Most of the airflow to the lungs occurs through the nasal cavity. Oral respiration is not physiologic; it is a learned action. The three physiologic functions of the nose are respiration, defense, and olfaction.[1] In respiration, airflow is modified by nasal resistance at the level of the nares and the nasal valves to allow efficient pulmonary ventilation. A major portion of the nasal airflow passes through the middle meatus. The passage of inspired air through the nasal cavity allows humidification and warming.[39]

1. Embryology

The development of the face, nose, and sinuses is complex but systematic. Thus, the occurrence of congenital lesions and malformations in these areas is quite logical and predictable, dependent on the time of prenatal insult. Face, nose, and sinus development is temporally and spatially related to the development of the optic nerve, globe, and corpus callosum, which accounts for the frequency of concurrent anomalies. The major features of the face develop in the fourth to eighth week of gestation owing to the growth, migration, and merging of a number of processes bordering on the stomodeum, which is a slitlike invagination of the ectoderm that marks the location of the mouth. The stomodeum is bordered superiorly by the unpaired median frontonasal prominence, laterally by the paired maxillary processes, and inferiorly by the paired mandibular processes, which are derivatives of the first branchial arch.[30] The various facial and palatal cleft syndromes can be explained by the failure of different processes to grow, migrate, and merge properly.[30]

Improper development of the frontonasal process or its failure to merge with adjacent processes results in a coherent series of malformations. Insufficient development of the frontonasal process may result in the absence of the intermaxillary segment, with a rectangular defect in the middle one third of the upper lip and upper incisors, the absence of the primary plate with a cleft secondary plate, and hypotelorism.

The nasal placodes are paired epithelial thickenings that arise near the lateral margins of the frontal prominence. Horseshoe-shaped elevations appear around the nasal placodes, which become recessed and by 5 weeks of gestation are referred to as nasal pits. The two sides of each horseshoe-shaped elevation are referred to as the nasomedial process and the nasolateral process. During the sixth week of gestation, the maxillary processes increase in size and push the enlarging nasomedial processes medially, where they merge with the frontal prominence to form the frontonasal prominence, from which arise the nasal and frontal bones, the cartilaginous nasal capsule, the central one third of the upper lip, the superior alveolar ridge, including incisors, and the primary plate of the hard palate, which is V shaped. The secondary plate is derived from the fusion of two palatal shelves arising from the maxillary process. The palatal shelves fuse in the midline and anteriorly with the primary plate. The lines of fusion of the palate appear Y shaped. The incisive foramina lie at the midpoint of the Y, marking the junction of the primary and secondary plates. As the palate is forming, the nasal septum grows downward and fuses with the hard palate. By the ninth week, the ventral three quarters of the nasal septum have fused with the hard palate. Next, the left and right nasal chambers separate from one another and from the oral cavity. Posteriorly, the palatal shelves do not fuse with the nasal septum or form the soft palate. The development of the nasal cavity is complete by the second month of fetal life. From the second to the sixth month of prenatal life, the nostrils are closed by epithelial plugs that recanalize to establish a patent nasal cavity. Failure to do so could account for the congenital stenoses and atresias that cause nasal airway obstruction, which are often seen in conjunction with craniofacial anomalies.[30]

Failure of the nasomedial processes to merge with the maxillary processes on one or both sides produces the typical unilateral or bilateral common (lateral) cleft lip (Fig. 2-29). Posterior extension of the cleft between the primary and secondary palates and further back between the left and right halves of the secondary palate produces the unilateral or bilateral common (lateral) cleft palate. Failure of the nasolateral process to merge with the maxillary process results in an oblique cleft extending from the inner canthus to the nose. This cleft may occur in association with a bilateral common cleft lip and palate. If the maxillary and mandibular processes do not merge, unilaterally or bilaterally, the result is a transverse facial cleft, also referred to as Wolf mouth or macrosomia. The truest midline cleft lip is secondary to failure of the two nasomedial processes to merge in the midline. Posterior extension of this cleft may result in a cleft superior alveolar ridge, diastasis of the medial incisors, double frenulum or upper lip, and a cleft primary palate. If the cleft extends more posteriorly, the secondary palate and uvula may be cleft.

Relevant to anesthetic practice is an awareness that the midline craniofacial dysraphism falls into two groups: an

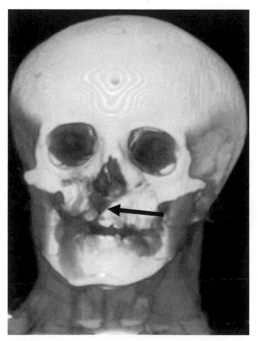

Figure 2-29 Cleft lip. Three-dimensional computed tomography reconstruction demonstrates a bone cleft of the maxilla, resulting in communication between the nasal and oral cavities.

inferior group, in which the clefting primarily affects the upper lip, with or without the nose, and a superior group, in which the clefting primarily affects the nose, with or without involvement of the forehead and the upper lip. It is the inferior group that is associated with basal encephalocele (i.e., sphenoidal, sphenoethmoid, and ethmoid encephaloceles), callosal agenesis, and optic nerve dysplasias. The superior group is characterized by hypertelorism, a broad nasal root, and a median cleft nose, with or without a median cleft lip. The superior group is also associated with an increased incidence of frontonasal and intraorbital encephaloceles (Fig. 2-30).[30] If the phenotypic features of possible encephalocele intruding into the nasal cavity are recognized in a patient, caution should be exercised when inserting a nasogastric tube or nasal airway.

The cartilage of the nasal capsule is the foundation of the upper part of the face. Eventually, nearly all the nasal capsule becomes ossified or atrophied. All that remains of the cartilage of the nasal capsule in adults is the anterior part of the nasal septum and the alar cartilages that surround the nostrils. The midline septal cartilage is continuous with the cartilaginous skull base. At birth, the lateral masses of the ethmoid are ossified but the septal cartilage and the cribriform plates are still cartilaginous. Another ossification center appears in the septal cartilage anterior to the cranial base and becomes the perpendicular plate of the ethmoid. In about the third to sixth year, the lateral masses of the ethmoid and the perpendicular plate become united across the roof of the nasal cavity by ossification of the cribriform plate, which unites with the vomer below somewhat later. Growth of the septal cartilage continues for a short time after craniofacial union is complete, which probably accounts for the common deflection of the nasal septum away from the midline.[30]

The external nose is pyramidal in shape. The cranial portion of the nose that joins the forehead is called the root. The lower free margin is known as the apex or tip. The upper midline margin near the root, which is supported by the nasal bones, is called the bridge. The curved ridge in the midline is called the dorsum, and the expanded lower margin of the nose is referred to as the alae. The caudal aspect of the midline nasal septum and the nasal alae form the boundaries of the nostrils, or nares, which are the external openings of the nose. There are two nasal bones, which articulate with the nasal process of the frontal bone, the perpendicular plate of the ethmoid bone, and the septal cartilage of the nose. The osseous opening of the nose is called the pyriform aperture. The lateral nasal cartilages attach to the upper edges of this aperture. The nasal cavities are separated in the midline by the nasal septum. The roof of the nasal cavity is formed by the cribriform plate of the ethmoid bone, and the floor is formed by the hard palate. The major portion of the nasal septum is formed by the perpendicular plate of the ethmoid posteriorly and the septal cartilage anteriorly. The vomer completes the posteroinferior portion of the septum. The nasal septum supports the dorsum of the nose. The paranasal sinuses open into the lateral nasal wall, from which three or four nasal turbinates or conchae project. The dominant structures of the lateral nasal wall are the inferior and the middle turbinates; the superior turbinates are usually small. The airspace beneath and lateral to each turbinate or concha is called the meatus, into which the paranasal sinuses open. Teleologically, the nasal septum separates the nasal fossa into two cavities so that one chamber can rest while the other chamber carries on the functions of the nose.

2. Imaging Anatomy

Cross-sectional imaging of the nose and paranasal sinuses allows one to examine the air passage from the nares to the nasopharynx. A dedicated examination of the nose and sinuses yields detailed information about this region (Fig. 2-31). However, routine brain or spine imaging allows incidental imaging of the sinuses and airway and a good assessment of the airway can be obtained (Fig. 2-32).

3. Imaging Pathology

From the imaging perspective, it is easy to appreciate how the small air passages or channels through the nasal vault flanked by the nasal septum and the turbinates are readily compromised. The spectrum of diseases affecting the airflow ranges from physiologic swelling of the turbinates to fixed structural abnormalities.

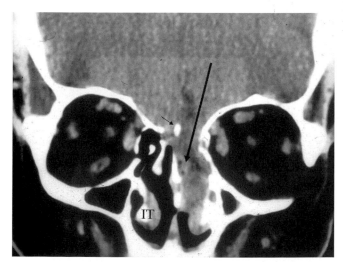

Figure 2-30 Frontonasal encephalocele. Coronal computed tomography demonstrates dehiscent left cribriform plate with soft tissue extending into the nasal cavity. Frontonasal encephalocele *(long arrow)*; crista galli *(short arrow)*; inferior turbinate, IT.

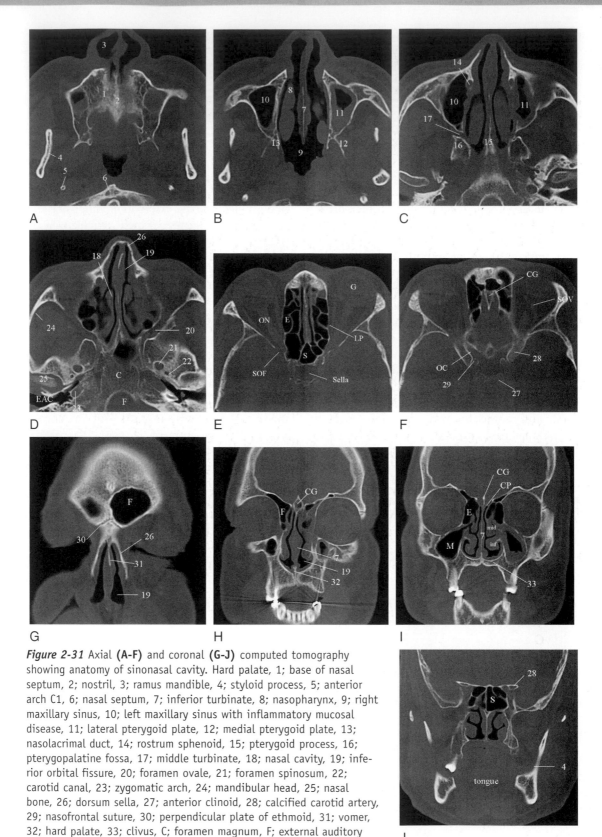

Figure 2-31 Axial **(A-F)** and coronal **(G-J)** computed tomography showing anatomy of sinonasal cavity. Hard palate, 1; base of nasal septum, 2; nostril, 3; ramus mandible, 4; styloid process, 5; anterior arch C1, 6; nasal septum, 7; inferior turbinate, 8; nasopharynx, 9; right maxillary sinus, 10; left maxillary sinus with inflammatory mucosal disease, 11; lateral pterygoid plate, 12; medial pterygoid plate, 13; nasolacrimal duct, 14; rostrum sphenoid, 15; pterygoid process, 16; pterygopalatine fossa, 17; middle turbinate, 18; nasal cavity, 19; inferior orbital fissure, 20; foramen ovale, 21; foramen spinosum, 22; carotid canal, 23; zygomatic arch, 24; mandibular head, 25; nasal bone, 26; dorsum sella, 27; anterior clinoid, 28; calcified carotid artery, 29; nasofrontal suture, 30; perpendicular plate of ethmoid, 31; vomer, 32; hard palate, 33; clivus, C; foramen magnum, F; external auditory canal, EAC; optic nerve, ON; ethmoid sinus, E; sphenoid sinus, S; globe, G; superior orbital fissure, SOF; crista galli, CG; superior ophthalmic vein, SOV; optic canal, OC; middle turbinate, mid; inferior turbinate, inf.

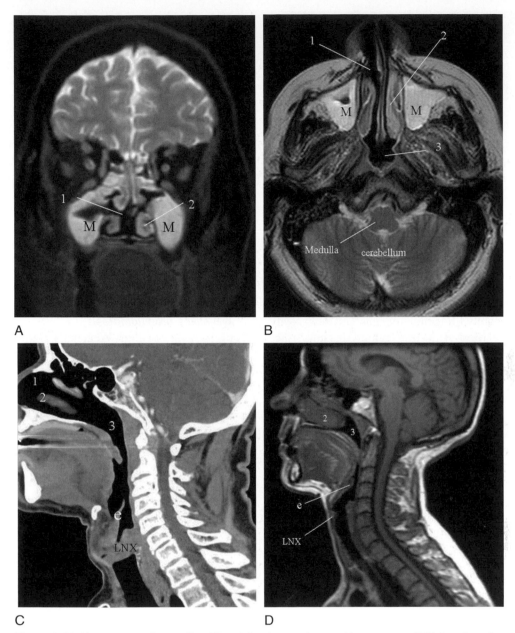

Figure 2-32 Airway on routine studies. T2-weighted coronal magnetic resonance (MR) imaging of the brain demonstrates hyperintense inflamed thickened mucosa of the maxillary sinuses **(A)**. T2-weighted axial MR imaging of the brain demonstrates sinus disease, clear nasal cavity and nasopharynx **(B)**. Sagittal reformation from computed tomography neck examination demonstrates clear airway from nose to trachea **(C)**. T1-weighted sagittal MR cervical spine examination demonstrating signal void (black) of the air column of the airway **(D)**. Nasal cavity, 1; inferior turbinate, 2; nasopharynx, 3; maxillary sinus with thickened mucosa, M; epiglottis, e; larynx, LNX.

a. Congenital and Developmental Abnormalities

i. Midface Anomalies Premature cranial synostosis may affect the development of the face and paranasal sinuses. Craniofacial dysostosis syndromes such as Crouzon's disease and Apert's syndrome are associated with facial anomalies. In Crouzon's disease, the most frequent form of craniofacial synostosis, bilateral coronal suture synostosis causes brachycephaly with shallow orbits and ocular proptosis. The midface is flat and the nasal passages are partially obstructed, causing mouth breathing. In Apert's syndrome, the midface hypoplasia malocclusion and anterior open-bite deformities are more severe than in Crouzon's disease. Midface anomalies such as hypoplastic syndromes and cleft lip or palate may cause airway obstruction at the nasopharyngeal level. Of all the cleft syndromes, the unilateral cleft lip and palate cause the most severe reduction in nasal airway area.[15,43]

ii. Choanal Stenosis or Atresia Because infants are obligate nasal breathers, they can experience severe airway obstruction with bilateral nasal airway disease. Congenital nasal airway obstruction most commonly occurs in the posterior nasal cavity, secondary to choanal atresia (Fig. 2-33). Nasal airway obstruction may also result from rhinitis,

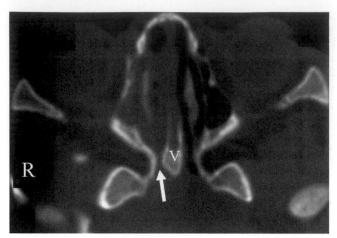

Figure 2-33 Choanal atresia. Axial computed tomography scan demonstrates posterior aperture stenosis on the right *(arrow)*. The vomer, V, is enlarged.

turbinate hypertrophy, congenital syphilis, and nasal cavity stenosis in association with the craniofacial anomalies and other syndromes.

Stenosis of the posterior nasal cavity (choanae) is probably more common than true atresia. The atresias may be bony, membranous, or both. Most atresias are unilateral and may remain undetected until late in life. Severe respiratory difficulty and the inability to insert a nasogastric tube more than 3 to 4 cm into the nose despite the presence of air in the trachea and the lungs suggests the diagnosis of atresia. About 75% of children with bilateral choanal stenosis or atresia have other congenital abnormalities, including Apert's, Treacher Collins, and fetal alcohol syndromes. Because the pathology is usually manifested as bone growth, CT is the imaging modality of choice. The major component of bone atresia is an abnormal widening of the vomer (Fig. 2-34).

b. Rhinosinusitis and Polyps

No imaging is required for work-up of uncomplicated rhinosinusitis. Normally, the sinus air abuts the bony sinus wall. Inflammatory sinus disease is characterized by increased water, therefore an increased T2 signal and a bright signal on T2-weighted imaging. In contrast, with increased cellularity, tumors generally exhibit an isointense signal. The most common local complication of inflammatory sinusitis is polyps and retention cysts.

The most common sinonasal pathologies that can affect the airway are easily recognizable on cross-sectional imaging. These are nasal polyps and an aerated turbinate, most often the middle turbinate, a concha bullosa. The presence of polyps may discourage an anesthesiologist from attempting nasal intubation (Figs. 2-35 and 2-36). Knowing which nasal cavity is narrowed by the presence of a concha bullosa helps to guide the selection of the nasal cavity to cannulate (Fig. 2-37).

c. Wegener's Granulomatosis

A necrotizing vasculitis, Wegener's granulomatosis usually affects the upper and lower respiratory tracts and causes a renal glomerulonephritis. It is probably autoimmune in origin. It most often involves the nasal septum first and may arise as a chronic nonspecific inflammatory process. This process becomes diffuse, and septal ulcerations and perforations occur. Secondary bacterial infection often complicates the clinical and imaging picture (Fig. 2-38).[37]

d. Trauma

Facial fractures are often classified using the Le Fort system and its variants. This system is based on experiments predicting the course of fractures on the basis of lines of weakness in the facial skeleton. Of all the facial fractures, nasal fractures are the most common and may involve the nasal bones or the cartilaginous structures.

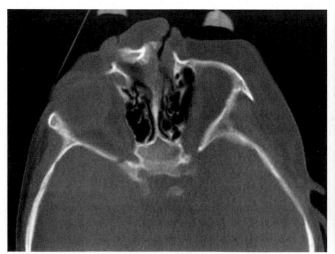
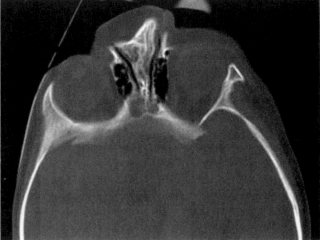

Figure 2-34 Congenital nasal deformity. Axial computed tomography scans demonstrate abnormal nasal bone architecture and soft tissue cleft and impact on nasal airways.

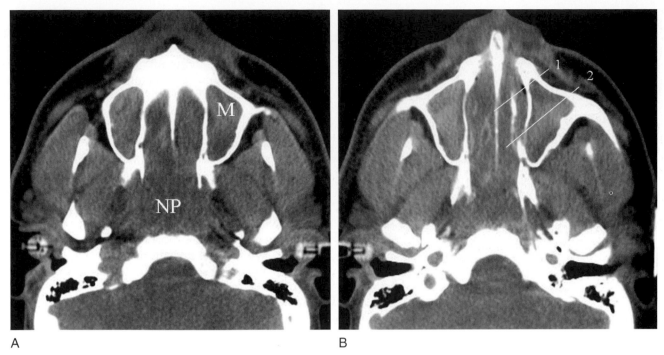

A B

Figure 2-35 Nasal polyps. Axial computed tomography scans (**A** and **B**) demonstrate complete obliteration of the nasal passageways and pharynx by soft tissue polyps, resulting in chronic maxillary sinus inflammatory changes. Nasal septum, 1; nasal cavity, 2; nasopharynx, NP; maxillary sinus, M.

If the nasal septum is fractured and a hematoma results, the vascular supply to the cartilage may be compromised, leading to cartilage necrosis. If the septal hematoma is not recognized and treated, it becomes an organized hematoma, causing an unyielding thickening of the septum and impaired breathing (Fig. 2-39). Without doubt, CT is the modality of choice for evaluating trauma to the facial structures. Three-dimensional reconstruction and surface rendering can also be performed to better highlight fracture deformities. Even if all the details of a complex facial fracture are not known, an oral airway is preferable to a nasal airway. However, in the case of mandibular fracture (Fig. 2-40), the nasal approach to intubation is preferred.

e. Tumors and Others
i. Malignant Tumors Carcinomas of the nasal cavity and the paranasal sinuses are rare and have a poor prognosis because they are frequently diagnosed in an advanced stage. They are often accompanied by inflammatory disease.

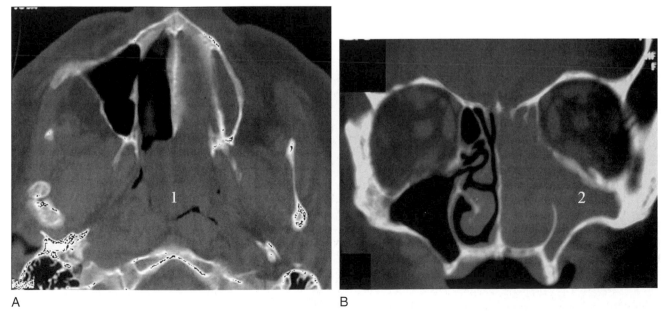

A B

Figure 2-36 Antrochoanal polyp. Axial (**A**) and coronal (**B**) computed tomography scans demonstrate soft tissue obliterating the left nasal cavity extending posteriorly into the nasopharynx, 1; and laterally into the left maxillary sinus, 2.

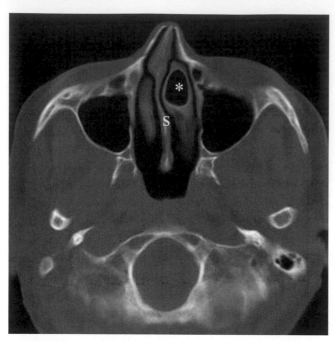

Figure 2-37 Concha bullosa. Axial computed tomography scan demonstrates pneumatization (asterisk) of the left middle turbinate and deviated septum, S.

MRI is superior to CT in differentiating tumor from inflammatory disease and therefore useful in delineating the tumor boundary from the often-associated inflammatory component. Inflammatory diseases involve a high water content; therefore, they have high T2-weighted intensity and appear bright on MRI. Nasal and paranasal tumors are generally cellular and have an intermediate-intensity signal on T2-weighted imaging (Fig. 2-41).[37,38] CT is useful for assessing bone involvement. The histology of the tumor can sometimes be suggested by the way in which the bone is affected: aggressive bone destruction is usually seen in squamous cell carcinoma, metastatic lung and breast cancers, and a few sarcomas and rare fibrous histiocytomas (Fig. 2-42).

ii. Nonmalignant Destructive Tumors An example of nonmalignant locally destructive tumor of the sinonasal cavity is juvenile nasopharyngeal angiofibroma. Juvenile nasopharyngeal angiofibroma is a benign hypervascular tumor found almost exclusively in young adolescent males. Most common presenting signs are unilateral nasal obstruction and spontaneous epistaxis. It usually arises at the sphenopalatine foramen at the lateral nasopharyngeal wall and is locally destructive over time.[37] The imaging characteristics consist of a nasal cavity and nasopharyngeal mass, widened pterygopalatine fossa, anterior displacement of the posterior wall of the maxillary sinus, and erosion of the medial pterygoid plate (Fig. 2-43). Treatment is surgical resection, often with preoperative embolization to decrease the blood supply.

f. Fibrous Dysplasia

Fibrous dysplasia, an idiopathic bone disorder, is not a tumor but can encroach on the airway and sinuses. Most patients are young at the time of diagnosis. There are monostotic and polyostotic forms. Craniofacial bones are more often involved in the polyostotic form (Fig. 2-44).[37]

B. ORAL CAVITY

The oral cavity, contiguous with the oropharynx, is the primary conduit to the gastrointestinal tract. The development of the mouth, along with the development of the face, is centered on a surface depression, the stomodeum, just below the developing brain. The ectoderm covering the forebrain extends into the stomodeum, where it lies adjacent to the foregut. The junctional zone between the ectoderm and the endoderm is the oropharyngeal membrane, which corresponds to Waldeyer's ring. Dissolution of the oropharyngeal membrane in the fourth gestational week results in establishing patency between the mouth and the foregut.[40]

The oral cavity is separated from the oropharynx by the circumvallate papillae, anterior tonsillar pillars, and soft palate. The anterior two thirds of the tongue (oral tongue), the floor of the mouth, gingivobuccal and buccomasseteric regions, maxilla, and mandible are considered oral cavity structures. The anatomic distinction between the oral cavity and the oropharynx has clinical importance. Malignancies, especially squamous cell carcinoma, in these two regions are different in their presentation and prognosis.

1. Imaging Anatomy

CT and MRI are used extensively for the evaluation of the oral cavity. The advantages of CT are the speed of data acquisition and the ability to detect calcifications pertinent in the evaluation of inflammatory diseases affecting the salivary glands. For evaluating the extent of tumor infiltration of the soft tissues, MRI is superior to CT but is easily degraded by motion artifacts (Fig. 2-45).

The tongue consists of two symmetrical halves separated by a midline lingual septum. Each half of the tongue is composed of muscular fibers, which are divided into extrinsic and intrinsic muscles. There are four intrinsic tongue muscles: the superior longitudinal muscle, inferior longitudinal muscle, transverse muscles, and vertical muscles. The intrinsic muscles receive motor innervation from the hypoglossal nerve (12th cranial nerve) and participate in the enunciation of various consonants. The intrinsic muscles are difficult to distinguish on CT. They are, however, well visualized on MRI, as each muscle bundle is surrounded by high-intensity fibrofatty tissues.

The muscles that originate externally to the tongue but have distal muscle fibers that interdigitate within the substance of the tongue are considered extrinsic muscles

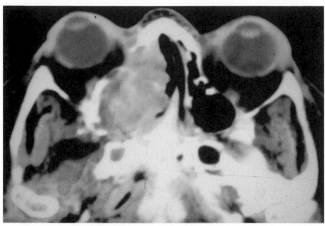

A

Figure 2-38 Wegener's and other septal pathologies narrowing anterior nasal cavity. Axial computed tomography scans (**A, B,** and **C**). **A,** A soft tissue mass invading the right nasal cavity and orbit is noted, diagnosed as Wegener's granuloma. **B,** A septal granuloma is noted associated with focal bone destruction. **C,** A ring-enhancing lesion of the anterior septum is noted, consistent with a septal abscess.

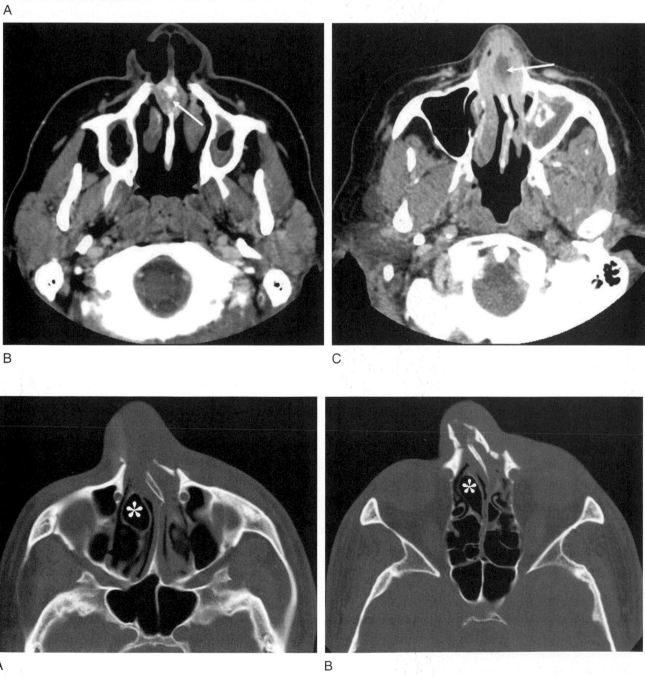

B

C

A

B

Figure 2-39 Nasal and septal fracture. Axial computed tomography scans (**A** and **B**) demonstrate comminuted fractures of the nasal bones bilaterally as well as a septal fracture. The nasal passages are further compromised by the incidental right concha bullosa *(asterisk)*.

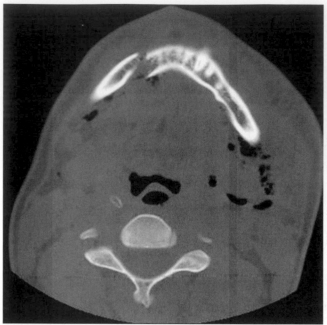

A

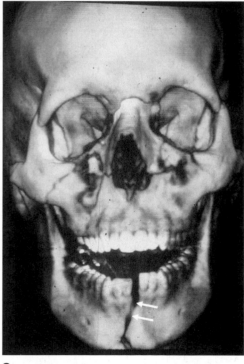

B

C

Figure 2-40 Mandibular fracture. Axial computed tomography (CT) **(A)** and **(B).** CT three-dimensional surface rendering **(C)** in a different patient. Axial CT scans demonstrate typically paired fractures involving the right parasymphyseal body **(A)** and left angle of the mandible. Note the extensive air within the soft tissues. In another patient **(C),** three-dimensional surface rendering demonstrates a midline fracture *(arrows)* of the mandible at the symphysis.

of the tongue. The main extrinsic muscles are the genioglossus, hyoglossus, and styloglossus. Sometimes the superior constrictors and the palatoglossus muscles are discussed with the extrinsic muscles of the tongue. The extrinsic muscles attach the tongue to the hyoid, mandible, and styloid process (Table 2-1).

Motor innervation comes from the hypoglossal nerve, which courses between the mylohyoid and hyoglossus muscles. The sensory input from the anterior tongue is by the lingual nerve, which is a branch of the trigeminal nerve (fifth cranial nerve). Special sensory taste fibers from the anterior two thirds of the tongue course with the lingual nerve before forming the chorda tympani nerve, which subsequently joins the facial nerve (seventh cranial nerve). The special sensory fibers from the posterior one third of the tongue (tongue base) are supplied by the glossopharyngeal nerve (ninth cranial nerve). The arterial blood supply to the tongue is from branches of the

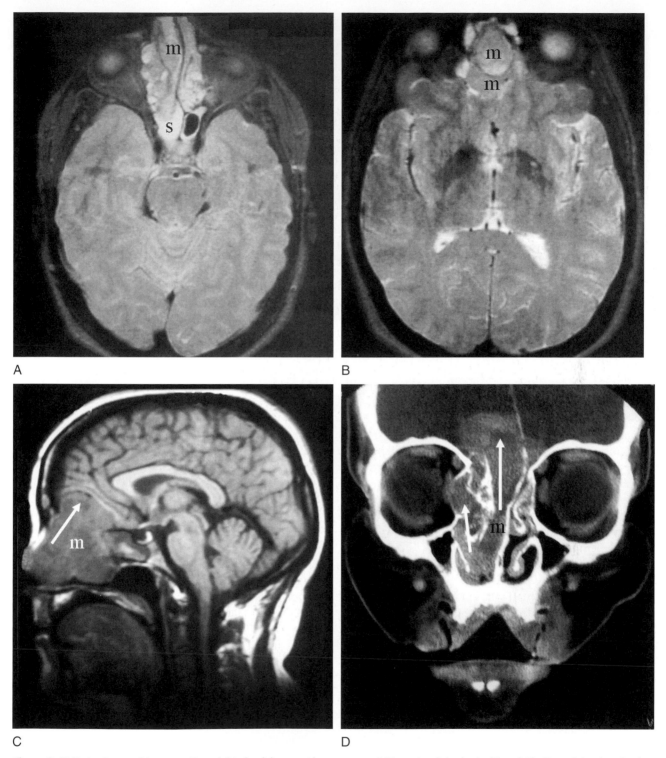

A

B

C

D

Figure 2-41 Esthesioneuroblastoma. T2-weighted axial magnetic resonance (MR) study of the brain (**A** and **B**). T1-weighted sagittal brain MR (**C**). Coronal computed tomography (CT) image of sinuses after contrast. Note the large isointense soft-tissue mass, m, in the nasal cavity (**A** and **B**) accompanied by obstructive inflammatory sinus disease of high T2 signal, s. The extension of the mass intracranially *(arrows)* is better appreciated on the sagittal T1 MR of the brain (**C**) and coronal CT with contrast **(D)**. Coronal CT better demonstrates bone destruction and also extension of the tumor to the right orbit.

lingual artery, which itself is a branch of the external carotid artery. Venous drainage is to the internal jugular vein (see Table 2-1).[46]

The floor of the mouth is considered to be the tissue layer between the mucosa of the floor of the mouth and the mylohyoid muscle sling. Additional support for the floor is provided by the paired anterior bellies of the digastric muscles and the geniohyoid muscles (Table 2-2). Caudal to the mylohyoid muscle and above the hyoid bone, this space is considered the suprahyoid neck. Through a gap between the free posterior border of the mylohyoid muscle and the hyoglossus muscle, the

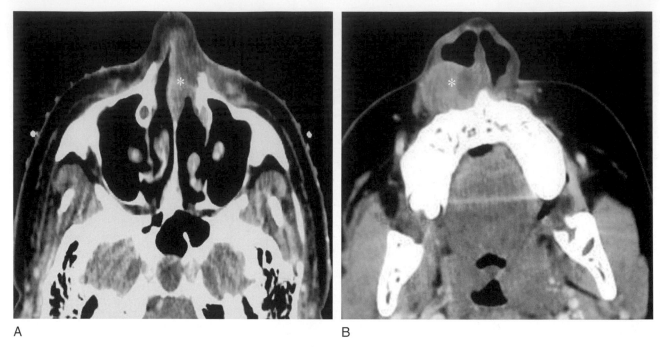

A

B

Figure 2-42 Lymphoma of the nasal septum. **A,** Axial computed tomography (CT) scan shows an infiltrating lesion of the anterior nasal septum (asterisk), extending into the left maxillary soft tissues. Rhabdomyosarcoma of the right nasal cavity and nasal ala. **B,** Axial CT scan demonstrates a soft-tissue mass (asterisk) effacing the right nostril.

submandibular gland wraps around the dorsal aspect of the mylohyoid muscle.

Several named spaces and regions in the oral cavity, such as the lingual artery and nerve, hypoglossal nerve, and salivary glands and ducts, are mentioned in brief because of their anatomic importance with respect to the structures contained within.[36] The *sublingual region* is below the mucosa of the floor of the mouth, superomedial to the mylohyoid muscle, and lateral to the genioglossus-geniohyoid muscles. It is primarily fat filled and is continuous with the submandibular region at the posterior margin of the mylohyoid muscle. The contents of this space include the sublingual gland and ducts, submandibular gland duct (Wharton's duct) and sometimes a portion of the hilum of the submandibular gland, anterior fibers of the hyoglossus muscle, and the lingual artery and vein. The hyoglossus muscle is an important surgical landmark (see Fig. 2-45 C). Lateral to this muscle, one can identify Wharton's duct, the hypoglossal nerve, and the lingual nerve, and the lingual artery and vein lie medially. Wharton's duct runs anteriorly from the gland, traveling with the hypoglossal and lingual (mandibular branch of the trigeminal nerve) nerves. Initially, it lies between the hyoglossus muscle and the mylohyoid muscle. More anteriorly, it lies between the genioglossus and mylohyoid muscles. The duct drains into the floor of the mouth, just lateral to the frenulum of the tongue.

The *submandibular space or fossa* is defined as the space inferior to the mylohyoid muscle, between the mandible and the hyoid bone. At the posterior margin of the mylohyoid muscle, the submandibular space is continuous with the sublingual space and the anterior aspect of the parapharyngeal space. This communication allows the spread of pathology. The submandibular space is primarily fat filled and contains the superficial portion of the submandibular gland and lymph nodes, lymphatic vessels, and blood vessels. The anterior bellies of the digastric muscle lie in the paramedian location in this space. Branches of the facial artery and vein course lateral to the anterior digastric muscle in the fat surrounding the submandibular gland. The artery lies deep to the gland, and the anterior facial vein is superficial. One important anatomic point is that pathology intrinsic to the submandibular gland displaces the facial vein laterally. Other masses lateral to the gland, including nodes, can be identified with the vein interposed between the gland and the mass.[44]

The *lips* are composed of orbicularis muscle, which is composed of muscle fibers from multiple facial muscles that insert into the lips and additional fibers proper to the lips. The innervation to the lips is from branches of the facial nerve (seventh cranial nerve). The vestibule of the mouth, or the *gingivobuccal region*, is the potential space separating the lips and cheeks from the gums and teeth. The parotid gland ducts and mucous gland ducts of the lips and cheek drain into this space, which is contiguous posteriorly with the oral cavity through the space between the last molar tooth and the ramus of the mandible.

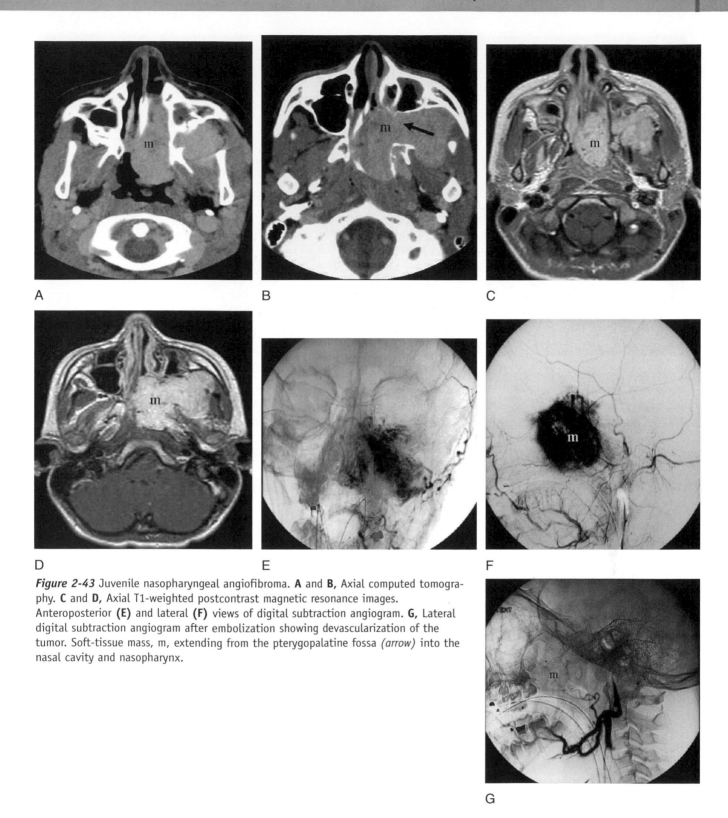

Figure 2-43 Juvenile nasopharyngeal angiofibroma. **A** and **B,** Axial computed tomography. **C** and **D,** Axial T1-weighted postcontrast magnetic resonance images. Anteroposterior **(E)** and lateral **(F)** views of digital subtraction angiogram. **G,** Lateral digital subtraction angiogram after embolization showing devascularization of the tumor. Soft-tissue mass, m, extending from the pterygopalatine fossa *(arrow)* into the nasal cavity and nasopharynx.

2. Imaging Pathology

a. Macroglossia

The tongue makes up the bulk of soft tissues in the oral cavity. Enlargement of the tongue, which is defined clinically as the protrusion of the tongue beyond the teeth or alveolar ridge in the resting position, compromises the oral airway and makes the insertion of airway devices challenging. Larsson and colleagues[24] defined the appearance of macroglossia on CT imaging as (1) base of the tongue more than 50 mm in the transverse dimension, (2) genioglossus muscle more than 11 mm in the transverse dimension, (3) midline cleft on the tongue surface, and (4) submandibular glands that are normal in size but bulging out of the platysma muscle owing to

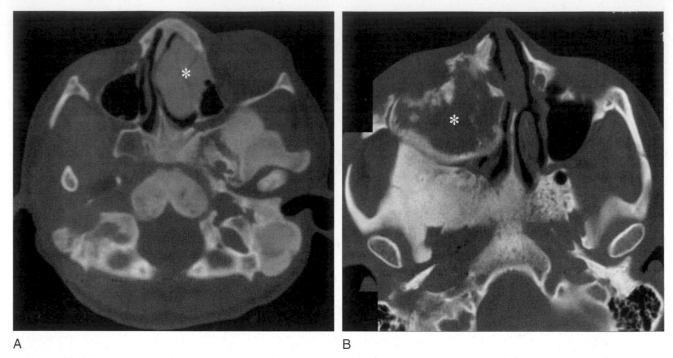

A   B

Figure 2-44 **A,** Fibrous dysplasia. **B,** Fibrous dysplasia with degeneration to osteosarcoma. **A,** Axial computed tomography (CT) demonstrates a mass obliterating the left nasal cavity with the typical "ground glass" appearance of fibrous dysplasia involving the left skull base. **B,** Axial CT scan from a different patient demonstrates malignant degeneration of fibrous dysplasia to osteosarcoma invading the right nasal cavity and orbit.

tongue enlargement. There are congenital and noncongenital causes of macroglossia. The congenital syndromes in which macroglossia can be seen are trisomy 21, Beckwith-Wiedemann syndrome, hypothyroidism, and mucopolysaccharidoses. The more common noncongenital causes are tumor of the tongue, lymphangioma, hemangioma, acromegaly, and amyloid (Figs. 2-46 and 2-47). Rarely, infection can result in macroglossia, especially in an immune compromised host (Fig. 2-48).

Posterior displacement of the tongue or glossoptosis may be observed with macroglossia, micro- or retrognathia, and neuromuscular disorders. It can also occur in normal patients in a minority of cases. The obvious complication is relative airway obstruction, which, if chronic, results in a compendium of complications.

b. Micrognathia and Retrognathia

Micrognathia is a term used to describe an abnormally small mandible. Retrognathia is defined as abnormal posterior placement of the mandible. These two findings often coexist. Abnormal growth or placement of the mandible can be caused by malformation, deformation, or connective tissue dysplasia.[33] The most familiar syndromic form featuring an abnormal mandible is in the Pierre Robin sequence. Other clinical entities include the Treacher Collins, Stickler, and DiGeorge syndromes. Thin-section CT with two- or three-dimensional reformation provides information regarding the size and proportions of the maxilla, nose, mandible, and airway.

Micrognathia and retrognathia not only contribute to airway obstruction; these features are also possible indicators of difficult direct laryngoscopy and endotracheal intubation that can lead to life-threatening complications (Figs. 2-49 and 2-50).

c. Exostosis

Hyperostosis of the hard palate or mandible is a benign disease, usually of no clinical significance. Most often these are small exostoses, which may arise from the oral surface of the hard palate (torus palatinus), from the alveolar portion of the maxilla in the molar region, along the lingual surface of the dental arch (torus maxillaries), or along the lingual surface of the mandible (torus mandibularis). Large lesions may restrict tongue motion and distort the airway, leading to speech disturbance.

d. Tumors

Only 7% of oral cavity lesions are malignant; however, most of these malignant tumors are squamous cell carcinoma. Other neoplasms include minor salivary gland tumors, lymphomas, and sarcomas. Risk factors for squamous cell carcinoma of the oral cavity include a long history of tobacco and alcohol use. Squamous cell carcinoma can arise anywhere in the oral cavity, but it has a predilection for the floor of the mouth, ventrolateral tongue, and soft palate complex including the retromolar trigone area and the anterior tonsillar pillar (Fig. 2-51). Most lesions are moderately advanced at the time of

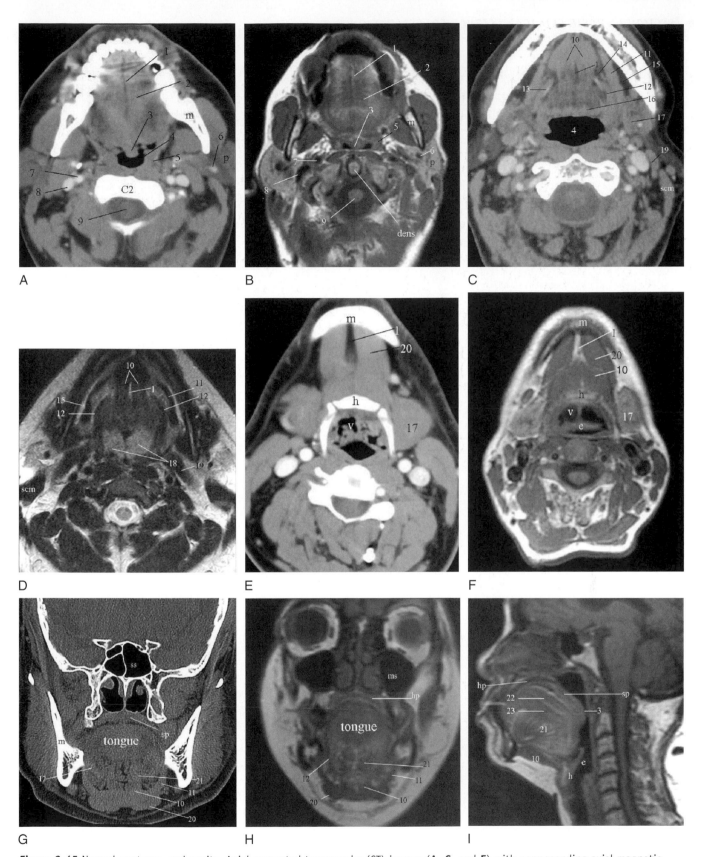

Figure 2-45 Normal anatomy, oral cavity. Axial computed tomography (CT) images (**A**, **C**, and **E**) with corresponding axial magnetic resonance (MR) scans (**B**, **D**, and **F**). Coronal CT **(G)** and coronal T1-weighted MR (T1-W) **(H)**. Sagittal T1-weighted MR **(I)**. Median raphe of tongue, 1—fat is low density on CT and bright on T1-W; tongue, 2—see transverse fibers of tongue better on MR; uvula, 3; oropharynx, 4; pharyngeal constrictor muscle, 5; retromandibular vein, 6; internal carotid artery, 7; internal jugular vein, 8; cervical cord, 9; paired geniohyoid muscles, 10; mylohyoid muscle, 11; hyoglossus muscle, 12; lingual artery and vein medial to hyoglossus muscle, 13; Wharton's duct, hypoglossal and lingual nerve lateral to hyoglossus muscle, 14; fat in sublingual space, 15; tongue base, 16; submandibular gland, 17; palatine tonsils narrowing oropharynx, 18; posterior belly of digastric muscle, 19; paired anterior belly of digastric muscle, 20; genioglossus muscle, 21; superior longitudinal muscle, 22; transverse muscle, 23; mandible, m; parotid gland, p; sternocleidomastoid muscle, scm; vallecula, v; epiglottis, e; body of hyoid bone, h; maxillary sinus, ms; sphenoid sinus, ss; hard palate, hp; soft palate, sp.

57

Table 2-1   **Muscles of the Tongue**

Muscle	Function	Innervation	Arterial Supply	Venous Drainage
INTRINSIC TONGUE MUSCLES		Motor: Hypoglossal n. (CN XII) Sensory: Anterior 2/3—lingual n. a branch of the mandibular branch (V3) of trigeminal n. (CN V) Sensory: Posterior 1/3— glossopharyngeal n. (CN IX) Taste: Anterior 2/3— chorda tympani n., branch of facial n. (CN VII) Taste: Posterior 1/3— glossopharyngeal n. (CN IX) Taste: Root and epiglottis-vagus n. (CN X)	Lingual a.—main supply Tonsillar branches and ascending palatine branches of the facial and ascending pharyngeal arteries	Dorsal lingual and deep lingual veins → internal jugular vein
Superior longitudinal m.	Shortens tongue Turns tip and sides up Renders dorsum of tongue concave			
Inferior longitudinal m.	Shortens tongue Pulls tip up Renders dorsum of tongue convex			
Transverse m.	Narrows and elongates tongue			
Vertical m.	Flattens and widens tongue			
EXTRINSIC TONGUE MUSCLES	Arise extrinsic to tongue but fibers interdigitate within tongue substance Provide attachment of tongue to hyoid, mandible, and styloid process			
Genioglossus m.	Anterior part depresses tongue Posterior part protrudes tongue			
Hyoglossus m.	Depresses and retracts tongue Important surgical landmark: CN V3, CN XII, and submandibular gland duct are lateral to muscle; lingual a. and v. are medial to muscle			
Styloglossus m.	Retracts and draws tongue edges up to create trough for swallowing			

a., artery; CN, cranial nerve; m., muscle; n., nerve; v., vein.

Table 2-2   **Principal Muscles of Floor of Mouth**

Muscles	Function	Innervation	Arterial Supply	Venous Drainage
Mylohyoid m.	Elevates hyoid bone and floor of mouth to aid in swallowing	Mylohyoid n., branch of inferior alveolar n., branch of mandibular division (V3) of trigeminal n. (CN V)	Lingual a.	External and internal jugular venous system
Geniohyoid m.	Elevates hyoid bone anteriorly and superiorly	Variable—CN XII, C1, and C2		
Digastric m. Anterior belly Posterior belly	Contributes to support of floor of mouth Raises the hyoid bone and tongue during swallowing	Anterior belly—mylohyoid n., branch of V3 Posterior belly—facial n. (CN VII)		

a., artery; CN, cranial nerve; m., muscle; n., nerve; v., vein.

presentation; 30% to 65% of patients with oral cavity squamous cell carcinoma have nodal involvement at the time of diagnosis. The tumors of the oral cavity are usually less aggressive than the squamous cell carcinomas arising from the oropharynx. Both CT and MRI are useful for assessing tumor extent and nodal involvement.[36]

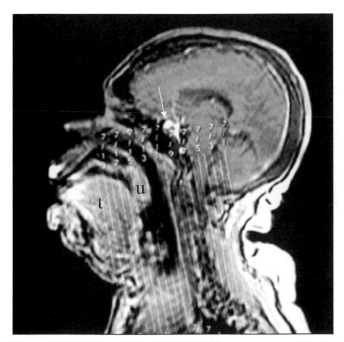

Figure 2-46 Acromegaly. Sagittal magnetic resonance scout demonstrates an enlarged protruding tongue, t, and prominent uvula, u, in a patient with a pituitary adenoma *(arrow)*.

C. PHARYNX

The pharynx is a musculomembranous tube extending from the skull base to the cervical esophagus. For ease of discussion, it is divided into three parts: the nasopharynx, oropharynx, and hypopharynx. Anatomically, the nasopharynx is defined from the skull base to the hard palate. The oropharynx extends from the hard palate to the hyoid bone and the hypopharynx from the hyoid bone to the caudal margin of the cricoid cartilage. Below the level of the cricoid cartilage, the cervical esophagus begins. The hypopharynx can be further subdivided into the pyriform sinus region, the posterior wall, the postcricoid regions, and the lateral surface of the aryepiglottic folds.

The pharyngeal musculature includes the three overlapping constrictor muscles, the superior, middle, and inferior pharyngeal constrictors, and the cricopharyngeus, salpingopharyngeus, stylopharyngeus, palatopharyngeus, tensor veli palatini, and levator veli palatini muscles. Innervation is primarily from the pharyngeal plexus of nerves, to which the vagus (10th cranial nerve) and glossopharyngeal nerve contribute. The vagus nerve primarily supplies motor innervation to the constrictors. The mandibular branch of the trigeminal nerve innervates the tensor veli palatini muscle. Sensory information travels along the glossopharyngeal nerve and the internal laryngeal branch of the superior laryngeal nerve, which arises from the vagus nerve. The arterial supply to the pharynx is from branches of the external carotid artery, including the ascending pharyngeal artery, tonsillar branches of the facial artery, and the palatine branches of the maxillary artery. Superior and inferior thyroid arteries

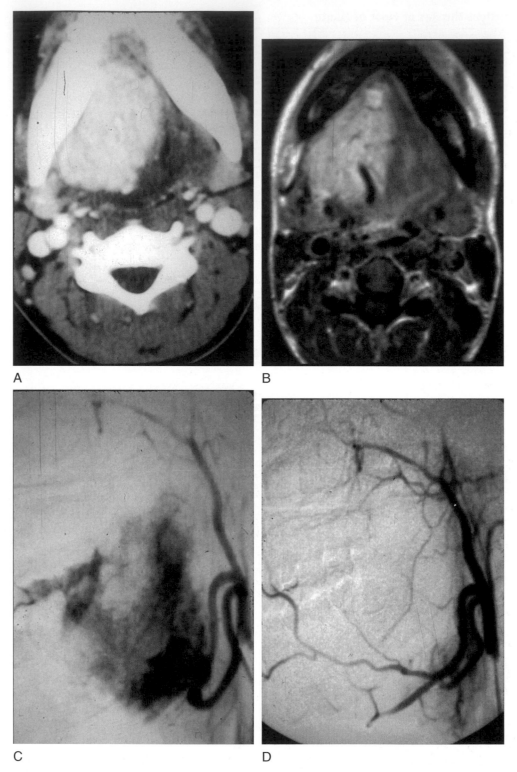

Figure 2-47 Tongue hemangioma. Contrast-enhanced computed tomography **(A)** and magnetic resonance **(B)** demonstrate an enhancing right tongue lesion, nearly filling the oral cavity. The vascularity of the lesion is further demonstrated in the lateral view of the right external carotid angiogram **(C).** The angiogram **(D)** after embolization shows devascularization of the tumor.

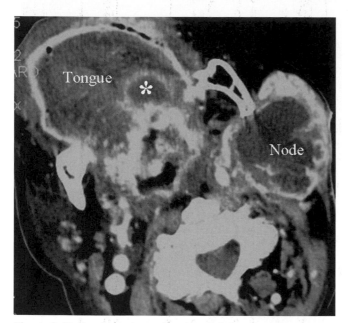

Figure 2-48 *Mycobacterium avium intracellulare*: immune compromised patient. Axial computed tomography with contrast demonstrates an irregular enhancement of lymph nodes and lymphoid tissue at the tongue base. The fungating tongue lesion *(asterisk)* compromises the oropharyngeal airway.

supply most of the lower pharynx. The primary venous drainage is through the superior and inferior thyroid veins and the pharyngeal veins into the internal jugular veins. The lymphatic drainage is complex and extensive to the jugular, retropharyngeal, posterior cervical, and paratracheal nodes (Table 2-3).[27,28]

Imaging studies of the pharynx most commonly include plain film x-rays, barium studies, CT, and MRI. In contrast to CT and MRI, a barium study is a dynamic imaging technique that can demonstrate the sequential contractions of the pharyngeal musculature during deglutition. It can show whether the pharyngeal wall is fixed or pliable and may detect mucosal lesions not apparent on CT or MRI. CT and MRI are most commonly done with the patient in the supine position and the neck in the neutral position. Intravenous contrast is recommended with CT for evaluation of lymphadenopathy. The inherent differences in signal intensity between tumor, fat, and muscle on MRI often allow accurate delineation of the tumor extent without gadolinium, which is the contrast agent commonly used in clinical practice.[28]

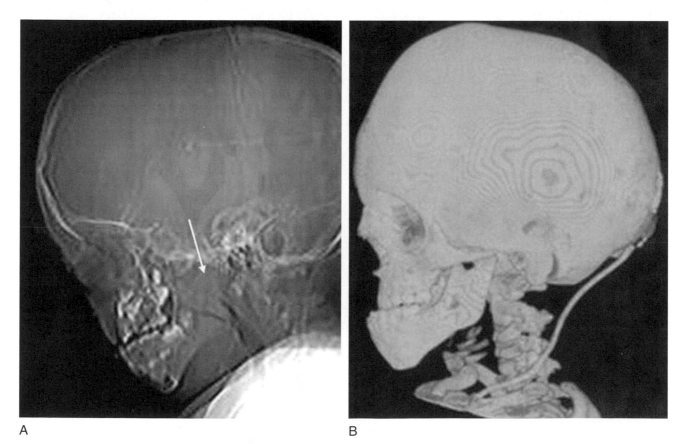

A

B

Figure 2-49 Midface regression syndrome. Two patients with Jackson-Weiss syndrome demonstrate maxillary regression on computed tomography scout **(A)** and three-dimensional surface rendering **(B).** Note the presence of a ventriculoperitoneal (V-P) shunt as hydrocephalus may result from the craniosynostosis associated with this syndrome. The mandible is hypoplastic and there is soft tissue obscuring the nasopharynx *(arrow).*

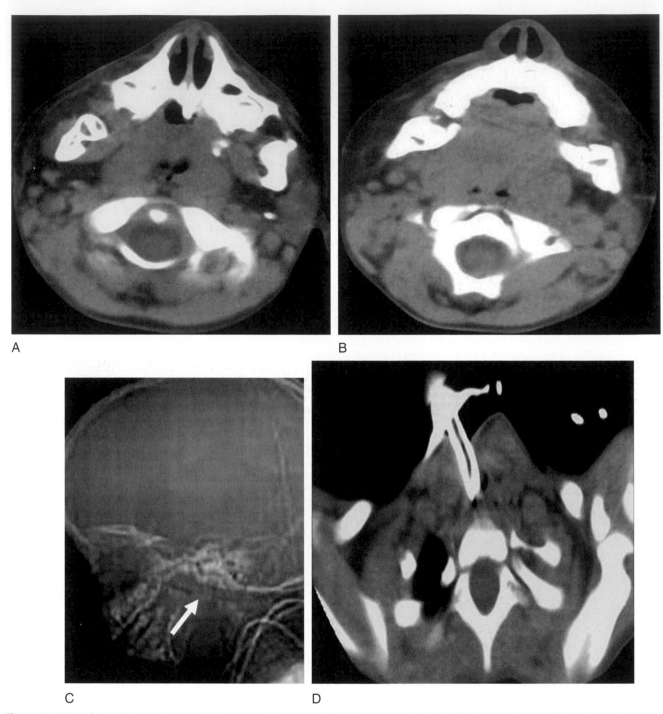

A

B

C

D

Figure 2-50 Treacher Collins syndrome. Axial computed tomography (CT) scans at the level of the nasopharynx **(A)** and oropharynx **(B)** demonstrate near obliteration of the airway by soft tissue, secondary to the facial microsomia. Lateral CT scout **(C)** demonstrates marked narrowing *(arrow)* of the airway. **D,** Axial CT scan at the thoracic inlet demonstrates the tracheostomy necessitated by this condition.

D. NASOPHARYNX

1. Imaging Anatomy

The nasopharynx is an epithelium-lined cavity that occupies the uppermost extent of the aerodigestive tract. The roof of the nasopharynx is formed cranially to caudally by the basisphenoid, basiocciput, and anterior aspect of the first two cervical vertebrae. The inferior aspect of the nasopharynx is formed by the hard palate, soft palate, and the ridge of pharyngeal musculature that opposes the soft palate when it is elevated (Passavant's ridge). The lateral nasopharyngeal walls are formed by the margins of the superior constrictor muscle. Anteriorly, the nasopharynx is in direct continuity with the nasal cavity through the posterior choanae. The nasopharynx

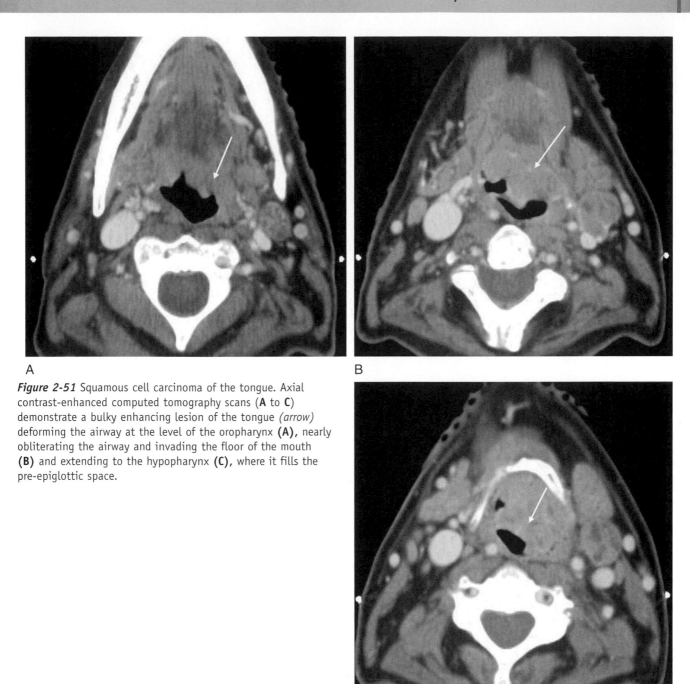

A

B

C

Figure 2-51 Squamous cell carcinoma of the tongue. Axial contrast-enhanced computed tomography scans (**A** to **C**) demonstrate a bulky enhancing lesion of the tongue *(arrow)* deforming the airway at the level of the oropharynx (**A**), nearly obliterating the airway and invading the floor of the mouth (**B**) and extending to the hypopharynx (**C**), where it fills the pre-epiglottic space.

is in direct communication with the middle ear cavity through the eustachian tubes (Fig. 2-52).

2. Imaging Pathology

a. Adenoidal Hypertrophy

The adenoids are lymphatic tissues, located in the upper posterior aspect of the nasopharynx. Prominent adenoids are typical in children; by the age of 2 to 3 years, the adenoids can fill the entire nasopharynx and extend posteriorly into the posterior choanae. Regression of the lymphoid tissue starts during adolescence and continues into later life. By the age of 30 to 40, adenoidal tissue is minimal, although normal adenoidal tissue may occasionally be seen in adults in their fourth and fifth decades of life. Adenoid tissues appear isodense to muscle on CT imaging (see Fig. 2-52*D*). On MRI, the adenoids are isointense to muscle on T1-weighted imaging and hyperintense on T2-weighted imaging. If prominent adenoidal tissue is seen in an adult, human immunodeficiency virus should be suspected.[28] Differentiation between lymphomatous involvement and hypertrophy of the adenoids is not possible on imaging, as both are hyperintense on T2-weighted imaging. Enlargement of the adenoids can cause partial obstruction of the nasopharyngeal airway and thus make insertion of a

Table 2-3 **Muscles of the Pharynx**

Muscle	Function	Innervation	Arterial Supply	Venous Drainage
Superior pharyngeal constrictor m.	Contracts the pharynx in swallowing	CN IX, X via pharyngeal plexus	Ascending pharyngeal a. branches	Pharyngeal plexus to pterygoid plexus and internal jugular and facial veins
Middle pharyngeal constrictor m.		Pharyngeal plexus (IX, X, sympathetic)	Ascending and palatine and tonsillar branches of facial a. Dorsal lingual branches of the lingual artery	
Inferior pharyngeal constrictor m.		Pharyngeal plexus (IX, X, sympathetic), external and recurrent laryngeal branches of CN X and CN XI	Pharyngeal branches of the maxillary a. (greater palatine, pharyngeal and artery of the pterygoid canal)	
Cricopharyngeus m.	Separates hypopharynx from cervical esophagus	Pharyngeal plexus (CN IX, X, and sympathetic)		
Palatoglossus m.	Forms anterior faucial arch Elevates posterior tongue	Pharyngeal plexus (sympathetic, IX, X, and cranial portion XI)		
Palatopharyngeus m.	Narrows oropharyngeal isthmus, elevates pharynx, closes off nasopharynx			
Stylopharyngeus m.	Raises and dilates pharynx	Glossopharyngeal (CN IX)		
Salpingopharyngeus m.	Raises nasopharynx, helps open eustachian tube during swallowing	Pharyngeal plexus (sympathetic, IX, X, and cranial portion XI)		
Levator veli palatini m.	Raises soft palate, helps open eustachian tube during swallowing			
Tensor veli palatini m.	Tenses soft palate and helps open eustachian tube during swallowing	Trigeminal (V_3)		

a., artery; CN, cranial nerve; m., muscle; n., nerve; v., vein.

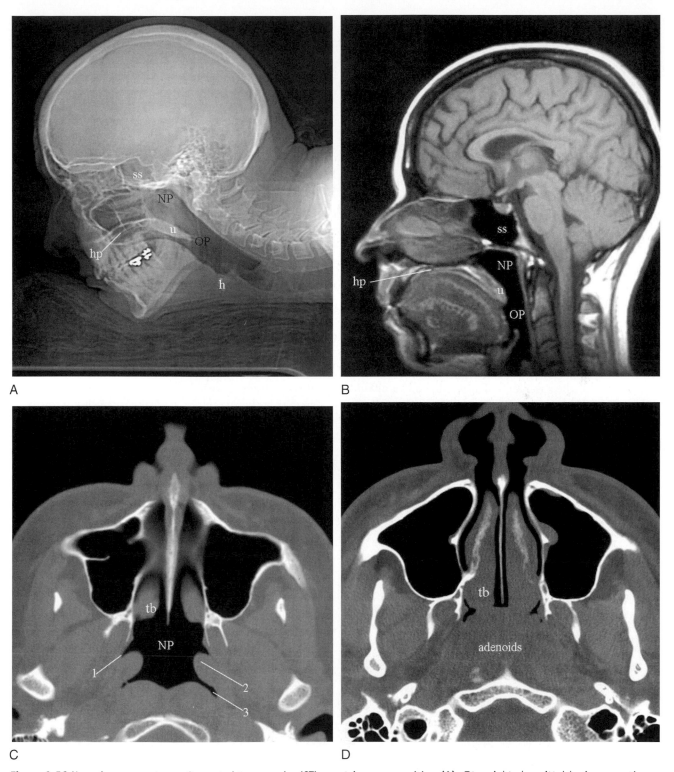

Figure 2-52 Nasopharynx anatomy. Computed tomography (CT) scout in prone position **(A)**. T1-weighted sagittal brain magnetic resonance **(B)**. Normal nasopharynx on axial CT scan **(C)** and prominent adenoids effacing the nasopharyngeal airway in **(D)**. Opening of the eustachian tube, 1; torus tubarius, 2; fossa of Rosenmüller, 3; turbinate, tb; sphenoid sinus, ss; hard palate, hp; uvula, u; hyoid, h; nasopharynx, NP; oropharynx, OP.

nasogastric tube difficult. They may also contribute to the symptom complex of sleep apnea.

b. Tornwaldt's Cyst

Tornwaldt's cyst is a not uncommon incidental finding on MRI. It is usually midline and located between the longus capitis muscles in the posterior nasopharynx. It is a developmental anomaly related to the ascension of the notochord back into the skull base, pulling a small tag of the developing nasopharyngeal mucosa with it and creating a midline pit or tract, which closes over and results in a midline cyst, usually after pharyngitis. These lesions usually have a high signal intensity on T1- and T2-weighted imaging, probably because of the high protein content of the cyst fluid. Tornwaldt's cyst is usually infected by anaerobic bacteria, which may empty into the nasopharynx and cause intermittent halitosis. The CT density of the cyst is similar to that of surrounding muscle and lymphoid tissue.

c. Infection and Abscess

Abscess in the parapharyngeal space may result from tonsillar infection or perforation of the pharynx, either iatrogenic or traumatic. The infection may extend from the skull base to the submandibular region and be difficult to differentiate from a neoplastic process. If large enough, it may compromise the airway. Infection spreading to

retropharyngeal nodes, suppurative adenitis, can also obliterate the nasopharynx airway (Fig. 2-53).

d. Tumors and Others

Squamous cell carcinoma of the nasopharynx is a relatively rare cancer that accounts for only 0.25% of all malignancies in North America. It has a high rate of incidence in Asia, however, where it is the most common tumor in males, accounting for 18% of cancers in China.[27] Squamous cell carcinoma accounts for 70% or more of the malignancies arising in the nasopharynx, and lymphomas account for approximately 20%. The remaining 10% are a variety of lesions, including adenocarcinoma, adenoid cystic carcinoma, rhabdomyosarcoma, melanoma, extramedullary plasmacytoma, fibrosarcoma, and carcinosarcoma. Risk factors for squamous cell carcinoma in the nasopharynx include the presence of immunoglobulin A antibodies against Epstein-Barr virus, human leukocyte antigen (HLA)-A2 and HLA-B-Sin histocompatibility loci, nitrosamines, polycyclic hydrocarbons, poor living conditions, and chronic sinonasal infections. The most common presentation is nodal disease. There is no correlation between primary tumor size and the presence of nodal disease. Imaging with CT and MRI is performed to map accurately the extent of the disease, not for histologic diagnosis (Fig. 2-54).

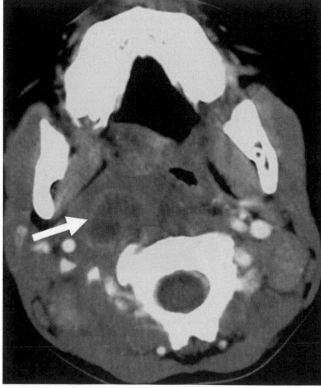

A

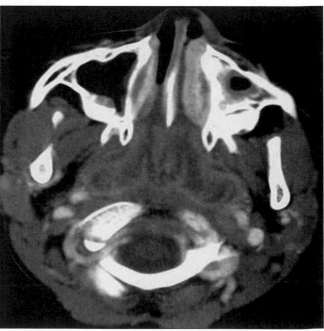

B

Figure 2-53 **A** and **B,** Suppurative adenitis. Axial computed tomography scans. **A,** A ring-enhancing mass *(arrow)* is noted in the right parapharyngeal space deviating the oropharynx. **B,** Bilateral bulky adenopathy is present with abscess formation obliterating the nasopharynx.

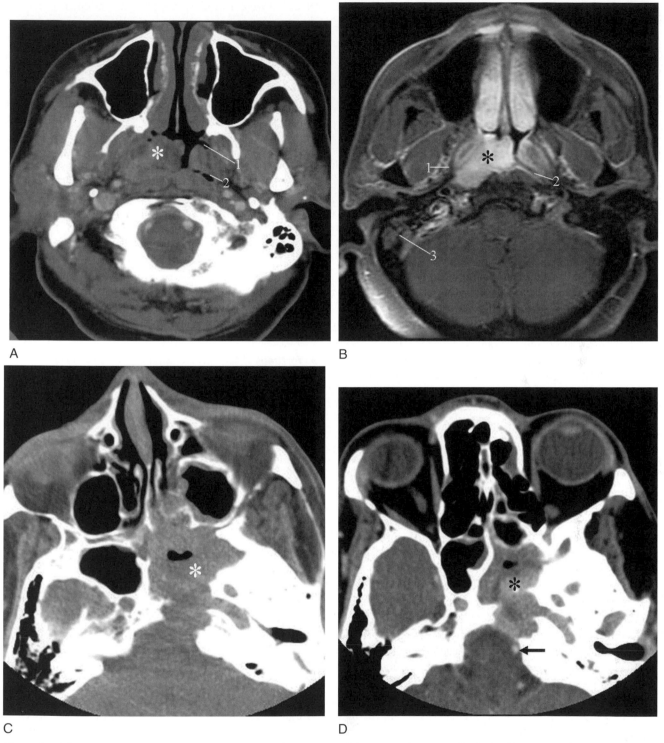

A

B

C

D

Figure 2-54 Squamous cell carcinoma of the right nasopharynx. **A,** Axial computed tomography (CT) with contrast demonstrates bulky soft tissue asymmetry in the nasopharynx with abnormal enhancement on the right. **B,** T1-weighted magnetic resonance with gadolinium confirms the right nasopharyngeal mass obstructing the eustachian canal and consequent opacification of the right mastoid air cells. **C,** Axial CT demonstrates squamous cell carcinoma extending from the soft tissues of the left nasopharynx to the posterior fossa of the brain with bone destruction of the skull base. **D,** Following contrast enhancement, note the proximity of this invasive lesion to the vertebral artery *(arrow)* at the foramen magnum. If these findings are not appreciated at the time of surgery, an errant nasogastric tube can easily enter the cranium and not only damage the brain stem but also injure the vertebral artery. Eustachian tube, 1; fossa of Rosenmüller, 2; opacified mastoid air cells, 3; mass (asterisk).

E. OROPHARYNX

1. Imaging Anatomy

The oropharynx is the region posterior to the oral cavity that includes the posterior one third of the tongue (tongue base), the palatine tonsils, the soft palate, and the oropharyngeal mucosa and constrictor muscles. The posterior pharyngeal wall is at the level of the second and third cervical vertebrae. Laterally, there are two mucosa-lined faucial arches; the anterior arch is formed by the mucosa of the palatoglossus muscle, and the posterior arch is formed by the palatopharyngeus muscle. The palatine tonsils are located between the two faucial arches, and the lingual tonsils reside at the base of the tongue. Both sets of tonsils vary in size and can encroach on the airway. The arterial supply to the oropharynx is mainly from the branches of the external carotid artery: the tonsillar branch of the facial artery, the ascending pharyngeal artery, the dorsal lingual arteries, and the internal maxillary and facial arteries. The venous drainage is primarily by the peritonsillar veins, which pierce the constrictor musculature and drain into the common facial vein and the pharyngeal plexus. Lymphatic drainage is mainly to the jugulodigastric chain from the skull base to the cricoid cartilage, the retropharyngeal nodes, the posterior triangle nodes from the level of the skull base to the cricoid cartilage, and sometimes the parotid nodes.

a. Tonsillar Hypertrophy

During the third and fourth fetal months, lymphoid tissues invade the pharyngeal region of the adenoid tonsils, the palatine region (palatine tonsils), and the root of the tongue (lingual tonsils).[40] The adenoids are located in the roof of the nasopharynx. As mentioned previously, enlargement of the palatine and lingual tonsils may compromise the airway (Fig. 2-55).

b. Tonsillitis and Peritonsillar Abscess

Acute bacterial tonsillitis is most commonly caused by beta-hemolytic streptococcus, staphylococcus, pneumococcus, or *Haemophilus*. It is usually a self-limiting disease; however, uncontrolled infection of the tonsils may result in a peritonsillar abscess or, rarely, in a tonsillar abscess. On CT imaging, the findings of acute or chronic tonsillitis are nonspecific. Focal homogeneous swelling of the palatine tonsils can be present and is difficult to differentiate from tumor. The imaging features of abscess formation are a low-density center and an enhancing rim of soft tissue (Fig. 2-56). Peritonsillar abscess is the accumulation of pus around the tonsils. The infection may extend to the retropharyngeal, parapharyngeal, or submandibular spaces.

c. Retropharyngeal Process

Infection of the retropharyngeal space is usually a result of an infection at a site whose primary drainage is to the retropharyngeal lymph nodes, such as the nose, sinuses, throat, tonsils, oral cavity, and middle ear. The lymph nodes enlarge and undergo suppuration and eventually rupture into the retropharyngeal space, creating an abscess. This can result from a penetrating injury or from cervical spine osteomyelitis or diskitis. Before the advent of antibiotics, retropharyngeal infection was potentially life threatening. A retropharyngeal space infection can extend from the skull base to the carina. On imaging, a retropharyngeal abscess expands the prevertebral space, with enhancement along its margins. Included in the differential diagnosis of a retropharyngeal abscess is tendinitis of the longus colli, which is characterized by inflammation of the tendinous insertion of the longus colli muscle with deposition of calcium hydroxyapatite crystals. An effusion may extend from the prevertebral space into the retropharyngeal space and mimic a retropharyngeal abscess. Post-traumatic hematoma may also increase the width of prevertebral space. In addition, cervical spine pathology can extend and enlarge the prevertebral space and cause the airway to deviate anteriorly.

d. Tortuous Internal or Common Carotid Artery

If the course of either the common carotid artery or the internal carotid artery is directed medially, bulging of the submucosa of the oropharynx or hypopharynx may result. In this less protected location, the artery is more vulnerable to trauma. Imaging is useful to prevent unnecessary biopsy of this pseudosubmucosal mass (Fig. 2-57).

e. Tumors and Others

Squamous cell carcinoma is the most common neoplasm of the oropharynx, and its predisposing factors include alcohol and tobacco use. The site of origin determines the spread of the tumor; the most common locations are the anterior and posterior tonsillar pillars, tonsillar fossa, soft palate, and base of the tongue (see Fig. 2-51*A* and *B*). Staging of tumor in the oropharynx is dependent on the size of the tumor and whether it has invaded adjacent structures. Other neoplasms include lymphoma, minor salivary gland tumors, and mesenchymal tumors.

F. HYPOPHARYNX

The classical boundary of the hypopharynx is defined as the segment of the pharynx extending from the level of the hyoid bone and the valleculae to the cricopharyngeus or the lower level of the cricoid cartilage. By definition, the cervical esophagus starts at the caudal end of the cricoid cartilage. The cricopharyngeus muscle acts as the superior esophageal sphincter. It arises from the lower aspect of the inferior constrictor muscle attached to the cricoid. The upper esophageal sphincter is normally closed until a specific volume and pressure in the hypopharynx trigger the relaxation of the cricopharyngeus muscle to allow a bolus of food to pass into the cervical esophagus. The cricopharyngeus muscle then closes to prevent reflux.[27]

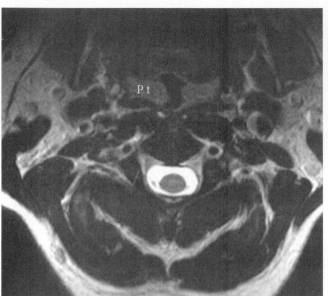

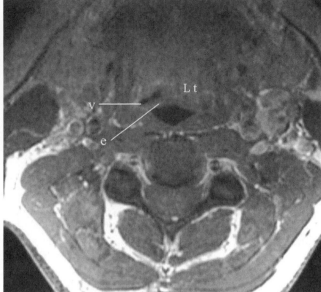

A

B

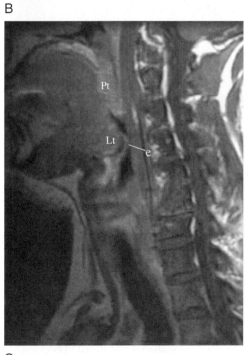

C

Figure 2-55 **A,** Palatine and lingual tonsils. T2-weighted axial magnetic resonance (MR) image demonstrates bilateral hyperintense palatine tonsils, Pt, effacing the oropharynx. **B,** T1-weighted axial MR shows enlarged lingual tonsils, Lt, effacing the vallecula, v. **C,** Routine T1-sagittal cervical spine study shows both palatine tonsils, Pt, and lingual tonsils, Lt, effacing the airway. The lingual tonsils push the epiglottis, e, dorsally.

1. Imaging Anatomy

The hypopharynx can be divided into four regions: the pyriform sinuses, the posterior wall of the hypopharynx, the postcricoid region, and the lateral surface of the aryepiglottic folds. The *pyriform sinus* is the anterolateral recess of the hypopharynx. The anterior pyriform sinus mucosa abuts on the posterior paraglottic space. The most caudal portion of each pyriform sinus lies at the level of the true vocal cord. The lateral aspect of the *aryepiglottic folds* forms the medial wall of the pyriform sinus (Fig. 2-58). This is considered a marginal zone because the aryepiglottic folds are considered part of both the hypopharynx and the supraglottic larynx.

Tumors involving the medial surface of the aryepiglottic folds behave like laryngeal tumors. The biologic behavior of tumors arising from the lateral surface of the aryepiglottic folds is similar to that of the more aggressive pharyngeal tumors. The lateral wall of the pyriform sinus is formed by the thyroid membrane and cartilage.

The *posterior hypopharyngeal wall* is continuous with the posterior wall of the oropharynx and begins at the level of the valleculae. It continues caudally as the posterior wall of the cricopharyngeus and the cervical esophagus. The retropharyngeal space lies behind the posterior pharyngeal wall. The anterior wall of the lower hypopharynx is referred to as the *postcricoid hypopharynx*: the larynx is

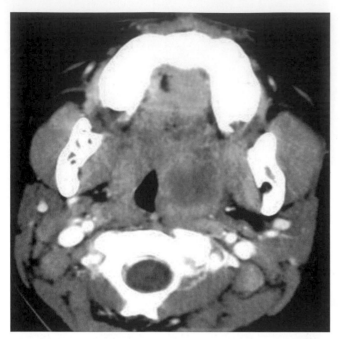

Figure 2-56 Tonsillar abscess. Axial computed tomography with contrast demonstrating a left tonsillar fluid collection compressing the oropharynx.

anterior and the hypopharynx is posterior to this soft tissue boundary. It extends from the level of the arytenoid cartilages to the lower cricoid cartilage. On imaging, the transition from the hypopharynx to the cervical esophagus is denoted by a change in the shape of the aerodigestive tract, from oval to round.

The arterial supply to the lower pharynx is mainly from the superior and inferior thyroid arteries. Venous drainage is by the superior and inferior thyroid veins and individual pharyngeal veins to the internal jugular vein.

2. Imaging Pathology

a. Pharyngitis

In immunocompetent patients, imaging is usually not required for the diagnosis or management of pharyngitis. In AIDS patients, imaging may be helpful to evaluate the extent of disease. Bacterial etiology is not the only concern; opportunistic infection with *Candida* or cytomegalovirus may involve the hypopharynx. These entities do not compromise the airway, but the mucosa is friable and susceptible to injuries from instrumentation.

b. Pharyngocele

A pharyngocele is a broad-based pouching of the pharyngeal mucosa of the upper pyriform sinus, which

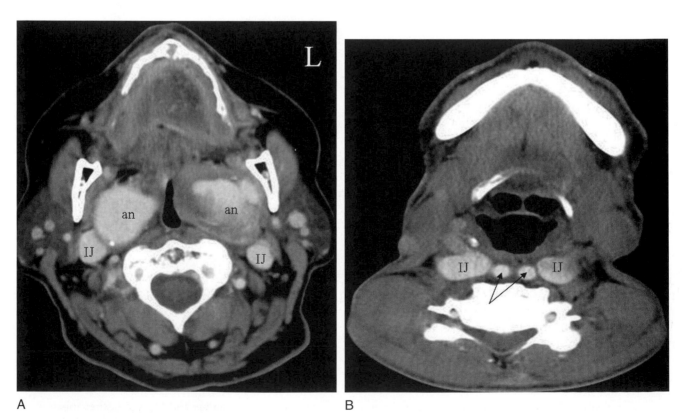

A

B

Figure 2-57 Anomalous course of carotids. **A,** Axial computed tomography (CT) with contrast shows bilateral carotid aneurysms, an, effacing the oropharynx. Note presence of thrombus in the lumen of the aneurysm on the left. **B,** Axial CT with contrast demonstrates medially deviated carotids, assuming a retropharyngeal location *(arrows)*. Internal jugular vein, IJ.

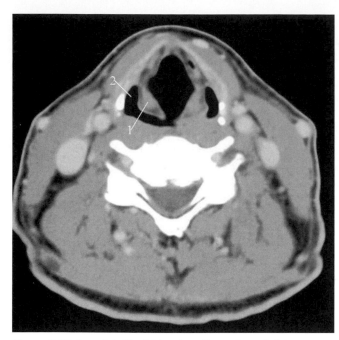

Figure 2-58 Aryepiglottic fold and pyriform sinus. Axial computed tomography at the level of hypopharynx. Aryepiglottic fold, 1; air-containing pyriform sinus, 2.

distends with phonation or during the Valsalva maneuver. These lesions are visible as air-filled structures on CT or as barium-filled areas on a barium swallow test.

c. Zenker's Diverticulum

It is postulated that dyssynergy of the cricopharyngeus muscle plays a role in the formation of this pulsion diverticulum of the hypopharynx. The diverticulum usually extends posteriorly and laterally, usually to the left, and may appear as an incidental, air-filled structure in the hypopharynx on CT and MRI. If alerted to the presence of a diverticulum, one should take more caution in the blind advancement of a nasogastric tube, which may take an errant course (Fig. 2-59).

d. Trauma

i. Hematomas Iatrogenic trauma caused by instrumentation or a foreign body may result in retropharyngeal hematoma. Hemophiliacs may be more susceptible to hematomas with minor trauma. The imaging finding is retropharyngeal or prevertebral soft-tissue swelling.

ii. Postradiation Changes The edema that occurs after radiation therapy may persist for many months or years and is reflective of a radiation-induced obliterative endarteritis. In cases of edema the pharyngeal and supraglottic mucosa is enlarged and hypodense on CT and the submucosa fat is thickened and streaky. The platysma muscle and skin are also thickened. The end result is fibrosis and loss of

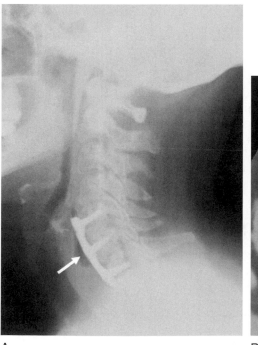

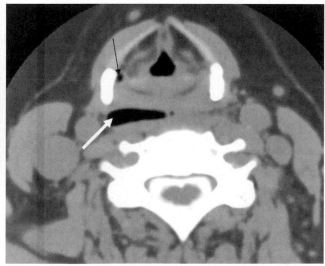

A   B

Figure 2-59 Zenker's diverticulum. **A,** Lateral cervical spine; soft-tissue technique demonstrates an air-filled structure in the hypopharynx *(white arrow)* in a patient after anterior fusion. **B,** Axial computed tomography at the level of the larynx shows the air-filled Zenker diverticulum to the right of midline *(white arrow)* and the tip of the right pyriform sinus *(black arrow)*.

elasticity of the soft tissues. This increased rigidity of the soft tissues should be taken into account during laryngoscopy for endotracheal intubation and selecting the correct size of a laryngeal mask airway.

e. Tumors and Others

i. Squamous Cell Carcinoma The hypopharynx is lined by stratified squamous epithelium, and the majority of tumors of the hypopharynx are squamous cell carcinomas (Fig. 2-60). The risk factors for squamous cell carcinoma of the hypopharynx include alcohol abuse, smoking, and previous radiation therapy. Patients with Plummer-Vinson syndrome have a higher incidence of postcricoid carcinoma. Extensive submucosal growth is common and can be appreciated only on imaging. The airway may be effaced and displaced. Most patients have metastases to the cervical nodes at presentation. Between 4% and 15% of patients with squamous cell carcinoma of the hypopharynx have a synchronous or metachronous second primary tumor.[28,42]

ii. Lymphomas Hodgkin's disease predominantly affects adolescents and young adults, whereas non-Hodgkin's lymphoma is a disease of older patients. In contrast to patients with Hodgkin's disease, patients with non-Hodgkin's lymphoma present with disease in extranodal sites, such as Waldeyer's ring. The imaging features of extranodal head and neck lymphoma are indistinguishable from those of squamous cell carcinoma. Lymphadenopathy in

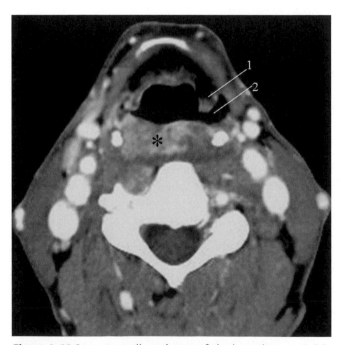

Figure 2-60 Squamous cell carcinoma of the hypopharynx. Axial computed tomography with contrast demonstrates an enhancing mass (asterisk) involving the posterior wall of the hypopharynx with deformity of the airway. Note the effacement of the right pyriform sinus. Aryepiglottic fold, 1; pyriform sinus, 2.

Hodgkin's disease can be quite large without affecting the airways.

iii. Minor Salivary Gland Tumors These tumors account for 2% to 3% of all malignancies of the extracranial head and neck.[28] The most common are adenoid cystic carcinoma, mucoepidermoid carcinoma, adenocarcinoma, malignant mixed tumor, acinic cell carcinoma, and pleomorphic adenoma. The soft palate is the most common site.

iv. Kaposi's Sarcoma This tumor occurs almost exclusively in AIDS patients and involves the hypopharynx less than the oral cavity.

G. LARYNX

The larynx provides a conduit to the lungs and allows vocalization. It has an outer supporting skeleton composed of a series of cartilages, fibrous sheets, muscles, and ligaments housing and protecting an inner mucosal tube, the endolarynx, with its recesses and mucosal folds. Between the cartilages and the mucosal surface lie the paraglottic and preepiglottic spaces, which contain loose areolar tissues, lymphatics, and muscles. Superiorly, the larynx is suspended from the hyoid bone, which is attached to the styloid process at the base of the skull by the stylohyoid ligament. Calcification of the stylohyoid ligament (see Fig. 2-13) has been proposed as a cause of difficult intubation.[35] Muscles attached to the hyoid bone elevate the larynx and move it ventrally, providing the primary protection from aspiration.[14]

The thyroid cartilage is the largest cartilage of the larynx. It is made up of two shieldlike laminae that fuse anteriorly to form the laryngeal prominence (Adam's apple). The angle of fusion is usually more acute and more prominent in males. Paired superior and inferior cornua project from the posterior margin of the thyroid cartilage. The superior thyroid cornua connects with the dorsal tip of the greater cornua of the hyoid bone by the thyrohyoid ligament. The inferior cornua articulates with the lateral facets of the cricoid cartilage to form the cricothyroid joint, where the thyroid cartilage rocks back and forth. Muscles that attach to the external surface of the thyroid cartilage include the sternothyroid and thyrohyoid muscles and the inferior pharyngeal constrictors. The thyrohyoid membrane bridges the gap between the upper surface of the thyroid cartilage and the hyoid bone. Likewise, the cricothyroid membrane spans the distance between the lower margin of the thyroid cartilage and the cricoid cartilage.

The cricoid cartilage, which is shaped like a signet ring with the larger part facing posteriorly, is the base of the larynx. On either side of the cricoid cartilage are facets, which articulate with the inferior horn of the thyroid cartilage. On the upper surface of the cricoid lamina are two paired articular facets, on which are situated the arytenoid cartilages.[46] The arytenoid cartilages are important surgical and imaging landmarks.[46] Each cartilage is pyramidal in shape. At the level of the base are two projections: the muscular process situated on the posterolateral margin and the vocal process located anteriorly. The superior process is the apex of the pyramid and is at the level of the false vocal cords. Small corniculate cartilage rests on the superior process. The muscular and vocal processes are at the level of the true vocal cords.

The arytenoid cartilages are important in maintaining airway patency and participate in vocalization by altering the opening of the glottis and the tension of the vocal cords. This is achieved by movements between the arytenoid and cricoid cartilages: adduction, abduction, anterior-posterior sliding, and medial-lateral sliding.

The endolarynx can be divided into three compartments for surgical planning. The false cord is the boundary between the supraglottic airway and the glottis. It includes the false vocal cords, epiglottis, aryepiglottic folds, and arytenoids. The glottis is defined by the laryngeal ventricle, true vocal cords, anterior and posterior commissure, and tissue 1 cm below the laryngeal ventricle. The subglottic larynx extends from 1 cm below the laryngeal ventricle to the lower margin of the cricoid cartilage.

Several structures in the endoskeleton of the larynx are worth describing. The epiglottis is a yellow elastic fibrocartilage; the tip defines the craniad margin of the supraglottic larynx. It has a flattened teardrop or leaf shape that tapers to an inferior point called the petiole of the epiglottis, where it attaches to the thyroid cartilage through the thyroepiglottic ligament. The superior and lateral edges are free. Most of the epiglottis extends behind the thyroid cartilage, and the tip may be above the hyoid bone and sometimes can be seen through the oral cavity. It is held in place and stabilized by the hyoepiglottic and thyroepiglottic ligaments. The hyoepiglottic ligament is a tough, fibrous, fanlike ligament extending from the ventral midline of the epiglottis to the dorsal margin of the hyoid cartilage. Immediately above the ligament are the pharyngeal recesses, the valleculae, situated just caudal to the tongue base. The epiglottis helps to guard against aspiration; during swallowing, the aryepiglottic folds pull the sides of the epiglottis down, thereby narrowing the entrance to the larynx.

The quadrangular membrane stretches anteriorly from the upper arytenoid and corniculate cartilages to the lateral margin of the epiglottis and contributes to the support of the epiglottis.[14] The superior free margin of this membrane forms the support for the aryepiglottic fold, which stretches from the upper margin of the arytenoids to the lateral margin of the epiglottis. The corniculate and cuneiform cartilages within the aryepiglottic fold help support the edge of each fold. These small, mucosa-covered cartilages are visualized on laryngoscopy as two small protuberances at the posterolateral border of the rima glottidis.

The aryepiglottic folds form the lateral margin of the vestibule of the supraglottic airway. The upper part of the aryepiglottic fold is the aryepiglottic muscle, which functions like a purse string to close the opening of the larynx when swallowing. Lateral to the aryepiglottic folds are the pyriform sinuses. The apex, or the most inferior aspect, of the pyriform sinus is at the level of the true vocal cords.

The inferior free margin of the quadrangular membrane forms the ventricular ligament, which extends anteriorly from the superior arytenoid cartilage to the inner lamina of the thyroid cartilage and supports the free edge of the false vocal cords. The false vocal cords are superior to the true vocal cords and are separated by a lateral pouching of the airway, the laryngeal ventricle.[14]

A second set of ligaments, the vocal ligaments, lies parallel and inferior to the ventricular ligament. It also extends from the vocal process of the arytenoid cartilage to the inner lamina of the thyroid just above the anterior commissure. The vocal ligament provides medial support for the true vocal cords. The space between the left and right vocal cords is referred to as the rima glottis, through which air passes to allow breathing and vocalization. Extending from the vocal ligament is another fibrous membrane, the conus elasticus, which attaches inferiorly to the upper inner margin of the cricoid cartilage. The conus spans part of the gap between the thyroid and cricoid cartilages.

The muscles of the larynx are categorized as intrinsic and extrinsic muscles. The intrinsic muscles regulate the aperture of the rima glottis: (1) the *thyroarytenoid* makes up the bulk of the true vocal cord and has a lateral and medial belly, (2) the *lateral cricoarytenoids* extend from the muscular process of the arytenoid cartilage to the upper lateral cricoid cartilage and function to adduct the cords, (3) the *posterior cricoarytenoids* extend from the muscular process of the arytenoid cartilage to the posterior surface of the cricoid cartilage and abduct the cords laterally, and (4) the *intra-arytenoid muscle* stretches from one arytenoid to the other and functions to adduct the vocal cords.

The extrinsic muscle is the *cricothyroid* muscle, which extends from the lower thyroid cartilage anteriorly to the upper cricoid cartilage. The contraction of this muscle pivots the thyroid cartilage forward around an axis through the cricothyroid joint, which stretches and tenses the vocal cords, thus affecting pitch in vocalization.[14]

The larynx is innervated primarily by branches of the vagus nerve.[46] The recurrent laryngeal nerve innervates all the intrinsic muscles of the larynx. When vocal cord paralysis is present and nerve damage is suspected, imaging should be tailored to follow the course of the recurrent laryngeal nerve in the neck and upper chest. The vagus nerve, after exiting the jugular foramen, passes vertically down the neck within the carotid sheath, between the internal jugular vein and the internal carotid artery (subsequently the common carotid artery) to the root of the neck. In front of the right subclavian artery, the recurrent laryngeal nerve branches from the vagus nerve, loops around the right subclavian artery, and ascends to the side of the trachea behind the common carotid artery, in the tracheoesophageal groove. On the left side, the recurrent laryngeal nerve arises at the level of the aortic arch. It loops around the arch at the point where ligamentum arteriosum is attached and ascends to the side of the trachea in the tracheoesophageal groove. The recurrent laryngeal nerve enters the larynx behind the cricothyroid joint and innervates all the muscles of the larynx except the cricothyroid muscle, which is an extrinsic muscle of the anterior larynx innervated by the external laryngeal branch of the superior laryngeal nerve, a branch of the vagus nerve in the neck. Sensory input from the laryngeal mucosa is by the internal laryngeal branch of the superior laryngeal nerve, which perforates the posterior lateral portion of the thyrohyoid membrane.[46]

The blood supply to the larynx is from branches of the external carotid artery: the superior and inferior laryngeal arteries. The superior laryngeal artery, a branch of the superior thyroid artery, travels with the internal branch of the superior laryngeal nerve. The inferior laryngeal artery, a branch of the inferior thyroid artery, which is a branch of the thyrocervical trunk, accompanies the recurrent laryngeal nerve into the larynx (Table 2-4).[46]

1. Imaging Anatomy

Prior to CT and MRI, examination of the larynx included laryngography and multidirectional tomography. Soft tissue film of the airway was a good survey study. Barium swallow, which is still used today, provides dynamic information about the swallowing mechanism and any dysfunction. CT and MRI allow visualization of structures deep to the mucosa (Fig. 2-61); however, breathing and swallowing movements made imaging of the larynx difficult. The faster CT scanning technology available today allows the entire neck to be scanned in a single breath-hold. Helical technology allows reformation of the airway in all three planes. MRI examination of the larynx has been inhibited by motion artifacts intrinsic and extrinsic to the larynx but has a greater ability than CT to separate out various soft tissue planes. Coronal and sagittal imaging on both CT and MRI is helpful in evaluating the spaces and mucosal folds. On a sagittal view, one can easily identify the hyoid bone, epiglottis, aryepiglottic folds, and vestibule, which is the space extending from the epiglottis to the level of the false vocal cords. At the level of the thyroid cartilage, a tiny slit of air is seen directed in the anterior-posterior direction. This is the laryngeal ventricle, which separates the false vocal cords from the true vocal cords (see Fig. 2-15). The vocal cords are not static structures, thus the difficulty in imaging. During normal respiration, the vocal cords are abducted and the inlet or the rima glottidis has a triangular shape. With maximal abduction during deep inspiration, the opening of the glottis adopts more of a diamond shape. The rima glottidis is narrowed during expiration and phonation.

Below the true vocal cords to the cricoid cartilage is the infraglottic cavity. The trachea begins below the level of the cricoid cartilage.

2. Imaging Pathology

a. Trauma

Fracture of the larynx, which usually occurs as a result of a vehicular accident, can involve the thyroid cartilage, cricoid cartilage, or both. Laryngotracheal separation is usually fatal. Dislocation of the arytenoids relative to the cricoid cartilage can be encountered. Malalignment of the thyroid cartilage and cricoid cartilage results in the dislocation of the cricothyroid joint. On imaging, the presence of air in the paraglottic soft tissues is an indication of laryngeal trauma (Fig. 2-62).

Foreign bodies may be the result of trauma but are more commonly due to ingestion or aspiration. The pyriform sinus is a common location for a foreign body. If the foreign body enters the larynx, it usually passes through to the trachea or bronchi.

Burn injury to the larynx can be due to the inhalation or ingestion of hot material. The supraglottic larynx is most likely to be involved and generalized edema can occur.

b. Vocal Cord Paralysis

Vocal cord paralysis may be characterized as either a superior laryngeal nerve deficit, recurrent laryngeal nerve deficit, or total vagus nerve deficit. Imaging should address the entire course of the vagus nerve and the recurrent laryngeal nerve when assessing vocal cord paralysis (Fig. 2-63).

The superior laryngeal nerve, through the external laryngeal branch, innervates only one muscle of the larynx—an extrinsic muscle, the cricothyroid muscle. This muscle extends between the thyroid and cricoid cartilages. As the muscle contracts, the anterior cricoid ring is pulled up toward the lower margin of the thyroid cartilage. This action rotates the upper cricoid lamina, and thus the arytenoids, posteriorly and puts tension on the true vocal cords. If one side is paralyzed, contraction of one muscle rotates the posterior cricoid to the contralateral paralyzed side.

More commonly, vocal cord paralysis is due to recurrent laryngeal nerve pathology. All of the laryngeal muscles, except for the cricothyroid muscle, are innervated by this nerve. Most findings are secondary to atrophy of the thyroarytenoid muscle, the muscle that contributes to the bulk of the true vocal cords. The vocal cords become thinner and more pointed, and the subglottic arch is lost. Compensatory enlargement of the ventricle and the pyriform sinus is seen.[14] In the more acute phase, the paralyzed cord appears flaccid and prolapses medially because of the lack of muscular tone in the thyroarytenoid muscle and demonstrates a lack of movement during breathing maneuvers and phonation.

Table 2-4 **Muscles of the Larynx**

Muscles	Function	Innervation	Arterial Supply	Venous Drainage
EXTRINSIC MUSCLES (MOVE THE LARYNX RELATIVE TO NECK)				
Sternothyroid m.	Depresses larynx and thyroid cartilage	Ansa cervicalis	Superior thyroid a.	Superior thyroid v. to internal jugular v.
Thyrohyoid m.	Depresses larynx and hyoid bone Elevates thyroid cartilage	C1		
Stylopharyngeus m.	Elevates and dilates pharynx	CN IX	Ascending pharyngeal a. branches	Internal jugular v.
Palatopharyngeus m.	Elevates pharynx	Pharyngeal plexus (CN IX, X, XI, sympathetic)		
INTRINSIC MUSCLES (MOVE LARYNGEAL CARTILAGES WITHIN LARYNX)				
Posterior cricoarytenoid m.	Draws muscular process of arytenoid posteriorly Pivots arytenoid cartilage Abducts vocal cords	Inferior laryngeal n., branch of recurrent laryngeal n., branch of vagus n. (CN X)	Superior laryngeal a., cricothyroid branch of the superior thyroid a. Penetrates the thyrohyoid membrane accompanied by internal branch of the superior laryngeal n.	Superior thyroid v. to internal jugular v. Inferior thyroid vein to left brachiocephalic v.
Arytenoideus m. (transverse m., oblique m.)	Draws arytenoids together, adducting the vocal cord		Laryngeal branch of the superior thyroid a.	
Aryepiglotticus	Draws epiglottis posteriorly and downward during swallowing			
Cricothyroid m.	Draws thyroid cartilage forward, lengthening vocal ligaments	External branch of superior laryngeal n., branch of vagus n. (CN X)	Cricothyroid branch of the superior thyroid a.	
Lateral cricoarytenoid m.	Draws muscular process of arytenoid cartilage anteriorly, which pivots arytenoid cartilage and adducts vocal cords	Inferior laryngeal n., branch of recurrent laryngeal n., branch of vagus n. (CN X)	Superior laryngeal a., cricothyroid branch of superior thyroid a.	
Thyroarytenoid	Draws arytenoid forward Relaxes and adducts vocal folds		Laryngeal branch of superior thyroid a.	
Thyroepiglottic m.	Draws epiglottis downward			
Vocalis m.	Relaxes vocal ligament			

a., artery; CN, cranial nerve; m., muscle; n., nerve; v., vein.

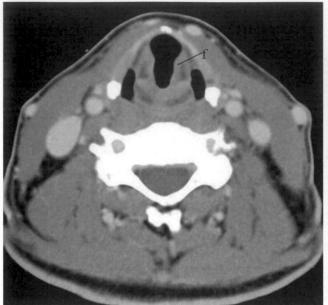

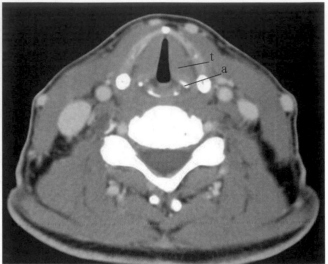

A

B

Figure 2-61 Normal larynx. Axial computed tomography (CT) scans at the level of the false cord **(A)** and true cord **(B).** The false cord (f) contains fat (dark on CT and bright on magnetic resonance [MR] T1-weighted imaging). The true cords, t, are at the level of the arytenoid cartilage, a, and contain no fat. Subglottic airway is ovoid in shape as shown in axial CT scan **(C).**

Continued

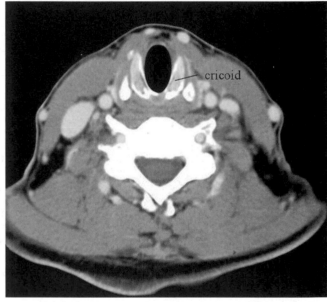

C

The posterior cricoarytenoid muscle stretches from the posterior surface of the cricoid to the lateral aspect of the muscular process of the arytenoids. This is the only muscle that rotates the vocal cords outward. Rarely, adductor paralysis affects all the muscles that adduct the cords, sparing the posterior cricoarytenoid muscle. Thus, the vocal cords remain in a lateral position. The cause of this abnormality is not well understood, but an intracranial pathology that affects only certain fibers of the recurrent laryngeal nerve has been postulated.

c. Congenital Lesions

The respiratory system is formed from an out-pouching of the primitive pharynx. The cells on each side of the entrance to the respiratory diverticulum become adherent and form the tracheoesophageal septum, separating the trachea from the primitive foregut. At one point in development, the laryngeal lumen is occluded and later recanalizes. The cartilages arise from the mesenchymal cells on either side of the respiratory tract, which then fuse in the midline to form the thyroid and cricoid cartilages. Congenital lesions are related to delays in the development and maturation of the respiratory system.

i. Laryngomalacia This entity represents a delay in the development of the laryngeal support system. The structures of the larynx are present but are not mature enough to keep the larynx open. The supraglottic larynx

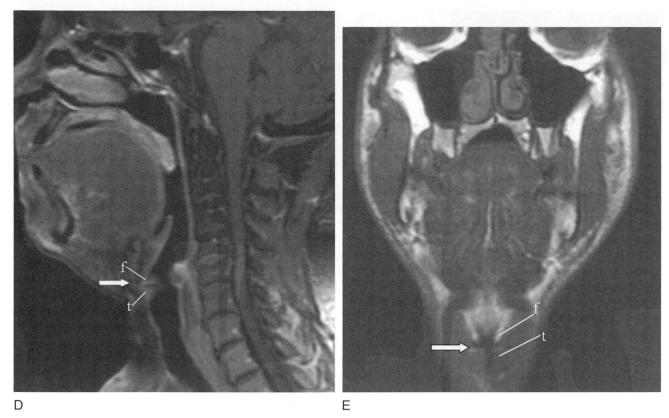

D

E

Figure 2-61, contd. T-1 weighted sagittal **(D)** and coronal **(E)** MR images demonstrate the false cord, f, separated from the true cord, t, by the laryngeal ventricle *(arrow)*.

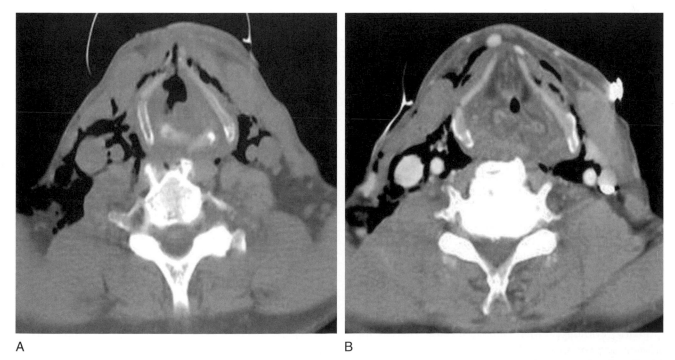

A

B

Figure 2-62 Laryngeal fracture. Precontrast **(A)** and postcontrast **(B)** axial computed tomography scans show extensive deep fascial emphysema as well as multiple fractures of the thyroid and cricoid cartilages.

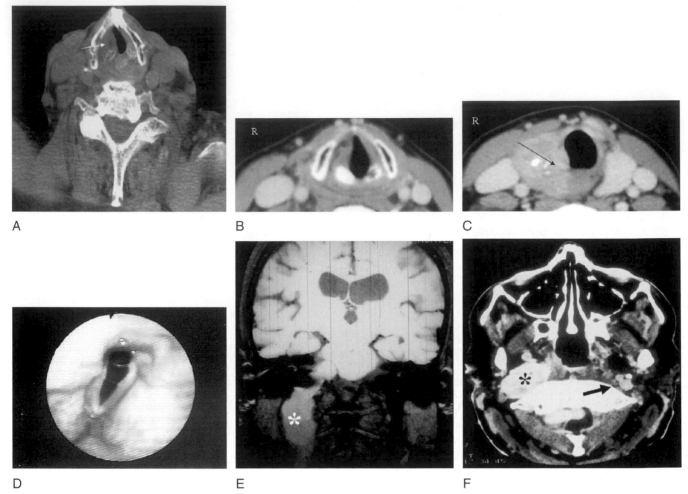

Figure 2-63 Causes of vocal cord paralysis in three different patients. Patient 1: Right vocal cord paralysis secondary to tumor inva-sion **(A)**. Axial computed tomography (CT) scan **(A)** demonstrates squamous cell carcinoma invasion of the right vocal cord, which is medially deviated. Patient 2: Right vocal cord paralysis secondary to tumor in the tracheoesophageal groove involving the recurrent laryngeal nerve **(B, C, and D)**. Axial contrast-enhanced CT scan **(B)** demonstrates a paralyzed right true vocal cord. In this case, dener-vation is due to neural compromise in the tracheoesophageal groove by papillary carcinoma of the right thyroid tumor **(C)**. Endoscopic visualization of the paralyzed right cord **(D)**. Patient 3: Contrast-enhanced coronal T1 magnetic resonance **(E)** and axial CT **(F)** scans demonstrate an enhancing vagus nerve schwannoma *(asterisk)* in a patient with known neurofibromatosis. Note the normal vagus nerve *(arrow)* within the contralateral carotid sheath, with the carotid artery and jugular vein. This patient presented with right vocal cord paralysis.

is affected, and the epiglottis may be floppy. As the carti-lages mature, the problem resolves.

ii. Webs and Atresias *Webs* can be seen at any level of the larynx, but they are usually at the level of the true vocal cords. Subglottic webs are sometimes associated with cricoid abnormalities. *Atresia* of the larynx results from a incomplete recanalization; there is no air passage to the trachea, which is present.

iii. Stenosis Stenosis of the larynx or the upper trachea may be caused by a congenital anomaly or by post-traumatic etiology, either iatrogenic or therapeutic. *Subglottic stenosis* is congenital soft tissue stenosis from the true cord down to the cricoid. The infant usually outgrows this problem, but sometimes a tracheostomy is needed.

The most common cause of stenosis is prolonged intuba-tion. Ingestion of caustic material can result in strictures of the posterior supraglottic airway. Both plain x-ray study and CT are good at assessing the extent and length of the stenotic segment.

iv. Clefts Rarely, incomplete fusion of the tracheoesophageal septum results in a laryngotracheal cleft. A laryngeal cleft can occur in isolation, but often there is an associated tracheal cleft.

d. Tumors and Others
i. Benign Tumors Benign masses encountered in the larynx include vocal cord nodules, juvenile papillomatosis, and other nonepithelial tumors such as hemangiomas, lipomas, leiomyomas, rhabdomyomas, chondromas, neural

tumors, paragangliomas, schwannomas, and granular cell tumors.

ii. Cysts and Laryngoceles Mucus-retention cysts can occur along any mucosal surface, but they are most common in the supraglottic larynx. Laryngoceles may be internal, external, or both. The common finding in a supraglottic mass is its connection with the laryngeal ventricle (Fig. 2-64).

iii. Malignant Neoplasms Most laryngeal tumors are malignant, and squamous cell carcinomas are the most common. These cancers arise on the mucosal surface and can be readily visualized by direct endoscopy. Imaging with CT and MRI is used to define the extent of the disease. Cross-sectional imaging is useful to assess the degree and direction of airway compromise (Fig. 2-65). Other cell types found are adenocarcinoma, verrucous carcinoma, and anaplastic carcinoma. More rare tumors are sarcoma, melanoma, lymphoma, leukemia, plasmacytoma, fibrous histiocytoma, and metastatic disease.

H. TRACHEA

The trachea is a tubular structure extending from the cricoid cartilage, at approximately the C6 level, to the carina, usually at the T5 or T6 level. It is a conduit between the larynx and the lungs and is composed of 16 to 20 incomplete hyaline cartilaginous rings bounded in a tight elastic connective tissue oriented longitudinally. The cartilage forms about two thirds of the circumference of the

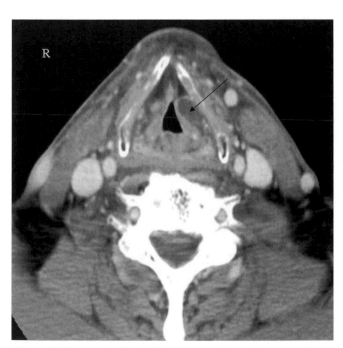

Figure 2-64 Laryngocele. Axial contrast-enhanced computed tomography scan demonstrates a fluid-filled internal laryngocele on the left *(arrow)*.

trachea; the posterior border is formed by a fibromuscular membrane. The trachea is approximately 10 to 13 cm in length (average length, 11 cm). The diameter of the tracheal lumen is dependent on the height, age, and gender of the subject. In men, the tracheal diameter ranges from 13 to 25 mm in the coronal imaging plane and from 13 to 27 mm in the sagittal imaging plane. In women, the dimensions are 10 to 21 mm in the coronal plane and 10 to 23 mm in the sagittal plane.[29,34] Cross-sectional area correlates best with height in children. The axial sections of the tracheal lumen assume the following vocal successive shapes: round, lunate, flattened, and elliptical. The luminal shape is also affected by the respiratory cycle, maneuvers, and body position. During rapid and deep inspiration, the thoracic portion of the trachea widens and the cervical portion narrows. The opposite occurs with expiration.

The innervation of the trachea is from the parasympathetic tracheal branches of the vagus nerve, the recurrent laryngeal nerve, and the sympathetic nerves. The trachea has a segmental blood supply from multiple branches of the inferior thyroidal arteries and bronchial arteries.

1. Imaging Anatomy

Radiologic evaluation of the trachea includes plain films of the neck and chest, CT, and MRI. A lateral view of the neck provides a good screening examination for the cervical trachea. CXR allows an initial assessment of the thoracic trachea and mediastinal structures. CT, and especially helical CT, is superior in the evaluation of the tracheal anatomy and pathology, as it allows direct visualization of the cross-sectional trachea. With multiplanar reconstruction, the degree and length of stenosis can be fully assessed. Virtual bronchoscopy, which is a three-dimensional reconstruction of helical CT data, allows navigation through the tracheobronchial tree through simulated bronchoscopy. MRI so far has limited use owing to the longer scanning time, intrinsic breathing motion artifacts, and limited resolution.

2. Imaging Pathology

Early detection of tracheal pathology is unusual because significant compromise of the airway can be present before symptoms manifest. At rest and during exertion, more than 75% and more than 50% of the luminal diameter, respectively, need to be occluded before symptoms of airway obstruction are manifested.[34] When symptoms are present, a superior mediastinal mass is often found on PA CXR. Also, the tracheal air column may be deviated or narrowed. Rarely, tracheal enlargement occurs as a result of tracheomalacia cystic fibrosis and Ehlers-Danlos complex. Pathology affecting the trachea can largely be classified into two groups as extrinsic and intrinsic diseases.

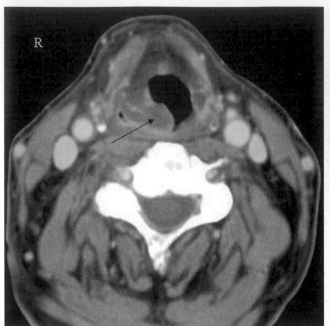

A

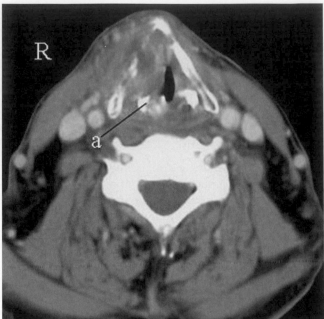

B

Figure 2-65 Laryngeal carcinoma. Axial contrast-enhanced computed tomography scans. In **A** to **C,** squamous cell carcinoma is noted extending from the right aryepiglottic fold, a, through the level of the arytenoids, to the cricoid, c, with cartilage destruction and invasion of the right vocal cord and strap muscles. The left thyroid cartilage, t, is intact and the right is destroyed by tumor.

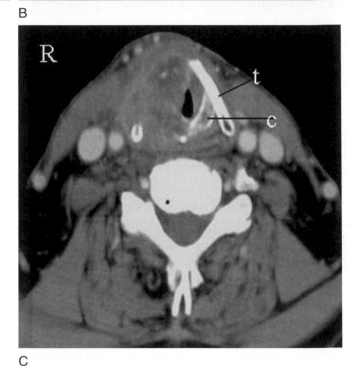

C

a. Extrinsic Tracheal Pathology

i. Thyroid Goiter One of the more common extrinsic pathologies affecting the cervical and substernal trachea is a goiter of the thyroid gland. The trachea is usually displaced laterally, and luminal compression is evident. Vocal cord paralysis, hoarseness, dyspnea, and dysphagia may be the presenting symptoms. These symptoms are all predictable and predicated by the location of the goiter with respect to the trachea, esophagus, and recurrent laryngeal nerve. The lateral and posterior extension of abnormal soft tissue with respect to the larynx displaces the airway anteriorly and laterally and may be a cause of difficult intubation (Fig. 2-66).

ii. Thyroid Carcinoma and Nodes As in the case of thyroid goiter, any mass involving or enlarging the thyroid gland can result in airway displacement and compression (Fig. 2-67). Enlarged lymph nodes secondary to lymphoma or metastatic disease can also cause extrinsic compression of the trachea.

iii. Vascular Rings and Slings Vascular rings encircle both the trachea and the esophagus with airway compression. The most common example is the double aortic arch. Vascular slings are noncircumferential vascular anomalies that may cause airway compromise. The trachea may be compressed posteriorly from a pulmonary artery sling,

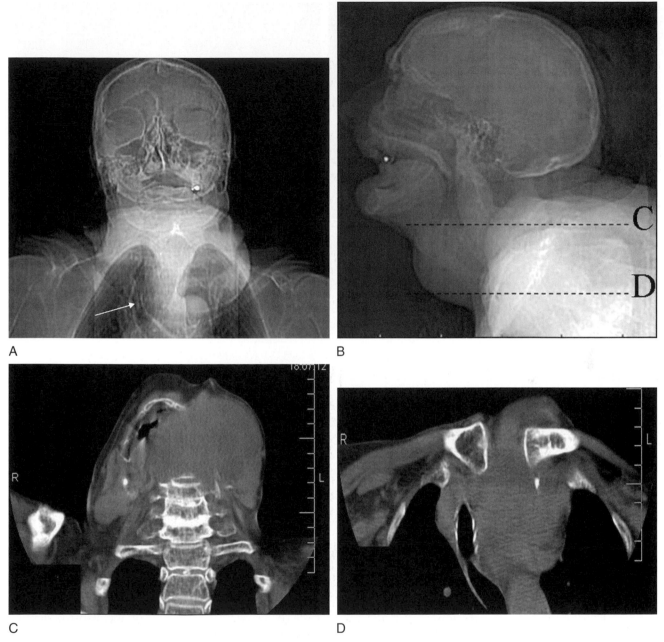

A

B

C

D

Figure 2-66 Goiter. **A** and **B,** Computed tomography anteroposterior and lateral scout films demonstrate a clinically obvious thyroid mass. Note the tracheal deviation in image **A** *(arrow)* and the anterior displacement of the airway in image **B**. Axial images **C** and **D** (referenced on the lateral scout) further demonstrate the mass effect on the airway from the level of the hyoid to the thoracic inlet.

where the left pulmonary artery arises from the right pulmonary artery. It can also be compressed from the front by the innominate artery or an aberrant left subclavian artery.

b. Intrinsic Tracheal Pathology

i. Trauma External injury to the trachea is more frequently a result of blunt trauma than of penetrating trauma and is often associated with significant other injuries to the chest, cervical spine, and great vessels. Pneumothorax, pneumomediastinum, and subcutaneous emphysema may be the presenting signs, in addition to endotracheal bleeding and airway compromise. Internal injuries such as chemical and thermal injury to the airway result in mucosal edema and subsequent airway compromise.

ii. Iatrogenic Injury A late complication of translaryngeal intubation is stenosis at the cuff site, tip, or stoma site of the tracheostomy. Cuff trauma is related to pressure necrosis, where the cuff pressure exceeds the capillary pressure. The incidence of this complication has decreased significantly with the introduction of the high-volume, low-pressure cuff, which is more pliable and can mold to the contours of the trachea. The blood supply to the anterior cartilages is more susceptible to pressure

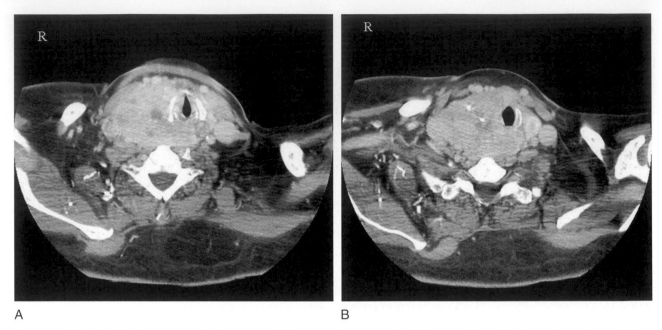

Figure 2-67 Tracheal displacement and effacement. Axial computed tomography (CT) scans (**A** and **B**) of a patient with medullary carcinoma of the thyroid. **A,** CT scan demonstrates the right thyroid mass displacing the airway anteriorly and to the contralateral side. **B,** The tumor has destroyed the cricoid cartilage on the right and abuts the subglottic airway.

effects, and anterior tracheal scarring may occur. With increased pressure, the posterior membranous part of the trachea can become affected, and the scarring becomes more circumferential. This type of injury is related to the position of the cuff and is seen radiographically as smooth tapering over one to two cartilage segments. Symptoms may arise from 2 weeks to months after extubation. Less common long-term complications of endotracheal intubation include tracheomalacia and tracheoesophageal fistula (TEF).[3,6]

Early tracheostomy complications are usually related to an abnormal angulation of the tube. In contrast to endotracheal intubation, tracheostomy is not affected by changes in head and neck position because it is not anchored at the nose or mouth. Angulation of the tracheostomy tube may result in increased airway resistance, difficulty in clearing secretions, erosion, and perforation of the trachea.

c. Non-neoplastic Tracheal Narrowing

The intrinsic pathology of diffuse tracheal narrowing, in addition to trauma secondary to the aspiration of heat, caustic or acid chemicals, radiation therapy, and intubation injury, would include unusual causes such as sarcoidosis, Wegener's granulomatosis, fungal infection, croup, and congenital causes (Fig. 2-68).

i. Tracheomalacia This entity is characterized by abnormal flaccidity of the trachea resulting in collapse of the thoracic tracheal segment during expiration. There is softening of the supporting cartilage and widening of the posterior

membranous wall, which may balloon anteriorly into the airway. Tracheomalacia can be categorized into primary intrinsic or secondary extrinsic forms. Patients may have minimal or severe symptoms dependent on the degree of airway obstruction.

ii. Congenital Stenosis (Subglottic or Tracheal) Congenital stenosis is uncommon and is usually associated with other congenital anomalies. The affected segment has rigid walls with a narrowed lumen, and the cartilages can be complete rings. The stenotic segment can be focal or affect the entire trachea. Symptoms usually arise within the first few weeks or months of age. Most patients are treated conservatively.

iii. Tracheoesophageal Fistula TEF is a common congenital anomaly, with an incidence of 1 in 3000 to 4000 births. TEF is often associated with esophageal atresia.[34] There are several forms of TEF. The most common is a proximal esophageal atresia with a distal TEF. This anomaly may be associated with severe neonatal respiratory distress and may require emergent tracheostomy. It is not uncommon to have more than one fistula present, and there may be other associated anomalies affecting the cardiovascular, gastrointestinal, renal, or central nervous system (Fig. 2-69).

d. Tumors and Others

Most benign tracheal neoplasms are found in pediatric patients. Squamous cell papilloma, fibroma, and hemangioma are the most common. In adults, the most common

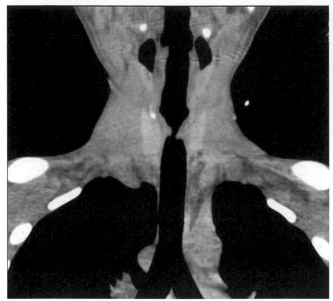

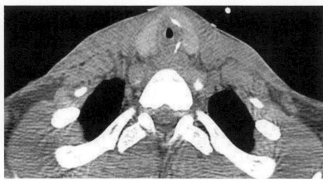

B

Figure 2-68 Tracheal stenosis. **A,** Coronal reformatted computed tomography (CT) image in a child demonstrates marked subglottic narrowing of the trachea. **B,** Axial CT in the same patient further defines the severity of narrowing.

A

benign tumors are chondroma, papilloma, fibroma, hemangioma, and granular cell myoblastoma.

Primary malignant neoplasms of the trachea are uncommon; laryngeal and bronchial primary tumors are much more common. In adults, however, primary neoplasms of the trachea are more common than benign tumors. The most common malignant tumor is squamous cell carcinoma.[34]

The trachea may be secondarily involved by metastatic disease, either from a remote primary tumor or by direct invasion, such as from a thyroid primary (Fig. 2-70).

V. CONCLUSION

As described in the preceding paragraphs, rapid technological advances in the field of radiology allow excellent visualization of airway structures and provide anesthesiologists with essential information to formulate a safe and effective anesthetic plan. However, radiology is not a part of the curriculum of any anesthesia residency training program; thus, most anesthesiologists do not know how to analyze the radiologic studies, such as MRI and CT, that are usually a part of the preoperative surgical evaluation.

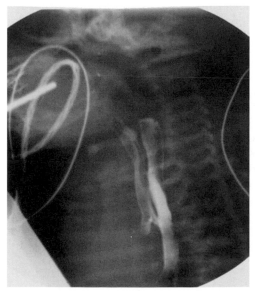

Figure 2-69 Tracheoesophageal fistula (TEF). Oblique radiograph from a swallow study with contrast outlines a classical H-type TEF. (Courtesy of Dr. Netta Marlyn Blitman, Montefiore Medical Center, Bronx, New York.)

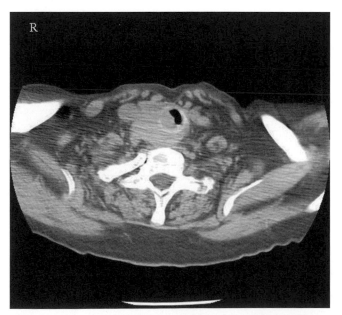

Figure 2-70 Tracheal invasion from follicular carcinoma of the thyroid. Axial computed tomography scan demonstrating a mass on the right deviating and invading the trachea.

We hope that by updating anesthesiologists on the principles of MRI and CT and illustrating how airway structures are displayed by these new imaging modalities we have provided clinicians with good basic skills in gathering clinically useful information from these imaging studies.

In addition, the authors wish that clinicians would not only incorporate the information from radiologic studies to provide better care to their patients but also consider using new imaging modalities as powerful research tools to study the airway.

REFERENCES

1. Bishop MJ, Weymuller EA Jr, Fink BR: Laryngeal effects of prolonged intubation. Anesth Analg 63:335-342, 1984.
2. Bougaki M, Sawamura S, Matsushita F, et al: Difficult intubation due to ossification of the anterior longitudinal ligament. Anaesthesia 59:303-304, 2004.
3. Calder I, Calder J, Crockard HA: Difficult direct laryngoscopy in patients with cervical spine disease. Anaesthesia 50:756-763, 1995.
4. Cattell HS, Filtzer DL: Pseudosubluxation and other normal variations of the cervical spine in children. J Bone Joint Surg Am 47:1295-1309, 1965.
5. Chou HC, Wu TL: Mandibulohyoid distance in difficult laryngoscopy. Br J Anaesth 71:335-339, 1993.
6. Crosby ET, Liu A: Review articles: The adult cervical spine: Implications for airway management. Can J Anaesth 37:77-93, 1990.
7. Curry TS III, Dowdey JE, Murry RC: Attenuation. In Christensen's Introduction to the Physics of Diagnostic Radiology, 3rd ed. Philadelphia, Lea & Febiger, 1984.
8. Curry TS III, Dowdey JE, Murry RC: Basic interactions between x rays and matter. In Christensen's Introduction to the Physics of Diagnostic Radiology, 3rd ed. Philadelphia, Lea & Febiger, 1984.
9. Curry TS III, Dowdey JE, Murry RC: Computed tomography. In Christensen's Introduction to the Physics of Diagnostic Radiology, 3rd ed. Philadelphia, Lea & Febiger, 1984.
10. Curry TS III, Dowdey JE, Murry RC: Nuclear magnetic resonance. In Christensen's Introduction to the Physics of Diagnostic Radiology, 3rd ed. Philadelphia, Lea & Febiger, 1984.
11. Curry TS III, Dowdey JE, Murry RC: Physical characteristics of x ray film and film processing. In Christensen's Introduction to the Physics of Diagnostic Radiology, 3rd ed. Philadelphia, Lea & Febiger, 1984.
12. Curry TS III, Dowdey JE, Murry RC: Production of x rays. In Christensen's Introduction to the Physics of Diagnostic Radiology, 3rd ed. Philadelphia, Lea & Febiger, 1984.
13. Curry TS III, Dowdey JE, Murry RC: Radiation. In Christensen's Introduction to the Physics of Diagnostic Radiology, 3rd ed. Philadelphia, Lea & Febiger, 1984.
14. Curtin HD: The larynx. In Som PS, Curtin HD (eds): Head and Neck Imaging, 4th ed. St. Louis, Mosby, 2003.
15. Drake AF, Davis JU, Warren DW: Nasal airway size in cleft and noncleft children. Laryngoscope 103:915-917, 1993.
16. Felson B: The mediastinum. In Chest Roentgenology. Philadelphia, WB Saunders, 1973.
17. Frerk CM, Till CBW, Bradley AJ: Difficult intubation: Thyromental distance and the atlanto-occipital gap. Anaesthesia 51:738-740, 1996.
18. Goodman LR, Putman CE: Intensive Care Radiology: Imaging of the Critically Ill. Philadelphia, WB Saunders, 1983, p 19.
19. Gutierrez FR: Mediastinum. In Sloan RM, Gutierrez FR, Fisher AJ (eds): Thoracic Imaging: A Practical Approach. New York, McGraw-Hill, 1999.
20. Hamberg LM, Rhea JT, Hunter GJ, Thrall JH: Multidetector row CT: Radiation dose characteristics. Radiology 226:762-772, 2003.
21. Harris JH Jr, Mirvis SE: The Radiology of Acute Cervical Spine Trauma, 3rd ed. Baltimore, Williams & Wilkins, 1996.
22. Hounsfield GN: Computed transverse axial scanning (tomography). Br J Radiol 46:1016-1022, 1973.
23. Keenan MA, Stiles CM, Kaufman RL: Acquired laryngeal deviation associated with cervical spine disease in erosive polyarticular arthritis: Use of the fiberoptic bronchoscope in rheumatoid disease. Anesthesiology 58:441-449, 1983.
24. Larsson SG, Benson L, Westmark P: Computed tomography of the tongue in primary amyloidosis. J Comput Assist Tomogr 10:836-840, 1986.
25. Manaligod JM, Bauman NM, Menezes AH, et al: Cervical vertebral anomalies in patients with anomalies of the head and neck. Ann Otol Rhinol Laryngol 108:925-933, 1999.
26. Miller MD, Gehweiler JA, Martinez S, et al: Significant new observations on cervical spine trauma. AJR 130:659-663, 1978.
27. Million RR, Cassisi NJ, Mancuso AA: Hypopharynx: Pharyngeal walls, pyriform sinus, postcricoid pharynx. In Million RR, Cassisi NJ (eds): Management of Head and Neck Cancer: A Multidisciplinary Approach. Philadelphia, Mosby, 1994, pp 505-532.
28. Mukherji SK: Pharynx. In Som PS, Curtin HD (eds): Head and Neck Imaging, 4th ed. St. Louis, Mosby, 2003.
29. Naidich DP, Webb R, Muller NL, et al: Airways. In Naidich DP et al (eds): Computed Tomography and Magnetic Resonance Imaging of the Thorax, 3rd ed. Philadelphia, Lippincott-Raven, 1999.
30. Naidich TP, Blaser SI, Bauer BS, et al: Embryology and congenital lesions of the midface. In Som PS, Curtin HD (eds): Head and Neck Imaging, 4th ed. St. Louis, Mosby, 2003.
31. Nichol HC, Zuck D: Difficult laryngoscopy—The "anterior" larynx and the atlanto-occipital gap. Br J Anaesth 55:141-143, 1983.
32. Noback GJ: The developmental topography of the larynx, trachea and lungs in the fetus, new-born, infant and child. Am J Dis Child 26:515-533, 1923.
33. Robson CD, Hudgins PA: Pediatric airway disease. In Som PS, Curtin HD (eds): Head and Neck Imaging, 4th ed. St. Louis, Mosby, 2003.

34. Sasson JP, Abdelrahman NG, Aquino S, et al: Trachea: Anatomy and pathology. In Som PS, Curtin HD (eds): Head and Neck Imaging, 4th ed. St. Louis, Mosby, 2003.

35. Sharwood-Smith GH: Difficulty in intubation—Calcified stylohyoid ligament. Anaesthesia 31:508-510, 1976.

36. Smoker WRK: The oral cavity. In Som PS, Curtin HD (eds): Head and Neck Imaging, 4th ed. St. Louis, Mosby, 2003.

37. Som PM, Brandwein MS: Tumors and tumor-like conditions. In Som PS, Curtin HD (eds): Head and Neck Imaging, 4th ed. St. Louis, Mosby, 2003.

38. Som PM, Shapiro MD, Biller HF, et al: Sinonasal tumors and inflammatory tissues: Differentiation with MR imaging. Radiology 167:803-808, 1988.

39. Som PM, Shugar JMA, Brandwein MS: Anatomy and physiology. In Som PS, Curtin HD (eds): Head and Neck Imaging, 4th ed. St. Louis, Mosby, 2003.

40. Som PM, Smoker WRK, Balboni A, et al: Embryology and anatomy of the neck. In Som PS, Curtin HD (eds): Head and Neck Imaging, 4th ed. St. Louis, Mosby, 2003.

41. Streitwieser DR, Knopp R, Wales LR, et al: Accuracy of the standard radiographic view in detecting cervical spine fractures. Ann Emerg Med 12:538-542, 1983.

42. Stringenz MA, Toohill RJ, Grossman TW: Association of laryngeal and pulmonary malignancies: a continuing challenge. Ann Otol Rhinol Laryngol 96:621-624, 1987.

43. Warren DW, Haurfield WM, Dalston ET, et al: Effects of cleft lip and palate on the nasal airway in children. Arch Otolaryngol Head Neck Surg 114:987-992, 1998.

44. Weissman, JL, Carrau R: Anterior facial vein and submandibular gland together: Predicting the histology of submandibular masses with CT or MR Imaging. Radiology 208:441-446, 1998.

45. White A, Kander PL: Anatomical factors in difficult direct laryngoscopy. Br J Anaesth 47:468-473, 1975.

46. Williams PL, Warwick R (eds): Gray's Anatomy, 36th ed. Philadelphia, WB Saunders, 1980.

47. Wilson TG. Some observations on the anatomy of the infantile larynx. Acta Otolaryngol 43:95-99, 1953.

3

PHYSICS AND MODELING OF THE AIRWAY

D. John Doyle
Kevin F. O'Grady

I. THE GAS LAWS

A. IDEAL GASES

Air is a fluid. Understanding the fundamentals of basic fluid mechanics is essential in grasping the concepts of airway flow. Because air is also a gas, it is important to understand the laws that govern its gaseous behavior. Gases are usually described in terms of pressure, volume, and temperature. Pressure is most often quantified clinically in terms of mm Hg (or torr), volume in mL, and temperature in Celsius. However, calculations often require conversion from one set of units to another and, therefore, can be quite tedious. We have included a small section at the end of the chapter to simplify these conversions.

Perhaps the most important law of gas flow in airways is the ideal (or perfect) gas law, which can be written as[45]:

$$PV = nRT \qquad (1)$$

where

P = pressure of gas (pascals or mm Hg)
V = volume of gas (m^3 or cm^3 or mL)
n = number of moles of the gas in volume V
R = gas constant (8.3143 J g-mol^{-1} K^{-1}, assuming P in pascals, V in m^3)
T = absolute temperature (in kelvins or K, 273.16 K = 0° C)

A mole of gas contains 6.023×10^{23} molecules, and this quantity is termed Avogadro's number. One mole of an ideal gas takes up 22.4138 liters at standard temperature and pressure (STP) (STP: 273.16 K at 1 atmosphere [760 mm Hg]).[45] Avogadro also stated that equal volumes of all ideal gases at the same temperature and pressure contain the same number of molecules.

The ideal gas law incorporates the laws of Boyle and Charles.[45] Boyle's law states that, at a constant temperature, the product of pressure and volume is equal to a constant, that is, P × V = constant (at constant T). Hence, P is proportional to 1/V. Gases do not obey Boyle's law at temperatures approaching their point of liquefaction (the state where the gas becomes a liquid). Boyle's law concerns perfect gases and is not obeyed by real gases over a wide range of pressures (see the next section for nonideal gases). However, at infinitely low pressures, all gases obey Boyle's law. Boyle's law does not apply to anesthetic gases and many other gases because of the van der Waals attraction between molecules (i.e., they are nonideal gases).

Charles' law states that, at a constant pressure, volume is proportional to temperature, that is, V is proportional to T (at constant P). Gay-Lussac's law states that, at a constant volume, pressure is proportional to temperature, that is, P ∝ T (at constant V).[45] Often, Charles' law and Gay-Lussac's law are shortened for convenience to Charles' law. When a gas obeys both Charles' law and Boyle's law, it is said to be an ideal gas and obeys the ideal gas law.

In clinical situations, gases are typically mixtures of several "pure" gases. Quantifiable properties of mixtures may be determined using Dalton's law of partial pressures. Dalton's law states that the pressure exerted by a mixture of gases is the sum of the pressures exerted by the individual pure gases[45,60]:

$$P_{total} = P_A + P_B + P_C + \dots + P_N \qquad (2)$$

where P_A, P_B, and P_C are the partial pressures of pure ideal gases.

B. NONIDEAL GASES: THE VAN DER WAALS EFFECT

Ideal gases have no forces of interaction. Real gases, however, have intramolecular attraction, which requires that the pressure-volume gas law be written as[45,60]:

$$\left(P + \frac{a}{V^2}\right) \times (V - b) = nRT \qquad (3)$$

where

P = pressure of gas (pascals or mm Hg)
V = volume of gas (m^3 or cm^3 or mL)
n = number of moles of the gas in volume V
R = gas constant (8.3143 J g-mol^{-1} K^{-1} assuming P in pascals, V in m^3)
T = absolute temperature (K)
a, b = physical constants for a given gas

The terms *a* and *b* for a given gas may be found in physical chemistry textbooks and other sources.[7,45,60,77] This formulation, provided by van der Waals, accounts for intramolecular forces fairly well.

C. DIFFUSION OF GASES

Clinically, diffusion of gases through a membrane is most applicable to gas flow across lung and placental membranes. The most commonly used relation to govern diffusion is Fick's first law of diffusion, which states that the rate of diffusion of a gas across a barrier is proportional to the concentration gradient for the gas. Fick's law may be expressed mathematically as[3]:

$$Flux = -D\frac{\Delta C}{\Delta X} \qquad (4)$$

where the flux is the number of molecules/cm^2/s crossing the membrane, ΔC is the concentration gradient (molecules/cm^3), ΔX is the diffusion distance (cm), and D is the diffusion coefficient (cm^2/s), whose value is generally inversely proportional to the gas's molecular weight as well as intrinsic properties of the membrane.

Because gases partially dissolve when they come into contact with liquid, Henry's law becomes important in some instances. It states that the mass of a gas dissolved in a given amount of liquid is proportional to the pressure of the gas at constant temperature. That is, gas concentration (in solvent) = constant × pressure (at constant T).[45]

D. PRESSURE, FLOW, AND RESISTANCE

The laws of fluid mechanics dictate an intricate relationship among pressure, flow, and resistance. Pressure is defined as a force per unit area and, as mentioned previously, is usually measured clinically as mm Hg or cm H_2O. However, it is most commonly measured scientifically in pascals (newtons force per square meter).

Flow (or the rate of flow) is equal to the change in pressure (pressure drop or pressure difference) divided by the resistance experienced by the fluid. For example, if the flow is 100 mL/s at a pressure difference of 100 mmHg, the resistance is 100 mm Hg/100 mL/s = 1 mmHg/mL/s. In *laminar* flow systems only, the resistance is constant, independent of the flow rate.[72,79]

An important relation that quantifies the relationship of pressure, flow, and resistance in laminar flow systems is given by the Hagen-Poiseuille equation. Poiseuille's law states that the fluid flow rate through a horizontal straight tube of uniform bore is proportional to the pressure gradient and the fourth power of the radius and is related inversely to the viscosity of the gas and the length of the tube. This law, *which is valid for laminar flow only*, may thus be stated as[72,79]:

$$\Delta P = \frac{8\,\mu L}{\pi^4} \times \text{Flow} \qquad (5)$$

where μ is the fluid viscosity (poise [g/cm · s]) and L is the length of the tube (cm). See Section II.A for further details.

When the flow rate exceeds a *critical velocity* (the flow velocity below which flow is laminar), the flow loses its laminar parabolic velocity profile, becomes disorderly, and is termed *turbulent* (Fig. 3-1). When turbulent flow exists, the relationship between pressure drop and flow is no longer governed by the Hagen-Poiseuille equation. Instead, the pressure gradient required (or the resistance encountered) during turbulent flow varies as the square of the flow rate. See Section II.B for further details.

Viscosity, μ, characterizes the resistance within a fluid to the flow of one layer of molecules over another (shear characteristics).[72] Blood viscosity is influenced primarily by hematocrit, so that at low hematocrit blood flow is easier—that is, blood is more dilute. The critical velocity at which turbulent flow begins depends on the ratio of viscosity (μ) to density (ρ), which is defined as the *kinematic viscosity* (ν), that is, $\nu = \mu/\rho$ (Section II.B.1 illustrates this in an example).[72,79,84] The units for viscosity are g/cm · s (poise). Typical units for kinematic viscosity are cm^2/s.

The viscosity of water is 0.01 poise at 25° C and 0.007 poise at 37° C. The viscosity of air is 183 micropoise at 18° C. Its density (dry) is 1.213 g/L.[80]

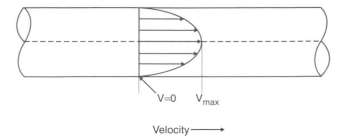

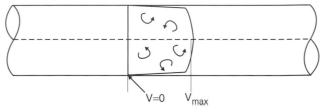

Figure 3-1 Laminar and turbulent flow. *Top,* Laminar flow in a long smooth pipe is characterized by smooth and steady flow with little or no fluctuations. Flow profile is parabolic in nature, with fluid traveling most quickly at the center of the tube and stationary at the edges. *Bottom,* Turbulent flow is characterized by fluctuating and agitated flow. Its flow profile is essentially flat with all fluid traveling at the same velocity except at tube edges.

Density is defined as mass per unit volume (g/cm^3 or g/mL). The density of water is 1 g/mL. The general relation for the density of a gas is given by:

$$D = D_0 \left(\frac{T_0 P}{T P_0} \right) \qquad (6)$$

where D_0 is a known density of the gas at temperature T_0 and pressure P_0 and D is the density of the gas at temperature T and pressure P. For dry air at 18° C and 760 mm Hg (or atmospheric pressure), D = 1.213 g/L.[77]

The fall in pressure at points of flow constriction (where the flow velocity is higher) is known as the Bernoulli effect (Fig. 3-2).[72,79] This phenomenon is used in apparatus employing the Venturi principle, for example, gas nebulizers, Venturi flowmeters, and some oxygen face masks. The lower pressure related to the Bernoulli effect sucks in (entrains) air to mix with oxygen.

One final consideration that is important in the study of the airway is Laplace's law for a sphere (Fig. 3-3). It states that, for a sphere with one air-liquid interface (e.g., an alveolus), the equation relating the transmural pressure difference, surface tension, and sphere radius is[67]:

$$P = \frac{2T}{R} \qquad (7)$$

where

P = transmural pressure difference (dynes/cm^2; 1 dyne/cm^2 = 0.1 Pa = 0.000751 torr)
T = surface tension (dynes/cm)
R = sphere radius (cm)

The key point in Laplace's law is that the smaller the sphere radius, the higher the transmural pressure.

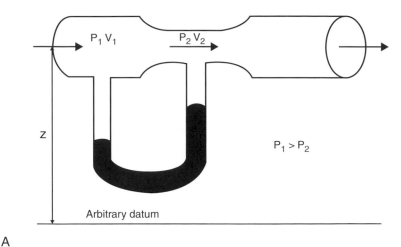

A

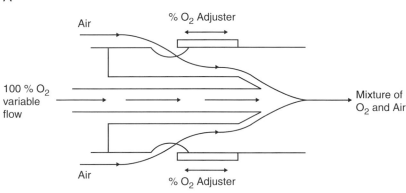

B

Figure 3-2 Bernoulli effect. **A,** Diagram shows fluid flow through a tube with varying diameters. At point of flow constriction, fluid pressure is less than at distal end of the tube, as indicated by height of the manometer fluid column. This effect is described by the Bernoulli equation. Note that, in the case of a horizontal pipe, Z_1 and $Z_2 = Z$, where Z_1 and Z_2 are distances between the centerline of the pipe at two different points and an arbitrary datum. **B,** A Venturi. The lower pressure caused by the Bernoulli effect entrains air to mix with oxygen.

However, real (in vivo) alveoli do *not* obey Laplace's law because of the action of pulmonary surfactant, which decreases the surface tension disproportionately compared with what is predicted using physical principles. When pulmonary surfactant is missing from the lungs, the lungs take on the behavior described by Laplace's law.

E. EXAMPLE: ANALYSIS OF TRANSTRACHEAL JET VENTILATION

Transtracheal jet ventilation (TTJV) has been used to oxygenate and ventilate patients who would otherwise perish because of a lost airway.[5] It is a temporizing measure until an airway can be secured. It is usually employed using equipment commonly available in the operating or emergency room and often using the 50 psi wall oxygen source.[5,10,47,70]

1. Analysis

The gas flow through a catheter depends on both the resistance of the catheter-connection hose assembly and the driving pressure applied to it. If the resistance of the catheter-connection hose assembly is R, the flow from the catheter is $F = P_d/R$, where P_d is the pressure difference between the ends of the catheter-connection assembly. R itself certainly depends on F when the flow becomes turbulent, but the preceding relationship still holds. However, P_d is very close to the driving pressure P applied to the ventilation catheter because the lung offers little relative back pressure. (At back pressures over 100 cm H_2O the lung is likely to burst, and P is often chosen to be 50 psi or about 3500 cm H_2O.) Thus, the preceding relationship may be simplified to $F = P/R$.

Next, TTJV is applied through a sequence of "jet pulses," each resulting in a given tidal volume (e.g., 500 mL). Then (ignoring entrained air effects) the delivered tidal volume = catheter flow × pulse duration. If we choose a catheter flow of 30 L/min, a jet pulse of 1 second duration results in a tidal volume of 30 L/min × 1/60 min = 0.5 L.

In a TTJV setup consisting of a 14-gauge Angiocath catheter connected to a regulated oxygen source by a 4.5-foot polyvinyl chloride (PVC) tube of 7/32 inch inside diameter (ID), for oxygen flows between 10 and

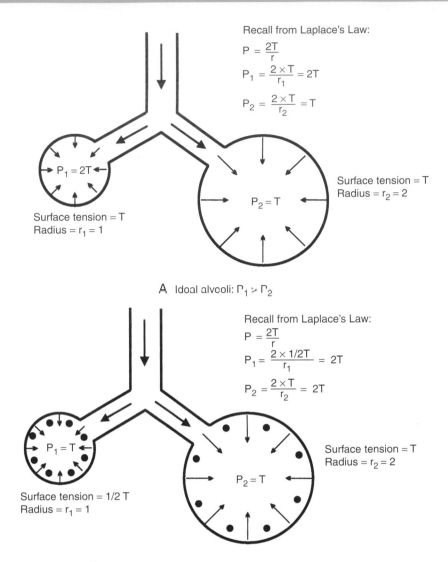

Recall from Laplace's Law:

$$P = \frac{2T}{r}$$

$$P_1 = \frac{2 \times T}{r_1} = 2T$$

$$P_2 = \frac{2 \times T}{r_2} = T$$

Surface tension = T
Radius = r_1 = 1

$P_1 = 2T$

Surface tension = T
Radius = r_2 = 2

$P_2 = T$

A Ideal alveoli: $P_1 > P_2$

Recall from Laplace's Law:

$$P = \frac{2T}{r}$$

$$P_1 = \frac{2 \times 1/2T}{r_1} = 2T$$

$$P_2 = \frac{2 \times T}{r_2} = 2T$$

Surface tension = 1/2 T
Radius = r_1 = 1

$P_1 = T$

Surface tension = T
Radius = r_2 = 2

$P_2 = T$

B Real alveoli: $P_1 = P_2$ with pulmonary surfactant

Figure 3-3 Laplace's law for a sphere. **A,** Laplace's law dictates that for two alveoli of unequal size but of equal surface tension, the smaller alveolus experiences a larger intra-alveolar pressure than the larger alveolus. This causes air to pass into the larger alveolus and causes the smaller alveolus to collapse. **B,** Collapse of smaller alveolus is prevented through action of pulmonary surfactant. Surfactant serves to decrease alveolar surface tension in the smaller alveolus, which results in equal pressures in both alveoli.

60 L/min, the resistance was relatively constant between 0.6 and 0.8 psi/L/min.[12]

Many systems for TTJV choose 50 psi for convenience (50 psi being the oxygen wall outlet pressure), although a regulator is very often used to permit lower pressures. However, 50 psi may not be an optimal pressure choice for TTJV. Using the preceding data, we can calculate the pressure required for TTJV for our tidal volume of 500 mL.

Assuming that the setup resistance is taken as 0.7 psi/L/min and the desired flow rate is 30 L/min (not an unreasonable assumption given the data), the driving pressure should be 0.7 × 30 = 21 psi. Similar analyses can be carried out for other arrangements from experiments to obtain resistance data.

II. GAS FLOW

A. LAMINAR FLOW

In laminar flow, fluid particles flow along smooth paths in layers, or laminas, with one layer gliding smoothly over an adjacent layer.[72] Any tendencies toward instability and turbulence are damped out by viscous shear forces that resist the relative motion of adjacent fluid layers. Under laminar flow conditions through a tube, the flow velocity is greatest at the center of the flow and zero at the inner edge of the tube (Fig. 3-4; see also Fig. 3-1). The flow profile has a parabolic shape. Under these conditions in a horizontal tube, the relation between flow, tube, and

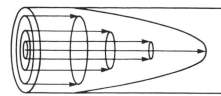

Figure 3-4 Laminar flow. Laminar gas flow through long straight tube of uniform bore has a velocity profile that is parabolic in shape, with the gas traveling most quickly at center of tube. Conceptually, it is helpful to view laminar gas flow as a series of concentric cylinders of gas, with the central cylinder moving most rapidly. (From Nunn JF: Nunn's Applied Respiratory Physiology, 4th ed. Stoneham, Mass, Butterworth-Heinemann, 1993.)

gas characteristics is given by the Hagen-Poiseuille equation[72,79,84]:

$$\dot{V} = \frac{\pi \Delta P r^4}{8 \mu L} \qquad (8)$$

where

$\dot{V}$ = flow rate [cm^3/s]
$\pi \approx 3.1416$
P = pressure gradient [pascals]
r = tube radius [cm]
L = tube length [cm]
μ = gas viscosity [$g/cm \cdot s$]

Typical units are shown in square brackets. The dot indicates rate of change. As V represents volume, $\dot{V}$ represents the *rate of change of volume* or *flow rate*. Another way in which the concept may be viewed is that, under conditions of laminar flow through a tube of known radius, the pressure difference across the tube is given by the following proportionality (note that this is essentially equation 5):

$$\Delta Pressure \propto \frac{Flow \times Viscosity \times Length}{Radius^4} \qquad (9)$$

That is, the pressure gradient through the airway increases proportionately with flow, viscosity, and tube length but increases exponentially as the tube radius decreases.

The conditions under which flow through a tube is predominantly laminar can be estimated from *critical flow* rates. The critical flow is the flow rate below which flow is predominantly laminar in a given airflow situation.

1. Laminar Flow Example

A tube of uniform bore is 1 cm in diameter and 3 m in length. A pressure difference of 5 mm H_2O exists between the ends of the tube, and air is the fluid flowing

through the tube. Assuming laminar flow, what flow rate should we expect to get?

Answer:

Using the centimeter-gram-second (CGS) system of units, we have:

r = 0.5 cm
L = 3000 cm
μ = 183 micropoise = 183×10^{-6} poise = 183×10^{-6} g/(cm $\cdot$ s)
ΔP = 0.5 cm H_2O = 490 dynes/cm^2

Using the Hagen-Poiseuille equation for laminar flow, we determine:

$$Flow = \frac{\pi \times 490 \times (0.5)^4}{8 \times 183 \times 10^{-6} \times 3000} = 219.06 \ cm^3/s \qquad (10)$$

B. TURBULENT FLOW

Flow in tubes below the critical flow rate remains mostly laminar. However, at flows above the critical flow rate, the flow becomes increasingly turbulent. Under turbulent flow conditions, the parabolic flow pattern is lost, and the resistance to flow increases with flow itself. Turbulence may also be created when sharp angles, changes in diameter, and branches are encountered (Fig. 3-5). The flow-pressure drop relationship is given approximately by[72,79]:

$$V \propto \sqrt{\Delta P} \qquad (11)$$

where

V = mean fluid velocity [cm/s]
P = pressure [pascals]

1. Reynolds Number Calculation Example

The Reynolds number (Re) represents the ratio of inertial forces to viscous forces.[72,79,81] It is useful because it characterizes the flow through a long, straight tube of uniform bore. It is a dimensionless number having the form:

$$Re = \frac{V \times D \times \rho}{\mu} = \frac{V \times D}{v} = \frac{2 \times \dot{V} \times \rho}{\pi \times r \times \mu} \qquad (12)$$

where

Re = Reynolds number
$\dot{V}$ = flow rate [mL/s]
ρ = density [g/mL]
μ = viscosity [poise or $g/cm \cdot s$]
r = radius [cm]
v = kinematic viscosity [cm^2/s] = μ/ρ
D = diameter [cm]
V = mean fluid velocity [cm/s]

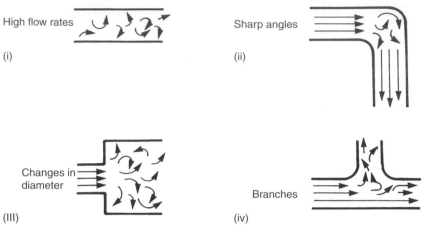

Figure 3-5 Turbulent flow. Four circumstances likely to produce turbulent flow. (From Nunn JF: Nunn's Applied Respiratory Physiology, 4th ed. Stoneham, Mass, Butterworth-Heinemann, 1993.)

Typical units are shown in brackets. For tubes that are long compared with their diameter (i.e., $L/D > 0.06 \times Re$),[79] the flow is laminar when Re is below 2000. Flow is turbulent at Re as low as 280 for shorter tubes.

When a tube's radius exceeds its length, it is an orifice; flow through an orifice is always turbulent. Under these conditions, the flow is influenced by density rather than the viscosity of the fluid.[30] This is why heliox (70% He, 30% O_2) flows better in a narrow edematous glottis: as the following data suggest, helium has a very low density and thus presents less resistance to flow through an orifice.

	Viscosity at 20° C	Density at 20° C
Helium	194.1 micropoise	0.179 g/L
Oxygen	210.8 micropoise	1.429 g/L

How can we predict whether a given gas flow through an endotracheal tube (ET) is laminar or turbulent? One approach is first to identify the physical conditions. For example, consider the case of a 6 mm ID ET 27 cm in length through which 1 L/min of air is passing. In this setting we have:

L = 27 cm
r = 0.3 cm (size 6 mm ET)
flow ($\dot{V}$) = 60 L/min = 1000 mL/s
viscosity (μ) = 183 micropoise = 183×10^{-6} g/cm · s (air at 18° C)
density (ρ) = 1.21 g/L = 0.001213 g/mL (dry air at 18° C)

With this information one can calculate the Reynolds number:

$$Re = \frac{2 \times 1000 \times 0.001213}{\pi \times 0.3 \times 183 \times 10^{-6}} = 1.41 \times 10^4 \qquad (13)$$

Because this number greatly exceeds 2000, flow is probably quite turbulent.

C. CRITICAL VELOCITY

The critical velocity is the point at which the transition from laminar to turbulent flow begins. The critical velocity is reached when Re becomes the critical Reynolds number Re_{crit}. Critical velocity, the flow velocity below which flow is laminar, is given by[79]:

$$V_{crit} = V_c = \frac{Re_{crit} \times \text{Viscosity}}{\text{Density} \times \text{Diameter}} \qquad (14)$$

where $Re_{crit} \approx 2000$ for circular tubes. As can be seen, the critical velocity is proportional to the viscosity of the gas and is related inversely to the density of the gas and the tube radius. Viscosity dimensions are force per unit area per second ($N \times s/m^2$). The critical velocity at which turbulent flow begins depends on the ratio of viscosity to density, that is, μ/ρ. This ratio is known as the *kinematic viscosity*, v, and has typical units of centimeters squared per second (cm^2/s). The actual measurement of viscosity of a fluid is carried out using a viscometer, which consists of two rotary cylinders with the test fluid flowing between.

1. Critical Velocity Calculation Example

Using the same data as in the previous Reynolds number calculation, we can calculate the critical velocity at which laminar flow starts to become turbulent:

$$V_c = \frac{(2000) \times (183 \times 10^{-6} \text{ poise})}{(0.001213 \text{ g/cm}^3) \times (2 \times 0.3 \text{ cm})} \qquad (15)$$

$$V_c = 502.8 \frac{\text{poise}}{(\text{g/cm}^3) \times \text{cm}} = 502.8 \frac{\text{cm}}{\text{s}}$$

D. FLOW THROUGH AN ORIFICE

Flow through an orifice (defined as involving flow through a tube whose length is smaller than its radius) is always somewhat turbulent.[30] Clinically, airway-obstructing conditions such as epiglottitis or swallowed obstructions are often best viewed as breathing through an orifice (Fig. 3-6). Under such conditions, the approximate flow across the orifice varies inversely with the square root of the gas density:

$$\dot{V} \propto \frac{1}{\sqrt{\text{Gas Density}}} \qquad (16)$$

This is in contrast to laminar flow conditions, in which gas flow varies inversely with gas viscosity. The viscosity values for helium and oxygen are similar, but their densities are very different (Table 3-1). Table 3-2 provides useful data to allow comparison of gas flow rates through an orifice.[63]

1. Helium-Oxygen Mixtures

The low density of helium allows it to play a significant clinical role in the management of some forms of airway obstruction.[13,38,44,69] For instance, Rudow and colleagues[63] described the use of helium-oxygen mixtures in a patient with severe airway obstruction related to a large thyroid mass (see "Clinical Vignettes" for details).

The usual available mixtures of helium and oxygen are 20% O_2:80% He and 30% O_2:70% He and are usually

Table 3-1 **Viscosity and Density Differences of Anesthetic Gases**[7,77]

	Viscosity at 300 K	Density at 20° C
Air	18.6 μPa × s	1.293 g/L
Nitrogen	17.9 μPa × s	1.250 g/L
Nitrous oxide	15.0 μPa × s	1.965 g/L
Helium	20.0 μPa × s	0.178 g/L
Oxygen	20.8 μPa × s	1.429 g/L

From Benumof JL: Airway Management: Principles and Practice. St. Louis, Mosby, 1996, p 53.

administered by a rebreathing face mask in patients who face an increased work-of-breathing effort because of the presence of airway pathology (e.g., edema) but in whom endotracheal intubation is preferably withheld at this time.

Although the use of helium-oxygen mixtures in patients with upper airway obstruction has met with considerable success, the hope that this approach would also work well for patients with severe asthma has not been borne out. In a systematic review of seven clinical trials involving 392 patients with acute asthma, the authors cautioned that "existing evidence does not provide support for the

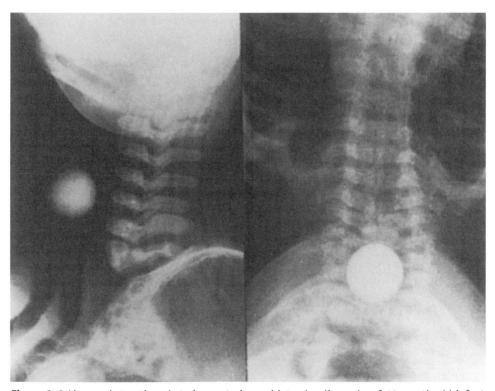

Figure 3-6 Airway obstruction. Anterior-posterior and lateral radiographs of 18-month-old infant who had swallowed a marble. Presence of this esophageal foreign body caused acute airway obstruction by causing extrinsic compression of the trachea. (From Badgwell JM, McLeod ME, Friedberg J: Airway obstruction in infants and children. Can J Anaesth 34:90, 1987.)

Table 3-2 **Gas Flow Rates through an Orifice**

	%	Density (g/L)	(Density)$^{-1/2}$	Relative Flow
Air	100	1.293	0.881	1.0
Oxygen	100	1.429	0.846	0.96
Helium (He)	100	0.179	2.364	2.68
He-oxygen	20/80	1.178	0.922	1.048
He-oxygen	60/40	0.678	1.215	1.381
He-oxygen	80/20	0.429	1.527	1.73

From Rudow M, Hill AB, Thompson NW, et al: Helium-oxygen mixtures in airway obstruction due to thyroid carcinoma. Can Anaesth Soc J 33:498, 1986.

administration of helium-oxygen mixtures to emergency department patients with moderate-to-severe acute asthma."[62] A similar study[31] noted that "heliox may offer mild-to-moderate benefits in patients with acute asthma within the first hour of use, but its advantages become less apparent beyond 1hr, as most conventionally treated patients improve to similar levels, with or without it," although the authors suggested that its effect "may be more pronounced in more severe cases." They concluded that "there are insufficient data on whether heliox can avert endotracheal intubation, or change intensive care and hospital admission rates and duration, or mortality."

2. Clinical Vignettes

Rudow and colleagues[63] provided the following story. A 78-year-old woman with both breast cancer and ophthalmic melanoma developed airway obstruction from a thyroid carcinoma that extended into her mediastinum and compressed her trachea. She had a 2-month history of worsening dyspnea, especially when positioned supine. On examination, inspiratory and expiratory stridor was present. Noted on the chest radiograph were a large superior mediastinal mass and pulmonary metastases. A solid mass was identified on a thyroid ultrasound scan. Computed tomography revealed a large mass at the thoracic inlet and extending caudally. Clinically, the patient was exhausted and in respiratory distress.

Almost instant relief was obtained by giving the patient a mixture of 78% He:22% O_2, with improvements in measured tidal volume and oxygenation. Later, a thyroidectomy was carried out to relieve the obstruction. Here, anesthesia was conducted by applying topical anesthesia to the airway with awake laryngoscopy and intubation performed in the sitting position. When the airway was secured using an armored tube, the patient was given a general anesthetic with an intravenous induction. Following the surgery, extubation occurred without complication.

Another interesting clinical vignette has been published by Khanlou and Eiger.[39] They presented the case of a 69-year-old woman in whom bilateral vocal cord paralysis developed after radiation therapy and in whom heliox was successfully used for temporary management of the resultant upper airway obstruction until she was able to receive a tracheostomy.

A final clinical vignette related to heliox is from Polaner,[58] who reported on the use of the laryngeal mask airway (LMA) and heliox in a 20:80 mixture for the administration of anesthesia to a 3-year-old boy with asthma and a large anterior mediastinal mass. Clinical management involved an unusual combination of management strategies: the child was kept in the sitting position, spontaneous ventilation with a halothane-in-heliox inhalation induction was used, and airway stimulation was minimized of by use of the LMA. However, the author cautioned that cases such as these can readily take a deadly turn, noting that "one must, of course, always be prepared to intervene with either manipulations of patient position in the event of airway compromise (including upright, lateral, and prone) or more aggressive strategies, such as rigid bronchoscopy and even median sternotomy (in the case of intractable cardiovascular collapse), or to allow the patient to awaken if critical airway or cardiovascular compromise becomes evident at any time during the course of the anesthesia."

E. PRESSURE DIFFERENCES

From the analysis of equations governing laminar flow and turbulent flow, the pressure drop along the noncompliant portion of the airway is given approximately by the Rohrer equation[24]:

$$\Delta P = K_1 \dot{V} + K_2 \dot{V}^2 \qquad (17)$$

where K_1 and K_2 are known as Rohrer constants. Physical interpretation of this equation is as follows: airway pressure is governed by the sum of two terms:

1. Effects proportional to gas flow (laminar flow effects)
2. Effects proportional to the square of the gas flow (turbulent flow effects)

It can be seen that the lowest pressure loss ΔP across the airway would be expected when $\dot{V}$ is small, that is, predominantly laminar flow. However, it is known that, under conditions of laminar flow, K_1 is largely influenced by viscosity and not density and K_2 (the turbulent term) is influenced primarily by density and not viscosity.

F. RESISTANCE TO GAS FLOW

When pressure readings are taken at each end of a horizontal tube with a fluid flowing through it, one notices that the pressure measurements at either end are not identical, the pressure at the distal end of the tube being less than the pressure at the proximal end (fluid flowing from the proximal to the distal end). In this case, the pressure loss is attributable to frictional losses incurred by the fluid when in contact with the inside of the tube. This is analogous to heat losses incurred by resistors in an electrical circuit (Fig. 3-7).

Frictional losses are irreversible; that is, the energy lost cannot be recovered by the fluid and is mostly lost

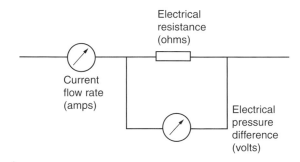

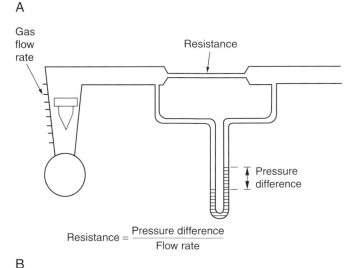

Figure 3-7 Electrical analogy of gas flow. Analogy between laminar gas flow and flow of electricity through a resistor. **A,** Gas: flow in volume/second (e.g., mL/s), pressure difference in force/area (e.g., dynes/cm²), and resistance described by Poiseuille's law. **B,** Electricity: flow in current (amperes), pressure difference in voltage (volts), and resistance described by Ohm's law. Note that for gases, pressure difference = flow rate × resistance, and for electricity, potential difference (voltage) = current × resistance. (From Nunn JF: Nunn's Applied Respiratory Physiology, 4th ed. Stoneham, Mass, Butterworth-Heinemann, 1993.)

as heat. Note that, if the tube is not horizontal, pressure differences are also attributable to height differences. The most common relation that describes the flow in a tube is the Bernoulli equation, which is valid for both laminar and turbulent flow[79]:

$$\frac{V_1^2}{2g} + \frac{P_1}{\rho g} + Z_1 = \frac{V_2^2}{2g} + \frac{P_2}{\rho g} + Z_2 + h_f \tag{18}$$

where

V = velocity [m/s]
g = gravitational constant [9.81 m/s² or 9.81 N/kg]
P = pressure [pascals or N/m²]
ρ = density of fluid [kg/m³]
Z = height from an arbitrary point (datum) [m]
h_f = frictional losses [m]

Typical units are shown in square brackets. Note that the preceding equation is in the units of meters and is termed "meters of head loss." This is typical of fluid mechanics equations. As mentioned previously, the Bernoulli equation is valid for both laminar and turbulent flow.

1. Endotracheal Tube Resistance

ETs, like all tubes, offer resistance to fluid flow (Fig. 3-8). However, ETs do not add external resistance to the normal airway but rather act as a substitute for the normal resistance of the airway from the mouth to the trachea, which accounts for 30% to 40% of normal airway resistance.[17] This is important because, although mechanical ventilators can overcome impedance to inspiratory flow during extended periods of artificial respiration, they do not augment passive exhalation. Resistance to exhalation through a long, small-diameter ET, which is compounded by turbulence, can seriously constrain ventilation rate and tidal volume.[8,78]

The use of the ET influences respiration in a number of ways. First, it decreases effective airway diameter and therefore increases the resistance to breathing. Resistance is further increased by the curved nature of the tube; resistance measurements are typically about 3% higher than if the tubes were straight.[76] Note that the passage from the mouth to the larynx is not a smooth curve and may create additional turbulence.

Second, studies show that intubated patients experience decreased peak flow rates (inspiratory and expiratory), decreased forced vital capacity, and forced expiratory volume in 1 second (FEV$_1$).[19] However, the tube may paradoxically increase peak flow rates during forced expiration through the prevention of dynamic compression of the trachea.[19] Finally, the tube may cause mechanical irritation of the larynx and trachea that may lead to a reflex constriction of the airway distal to the tube.[53]

The combination of tube and connector may cause higher resistance than the tube alone. Moreover, because

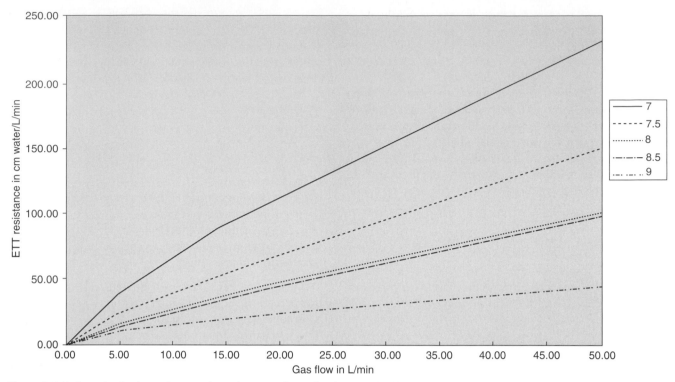

Figure 3-8 Endotracheal tube resistance dependence on flow. The data provided by Hicks in Table 3-3 can be used to show that endotracheal tube resistance increases nonlinearly with flow (because of turbulence effects). For pure laminar flow, resistance would be constant, regardless of flow.

of turbulence at component connections, the total resistance of a system is not necessarily the sum of the resistances of its component parts, especially where sharp-angled connectors are used (see Fig. 3-5).[26,39] In addition, humidified gases contribute to slightly higher resistances because of the increased density of moist gas.[1] The resistance of single-lumen tubes is generally lower than that of double-lumen tubes.[1]

The resistance associated with ETs may be reduced by increasing tube diameter, decreasing tube length, or decreasing the gas density (hence the occasional use of helium-oxygen mixtures). It has been suggested that the presence of the ET may double the work of breathing in chronically intubated adults and lead to respiratory failure in some infants.[76] Therefore, it is important to use as large an ET as is practical in patients who exhibit respiratory dysfunction.

ET resistance can be measured in the laboratory using differential pressure and flow measurement techniques,[32,48] the most common method of which is described by Gaensler and colleagues.[18] Theoretical estimates of resistance under laminar flow conditions can also be obtained using the Poiseuille equation. In vivo resistance measurements are generally higher than in vitro measurements of ET, perhaps because of secretions, head or neck position, tube deformation, or increased turbulence.[20,80]

Airway resistance may be established from first principles using Poiseuille's law when the gas flow is laminar. When gas flow is turbulent, resistance is no longer independent of material properties, and *empirical*

measurements become the only feasible means of characterizing resistance. Intrinsic airway resistance is determined by measuring the transairway pressure, that is, the pressure drop between the airway opening and the alveoli. The following relationship applies[28]:

$$R = \frac{P_{airway} - P_{alveolar}}{\dot{V}} \tag{19}$$

where

R = airway resistance [cm H_2O/L/s]
P_{airway} = proximal airway pressure [cm H_2O]
$P_{alveolar}$ = alveolar pressure [cm H_2O]
$\dot{V}$ = gas flow rate [L/s]

Typical units used are shown in brackets. In clinical practice, airway resistance is easiest to determine using a whole-body plethysmograph. Unfortunately, it is an apparatus unsuitable for critically ill patients.

An alternative method of presenting airway resistance is provided by Hicks,[28] in which the following equation and constants are used:

$$\Delta P = a\dot{V}^b \tag{20}$$

where

ΔP = pressure difference [cm H_2O]
$\dot{V}$ = gas flow [L/min]
a, b = empirical constants provided in Table 3-3

Table 3-3 **Coefficients for Airway Resistance Computations**

Tube	a	b
7.0	9.78	1.81
7.5	7.73	1.75
8.0	5.90	1.72
8.5	4.61	1.78
9.0	3.90	1.63

From Hicks GH: Monitoring respiratory mechanics. Probl Respir Care 2:191, 1989.

Figure 3-8 depicts the effect of tube diameter and flow rate on ET resistance. Note that resistance is increased as a result of increasing turbulence caused by decreasing ET diameter and increasing flow rate.

Clinically, the issue of ET resistance is perhaps most important in pediatrics and during T-piece trials. In a laboratory study, Manczur and coworkers[46] sought to determine the resistances of ETs commonly used in neonatal and pediatric intensive care units. They examined straight tubes with IDs between 2.5 and 6 mm and shouldered (Cole) tubes with ID/outer diameter between 2.5/4 and 3.5/5 mm. Predictably, they found that resistance increased as ET diameter decreased. The resistances of the 6 mm ID ET were 3.1 $H_2O/L/s$ and 4.6 cm $H_2O/L/s$, respectively, at flows of 5 and 10 L/min, and the resistances of the 2.5 mm ID ET were 81.2 $H_2O/L/s$ and 139.4 cm $H_2O/L/s$, respectively. They noted that shortening an ET to a length appropriate for the patient (e.g., a 4.0 mm ID, 20.7 to 11.3 cm) reduced its resistance on average by 22%. Finally, they noted that the resistance of a Cole tube was "about 50% lower than that of a straight tube with an ID corresponding to the narrow part of the shouldered tube."

Using an acoustic reflection research method, Straus and associates[71] sought to study the influence of the ET resistance during T-piece trials by comparing the work of breathing of 14 successfully extubated patients at the end of a 2-hour trial and after extubation. They found that the work of breathing of the patients was identical in both groups and that there was no significant difference between the beginning and the end of the T-piece trial. The work caused by the ET amounted to about 11.0% of the total work of breathing, and the supraglottic airway resistance was significantly smaller than the ET resistance. They concluded that "a 2hr trial of spontaneous breathing through an ET well mimics the work of breathing performed after extubation, in patients who pass a weaning trial and do not require reintubation."

III. WORK OF BREATHING

Breathing comprises a two-part cycle: inspiration and expiration. During normal breathing, inspiration is an active, energy-consuming process and expiration is ordinarily a passive process in which the diaphragm and intercostal muscles relax (Figs. 3-9 and 3-10). However, expiration becomes an active process during forced expiration, as during exercise or during expiration against a resistance load. Several studies have examined the work of breathing in some clinical settings.[4,16,51,54,57,68]

Considering only normal breathing, the work of breathing is given by:

$$\text{Work} = \text{force} \times \text{distance}$$

$$\text{Force} = \text{pressure} \times \text{area}$$

$$\text{Distance} = \text{volume/area}$$

$$\text{Work} = (\text{pressure} \times \text{area}) \times (\text{volume/area}) = \text{pressure} \times \text{volume}$$

Because the air pressure in the lung varies with lung volume and pressure measurements are obtained distal to the end of the ET, work may be expressed as[6]:

$$\text{WORK}_{\text{INSPIRATION}} = \int_{\text{FRC}}^{\text{FRC+TV}} P\,dV \qquad (21)$$

where

P = airway pressure [cm H_2O]
dV = (infinitesimal) volume of gas added to the lung [mL]
FRC = functional residual capacity of the lungs [mL]
TV = tidal volume breathed in during respiration [mL]

When the pressure varies as a function of time, the preceding equation may be integrated in the following manner:

$$\text{LET } dV = \frac{dV}{dt} \times dt = \dot{V}\,dt \qquad (22)$$

Changing the limits of integration yields:

$$\text{WORK}_{\text{INSPIRATION}} = \int_{t_1}^{t_2} P(t)\,\dot{V}(t)\,dt \qquad (23)$$

where

t_1 = time at the beginning of inspiration [s]
t_2 = time at the end of inspiration [s]
P = pressure measured at a point of interest in the airway (e.g., at the tip of the ET or at the carina) [cm H_2O]
$\dot{V}$ = flow [mL/s]

The preceding equation is cumbersome to integrate quickly. However, it is sometimes reasonable to assume that the pressure during inspiration remains fairly constant. Under these circumstances, integration of the original work equation during constant-pressure inspiration yields the following approximation:

$$\text{WORK}_{\text{INSPIRATION}} = P_{\text{AVE}} \times \text{TV} \qquad (24)$$

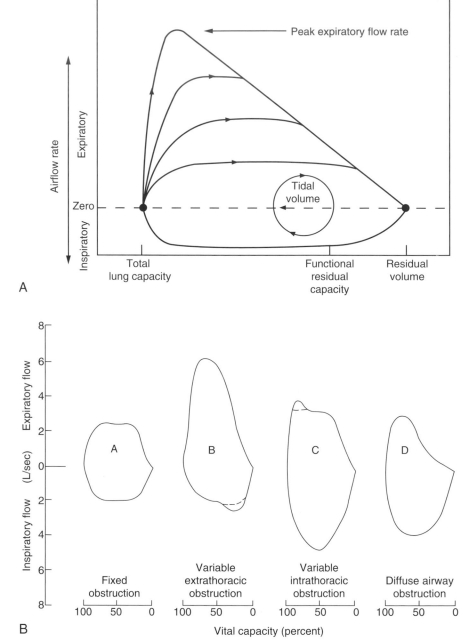

Figure 3-9 Flow-volume curves. **A,** A flow-volume curve consists of a plot of gas flow against lung volume. Shown here are four loops corresponding to four different levels of expiratory effort. As can be seen, peak expiratory flow is effort dependent, but toward the end of expiration the curves converge (flow limited by dynamic airway collapse). From a diagnostic viewpoint, the expiratory portion of the loop is of more value than the inspiratory portion. **B,** Maximum inspiratory and expiratory flow-volume curves (flow-volume loops) in four types of airway obstruction. (**A,** From Nunn JF: Nunn's Applied Respiratory Physiology, 4th ed. Stoneham, Mass, Butterworth-Heinemann, 1993; **B,** from Gal TJ: Anesthesia, 2nd ed. New York, Churchill Livingstone, 1986.)

where
P_{AVE} = mean airway pressure during inspiration [cm H_2O]
TV = tidal volume of inspiration [mL]

During anesthesia, an ET is often inserted, and additional energy is required to overcome the friction effects of the ET. The added work of breathing presented by an ET is given by:

$$WORK_{ETT} = \int_{FRC}^{FRC+TV} \Delta P \, dV \qquad (25)$$

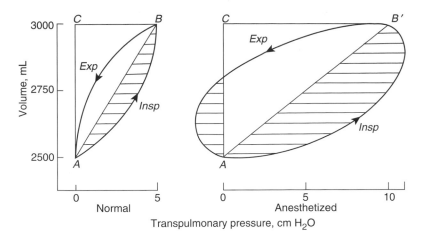

Figure 3-10 The work of breathing. Lung volume plotted against transpulmonary pressure in a pressure-volume diagram for an awake *(normal)* and an anesthetized patient. Total area within the oval and triangles has the dimensions of pressure multiplied by volume and represents the total work of breathing. Hatched area to the right of lines *AB* and *AB'* represents active inspiratory work necessary to overcome resistance to airflow during inspiration *(Insp)*. The hatched area to the left of the triangle *AB'C* represents active expiratory work necessary to overcome resistance to airflow during expiration *(Exp)*. Expiration is passive in the normal subject because sufficient potential energy is stored during inspiration to produce expiratory airflow. The fraction of total inspiratory work necessary to overcome elastic resistance is shown by triangles *ABC* and *AB'C*. The anesthetized patient has decreased compliance and increased elastic resistance work (triangle *AB'C*) compared with the normal patient's compliance and elastic resistance work (triangle *ABC*). The anesthetized patient shown has increased airway resistance to both inspiratory and expiratory work. (From Benumof JL: Anesthesia, 2nd ed. New York, Churchill Livingstone, 1986.)

where ΔP is the pressure drop across the tube. Often, the pressure gradient ΔP is relatively constant during inspiration, and hence:

$$WORK_{ETT} = \Delta P \int_{FRC}^{FRC+TV} dV = \Delta P \times \Delta V \quad (26)$$

where

ΔP = pressure drop across ET during inspiration [mm Hg]
ΔV = volume added to lungs = tidal volume [mL]

Hence, the total work done, measured in joules (kg $\times$ m^2/s^2), is:

$$WORK_{TOTAL} = WORK_{ET} + WORK_{INSPIRATION} \quad (27)$$

IV. PULMONARY BIOMECHANICS

A. THE RESPIRATORY MECHANICS EQUATION

Approximately 3% of the body's total energy is required to maintain normal respiratory function.[67] Energy is required to overcome three main forces: (1) the elastic resistance of the lungs, which restores the lungs to their original size after inflation; (2) the force required to move the rib cage, diaphragm, and appropriate visceral contents; and (3) the dissipative resistance of the airway and any breathing apparatus.[29] The respiratory system is commonly modeled as the frictional airway R_L that is in series with the lung compliance C_L. Such a model is analogous to a resistor and capacitor in series that form a resistive-capacitive (RC) circuit (Fig. 3-11).

A transmural (P_{TM}) pressure gradient exists between the airway at the mouth (at atmospheric pressure) and the pressure inside the pleural cavity. This pressure gradient is responsible for the lungs "hugging" the thoracic cavity as the chest enlarges during inspiration. The presence of an external breathing apparatus causes a further pressure loss (P_{EXT}). Hence, the total pressure drop between the atmosphere and the pleural cavity is given by the respiratory mechanics equation and may be modeled as[29]:

$$P_{TOTAL} = P_{EXT} + P_{TM} = P_{EXT}\dot{V} + \frac{V}{C_L} + R_L\dot{V} \quad (28)$$

$$P_{EXT} = P_{EXT}\dot{V} \quad (29)$$

$$P_{TM} = \frac{V}{C_L} + R_L\dot{V} \quad (30)$$

where

P_{TOTAL} = pressure drop between atmosphere and pleural cavity
P_{EXT} = pressure drop across external breathing apparatus
P_{TM} = transmural pressure gradient
R_{EXT} = external apparatus resistance (e.g., an ET)
$\dot{V} = dV/dt$ = gas flow rate into the lungs
C_L = lung compliance

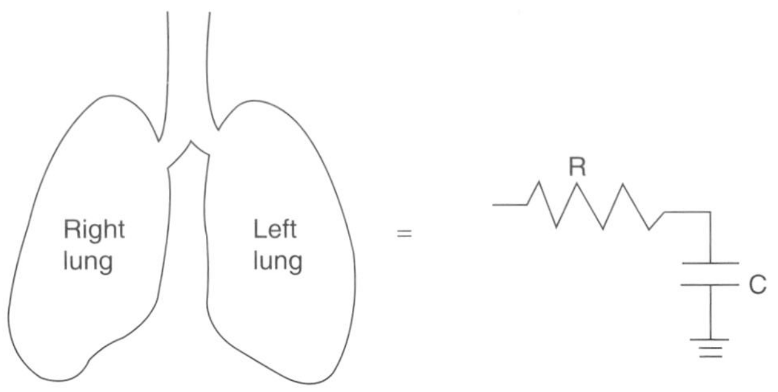

$$R = \text{Resistance} = \frac{\text{Pressure change}}{\text{Flow rate}}$$

$$C = \text{Compliance} = \frac{\text{Volume change}}{\text{Pressure change}}$$

Figure 3-11 Resistance-compliance (RC) model of the lungs. Resistance of lungs to airflow and natural ability to resist stretch (or compliance) enable lungs to be modeled as an electric circuit. A resistor of resistance R placed in series with a capacitor of charge C is a simple and convenient analogy upon which to base pulmonary biomechanics.

R_L = airway resistance
V = volume of gas above the FRC in the lungs

Thus, the pressure required to inflate the lungs depends on both the lung compliance and gas flow rate. The time required to inflate the lungs is measured in terms of a pulmonary time constant. This time constant (t) is simply the product $R_L \times C_L$. However, determination of the time constant is not a trivial matter, and attention is now turned to that determination.

1. The Pulmonary Time Constant

Using the previous formula in the case that no external resistance exists, one can show that, during passive expiration, the volume in the lungs in excess of FRC takes on the form[83]:

$$V = V_0 e^{-t/\tau} \tag{31}$$

where V_0 is the volume taken in during inspiration and $\tau = R_L C_L$ is the time constant for the lungs. Flow from the lungs is obtained by differentiating this equation with respect to time:

$$\dot{V} = \frac{dV}{dt} = V_0 \frac{d\left(e^{-t/\tau}\right)}{dt} = V_0 e^{-t/\tau}\left(-\frac{1}{\tau}\right) = -\frac{V_0}{\tau}e^{-t/\tau} \tag{32}$$

Tau (τ) may be now estimated by dividing the preceding equation by the first one:

$$\frac{\dot{V}}{V} = \frac{V_0 e^{-t/\tau}\left(-\dfrac{1}{\tau}\right)}{V_0 e^{-t/\tau}} = -\frac{1}{\tau} \tag{33}$$

Tau (τ) can be estimated as the negative of the reciprocal of the average slope of the plot of flow ($\dot{V}$) against volume (V) during expiration. Another means of estimating τ is by taking the natural logarithm of the volume equation $V = V_0 e^{-t/\tau}$.

Tau can also be estimated as the negative of reciprocal of the average slope of the natural logarithm of the lung volume plotted against time.

$$\ln V = \ln\left(V_0\right) - \frac{t}{\tau} = \frac{d\left(\ln V\right)}{dt} = -\frac{1}{\tau} \tag{34}$$

2. Determination of Rohrer's Constants

A more complete approach to modeling the pressure-flow relationship of the respiratory system assumes that a single time constant τ may be inadequate to describe pulmonary biomechanics in some situations and goes from the classical form[24]:

$$\frac{V}{\dot{V}} = -\tau = C_L \times R_L \tag{35}$$

to a more elaborate form of:

$$\frac{V}{\dot{V}} = -C_L\left(K_1 + K_2\dot{V}\right) \tag{36}$$

where K_1 and K_2 are known as Rohrer's constants and $(K_1 + K_2)$ is a form of R_L. In this situation, the resistance of the pulmonary system is not assumed to be constant but rather is assumed to be flow dependent:

$$R = K_1 + K_2\dot{V} \tag{37}$$

When this equation is expressed as:

$$\frac{V}{C_L\dot{V}} = -\left(K_1 + K_2\dot{V}\right) \tag{38}$$

K_1 and K_2 may be determined as the intercept and slope, respectively, of a plot of $V/C_L\dot{V}$ against $\dot{V}$.

3. Compliance

Pulmonary compliance measurements reflect the elastic properties of the lungs and thorax and are influenced by factors such as degree of muscular tension, degree of interstitial lung water, degree of pulmonary fibrosis, degree of lung inflation, and alveolar surface tension.[52] Total respiratory system compliance is given by[28]:

$$C = \frac{\Delta V}{\Delta P} \tag{39}$$

where
ΔV = change in lung volume
ΔP = change in airway pressure

This total compliance may be related to lung compliance and thoracic (chest wall) compliance by the relation:

$$\frac{1}{C_T} = \frac{1}{C_L} + \frac{1}{C_{Th}} \qquad (40)$$

where

C_T = total compliance (typically 100 mL/cm H_2O)
C_L = lung compliance (typically 200 mL/cm H_2O)
C_{Th} = thoracic compliance (typically 200 mL/cm H_2O)

Values in parentheses are some typical normal adult values that can be used for modeling purposes.[28] Elastance is the reciprocal of compliance and offers notational advantage over compliance in some physiologic problems. However, its use has not been popular in clinical practice.

Compliance may be estimated using the pulmonary time constant τ. If a linear resistance of known value ΔR is added to the patient's airway, the time constant will change, becoming[24]:

$$\tau' = (R_L + \Delta R) \times C_L = \tau + C_L \times \Delta R = \tau + \Delta\tau \qquad (41)$$

Thus, if ΔR is known and τ and τ' are determined experimentally, one can solve for C_L and then for R_L:

$$C_L = \frac{\tau' - \tau}{\Delta R} = \frac{\Delta\tau}{\Delta R} \qquad R_L = \tau \times \frac{\Delta R}{\Delta\tau} = \frac{\tau \times \Delta R}{\tau' - \tau} \qquad (42)$$

B. AN ADVANCED FORMULATION OF THE RESPIRATORY MECHANICS EQUATION

An alternative equation, the advanced respiratory mechanics equation, to the elementary respiratory mechanics equation may be used to describe the physical behavior of the lungs. The original formulation of the equation was carried out by Rohrer during World War I, but the first completely correct formulation is due to Gaensler and colleagues[18] and is of the form:

$$P = \frac{V}{C} + K_1\dot{V} + K_2\dot{V}^2 \qquad (43)$$

where

P = airway pressure
V = lung volume
$\dot{V}$ = gas flow rate into (out of) lung
C = compliance of the pulmonary system
K_1, K_2 = empirical Rohrer's constants

This equation is more advanced than the elementary respiratory mechanics equation because it is able to account for flow losses attributable to turbulence. Because turbulent flow conditions are most likely to exist during anesthesia, the $\dot{V}^2$ term is very important in accurately quantifying the pressure losses of respiration. In addition,

it combines the resistance losses into the constants K_1 and K_2, which requires only empirical determination.

V. ANESTHESIA AT MODERATE ALTITUDE

The parameters that govern the administration of anesthesia are altered slightly when the elevation above sea level is increased. Generally, a change in the atmospheric (or barometric) pressure is responsible for these differences. This section briefly examines the consequences of a moderate change in altitude.

The approximate alveolar gas equation is a useful tool in quantifying the differences that occur at higher elevations[43]:

$$P_{AO_2} = P_{IO_2} - \frac{P_{aCO_2}}{R} \qquad P_{IO_2} = (P_B - 47) \times F_{IO_2} \qquad (44)$$

where

P_{AO_2} = alveolar oxygen tension
P_{IO_2} = inspired oxygen tension partial pressure
P_{aCO_2} = arterial carbon dioxide tension
$R = 0.8 \rightarrow$ gas exchange coefficient: CO_2 produced/O_2 consumed
P_B = barometric pressure (760 mm Hg at sea level)
47 = water vapor pressure at 37° C
F_{IO_2} = fraction of inspired oxygen = 0.21 at all altitudes (room air)

All tensions are in mm Hg (torr).

A. ALTERED PARTIAL PRESSURE OF GASES

The effect of altitude is very apparent on the partial pressure of administered gases. The partial pressure of oxygen is given by $P_{IO_2} = (P_B - P_{H_2O}) \times 0.21$. At 1524 m (5000 ft) above sea level, P_{IO_2} is reduced to 128 mm Hg from 158 mm Hg at sea level, so that the maximum P_{AO_2} is about 83 mm Hg (assuming $P_{aCO_2} = 36$).[33] At 3048 m (10,000 ft), P_{IO_2} is 111 mm Hg, and the maximum P_{AO_2} is 65 mm Hg.[33] In order to counteract the effects of the hypoxia, ventilation is increased, so that at 5000 ft $P_{aCO_2} = 36$ mm Hg, and, at 3048 m, $P_{aCO_2} = 34$ mm Hg on average.[33] The effectiveness of N_2O decreases with altitude because of an absolute reduction of its partial pressure (tension).

B. OXYGEN ANALYZERS

There are five main types of oxygen analyzers: paramagnetic, fuel cell, oxygen electrodes, mass spectrometers, and Raman spectrographs. All respond to oxygen partial pressure (not concentration) so that the output changes with barometric pressure. At 1524 m, an analyzer set to measure 21% O_2 at sea level reads 17.4%. If these devices were to calculate the amount of oxygen in terms of partial pressure, the scale readings would reflect the true state of oxygen availability, but clinical practice dictates that a percentage scale be used anyway.

C. CO₂ ANALYZERS AND VAPOR ANALYZERS

Absorption of infrared radiation by gas is the usual analytic method to determine the amount of CO_2 in a gas mixture, although other methods (e.g., Raman spectrographs) work well. This type of method measures partial pressures, not percentages. To operate accurately, these machines must either be calibrated using known CO_2 concentrations at the correct barometric pressure or have the scale converted to read partial pressures.

Similar arguments apply to modern vapor analyzers, all of which respond to partial pressures, not concentrations, despite the fact that the output of these devices, by clinical custom, is usually calculated in percentages.

D. VAPORS AND VAPORIZERS

Practically speaking, the saturated vapor pressure of a volatile agent depends only on its temperature. Thus, at a given temperature, the concentration of a given mass of vapor increases as barometric pressure decreases, but its partial pressure remains unchanged. Similarly, the output of calibrated vaporizers is altered with changes in barometric pressure. Only the concentration of the vapor changes; the partial pressure remains the same, as does the patient's response at a given setting as compared with sea level. This assumes that the vaporizer characteristics do not change with altered density and viscosity of the carrier gases.

E. FLOWMETERS

Most flowmeters measure the drop in pressure that occurs when a gas passes through a resistance and correlate this pressure drop to flow. The pressure drop is dependent on gas density and viscosity. When the resistance is an orifice, resistance depends primarily on gas density. For laminar flow through a tube, viscosity determines resistance (Hagen-Poiseuille equation). Some flowmeters employ a floating ball or bobbin supported by the stream of gas in a tapered tube. The float is fluted so that it remains in the center of the flow. At low flow, the device depends primarily on laminar flow, and, as the float moves up the tube, the resistance behaves progressively more like an orifice. The density of a gas changes, of course, with barometric pressure, but the viscosity changes little, being primarily dependent on temperature. Gas flow through an orifice is inversely proportional to the square root of gas density, so that, as the density falls, flow increases (orifice size constant). Thus, at high altitude, the actual flowmeter flow is greater than that indicated by the float position:

$$\text{Actual flow} = \text{Nominal flow} \times \sqrt{\frac{760 \text{ mm Hg}}{P_B}} \quad (45)$$

F. FLOWMETER CALIBRATION

The calibration of standard flowmeters, such as the Thorpe tube, depends on gas properties. Usually, a particular flowmeter is calibrated for a particular gas, such as oxygen or air. The factor used to convert nominal flow measurements to actual flow measurements is given by[43]:

$$k = \frac{\sqrt{GMW_A}}{\sqrt{GMW_B}} \quad (46)$$

where A is the gas for which the flowmeter is originally designed, B is the gas actually used, and GMW is the gram molecular weight of the gas in question. A list of common anesthetic gases and their respective GMWs are presented in Table 3-4.

Example Calculation 1

Determine the actual flow rate of a 70%:30% helium-oxygen mixture if it is passed through an oxygen flowmeter that reads 10 L/min.

Answer:

$$GMW_{O_2} = 32 \text{ g/gmol} \quad (47)$$

$$GMW_{heliox} = 0.3(32) + 0.7(4) = 12.4 \text{ g/gmol} \quad (48)$$

The actual flow rate of heliox is given by:

$$\begin{aligned}
\text{Actual flow rate} &= 10 \times \frac{\sqrt{GMW}_{O_2}}{\sqrt{GMW}_{Heliox}} \\
&= 10 \times \frac{\sqrt{32}}{\sqrt{12.4}} = 16.1 \text{ L/min}
\end{aligned} \quad (49)$$

Table 3-4   **Gram Molecular Weights (GMWs) for Some Common and Anesthetic Gases**

Name	Symbol	GMW
Hydrogen	H	1.00797
Helium	He	4.0026
Nitrogen (molecular)	N_2	28.0134
Oxygen (molecular)	O_2	31.9988
Neon	Ne	20.183
Argon	Ar	39.948
Xenon	Xe	131.30
Halothane	$CF_3CClBrH$	197
Isoflurane	$CF_2H\text{-}O\text{-}CHClCF_3$	184.5
Enflurane	$CF_2H\text{-}O\text{-}CF_2CFHCl$	184.5
Nitrous oxide	N_2O	44.013

From Benumof JL: Airway Management: Principles and Practice. St. Louis, Mosby, 1996, p 61.

Example Calculation 2

Determine the appropriate multiplier if oxygen is passed through an airflow meter.

Answer:

$$\text{Multiplier} = \frac{\sqrt{GMW_{AIR}}}{\sqrt{GMW_{O_2}}} = \frac{\sqrt{0.21(32) + 0.79(28)}}{\sqrt{32}} = 0.95 \quad (50)$$

G. ANESTHETIC IMPLICATIONS

At 3048 m (10,000 ft), a 30% O_2 mixture has the same partial pressure as a 20% O_2 mixture at sea level.[33] In addition, the reduction in partial pressure of N_2O that occurs seriously impairs the effectiveness of the agent, and it may be of no benefit to administer. The concept of minimum alveolar concentration (MAC) does not apply at higher altitudes and should be substituted by the concept of minimal alveolar partial pressure (MAPP) (Table 3-5). The use of this concept would eliminate many of the problems identified earlier.

VI. ESTIMATION OF GAS RATES

A. ESTIMATION OF CARBON DIOXIDE PRODUCTION RATE

The carbon dioxide production rate ($\dot{V}_{CO_2}$) of a patient may be estimated in the following manner. The CO_2 production rate can be described as the product of the amount of CO_2 produced per breath and the number of breaths per minute. The CO_2 production rate hence has typical units of milliliters per minute (mL/min). Hence, $\dot{V}_{CO_2}$ may be expressed as:

$$\dot{V}_{CO_2} = CO_2 \text{ produced per breath} \times \text{number of} \\ \text{breaths per minute (BPM)} \quad (51)$$

$$\dot{V}_{CO_2} = V_{CO_2} \times BPM \quad (52)$$

The amount of CO_2 produced per breath is calculated as follows:

$$V_{CO_2} = \int_{t=0}^{t=t_{end\ expiration}} C_{CO_2}(t) \times Q(t) \times \gamma\, dt \quad (53)$$

where

$C_{CO_2}(t)$ = capnogram signal [mm Hg]
$Q(t)$ = gas flow rate signal [mL/min]
γ = scaling factor to switch dimensions from mm Hg to concentration % = 100%/(760 mm Hg) = 0.1312

B. ESTIMATION OF OXYGEN CONSUMPTION RATE

The oxygen consumption rate may be estimated in a manner very similar to that of $\dot{V}_{CO_2}$. The oxygen consumption rate can be expressed as the product of oxygen consumed per breath and the number of breaths per minute. Mathematically, this may be written as:

$$\dot{V}_{O_2} = O_2 \text{ consumed per breath} \times \\ \text{number of breaths per minute} \quad (54)$$

$$\dot{V}_{O_2} = V_{O_2} \times BPM \quad (55)$$

The amount of O_2 consumed per breath can now be expressed as:

$$V_{O_2} = \int_{t=0}^{t=t_{end\ expiration}} (P_{IO_2} - C_{O_2}) \times Q(t) \times \gamma\, dt \quad (56)$$

where

P_{IO_2} = inspiratory oxygen pressure = $(PB - 47) \times F_{IO_2}$ [mm Hg]
$C_{O_2}(t)$ = oxygen signal [mm Hg]
Q = gas flow rate signal [mL/min]
γ = scaling factor = 0.1312

Table 3-5 **Variations in Minimum Alveolar Concentration (MAC) That Occur at Various Altitude Levels, with the Comparative Values for Minimal Partial Pressure (MAPP)**

	MAC (%)			MAPP	
Agent	Sea level	5000 ft	10,000 ft	(kPa)	(mm Hg)
Nitrous oxide	105.0	126.5	152.2	106.1	798.0
Ethyl ether	1.92	2.31	2.78	1.94	14.6
Halothane	0.75	0.90	1.09	0.76	5.7
Enflurane	1.68	2.02	2.43	1.70	12.8
Isoflurane	1.2	1.45	1.73	1.22	9.1

MAPP = MAC × 0.01 × 760 mm Hg.
Adapted from James MFM, White JF: Anesthetic considerations at moderate altitude. Anesth Analg 63:1097, 1984.

C. INTERPRETATION OF CARBON DIOXIDE PRODUCTION AND OXYGEN CONSUMPTION RATES

The rates $\dot{V}_{O_2}$ and $\dot{V}_{CO_2}$ are linked by the respiratory exchange coefficient RQ (RQ = $\dot{V}_{CO_2}/\dot{V}_{O_2}$), which is governed largely by diet, some diets producing less CO_2 than others (RQ smaller). Typically, RQ = 0.8. $\dot{V}_{O_2}$ and $\dot{V}_{CO_2}$ both go up with increases in metabolism, perhaps related to one of several factors (e.g., fever, sepsis, light anesthesia, shivering, malignant hyperthermia, thyroid storm). Decreases in $\dot{V}_{CO_2}$ and $\dot{V}_{O_2}$ may be due to many causes as well (e.g., hypothermia, deep anesthesia, hypothyroidism).

VII. MATHEMATICAL MODELING RELATED TO THE AIRWAY

A. OVERVIEW

In this section, the role of "ready-to-use" numeric analysis software for physiologic model building is discussed, using the respiratory system as a basis for discussion. Using well-established physiologic principles, it can be shown that some "what if" physiologic questions can be answered. These questions could not have been answered in the past because of experimental complexity or because of ethical considerations. Because the model is based upon simple equations accepted by the physiologic community, the results obtained are directly credible, and many of the difficulties of direct experimentation are avoided.

The model concept is explored through a discussion of four oxygen transport problems, some of which are too complex in experimental design for empirical study to be practical. However, considerable insight can be obtained using numerical methods alone.

B. BACKGROUND

Some physiologic systems are especially well suited to physiologic modeling. For example, physiologic modeling of the cardiopulmonary system may be performed to examine issues such as the determinants of pulmonary gas exchange. For instance, both Doyle[11] and Viale and coauthors[75] have written custom software to explore the determinants of the arterial-alveolar oxygen tension ratio, and Torda[73] has explored the determinants of the alveolar-arterial oxygen tension difference in a similar manner. Prior to the common use of digital computers, graphic techniques were sometimes used for solving respiratory physiologic models, early work by Kelman and colleagues on the influence of cardiac output on arterial oxygenation being a well-known example.[36] Central to the construction of such a mathematic model is the existence of a number of equations relating physiologic parameters. Examples of physiologic relationships in the respiratory system well described by equations include (1) the alveolar gas equation,[43,55] (2) the pulmonary shunt equation,[34] (3) the blood oxygen content equation,[34] and (4) various equations describing the oxyhemoglobin dissociation curve.[2,37,42,64,65]

C. PROBLEMS IN MODEL SOLVING

Although many physiologic problems are readily solved by direct analytic methods, frequently their solution is hampered by nonlinearities, self-referencing (circular) equations, or other complexities. (An example of a nonlinearity is the equation $y = x^2$; an example of a self-referencing equation set is the equation pair $y = 1/x$; $x = y + 1$.) Experience has shown that early conventional spreadsheet programs were poorly equipped to solve systems of this kind because they are not generally designed for iterative equation-solving methods. Newer spreadsheets usually contain an iterative solver of some kind.

Some authors have applied successive approximation methods with custom-written software to solve equation sets of this kind.[11] However, this approach may involve considerable effort, even by experienced computer programmers. Furthermore, many physiologists have limited experience and training in writing computer programs. In the next section we show how equation-solving computer programs can be used to advantage to solve complex physiologic modeling equations. TK SOLVER is the equation-solver package used in most of the examples shown in the following, but many other packages could also have been used.

D. DESCRIPTION OF TK SOLVER

TK SOLVER (the TK stands for "tool kit") is a software package for equation solving.[57-61] Although intended primarily for engineering applications, TK SOLVER functions well in a variety of other application areas. On start-up, TK SOLVER displays 2 "sheets" or tables out of a total of 13 (Fig. 3-12). The Variable Sheet is presented on the top "window," and the Rule Sheet goes on the bottom. Equations are then entered in the Rule Sheet using a built-in editor; the variables associated with the equations are then automatically entered in the variable sheet by TK SOLVER. Errors such as unmatched parentheses are automatically detected. (Figure 3-12 shows sample Rule and Variable Sheets for a pulmonary exchange model.)

Once the equations are entered, TK SOLVER is ready to find solutions. In some cases, the equation set can be solved in "direct-solver" mode, but complex equation sets generally must be solved in "iterative-solver" mode on the basis of initial guesses for all variables. A discussion of the methods used to obtain solutions is presented by Konopasek and Jayaraman.[40] A book reviewing TK SOLVER from a user's viewpoint is also available.[41]

```
========================= RULE SHEET =============================

S  Rule
--------
    PaO2=PAO2-(Cav*(Z/(1-Z))-1.34*Hb*(ScO2-SaO2))/0.0031
    SaO2=PaO2^a/(PaO2^a+P50^a)
    ScO2=PAO2^a/(PAO2^a+P50^a)
    Cav=VO2/(10*CO)
    Sav=(Cav-0.0031*(PaO2-PvO2))/(1.34*Hb)
    SvO2=SaO2-Sav
    PvO2=P50*(SvO2/(1-SvO2))^(1/a)
    CaO2=1.34*Hb*SaO2+0.0031*PaO2
    CvO2=CaO2-Cav
    CcO2=1.34*Hb*ScO2+0.0031*PAO2

======================== VARIABLE SHEET ==========================

St  Input   Name    Output     Unit    Comment
----------  ----    -------    ----    --------
    50      PAO2                mmHg    Alveolar Oxygen Tension
            PaO2    46.602925   mmHg    Arterial Oxygen Tension
            PvO2    29.722228   mmHg    Mixed Venous Oxygen Tension
            SaO2    .80944994   none    Arterial Saturation (%)
            ScO2    .83656560   none    End Pulmonary Capillary Saturation (%)
            SvO2    .56329721   none    Mixed Venous Saturation (%)
            Sav     .24615273   none    Arterio-Venous Saturation Difference
    250     vo2                 ml/min  Oxygen Consumption
    5       co                  L/min   Cardiac Output
    .1      z                   none    Pulmonary Shunt Fraction
            Cav     5           vol%    Arterio-venous O2 Content Diff
    15      Hb                  g/dl    Hemoglobin Concentration
    2.65    a                   none    Hill's coefficient
    27      P50                 mmHg    PO2 for 50% Saturation
            CaO2    16.414413   vol%    Arterial Oxygen Content
            CvO2    11.414413   vol%    Mixed Venous Oxygen Content
            CcO2    16.969968   vol%    End Pulmonary Capillary Oxygen Content
```

Figure 3-12 Sample TK SOLVER sheets. *Top*, TK SOLVER Rule Sheet; *bottom*, TK SOLVER Variable Sheet. In this case, equations relate factors that determine arterial oxygen tension (Pa_{O_2}). All variables are defined in comment section of variable sheet. First equation in the Rule Sheet is from Torda[73] and Doyle.[11] Second and third equations are Hill equation.

E. EXAMPLE 1: APPLICATION OF MATHEMATICAL MODELING TO THE STUDY OF GAS EXCHANGE INDICES

Gas exchange indices are commonly used in anesthesia and critical care medicine to assess pulmonary function from an oxygen transport viewpoint. Although the determination of pulmonary shunt would be viewed by many as a "gold standard" preferable to any index, measurement of true pulmonary shunt requires pulmonary artery catheterization—a relatively expensive and risky procedure that is not always clinically warranted. Four gas exchange indices that are in common use are:

1. Alveolar-arterial oxygen tension difference $(P[A-a]O_2)$[15,35,41,73]
2. Arterial-alveolar oxygen tension ratio (a/A PO_2)[11,21,22,66,75]
3. Respiratory index (RI) = $P[A-a]O_2/PA_{O_2}$[23,56]
4. Pa_{O_2}/FI_{O_2} ratio[26]

The importance of these indices and the controversies surrounding their use in clinical practice are reflected in the many publications concerning their use and limitations.[9,26,27,59,82]

1. Analysis

The pulmonary shunt equation is used as a foundation upon which arterial oxygenation and gas exchange indices can be studied. It may be expressed as:

$$\frac{Qs}{Qt} = \frac{Cc'_{O_2} - Ca_{O_2}}{Cc'_{O_2} - C\overline{v}_{O_2}} \qquad (57)$$

where

Cc'_{O_2} = end-pulmonary capillary oxygen content
Ca_{O_2} = arterial oxygen content
$C\overline{v}_{O_2}$ = mixed venous oxygen content

By algebraic manipulation of the shunt equation, it is possible to relate arterial oxygen tension to its influencing factors[11,73]:

$$Pao_2 = PAO_2 - \frac{Ca-\bar{v}o_2 \times \dfrac{\dfrac{Qs}{Qt}}{1-\dfrac{Qs}{Qt}} - 1.34 \times (Sc'o_2 - Sao_2) \times Hb}{0.0031}$$

(58)

where PAO_2 (mm Hg) is the alveolar oxygen tension; $Ca-\bar{v}o_2$ (vol%) is the arterial-mixed venous oxygen content difference (= $CaO_2 - Co_2$), $Sc'o_2$ is end-pulmonary capillary fractional saturation, Sao_2 is the arterial saturation, and Hb is the blood hemoglobin concentration (g/dL). The full alveolar gas equation is used to determine PAO_2:

$$PAo_2 = \left(P_B - P_{H_2O}\right) \times Fio_2 - Paco_2 \times \left(Fio_2 + \frac{1 - Fio_2}{R}\right)$$ (59)

where P_B is the barometric pressure (assumed to be 760 mm Hg), P_{H_2O} is the patient's water vapor pressure (assumed to be 47 mm Hg), $Paco_2$ is the arterial CO_2 tension (usually assumed to be 40 mm Hg), and R is the gas exchange ratio (assumed to be 0.8).

Equation (58) does not explicitly show the influence of P_{50} on arterial oxygen tension; such influences are mediated indirectly, principally through the Sao_2 term. To make explicit the influence of Pao_2 and P_{50} on Sao_2, we use the relationship given by Hill[64]:

$$Sao_2 = \frac{Pao_2^n}{Pao_2^n + P_{50}^n}$$ (60)

where n is an empirical constant (generally taken as 2.65). A similar expression relates PAO_2, P_{50}, and $Sc'o_2$.

The arterial oxygen tension, the alveolar-arterial oxygen tension difference, and the arterial-alveolar oxygen tension ratio can then be obtained using equations (58), (59), and (60) for specific choices of physiologic variables. Unfortunately, equation (58) is not easily solved because it requires the solution of two simultaneous nonlinear equations (i.e., equations 58 and 60). In the past, a custom, computer-based successive approximation method was employed to obtain a solution. This amounted to iteratively making successively more accurate estimates of Pao_2 levels that met both equations (58) and (60). In the case of Doyle,[11] equation (58) was solved in this way to an accuracy of 0.1 mm Hg for various values of Hb, $Ca-\bar{v}o_2$, Fio_2, $Paco_2$, and Qs/Qt. The process is considerably simplified when TK SOLVER is used, as can be seen by examining the equation sheets presented in Figure 3-12.

F. EXAMPLE 2: THEORETICAL STUDY OF HEMOGLOBIN CONCENTRATION EFFECTS ON GAS EXCHANGE INDICES

It is of both theoretical and clinical interest to know what changes in gas exchange indices might be expected with changes in blood hemoglobin concentration when other physiologic parameters are kept constant. Figure 3-13 shows the results of varying hemoglobin concentration with the following parameters held constant: alveolar oxygen tension (PAO_2) = 100 mm Hg; cardiac output (CO) = 5 L/min; oxygen consumption ($\dot{V}o_2$) = 250 mL/min; shunt fraction (Qs/Qt) = 0.1; P_{50} (oxygen tension corresponding to 50% hemoglobin saturation) = 27 mm Hg.

As can be seen in Figure 3-13, increasing blood hemoglobin concentration would be expected to improve arterial oxygen tension and improve the gas exchange indices under study. Such data would be almost impossible to obtain experimentally because of the difficulty of varying blood hemoglobin concentration independent of other physiologic factors such as cardiac output.

G. EXAMPLE 3: MODELING THE OXYGENATION EFFECTS OF P_{50} CHANGES AT ALTITUDE

It is well known that the oxyhemoglobin dissociation curve may shift in response to physiologic changes. For example, acidosis, hypercarbia, increased temperature, and increased levels of 2,3-diphosphoglycerate (2,3-DPG) all shift the curve to the right, reducing hemoglobin affinity for oxygen and thereby facilitating its release into tissues. Also, with chronic anemia, intraerythrocyte 2,3-DPG levels increase, yielding a right-shifted oxyhemoglobin curve.[74] Because such a shift apparently increases oxygen release into tissues, teleologically it would also appear to be an appropriate response to high-altitude hypoxemia. In fact, however, the opposite appears to be true. Animals that have successfully adapted to high-altitude hypoxemia have left-shifted curves,[14,49] as do Sherpas.[25,50] In this example, we use computer modeling to develop a possible explanation for this finding.

It is proposed here that the reason that a left-shifted curve is beneficial in high-altitude hypoxemia is that it increases arterial oxygen content by virtue of increasing end-pulmonary capillary oxygen content. To demonstrate this, first suppose that a person has a pulmonary shunt fraction Qs/Qt. Then, from rearranging the preceding shunt equation, we can show that:

$$Cao_2 = Cc'o_2 - \frac{\dfrac{Qs}{Qt}}{1-\dfrac{Qs}{Qt}} \times Ca\bar{v}o_2$$ (61)

Thus, at constant pulmonary shunt and arteriovenous oxygen content difference, increases in end-pulmonary

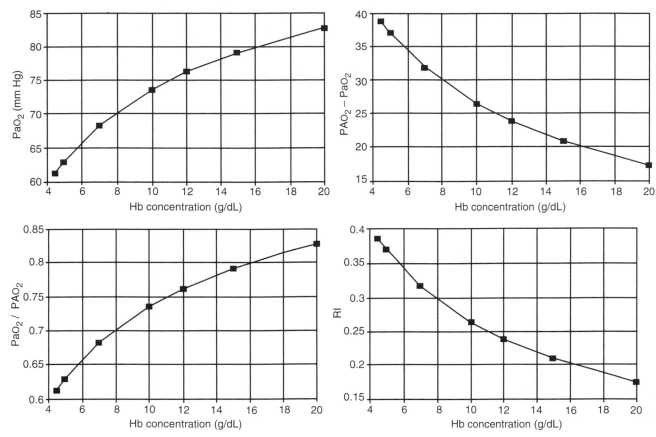

Figure 3-13 Effect of hemoglobin concentration on various gas exchange indices according to TK SOLVER model. *Top left,* Effect on arterial oxygen tension (PaO$_2$); *top right,* effect on alveolar-arterial oxygen tension difference (PAO$_2$ – PaO$_2$); *bottom left,* effect on arterial-alveolar oxygen tension ratio (PaO$_2$/PAO$_2$); *bottom right,* effect on the respiratory index (RI).

capillary oxygen content increase arterial oxygen content.

Now the end-pulmonary capillary oxygen content, Cc'O$_2$, consists of two terms, the first being the oxygen bound to hemoglobin and the second the oxygen dissolved in plasma:

$$Cc'O_2 = 1.34 \, Hb \, Sc'O_2 + 0.0031 \, PAO_2 \qquad (62)$$

where

Hb = hemoglobin concentration [g/dL]
Sc'O$_2$ = end-pulmonary capillary hemoglobin saturation
PAO$_2$ = alveolar oxygen tension [mm Hg]

PAO$_2$ is determined only by the alveolar gas equation and is independent of the oxyhemoglobin curve position.[34] Thus, the dissolved oxygen portion of Cc'O$_2$ is also independent of the curve position. However, the Sc'O$_2$ term does vary with curve position and increases with a left-shifted curve. Thus, Cc'O$_2$ also increases with a left shift and takes on a maximum value of:

$$[Cc'O_2]_{max} = 1.34 \, Hb + 0.0031 \, PAO_2 \qquad (63)$$

This analysis demonstrates that a left-shifted curve increases arterial oxygen content by increasing end-pulmonary capillary oxygen content.

1. Situation A

Consider a patient with high-altitude hypoxemia as a result of an alveolar oxygen tension (PAO$_2$) of 50 mm Hg. With a cardiac output of 5 L/min, hemoglobin concentration (Hb) of 15 g/dL, oxygen consumption (V̇O$_2$) of 250 mL/min, and shunt fraction (Qs/Qt) of 0.1, it can be shown (Table 3-6) that CaO$_2$ goes from 16.41 vol% with a P$_{50}$ of 27 mm Hg to 18.44 vol% with a P$_{50}$ of 18 mm Hg, a significant increase.

2. Situation B

Consider a patient with a large pulmonary shunt (Qs/Qt = 0.4), a normal alveolar oxygen tension (PAO$_2$ = 100 mm Hg), and other parameters as in situation A. Here CaO$_2$ goes from 16.47 vol% with a P$_{50}$ of 27 mm Hg to 16.87 vol% with a P$_{50}$ of 18 mm Hg, an insignificant change.

Figure 3-14 illustrates this concept in more detail, where the two examples are studied for P$_{50}$ values 10 to 50.

The numbers provided in situations A and B and in Figure 3-14 were obtained using the preceding mathematical computer model of the oxyhemoglobin dissociation curve. Hill's equation relating saturation, tension,

Table 3-6 **Oxygenation effects of P_{50} Changes at Altitude**

Oxygen Variable	Altitude Case*		Shunt Case	
	$P_{50} = 27$	$P_{50} = 18$	$P_{50} = 27$	$P_{50} = 18$
Pa_{O_2}	46.6	43.3	46.9	33.1
$P\bar{v}_{O_2}$	29.7	23.3	29.8	20.6
Sa_{O_2}	0.809	0.911	0.812	0.834
$S\bar{v}_{O_2}$	0.563	0.665	0.566	0.587
Sc_{O_2}	0.837	0.937	0.970	0.989
Ca_{O_2}	16.41	18.44	16.47	16.87
Cv_{O_2}	11.41	13.44	11.47	11.87
Cc'_{O_2}	16.99	19.00	19.80	20.20

*Detailed figures for altitude case ($PA_{O_2} = 50$ mm Hg) and for shunt case ($Qs/Qt = 0.4$). Other parameters are given in the text. Note that a shift from a P_{50} of 27 to a P_{50} of 18 significantly increases arterial oxygen content (Ca_{O_2}) in the altitude case but not in the shunt case.
From Benumof JL: Airway Management: Principles and Practice. St. Louis, Mosby, 1996, p 67.

and P_{50}[64] was used in conjunction with Doyle's equation for arterial oxygen tension[11] and solved using TK SOLVER.

These two example situations demonstrate that a left shift to the oxyhemoglobin dissociation curve significantly improves arterial oxygen content in the case of high-altitude hypoxemia but not in the case of large shunts. This observation is consistent with the fact that, with right-to-left shunts, such as those in cyanotic heart disease,

a right-shifted curve is the general finding.[37] In the latter case, a left-shifted curve is not beneficial because only a trivial improvement in end-pulmonary capillary oxygen content (and thus arterial oxygen content) is obtained. Teleologically, it may be argued that in the presence of hypoxemia, at approximately equal arterial contents, the body prefers higher oxygen tensions (right shift preferred), but if arterial oxygen content can be significantly improved, despite a decrease in oxygen tension, a left shift is preferred.

H. EXAMPLE 4: MATHEMATICAL/COMPUTER MODEL FOR EXTRACORPOREAL MEMBRANE OXYGENATION

Extracorporeal membrane oxygenation (ECMO) is sometimes used to treat respiratory failure refractory to more conservative measures.[81] Unfortunately, clinical experience with ECMO is limited, so that even clinicians familiar with ECMO may disagree about its potential benefits in a particular clinical setting. This is especially true when the patient has a high cardiac output (e.g., 20 L/min) and the ECMO pump is limited to much smaller flows (e.g., 5 L/min). In this example, we describe how a computer model may be designed to facilitate management decisions for patients being considered for venovenous ECMO.

A mathematic model of the venovenous ECMO situation may be developed on the basis of the shunt equation,[75] the Hill model for the oxyhemoglobin dissociation curve,[73] Doyle's equation for arterial oxygen tension as a function of cardiorespiratory parameters,[36] and

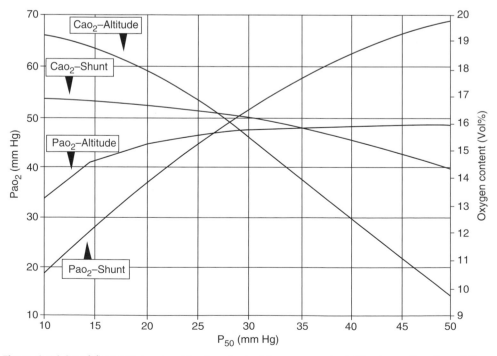

Figure 3-14 Arterial oxygen tension (Pa_{O_2}) and arterial oxygen content (Ca_{O_2}) as a function of P_{50} for cases depicted in situations A and B. Notice that in altitude hypoxemia case a decrease in P_{50} (left-shifted curve) significantly increases oxygen content but not in the shunt hypoxemia case. (From Doyle DJ: Simulation in medical education: Focus on anesthesiology. Can J Anaesth 39:A89, 1992.)

the schematic diagram for venovenous ECMO shown in Figure 3-15. The relevant equations are given in Figure 3-16. The model may be solved for various hypothetical clinical circumstances using an equation solver package. In this instance, we used EUREKA, a DOS-based commercial computer software package for solving systems of equations.

Some sample results are shown in Figure 3-17. Here, the patient's parameters are CO = 5 L/min; $\dot{V}O_2$ = 250 mL/min; Hb = 15 g/dL; Qs/Qt = 0.5; PAO_2 = 200 mm Hg; and an oxygenator oxygen tension output that results in complete hemoglobin saturation.

I. DISCUSSION

Many questions in physiology are not easily answered by direct experimentation, either because it is impractical, or impossible, to control all the pertinent variables or because of ethical considerations. In the case of studying the influence of blood hemoglobin concentration on pulmonary

gas exchange indices, it would be difficult to control rigorously cardiac output, total body oxygen consumption, and other variables to study the issue experimentally. The approach presented here offers several advantages.

1. It relies on well-established physiologic relationships (e.g., alveolar gas equation, pulmonary shunt equation).
2. It permits insight into physiologic issues not generally attainable in other ways.
3. It is inexpensive.
4. It potentially reduces the need to carry out animal experimentation.

Three drawbacks to the method exist:

1. The method is no better than the equations upon which it is based.
2. The method may not be convincing to some physiologists who may be satisfied only by confirmatory experimental results.
3. Errors can occur in model building.

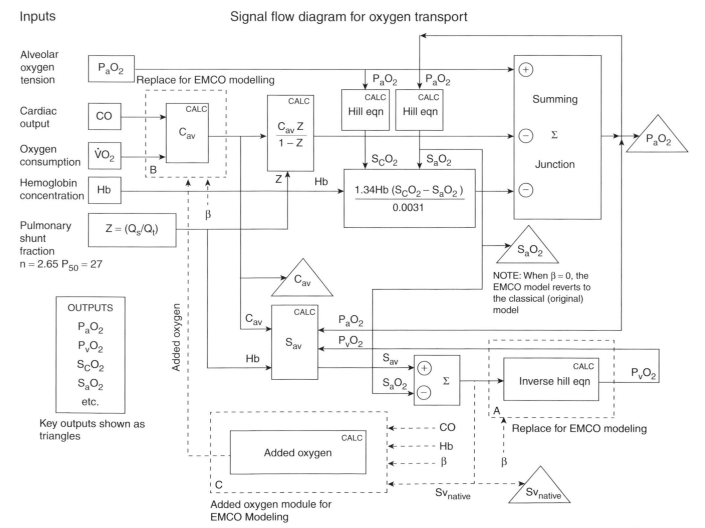

Figure 3-15 Schematic diagram for venovenous extracorporeal membrane oxygenation (ECMO) model. Schematic conceptual diagram for venovenous ECMO. Nomenclature: SVO$_2$, mixed oxygen saturation; Sao$_2$, arterial oxygen saturation; Sco$_2$, end pulmonary capillary oxygen saturation; Qs/Qt (Z), pulmonary shunt fraction; CO, cardiac output; $\dot{V}$O$_2$, oxygen consumption; PAO$_2$, alveolar oxygen tension (mm Hg); Pao$_2$, arterial oxygen tension (mm Hg); Hb, hemoglobin concentration (g/dL).

```
alpha=2.65      ; Hill's constant
beta= 0.75        ; beta is the ratio of ECMO flow to cardiac output
CO=5             ; cardiac output
Hb=15            ; hemoglobin concentration
VO2=250         ; oxygen consumption
PAO2=200       ; alveolar oxygen tension
Z=0.6             ; pulmonary shunt
; P50=27           ; a resonable value for P50
; consider oxygen added to body by ECMO machine
; addedO2 = beta*CO*10*(1.34*Hb*(1-SvO2native))
Cav=(VO2 - (beta*CO*13.4*Hb*(1-SvO2native)))/(10*CO)
SvO2=SaO2 - (Cav - 0.0031*(PaO2-PvO2))/(1.34*Hb)
PaO2=PAO2 - (Cav*(Z/(1-Z)) - 1.34*Hb*(SAO2-SaO2))/0.0031
PaO2:=85
SvO2native:=0.7
Cav:=0.8
SAO2=PAO2^alpha / (PAO2^alpha + 27^alpha)  ; Hill's equation
SaO2=PaO2^alpha / (PaO2^alpha + 27^alpha)  ; Hill's equation
PvO2=27*(SvO2 /(1-SvO2))^(1/alpha)  ; augmented mixed-venous PO2
PvO2native=27*(SvO2native/(1-SvO2native))^(1/alpha)
SvO2native=(SvO2-beta)/(1-beta)     ; SvO2 entering ECMO
PvO2>=PvO2native
PAO2>PaO2 >0
SvO2>=SvO2native>0
SvO2native<1
```

Figure 3-16 Equations for venovenous extracorporeal membrane oxygenation (ECMO) model. Equations for venovenous ECMO problem, this time using EUREKA, an equation solver similar to TK SOLVER but somewhat easier to learn. First seven lines indicate the values of physiologic parameters that are held constant. Next three lines are comments to user and are not used by EUREKA. Lines 11 to 13 and 17 to 21 list basic equations to be solved. Lines 22 to 25 give some physiologic constraints that cannot be violated (e.g., arterial oxygen tension must be less than alveolar oxygen tension). Lines 14 to 16 provide initial estimates for EUREKA's iterative solver. (EUREKA is also available in a shareware version known as Mercury, which runs under MS-DOS.) (Adapted from Doyle DJ: Computer model for veno-veno extracorporeal membrane oxygenation. Can J Anaesth 39:A34, 1992.)

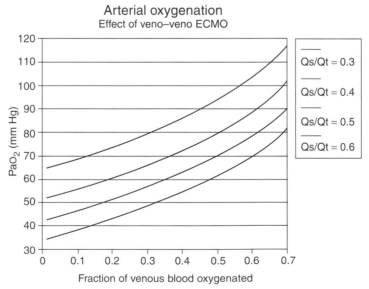

Figure 3-17 Sample results for venovenous extracorporeal membrane oxygenation (ECMO) model for various levels of relative flow through ECMO oxygenator. Plot of arterial oxygen tension (PaO_2) as function of fraction of venous blood that passes through ECMO oxygenator for various values of pulmonary shunt fraction (Qs/Qt [Z]). (Adapted from Doyle DJ: Computer model for veno-veno extracorporeal membrane oxygenation. Can J Anaesth 39:A34, 1992.)

One potential difficulty with such modeling methods is that the results obtained depend critically on the equations used. In cases in which the equations are known from first principles (e.g., alveolar gas equation, pulmonary shunt equation), this is not an issue, but where an equation is empirical, alternative equations may possibly produce different results. An example here is the equation for the oxyhemoglobin dissociation curve, which has many competing formulations.[2,37,42,64,65] In this example we used the formulation given by Hill.[64]

J. UTILITY

Where can such a model be useful? In a particular patient with severe adult respiratory distress syndrome and resulting severe hypoxemia, clinicians might be interested in knowing, for instance, how ECMO would be expected to improve oxygenation. From pulmonary artery catheterization and arterial blood samples one can obtain the following and other data relevant to carrying out oxygen transport modeling:

1. Hemoglobin concentration
2. Cardiac output
3. P_{50} on dissociation curve
4. Arterial and mixed venous (arterial blood gas) data

On the basis of a model constructed for that time point, one could explore, for example, the effect of augmenting cardiac output and mixed venous oxygen tension in the ECMO situation. Without a model to describe this problem, the best we can do is fit empirical curves to experimental data. However, with a model, one can easily ask "what if" questions: for example, what happens when the ratio of pump oxygenator flow to cardiac output is set at a particular value.[74]

A good example is one question in respiratory physiology: How does a patient's alveolar-arterial oxygen tension difference change with reduced inspired oxygen tension? The first attempt at this question used pulse oximetry to infer arterial oxygen tension in volunteers subjected to controlled hypoxia by rebreathing.[14] A subsequent study took a more direct approach by cannulating the radial artery of elderly respiratory patient volunteers and drawing off serial arterial blood samples as the patients were subjected to hypoxemia in a hypobaric chamber.[49] The latter study is sufficiently invasive (and even, perhaps, sufficiently risky) that many hospital ethics committees would not approve it under existing guidelines.

Where more than one set of equations exists to describe a physiologic relationship, one can explore the effect of equation choice. One would expect, however, that, if several equations existed that all did a good job of representing the underlying data, equation choice would not have a great influence on the results obtained. In the case of a few days (or even a few hours), one can obtain meaningful information about the interaction of several physiologic variables, provided that the relationships

describing the variables are available in equation form. By contrast, actual experimentation takes time, funds, and effort that may not always be available. In fields such as oxygen transport, many relevant equations are simple well-known physiologic principles written in equation form, such as the following:

1. Alveolar gas equation
2. Pulmonary shunt equation
3. Oxyhemoglobin dissociation curve
4. Oxygen transport parameter definitions

To the extent that one accepts these physiologic principles, the results obtained should also be credible (provided that model design and implementation have been done correctly). In this respect, three issues exist:

1. How meaningful are the equations used? Are they a mathematical form of a well-known physiologic principle?
2. How accurate are the equations in describing the data they are based on?
3. Has the model been appropriately designed and implemented?

K. SOFTWARE

Several platforms exist to do such computations in the IBM-PC environment. TK SOLVER is still available (in a "Plus" form) from software distributors but does not have the market share of MATHCAD, a widely available, popular mathematic modeling package with strong graphical features. MATHCAD has equation-solving features similar to those of TK SOLVER that would make it appropriate for mathematic model building. Another suitable package would be Mercury, a shareware equation solver derived from EUREKA (Borland). All these packages take some effort to master. In particular, the manner in which each package handles convergence to solution greatly affects ease of use and reliability. In general, the three packages mentioned (TK SOLVER, MATHCAD, and Mercury) work reasonably well with some effort. However, it is more difficult to do this modeling using ordinary computer spreadsheets (e.g., early releases of Lotus 1-2-3): first, because it is somewhat awkward for working with equations; and, second, because most spreadsheets are not set up to handle complicated iterative equation solving.

TK SOLVER is available from Universal Technical Systems, Inc., 1220 Rock Street, Rockford, Illinois, USA. Tel: (815) 963-2220 Fax: (815) 963-8884.

L. COMPUTATIONAL FLOW DIAGRAMS

The representation of mathematic models for complex physiologic systems can sometimes be facilitated by representing the relevant equations using a computational flow diagram. The concept is most easily understood by reviewing the examples mentioned previously.

Example 1. Computation of the alveolar-arterial oxygen tension gradient
Example 2. Computation of alveolar oxygen tension
Example 3. Computation of arterial oxygen tension
Example 4. Modeling the effects of venovenous ECMO

Note that where the examples involve feedback (examples 3 and 4), special iterative methods are necessary to obtain a solution. Not all spreadsheets are able to do this.

VIII. SELECTED DIMENSIONAL EQUIVALENTS

Discussions regarding physics in anesthesia may be confusing because of the variety of units used in the clinical literature. The following list is a compilation of the units and their equivalents that one is likely to encounter.

Length

1 m = 3.2808 ft = 39.37 in
1 ft = 0.3048 m
1 m = 100 cm = 1000 mm = 1,000,000 μm = 10,000,000 Å = 10^{-3} km
1 km = 0.621 mi
1 in = 2.54 cm = 0.254 m

Volume

1 US gal = 0.133 68 ft^3 = 3.785 541 L
1 Imp gal = 4.546 092 L
1 m^3 = 1000 L
1 mL = 1 cm^3

Mass

1 kg = 1000 g = 2.2046 lbm = 0.068 521 slugs
1 lbm = 0.453 592 kg
1 slug = 1 lbf $\times$ s^2/ft = 32.174 lbm

Force

1 lbf = 4.448 222 N = 4.448 $\times$ 10^5 dynes
1 N = 1 kg $\times$ m/s^2 = 10,000 dynes = 10,000 g $\times$ cm/s^2

Pressure

1 N/m^2 = 10 dynes/cm^2 = 1 Pa = 0.007 501 mm Hg
1 atmosphere = 1013.25 millibars = 760 mm Hg = 101 325 Pa = 14.696 lbf/in^2
1 cm H_2O = 0.735 mm Hg
1 lbf/in^2 = 51.71 mm Hg
1 dyne/cm^2 = 0.1 Pa = 145.04 $\times$ 10^{-7} lbf/in^2
1 bar = 10^5 N/m^2 = 14.504 lbf/in^2 = 10^6 dynes/cm^2

Viscosity

1 kg/(m $\times$ s) = 1 N $\times$ s/m^2 = 0.6729 lbm/(ft $\times$ s) = 10 poise

Energy

1 joule (J) = 1 kg $\times$ m^2/s^2
1 Btu = 778.16 ft $\times$ lbf = 1055.056 J = 252 cal = 1.055 $\times$ 10^{10} ergs
1 cal = 4.1868 J

Power

1 watt (W) = 1 kg $\times$ m^2/s^3 = 1 J/s
1 hp = 550 ft $\times$ lbf/s = 745.699 W

REFERENCES

1. Aalto-Setala M, Heinonen J: Resistance to gas-flow of endobronchial tubes. Ann Chir Gynaecol Fenn 62:271, 1973.
2. Aberman A, Cavanilles JM, Trotter J, et al: An equation for the oxygen-hemoglobin dissociation curve. J Appl Physiol 35:750, 1973.
3. Askeland DR: The Science and Engineering of Materials, 2nd ed. Boston, PWS-Kent, 1989.
4. Beatty PC, Healy TE: The additional work of breathing through Portex Polar Blue-Line preformed paediatric tracheal tubes. Eur J Anaesthesiol 9:77, 1992.
5. Benumof JL, Scheller MS: The importance of transtracheal jet ventilation in the management of the difficult airway. Anesthesiology 71:769, 1989.
6. Bolder PM, Healy TEJ, Bolder AR, et al: The extra work of breathing through adult endotracheal tubes. Anesth Analg 65:853, 1986.
7. Boltz RE, Tuve GL (eds): CRC Handbook of Tables for Applied Engineering Science, 2nd ed. Cleveland, CRC Press, 1973.
8. Boretos JW, Battig CG, Goodman L: Decreased resistance to breathing through a polyurethane pediatric endotracheal tube. Anesth Analg 51:292, 1972.
9. Covell HD, Nessan VJ, Tuttle WK: Oxygen derived variables in acute respiratory failure. Crit Care Med 11:646, 1983.
10. Delaney WA, Kaiser RE: Percutaneous transtracheal jet ventilation made easy. Anesthesiology 74:952, 1991.
11. Doyle DJ: Arterial/alveolar oxygen tension ratio: A critical appraisal. Can Anaesth Soc J 33:471, 1986.
12. Doyle DJ, Zawacki J: Importance of catheter resistance in transtracheal jet ventilation. Can J Anaesth 40:A37, 1993.
13. Duncan PG: Efficacy of helium-oxygen mixtures in the management of severe viral and postintubation croup. Can Anaesth Soc J 26:206, 1979.
14. Eaton JW, Skelton TD, Berger E: Survival at extreme altitude: Protective effect of increased hemoglobin-oxygen affinity. Science 183:743, 1974.
15. Farhi LE, Rahn HA: A theoretical analysis of the alveolar-arterial O_2 difference with special reference to the distribution effect. J Appl Physiol 7:699, 1955.
16. Fawcett WJ, Ooi R, Riley B: The work of breathing through large-bore intravascular catheters. Anesthesiology 76:323, 1992.

17. Ferris BG, Mead J, Opie LH: Partitioning of respiratory flow resistance in man. J Appl Physiol 19:653, 1964.

18. Gaensler EA, Maloney JV, Bjork VO: Bronchospirometry. II. Experimental observations and theoretical considerations of resistance breathing. J Lab Clin Med 39:935, 1952.

19. Gal TJ: Pulmonary mechanics in normal subjects following endotracheal intubation. Anesthesiology 52:27, 1980.

20. Gal TJ, Suratt PM: Resistance to breathing in healthy subjects following endotracheal intubation under topical anesthesia. Anesth Analg 59:270, 1980.

21. Gilbert R, Auchincloss JH, Kuppinger M, et al: Stability of the arterial/alveolar oxygen partial pressure ratio: Effects of low ventilation/perfusion regions. Crit Care Med 7:267, 1979.

22. Gilbert R, Keighley JF: The arterial/alveolar oxygen tension ratio: An index of gas exchange applicable to varying inspired oxygen concentrations. Am Rev Respir Dis 109:142, 1974.

23. Goldfarb MA, Ciurej TF, McAslan TC, et al: Tracking respiratory therapy in the trauma patient. Am J Surg 129:255, 1975.

24. Gottfried SP, Emili JM: Noninvasive monitoring of respiratory mechanics. In Nochomovitz ML, Cherniac NS (eds): Noninvasive Respiratory Monitoring. New York, Churchill Livingstone, 1986.

25. Hebbel RP, Eaton JW, Kronenberg RS, et al: Human llamas: Adaptation to altitude in subjects with high hemoglobin oxygen affinity. J Clin Invest 62:593, 1978.

26. Hegyi T, Hiatt IM: Respiratory index: A simple evaluation of severity of idiopathic respiratory distress syndrome. Crit Care Med 7:500, 1979.

27. Herrick IA, Champion LK, Froese AB: A clinical comparison of indices of pulmonary gas exchange with changes in the inspired oxygen concentration. Can J Anaesth 37:69, 1990.

28. Hicks GH: Monitoring respiratory mechanics. Probl Respir Care 2:191, 1989.

29. Hill DW: Physics Applied to Anaesthesia, 3rd ed. London, Butterworths, 1976.

30. Hill DW: Physics applied to anaesthesia. VI. Gases and vapours. Br J Anaesth 38:753, 1966.

31. Ho AM, Lee A, Karmakar MK, et al: Heliox vs air-oxygen mixtures for the treatment of patients with acute asthma: A systematic overview. Chest 123:882, 2003.

32. Holst M, Striem J, Hedenstierna G: Errors in tracheal pressure recording in patients with a tracheostomy tube: A model study. Intensive Care Med 16:384, 1990.

33. James MFM, White JF: Anesthetic considerations at moderate altitude. Anesth Analg 63:1097, 1984.

34. Jones N: Blood Gases and Acid-Base Physiology. New York, Thieme-Stratton, 1980.

35. Kanber GJ, King FW, Eschar YR, et al: The alveolar-arterial oxygen gradient in young and elderly men during air and oxygen breathing. Am Rev Respir Dis 97:376, 1968.

36. Kelman GR, Nunn JF, Prys-Roberts C: The influence of cardiac output on arterial oxygenation: A theoretical study. Br J Anesth 39:450, 1967.

37. Kelman GR: Digital computer subroutine for the conversion of oxygen tension into saturation. J Appl Physiol 21:1375, 1966.

38. Kemper KJ, Ritz RH, Benson MS, Bishop MS: Helium-oxygen mixture in the treatment of postextubation stridor in pediatric trauma patients, Crit Care Med 19:356, 1991.

39. Khanlou H. Eiger G: Safety and efficacy of heliox as a treatment for upper airway obstruction due to radiation-induced laryngeal dysfunction. Heart Lung 30:146, 2001.

40. Konopasek M, Jayaraman S: Constant and declarative languages for engineering applications: The TK Solver contribution. Proc IEEE 73:1791, 1985.

41. Konopasek M, Jayaraman S: The TK Solver Book: A Guide to Problem-Solving in Science, Engineering, Business and Education. Berkeley, Calif, Osborne/McGraw-Hill, 1984.

42. Lobdell DD: An invertible simple equation for computation of blood O_2 dissociation relations. J Appl Physiol 50:971, 1981.

43. Lough MD, Chathurn R, Schrock WA: In Handbook of Respiratory Care. Chicago, Year Book, 1983.

44. Lu TS, Ohmura A, Wong KC, et al: Helium-oxygen in treatment of upper airway obstruction. Anesthesiology 45:678, 1976.

45. Mahan BM, Myers RJ: University Chemistry, 4th ed. Don Mills, Ontario, Benjamin/Cummings, 1987.

46. Manczur T, Greenough A, Nicholson GP, Rafferty GF: Resistance of pediatric and neonatal endotracheal tubes: Influence of flow rate, size, and shape. Crit Care Med 28:1595, 2000.

47. Meyer PD: Emergency transtracheal jet ventilation. Anesthesiology 73:787, 1990.

48. Michels A, Landser FJ, Cauberghs M, et al: Measurement of total respiratory impedance via the endotracheal tube: A model study. Bull Eur Physiopathol Respir 22:615, 1986.

49. Monge C, Wittembury J: Increased hemoglobin-oxygen affinity at extremely high altitudes. Science 186:843, 1974.

50. Morpurgo G, Arese P, Bosia A, et al: Sherpas living permanently at high altitude: A new pattern of adaptation. Proc Natl Acad Sci USA 73:747, 1976.

51. Mullins JB, Templer JW, Kong J, et al: Airway resistance and work of breathing in tracheostomy tubes. Laryngoscope 103:1367, 1993.

52. Murray JF: The Normal Lung: The Basis for Diagnosis and Treatment of Pulmonary Disease, 2nd ed. Philadelphia, WB Saunders, 1986.

53. Nadel JA: Mechanisms controlling airway size. Arch Environ Health 7:179, 1963.

54. Ooi R, Fawcett WJ, Soni N, et al: Extra inspiratory work of breathing imposed by cricothyrotomy devices. Br J Anaesth 70:17, 1993. Erratum in: Br J Anaesth 70:494, 1993.

55. Pappenheimer JR, Comroe JH, Cournand A, et al: Standardization of definitions and symbols in respiratory physiology. Fed Proc 34:315, 1950.

56. Perez LV, Boix JH, Salom JV, et al: Clinical use of the arterial/alveolar oxygen tension ratio. Crit Care Med 11:999, 1983.

57. Petros AJ, Lamond CT, Bennett D: The Bicore pulmonary monitor: A device to assess the work of breathing while weaning from mechanical ventilation. Anaesthesia 48:985, 1993.

58. Polaner DM: The use of heliox and the laryngeal mask airway in a child with an anterior mediastinal mass. Anesth Analg 82:208, 1996.

59. Rasanen J, Downs JB, Malec DJ, et al: Oxygen tensions and oxyhemoglobin saturations in the assessment of pulmonary gas exchange. Crit Care Med 15:1058, 1987.

60. Reynolds WC, Perkins HC: Engineering Thermodynamics, 2nd ed. New York, McGraw-Hill, 1977.

61. Rodgers E: TK Solver: A new concept in problem solving software. PC World 1(4):93, 1983.

62. Rodrigo GJ, Rodrigo C, Pollack CV, Rowe B: Use of helium-oxygen mixtures in the treatment of acute asthma: A systematic review. Chest 123:891, 2003.

63. Rudow M, Hill AB, Thompson NW, et al: Helium-oxygen mixtures in airway obstruction due to thyroid carcinoma. Can Anaesth Soc J 33:498, 1986.

64. Schnider AJ, Stockman JA, Oski FA: Transfusion nomogram: An application of physiology to clinical decisions regarding the use of blood. Crit Care Med 9:469, 1981.

65. Severinghaus JW: Simple accurate equation for human blood O_2 dissociation computations. J Appl Physiol 46:599, 1979.

66. Shapiro AR, Virgilio RW, Peters RM: Interpretation of alveolar-arterial oxygen tension difference. Surg Gynecol Obstet 144:547, 1977.

67. Sherwood L: Human Physiology: From Cells to Systems, 2nd ed. St Paul, Minn, West Publishing, 1993.

68. Shikora SA, Bistrian BR, Borlase BC, et al: Work of breathing: Reliable predictor of weaning and extubation. Crit Care Med 18:157, 1990.

69. Skyrinskas GJ, Hyland RH, Hutcheon MA: Using helium-oxygen mixtures in the management of acute upper airway obstruction. Can Med Assoc J 128:555, 1983.

70. Sprague DH: Transtracheal jet oxygenator from capnographic monitoring components. Anesthesiology 73:788, 1990.

71. Straus C, Louis B, Isabey D, et al: Contribution of the endotracheal tube and the upper airway to breathing workload. Am J Respir Crit Care Med 157:23, 1998.

72. Streeter VL, Wylie EB: Fluid Mechanics, 8th ed. New York, McGraw-Hill, 1985.

73. Torda TA: Alveolar-arterial oxygen tension difference: A critical look. Anaesth Intensive Care 9:326, 1981.

74. Torrance J, Jacobs P, Restrepo A, et al: Intraerythrocytic adaptation to anemia. N Engl J Med 283:165, 1970.

75. Viale JP, Carlisle CJ, Annat G, et al: Arterial-alveolar oxygen partial pressure ratio: A theoretical reappraisal. Crit Care Med 14:153, 1986.

76. Wall MA: Infant endotracheal tube resistance: Effects of changing length, diameter, and gas density. Crit Care Med 8:38, 1980.

77. Weast RC (ed): CRC Handbook of Chemistry and Physics: Student Edition. Boca Raton, Fla, CRC Press, 1988.

78. Weissman C, Askanazi J, Rosenbaum SH, et al: Response to tubular airway resistance in normal subjects and postoperative patients. Anesthesiology 64:353, 1986.

79. White FM: Fluid Mechanics, 2nd ed. New York, McGraw Hill, 1986.

80. Wright PE, Marini JJ, Bernard GR: In vitro versus in vivo comparison of endotracheal tube airflow resistance. Am Rev Respir Dis 140:10, 1989.

81. Zapol W, Snider MT, Hill JD, et al: Extracorporeal membrane oxygenation in severe acute respiratory failure: A randomized prospective study. JAMA 242:2193, 1979.

82. Zetterstrom H: Assessment of the efficiency of pulmonary oxygenation: The choice of oxygenation index. Acta Anaesthesiol Scand 32:579, 1988.

83. Zin WA, Pengelly LD, Millic-Emili J: Single breath method for measurement of respiratory mechanics in anaesthetized animals. J Appl Physiol 52:1266, 1982.

84. Zuck D: Osborne Reynolds, 1842-1912, and the flow of fluids through tubes. Br J Anaesth 43:1175, 1971.

4

PHYSIOLOGY OF THE AIRWAY*

William C. Wilson
Jonathan L. Benumof

*Adapted from Miller: Anesthesia, 6th ed. Philadelphia, Churchill Livingstone Elsevier, 2004, pp 679-722.

I. RESPIRATORY PHYSIOLOGY

Anesthesiologists require an extensive knowledge of respiratory physiology to care for patients in the operating room and the intensive care unit. Mastery of the normal respiratory physiologic processes is a prerequisite to understanding the mechanisms of impaired gas exchange that occur during anesthesia and surgery and with disease. This chapter is divided into two sections. The first section reviews the normal (gravity-determined) distribution of perfusion and ventilation, the major nongravitational determinants of resistance to perfusion and ventilation, transport of respiratory gases, and the pulmonary reflexes and special functions of the lung. In the second section of this chapter, these processes and concepts are discussed in relation to the general mechanisms of impaired gas exchange during anesthesia and surgery.

A. NORMAL (GRAVITY-DETERMINED) DISTRIBUTION OF PERFUSION, VENTILATION, AND THE VENTILATION-PERFUSION RATIO

1. Distribution of Pulmonary Perfusion

Contraction of the right ventricle imparts kinetic energy to the blood in the main pulmonary artery. As the kinetic energy in the main pulmonary artery is dissipated in climbing a vertical hydrostatic gradient, the absolute pressure in the pulmonary artery (Ppa) decreases by 1 cm H_2O per centimeter of vertical distance up the lung (Fig. 4-1). At some height above the heart, Ppa becomes zero (atmospheric), and still higher in the lung, Ppa becomes negative.[197] In this region, alveolar pressure (PA) then exceeds Ppa and pulmonary venous pressure (Ppv), which is very negative at this vertical height. Because the pressure outside the vessels is greater than the pressure inside the vessels, the vessels in this region of the lung are collapsed, and no blood flow occurs (zone 1, PA > Ppa > Ppv). Because there is no blood flow, no gas exchange is possible, and the region functions as alveolar dead space, or "wasted" ventilation. Little or no zone 1 exists in the lung under normal conditions,[148] but the amount of zone 1 lung may be greatly increased if Ppa is reduced, as in oligemic shock, or if PA is increased, as in the application of excessively large tidal volumes or levels of positive end-expiratory pressure (PEEP) during positive-pressure ventilation.

Further down the lung, absolute Ppa becomes positive, and blood flow begins when Ppa exceeds PA (zone 2, Ppa > PA > Ppv). At this vertical level in the lung, PA exceeds Ppv, and blood flow is determined by the mean Ppa − PA difference rather than by the more conventional Ppa − Ppv difference (see later).[141] The zone 2 blood flow–alveolar pressure relationship has the same physical characteristics as a waterfall flowing over a dam. The height of the upstream river (before reaching the dam) is equivalent to Ppa, and the height of the dam is equivalent to PA. The rate of water flow over the dam is proportional to only the difference between the height of the upstream river and the dam (Ppa − PA), and it does not matter how far below the dam the downstream riverbed (Ppv) is. This phenomenon has various names, including the waterfall, Starling resistor, weir (dam made by beavers), and "sluice" effect. Because mean Ppa increases down this region of the lung but mean PA is relatively constant, the mean driving pressure (Ppa − PA) increases linearly, and therefore mean blood flow increases linearly.

The four zones of the lung

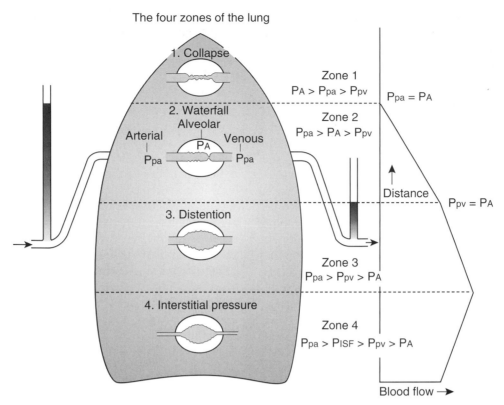

Figure 4-1 Schematic diagram showing the distribution of blood flow in the upright lung. In zone 1, alveolar pressure (PA) exceeds pulmonary artery pressure (Ppa), and no flow occurs because the intra-alveolar vessels are collapsed by the compressing alveolar pressure. In zone 2, Ppa exceeds PA, but PA exceeds pulmonary venous pressure (Ppv). Flow in zone 2 is determined by the Ppa-PA difference (Ppa − PA) and has been likened to an upstream river waterfall over a dam. Because Ppa increases down zone 2 whereas PA remains constant, perfusion pressure increases, and flow steadily increases down the zone. In zone 3, Ppv exceeds PA, and flow is determined by the Ppa-Ppv difference (Ppa − Ppv), which is constant down this portion of the lung. However, transmural pressure across the wall of the vessel increases down this zone, so the caliber of the vessels increases (resistance decreases), and therefore flow increases. Finally, in zone 4, pulmonary interstitial pressure becomes positive and exceeds both Ppv and PA. Consequently, flow in zone 4 is determined by the Ppa–interstitial pressure difference (Ppa − PISF). (Redrawn with modification from West JB: Ventilation/Blood Flow and Gas Exchange, 4th ed. Oxford, Blackwell Scientific, 1970.)

However, respiration and pulmonary blood flow are cyclic phenomena. Therefore, absolute instantaneous Ppa, Ppv, and PA are changing continuously, and the relationships among Ppa, Ppv, and PA are dynamically determined by the phase lags between the cardiac and respiratory cycles. Consequently, a given point in zone 2 may actually be in either a zone 1 or a zone 3 condition at a given moment, depending on whether the patient is in respiratory systole or diastole or in cardiac systole or diastole.

Still lower in the lung, there is a vertical level at which Ppv becomes positive and also exceeds PA. In this region, blood flow is governed by the pulmonary arteriovenous pressure difference (Ppa − Ppv) (zone 3, Ppa > Ppv > PA), for here both these vascular pressures exceed PA, and the capillary systems are thus permanently open and blood flow is continuous. In descending zone 3, gravity causes both absolute Ppa and Ppv to increase at the same rate, so perfusion pressure (Ppa − Ppv) is unchanged. However, the pressure outside the vessels, namely, pleural pressure (Ppl), increases less than Ppa and Ppv, so the

transmural distending pressures (Ppa − Ppl and Ppv − Ppl) increase down zone 3, the vessel radii increase, vascular resistance decreases, and blood flow therefore increases further.

Finally, whenever pulmonary vascular pressures (Ppa) are extremely high, as they are in a severely volume-overloaded patient, in a severely restricted and constricted pulmonary vascular bed, in an extremely dependent lung (far below the vertical level of the left atrium), and in patients with pulmonary embolism or mitral stenosis, fluid may transude out of the pulmonary vessels into the pulmonary interstitial compartment. In addition, pulmonary interstitial edema can be caused by extremely negative Ppl and perivascular hydrostatic pressure, such as may occur in a vigorously spontaneously breathing patient with an obstructed airway (upper airway masses [tumors, hematoma, abscess, edema], laryngospasm [most common], strangulation, infectious processes [epiglottitis, pharyngitis, croup], and vocal cord paralysis), by rapid reexpansion of lung, and by the application of very negative Ppl during thoracentesis.[21,121] Transuded pulmonary interstitial fluid may significantly alter the distribution of pulmonary blood flow.

When the flow of fluid into the interstitial space is excessive and the fluid cannot be cleared adequately by the lymphatics, it accumulates in the interstitial connective tissue compartment around the large vessels and airways and forms peribronchial and periarteriolar edema fluid cuffs. The transuded pulmonary interstitial fluid fills the pulmonary interstitial space and may eliminate the normally present negative and radially expanding interstitial tension on the extra-alveolar pulmonary vessels. Expansion of the pulmonary interstitial space by fluid causes pulmonary interstitial pressure (PISF) to become positive and exceed Ppv (zone 4, Ppa > PISF > Ppv > PA).[194,196] In addition, the vascular resistance of extra-alveolar vessels may be increased at a very low lung volume (i.e., residual volume); at such volumes the tethering action of the pulmonary tissue on the vessels is also lost, and as a result, PISF increases positively (see the lung volume discussion later).[88,89] Consequently, zone 4 blood flow is governed by the arteriointerstitial pressure difference (Ppa – PISF), which is less than the Ppa – Ppv difference, and therefore zone 4 blood flow is less than zone 3 blood flow. In summary, zone 4 is a region of the lung from which a large amount of fluid has transuded into the pulmonary interstitial compartment or is possibly at a very low lung volume. Both these circumstances produce positive interstitial pressure, which causes compression of extra-alveolar vessels, increased extra-alveolar vascular resistance, and decreased regional blood flow.

It should be evident that as Ppa and Ppv increase, three important changes take place in the pulmonary circulation, namely, recruitment or opening of previously unperfused vessels, distention or widening of previously perfused vessels, and transudation of fluid from very distended vessels.[119,142] Thus, as mean Ppa increases, zone 1 arteries may become zone 2 arteries, and as mean Ppv increases, zone 2 veins may become zone 3 veins. The increase in both mean Ppa and Ppv distends zone 3 vessels according to their compliance and decreases the resistance to flow through them. Zone 3 vessels may become so distended that they leak fluid and become converted to zone 4 vessels. In general, recruitment is the principal change as Ppa and Ppv increase from low to moderate levels, distention is the principal change as Ppa and Ppv increase from moderate to high levels, and transudation is the principal change when Ppa and Ppv increase from high to very high levels.

2. Distribution of Ventilation

Gravity also causes differences in vertical Ppl, which in turn causes differences in regional alveolar volume, compliance, and ventilation. The vertical gradient of Ppl can best be understood by imagining the lung as a plastic bag filled with semifluid contents; in other words,

it is a viscoelastic structure. Without the presence of a supporting chest wall, the effect of gravity on the contents of the bag would cause the bag to bulge outward at the bottom and inward at the top (it would assume a globular shape). With the lung inside the supporting chest wall, the lung cannot assume a globular shape. However, gravity still exerts a force on the lung to assume a globular shape; this force creates relatively more negative pressure at the top of the pleural space (where the lung pulls away from the chest wall) and relatively more positive pressure at the bottom of the lung (where the lung is compressed against the chest wall) (Fig. 4-2). The density of the lung determines the magnitude of this pressure gradient. Because the lung has about one fourth the density of water, the gradient of Ppl (in cm H_2O) is about one fourth the height of the upright lung (30 cm). Thus, Ppl increases positively by $30/4 = 7.5$ cm H_2O from the top to the bottom of the lung.[84]

Because PA is the same throughout the lung, the Ppl gradient causes regional differences in transpulmonary distending pressure (PA – Ppl). Ppl is most positive (least negative) in the dependent basilar lung regions, so alveoli in these regions are more compressed and are therefore considerably smaller than the superior, relatively noncompressed apical alveoli (there is an approximately fourfold volume difference).[124] If regional differences in alveolar volume are translated to a pressure-volume curve for normal lung (Fig. 4-3), the dependent small alveoli are on the midportion and the nondependent

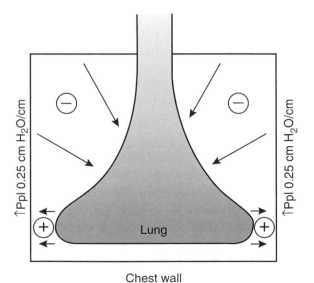

Figure 4-2 Schematic diagram of the lung within the chest wall showing the tendency of the lung to assume a globular shape because of gravity and the lung's viscoelastic nature. The tendency of the top of the lung to collapse inward creates a relatively negative pressure at the apex of the lung, and the tendency of the bottom of the lung to spread outward creates a relatively positive pressure at the base of the lung. Thus, alveoli at the top of the lung tend to be held open and are larger at end exhalation, whereas those at the bottom tend to be smaller and compressed at end exhalation. Pleural pressure increases by 0.25 cm H_2O per centimeter of lung dependence.

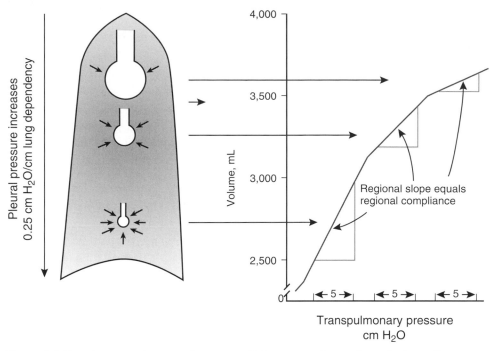

Figure 4-3 Pleural pressure increases by 0.25 cm H_2O every centimeter down the lung. The increase in pleural pressure causes a fourfold decrease in alveolar volume from the top of the lung to the bottom. The caliber of the air passages also decreases as lung volume decreases. When regional alveolar volume is translated over to a regional transpulmonary pressure–alveolar volume curve, small alveoli are on a steep (large slope) portion of the curve, and large alveoli are on a flat (small slope) portion of the curve. Because the regional slope equals regional compliance, the dependent small alveoli normally receive the largest share of the tidal volume. Over the normal tidal volume range (lung volume increases by 500 mL from 2500 mL [normal functional residual capacity] to 3000 mL), the pressure-volume relationship is linear. The lung volume values in this diagram are derived from the upright position.

large alveoli are on the upper portion of the S-shaped pressure-volume curve. Because the different regional slopes of the composite curve are equal to the different regional lung compliance values, dependent alveoli are relatively compliant (steep slope), and nondependent alveoli are relatively noncompliant (flat slope). Thus, most of the tidal volume (VT) is preferentially distributed to dependent alveoli because they expand more per unit pressure change than nondependent alveoli do.

3. Distribution of the Ventilation-Perfusion Ratio

Both blood flow and ventilation (both on the left-hand vertical axis of Fig. 4-4) increase linearly with distance down the normal upright lung (horizontal axis, reverse polarity).[195] Because blood flow increases from a very low value and more rapidly than ventilation does with distance down the lung, the ventilation-perfusion ($\dot{V}A/\dot{Q}$) ratio (right-hand vertical axis) decreases rapidly at first and then more slowly.

The $\dot{V}A/\dot{Q}$ ratio best expresses the amount of ventilation relative to perfusion in any given lung region. Thus, alveoli at the base of the lung are overperfused in relation to their ventilation ($\dot{V}A/\dot{Q} < 1$). Figure 4-5 shows the calculated ventilation ($\dot{V}A$) and blood flow ($\dot{Q}$) in liters per minute, the $\dot{V}A/\dot{Q}$ ratio, and the alveolar

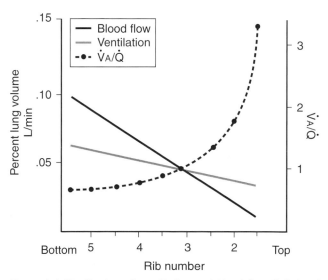

Figure 4-4 Distribution of ventilation and blood flow (left-hand vertical axis) and the ventilation-perfusion ratio ($\dot{V}A/\dot{Q}$, right-hand vertical axis) in normal upright lung. Both blood flow and ventilation are expressed in liters per minute per percentage of alveolar volume and have been drawn as smoothed-out linear functions of vertical height. The closed circles mark the $\dot{V}A/\dot{Q}$ ratios of horizontal lung slices (three of which are shown in Fig. 4-5). A cardiac output of 6 L/min and a total minute ventilation of 5.1 L/min were assumed. (Redrawn with modification from West JB: Ventilation/Blood Flow and Gas Exchange, 4th ed. Oxford, Blackwell Scientific, 1970.)

partial pressure of oxygen ($P_{A}O_2$) and partial pressure of carbon dioxide ($P_{A}CO_2$) in mm Hg for horizontal slices from the top (7% of lung volume), middle (11% of lung volume), and bottom (13% of lung volume) of the lung.[193] $P_{A}O_2$ increases by more than 40 mm Hg from 89 mm Hg at the base to 132 mm Hg at the apex, whereas P_{CO_2} decreases by 14 mm Hg from 42 mm Hg at the bottom to 28 mm Hg at the top. Thus, in keeping with the regional $\dot{V}A/\dot{Q}$ ratio, the bottom of the lung is relatively hypoxic and hypercapnic compared with the top of the lung.

$\dot{V}A/\dot{Q}$ inequalities have different effects on arterial P_{CO_2} ($PaCO_2$) than on arterial P_{O_2} (PaO_2). Blood passing through underventilated alveoli tends to retain its CO_2 and does not take up enough O_2; blood traversing over-ventilated alveoli gives off an excessive amount of CO_2 but cannot take up a proportionately increased amount of O_2 because of the flatness of the oxygen-hemoglobin (oxy-Hb) dissociation curve in this region (see Fig. 4-25). Hence, a lung with uneven $\dot{V}A/\dot{Q}$ relationships can eliminate CO_2 from the overventilated alveoli to compensate for the underventilated alveoli. Thus, with uneven $\dot{V}A/\dot{Q}$ relationships, $P_{A}CO_2$-to-$PaCO_2$ gradients are small, and PaO_2-to-$P_{A}O_2$ gradients are usually large.

In 1974, Wagner and colleagues[183] described a method of determining the continuous distribution of $\dot{V}A/\dot{Q}$ ratios within the lung based on the pattern of elimination of a series of intravenously infused inert gases. Gases of differing solubility are dissolved in physiologic saline solution and infused into a peripheral vein until a steady state is achieved (20 minutes). Toward the end of the infusion period, samples of arterial and mixed expired gas are collected, and total ventilation and cardiac output ($\dot{Q}T$) are measured. For each gas, the ratio of arterial to mixed venous concentration (retention) and the ratio of expired to mixed venous concentration (excretion) are calculated, and retention-solubility and excretion-solubility curves are drawn. The retention- and excretion-solubility curves can be regarded as fingerprints of the particular distribution of $\dot{V}A/\dot{Q}$ ratios that give rise to them.

Figure 4-6 shows the type of distributions found in young, healthy subjects breathing air in the semirecumbent position.[192] The distributions of both ventilation and blood flow are relatively narrow. The upper and lower 9% limits shown (vertical interrupted lines) correspond to $\dot{V}A/\dot{Q}$ ratios of 0.3 and 2.1, respectively. Note that these young, healthy subjects had no blood flow perfusing areas with very low $\dot{V}A/\dot{Q}$ ratios, nor did they have any blood flow to unventilated or shunted areas ($\dot{V}A/\dot{Q} = 0$) or unperfused areas ($\dot{V}A/\dot{Q} = 8$). Figure 4-6 also shows $P_{A}O_2$ and $P_{A}CO_2$ in respiratory units with different $\dot{V}A/\dot{Q}$ ratios. Within the 95% range of $\dot{V}A/\dot{Q}$ ratios (0.3 to 2.1), P_{O_2} ranges from 60 to 123 mm Hg, whereas the corresponding P_{CO_2} range is 44 to 33 mm Hg.

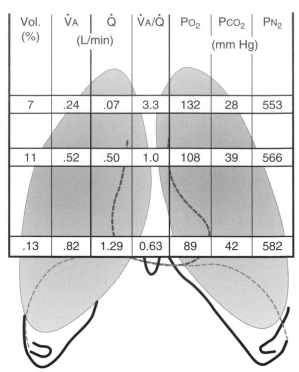

Vol. (%)	$\dot{V}A$	$\dot{Q}$	$\dot{V}A/\dot{Q}$	P_{O_2}	P_{CO_2}	P_{N_2}
	(L/min)			(mm Hg)		
7	.24	.07	3.3	132	28	553
11	.52	.50	1.0	108	39	566
.13	.82	1.29	0.63	89	42	582

Figure 4-5 Ventilation-perfusion ratio ($\dot{V}A/\dot{Q}$) and the regional composition of alveolar gas. Values for regional flow ($\dot{Q}$), ventilation ($\dot{V}A$), P_{O_2}, and P_{CO_2} were derived from Figure 4-4. P_{N_2} was obtained by what remains from total gas pressure (which, including water vapor, equals 760 mm Hg). The volumes [Vol. (%)] of the three lung slices are also shown. When compared with the top of the lung, the bottom of the lung has a low $\dot{V}A/\dot{Q}$ ratio and is relatively hypoxic and hypercapnic. (Redrawn from West JB: Regional differences in gas exchange in the lung of erect man. J Appl Physiol 17:893, 1962.)

B. NONGRAVITATIONAL DETERMINANTS OF PULMONARY VASCULAR RESISTANCE AND BLOOD FLOW DISTRIBUTION

1. Passive Processes

a. Cardiac Output

The pulmonary vascular bed is a high-flow, low-pressure system in health. As $\dot{Q}T$ increases, pulmonary vascular pressures increase minimally.[55] However, increases in $\dot{Q}T$ distend open vessels and recruit previously closed vessels. Accordingly, pulmonary vascular resistance (PVR) drops because the normal pulmonary vasculature is quite distensible (and partly because of the addition of previously unused vessels to the pulmonary circulation). As a result of the distensibility of the normal pulmonary circulation, an increase in Ppa increases the radius of the pulmonary vessels, which causes PVR to decrease (Fig. 4-7). Conversely, the opposite effect occurs within the pulmonary vessels during a decrease in $\dot{Q}T$. As $\dot{Q}T$ decreases, pulmonary vascular pressures decrease, the radii of the pulmonary vessels are reduced, and PVR consequently increases. The pulmonary vessels of patients with significant pulmonary hypertension are less distensible and act more like rigid pipes. In this setting, Ppa increases much more sharply with any increase

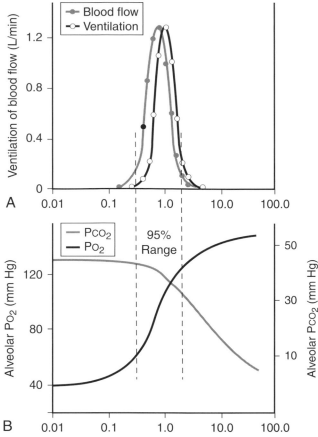

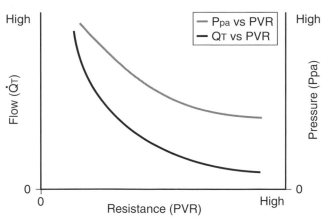

Figure 4-7 Passive changes in pulmonary vascular resistance (PVR) as a function of pulmonary artery pressure (Ppa) and pulmonary blood flow ($\dot{Q}T$) (PVR = Ppa/$\dot{Q}T$). As $\dot{Q}T$ increases, Ppa also increases, but to a lesser extent, and PVR decreases. As $\dot{Q}T$ decreases, Ppa also decreases, but to a lesser extent, and PVR increases. (Redrawn with modification from Fishman AP: Dynamics of the pulmonary circulation. In Hamilton WF [ed]: Handbook of Physiology, section 2. Circulation, vol 2. Baltimore, Williams & Wilkins, 1963, p 1667.)

Figure 4-6 A, Average distribution of ventilation-perfusion ratios ($\dot{V}A/\dot{Q}$) in normal young semirecumbent subjects. The 95% range covers from 0.3 to 2.1 (between *dashed lines*). **B,** Corresponding variations in P_{O_2} and P_{CO_2} in alveolar gas. (Redrawn from West JB: Blood flow to the lung and gas exchange. Anesthesiology 41:124, 1974.)

in $\dot{Q}T$ because PVR in these stiff vessels does not decrease significantly due to minimal expansion of their radii.

Understanding the relationship among Ppa, PVR, and $\dot{Q}T$ during passive events is a prerequisite to recognition of active vasomotion in the pulmonary circulation (see the next section). Active vasoconstriction occurs whenever $\dot{Q}T$ decreases and Ppa either remains constant or increases. Increased Ppa and PVR have been found to be "a universal feature of acute respiratory failure."[207] Active pulmonary vasoconstriction can increase Ppa and Ppv, thereby contributing to the formation of pulmonary edema, and in that way has a role in the genesis of adult respiratory distress syndrome (ARDS). Active vasodilation occurs whenever $\dot{Q}T$ increases and Ppa either remains constant or decreases. When deliberate hypotension is achieved with sodium nitroprusside, $\dot{Q}T$ often remains constant or increases, but Ppa decreases, and therefore so does PVR.

b. Lung Volume
Lung volume and PVR have an asymmetric U-shaped relationship because of the varying effect of lung volume on intra- and extra-alveolar vessels, which in both cases

is minimal at functional residual capacity (FRC). FRC is defined as the amount of volume (gas) in the lungs at end exhalation during normal tidal breathing. Ideally, this means that the patient is inspiring a normal V_T, with minimal or no muscle activity or pressure difference between the alveoli and atmosphere at end exhalation. Total PVR is increased when lung volume is either increased or decreased from FRC (Fig. 4-8).[29,166,201] The increase in total PVR above FRC is due to alveolar compression of small intra-alveolar vessels, which results in an increase in small-vessel PVR (i.e., creation of zone 1 or zone 2).[16] As a relatively small mitigating or counterbalancing effect to the compression of small vessels, the large extra-alveolar vessels may be expanded by the increased tethering of interstitial connective tissue at high lung volumes (and with spontaneous ventilation only—the negativity of perivascular pressure at high lung volumes). The increase in total PVR below FRC is due to an increase in the PVR of large extra-alveolar vessels (passive effect). The increase in large-vessel PVR is partly due to mechanical tortuosity or kinking of these vessels (passive effect). However, small or grossly atelectatic lungs become hypoxic, and it has been shown that the mechanism of increased large-vessel PVR in these lungs is due mainly to an active vasoconstrictive mechanism known as hypoxic pulmonary vasoconstriction (HPV).[12] The effect of HPV (discussed in greater detail in the next section) is significant whether the chest is open or closed and whether ventilation is by positive pressure or spontaneous.[145]

2. Active Processes
Four major categories of active processes affect the pulmonary vascular tone of normal patients: (1) local tissue

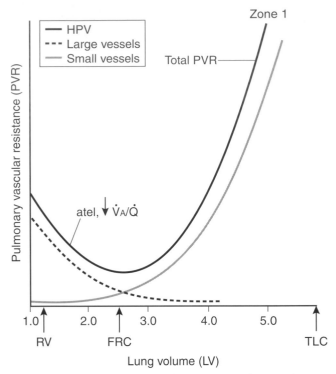

Figure 4-8 Total pulmonary vascular resistance relates to lung volume as an asymmetric U-shaped curve. The trough of the curve occurs when lung volume equals functional residual capacity (FRC). Total pulmonary resistance is the sum of the resistance in small vessels (increased by increasing lung volume) and the resistance in large vessels (increased by decreasing lung volume). The end point for increasing lung volume (toward total lung capacity [TLC]) is the creation of zone 1 conditions, and the end point for decreasing lung volume (toward residual volume [RV]) is the creation of low ventilation-perfusion ($\dot{V}_A/\dot{Q}$) and atelectatic (atel) areas that demonstrate hypoxic pulmonary vasoconstriction (HPV). The curve represents a composite of data from references 13, 19, and 21.

(endothelial and smooth muscle)–derived autocrine or paracrine products, which act on smooth muscle (Table 4-1); (2) alveolar gas concentrations (chiefly hypoxia), which also act on smooth muscle; (3) neural influences; and (4) humoral (or hormonal) effects of circulating products within the pulmonary capillary bed. The neural and humoral effects work by means of either receptor-mediated mechanisms involving the autocrine/paracrine molecules listed in Table 4-1 or related mechanisms ultimately affecting the smooth muscle cell.[4] These four interrelated systems, each affecting pulmonary vascular tone, are briefly reviewed in sequence.

a. Tissue (Endothelial and Smooth Muscle–Derived) Products

The pulmonary vascular endothelium synthesizes, metabolizes, and converts a multitude of vasoactive mediators and plays a central role in the regulation of PVR. However, the main effecter site of pulmonary vascular tone is the pulmonary vascular smooth muscle cell (which both senses and produces multiple pulmonary vasoactive compounds).[1] The autocrine/paracrine molecules listed in Table 4-1 are all actively involved in the regulation of pulmonary vascular tone during various conditions. Numerous additional compounds bind to receptors on the endothelial or smooth muscle cell membranes and modulate the levels (and effects) of these vasoactive molecules.

Nitric oxide (NO) is the predominant (but not the only) endogenous vasodilatory compound. It was discovered to be the long-sought-after endothelium-derived relaxant factor (EDRF) over a decade ago by Palmer and colleagues.[137] Since then, a massive amount of laboratory and clinical research has demonstrated the ubiquitous nature of NO and its predominant role in vasodilation of both pulmonary and systemic blood vessels.[184] In the pulmonary endothelial cell, L-arginine is converted to L-citrulline (by means of NO synthase [NOS]) to produce the small, yet highly reactive NO molecule.[132] Because of its small size, NO can diffuse freely across membranes into the smooth muscle cell, where it binds to the heme moiety of guanylate cyclase (which converts guanosine triphosphate to cyclic guanosine monophosphate [cGMP]).[126] cGMP activates protein kinase G, which dephosphorylates the myosin light chains of pulmonary vascular smooth muscle cells and thereby causes vasodilation.[126] NOS exists in two forms: constitutive (cNOS) and inducible (iNOS). cNOS is permanently expressed in some cells, including pulmonary vascular endothelial cells, and produces short bursts of NO in response to changing levels of calcium and calmodulin and shear stress. The cNOS enzyme is also stimulated by linked membrane-based receptors that bind numerous molecules in the blood (e.g., acetylcholine, bradykinin).[126] In contrast, iNOS is usually produced only as a result of inflammatory mediators and cytokines and, when stimulated, produces large quantities of NO for an extended duration.[126] There is now ample and long-standing evidence that NO is produced in normal lungs and contributes to the maintenance of low PVR.[27,170]

Endothelin-1 (ET-1) is a pulmonary vasoconstrictor.[85] The endothelins are 21-amino-acid peptides produced by a variety of cells. ET-1 is the only family member produced in pulmonary endothelial cells, and it is also produced in vascular smooth muscle cells.[85] ET-1 exerts its major vascular effects through activation of two distinct G protein–coupled receptors (ETA and ETB). ETA receptors are found in the medial smooth muscle layers of the pulmonary (and systemic) blood vessels and in atrial and ventricular myocardium.[85] When stimulated, ETA receptors induce vasoconstriction and cellular proliferation by increasing intracellular calcium.[205] ETB receptors are localized on endothelial cells and some smooth muscle cells.[134] Activation of ETB receptors stimulates the release of NO and prostacyclin, thereby promoting pulmonary vasodilation and inhibiting apoptosis.[132] In addition, the ET-1 receptor antagonist

Table 4-1 **Local Tissue (Autocrine/Paracrine) Molecules Involved in Active Control of Pulmonary Vascular Tone**

Molecule	Subtype (Abbreviation)	Site of Origin	Site of Action	Response
Nitric oxide	NO	Endothelium	Sm. muscle	Vasodilation
Endothelin	ET-1	Endothelium	Sm. muscle (ETA receptor)	Vasoconstriction
	ET-1	Endothelium	Endothelium (ETB receptor)	Vasodilation
Prostaglandin	PGI_2	Endothelium	Endothelium	Vasodilation
Prostaglandin	$PGF_{2\alpha}$	Endothelium	Sm. muscle	Vasoconstriction
Thromboxane	TXA_2	Endothelium	Sm. muscle	Vasoconstriction
Leukotriene	LTB_4-LTE_4	Endothelium	Sm. muscle	Vasoconstriction

ETA receptor, endothelin-1 receptor located on the smooth muscle cell membrane; ETB receptor, endothelin-1 receptor located on the endothelial cell membrane; Sm. muscle, pulmonary arteriole smooth muscle cell.

bosentan showed modest improvement in the treatment of pulmonary hypertension.[32] The more selective ETA receptor antagonist sitaxsentan showed additional benefit in improving pulmonary hypertension.[5] However, both ET-1 receptor antagonists (bosentan and sitaxsentan) are associated with an increased risk of liver toxicity.[154] In summary, it appears that there is a normal balance between NO and ET-1, with a slight predominance toward NO production and vasodilation in health.

Similarly, various eicosanoids are elaborated by the pulmonary vascular endothelium, with a balance toward the vasodilatory compounds in health. Prostaglandin I_2 (PGI_2), now known as epoprostenol (previously known as prostacyclin), causes vasodilation and is continuously elaborated in small amounts in healthy endothelium. In contrast, thromboxane A_2 and leukotriene B_4 are elaborated under pathologic conditions and are thought to be involved in the pathophysiology of pulmonary artery hypertension (PAH) associated with sepsis and reperfusion injury.[4]

Therapeutically, epoprostenol has been used successfully to decrease PVR in patients with chronic PAH when infused[7] or inhaled.[135] Currently, the synthetic PGI_2 iloprost is now the most commonly used inhaled eicosanoid for reduction of PVR in patients with PAH.[135] Interestingly, most patients with chronic PAH are unresponsive to an acute vasodilator challenge with short-acting agents such as epoprostenol, adenosine, or NO.[98] However, long-term administration of epoprostenol has been shown to decrease PVR in these patients despite their initial nonresponsiveness.[122] Furthermore, some patients with previously severe PAH have been weaned from epoprostenol after long-term administration, with dramatically decreased PVR and improved exercise tolerance.[98] The vascular remodeling required to provide such a dramatic reduction in PVR is probably due to mechanisms besides simple local vasodilation, as predicted by Fishman in an editorial in 1998.[58] One such mechanism that appears important is the fact that long-term epoprostenol administration increases the clearance of ET-1 (a potent vasoconstrictor and mitogen).[102]

b. Alveolar Gases

Hypoxia-induced vasoconstriction in pulmonary vessels constitutes a fundamental difference from all other systemic blood vessels (which vasodilate in the presence of hypoxia). Alveolar hypoxia of in vivo and in vitro whole lung, unilateral lung, lobe, or lobule of lung results in localized pulmonary vasoconstriction. This phenomenon is widely referred to as "hypoxic pulmonary vasoconstriction" and was first described nearly 60 years ago by Von Euler and Liljestrand.[181] The HPV response is present in all mammalian species and serves as an adaptive mechanism for diverting blood flow away from poorly ventilated to better ventilated regions of the lung and thereby improving $\dot{V}_A/\dot{Q}$ ratios.[41] The HPV response is also critical for fetal development by minimizing perfusion of the unventilated lung.

The HPV response occurs primarily in pulmonary arterioles of about 200 μm internal diameter in humans (60 to 700 μm internal diameter, depending on the species).[191] These vessels are advantageously situated anatomically in close relation to small bronchioles and alveoli, which permits rapid and direct detection of alveolar hypoxia. Indeed, blood may actually become oxygenated in small pulmonary arteries because of the ability of oxygen to diffuse directly across the small distance between the contiguous air spaces and vessels.[152] This direct access that gas in the airways has to small arteries makes possible a rapid and localized vascular response to changes in gas composition.

The oxygen tension at the HPV stimulus site (P_{SO_2}) is a function of both P_{AO_2} and mixed venous O_2 pressure ($P\bar{v}_{O_2}$).[117] The P_{SO_2}-HPV response is sigmoid, with a 50% response when P_{AO_2}, $P\bar{v}_{O_2}$, and P_{SO_2} are approximately 30 mm Hg. Usually, P_{AO_2} has a much greater effect than $P\bar{v}_{O_2}$ does because O_2 uptake is from the alveolar space to the blood in the small pulmonary arteries.[117]

Over the last 50 years, numerous theories were developed to explain the mechanism of HPV.[15,23,56,181] Many vasoactive substances have been proposed as mediators of HPV (e.g., leukotrienes, prostaglandins, catecholamines, serotonin, histamine, angiotensin, bradykinin, and ET-1), but none has been identified as the primary mediator. In 1992, Xuan proposed that NO has a pivotal role in modulating PVR.[204] NO has involvement, but not precisely the way that Xuan first proposed. There are multiple sites of oxygen sensing with variable contributions from the NO, ET-1, and eicosanoid systems (described earlier). In vivo, HPV is currently thought to result from the synergistic action of molecules produced in both endothelial cells and smooth muscle cells.[71] However, HPV can proceed in the absence of intact endothelium, suggesting that the primary oxygen sensor is in the smooth muscle cell and that endothelium-derived molecules modulate only the primary HPV response.

The precise mechanism of HPV is still under investigation. However, current data support a mechanism involving the smooth muscle mitochondrial electron transport chain as the HPV sensor (Fig. 4-9).[189] In addition, reactive oxygen species (possibly H_2O_2 or superoxide) are released from complex III of the electron transport chain and probably serve as second messengers to increase calcium in pulmonary artery smooth muscle cells during acute hypoxia.[188] However, alternative (less likely) mechanisms are still being investigated.[164] One alternative hypothesis suggests that smooth muscle microsomal reduced nicotinamide adenine dinucleotide phosphate (NADPH) oxidoreductase or sarcolemmal NADPH oxidase is the sensing mechanism.[164] Another, previously popular theory posited that voltage-sensitive potassium (K_V) channels were required for the HPV response. However, K_V channels are no longer believed to be "obligate" but instead are thought to be attenuators because a study demonstrated that inhibition of K_V channels failed to inhibit the HPV response.[164]

In summary, HPV is probably due to a direct action of alveolar hypoxia on pulmonary smooth muscle cells, sensed by the mitochondrial electron transport chain, with reactive oxygen species (probably H_2O_2 or superoxide) serving as second messengers to increase calcium and smooth muscle vasoconstriction. The endothelium-derived products serve to both potentiate (ET-1) and attenuate (NO, PGI_2) the HPV response. Additional mechanisms (humoral, neurogenic influences) may also modulate the baseline pulmonary vascular tone and affect the magnitude of the HPV response.

Elevated Pa_{CO_2} has a pulmonary vasoconstrictor effect. Both respiratory acidosis and metabolic acidosis augment HPV, whereas alkalosis (both respiratory and metabolic) causes pulmonary vasodilation and serves to reduce HPV.

The clinical effects of HPV can be classified under three basic mechanisms in humans. First, life at high altitude or whole-lung respiration of a low inspired concentration of O_2 (FI_{O_2}) increases Ppa. This is true for newcomers to high altitude, for the acclimatized, and for natives.[56] The vasoconstriction is considerable, and in healthy people breathing 10% O_2, Ppa doubles whereas pulmonary wedge pressure remains constant.[47]

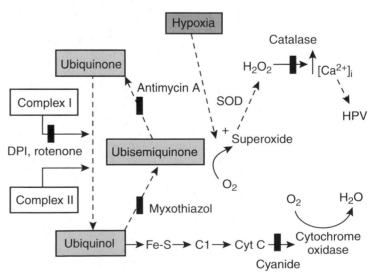

Figure 4-9 Schematic model of the mitochondrial O_2-sensing and effector mechanism probably responsible for hypoxic pulmonary vasoconstriction (HPV). In this model, reactive O_2 species (ROS) are released from electron transport chain complex III and act as second messengers in the hypoxia-induced calcium (Ca^{2+}) increase and resultant HPV. The *solid arrows* represent electron transfer steps; *solid bars* show sites of electron chain inhibition. Normal mitochondrial electron transport involves the movement of reducing equivalents generated in the Krebs cycle through complex I or II and then through complex III (ubiquinone) and IV (cytochrome oxidase). The Q cycle converts the dual electron transfer in complex I and II into a single electron transfer step used in complex IV. The ubisemiquinone (a free radical) created in this process can generate superoxide, which in the presence of superoxide dismutase (SOD) produces H_2O_2, the probable mediator of the hypoxia-induced increased Ca^{2+} and HPV. This process is amplified during hypoxia. (DPI, diphenyleneiodonium. DPI, rotenone, and myxothiazol [not shown in figure] are inhibitors of the proximal portion of the electron transport chain.) (From Waypa GB, Marks JD, Mack MM, et al: Mitochondrial reactive oxygen species trigger calcium increases during hypoxia in pulmonary artery myocytes. Circ Res 91:719, 2002.)

The increased Ppa increases perfusion of the apices of the lung (recruitment of previously unused vessels), which results in gas exchange in a region of lung not normally used (i.e., zone 1). Thus, with a low F_{IO_2}, Pa_{O_2} is greater and the alveolar-arterial O_2 tension difference and the V_D/V_T ratio are less than would be expected or predicted on the basis of a normal (sea level) distribution of ventilation and blood flow. High-altitude pulmonary hypertension is an important component in the development of mountain sickness subacutely (hours to days) and cor pulmonale chronically (weeks to years).[59] In fact, there is now good evidence that in patients with chronic obstructive pulmonary disease, even nocturnal episodes of arterial O_2 desaturation (caused by episodic hypoventilation) are accompanied by elevations in Ppa and may account for or lead to sustained pulmonary hypertension and cor pulmonale.[24]

Second, hypoventilation (low $\dot{V}_A/\dot{Q}$ ratio), atelectasis, or nitrogen ventilation of any region of the lung (one lung, lobe, lobule) generally causes a diversion of blood flow away from the hypoxic to the nonhypoxic lung (40% to 50%, 50% to 60%, 60% to 70%, respectively) (Fig. 4-10).[208] The regional vasoconstriction and blood flow diversion are of great importance in minimizing transpulmonary shunting and normalizing regional $\dot{V}_A/\dot{Q}$ ratios during disease of one lung, one-lung anesthesia (see Chapter 24), inadvertent intubation of a main stem bronchus, and lobar collapse.

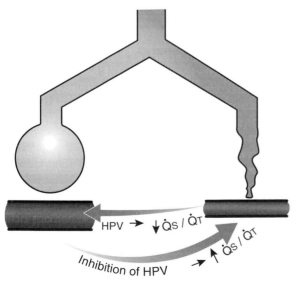

Figure 4-10 Schematic drawing of regional hypoxic pulmonary vasoconstriction (HPV); one-lung ventilation is a common clinical example of regional HPV. HPV in the hypoxic atelectatic lung causes redistribution of blood flow away from the hypoxic lung to the normoxic lung, thereby diminishing the amount of shunt flow ($\dot{Q}_S/\dot{Q}_T$) that can occur through the hypoxic lung. Inhibition of hypoxic lung HPV causes an increase in the amount of shunt flow through the hypoxic lung, thereby decreasing Pa_{O_2}.

Third, in patients who have chronic obstructive pulmonary disease, asthma, pneumonia, or mitral stenosis but not bronchospasm, administration of pulmonary vasodilator drugs such as isoproterenol, sodium nitroprusside, and nitroglycerin causes a decrease in Pa_{O_2} and PVR and an increase in right-to-left transpulmonary shunting.[11] The mechanism for these changes is thought to be deleterious inhibition of preexisting and, in some lesions, geographically widespread HPV without concomitant and beneficial bronchodilation.[11] In accordance with the latter two lines of evidence (one-lung or regional hypoxia and vasodilator drug effects on whole-lung or generalized disease), HPV is thought to divert blood flow away from hypoxic regions of the lung, thereby serving as an autoregulatory mechanism that protects Pa_{O_2} by favorably adjusting regional $\dot{V}_A/\dot{Q}$ ratios. Factors that inhibit regional HPV are extensively discussed elsewhere.[9,10]

c. Neural Influences on Pulmonary Vascular Tone

The three systems used to innervate the pulmonary circulation are the same ones that innervate the airways: the sympathetic, parasympathetic, and nonadrenergic noncholinergic (NANC) systems.[4]

Sympathetic (adrenergic) fibers originate from the first five thoracic nerves and enter the pulmonary vessels as branches from the cervical ganglia, as well as from a plexus of nerves arising from the trachea and main stem bronchi. These nerves act mainly on pulmonary arteries down to a diameter of 60 μm.[4] Sympathetic fibers cause pulmonary vasoconstriction through α_1-receptors. However, the pulmonary arteries also contain vasodilatory α_2-receptors and β_2-receptors. The α_1-adrenergic response predominates during sympathetic stimulation, as occurs during pain, fear, and anxiety.[4]

The parasympathetic (cholinergic) nerve fibers originate from the vagus nerve and cause pulmonary vasodilation through an NO-dependent process.[4] Binding of acetylcholine to a muscarinic (M_3) receptor on the endothelial cell increases intracellular calcium and stimulates cNOS.[4]

NANC nerves cause pulmonary vasodilation through NO-mediated systems by using vasoactive intestinal peptide as the neurotransmitter. The functional significance of this system is still under investigation.[4]

d. Humoral Influences on Pulmonary Vascular Tone

Numerous molecules are released into the circulation that either affect pulmonary vascular tone (by binding to pulmonary endothelial receptors) or are acted on by the pulmonary endothelium and subsequently become activated or inactivated (Table 4-2). The entire topic of nonrespiratory function of the lung is fascinating but beyond the scope of this chapter. Here, we highlight the

Table 4-2 **Effect of Compounds Passing through Pulmonary Circulation**

Molecule	Activated	Unchanged	Inactivated
Amines		Dopamine Epinephrine Histamine	5-Hydroxytryptamine Norepinephrine
Peptides	Angiotensin I	Angiotensin II Oxytocin Vasopressin	Bradykinin Atrial natriuretic peptide Endothelins
Eicosanoids	Arachidonic acid	PGI_2 PGA_2	PGD_2 PGE_1, PGE_2 $PGF_{2\alpha}$ Leukotrienes
Purine derivatives			Adenosine ATP, ADP, AMP

ADP, adenosine diphosphate; AMP, adenosine monophosphate; ATP, adenosine triphosphate; PG, prostaglandin.
Modified from Lumb AB: Non-respiratory functions of the lung. In Lumb AB (ed): Nunn's Applied Respiratory Physiology, 5th ed. London, Butterworths, 2000, p 309.

effects that circulating molecules have on pulmonary vascular tone.

Although we understand the basic effect that various circulating factors have on pulmonary vascular tone, it is unlikely that these compounds are modulators of normal pulmonary vascular tone. However, they have marked effects on pulmonary vascular tone during disease (e.g., acquired respiratory distress syndrome, sepsis).

Endogenous catecholamines (epinephrine and norepinephrine) bind to both α_1 (vasoconstrictor) and β_2 (vasodilator) receptors on the pulmonary endothelium but, when elaborated in high concentration, have a predominant α_1 (vasoconstrictor) effect. The same is true for exogenously administered catecholamines.

Other amines (e.g., histamine, serotonin) are elaborated systemically or locally after various challenges and have variable effects on PVR. Histamine can be released from mast cells, basophils, and elsewhere. When histamine binds directly to H_1 receptors on endothelium, NO-mediated vasodilation occurs (as seen after epinephrine-induced pulmonary vasoconstriction). Direct stimulation of H_2 receptors on smooth muscle cell membranes also causes vasodilation. In contrast, stimulation of H_1 receptors on the smooth muscle membrane results in vasoconstriction. Serotonin (5-hydroxytryptamine) is a potent vasoconstrictor that can be elaborated from activated platelets (e.g., after pulmonary embolism) and lead to acute severe pulmonary hypertension.[51]

Numerous peptides circulate and cause either pulmonary vasodilation (e.g., substance P, bradykinin, and vasopressin [a systemic vasoconstrictor]) or vasoconstriction (e.g., neurokinin A and angiotensin). These peptides produce clinically detectable effects on PVR only when administered in high concentration (e.g., exogenous administration or in disease).

Two other classes of molecules must be mentioned for completeness, eicosanoids (vasoactive effects discussed earlier) and purine nucleosides (which are similarly highly vasoactive).[4] Adenosine is a pulmonary vasodilator in normal subjects, whereas adenosine triphosphate (ATP) has a variable "normalizing effect," depending on baseline pulmonary vascular tone.[153]

3. Alternative (Nonalveolar) Pathways of Blood Flow through the Lung

Blood can use several possible pathways to travel from the right side of the heart to the left without being fully oxygenated or oxygenated at all. Blood flow through poorly ventilated alveoli (low-$\dot{V}A/\dot{Q}$ regions at an FIO_2 < 0.3 have a right-to-left shunt effect on oxygenation) and blood flow through nonventilated alveoli (atelectatic or consolidated regions; $\dot{V}A/\dot{Q} = 0$ at all FIO_2 values) are sources of right-to-left shunting. Low-$\dot{V}A/\dot{Q}$ and atelectatic lung units occur in conditions in which FRC is less than the closing capacity (CC) of the lung (see "Lung Volumes, Functional Residual Capacity, and Closing Capacity").

Several right-to-left blood flow pathways through the lungs and heart do not pass by or involve the alveoli at all. The bronchial and pleural circulations originate from systemic arteries and empty into the left side of the heart without being oxygenated; these circulations constitute the 1% to 3% true right-to-left shunt normally present. With chronic bronchitis, the bronchial circulation may carry 10% of the cardiac output, and with pleuritis, the pleural circulation may carry 5% of the cardiac output. Consequently, as much as a 10% and a 5% obligatory right-to-left shunt may be present, respectively, under these conditions. Intrapulmonary arteriovenous anastomoses are normally closed, but in the presence of acute pulmonary hypertension, such as may be caused by a pulmonary embolus, they may open and result in a direct increase in right-to-left shunting. The foramen ovale is patent in 20% to 30% of individuals, but it normally remains functionally closed because left atrial pressure exceeds right atrial pressure. However, any condition that causes right atrial pressure to be greater than left atrial pressure may produce a right-to-left shunt, with resultant hypoxemia and possible paradoxical embolization. Such conditions include the use of high levels of PEEP, pulmonary embolization, pulmonary hypertension, chronic obstructive pulmonary disease, pulmonary valvular stenosis, congestive heart failure, and postpneumonectomy states.[73] Indeed, even such common events as mechanical ventilation[90] and reaction to the presence of an endotracheal tube (ET) during the excitement phase of emergence from anesthesia[128] have caused right-to-left shunting across a patent foramen ovale (PFO) and severe arterial desaturation (with the potential for paradoxical embolization).[128]

Transesophageal echocardiography (TEE) has been demonstrated to be the most sensitive modality for diagnosing a PFO in anesthetized patients with elevated right atrial pressure.[43] Esophageal to mediastinal to bronchial to pulmonary vein pathways have been described and may explain in part the hypoxemia associated with portal hypertension and cirrhosis. There are no known conditions that selectively increase thebesian channel blood flow (thebesian vessels nourish the left ventricular myocardium and originate and empty into the left side of the heart).

C. OTHER (NONGRAVITATIONAL) IMPORTANT DETERMINANTS OF PULMONARY COMPLIANCE, RESISTANCE, LUNG VOLUME, AND VENTILATION

1. Pulmonary Compliance

For air to flow into the lungs, a pressure gradient (ΔP) must be developed to overcome the elastic resistance of the lungs and chest wall to expansion. These structures are arranged concentrically, and their elastic resistance is therefore additive. The relationship between ΔP and the resultant volume increase (ΔV) of the lungs and thorax is independent of time and is known as total compliance (CT), as expressed in the following equation:

$$CT \ (L/cm \ H_2O) = \Delta V \ (L)/\Delta P \ (cm \ H_2O) \qquad (1)$$

The CT of lung plus chest wall is related to the individual compliance of the lungs (CL) and chest wall (CCW) according to the following expression:

$$1/CT = 1/CL + 1/CCW \ [or \ CT = (CL)(CCW)/CL + CCW] \qquad (2)$$

Normally, CL and CCW each equal 0.2 L/cm H_2O; thus, CT = 0.1 L/cm H_2O. To determine CL, ΔV and the transpulmonary pressure gradient (PA – Ppl, the ΔP for the lung) must be known; to determine CCW,

ΔV and the transmural pressure gradient (Ppl – $P_{ambient}$, the ΔP for the chest wall) must be known; and to determine CT, ΔV and the transthoracic pressure gradient (PA – $P_{ambient}$, the ΔP for the lung and chest wall together) must be known. In clinical practice, only CT is measured, which can be done dynamically or statically, depending on whether a peak or plateau inspiratory ΔP (respectively) is used for the CT calculation.

During a positive- or negative-pressure inspiration of sufficient duration, transthoracic ΔP first increases to a peak value and then decreases to a lower plateau value. The peak transthoracic pressure value is due to the pressure required to overcome both elastic and airway resistance (see "Airway Resistance"). Transthoracic pressure decreases to a plateau value after the peak value because with time, gas is redistributed from stiff alveoli (which expand only slightly and therefore have only a short inspiratory period) into more compliant alveoli (which expand a great deal and therefore have a long inspiratory period). Because the gas is redistributed into more compliant alveoli, less pressure is required to contain the same amount of gas, which explains why the pressure decreases. In practical terms, dynamic compliance is the volume change divided by the peak inspiratory transthoracic pressure, and static compliance is the volume change divided by the plateau inspiratory transthoracic pressure. Therefore, static CT is usually greater than dynamic CT because the former calculation uses a smaller denominator (lower pressure) than the latter. However, if the patient is receiving PEEP, this pressure must first be subtracted from the peak or plateau pressure before calculating thoracic compliance (i.e., compliance = volume delivered/peak or plateau pressure – PEEP).

PA deserves special comment. The alveoli are lined with a layer of liquid. The lining of a curved surface (sphere or cylinder, such as the alveoli, bronchioles, and bronchi) with liquid creates a surface tension that tends to make the surface area that is exposed to the atmosphere as small as possible. Simply stated, water molecules crowd much closer together on the surface of a curved layer of water than elsewhere in the fluid. As lung or alveolar size decreases, the degree of curvature and the retractive surface tension increase.

According to the Laplace expression (equation 3), the pressure in an alveolus (P, in dynes per square centimeter) is higher than ambient pressure by an amount that depends on the surface tension of the lining liquid (T, in dynes per centimeter) and the radius of curvature of the alveolus (R, in centimeters). This relationship is expressed in the following equation:

$$P = 2T/R \qquad (3)$$

Although surface tension contributes to the elastic resistance and retractive forces of the lung, two difficulties must be resolved. First, the pressure inside small alveoli should be higher than that inside large alveoli, a conclusion that stems directly from the Laplace equation

(R in the denominator). From this reasoning, one would expect a progressive discharge of each small alveolus into a larger one until eventually only one gigantic alveolus would be left (Fig. 4-11A). The second problem concerns the relationship between lung volume and transpulmonary ΔP (PA − Ppl). Theoretically, the retractive forces of the lung should increase as lung volume decreases. If this were true, lung volume should decrease in a vicious circle, with an increasingly progressive tendency to collapse as lung volume diminishes.

These two problems are resolved by the fact that the surface tension of the fluid lining the alveoli is variable and decreases as its surface area is reduced. The surface tension of alveolar fluid can reach levels that are well below the normal range for body fluids such as water and plasma. When an alveolus decreases in size, the surface tension of the lining fluid falls to an extent greater than the corresponding reduction in radius, and as a result, the transmural pressure gradient (equal to 2T/R) diminishes. This explains why small alveoli do not discharge their contents into large alveoli (Fig. 4-11B) and why the elastic recoil of small alveoli is less than that of large alveoli.

The substance responsible for the reduction (and variability) in alveolar surface tension is secreted by the intra-alveolar type II pneumocyte and is a lipoprotein called surfactant, which floats as a 50-Å-thick film on the surface of the fluid lining the alveoli. When the surface film is reduced in area and the concentration of surfactant at the surface is increased, the surface-reducing pressure is increased and counteracts the surface tension of the fluid lining the alveoli.

2. Airway Resistance

For air to flow into the lungs, ΔP (pressure gradient) must also be developed to overcome the nonelastic airway resistance of the lungs to airflow. The relationship between ΔP and the rate of airflow ($\dot{V}$) is known as airway resistance (R):

$$R\left(cm\ H_2O/L/sec\right)=\frac{\Delta P\left(cm\ H_2O\right)}{\Delta \dot{V}\left(L/sec\right)} \tag{4}$$

The ΔP along the airway depends on the caliber of the airway and the rate and pattern of airflow. There are three main patterns of airflow. Laminar flow occurs when the gas passes down parallel-sided tubes at less than a certain critical velocity. With laminar flow, the pressure drop down the tube is proportional to the flow rate and may be calculated from the equation derived by Poiseuille:

$$\Delta P = \dot{V} \times 8\ L \times \mu/\pi r^4 \tag{5}$$

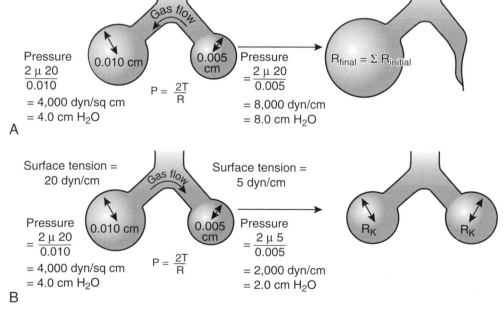

Figure 4-11 Relationship between surface tension (T), alveolar radius (R), and alveolar transmural pressure (P). The left side of the diagrams shows the starting condition. The right side of the diagrams shows the expected result in alveolar size (using the Laplace equation to calculate the starting pressure). In the upper example **(A)**, the surface tension in the fluid lining both the large and the small alveolus is the same (no surfactant). Accordingly, the direction of gas flow is from the higher pressure small alveolus to the lower pressure large alveolus, which results in one large alveolus ($R_{final} = \Sigma R_{initial}$). In the bottom example **(B)**, the expected changes in surface tension when surfactant lines the alveolus are shown (less tension in the smaller alveolus). The direction of gas flow is from the larger alveolus to the smaller alveolus until the two alveoli are of equal size and are volume stable (R_K). K, constant; ΣR, sum of all individual radii.

In equation (5), ΔP is the pressure drop (in cm H_2O), $\dot{V}$ is the volume flow rate (in mL/sec), μ is viscosity (in poises), L is the length of the tube (in cm), and r is the radius of the tube (in cm).

When flow exceeds the critical velocity, it becomes turbulent. The significant feature of turbulent flow is that the pressure drop along the airway is no longer directly proportional to the flow rate but is proportional to the square of the flow rate according to equation (6) for turbulent flow:

$$\Delta P = \dot{V}^2 pfL/4\pi^2 r^5 \qquad (6)$$

In equation (6), p is the density of the gas (or liquid), and f is a friction factor that depends on the roughness of the tube wall.[175] Thus, with increases in turbulent flow (and/or orifice flow; see the next paragraph), ΔP increases much more than $\dot{V}$, and therefore airway resistance (R) also increases more, as predicted by equation (4).

Orifice flow occurs at severe constrictions such as a nearly closed larynx or a kinked ET. In these situations, the pressure drop is also proportional to the square of the flow rate, but density replaces viscosity as the important factor in the numerator. This explains why a low-density gas such as helium diminishes the resistance to flow (by threefold in comparison with air) in severe obstruction of the upper airway.

Because the total cross-sectional area of the airways increases as branching occurs, the velocity of airflow decreases distal in the airways; laminar flow is therefore chiefly confined to the airways below the main bronchi. Orifice flow occurs at the larynx, and flow in the trachea is turbulent during most of the respiratory cycle. By viewing the components that constitute each of the preceding airway pressure equations, one can see that many factors may obviously affect the pressure drop down the airways during respiration. However, variations in diameter of the smaller bronchi and bronchioles are particularly critical (bronchoconstriction may convert laminar flow to turbulent flow), and the pressure drop along the airways may become much more closely related to the flow rate.

3. Different Regional Lung Time Constants

Thus far, the compliance and airway resistance properties of the chest have been discussed separately. In the following analysis, pressure at the mouth is assumed to increase suddenly to a fixed positive value[109] (Fig. 4-12) that overcomes both elastic and airway resistance and to be maintained at this value during inflation of the lungs. The ΔP required to overcome nonelastic airway resistance is the difference between the fixed mouth pressure and the instantaneous height of the dashed line in Figure 4-12 and is proportional to the flow rate during most of the respiratory cycle. Thus, the ΔP required to overcome nonelastic airway resistance is maximal initially but then decreases exponentially (Fig. 4-12A, hatched lines).

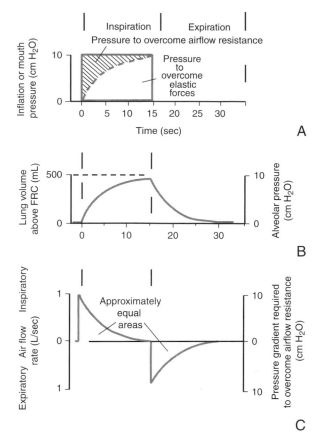

Figure 4-12 Artificial ventilation by intermittent application of constant pressure (square wave) followed by passive expiration. The pressure required to overcome airway resistance (*hatched lines*, **A**) and the airflow rate (of equation 4, **C**) are proportional to one another and decrease exponentially (assuming that resistance to airflow is constant). The pressure required to overcome the elastic forces (height of the *dashed line*, **A**) and lung volume **(B)** are proportional to one another and increase exponentially. Values shown are typical for an anesthetized supine paralyzed patient: total dynamic compliance, 50 mL/cm H_2O; pulmonary resistance, 3 cm H_2O/L/sec; apparatus resistance, 7 cm H_2O/L/sec; total resistance, 10 cm H_2O/L/sec; time constant, 0.5 second. (Redrawn from Lumb AB: Artificial ventilation. In Lumb AB [ed]: Nunn's Applied Respiratory Physiology, 5th ed. London, Butterworths, 2000, p 590.)

The rate of filling therefore also declines in an approximately exponential manner. The remainder of the pressure gradient overcomes the elastic resistance (the instantaneous height of the dashed line in Fig. 4-12A) and is proportional to the change in lung volume. Thus, the ΔP required to overcome elastic resistance is minimal initially but then increases exponentially, as does lung volume. Alveolar filling ceases (lung volume remains constant) when the pressure resulting from the retractive elastic forces balances the applied (mouth) pressure (see Fig. 4-12A, dashed line).

Because only a finite time is available for alveolar filling and because alveolar filling occurs in an exponential manner, the degree of filling obviously depends on the duration of the inspiration. The rapidity of change in an exponential curve can be described by its time constant τ, which is the time required to complete 63% of an exponentially changing function if the total time allowed for the function change is unlimited ($2\tau = 87\%$, $3\tau = 95\%$, and $4\tau = 98\%$). For lung inflation, $\tau = CT \times R$; normally, $CT = 0.1$ L/cm H_2O, $R = 2.0$ cm $H_2O/L/sec$, $\tau = 0.2$ second, and $3\tau = 0.6$ second.

When this equation is applied to individual alveolar units, the time taken to fill such a unit clearly increases as airway resistance increases. The time to fill an alveolar unit also increases as compliance increases because a greater volume of air is transferred into a more compliant alveolus before the retractive force equals the applied pressure. The compliance of individual alveoli differs from top to bottom of the lung, and the resistance of individual airways varies widely depending on their length and caliber. Therefore, various time constants for inflation exist throughout the lung.

4. Pathways of Collateral Ventilation

Collateral ventilation is another nongravitational determinant of the distribution of ventilation. Four pathways of collateral ventilation are known. First, interalveolar communications (pores of Kohn) exist in most species; they may range from 8 to 50 per alveolus and may increase with age and with the development of obstructive lung disease. Their precise role has not been defined, but they probably function to prevent hypoxia in neighboring but obstructed lung units. Second, distal bronchiolar to alveolar communications are known to exist (channels of Lambert), but their function in vivo is speculative (may be similar to the pores of Kohn). Third, respiratory bronchiole-to-terminal bronchiole connections have been found in adjacent lung segments (channels of Martin) in healthy dogs and in humans with lung disease. Fourth, interlobar connections exist; the functional characteristics of interlobar collateral ventilation through these connections have been described in dogs,[159] and they have been observed in humans as well.[96]

5. Work of Breathing

The pressure-volume characteristics of the lung also determine the work of breathing. Because

$$\begin{aligned}
\text{Work} &= \text{force} \times \text{distance} \\
\text{Force} &= \text{pressure} \times \text{area} \qquad (7) \\
\text{Distance} &= \text{volume/area}
\end{aligned}$$

work is defined by the equation

$$\begin{aligned}
\text{Work} &= (\text{pressure} \times \text{area})(\text{volume/area}), \\
\text{Work} &= \text{pressure} \times \text{volume} \qquad (8)
\end{aligned}$$

and ventilatory work may be analyzed by plotting pressure against volume.[143] In the presence of increased airway resistance or decreased CL, increased transpulmonary pressure is required to achieve a given VT with a

consequent increase in the work of breathing. The metabolic cost of the work of breathing at rest constitutes only 1% to 3% of the total O_2 consumption in healthy subjects, but it is increased considerably (up to 50%) in patients with pulmonary disease.

Two different pressure-volume diagrams are shown in Figure 4-13. During normal inspiration (left graph), transpulmonary pressure increases from 0 to 5 cm H_2O while 500 mL of air is drawn into the lung. Potential energy is stored by the lung during inspiration and is expended during expiration; as a consequence, the entire expiratory cycle is passive. The hatched area plus the triangular area ABC represents pressure multiplied by volume and is the work of breathing. Line AB is the lower section of the pressure-volume curve of Figure 4-13. The triangular area ABC is the work required to overcome elastic forces (CT), whereas the hatched area is the work required to overcome airflow or frictional resistance (R). The graph on the right applies to an anesthetized patient with diffuse obstructive airway disease resulting from the

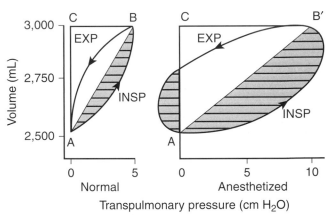

Figure 4-13 Lung volume plotted against transpulmonary pressure in a pressure-volume diagram for an healthy awake (normal) and an anesthetized patient. The lung compliance of the awake patient (slope of line AB = 100 mL/cm H_2O) equals that shown for the small dependent alveoli in Figure 4-3. The lung compliance of the anesthetized patient (slope of line AB' = 50 mL/cm H_2O) equals that shown for the medium midlung alveoli in Figure 4-3 and for the anesthetized patient in Figure 4-12. The total area within the oval and triangles has the dimensions of pressure multiplied by volume and represents the total work of breathing. The hatched area to the right of lines AB and AB' represents the active inspiratory work necessary to overcome resistance to airflow during inspiration (INSP). The hatched area to the left of the triangle AB'C represents the active expiratory work necessary to overcome resistance to airflow during expiration (EXP). Expiration is passive in the healthy subject because sufficient potential energy is stored during inspiration to produce expiratory airflow. The fraction of total inspiratory work necessary to overcome elastic resistance is shown by the triangles ABC and AB'C. The anesthetized patient has decreased compliance and increased elastic resistance work (triangle AB'C) compared with the healthy patient's compliance and elastic resistance work (triangle ABC). The anesthetized patient represented in this figure has increased airway resistance to both inspiratory and expiratory work.

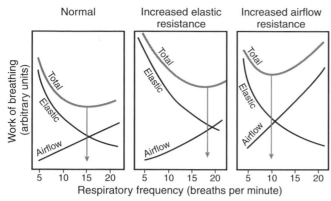

Figure 4-14 The diagrams show the work done against elastic and airflow resistance separately and summated to indicate the total work of breathing at different respiratory frequencies. The total work of breathing has a minimum value at about 15 breaths/min under normal circumstances. For the same minute volume, minimum work is performed at higher frequencies with stiff (less compliant) lungs and at lower frequencies when airflow resistance is increased. (Redrawn with modification from Lumb AB: Pulmonary ventilation: Mechanisms and the work of breathing. In Lumb AB [ed]: Nunn's Applied Respiratory Physiology, 5th ed. London, Butterworths, 2000, p 128.)

accumulation of mucous secretions. There is a marked increase in both the elastic (triangle AB'C) and airway (hatched area) resistive components of respiratory work. During expiration, only 250 mL of air leaves the lungs during the passive phase when intrathoracic pressure reaches the equilibrium value of 0 cm H_2O. Active effort-producing work is required to force out the remaining 250 mL of air, and intrathoracic pressure actually becomes positive.

For a constant minute volume, the work done against elastic resistance is increased when breathing is deep and slow. On the other hand, the work done against airflow resistance is increased when breathing is rapid and shallow. If the two components are summated and the total work

is plotted against respiratory frequency, there is an optimal respiratory frequency at which the total work of breathing is minimal (Fig. 4-14).[110] In patients with diseased lungs in which elastic resistance is high (pulmonary fibrosis, pulmonary edema, infants), the optimum frequency is increased, and rapid, shallow breaths are favored. As with other muscles, respiratory muscles can become fatigued, especially with rapid, shallow breathing.[129] When airway resistance is high (asthma, obstructive lung disease), the optimum frequency is decreased, and slow, deep breaths are favored. Although the optimum frequency is slow (allowing a prolonged expiratory phase), a rapid shallow breathing pattern also develops in these patients when fatigued and further exacerbates their primary (airway resistance) problem.[129]

6. Lung Volumes, Functional Residual Capacity, and Closing Capacity

a. Lung Volumes and Functional Residual Capacity

FRC is defined as the volume of gas in the lung at the end of a normal expiration when there is no airflow and PA equals ambient pressure. Under these conditions, expansive chest wall elastic forces are exactly balanced by retractive lung tissue elastic forces (Fig. 4-15).[165]

The expiratory reserve volume is part of FRC; it is the additional gas beyond the end-tidal volume that can be consciously exhaled and result in the minimum volume of lung possible, known as residual volume. Thus, FRC equals residual volume plus the expiratory reserve volume (Fig. 4-16). With regard to the other lung volumes shown in Figure 4-16, VT, vital capacity, inspiratory capacity, inspiratory reserve volume, and expiratory reserve volume can all be measured by simple spirometry. Total lung capacity (TLC), FRC, and residual volume all contain a fraction (residual volume) that cannot be measured by simple spirometry. However, if one of these three volumes is measured, the others can easily be derived because the

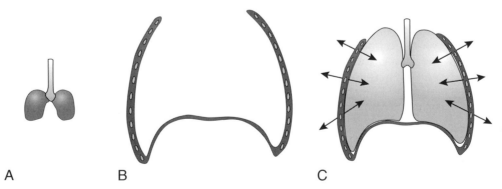

Figure 4-15 A, The resting state of normal lungs when they are removed from the chest cavity; that is, elastic recoil causes total collapse. **B,** The resting state of a normal chest wall and diaphragm when the thoracic apex is open to the atmosphere and the thoracic contents are removed. **C,** The lung volume that exists at the end of expiration is the functional residual capacity (FRC). At FRC, the elastic forces of the lung and chest walls are equal and in opposite directions. The pleural surfaces link these two opposing forces. (Redrawn with modification from Shapiro BA, Harrison RA, Trout CA: The mechanics of ventilation. In Clinical Application of Respiratory Care, 3rd ed. Chicago, Year Book, 1985, p 57.)

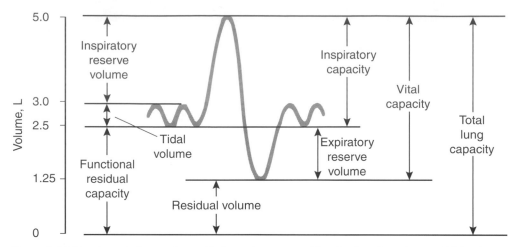

Figure 4-16 The dynamic lung volumes that can be measured by simple spirometry are tidal volume, inspiratory reserve volume, expiratory reserve volume, inspiratory capacity, and vital capacity. The static lung volumes are residual volume, functional residual capacity, and total lung capacity. Static lung volumes cannot be measured by simple spirometry and require separate methods of measurement (e.g., inert gas dilution, nitrogen washout, or whole-body plethysmography).

other lung volumes, which relate these three volumes to one another, can be measured by simple spirometry.

Residual volume, FRC, and TLC can be measured by any of three techniques: (1) nitrogen washout, (2) inert gas dilution, and (3) total-body plethysmography. The first method, the nitrogen washout technique, is based on measuring expired nitrogen concentrations before and after breathing pure O_2 for several minutes and thus calculating the total quantity of nitrogen eliminated. Thus, if 2 L of nitrogen is eliminated and the initial alveolar nitrogen concentration was 80%, the initial volume of the lung was 2.5 L. The second method, the inert gas dilution technique, uses the wash-in of an inert tracer gas such as helium. If 50 mL of helium is introduced into the lungs and, after equilibration, the helium concentration is found to be 1%, the volume of the lung is 5 L. The third method, the total-body plethysmography technique, uses Boyle's law (i.e., $P_1V_1 = P_2V_2$, where P_1 = initial pressure, V_1 = initial volume). The subject is confined within a gas-tight box (plethysmograph) so that changes in the volume of the body during respiration may be readily determined as a change in pressure within the sealed box. Although each technique has technical limitations, all are based on sound physical and physiologic principles and provide accurate results in normal patients. Disparity between FRC as measured in the body plethysmograph and by the helium dilution method is often used as a way of detecting large, nonventilating air-trapped blebs.[36] Obviously, there are difficulties in applying the body plethysmograph to anesthetized patients.

b. Airway Closure and Closing Capacity

As discussed earlier in the section on the distribution of ventilation, Ppl increases from the top to the bottom of the lung and determines regional alveolar size, compliance, and ventilation. Of even greater importance to the

anesthesiologist is the recognition that these gradients in Ppl may lead to airway closure and collapse of alveoli.

i. Patient with Normal Lungs Figure 4-17A illustrates the normal resting end-expiratory (FRC) position of the lung–chest wall combination. The distending transpulmonary and the intrathoracic air passage transmural ΔP is 5 cm H_2O, and the airways remain patent. During the middle of a normal inspiration (Fig. 4-17B), there is an increase in transmural ΔP (to 6.8 cm H_2O) that encourages distention of the intrathoracic air passages. During the middle of a normal expiration (Fig. 4-17C), expiration is passive; Pa is attributable only to the elastic recoil of the lung (2 cm H_2O), and there is a decrease (to 5.2 cm H_2O) but still a favorable (distending) intraluminal transmural ΔP. During the middle of a severe forced expiration (Fig. 4-17D), Ppl increases far higher than atmospheric pressure and is communicated to the alveoli, which have a pressure that is still higher because of the elastic recoil of the alveolar septa (an additional 2 cm H_2O).

At high gas flow rates, the pressure drop down the air passage is increased, and there is a point at which intraluminal pressure equals either the surrounding parenchymal pressure or Ppl; that point is termed the equal pressure point (EPP). If the EPP occurs in small intrathoracic air passages (distal to the 11th generation, the airways have no cartilage and are called bronchioles), they may be held open at that particular point by the tethering effect of the elastic recoil of the immediately adjacent or surrounding lung parenchyma. If the EPP occurs in large extrathoracic air passages (proximal to the 11th generation, the airways have cartilage and are called bronchi), they may be held open at that particular point by their cartilage. Downstream of the EPP (in either small or large airways), transmural ΔP is reversed (−6 cm H_2O), and airway closure occurs. Thus, the patency of airways

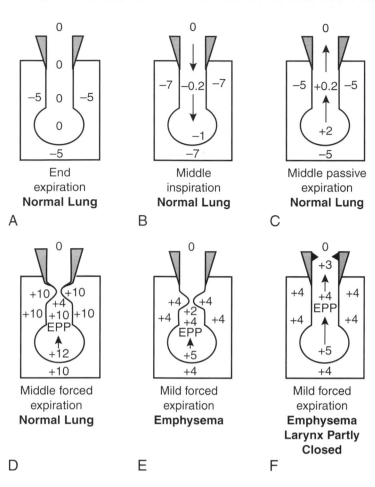

Figure 4-17 Pressure gradients across the airways. The airways consist of a thin-walled intrathoracic portion (near the alveoli) and a more rigid (cartilaginous) intrathoracic and extrathoracic portion. During expiration, the pressure from elastic recoil is assumed to be +2 cm H_2O in normal lungs (**A** to **D**) and +1 cm H_2O in abnormal lungs (**E** and **F**). The total pressure inside the alveolus is pleural pressure plus elastic recoil. The *arrows* indicate the direction of airflow. EPP, equal pressure point. See the text for an explanation. (Redrawn with modification from Benumof JL: Anesthesia for Thoracic Surgery, 2nd ed. Philadelphia, WB Saunders, 1995, Chapter 8.)

distal to the 11th generation is a function of lung volume, and the patency of airways proximal to the 11th generation is a function of intrathoracic (pleural) pressure. In extrathoracic bronchi with cartilage, the posterior membranous sheath appears to give first by invaginating into the lumen.[113] If lung volume were abnormally decreased (for example, because of splinting) and expiration were still forced, the caliber of the airways would be relatively reduced at all times, which would cause the EPP and point of collapse to move progressively from larger to smaller air passages (closer to the alveolus).

In adults with normal lungs, airway closure may still occur even if exhalation is not forced, provided that residual volume is approached closely enough. Even in patients with normal lungs, as lung volume decreases toward residual volume during expiration, small airways (0.5 to 0.9 mm in diameter) show a progressive tendency to close, whereas larger airways remain patent.[28,38] Airway closure occurs first in the dependent lung regions (as directly observed by computed tomography)[27] because the distending transpulmonary pressure is less and the volume change during expiration is greater. Airway closure is most likely to occur in the dependent regions of the lung whether the patient is in the supine or the lateral decubitus position[27] and whether ventilation is spontaneous or positive-pressure ventilation.[173,174]

ii. Patients with Abnormal Lungs Airway closure occurs with milder active expiration, lower gas flow rates, and higher lung volumes and occurs closer to the alveolus in patients with emphysema, bronchitis, asthma, and pulmonary interstitial edema. In all four conditions, the increased airway resistance causes a larger decrease in pressure from the alveoli to the larger bronchi, thereby creating the potential for negative intrathoracic transmural ΔP and narrowed and collapsed airways. In addition, the structural integrity of the conducting airways may be diminished because of inflammation and scarring, and therefore these airways may close more readily for any given lung volume or transluminal ΔP.

In emphysema, the elastic recoil of the lung is reduced (to 1 cm H_2O in Fig. 4-17E), the air passages are poorly supported by the lung parenchyma, the point of airway resistance is close to the alveolus, and transmural ΔP can become negative quickly. Therefore, during only a mild forced expiration in an emphysematous patient, the EPP and the point of collapse are near the alveolus (see Fig. 4-17E). The use of pursed-lip or grunting expiration (the equivalents of partly closing the larynx during expiration), PEEP, and continuous positive airway pressure in an emphysematous patient restores a favorable (distending) intrathoracic transmural air ΔP (Fig. 4-17F). In bronchitis, the airways are structurally weakened and may close when only a small negative transmural ΔP is present (as with mild forced expiration). In asthma, the middle-sized airways are narrowed by bronchospasm, and if expiration is forced, they are further narrowed by a negative transmural ΔP. Finally, with pulmonary interstitial edema, perialveolar interstitial edema compresses the alveoli and acutely decreases FRC; the peribronchial edema fluid cuffs (within the connective tissue sheaths around the larger arteries and bronchi) compress the bronchi and acutely increase closing volume.[22,74,76]

iii. Measurement of Closing Capacity CC is a sensitive test of early small-airway disease and is performed by having the patient exhale to residual volume (Fig. 4-18).[111] As inhalation from residual volume toward TLC is begun, a bolus of tracer gas (xenon 133, helium) is injected into the inspired gas. During the initial part of this inhalation from residual volume, the first gas to enter the alveolus is the VD gas and the tracer bolus. The tracer gas enters only alveoli that are already open (presumably the apices of the lung) and does not enter alveoli that are already

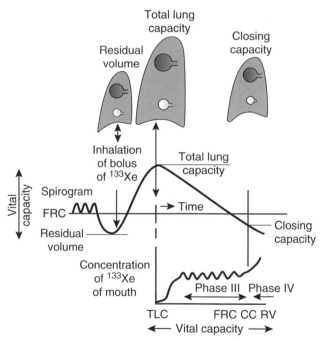

Figure 4-18 Measurement of closing capacity with the use of a tracer gas such as xenon 133 (^{133}Xe). The bolus of tracer gas is inhaled near residual volume and, because of airway closure in the dependent lung, is distributed only to nondependent alveoli whose air passages are still open. During expiration, the concentration of tracer gas becomes constant after the dead space is washed out. This plateau (phase III) gives way to a rising concentration of tracer gas (phase IV) when there is once again closure of the dependent airways because the only contribution made to expired gas is by the nondependent alveoli with a high ^{133}Xe concentration. CC, closing capacity; FRC, functional residual volume; RV, residual volume; TLC, total lung capacity. (Redrawn with modification from Lumb AB: Respiratory system resistance: Measurement of closing capacity. In Lumb AB [ed]: Nunn's Applied Respiratory Physiology, 5th ed. London, Butterworths, 2000, p 79.)

closed (presumably the bases of the lung). As the inhalation continues, the apical alveoli complete filling and the basilar alveoli begin to open and fill, but with gas that does not contain any tracer gas.

A differential tracer gas concentration is thus established, with the gas in the apices having a higher tracer concentration (see Fig. 4-18) than that in the bases (see Fig. 4-18). As the subject exhales and the diaphragm ascends, a point is reached at which the small airways just above the diaphragm start to close and thereby limit airflow from these areas. The airflow now comes more from the upper lung fields, where the alveolar gas has a much higher tracer concentration, which results in a sudden increase in the tracer gas concentration toward the end of exhalation (phase IV of Fig. 4-18).

Closing volume (CV) is the difference between the onset of phase IV and residual volume; because it represents part of a vital capacity maneuver, it is expressed as a percentage of vital lung capacity. CV plus residual volume is known as CC and is expressed as a percentage of TLC. Smoking, obesity, aging, and the supine position increase CC.[151] In healthy individuals at a mean age of 44 years, CC = FRC in the supine position, and at a mean age of 66 years, CC = FRC in the upright position.[105]

iv. Relationship between Functional Residual Capacity and Closing Capacity The relationship between FRC and CC is far more important than consideration of FRC or CC alone because it is this relationship that determines whether a given respiratory unit is normal or atelectatic or has a low $\dot{V}A/\dot{Q}$ ratio. The relationship between FRC and CC is as follows. When the volume of the lung at which some airways close is greater than the whole of VT, lung volume never increases enough during tidal inspiration to open any of these airways. Thus, these airways stay closed during the entire tidal respiration. Airways that are closed all the time are equivalent to atelectasis (Fig. 4-19). If the CV of some airways lies within VT, as lung volume increases during inspiration, some previously closed airways open for a short time until lung volume recedes once again below the CV of these airways. Because these opening and closing airways are open for a shorter time than normal airways are, they have less chance or time to participate in fresh gas exchange, a circumstance equivalent to a low-$\dot{V}A/\dot{Q}$ region. If the CC of the lung is below the whole of tidal respiration, no airways are closed at any time during tidal respiration; this is a normal circumstance. Anything that decreases FRC relative to CC or increases CC relative to FRC converts normal areas to low-$\dot{V}A/\dot{Q}$ and atelectatic areas,[38] which causes hypoxemia.

Mechanical intermittent positive-pressure breathing (IPPB) may be efficacious because it can take a previously spontaneously breathing patient with a low-$\dot{V}A/\dot{Q}$ relationship (in which CC is greater than FRC but still within VT, as depicted in Fig. 4-20, right panel) and increase the amount of inspiratory time that some

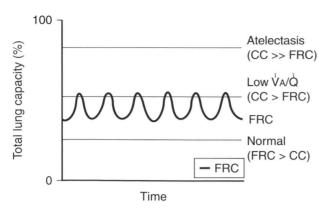

Figure 4-19 Relationship between functional residual capacity (FRC) and closing capacity (CC). FRC is the amount of gas in the lungs at end exhalation during normal tidal breathing, shown by the level of each trough of the sine wave tidal volume. CC is the amount of gas that must be in the lungs to keep the small conducting airways open. This figure shows three different CCs, as indicated by the three different straight lines. See the text for an explanation of why the three different FRC-CC relationships depicted result in normal or low ventilation-perfusion ($\dot{V}_A/\dot{Q}$) relationships or atelectasis. The abscissa is time. (Redrawn from Benumof JL: Anesthesia for Thoracic Surgery, 2nd ed. Philadelphia, WB Saunders, 1995, Chapter 8.)

previously closed (at end-exhalation) airways spend in fresh gas exchange and thereby increase the $\dot{V}_A/\dot{Q}$ relationship (Fig. 4-20, middle panel). However, if PEEP is added to IPPB, PEEP increases FRC to or above a lung volume greater than CC, thereby restoring a normal FRC-to-CC relationship so that no airways are closed at any time during the tidal respiration depicted in Figure 4-20 (left panel) (IPPB + PEEP). Thus, anesthesia-induced atelectasis (computed tomography shows crescent-shaped

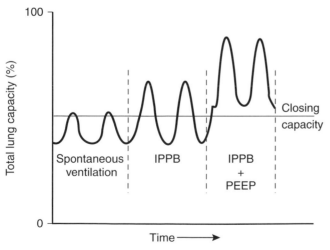

Figure 4-20 Relationship of functional residual capacity (FRC) to closing capacity (CC) during spontaneous ventilation, intermittent positive-pressure breathing (IPPB), and IPPB and positive end-expiratory pressure (IPPB + PEEP). See the text for an explanation of the effect of the two ventilatory maneuvers (IPPB and PEEP) on the relationship of FRC to CC. The abscissa is time.

densities) in the dependent regions of patients' lungs has not been reversed with IPPB alone but has been reversed with IPPB plus PEEP (5 to 10 cm H_2O).[27]

D. OXYGEN AND CARBON DIOXIDE TRANSPORT

1. Alveolar and Dead Space Ventilation and Alveolar Gas Tensions

In normal lungs, approximately two thirds of each breath reaches perfused alveoli to take part in gas exchange. This constitutes the effective or alveolar ventilation ($\dot{V}_A$). The remaining third of each breath takes no part in gas exchange and is therefore termed the total (or physiologic) dead space ventilation ($\dot{V}_D$). The relationship is as follows: alveolar ventilation ($\dot{V}_A$) = frequency (f) ($V_T - V_D$). The physiologic (or total) dead space ventilation ($V_{D_{physiologic}}$) may be further divided into two components: a volume of gas that ventilates the conducting airways, the anatomic dead space ($V_{D_{anatomic}}$), and a volume of gas that ventilates unperfused alveoli, the alveolar dead space ($V_{D_{alveolar}}$). Clinical examples of $V_{D_{alveolar}}$ ventilation include zone 1, pulmonary embolus, and destroyed alveolar septa, and such ventilation therefore does not participate in gas exchange. Figure 4-21 shows a two-compartment model of the lung in which the anatomic and alveolar dead space compartments have been combined into the total (physiologic) dead space compartment; the other compartment is the alveolar ventilation compartment, whose idealized $\dot{V}_A/\dot{Q}$ ratio is 1.0.

The anatomic dead space varies with lung size and is approximately 2 mL/kg of body weight (150 mL in a 70-kg adult). In a normal healthy adult lying supine, anatomic dead space and total (physiologic) dead space are approximately equal to each other because alveolar dead space is normally minimal. In the erect posture, the uppermost alveoli may not be perfused (zone 1), and alveolar dead space may increase from a negligible amount to 60 to 80 mL.

Figure 4-21 illustrates that in a steady state, the volume of CO_2 entering the alveoli ($\dot{V}_{CO_2}$) is equal to the volume of CO_2 eliminated in the expired gas ($\dot{V}_E$)($F_{E_{CO_2}}$). Thus $\dot{V}_{CO_2} = (\dot{V}_E)(F_{E_{CO_2}})$. However, the expired gas volume consists of alveolar gas ($\dot{V}_A$) ($F_{A_{CO_2}}$) and $\dot{V}_D$ gas ($\dot{V}_D$)($F_{I_{CO_2}}$). Thus, $\dot{V}_{CO_2} = (\dot{V}_A)$ ($F_{A_{CO_2}}$) + ($\dot{V}_D$)($F_{I_{CO_2}}$). Setting the first equation equal to the second equation and using the relationship $\dot{V}_E = \dot{V}_A + \dot{V}_D$, subsequent algebraic manipulation, including setting $P_{A_{CO_2}}$ equal to Pa_{CO_2}, results in the modified Bohr equation:

$$V_D/V_T = (Pa_{CO_2} - P_{E_{CO_2}})/Pa_{CO_2} \qquad (9)$$

The $P_{E_{CO_2}}$ value may be obtained by measuring exhaled CO_2 in a large (Douglas) bag, or, more commonly, end-tidal P_{CO_2} ($P_{ET_{CO_2}}$) can be used as a surrogate. In severe lung disease, physiologic V_D/V_T provides a useful expression of the inefficiency of ventilation. In a healthy adult, this ratio is usually less than 30%; that is,

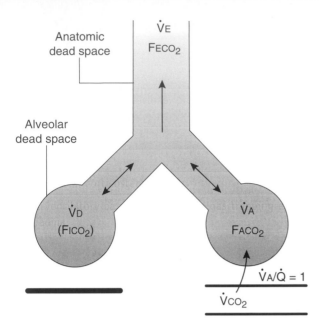

V_D = Total dead space
 = Anatomic + alveolar dead space

Figure 4-21 Two-compartment model of the lung in which the anatomic and alveolar dead space compartments have been combined into the total (physiologic) dead space ($\dot{V}_D$). F_{ACO_2} = alveolar CO_2 fraction; F_{ECO_2} = mixed expired CO_2 fraction; F_{ICO_2} = inspired CO_2 fraction; $\dot{V}_A$ = alveolar ventilation; $\dot{V}_A/\dot{Q}$ = 1 means ventilation and perfusion are equal in liters per minute; $\dot{V}_{CO_2}$ = carbon dioxide production; $\dot{V}_E$ = expired minute ventilation. Normally, the amount of CO_2 eliminated at the airway ($\dot{V}_E \times F_{ECO_2}$) equals the amount of CO_2 removed by alveolar ventilation ($\dot{V}_A \times F_{ACO_2}$) because there is no CO_2 elimination from alveolar dead space ($F_{ICO_2} = 0$).

ventilation is more than 70% efficient. In a patient with obstructive airway disease, V_D/V_T may increase to 60% to 70%. Under these conditions, ventilation is obviously grossly inefficient. Figure 4-22 shows the relationship between minute ventilation ($\dot{V}_E$) and Pa_{CO_2} for several V_D/V_T values. As $\dot{V}_E$ decreases, Pa_{CO_2} increases for all V_D/V_T values. As V_D/V_T increases, a given decrease in $\dot{V}_E$ causes a much greater increase in Pa_{CO_2}. If Pa_{CO_2} is to remain constant while V_D/V_T increases, $\dot{V}_E$ must increase.

The alveolar concentration of a gas is equal to the difference between the inspired concentration of a gas and the ratio of the output (or uptake) of the gas to $\dot{V}_A$. Thus, for gas X during dry conditions, $P_{AX} = (P_{dry atm})(F_{IX}) \pm \dot{V}_X$ (output or uptake)$/\dot{V}_A$, where P_{AX} = alveolar partial pressure of gas X, F_{IX} = inspired concentration of gas X, $P_{dry atm}$ = dry atmospheric pressure = $P_{wet atm} - PH_2O = 760 - 47 = 713$ mm Hg, $\dot{V}_X$ = output or uptake of gas X, and $\dot{V}_A$ = alveolar ventilation.

For CO_2, $Pa_{CO_2} = 713(F_{ICO_2} + \dot{V}_{CO_2}/\dot{V}_A)$. Because $F_{ICO_2} = 0$ and using standard conversion factors:

$$P_{ACO_2} = 713[\dot{V}_{CO_2} \text{ (mL/min STPD)}/\dot{V}_A \text{ (L/min/BTPS)(0.863)]} \qquad (10)$$

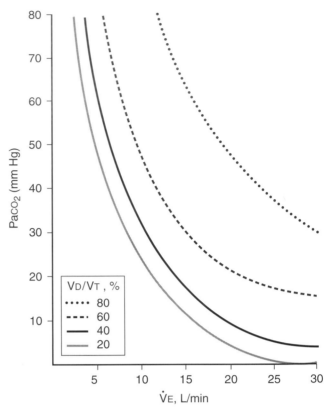

Figure 4-22 The relationship between alveolar ventilation and PA_{O_2} and Pa_{O_2} for a group of different O_2 consumption ($\dot{V}_{O_2}$) and CO_2 production ($\dot{V}_{CO_2}$) values is derived from equations (10) and (11) in the text and is hyperbolic. As alveolar ventilation increases, PA_{O_2} and Pa_{CO_2} approach inspired concentrations. Decreases in alveolar ventilation to less than 4 L/min are accompanied by precipitous decreases in PA_{O_2} and increases in Pa_{CO_2}.

Where BTPS = body temperature and pressure, saturated (i.e., 37° C, $PH_2O = 47$ mmHg) and STPD = standard temperature and pressure, dry.

For example, 36 mm Hg = (713)(200/4000).
For O_2,

$$P_{AO_2} = 713[F_{IO_2} - \dot{V}_{O_2} \text{ (mL/min)}/\dot{V}_A \text{ (mL/min)}] \qquad (11)$$

For example, 100 mm Hg = 713(0.21 − 225/3200). Figure 4-23 shows the hyperbolic relationships expressed in equations (10) and (11) between Pa_{CO_2} and $\dot{V}_A$ (see Fig. 4-22) and between PA_{O_2} and $\dot{V}_A$ for different levels of $\dot{V}_{CO_2}$ and $\dot{V}_{O_2}$, respectively. Pa_{CO_2} is substituted for PA_{CO_2} because PA_{CO_2}-to-Pa_{CO_2} gradients are small (as opposed to PA_{O_2}-to-Pa_{O_2} gradients, which can be large). Note that as $\dot{V}_A$ increases, the second term of the right side of equations (10) and (11) approaches zero and the composition of the alveolar gas approaches that of the inspired gas. In addition, it should be noted from Figure 4-22 through Figure 4-24 that because anesthesia is usually administered with an oxygen-enriched gas mixture, hypercapnia is a more common result of hypoventilation than hypoxemia is.

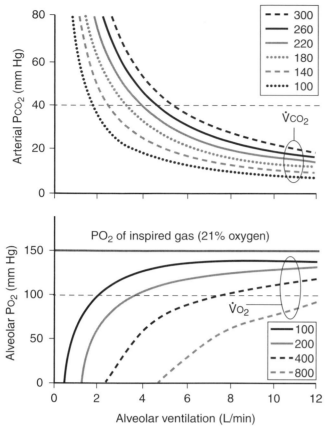

Figure 4-23 Relationship between minute ventilation ($\dot{V}_E$, L/min) and Pa_{CO_2} for a family of ratios of total dead space to tidal volume (V_D/V_T). These curves are hyperbolic (see equation 10) and rise steeply at low $\dot{V}_E$ values.

2. Oxygen Transport

a. Overview

The principal function of the heart and lungs is supporting O_2 delivery to and CO_2 removal from the tissues in accordance with metabolic requirements while maintaining arterial blood O_2 and CO_2 partial pressures within a narrow range. The respiratory and cardiovascular systems are series linked to accomplish this function over a wide range of metabolic requirements, which may increase 30-fold from rest to heavy exercise. The functional links in the oxygen transport chain are as follows: (1) ventilation and distribution of ventilation with respect to perfusion, (2) diffusion of O_2 into blood, (3) chemical reaction of O_2 with Hb, (4) $\dot{Q}_T$ of arterial blood, and (5) distribution of blood to tissues and release of O_2 (Table 4-3). The system is seldom stressed except at exercise, and the earliest symptoms of cardiac or respiratory diseases are often seen only during exercise.

The maximum functional capacity of each link can be determined independently. Table 4-3 lists these measured functional capacities for healthy, young men. Because theoretical maximal O_2 transport at the ventilatory step or the diffusion and chemical reaction steps (about 6 L/min in healthy humans at sea level) exceeds the O_2 transportable by the maximum cardiac output

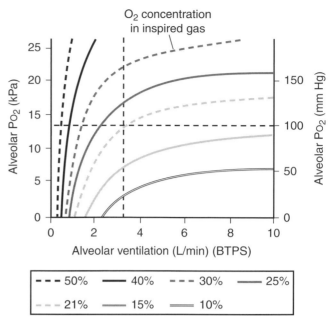

Figure 4-24 For any given O_2 concentration in inspired gas, the relationship between alveolar ventilation and PA_{O_2} is hyperbolic. As the inspired O_2 concentration is increased, the amount that alveolar ventilation must decrease to produce hypoxemia is greatly increased. BTPS, body temperature, ambient pressure, saturated. (Redrawn from Lumb AB: Respiratory system resistance: Measurement of closing capacity. In Lumb AB [ed]: Nunn's Applied Respiratory Physiology, 5th ed. London, Butterworths, 2000, p 79.)

and distribution steps, the limit to O_2 transport is the cardiovascular system. Respiratory diseases would not be expected to limit maximum O_2 transport until functional capacities are reduced nearly 40% to 50%.

b. Oxygen-Hemoglobin Dissociation Curve

As a red blood cell (RBC) passes by the alveolus, O_2 diffuses into plasma and increases PA_{O_2}. As PA_{O_2} increases, O_2 diffuses into the RBC and combines with Hb. Each Hb molecule consists of four heme molecules attached to a globin molecule. Each heme molecule consists of glycine, α-ketoglutaric acid, and iron in the ferrous (Fe^{2+}) form. Each ferrous ion has the capacity to bind with one O_2 molecule in a loose, reversible combination. As the ferrous ions bind to O_2, the Hb molecule begins to become saturated.

The oxy-Hb dissociation curve relates the saturation of Hb (rightmost *y* axis in Fig. 4-25) to PA_{O_2}. Hb is fully saturated (100%) by a P_{O_2} of about 700 mm Hg. The normal arterial point on the right side and flat part of the oxy-Hb curve in Figure 4-25 is 95% to 98% saturated by a Pa_{O_2} of about 90 to 100 mm Hg. When P_{O_2} is less than 60 mm Hg (90% saturation), saturation falls steeply, and the amount of Hb uncombined with O_2 increases greatly for a given decrease in P_{O_2}. Mixed venous blood has a P_{O_2} ($P\bar{v}_{O_2}$) of about 40 mm Hg and is approximately 75% saturated, as indicated by the middle of the three points on the oxy-Hb curve in Figure 4-25.

Table 4-3 **Functional Capacities and Potential Maximum O_2 Transport of Each Link in the O_2 Transport Chain in Normal Humans* at Sea Level**

Link in Chain	Functional Capacity in Normal Humans	Theoretical Maximum O_2 Transport Capacity
Ventilation	200 L/min (MVV)	$0.030 \times MVV = 6.0$ L O_2/min
Diffusion and chemical reaction		$DLO_2 = 6.1$ L O_2/min
CO	20 L/min	
O_2 extraction	75%	$0.16 \times CO = 3.2$ L O_2/min
(a-v O_2 difference)	(16 mL O_2/100 mL or 0.16)	

*Hemoglobin = 15 g/dL; physiologic dead space in percentage of tidal volume = 0.25; partial alveolar pressure of oxygen > 110 mm Hg.
CO, cardiac output; MVV, maximum voluntary ventilation.
From Cassidy SS: Heart-lung interactions in health and disease. Am J Med Sci 30:451-461, 1987.

The oxy-Hb curve can also relate the O_2 content (CO_2) (vol%, mL of O_2/0.1 L of blood; second most right *y* axis in Fig. 4-25) to PO_2. Oxygen is carried in solution in plasma, 0.003 mL of O_2/mm Hg PO_2/0.1 L, and is combined with Hb, 1.39 mL of O_2/g of Hb, to the extent (percentage) that Hb is saturated. Thus,

$$CO_2 = (1.39)(Hb)(\text{percent saturation}) + 0.003(PO_2) \quad (12)$$

For a patient with an Hb content of 15 g/0.1 L, PAO_2 of 100 mm Hg, and $P\bar{v}O_2$ of 40 mm Hg, the arterial O_2 content (CaO_2) = $(1.39)(15)(1) + (0.003)(100) =$ $20.9 + 0.3 = 21.2$ mL of O_2/0.1 L; the mixed venous O_2 content ($C\bar{v}O_2$) = $(1.39)(15)(0.75) + (0.003)(40) = 15.6 + 0.1 = 15.7$ mL of O_2/0.1 L. Thus, the normal arteriovenous O_2 content difference is approximately 5.5 mL/0.1 L.

Note that equation (12) uses the constant 1.39, which means that 1 g of Hb can carry 1.39 mL of oxygen. Controversy exists over the magnitude of this number. Originally, 1.34 had been used,[60] but with determination of the molecular weight of Hb (64,458), the theoretical value of 1.39 became popular.[176] After extensive human studies, Gregory[68] observed in 1974 that the applicable value was 1.31 mL O_2/g of Hb in human adults.

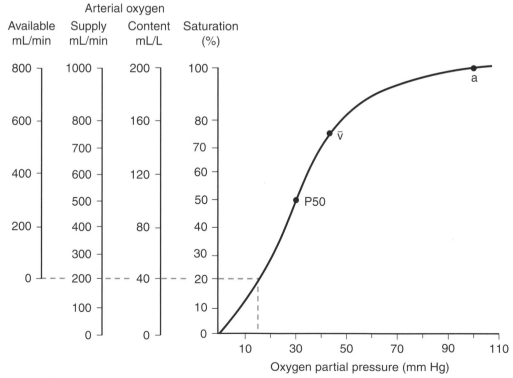

Figure 4-25 Oxygen-hemoglobin dissociation curve. Four different ordinates are shown as a function of oxygen partial pressure (the abscissa). In order from right to left, they are saturation (%), O_2 content (mL of O_2/0.1 L of blood), O_2 supply to peripheral tissues (mL/min), and O_2 available to peripheral tissues (mL/min), which is O_2 supply minus the approximately 200 mL/min that cannot be extracted below a partial pressure of 20 mm Hg. Three points are shown on the curve: a, normal arterial pressure; $\bar{v}$, normal mixed venous pressure; and P50, the partial pressure (27 mm Hg) at which hemoglobin is 50% saturated.

That the clinically measured CO_2 is lower than the theoretical 1.39 is probably due to the small amount of methemoglobin (Met-Hb) and carboxyhemoglobin (CO-Hb) normally present in blood.

The oxy-Hb curve can also relate O_2 transport (L/min) to the peripheral tissues (see the third most right *y* axis in Fig. 4-25) to PO_2. This value is obtained by multiplying the O_2 content by $\dot{Q}T$ (O_2 transport = $\dot{Q}T \times CaO_2$). To do this multiplication, one must convert the content unit of mL/0.1 L to mL/L by multiplying the usual O_2 content by 10 (results in mL of O_2/L of blood); subsequent multiplication of mL/L against $\dot{Q}T$ in L/min yields mL/min. Thus, if $\dot{Q}T$ = 5 L/min and CaO_2 = 20 mL of O_2/0.1 L, the arterial point corresponds to 1000 mL O_2/min going to the periphery, and the venous point corresponds to 750 mL O_2/min returning to the lungs, with $\dot{V}O_2$ = 250 mL/min.

The oxy-Hb curve can also relate the O_2 actually available to the tissues (see leftmost *y* axis in Fig. 4-25) as a function of PO_2. Of the 1000 mL/min of O_2 normally going to the periphery, 200 mL/min of O_2 cannot be extracted because it would lower PO_2 below the level (see the rectangular dashed line in Fig. 4-25) at which organs such as the brain can survive; the O_2 available to tissues is therefore 800 mL/min. This amount is approximately three to four times the normal resting $\dot{V}O_2$. When $\dot{Q}T$ = 5 L/min and arterial saturation is less than 40%, the total flow of O_2 to the periphery is reduced to 400 mL/min; the available O_2 is now 200 mL/min and O_2 supply just equals O_2 demand. Consequently, with low arterial saturation, tissue demand can be met only by an increase in $\dot{Q}T$ or, in the longer term, by an increase in Hb concentration.

The affinity of Hb for O_2 is best described by the PO_2 level at which Hb is 50% saturated (P50) on the oxy-Hb curve. The normal adult P50 is 26.7 mm Hg (see the point on the left side and steep portion of the oxy-Hb curve in Fig. 4-24).

The effect of a change in PO_2 on Hb saturation is related to both P50 and the portion of the oxy-Hb curve at which the change occurs.[86] In the region of normal PaO_2 (75 to 100 mm Hg), the curve is relatively horizontal, and shifts of the curve have little effect on saturation. In the region of mixed venous PO_2, where the curve is relatively steep, a shift of the curve leads to a much greater difference in saturation. A P50 lower than 27 mm Hg describes a left-shifted oxy-Hb curve, which means that at any given PO_2, Hb has a higher affinity for O_2 and is therefore more saturated than normal. This lower P50 may require higher than normal tissue perfusion to produce the normal amount of O_2 unloading. Causes of a left-shifted oxy-Hb curve are alkalosis (metabolic and respiratory—the Bohr effect), hypothermia, abnormal and fetal Hb, carboxyhemoglobin, methemoglobin, and decreased RBC 2,3-diphosphoglycerate (2,3-DPG) content (which may occur with the transfusion of old acid citrate-dextrose–stored blood; storage of blood in citrate-phosphate-dextrose minimizes changes in 2,3-DPG with time).[86]

A P50 higher than 27 mm Hg describes a right-shifted oxy-Hb curve, which means that at any given PO_2, Hb has a low affinity for O_2 and is less saturated than normal. This higher P50 may allow a lower tissue perfusion than normal to produce the normal amount of O_2 unloading. Causes of a right-shifted oxy-Hb curve are acidosis (metabolic and respiratory—the Bohr effect), hyperthermia, abnormal Hb, increased RBC 2,3-DPG content, and inhaled anesthetics (see later).[86]

Abnormalities in acid-base balance result in alteration of 2,3-DPG metabolism to shift the oxy-Hb curve to its normal position. This compensatory change in 2,3-DPG requires between 24 and 48 hours. Thus, with acute acid-base abnormalities, O_2 affinity and the position of the oxy-Hb curve change. However, with more prolonged acid-base changes, the reciprocal changes in 2,3-DPG levels shift the oxy-Hb curve and therefore O_2 affinity back toward normal.[86]

Many inhaled anesthetics have been shown to shift the oxy-Hb dissociation curve to the right.[66] Isoflurane shifts P50 to the right by 2.6 ± 0.07 mm Hg at a vapor pressure of approximately 1 minimum alveolar concentration (MAC) (1.25%).[93] On the other hand, high-dose fentanyl, morphine, and meperidine do not alter the position of the curve.

c. Effect of $\dot{Q}s/\dot{Q}T$ on PaO_2

PAO_2 is directly related to FIO_2 in normal patients. PAO_2 and FIO_2 also correspond to PaO_2 when there is little to no right-to-left transpulmonary shunt ($\dot{Q}s/\dot{Q}T$). Figure 4-26 shows the relationship between FIO_2 and PaO_2 for a family of right-to-left transpulmonary shunts ($\dot{Q}s/\dot{Q}T$); the calculations assume a constant and normal $\dot{Q}T$ and $PaCO_2$. With no $\dot{Q}s/\dot{Q}T$, a linear increase in FIO_2 results in a linear increase in PAO_2 (solid straight line). As the shunt is increased, the $\dot{Q}s/\dot{Q}T$

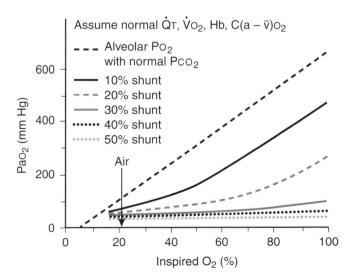

Figure 4-26 Effect of changes in inspired oxygen concentration on PaO_2 for various right-to-left transpulmonary shunts. Cardiac output ($\dot{Q}T$), hemoglobin (Hb), oxygen consumption ($\dot{V}O_2$), and arteriovenous oxygen content differences [$C(a-\bar{v})O_2$] are assumed to be normal.

lines relating F_{IO_2} to P_{aO_2} become progressively flatter.[104] With a shunt of 50% of $\dot{Q}_T$, an increase in F_{IO_2} results in almost no increase in P_{aO_2}. The solution to the problem of hypoxemia secondary to a large shunt is not increasing the F_{IO_2} but rather causing a reduction in the shunt (fiberoptic bronchoscopy, PEEP, patient's positioning, antibiotics, suctioning, diuretics).

d. Effect of $\dot{Q}_T$ and $\dot{V}_{O_2}$ on C_{aO_2}

In addition to an increased $\dot{Q}_S/\dot{Q}_T$, C_{aO_2} is decreased by decreased $\dot{Q}_T$ (for a constant $\dot{V}_{O_2}$) and by increased $\dot{V}_{O_2}$ (for a constant $\dot{Q}_T$). In either case (decreased $\dot{Q}_T$ or increased $\dot{V}_{O_2}$), along with a constant right-to-left shunt, the tissues must extract more O_2 from blood per unit blood volume, and therefore, $C\bar{v}_{O_2}$ must primarily decrease (Fig. 4-27). When blood with lower $C\bar{v}_{O_2}$ passes through whatever shunt exists in the lung and remains unchanged in its $\dot{V}_{O_2}$, it must inevitably mix with oxygenated end-pulmonary capillary blood (c' flow) and secondarily decrease C_{aO_2} (see Fig. 4-27).

The amount of O_2 flowing through any given particular lung channel per minute, as depicted in Figure 4-27, is a product of blood flow times the O_2 content of that blood. Thus, from Figure 4-27, $\dot{Q}_T \times C_{aO_2} = \dot{Q}_{c'} \times C_{c'O_2} + \dot{Q}_S \times C\bar{v}_{O_2}$. With $\dot{Q}_{c'} = \dot{Q}_T - \dot{Q}_S$ and further algebraic manipulation.[95]

$$\dot{Q}_S/\dot{Q}_T = C_{c'O_2} - C_{aO_2} / C_{c'O_2} - C\bar{v}_{O_2} \qquad (13)$$

The larger the intrapulmonary shunt, the greater is the decrease in C_{aO_2} because more venous blood with lower $C\bar{v}_{O_2}$ can admix with end-pulmonary capillary blood (see Fig. 4-37).[19,144] Thus, $P_{(A-a)O_2}$ is a function both of the size of the $\dot{Q}_S/\dot{Q}_T$ and of what is flowing through the $\dot{Q}_S/\dot{Q}_T$, namely, $C\bar{v}_{O_2}$, and $C\bar{v}_{O_2}$ is a primary function of $\dot{Q}_T$ and $\dot{V}_{O_2}$. Figure 4-28 shows the equivalent circuit of the pulmonary circulation in a patient with a 50% shunt, a normal $C\bar{v}_{O_2}$ of 15 vol%, and a moderately low C_{aO_2} of 17.5 vol%. Decreasing $\dot{Q}_T$ or increasing $\dot{V}_{O_2}$, or both, causes a larger primary decrease in $C\bar{v}_{O_2}$ to 10 vol% and a smaller but still significant secondary decrease in C_{aO_2} to 15 vol%; the ratio of change in $C\bar{v}_{O_2}$ to C_{aO_2} in this example of 50% $\dot{Q}_S/\dot{Q}_T$ is 2:1.

If a decrease in $\dot{Q}_T$ or an increase in $\dot{V}_{O_2}$ is accompanied by a decrease in $\dot{Q}_S/\dot{Q}_T$, there may be no change in P_{aO_2} (a decreasing effect on P_{aO_2} is offset by an increasing effect on P_{aO_2}) (Table 4-4). These changes sometimes occur in diffuse lung disease. If a decrease in $\dot{Q}_T$ or an increase in $\dot{V}_{O_2}$ is accompanied by an increase in $\dot{Q}_S/\dot{Q}_T$, P_{aO_2} may be greatly decreased (a decreasing effect on P_{aO_2} is compounded by another decreasing effect on P_{aO_2}) (see Table 4-4). These changes sometimes occur in regional ARDS and atelectasis.[33]

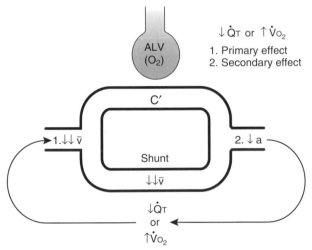

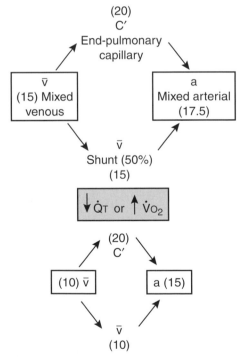

Figure 4-27 Effect of a decrease in cardiac output or an increase in oxygen consumption on mixed venous and arterial oxygen content. Mixed venous blood ($\bar{v}$) either perfuses ventilated alveolar (ALV O_2) capillaries and becomes oxygenated end-pulmonary capillary blood (c') or perfuses whatever true shunt pathways exist and remains the same in composition (desaturated). These two pathways must ultimately join together to form mixed arterial (a) blood. If cardiac output ($\dot{Q}_T$) decreases or oxygen consumption ($\dot{V}_{O_2}$) increases, or both, the tissues must extract more oxygen per unit volume of blood than under normal conditions. Thus, the primary effect of a decrease in $\dot{Q}_T$ or an increase in $\dot{V}_{O_2}$ is a decrease in mixed venous oxygen content. The mixed venous blood with a decreased oxygen content must flow through the shunt pathway as before (which may remain constant in size) and lower the arterial content of oxygen. Thus, the secondary effect of a decrease in $\dot{Q}_T$ or an increase in $\dot{V}_{O_2}$ is a decrease in arterial oxygen content.

Figure 4-28 The equivalent circuit of the pulmonary circulation in a patient with a 50% right-to-left shunt. Oxygen content is in mL/100 mL of blood (vol%). A decrease in cardiac output ($\dot{Q}_T$) or an increase in O_2 consumption ($\dot{V}_{O_2}$) can cause a decrease in mixed venous oxygen content (from 15 to 10 vol% in this example), which in turn causes a decrease in the arterial content of oxygen (from 17.5 to 15.0 vol%). In this 50% shunt example, the decrease in mixed venous oxygen content was twice the decrease in arterial oxygen content.

Table 4-4 **Cardiac Output ($\dot{Q}T$), Shunt ($\dot{Q}s/\dot{Q}T$), and Venous ($P\bar{v}o_2$) and Arterial (Pao_2) Oxygenation**

Changes	Clinical Situation
If $\dot{Q}T \downarrow \rightarrow \downarrow P\bar{v}o_2$ and $\dot{Q}s/\dot{Q}T = K \rightarrow Pao_2 \downarrow$	Decreased cardiac output, stable shunt
If $\dot{Q}T \downarrow \rightarrow \downarrow P\bar{v}o_2$ and $\dot{Q}s/\dot{Q}T \downarrow \rightarrow Pao_2 = K$	Application of PEEP in ARDS
If $\dot{Q}T \downarrow \rightarrow \downarrow P\bar{v}o_2$ and $\dot{Q}s/\dot{Q}T \uparrow \rightarrow Pao_2 \downarrow\downarrow$	Shock combined with ARDS or atelectasis

ARDS, adult respiratory distress syndrome; K, constant; PEEP, positive end-expiratory pressure; $\downarrow$, decrease; $\uparrow$, increase.

e. Fick Principle

The Fick principle allows calculation of $\dot{V}o_2$ and states that the amount of O_2 consumed by the body ($\dot{V}o_2$) is equal to the amount of O_2 leaving the lungs ($\dot{Q}T$) (Cao_2) minus the amount of O_2 returning to the lungs ($\dot{Q}T$)($C\bar{v}o_2$). Thus

$$\dot{V}o_2 = (\dot{Q}T)(Cao_2) - (\dot{Q}T)(C\bar{v}o_2) = \dot{Q}T(Cao_2 - C\bar{v}o_2)$$

Condensing the content symbols yields the usual expression of the Fick equation:

$$\dot{V}o_2 = (\dot{Q}T)[C(a\text{-}\bar{v})o_2] \qquad (14)$$

This equation states that O_2 consumption is equal to $\dot{Q}T$ times the arteriovenous O_2 content difference. Normally, $(5 \text{ L/min})(5.5 \text{ mL})/0.1 \text{ L} = 0.27 \text{ L/min}$ (see "Oxygen-Hemoglobin Dissociation Curve").

$$\dot{V}o_2 = \dot{V}E(Fio_2) - \dot{V}E(Feo_2) = \dot{V}E(Fio_2 - Feo_2) \qquad (15)$$

Similarly, the amount of O_2 consumed by the body ($\dot{V}o_2$) is equal to the amount of O_2 brought into the lungs by ventilation ($\dot{V}I$)(Fio_2) minus the amount of O_2 leaving the lungs by ventilation ($\dot{V}E$)(Feo_2), where $\dot{V}E$ is expired minute ventilation and Feo_2 is the mixed expired O_2 fraction.

Thus, $\dot{V}o_2 = (\dot{V}I)(Fio_2) - (\dot{V}E)(Feo_2)$. Because the difference between $\dot{V}I$ and $\dot{V}E$ is due to the difference between $\dot{V}o_2$ (normally 250 mL/min) and $\dot{V}co_2$ (normally 200 mL/min) and is only 50 mL/min (see later), $\dot{V}I$ essentially equals $\dot{V}E$.

Normally, $\dot{V}o_2 = 5.0 \text{ L/min}(0.21 - 0.16) = 0.25 \text{ L/min}$. In determining $\dot{V}o_2$ in this way, $\dot{V}E$ can be measured with a spirometer, Fio_2 can be measured with an O_2 analyzer or from known fresh gas flows, and Feo_2 can be measured by collecting expired gas in a bag for a few minutes. A sample of the mixed expired gas is used to measure Peo_2. To convert Peo_2 to Feo_2, one simply divides Peo_2 by dry atmospheric pressure: $Peo_2/713 = Feo_2$.

In addition, the Fick equation is useful in understanding the impact of changes in $\dot{Q}T$ on Pao_2 and $P\bar{v}o_2$. If $\dot{V}o_2$ remains constant (K) and $\dot{Q}T$ decreases ($\downarrow$), the arteriovenous O_2 content difference has to increase ($\uparrow$):

$$\dot{V}o_2 = K = (\downarrow)\dot{Q}T \times (\uparrow)C(a\text{-}\bar{v})o_2$$

The $C(a\text{-}\bar{v})o_2$ difference increases because a decrease in $\dot{Q}T$ causes a much larger and primary decrease in $C\bar{v}o_2$ versus a smaller and secondary decrease in Cao_2:

$$(\uparrow)C(a\text{-}\bar{v})o_2 = C(\downarrow a - \downarrow\downarrow\bar{v})o_2 \text{[144]}$$

Thus, $C\bar{v}o_2$ and $P\bar{v}o_2$ are much more sensitive indicators of $\dot{Q}T$ because they change more with changes in $\dot{Q}T$ than Cao_2 (or Pao_2) does (see Figs. 4-27 and 4-37).

3. Carbon Dioxide Transport

The amount of CO_2 circulating in the body is a function of both CO_2 elimination and production. Elimination of CO_2 depends on pulmonary blood flow and alveolar ventilation. Production of CO_2 ($\dot{V}co_2$) parallels O_2 consumption ($\dot{V}o_2$) according to the respiratory quotient (RQ):

$$RQ = \frac{\dot{V}co_2}{\dot{V}o_2} \qquad (16)$$

Under normal resting conditions, R is 0.8; that is, only 80% as much CO_2 is produced as O_2 is consumed. However, this value changes as the nature of the metabolic substrate changes. If only carbohydrate is used, the respiratory quotient is 1.0. Conversely, with the sole use of fat, more O_2 combines with hydrogen to produce water, and the R value drops to 0.7.

CO_2 is transported from mitochondria to the alveoli in a number of forms. In plasma, CO_2 exists in physical solution, hydrated to carbonic acid (H_2CO_3), and as bicarbonate (HCO_3^-). In the RBC, CO_2 combines with Hb as carbaminohemoglobin (Hb-CO_2). The approximate values of H_2CO_3 ($H_2O + CO_2$), HCO_3^-, and Hb-CO_2 relative to the total CO_2 transported are 7%, 80%, and 13%, respectively.

In plasma, CO_2 exists both in physical solution and as H_2CO_3:

$$H_2O + CO_2 \Leftrightarrow H_2CO_3 \qquad (17)$$

The CO_2 in solution can be related to Pco_2 by the use of Henry's law.[80]

$$Pco_2 \times \alpha = [CO_2] \text{ in solution} \qquad (18)$$

where α is the solubility coefficient of CO_2 in plasma (0.03 mmol/L/mm Hg at 37° C). However, the major fraction of CO_2 produced passes into the RBC. As in plasma,

CO_2 combines with water to produce H_2CO_3. However, unlike the slow reaction in plasma, in which the equilibrium point lies toward the left, the reaction in an RBC is catalyzed by the enzyme carbonic anhydrase. This zinc-containing enzyme moves the reaction to the right at a rate 1000 times faster than in plasma. Furthermore, nearly 99.9% of the H_2CO_3 dissociates to HCO_3^- and hydrogen ions (H^+):

$$H_2O + CO_2 \xrightarrow[H_2CO_3 \rightarrow H^+ + HCO_3^-]{\text{carbonic anhydrase}} H_2CO_3 \qquad (19)$$

The H^+ produced from H_2CO_3 in the production of HCO_3^- is buffered by Hb ($H^+ + Hb \Leftrightarrow HHb$). The HCO_3^- produced passes out of the RBC into plasma to perform its function as a buffer. To maintain electrical neutrality within the RBC, chloride ion (Cl^-) moves in as HCO_3^- moves out (Cl^- shift). Finally, CO_2 can combine with Hb in the erythrocyte (to produce $Hb\text{-}CO_2$). Again, as in HCO_3^- release, an H^+ ion is formed in the reaction of CO_2 and Hb. This H^+ ion is also buffered by Hb.

4. Bohr and Haldane Effects

Just as the percent saturation of Hb with O_2 is related to Po_2 (described by the oxy-Hb curve), so is the total CO_2 in blood related to Pco_2. In addition, Hb has variable affinity for CO_2; it binds more avidly in the reduced state than as oxy-Hb.[86] The Bohr effect describes the effect of Pco_2 and [H^+] ions on the oxy-Hb curve. Hypercapnia and acidosis both shift the curve to the right (reducing the oxygen-binding affinity of hemoglobin), and hypocapnia and alkalosis both shift the curve to the left. Conversely, the Haldane effect describes the shift in the CO_2 dissociation curve caused by oxygenation of Hb. Low Po_2 shifts the CO_2 dissociation curve to the left so that the blood is able to pick up more CO_2 (as occurs in capillaries of rapidly metabolizing tissues). Conversely, oxygenation of Hb (as occurs in the lungs) reduces the affinity of Hb for CO_2, and the CO_2 dissociation curve is shifted to the right, thereby increasing CO_2 removal.

E. PULMONARY MICROCIRCULATION, PULMONARY INTERSTITIAL SPACE, AND PULMONARY INTERSTITIAL FLUID KINETICS (PULMONARY EDEMA)

The ultrastructural appearance of an alveolar septum[57] is depicted schematically in Figure 4-29. Capillary blood is separated from alveolar gas by a series of anatomic layers: capillary endothelium, endothelial basement membrane, interstitial space, epithelial basement membrane, and alveolar epithelium (of the type I pneumocyte).

On one side of the alveolar septum (the thick, upper [see Fig. 4-29], fluid- and gas-exchanging side), the epithelial and endothelial basement membranes are separated

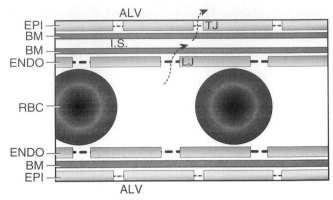

Figure 4-29 Schematic summary of the ultrastructure of a pulmonary capillary. The upper side of the capillary has the endothelial and epithelial basement membranes separated by an interstitial space, whereas the lower side contains only fused endothelial and epithelial basement membranes. The *dashed arrows* indicate a potential pathway for fluid to move from the intravascular space to the interstitial space (through loose junctions in the endothelium) and from the interstitial space to the alveolar space (through tight junctions in the epithelium). ALV, alveolus; BM, basement membrane; ENDO, endothelium; EPI, epithelium; IS, interstitial space; LJ, loose junction; RBC, red blood cell; TJ, tight junction. (Redrawn from Fishman AP: Pulmonary edema: The water-exchanging function of the lung. Circulation 46:390, 1972.)

by a space of variable thickness containing connective tissue fibrils, elastic fibers, fibroblasts, and macrophages. This connective tissue is the backbone of the lung parenchyma; it forms a continuum with the connective tissue sheaths around the conducting airways and blood vessels. Thus, the pericapillary perialveolar interstitial space is continuous with the interstitial tissue space that surrounds terminal bronchioles and vessels, and both spaces constitute the connective tissue space of the lung. There are no lymphatics in the interstitial space of the alveolar septum. Instead, lymphatic capillaries first appear in the interstitial space surrounding terminal bronchioles, small arteries, and veins.[115]

The opposite side of the alveolar septum (the thin, down [see Fig. 4-29], gas-exchanging-only side) contains only fused epithelial and endothelial basement membranes. The interstitial space is thus greatly restricted on this side because of fusion of the basement membranes. Interstitial fluid cannot separate the endothelial and epithelial cells from one another, and as a result the space and distance barrier to fluid movement from the capillary to the alveolar compartment is reduced and composed of only the two cell linings with their associated basement membranes.[190]

Between the individual endothelial and epithelial cells are holes or junctions that provide a potential pathway for fluid to move from the intravascular space to the interstitial space and finally from the interstitial space to the alveolar space. The junctions between endothelial cells are relatively large and are therefore termed loose;

the junctions between epithelial cells are relatively small and are therefore termed tight. Pulmonary capillary permeability (K) is a direct function of and essentially equivalent to the size of the holes in the endothelial and epithelial linings.

To understand how pulmonary interstitial fluid is formed, stored, and cleared, it is necessary first to develop the concepts that (1) the pulmonary interstitial space is a continuous space between the periarteriolar and peribronchial connective tissue sheath and the space between the endothelial and epithelial basement membranes in the alveolar septum and (2) the space has a progressively negative distal-to-proximal ΔP.

The concepts of a continuous connective tissue sheath–alveolar septum interstitial space and a negative interstitial space ΔP are prerequisite to understanding interstitial fluid kinetics (Fig. 4-30). After entering the lung parenchyma, both the bronchi and arteries run within a connective tissue sheath that is formed by an invagination of the pleura at the hilum and ends at the level of the bronchioles (Fig. 4-30A). Thus, there is a potential perivascular and peribronchial space, respectively, between the arteries and the bronchi and the connective tissue sheath. The negative pressure in the pulmonary tissues surrounding the perivascular connective tissue sheath exerts a radial outward traction force on the sheath. This radial traction creates negative pressure within the sheath that is transmitted to the bronchi and arteries and tends to hold them open and increase their diameters (see Fig. 4-30).[190] The alveolar septum interstitial space is the space between the capillaries and alveoli (or, more precisely, the space between the endothelial and epithelial basement membranes) and is continuous with the interstitial tissue space that surrounds the larger arteries and bronchi (see Fig. 4-30A). Studies indicate that the alveolar interstitial pressure is also uniquely negative but not as much as the negative interstitial space pressure around the larger arteries and bronchi.[72]

The forces governing net transcapillary–interstitial space fluid movement are as follows. The net transcapillary flow of fluid (F) out of pulmonary capillaries (across the endothelium and into the interstitial space) is equal to the difference between pulmonary capillary hydrostatic pressure (P_{inside}) and interstitial fluid hydrostatic pressure ($P_{outside}$) and the difference between capillary colloid oncotic pressure (π_{inside}) and interstitial colloid oncotic pressure ($\pi_{outside}$). These four forces produce a steady-state fluid flow (F) during a constant capillary permeability (K) as predicted by the Starling equation:

$$F = K[(P_{inside} - P_{outside}) - (\pi_{inside} - \pi_{outside})] \qquad (20)$$

K is a capillary filtration coefficient expressed in mL/min/mm Hg/100 g. The filtration coefficient is the product of the effective capillary surface area in a given mass of tissue and the permeability per unit surface area of the capillary wall to filter the fluid. Under normal circumstances and at a vertical height in the lung that is

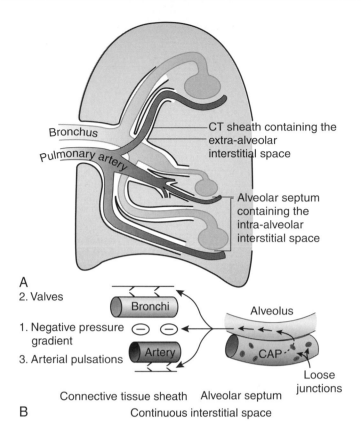

A
2. Valves

1. Negative pressure gradient

3. Arterial pulsations

Connective tissue sheath — Alveolar septum
B   Continuous interstitial space

Figure 4-30 **A,** Schematic diagram of the concept of a continuous connective tissue (CT) sheath–alveolar septum interstitial space. The entry of the main stem bronchi and pulmonary artery into the lung parenchyma invaginates the pleura at the hilum and forms a surrounding connective tissue sheath. The connective tissue sheath ends at the level of the bronchioles. The space between the pulmonary arteries and bronchi and the interstitial space is continuous with the alveolar septum interstitial space. The alveolar septum interstitial space is contained within the endothelial and epithelial basement membranes of the capillaries and alveoli, respectively. **B,** Schematic diagram showing how interstitial fluid moves from the alveolar septum interstitial space (no lymphatics) to the connective tissue interstitial space (lymphatic capillaries first appear). The mechanisms are a negative-pressure gradient (sump), the presence of one-way valves in the lymphatics, and the massaging action of arterial pulsations. (Redrawn with modification from Benumof JL: Anesthesia for Thoracic Surgery, 2nd ed. Philadelphia, WB Saunders, 1995, Chapter 8.)

at the junction of zones 2 and 3, intravascular colloid oncotic pressure (≈ 26 mm Hg) acts to keep water in the capillary lumen, and working against this force, pulmonary capillary hydrostatic pressure (≈ 10 mm Hg) acts to force water across the loose endothelial junctions into the interstitial space. If these were the only operative forces, the interstitial space and, consequently, the alveolar surfaces would be constantly dry and there would be no lymph flow. In fact, alveolar surfaces are moist, and lymphatic flow from the interstitial compartment is constant (≈ 500 mL/day). This can be explained in part by $\pi_{outside}$ (≈ 8 mm Hg) and in part by the negative $P_{outside}$ (−8 mm Hg).

Negative (subatmospheric) interstitial space pressure would promote, by suction, a slow loss of fluid across the endothelial holes.[168] Indeed, extremely negative pleural (and perivascular hydrostatic) pressure, such as may occur in a vigorously, spontaneously breathing patient with an obstructed airway, can cause pulmonary interstitial edema (Table 4-5).[136] Relative to the vertical level of the junction of zones 2 and 3, as lung height decreases (lung dependence), absolute P_{inside} increases, and fluid has a propensity to transudate; as lung height increases (lung nondependence), absolute P_{inside} decreases, and fluid has a propensity to be reabsorbed. However, fluid transudation induced by an increase in P_{inside} is limited by a concomitant dilution of proteins in the interstitial space and therefore a decrease in $\pi_{outside}$.[171] Any change in the size of the endothelial junctions, even if the foregoing four forces remain constant, changes the magnitude and perhaps even the direction of fluid movement; increased size of endothelial junctions (increased permeability) promotes transudation, whereas decreased size of endothelial junctions (decreased permeability) promotes reabsorption.

No lymphatics are present in the interstitial space of the alveolar septum. The lymphatic circulation starts as blind-ended lymphatic capillaries, first appearing in the interstitial space sheath surrounding terminal bronchioles and small arteries, and ends at the subclavian veins. Interstitial fluid is normally removed from the alveolar interstitial space into the lymphatics by a sump (pressure gradient) mechanism, which is caused by the presence of more negative pressure surrounding the larger arteries and bronchi.[141,172] The sump mechanism is aided by the presence of valves in the lymph vessels. In addition, because the lymphatics run in the same sheath as the pulmonary arteries, they are exposed to the massaging action of arterial pulsations. The differential negative pressure, the lymphatic valves, and the arterial pulsations all help propel the lymph proximally toward the hilum

Table 4-5 Causes of Extremely Negative Pulmonary Interstitial Fluid Pressure ($P_{outside}$) in Pulmonary Edema

Vigorous spontaneous ventilation against an obstructed airway
Laryngospasm
Infection, inflammation, edema
Upper airway mass (e.g., tumor, hematoma, abscess, foreign body)
Vocal cord paralysis
Strangulation
Rapid reexpansion of lung
Vigorous pleural suctioning (thoracentesis, chest tube)

through the lymph nodes (pulmonary to bronchopulmonary to tracheobronchial to paratracheal to scalene and cervical nodes) to the central venous circulation depot (Fig. 4-30B). An increase in central venous pressure, which is the backpressure for lymph to flow out of the lung, would decrease lung lymph flow and perhaps promote pulmonary interstitial edema.

If the rate of entry of fluid into the pulmonary interstitial space exceeds the capability of the pulmonary interstitial space to clear the fluid, the pulmonary interstitial space fills with fluid; the fluid, now under an increased and positive driving force (P_{ISF}), crosses the relatively impermeable epithelial wall holes and the alveolar space fills. Intra-alveolar edema fluid additionally causes alveolar collapse and atelectasis, thereby promoting further accumulation of fluid.

II. RESPIRATORY FUNCTION DURING ANESTHESIA

Arterial oxygenation is impaired in most patients during anesthesia with either spontaneous or controlled ventilation.[77,107,116,133,177,199] In otherwise normal patients, it is generally accepted that the impairment in arterial oxygenation during anesthesia is more severe in elderly persons,[70,108] obese people,[180] and smokers.[48] In various studies of healthy young to middle-aged patients under general anesthesia, venous admixture (shunt) has been found to average 10%, and the scatter in $\dot{V}A/\dot{Q}$ ratios is small to moderate,[108,150] whereas in patients with a more marked deterioration in preoperative pulmonary function, general anesthesia causes considerable widening of the $\dot{V}A/\dot{Q}$ distribution and large increases in both low-$\dot{V}A/\dot{Q}$ ($0.005 < \dot{V}A/\dot{Q} < 0.1$) (underventilated) regions and shunting.[48,70,178] The magnitude of shunting correlates closely with the degree of atelectasis.[70,178]

In addition to the foregoing generalizations concerning respiratory function during anesthesia, the effect of a given anesthetic on respiratory function depends on the depth of general anesthesia, the patient's preoperative respiratory condition, and the presence of special intraoperative anesthetic and surgical conditions.

A. EFFECT OF ANESTHETIC DEPTH ON RESPIRATORY PATTERN

The respiratory pattern is altered by the induction and deepening of anesthesia. When the depth of anesthesia is inadequate (less than MAC), the respiratory pattern may vary from excessive hyperventilation and vocalization to breath holding. As anesthetic depth approaches or equals MAC (light anesthesia), irregular respiration progresses to a more regular pattern that is associated with a larger than normal VT. However, during light but deepening anesthesia, the approach to a more regular respiratory pattern may be interrupted by a pause at the end of inspiration (a "hitch" in inspiration), followed by a relatively prolonged and active expiration in which the patient seems to exhale forcefully rather than passively. As anesthesia deepens to moderate levels, respiration becomes faster and more regular but shallower. The respiratory pattern is a sine wave losing the inspiratory hitch and lengthened expiratory pause. There is little or no inspiratory or expiratory pause, and the inspiratory and expiratory periods are equivalent. Intercostal muscle activity is still present, and there is normal movement of the thoracic cage with lifting of the chest during inspiration.

The respiratory rate is generally slower and the V_T larger with nitrous oxide–narcotic anesthesia than with anesthesia involving halogenated drugs. During deep anesthesia with halogenated drugs, increasing respiratory depression is manifested by increasingly rapid and shallow breathing (panting). On the other hand, with deep nitrous oxide–narcotic anesthesia, respirations become slower but may remain deep. In the case of very deep anesthesia with all inhaled drugs, respirations often become jerky or gasping in character and irregular in pattern. This situation results from loss of the active intercostal muscle contribution to inspiration. As a result, a rocking boat movement occurs in which there is out-of-phase depression of the chest wall during inspiration, flaring of the lower chest margins, and billowing of the abdomen. The reason for this type of movement is that inspiration is dependent solely on diaphragmatic effort. Independent of anesthetic depth, similar chest movements may be simulated by upper and lower airway obstruction and by partial paralysis.

B. EFFECT OF ANESTHETIC DEPTH ON SPONTANEOUS MINUTE VENTILATION

Despite the variable changes in respiratory pattern and rate as anesthesia deepens, overall spontaneous $\dot{V}_E$ progressively decreases. The normal awake response to breathing CO_2 (the *x* axis in Fig. 4-31 shows an increasing end-tidal concentration of CO_2) causes a linear increase in $\dot{V}_E$ (see the *y* axis in Fig. 4-31). In Figure 4-31 the slope of the line relating $\dot{V}_E$ to the end-tidal CO_2 concentration in awake individuals is 2 L/min/mm Hg. (In healthy individuals, the variation in the slope of this response is large.) Figure 4-31 also shows that increasing halothane concentration displaces the end-tidal CO_2 ventilation-response curve progressively to the right (meaning that at any CO_2 concentration, ventilation is less than before), decreases the slope of the curve, and shifts the apneic threshold to a higher end-tidal CO_2 concentration level.[130] Similar alterations are observed with narcotics and other halogenated anesthetics.[67] Figures 4-22 to 4-24 show that decreases in $\dot{V}_E$ cause increases in $PaCO_2$ and decreases in PaO_2. The relative increase in $PaCO_2$ caused by depression of $\dot{V}_E$ (<1.24 MAC) by halogenated anesthetics is enflurane > desflurane = isoflurane > sevoflurane > halothane. At higher concentrations,

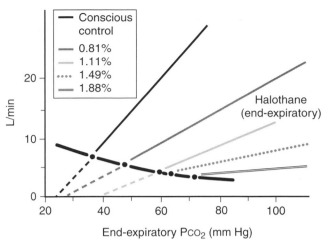

Figure 4-31 In conscious controls *(heavy solid line)*, increasing end-expiratory PCO_2 increases pulmonary minute volume. The *dashed line* is an extrapolation of the CO_2 response curve to zero ventilation and represents the apneic threshold. An increase in anesthetic (halothane) concentration (end-expiratory concentration) progressively diminishes the slope of the CO_2 response curve and shifts the apneic threshold to a higher PCO_2. The *heavy line interrupted by dots* shows the decrease in minute ventilation and the increase in PCO_2 that occur with increasing depth of anesthesia. (Redrawn with modification from Munson ES, Larson CP Jr, Babad AA, et al: The effects of halothane, fluroxene and cyclopropane on ventilation: A comparative study in man. Anesthesiology 27:716, 1966.)

desflurane causes increasing ventilatory depression and becomes similar to enflurane, and sevoflurane becomes similar to isoflurane.

C. EFFECT OF PREEXISTING RESPIRATORY DYSFUNCTION

Anesthesiologists are frequently required to care for (1) patients with acute chest disease (pulmonary infection, atelectasis) or systemic diseases (sepsis, cardiac and renal failure, multiple trauma) who require emergency operations, (2) heavy smokers with subtle pathologic airway and parenchymal conditions and hyperreactive airways, (3) patients with classical emphysematous and bronchitic problems, (4) obese people susceptible to decreases in FRC during anesthesia,[37] (5) patients with chest deformities, and (6) extremely old patients.

The nature and magnitude of these preexisting respiratory conditions determine, in part, the effect of a given standard anesthetic on respiratory function. For example, in Figure 4-32, the FRC-CC relationship is depicted for normal, obese, bronchitic, and emphysematous patients. In a healthy patient, FRC exceeds CC by approximately 1 L. In the latter three respiratory conditions, CC is 0.5 to 0.75 L less than FRC. If anesthesia causes a 1-L decrease in FRC, a healthy patient has no change in the qualitative relationship between FRC and CC.

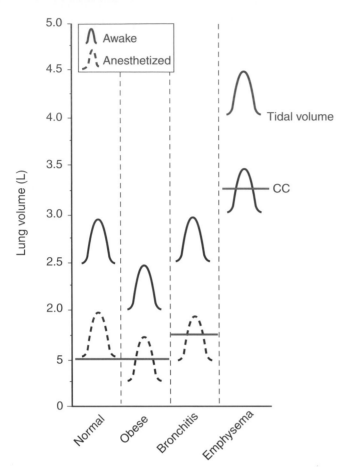

Figure 4-32 The lung volume (ordinate) at which tidal volume is breathed decreases (by 1 L) from the awake state to the anesthetized state. Functional residual capacity (FRC), which is the volume of lung existing at the end of tidal volume, therefore also decreases (by 1 L) from the awake to the anesthetized state. In healthy, obese, bronchitic, and emphysematous patients, the awake FRC considerably exceeds the closing capacity (CC). In obese, bronchitic, and emphysematous patients, the anesthetized state causes FRC to be less than CC. In healthy patients, anesthesia causes FRC to equal CC.

In patients with special respiratory conditions, a 1-L decrease in FRC causes CC to exceed FRC and changes the previous marginally normal FRC-CC relationship to either a grossly low $\dot{V}A/\dot{Q}$ or an atelectatic FRC-CC relationship. Similarly, patients with chronic bronchitis, who have copious airway secretions, may suffer more from an anesthetic-induced decrease in mucus velocity flow than other patients. Finally, if an anesthetic inhibits HPV, the drug may increase shunting more in patients with preexisting HPV than in those without preexisting HPV. Thus, the effect of a standard anesthetic can be expected to produce varying degrees of respiratory change in patients who have different degrees of preexisting respiratory dysfunction.

D. EFFECT OF SPECIAL INTRAOPERATIVE CONDITIONS

Some special intraoperative conditions (such as surgical position, massive blood loss, and surgical retraction on the lung) may cause impaired gas exchange. For example, some of the surgical positions (i.e., the lithotomy, jackknife, and kidney rest positions) and surgical exposure requirements may decrease QT, may cause hypoventilation in a spontaneously breathing patient, and may reduce FRC. The type and severity of preexisting respiratory dysfunction, as well as the number and severity of special intraoperative conditions that can embarrass respiratory function, magnify the respiratory depressant effects of any anesthetic.

E. MECHANISMS OF HYPOXEMIA DURING ANESTHESIA

1. Malfunction of Equipment

a. Mechanical Failure of Anesthesia Apparatus to Deliver Oxygen to the Patient

Hypoxemia resulting from mechanical failure of the O_2 supply system (also see Chapter 13) or the anesthesia machine is a recognized hazard of anesthesia. Disconnection of the patient from the O_2 supply system (usually at the juncture of the ET and the elbow connector) is by far the most common cause of mechanical failure to deliver O_2 to the patient. Other reported causes of failure of the O_2 supply during anesthesia include the following: an empty or depleted O_2 cylinder, substitution of a nonoxygen cylinder at the O_2 yoke because of absence or failure of the pin index, an erroneously filled O_2 cylinder, insufficient opening of the O_2 cylinder (which hinders free flow of gas as pressure decreases), failure of gas pressure in a piped O_2 system, faulty locking of the piped O_2 system to the anesthesia machine, inadvertent switching of the Schrader adapters on piped lines, crossing of piped lines during construction, failure of a reducing valve or gas manifold, inadvertent disturbance of the setting of the O_2 flowmeter, use of the fine O_2 flowmeter instead of the coarse flowmeter, fractured or sticking flowmeters, transposition of rotameter tubes, erroneous filling of a liquid O_2 reservoir with nitrogen, and disconnection of the fresh gas line from machine to in-line hosing.[50,52,120,169,186] Monitoring of the inspired O_2 concentration with an in-line F_{IO_2} analyzer and monitoring of airway pressure should detect most of these causes of failure to deliver O_2 to the patient.[50,52,120,169,186]

b. Mechanical Failure of the Endotracheal Tube: Intubation of the Main Stem Bronchus

Esophageal intubation results in almost no ventilation. Virtually all other mechanical problems (except disconnection) with ETs (such as kinking, blockage of secretions, and herniated or ruptured cuffs) cause an increase in airway resistance that may result in hypoventilation. Intubation of a main stem bronchus (also see Chapter 6) results in absence of ventilation of the contralateral lung. Although potentially minimized by HPV, some perfusion to the contralateral lung always remains, and shunting increases and PaO_2 decreases. A tube previously well positioned in the trachea may enter a bronchus after the patient or the patient's head is turned or moved into a new position.[118] Flexion of the head causes the tube to migrate deeper (caudad) into the trachea, whereas extension of the head causes cephalad (outward) migration of the ET.[118] A high incidence of main stem bronchial intubation after the institution of a 30-degree Trendelenburg position has been reported.[78] Cephalad shift of the carina and mediastinum during the Trendelenburg position caused the previously "fixed" ET to migrate into a main stem bronchus. Main stem bronchial intubation may obstruct the ipsilateral upper lobe in addition to the contralateral lung.[75,162] Infrequently, the right upper bronchus or one of its segmental bronchi branches from the lateral wall of the trachea and may be occluded by a properly positioned ET.

2. Hypoventilation

Patients under general anesthesia may have a reduced spontaneous V_T for two reasons. First, increased work of breathing can occur during general anesthesia as a result of increased airway resistance and decreased C_L. Airway resistance may be increased because of reduced FRC, endotracheal intubation, the presence of external breathing apparatus and circuitry, and possible airway obstruction in patients whose tracheas are not intubated.[20,123,202] C_L is reduced as a result of some (or all) of the factors that can decrease FRC.[111] Second, patients may have a decreased drive to breathe spontaneously during general anesthesia (decreased chemical control of breathing) (see Fig. 4-31).

Decreased V_T may cause hypoxemia in two ways.[199] First, shallow breathing may promote atelectasis and cause a decrease in FRC (see "Ventilation Pattern [Rapid Shallow Breathing]").[7,8] Second, decreased $\dot{V}_E$ decreases the overall $\dot{V}_A/\dot{Q}$ ratio of the lung, which decreases Pa_{O_2} (see Figs. 4-23 and 4-24).[199] This is likely to occur with spontaneous ventilation during moderate to deep levels of anesthesia, in which the chemical control of breathing is significantly altered.

3. Hyperventilation

Hypocapnic alkalosis (hyperventilation) may result in decreased Pa_{O_2} by several mechanisms: decreased $\dot{Q}_T$[95,144] and increased $\dot{V}_{O_2}$[30,94] (see "Decreased Cardiac Output and Increased Oxygen Consumption"), a left-shifted oxy-Hb curve (see "Oxygen-Hemoglobin Dissociation Curve"), decreased HPV[14] (see "Inhibition of Hypoxic Pulmonary Vasoconstriction"), and increased airway resistance and decreased compliance[39] (see "Increased Airway Resistance").

4. Decrease in Functional Residual Capacity

Induction of general anesthesia is consistently accompanied by a significant (15% to 20%) decrease in FRC,[27,38,45]

which usually causes a decrease in compliance.[111] The maximum decrease in FRC appears to occur within the first few minutes of anesthesia[27,46] and, in the absence of any other complicating factor, does not seem to decrease progressively during anesthesia. During anesthesia, the reduction in FRC is of the same order of magnitude whether ventilation is spontaneous or controlled. Conversely, in awake patients, FRC is only slightly reduced during controlled ventilation.[198] In obese patients, the reduction in FRC is far more pronounced than in normal patients, and the decrease is inversely related to the body mass index (BMI).[140] The reduction in FRC continues into the postoperative period.[2] For individual patients, the reduction in FRC correlates well with the increase in the alveolar-arterial Po_2 gradient during anesthesia with spontaneous breathing,[81] during anesthesia with artificial ventilation,[198] and in the postoperative period.[2] The reduced FRC may be restored to normal or above normal by the application of PEEP.[28,203] The following discussion considers all possible causes of reduced FRC.

a. Supine Position

Anesthesia and surgery are usually performed with the patient in the supine position. In changing from the upright to the supine position, FRC decreases by 0.5 to 1.0 L[27,38,45] because of a 4-cm cephalad displacement of the diaphragm by the abdominal viscera (Fig. 4-33). Pulmonary vascular congestion may also contribute to the decrease in FRC in the supine position, particularly in patients who experienced orthopnea preoperatively. These FRC changes are magnified in obese patients, with the decrement directly related to BMI.[140]

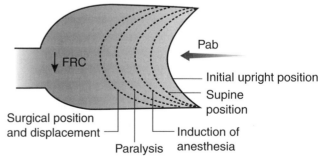

Progressive Cephalad Displacement of the Diaphragm

Figure 4-33 Anesthesia and surgery may cause a progressive cephalad displacement of the diaphragm. The sequence of events involves assumption of the supine position, induction of anesthesia, establishment of paralysis, assumption of several surgical positions, and displacement by retractors and packs. Cephalad displacement of the diaphragm results in decreased functional residual capacity (↓ FRC). Pab, pressure of abdominal contents. (Redrawn with modification from Benumof JL: Anesthesia for Thoracic Surgery, 2nd ed. Philadelphia, WB Saunders, 1995, Chapter 8.)

b. Induction of General Anesthesia: Change in Thoracic Cage Muscle Tone

At the end of a normal (awake) exhalation, there is slight tension in the inspiratory muscles and no tension in the expiratory muscles. Thus, at the end of a normal exhalation, there is a force tending to maintain lung volume and no force decreasing lung volume. After induction of general anesthesia, there is a loss of inspiratory tone and an appearance of end-expiratory tone in the abdominal expiratory muscles at the end of exhalation. The end-expiratory tone in the abdominal expiratory muscles increases intra-abdominal pressure, forces the diaphragm cephalad, and decreases FRC (see Fig. 4-33).[46,63] Thus, after the induction of general anesthesia, there is loss of the force tending to maintain lung volume and gain of the force tending to decrease lung volume. Indeed, Innovar (droperidol and fentanyl citrate) may increase tone in expiratory muscles to such an extent that the reduction in FRC with Innovar anesthesia alone is greater than that with Innovar plus paralysis induced by succinylcholine.[63,92]

With emphysema, exhalation may be accompanied by pursing the lips or grunting (partially closed larynx). An emphysematous patient exhales in either of these ways because both these maneuvers cause an expiratory retardation that produces PEEP in the intrathoracic air passage and decreases the possibility of airway closure and a decrease in FRC (see Fig. 4-17F). Endotracheal intubation bypasses the lips and glottis and may abolish the normally present pursed-lip or grunting exhalation and in that way contributes to airway closure and loss of FRC in some spontaneously breathing patients.

c. Paralysis

In an upright subject, FRC and the position of the diaphragm are determined by the balance between lung elastic recoil pulling the diaphragm cephalad and the weight of the abdominal contents pulling it caudad.[31] There is no transdiaphragmatic pressure gradient.

The situation is more complex in the supine position. The diaphragm separates two compartments of markedly different hydrostatic gradients. On the thoracic side, pressure increases by approximately 0.25 cm H_2O/cm of lung height,[5,6] and on the abdominal side, it increases by 1.0 cm H_2O/cm of abdominal height,[31] which means that in horizontal postures, progressively higher transdiaphragmatic pressure must be generated toward dependent parts of the diaphragm to keep the abdominal contents out of the thorax. In an unparalyzed patient, this tension is developed either by passive stretch and changes in shape of the diaphragm (causing an increased contractile force) or by neurally mediated active tension. With acute muscle paralysis, neither of these two mechanisms can operate, and a shift of the diaphragm to a more cephalad position occurs (see Fig. 4-33).[125] The latter position must express the true balance of forces on the diaphragm, unmodified by any passive or active muscle activity.

The cephalad shift in the FRC position of the diaphragm as a result of expiratory muscle tone during general anesthesia is equal to the shift observed during paralysis (awake or anesthetized patients).[46,64] The equal shift suggests that the pressure on the diaphragm caused by an increase in expiratory muscle tone during general anesthesia is equal to the pressure on the diaphragm caused by the weight of the abdominal contents during paralysis. It is quite probable that the magnitude of these changes in FRC related to paralysis also depends on body habitus.

d. Light or Inadequate Anesthesia and Active Expiration

Induction of general anesthesia can result in increased expiratory muscle tone,[63] but the increased expiratory muscle tone is not coordinated and does not contribute to the exhaled volume of gas. In contrast, spontaneous ventilation during light general anesthesia usually results in a coordinated and moderately forceful active exhalation and larger exhaled volumes. Excessively inadequate anesthesia (relative to a given stimulus) results in very forceful active exhalation, which may produce exhaled volumes of gas equal to an awake expiratory vital capacity.

As during an awake expiratory vital capacity maneuver, forced expiration during anesthesia raises intrathoracic and alveolar pressure considerably above atmospheric pressure (see Fig. 4-17). This increase in pressure results in rapid outflow of gas, and because part of the expiratory resistance lies in the smaller air passages, a drop in pressure occurs between the alveoli and the main bronchi. Under these circumstances, intrathoracic pressure rises considerably above the pressure within the main bronchi. Collapse occurs if this reversed pressure gradient is sufficiently high to overcome the tethering effect of the surrounding parenchyma on the small intrathoracic bronchioles or the structural rigidity of cartilage in the large extrathoracic bronchi. Such collapse occurs in a normal subject during a maximal forced expiration and is responsible for the associated wheeze in both awake and anesthetized patients.[42]

In a paralyzed, anesthetized patient, the use of a subatmospheric expiratory pressure phase is analogous to a forced expiration in a conscious subject; the negative phase may set up the same adverse ΔP, which can cause airway closure, gas trapping, and a decrease in FRC. An excessively rapidly descending bellows of a ventilator during expiration has caused subatmospheric expiratory pressure and resulted in wheezing.[185]

e. Increased Airway Resistance

The overall reduction in all components of lung volume during anesthesia results in reduced airway caliber, which increases airway resistance and any tendency toward

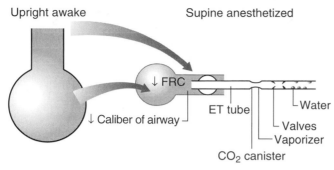

Figure 4-34 An anesthetized patient in the supine position has increased airway resistance as a result of decreased functional residual capacity (FRC), decreased caliber of the airways, endotracheal intubation, and connection of the ET to the external breathing apparatus and circuitry. ↓ = decreased. (Redrawn with modification from Benumof JL: Anesthesia for Thoracic Surgery, 2nd ed. Philadelphia, WB Saunders, 1995, Chapter 8.)

airway collapse (Fig. 4-34). The relationship between airway resistance and lung volume is well established (Fig. 4-35). The decreases in FRC caused by the supine position (≈ 0.8 L) and induction of anesthesia (≈ 0.4 L) are often sufficient to explain the increased resistance seen in a healthy anesthetized patient.[123]

In addition to this expected increase in airway resistance in anesthetized patients, there are a number of special potential sites of increased airway resistance,

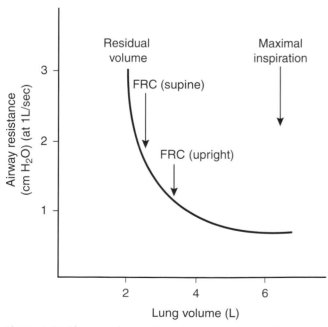

Figure 4-35 Airway resistance is an increasing hyperbolic function of decreasing lung volume. Functional residual capacity (FRC) decreases when changing from the upright to the supine position. (Redrawn with modification from Lumb AB: Respiratory system resistance. In Lumb AB [ed]: Nunn's Applied Respiratory Physiology, 5th ed. London, Butterworths, 2000, p 67.)

including the ET (if present), the upper and lower airway passages, and the external anesthesia apparatus. Endotracheal intubation reduces the size of the trachea, usually by 30% to 50% (see Fig. 4-34). Pharyngeal obstruction, which can be considered to be a normal feature of unconsciousness, is most common. A minor degree of this type of obstruction occurs in snoring. Laryngospasm and obstructed ETs (secretions, kinking, herniated cuffs) are not uncommon and may be life threatening.

The respiratory apparatus often causes resistance that is considerably higher than the resistance in the normal human respiratory tract (see Fig. 4-34).[111] When certain resistors such as those shown in Figure 4-34 are joined in a series to form an anesthetic gas circuit, they generally add to produce larger resistance (as with resistance in series in an electrical circuit). The increase in resistance associated with commonly used breathing circuits and ETs may impose an additional work of breathing that is two to three times normal.[20]

f. Supine Position, Immobility, and Excessive Intravenous Fluid Administration

Patients undergoing anesthesia and surgery are often kept supine and immobile for long periods. Thus, some of the lung may be continually dependent and below the left atrium and therefore in zone 3 or 4 condition. Being in a dependent position, the lung is predisposed to accumulation of fluid. Coupled with excessive fluid administration, conditions sufficient to promote transudation of fluid into the lung are present and result in pulmonary edema and decreased FRC. When mongrel dogs were placed in a lateral decubitus position and anesthetized for several hours (Fig. 4-36, bottom horizontal axis), expansion of the extracellular space with fluid (top horizontal axis) caused the P_{O_2} (left-hand axis) of blood draining the dependent lung (closed circles) to decrease precipitously to mixed venous levels (no O_2 uptake).[149] Blood draining the nondependent lung maintained its P_{O_2} for a period, but in the presence of the extracellular fluid expansion, it also suffered a decline in P_{O_2} after 5 hours. Transpulmonary shunting (right-hand axis) progressively increased. If the animals were turned every hour (and received the same fluid challenge), only the dependent lung, at the end of each hour period, suffered a decrease in oxygenation. If the animals were turned every half-hour and received the same fluid challenge, neither lung suffered a decrease in oxygenation. In patients who undergo surgery in the lateral decubitus position (e.g., pulmonary resection, in which they have or will have a restricted pulmonary vascular bed) and receive excessive intravenous fluids, the risk of the dependent lung becoming edematous is certainly increased. These considerations also explain, in part, the beneficial effect of a continuously rotating (side-to-side) bed on the incidence of pulmonary complications in critically ill patients.[65]

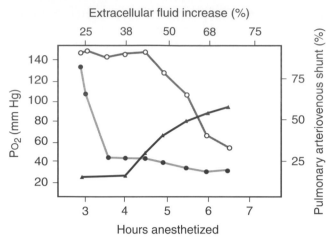

Figure 4-36 Mongrel dogs anesthetized with pentobarbital (bottom axis), placed in a lateral decubitus position, and subjected to progressive extracellular fluid expansion (top axis) have a marked decrease in the Po2 (left vertical axis) of blood draining the dependent lung (solid circles) and a smaller, much slower decrease in the Po2 of blood draining the nondependent lung (open circles). The pulmonary arteriovenous shunt (right vertical axis) rises progressively (triangles). (Redrawn from Ray JF, Yost L, Moallem S, et al: Immobility, hypoxemia, and pulmonary arteriovenous shunting. Arch Surg 109:537, 1974.)

g. High Inspired Oxygen Concentration and Absorption Atelectasis

General anesthesia is usually administered with an increased F_{IO_2}. In patients who have areas of moderately low $\dot{V}_A/\dot{Q}$ ratios (0.1 to 0.01), administration of F_{IO_2} greater than 0.3 adds enough O_2 into the alveolar space in these areas to eliminate the shuntlike effect that they have, and total measured right-to-left shunting decreases. However, when patients with a significant amount of blood flow perfusing lung units with very low $\dot{V}_A/\dot{Q}$ ratios (0.01 to 0.0001) have a change in F_{IO_2} from room air to 1.0, the very low $\dot{V}_A/\dot{Q}$ units virtually disappear, and a moderately large right-to-left shunt appears.[182,183,192] In these studies, the increase in shunting was equal to the amount of blood flow previously perfusing the areas with low $\dot{V}_A/\dot{Q}$ ratios during the breathing of air. Thus, in these studies the effect of breathing O_2 was to convert units that had low $\dot{V}_A/\dot{Q}$ ratios into shunt units. The pathologic basis for these data is the conversion of low-$\dot{V}_A/\dot{Q}$ units into atelectatic units.

The cause of the atelectatic shunting during O_2 breathing is presumably a large increase in O_2 uptake by lung units with low $\dot{V}_A/\dot{Q}$ ratios.[26,182] A unit that has a low $\dot{V}_A/\dot{Q}$ ratio during breathing of air will have a low P_{AO_2}. When an enriched O_2 mixture is inspired, P_{AO_2} rises, and the rate at which O_2 moves from alveolar gas to capillary blood increases greatly. The O_2 flux may increase so much that the net flow of gas into blood

exceeds the inspired flow of gas, and the lung unit becomes progressively smaller. Collapse is most likely to occur if F_{IO_2} is high, the $\dot{V}_A/\dot{Q}$ ratio is low, the time of exposure of the unit with low $\dot{V}_A/\dot{Q}$ to high F_{IO_2} is long, and $C\bar{v}_{O_2}$ is low. Thus, given the right $\dot{V}_A/\dot{Q}$ ratio and time of administration, an F_{IO_2} as low as 50% can produce absorption atelectasis.[26,182] This phenomenon is of considerable significance in the clinical situation for two reasons. First, enriched O_2 mixtures are often used therapeutically, and it is important to know whether this therapy is causing atelectasis. Second, the amount of shunt is often estimated during breathing of 100% O_2, and if this maneuver results in additional shunt, the measurement is hard to interpret.

h. Surgical Position

i. Supine Position In the supine position, the abdominal contents force the diaphragm cephalad and reduce FRC.[38,46,63,64] The Trendelenburg position allows the abdominal contents to push the diaphragm further cephalad so that the diaphragm must not only ventilate the lungs but also lift the abdominal contents out of the thorax. The result is a predisposition to decreased FRC and atelectasis.[167] The Trendelenburg position–related decrease in FRC is exacerbated in obese patients.[140] Increased pulmonary blood volume and gravitational force on the mediastinal structures are additional factors that may decrease pulmonary compliance and FRC. In the steep Trendelenburg position, most of the lung may be below the left atrium and therefore in a zone 3 or 4 condition. In this condition, the lung may be susceptible to the development of pulmonary interstitial edema. Thus, patients with elevated Ppa, such as those with mitral stenosis, do not tolerate the Trendelenburg position well.[103]

ii. Lateral Decubitus Position In the lateral decubitus position, the dependent lung experiences a moderate decrease in FRC and is predisposed to atelectasis, whereas the nondependent lung may have increased FRC. The overall result is usually a slight to moderate increase in total-lung FRC.[112] The kidney and lithotomy positions also cause small decreases in FRC above that caused by the supine position. The prone position may increase FRC moderately.[112]

i. Ventilation Pattern (Rapid Shallow Breathing)

Rapid shallow breathing is often a regular feature of anesthesia. Monotonous shallow breathing may cause a decrease in FRC, promote atelectasis, and decrease compliance.[7,8,87] These changes with rapid shallow breathing are probably due to progressive increases in surface tension.[87] Initially, these changes may cause hypoxemia with normocapnia and may be prevented or reversed (or both) by periodic large mechanical inspirations, spontaneous sighs, PEEP, or a combination of these techniques.[69,87,179]

j. Decreased Removal of Secretions (Decreased Mucociliary Flow)

Tracheobronchial mucous glands and goblet cells produce mucus, which is swept by cilia up to the larynx, where it is swallowed or expectorated. This process clears inhaled organisms and particles from the lungs. The secreted mucus consists of a surface gel layer lying on top of a more liquid sol layer in which the cilia beat. The tips of the cilia propel the gel layer toward the larynx (upward) during the forward stroke. As the mucus streams upward and the total cross-sectional area of the airways diminishes, absorption takes place from the sol layer to maintain a constant depth of 5 mm.[206]

Poor systemic hydration and low inspired humidity reduce mucociliary flow by increasing the viscosity of secretions and slowing the ciliary beat.[3,62,83] Mucociliary flow varies directly with body or mucosal temperature (low inspired temperature) over a range of 32° C to 42° C.[40,82] High FIO_2 decreases mucociliary flow.[158] Inflation of an ET cuff suppresses tracheal mucus velocity,[157] an effect that occurs within 1 hour, and apparently it does not matter whether a low- or high-compliance cuff is used. Passage of an uncuffed tube through the vocal cords and keeping it in situ for several hours does not affect tracheal mucus velocity.[157]

The mechanism for suppression of mucociliary clearance by the ET cuff is speculative. In the report of Sackner and colleagues,[157] mucus velocity was decreased in the distal portion of the trachea, but the cuff was inflated in the proximal portion. Thus, the phenomenon cannot be attributed solely to damming of mucus at the cuff site. One possibility is that the ET cuff caused a critical increase in the thickness of the layer of mucus proceeding distally from the cuff. Another possibility is that mechanical distention of the trachea by the ET cuff initiated a neurogenic reflex arc that altered mucous secretions or the frequency of ciliary beating.

Other investigators have shown that when all the foregoing factors are controlled, halothane reversibly and progressively decreases but does not stop mucus flow over an inspired concentration of 1 to 3 MAC.[61] The halothane-induced depression of mucociliary clearance was probably due to depression of the ciliary beat, an effect that caused slow clearance of mucus from the distal and peripheral airways. In support of this hypothesis is the finding that cilia are morphologically similar throughout the animal kingdom, and in clinical dosages, inhaled anesthetics, including halothane, have been found to cause reversible depression of the ciliary beat of protozoa.[133]

5. Decreased Cardiac Output and Increased Oxygen Consumption

Decreased $\dot{Q}T$ in the presence of constant O_2 consumption ($\dot{V}O_2$), increased $\dot{V}O_2$ in the presence of a constant $\dot{Q}T$, and decreased $\dot{Q}T$ and increased $\dot{V}O_2$ must all result in lower $C\bar{v}O_2$. Venous blood with lowered $C\bar{v}O_2$ then flows through whichever shunt pathways exist, mixes with the oxygented end-pulmonary capillary blood, and lowers CaO_2 (see Figs. 4-27 and 4-28). Figure 4-37 shows these relationships quantitatively for several different intrapulmonary shunts.[19,144] The larger the intrapulmonary shunt, the greater the decrease in CaO_2 because more venous blood with lower $C\bar{v}O_2$ can admix with end-pulmonary capillary blood. Decreased $\dot{Q}T$ may occur with myocardial failure and hypovolemia; the specific causes of these two conditions are beyond the scope of this chapter. Increased $\dot{V}O_2$ may occur with excessive stimulation of the sympathetic nervous system, hyperthermia, or shivering and can further contribute to impaired oxygenation of arterial blood.[147]

6. Inhibition of Hypoxic Pulmonary Vasoconstriction

Decreased regional PaO_2 causes regional pulmonary vasoconstriction, which diverts blood flow away from hypoxic regions of the lung to better ventilated normoxic regions. The diversion of blood flow minimizes venous admixture from the underventilated or nonventilated lung regions. Inhibition of regional HPV could impair arterial oxygenation by permitting increased venous admixture from hypoxic or atelectatic areas of the lung (see Fig. 4-9).

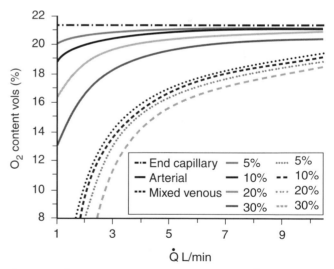

Figure 4-37 Effects of changes in cardiac output ($\dot{Q}$) on the O_2 content of end-pulmonary capillary, arterial, and mixed venous blood for a group of different transpulmonary right-to-left shunts. The magnitude of the right-to-left shunt is indicated by the various numbered percent symbols for arterial *(solid line)* and mixed venous *(dashed line)* blood; the oxygen content of end-capillary blood is unaffected by the degree of shunting. Note that a decrease in $\dot{Q}$ results in a greater decrease in the arterial content of O_2 the larger the shunt. (Redrawn from Kelman GF, Nunn JF, Prys-Roberts C, et al: The influence of the cardiac output on arterial oxygenation: A theoretical study. Br J Anaesth 39:450, 1967.)

Because the pulmonary circulation is poorly endowed with smooth muscle, any condition that increases the pressure against which the vessels must constrict (i.e., Ppa) decreases HPV. Numerous clinical conditions can increase Ppa and therefore decrease HPV. Mitral stenosis,[17] volume overload,[17] low (but greater than room air) F_{IO_2} in nondiseased lung,[159] a progressive increase in the amount of diseased lung,[159] thromboembolism,[159] hypothermia,[18] and vasoactive drugs[9] can all increase Ppa. Direct vasodilating drugs (such as isoproterenol, nitroglycerin, and sodium nitroprusside),[9,47] inhaled anesthetics,[10] and hypocapnia[9,14] can directly decrease HPV. The selective application of PEEP to only the nondiseased lung can selectively increase PVR in the nondiseased lung and may divert blood flow back into the diseased lung.[13]

7. Paralysis

In the supine position, the weight of the abdominal contents pressing against the diaphragm is greatest in the dependent or posterior part of the diaphragm and least in the nondependent or anterior part of the diaphragm. In an awake patient breathing spontaneously, active tension in the diaphragm is capable of overcoming the weight of the abdominal contents, and the diaphragm moves most in the posterior portion (because the posterior of the diaphragm is stretched higher into the chest, it has the smallest radius of curvature, and therefore it contracts most effectively) and least in the anterior portion. This circumstance is healthy because the greatest amount of ventilation occurs in areas with the most perfusion (posteriorly or dependently), and the least amount occurs in areas with the least perfusion (anteriorly or nondependently). During paralysis and positive-pressure breathing, the passive diaphragm is displaced by the positive pressure preferentially in the anterior nondependent portion (where there is the least resistance to diaphragmatic movement) and is displaced minimally in the posterior dependent portion (where there is the most resistance to diaphragmatic movement). This circumstance is unhealthy because the greatest amount of ventilation now occurs in areas with the least perfusion, and the least amount occurs in areas with the most perfusion.[64] However, the magnitude of the change in the diaphragmatic motion pattern with paralysis varies with body position.[64,100]

8. Right-to-Left Interatrial Shunting

Acute arterial hypoxemia from a transient right-to-left shunt through a PFO has been described, particularly during emergence from anesthesia.[128] However, unless a real-time technique of imaging the cardiac chambers is used (e.g., TEE with color flow Doppler imaging),[43] it is difficult to document an acute and transient right-to-left intracardiac shunt as a cause of arterial hypoxemia. Nonetheless, right-to-left shunting through a PFO has been described in virtually every conceivable clinical

situation that afterloads the right side of the heart and increases right atrial pressure. When right-to-left shunting through a PFO is identified, administration of inhaled NO can decrease PVR and functionally close the PFO.[53]

9. Involvement of Mechanisms of Hypoxemia in Specific Diseases

In any given pulmonary disease, many of the mechanisms of hypoxemia listed earlier may be involved.[199] Pulmonary embolism (air, fat, thrombi) (Fig. 4-38) and the evolution of ARDS (Fig. 4-39) are used to illustrate this point. A significant pulmonary embolus can cause severe increases in pulmonary artery pressure, and these increases can result in right-to-left transpulmonary shunting through opened arteriovenous anastomoses and the foramen ovale (possible in 20% of patients), pulmonary edema in nonembolized regions of the lung, and inhibition of HPV. The embolus may cause hypoventilation through increased dead space ventilation. If the embolus contains platelets, serotonin may be released, and such release can cause hypoventilation as a result of bronchoconstriction and pulmonary edema as a result of increased pulmonary capillary permeability. Finally, the pulmonary embolus can increase PVR (by platelet-induced serotonin release,[4] among other etiologies) and decrease cardiac output.

After major hypotension, shock, blood loss, sepsis, and other conditions, noncardiogenic pulmonary edema may occur and lead to acute respiratory failure or ARDS.[187] The syndrome can evolve during and after anesthesia and has the hallmark characteristics of decreased FRC and compliance and hypoxemia. After shock and trauma, plasma levels of serotonin, histamine, kinins, lysozymes,

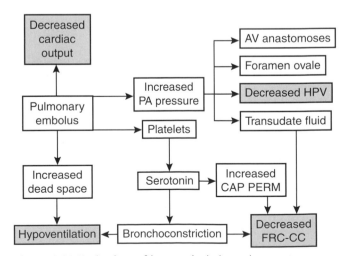

Figure 4-38 Mechanisms of hypoxemia during pulmonary embolism. See the text for an explanation of the pathophysiologic flow diagram. AV, arteriovenous; CAP PERM, capillary permeability; CC, closing capacity; FRC, functional residual capacity; HPV, hypoxic pulmonary vasoconstriction; PA, pulmonary artery. (Redrawn with modification from Benumof JL: Anesthesia for Thoracic Surgery, 2nd ed. Philadelphia, WB Saunders, 1995, Chapter 8.)

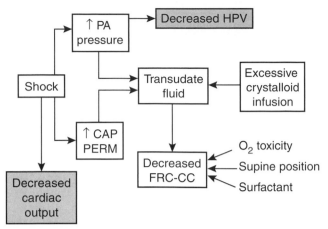

Figure 4-39 Mechanisms of hypoxemia during adult respiratory distress syndrome. See the text for an explanation of the pathophysiologic flow diagram. CAP PERM, capillary permeability; CC, closing capacity; FRC, functional residual capacity; HPV, hypoxic pulmonary vasoconstriction; PA, pulmonary artery. (Redrawn with modification from Benumof JL: Anesthesia for Thoracic Surgery, 2nd ed. Philadelphia, WB Saunders, 1995, Chapter 8.)

reactive oxygen species, fibrin degradation products, products of complement metabolism, and fatty acids all increase. Sepsis and endotoxemia may be present. Increased levels of activated complement activate neutrophils into chemotaxis in patients with trauma and pancreatitis; activated neutrophils can damage endothelial cells. These factors, along with pulmonary contusion (if it occurs), may individually or collectively increase pulmonary capillary permeability. After shock, acidosis, increased circulating catecholamines and sympathetic nervous system activity, leukotriene and prostaglandin release, histamine release, microembolism (with serotonin release), increased intracranial pressure (with head injury), and alveolar hypoxia may occur and may individually or collectively, particularly after resuscitation, cause a moderate increase in Ppa. After shock, the normal compensatory response to hypovolemia is movement of a protein-free fluid from the interstitial space into the vascular space to restore vascular volume. Dilution of vascular proteins by protein-free interstitial fluid can cause decreased capillary colloid oncotic pressure. Increased pulmonary capillary permeability and Ppa along with decreased capillary colloid oncotic pressure results in fluid transudation and pulmonary edema. In addition, decreased $\dot{Q}T$, inhibition of HPV, immobility, the supine position, excessive fluid administration, and an excessively high FIO_2 can contribute to the development of ARDS.

F. MECHANISMS OF HYPERCAPNIA AND HYPOCAPNIA DURING ANESTHESIA

1. Hypercapnia

Hypoventilation, increased dead space ventilation, increased CO_2 production, and inadvertent switching off of a CO_2 absorber can all cause hypercapnia (Fig. 4-40).

2. Hypoventilation

Patients spontaneously hypoventilate during anesthesia because it is more difficult to breathe (abnormal surgical position, increased airway resistance, decreased compliance) and they are less willing to breathe (decreased respiratory drive because of anesthetics). Hypoventilation results in hypercapnia (see Figs. 4-22 and 4-23).

3. Increased Dead Space Ventilation

A decrease in Ppa, as during deliberate hypotension,[49] may cause an increase in zone 1 and alveolar dead space ventilation. An increase in airway pressure (as with PEEP) may also cause an increase in zone 1 and alveolar dead space ventilation. Pulmonary embolism, thrombosis, and vascular obliteration (kinking, clamping, blocking of the pulmonary artery during surgery) may increase the amount of lung that is ventilated but unperfused. Vascular obliteration may be responsible for the increase in dead space ventilation with age (VD/VT% = 33 + age/3). Rapid short inspirations may be distributed preferentially to noncompliant (short time constant for inflation) and badly perfused alveoli, whereas slow inspiration allows time for distribution to more compliant (long time constant for inflation) and better perfused alveoli. Thus, rapid, short inspirations may have a dead space ventilation effect.

The anesthesia apparatus increases total dead space (VD/VT) for two reasons. First, the apparatus simply increases the anatomic dead space. Inclusion of normal apparatus dead space increases the total VD/VT ratio from 33% to about 46% in intubated patients and to about 64% in patients breathing through a mask.[91] Second, anesthesia circuits cause rebreathing of expired gases, which is equivalent to dead space ventilation. The rebreathing classification by Mapleson is widely accepted. The order of increasing rebreathing (decreasing clinical merit) during spontaneous ventilation with Mapleson circuits is A (Magill), D, C, and B. The order of increasing rebreathing (decreasing clinical merit) during controlled ventilation is D, B, C, and A. There is no rebreathing in system E (Ayre's T-piece) if the patient's respiratory diastole is long enough to permit washout with a given fresh gas flow (common event) or if the fresh gas flow is greater than the peak inspiratory flow rate (uncommon event).

The effects of an increase in dead space can usually be counteracted by a corresponding increase in the respiratory $\dot{V}E$. If, for example, the $\dot{V}E$ is 10 L/min and the VD/VT ratio is 30%, alveolar ventilation is 7 L/min. If a pulmonary embolism occurred and resulted in an increase in the VD/VT ratio to 50%, $\dot{V}E$ would need to be increased to 14 L/min to maintain an alveolar ventilation of 7 L/min (14 L/min × 0.5).

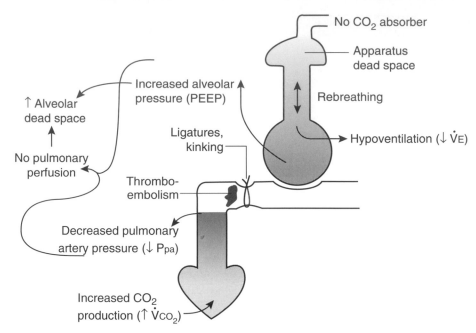

Figure 4-40 Schematic diagram of the causes of hypercapnia during anesthesia. An increase in carbon dioxide (CO_2) production ($\dot{V}_{CO_2}$) increases Pa_{CO_2} with a constant minute ventilation ($\dot{V}_E$). Several events can increase alveolar dead space: a decrease in pulmonary artery pressure (Ppa), the application of positive end-expiratory pressure (PEEP), thromboembolism, and mechanical interference with pulmonary arterial flow (ligatures and kinking of vessels). Most commonly in trauma, surgery, and critical care, hypovolemia due to hemorrhage or third spacing leads to increased alveolar dead space and consequent increased Pa_{CO_2}. A decrease in $\dot{V}_E$ causes an increase in Pa_{CO_2} with a constant $\dot{V}_{CO_2}$. It is possible for some anesthesia systems to cause rebreathing of CO_2. Finally, the anesthesia apparatus may increase the anatomic dead space, and inadvertent switching off of a CO_2 absorber in the presence of low fresh gas flow can increase Pa_{CO_2}. ↑ = increased; ↓ = decreased. (Redrawn with modification from Benumof JL: Anesthesia for Thoracic Surgery, 2nd ed. Philadelphia, WB Saunders, 1995, Chapter 8.)

4. Increased Carbon Dioxide Production

All the causes of increased O_2 consumption also increase CO_2 production: hyperthermia, shivering, catecholamine release (light anesthesia), hypertension, and thyroid storm. If $\dot{V}_E$, total dead space, and $\dot{V}_A/\dot{Q}$ relationships are constant, an increase in CO_2 production results in hypercapnia.

5. Inadvertent Switching Off of a Carbon Dioxide Absorber

Many factors, such as patients' ventilatory responsiveness to CO_2 accumulation, fresh gas flow, circle system design, and CO_2 production, determine whether hypercapnia results from accidental switching off or depletion of a circle CO_2 absorber. However, high fresh gas flows (≥–5 L/min) minimize the problem with almost all systems for almost all patients.

6. Hypocapnia

The mechanisms of hypocapnia are the reverse of those that produce hypercapnia. Thus, all other factors being equal, hyperventilation (spontaneous or controlled ventilation), decreased V_D ventilation (change from a mask airway to an ET airway, decreased PEEP, increased Ppa, or decreased rebreathing), and decreased CO_2 production (hypothermia, deep anesthesia, hypotension) lead to hypocapnia. By far the most common mechanism of hypocapnia is passive hyperventilation by mechanical means.

G. PHYSIOLOGIC EFFECTS OF ABNORMALITIES IN RESPIRATORY GASES

1. Hypoxia

The end products of aerobic metabolism (oxidative phosphorylation) are CO_2 and water, both of which are easily diffusible and lost from the body. The essential feature of hypoxia is the cessation of oxidative phosphorylation when mitochondrial Po_2 falls below a critical level. Anaerobic pathways, which produce energy (ATP) inefficiently, are then used. The main anaerobic metabolites are hydrogen and lactate ions, which are not easily excreted. They accumulate in the circulation, where they may be quantified in terms of the base deficit and the lactate-pyruvate ratio.

Because the various organs have different blood flow and O_2 consumption rates, the manifestations and clinical diagnosis of hypoxia are usually related to symptoms arising from the most vulnerable organ. This organ is generally the brain in an awake patient and the heart in

Table 4-6 **Cardiovascular Response to Hypoxemia**

Hemodynamic Variable O$_2$ Saturation (%)	HR	BP	SV	CO	SVR	Predominant Response
>80	↑	↑	↑	↑	No change	Reflex, excitatory
60-80	↑Baroreceptor	↓	No change	No change	↓	Local, depressant > reflex, excitatory
<60	↓	↓	↓	↓	↓	Local, depressant

BP, systemic blood pressure; CO, cardiac output; HR, heart rate; SV, stroke volume; SVR, systemic vascular resistance; ↑ increase; ↓ decrease.

an anesthetized patient (see later), but in special circumstances it may be the spinal cord (aortic surgery), kidney (acute tubular necrosis), liver (hepatitis), or limb (claudication, gangrene).

The cardiovascular response to hypoxemia[79,155,156] is a product of both reflex (neural and humoral) and direct effects (Table 4-6). The reflex effects occur first and are excitatory and vasoconstrictive. The neuroreflex effects result from aortic and carotid chemoreceptor, baroreceptor, and central cerebral stimulation, and the humoral reflex effects result from catecholamine and renin-angiotensin release. The direct local vascular effects of hypoxia are inhibitory and vasodilatory and occur late. The net response to hypoxia in a subject depends on the severity of the hypoxia, which determines the magnitude and balance between the inhibitory and excitatory components; the balance may vary according to the type and depth of anesthesia and the degree of preexisting cardiovascular disease.

Mild arterial hypoxemia (arterial saturation less than normal but still 80% or higher) causes general activation of the sympathetic nervous system and release of catecholamines. Consequently, the heart rate, stroke volume, $\dot{Q}_T$, and myocardial contractility (as measured by a shortened pre-ejection period [PEP], left ventricular ejection time [LVET], and a decreased PEP/LVET ratio) are increased (Fig. 4-41).[161] Changes in systemic vascular resistance are usually slight. However, in patients under anesthesia with β-blockers, hypoxia (and hypercapnia when present) may cause circulating catecholamines to have only an α-receptor effect, the heart may be unstimulated (even depressed by a local hypoxia effect), and systemic vascular resistance may be increased. Consequently, $\dot{Q}_T$ may be decreased in these patients. With moderate hypoxemia (arterial O$_2$ saturation of 60% to 80%), local vasodilation begins to predominate and systemic vascular resistance and blood pressure (BP) decrease, but the heart rate may continue to be increased because of a systemic hypotension-induced stimulation of baroreceptors. Finally, with severe hypoxemia (arterial saturation < 60%), local depressant effects dominate and BP falls rapidly, the pulse slows, shock develops, and the heart either fibrillates or becomes asystolic. Significant preexisting hypotension converts a mild hypoxemic hemodynamic profile into a moderate hypoxemic hemodynamic profile and converts

a moderate hypoxemic hemodynamic profile into a severe hypoxemic hemodynamic profile. Similarly, in well-anesthetized or sedated patients (or both), early sympathetic nervous system reactivity to hypoxemia may be reduced and the effects of hypoxemia may be expressed only as bradycardia with severe hypotension and, ultimately, circulatory collapse.[44]

Hypoxemia may also promote cardiac dysrhythmias, which may in turn potentiate the already mentioned deleterious cardiovascular effects. Hypoxemia-induced dysrhythmias may be caused by multiple mechanisms; the mechanisms are interrelated because they all cause a decrease in the myocardial O$_2$ supply-demand ratio,

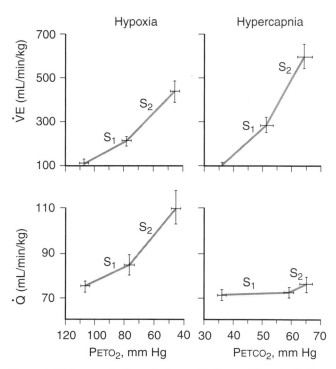

Figure 4-41 Changes in the minute ventilation and the circulation of healthy awake humans during progressive isocapnic hypoxia and hyperoxic hypercapnia. PETCO_2, end-tidal PCO_2; PETO_2, end-tidal PO_2; $\dot{Q}$, cardiac output; S$_1$, slope during the first phase of slowly increasing ventilation and/or circulation; S$_2$, slope during the second phase of sharply increasing ventilation and/or circulation; $\dot{V}_E$, expired minute ventilation. (Redrawn from Serebrovskaya TV: Comparison of respiratory and circulatory human responses to progressive hypoxia and hypercapnia. Respiration 59:35, 1992.)

which in turn increases myocardial irritability. First, arterial hypoxemia may directly decrease the myocardial O_2 supply. Second, early tachycardia may result in increased myocardial O_2 consumption, and decreased diastolic filling time may lead to decreased myocardial O_2 supply. Third, early increased systemic BP may cause an increased afterload on the left ventricle, which increases left ventricular O_2 demand. Fourth, late systemic hypotension may decrease myocardial O_2 supply because of decreased diastolic perfusion pressure. Fifth, coronary blood flow reserve may be exhausted by a late, maximally increased coronary blood flow as a result of maximal coronary vasodilation.[106] The level of hypoxemia that causes cardiac dysrhythmias cannot be predicted with certainty because the myocardial O_2 supply-demand relationship in a given patient is not known (i.e., the degree of coronary artery atherosclerosis may not be known). However, if a myocardial area (or areas) become hypoxic or ischemic, or both, unifocal or multifocal premature ventricular contractions, ventricular tachycardia, and ventricular fibrillation may occur.

The cardiovascular response to hypoxia includes a number of other important effects. Cerebral blood flow increases (even if hypocapnic hyperventilation is present). Ventilation is stimulated no matter why hypoxia exists (see Fig. 4-41). The pulmonary distribution of blood flow is more homogeneous because of increased pulmonary artery pressure. Chronic hypoxia causes an increased Hb concentration and a right-shifted oxy-Hb curve (as a result of either an increase in 2,3-DPG or acidosis), which tends to raise tissue P_{O_2}.

2. Hyperoxia (Oxygen Toxicity)

The dangers associated with the inhalation of excessive O_2 are multiple. Exposure to high O_2 tension clearly causes pulmonary damage in healthy individuals.[101,200] A dose-time toxicity curve for humans is available from a number of studies.[34,101,200] Because the lungs of normal human volunteers cannot be directly examined to determine the rate of onset and the course of toxicity, indirect measures such as the onset of symptoms have been used to construct dose-time toxicity curves. Examination of the curve indicates that 100% O_2 should not be administered for more than 12 hours, 80% O_2 should not be administered for more than 24 hours, and 60% O_2 should not be administered for more than 36 hours.[34,101,200] No measurable changes in pulmonary function or blood-gas exchange occur in humans during exposure to less than 50% O_2, even for long periods.[34] Nevertheless, it is important to note that in the clinical setting, these dose-time toxicity relationships are often generally obscured[99] because of the complex multivariable nature of the clinical setting.

The dominant symptom of O_2 toxicity in human volunteers is substernal distress, which begins as mild irritation in the area of the carina and may be accompanied by occasional coughing.[127] As exposure continues, the pain becomes more intense, and the urge to cough and to deep-breathe also becomes more intense. These symptoms progress to severe dyspnea, paroxysmal coughing, and decreased vital capacity when the F_{IO_2} has been 1.0 for longer than 12 hours. At this point, recovery of mechanical lung function usually occurs within 12 to 24 hours, but more than 24 hours may be required in some individuals.[34] As toxicity progresses, other pulmonary function studies such as compliance and blood gases deteriorate. Pathologically, in animals, the lesion progresses from tracheobronchitis (exposure for 12 hours to a few days), to involvement of the alveolar septa with pulmonary interstitial edema (exposure for a few days to 1 week), to pulmonary fibrosis of the edema (exposure for > 1 week).[131]

Ventilatory depression may occur in patients who, by reason of drugs or disease, have been ventilating in response to a hypoxic drive. By definition, ventilatory depression resulting from removal of a hypoxic drive by increasing the inspired O_2 concentration causes hypercapnia but does not necessarily produce hypoxia (because of the increased F_{IO_2}).

Absorption atelectasis was presented earlier (see "High Inspired Oxygen Concentration and Absorption Atelectasis"). Retrolental fibroplasia, an abnormal proliferation of the immature retinal vasculature of a prematurely born infant, can occur after exposure to hyperoxia. Extremely premature infants are most susceptible to retrolental fibroplasia (i.e., those < 1.0 kg in birth weight and 28 weeks' gestation). The risk of retrolental fibroplasia exists whenever F_{IO_2} causes Pa_{O_2} to be greater than 80 mm Hg for more than 3 hours in an infant whose gestational age plus life age combined is less than 44 weeks. If the ductus arteriosus is patent, arterial blood samples should be drawn from the right radial artery (umbilical or lower extremity Pa_{O_2} is lower than the Pa_{O_2} to which the eyes are exposed because of ductal shunting of unoxygenated blood).

The mode of action of O_2 toxicity in tissues is complex, but interference with metabolism seems to be widespread. Most important, many enzymes, particularly those with sulfhydryl groups, are inactivated by O_2-derived free radicals.[99] Neutrophil recruitment and release of mediators of inflammation occur next and greatly accelerate the extent of endothelial and epithelial damage and impairment of the surfactant systems.[99] The most acute toxic effect of O_2 in humans is a convulsive effect, which occurs during exposure to pressures in excess of 2 atm absolute.

High inspired O_2 concentrations can be of use therapeutically. Clearance of gas loculi in the body may be greatly accelerated by the inhalation of 100% O_2. Inhalation of 100% O_2 creates a large nitrogen gradient from the gas space to the perfusing blood. As a result, nitrogen leaves the gas space and the space diminishes in size. Administration of O_2 to remove gas may be used to ease intestinal gas pressure in patients with intestinal obstruction, decrease the size of an air embolus, and aid in the absorption of pneumoperitoneum, pneumocephalus, and pneumothorax.

3. Hypercapnia

The effects of CO_2 on the cardiovascular system are as complex as those of hypoxia. Like hypoxemia, hypercapnia appears to cause direct depression of both cardiac muscle and vascular smooth muscle, but at the same time it causes reflex stimulation of the sympathoadrenal system, which compensates to a greater or lesser extent for the primary cardiovascular depression (see Fig. 4-41).[106,156] With moderate to severe hypercapnia, a hyperkinetic circulation results with increased $\dot{Q}T$ and systemic BP (see Fig. 4-41).[161] Even in patients under halothane anesthesia, plasma catecholamine levels increase in response to increased CO_2 levels in much the same way as in conscious subjects. Thus, hypercapnia, like hypoxemia, may cause increased myocardial O_2 demand (tachycardia, early hypertension) and decreased myocardial O_2 supply (tachycardia, late hypotension).

Table 4-7 summarizes the interaction of anesthesia with hypercapnia in humans; increased $\dot{Q}T$ and decreased systemic vascular resistance should be emphasized.[114,146] The increase in $\dot{Q}T$ is most marked during anesthesia with drugs that enhance sympathetic activity and least marked with halothane and nitrous oxide. The decrease in systemic vascular resistance is most marked during enflurane anesthesia and hypercapnia. Hypercapnia is a potent pulmonary vasoconstrictor even after the inhalation of 3% isoflurane for 5 minutes.[114]

Dysrhythmias have been reported in unanesthetized humans during acute hypercapnia, but they have seldom been of serious import. A high $PaCO_2$ level is, however, more dangerous during general anesthesia. With halothane anesthesia, dysrhythmias frequently occur above a $PaCO_2$ arrhythmic threshold that is often constant for a particular patient. Furthermore, halothane, enflurane, and isoflurane have been shown to prolong the QT_C interval in humans, thereby increasing the risk

for torsades de pointes ventricular tachycardia, which in turn is notorious for decompensating into ventricular fibrillation.[160]

The maximum stimulatory respiratory effect is attained by a $PaCO_2$ of about 100 mm Hg. With a higher $PaCO_2$, stimulation is reduced, and at extremely high levels, respiration is depressed and later ceases altogether. The PCO_2 ventilation-response curve is generally displaced to the right, and its slope is reduced by anesthetics and other depressant drugs.[163] With profound anesthesia, the response curve may be flat or even sloping downward, and CO_2 then acts as a respiratory depressant. In patients with ventilatory failure, CO_2 narcosis occurs when $PaCO_2$ rises to greater than 90 to 120 mm Hg. A 30% CO_2 concentration is sufficient for the production of anesthesia, and this concentration causes total but reversible flattening of the electroencephalogram.[35] As expected, hypercapnia causes bronchodilation in both healthy persons and patients with lung disease.[138]

Quite apart from the effect of CO_2 on ventilation, it exerts two other important effects that influence the oxygenation of the blood.[199] First, if the concentration of nitrogen (or other inert gas) remains constant, the concentration of CO_2 in alveolar gas can increase only at the expense of O_2, which must be displaced. Thus, PAO_2 and PaO_2 may decrease. Second, hypercapnia shifts the oxy-Hb curve to the right, thereby facilitating tissue oxygenation.[86]

Chronic hypercapnia results in increased resorption of bicarbonate by the kidneys, which further raises the plasma bicarbonate level and constitutes a secondary or compensatory metabolic alkalosis. The decrease in renal resorption of bicarbonate in patients with chronic hypocapnia results in a further fall in plasma bicarbonate and produces a secondary or compensatory metabolic acidosis. In each case, arterial pH returns toward the normal value, but the bicarbonate ion concentration departs even further from normal.

Hypercapnia is accompanied by leakage of potassium from cells into plasma. Much of the potassium comes from the liver, probably from glucose release and mobilization,

Table 4-7 **Cardiovascular Responses to Hypercapnia ($PaCO_2$ = 60-83 mm Hg) during Various Types of Anesthesia (1 MAC Equivalent Except for Nitrous Oxide)***

Anesthesia	Heart Rate	Contractility	Cardiac Output	Systemic Vascular Resistance
Conscious	↑↑	↑↑	↑↑↑	↓
Nitrous oxide	0	↑	↑↑	↓↓
Halothane	0	↑	↑	↓
Isoflurane	↑↑	↑↑↑	↑↑↑	↓

*The increase in the partial arterial pressure of carbon dioxide ($PaCO_2$) in conscious subjects was 11.5 mm Hg from a normal level of 38 mm Hg.
↑, <10% increase; ↑↑, 10%-25% increase; ↑↑↑, >25% increase; 0, no change; ↓, <10% decrease; ↓↓, 10-25% decrease; ↓↓↓, >25% decrease; MAC, minimum alveolar concentration for adequate anesthesia in 50% of subjects.

which occur in response to the rise in plasma catecholamine levels.[54] Because the plasma potassium level takes an appreciable time to return to normal, repeated bouts of hypercapnia at short intervals result in a stepwise rise in plasma potassium. Finally, hypercapnia can predispose the patient to other complications in the operating room (e.g., the oculocephalic response is far more common during hypercapnia than during eucapnia).[97]

4. Hypocapnia

In this section, hypocapnia is considered to be produced by passive hyperventilation (by the anesthesiologist or ventilator). Hypocapnia may cause a decrease in $\dot{Q}T$ by three separate mechanisms. First, if it is present, an increase in intrathoracic pressure decreases cardiac output. Second, hypocapnia is associated with withdrawal of sympathetic nervous system activity, and such withdrawal can decrease the inotropic state of the heart. Third, hypocapnia can increase pH, and the increased pH can decrease ionized calcium, which may in turn decrease the inotropic state of the heart. Hypocapnia

with alkalosis also shifts the oxy-Hb curve to the left, which increases Hb affinity for O_2 and thus impairs O_2 unloading at the tissue level. The decrease in peripheral flow and the impaired ability to unload O_2 to the tissues are compounded by an increase in whole-body O_2 consumption as a result of increased pH-mediated uncoupling of oxidation from phosphorylation.[139] A Pa_{CO_2} of 20 mm Hg increases tissue O_2 consumption by 30%. Consequently, hypocapnia may simultaneously increase tissue O_2 demand and decrease tissue O_2 supply. Thus, to have the same amount of O_2 delivery to the tissues, $\dot{Q}T$ or tissue perfusion has to increase at a time when it may not be possible to do so. The cerebral effects of hypocapnia may be related to a state of cerebral acidosis and hypoxia because hypocapnia may cause a selective reduction in cerebral blood flow and also shifts the oxy-Hb curve to the left.[25]

Hypocapnia may cause $\dot{V}A/\dot{Q}$ abnormalities by inhibiting HPV or by causing bronchoconstriction and decreased C_L. Finally, passive hypocapnia promotes apnea.

REFERENCES

1. Aaronson PI, Robertson TP, Ward JP: Endothelium-derived mediators and hypoxic pulmonary vasoconstriction. Respir Physiol Neurobiol 132:107, 2002.
2. Alexander JI, Spence AA, Parikh RK, et al: The role of airway closure in postoperative hypoxemia. Br J Anaesth 45:34, 1973.
3. Bang BG, Bang FB: Effect of water deprivation on nasal mucous flow. Proc Soc Exp Biol Med 106:516, 1961.
4. Barnes PJ, Liu SF: Regulation of pulmonary vascular tone. Pharmacol Rev 47:87, 1995.
5. Barst RJ, Rich S, Widlitz A, et al: Clinical efficacy of sitaxsentan, an oral endothelin-A receptor antagonist, in patients with pulmonary arterial hypertension. Chest 121:1860, 2002.
6. Barst RJ, Rubin LJ, Long WA, et al: A comparison of continuous intravenous epoprostenol (prostacyclin) with conventional therapy for primary pulmonary hypertension. The Primary Pulmonary Hypertension Study Group. N Engl J Med 334:296, 1996.
7. Bendixen HH, Bullwinkel B, Hedley-Whyte J, et al: Atelectasis and shunting during spontaneous ventilation in anesthetized patients. Anesthesiology 25:297, 1964.
8. Bendixen HH, Hedley-Whyte J, Chir B, et al: Impaired oxygenation in surgical patients during general anesthesia with controlled ventilation. N Engl J Med 269:991, 1963.
9. Benumof JL: Anesthesia for Thoracic Surgery, 2nd ed. Philadelphia, WB Saunders, 1995, Chapter 4.
10. Benumof JL: Anesthesia for Thoracic Surgery, 2nd ed. Philadelphia, WB Saunders, 1995, Chapter 8.
11. Benumof JL: Hypoxic pulmonary vasoconstriction and sodium nitroprusside perfusion. Anesthesiology 50:481, 1979.
12. Benumof JL: Mechanism of decreased blood flow to the atelectatic lung. J Appl Physiol 46:1047, 1978.
13. Benumof JL: One lung ventilation: Which lung should be PEEPed? Anesthesiology 56:161, 1982.
14. Benumof JL, Mathers JM, Wahrenbrock EA: Cyclic hypoxic pulmonary vasoconstriction induced by concomitant carbon dioxide changes. J Appl Physiol 41:466, 1976.
15. Benumof JL, Mathers JM, Wahrenbrock EA: The pulmonary interstitial compartment and the mediator of hypoxic pulmonary vasoconstriction. Microvasc Res 15:69, 1978.
16. Benumof JL, Rogers SN, Moyce PR, et al: Hypoxic pulmonary vasoconstriction and regional and whole lung PEEP in the dog. Anesthesiology 52:503, 1979.
17. Benumof JL, Wahrenbrock EA: Blunted hypoxic pulmonary vasoconstriction by increased lung vascular pressures. J Appl Physiol 38:846, 1975.
18. Benumof JL, Wahrenbrock EA: Dependency of hypoxic pulmonary vasoconstriction on temperature. J Appl Physiol 42:56, 1977.
19. Berggren SM: The oxygen deficit of arterial blood caused by non-ventilating parts of the lung. Acta Physiol Scand Suppl 4:11, 1942.
20. Bersten AD, Rutten AJ, Vedig AE, et al: Additional work of breathing imposed by endotracheal tube, breathing circuits and intensive care ventilators. Crit Care Med 17:671, 1989.
21. Bhavani-Shankar K, Hart NS, Mushlin PS: Negative pressure induced airway and pulmonary injury. Can J Anaesth 44:78, 1997.
22. Biddle TL, Yu PN, Hodges M, et al: Hypoxemia and lung water in acute myocardial infarction. Am Heart J 92:692, 1976.

23. Bohr D: The pulmonary hypoxic response. Chest 71(Suppl):244, 1977.
24. Boysen PG, Block AJ, Wynne JW, et al: Nocturnal pulmonary hypertension in patients with chronic obstructive pulmonary disease. Chest 76:536, 1979.
25. Brian JE Jr: Carbon dioxide and the cerebral circulation. Anesthesiology 88:1365, 1998.
26. Briscoe WA, Cree EM, Filler J, et al: Lung volume, alveolar ventilation and perfusion interrelationships in chronic pulmonary emphysema. J Appl Physiol 15:785, 1960.
27. Brismer B, Hedenstierna G, Lundquist H, et al: Pulmonary densities during anesthesia with muscular relaxation: A proposal of atelectasis. Anesthesiology 62:422, 1985.
28. Burger EJ Jr, Macklem P: Airway closure: Demonstration by breathing 100% O_2 at low lung volumes and by N_2 washout. J Appl Physiol 25:139, 1968.
29. Burton AC, Patel DJ: Effect on pulmonary vascular resistance of inflation of the rabbit lungs. J Appl Physiol 12:239, 1958.
30. Cain SM: Increased oxygen uptake with passive hyperventilation of dogs. J Appl Physiol 28:4, 1970.
31. Campbell EJM, Agostini E, David JN: The Respiratory Muscles: Mechanics and Neural Control, 2nd ed. Philadelphia, WB Saunders, 1970.
32. Channick RN, Simonneau G, Sitbon O, et al: Effects of the dual endothelin-receptor antagonist bosentan in patients with pulmonary hypertension: A randomized placebo-controlled study. Lancet 358:1119, 2001.
33. Cheney FW, Colley PS: The effect of cardiac output on arterial blood oxygenation. Anesthesiology 52:496, 1980.
34. Clark JM: Pulmonary limits of oxygen tolerance in man. Exp Lung Res 14:897, 1988.
35. Clowes GHA, Hopkins AL, Simeone FA: A comparison of the physiological effects of hypercapnia and hypoxia in the production of cardiac arrest. Ann Surg 142:446, 1955.
36. Comroe JH, Forster RE, Dubois AB, et al: The Lung, 2nd ed. Chicago, Year Book, 1962.
37. Couture J, Picken J, Trop D, et al: Airway closure in normal, obese, and anesthetized supine subjects. FASEB J 29:269, 1970.
38. Craig DB, Wahba WM, Don HF, et al: "Closing volume" and its relationship to gas exchange in seated and supine positions. J Appl Physiol 31:717, 1971.
39. Cutillo A, Omboni E, Perondi R, et al: Effect of hypocapnia on pulmonary mechanics in normal subjects and in patients with chronic obstructive lung disease. Am Rev Respir Dis 110:25, 1974.
40. Dalhamn T: Mucous flow and ciliary activity in the tracheas of rats exposed to respiratory irritant gases. Acta Physiol Scand Suppl 36:123, 1956.
41. Dawson CA: The role of pulmonary vasomotion in physiology of the lung. Physiol Rev 64:544, 1984.
42. Dekker E, Defares JG, Heemstra H: Direct measurement of intrabronchial pressure: Its application to the location of the check-valve mechanism. J Appl Physiol 13:35, 1958.
43. Dittrich HC, McCann HA, Wilson WC, et al: Identification of interatrial communication in patients with elevated right atrial pressure using surface and transesophageal contrast echocardiography. J Am Coll Cardiol 21(Suppl):135A, 1993.
44. Dohzaki S, Ohtsuka H, Yamamura T, et al: Comparative effects of volatile anesthetics on the sympathetic activity to acute hypoxemia or hypercarbia in dogs. Anesth Analg 70:S87, 1990.
45. Don H: The mechanical properties of the respiratory system during anesthesia. Int Anesthesiol Clin 15:113, 1977.
46. Don HF, Wahba M, Cuadrado L, et al: The effects of anesthesia and 100 percent oxygen on the functional residual capacity of the lungs. Anesthesiology 32:521, 1970.
47. Doyle JT, Wilson JS, Warren JV: The pulmonary vascular responses to short-term hypoxia in human subjects. Circulation 5:263, 1952.
48. Dueck R, Young I, Clausen J, et al: Altered distribution of pulmonary ventilation and blood flow following induction of inhalational anesthesia. Anesthesiology 52:113, 1980.
49. Eckenhoff JE, Enderby GEH, Larson A, et al: Pulmonary gas exchange during deliberate hypotension. Br J Anaesth 35:750, 1963.
50. Eger EI II, Epstein RM: Hazards of anesthetic equipment. Anesthesiology 25:490, 1964.
51. Elliott CG: Pulmonary physiology during pulmonary embolism. Chest 101:163S, 1992.
52. Epstein RM, Rackow H, Lee ASJ, et al: Prevention of accidental breathing of anoxic gas mixture during anesthesia. Anesthesiology 23:1, 1962.
53. Fellahi JL, Mourgeon E, Goarin JP, et al: Inhaled nitric oxide–induced closure of a patent foramen ovale in an adult patient with acute respiratory distress syndrome and life-threatening hypoxemia. Anesthesiology 83:635, 1995.
54. Fenn WO, Asano T: Effects of carbon dioxide inhalation on potassium liberation from the liver. Am J Physiol 185:567, 1956.
55. Fishman AP: Dynamics of the pulmonary circulation. In Hamilton WF (ed): Handbook of Physiology, section 2. Circulation, vol 2. Baltimore, Williams & Wilkins, 1963, p 1667.
56. Fishman AP: Hypoxia on the pulmonary circulation: How and where it works. Circ Res 38:221, 1976.
57. Fishman AP: Pulmonary edema: The water-exchanging function of the lung. Circulation 46:390, 1972.
58. Fishman AP: Pulmonary hypertension—beyond vasodilator therapy. N Engl J Med 338:321, 1998.
59. Fishman AP: State of the art: Chronic cor pulmonale. Am Rev Respir Dis 114:775, 1976.
60. Föex P, Prys-Roberts C, Hahn CEW, et al: Comparison of oxygen content of blood measured directly with values derived from measurement of oxygen tension. Br J Anaesth 42:803, 1970.
61. Forbes AR: Halothane depresses mucociliary flow in the trachea. Anesthesiology 45:59, 1976.
62. Forbes AR: Humidification and mucous flow in the intubated trachea. Br J Anaesth 45:874, 1973.
63. Freund F, Roos A, Dodd RB: Expiratory activity of the abdominal muscles in man during general anesthesia. J Appl Physiol 19:693, 1964.
64. Froese AB, Bryan CA: Effects of anesthesia and paralysis on diaphragmatic mechanics in man. Anesthesiology 41:242, 1974.

65. Gentilello L, Thompson DA, Tonnesen AS, et al: Effect of a rotating bed on the incidence of pulmonary complications in critically ill patients. Crit Care Med 16:783, 1988.

66. Gilles IDS, Bard BD, Norman J: The effect of anesthesia on the oxyhemoglobin dissociation curve. Br J Anaesth 42:561, 1970.

67. Green WB Jr: The ventilatory effects of sevoflurane. Anesth Analg 81:S23, 1995.

68. Gregory IC: The oxygen and carbon monoxide capacities of foetal and adult blood. J Physiol 236:625, 1974.

69. Grim PS, Freund PR, Cheney FW: Effect of spontaneous sighs on arterial oxygenation during isoflurane anesthesia in humans. Anesth Analg 66:839, 1987.

70. Gunnarsson L, Tokics L, Gustavsson H, et al: Influence of age on atelectasis formation and gas exchange impairment during general anesthesia. Br J Anaesth 66:423, 1991.

71. Gurney AM: Multiple sites of oxygen sensing and their contributions to hypoxic pulmonary vasoconstriction. Respir Physiol Neurobiol 132:43, 2002.

72. Guyton AC: A concept of negative interstitial pressure based on pressures in implanted perforated capsules. Circ Res 12:399, 1963.

73. Hagen PT, Scholz DG, Edwards WD: Incidence and size of patent foramen ovale during the first ten decades of life: An autopsy study of 965 normal hearts. Mayo Clin Proc 59:17, 1984.

74. Hales CA, Kazemi H: Small airways function in myocardial infarction. N Engl J Med 290:761, 1974.

75. Halpern NA, Siegal RE, Papadakos PJ, et al: Right upper lobe collapse following uneventful endotracheal intubation. J Cardiothorac Vasc Anesth 3:620, 1989.

76. Harken AH, O'Connor NE: The influence of clinically undetectable edema on small airway closure in the dog. Ann Surg 184:183, 1976.

77. Hedenstierna G: Gas exchange during anaesthesia. Br J Anaesth 64:507, 1990.

78. Heinonen J, Takki S, Tammisto T: Effect of the Trendelenburg tilt and other procedures on the position of endotracheal tubes. Lancet 1:850, 1969.

79. Heistad DD, Abboud FM: Circulatory adjustments to hypoxia: Dickinson W. Richards Lecture. Circulation 61:463, 1980.

80. Henry W: Experiments on the quantity of gases absorbed by water at different temperatures and under different pressures. Philos Trans R Soc 93:29, 1803.

81. Hickey RF, Visick W, Fairley HB, et al: Effects of halothane anesthesia on functional residual capacity and alveolar-arterial oxygen tension difference. Anesthesiology 38:20, 1973.

82. Hill L: The ciliary movement of the trachea studies in vitro. Lancet 2:802, 1928.

83. Hirsch JA, Tokayer JL, Robinson MJ, et al: Effects of dry air and subsequent humidification on tracheal mucous velocity in dogs. J Appl Physiol 39:242, 1975.

84. Hoppin FG Jr, Green ID, Mead J: Distribution of pleural surface pressure. J Appl Physiol 27:863, 1969.

85. Hosada K, Nakao K, Arai H, et al: Cloning and expression of human endothelin-1 receptor cDNA. FEBS Lett 287:23, 1991.

86. Hsia CCW: Respiratory function of hemoglobin. N Engl J Med 338:239, 2003.

87. Huang YC, Weinmann GG, Mitzner W: Effect of tidal volume and frequency on the temporal fall in lung compliance. J Appl Physiol 65:2040, 1988.

88. Hughes JM, Glazier JB, Maloney JE, et al: Effect of extra-alveolar vessels on the distribution of pulmonary blood flow in the dog. J Appl Physiol 25:701, 1968.

89. Hughes JMB, Glazier JB, Maloney JE, et al: Effect of lung volume on the distribution of pulmonary blood flow in man. Respir Physiol 4:58, 1968.

90. Jaffe RA, Pinto FJ, Schnittger I, et al: Intraoperative ventilator-induced right-to-left intracardiac shunt. Anesthesiology 75:153, 1991.

91. Kain ML, Panday J, Nunn JF: The effect of intubation on the dead space during halothane anaesthesia. Br J Anaesth 41:94, 1969.

92. Kallos T, Wyche MQ, Garman JK: The effect of Innovar on functional residual capacity and total chest compliance. Anesthesiology 39:558, 1973.

93. Kambam JR: Effect of isoflurane on P_{50} and on PO_2 measurement. Anesthesiol Rev 14:40, 1987.

94. Karetzky MS, Cain SM: Effect of carbon dioxide on oxygen uptake during hyperventilation in normal man. J Appl Physiol 28:8, 1970.

95. Kelman GF, Nunn JF, Prys-Roberts C, et al: The influence of the cardiac output on arterial oxygenation: A theoretical study. Br J Anaesth 39:450, 1967.

96. Kent EM, Blades B: The surgical anatomy of the pulmonary lobes. J Thorac Surg 12:18, 1941.

97. Kil HK: Hypercapnia is an important adjuvant factor of oculocardiac reflex during strabismus surgery. Anesth Analg 91:1044, 2000.

98. Kim NH, Channick RN, Rubin LJ: Successful withdrawal of long-term epoprostenol therapy for pulmonary arterial hypertension. Chest 124:1612, 2003.

99. Klein J: Normobaric pulmonary oxygen toxicity. Anesth Analg 70:195, 1990.

100. Krayer S, Rehder K, Vettermann, et al: Position and motion of the human diaphragm during anesthesia-paralysis. Anesthesiology 70:891, 1989.

101. Lambertsen CJ: Effects of oxygen at high partial pressure. In Fenn WO, Rahn H (eds): Handbook of Physiology, section 3. Respiration, vol 2. Baltimore, Williams & Wilkins, 1965, p 1027.

102. Langleben D, Barst RJ, Badesch D, et al: Continuous infusion of epoprostenol improves the net balance between pulmonary endothelin-1 clearance and release in primary pulmonary hypertension. Circulation 99:3266, 1999.

103. Laver MB, Hallowell P, Goldblatt A: Pulmonary dysfunction secondary to heart disease: Aspects relevant to anesthesia and surgery. Anesthesiology 33:161, 1970.

104. Lawler PGP, Nunn JF: A re-assessment of the validity of the iso-shunt graph. Br J Anaesth 56:1325, 1984.

105. Leblanc P, Ruff F, Milic-Emili J: Effects of age and body position on "airway closure" in man. J Appl Physiol 28:448, 1970.

106. Lehot JJ, Leone BJ, Föex P: Effects of altered P_{AO_2} and $Paco_2$ on left ventricular function and coronary hemodynamics of sheep. Anesth Analg 72:737, 1991.

107. Lumb AB: Anaesthesia. In Lumb AB (ed): Nunn's Applied Respiratory Physiology, 5th ed. London, Butterworths, 2000, p 420.

108. Lumb AB: Anaesthesia: Ventilation/perfusion relationships: Effect of age. In Lumb AB (ed): Nunn's Applied Respiratory Physiology, 5th ed. London, Butterworths, 2000, p 445.

109. Lumb AB: Artificial ventilation. In Lumb AB (ed): Nunn's Applied Respiratory Physiology, 5th ed. London, Butterworths, 2000, p 590.

110. Lumb AB: Pulmonary ventilation: Mechanisms and the work of breathing. In Lumb AB (ed): Nunn's Applied Respiratory Physiology, 5th ed. London, Butterworths, 2000, p 128.

111. Lumb AB: Respiratory system resistance. In Lumb AB (ed): Nunn's Applied Respiratory Physiology, 5th ed. London, Butterworths, 2000, p 67.

112. Lumb AB, Nunn JF: Respiratory function and ribcage contribution to ventilation in body positions commonly used during anesthesia. Anesth Analg 73:422, 1991.

113. Macklem PT, Fraser RG, Bates DV: Bronchial pressures and dimensions in health and obstructive airway disease. J Appl Physiol 18:699, 1983.

114. Magnus L, Wattwil T, Olsson JG: Circulatory effects of isoflurane during acute hypercapnia. Anesth Analg 66:1234, 1987.

115. Mallick A, Bodenham AR: Disorders of the lymph circulation: Their relevance to anesthesia and intensive care. Br J Anaesth 91:265, 2003.

116. Marshall BE, Wyche MO: Hypoxemia during and after anesthesia. Anesthesiology 37:178, 1972.

117. Marshall C, Marshall BE: Site and sensitivity for stimulation of hypoxic pulmonary vasoconstriction. J Appl Physiol 55:711, 1983.

118. Martin JT: Positioning in Anesthesia and Surgery. Philadelphia, WB Saunders, 1978.

119. Maseri A, Caldini P, Harward P, et al: Determinants of pulmonary vascular volume: Recruitment versus distensibility. Circ Res 31:218, 1972.

120. Mazze RI: Therapeutic misadventures with oxygen delivery systems: The need for continuous in-line oxygen monitors. Anesth Analg 51:787, 1972.

121. McConkey PP: Postobstructive pulmonary oedema: A case series and review. Anaesth Intensive Care 28:72, 2000.

122. McLaughlin VV, Genthner DE, Panella MM, et al: Reduction in pulmonary vascular resistance with long-term epoprostenol (prostacyclin) therapy in primary pulmonary hypertension. N Engl J Med 338:273, 1998.

123. Mead J, Agostoni E: Dynamics of breathing. In Fenn WO, Rahn H (eds): Handbook of Physiology, section 3. Respiration, vol 1. Baltimore, Williams & Wilkins, 1964, p 411.

124. Milic-Emili J, Henderson JAM, Dolovich MB, et al: Regional distribution of inspired gas in the lung. J Appl Physiol 21:749, 1966.

125. Milic-Emili J, Mead J, Tanner JM: Topography of esophageal pressure as a function of posture in man. J Appl Physiol 19:212, 1964.

126. Moncada S, Higgs A: The L-arginine–nitric oxide pathway. N Engl J Med 329:2002, 1993.

127. Montgomery AB, Luce JM, Murray JF: Retrosternal pain is an early indicator of oxygen toxicity. Am Rev Respir Dis 139:1548, 1989.

128. Moorthy SS, Haselby KA, Caldwell RL, et al: Transient right-left interatrial shunt during emergence from anesthesia: Demonstration by color flow Doppler mapping. Anesth Analg 68:820, 1989.

129. Moxham J: Respiratory muscle fatigue: Mechanisms, evaluation and therapy. Br J Anaesth 65:43, 1990.

130. Munson ES, Larson CP Jr, Babad AA, et al: The effects of halothane, fluroxene and cyclopropane on ventilation: A comparative study in man. Anesthesiology 27:716, 1966.

131. Nash G, Blennerhasset JB, Pontoppidan H: Pulmonary lesions associated with oxygen therapy and artificial ventilation. N Engl J Med 276:368, 1967.

132. Niwa Y, Nagata N, Oka M, et al: Production of nitric oxide from endothelial cells by 31-amino-acid length endothelin-1, a novel vasoconstrictive product by human chymase. Life Sci 67:1103, 2000.

133. Nunn JF, Bergman NA, Coleman AJ: Factors influencing the arterial oxygen tension during anaesthesia with artificial ventilation. Br J Anaesth 37:898, 1965.

134. Ogawa Y, Nakao K, Arai H, et al: Molecular cloning of a non-isopeptide-selective human endothelin receptor. Biochem Biophys Res Commun 178:248, 1991.

135. Olschewski H, Rohde B, Behr J, et al: Pharmacodynamics and pharmacokinetics of inhaled iloprost, aerosolized by three different devices, in severe pulmonary hypertension. Chest 124:1294, 2003.

136. Oswalt CE, Gates GA, Holmstrom EMG: Pulmonary edema as a complication of acute airway obstruction. Rev Surg 34:364, 1977.

137. Palmer RM, Ferrige AG, Moncada A: Nitric oxide release accounts for the biological activity of endothelium-derived relaxing factor. Nature 327:524, 1987.

138. Parson PE, Grunstein MM, Fernandez E: The effects of acute hypoxia and hypercapnia on pulmonary mechanics in normal subjects and patients with chronic pulmonary disease. Chest 96:96, 1989.

139. Patterson RW: Effect of $Paco_2$ on O_2 consumption during cardiopulmonary bypass in man. Anesth Analg 55:269, 1976.

140. Pelosi P, Croci M, Ravagnan I, et al: The effects of body mass on lung volumes, respiratory mechanics, and gas exchange during general anesthesia. Anesth Analg 87:654, 1998.

141. Permutt S, Bromberger-Barnea B, Bane HN: Alveolar pressure, pulmonary venous pressure and the vascular waterfall. Med Thorac 19:239, 1962.

142. Permutt S, Caldini P, Maseri A, et al: Recruitment versus distensibility in the pulmonary vascular bed. In Fishman AP, Hecht H (eds): The Pulmonary Circulation and Interstitial Space. Chicago, University of Chicago Press, 1969, p 375.

143. Peters RM: Work of breathing following trauma. J Trauma 8:915, 1968.

144. Philbin DM, Sullivan SF, Bowman FO, et al: Post-operative hypoxemia: Contribution of the cardiac output. Anesthesiology 32:136, 1970.

145. Pirlo AF, Benumof JL, Trousdale FR: Atelectatic lobe blood flow: Open vs. closed chest, positive pressure vs. spontaneous ventilation. J Appl Physiol 50:1022, 1981.

146. Prys-Roberts C: Hypercapnia. In Gray TC, Nunn JF, Utting JE (eds): General Anaesthesia, 4th ed. London, Butterworths, 1980, p 435.

147. Prys-Roberts C: The metabolic regulation of circulatory transport. In Scurr C, Feldman S (eds): Scientific Foundation of Anesthesia. Philadelphia, FA Davis, 1970, p 87.

148. Puri GD, Venkataranan RK, Singh H, et al: Physiological dead space and arterial to end-tidal CO_2 difference under controlled normocapnic ventilation in young anaesthetized subjects. Indian J Med Res 94:41, 1991.

149. Ray JF, Yost L, Moallem S, et al: Immobility, hypoxemia, and pulmonary arteriovenous shunting. Arch Surg 109:537, 1974.

150. Rehder K, Knopp TH, Sessler AD, et al: Ventilation-perfusion relationships in young healthy awake and anesthetized-paralyzed man. J Appl Physiol 47:745, 1979.

151. Rehder K, Marsh HM, Rodarte JR, et al: Airway closure. Anesthesiology 47:40, 1977.

152. Reid L: Structural and functional reappraisal of the pulmonary arterial system. In The Scientific Basis of Medicine Annual Reviews. London, Athlone Press, 1968.

153. Reid PG, Fraser A, Watt A, et al: Acute haemodynamic effects of adenosine in conscious man. Eur Heart J 11:1018, 1990.

154. Rich S, McLaughlin VV: Endothelin receptor blockers in cardiovascular disease. Circulation 108:2184, 2003.

155. Roberts JG: The effect of hypoxia on the systemic circulation during anaesthesia. In Prys-Roberts E (ed): The Circulation in Anaesthesia: Applied Physiology and Pharmacology. Oxford, Blackwell Scientific, 1980, p 311.

156. Rothe CF, Flanagan AD, Maass-Moreno R: Reflex control of vascular capacitance during hypoxia, hypercapnia, or hypoxic hypercapnia. Can J Physiol Pharmacol 68:384, 1990.

157. Sackner MA, Hirsch J, Epstein S: Effect of cuffed endotracheal tubes on tracheal mucous velocity. Chest 68:774, 1975.

158. Sackner MA, Landa J, Hirsch J, et al: Pulmonary effects of oxygen breathing. Ann Intern Med 82:40, 1975.

159. Scanlon TS, Benumof JL: Demonstration of interlobar collateral ventilation. J Appl Physiol 46:658, 1979.

160. Schmeling WT, Warltier DC, McDonald DJ, et al: Prolongation of the QT interval by enflurane, isoflurane, and halothane in humans. Anesth Analg 72:137, 1991.

161. Serebrovskaya TV: Comparison of respiratory and circulatory human responses to progressive hypoxia and hypercapnia. Respiration 59:35, 1992.

162. Seto K, Goto H, Hacker D, et al: Right upper lobe atelectasis after inadvertent right main bronchial intubation. Anesth Analg 62:851, 1983.

163. Severinghaus JW, Larson CP: Respiration in anesthesia. In Fenn WO, Rahn H (eds): Handbook of Physiology, section 3. Respiration, vol 2. Baltimore, Williams & Wilkins, 1965, p 1219.

164. Sham JSK: Hypoxic pulmonary vasoconstriction: Ups and downs of reactive oxygen species. Circ Res 91:649, 2002.

165. Shapiro BA, Harrison RA, Trout CA: The mechanics of ventilation. In Clinical Application of Respiratory Care, 3rd ed. Chicago, Year Book, 1985, p 57.

166. Simmons DH, Linde CM, Miller JH, et al: Relation of lung volume and pulmonary vascular resistance. Circ Res 9:465, 1961.

167. Slocum HC, Hoeflich EA, Allen CR: Circulatory and respiratory distress from extreme positions on the operating table. Surg Gynecol Obstet 84:1065, 1947.

168. Smith-Erichsen N, Bo G: Airway closure and fluid filtration in the lung. Br J Anaesth 51:475, 1979.

169. Sprague DH, Archer GW: Intraoperative hypoxia from an erroneously filled liquid oxygen reservoir. Anesthesiology 42:360, 1975.

170. Stamler JS, Loh E, Roddy M-A, et al: Nitric oxide regulated basal systemic and pulmonary vascular resistance in healthy humans. Circulation 89:2035, 1994.

171. Staub NC: Pulmonary edema: Physiologic approaches to management. Chest 74:559, 1978.

172. Staub NC: "State of the art" review: Pathogenesis of pulmonary edema. Am Rev Respir Dis 109:358, 1974.

173. Strandberg A, Hedenstierna G, Tokics L, et al: Densities in dependent lung regions during anaesthesia: Atelectasis or fluid accumulation? Acta Anaesthesiol Scand 30:256, 1986.

174. Strandberg A, Tokics L, Brismar B, et al: Atelectasis during anesthesia and in the postoperative period. Acta Anaesthesiol Scand 30:154, 1986.

175. Sykes MK: The mechanics of ventilation. In Scurr C, Feldman S (eds): Scientific Foundations of Anesthesia. Philadelphia, FA Davis, 1970, p 174.

176. Sykes MK, Adams AP, Finley WEI, et al: The cardiorespiratory effects of hemorrhage and overtransfusion in dogs. Br J Anaesth 42:573, 1970.

177. Sykes MK, Young WE, Robinson BE: Oxygenation during anaesthesia with controlled ventilation. Br J Anaesth 37:314, 1965.

178. Tokics L, Hedenstierna G, Strandberg A, et al: Lung collapse and gas exchange during general anesthesia: Effects of spontaneous breathing, muscle paralysis and positive end-expiratory pressure. Anesthesiology 66:157, 1987.

179. Tweed WA, Phua WT, Chong KY, et al: Large tidal volume ventilation improves pulmonary gas exchange during lower abdominal surgery in Trendelenburg's position. Can J Anaesth 38:989, 1991.

180. Vaughan RW, Wise L: Intraoperative arterial oxygenation in obese patients. Ann Surg 184:35, 1976.

181. Von Euler US, Liljestrand G: Observations on the pulmonary arterial blood pressure in the cat. Acta Physiol Scand 12:301, 1946.

182. Wagner PD, Laravuso RB, Uhl RR, et al: Continuous distributions of ventilation-perfusion ratios in normal

subjects breathing air and 100% O_2. J Clin Invest 54:54, 1974.

183. Wagner PD, Saltzman HA, West JB: Measurement of continuous distributions of ventilation-perfusion ratios: Theory. J Appl Physiol 36:588, 1974.

184. Wang T, El Kebir D, Blaise G: Inhaled nitric oxide in 2003: A review of its mechanisms of action. Can J Anaesth 50:839, 2003.

185. Ward CF, Gagnon RL, Benumof JL: Wheezing after induction of general anesthesia: Negative expiratory pressure revisited. Anesth Analg 58:49, 1979.

186. Ward CS: The prevention of accidents associated with anesthetic apparatus. Br J Anaesth 40:692, 1968.

187. Ware LB, Matthay MA: Acute respiratory distress syndrome. N Engl J Med 342:1334, 2000.

188. Waypa GB, Marks JD, Mack MM, et al: Mitochondrial reactive oxygen species trigger calcium increases during hypoxia in pulmonary artery myocytes. Circ Res 91:719, 2002.

189. Waypa GB, Schumacker PT: O_2 sensing in hypoxic pulmonary vasoconstriction: The mitochondrial door re-opens. Respir Physiol Neurobiol 132:81, 2002.

190. Weibel ER: Morphological basis of alveolar-capillary gas exchange. Physiol Rev 53:419, 1973.

191. Weir EK, Archer SL: The mechanism of acute hypoxic pulmonary vasoconstriction: The tale of two channels. FASEB J 9:183, 1995.

192. West JB: Blood flow to the lung and gas exchange. Anesthesiology 41:124, 1974.

193. West JB: Regional differences in gas exchange in the lung of erect man. J Appl Physiol 17:893, 1962.

194. West JB (ed): Regional Differences in the Lung. Orlando, Fla, Academic Press, 1977.

195. West JB: Ventilation/Blood Flow and Gas Exchange, 4th ed. Oxford, Blackwell Scientific, 1970.

196. West JB, Dollery CT, Heard BE: Increased pulmonary vascular resistance in the dependent zone of the isolated dog lung caused by perivascular edema. Circ Res 17:191, 1965.

197. West JB, Dollery CT, Naimark A: Distribution of blood flow in isolated lung: Relation to vascular and alveolar pressures. J Appl Physiol 19:713, 1964.

198. Westbrook PR, Stubbs SE, Sessler AD, et al: Effects of anesthesia and muscle paralysis on respiratory mechanics in normal man. J Appl Physiol 34:81, 1973.

199. Wilson WC, Shapiro B: Perioperative hypoxia: The clinical spectrum and current oxygen monitoring methodology. Anesthesiol Clin North Am 19:769, 2001.

200. Winter PM, Smith G: The toxicity of oxygen. Anesthesiology 37:210, 1972.

201. Wittenberger JL, McGregor M, Berglund E, et al: Influence of state of inflation of the lung on pulmonary vascular resistance. J Appl Physiol 15:878, 1960.

202. Wright PE, Marini JJ, Bernard GR: In vitro versus in vivo comparison of endotracheal tube airflow resistance. Am Rev Respir Dis 140:10, 1989.

203. Wyche MQ, Teichner RL, Kallos T, et al: Effects of continuous positive-pressure breathing on functional residual capacity and arterial oxygenation during intra-abdominal operation. Anesthesiology 38:68, 1973.

204. Xuan DAT: Endothelial modulation of pulmonary vascular tone. Eur Respir J 5:757, 1992.

205. Yang Z, Krasnici N, Luscher TF: Endothelin-1 potentiates human smooth muscle cell growth to PDGF: Effects of ETA and ETB receptor blockade. Circulation 100:5, 1999.

206. Yeaker H: Tracheobronchial secretions. Am J Med 50:493, 1971.

207. Zapol WM, Snider MT: Pulmonary hypertension in severe acute respiratory failure. N Engl J Med 296:476, 1977.

208. Zasslow MA, Benumof JL, Trousdale FR: Hypoxic pulmonary vasoconstriction and the size of the hypoxic compartment. J Appl Physiol 53:626, 1982.

5

AIRWAY PHARMACOLOGY

David O. Warner

I. INTRODUCTION

Many drugs can affect airway function. Agents such as bronchodilators may be administered specifically to produce therapeutic effects on the airways. Other drugs, primarily targeted to other organ systems, may also affect the airways. For example, many general anesthetic agents profoundly depress the function of the striated muscles of the upper airway, requiring that much of modern anesthetic practice be directed toward maintaining airway patency. Numerous drugs used in anesthetic practice may also affect the smooth muscle of the lower airway. Thus, an understanding of the pharmacology of drugs with effects on the airways is critical to optimal airway management and the safe conduct of anesthesia.

This chapter reviews the pharmacology of drugs commonly administered in the perioperative period that may affect the airways. Both the upper airway (from nares to glottis) and the lower airway (from glottis to terminal bronchiole) are considered.

II. UPPER AIRWAY

A. CLINICAL CONCERNS

Two aspects of upper airway function are of primary clinical concern. First, the coordinated activity of the striated muscles of the upper airway is critical to maintain airway patency. Sedation and anesthesia interfere with this activity, and the integrity of the upper airway may be compromised. Second, artificial support of the upper airway, such as that provided by an endotracheal tube (ET), is often required to manage this problem. It is often necessary to provide topical anesthesia of the upper airway to permit such instrumentation.

B. PHARMACOLOGIC EFFECTS ON THE FUNCTION OF UPPER AIRWAY MUSCLES

1. Physiology of the Upper Airway

The patency of the upper airway is controlled by a complex arrangement of muscles.[266,274] Gas enters and exits the airways through either the mouth or the nose, as controlled by the muscles of the soft palate. An intricate system of pharyngeal constrictors and muscles that insert on the tongue and hyoid bone regulates pharyngeal caliber, allowing the pharynx to serve multiple functions, including the conduct of respiratory gases, deglutition, and speech. The position and caliber of the larynx are controlled by muscles both intrinsic and extrinsic to the laryngeal cartilages.

During breathing, activity in several upper airway muscles is crucial to maintain upper airway patency. Many upper airway muscles that surround the pharynx demonstrate phasic activity during inspiration. These muscles include the genioglossus, stylopharyngeus,

and styloglossus muscles.[231] All of them help maintain pharyngeal patency during the negative upper airway pressures generated by inspiratory flow. In the absence of their activity, even modest negative upper airway pressures can markedly narrow the upper airway of healthy subjects (Fig. 5-1).[281]

Laryngeal muscles are also important in the maintenance of airway patency during breathing. The glottis widens during inspiration and narrows during expiration in human subjects, primarily because of phasic activation of the posterior cricoarytenoid muscle, a vocal cord abductor.[23-25,149] This activity decreases during expiration; the resulting glottic narrowing may serve to retard and control expiratory flow.[25,72] Phasic expiratory activity in vocal cord adductors such as the thyroarytenoids also controls expiratory flow.[124] Other laryngeal muscles such as the cricothyroid muscle may also demonstrate respiratory activity.[280] Although the interaction among these muscles is not fully understood, it is likely that the coordinated activity of all these muscles is necessary to maintain normal upper airway caliber.

There are two characteristics that distinguish the control of upper airway muscles (Fig. 5-2). First, afferent information plays an important role in the control of these muscles. Receptors in both the lung and the walls

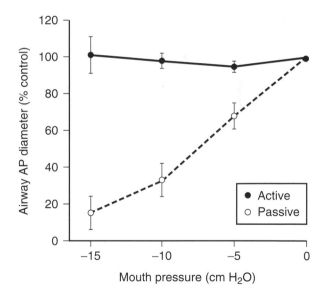

Figure 5-1 Anterior-posterior (AP) diameter of the upper airway of six human subjects during negative mouth pressure generated by inspiring against an externally occluded airway ("active" upper airway muscles) or external suction at the mouth during voluntary glottic closure with no inspiratory effort ("passive" upper airway muscles). Note that active muscles are required to prevent airway narrowing during negative mouth pressures, such as those generated by inspiratory effort. These data demonstrate that upper airway muscle activity is crucial to the maintenance of upper airway patency. Values are mean ± SE. (Modified from Wheatley JR, Kelly WT, Tully A, Engel LA: Pressure-diameter relationships of the upper airway in awake supine subjects. J Appl Physiol 70:2242, 1991.)

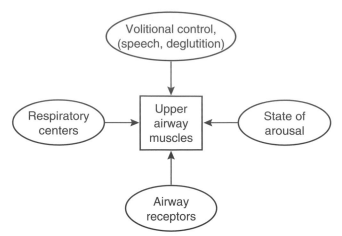

Figure 5-2 Influences modulating the activity of upper airway muscles. (From Benumof JL [ed]: Airway Management: Principles and Practice, 1st ed. St. Louis, Mosby, 1996, p 76.)

of the upper airway provide the bulk of this sensory information. These receptors, which respond to changes in airway pressure and a variety of mechanical and chemical stimuli (including volatile anesthetics),[190] play an important role in modulating the activities of upper airway muscles. They mediate reflex closure of the glottis, involving contraction of multiple upper airway muscles, which serves an important protective function to prevent aspiration of material into the lungs.[220,230] Second, the activity of upper airway muscles is very dependent on the state of arousal.[202] The most familiar example of this dependence is the increase in upper airway resistance that accompanies natural sleep, which often produces an audible manifestation (snoring).[126]

2. Effects of Anesthesia and Sedation

In most experimental animal preparations, anesthesia and sedation depress the activity of upper airway muscles.[112,123,190,191,196] Several reports have documented that the sensitivity of upper airway muscles to anesthetic-induced depression differs from that of other respiratory muscles such as the diaphragm.[123,190,191,196] Halothane, enflurane, diazepam, and thiopental all produce a greater depression of hypoglossal nerve activity than phrenic nerve activity in paralyzed, ventilated, vagotomized cats.[190,191] Measurements of respiratory muscle activity in intact anesthetized cats breathing spontaneously show similar results; electromyogram activity in the diaphragm is more resistant to depression by halothane than that in the genioglossus muscle (Fig. 5-3).[196] This differential suppression may be less pronounced after ketamine administration,[123,191,224] suggesting that it is not a property common to all general anesthetics. Other reports have also noted an apparent preservation of upper airway motoneuron activities in animals anesthetized with ketamine.[112,224] This observation is consistent with the clinical impression that upper airway patency is better

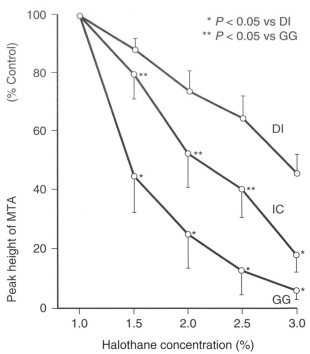

Figure 5-3 Phasic inspiratory muscle activity, expressed as the peak height of a moving time average (MTA) value of the electromyogram, during halothane anesthesia in cats. Note that the genioglossus (GG), an upper airway muscle, is most sensitive to anesthetic-induced depression, followed by the internal intercostal muscle (IC, a muscle of the rib cage) and the diaphragm (DI). *$P < .05$ compared with DI. Values are mean ± SEM. (From Ochiai R, Guthrie RD, Motoyama EK: Effects of varying concentrations of halothane on the activity of the genioglossus, intercostals, and diaphragm in cats: An electromyographic study. Anesthesiology 70:812, 1989.)

preserved with ketamine anesthesia,[63] although firm experimental evidence to support this assertion is lacking. In human subjects, even relatively low-dose isoflurane (0.4%) causes profound depression of upper airway motor activity.[68]

Because the activity of upper airway motoneurons is highly dependent on inputs from the reticular activating system (see Fig. 5-2), it is possible that the sensitivity of this activity to anesthetics is related to anesthetic-induced depression of the reticular activating system. In other words, anesthetic effects may be mediated not only by a direct effect on motoneurons but also indirectly through changes in the state of arousal. Consistent with this idea, some of the changes in upper airway activity caused by anesthesia mimic those seen during some stages of natural sleep, although there are also important differences that depend on sleep state.[126]

Alterations in airway reflexes that normally protect the laryngeal inlet may also affect perioperative upper airway function. These reflexes are impaired by many anesthetic drugs,[180,189] including the benzodiazepines.[65,180] The mechanism of this depression is unknown. Paradoxically, reflex irritability is apparently increased during some stages of anesthesia and may produce laryngospasm; this phenomenon, although clinically significant, is poorly understood.[220,230] This reflex irritability requires that great care be exercised to minimize airway stimulation during the induction of and emergence from anesthesia. Of interest, the inhalation of volatile anesthetics, especially the ethers, may initially stimulate airway receptors, leading to coughing, alterations in respiratory pattern, and cardiovascular stimulation.[53,190,229] This reflex irritability significantly limits the use of agents such as desflurane and isoflurane as inhalation induction agents.[254] Another ether, sevoflurane, is apparently less irritating and is more suitable for this purpose.[53,182]

How changes in the activity of upper airway muscles produced by anesthesia and sedation may influence upper airway caliber is uncertain. On the basis of early studies in human subjects, it is often assumed that anesthesia and sedation cause a posterior displacement of the tongue, which produces airway obstruction at an oropharyngeal level.[176,227] However, a more recent study using ultrasonography could not confirm this finding.[1] In the absence of airflow, the most consistent site of obstruction is at the nasopharyngeal level, where the soft palate becomes approximated to the posterior pharynx (Fig. 5-4).[166,183,219] This site is also susceptible to obstruction in patients with obstructive sleep apnea.[122,236] The epiglottis and supralaryngeal tissues may also participate in upper airway narrowing.[20] Under these conditions, efforts by the diaphragm and other respiratory muscles of the chest wall actually encourage upper airway collapse. These inspiratory efforts decrease airway pressures and produce narrowing at multiple levels, including the base of the tongue.[183]

There is not a consistent relationship between phasic electromyogram activity of upper airway muscles and upper airway resistance. Drummond found that thiopental produced alterations in the amount and pattern of activity in neck and tongue muscles measured with surface electrodes in human subjects.[64] However, reductions in activity could not be related directly to the onset of airway obstruction; rather, activity was often increased, presumably in an attempt to overcome partial obstruction. Also, although benzodiazepines appear to increase upper airway resistance in human subjects,[175] they decrease genioglossus activity only in older subjects,[157] not in younger subjects. Thus, airway obstruction may be caused not by a simple diminution of activity but by disruption of the normal coordination of activity of muscles controlling different segments of the airways.[9]

It is possible that anesthetics could produce tonic activity in upper airway constrictors, which would explain the clinical observation that pharmacologic paralysis frequently decreases upper airway resistance following induction of anesthesia with thiopental. Factors not directly involving the upper airway muscles may also affect upper airway resistance during anesthesia. For example, the position of the head and neck may change as normal

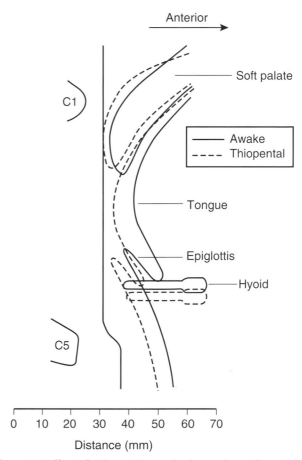

Figure 5-4 Effect of thiopental anesthesia on airway dimensions. Note that the primary site of obstruction is at the level of the soft palate. (Modified from Nandi PR, Charlesworth CH, Taylor SJ, et al: Effect of general anaesthesia on the pharynx. Br J Anaesth 66:157, 1991.)

postural muscle tone decreases with the onset of anesthesia. Decreases in the functional residual capacity produced by anesthesia may also increase upper airway resistance.[14,68]

3. Effects of Neuromuscular Blockade

Drugs that block the neuromuscular junction are frequently used in clinical practice to inhibit respiratory muscle function, both to facilitate endotracheal intubation and to eliminate respiratory efforts during mechanical ventilation. These drugs may affect the respiratory muscles differently than other skeletal muscles. This observation becomes clinically relevant during partial neuromuscular blockade with nondepolarizing agents, a situation frequently encountered in the postanesthesia recovery area.

Greater doses of vecuronium,[57,154,155] atracurium,[154] and pancuronium[56] are required to achieve a given degree of neuromuscular block in the diaphragm compared with the adductor pollicis, although the onset of block is more rapid in the diaphragm. This relative sparing of the diaphragm permits the maintenance of respiratory effort even during complete paralysis of peripheral muscles (Fig. 5-5).[88,89] The adductor muscles of the larynx may be even more resistant to the effects of nondepolarizing drugs than the diaphragm.[56] However, other upper airway muscles may not behave similarly. The susceptibility of the masseter to block appears to be equal to or greater than that of the adductor pollicis. The mechanisms responsible for this differential sensitivity are unknown. Nevertheless, it is apparent that upper airway patency may be compromised at levels of paralysis that otherwise permit maintenance of normal ventilation (see Fig. 5-5).[208]

This differential sensitivity may assume great clinical importance in the postoperative period. If residual neuromuscular blockade is present, the patient with an ET or other airway support in place may be able to maintain adequate ventilation. However, when the ET is removed, upper airway obstruction may develop. For this reason, adequacy of the reversal of neuromuscular blockade must always be assured before removal of artificial airway support.

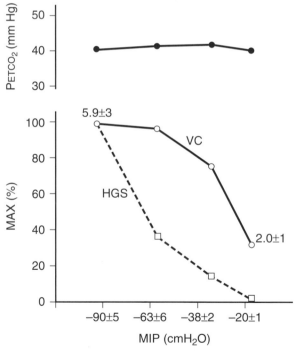

Figure 5-5 Handgrip strength (HGS), vital capacity (VC, with absolute values noted at the extremes of measurement), and end-tidal CO_2 (P_{ETCO_2}) as a function of maximum inspiratory pressure (MIP) developed at the mouth during maximum inspiration against an occluded airway at rest and during increasing degrees of paralysis with *d*-tubocurarine in human subjects. Mandibular elevation was necessary at MIP $\geq -39 \pm 5$ cm H_2O to prevent upper airway obstruction. This study demonstrates that ventilation can be maintained by the diaphragm at levels of neuromuscular blockade that cause upper airway collapse. (From Pavlin EG, Holle RH, Schoene RB: Recovery of airway protection compared with ventilation in humans after paralysis with curare. Anesthesiology 70:381, 1989.)

4. Effects of Hypoxia and Hypercarbia

Like the diaphragm and other chest wall muscles, the upper airway muscles also respond to the stresses of hypoxia and hypercarbia.[201] In humans, the inspiratory activity of the upper airway muscles initially increases with both hypoxia and hypercarbia, presumably to maintain airway patency during concurrent increases in minute ventilation.[199] However, these increases cannot be sustained during prolonged hypoxia,[197,228] and airway patency may be compromised.

C. PHARMACOLOGIC EFFECTS ON SENSORY FUNCTION

The upper airway is richly endowed with sensory nerves that normally serve as the afferent limbs of powerful reflexes that protect the airways from the aspiration of foreign material. To instrument the upper airway, this sensory function must be attenuated. This topic is fully covered in Chapter 6; here we briefly review the pharmacology of local anesthetics commonly used to provide topical airway anesthesia.

1. Agents

Local anesthetics reversibly block nerve conduction, disrupting the propagation of action potentials by binding to sodium channels and interfering with their function.[45] Chemically, local anesthetics usually consist of a lipophilic group connected to an ionizable group (usually a tertiary amine) by either an ester or amide link (Fig. 5-6).[46]

They are weak bases and are usually formulated as salts. Local anesthetics are metabolized in the liver (amides) or plasma (esters) to water-soluble metabolites and excreted in the urine. Adequate drug diffusion through mucous membranes to the sensory nerves is necessary for topical efficacy. Almost every local anesthetic agent has some effects when applied to the mucous membranes of the upper airways, although some are too irritating or toxic for this use.

Lidocaine remains the prototypic agent for topical use. Available formulations for upper airway use include a 2% viscous gel and solutions ranging in concentration from 2% to 10%; use of a eutectic mixture with prilocaine has also been reported to provide airway anesthesia.[152] There are few data concerning any dose-response relationship for intensity or duration of anesthesia within these ranges of concentration. The duration of action is quite variable, ranging from approximately 10 to 30 minutes.

Benzocaine is poorly soluble in water and thus is poorly absorbed into the systemic circulation. It is available in 20% solution for topical use. Chemically, it differs from most other local anesthetics in that it is an ester of *p*-aminobenzoic acid that lacks a terminal amino group (see Fig. 5-6). The duration of action is from approximately 10 to 30 minutes.

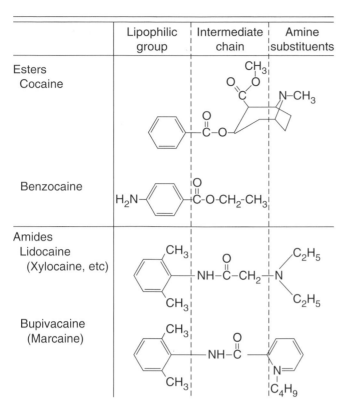

	Lipophilic group	Intermediate chain	Amine substituents
Esters Cocaine			
Benzocaine			
Amides Lidocaine (Xylocaine, etc)			
Bupivacaine (Marcaine)			

Figure 5-6 Structure of local anesthetics used for topical airway anesthesia. (From Benumof JL [ed]: Airway Management: Principles and Practice, 1st ed. St. Louis, Mosby, 1996, p 80.)

Bupivacaine has been used for topical airway anesthesia in concentrations ranging from 1% to 4%. In animal models, these concentrations provide durations of anesthesia that exceed those provided by lidocaine (up to 75 minutes).[82] However, the potential for toxicity from drug that is systemically absorbed has limited enthusiasm for this application.

Sodium benzonatate is a nonopioid antitussive that is a long-chain polyglycol derivative of procaine. When applied orally, it provides rapid topical anesthesia suitable for awake oral intubation.[174]

Cocaine, in solutions from 1% to 10%, provides excellent topical anesthesia. It has the advantage of providing vasoconstriction because of its sympathomimetic actions, which may be useful in preventing epistaxis during nasotracheal intubation. However, its potential to be abused limits its clinical use.

Dyclonine produces excellent topical airway anesthesia (up to 1% spray). Of interest, despite this excellent airway anesthesia, it does not appear to be as effective as lidocaine in reducing airway reflex responses to interventions such as bronchoscopy (see Section III.D.5).

2. Systemic Absorption and Toxicity

Varying amounts of local anesthetic are absorbed into the systemic circulation when topically applied. Most reports show that systemic absorption of topically applied lidocaine

is limited. Chinn and colleagues[37] found plasma lidocaine levels of 0.44 μg/mL after inhalation of 400 mg of nebulized lidocaine. Similarly, Baughman and associates[12] found that patients breathing 4 mg/kg aerosolized lidocaine developed plasma levels of less than 0.5 μg/mL. Oral lidocaine produced even lower plasma levels,[97] probably because much of the dose is swallowed and subjected to first-pass metabolism by the liver. Lidocaine applied directly to the trachea and bronchi results in higher plasma levels. Viegas and Stoelting[271] found plasma levels of 1.7 μg/mL 9 minutes after tracheal installation of 2 mg/kg lidocaine; similar results have been reported by others.[49,210] Sutherland and Williams[250] utilized a standardized topical anesthesia protocol for awake fiberoptic intubation, combining 4% lidocaine aerosol, topical 2% viscous lidocaine gel, and direct installation of lidocaine through the bronchoscope. Despite a large total dose of lidocaine (5.3 ± 2.1 mg/kg), the mean peak arterial plasma lidocaine concentration was low (0.6 ± 2.1 μg/mL). All of these levels are well below the reported toxic range for lidocaine (>5 to 6 μg/mL), so that the administration of doses less than the commonly cited limit for parenteral administration of lidocaine (4 mg/mL) should be associated with minimal risk of toxicity.[151,206] However, gargling of large volumes (0.3 mL/kg) of 2% lidocaine may be associated with peak lidocaine concentrations approaching a potentially toxic level.[163] Few studies have been done specifically in children, but Sitbon and coauthors[244] suggested that up to 2.6 mg/kg topical lidocaine produces minimal plasma levels. Swallowed lidocaine in the setting of topical airway anesthesia can cause nausea and vomiting.[18]

Prominent toxic reactions related to systemic absorption involve the central nervous system, ranging from irritability to convulsions, and the cardiovascular system, leading in the extreme to cardiovascular collapse. Allergic reactions to amide local anesthetics are extremely rare. Ester agents are metabolized to *p*-aminobenzoic acid derivatives, which may produce hypersensitivity reactions in some patients. Absorbed benzocaine may produce methemoglobinemia[216,263]; because absorption is variable, the threshold dose needed to produce this complication is unclear. Methemoglobinemia is detectable by pulse oximetry, although its magnitude may be underestimated.[4,6] Treatment includes supplemental oxygen and intravenous methylene blue. Benzocaine should probably be avoided in infants and in patients with anemia or other disorders in which oxygen transport may be impaired.[234]

3. Effects of Topical Anesthesia on Upper Airway Patency

Topical anesthesia may also affect upper airway patency because upper airway reflex mechanisms play an important role in its maintenance. Topical anesthesia of the upper airway can produce airway obstruction in both healthy subjects[170] and subjects with obstructive sleep apnea.[33,79] Furthermore, instrumentation of the upper airway is often facilitated by the use of sedatives such as benzodiazepines, which themselves may depress upper airway muscle function. Thus, airway patency must be carefully monitored until an artificial airway is secured or until the effects of local anesthesia and sedation have dissipated.

III. LOWER AIRWAYS

A. CLINICAL CONCERNS

Although the physiologic function of airway smooth muscle remains obscure, there is no doubt that its constriction can produce serious morbidity in the perioperative period. Airway instrumentation during perioperative airway management is a potent stimulus for reflex bronchoconstriction. Other interventions, such as the administration of drugs that may release histamine or other inflammatory mediators, may also trigger bronchospasm. Patients with diseases characterized by heightened airway reactivity, such as asthma and some forms of chronic obstructive pulmonary disease, are thought to be at particular risk for the development of perioperative bronchoconstriction.[238] Asthma is one of the most common chronic diseases, affecting over 10 million Americans, and its incidence continues to increase.[291] Thus, proper management of drugs affecting lower airway function continues to be an important factor in perioperative airway management. It is also important to realize that many instances of perioperative bronchospasm occur in patients without any history of heightened airway reactivity.[35,83,200] Principal concerns include optimization of preoperative therapy for patients with hyperreactive airways and the prevention and treatment of intraoperative and postoperative bronchospasm. Achievement of these goals requires a thorough understanding of the pharmacology of drugs with primary actions on the lower airways. This section reviews the clinical pharmacology of each class of agents and then discusses their rational use in perioperative airway management.

B. DRUGS THAT ATTENUATE THE INFLAMMATORY RESPONSE

Until recently, asthma and other diseases characterized by heightened airway reactivity were regarded as manifestations of abnormalities of airway smooth muscle. However, current understanding regards asthma as a chronic inflammatory disease of the airways.[10,125] This inflammation causes symptoms of reversible airway obstruction, as inflammatory mediators constrict airway smooth muscle (Fig. 5-7). Furthermore, chronic inflammation thickens the airway wall, narrowing the airway and amplifying the effects of smooth muscle shortening. The appreciation of the importance of inflammation to the pathogenesis of asthma has shifted the emphasis of therapeutic strategies from bronchodilators per se, which act directly to relax

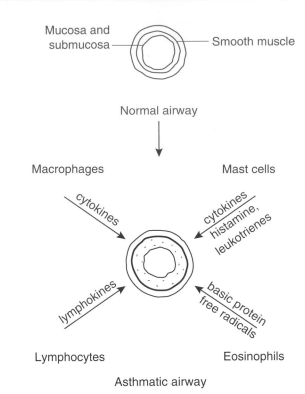

Figure 5-7 Changes in the cross-sectional anatomy of normal and asthmatic airways, with some of the inflammatory cell types and mediators that may be responsible for these changes. Note the thickening of the smooth muscle and submucosa, associated with infiltration of inflammatory cells. (From Benumof JL [ed]: Airway Management: Principles and Practice, 1st ed. St. Louis, Mosby, 1996, p 81.)

smooth muscle, to drugs that ameliorate the inflammatory response.

1. Cromolyn Sodium and Nedocromil

a. Mechanism of Action

Cromolyn sodium (disodium cromoglycate) and nedocromil prevent the release of inflammatory mediators from various cell types associated with asthma.[118,205,256] One effect of potential benefit is thought to be suppression of immunoglobulin E–provoked mediator release from lung mast cells. These drugs may also have multiple other anti-inflammatory actions, such as inhibition of the release of other mediators from several other types of inflammatory cells. Pretreatment with these agents inhibits bronchospasm produced by antigen and by exercise, concurrently attenuating the production of chemotactic factors associated with mast cell activation.

b. Pharmacokinetics, Toxicity

These drugs are poorly absorbed and are administered by inhalation of powdered drug through a metered-dose inhaler. Absorbed drug is not significantly metabolized and is excreted in urine and bile. Significant side effects and toxicity are rare and include oropharyngeal irritation or symptoms such as cough, caused by the direct irritant effect of the powder. Anaphylaxis is rare but has been reported.

c. Clinical Use

Because of their mechanism of action, these drugs are useful only in the prevention of bronchospasm, not in the treatment of established bronchospasm. They may be useful both as a single preventive treatment before exercise or exposure to antigens and as chronic therapy. Efficacy in individual patients varies widely, and at present a therapeutic trial is the only way of determining which patients will benefit. Although nedocromil is more potent in preventing some forms of acute bronchoconstriction in some studies, its efficacy in clinical use does not appear to differ significantly from that of cromolyn sodium.[205] Neither agent has been studied as an adjunct to airway management in the perioperative period.

2. Corticosteroids

a. Mechanism of Action

These drugs are the most effective anti-inflammatory agents for the treatment of asthma.[7,8,229] The multiple possible sites of action in interrupting inflammation probably account for their usefulness in all forms of asthma. After binding to receptors within the cytoplasm, corticosteroids are translocated to the nucleus, where they regulate the function of steroid-responsive genes (Fig. 5-8). This regulation may increase or decrease the formation of specific proteins.[171]

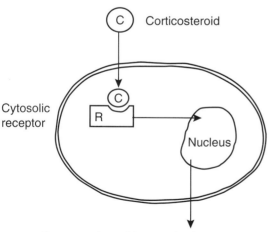

Decreased cytokine production
Reduced number of mast cells
Reduced plasma exudation from pulmonary vessels
Inhibited secretion of mucus glycoprotein
Increased sensitivity to β_2 agonists

Figure 5-8 Possible mechanisms of action of corticosteroids in asthma. Corticosteroid bind to cytosolic receptors, which are translated into the nucleus, where they control gene expression and regulate the activity of many cell types. (From Benumof JL [ed]: Airway Management: Principles and Practice, 1st ed. St. Louis, Mosby, 1996, p 82.)

In particular, corticosteroids may inhibit the formation of several cytokines that are important mediators of the inflammatory response; this effect may be most important on T lymphocytes.[104] This inhibition may lead to reductions in the numbers of mast cells[150] and decreases in neutrophil survival.[111] Corticosteroids may also reduce plasma exudation from pulmonary vessels[21] and inhibit the secretion of mucus glycoprotein.[237] As a result of these actions, corticosteroids reduce the immediate and late-phase responses to allergens[40] and also reduce nonspecific airway reactivity when administered chronically.[10] Chronic administration improves airway wall inflammation assessed by bronchial biopsy.[161] Corticosteroids may also have actions in addition to direct effects on inflammation. For example, they increase the number of β receptors and so may increase sensitivity to β_2 receptor agonists.[84]

b. Pharmacokinetics

Corticosteroids may be administered by oral, parenteral, or inhaled routes.[96] Oral absorption is rapid and complete. Parenteral administration may be necessary to administer high doses or if the patient cannot take oral medications. The use of inhaled corticosteroids represents a significant advance in asthma therapy, as high local concentrations of steroids can be achieved in the airway while minimizing the side effects associated with systemic administration. These topical steroids have enhanced topical anti-inflammatory potency (related to high affinity for glucocorticoid receptors) with low systemic potency (reflecting their rapid biotransformation in the liver into inactive metabolites).[259] Examples of these compounds include *beclomethasone dipropionate*, *triamcinolone acetonide*, *fluticasone*, and *flunisolide* (Table 5-1). There is little evidence for clinically significant differences in efficacy among the currently available agents. These agents are rapidly and extensively absorbed from the lung and the gut.[259] Drug absorbed from the gut is subject to first-pass hepatic metabolism and largely inactivated.[226] However, that absorbed from the lung is active systemically. Many preparations are available, including inhalers that do not utilize fluorocarbon propellants.

Like endogenous cortisol, these compounds are significantly protein bound. They are removed from the

Table 5-1   Aerosol Corticosteroids

Generic	Brands	Dose per Puff (μg)
Beclomethasone	Beclovent, Vanceril	42
Budesonide	Pulmicort	200
Triamcinolone acetonide	Azmacort	100
Fluticasone	Flovent	220
Flunisolide	AeroBid	250

circulation by the liver, where they are reduced and conjugated to form water-soluble compounds that are excreted into the urine.

c. Adverse Effects

Prolonged use of systemic corticosteroids can produce weight gain, muscle wasting, growth retardation, cataracts, diabetes, osteoporosis, avascular necrosis of the hip, and other well-known side effects. In low dose, inhaled corticosteroids are usually free of such clinical effects. However, even low doses may cause detectable abnormalities in sensitive assays of hypothalamic-pituitary-adrenal axis function, such as 24-hour free urinary cortisol output (Fig. 5-9).[260] The clinical significance of these changes is uncertain. High-dose therapy produces more profound suppression of adrenal activity, with decreases in morning serum cortisol and peripheral eosinophil count.[260] The definition of "low" and "high" doses varies among agents. For most formulations, a total daily dose less than 16 to 20 "puffs" of a metered-dose inhaler constitutes a low dose (e.g., approximately 600 to 800 μg daily of beclomethasone). There is little evidence to support the need for preoperative systemic corticosteroid supplementation in the patient receiving low-dose inhaled corticosteroids.[141] Local effects of inhaled corticosteroids include oropharyngeal candidiasis and dysphonia.[261]

d. Clinical Use

Inhaled corticosteroids are often considered as first-line therapy for the chronic management of newly diagnosed asthma.[10,125] More severe asthma may require the chronic use of systemic corticosteroids. Oral doses equivalent to 60 mg of prednisone daily may be required, with dose decreased gradually as tolerated. High-dose inhaled corticosteroids (doses greater than the equivalent of 1 mg daily of beclomethasone) may also be effective in more severe asthma, with fewer systemic side effects. Systemic therapy is effective in the treatment of acute exacerbations of asthma, with parenteral administration sometimes required. No good dose-response data for the use of steroids in asthma exacerbations or status asthmaticus exist, but there is little evidence that doses greater than the equivalent of 60 mg of prednisone every 6 hours confer additional benefit.[225] Several hours may be necessary for clinical benefit to occur after administration. If patients are switched from parenteral to inhaled corticosteroids, this transition must be made gradually to prevent symptoms of steroid withdrawal and severe asthma relapse.[259]

3. Methylxanthines

a. Chemistry and Mechanism of Action

Caffeine, *theophylline*, and *theobromine* are methylated xanthines and are found naturally. Their solubility is low and is enhanced by the formation of complexes with other compounds. *Aminophylline* is a complex of theophylline and ethylenediamine. Other preparations such as salts of theophylline (e.g., *oxtriphylline*) or covalently modified derivatives (e.g., *dyphylline*) also find clinical use.

Theophylline and other methylxanthines have multiple mechanisms of action, and the effect of primary importance remains controversial (Table 5-2).[172] Traditionally, theophylline was thought to work primarily by inhibiting phosphodiesterases that metabolize cyclic adenosine monophosphate (cAMP). This inhibition would increase intracellular cAMP, causing bronchodilation. However, the drug concentrations needed to demonstrate this effect in vitro exceed those present at therapeutic levels

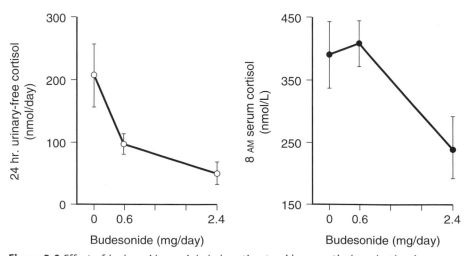

Figure 5-9 Effect of budesonide, an inhaled corticosteroid, on cortisol production in 10 subjects. Evidence of adrenal suppression resulting from the systemic absorption of budesonide is seen in the most sensitive index of cortisol production (24-hour urinary free cortisol) even at relatively low doses of inhaled corticosteroid. (Adapted from Toogood JH, Crilly RG, Jones G, et al: Effect of high-dose inhaled budesonide on calcium and phosphate metabolism and the risk of osteoporosis. Am Rev Respir Dis 138:57, 1988.)

Table 5-2 **Possible Mechanisms of Action of Methylxanthines**

Inhibition of phosphodiesterase
Antagonism of adenosine
Stimulation of endogenous catecholamine release
Anti-inflammatory actions
Improved mucociliary clearance
Stimulation of ventilatory drive
Increased diaphragm contractility
Diuresis
Positive inotropy
Reductions in preload and afterload

in vivo,[215] other phosphodiesterase inhibitors are not efficacious in asthma,[212] and theophylline-induced relaxation of airway smooth muscle in vitro occurs without changes in intracellular cAMP levels.[146] Inhibition of cyclic guanine monophosphate (cGMP) phosphodiesterase by theophylline, demonstrable in vitro,[179] also does not appear to contribute to clinical effects. Other mechanisms demonstrable in laboratory preparations, including antagonism of adenosine and stimulation of endogenous catecholamine release, also do not appear significant to the clinical action of theophylline.[160,162] Some evidence supports an anti-inflammatory role for theophylline in asthma.[172] Xanthines reduce the activity of many of the inflammatory cells implicated in the pathogenesis of asthma.[207] Theophylline increases the activity and numbers of suppressor T cells, which may play an important role in airway inflammation.[239] This indirect evidence awaits confirmation.

Some of the therapeutic actions of methylxanthines may be due to actions other than the relaxation of smooth muscle. These drugs may improve mucociliary clearance, stimulate ventilatory drive,[249] and increase diaphragm contractility,[5,67] actions that may all be beneficial in the patient with reactive airway disease. They also have significant cardiovascular effects, including direct positive chronotropic and inotropic effects on the heart, reductions in preload and afterload, and diuresis,[42] which may be beneficial in patients with cardiovascular disease.

b. Pharmacokinetics

The methylxanthines are readily absorbed after oral administration. Aminophylline, containing 85% anhydrous theophylline by weight, is used for intravenous administration because of greater aqueous solubility.[218] Methylxanthines are eliminated primarily by hepatic metabolism.[109] The plasma clearance varies widely even among healthy subjects; the half-life ranges from approximately 3 hours in children to 8 hours in adults. The half-life may be prolonged in patients with

hepatic disease or low cardiac output and may be reduced in smokers.

c. Toxicity

Areas of primary concern include the central nervous and cardiovascular systems. Central nervous system effects include stimulation, insomnia, and tremor, leading to convulsions at toxic plasma levels (considered to be >20 μg/mL). In the cardiovascular system, toxic levels may produce ventricular and atrial dysrhythmias. Methylxanthines may also produce gastrointestinal disturbances ranging from epigastric discomfort to nausea and vomiting.

d. Clinical Use

Given recent therapeutic advances in other drugs used in asthma, some have questioned the continued role of methylxanthines in the management of patients with reactive airways.[187] However, when properly used, these drugs remain safe and efficacious for the chronic management of asthma and some patients with chronic obstructive pulmonary disease.[269]

A multitude of methylxanthine preparations are available for clinical use. Most vary the physical preparation of theophylline rather than chemically modify it. Several microcrystalline forms of anhydrous theophylline are available to enhance rapid and reliable absorption. Sustained-release forms are also currently popular, providing dosing convenience and (perhaps) less fluctuation in blood levels. Regardless of the preparation chosen, plasma concentrations of theophylline should be monitored to ensure that levels are in the therapeutic range (approximately 5 to 20 μg/mL).

Aminophylline is usually given to patients requiring parenteral administration of methylxanthines. The initial loading dose is approximately 5 mg/kg, administered over 30 minutes to minimize toxicity. After this loading dose, an infusion of 0.7 mg/kg/hr provides therapeutic levels in most patients. This loading dose and rate may need to be increased in smokers and decreased in patients with liver disease or congestive heart failure. All dose recommendations are guidelines, and patients must be monitored with plasma theophylline concentrations.

4. Leukotriene Inhibitors

a. Mechanism of Action

In inflammation, arachidonic acid may be transformed through the enzyme 5-lipoxygenase into a series of compounds known as the leukotrienes.[62] These compounds may mediate some features of human asthma, including smooth muscle contraction and airway edema. Two classes of compounds have been developed to manipulate this pathway. Antagonists of the leukotriene receptor (*montelukast* [*Singulair*], *zafirlukast* [*Accolate*]) act at receptors on cells, and 5-lipoxygenase inhibitors (*zileuton* [*Zyflo*]) block leukotriene synthesis.

The increased use of sympathomimetic agents has been implicated as one of the factors responsible for this paradox.

Several studies have shown that sole therapy with β_2-agonists over treatment times ranging from 15 days to 1 year may actually enhance airway reactivity.[148,267,268] Others have found that the regular use of inhaled β_2-agonist bronchodilators is associated with an increased risk of death or near death in asthmatics.[13,247] Whether β_2-agonists are responsible for this increased risk or whether their use is simply a marker for severe asthma remains to be determined. It has been suggested that the chronic use of β_2-agonists may relieve symptoms without treating the underlying chronic inflammatory process that is apparently responsible for asthma.[203] This process can lead to irreversible thickening of the airway wall, which ultimately worsens hyperreactivity. Others have questioned this association.[169] Although this hypothesis is speculative and a cause-and-effect relationship between the use β_2-agonists and worsening of asthma has not been established, heavy use of these agents should alert the clinician to the possibility of an increased incidence of severe perioperative bronchospasm.

3. Muscarinic Antagonists

a. Mechanism of Action

These drugs compete with acetylcholine for binding at the muscarinic receptor. At least three subtypes of muscarinic receptors are present in human airways (Fig. 5-11).[11] Muscarinic receptors of the M_3 subtype produce contraction of airway smooth muscle, vasodilation, and mucus secretion; antagonism of these effects may be beneficial. M_1 subtype muscarinic receptors facilitate ganglionic transmission in parasympathetic pathways innervating airway smooth muscle, and antagonism of this effect should also be beneficial. M_2 subtype muscarinic receptors inhibit the release of acetylcholine from postganglionic nerves; antagonism of this effect may increase acetylcholine release and thus actually increase airway responsiveness. The net effect of muscarinic antagonists depends on the balance of these physiologic effects and on the mechanisms causing bronchoconstriction. For example, these agents should improve or prevent reflex bronchospasm mediated by parasympathetic activation. Conversely, they may have little effect on bronchospasm produced by release of inflammatory mediators (i.e., anaphylactoid or anaphylactic responses to drugs). Because mechanisms producing bronchospasm may vary widely among patients, so also does the efficacy of these agents.

b. Specific Agents

Atropine, the prototypic muscarinic antagonist, may decrease airway resistances and attenuate airway reactivity when given parenterally or when inhaled. Systemic side effects have limited its use specifically as a bronchodilator.

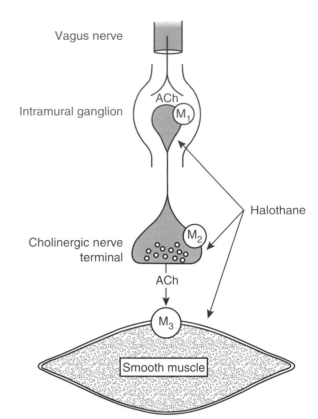

Figure 5-11 Demonstrated sites of action of halothane on the vagal motor pathway. Halothane depresses ganglionic transmission and acetylcholine (ACh) release from cholinergic nerve terminals and directly depresses smooth muscle cell contractility. Also shown are the locations of muscarinic receptor subtypes in the vagal motor pathway. M_1 receptors facilitate ganglionic transmission, M_2 receptors inhibit release of ACh, and M_3 receptors mediate smooth muscle contraction. (From Benumof JL [ed]: Airway Management: Principles and Practice, 1st ed. St. Louis, Mosby, 1996, p 87.)

Ipratropium bromide is a quaternary ammonium derivative of atropine. Because it is poorly absorbed and does not readily cross the blood-brain barrier, it can be administered at higher dose and with few systemic side effects compared with atropine. It does not appear to be as efficacious as β_2-agonists in asthmatics. However, in patients with chronic obstructive pulmonary disease that includes a reversible component of bronchospasm, ipratropium may have benefits over β_2-agonists, including a longer duration of action and efficacy in some patients in whom β_2-agonists have little effect.[27] It is available as a metered-dose inhaler (18 μg/puff). The usual dose is two puffs four times daily.

D. ANESTHETICS AND ANESTHETIC ADJUVANTS

Many other drugs administered during the perioperative period may affect the function of the lower airways. Some effects may be beneficial, others deleterious.

1. General Anesthetics

Just as most anesthetic agents depress the activity of the striated muscles of the upper airways, most also depress contractility of the smooth muscle of the lower airways. This side effect can prove useful in the perioperative management of patients with reactive airways. On the other hand, to the extent that normal tone in airway smooth muscle helps regulate the matching of ventilation to perfusion, this suppression of normal airway smooth muscle tone may contribute to impaired gas exchange in the perioperative period.

a. Volatile Anesthetics

Volatile anesthetics are potent bronchodilators. They reduce responses to bronchoconstricting stimuli in both humans and animals.[115,117,270,272,276] They also reduce baseline airway resistances in animals.[29,278] Effects on baseline airway resistances in human subjects are more difficult to interpret because of confounding influences such as endotracheal intubation and decreases in lung volume associated with general anesthesia, but it appears that these agents may also reduce resting airway smooth muscle tone in humans.[110,156] Because of these bronchodilating effects, volatile anesthetics have been used to treat status asthmaticus, although their efficacy in this condition is not firmly established.[132,195] Multiple mechanisms contribute to the relaxation of airway smooth muscle produced by volatile anesthetics. These agents attenuate reflex bronchoconstriction in part by depressing neural pathways that mediate these reflexes.[28,147,235,276] This action has been localized in the vagal motor pathway to a depression of parasympathetic ganglionic transmission and, at higher concentrations of volatile anesthetic, attenuation of acetylcholine release from postganglionic nerves (see Fig. 5-11).[28] These agents may also depress afferent and central integrative portions of airway reflex pathways.

Volatile anesthetics also produce dose-dependent bronchodilation by directly relaxing airway smooth muscle.[276,289] Several mechanisms contribute to this direct relaxation (Fig. 5-12). Halothane attenuates increases in intracellular calcium concentration during the initiation of airway smooth muscle contraction[134] and decreases intracellular calcium concentration during the maintenance of airway smooth muscle contraction.[287,288] Effects during force initiation imply a depression of pathways that mobilize calcium from intracellular stores, whereas effects during force maintenance imply a depression of extracellular calcium influx through calcium channels. Evidence for both mechanisms exists in vascular smooth muscle[32,242] and in the airways.[275] In addition to these effects on intracellular calcium, volatile anesthetics decrease the amount of force developed by the smooth muscle for a given level of intracellular calcium (i.e., halothane depresses the calcium sensitivity of the airway smooth muscle).[2,133,135] This action does not occur with intravenous anesthetics.[107] These effects of

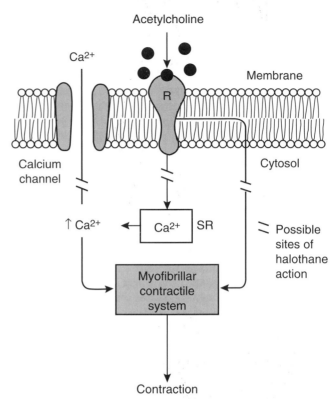

Figure 5-12 Sites of halothane action in depressing smooth muscle contractility. Halothane may block calcium influx, impair intracellular calcium release from the sarcoplasmic reticulum (SR), or disrupt mechanisms that sensitize the myofibrillar contractile system to calcium. (From Benumof JL [ed]: Airway Management: Principles and Practice, 1st ed. St. Louis, Mosby, 1996, p 88.)

volatile anesthetics on airway smooth muscle are mediated not by airway epithelium,[232] β-adrenergic effects,[276] or pertussis-sensitive G proteins[177] but rather by inhibition of receptor–G protein coupling.[137]

The relative importance of neurally mediated and direct effects of volatile anesthetics to their bronchodilating actions depends on the mechanism producing bronchoconstriction.[276] During reflex bronchoconstriction, such as that produced in response to airway instrumentation, depression of neural pathways is most significant. During bronchoconstriction produced by the release of mediators from inflammatory cells, such as during anaphylactic or anaphylactoid reactions, direct effects would assume greater importance.

Although most volatile agents produce bronchodilation, some differences among agents have been identified. The ability of halothane, enflurane, and isoflurane to attenuate neurally mediated increases in pulmonary resistance produced by electrical stimulation of the vagus nerve does not differ in animals at any concentrations of volatile anesthetic (Fig. 5-13).[270] However, halothane has been shown to be more effective than isoflurane in dilated histamine-constricted airways at concentrations less than 1.2 minimum alveolar concentration (MAC).[31] Above this

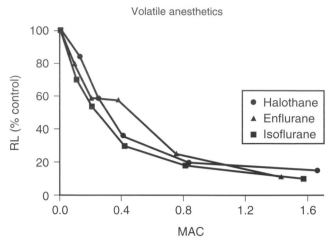

Figure 5-13 Response of pulmonary resistance (RL) to vagus nerve stimulation in dogs as a function of expired anesthetic concentration expressed in minimum alveolar concentration (MAC). All volatile agents studied profoundly depress this response. (From Benumof JL [ed]: Airway Management: Principles and Practice, 1st ed. St. Louis, Mosby, 1996, p 89.)

concentration, effects were similar. This result is consistent with another study finding that halothane causes greater relaxation of isolated airway smooth muscle compared with isoflurane at similar MAC concentrations.[289] In clinical practice, the ethers isoflurane and desflurane are more irritating than the hydrocarbon halothane.[254] This stimulation of airway receptors may produce coughing, breath-holding, and laryngospasm, limiting the usefulness of these agents for the induction of anesthesia by inhalation. For desflurane, stimulation of airway receptors may also be responsible for the hypertension and tachycardia observed after its acute administration.[69] It may also explain the lack of effect of desflurane on postintubation pulmonary resistance seen in one study, in contrast to sevoflurane, which produced bronchodilation.[94] Indeed, airway irritation by sevoflurane appears to be minimal, making it a more suitable agent for inhalation induction.[182]

In addition to these effects on airway smooth muscle, the volatile anesthetics may depress mucociliary function. Although some of this effect may be attributed to the inhalation of dry gases, halothane and other anesthetics may interfere with ion transport in airway epithelial cells and directly depress ciliary function.[80,81,164,214] Both effects may impair the ability of the airways to clear secretions and contribute to postoperative respiratory complications.

b. Intravenous Anesthetics

The intravenous anesthetics may also affect airway reactivity. The barbiturates depress neural portions of the airway reflex pathway in animals, including centers in the central nervous system and parasympathetic ganglia in the vagal motor pathway.[120,128,245] Reported effects of barbiturates directly on the smooth muscle have varied, ranging from relaxation to no effect to constriction.[70,78,198] Thiopental produced a dose-dependent constriction of guinea pig trachea.[158] This constriction was not observed with oxybarbiturates such as methohexital[50] and was shown to be caused by thromboxane A$_2$ (Fig. 5-14). Thiopental has also been reported to cause bronchospasm[213] by releasing histamine[39]; other studies have not demonstrated an association between bronchospasm and barbiturate administration.[200,238] Although thiopental releases histamine from skin mast cells, this effect has not been experimentally demonstrated in the lung.[158]

Ketamine also depresses neural airway reflex pathways and directly relaxes airway smooth muscle by mechanisms that are unknown.[209,283] Ketamine-induced release of endogenous catecholamines may also contribute to its bronchodilating effects.[116] Ketamine has been used successfully to treat status asthmaticus,[76,129,222] although, as with volatile anesthetics, its efficacy for this indication is not fully established.

Propofol also blunts airway reflexes, as propofol induction of anesthesia permits insertion of the laryngeal mask airway without apparent reflex responses.[282] Both healthy subjects and asthmatics wheeze less when induced with propofol compared with thiopental,[213] and similar differential effects have been noted for the response of respiratory system resistance to endotracheal intubation.[285] In laboratory studies, propofol relaxed airway smooth muscle both by direct effects on the muscle[36,209] and by inhibiting reflex activity.[30,171]

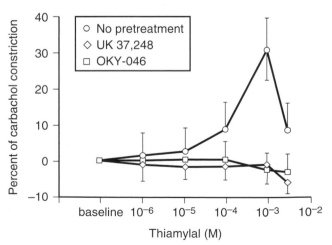

Figure 5-14 Contraction of a segment of guinea pig trachea, expressed as a percentage of a maximal contraction to carbachol, produced by thiamylal in the absence or presence of two thromboxane synthase inhibitors. These results suggest that thiobarbiturates can produce airway constriction mediated by the production of thromboxane. (From Curry C, Lenox WC, Spannhake EW, Hirshman CA: Contractile responses of guinea pig trachea to oxybarbiturates and thiobarbiturates. Anesthesiology 75:679, 1991.)

2. Neuromuscular Blocking Drugs

There are at least three properties of neuromuscular blocking drugs that could affect airway function.

Some agents, including tubocurarine, atracurium, and mivacurium, can produce a dose-dependent release of histamine, which could constrict airway smooth muscle. Atracurium enhances increases in pulmonary resistance caused by vagus nerve stimulation in the dog,[270] although it is not known whether histamine release is responsible for this effect. There are case reports of bronchospasm following atracurium administration,[241] and one study found a mild transient decrease in specific airways conductance (the reciprocal of airway resistance) after atracurium (but not tubocurarine).[243] Other studies have also found no effect of tubocurarine on airway tone.[47,93]

Some neuromuscular blocking drugs act as competitive antagonists at muscarinic receptors and so can affect airway reactivity. Pancuronium, but not vecuronium, at lower doses (less than 0.14 mg/kg) also enhances increases in pulmonary resistance caused by vagus nerve stimulation in the dog,[270] probably by blocking prejunctional M_2 subtype muscarinic receptors that normally inhibit acetylcholine release from postganglion parasympathetic nerves. It is not known whether this action is clinically significant. However, it appears that this effect may contribute to the severe bronchospasm produced by rapacuronium, which was subsequently withdrawn from clinical practice.[121]

Finally, because succinylcholine is closely related to acetylcholine, it potentially can occupy muscarinic receptors and interact with cholinesterases and so affect airway reactivity. Succinylcholine increases smooth muscle tone in the trachea of dogs.[144] The increase in tracheal tone appears to be mediated by parasympathetic stimulation, as it is abolished by vagotomy, and is not present in studies of excised airway smooth muscle. Succinylcholine increases peripheral airway reactivity to acetylcholine,[139] perhaps by competing for plasma cholinesterase. Although case reports have attributed bronchospasm to succinylcholine,[15,140,167] the widespread clinical use of succinylcholine in asthmatic patients makes the clinical significance of these observations uncertain.

Reversal of neuromuscular blockade by neostigmine and other cholinesterase inhibitors could theoretically cause bronchospasm. However, when coadministered with the anticholinergic drug atropine or glycopyrrolate, neostigmine does not significantly change specific airway conductance.[106]

3. Narcotics

Opioids may have several effects on airway function. Opioid administration may release histamine, which could potentially produce bronchoconstriction. However, this effect has not been demonstrated. There is evidence in animals that opioid receptors may inhibit cholinergic neurotransmission in the airways of some species.[258]

Opioids may also inhibit tachykinin release from sensory nerves and other aspects of sensory nerve function.[11] These actions suggest that opioids should reduce airway reactivity, and evidence exists that morphine can attenuate vagally mediated bronchoconstriction in asthmatics.[73] However, fentanyl and morphine have been found to increase baseline tracheal smooth muscle tone as measured by tracheal cuff pressures in humans anesthetized with thiopental and nitrous oxide.[290] This increase could be abolished by atropine, suggesting an increase in vagal nerve activity. Two other studies have also documented apparent increases in airway resistance caused by fentanyl during barbiturate (but not propofol) anesthesia in humans[38,41] that could be partially blocked by atropine. The clinical significance of these findings is uncertain. Thus, there is currently little evidence to suggest that the use of these agents should be restricted in patients with reactive airways.

4. Benzodiazepines

Receptors for the neurotransmitter γ-aminobutyric acid (GABA) are present in airway nerves and may modulate neurotransmission.[251] Thus, benzodiazepines, which modulate neurotransmission mediated by GABA, have the potential to attenuate reflex bronchoconstriction. In addition, benzodiazepines may relax airway smooth muscle by a direct effect.[145] Finally, the benzodiazepines produce bronchodilation in dogs by actions on centers in the central nervous system that control airway smooth muscle tone.[108] As with the narcotics, the clinical significance of these effects is unknown, but they suggest at least that these agents should not contribute to increases in airway smooth muscle tone and may be beneficial.

5. Lidocaine

Given intravenously, lidocaine antagonizes both irritant (reflex) and, to a lesser extent, antigen-induced bronchospasm in dogs with hyperreactive airways.[58,60] However, not all of this effect can be attributed to attenuation of airway reflexes, as airway anesthesia produced by dyclonine, unlike lidocaine and ropivacaine, does not affect histamine reactivity in humans.[98] Lidocaine also directly relaxes airway smooth muscle in high concentrations,[61,138] although it is not clear that this effect occurs at concentrations of lidocaine achieved in vivo. Intravenous lidocaine has been employed, apparently successfully, to treat intraoperative bronchospasm.[26] Inhaled lidocaine attenuates reflex-induced bronchoconstriction, presumably by interrupting reflex afferents.[59] However, Downes and Hirshman[59] found that nebulized lidocaine was ineffective in antagonizing antigen-induced bronchoconstriction in dogs, and lidocaine can also produce bronchoconstriction in dogs.[113] Also, several reports have documented significant bronchoconstriction in asthmatics following nebulized lidocaine (Fig. 5-15)[77,168,173,217]; lower

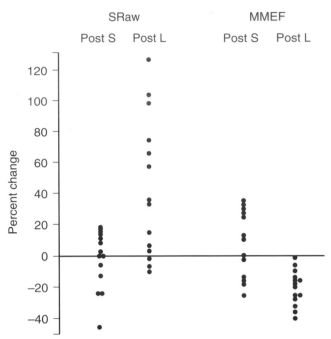

Figure 5-15 Changes in specific airway resistance (SRaw) and maximal midexpiratory flows (MMEF) after inhalation of nebulized saline (S) or 1% lidocaine (L). Note that lidocaine tended to increase SRaw and decrease MMEF, suggestive of bronchoconstriction. (From Miller WC, Awe R: Effect of nebulized lidocaine on reactive airways. Am Rev Respir Dis 111:739, 1975.)

concentrations of lidocaine may minimize this irritation while maintaining adequate topical anesthesia.[99] Bronchoconstriction can be reversed with aerosolized atropine or isoproterenol[77] and probably represents a reflex bronchoconstriction produced by the locally irritating effects of aerosol administered to the airways. Indeed, a combination of lidocaine and β-adrenergic agents has been shown to attenuate dramatically airway responses to bronchoscopy.[100]

These bronchoconstrictor effects raise concerns regarding the use of topical lidocaine to permit airway manipulation in awake patients with heightened airway reactivity. However, it is likely that the stimulus for reflex bronchospasm produced by manipulation of an unanesthetized airway would far exceed any bronchoconstricting effects of the lidocaine aerosol itself. Thus, topical lidocaine can be employed in these patients when necessary, with the recognition that lidocaine aerosol may initially cause some degree of bronchoconstriction.[168,217] These reports also call into question the practice of utilizing intratracheal lidocaine as an adjunct to endotracheal intubation in asthmatics following the induction of general anesthesia.

6. Antihistamines

Many atopic patients utilize antihistamines. These drugs are also used in the perioperative period to reduce the volume and acidity of gastric secretions by actions on the

H_2 subtype histamine receptor. At least three subtypes of histamine receptors are present in the lung.[9] Specific antagonists of H_1 subtype receptors, which mediate bronchoconstriction, can reduce airway reactivity in some asthmatic subjects.[43] Some studies have found that antagonists of the H_2 subtype receptor, such as cimetidine and ranitidine, can increase airway reactivity.[184,252] Others studies have not been able to confirm this finding.[71,192] This increase in reactivity was originally thought to result from block of receptors that inhibited airway neural transmission. However, it is now clear that neural transmission is modulated by H_3 subtype receptors,[9] so that the mechanisms by which cimetidine and other H_2 agonists might increase airway reactivity are unclear. Clinically, bronchospasm has not been attributed to the use of these agents in the perioperative period, and they may be utilized in asthmatic patients when appropriate.

E. RESPIRATORY GASES

Several respiratory gases may have important effects on lower airway function.

1. Carbon Dioxide

In general, both hypocapnia and hypercapnia cause bronchoconstriction in the lung. Hypocapnic bronchoconstriction is probably caused at least in part by a direct effect on smooth muscle, as it is present after vagotomy or atropine under most conditions.[193,233] The mechanism for this direct effect is not known but may involve changes in intracellular pH.[284] This response may assist in the matching of ventilation to perfusion, diverting gas flow away from overventilated regions of the lung.[55] Of interest, halothane attenuates hypocapnic bronchoconstriction by directly affecting smooth muscle.[44,153] The attenuation of this normal homeostatic mechanism may contribute to the ventilation-perfusion mismatch observed during halothane anesthesia.

Hypercapnia produces airway constriction in intact animals by reflex mechanisms, as this bronchoconstriction can be eliminated by vagotomy.[181] In denervated airway smooth muscle, hypercapnia directly relaxes airway smooth muscle.[153,248,264]

2. Oxygen

The effect of hypoxia on the lower airways is controversial. Most studies in humans show that hypoxia does not affect pulmonary resistance, although concurrent changes in lung volume may make these results difficult to interpret. Hypoxia has been reported to increase pulmonary resistance in dogs. One study suggests that hypoxia in fact produces bronchodilation,[279] a finding consistent with in vitro studies showing a direct relaxing effect of hypoxia in isolated tissues mediated by opening of potassium channels.[159] Hypoxia may also enhance airway reactivity without changing baseline lung resistance, perhaps by increasing the synthesis of leukotrienes.[51]

3. Nitrogen Oxides

Nitrogen oxides (NO_x) are ubiquitous endogenous compounds with important physiologic roles in virtually every vertebrate organ system. Since the proposal that endothelium-derived relaxing factor, a crucial mediator of vascular tone, was the nitric oxide free radical, interest in these compounds has increased exponentially. These compounds may play an important role in the pathogenesis of many diseases affecting the lungs, including asthma, the adult respiratory distress syndrome, and pulmonary hypertension.[92] The family of nitrogen oxides contains elemental nitrogen in one of five oxidation states and includes nitroxyl anion (NO^-), the nitric oxide free radical ($NO\cdot$), nitrite (NO_2^-), nitrogen dioxide ($NO_2\cdot$) and nitrate (NO_3^-).

The metabolic machinery needed to synthesize nitrogen oxides, based on the enzyme nitric oxide synthase (NOS), is present in the lung. Nitrogen oxides can be classified as respiratory gases, as they are present in the expired gas of normal subjects.[103] NOS has been found in alveolar macrophages.[136] Other possible sources in the lung include mast cells, neurons, airway epithelium, vascular endothelium, and airway smooth muscle.[92]

Nitroso compounds such as nitroglycerin, which act as nitric oxide donors, have been studied for many years as therapy for bronchospasm with varying results.[95] In isolated preparations, a variety of these compounds directly relax airway smooth muscle.[102] The mechanism of action appears to be primarily activation of guanylyl cyclase, which increases cGMP concentrations and relaxes the muscle.[130] However, other mechanisms may also operate. $NO\cdot$ may also play a role in the NANC system innervating airway smooth muscle.[16,17] Studies of intact animals and humans have shown that inhaled $NO\cdot$ can produce bronchodilation,[66,119] although the effect in humans is modest (Fig. 5-16). Also, inhibition of endogenous NOS enhances airway reactivity,[240] suggesting its role in modifying baseline airway tone.

As in other vascular beds, where it serves as an endothelium-derived relaxing factor, $NO\cdot$ may play an important role in the regulation of pulmonary vascular tone.[85] For example, it has been proposed as mediator of the regional matching of ventilation and perfusion. Disruption of its function may contribute to the hypoxemia observed in a variety of pulmonary diseases. Inhalation of exogenous $NO\cdot$ can improve oxygenation in diseases such as adult respiratory distress syndrome.[223] This therapy can also act as a selective pulmonary vasodilator because rapid scavenging by hemoglobin prevents any absorbed $NO\cdot$ from reaching the systemic circulation.[85,211]

Although the therapeutic effects of these compounds are promising, any potentially beneficial effects must be balanced against the potential for these highly reactive

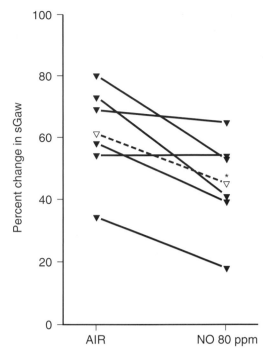

Figure 5-16 Change in specific airway conductance (sGaw) produced by methacholine challenge in asthmatic subjects breathing air or 80 parts per million (ppm) nitric oxide (NO). Individual data are shown with closed symbols; open symbols represent mean values. NO produced a small but significant decrease in the response to methacholine. (From Högman M, Frostell CG, Hedenstrom H, Hedenstierna G: Inhalation of nitric oxide modulates adult human bronchial tone. Am Rev Respir Dis 148:1474, 1993.)

compounds to stimulate airway inflammation and edema.[178] Indeed, these compounds may be important mediators of lung inflammation and are found in increased concentration in the expired gas of asthmatics.[91] In general, although there is no doubt that inhaled NO can improve measures of acute physiology (e.g., oxygenation in acute lung injury), it often does not. Further, evidence that its use improves meaningful measures of longer term outcome is still lacking.[186]

IV. APPROACH TO THE PERIOPERATIVE AIRWAY MANAGEMENT OF THE PATIENT WITH INCREASED AIRWAY REACTIVITY

A detailed discussion of all aspects of the perioperative management of patients with reactive airway diseases such as asthma and some forms of chronic obstructive pulmonary disease is beyond the scope of this chapter and is the subject of several reviews.[87,114] This section is instead limited to an extension of previously discussed pharmacologic principles to the airway management of these patients. Primary areas of concern include prophylaxis to prevent bronchospasm and pharmacologic therapy of established bronchospasm. Of course, these principles also apply to patients without a history of increased airway reactivity, who may also develop perioperative bronchospasm.[35,83,200] The significance and potential seriousness of perioperative bronchospasm should not be minimized. However, large series have demonstrated that most patients with reactive airway disease in fact do quite well in the perioperative period.[277]

A. INHALATION THERAPY

Inhalation therapy with anti-inflammatory agents and bronchodilators has the advantage of producing the greatest local effect on airway smooth muscle with less potential for systemic toxicity. In other words, the ratio between therapeutic effect and side effects such as cardiovascular or central nervous system stimulation may be lower for oral and parenteral formulations than for the inhaled methods of administration. Delivery of drug to the airway mucosa by inhalation therapy depends on many factors, including the pattern of breathing, the geometry of lungs and airways (often altered in patients with lung disease), and the size of the aerosol particles. Particles below approximately 1 μm in size generally do not strike the mucosa and are exhaled, whereas the inertia of particles greater than approximately 5 μm causes them to be deposited in the delivery devices and the upper airway (Fig. 5-17).[22] Because much of the delivered dose may be contained in these larger particles, only approximately 10% to 20% of the delivered dose actually reaches the

lung under optimal conditions in patients whose tracheas are not intubated.[54,143] The deposition of particles in the lung can be enhanced by breath holding in inspiration following drug inhalation.[188] The deposition of larger particles in the oropharynx, which are systemically absorbed and may cause side effects, can be reduced by the use of "spacer" devices between the mouth and the drug delivery systems.[143] These devices slow aerosol flow and encourage impaction of these large particles in the spacer rather than in the mouth.

In the perioperative period, it may be necessary to deliver aerosols through an ET. Delivery devices include jet nebulizers, more sophisticated ultrasonic nebulizers, and metered-dose inhalers using fluorocarbon propellants, which are connected to the ET by a variety of adapters.[19,48,86,194,255] Several studies have shown that the efficiency of drug delivery is less than that achieved in nonintubated patients, with most of the delivered dose being deposited in the breathing circuit and ET. As little as 1% to 2% of the delivered dose actually reaches the lungs with some systems, with most averaging between 3% and 10% delivery.[19,48,86,194,255] Delivery to the lungs can be enhanced by actuating metered-dose inhalers during inspiratory flow,[48] by increasing tidal volume and prolonging inspiration, and by using larger diameter ETs.[194,255] Ultrasonic nebulizers may promote more efficient delivery by providing a more consistent and appropriate particle size.[255] However, it is still necessary to increase the delivered dose (e.g., by giving more puffs of metered-dose inhalers) to provide an equivalent dose of drug to the lung during mechanical ventilation compared with inhalation during spontaneous breathing.

B. PROPHYLAXIS OF BRONCHOSPASM _(Table 5-4)_

Based on the understanding of asthma as a chronic inflammatory disease, preoperative pharmacotherapy should strive to minimize airway inflammation. A stepwise approach based on the adequacy of control as assessed by symptoms and spirometric values such as peak expiratory flow is currently recommended (Table 5-5). For mild, intermittent asthma, short-acting β2-agonists as necessary often suffice. With moderate symptoms, chronic therapy with inhaled anti-inflammatory agents such as corticosteroids or cromolyn is instituted. As a next step, the dose of inhaled corticosteroids can be increased and a long-acting bronchodilator such as salmeterol added. For severe asthma, defined in part as a limitation of activities with severe exacerbations despite medication, systemic corticosteroids may be necessary. With each step, inhaled β2-agonists can be used as necessary but should not be taken more than three or four times daily. It would seem prudent to postpone elective surgery until optimal control is achieved, as supported by current evidence.[277]

Patients receiving chronic inhaled or systemic corticosteroids should receive these drugs until immediately before surgery. Patients taking systemic corticosteroids

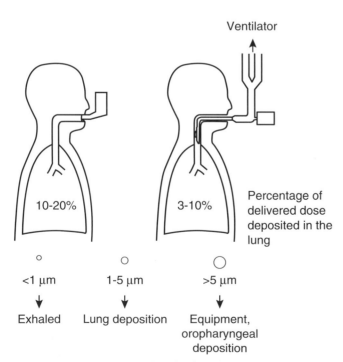

Figure 5-17 Factors controlling the deposition of inhaled aerosol particles, including route of administration (spontaneous inhalation versus delivery by positive pressure through an endotracheal tube) and particle size. (From Benumof JL [ed]: Airway Management: Principles and Practice, 1st ed. St. Louis, Mosby, 1996, p 94.)

Table 5-4 **Prophylaxis of Perioperative Bronchospasm**

Optimal preoperative pharmacotherapy, continued up to the morning of surgery
Adequate corticosteroid preparation
Adequate preoperative anxiolysis
Inhaled β_2-agonists or muscarinic antagonists immediately before induction
Regional anesthesia if feasible
General anesthetic techniques based on the volatile anesthetics
Adequate anesthesia of the airway before instrumentation
Intravenous lidocaine, narcotics, propofol, and ketamine as adjuncts

should receive an increased dose preoperatively, both to ensure adequate protection against adrenocortical suppression and to ensure that airway inflammation is minimized. Because asthma may be exacerbated by emotional distress, adequate preoperative anxiolysis should be provided. The administration of an inhaled β_2-agonist immediately before anesthetic induction may be helpful. The use of inhaled muscarinic antagonists also attenuates reflex bronchospasm by approximately the same amount as β_2-agonists if given before intubation.[142,286]

Tradition favors the use of regional anesthetic techniques in these patients when feasible, to avoid the upper airway instrumentation often required during general anesthesia. However, firm evidence demonstrating improved perioperative outcomes is lacking. If awake airway manipulation is necessary, every effort must be made to ensure adequate topical airway anesthesia, with the recognition that this topical anesthesia may tend to increase airway resistances in these patients. Avoidance of endotracheal intubation is preferable.

Because of their excellent bronchodilating properties, volatile anesthetics are the foundation of general anesthetic techniques. As previously discussed, halothane, enflurane, and isoflurane are equally efficacious in attenuating neurally mediated bronchoconstriction in animals; available evidence suggests that sevoflurane is also efficacious, but perhaps not desflurane, at least acutely. Although halothane may be a more potent bronchodilator under some experimental conditions and has the advantage of being less pungent, Forrest and colleagues[83] found no difference in the incidence of bronchospasm among patients anesthetized with halothane, enflurane, or isoflurane in a large multicenter study. However, the incidence of bronchospasm was increased in patients anesthetized with fentanyl-N_2O, confirming the usefulness of volatile anesthetics. For the intravenous induction of anesthesia, thiopental has been implicated in causing bronchospasm; ketamine and propofol are useful alternatives.

Regardless of the technique employed, the most important principle to prevent bronchospasm is to provide adequate anesthesia of the airway before instrumentation. One useful technique is to induce anesthesia with an intravenous agent, then ventilate the lungs with a volatile anesthetic over a period of time to allow significant uptake (at least 10 minutes). Other adjuncts, such as intravenous lidocaine[101] and narcotics, may also be useful in attenuating airway reflexes, although the effectiveness of the former is not established.[165] Intratracheal lidocaine should be avoided during induction, as any aerosol instilled into the trachea may itself cause bronchospasm. Extubation of the trachea during deep levels of anesthesia may be desirable, although this approach should be avoided if there are any doubts about the ability to maintain airway patency. Again, adjuncts such as intravenous lidocaine and narcotics may be useful in blunting airway reflexes during emergence. Other strategies have included lidocaine sprayed into the ET[131] or instilled into the ET cuff, from which it diffuses to the trachea.[3,74,246]

Table 5-5 **Asthma Therapy**

Intermittent (Mild)	Persistent		Persistent (Severe)
Step 1	**Step 2 (Mild)**	**Step 3 (Moderate)**	**Step 4**
β_2-Agonist prn or cromolyn prn	Long term (one of the following): Inhaled corticosteroids OR cromolyn/nedocromil Theophylline (not preferred) Leukotriene inhibitors Quick relief: short-acting β_2-agonist	Long term: inhaled corticosteroids, AND long-acting bronchodilator (β_2-agonists, theophylline, leukotriene inhibitor) Quick relief: short-acting β_2-agonist	Long term: inhaled corticosteroids (high dose), AND long-acting bronchodilators; AND oral corticosteroids Quick relief: short-acting β_2-agonist

Table 5-6 **Treatment of Perioperative Bronchospasm**

Confirm diagnosis
Deepen anesthesia with a volatile agent
Consider ketamine, IV lidocaine, propofol to deepen anesthesia further
Use inhaled β₂-agonists
Avoid aminophylline
Use parenteral corticosteroids
Adjust ventilatory parameters to avoid gas trapping and barotrauma

C. TREATMENT OF BRONCHOSPASM *(Table 5-6)*

The proper diagnosis of bronchospasm is paramount. Although it is usually not difficult in the awake patient, many other conditions may mimic bronchospasm in the anesthetized patient. Signs include wheezing, diminished breath sounds, prolonged expiration, and increased airway pressures during positive-pressure ventilation. Common conditions that must be excluded include mechanical airway obstruction at any site, tension pneumothorax, aspiration, and pulmonary edema.

When the diagnosis is firmly established, the first consideration is to increase anesthetic depth by increasing the inspired concentration of volatile anesthetic. Intravenous adjuncts such as ketamine, propofol, and lidocaine may also be useful. The role of intravenous aminophylline in treating intraoperative bronchospasm is limited. In an animal model of asthma, aminophylline provided no additional protection against airway constriction beyond that provided by halothane.[34] Further, aminophylline may produce dysrhythmias, especially when combined with volatile anesthetics (especially halothane) and the hypercarbia that may accompany bronchospasm. Unlike aminophylline, β₂-agonists did provide benefit beyond that afforded by the volatile anesthetics in an animal model of asthma.[257] Inhaled β₂-agonists may be nebulized into the ET, recognizing that doses well above those required in ambulatory patients may be needed to compensate for decreased efficiency of drug delivery to the lung. Intravenous adrenergic agonists such as epinephrine may be necessary, particularly as inadequate tidal volumes may preclude significant delivery of inhaled drugs to the lung. Parenteral corticosteroids may be administered, but several hours are required for significant benefit. Parameters of mechanical ventilation may need to be altered to minimize airway pressures and prolong expiration to minimize gas trapping.

REFERENCES

1. Abernethy LJ, Allan PL, Drummond GB: Ultrasound assessment of the position of the tongue during induction of anaesthesia. Br J Anaesth 65:744, 1990.
2. Akao M, Hirasaki A, Jones KA, et al: Halothane reduces myofilament Ca²⁺ sensitivity during muscarinic receptor stimulation of airway smooth muscle. Am J Physiol 271:L719, 1996.
3. Altintas F, Bozkurt P, Kaya G, Akkan G: Lidocaine 10% in the endotracheal tube cuff: Blood concentrations, haemodynamic and clinical effects. Eur J Anaesthesiol 17:436, 2000.
4. Anderson ST, Hajduczek J, Barker SJ: Benzocaine-induced methemoglobinemia in an adult: Accuracy of pulse oximetry with methemoglobinemia. Anesth Analg 67:1099, 1988.
5. Aubier M, De Troyer A, Sampson M, et al: Aminophylline improves diaphragmatic contractility. N Engl J Med 305:249, 1981.
6. Barker SJ, Tremper KK, Hyatt J: Effects of methemoglobinemia on pulse oximetry and mixed venous oximetry. Anesthesiology 70:112, 1989.
7. Barnes PJ: A new approach to the treatment of asthma. N Engl J Med 321:1517, 1989.
8. Barnes PJ: Effect of corticosteroids on airway hyperresponsiveness. Am Rev Respir Dis 141:S70, 1990.
9. Barnes PJ: Histamine receptors in the lung. Agents Actions Suppl 33:103, 1991.
10. Barnes PJ: Modulation of neurotransmission in airways. Physiol Rev 72:699, 1992.
11. Bartlett D Jr, Leiter JC, Knuth SL: Control and actions of the genioglossus muscle. In Issa FG, Suratt PM, Remmers JE (eds): Sleep and Respiration. New York, Wiley-Liss, 1990.
12. Baughman VL, Laurito CE, Polek WV: Lidocaine blood levels following aerosolization and intravenous administration. J Clin Anesth 4:325, 1992.
13. Beasley R, Pearce N, Crane J, et al: Asthma mortality and inhaled beta agonist therapy. Aust N Z J Med 21:753, 1991.
14. Begle RL, Badr S, Skatrud JB, Dempsey JA: Effect of lung inflation on pulmonary resistance during NREM sleep. Am Rev Respir Dis 141:854, 1990.
15. Bele-Binda N, Valeri F: A case of bronchospasm induced by succinylcholine. Can Anaesth Soc J 18:116, 1971.
16. Belvisi MG, Stretton D, Barnes PJ: Nitric oxide as an endogenous modulator of cholinergic neurotransmission in guinea-pig airways. Eur J Pharmacol 198:219, 1991.
17. Belvisi MG, Stretton CD, Yacoub M, Barnes PJ: Nitric oxide is the endogenous neurotransmitter of bronchodilator nerves in humans. Eur J Pharmacol 210:221, 1992.
18. Benumof JL, Feroe D: Swallowing topically administered 4% lidocaine results in nausea and vomiting. Am J Anesthesiol 25:150, 1998.
19. Bishop MJ, Larson RP, Buschman DL: Metered dose inhaler aerosol characteristics are affected by the endotracheal tube actuator/adapter used. Anesthesiology 73:1263, 1990.

20. Boidin MP: Airway patency in the unconscious patient. Br J Anaesth 57:306, 1985.

21. Boschetto P, Rogers DF, Fabbri LM, Barnes PJ: Corticosteroid inhibition of airway microvascular leakage. Am Rev Respir Dis 143:605, 1991.

22. Brain JD, Valberg PA: Deposition of aerosol in the respiratory tract. Am Rev Respir Dis 120:1325, 1979.

23. Brancatisano T, Collett PW, Engel LA: Respiratory movements of the vocal cords. J Appl Physiol 54:1269, 1983.

24. Brancatisano A, Dodd DS, Engel LA: Posterior cricoarytenoid activity and glottic size during hyperpnea in humans. J Appl Physiol 71:977, 1991.

25. Brancatisano TP, Dodd DS, Engel LA: Respiratory activity of posterior cricoarytenoid muscle and vocal cords in humans. J Appl Physiol 57:1143, 1984.

26. Brandus V, Joffe S, Benoit CV, Wolff WI: Bronchial spasm during general anaesthesia. Can Anaesth Soc J 17:269, 1970.

27. Braun SR, Levy SF: Comparison of ipratropium bromide and albuterol in chronic obstructive pulmonary disease: A three-center study. Am J Med 91:28S, 1991.

28. Brichant JF, Gunst SJ, Warner DO, Rehder K: Halothane, enflurane, and isoflurane depress the peripheral vagal motor pathway in isolated canine tracheal smooth muscle. Anesthesiology 74:325, 1991.

29. Brown RH, Mitzner W, Zerhouni E, Hirshman CA: Direct in vivo visualization of bronchodilation induced by inhalational anesthesia using high-resolution computed tomography. Anesthesiology 78:295, 1993.

30. Brown RH, Wagner EM: Mechanisms of bronchoprotection by anesthetic induction agents: Propofol versus ketamine. Anesthesiology 90:822, 1999.

31. Brown RH, Zerhouni EA, Hirshman CA: Comparison of low concentrations of halothane and isoflurane as bronchodilators. Anesthesiology 78:1097, 1993.

32. Buljubasic N, Rusch NJ, Marijic J, et al: Effects of halothane and isoflurane on calcium and potassium channel currents in canine coronary arterial cells. Anesthesiology 76:990, 1992.

33. Chadwick GA, Crowley P, Fitzgerald MX, et al: Obstructive sleep apnea following topical oropharyngeal anesthesia in loud snorers. Am Rev Respir Dis 143:810, 1991.

34. Cheek DBC, Beebe BW, Downes H, et al: Aminophylline does not inhibit bronchoconstriction during halothane anesthesia. Anesthesiology 65:A270, 1986.

35. Cheney FW, Posner KL, Caplan RA: Adverse respiratory events infrequently leading to malpractice suits. A closed claims analysis. Anesthesiology 75:932, 1991.

36. Cheng EY, Mazzeo AJ, Bosnjak ZJ, et al: Direct relaxant effects of intravenous anesthetics on airway smooth muscle. Anesth Analg 83:162, 1996.

37. Chinn WM, Zavala DC, Ambre J: Plasma levels of lidocaine following nebulized aerosol administration. Chest 71:346, 1977.

38. Cigarini I, Bonnet F, Lorino AM, et al: Comparison of the effects of fentanyl on respiratory mechanics under propofol or thiopental anaesthesia. Acta Anaesthesiol Scand 34:253, 1990.

39. Clarke RS, Dundee J, Garrett FT, et al: Adverse reactions to intravenous anaesthetics. Br J Anaesth 47:575, 1975.

40. Cockcroft DW, Murdock KY: Comparative effects of inhaled salbutamol, sodium cromoglycate, and beclomethasone dipropionate on allergen-induced early asthmatic responses, late asthmatic responses, and increased bronchial responsiveness to histamine. J Allergy Clin Immunol 79:743, 1987.

41. Cohendy R, Lefrant JY, Laracine M, et al: Effect of fentanyl on ventilatory resistances during barbiturate general anaesthesia. Br J Anaesth 69:595, 1992.

42. Cohn JN, Franciosa JA: Vasodilator therapy of cardiac failure (second of two parts). N Engl J Med 297:254, 1977.

43. Cookson WO: Bronchodilator action of the anti-histaminic terfenadine. Br J Clin Pharmacol 24:120, 1987.

44. Coon RL, Kampine JP: Hypocapnic bronchoconstriction and inhalation anesthetics. Anesthesiology 43:635, 1975.

45. Courtney KR: Mechanism of frequency-dependent inhibition of sodium currents in frog myelinated nerve by the lidocaine derivative GEA 968. J Pharmacol Exp Ther 195:225, 1975.

46. Covino BG: Pharmacology of local anaesthetic agents. Br J Anaesth 58:701, 1986.

47. Crago RR, Bryan AC, Laws AK, Winestock AE: Respiratory flow resistance after curare and pancuronium, measured by forced oscillations. Can Anaesth Soc J 19:607, 1972.

48. Crogan SJ, Bishop MJ: Delivery efficiency of metered dose aerosols given via endotracheal tubes. Anesthesiology 70:1008, 1989.

49. Curran J, Hamilton C, Taylor T: Topical analgesia before endotracheal intubation. Anaesthesia 30:765, 1975.

50. Curry C, Lenox WC, Spannhake EW, Hirshman CA: Contractile responses of guinea pig trachea to oxybarbiturates and thiobarbiturates. Anesthesiology 75:679, 1991.

51. D'Brot J, Ahmed T: Hypoxia-induced enhancement of nonspecific bronchial reactivity: Role of leukotrienes. J Appl Physiol 65:194, 1988.

52. de Lanerolle P, Nishikawa M, Yost DA, Adelstein RS: Increased phosphorylation of myosin light chain kinase after an increase in cyclic AMP in intact smooth muscle. Science 223:1415, 1984.

53. Doi M, Ikeda K: Airway irritation produced by volatile anaesthetics during brief inhalation: Comparison of halothane, enflurane, isoflurane and sevoflurane. Can J Anaesth 40:122, 1993.

54. Dolovich M, Ruffin R, Corr D, Newhouse MT: Clinical evaluation of a simple demand inhalation MDI aerosol delivery device. Chest 84:36, 1983.

55. Domino KB, Swenson ER, Polissar NL, et al: Effect of inspired CO_2 on ventilation and perfusion heterogeneity in hyperventilated dogs. J Appl Physiol 75:1306, 1993.

56. Donati F, Meistelman C, Plaud B: Vecuronium neuromuscular blockade at the adductor muscles of the larynx and adductor pollicis. Anesthesiology 74:833, 1991.

57. Donati F, Meistelman C, Plaud B: Vecuronium neuromuscular blockade at the diaphragm, the orbicularis oculi, and adductor pollicis muscles. Anesthesiology 73:870, 1990.

58. Downes H, Gerber N, Hirshman CA: I.V. lignocaine in reflex and allergic bronchoconstriction. Br J Anaesth 52:873, 1980.

59. Downes H, Hirshman CA: Lidocaine aerosols do not prevent allergic bronchoconstriction. Anesth Analg 60:28, 1981.

60. Downes H, Hirshman CA, Leon DA: Comparison of local anesthetics as bronchodilator aerosols. Anesthesiology 58:216, 1983.

61. Downes H, Loehning RW: Local anesthetic contracture and relaxation of airway smooth muscle. Anesthesiology 47:430, 1977.

62. Drazen JM, Israel E, O'Byrne PM: Treatment of asthma with drugs modifying the leukotriene pathway. N Engl J Med 340:197, 1999.

63. Drummond GB: Comparison of sedation with midazolam and ketamine: Effects on airway muscle activity. Br J Anaesth 76:663, 1996.

64. Drummond GB: Influence of thiopentone on upper airway muscles. Br J Anaesth 63:12, 1989.

65. Drummond GB: Upper airway reflexes [editorial; comment]. Br J Anaesth 1993;70:121, 1989.

66. Dupuy PM, Shore SA, Drazen JM, et al: Bronchodilator action of inhaled nitric oxide in guinea pigs. J Clin Invest 90:421, 1992.

67. Dureuil B, Desmonts JM, Mankikian B, Prokocimer P: Effects of aminophylline on diaphragmatic dysfunction after upper abdominal surgery. Anesthesiology 62:242, 1985.

68. Eastwood PR, Szollosi I, Platt PR, Hillman DR: Collapsibility of the upper airway during anesthesia with isoflurane. Anesthesiology 97:786, 2002.

69. Ebert TJ, Muzi M: Sympathetic hyperactivity during desflurane anesthesia in healthy volunteers. A comparison with isoflurane. Anesthesiology 79:444, 1993.

70. Edney SM, Downes H: Contractor effect of barbiturates on smooth muscle. Arch Int Pharmacodyn Ther 217:180, 1975.

71. Eiser NM, Mills J, Snashall PD, Guz A: The role of histamine receptors in asthma. Clin Sci (Lond) 60:363, 1981.

72. England SJ, Bartlett D Jr: Changes in respiratory movements of the human vocal cords during hyperpnea. J Appl Physiol 52:780, 1982.

73. Eschenbacher WL, Bethel RA, Boushey HA, Sheppard D: Morphine sulfate inhibits bronchoconstriction in subjects with mild asthma whose responses are inhibited by atropine. Am Rev Respir Dis 130:363, 1984.

74. Fagan C, Frizelle HP, Laffey J, et al: The effects of intracuff lidocaine on endotracheal-tube-induced emergence phenomena after general anesthesia. Anesth Analg 91:201, 2000.

75. Felbel J, Trockur B, Ecker T, et al: Regulation of cytosolic calcium by cAMP and cGMP in freshly isolated smooth muscle cells from bovine trachea. J Biol Chem 263:16764, 1988.

76. Fischer MM: Ketamine hydrochloride in severe bronchospasm. Anaesthesia 32:771, 1977.

77. Fish JE, Peterman VI: Effects of inhaled lidocaine on airway function in asthmatic subjects. Respiration 37:201, 1979.

78. Fletcher SW, Flacke W, Alper MH: The actions of general anesthetic agents on tracheal smooth muscle. Anesthesiology 29:517, 1968.

79. Fogel RB, Malhotra A, Shea SA, et al: Reduced genioglossal activity with upper airway anesthesia in awake patients with OSA. J Appl Physiol 88:1346, 2000.

80. Forbes AR: Halothane depresses mucociliary flow in the trachea. Anesthesiology 45:59, 1976.

81. Forbes AR, Gamsu G: Depression of lung mucociliary clearance by thiopental and halothane. Anesth Analg 58:387, 1979.

82. Ford DJ, Singh P, Watters C, Raj PP: Duration and toxicity of bupivacaine for topical anesthesia of the airway in the cat. Anesth Analg 63:1001, 1984.

83. Forrest JB, Rehder K, Cahalan MK, Goldsmith CH: Multicenter study of general anesthesia. III. Predictors of severe perioperative adverse outcomes. Anesthesiology 76:3, 1992. Erratum in: Anesthesiology 77:222, 1992.

84. Fraser CM, Venter JC: Beta-adrenergic receptors. Relationship of primary structure, receptor function, and regulation. Am Rev Respir Dis 141:S22, 1990.

85. Frostell C, Fratacci MD, Wain JC, et al: Inhaled nitric oxide. A selective pulmonary vasodilator reversing hypoxic pulmonary vasoconstriction. Circulation 83:2038, 1991.

86. Fuller HD, Dolovich MB, Posmituck G, et al: Pressurized aerosol versus jet aerosol delivery to mechanically ventilated patients. Comparison of dose to the lungs. Am Rev Respir Dis 141:440, 1990.

87. Gal TJ: Bronchial hyperresponsiveness and anesthesia: Physiologic and therapeutic perspectives. Anesth Analg 78:559, 1994.

88. Gal TJ, Goldberg SK: Diaphragmatic function in healthy subjects during partial curarization. J Appl Physiol 48:921, 1980.

89. Gal TJ, Goldberg SK: Relationship between respiratory muscle strength and vital capacity during partial curarization in awake subjects. Anesthesiology 54:141, 1981.

90. Gao Y, Vanhoutte PM: Attenuation of contractions to acetylcholine in canine bronchi by an endogenous nitric oxide-like substance. Br J Pharmacol 109:887, 1993.

91. Gaston B, Drazen J: Expired nitric oxide (NO) concentrations are elevated in patients with reactive airways disease. Endothelium 1:s87, 1993.

92. Gaston B, Drazen JM, Loscalzo J, Stamler JS: The biology of nitrogen oxides in the airways. Am J Respir Crit Care Med 149:538, 1994.

93. Gerbershagen HU, Bergman NA: The effect of d-tubocurarine on respiratory resistance in anesthetized man. Anesthesiology 28:981, 1967.

94. Goff MJ, Arain SR, Ficke DJ, et al: Absence of bronchodilation during desflurane anesthesia: A comparison to sevoflurane and thiopental. Anesthesiology 93:404, 2000.

95. Goldstein JA: Nitroglycerin therapy of asthma. Chest 85:449, 1984.

96. Greenberger PA: Corticosteroids in asthma. Rationale, use, and problems. Chest 101:418S, 1992.

97. Greenblatt DJ, Benjamin DM, Willis CR, et al: Lidocaine plasma concentrations following administration of intraoral lidocaine solution. Arch Otolaryngol 111:298, 1985.

98. Groeben H, Grosswendt T, Silvanus M, et al: Lidocaine inhalation for local anaesthesia and attenuation of bronchial hyper-reactivity with least airway irritation. Effect of three different dose regimens. Eur J Anaesthesiol 17:672, 2000.

99. Groeben H, Grosswendt T, Silvanus MT, et al: Airway anesthesia alone does not explain attenuation of histamine-induced bronchospasm by local anesthetics: A comparison of lidocaine, ropivacaine, and dyclonine. Anesthesiology 94:423; discussion 5A, 2001.

100. Groeben H, Schlicht M, Stieglitz S, et al: Both local anesthetics and salbutamol pretreatment affect reflex bronchoconstriction in volunteers with asthma undergoing awake fiberoptic intubation. Anesthesiology 97:1445, 2002.

101. Groeben H, Silvanus MT, Beste M, Peters J: Both intravenous and inhaled lidocaine attenuate reflex bronchoconstriction but at different plasma concentrations. Am J Respir Crit Care Med 159:530, 1999.

102. Gruetter CA, Childers CE, Bosserman MK, et al: Comparison of relaxation induced by glyceryl trinitrate, isosorbide dinitrate, and sodium nitroprusside in bovine airways. Am Rev Respir Dis 139:1192, 1989.

103. Gustafsson LE, Leone AM, Persson MG, et al: Endogenous nitric oxide is present in the exhaled air of rabbits, guinea pigs and humans. Biochem Biophys Res Commun 181:852, 1991.

104. Guyre PM, Girard MT, Morganelli PM, Manganiello PD: Glucocorticoid effects on the production and actions of immune cytokines. J Steroid Biochem 30:89, 1988.

105. Habib MP, Campbell SC, Shon BY, Pinnas JL: A comparison of albuterol and metaproterenol nebulizer solutions. Ann Allergy 58:421, 1987.

106. Hammond J, Wright D, Sale J: Pattern of change of bronchomotor tone following reversal of neuromuscular blockade. Comparison between atropine and glycopyrrolate. Br J Anaesth 55:955, 1983.

107. Hanazaki M, Jones KA, Warner DO: Effects of intravenous anesthetics on Ca^{2+} sensitivity in canine tracheal smooth muscle. Anesthesiology 92:133, 2000.

108. Haxhiu MA, van Lunteren E, Cherniack NS, Deal EC: Benzodiazepines acting on ventral surface of medulla cause airway dilation. Am J Physiol 257:R810, 1989.

109. Hendeles L, Weinberger M, Bighley L: Disposition of theophylline after a single intravenous infusion of aminophylline. Am Rev Respir Dis 118:97, 1978.

110. Heneghan CP, Bergman NA, Jordan C, et al: Effect of isoflurane on bronchomotor tone in man. Br J Anaesth 58:24, 1986.

111. Her E, Frazer J, Austen KF, Owen WF Jr: Eosinophil hematopoietins antagonize the programmed cell death of eosinophils. Cytokine and glucocorticoid effects on eosinophils maintained by endothelial cell-conditioned medium. J Clin Invest 88:1982, 1991.

112. Hershenson M, Brouillette RT, Olsen E, Hunt CE: The effect of chloral hydrate on genioglossus and diaphragmatic activity. Pediatr Res 18:516, 1984.

113. Hirota K, Hashimoto Y, Sato T, et al: Bronchoconstrictive and relaxant effects of lidocaine on the airway in dogs. Crit Care Med 29:1040, 2001.

114. Hirshman CA, Bergman NA: Factors influencing intrapulmonary airway calibre during anaesthesia. Br J Anaesth 65:30, 1990.

115. Hirshman CA, Bergman NA: Halothane and enflurane protect against bronchospasm in an asthma dog model. Anesth Analg 57:629, 1978.

116. Hirshman CA, Downes H, Farbood A, Bergman NA: Ketamine block of bronchospasm in experimental canine asthma. Br J Anaesth 51:713, 1979.

117. Hirshman CA, Edelstein G, Peetz S, et al: Mechanism of action of inhalational anesthesia on airways. Anesthesiology 56:107, 1982.

118. Hoag JE, McFadden ER Jr: Long-term effect of cromolyn sodium on nonspecific bronchial hyperresponsiveness: A review. Ann Allergy 66:53, 1991.

119. Hogman M, Frostell CG, Hedenstrom H, Hedenstierna G: Inhalation of nitric oxide modulates adult human bronchial tone. Am Rev Respir Dis 148:1474, 1993.

120. Holtzman MJ, Hahn HL, Sasaki K, et al: Selective effect of general anesthetics on reflex bronchoconstrictor responses in dogs. J Appl Physiol 53:126, 1982.

121. Hou VY, Hirshman CA, Emala CW: Neuromuscular relaxants as antagonists for M2 and M3 muscarinic receptors. Anesthesiology 88:744, 1998.

122. Hudgel DW, Hendricks C: Palate and hypopharynx— Sites of inspiratory narrowing of the upper airway during sleep. Am Rev Respir Dis 138:1542, 1988.

123. Hwang JC, St. John WM, Bartlett D Jr: Respiratory-related hypoglossal nerve activity: Influence of anesthetics. J Appl Physiol 55:785, 1983.

124. Insalaco G, Kuna ST, Cibella F, Villeponteaux RD: Thyroarytenoid muscle activity during hypoxia, hypercapnia, and voluntary hyperventilation in humans. J Appl Physiol 69:268, 1990.

125. International consensus report on diagnosis and treatment of asthma. National Heart, Lung, and Blood Institute, National Institutes of Health. Bethesda, Maryland 20892. Publication no. 92-3091, March 1992. Eur Respir J 5:601, 1992.

126. Iscoe SD: Central control of the upper airway. In Mathew OP, Sant'Ambrogio G (eds): Respiratory Function of the Upper Airway. New York, Marcel Dekker, 1988, p 125.

127. Ito Y, Tajima K: Dual effects of catecholamines on pre- and post-junctional membranes in the dog trachea. Br J Pharmacol 75:433, 1982.

128. Jackson DM, Richards IM: The effects of pentobarbitone and chloralose anaesthesia on the vagal component of bronchoconstriction produced by histamine aerosol in the anaesthetized dog. Br J Pharmacol 61:251, 1977.

129. Jahangir SM, Islam F, Aziz L: Ketamine infusion for postoperative analgesia in asthmatics: A comparison with intermittent meperidine. Anesth Analg 76:45, 1993.

130. Jansen A, Drazen J, Osborne JA, et al: The relaxant properties in guinea pig airways of S-nitrosothiols. J Pharmacol Exp Ther 261:154, 1992.

131. Jee D, Park SY: Lidocaine sprayed down the endotracheal tube attenuates the airway-circulatory reflexes by local anesthesia during emergence and extubation. Anesth Analg 96:293, table of contents, 2003.

132. Johnston RG, Noseworthy TW, Friesen EG, et al: Isoflurane therapy for status asthmaticus in children and adults. Chest 97:698, 1990.

133. Jones KA, Hirasaki A, Bremerich DH, et al: Halothane inhibits agonist-induced potentiation of rMLC phosphorylation in permeabilized airway smooth muscle. Am J Physiol 273:L80, 1997.

134. Jones KA, Housmans PR, Warner DO, et al: Halothane alters cytosolic calcium transient in tracheal smooth muscle. Am J Physiol 265:L80, 1993.

135. Jones KA, Wong GY, Lorenz RR, et al: Effects of halothane on the relationship between cytosolic calcium and force in airway smooth muscle. Am J Physiol 266:L199, 1994.

136. Jorens PG, Van Overveld FJ, Bult H, et al: L-Arginine-dependent production of nitrogen oxides by rat pulmonary macrophages. Eur J Pharmacol 200:205, 1991.

137. Kai T, Jones KA, Warner DO: Halothane attenuates calcium sensitization in airway smooth muscle by inhibiting G-proteins. Anesthesiology 89:1543, 1998.

138. Kai T, Nishimura J, Kobayashi S, et al: Effects of lidocaine on intracellular Ca^{2+} and tension in airway smooth muscle. Anesthesiology 78:954, 1993.

139. Kaise A, Weinmann GG, Levitt RC, Hirshman CA: Succinylcholine potentiates responses to intravenous acetylcholine in the canine lung periphery. J Appl Physiol 69:1137, 1990.

140. Katz AM, Mulligan PG: Bronchospasm induced by suxamethonium. A case report. Br J Anaesth 44:1097, 1972.

141. Kehlet H, Binder C: Adrenocortical function and clinical course during and after surgery in unsupplemented glucocorticoid-treated patients. Br J Anaesth 45:1043, 1973.

142. Kil HK, Rooke GA, Ryan-Dykes MA, Bishop MJ: Effect of prophylactic bronchodilator treatment on lung resistance after endotracheal intubation. Anesthesiology 81:43, 1994.

143. Kim CS, Eldridge MA, Sackner MA: Oropharyngeal deposition and delivery aspects of metered-dose inhaler aerosols. Am Rev Respir Dis 135:157, 1987.

144. Koga Y, Downes H, Leon DA, Hirshman CA: Mechanism of tracheal constriction by succinylcholine. Anesthesiology 55:138, 1981.

145. Koga Y, Sato S, Sodeyama N, et al: Comparison of the relaxant effects of diazepam, flunitrazepam and midazolam on airway smooth muscle. Br J Anaesth 69:65, 1992.

146. Kolbeck RC, Speir WA Jr, Carrier GO, Bransome ED Jr: Apparent irrelevance of cyclic nucleotides to the relaxation of tracheal smooth muscle induced by theophylline. Lung 156:173, 1979.

147. Korenaga S, Takeda K, Ito Y: Differential effects of halothane on airway nerves and muscle. Anesthesiology 60:309, 1984.

148. Kraan J, Koeter GH, vd Mark TW, et al: Changes in bronchial hyperreactivity induced by 4 weeks of treatment with antiasthmatic drugs in patients with allergic asthma: A comparison between budesonide and terbutaline. J Allergy Clin Immunol 76:628, 1985.

149. Kuna ST, Smickley JS, Insalaco G: Posterior cricoarytenoid muscle activity during wakefulness and sleep in normal adults. J Appl Physiol 68:1746, 1990.

150. Laitinen LA, Laitinen A, Haahtela T: A comparative study of the effects of an inhaled corticosteroid, budesonide, and a beta 2-agonist, terbutaline, on airway inflammation in newly diagnosed asthma: A randomized, double-blind, parallel-group controlled trial. J Allergy Clin Immunol 90:32, 1992.

151. Langmack EL, Martin RJ, Pak J, Kraft M: Serum lidocaine concentrations in asthmatics undergoing research bronchoscopy. Chest 117:1055, 2000.

152. Larijani GE, Cypel D, Gratz I, et al: The efficacy and safety of EMLA cream for awake fiberoptic endotracheal intubation. Anesth Analg 91:1024, 2000.

153. Lau HP, Sayiner A, Warner DO, et al: Halothane alters the response of isolated airway smooth muscle to carbon dioxide. Respir Physiol 87:255, 1992.

154. Laycock JR, Donati F, Smith CE, Bevan DR: Potency of atracurium and vecuronium at the diaphragm and the adductor pollicis muscle. Br J Anaesth 61:286, 1988.

155. Lebrault C, Chauvin M, Guirimand F, Duvaldestin P: Relative potency of vecuronium on the diaphragm and the adductor pollicis. Br J Anaesth 63:389, 1989.

156. Lehane JR, Jordan C, Jones JG: Influence of halothane and enflurane on respiratory airflow resistance and specific conductance in anaesthetized man. Br J Anaesth 52:773, 1980.

157. Leiter JC, Knuth SL, Krol RC, Bartlett D Jr: The effect of diazepam on genioglossal muscle activity in normal human subjects. Am Rev Respir Dis 132:216, 1985.

158. Lenox WC, Mitzner W, Hirshman CA: Mechanism of thiopental-induced constriction of guinea pig trachea. Anesthesiology 72:921, 1990.

159. Lindeman KS, Fernandes LB, Croxton TL, Hirshman CA: Role of potassium channels in hypoxic relaxation of porcine bronchi in vitro. Am J Physiol 266:L232, 1994.

160. Londos C, Wolff J: Two distinct adenosine-sensitive sites on adenylate cyclase. Proc Natl Acad Sci USA 74:5482, 1977.

161. Lundgren R, Soderberg M, Horstedt P, Stenling R: Morphological studies of bronchial mucosal biopsies from asthmatics before and after ten years of treatment with inhaled steroids. Eur Respir J 1:883, 1988.

162. Lunell E, Svedmyr N, Andersson KE, Persson CG: A novel bronchodilator xanthine apparently without adenosine receptor antagonism and tremorogenic effect. Eur J Respir Dis 64:333, 1983.

163. Mainland PA, Kong AS, Chung DC, et al: Absorption of lidocaine during aspiration anesthesia of the airway. J Clin Anesth 13:440, 2001.

164. Manawadu BR, Mostow SR, LaForce FM: Impairment of tracheal ring ciliary activity by halothane. Anesth Analg 58:500, 1979.

165. Maslow AD, Regan MM, Israel E, et al: Inhaled albuterol, but not intravenous lidocaine, protects against intubation-induced bronchoconstriction in asthma. Anesthesiology 93:1198, 2000.

166. Mathru M, Esch O, Lang J, et al: Magnetic resonance imaging of the upper airway. Effects of propofol anesthesia and nasal continuous positive airway pressure in humans. Anesthesiology 84:273, 1996.

167. Matthews MD, Ceglarski JZ, Pabari M: Anaphylaxis to suxamethonium—A case report. Anaesth Intensive Care 5:235, 1977.

168. McAlpine LG, Thomson NC: Lidocaine-induced bronchoconstriction in asthmatic patients. Relation to histamine airway responsiveness and effect of preservative. Chest 96:1012, 1989.

169. McFadden ER Jr: The beta 2-agonist controversy revisited. Ann Allergy Asthma Immunol 75:173, 1995.

170. McNicholas WT, Coffey M, McDonnell T, et al: Upper airway obstruction during sleep in normal subjects after selective topical oropharyngeal anesthesia. Am Rev Respir Dis 135:1316, 1987.

171. Miesfeld RL: Molecular genetics of corticosteroid action. Am Rev Respir Dis 141:S11, 1990.

172. Milgrom H, Bender B: Current issues in the use of theophylline. Am Rev Respir Dis 147:S33, 1993.

173. Miller WC, Awe R: Effect of nebulized lidocaine on reactive airways. Am Rev Respir Dis 111:739, 1975.

174. Mongan PD, Culling RD: Rapid oral anesthesia for awake intubation. J Clin Anesth 4:101, 1992.

175. Montravers P, Dureuil B, Desmonts JM: Effects of IV midazolam on upper airway resistance. Br J Anaesth 68:27, 1992.

176. Morikawa S, Safar P, DeCarlo J: Influence of the head-jaw position upon upper airway patency. Anesthesiology 22:265, 1961.

177. Morimoto N, Yamamoto K, Jones KA, Warner DO: Halothane and pertussis toxin-sensitive G proteins in airway smooth muscle. Anesth Analg 78:328, 1994.

178. Morrow PE: Toxicological data on NOx: An overview. J Toxicol Environ Health 13:205, 1984.

179. Murad F: Effects of phosphodiesterase inhibitors and the role of cyclic nucleotides in smooth-muscle relaxation. In Andersson KE, Persson CGA (eds): Anti-Asthma Xanthines and Adenosine. Amsterdam, Excerpta Medica, 1985, p 297.

180. Murphy PJ, Langton JA, Barker P, Smith G: Effect of oral diazepam on the sensitivity of upper airway reflexes. Br J Anaesth 70:131, 1993.

181. Nadel JA, Widdicombe JG: Effect of changes in blood gas tensions and carotid sinus pressure on tracheal volume and total lung resistance to airflow. J. Physiol 163:13, 1962.

182. Naito Y, Tamai S, Shingu K, et al: Comparison between sevoflurane and halothane for paediatric ambulatory anaesthesia. Br J Anaesth 67:387, 1991.

183. Nandi PR, Charlesworth CH, Taylor SJ, et al: Effect of general anaesthesia on the pharynx. Br J Anaesth 66:157, 1991.

184. Nathan RA, Segall N, Glover GC, Schocket AL: The effects of H1 and H2 antihistamines on histamine inhalation challenges in asthmatic patients. Am Rev Respir Dis 120:1251, 1979.

185. Nelson HS: Adrenergic therapy of bronchial asthma. J Allergy Clin Immunol 77:771, 1986.

186. Nevin BJ, Broadley KJ: Nitric oxide in respiratory diseases. Pharmacol Ther 95:259, 2002.

187. Newhouse MT: Is theophylline obsolete? Chest 98:1, 1990.

188. Newman SP, Pavia D, Moren F, et al: Deposition of pressurised aerosols in the human respiratory tract. Thorax 36:52, 1981.

189. Nishino T, Hiraga K, Yokokawa N: Laryngeal and respiratory responses to tracheal irritation at different depths of enflurane anesthesia in humans. Anesthesiology 73:46, 1990.

190. Nishino T, Kohchi T, Yonezawa T, Honda Y: Responses of recurrent laryngeal, hypoglossal, and phrenic nerves to increasing depths of anesthesia with halothane or enflurane in vagotomized cats. Anesthesiology 63:404, 1985.

191. Nishino T, Shirahata M, Yonezawa T, Honda Y: Comparison of changes in the hypoglossal and the phrenic nerve activity in response to increasing depth of anesthesia in cats. Anesthesiology 60:19, 1984.

192. Nogrady SG, Bevan C: H2 receptor blockade and bronchial hyperreactivity to histamine in asthma. Thorax 36:268, 1981.

193. O'Cain CF, Hensley MJ, McFadden ER Jr, Ingram RH Jr: Pattern and mechanism of airway response to hypocapnia in normal subjects. J Appl Physiol 47:8, 1979.

194. O'Doherty MJ, Thomas SH, Page CJ, et al: Delivery of a nebulized aerosol to a lung model during mechanical ventilation. Effect of ventilator settings and nebulizer type, position, and volume of fill. Am Rev Respir Dis 146:383, 1992.

195. O'Rourke PP, Crone RK: Halothane in status asthmaticus. Crit Care Med 10:341, 1982.

196. Ochiai R, Guthrie RD, Motoyama EK: Effects of varying concentrations of halothane on the activity of the genioglossus, intercostals, and diaphragm in cats: An electromyographic study. Anesthesiology 70:812, 1989.

197. Okabe S, Hida W, Kikuchi Y, et al: Upper airway muscle activity during sustained hypoxia in awake humans. J Appl Physiol 75:1552, 1993.

198. Okumura F, Denborough MA: Effects of anaesthetics on guineapig tracheal smooth muscle. Br J Anaesth 52:199, 1980.

199. Oliven A, Odeh M, Gavriely N: Effect of hypercapnia on upper airway resistance and collapsibility in anesthetized dogs. Respir Physiol 75:29, 1989.

200. Olsson GL: Bronchospasm during anaesthesia. A computer-aided incidence study of 136,929 patients. Acta Anaesthesiol Scand 31:244, 1987.

201. Onal E, Lopata M, O'Connor TD: Diaphragmatic and genioglossal electromyogram responses to CO_2 rebreathing in humans. J Appl Physiol 50:1052, 1981.

202. Orem J, Lydic R, Norris P: Experimental control of the diaphragm and laryngeal abductor muscles by brain stem arousal systems. Respir Physiol 38:203, 1977.

203. Page CP: Beta agonists and the asthma paradox. J Asthma 30:155, 1993.

204. Palmer JB, Cuss FM, Barnes PJ: VIP and PHM and their role in nonadrenergic inhibitory responses in isolated human airways. J Appl Physiol 61:1322, 1986.

205. Parish RC, Miller LJ: Nedocromil sodium. Ann Pharmacother 27:599, 1993.

206. Parkes SB, Butler CS, Muller R: Plasma lignocaine concentration following nebulization for awake intubation. Anaesth Intensive Care 25:369, 1997.

207. Pauwels R, Persson CGA: Xanthines. Lung Biol Health Dis 49:503, 1991.

208. Pavlin EG, Holle RH, Schoene RB: Recovery of airway protection compared with ventilation in humans after paralysis with curare. Anesthesiology 70:381, 1989.

209. Pedersen CM, Thirstrup S, Nielsen-Kudsk JE: Smooth muscle relaxant effects of propofol and ketamine in isolated guinea-pig trachea. Eur J Pharmacol 238:75, 1993.

210. Pelton DA, Daly M, Cooper PD, Conn AW: Plasma lidocaine concentrations following topical aerosol application to the trachea and bronchi. Can Anaesth Soc J 17:250, 1970.

211. Pepke-Zaba J, Higenbottam TW, Dinh-Xuan AT, et al: Inhaled nitric oxide as a cause of selective pulmonary vasodilatation in pulmonary hypertension. Lancet 338:1173, 1991.

212. Persson CGA: The profile of action of enprofylline, or why adenosine antagonism seems less desirable with xanthine antiasthmatic. In Morley J, Rainsford KD (eds): Pharmacology of Asthma. Basel, Birkhauser, 1983, p 412.

213. Pizov R, Brown RH, Weiss YS, et al: Wheezing during induction of general anesthesia in patients with and without asthma. A randomized, blinded trial. Anesthesiology 82:1111, 1995.

214. Pizov R, Takahashi M, Hirshman CA, Croxton T: Halothane inhibition of ion transport of the tracheal epithelium. A possible mechanism for anesthetic-induced impairment of mucociliary clearance. Anesthesiology 76:985, 1992.

215. Polson JB, Krzanowski JJ, Anderson WH, et al: Analysis of the relationship between pharmacological inhibition of cyclic nucleotide phosphodiesterase and relaxation of canine tracheal smooth muscle. Biochem Pharmacol 28:1391, 1979.

216. Potter JL, Hillman JV: Benzocaine-induced methemoglobinemia. JACEP 8:26, 1979.

217. Prakash GS, Sharma SK, Pande JN: Effect of 4% lidocaine inhalation in bronchial asthma. J Asthma 27:81, 1990.

218. Rall TW: Central nervous system stimulants. In Gilman AG, Goodman LS, Gilman A (eds): The Pharmacological Basis of Therapeutics. New York, Macmillan, 1980, p 592.

219. Reber A, Wetzel SG, Schnabel K, et al: Effect of combined mouth closure and chin lift on upper airway dimensions during routine magnetic resonance imaging in pediatric patients sedated with propofol. Anesthesiology 90:1617, 1999.

220. Rex MA: A review of the structural and functional basis of laryngospasm and a discussion of the nerve pathways involved in the reflex and its clinical significance in man and animals. Br J Anaesth 42:891, 1970.

221. Richardson J, Beland J: Nonadrenergic inhibitory nervous system in human airways. J Appl Physiol 41:764, 1976.

222. Rock MJ, Reyes de la Rocha S, L'Hommedieu CS, Truemper E: Use of ketamine in asthmatic children to treat respiratory failure refractory to conventional therapy. Crit Care Med 14:514, 1986.

223. Rossaint R, Falke KJ, Lopez F, et al: Inhaled nitric oxide for the adult respiratory distress syndrome. N Engl J Med 328:399, 1993.

224. Rothstein RJ, Narce SL, deBerry-Borowiecki B, Blanks RH: Respiratory-related activity of upper airway muscles in anesthetized rabbit. J Appl Physiol 55:1830, 1983.

225. Rowe BH, Keller JL, Oxman AD: Effectiveness of steroid therapy in acute exacerbations of asthma: A meta-analysis. Am J Emerg Med 10:301, 1992.

226. Ryrfeldt A, Andersson P, Edsbacker S, et al: Pharmacokinetics and metabolism of budesonide, a selective glucocorticoid. Eur J Respir Dis Suppl 122:86, 1982.

227. Salomone RJ, Van Lunteren E: Effects of hypoxia and hypercapnia on geniohyoid contractility and endurance. J Appl Physiol 71:709, 1991.

228. Sant'Ambrogio FB, Anderson JW, Nishino T, Sant'Ambrogio G: Effects of halothane and isoflurane in the upper airway of dogs during development. Respir Physiol 91:237, 1993.

229. Safar P, Escarrage LA, Chang F: Upper airway obstruction in the unconscious patient. J Appl Physiol 14:760, 1959.

230. Sasaki CT, Buckwalter J: Laryngeal function. Am J Otolaryngol 5:281, 1984.

231. Sauerland EK, Harper RM: The human tongue during sleep: Electromyographic activity of the genioglossus muscle. Exp Neurol 51:160, 1976.

232. Sayiner A, Lorenz RR, Warner DO, Rehder K: Bronchodilation by halothane is not modulated by airway epithelium. Anesthesiology 75:75, 1991.

233. Severinghaus JW, Swenson EW, Finley TN, et al: Unilateral hypoventilation produced in dogs by occluding one pulmonary artery. J Appl Physiol 16:53, 1961.

234. Severinghaus JW, Xu FD, Spellman MJ Jr: Benzocaine and methemoglobin: Recommended actions. Anesthesiology 74:385, 1991.

235. Shah MV, Hirshman CA: Mode of action of halothane on histamine-induced airway constriction in dogs with reactive airways. Anesthesiology 65:170, 1986.

236. Shepard JW Jr, Thawley SE: Localization of upper airway collapse during sleep in patients with obstructive sleep apnea. Am Rev Respir Dis 141:1350, 1990.

237. Shimura S, Sasaki T, Ikeda K, et al: Direct inhibitory action of glucocorticoid on glycoconjugate secretion from airway submucosal glands. Am Rev Respir Dis 141:1044, 1990.

238. Shnider SM, Papper EM: Anesthesia for the asthmatic patient. Anesthesiology 22:886, 1961.

239. Shohat B, Volovitz B, Varsano I: Induction of suppressor T cells in asthmatic children by theophylline treatment. Clin Allergy 13:487, 1983.

240. Shore SA, Romero L: Effect of a nitric oxide synthase inhibitor on bronchoconstriction induced by intravenous histamine. Am Rev Respir Dis 147:A445, 1993.

241. Siler JN, Mager JG Jr, Wyche MQ Jr: Atracurium: Hypotension, tachycardia and bronchospasm. Anesthesiology 62:645, 1985.

242. Sill JC, Uhl C, Eskuri S, et al: Halothane inhibits agonist-induced inositol phosphate and Ca^{2+} signaling in A7r5 cultured vascular smooth muscle cells. Mol Pharmacol 40:1006, 1991.

243. Simpson DA, Wright DJ, Hammond JE: Influence of tubocurarine, pancuronium and atracurium on bronchomotor tone. Br J Anaesth 57:753, 1985.

244. Sitbon P, Laffon M, Lesage V, et al: Lidocaine plasma concentrations in pediatric patients after providing airway topical anesthesia from a calibrated device. Anesth Analg 82:1003, 1996.

245. Skoogh BE, Holtzman MJ, Sheller JR, Nadel JA: Barbiturates depress vagal motor pathway to ferret trachea at ganglia. J Appl Physiol 53:253, 1982.

246. Soltani HA, Aghadavoudi O: The effect of different lidocaine application methods on postoperative cough and sore throat. J Clin Anesth 14:15, 2002.

247. Spitzer WO, Suissa S, Ernst P, et al: The use of beta-agonists and the risk of death and near death from asthma. N Engl J Med 326:501, 1992.

248. Sterling GM, Holst PE, Nadel JA: Effect of CO_2 and pH on bronchoconstriction caused by serotonin vs. acetylcholine. J Appl Physiol 32:39, 1972.

249. Stroud MWI, Lambertsen CJ, Ewing JH, et al: The effects of aminophylline and meperidine alone and in combination on the respiratory response to carbon dioxide inhalation. J Pharmacol Exp Ther 114:461, 1955.

250. Sutherland AD, Williams RT: Cardiovascular responses and lidocaine absorption in fiberoptic-assisted awake intubation. Anesth Analg 65:389, 1986.

251. Tamaoki J, Graf PD, Nadel JA: Effect of gamma-aminobutyric acid on neurally mediated contraction of guinea pig trachealis smooth muscle. J Pharmacol Exp Ther 243:86, 1987.

252. Tashkin DP, Ungerer R, Wolfe R, et al: Effect of orally administered cimetidine on histamine- and antigen-induced bronchospasm in subjects with asthma. Am Rev Respir Dis 125:691, 1982.

253. Tattersfield AE: Clinical pharmacology of long-acting beta-receptor agonists. Life Sci 52:2161, 1993.

254. Taylor RH, Lerman J: Induction, maintenance and recovery characteristics of desflurane in infants and children. Can J Anaesth 39:6, 1992.

255. Thomas SH, O'Doherty MJ, Page CJ, et al: Delivery of ultrasonic nebulized aerosols to a lung model during mechanical ventilation. Am Rev Respir Dis 148:872, 1993.

256. Thomson NC: Nedocromil sodium: An overview. Respir Med 83:269, 1989.

257. Tobias JD, Hirshman CA: Attenuation of histamine-induced airway constriction by albuterol during halothane anesthesia. Anesthesiology 72:105, 1990.

258. Toda N, Hatano Y: Contractile responses of canine tracheal muscle during exposure to fentanyl and morphine. Anesthesiology 53:93, 1980.

259. Toogood JH: Complications of topical steroid therapy for asthma. Am Rev Respir Dis 141:S89, 1990.

260. Toogood JH, Crilly RG, Jones G, et al: Effect of high-dose inhaled budesonide on calcium and phosphate metabolism and the risk of osteoporosis. Am Rev Respir Dis 138:57, 1988.

261. Toogood JH, Jennings B, Greenway RW, Chuang L: Candidiasis and dysphonia complicating beclomethasone treatment of asthma. J Allergy Clin Immunol 65:145, 1980.

262. Torphy TJ, Hay DWP: Biochemical regulation of airway smooth muscle tone: An overview. In Agrawal DK, Townley RG (eds): Airway Smooth Muscle: Modulation of Receptors and Response. Boca Raton, Fla, CRC Press, 1990.

263. Townes PL, Geertsma MA, White MR: Benzocaine-induced methemoglobinemia. Am J Dis Child 131:697, 1977.

264. Twort CH, Cameron IR: Effects of PCO_2, pH and extracellular calcium on contraction of airway smooth muscle from rats. Respir Physiol 66:259, 1986.

265. Uddman R, Sundler F: Neuropeptides in the airways: A review. Am Rev Respir Dis 136:S3, 1987.

266. Van Lunteren E, Strohl KP: Striated respiratory muscles of the upper airways. Lung Biol 35:87, 1988.

267. Van Schayck CP, Graafsma SJ, Visch MB, et al: Increased bronchial hyperresponsiveness after inhaling salbutamol during 1 year is not caused by subsensitization to salbutamol. J Allergy Clin Immunol 86:793, 1990.

268. Vathenen AS, Knox AJ, Higgins BG, et al: Rebound increase in bronchial responsiveness after treatment with inhaled terbutaline. Lancet 1:554, 1988.

269. Vaz Fragoso CA, Miller MA: Review of the clinical efficacy of theophylline in the treatment of chronic obstructive pulmonary disease. Am Rev Respir Dis 147:S40, 1993.

270. Vettermann J, Beck KC, Lindahl SG, et al: Actions of enflurane, isoflurane, vecuronium, atracurium, and pancuronium on pulmonary resistance in dogs. Anesthesiology 69:688, 1988.

271. Viegas O, Stoelting RK: Lidocaine in arterial blood after laryngotracheal administration. Anesthesiology 43:491, 1975.

272. Waltemath CL, Bergman NA: Effects of ketamine and halothane on increased respiratory resistance provoked by ultrasonic aerosols. Anesthesiology 41:473, 1974.

273. Ward JK, Belvisi MG, Fox AJ, et al: Modulation of cholinergic neural bronchoconstriction by endogenous nitric oxide and vasoactive intestinal peptide in human airways in vitro. J Clin Invest 92:736, 1993.

274. Warner DO: Respiratory muscle function. In Biebuyck JF, Lynch C III, Maze M, et al (eds): Anesthesia: Biologic Foundations. New York, Raven Press, 1994, p 1395.

275. Warner DO, Jones KA, Lorenz RR, Pabelick CM: Muscarinic receptor stimulation modulates the effect of halothane on Mn^{2+} influx in airway smooth muscle. Am J Physiol 273:C868, 1997.

276. Warner DO, Vettermann J, Brichant JF, Rehder K: Direct and neurally mediated effects of halothane on pulmonary resistance in vivo. Anesthesiology 72:1057, 1990.

277. Warner DO, Warner MA, Barnes RD, et al: Perioperative respiratory complications in patients with asthma. Anesthesiology 85:460, 1996.

278. Watney GC, Jordan C, Hall LW: Effect of halothane, enflurane and isoflurane on bronchomotor tone in anaesthetized ponies. Br J Anaesth 59:1022, 1987.

279. Wetzel RC, Herold CJ, Zerhouni EA, Robotham JL: Hypoxic bronchodilation. J Appl Physiol 73:1202, 1992.

280. Wheatley JR, Kelly WT, Tully A, Engel LA: Pressure-diameter relationships of the upper airway in awake supine subjects. J Appl Physiol 70:2242, 1991.

281. Wheatley JR, Brancatisano A, Engel LA: Respiratory-related activity of cricothyroid muscle in awake normal humans. J Appl Physiol 70:2226, 1991.

282. Wilkins CJ, Cramp PG, Staples J, Stevens WC: Comparison of the anesthetic requirement for tolerance of laryngeal mask airway and endotracheal tube. Anesth Analg 75:794, 1992.

283. Wilson LE, Hatch DJ, Rehder K: Mechanisms of the relaxant action of ketamine on isolated porcine trachealis muscle. Br J Anaesth 71:544, 1993.

284. Wray S: Smooth muscle intracellular pH: Measurement, regulation, and function. Am J Physiol 254:C213, 1988.

285. Wu RS, Wu KC, Sum DC, Bishop MJ: Comparative effects of thiopentone and propofol on respiratory resistance after tracheal intubation. Br J Anaesth 77:735, 1996.
286. Wu RS, Wu KC, Wong TK, et al: Effects of fenoterol and ipratropium on respiratory resistance of asthmatics after tracheal intubation. Br J Anaesth 84:358, 2000.
287. Yamakage M: Direct inhibitory mechanisms of halothane on canine tracheal smooth muscle contraction. Anesthesiology 77:546, 1992.
288. Yamakage M, Kohro S, Kawamata T, Namiki A: Inhibitory effects of four inhaled anesthetics on canine tracheal smooth muscle contraction and intracellular Ca^{2+} concentration. Anesth Analg 77:67, 1993.
289. Yamamoto K, Morimoto N, Warner DO, et al: Factors influencing the direct actions of volatile anesthetics on airway smooth muscle. Anesthesiology 78:1102, 1993.
290. Yasuda I, Hirano T, Yusa T, Satoh M: Tracheal constriction by morphine and by fentanyl in man. Anesthesiology 49:117, 1978.
291. Yunginger JW, Reed CE, O'Connell EJ, et al: A community-based study of the epidemiology of asthma. Incidence rates, 1964-1983. Am Rev Respir Dis 146:888, 1992.

6

PHYSIOLOGIC AND PATHOPHYSIOLOGIC RESPONSES TO INTUBATION

Steven A. Deem
Michael J. Bishop
Robert F. Bedford

I. BACKGROUND

Laryngoscopy, endotracheal intubation, and other airway manipulations (i.e., placement of a Combitube or laryngeal mask airway [LMA]) are noxious stimuli that induce profound changes in cardiovascular physiology, primarily through reflex responses. Although these responses may be of short duration and of little consequence in healthy individuals, serious complications may occur in patients with underlying coronary artery disease,[90,144] reactive airways,[35,108] or intracranial neuropathology.[41,140]

II. CARDIOVASCULAR RESPONSES DURING AIRWAY MANIPULATION

A. THE CARDIOVASCULAR REFLEXES

The cardiovascular responses to noxious airway manipulation are initiated by proprioceptors responding to tissue irritation in the supraglottic region and trachea.[143] Located in close proximity to the airway mucosa, these proprioceptors consist of mechanoreceptors with small-diameter myelinated fibers, slowly adapting stretch receptors with large-diameter myelinated fibers, and polymodal endings of nonmyelinated nerve fibers.[130] (The superficial location of the proprioceptors and their nerves is the reason that topical local anesthesia of the airway is such an effective means of blunting cardiovascular responses to airway interventions.) The glossopharyngeal and vagal afferent nerves transmit these impulses to the brain stem, which, in turn, causes widespread autonomic activation through both the sympathetic and parasympathetic nervous systems. Bradycardia, often elicited in infants and small children during laryngoscopy or intubation, is the autonomic equivalent of the laryngospasm response. Although seen only rarely in adults, this reflex results from an increase in vagal tone at the sinoatrial node and is virtually a monosynaptic response to a noxious stimulus in the airway.

In adults and adolescents, the more common response to airway manipulation is hypertension and tachycardia, mediated by the cardioaccelerator nerves and sympathetic chain ganglia. This response includes widespread release of norepinephrine from adrenergic nerve terminals and secretion of epinephrine from the adrenal medulla.[63] Some of the hypertensive response to endotracheal intubation also results from activation of the renin-angiotensin system, with release of renin from the renal juxtaglomerular apparatus, which is innervated by β-adrenergic nerve terminals.

In addition to activation of the autonomic nervous system, laryngoscopy and endotracheal intubation result in stimulation of the central nervous system (CNS), as evidenced by increases in electroencephalographic activity, cerebral metabolic rate, and cerebral blood flow (CBF).[96]

In patients with compromised intracranial compliance, the increase in CBF may result in elevated intracranial pressure (ICP), which, in turn, may result in herniation of brain contents and severe neurologic compromise (see later).

The effects of endotracheal intubation on the pulmonary vasculature are probably less well understood than the responses elicited in the systemic circulation. They are often coupled with changes in airway reactivity associated with intubation. Thus, acute bronchospasm or a main stem bronchial intubation results in a marked maldistribution of perfusion to poorly ventilated lung units, causing desaturation of pulmonary venous blood and subsequent reduction in systemic arterial oxygen tension. In addition, institution of positive end-expiratory pressure (PEEP) following endotracheal intubation causes a reduction in cardiac output related to impaired venous return to the left heart from the pulmonary circulation. The impact of these changes can be profound in patients with severely compromised myocardial function or intravascular volume depletion.

B. INTUBATION IN THE PRESENCE OF CARDIOVASCULAR DISEASE

The neuroendocrine responses to airway manipulation that result in hypertension and tachycardia can cause a variety of complications in patients with cardiac disease. Probably the most common adverse cardiovascular problem related to intubation is myocardial ischemia in patients with coronary artery insufficiency. Because two of the major determinants of myocardial oxygen demand are heart rate and blood pressure,[90] the increase in myocardial oxygen demand created by the hypertensive-tachycardic response to endotracheal intubation must be met by an increase in the flow of oxygenated blood through the coronary circulation. However, when one or more occlusive coronary lesions result in relatively fixed coronary blood flow, the ability to increase myocardial blood flow during periods of increased demand is minimal, and an abrupt increase in myocardial oxygen demand can result in tissue ischemia that may lead either to myocardial dysfunction or to overt tissue infarction. Furthermore, cardiac ischemia induced by arterial hypertension may be compounded by an increase in left ventricular end-diastolic pressure, resulting in further compromise of perfusion to subendocardial tissues. This set of circumstances is responsible for episodes of electrocardiographic ST-segment depression and increased pulmonary artery diastolic pressure that may be seen when endotracheal intubation is performed in patients with arteriosclerosis; occasionally, these episodes presage the occurrence of a perioperative myocardial infarction.[144]

Patients with vascular anomalies that cause weakening of the lining of major arteries are also at risk during endotracheal intubation. In particular, the integrity of cerebral and aortic aneurysms is largely a function of transmural pressure. A sudden increase in blood pressure can lead to rupture of the affected vessel and abrupt deterioration in the patient's status. Leaking aortic aneurysms are partially tamponaded by intra-abdominal pressure but can suddenly expand into the retroperitoneal space during arterial hypertension. The results are both significant blood loss for the anesthesiologist to replace and additional technical problems for the surgeon trying to resect the lesion and insert a vascular prosthesis.

C. IMPLICATIONS FOR PATIENTS WITH NEUROVASCULAR DISEASE

Intracranial aneurysms and arteriovenous malformations (AVMs) often arise with a small "sentinel" hemorrhage that serves as a warning of worse things to come. During subsequent periods of elevated arterial pressure these lesions are likely to rebleed, resulting in sudden and permanent neurologic injury. Many neurosurgeons and interventional neuroradiologists attempt to stabilize cerebral aneurysms and AVMs soon after hospitalization in an effort to minimize the risk of rebleeding. This means that the patient presents for anesthesia at a time when the clot tamponading the aneurysm or AVM is particularly delicate, and a small increase in arterial transmural pressure may cause rerupture. One of the times this is most likely to occur is when arterial pressure and pulse rate are increased in response to endotracheal intubation.[41] Thus, neurosurgical anesthesiologists pay meticulous attention to attenuating these responses during the course of anesthetic induction and endotracheal intubation.

D. INTUBATION IN NEUROPATHOLOGIC DISORDERS

Reflex responses to endotracheal intubation are also a potential hazard to patients with compromised intracranial compliance resulting from neuropathologic processes such as intracranial mass lesions, brain edema, or acute hydrocephalus. Uncontrolled coughing can result in a marked increase in intrathoracic and intra-abdominal pressure that is transmitted as increased cerebrospinal fluid pressure and may result in impairment of cerebral perfusion. In patients with impaired cerebral autoregulation (brain trauma, cerebrovascular accidents, neoplasms), the normal tendency for CBF to remain constant over the mean blood pressure from 50 to 150 mm Hg is lost. When endotracheal intubation causes an increase in arterial pressure, there is a marked increase in CBF and cerebral blood volume, which, in turn, can cause dangerous increases in ICP.[140] This effect is magnified by the fact that noxious stimuli such as airway manipulation result in increased CBF, which summates with the hypertensive blood pressure response, occasionally causing profound increases in ICP (Fig. 6-1).

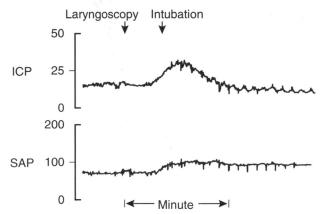

Figure 6-1 Increases in systemic arterial pressure (SAP) and intracranial pressure (ICP) in response to endotracheal intubation in a patient with a small brain tumor. Note the minimal response to rigid laryngoscopy. There is a sustained increase in SAP but only a transient increase in ICP, which returns to normal as cerebrovascular autoregulation becomes operative. (From Bedford RF: Circulatory responses to tracheal intubation. Probl Anesth 2:201, 1988.)

E. NEUROMUSCULAR BLOCKING DRUGS AND CARDIOVASCULAR RESPONSES

Endotracheal intubation is usually performed in the presence of neuromuscular blockade in order to facilitate laryngoscopy and minimize glottic closure and cough reflexes. Accordingly, it is appropriate to consider the cardiovascular and cerebrovascular responses to the administration of the neuromuscular blocking agents. Indeed, the hypertensive-tachycardic response to endotracheal intubation was not identified until neuromuscular blocking agents were introduced into clinical practice because, before this time, intubation was performed only under such deep levels of anesthesia that relatively little cardiovascular response was generated.[84]

The depressor effects of benzylisoquinolinium relaxants (atracurium and mivacurium) are mediated by histamine release.[2] This effect could be looked upon as a potential antagonist to the pressor response from laryngoscopy and endotracheal intubation. In the case of patients at risk for intracranial hypertension, however, histamine-induced cerebral vasodilation may produce increases in ICP even as the blood pressure falls.[158] By contrast, pancuronium, rocuronium, and to a lesser extent vecuronium may initiate a hyperdynamic cardiovascular state that can potentiate the cardiovascular responses seen after endotracheal intubation in lightly anesthetized patients. The greater cardiovascular stability and rapidity of onset afforded by intubating doses of rocuronium are the reason for its current widespread use for intubation in operations expected to last longer than an hour.[65]

Succinylcholine is the muscle relaxant used most commonly to facilitate endotracheal intubation for brief-duration anesthetics. Although occasionally associated with bradycardia in children, it is a cardiovascular stimulant in adults. This phenomenon is often associated with activation of the electroencephalogram,[105] and patients with brain tumors may sustain marked increases in ICP following succinylcholine,[105] particularly when intracranial compliance is compromised and cerebrovascular autoregulation is impaired. Studies in dogs indicate that succinylcholine increases afferent CNS input as a result of activation of muscle spindles at the time of muscle fasciculations.[87] However, the effect of succinylcholine on ICP in patients is less clear. Succinylcholine administered to intubated patients being treated for intracranial hypertension of various causes had no effect on ICP, cerebral perfusion pressure, or CBF.[86] But succinylcholine administered to patients with brain tumors resulted in a mean 5- to 12-torr increase in ICP with no significant effect on cerebral perfusion pressure.[101,152] The increase in ICP could be prevented by pretreatment with metocurine[152] or vecuronium.[101] Thus, given the wide availability of alternative neuromuscular blocking agents, succinylcholine should be considered a second-line agent for intubation of patients with poor intracranial compliance and should ideally be used only after pretreatment with a nondepolarizing agent.

F. CARDIOPULMONARY CONSEQUENCES OF POSITIVE-PRESSURE VENTILATION

Positive-pressure ventilation is usually instituted immediately after successful endotracheal intubation. It results in an increase in mean intrathoracic pressure, which, in turn, impairs cardiac filling and results in a decrease in cardiac output and arterial pressure. Patients with decreased intravascular volume or impaired myocardial contractility are particularly sensitive to this phenomenon, and it is not uncommon for a patient to become acutely hypotensive shortly after endotracheal intubation and institution of positive-pressure ventilation. In some instances, the hypotension is worsened by intravascular volume depletion secondary to surgical bowel preparation or vigorous diuretic therapy. In other cases, the hypovolemia may be part of the disease process that has brought the patient to the operating room, that is, active bleeding or extravascular fluid accumulation in the peritoneal cavity. Thus, one common clinical scenario is a patient who may respond to endotracheal intubation with a brisk increase in blood pressure and who then suddenly develops acute hypotension as positive-pressure ventilation is instituted. In such a situation, rapid use of the head-down position to augment venous return, discontinuation of potent anesthetic agent, and prompt instillation of appropriate vascular volume expanders usually suffice to correct the situation. Patients with suspected coronary artery disease might respond more favorably to judicious administration of an α-adrenergic agent such as phenylephrine, which may increase diastolic pressure and maintain coronary filling pressures. Usually, the adrenergic stimulus of

the surgical incision then suffices to maintain arterial pressure for the duration of the operation.

III. PREVENTION OF CARDIOVASCULAR RESPONSES

A. TECHNICAL CONSIDERATIONS: MINIMIZING STIMULATION OF AIRWAY PROPRIOCEPTORS

As a general rule, cardiovascular responses to airway maneuvers can be minimized by limiting airway proprioceptor stimulation, starting with manipulation of the larynx itself. For instance, cricoid cartilage pressure with a posterior force of 4.5 kg is widely used to prevent regurgitation of gastric contents or to facilitate laryngeal visualization. In a double-blind study, cricoid pressure resulted in a significantly greater heart rate and blood pressure response to endotracheal intubation than occurred in patients whose cricoid area was gently palpated.[129] This is a little-recognized effect of cricoid pressure that should be considered when estimating the risk-benefit ratio of this procedure in individual patients.

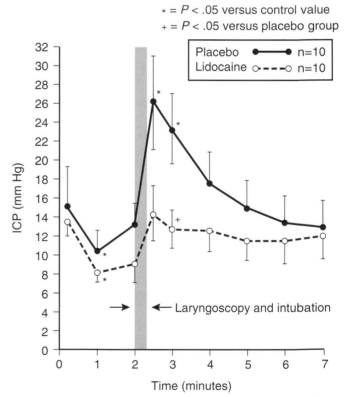

Figure 6-2 Impact of intravenous lidocaine, 1.5 mg/kg, on the intracranial pressure (ICP) response to tracheal intubation in patients with brain tumor after a rapid-sequence intubation with thiopental, 3 mg/kg IV, and succinylcholine, 1.5 mg/kg IV. (From Bedford R: Intracranial pressure response to endotracheal intubation: Efficacy of intravenous lidocaine pretreatment for patients with brain tumors. In Shulman K, Marmarou A, Miller JD, et al [eds]: Intracranial Pressure IV. New York, Springer-Verlag, 1980, pp 595-598.)

Laryngoscopy itself is a moderately stimulating procedure (Fig. 6-2), and use of a straight blade (Miller) with elevation of the vagally innervated posterior aspect of the epiglottis results in significantly higher arterial pressure than does use of a curved blade (Macintosh or McCoy).[113] However, the act of passing an endotracheal tube (ET) is far more hemodynamically stimulating than just laryngoscopy and, surprisingly, use of a lighted intubation stylet fails to prevent hemodynamic stimulation when the ET is advanced past the vocal cords.[156]

Insertion of a conventional LMA after induction of general anesthesia with thiopental or propofol and fentanyl has been shown to cause less cardiovascular and endocrine response than laryngoscopy and endotracheal intubation.[15,115,166,167] The LMA has the advantage of avoiding the vagally mediated infraglottic stimulation entailed by the use of a laryngoscope, thus enabling lighter levels of general anesthesia. Furthermore, because muscle relaxation is not required for airway control, spontaneously initiated ventilation is possible, with avoidance of the adverse hemodynamic consequences of positive-pressure ventilation. In contrast, endotracheal intubation using the intubating LMA resulted in a similar hemodynamic and endocrine response to direct laryngoscopy and intubation after propofol induction.[27]

Thus, if endotracheal intubation is necessary, there does not appear to be a hemodynamic advantage to instrumenting the airway with the LMA-Fastrach (intubating LMA).

It should be emphasized that the hypertensive, tachycardic response to endotracheal intubation is a manifestation of insufficient anesthesia. The first line of prevention should be induction of a sufficient depth of anesthesia before endotracheal intubation is performed. Patients with ischemic coronary artery disease, arterial vascular anomalies, and compromised intracranial compliance require special management and meticulous hemodynamic monitoring in order to optimize their care during this most stressful of anesthetic procedures.

B. TOPICAL AND REGIONAL ANESTHESIA

Topical anesthesia to the upper airway is effective in blunting hemodynamic responses to endotracheal intubation,[154,155] but almost invariably, topical anesthesia of the airway has proved to be less effective than systemic administration of lidocaine. During general anesthesia, rigid laryngoscopy and instillation of lidocaine solution initiate the same adverse reflexes caused by placement of an ET (Figs. 6-3 and 6-4).[169] Furthermore, laryngotracheal spray of lidocaine solution may, in itself, produce

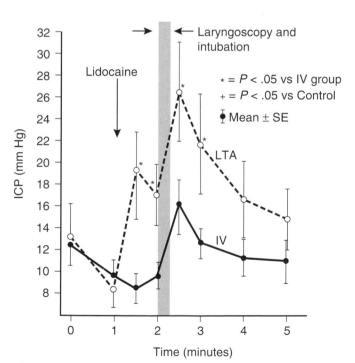

Figure 6-3 Comparison of effects of intravenous (IV) and intratracheal (LTA) lidocaine, 1.5 mg/kg, on the intracranial pressure (ICP) response to laryngoscopy and endotracheal intubation in 22 patients with brain tumor. Note early elevation of ICP from intratracheal lidocaine instillation followed by augmented response from intubation. (From Hamill JF, Bedford RF, Weaver DC, Colohan AR: Lidocaine before endotracheal intubation: Intravenous or laryngotracheal? Anesthesiology 55:578, 1981.)

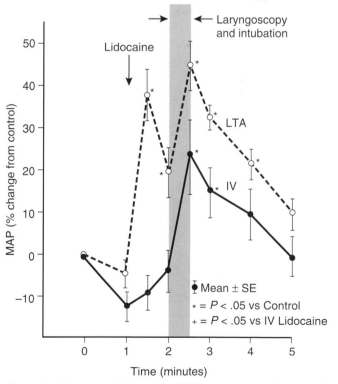

Figure 6-4 Mean arterial pressure (MAP) response to endotracheal intubation after either intravenous or intratracheal lidocaine instillation, as in Figure 6-3. (From Hamill JF, Bedford RF, Weaver DC, Colohan AR: Lidocaine before endotracheal intubation: Intravenous or laryngotracheal? Anesthesiology 55:578, 1981.)

profound cardiovascular stimulation in adults, or in children it may produce the same sort of bradycardic response associated with endotracheal intubation.[102] If topical lidocaine is administered to the upper airway, there should be an intervening period of at least 2 minutes to allow initiation of anesthetic effect before airway instrumentation begins.[157]

Excellent topical anesthesia of the airway performed before awake flexible fiberoptic endotracheal intubation was responsible for reports suggesting that there was less cardiovascular stimulation after this procedure than after intubation with a rigid laryngoscope.[64] Subsequent studies performed under general anesthesia, however, have demonstrated that there is no difference between the two modes of intubation with regard to hemodynamic impact, probably because the more profound stimulus results from placement of the ET below the level of the glottis.[40,135,145,146]

Although topical anesthesia of the airway appears to be of limited benefit, regional nerve blocks involving the sensory pathways from the airway prevent hemodynamic responses to intubation. The superior laryngeal nerve innervates the superior surface of the larynx, and the glossopharyngeal nerve innervates the oropharynx. Depositing local anesthetic on each cornu of the hyoid bone can block the superior laryngeal nerve. Blockade of the glossopharyngeal nerve at the tonsillar pillars (sensory distribution above the level of the epiglottis) potentiates this effect by decreasing the stimulus of laryngoscopy.[128] The inferior surfaces of the larynx and trachea require topical anesthesia, however, as these surfaces are innervated by the recurrent laryngeal nerve and the vagus, which cannot be directly blocked. With the preceding combination, awake patients exhibit little response as the ET is inserted.

C. INHALATIONAL ANESTHETICS

Defining the anesthetic dose requirement for effectively blocking (or even blunting) hemodynamic and ICP responses to endotracheal intubation has remained an elusive goal. Airway maneuvers are typically brief interventions that produce short-lived responses during a dynamic perioperative period, with drug concentrations rapidly fluctuating both in blood and at effect sites. Agents that are capable of preventing responses may also produce profound cardiovascular depression before and after the stimulation of endotracheal intubation. Accordingly, there are relatively few well-controlled dose-response studies, and those that are available often give information that is not useful for the clinical practitioner.

For inhalational anesthetics, endotracheal intubation in the 1 minimum alveolar concentration (MAC) dose range results in marked cardiovascular stimulation during halothane-N_2O and N_2O-morphine anesthetic techniques.[7] It should not be surprising that 1 MAC is insufficient because it is known that approximately 1.5 to 1.6 MAC is needed to block the adrenergic and cardiovascular responses to a simple surgical skin incision (MAC-BAR).[126]

However, the dose of anesthetic required to prevent coughing during endotracheal intubation with sevoflurane may exceed MAC by a factor of 2.86 in adults,[83] although this factor appears to be close to 1.3 in children.[111] Accordingly, it appears that the dose of volatile anesthetic required to block the cardiovascular response to endotracheal intubation must be inordinately high, resulting in profound cardiovascular depression prior to endotracheal intubation.[172] From a cerebrovascular viewpoint, this approach is totally impractical because high doses of volatile anesthetics cause cerebral vasodilation and marked increases in ICP in patients with compromised intracranial compliance. Furthermore, from a cardiovascular point of view, the arterial hypotension and reduced cerebral perfusion pressure before intubation would be entirely unacceptable for all but the most fit patients.

D. INTRAVENOUS AGENTS

Propofol, barbiturates, and benzodiazepines are all associated with profound hypotension at doses that suppress the hemodynamic and ICP responses to intubation.[50,106,124] In the case of etomidate, the effective dose for blocking cardiovascular response to intubation can be identified by a burst-suppression pattern on the cortical surface electroencephalogram, indicating fairly deep cerebral depression.[104] Because etomidate supports blood pressure at such deep levels of anesthesia, it is probably the only contemporary agent that, by itself, can achieve suppression of cardiovascular responses without first producing undue arterial hypotension and compromise of coronary and cerebral perfusion.

As it is clinically impractical to achieve sufficient anesthetic depth for preventing a hyperdynamic response to intubation solely with an intravenous (IV) or inhalational agent (etomidate excepted), a wide variety of anesthetic drug combinations or adjuvants, or both, have been employed in an attempt to potentiate anesthetic effects while minimizing hemodynamic depression.

Opioids are the adjuvants that are most widely utilized to potentiate the relatively light anesthetic techniques used in contemporary practice. In the case of fentanyl, however, it should be remembered that the drug does not achieve peak CNS effect until 10 minutes after bolus IV injection.[11] Fentanyl appears to give a graded response to blunting hemodynamic responses: 2 µg/kg IV several minutes before induction only partially prevents hypertension and tachycardia during a rapid-sequence intubation with thiopental and succinylcholine. In this situation, 6 µg/kg is considerably more effective.[79] Chen[24] noted almost complete suppression of the hemodynamic response to intubation at both 11 and 15 µg/kg IV fentanyl, whereas higher doses (30 to 75 µg/kg IV) allowed only a very occasional response to intubation. In doses that prevent a hemodynamic response to intubation, however, fentanyl is not a short-acting agent, and the risk of prolonged postoperative respiratory depression must be weighed against the advantages of perioperative cardiovascular stability. With this risk in mind, it has been observed that pretreatment with IV fentanyl, 2 µg/kg, given 10 minutes before intubation during an infusion of propofol sufficient to reduce the bispectral index score to 45 prevented a significant increase in heart rate or blood pressure compared with awake preanesthetic values.[96] Similar results were observed when intubation was performed after fentanyl, 2 µg/kg, and propofol bolus doses of 2.0 to 3.5 mg/kg.[96]

Fentanyl and propofol require 6.4 and 2.9 minutes, respectively, to achieve effect-site equilibrium after IV bolus administration. Thus, laryngoscopy and intubation should be timed to coincide with the peak effect of these agents in order to minimize hemodynamic stimulation.[96]

Opioids with shorter onset and offset times have some advantages over fentanyl for modulating circulatory responses to intubation. Alfentanil has a smaller steady-state distribution volume and shorter terminal elimination half-life than fentanyl.[137] Ausems and colleagues[4] demonstrated that an alfentanil plasma concentration of 600 ng/mL effectively prevented hemodynamic responses to intubation during induction of nitrous oxide anesthesia. This was achieved by a 30-second infusion of alfentanil, 150 µg/kg. During this induction period, nitrous oxide and succinylcholine were also administered. Only 5 of the 35 patients sustained an increase in heart rate or blood pressure greater than 15% above preinduction values.

Remifentanil has been found to be highly effective in preventing hemodynamic responses to intubation, albeit always with the cost of impressive bradycardia or hypotension, or both, before and after airway manipulation.[159] Many studies have used vagolytic agents to avoid bradycardia, at the risk of an elevated heart rate response following intubation. Remifentanil's half-time for equilibration between blood and effect site is 1.3 minutes,[51] and it has a brief half-life of 3 to 5 minutes because of hydrolysis by tissue and blood esterases.[77] Typical remifentanil doses used for blunting hemodynamic responses are infusion rates of 0.25 to 1.0 µg/kg/min in association with cautious propofol administration and nondepolarizing neuromuscular blockade.[91] For rapid-sequence intubation with thiopental and succinylcholine, the optimal dose of remifentanil appears to be 1.0 µg/kg administered over 30 seconds, with laryngoscopy performed 1 minute after induction. A bolus dose of 1.25 µg/kg was associated with unsatisfactory bradycardia, whereas 0.5 µg/kg resulted in excessive cardiovascular stimulation.[116]

IV lidocaine may also blunt hemodynamic and cerebrovascular responses to intubation. When given in an IV bolus of 1.5 mg/kg, it adds approximately 0.3 MAC of anesthetic potency.[69] Significant reductions in hemodynamic response to endotracheal intubation have been noted when lidocaine (3 mg/kg) was used as an adjunct to high-dose fentanyl anesthesia[78] as well as during other light anesthetic techniques such as those involving thiopental-N_2O-O_2.[1] However, smaller doses of lidocaine (1.5 mg/kg) do not appear to be effective in reducing the hemodynamic response to laryngoscopy and endotracheal intubation.[99,148]

The general anesthetic properties of lidocaine tend to reduce the cerebral metabolic rate for oxygen and CBF, thus lowering ICP in patients with compromised intracranial compliance.[8] Furthermore, lidocaine effectively prevents increases in ICP when used as an adjunct prior to endotracheal intubation in patients susceptible to intracranial hypertension (see Fig. 6-2).[6]

With regard to the patient at risk for intracranial hypertension, it is important that agents used to control cardiovascular responses to intubation also have a minimal adverse impact on ICP. During anesthesia induction, therefore, most neuroanesthetists utilize an IV sleep dose of barbiturate, propofol, or etomidate, followed by small doses of opioid (fentanyl 1 to 2 µg/kg IV), IV lidocaine (1.5 mg/kg), and hyperventilation to a partial pressure of carbon dioxide in arterial blood ($PaCO_2$) of approximately 30 mm Hg while an intubating dose of nondepolarizing muscle relaxant takes effect. Often, an adrenergic blocking agent such as labetalol (5 to 10 mg IV) or esmolol (50 to 100 mg IV) is also given prior to endotracheal intubation. Agents that act as cerebral vasodilators, such as volatile anesthetics, nitroglycerin, nitroprusside, or hydralazine, are generally avoided if there is a serious risk of intracranial hypertension.

F. NONANESTHETIC ADJUVANT AGENTS

A final means for modifying the cardiovascular responses to endotracheal intubation is to administer prophylactically vasoactive substances that directly affect the cardiovascular system. This approach was introduced in 1960 by DeVault and coworkers,[32] who found that pretreatment with phentolamine, 5 mg IV, prevented the hypertensive and tachycardic response to endotracheal intubation during a light barbiturate-succinylcholine anesthetic technique. Subsequently, a large number of articles appeared advocating the use of various vasodilators and adrenergic blocking agents as pretreatment before endotracheal intubation. Among those described are diltiazem, verapamil, and nicardipine[3,42,43,97]; hydralazine[30]; nitroprusside[153]; nitroglycerin[48]; labetalol[162]; esmolol[3,53,100,142]; and clonidine.[49,98] Virtually all of these agents appear to be somewhat effective compared with placebo, particularly when used in high doses. Esmolol is the best studied of the group, and in a large, multicenter, placebo-controlled trial esmolol at a dose of 100 or 200 mg suppressed the hemodynamic response to endotracheal intubation, particularly when combined with a moderate-dose opiate.[100] However, esmolol doses of 200 mg were associated with a doubling of the incidence of hypotension compared with placebo. In another study, smaller doses of esmolol (1 mg/kg) had no effect on the hemodynamic response to laryngoscopy and intubation compared with placebo.[3]

The optimal use of any of these agents is undefined, although their use as adjuncts to rapid-sequence induction in high-risk patients may be reasonable, with the caveat that sufficiently high doses must be used to achieve the desired effect.

IV. AIRWAY EFFECTS OF ENDOTRACHEAL INTUBATION

A. UPPER AIRWAY REFLEXES

Because the upper airway protects the respiratory gas exchange surface from noxious substances, it is appropriate that the nose, mouth, pharynx, larynx, trachea, and carina have an abundance of sensory nerve endings and brisk motor responses. Anesthesiologists are especially familiar with the glottic closure reflex (laryngospasm), which is invariably encountered early in their training. The sneeze, cough, and swallow reflexes are equally important upper airway reflexes.

Afferent pathways for laryngospasm and the cardiovascular responses to endotracheal intubation are initiated by the glossopharyngeal nerve when stimuli occur superior to the anterior surface of the epiglottis and by the vagus nerve when stimuli occur from the level of the posterior epiglottis down into the lower airway. Because the laryngeal closure reflex is mediated by vagal efferents to the glottis, it is virtually a monosynaptic response, occurring primarily when a patient is lightly anesthetized as vagally innervated sensory endings in the upper airway are stimulated and conscious respiratory efforts cannot override the reflex.

B. DEAD SPACE

Patients with severe chronic lung disease may find it easier to breathe following intubation or a tracheostomy. The improvement is most likely due to reduced dead space. The normal extrathoracic anatomic dead space, based on cadaver measurements, is approximately 70 to 75 mL.[114] The exact volume of the ET is easily calculated as the volume (V) of a cylinder using the formula $V = r^2 l$, where r is the radius of the tube and l is the length. Thus, an 8-mm inner diameter (ID) ET that is 25 cm in length has a volume of 12.6 mL. Intubation would therefore result in a reduction in dead space of approximately 60 mL.

Tracheostomy tubes are shorter than oral ETs and have an even smaller dead space, although the difference as a proportion of tidal volume is negligible. In healthy individuals, such a reduction in dead space is negligible compared with the normal tidal volume, thus offering little benefit. In a patient with severe restrictive lung disease such as in end-stage kyphoscoliosis, tidal volume may be as low as 100 mL. Thus, intubation can confer a major benefit. Similarly, patients with emphysema changed from mouth breathing to tracheostomy demonstrate a reduction in minute volume required and a decrease in total body oxygen consumption, presumably related to a decreased work of breathing.[29] The decreased volume required probably more than compensates for the slight increase in resistance (see later).

The decreases in dead space described refer only to the volume of the tracheal tube alone and would be applicable only during T-piece breathing. Any extensions or Y-pieces added to the breathing circuit and attached to the ET must also be added to the total.

C. UPPER AIRWAY RESISTANCE

Anesthesiologists are well aware that in most anesthetized patients, adequate ventilation can be maintained with an ET as small as 6 mm ID in place. Intensivists caring for a patient with respiratory failure, however, often insist that a minimum ET ID be 8 mm. It should be recognized that these tube sizes are each appropriate for the clinical situations described. The high resistance of the 6-mm ET is inconsequential for the low minute ventilation required under general anesthesia. By contrast, the high flow rates required for a patient with respiratory failure may render the resistance of a small ET prohibitive.

The ET creates a mechanical burden for a spontaneously breathing patient in the form of a fixed upper airway resistance because it decreases airway caliber and increases resistance to breathing. Gas flow across an ET is determined by the pressure difference across the tube and the resistance of the ET. Gas flows whenever there is a pressure difference across the ET, whether caused by subatmospheric pressure generated during spontaneous breathing or by positive pressure generated from a mechanical ventilator.

The apparent resistance of an ET is influenced both by the shape of the tube and by two types of friction: the friction among the gas molecules and the friction between the tube wall and the gas molecules.[60,72] Irregular surfaces created by secretions or by ridges from wire reinforcement may create greater friction and greater resistance.[80] Tracheal tubes or tracheostomies have a higher resistance than the normal upper respiratory tract.[23,171] The relationship between pressure difference and flow rate depends on the nature of the flow: laminar, turbulent, or a mixture of the two. In an ET, turbulent flow predominates. During turbulent flow, the measured resistance is not a constant but varies with flow rate, becoming markedly higher at high flow rates. Instead of the laminar flow relationship of pressure being directly proportional to flow, the pressure required to move the gas through an ET with turbulent flow is proportional to the square of the flow. The relationship is thus described by a parabolic curve as in Figure 6-5. The apparent resistance of a tube is proportional to the fourth power of the radius during laminar flow (Poiseuille's law) but the fifth power during turbulent flow. Assuming turbulent flow, the relative resistance of a 6-mm ET versus an

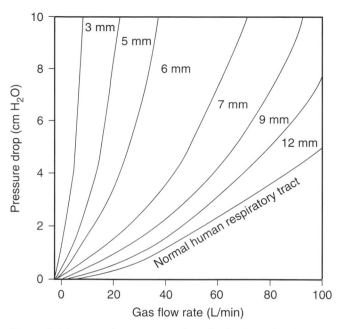

Figure 6-5 Pressure drop across endotracheal tubes of various sizes at flow rates from 0 to 100 L/min. Note the wide disparity between 6- and 7-mm tubes as flow rate increases to the range typically seen in patients with respiratory failure. (Adapted from Nunn JF: Applied Respiratory Physiology. London, Butterworths, 1987.)

8-mm ET would be $(4^5/3^5)$, or 4.2-fold as great. However, as flow patterns are not entirely predictable, exact respiratory pressure-flow relationships may not be predictable without empirical determination. Such determinations are depicted in Figure 6-5. The slope of the pressure-flow graph is the apparent resistance. The parabolic shape of the graphs demonstrates the primarily turbulent nature of the flow through an ET.

Although the resistance of the ET may be severalfold greater than the resistance of the normal human upper airway, this is of relatively little consequence at low minute ventilation.[28] With a typical peak inspiratory flow of 25 to 30 L/min, approximately 0.5 cm H_2O pressure must be generated to overcome the resistance of the upper respiratory tract. This represents approximately 10% of the total work of breathing. Even a doubling or tripling of that resistance by placement of an ET does not result in a clinically worrisome increase in the total work of breathing.[13]

As flow rates increase, however, flow becomes more turbulent and tube resistance may then become a problem. For flow rates above 15 L/min, flow through any tube less than 10 mm in diameter becomes turbulent.[67] At the high flows required by patients in respiratory failure, however, the resistance of smaller tubes becomes prohibitive.[141] At the time of weaning patients with respiratory failure from mechanical ventilation, tube size often becomes a critical factor, with a common question being whether to change from a 7- to an 8-mm ET.

As Figure 6-5 demonstrates, the difference between the two is negligible at flows below 40 L/min. At a flow of 60 L/min, however, the difference of 3 cm H_2O pressure becomes consequential. Theoretically, the patient's native airway should have less resistance than an ET of any size. However, a patient who has been intubated for an extended period of time may not have a normal upper airway. Indeed, some evidence suggests that work of breathing may actually increase after extubation, perhaps because of high upper airway resistance.[75,110] Thus, if the patient is close to successful weaning, a reasonable approach may be to attempt extubation rather than to change ETs, recognizing that the need for reintubation is a possibility. Alternatively, pressure support ventilation can be used to compensate for the added work of breathing through the smaller tube until extubation is warranted.[17]

Tracheostomy tubes have lower resistance than ETs of comparable diameters because they are shorter. However, there is little, if any, difference in the work of breathing imposed by fresh tracheostomy tubes and ETs of comparable internal diameter.[164] On the other hand, tracheostomy does appear to decrease the work of breathing in patients who have undergone prolonged intubation and mechanical ventilation. This paradox may be explained by a reduction in the internal diameter of ETs over time, perhaps related to inspissated secretions or conformational changes.[33] The latter finding may explain the observation that patients being weaned from mechanical ventilation are sometimes more rapidly weaned after a tracheostomy is performed,[31] although it may also reflect the increased comfort of clinicians in discontinuing ventilatory support when the airway is secured.

D. LOWER AIRWAY RESISTANCE

Bronchospasm after induction of anesthesia is a relatively uncommon but well-recognized event and is probably related to a reflex response to endotracheal intubation. Several studies provide some evidence regarding the frequency of bronchospasm. The American Society of Anesthesiologists closed claims study has been reviewing malpractice claims since 1985. Adverse respiratory events were involved in 762 of 2046 claims, with bronchospasm accounting for 2% of the cases.[21,25] Only half of the patients had a prior history of asthma or obstructive lung disease. Bronchospasm occurred during induction in 70% of the cases, supporting the possibility that intubation is a trigger. Tiret and coauthors studied complications at the time of induction and noted that bronchospasm accounted for 5.3% of fatal or near-fatal peri-induction complications.[160] The study with the largest denominator was reported by Olsson,[117] who reported 246 cases of bronchospasm out of a total of 136,929 for an incidence of 1.7 per 1000 patients. However, the exact number undoubtedly depends substantially on the population of patients. The incidence of malpractice claims for bronchospasm has decreased in recent years

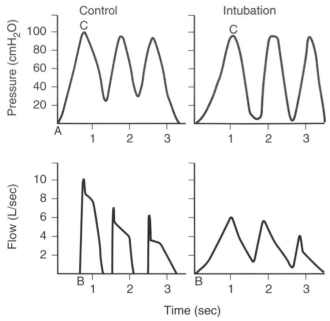

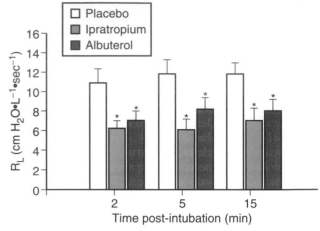

Figure 6-6 Pressure (**A**) and flow (**B**) curves generated during a burst of three successive coughs (C) by a volunteer prior to and following tracheal intubation. Note that the flow and pressures generated are only modestly diminished after intubation. (From Gal TJ: How does tracheal intubation alter respiratory mechanics. Probl Anesth 2:191, 1988.)

Figure 6-7 Lung resistance at 2, 5, and 15 minutes following intubation in patients pretreated with either a placebo, the β-adrenergic agonist albuterol, or the anticholinergic drug ipratropium bromide. Either drug markedly diminished lung resistance for at least 15 minutes after tracheal intubation under thiopental-narcotic anesthesia. (From Kil HK, Rooke GA, Ryan-Dykes MA, Bishop MJ: Effect of prophylactic bronchodilator treatment on lung resistance after tracheal intubation. Anesthesiology 81:43, 1994.)

(F. W. Cheney, personal communication), possibly because of the increasing use of propofol as an induction agent. Propofol is more effective at preventing postintubation bronchospasm than thiopental (see later).

Although the incidence of overt clinical bronchospasm is low, a reflex increase in airway resistance may occur much more often. Receptors in the larynx and upper trachea may cause large airway constriction distal to the tube, which, in turn, may extend to the smaller peripheral airways.[107] Support for this hypothesis comes from the work of Gal, who found an increase in lower airway resistance in a series of volunteers whose tracheas were intubated following topical anesthesia (Fig. 6-6).[45]

Bronchoconstriction also occurs after endotracheal intubation of healthy subjects who have received thiopental-narcotic anesthesia.[81] In a series of patients treated prior to anesthesia with either a β-adrenergic agonist (albuterol) or an inhaled anticholinergic agent (ipratropium bromide), measured airway resistance following intubation is markedly lower than in placebo-treated patients (Fig. 6-7).

Increases in airway resistance may result from changes in intrinsic smooth muscle tone, airway edema, or intraluminal secretions. These factors are, in turn, controlled by a series of intracellular and extracellular events including neural and hormonal factors. Rapid changes in airway caliber following airway instrumentation are thought to result largely from parasympathetic nervous system activation of airway smooth muscle.[14,71] Cholinergic innervation predominates in the larger central airways, with efferent nerves arising in the vagal nuclei of the brain stem and synapsing with ganglia in the airway walls. Postganglionic parasympathetic nerves release acetylcholine, activating muscarinic receptors on airway smooth muscle, which lead to smooth muscle constriction. Such responses can be blocked by muscarinic blockade, using either systemic or inhaled anticholinergic agents.

Tracheal intubation may also induce bronchospasm by causing coughing. A cough reduces lung volume, which, in turn, markedly increases bronchoconstriction in response to a stimulus.[34] In the patient with known reactive airways, preventing coughing at the time of endotracheal intubation by using either a deep level of anesthetic or a muscle relaxant may help to minimize the likelihood of bronchospasm.

E. ENDOTRACHEAL TUBE RESISTANCE AND EXHALATION

In normal patients breathing at moderately elevated minute ventilation, exhalation is usually completed well before the next inhalation begins. By contrast, patients with obstructive airway disease may not complete full exhalation prior to the start of the next inhalation. In this situation, inhalation begins before exhalation to functional residual capacity (FRC), resulting in persistent positive pressure in the alveoli. This phenomenon has been called auto-PEEP or dynamic hyperinflation and results in air trapping, elevated intrathoracic pressure, and hemodynamic compromise.[92]

Auto-PEEP most commonly occurs in patients with obstructive lung disease and high minute ventilation, but it may also rarely occur in patients with relatively normal airways who are ventilated at very high minute ventilation. This has been observed in patients with burns or sepsis, who may require as much as 30 to 40 L of minute ventilation. Under these circumstances, the resistance of the ET may limit expiratory flow so that full exhalation does not occur. This has been demonstrated experimentally, with the magnitude of the auto-PEEP correlating directly with the resistance of the ET.[138] Under anesthesia, major resistance to exhalation by the ET is of no consequence in routine cases and is only rarely seen in critically ill patients. However, low levels of auto-PEEP related to tube resistance probably occur frequently in patients with high minute ventilation[31] or during single-lung ventilation with a double-lumen ET.

F. FUNCTIONAL RESIDUAL CAPACITY

The effect of endotracheal intubation on FRC has been a subject of considerable controversy. Intensivists are well aware of patients recovering from respiratory failure in whom oxygenation has improved following extubation. The improvement has been attributed to "physiologic PEEP"—the presumption that there is normally a small positive pressure created by the glottis, which, in turn, leads to breathing at a higher lung volume. The assumption is that an ET removes the glottic barrier and may, therefore, lower lung volume. The existence of positive intratracheal pressure, however, has never been documented and, in a study of volunteers who underwent awake intubation, no consistent change in FRC could be measured.[46,47,125]

By contrast, a different conclusion was reached in a series of patients just before and after extubation following recovery from respiratory failure. In this situation, both FRC and PaO_2 were found to increase following extubation, supporting the concept that the presence of an ET tends to decrease FRC.[123] Resolution of these disparate results is suggested by a study in which normal rabbits did not demonstrate a difference in oxygenation or tracheal pressure following intubation but, after respiratory failure was induced, endotracheal intubation worsened oxygenation.[147] These results suggest that the rabbits compensated for respiratory failure by using glottic closure to maintain a positive intratracheal pressure and that the effect of an ET on FRC depends on the underlying respiratory state.

G. COUGH

Although it is widely recognized that cough efficiency is reduced whenever an ET is in place, it is a common observation that a disconnected ET is likely to produce a plug of sputum when the patient is stimulated to cough. In awake intubated volunteers, peak airway flow was reduced but still adequate to enable secretion clearance.[44] The ET, however, prevented collapse of the trachea by acting as a stent. Thus, although secretions could be moved to the central airways, the ET prevented maximum efficiency of expectoration. Large airway collapse is important for producing maximum force against secretions, and this explains why moving secretions from the trachea out through the ET often requires assistance with a suction catheter.

H. HUMIDIFICATION OF GASES

Under normal circumstances, the upper airway warms, humidifies, and filters between 7000 and 10,000 L of inspired air daily, adding up to 1 L of moisture to the gases. When the upper airway is bypassed following intubation, the gas must be warmed and humidified in the trachea if it is not adequately humidified prior to inhalation. In an anesthetized patient breathing dry gases, up to 10% of the average metabolic rate may be required to perform these tasks.[10] Delivery of cool, dry gases may also have a significant effect on mucociliary transport, a critical defense mechanism of the respiratory tract. Inhalation of unconditioned gas rapidly leads to abnormal mucosal ciliary motion, with subsequent encrustation and inspissation of tracheal secretions.[22,85] These changes occur as early as 30 minutes after intubation and, theoretically, may lead to an increase in postoperative complications in patients with limited chest excursion. Accordingly, assurance of adequate gas conditioning should be standard in all but very brief endotracheal intubations.

V. CONTROL AND TREATMENT OF THE RESPIRATORY RESPONSES TO AIRWAY INSTRUMENTATION

A. PREVENTING UPPER AIRWAY RESPONSES

Cough and laryngospasm in response to intubation appear to be sound protective reflexes by the body. Under most circumstances, the body needs to prevent further intrusion by a foreign body and to expel it from the airway. These responses can be troublesome, however, during induction of anesthesia or at the time of extubation. Cough can lead to bronchospasm as lung volume is reduced and can also result in desaturation as the lung volume drops to residual volume. Laryngospasm may result in life-threatening abnormalities of blood gases. Consequently, the anesthesiologist routinely tries to prevent these responses using medications delivered topically, by inhalation, or intravenously.

Inhibition of upper airway reflexes can certainly be accomplished by performing endotracheal intubation after the administration of neuromuscular blocking agents. However, both laryngeal and tracheal reflexes are difficult to inhibit by deep levels of general anesthesia alone.[112] Thus, when circumstances preclude the use of neuromuscular blockade, the clinician must give consideration to how best to prevent discomfort, gagging, coughing, and laryngospasm during endotracheal intubation, through either avoidance of endotracheal intubation, the use of regional and topical anesthesia, very deep general anesthesia, or a combination of all modalities.

1. Technical Considerations: Minimizing Airway Stimulation

Although placement of the LMA is likely to be less noxious than direct laryngoscopy and endotracheal intubation, it remains a highly stimulating procedure. For example, Scanlon and colleagues found a 60% incidence of gagging, 30% incidence of laryngospasm, and 19% incidence of coughing when the LMA was placed after induction with thiopental 5 mg/kg.[134] Induction with propofol 2.5 mg/kg reduced these events by about two thirds but did not ablate them. Thus, instrumentation of the upper airway by any technique elicits protective reflexes that must be obtunded with local or general anesthesia, or both.

2. Regional and Topical Anesthesia

The surfaces of the mouth and nose are easily anesthetized with topical anesthetic sprays or gels. Lidocaine is as effective as cocaine and less toxic and can be combined with a vasoconstrictor to give equivalent intubating conditions.[55,59,139] Administration of an antisialagogue 30 to 60 minutes before application of the topical anesthetic results in better anesthesia as well as better intubating conditions. The lack of secretions probably minimizes dilution of the applied anesthetic and also results in better intubating conditions.

The mouth and pharynx derive their sensory innervation from the trigeminal and glossopharyngeal nerves. The supraglottic larynx derives its sensory innervation from the superior laryngeal nerve, a branch of the vagus, and intubation can be facilitated by blocking it bilaterally.[56] The nerve block relies on the consistent relationship of the superior laryngeal nerve to the lateral horns of the hyoid bone. When combined with topical anesthesia of the nose or mouth and adequate anesthesia of the infraglottic larynx, the nerve block provides excellent intubating conditions and most patients accept a tube without cough, gag, or laryngospasm. Despite the success of this block, equal success in blunting upper airway reflexes can be achieved by careful spraying of the larynx with topical anesthesia. A nasal trumpet helps ensure that solution reaches the larynx. Topical anesthesia spares the patient two injections.

The infraglottic larynx derives sensory innervation from the recurrent laryngeal nerves, which run along the posterolateral surfaces of the trachea. Again, topical anesthesia rather than nerve block is the method of choice for obtunding reflexes. Injection of several milliliters of 4% lidocaine through the cricothyroid membrane routinely results in excellent blockade of sensation.

The efficacy of topical and nerve block anesthesia at suppressing airway reflexes during intubation is evident. Several studies document that topical anesthesia applied preoperatively (for brief cases) or intraoperatively can suppress cough and laryngospasm at the time of extubation.[163] A randomized study of patients undergoing tonsillectomy found that the incidence of stridor or laryngospasm at the time of extubation could be reduced from 12% to 3% by application of topical lidocaine at the time of intubation.[149] The LITA endotracheal tube (Laryngotracheal Instillation of Topical Anesthetic, Sheridan Corp, Argyle, NY) contains a small channel that can be used to spray the upper airway while an ETT is in place. Using this method to spray the ETT prior to extubation, coughs were reduced by more than 60% and the severity of the coughing decreased.[54]

3. Intravenous Agents

Given a high enough dose, virtually all agents used as IV anesthetics suppress the cough response to intubation. However, different agents appear to vary in their ability to inhibit upper airway reflexes when judged on the basis of equal potency in depressing consciousness and in depressing the cardiovascular system. Propofol-narcotic anesthesia may be adequate for intubating the trachea in some patients[136] even without the use of muscle relaxants. On the other hand, ketamine clinically appears to enhance laryngeal reflexes at doses that provide adequate anesthesia for surgery.

IV lidocaine is frequently used to prevent cough or laryngospasm, or both, at the time of intubation or extubation. Although the studies are not uniform in documenting efficacy, the preponderance of evidence supports the use of lidocaine.[151,170] Studies that did not document efficacy are sometimes flawed by the lack of documentation that adequate serum levels were reached. The maximal efficacy of IV lidocaine occurs 1 to 3 minutes after injection and requires a dose of 1.5 mg/kg or greater. This corresponded to a plasma level in excess of 4 g/mL.

The ability of IV lidocaine to suppress cough appears to be due to factors beyond induction of general anesthesia because cough suppression occurs at levels routinely seen in awake patients being treated with the drug. A comparison of the antitussive effects of lidocaine compared with meperidine and thiopental demonstrated that severe respiratory depression occurs with the latter drugs to achieve the same antitussive efficacy that can be achieved with lidocaine with virtually no respiratory depression.[150]

Whether IV lidocaine suppresses laryngospasm remains controversial. A study in which tonsillectomy patients were given 2 mg/kg IV lidocaine and then extubated 1 minute later found suppression of laryngospasm.[5] Another study of tonsillectomy patients given 1.5 mg/kg found no clear effect.[89] A major difference in the latter study was the authors' design of not extubating the patient until swallowing had begun. Thus, there may have been a significant difference in the anesthetic depth at which the children were extubated.

B. PREVENTING BRONCHOCONSTRICTION

Following endotracheal intubation, bronchoconstriction appears to result routinely. As noted earlier, in healthy subjects it appears to be of moderate degree. However, the exaggerated response seen in patients with hyperactive airways may be life threatening. Prevention or treatment of this response can be performed using topical or IV agents. Inhaled anesthetic agents also inhibit the response, whether because of direct absorption by smooth muscle or by inhibition of reflexes.

Bronchospasm after intubation may be cholinergically mediated. Afferent parasympathetic fibers travel to bronchial smooth muscle and then result in bronchoconstriction by stimulation of the M_3 cholinergic receptors on bronchial smooth muscle. Following release of acetylcholine at the M_3 receptor, the acetylcholine stimulates the M_3 muscarinic receptor, which is an inhibitory receptor that limits further release of acetylcholine. Alterations of M_2 receptor function may contribute to bronchospasm by interfering with this feedback loop.

1. Technical Considerations: Minimizing Airway Stimulation

Avoidance of endotracheal intubation is the most logical first step in terms of limiting airway irritation and bronchoconstriction. If general anesthesia is required, the LMA may be preferable to the ET in terms provocation of bronchospasm, but as alluded to earlier, the LMA does not prevent coughing in the absence of neuromuscular blockade.[134] However, the LMA does appear to result in reduced lower airway resistance when compared with intubation after induction of general anesthesia.[9,82] This difference is assumed to be due to induction of reversible bronchospasm by the ET.[9,82] In addition, use of the LMA resulted in fewer pulmonary complications and improved pulmonary function when compared with endotracheal intubation in former premature infants with bronchopulmonary dysplasia[39] and adults without lung disease.[109]

2. Topical Anesthesia

The studies of Gal and Suratt[47] demonstrated a doubling of lower airway resistance following endotracheal intubation of awake volunteers under topical anesthesia. The bronchoconstrictive response must indeed be a powerful one if local anesthesia sufficient to permit volunteers to be intubated was not sufficient to prevent the reflex bronchoconstriction. A study of awake fiberoptic intubation in asthmatics demonstrated a marked decrease in forced expiratory volume in 1 second (FEV_1) after intubation.

This decrease was somewhat mitigated by topical lidocaine, although lidocaine was not as effective as albuterol in preventing the bronchoconstriction.[57] However, a lidocaine aerosol given to dogs prior to a challenge with inhaled citric acid did not attenuate the response to this irritant.[37] The aerosol itself produces a slight increase in lung resistance, and the efficacy of the inhaled aerosol lidocaine may be due in part to IV absorption of the drug. Given these considerations and the time required to administer the aerosol compared with the immediacy and efficacy of IV drugs or other inhaled drugs, aerosolized lidocaine is probably a poor choice for the attenuation of bronchoconstriction associated with endotracheal intubation.

3. Intravenous Agents

A variety of drugs have been studied for their bronchodilating properties. Although IV β-agonists clearly produce bronchodilation, there is no benefit from parenteral administration of these drugs rather than inhalational administration. Among anesthetic induction agents, considerable experimental evidence suggests that ketamine has both direct and indirect relaxant effects on airway smooth muscle through non–β-receptor mechanisms.[18,20,68,73,120,132] However, the clinical data supporting the use of ketamine for the prevention or treatment of bronchospasm are largely anecdotal[131] or in more rigorous trials unimpressive.[66,74,88] This may be related to reluctance to use ketamine at high doses routinely because of its side effects, including dysphoria and sympathetic stimulation, rather than a lack of benefit of the drug.

Propofol, midazolam, and etomidate all relax airway smooth muscle in vitro, although generally at higher site concentrations than would be used clinically.[26,62,95,118,121] In contrast, barbiturates may have direct bronchoconstricting effects.[119] Propofol may also have indirect effects on airway constriction, perhaps through inhibition of vagal tone.[18,70] Clinically, propofol has been shown to be superior to the barbiturates and etomidate in reducing wheezing and airway resistance in both asthmatic and nonasthmatic subjects.[38,122,168] When asthmatic subjects were induced with thiopental, methohexital, or propofol at equipotent doses, none of the asthmatic patients wheezed after endotracheal intubation if propofol was used, whereas both of the barbiturates were associated with a significant incidence of wheezing (Fig. 6-8).[122]

IV lidocaine administered to dogs at blood levels of 1.5 to 2.5 μg/mL substantially inhibited the response to an irritative citric acid aerosol.[36] In human subjects with bronchial hyperreactivity, IV lidocaine reduced the bronchoconstrictor response to histamine challenge and had an additive effect with albuterol in reducing this response.[58] However, a double-blind, placebo-controlled trial of IV lidocaine (1.5 mg/kg) or inhaled albuterol in asthmatics found that albuterol but not lidocaine prevented postintubation bronchoconstriction.[93]

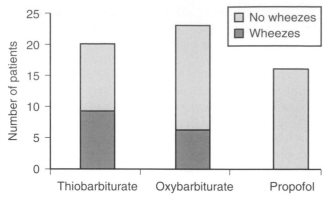

Figure 6-8 Incidence of wheezing following tracheal intubation in asthmatics when induction is performed with either an oxybarbiturate, a thiobarbiturate, or propofol ($P < .05$ for either thiobarbiturate or oxybarbiturate versus propofol). (From Pizow R, Brown RH, Weiss YS, et al: Wheezing during induction of general anesthesia in patients with and without asthma. A randomized, blinded trial. Anesthesiology 81:1111, 1995.)

A combination of the two agents was not studied. Thus, the utility of IV lidocaine in preventing postintubation bronchospasm is not clear, but it appears to be of little benefit when used without the concomitant administration of an inhaled β-agonist.

The role of theophylline in preventing the bronchoconstrictive response to endotracheal intubation has not been studied. However, in most studies of the treatment of patients with bronchospasm, theophylline appeared to add little to inhaled β-agonists, nor did it supplement the bronchodilating effects of inhaled halothane.[161]

4. Inhaled Agents

All of the volatile anesthetics have direct and perhaps indirect relaxant effects on airway smooth muscle in experimental models.[16,72,94,103,165] Although differences in the potency of these agents are present in vitro, the clinical importance of these differences is unclear.[19,94,165] In adult patients, sevoflurane was more effective than isoflurane, desflurane, and halothane in reducing airway

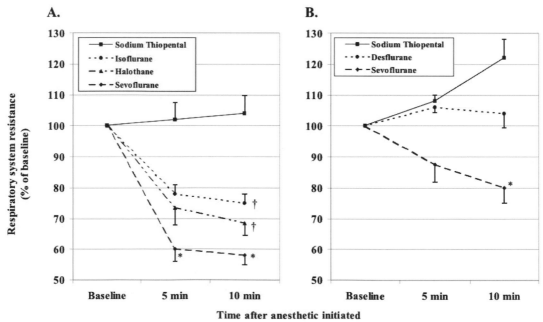

Figure 6-9 Respiratory system resistance (percent of baseline) during maintenance anesthesia. **A,** Isoflurane, halothane, or sevoflurane compared with thiopental 0.25 mg/kg/min plus 50% nitrous oxide. *$P < .05$ versus isoflurane, halothane, and thiopental. †$P < .05$ versus thiopental. **B,** Desflurane or sevoflurane compared with thiopental 0.25 mg/kg/min. *$P < .05$ versus desflurane and thiopental. (**A,** Adapted from Rooke GA, Choi JH, Bishop MJ: The effect of isoflurane, halothane, sevoflurane, and thiopental/ nitrous oxide on respiratory system resistance after tracheal intubation. Anesthesiology 86:1294, 1997; **B,** from Goff MJ, Arain SR, Ficke DJ, et al: Absence of bronchodilation during desflurane anesthesia: A comparison to sevoflurane and thiopental. Anesthesiology 93:404, 2000.)

resistance after endotracheal intubation,[52,127] but it did not prevent an increase in airway resistance after intubation of asthmatic children.[61] However, given the available data, sevoflurane is probably the volatile agent of choice and desflurane a poor choice for use in high-risk patients (Fig. 6-9).

There are no prospective, controlled studies comparing deep inhalation anesthesia with IV induction with bronchoprotective agents such as ketamine or propofol in high-risk patients. Achieving a deep plane of anesthesia with a bronchoprotective agent prior to intubation is probably the most important point in preventing severe bronchospasm in high-risk patients rather than the choice of IV versus inhalation induction techniques.

Pretreatment of patients with either inhaled β_2-adrenergic agonists or an inhaled anticholinergic markedly reduced lung resistance following endotracheal intubation[81,133] and should be used routinely in patients known to have bronchospasm.

5. Choice of Neuromuscular Blocking Drug

The choice of muscle relaxants can influence bronchial tone after endotracheal intubation. Rapacuronium was withdrawn from the market after a number of reports of severe bronchospasm, most likely related to antagonism at the M_2 receptor.[76] Mivacurium releases significant amounts of histamine and leads to mast cell degranulation and should be used extremely cautiously if at all in patients with a history of atopy or asthma.[12] Studies in France and Norway have suggested a high incidence of anaphylaxis with rocuronium, although this does not appear to be supported in literature from other countries.

REFERENCES

1. Abou-Madi M, Keszler H, Yacoub J: Cardiovascular reactions to laryngoscopy and tracheal intubation following small and large intravenous doses of lidocaine. Can Anaesth Soc J 24:12, 1977.
2. Ali HH, Lien CA, Witkowski T, et al: Efficacy and safety of divided dose administration of mivacurium for a 90-second tracheal intubation. J Clin Anesth 8:276, 1996.
3. Atlee JL, Dhamee MS, Olund TL, George V: The use of esmolol, nicardipine, or their combination to blunt hemodynamic changes after laryngoscopy and tracheal intubation. Anesth Analg 90:280, 2000.
4. Ausems ME, Hug CC Jr, Stanski DR, Burm AG: Plasma concentrations of alfentanil required to supplement nitrous oxide anesthesia for general surgery. Anesthesiology 65:362, 1986.
5. Baraka A: Intravenous lidocaine controls extubation laryngospasm in children. Anesth Analg 57:506, 1978.
6. Bedford R: Intracranial pressure response to endotracheal intubation: Efficacy of intravenous lidocaine pretreatment for patients with brain tumors. In Shulman K, Marmarou A, Miller JD, et al (eds): Intracranial Pressure IV. New York, Springer-Verlag, 1980, pp 595-598.
7. Bedford R, Marshall W: Cardiovascular response to endotracheal intubation during four anesthetic techniques. Acta Anaesthesiol Scand 28:563, 1984.
8. Bedford R, Persing JA, Pobereskin L, Butler A: Lidocaine or thiopental for rapid control of intracranial hypertension? Anesth Analg 58:435, 1980.
9. Berry A, Brimacombe J, Keller C, Verghese C: Pulmonary airway resistance with the endotracheal tube versus laryngeal mask airway in paralyzed anesthetized adult patients. Anesthesiology 90:395, 1999.
10. Bickler P, Sessler D: Efficiency of airway heat and moisture exchangers in anesthetized humans. Anesth Analg 71:415, 1990.
11. Billard V, Moulla F, Bourgain JL, et al: Hemodynamic response to induction and intubation. Propofol/fentanyl interaction. Anesthesiology 81:1384, 1994.
12. Bishop MJ, O'Donnell JT, Salemi JR: Mivacurium and bronchospasm. Anesth Analg 97:484, 2003.
13. Bolder PM, Healy TE, Bolder AR, et al: The extra work of breathing through adult endotracheal tubes. Anesth Analg 65:853, 1986.
14. Boushey HA, Holtzman MJ, Sheller JR, Nadel JA: Bronchial hyperreactivity. Am Rev Respir Dis 121:89, 1980.
15. Braude N, Clements EA, Hodges UM, Andrews BP: The pressor response and laryngeal mask insertion. A comparison with tracheal intubation. Anaesthesia 44:551, 1989.
16. Brichant JF, Gunst SJ, Warner DO, Rehder K: Halothane, enflurane, and isoflurane depress the peripheral vagal motor pathway in isolated canine tracheal smooth muscle. Anesthesiology 74:325, 1991.
17. Brochard L, Rua F, Lorino H, et al: Inspiratory pressure support compensates for the additional work of breathing caused by the endotracheal tube. Anesthesiology 75:739, 1991.
18. Brown RH, Wagner EM: Mechanisms of bronchoprotection by anesthetic induction agents: Propofol versus ketamine. Anesthesiology 90:822, 1999.
19. Brown RH, Zerhouni EA, Hirshman CA: Comparison of low concentrations of halothane and isoflurane as bronchodilators. Anesthesiology 78:1097, 1993.
20. Cabanas A, Souhrada JF, Aldrete JA: Effects of ketamine and halothane on normal and asthmatic smooth muscle of the airway in guinea pigs. Can Anaesth Soc J 27:47, 1980.
21. Caplan RA, Posner KL, Ward RJ, Cheney FW: Adverse respiratory events in anesthesia: A closed claims analysis. Anesthesiology 72:828, 1990.
22. Casthely P, Chalon J: Tracheobronchial cytologic changes during prolonged cannulation. Anesth Analg 59:759, 1980.
23. Cavo J, Ogura JH, Sessions DG, Nelson JR: Flow resistance in tracheotomy tubes. Ann Otol Rhinol Laryngol 82:827, 1973.
24. Chen C: Fentanyl dosage for suppression of circulatory response to laryngoscopy and endotracheal intubation. Anesthesiol Rev 13:37, 1986.

25. Cheney FW, Posner KL, Caplan RA: Adverse respiratory events infrequently leading to malpractice suits. A closed claims analysis. Anesthesiology 75:932, 1991.

26. Cheng EY, Mazzeo AJ, Bosnjak ZJ, et al: Direct relaxant effects of intravenous anesthetics on airway smooth muscle. Anesth Analg 83:162, 1996.

27. Choyce A, Avidan MS, Harvey A, et al: The cardiovascular response to insertion of the intubating laryngeal mask airway. Anaesthesia 57:330, 2002.

28. Colgan F, Lian J, Borrow R: Non-invasive assessment by capacitance respirometry of respiration before and after extubation. Anesth Analg 54:807, 1975.

29. Cullen J: An evaluation of tracheostomy in pulmonary emphysema. Ann Intern Med 58:953, 1963.

30. Davies MJ, Cronin K, Cowie R: The prevention of hypertension at intubation. A controlled study of intravenous hydralazine on patients undergoing intracranial surgery. Anaesthesia 36:147, 1981.

31. Davis K Jr, Campbell RS, Johannigman JA, et al: Changes in respiratory mechanics after tracheostomy. Arch Surg 134:59, 1999.

32. DeVault M, Greifenstein F, Harris LJ: Circulatory responses to endotracheal intubation in light general anesthesia—The effect of atropine and phentolamine. Anesthesiology 21:360, 1960.

33. Diehl JL, El Atrous S, Touchard D, et al: Changes in the work of breathing induced by tracheotomy in ventilator-dependent patients. Am J Respir Crit Care Med 159:383, 1999.

34. Ding D, Martin J, Macklem P: Effects of lung volume on maximal methacholine-induced bronchoconstrictions in normal humans. J Appl Physiol 62:1324, 1987.

35. Dohi S, Gold M: Pulmonary mechanics during general anesthesia. Br J Anaesth 51:205, 1979.

36. Downes H, Gerber N, Hirshman C: I.V. lignocaine in reflex and allergic bronchoconstriction. Br J Anaesth 52:873, 1980.

37. Downes H, Hirshman CA: Lidocaine aerosols do not prevent allergic bronchoconstriction. Anesth Analg 60:28, 1981.

38. Eames WO, Rooke GA, Wu RS, Bishop MJ: Comparison of the effects of etomidate, propofol, and thiopental on respiratory resistance after tracheal intubation. Anesthesiology 84:1307, 1996.

39. Ferrari LR, Goudsouzian NG: The use of the laryngeal mask airway in children with bronchopulmonary dysplasia. Anesth Analg 81:310, 1995.

40. Finfer S, MacKenzie SI, Saddler JM, Watkins TG: Cardiovascular responses to tracheal intubation: A comparison of direct laryngoscopy and fiberoptic intubation. Anaesth Intensive Care 17:44, 1989.

41. Fox EJ, Sklar GS, Hill CH, et al: Complications related to the pressor response to endotracheal intubation. Anesthesiology 47:524, 1977.

42. Fujii Y, Kihara S, Takahashi S, et al: Calcium channel blockers attenuate cardiovascular responses to tracheal extubation in hypertensive patients. Can J Anaesth 45:655, 1998.

43. Fujii Y, Saitoh Y, Takahashi S, Toyooka H: Diltiazem-lidocaine combination for the attenuation of cardiovascular responses to tracheal intubation in hypertensive patients. Can J Anaesth 45:933, 1998.

44. Gal T: Effects of endotracheal intubation on normal cough performance. Anesthesiology 52:324, 1980.

45. Gal T: Pulmonary mechanics in normal subjects following endotracheal intubation. Anesthesiology 52:27, 1980.

46. Gal T, Arora N: Respiratory mechanics in supine subjects during progressive partial curarization. J Appl Physiol 52:57, 1982.

47. Gal T, Suratt P: Resistance to breathing in healthy subjects after endotracheal intubation under topical anesthesia. Anesthesiology 59:270, 1980.

48. Gallagher JD, Moore RA, Jose AB, et al: Prophylactic nitroglycerin infusions during coronary artery bypass surgery. Anesthesiology 64:785, 1986.

49. Ghignone M, Quintin L, Duke PC, et al: Effects of clonidine on narcotic requirements and hemodynamic response during induction of fentanyl anesthesia and endotracheal intubation. Anesthesiology 64:36, 1986.

50. Giffin JP, Cottrell JE, Shwiry B, et al: Intracranial pressure, mean arterial pressure, and heart rate following midazolam or thiopental in humans with brain tumors. Anesthesiology 60:491, 1984.

51. Glass PS, Hardman D, Kamiyama Y, et al: Preliminary pharmacokinetics and pharmacodynamics of an ultra-short-acting opioid: Remifentanil (gi87084b). Anesth Analg 77:1031, 1993.

52. Goff MJ, Arain SR, Ficke DJ, et al: Absence of bronchodilation during desflurane anesthesia: A comparison to sevoflurane and thiopental. Anesthesiology 93:404, 2000.

53. Gold MI, Brown M, Coverman S, Herrington C: Heart rate and blood pressure effects of esmolol after ketamine induction and intubation. Anesthesiology 64:718, 1986.

54. Gonzalez RM, Bjerke RJ, Drobycki T, et al: Prevention of endotracheal tube-induced coughing during emergence from general anesthesia. Anesth Analg 79:792, 1994.

55. Goodell J, Gilroy G, Huntress J: Reducing cocaine solution use by promoting the use of a lidocaine-phenylephrine solution. Am J Hosp Pharm 45:2510, 1988.

56. Gotta A, Sullivan C: Anaesthesia of the upper airway using topical anaesthetic and superior laryngeal nerve block. Br J Anaesth 53:1055, 1981.

57. Groeben H, Schlicht M, Stieglitz S, et al: Both local anesthetics and salbutamol pretreatment affect reflex bronchoconstriction in volunteers with asthma undergoing awake fiberoptic intubation. Anesthesiology 97:1445, 2002.

58. Groeben H, Silvanus MT, Beste M, Peters J: Combined intravenous lidocaine and inhaled salbutamol protect against bronchial hyperreactivity more effectively than lidocaine or salbutamol alone. Anesthesiology 89:862, 1998.

59. Gross J, Hartigan M, Schaffer D: A suitable substitute for 4% cocaine before blind nasotracheal intubation: 3% lidocaine–0.25% phenylephrine nasal spray. Anesth Analg 63:915, 1984.

60. Habib M: Physiologic implications of artificial airways. Chest 96:180, 1989.

61. Habre W, Scalfaro P, Sims C, et al: Respiratory mechanics during sevoflurane anesthesia in children with and without asthma. Anesth Analg 89:1177, 1999.

62. Hashiba E, Sato T, Hirota K, et al: The relaxant effect of propofol on guinea pig tracheal muscle is independent of airway epithelial function and beta-adrenoceptor activity. Anesth Analg 89:191, 1999.

63. Hassan HG, el-Sharkawy TY, Renck H, et al: Hemodynamic and catecholamine responses to laryngoscopy with vs. without endotracheal intubation. Acta Anaesthesiol Scand 35:442, 1991.

64. Hawkyard SJ, Morrison A, Doyle LA, et al: Attenuating the hypertensive response to laryngoscopy and endotracheal intubation using awake fibreoptic intubation. Acta Anaesthesiol Scand 36:1, 1992.

65. Heier T, Caldwell JE: Rapid tracheal intubation with large-dose rocuronium: A probability-based approach. Anesth Analg 90:175, 2000.

66. Hemmingsen C, Nielsen PK, Odorico J: Ketamine in the treatment of bronchospasm during mechanical ventilation. Am J Emerg Med 12:417, 1994.

67. Hill D: Properties of liquids, gases and vapours. Physics Applied to Anaesthesia, 4th ed. London, Butterworth, 1980, p 174.

68. Hill GE, Anderson JL, Whitten CW: Ketamine inhibits agonist-induced cAMP accumulation increase in human airway smooth muscle cells. Can J Anaesth 46:1172, 1999.

69. Himes RJ, DiFazio C, Burney R: Effects of lidocaine on the anesthetic requirements for nitrous oxide and halothane. Anesthesiology 47:437, 1977.

70. Hirota K, Sato T, Hashimoto Y, et al: Relaxant effect of propofol on the airway in dogs. Br J Anaesth 83:292, 1999.

71. Hirshman C: Airway reactivity in humans. Anesthesiology 58:170, 1983.

72. Hirshman C, Bergman M: Factors influencing intrapulmonary airway calibre during anaesthesia. Br J Anaesth 65:30, 1990.

73. Hirshman CA, Downes H, Farbood A, Bergman NA: Ketamine block of bronchospasm in experimental canine asthma. Br J Anaesth 51:713, 1979.

74. Howton JC, Rose J, Duffy S, et al: Randomized, double-blind, placebo-controlled trial of intravenous ketamine in acute asthma. Ann Emerg Med 27:170, 1996.

75. Ishaaya AM, Nathan SD, Belman MJ: Work of breathing after extubation. Chest 107:204, 1995.

76. Jooste E, Klafter F, Hirshman CA, Emala CW: A mechanism for rapacuronium-induced bronchospasm: M2 muscarinic receptor antagonism. Anesthesiology 98:906, 2003.

77. Kapila A, Glass PS, Jacobs JR, et al: Measured context-sensitive half-times of remifentanil and alfentanil. Anesthesiology 83:968, 1995.

78. Kasten GW, Owens E: Evaluation of lidocaine as an adjunct to fentanyl anesthesia for coronary artery bypass graft surgery. Anesth Analg 65:511, 1986.

79. Kautto H: Attenuation of the circulatory response to laryngoscopy and intubation by fentanyl. Acta Anaesth Scand 26:217, 1982.

80. Kil HK, Bishop MJ: Head position and oral vs nasal route as factors determining endotracheal tube resistance. Chest 105:1794, 1994.

81. Kil HK, Rooke GA, Ryan-Dykes MA, Bishop MJ: Effect of prophylactic bronchodilator treatment on lung resistance after tracheal intubation. Anesthesiology 81:43, 1994.

82. Kim ES, Bishop MJ: Endotracheal intubation, but not laryngeal mask airway insertion, produces reversible bronchoconstriction. Anesthesiology 90:391, 1999.

83. Kimura T, Watanabe S, Asakura N, et al: Determination of end-tidal sevoflurane concentration for tracheal intubation and minimum alveolar anesthetic concentration in adults. Anesth Analg 79:378, 1994.

84. King B: Reflex circulatory responses to direct laryngoscopy and tracheal intubation performed during general anesthesia. Anesthesiology 12:556, 1951.

85. Klainer A, Turndorf H: Surface alterations due to endotracheal intubation. Am J Med 58:674, 1975.

86. Kovarik WD, Mayberg TS, Lam AM, et al: Succinylcholine does not change intracranial pressure, cerebral blood flow velocity, or the electroencephalogram in patients with neurologic injury. Anesth Analg 78:469, 1994.

87. Lanier W, Milde J, Michenfelder J: Cerebral stimulation following succinylcholine in dogs. Anesthesiology 64:551, 1986.

88. Lau TT, Zed PJ: Does ketamine have a role in managing severe exacerbation of asthma in adults? Pharmacotherapy 21:1100, 2001.

89. Leicht P, Wisborg T, Chraemmer-Jorgensen B: Does intravenous lidocaine prevent laryngospasm after extubation in children? Anesth Analg 64:1193, 1985.

90. Loeb HS, Saudye A, Croke RP, et al: Effects of pharmacologically-induced hypertension on myocardial ischemia and coronary hemodynamics in patients with fixed coronary obstruction. Circulation 57:41, 1978.

91. Maguire AM, Kumar N, Parker JL, et al: Comparison of effects of remifentanil and alfentanil on cardiovascular response to tracheal intubation in hypertensive patients. Br J Anaesth 86:90, 2001.

92. Marini J, Pepe P: Occult positive end-expiratory pressure in mechanically ventilated patients with airflow obstruction. Am Rev Respir Dis 126:166, 1982.

93. Maslow AD, Regan MM, Israel E, et al: Inhaled albuterol, but not intravenous lidocaine, protects against intubation-induced bronchoconstriction in asthma. Anesthesiology 93:1198, 2000.

94. Mazzeo AJ, Cheng EY, Bosnjak ZJ, et al: Differential effects of desflurane and halothane on peripheral airway smooth muscle. Br J Anaesth 76:841, 1996.

95. Mehr EH, Lindeman KS: Effects of halothane, propofol, and thiopental on peripheral airway reactivity. Anesthesiology 79:290, 1993.

96. Mi WD, Sakai T, Takahashi S, Matsuki A: Haemodynamic and electroencephalograph responses to intubation during induction with propofol or propofol/fentanyl. Can J Anaesth 45:19, 1998.

97. Mikawa K, Nishina K, Maekawa N, Obara H: Comparison of nicardipine, diltiazem and verapamil for controlling the cardiovascular responses to tracheal intubation. Br J Anaesth 76:221, 1996.

98. Mikawa K, Nishina K, Maekawa N, et al: Attenuation of the catecholamine response to tracheal intubation with oral clonidine in children. Can J Anaesth 42:869, 1995.

99. Miller CD, Warren SJ: IV lignocaine fails to attenuate the cardiovascular response to laryngoscopy and tracheal intubation. Br J Anaesth 65:216, 1990.

100. Miller DR, Martineau RJ, Wynands JE, Hill J: Bolus administration of esmolol for controlling the haemodynamic response to tracheal intubation: The Canadian Multicentre Trial. Can J Anaesth 38:849, 1991.

101. Minton MD, Grosslight K, Stirt JA, Bedford RF: Increases in intracranial pressure from succinylcholine: Prevention by prior nondepolarizing blockade. Anesthesiology 65:165, 1986.

102. Mirakhur R: Bradycardia with laryngeal spraying in children. Acta Anaesth Scand 26:130, 1982.

103. Mitsuhata H, Saitoh J, Shimizu R, et al: Sevoflurane and isoflurane protect against bronchospasm in dogs. Anesthesiology 81:1230, 1994.

104. Modica PA, Tempelhoff R: Intracranial pressure during induction of anaesthesia and tracheal intubation with etomidate-induced EEG burst suppression. Can J Anaesth 39:236, 1992.

105. Mori K, Iwabuchi K, Fujita M: The effects of depolarizing muscle relaxants on the electroencephalogram and the circulation during halothane anaesthesia in man. Br J Anaesth 45:604, 1973.

106. Moss E, Powell D, Gibson RM, McDowall DG: Effects of tracheal intubation on intracranial pressure following induction of anaesthesia with thiopentone or althesin in patients undergoing neurosurgery. Br J Anaesth 50:353, 1978.

107. Nadel J: Mechanisms controlling airway size. Arch Environ Health 158:179, 1963.

108. Nadel J, Widdicombe J: Reflex effects of upper airway irritation on total lung resistance and blood pressure. J Appl Physiol 17:861, 1962.

109. Natalini G, Franceschetti ME, Pletti C, et al: Impact of laryngeal mask airway and tracheal tube on pulmonary function during the early postoperative period. Acta Anaesthesiol Scand 46:525, 2002.

110. Nathan SD, Ishaaya AM, Koerner SK, Belman MJ: Prediction of minimal pressure support during weaning from mechanical ventilation. Chest 103:1215, 1993.

111. Nishina K, Mikawa K, Shiga M, et al: Oral clonidine premedication reduces minimum alveolar concentration of sevoflurane for tracheal intubation in children. Anesthesiology 87:1324, 1997.

112. Nishino T, Kochi T, Ishii M: Differences in respiratory reflex responses from the larynx, trachea, and bronchi in anesthetized female subjects. Anesthesiology 84:70, 1996.

113. Nishiyama T, Higashizawa T, Bito H, et al: [Which laryngoscope is the most stressful in laryngoscopy; Macintosh, Miller, or McCoy?]. Masui 46:1519, 1997.

114. Nunn J, Campbell E, Peckett B: Anatomical subdivisions of the volume of respiratory dead space and effect of position of the jaw. J Appl Physiol 14:174, 1959.

115. Oczenski W, Krenn H, Dahaba AA, et al: Hemodynamic and catecholamine stress responses to insertion of the Combitube, laryngeal mask airway or tracheal intubation. Anesth Analg 88:1389, 1999.

116. O'Hare R, McAtamney D, Mirakhur RK, et al: Bolus dose remifentanil for control of haemodynamic response to tracheal intubation during rapid sequence induction of anaesthesia. Br J Anaesth 82:283, 1999.

117. Olsson G: Bronchospasm during anaesthesia. A computer-aided incidence study of 136,929 patients. Acta Anaesthesiol Scand 31:244, 1987.

118. Ouedraogo N, Marthan R, Roux E: The effects of propofol and etomidate on airway contractility in chronically hypoxic rats. Anesth Analg 96:1035, table of contents, 2003.

119. Ouedraogo N, Roux E, Forestier F, et al: Effects of intravenous anesthetics on normal and passively sensitized human isolated airway smooth muscle. Anesthesiology 88:317, 1998.

120. Pabelick CM, Jones KA, Street K, et al: Calcium concentration-dependent mechanisms through which ketamine relaxes canine airway smooth muscle. Anesthesiology 86:1104, 1997.

121. Pedersen CM, Thirstrup S, Nielsen-Kudsk JE: Smooth muscle relaxant effects of propofol and ketamine in isolated guinea-pig trachea. Eur J Pharmacol 238:75, 1993.

122. Pizov R, Brown RH, Weiss YS, et al: Wheezing during induction of general anesthesia in patients with and without asthma. A randomized, blinded trial. Anesthesiology 82:1111, 1995.

123. Quan S, Falltrick R, Schlobohm R: Extubation from ambient or expiratory positive airway pressure in adults. Anesthesiology 55:53, 1984.

124. Ravussin P, Guinard JP, Ralley F, Thorin D: Effect of propofol on cerebrospinal fluid pressure and cerebral perfusion pressure in patients undergoing craniotomy. Anaesthesia 43(Suppl):37, 1988.

125. Rodenstein D, Stanescue D, Francis C: Demonstration of failure of body plethysmography in airway obstruction. Appl Physiol 52:949, 1982.

126. Roizen MF, Horrigan R, Frazer B: Anesthetic doses that block adrenergic (stress) and cardiovascular responses to incision–MAC BAR. Anesthesiology 54:390, 1981.

127. Rooke GA, Choi JH, Bishop MJ: The effect of isoflurane, halothane, sevoflurane, and thiopental/nitrous oxide on respiratory system resistance after tracheal intubation. Anesthesiology 86:1294, 1997.

128. Rovenstine E, Papper E: Glossopharyngeal nerve block. Am J Surg 75:713, 1948.

129. Saghaei M, Masoodifar M: The pressor response and airway effects of cricoid pressure during induction of general anesthesia. Anesth Analg 93:787, 2001.

130. Sant'Ambrogio G: Nervous receptors of the tracheobronchial tree. Annu Rev Physiol 49:611, 1987.

131. Sarma VJ: Use of ketamine in acute severe asthma. Acta Anaesthesiol Scand 36:106, 1992.

132. Sato T, Matsuki A, Zsigmond EK, Rabito SF: Ketamine relaxes airway smooth muscle contracted by endothelin. Anesth Analg 84:900, 1997.

133. Scalfaro P, Sly PD, Sims C, Habre W: Salbutamol prevents the increase of respiratory resistance caused by tracheal intubation during sevoflurane anesthesia in asthmatic children. Anesth Analg 93:898, 2001.

134. Scanlon P, Carey M, Power M, Kirby F: Patient response to laryngeal mask insertion after induction of anaesthesia with propofol or thiopentone. Can J Anaesth 40:816, 1993.

135. Schaefer H, Marsch S: Comparison of orthodox with fiberoptic orotracheal intubation under total IV anaesthesia. Br J Anaesth 66:608, 1991.

136. Scheller M, Zornow M, Saidman L: Tracheal intubation without use of muscle relaxants: A technique using propofol and varying doses of alfentanil. Anesth Analg 75:788, 1992.

137. Scott JC, Ponganis KV, Stanski DR: EEG quantitation of narcotic effect: The comparative pharmacodynamics of fentanyl and alfentanil. Anesthesiology 62:234, 1985.

138. Scott L, Benson M, Bishop M: Relationship of endotracheal tube size to auto-PEEP at high minute ventilation. Respir Care 31:1080, 1986.

139. Sessler CN, Vitaliti JC, Cooper KR, et al: Comparison of 4% lidocaine/0.5% phenylephrine with 5% cocaine: Which dilates the nasal passage better? Anesthesiology 64:274, 1986.

140. Shapiro HM, Wyte SR, Harris AB, Galindo A: Acute intraoperative intracranial hypertension in neurosurgical patients: Mechanical and pharmacologic factors. Anesthesiology 37:399, 1972.

141. Shapiro M, Wilson RK, Casar G, et al: Work of breathing through different sized endotracheal tubes. Crit Care Med 14:1028, 1986.

142. Sharma S, Mitra S, Grover VK, Kalra R: Esmolol blunts the haemodynamic responses to tracheal intubation in treated hypertensive patients. Can J Anaesth 43:778, 1996.

143. Shribman AJ, Smith G, Achola KJ: Cardiovascular and catecholamine responses to laryngoscopy with and without tracheal intubation. Br J Anaesth 59:295, 1987.

144. Slogoff S, Keats A: Does perioperative myocardial ischemia lead to postoperative myocardial infarction? Anesthesiology 55:212, 1981.

145. Smith J: Heart rate and arterial pressure changes during fiberoptic tracheal intubation under general anesthesia. Anaesthesia 43:629, 1988.

146. Smith J, Mackenzie A, Scott-Knight V: Comparison of two methods of fiber-scope-guided tracheal intubation. Br J Anaesth 66:546, 1991.

147. Smith RA, Venus B, Johnson MT, Carter C: Influence of glottic mechanism on pulmonary function after acute lung injury. Chest 98:206, 1990.

148. Splinter WM: Intravenous lidocaine does not attenuate the haemodynamic response of children to laryngoscopy and tracheal intubation. Can J Anaesth 37:440, 1990.

149. Staffel JG, Weissler MC, Tyler EP, Drake AF: The prevention of postoperative stridor and laryngospasm with topical lidocaine. Arch Otolaryngol Head Neck Surg 117:1123, 1991.

150. Steinhaus J, Gaskin L: A study of intravenous lidocaine as a suppressant of cough reflex. Anesthesiology 24:285, 1963.

151. Steinhaus J, Howland D: Intravenously administered lidocaine as a supplement to nitrous oxide thiobarbiturate anesthesia. Anesth Analg 37:40, 1958.

152. Stirt JA, Grosslight KR, Bedford RF, Vollmer D: "Defasciculation" with metocurine prevents succinylcholine-induced increases in intracranial pressure. Anesthesiology 67:50, 1987.

153. Stoelting R: Attenuation of blood pressure response to laryngoscopy and tracheal intubation with sodium nitroprusside. Anesth Analg 58:116, 1979.

154. Stoelting RK: Circulatory changes during direct laryngoscopy and tracheal intubation: Influence of duration of laryngoscopy with or without prior lidocaine. Anesthesiology 47:381, 1977.

155. Stoelting RK: Circulatory response to laryngoscopy and tracheal intubation with or without prior oropharyngeal viscous lidocaine. Anesth Analg 56:618, 1977.

156. Takahashi S, Mizutani T, Miyabe M, Toyooka H: Hemodynamic responses to tracheal intubation with laryngoscope versus lightwand intubating device (Trachlight) in adults with normal airway. Anesth Analg 95:480, table of contents, 2002.

157. Takita K, Morimoto Y, Kemmotsu O: Tracheal lidocaine attenuates the cardiovascular response to endotracheal intubation. Can J Anaesth 48:732, 2001.

158. Tarkkanen L, Laitinen L, Johansson G: Effects of d-tubocurarine on intracranial pressure and thalamic electrical impedance. Anesthesiology 40:247, 1974.

159. Thompson JP, Hall AP, Russell J, et al: Effect of remifentanil on the haemodynamic response to orotracheal intubation. Br J Anaesth 80:467, 1998.

160. Tiret L, Desmonts JM, Hatton F, Vourc'h G: Complications associated with anaesthesia—A prospective survey in France. Can Anaesth Soc J 33:336, 1986.

161. Tobias J, Lubos K, Hirshman C: Aminophylline does not attenuate histamine-induced airway constriction during halothane anesthesia. Anesthesiology 71:723, 1989.

162. Van Aken H, Puchstein C, Hidding J: The prevention of hypertension at intubation. Anaesthesia 37:82, 1982.

163. Viguera M, Diakum TA, Shelsky R, et al: [Efficacy of topical administration of lidocaine through a Malinckrodt Hi-Lo Jet tube in lessening cough during recovery from general anesthesia]. Rev Esp Anestesiol Reanim 39:316, 1992.

164. Vines D, Peters J, Merritt J, et al: A comparison of total patient work of breathing (TPWOB) between 8.0 endotracheal tubes (ETT) and tracheostomy tubes (TT) during spontaneous breathing in a lung model. Am J Respir Crit Care Med 167:A460, 2003.

165. Wiklund CU, Lim S, Lindsten U, Lindahl SG: Relaxation by sevoflurane, desflurane and halothane in the isolated guinea-pig trachea via inhibition of cholinergic neurotransmission. Br J Anaesth 83:422, 1999.

166. Wilson IG, Fell D, Robinson SL, Smith G: Cardiovascular responses to insertion of the laryngeal mask. Anaesthesia 47:300, 1992.

167. Wood ML, Forrest ET: The haemodynamic response to the insertion of the laryngeal mask airway: A comparison with laryngoscopy and tracheal intubation. Acta Anaesthesiol Scand 38:510, 1994.

168. Wu RS, Wu KC, Sum DC, Bishop MJ: Comparative effects of thiopentone and propofol on respiratory resistance after tracheal intubation. Br J Anaesth 77:735, 1996.

169. Youngberg J, Graybar G, Hutchings D: Comparison of intravenous and topical lidocaine in attenuating the cardiovascular responses to endotracheal intubation. South Med J 76:1122, 1983.

170. Yukioka H, Hayashi M, Terai T, Fujimori M: Intravenous lidocaine as a suppressant of coughing during tracheal intubation in elderly patients. Anesth Analg 77:309, 1993.

171. Yung M, Snowdon S: Respiratory resistance of tracheostomy tubes. Arch Otolaryngol 110:591, 1984.

172. Zbinden AM, Petersen-Felix S, Thomson DA: Anesthetic depth defined using multiple noxious stimuli during isoflurane/oxygen anesthesia. II. Hemodynamic responses. Anesthesiology 80:261, 1994.

THE DIFFICULT AIRWAY: DEFINITION, RECOGNITION, AND THE ASA ALGORITHM

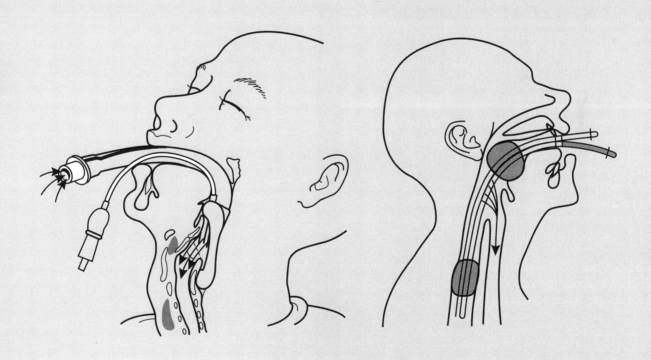

7

DEFINITION AND INCIDENCE OF THE DIFFICULT AIRWAY

P. Allan Klock, Jr.
Jonathan L. Benumof

I. INTRODUCTION

The fundamental responsibility of an anesthesiologist is to maintain adequate gas exchange in the patient. For this to be done, the patient's airway must be managed so that it is almost continuously patent. Failure to maintain a patent airway for more than a few minutes results in brain damage or death. Thus, it is not surprising that the 1990 closed claims analysis showed that more than 85% of all respiratory event–related closed malpractice claims involved a brain-damaged or dead patient.[6] Intubation difficulties and problems with airway management during emergence remain among the leading causes of serious intraoperative problems,[13] and it has been estimated that inability to manage successfully very difficult airways (DAs) is responsible for as many as 30% of deaths totally attributable to anesthesia.[3,5]

In any patient, the greater the degree of difficulty in maintaining airway patency, the greater the risk of brain damage or death. Before discussing the specific management of a DA (Chapters 8 to 43), we must (1) define what is meant by a DA, (2) classify the degrees of difficulty in maintaining a patent airway, (3) determine the incidence of each degree of airway difficulty, and (4) determine the incidence of major and minor complications as a function of the degree of airway difficulty. In this discussion, it is always assumed that a reasonably well-trained anesthesiologist is attempting to maintain airway patency.

II. DEFINITION AND CLASSIFICATION OF AIRWAY DIFFICULTY

There are three common ways to maintain airway patency and gas exchange. First, inspired gas is delivered to the face through a mask that is sealed to the patient's face, while the natural airway from the face to the vocal cords is kept patent with or without external jaw thrust maneuvers or internal upper airway devices (mask ventilation) (Chapter 14). Second, inspired gas is delivered through a supraglottic airway, such as the laryngeal mask airway. Because these devices are extensively described in Chapters 21 and 22, they are not specifically considered in this chapter. Third, the airway is kept open to inspired gas by a tube passed from the environment to some point below the vocal cords (endotracheal intubation).

Difficult mask ventilation is a condition in which it is not possible for the anesthesiologist to provide adequate face mask ventilation because of one or more of the following problems: inadequate mask seal, excessive gas leak, or excessive resistance to the ingress or egress of gas. There are two main reasons for inadequate face mask ventilation: inability to establish an adequate seal between the face and the mask and inadequate patency of the airway in either the nasopharynx, oropharynx, hypopharynx, larynx, or trachea. These manifest, respectively, as either a large leak that prevents generation of adequate pressure in the breathing circuit or inability to move air into the lungs despite an adequate driving pressure.

Langeron and colleagues designed a study to determine predictors of difficult mask ventilation by requesting the anesthesiologist to rate face mask ventilation as difficult when it was "clinically relevant and could have led to potential problems if mask ventilation had to be maintained for a longer time."[18] This study listed six reasons for difficult mask ventilation: (1) inability for the unassisted anesthesiologist to maintain oxygen saturation as measured by pulse oximetry (SpO_2) to greater than 92% using 100% oxygen and positive-pressure mask ventilation, (2) important gas flow leak by the face mask, (3) necessity to increase the gas flow to greater than 15 L/min and to use the oxygen flush valve more than twice, (4) no perceptible gas movement, (5) necessity to perform a two-handed mask ventilation technique, and (6) change of operator required.[5] El-Ganzouri and associates, on the other hand, defined difficult ventilation as "inability to obtain chest excursion sufficient to maintain a clinically acceptable capnogram waveform despite optimal head and neck positioning and use of muscle paralysis, use of an oral airway, and optimal application of a face mask by anesthesia personnel."[12]

Methods used to improve airway patency include the triple airway maneuver (TAM; T = tilt head, A = advance mandible, and M = mouth open) as well as insertion of oral and nasal airways. If there is an inadequate mask seal, the anesthesiologist may choose a different face mask, use a two-hand or two-person technique, insert bolsters between the alveolar ridge and the cheeks, or employ other methods to improve the interface between the face and the mask. Because of the multiple modes of mask ventilation failure, there is no agreed-upon classification system to describe inadequate mask ventilation.

In terms of degree of difficulty, face mask ventilation can range from zero to infinite (Fig. 7-1, *top*). Zero difficulty means that no external effort or internal upper airway device is required to maintain airway patency; that is, mask ventilation is extremely easy and occurs through the natural airway. Among the specific, reproducible, and progressive degrees of mask ventilation difficulty are (1) application of one-person jaw thrust and mask seal, (2) insertion of an oropharyngeal or nasopharyngeal airway, (3) one-person jaw thrust and insertion of one or both airways, and (4) two-person jaw thrust and mask seal and insertion of both airways. Whenever an airway is used, it is likely that jaw thrust will also be used, and therefore these indices of difficulty are shown in Figure 7-1 as occurring together. An infinite degree of

DEFINITION OF DIFFERENT DEGREES OF A DIFFICULT AIRWAY

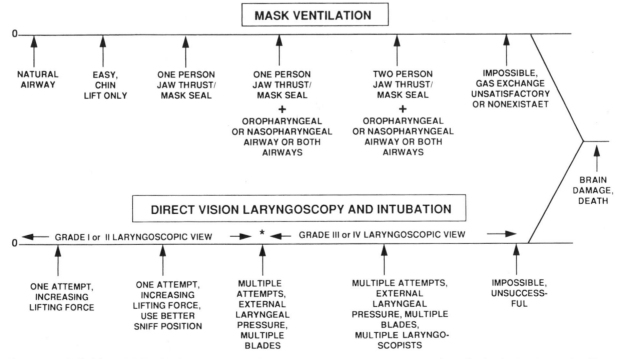

Figure 7-1. Definition of difficult airway. Airway refers to either mask ventilation or endotracheal tube intubation by direct vision laryngoscope. The degree of difficulty can range from zero, which is extremely easy, to infinity, which is impossible. When both mask ventilation and direct vision laryngoscopy are impossible and no other maneuver is successful, brain damage or death, or both, will ensue. Between these extremes, there are several well-defined, commonly encountered degrees of difficulty. Grade of laryngoscopic view is represented as an approximate continuum above the discrete progressive indices of laryngoscopic difficulty. (From Benumof JL: Management of the difficult adult airway. With special emphasis on awake tracheal intubation. Anesthesiology 75:1087, 1991.)

mask ventilation difficulty means that, despite maximal two-person external effort and full use of oropharyngeal and nasopharyngeal airways, adequate airway patency cannot be maintained; that is, mask ventilation is impossible. Of course, in any given patient the degree of difficulty with mask ventilation may change with time.

When two persons combine to effect jaw thrust and mask seal, they must interact in an additive-synergistic way. Ideally, the primary anesthesiologist stands at the patient's head and initiates jaw thrust with the left hand at the angle of the left mandible and left-sided mask seal, while the right hand compresses the reservoir bag. The standard position for the primary anesthesiologist appears in Figure 7-2. The secondary (helping) person stands at the patient's side, at the level of the patient's shoulder, facing the primary anesthesiologist. The right hand of the secondary anesthesiologist should cover the left hand of the primary anesthesiologist and contribute to left-sided jaw thrust and mask seal, and the left hand of the secondary person should initiate right-sided jaw thrust and mask seal. In this way, all four hands are doing something important without interfering with one another, and there is almost no redundant effort. With this positioning, the secondary person can continuously watch the monitors, provide external laryngeal manipulation to the patient, and hand equipment to the primary anesthesiologist.

Tracheal intubation is described as difficult when it requires multiple attempts, in the presence or absence of tracheal pathology. The difficulty of intubation under direct vision can also range from zero to infinity (see Fig. 7-1, *bottom*). Zero difficulty means that an endotracheal tube (ET) can be inserted into a fully visualized laryngeal aperture (Fig. 7-3, grade I laryngoscopic view[8,24]) with

little effort. The several specific, reproducible, and progressive degrees of intubation difficulty arise from visualization of progressively less of the laryngeal aperture (see Figs. 7-1 and 7-3, grade II and III laryngoscopic views[8,24]). As the view worsens, increasing anterior lifting force with the laryngoscope blade, optimal sniff position, multiple attempts, external laryngeal manipulation (see Chapter 16 and Fig. 16-10), multiple blades, and laryngoscopists may be required to achieve intubation. External laryngeal manipulation (see Chapter 16 and Fig. 16-10) may be required to push the larynx more posteriorly and cephalad for a better view (thereby decreasing the laryngoscopic view from a higher to a lower grade). Similarly, it should be recognized that anatomy that results in a high-grade laryngoscopic view for an inexperienced individual with a given laryngoscopic blade may result in a lower laryngoscopic grade for a more experienced or skillful individual with perhaps a different blade. Whenever multiple attempts are required, it is likely that external laryngeal manipulation will also be applied; therefore, these indices of difficulty are shown occurring together. Although a severe

Laryngoscopic View Grading System

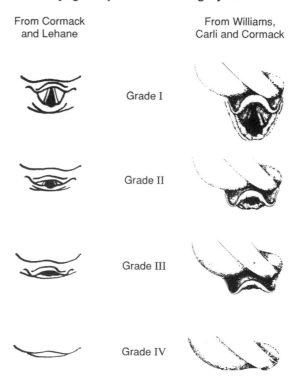

From Cormack and Lehane   From Williams, Carli and Cormack

Grade I

Grade II

Grade III

Grade IV

Figure 7-3. Four grades of laryngoscopic view. Grade I is visualization of entire laryngeal aperture; grade II is visualization of just the posterior portion of laryngeal aperture; grade III is visualization of only the epiglottis; and grade IV is visualization of just the soft palate. It is assumed that care has been taken to get the best possible view of the vocal cords (see text). (*Left,* Adapted from Cormack RS, Lehane J: Difficult tracheal intubation in obstetrics. Anaesthesia 39:1105, 1984; *right,* adapted from Williams KN, Carli F, Cormack RS: Unexpected, difficult laryngoscopy: A prospective survey in routine general surgery. Br J Anaesth 66:38, 1991.)

TWO-PERSON MAXIMUM MASK VENTILATION EFFORT

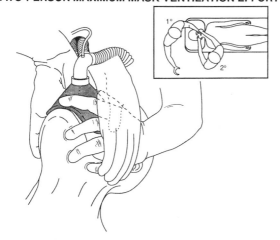

Figure 7-2. Optimal two-person mask ventilation effort. Primary anesthesiologist stands at head of patient and uses left and right hands in standard-classical fashion. Secondary (helping) person stands facing the primary anesthesiologist at level of patient's shoulder and uses right hand to help achieve left-sided jaw thrust and mask seal, while left hand achieves right-sided jaw thrust and mask seal. (From Benumof J.L.: Airway Management: Principles and Practice. St. Louis, Mosby, 1996.)

grade III (tip of epiglottis) or a grade IV (just soft palate) laryngoscopic view[8,24] (see Figs. 7-1 and 7-3) may result in a successful "blind" intubation, these views more often make intubation impossible. An infinitely difficult intubation (DI) means that the trachea cannot be intubated under direct vision, despite full paralysis and optimal head and neck positioning; very forceful anterior elevation of the laryngoscope blade; use of multiple attempts, laryngoscope blades, and laryngoscopists; and external posterior and cephalad displacement of the larynx; that is, endotracheal intubation through a nonvisualized larynx is impossible. Of course, in any given patient, the degree of endotracheal intubation difficulty can be independent of the degree of mask ventilation difficulty and can progressively increase and approach the impossible extreme. Failed intubation is defined as the inability to place the ET after multiple intubation attempts.

Difficult laryngoscopy is described as not being able to visualize any portion of the vocal cords after multiple attempts at conventional laryngoscopy, and many investigators include grades III and IV or grade IV alone, according to the Cormack-Lehane original grading of the rigid laryngoscopic view. For studies of difficult laryngoscopy to be reliable and for the preceding laryngoscopic grading system to be helpful, the reported grades must describe the best view that was obtained, which, in turn, depends on the best possible performance of laryngoscopy. The components of best performance of laryngoscopy consist of the optimal sniff position, good complete muscle relaxation, firm forward traction on the laryngoscope, and, if necessary, firm external laryngeal manipulation. For example, the application of external laryngeal pressure may reduce the incidence of grade III view from 9% to 5.4 to 1.3%.[28] In doubtful cases, the anesthesiologist, while performing laryngoscopy with the left hand, should quickly apply external pressure over the hyoid-thyroid-cricoid cartilages with the right hand. The pressure point that affords the best laryngeal view can be determined in just several seconds. Having found the position that gives the best view, the laryngoscopist should ask the assistant to press carefully on exactly the same spot. Reproducing the identical external laryngeal pressure by the assistant must be directed by the laryngoscopist, even if the assistant is fully trained. The best performance of laryngoscopy avoids awkward high-arm postures, positioning the laryngoscope blade over part of the tongue, gripping the laryngoscope at the junction of the handle and blade with rotation about a horizontal axis, choosing the wrong blade size or shape, and wrong blade placement. Theoretically, if the preceding components of best performance of laryngoscopy are used and the pitfalls avoided, all laryngoscopists (novice and expert) should have close to the same laryngoscopic view.

Difficult laryngoscopy (a grade III or IV view)[8,24] is synonymous with DI in the majority of patients. However, endotracheal intubation depends slightly more on the skill of the individual than does laryngoscopy, and therefore the degrees of difficulty with laryngoscopy and endotracheal intubation may be inconsistent. Consequently, studies of the incidence of difficult endotracheal intubation depend on the dexterity of the intubationists, which makes variability in results inevitable. For example, in a study of respiratory complications associated with endotracheal intubation, Asai and colleagues had three patients with Cormack and Lehane grade IV laryngoscopic views. One patient was easy to intubate, one was "moderately difficult" to intubate, and one was "difficult" to intubate.[2] Of the 68 patients reported to have a grade III laryngoscopic view in the same study, 5 (7%) were difficult to intubate, 50 (74%) were moderately difficult to intubate, and 13 (19%) were easy to intubate.[2]

There are four relatively uncommon scenarios that explain some of the discordance between difficult laryngoscopy and DI. First, some patients with a grade II view have a trachea that may be intubated at the first or second attempt if the distal end of the ET is appropriately curved by a malleable stylet (hockey stick shape) or a small curved introducer is used (e.g., a gum elastic bougie). Second, grade III laryngoscopic views have been variously described as seeing only the palate and all of the epiglottis[8,27,28] or as seeing only the palate and just the tip of the epiglottis.[24,27] These different definitions of grade III may respond differently to adjustments, such as optimal external laryngeal pressure, and therefore may differ initially and subsequently with respect to difficulty of endotracheal intubation. Third, a grade III view with a curved blade placed in the vallecula (because of a long floppy epiglottis) may be a grade I or II view if either a curved or straight blade is placed posterior to the epiglottis and lifted anteriorly. Fourth, pathologic conditions, such as laryngeal web, laryngeal tumors, or tracheal stenosis, may disassociate ease of laryngoscopy from difficulty of endotracheal intubation.

III. INCIDENCE OF EACH DEGREE OF AIRWAY DIFFICULTY

The incidence of difficulty with laryngoscopy or intubation in the general surgical population varies greatly depending on its degree (Table 7-1). A grade II or III laryngoscopic view requiring multiple attempts or blades or both (and presumably external laryngeal pressure) is relatively common and is found in 100 to 1800 of 10,000 patients, or 1% to 18%.[1,8,9,14,22] As the degree of difficulty increases to a definite grade III laryngoscopic view, the incidence ranges from 100 to 400 of 10,000 patients, or 1% to 4%.[7,16,23-26,28] The incidence of failed endotracheal intubation (presumably a severe grade III or grade IV view) ranges from 5 to 35 of 10,000 patients, or 0.05% to 0.35%[3,8,15,19,20,24-26]; the high and low ends of this range are associated with obstetric and other surgical patients, respectively.

Table 7-1 **Incidence of Difficult Intubation According to Degree of Difficulty**

Degree of Difficulty with Intubation (Fig. 7-1)	Range of Incidence Per 10,000	%	Reference
Endotracheal tube (ET) intubation successful but multiple attempts and/or blades may be required; probable grade II or III	100-1800	1-18	1, 8, 9,14, 21-23
ET intubation successful but multiple attempts and/or blades and/or laryngoscopists required; grade III	100-400	1-4	7, 15, 16, 23, 24, 26, 28
ET intubation not successful; grade III or IV	5-35	0.05-0.35	4, 8, 15, 19, 20, 24, 26
Cannot ventilate by mask plus cannot intubate; transtracheal jet ventilation, tracheostomy, brain damage, or death	0.01-2.0	0.0001-0.02	4, 5, 11, 17, 25

From Benumof JL: Airway Management: Principles and Practice. St. Louis, Mosby, 1996, p 124.

There are considerably fewer data with regard to difficult face mask ventilation. There is no standard definition of difficult mask ventilation, and each study needs to be read carefully to determine the definition used. As previously mentioned, Langeron and colleagues measured difficulty in mask ventilation as the primary outcome and rated face mask ventilation as difficult when it was "clinically relevant and could have led to potential problems if mask ventilation had to be maintained for a longer time"; they reported a 5% incidence of difficult mask ventilation with 1 out of 1502 patients being impossible to ventilate with a face mask.[18] One of the significant findings in this study is that difficult mask ventilation conferred a 4-fold increased risk for DI and 12-fold increase in the risk for an impossible intubation.[18] Other large prospective studies have reported incidences of difficult mask ventilation as 0.07%,[12] 0.9%,[23] and 1.4%,[2] although this was not the primary outcome being assessed.

The incidence of completely failed mask ventilation *and* ET intubation can be estimated because such an airway failure combination heretofore frequently resulted in brain damage or death and has ranged from 0.01 to 2.0 of 10,000 patients.[3,5,11,17,25] Fortunately, the incidence of brain damage, cardiac arrest, and death appears to be decreasing.[11,17]

IV. INCIDENCE OF COMPLICATIONS WITH EACH DEGREE OF AIRWAY DIFFICULTY

Anesthesia in a patient with a DA can lead to direct airway trauma and morbidity from hypoxia and hypercarbia. Management of the DA sometimes involves the application of more physical force to the patient's airway than is normally used, which can cause direct airway trauma. The most common consequence is probably a chipped or broken tooth. Direct trauma may involve any part of the face, teeth, and upper airway, resulting in hemorrhage, lacerations, and subsequent tissue emphysema and infection, fracture-subluxation of the cervical spine, and trauma to the eye. Much of the morbidity specifically attributable to managing a DA comes from an interruption of gas exchange (hypoxia and hypercapnia), which may cause brain damage and cardiovascular activation or depression. Directly mediated reflexes (laryngovagal [airway spasm, apnea, bradycardia, dysrhythmia, or hypotension] and laryngospinal [coughing, vomiting, or bucking]) provide the final source of morbidity. Both direct trauma and morbidity from airway obstruction can range from minor (trivial or nuisance value) to major (life threatening or death).

The more difficult the airway is to manage, the greater are the use of physical force, the number of attempts to establish the airway, and the incidence of complications. Only one study[19] has directly addressed this question, and its data strongly support this premise. In this study, the incidence of relatively minor upper airway complications (posterior pharyngeal and lip lacerations and bruises) with laryngoscopy and intubation under direct vision in patients with normal airways was 5%.[16] In patients in whom endotracheal intubation was anticipated to be difficult, the incidence of minor trauma to the upper airway increased to 17%.[16] In patients in whom endotracheal intubation was actually found to be difficult (multiple attempts at laryngoscopy but ultimately successful), the incidence of upper airway complications was 63%. These findings may seem contrary to the closed claims analysis of airway injury during anesthesia, which revealed that only 39% of the 266 airway injury claims were associated with DI.[10] However, these findings are consistent if one considers that a very low incidence of injury with routine airway management together with a much higher risk of injury with the infrequently occurring DAs would combine for a final product in which the majority of injuries are associated with cases in which the intubation was not difficult. Of course, when an airway has been impossible to manage, the incidence of complications may further increase because of the inclusion of some cases of brain damage or death.[25]

REFERENCES

1. Aro L, Takki S, Aromaa U: Technique for difficult intubation. Br J Anaesth 43:1081, 1971.

2. Asai T, Koga K, Vaughan RS: Respiratory complications associated with tracheal intubation and extubation. Br J Anaesth 80:767, 1998.

3. Bellhouse CP: An angulated laryngoscope for routine and difficult tracheal intubation. Anesthesiology 69:126, 1988.

4. Bellhouse CP, Doré C: Criteria for estimating likelihood of difficulty of endotracheal intubation with the Macintosh laryngoscope. Anaesth Intensive Care 16:329, 1988.

5. Benumof JL, Scheller MS: The importance of transtracheal jet ventilation in the management of the difficult airway. Anesthesiology 71:769, 1989.

6. Caplan RA, Posner KL, Ward RJ, et al: Adverse respiratory events in anesthesia: A closed claims analysis. Anesthesiology 72:828, 1990.

7. Cohen SM, Laurito CE, Segil LJ: Oral exam to predict difficult intubations: A large prospective study [abstract]. Anesthesiology 71:A937, 1989.

8. Cormack RS, Lehane J: Difficult tracheal intubation in obstetrics. Anaesthesia 39:1105, 1984.

9. Deller A, Schreiber MN, Gramer J, et al: Difficult intubation: Incidence and predictability. A prospective study of 8,284 adult patients [abstract]. Anesthesiology 73:A1054, 1990.

10. Domino KB, Posner KL, Caplan RA, et al: Airway injury during anesthesia: A closed claims analysis. Anesthesiology 91:1703, 1999.

11. Eichhorn JH: Documenting improved anesthesia outcome. J Clin Anesth 3:351, 1991.

12. El-Ganzouri AR, McCarthy RJ, Tuman KJ, et al: Preoperative airway assessment: Predictive value of a multivariate risk index. Anesth Analg 82:1197, 1996.

13. Fasting S, Gisvold SE: Serious intraoperative problems—A five-year review of 83,844 anesthetics. Can J Anaesth 49:545, 2002.

14. Finucane BT, Santora AH: Difficult Intubation. Principles of Airway Management, 2nd ed. St. Louis, Mosby–Year Book, 1996, p 187.

15. Glassenberg R, Vaisrub N, Albright G: The incidence of failed intubation in obstetrics: Is there an irreducible minimum [abstract]? Anesthesiology 73:A1062, 1990.

16. Hirsch IA, Reagan JO, Sullivan N: Complications of direct laryngoscopy: A prospective analysis. Anesthesiol Rev 17:34, 1990.

17. Keenan RL, Boyan CP: Decreasing frequency of anesthetic cardiac arrests. J Clin Anesth 3:354, 1991.

18. Langeron O, Masso E, Huraux C, et al: Prediction of difficult mask ventilation. Anesthesiology 92:1229, 2000.

19. Lyons G: Failed intubation, six years' experience in a teaching maternity unit. Anaesthesia 40:759, 1985.

20. Lyons G, MacDonald R: Difficult intubation in obstetrics [letter]. Anaesthesia 40:1016, 1985.

21. Mallampati SR, Gatt SP, Gugino LD, et al: A clinical sign to predict difficult tracheal intubation: A prospective study. Can Anaesth Soc J 32:429, 1985.

22. Phillips OC, Duerksen RL: Endotracheal intubation: A new blade for direct laryngoscopy. Anesth Analg 52:691, 1973.

23. Rose DK, Cohen MM: The airway: Problems and predictions in 18,500 patients. Can J Anaesth 41:372, 1994.

24. Samsoon GLT, Young JRB: Difficult tracheal intubation: A retrospective study. Anaesthesia 42:487, 1987.

25. Tunstall ME: Failed intubation in the parturient [editorial]. Can J Anaesth 36:611, 1989.

26. Williams KN, Carli F, Cormack RS: Unexpected, difficult laryngoscopy: A prospective survey in routine general surgery. Br J Anaesth 66:38, 1991.

27. Williamson R: Grade III laryngoscopy—Which is it? Anaesthesia 43:424, 1988.

28. Wilson ME, Spiegelhalter D, Robertson JA, et al: Predicting difficult intubation. Br J Anaesth 61:211, 1988.

8

EVALUATION AND RECOGNITION OF THE DIFFICULT AIRWAY

Allan P. Reed

I. INTRODUCTION

Identification of the difficult airway, before manipulation, is the Holy Grail of clinical management. The landmark article of Cass and colleagues, 50 years ago, underscores this point.[23] It is the first step in preparing for patient care. Selection of airway devices, techniques, and procedures all pivot on airway evaluation. Absent reliable data, practitioners fall back upon experience or, worse, luck.[6] Experience is not a bad teacher, but it is second best to knowledge based on firm scientific principles.

The medical literature boasts a plethora of articles discussing predictors of difficult intubation but relatively few explaining predictors of difficult face mask ventilation. Among all of them, practitioners seek to determine which criteria are dependable and which are not. Having established a basis upon which to predict difficult mask ventilation or tracheal intubation, or both, it becomes possible to select modes of airway management that optimize patients' safety and comfort.

Generally, failed tracheal intubation occurs once in every 2230 attempts.[83] For the average anesthesiologist in the United States, that represents one failed intubation every other year. The incidence is small, but the potential consequences of difficult airway management are of major importance. Failed ventilation accounted for 44% of intraoperative cardiac arrests reported by Keenan and Boyan.[51] Thirty-four percent of liability claims identified by Caplan and coauthors were based on adverse respiratory events,[20] of which, three quarters were judged to be preventable.[24]

On a worldwide scale, difficulty managing the airway occurs infrequently. From a scientific point of view, investigating such events is difficult. The number of patients studied must be very large. Patients entered into each study must be divided into several groups because of the numerous factors that influence airway management. Each group must contain a sufficient number of patients, all of whom share one or more characteristics. Additional problems relate to the intubators' expertise. Different skill levels among various operators introduce another variable into identifying difficult or failed intubations. Ideally, laryngoscopy as a procedure should be performed by a limited number of investigators. Other factors that must be controlled include the type of laryngoscope, the laryngoscope blade, the intubating position (literature has questioned the importance of the sniffing position),[1] the degree of muscle relaxation achieved, and the presence of a qualified assistant. Control groups are also desirable.

Many classical terms are poorly defined. "High arched palate" and "anterior larynx" are concepts that have meaning to practitioners but are not well characterized. Consequently, they must be delineated in order to be measured and introduced into clinical studies. Radiographs and other imaging techniques have been advocated to predict difficult intubation but are too expensive and inconvenient for patients to undergo as screening tests. Highly specialized techniques such as acoustic reflectometry are of dubious reliability.[65] More quantitative, noninvasive measurements such as those with the laryngeal indices caliper,[79] bubble inclinometer,[78] and goniometer offer the potential for accurate measurements but have never found their way into clinical practice.

This chapter reviews the current state of the art regarding predictability of difficult mask airway management and difficult traditional laryngoscopy. Historically, these procedures were performed with anesthesia face masks in the case of mask ventilation and with Macintosh or Miller blades in the case of laryngoscopy. The ensuing discussion observes these limitations. The application of supraglottic ventilatory devices and alternative intubation techniques are addressed in other chapters.

The airway begins at the nose and mouth and ends at the alveoli. The airway is easily separated into upper and lower divisions. This chapter focuses on the upper airway, which encompasses the nose, mouth, nasopharynx, oropharynx, laryngopharynx, and larynx. In this chapter, all references to the airway refer to the upper airway.

II. DIFFICULT MASK VENTILATION

In this author's opinion, *the single most reliable predictor of a difficult airway is a history of difficult airway.* The contrapositive is not necessarily true. A history of problem-free airway management is suggestive of future ease but not a guarantee. Many factors that contribute to difficulty are progressive. Examples of such problems include rheumatoid arthritis and obesity. An airway history should be elicited from all patients. Review of prior anesthesia records is frequently helpful. They may describe previously encountered problems, failed therapies, and successful solutions.[3]

Difficult face mask ventilation occurs when a practitioner cannot provide sufficient gas exchange because of inadequate mask seal, large volume leaks, or excessive resistance to the ingress or egress of gas.[3] This occurs with an incidence between 0.08% and 5%.[35,54] The wide range is probably due to conflicting definitions of difficult mask airway.[82] Risk factors for difficult mask ventilation include full beard, massive jaw, edentulousness, skin sensitivity (burns, epidermolysis bullosa, fresh skin grafts),

facial dressings, obesity, age older than 55 years, and a history of snoring.[54] Other criteria that suggest the possibility of difficult face mask ventilation include large tongue, heavy jaw muscles, history of sleep apnea, poor atlanto-occipital extension, some types of pharyngeal pathology, facial burns, and facial deformities[42] as seen in Table 8-1. Multiple types of pharyngeal problems can produce difficult face mask ventilation. They include lingual tonsil hypertrophy,[67] lingual tonsillar abscess, lingual thyroid,[17] and thyroglossal cyst.[43,46,59,74] Many abnormalities cannot be diagnosed by classical airway examination techniques. The presence of any one factor is suggestive of difficult mask ventilation, and as factors increase in number, the likelihood of difficulty increases. A greater than normal mandibulohyoid distance has been associated with obstructive sleep apnea, the pathophysiology of which may be related to difficult mask ventilation.[25,26,77]

Traditional face mask airway management is generally safe and effective. In the unusual instances when it is not, tracheal intubation remains the fallback option. Although this scheme works well in most cases, approximately 15% of difficult intubations are also difficult mask airways.[100]

Table 8-1 Risk Factors for Difficult Mask Ventilation

Obesity
Beards
Edentulousness
History of snoring
History of obstructive sleep apnea
Skin sensitivity (burns, epidermolysis bullosa, fresh skin grafts)
Massive jaw
Heavy jaw muscles
Age older than 55 years
Large tongue
Poor atlanto-occipital extension
Pharyngeal pathology
Lingual tonsil hypertrophy
Lingual tonsil abscess
Lingual thyroid
Thyroglossal cyst
Facial dressings
Facial burns
Facial deformities

III. DIFFICULT INTUBATION

A. SNIFFING POSITION

Difficult tracheal intubation occurs when multiple attempts at endotracheal intubation are required.[3] The presence or absence of airway pathology does not influence its definition. Traditional laryngoscopy is performed in order to visualize the laryngeal opening. The observing laryngoscopist is situated outside the airway, above the patient's head. To see through the airway, light must travel from the glottic opening to the laryngoscopist's eye. Because light generally travels in straight lines, the technique requires an uninterrupted linear path between larynx and observer. Most of the manipulations performed attempt to satisfy this criterion.

The airway contains three visual axes. They are the long axes of the mouth, oropharynx, and larynx. In the neutral position, these axes form acute and obtuse angles with one another (Fig. 8-1). Light cannot bend around these angles under normal circumstances. In order to bring all three axes into better alignment, McGill suggested the "sniffing the morning air" position.[61] The true sniffing position has two components—cervical flexion and atlanto-occipital extension. Cervical flexion approximates the pharyngeal and laryngeal axes. Atlanto-occipital extension brings the oral axis into better alignment with the other two. Normal atlanto-occipital extension measures 35 degrees.[64] With optimal alignment of the airway's visual axes, it becomes possible to look through the airway into the laryngeal opening. A reduced atlanto-occipital gap or prominent C1 spinous processes impair laryngoscopy,[15,98] if vigorous attempts at extension are performed, because the trachea bows and the larynx is forced anteriorly.[15]

Inability to assume the sniffing position is a predictor of difficult intubation. Examples of problems that prevent the sniffing position are cervical vertebral arthritis, cervical ankylosing spondylitis, unstable cervical fractures, protruding cervical discs, atlantoaxial subluxation, cervical fusions, cervical collars, and halo frames. Morbidly obese patients sometimes have posterior neck fat pads that prevent atlanto-occipital extension.

The ability to achieve the sniffing position is easily tested. One simply has the patient flex the lower cervical vertebrae and extend at the atlanto-occipital joint. Pain, tingling, numbness, or inability to achieve these maneuvers predicts difficult intubation.[101] The benefits of the sniffing position have been dogma for more than 70 years, but Adnet and colleagues[1] and Chou and Wu[27] have questioned its utility.

B. MOUTH OPENING

Mouth opening is important because it determines the available space for placing and manipulating laryngoscopes

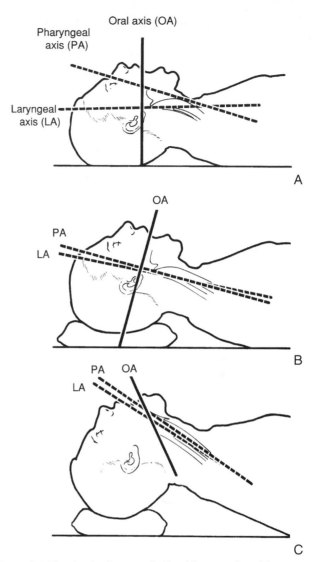

Figure 8-1 Visual axis diagram. **A,** Head in neutral position. None of the three visual axes align. **B,** Elevation of the head approximates the laryngeal and pharyngeal axes. **C,** Extension at the atlanto-occipital joint brings the visual axis of the mouth into better alignment with those of the larynx and pharynx. (From Stone DJ, Gal TJ: Airway management. In Miller RJ [ed]: Anesthesia, 5th ed. Philadelphia, Churchill Livingstone, 2000, p 1419.)

as well as tracheal tubes.[13,33] A small mouth opening may not accommodate either. Mouth opening also provides room to see through the uppermost part of the airway. Mouth opening relies on the temporomandibular joint (TMJ), which works in two ways. It has a hingelike movement and a gliding motion. The gliding motion is known as translation. The hingelike movement allows the mandible to pivot on the maxilla. The more the mandible swings away from the maxilla, the bigger the mouth opening.

The adequacy of mouth opening is assessed by measuring the interincisor distance. An interincisor distance of 3 cm provides sufficient space for intubation, absent other complicating factors. This corresponds approximately to two finger breadths.[2] The two finger breadth test is performed by placing the examiner's second and third digits between the patient's central incisors. If they fit, there should be adequate room to perform laryngoscopy. If they do not fit, laryngoscopy may be difficult. Factors that interfere with mouth opening include masseter muscle spasm, TMJ dysfunction, and various integumentary aliments. Skin problems that adversely effect mouth opening include burn scar contractures and progressive systemic sclerosis. Masseter muscle spasm can be relieved by induction of anesthesia and administration of muscle relaxants. Mechanical problems at the TMJ remain unaltered by medications. Some patients demonstrate adequate mouth opening when awake but not after anesthesia induction.[75] The problem can often be relieved by pulling the mandible forward. A mouth opening that was sufficient for a previous anesthetic may not be after temporal neurosurgical procedures.[49]

C. DENTITION

Instrumentation of the airway places teeth at risk for damage. Multiple problems result from dental injury. Teeth may be dislodged or broken. Such teeth cannot be used for chewing, may be painful, and are costly to repair. Beyond these issues, broken teeth can fall into the trachea, migrate to the lung, and predispose to abscesses. Poor dentition is at risk for damage as the mouth is opened and as the laryngoscope blade is employed. Teeth that can be extracted easily with digital pressure should probably be removed. During laryngoscopy, in the presence of poor dentition, extra efforts are made to avoid placing pressure on maxillary incisors. In doing so, laryngoscopes are manipulated into less than ideal positions for visualizing the larynx, resulting in poor visualization of the glottis.

Prominent maxillary incisors complicate laryngoscopy in another way. They protrude into the mouth and block the line of sight to the larynx. In order to overcome this problem, laryngoscopists must adjust their line of sight. To accomplish this, the observer's eye is brought to a new position that is higher than the original one. The laryngoscopist then looks tangentially over the protruding maxillary incisor. Two new points of observation exist in the adjusted line of sight and determine a new line of sight. The new line of sight brings the laryngoscopist's view to a more posterior laryngopharyngeal position. The result is a view that is posterior to the larynx. Consequently, the larynx is not visualized and a difficult laryngoscopy is produced. In much the same way, edentulous patients tend to be easy to intubate because the laryngoscopist can adjust the line of sight to a more advantageous angle.

D. TONGUE

The tongue occupies space in the mouth and oropharynx. The base of tongue resides close to the glottic aperture.

During traditional direct laryngoscopy, the base of tongue falls posteriorly, obstructing the line of sight into the glottis. Visualizing the larynx requires displacing the base of tongue anteriorly so that the line of sight to the glottis is restored. The tongue is frequently displaced with a hand-held rigid laryngoscope, to which Macintosh and Miller blades are most commonly attached. These laryngoscopes push the tongue anteriorly and, in so doing, move it from a posterior obstructing position to a new anterior nonobstructing position. The new position is within the mandibular space. The mandibular space is the area between the two rami of the mandible. Even with the tongue maximally displaced into the mandibular space, visualization of the larynx is sometimes inadequate.

Usually, a normal size tongue fits easily into a normal size mandibular space. A large tongue fits poorly into a normal size mandibular space. After filling the space, a large tongue still occupies some of the oropharyngeal airway and obstructs it. For this reason, large tongue (macroglossia) is a predictor of difficult intubation. Similarly, a normal size tongue fits poorly into a small mandibular space.[102] It, too, occupies some of the oropharyngeal airway, thereby obstructing the line of sight. Consequently, a small mandible (micrognathia) is a predictor of difficult intubation. In essence, a tongue that is large compared with the size of the mouth (oropharynx) and mandible takes up excessive space in the oropharynx and interferes with visualization. The base of tongue resides so close to the larynx that inability to displace it adequately anteriorly creates another problem. As the base of tongue hangs down over the larynx, the glottis is hidden from view. The glottic aperture is then anatomically anterior to the base of tongue. Hence, the term anterior larynx. Under such circumstances, the larynx is anterior to the base of tongue and cannot be seen because the tongue hides it. In this manner, glottic and supraglottic masses can create difficult intubation if they force the base of tongue posteriorly. Some of the masses that may be encountered are lingual tonsils,[40,67] epiglottic cysts,[59] and thyroglossal duct cysts.

After filling the mandibular space with the tongue, additional pressure on the laryngoscope blade lifts the mandible anteriorly. In this setting, mandibular displacement is dependent upon the TMJ. In addition to its hingelike motion, the TMJ works in a gliding (translational) movement. It is the gliding motion that allows the mandible to slide anteriorly across the maxilla. If the joint does not translate, the mandible cannot be displaced anteriorly and the tongue cannot be moved out of the line of sight.

Recognizing the implications of tongue size for successful laryngoscopy, Mallampati and colleagues[58] in 1985 and Samsoon and Young[83] in 1987 devised classification systems to predict difficult laryngoscopy utilizing this concept. A difficult laryngoscopy occurs when it is not possible to visualize any portion of the vocal cords.[3] Mallampati and Samsoon reasoned that a large tongue could be identified upon visual inspection of the open mouth. Both classification systems relate the size of the tongue to the oropharyngeal structures identified. A normal size tongue allows visualization of certain oropharyngeal structures. As the tongue size increases, some structures become hidden from view. Consequently, both investigators proposed systems that reasoned backward from this premise.

Application of the Mallampati or Samsoon classification system is easy and painless. The patient is seated in the neutral position. The mouth is opened as wide as possible and the tongue is protruded as far as possible. Phonation is discouraged because it raises the soft palate and allows visualization of additional structures.[89] The observer looks for specified anatomic landmarks. They are the fauces, pillars, uvula, and soft palate. The Mallampati classification system utilizes three groups and the Samsoon classification system employs four groups (Fig. 8-2). Both systems suggest that as the tongue size increases, fewer structures are visualized and laryngoscopy becomes more difficult. Mallampati scores tend to be higher in pregnant patients than nonpregnant ones.[70]

Just as the size of tongue can be estimated, so, too, can the size of the mandible. The patient's head is extended at the atlanto-occipital joint. The mentum of the mandible and the thyroid cartilage are identified. The "Adam's apple" (thyroid notch) is the most superficial structure in the neck and serves as a good landmark for the thyroid cartilage. The vocal cords lie just caudad to the thyroid notch. The distance between the thyroid cartilage and mentum (thyromental distance) is measured in one of three ways. The measurement can be made with a set of spacers, with a small pocket ruler, or with the observer's fingers. The normal thyromental distance is 6.5 cm. A thyromental distance greater than 6 cm is predictive of easy intubation. A thyromental distance of 6 cm or less is suggestive of difficult intubation.[69] Often, rulers are not present at the bedside. Absent an available ruler, practitioners can judge the thyromental distance with their own fingers. The width of one's middle three fingers frequently approximates 6 cm, and the thyromental distance can be compared with the fingers' span. In that way, clinically relevant approximations can be taken into account when examining patients for the purpose of predicting difficult intubation.

The usefulness of predicting difficult intubation on the basis of thyromental distance has been challenged.[18,26,28,45,92] Data from Rocke and colleagues[81] in 1992 and El-Ganzouri and coworkers[35] in 1996 indicate that thyromental distance (receding mandible) offers a 7% or less probability of predicting difficult intubation.[35,81] Chou and Wu[26] in 1993 and Brodsky and associates[16] in 2002 pointed out patients whose thyromental distances were well in excess of 6.5 cm and who turned out to have a difficult intubation. Similar measurements and predictions have been made utilizing the hyoid bone and mandible as well as the sternum and mentum.[26,84] Chou and Wu suggested that a long mandibulohyoid distance predicts a large hypopharyngeal tongue, which hides the glottis during laryngoscopy and thereby produces a difficult intubation.[26] They reasoned that the tongue is hinged to the hyoid bone, so that a long hyomandibular length represents a caudad-lying tongue. With the base of tongue positioned farther inferiorly, it occupies more space in the oropharyngeal airway. Consequently, it obstructs the laryngoscopist's line of site. The hyoid bone is more difficult to feel than the thyroid cartilage and is often impossible to locate.[56] The sternum and mentum are generally easy to find, but the sternomental distance has not been substantiated as a good predictor of difficult intubation by other investigators.

The ability to translate the temporomandibular joint is easily assessed before induction. The patient is simply asked to place the mandibular incisors (bottom teeth) in front of the maxillary incisors (upper teeth). Inability to perform this simple task usually results from one of two sources. First, the TMJ may not glide, predicting difficult intubation.[19] Second, some patients find it difficult to coordinate the maneuver, in which case there is no implication for difficult intubation.

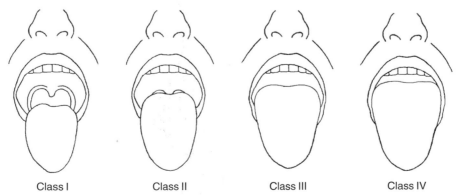

Class I   Class II   Class III   Class IV

Figure 8-2 Samsoon classification system. The oropharynx is divided into four classes on the basis of the structures visualized. Class I, soft palate, fauces, uvula, pillars. Class II, soft palate, fauces, uvula. Class III, soft palate, base of uvula. Class IV, soft palate not visible. (From Mallampati SR: Recognition of the difficult airway. In Benumof JL [ed]: Airway Management-Principles and Practice. St. Louis, Mosby, 1996, p 132.)

The upper lip bite test was proposed as a modification of the temporomandibular displacement test.[52] The upper lip bite test is performed by asking the patient to move the mandibular incisors as high on the upper lip as possible. The maneuver is similar to biting the lip. Contact of the teeth above or on the vermilion border is thought to predict adequate laryngoscopic views. Inability to touch the vermilion boarder with the mandibular teeth is thought to predict poor laryngoscopic views. Both the TMJ translation test and the upper lip bite test assess TMJ glide, which is an important consideration during laryngoscopy. Table 8-2 summarizes a quick, easy, bedside scheme for predicting difficult intubation.

IV. SPECIAL SITUATIONS

A. MORBID OBESITY

The Centers for Disease Control and Prevention currently define morbid obesity (MO) in terms of body mass index (BMI). BMI is calculated as a ratio between weight in kilograms and height in meters squared:

$$BMI = weight\ in\ kg/(height\ in\ m)^2$$

A BMI of 20 to 25 is normal, a BMI of 25 to 30 is overweight, a BMI of 30 to 40 is obese, and a BMI of more than 40 is morbidly obese. Other definitions of MO have fallen into disfavor.

Morbidly obese patients frequently suffer from upper airway obstruction, which may present as obstructive sleep apnea. During normal inspiration, the diaphragm descends and the chest wall expands, resulting in creation of negative intrathoracic pressure (subatmospheric pressure). Negative intrathoracic pressure is transmitted along the entire airway, including the upper airway. Soft tissues are drawn into the airway as if it were imploding. Under normal circumstances, obstruction is prevented by contraction of three sets of dilator muscles. The tensor palatini prevents airway obstruction by the soft palate at the nasopharynx. The genioglossus pulls the tongue anteriorly to open the oropharynx. The hyoid muscles pull the epiglottis forward and upward to prevent obstruction at the laryngopharynx. In healthy young patients, these muscles prevent obstruction during sleep. As patients age, the dilator muscles become less efficacious and there is a tendency for partial obstruction to occur.

In patients with MO, adipose tissue deposits in the lateral pharyngeal walls. These deposits are not fixed to bone and are highly mobile. They protrude into the airway, narrowing it, and are drawn farther into the airway during periods of negative airway pressure. Consequently, excess adipose tissue tends to obstruct the airway even more during inspiration. In these ways, reduced dilator muscle function or pharyngeal adipose depositions predispose to obstructive sleep apnea. See Chapter 40 for further details. Clinically, obstructive sleep apnea is implied by a history of heavy snoring, daytime somnolence, impaired memory, inability to concentrate, and frequent accidents. Associated findings include hypoxemia, polycythemia, systemic hypertension, pulmonary hypertension, and hypercarbia. Definitive diagnosis is made by polysomnography in sleep laboratories. During sleep, patients experience 5 or more episodes per hour of apnea, lasting at least 10 seconds, or 15 or more episodes per hour of hypopnea (50% decrease in airflow). Both are frequently associated with decreases in pulse oximetry of 4% or greater. Risk factors for obstructive sleep apnea are male gender, middle age or older, obesity, evening alcohol consumption, and drug-induced sleep.

Hypopnea or apnea occurs as the pharynx is obstructed. Partial obstruction leads to hypopnea and total obstruction produces apnea. Normally, dilator muscles prevent obstruction, but they do so less successfully with increasing

Table 8-2   **Generally Accepted Predictors of Difficult Intubation**

Criteria	Suggestion of Difficult Intubation
History of difficult intubation	
Length of upper incisors	Relatively long
Interincisor distance	Less than two finger breadths or less than 3 cm
Overbite	Maxillary incisors override mandibular incisors
Temporomandibular joint translation	Inability to extend mandibular incisors anterior to maxillary incisors
Mandibular space	Small, indurated, encroached upon by mass
Cervical vertebral range of motion	Cannot touch chin to chest or cannot extend neck
Thyromental distance	Less than three finger breadths (less than 6 cm)
Mallampati-Samsoon classification	Mallampati III/Samsoon IV—relatively large tongue, uvula not visible
Neck	Short, thick

Adapted from American Society of Anesthesiologists Task Force on Difficult Airway Management: Practice guidelines for management of the difficult airway. Anesthesiology 98:1269, 2003.

age and obesity. As airflow to the alveoli diminishes, hypoxemia and possibly hypercarbia develop. Both result in enhanced sympathetic outflow and patients awaken. In the awake state, dilator activity increases and airway patency is restored. Patients then fall asleep and the cycle is repeated numerous times. Rapid-eye-movement sleep is achieved poorly, and patients remain tired during the day.

Treatment frequently centers around continuous positive airway pressure, but not all patients tolerate the mask. Alternative therapies include oral appliances to move the tongue anteriorly and nocturnal oxygen. Surgical options exist. Examples include uvulopalatopharyngoplasty, genioglossus advancement, maxillomandibular advancement, and tracheostomy.

Although time to oxyhemoglobin desaturation is not a predictor of difficult intubation, it is an important consideration. The longer one has to perform laryngoscopy, the greater the likelihood of success. Rapid hemoglobin desaturation limits that time and thereby reduces the chance of tracheal intubation. A patient with MO with a BMI of 40 kg/m^2, breathing room air, who becomes apneic, desaturates to an oxygen saturation in arterial blood (SaO$_2$) of 90% in approximately 1 minute and then rapidly desaturates to an SaO$_2$ of 60% in the next minute. In contrast is the same patient breathing 100% oxygen before induction of anesthesia. After successful preoxygenation, this patient's SaO$_2$ does not fall to 90% for approximately $2\frac{1}{2}$ minutes and does not reach an SaO$_2$ of 60% for an additional $1\frac{1}{2}$ minutes.[10,37] The data show that successful oxygenation prior to induction of anesthesia extends the period of time until oxyhemoglobin desaturation takes place. Consequently, preoxygenation provides a longer period for laryngoscopy, which should increase the chances of successful intubation.

Preoxygenation may be thought of as denitrogenation. During preoxygenation, patients breath 100% oxygen. Air, which is mostly nitrogen, is washed out of alveoli and replaced with oxygen. This process stores oxygen in all open alveoli, including those constituting the functional residual capacity (FRC). The more oxygen contained in the FRC, the more time before oxyhemoglobin desaturation and the greater the period for laryngoscopy. The FRC in patients with MO is reduced. Consequently, less oxygen is stored. After preoxygenation of a 70-kg adult, following induction of anesthesia, SaO$_2$ does not fall to 90% for approximately 8 minutes and does not fall to 60% for almost 10 minutes. After preoxygenation of a morbidly obese patient weighing 127 kg, following induction of anesthesia, SaO$_2$ falls to 90% in approximately $2\frac{1}{2}$ minutes and falls to 60% in almost 4 minutes.

Evaluation before airway manipulation requires a history and physical examination. Important aspects of the history include previous airway difficulties and the patient's weight at that time. A present-day airway examination is also necessary.

Although obstructive sleep apnea pathology and pathophysiology predispose to difficult face mask ventilation and intubation, the true incidence of problems resulting from MO is undefined. The popularity of bariatric surgery has brought numerous morbidly obese patients to the operating room. Because they receive face mask ventilation infrequently, there is little practical experience to refute classical teachings about such ventilation. It is reasonable to expect fat cheeks, a short immobile neck, a large tongue, and pharyngeal adipose deposits to complicate face mask ventilation. Nevertheless, Brodsky and colleagues reported a morbidly obese patient with a BMI of 43 kg/m^2 and obstructive sleep apnea who was ventilated easily by face mask.[16] This experience serves to document the clinical findings of many practitioners. Along the same lines, considerable experience with laryngoscopy in morbidly obese patients has developed. Absent findings to the contrary, most morbidly obese patients are easy to intubate. In other words, MO does not appear to be an independent predictor of difficult intubation.[16,81] The presence of other difficult intubation predictors suggests potential problems.[97]

B. PREGNANCY

Airway management is one of the most important factors contributing to maternal mortality.[76,80] See Chapter 34 for further details. Airway difficulties pose a risk of pulmonary aspiration and hypoxic cardiopulmonary arrest. Rocke and associates reported some degree of difficulty during intubation in almost 8% of full-term pregnant patients undergoing cesarean section.[81]

Pregnant patients are generally young and have full dentition. Prominent maxillary incisors obstruct the line of sight as discussed previously. Furthermore, many present with reduced interincisor distances because of TMJ dysfunction or other etiologies. Reduced interincisor distances limit the space available for visualization and manipulation of instruments in the mouth.

Pregnant patients suffer from generalized soft tissue swelling. They all gain weight and often reach MO proportions. Short fat necks tend to prevent achieving proper sniffing position, which impairs aligning the visual axes of the mouth, pharynx, and larynx. Redundant pharyngeal tissues may fall into the airway during traditional laryngoscopy, obstructing the line of sight. Tissue edema can produce so much mucosal swelling that landmarks such as epiglottis and arytenoids are hard to distinguish. The breasts may be so engorged that they interfere with placement of a laryngoscope handle.[50] As the space between mandible and chest diminishes, less room is available for the assistant's hand to provide cricoid pressure. In fact, the assistant's hand may take up space needed to open the mouth, thereby preventing adequate mouth opening. Sufficient mouth opening is required to see through the airway as well as insert and manipulate equipment.

Tongue swelling produces macroglossia. Macroglossia prevents sufficient displacement into the mandibular space so that the line of sight is obstructed. It has been suggested that straining could exacerbate the Mallampati-Samsoon classification.[36]

Overzealous left lateral uterine displacement can tilt the torso and neck, altering the airway position in relation to the cervical spine. Cricoid pressure may exacerbate this problem by displacing the airway laterally, occluding it,[55] or angulating the larynx.

Swelling of the supraglottic airway interferes with face mask ventilation as well as complicating laryngoscopy and intubation. As the upper airway becomes edematous, it also becomes more friable. Instrumentation of such airways frequently leads to bleeding, which further complicates face mask ventilation and tracheal intubation.[31]

Parturients, especially obese parturients, suffer from reduced FRC.[5,11] All pregnant women experience an increase in oxygen consumption of approximately 20%. Consequently, periods of apnea, such as during laryngoscopy under general anesthesia, predispose to desaturation much more quickly than in their nonpregnant and nonobese counterparts.[4,7] Rapid oxyhemoglobin desaturation reduces time for laryngoscopy and detracts from the successful completion of intubation.

Other factors tend to impair successful laryngoscopy. Anxiety on the part of inexperienced physicians has led to intubation attempts prior to achieving adequate conditions. Laryngoscopy under general anesthesia requires adequate depth of anesthesia and profound muscle relaxation.[21,62] Absent one or both of these conditions, the chances of success are markedly reduced. The result is poor mouth opening, reduced interincisor distance, retching, vomiting, and aspiration. Well-intentioned, novice assistants degrade intubating conditions or fail to enhance them.[62] The Report on Confidential Enquiries into Maternal Deaths in England and Wales pointed to failure to provide cricoid pressure, poorly applied cricoid pressure, or release of cricoid pressure during a vomiting episode as major contributors to maternal morbidity and mortality.[76]

The application of cricoid pressure during active vomiting has been controversial. Sellick's original description of cricoid pressure called for release of the maneuver during vomiting episodes.[85] A single case report described an elderly woman who vomited during application of cricoid pressure and who suffered an esophageal rupture.[72] In this patient, other factors could have contributed to or caused the rupture. Nevertheless, some have recommended relinquishing cricoid pressure during vomiting episodes on the basis of this occurrence. Sellick has retracted his initial recommendation, and others have supported the maintenance of cricoid pressure during active vomiting.[86,95,99] They believe that the risk of aspiration pneumonia is greater than the risk of esophageal rupture.[86,99] Furthermore, cricoid pressure sometimes pushes the entire neck posteriorly, resulting in forward flexion of the head on the neck. Consequently, the advantages of the sniffing position are lost and laryngoscopy becomes more difficult. To correct this problem,

bimanual cricoid pressure has been suggested by Crowley and Giesecke.[32] To accomplish this maneuver, the assistant's left hand supports the patient's neck from underneath as the assistant's right hand places pressure on the cricoid cartilage.

C. LINGUAL TONSIL HYPERTROPHY

Over 11½ years, Ovassapian and colleagues[67] analyzed 33 patients who presented unanticipated difficult intubations. Before induction of anesthesia, none of these patients were thought to pose a significant likelihood of difficulty on the basis of careful preanesthetic airway examinations. Of the 33 patients, 15 had normal airway examinations. Among those 15 patients, 3 had BMIs of 31 to 40. The remaining 18 patients presented with varying predictors of difficult intubation but were judged to have been at low risk for poor laryngoscopic views. Following induction, all turned out to have difficult intubations in the hands of experienced attending anesthesiologists. They subsequently underwent flexible fiberoptic pharyngoscopy for pharyngeal assessments. All 33 demonstrated lingual tonsil hypertrophy.

Lingual tonsils are lymph tissues located at the base of the tongue. They usually experience hypertrophy bilaterally but may do so unilaterally. Enlarged lingual tonsils can push the epiglottis posteriorly, obstructing the line of sight and preventing anterior displacement of the base of tongue. They sometimes encroach on the vallecula, preventing optimal location of curved laryngoscope blades. They can distort the epiglottis so that it covers the glottic opening or is difficult to recognize. Not only do hypertrophied lingual tonsils prevent elevating the base of tongue from the line of sight, they also have a tendency to bleed, complicating intubation even further.[44,91]

Lingual tonsil hypertrophy cannot be identified by classical airway examinations to predict difficult intubation. It is often asymptomatic, and its suggestive symptoms are nonspecific. They include sore throat, dysphagia, snoring, obstructive sleep apnea, and sensations of fullness or lumps in the throat. Most patients have a history of palatine tonsillectomy or adenoidectomy.[40] Lingual tonsil hypertrophy has been associated with airway obstruction and obstructive sleep apnea.[14,34,48,66] Other pharyngeal problems that can complicate laryngoscopy include acute lingual tonsillitis,[14] lingual tonsillar abscesses, lingual thyroids,[17] and thyroglossal cysts.[43,46,59] These structures reside at the base of tongue, a location that is hidden from view during routine physical examination.

D. BURNS

Thermal burns of the head and neck complicate airway management in several ways. See Chapter 41 for further details. Burn patients with coexisting airway problems experience approximately 50% greater mortality. Thermal damage to the upper airway results in massive swelling within 2 to 24 hours. Edematous mucosa encroaches on the airway lumen to create severe narrowing or even occlusion. A narrowed upper airway reduces the amount of air drawn into the lungs. An occluded upper airway prevents any oxygen from reaching the alveoli. Both result in hypoxia. As the mucosa swells, traditional laryngoscopy becomes difficult or impossible. So much edema can collect in the mucosa that landmarks may be unrecognizable. For these reasons, it is sometimes best to perform tracheal intubation early in the care of burn patients, before swelling creates hypoxia and difficult intubation.[90]

Airway burns are suggested by occurrence of fire in a closed space; stridor; hoarseness; dyspnea; singed nasal hairs; and carbonaceous material in the mouth, nares, or pharynx. The risk of airway compromise and difficult intubation in the near future is significant. Elective prophylactic intubation is indicated for such patients.

For those who survive the acute burn period, chronic airway problems occur frequently. Burn tissue heals by formation of scar, which is nonelastic. Scars over the face and neck limit mobility of the TMJ and cervical vertebrae. The result is a small mouth opening and inability to achieve sniffing position. Scar release under local anesthesia may be helpful to restore mobility to these important joints and allow improved intubating conditions.

E. ACROMEGALY

Acromegaly results from excess growth hormone, which is frequently produced by pituitary tumors. One screening test for acromegaly involves administration of 75 to 100 g of glucose. If plasma growth hormone concentrations do not fall after 1 to 2 hours, acromegaly is suspected. High plasma growth hormone levels may indicate acromegaly. Skull radiographs and computed tomography (CT) scans showing an enlarged sella turcica suggest anterior pituitary adenomas.

Typical acromegalic features include enlarged nose, big tongue, thick mandible, full lips, elevated nasolabial folds, and prominent frontal sinuses. These patients appear to experience overgrowth of mucosa and soft tissues of the pharynx, larynx, and vocal cords.[12,53] Many experience sleep apnea.[41,71] Early in the disease process, joint spaces may be widened, but later on they develop arthritis with limited range of motion. This frequently occurs at the TMJ, resulting in a small mouth opening, and may occur in cricoarytenoid joints. Overgrowth of tissues can produce vocal cord abnormalities resulting in hoarseness or recurrent laryngeal nerve paralysis.

These features predispose to difficult mask ventilation and difficult laryngoscopy. Large tongues and epiglottides produce upper airway obstruction and make laryngoscopy difficult. Big mandibles increase the distance between teeth and vocal cords, necessitating longer laryngoscope blades. Thickened vocal cords and subglottic narrowing may require smaller tracheal tubes than would otherwise be selected. Nasal turbinate enlargement may obstruct the nasal airway and prevent passage of tubes. Dyspnea on exertion, stridor, or hoarseness may suggest laryngeal abnormalities that can complicate intubation.

F. EPIGLOTTITIS

Epiglottitis (supraglottitis) is due to a potentially life-threatening infection that causes upper airway swelling and obstruction. Formerly, the most common etiology was *Haemophilus influenza* type B (HIB). The disease usually occurred in children between 2 and 8 years of age. Since the widespread use of HIB vaccine, it is an unusual finding in the pediatric population. Nevertheless, epiglottitis still occurs in immunosuppressed adults. Common presenting signs include sore throat and dysphagia. Other signs and symptoms include drooling, inspiratory stridor, high fever, rapid deterioration to respiratory distress, pharyngitis, tachypnea, cyanosis, lethargy, and tripod positioning. These patients are most comfortable sitting up, extending the neck, and leaning forward. The "muffled voice" is an infrequent finding.[68] Lateral radiographs of the neck classically demonstrate a swollen epiglottis. Mild adult forms may be treated with observation for exacerbation of respiratory function.[30,60,63] Severe cases with respiratory compromise require airway management, which usually means tracheal intubation and antibiotics.

Instrumentation of the airway can result in total airway obstruction and is contraindicated in the awake patient. Only deep general anesthesia is likely to protect against exacerbation of airway obstruction during intubation. Prior to induction of anesthesia, preparations are made for immediate tracheostomy if required. Intravenous access is obtained before or just after induction of anesthesia. Despite the fever, glycopyrrolate is administered to dry secretions, which are generally copious and hinder laryngoscopy. Inhalation induction with sevoflurane or halothane is begun in the sitting position. After loss of consciousness, patients are placed supine to deepen the level of anesthesia. Assisted ventilation by bag and mask is frequently necessary to maintain airway patency. Supraglottic swelling, copious secretions, and reactive upper airway combine to make mask ventilation and laryngoscopy difficult. Deep inhalation anesthesia allows high concentrations of inspired oxygen. When appropriate, laryngoscopy and intubation are performed. Elective extubation usually takes place 2 to 4 days later.

G. ACUTE SUBMANDIBULAR SPACE CELLULITIS

Acute submandibular space cellulitis (Ludwig's angina) can progress rapidly to a life-threatening situation. It generally begins as a mixed flora infection around the mandibular molars. Aerobic and anaerobic pathogens are involved. The floor of the mouth swells and forces the tongue into the airway, creating upper airway obstruction. Extension to sublingual and hypopharyngeal areas produces tongue and pharyngeal swelling.[8,87] This mechanism is exacerbated in the supine position, and patients often cannot tolerate lying flat. Inability to assume the supine position precludes CT scanning, but the diagnosis can be confirmed with lateral neck soft tissue radiographs. Potential exists for infection to track down the airway and into the mediastinum, creating significant edema and swelling throughout the airway.

Submandibular cellulitis brings infection and edema fluid into the submandibular space, effectively reducing the area into which the tongue can be displaced during laryngoscopy. The swollen tongue fits poorly into the already reduced submandibular space, so that it cannot be elevated out of the line of sight during laryngoscopy. Swelling throughout the airway reduces space for visualization. It also distorts and hides landmarks needed for successful intubation. Many cases require awake tracheostomy under local anesthesia because traditional laryngoscopy fails to expose the larynx. Awake fiberoptic intubation may also be considered appropriate in these patients.

H. RHEUMATOID ARTHRITIS

Synovitis of the TMJ leads to reduced mandibular motion. Consequently, mouth opening is small. This hampers laryngoscopy by limiting the amount of space available to insert a laryngoscope and tracheal tube. Once these devices are placed, their manipulation is impaired by a small mouth opening. Severe forms of Still's disease (juvenile rheumatoid arthritis) can involve the TMJ of children, leading to poor mandibular development (micrognathia). Micrognathia is probably related to a small mandibular space. The small mandibular space does not accommodate a normal size tongue during laryngoscopy. Consequently, the tongue is not displaced anteriorly out of the line of sight. It hangs down into the airway and obstructs visualization of the larynx.

Cervical spine arthritis limits the neck's range of motion. Consequently, patients neither flex the lower cervical vertebrae nor extend the atlanto-occipital joint (sniffing position). Inability to perform these maneuvers prevents visual axis alignment of the mouth, pharynx, and larynx. Consequently, laryngoscopy may be difficult and fiberoptic intubation may be considered. In addition, atlanto-axial subluxation and separation of the atlanto-odontoid articulation can result. The diagnosis is made with lateral neck radiographs. When this occurs, the odontoid process is free to enter the foramen magnum and impinge on the spinal cord or vertebral arteries. Often the odontoid process is eroded, reducing the risk of spinal cord or vertebral artery compression. Cervical flexion deformities can render the neck totally immobile, impairing mask ventilation and laryngoscopy.

Cricoarytenoid arthritis may arise with hoarseness, pain on swallowing, dyspnea, stridor, and tenderness over the larynx. The arytenoids are edematous and fixed in adduction. Swelling may be so severe that the glottis is obscured.[96] The vocal cords move poorly,[39] which makes the larynx much more difficult to identify.[96]

V. RELIABILITY OF PREDICTION CRITERIA

Although intuitively it makes sense to perform and is consistent with best medical practices, airway evaluation frequently falls short of its intended goal.[3] Numerous rating systems based on recognized prediction criteria have been investigated. Most suffer from recurrent problems.[103] The first problem is nomenclature. A standardized definition of the difficult airway did not exist until 1993.[88] At that time, it was explained as a situation in which a conventionally trained anesthesiologist experienced difficulty with mask ventilation, difficulty with tracheal intubation, or both. For years, individual investigators needed to establish their own definition of difficult intubation each time studies were conducted. Consequently, the endpoints of their work were not necessarily comparable to other investigations in the field. Multiple meanings of the term difficult intubation prevented comparative analysis of studies.

In 1993 the American Society of Anesthesiologists (ASA) Committee on Practice Guidelines for Management of the Difficult Airway offered a generally acceptable definition.[88] Ten years later the definition was altered slightly. In 2003, "difficult tracheal intubation" referred to any intubation that requires multiple attempts.[3] This is a good clinical definition but lacks the precision required for scientific investigation. For example, some practitioners may perform a single laryngoscopy and, on the basis of the view obtained, elect to forgo further attempts at laryngoscopy. Such cases may be handled with supraglottic ventilatory devices, regional anesthesia, or other techniques. This situation does not meet the definition of difficult intubation when, in fact, it would have if one more attempt at intubation was made. Thus, the ASA's definition serves as a good clinical understanding of difficult intubation but lacks the rigid, encompassing concerns required for scientific investigation. "Failed intubation" is an easier term to understand. A failed intubation exists when laryngoscopists give up and admit that traditional intubation will not be successful. The endpoint is clear and occurs with an incidence of 1 in 280 in obstetric patients and 1 in 2230 in the general operating room population.[83]

The second problem is identifying features that predict difficult intubation. This is frequently accomplished by attempting to recognize characteristics found in patients who have proved to have difficult intubations. The problem with such an approach is the lack of information about the same characteristics in patients who have easy intubations. As Turkan and colleagues pointed out, we do not even know the normal values for many prediction criteria.[93] A better method is to apply multivariate analysis to populations of patients in a prospective manner. In that way, a single factor can be compared in difficult and easy intubations. Various rating systems attempt to combine multiple predictors into a formula. To date, none are satisfactory.

The third problem is validating the tests, once they are promulgated. Validation tests performed on the same population of patients used to identify them are misleading. This is like counting the number of envelopes in a particular mailbox, predicting that all mailboxes contain that number of envelopes, and then validating the prediction by recounting the envelopes in the same mailbox. Validation must be performed by counting the envelopes in multiple different mailboxes. In the same way, validation of difficult intubation predictors must be performed in multiple other populations of patients. The experimental sample of patients cannot be used to validate experimental results. Different sample populations are needed for that.

The fourth problem is experimental methods. Individual practitioners differ in many ways. Any given patient, on any given day, may be difficult to intubate for one laryngoscopist and not for another. Clinical practice has shown that a particular patient who is difficult to intubate in the hands of one laryngoscopist may be successfully intubated by another laryngoscopist. In this way, experimental designs utilizing more than one laryngoscopist introduce a source of variation, which detracts from attempts to control experimental conditions. Relying on a single laryngoscopist obviates this problem but limits the number of patients who can be enrolled into a single study. Another source of experimental error is observer variation. Just as laryngoscopists differ, so do observers.[47,56] Observations performed by different experimenters are subject to variations and introduce another source of erroneous data. The best way to prevent this problem is to have all observations be performed by a single experimenter. This, too, may limit the number of patients enrolled in a single study.

Statistical tests for assessing the usefulness of criteria involve sensitivity and positive predictive value. Sensitivity is the ratio of difficult intubation patients correctly identified compared with all the difficult intubation patients within the entire population of patients. For example, take a population of patients in which five people are difficult to intubate. If a particular predictor of difficult intubation correctly identifies all five patients, its sensitivity is 100%. A sensitivity of 100% means that all the difficult intubation patients are identified by the test. If the test correctly identifies only two of the five patients, its sensitivity is two fifths or 40%. Positive predictive value is the probability that difficult intubation patients identified by the test are, in fact, difficult to intubate. If the test predicts that five patients will be difficult to intubate and all five of those patients are difficult to intubate, its positive predictive value is 100%. A positive predictive value of 100% means that if the test says that any particular patient will be difficult to intubate, that patient will be difficult to intubate. If the test predicts that 10 patients will be difficult to intubate but only 5 of them are difficult to intubate, its predictive value is 5/10, 50%.

Unfortunately, statistical tests such as sensitivity and positive predictive value, applied to classical prediction criteria, have yielded disappointing results.[35,103]

In 1984 Cormack and Lehane described a grading system for comparing laryngoscopic views (Fig. 8-3).[29] Cormack-Lehane grade I views demonstrate the entire glottic opening. Grade II views show the posterior laryngeal aperture but not the anterior portion. Grade III views allow visualization of the epiglottis but not any part of the larynx. Grade IV views allow the laryngoscopist to see the soft palate but not the epiglottis. Early evidence indicated

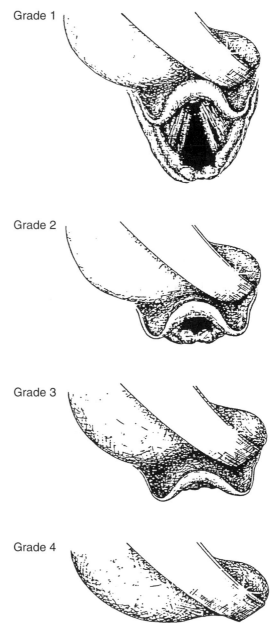

Figure 8-3 Cormack-Lehane grading system. Four laryngoscopic grades are identified. Grade I, Most of the glottis is visible. Grade II, Only the posterior extremity of the glottis is visible. Grade III, Only the epiglottis is seen. Grade IV, The epiglottis is not seen. (From Cormack RS, Lehane J: Difficult tracheal intubation in obstetrics. Anaesthesia 39:1105, 1984.)

a good correlation between Mallampati-Samsoon classes and laryngoscopic grades.[58,83] In other words, as the Mallampati-Samsoon classes increased in number, the prediction was that corresponding laryngoscopic grades would increase in number for any given patient. This concept formed the basis for using Mallampati-Samsoon classes to predict difficult intubation. In 1992, Rocke and coworkers disproved that relationship.[81] They investigated several classical predictors of difficult intubation and demonstrated that none of the ones studied were reliable predictors of difficult intubation (Fig. 8-4). Classical prediction criteria essentially deal with surface anatomy. They screen for some factors that are associated with difficult intubation but fail to address others. Some potential problems are hidden from surface anatomy examinations. Glottic and supraglottic abnormalities such as lingual tonsil hypertrophy[57,67] or epiglottic prolapse into the glottic opening[73] cannot be diagnosed by standard physical examinations for predicting difficult intubation. Pathophysiologic factors such as mobile TMJ discs or disc fragments can produce severely limited mouth opening following induction of anesthesia when none existed before.[57] Precise measurements of atlantoaxial motion sometimes fail to predict difficult intubation.[94] Supraglottic, glottic, or subglottic pathology may be unrecognized by standard tests but complicate intubation nonetheless.[22] As of this writing, *no single factor reliably predicts difficult intubation. As more and more*

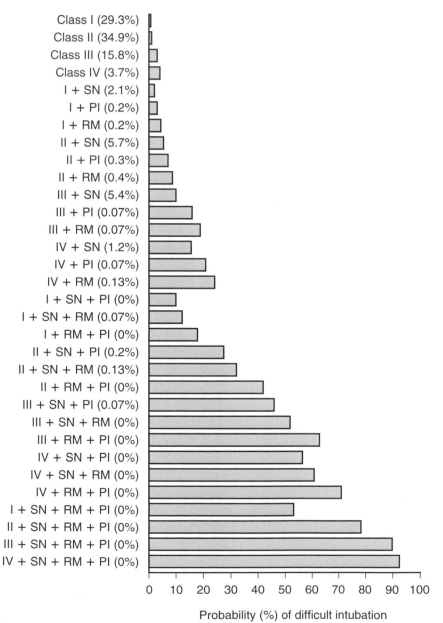

Figure 8-4 Probability of difficult intubation. PI, protruding incisors; RM, receding mandible; SN, short neck. (From Rocke DA, Murray WB, Rout CC, Gouws E: Relative risk analysis of factors associated with difficult intubation in obstetric anesthesia. Anesthesiology 77:67, 1992.)

predictors of difficult intubation are found in the same patient, at the same time, the likelihood of difficult intubation increases.[9,38,56,92,101]

VI. CONCLUSION

The first consideration in caring for patients is maintaining airway patency. In many cases, that is a hard goal to achieve. Predicting the difficult airway is important because it allows appropriate management planning. It is hoped that heightened awareness and altered treatment strategies will prevent some of the untoward events associated with treating patients with difficult airways. At present, no single factor reliably predicts difficult intubation. Consequently, prediction of difficult intubation relies on various tests, the results of which are taken into account. After assimilating the data, practitioners assess the information and compare it with similar situations that have been encountered previously. In other words, clinical judgments are made on the basis of previous experience.

New tests are sorely needed. They should be painless. Patients do not tolerate discomfort for the sake of difficult airway screening. The tests should be quick, simple to apply, and require little or no equipment. Practitioners need to perform these tests on each patient. Complex procedures, cumbersome equipment, and difficult calculations will dissuade many physicians and nurses from using tests. They should be bedside procedures. It is impractical to send ambulatory surgery patients, day of admission surgery patients, or emergency patients to distant places for high-technology, expensive imaging studies. The tests should be objective, with little inter-examiner variation,[47,82] and reproducible. They should be reliable.[35,92] High degrees of sensitivity and positive predictive value are crucial.

Classical prediction criteria deal primarily with surface anatomy and fail to address issues such as lingual tonsils, epiglottic cysts, and other soft tissue pathology. For this reason, *despite outward appearances, a history of difficult intubation may be the most reliable predictor of future difficult intubations.* A history of prior difficult intubation is generally elicited in one of two ways—orally or in writing. Frequently, patients discuss prior intubation difficulties during the preanesthetic interview. Alternatively, this information may be elicited in old records of patients, written letters, or through the Medic Alert National Registry. The Medic Alert Registry provides patients with bracelets and cards that identify their basic medical problem. More information is generally available through an emergency phone number provided to each registrant.

Until the ideal predictive criteria are discovered, we will continue to rely on imperfect tests and identification of circumstances that are recognized as associated with difficult airways.

REFERENCES

1. Adnet F, Borron SW, Dumas JL, et al: Study of the 'sniffing position' by magnetic resonance imaging. Anesthesiology 94:83, 2001.
2. Aiello G, Metcalf I: Anesthetic implications of temporomandibular joint disease. Can J Anaesth 39:610, 1992.
3. American Society of Anesthesiologists Task Force on Difficult Airway Management: Practice guidelines for management of the difficult airway. Anesthesiology 98:1269, 2003.
4. Archer GW, Marx GF: Arterial oxygen tension during apnoea in parturient women. Br J Anaesth 46:358, 1992.
5. Awe RJ, Nicotra MB, Newsome TD, et al: Arterial oxygenation and alveolar-arterial gradients in term pregnancy. Obstet Gynecol 53:182, 1979.
6. Bannister FB, MacBeth RG: Direct laryngoscopy and tracheal intubation. Lancet 18:651, 1944.
7. Baraka AS, Hanna MT, Samar SI, et al: Preoxygenation of pregnant and nonpregnant women in the head-up versus supine position. Anesth Analg 75:757, 1992.
8. Barkin RM, Bonis SL, Elghammer RM, Todd JK: Ludwig's angina in children. J Pediatr 87:563, 1975.
9. Bellhouse CP, Dore C: Criteria for estimating likelihood of difficulty of endotracheal intubation with the Macintosh laryngoscope. Anaesth Intensive Care 16:329, 1988.
10. Benumof JL, Dagg R, Benumof R: Critical hemoglobin desaturation will occur before return to an unparalyzed state following 1 mg/kg of intravenous succinylcholine. Anesthesiology 87:979, 1997.
11. Bevan DR, Holdcroft A, Loh L, et al: Closing volume and pregnancy. Br Med J 1:13, 1974.
12. Bhatia ML: Laryngeal manifestations in acromegaly. J Laryngol Otol 80:412, 1966.
13. Block C, Brechner VL: Unusual problems in airway management. II. The influence of the temporomandibular joint, the mandible, and associated structures on tracheal intubation. Anesth Analg 50:114, 1971.
14. Bourne RA, Cameron PA, Dziukas L: Respiratory obstruction with lingual tonsillitis. Anaesth Intensive Care 20:367, 1992.
15. Brechner VL: Unusual problems in the management of airways. I. Flexion-extension mobility of the cervical vertebrae. Anesth Analg 47:362, 1968.
16. Brodsky JB, Lemmens HJ, Rock-Utne JG, et al: Morbid obesity and tracheal intubation. Anesth Analg 94:732, 2002.
17. Buckland RW, Pedley J: Lingual thyroid: A threat to the airway. Anaesthesia 55:1103, 2000.
18. Butler PJ, Dhara SS: Prediction of difficult laryngoscopy: An assessment of thyromental distance and Mallampati predictive tests. Anaesth Intensive Care 20:139, 1992.
19. Calder I, Calder J, Crockard HA: Difficult direct laryngoscopy in patients with cervical spine disease. Anaesthesia 50:756, 1995.
20. Caplan RA, Posner KL, Ward FJ, et al: Adverse respiratory events in anesthesia: A closed claims analysis. Anesthesiology 72:828, 1990.

21. Carnie JC, Street MK, Kumar B: Emergency intubation of the trachea facilitated by suxamethonium: Observations in obstetric and general surgical patients. Br J Anaesth 58:498, 1986.

22. Carroll CDC, Saunders NC: Respiratory papillomatosis: A rare cause of collapse in a young adult presenting to the emergency department. Emerg Med J 19:362, 2002.

23. Cass NM, James NR, Lines V: Difficult direct laryngoscopy complicating intubation for anaesthesia. Br Med J 1:488, 1956.

24. Cheney FW, Posner KL, Caplan RA: Adverse respiratory events infrequently leading to malpractice suits: A closed claims analysis. Anesthesiology 75:932, 1991.

25. Chou HC, Wu TL: Large hypopharyngeal tongue: A shared anatomic abnormality for difficult mask ventilation, difficult intubation, and obstructive sleep apnea. Anesthesiology 94:936, 2001.

26. Chou HC, Wu TL: Mandibulohyoid distance in difficult laryngoscopy. Br J Anaesth 71:335, 1993.

27. Chou HC, Wu TL: Rethinking the three axes alignment theory for direct laryngoscopy. Acta Anaesthesiol Scand 45:261, 2001.

28. Chou HC, Wu TL: Thyromental distance: Should we redefine its role in predicting difficult laryngoscopy? Acta Anaesthesiol Scand 42:136, 1998.

29. Cormack RS, Lehane J: Difficult tracheal intubation in obstetrics. Anaesthesia 39:1105, 1984.

30. Crosby E, Reid D: Acute epiglottitis in the adult: Is intubation mandatory? Can J Anaesth 38:914, 1991.

31. Crowhurst JA: Failed intubation management at caesarean section. Anaesth Intensive Care 19:305, 1991.

32. Crowley DS, Giesecke AH: Bimanual cricoid pressure. Anaesthesia 45:588, 1990.

33. De Beer DAH, Williams DG, Mackersie A: An unexpected difficult laryngoscopy. Paediatr Anaesth 12:645, 2002.

34. Dindzans LJ, Irvine BWH, Haydern RE: An unusual cause of airway obstruction. 13:252, 1984.

35. El-Ganzouri AR, McCarthy RJ, Tuman KI, et al: Preoperative airway assessment: Predictive value of a multivariate risk index. Anesth Analg 82:1197, 1996.

36. Farcon EL, Kim MH, Marx GF: Changing Mallampati score during labour. Can J Anaesth 41:50, 1994.

37. Farmery AD, Roe PG: A model to describe the rate of oxyhaemoglobin desaturation during apnoea. Br J Anaesth 76:284, 1996.

38. Frerk CM: Predicting difficult intubation. Anaesthesia 46:1005, 1991.

39. Fultran ND, Sherris D, Norante JD: Cricoarytenoid arthritis in children. Otolaryngol Head Neck Surg 104:366, 1990.

40. Golding-Wood DG, Whittet HB: The lingual tonsil—A neglected symptomatic structure? J Laryngol Otol 103:922, 1989.

41. Grunstein RR: Central sleep apnea is associated with increased ventilatory response to carbon dioxide and hypersecretion of growth hormone in patients with acromegaly. Am J Respir Crit Care Med 150:496, 1994.

42. Hagberg C, Boin MH: Management of the airway: Complications. In Benumof JL, Saidman LJ (eds): Anesthesia and Perioperative Complications, 2nd ed. St. Louis, Mosby, 1999, p 4.

43. Henderson LT, Denneny JC III, Teichgraeber J: Airway-obstructing epiglottic cyst. Ann Otol Rhinol Laryngol 94:473, 1985.

44. Henderson K, Abernathy S, Bays T: Lingual tonsillar hypertrophy: The anesthesiologist's view. Anesth Analg 79:814, 1994.

45. Jacobson J, Jenson E, Waldau T, Poulsen TD: Preoperative evaluation of intubation conditions in patients scheduled for elective surgery. Acta Anaesthesiol Scand 40:421, 1996.

46. Kamble VA, Lilly RB, Gross JB: Unanticipated difficult intubation as a result of an asymptomatic vallecular cyst. Anesthesiology 91:872, 1999.

47. Karkouti K, Rose DK, Ferris LE, et al: Inter-observer reliability of ten tests used for predicting difficult intubation. Can J Anaesth 43:554, 1996.

48. Kashyap A, Farid A, Aldridge R, King AB: Lingual tonsil causing airway obstruction. Ear Nose Throat J 73:830, 1994.

49. Kawaguchi M, Sakamoto T, Furuya H, et al: Pseudoankylosis of the mandible after supratentorial craniotomy. Anesth Analg 83:731, 1996.

50. Kay NH: Mammomegaly and intubation. Anaesthesia 37:221, 1982.

51. Keenan RL, Boyan CP: Cardiac arrest due to anesthesia. JAMA 252:2373, 1985.

52. Khan ZH, Kashfi A, Ebrahimkhani E: A comparison of the upper lip bite test (a simple new technique) with modified Mallampati classification in predicting difficulty in endotracheal intubation: A prospective blinded study. Anesth Analg 96:595, 2003.

53. Kitahata LM: Airway difficulties associated with anaesthesia in acromegaly. Br J Anaesth 43:1187, 1971.

54. Langeron O, Masso E, Huraux C, et al: Prediction of difficult mask ventilation. Anesthesiology 92:1229, 2000.

55. Lawes EG, Duncan PW, Bland B, et al: The cricoid yoke—A device for providing consistent and reproducible cricoid pressure. Br J Anaesth 58:925, 1986.

56. Lewis M, Keramati S, Benumof JL, Berry CC: What is the best way to determine oropharyngeal classification and mandibular space length to predict difficult laryngoscopy? Anesthesiology 81:69, 1994.

57. Lim BSL, Andrews R: Unexpected difficult intubation in a patient with normal airway on assessment. Anaesth Intensive Care 29:642, 2001.

58. Mallampati SR, Gatt SP, Gugino LD, et al: A clinical sign to predict difficult tracheal intubation: A prospective study. Can J Anaesth 32:429, 1985.

59. Mason DG, Wark KJ: Unexpected difficult intubation: Asymptomatic epiglottic cysts as a cause of upper airway obstruction during anaesthesia. Anaesthesia 42:407, 1987.

60. Mayo-Smith MF, Hirsch PJ, Wodzinski SF: Acute epiglottitis in adults. N Engl J Med 314:1133, 1986.

61. McGill IW: Technique in endotracheal anaesthesia. Br Med J 2:817, 1930.

62. Morgan M: The confidential inquiry into maternal deaths. Anaesthesia 41:689, 1986.

63. Muller BJ, Fliegel JE: Acute epiglottitis in a 79-year old man. Can Anaesth Soc J 32:415, 1985.

64. Nichol HC, Zuck D: Difficult laryngoscopy—The 'anterior' larynx and the atlanto-occipital gap. Br J Anaesth 55:141, 1983.

65. Ochroch EA, Eckmann DM: Clinical application of acoustic reflectometry in predicting the difficult airway. Anesth Analg 95:645, 2002.

66. Olsen KD, Suh KW, Staats BA: Surgically correctable causes of sleep apnea syndrome. Otolaryngol Head Neck Surg 89:726, 1981.

67. Ovassapian A, Glassenberg R, Randel GI, et al: The unexpected difficult airway and lingual tonsil hyperplasia—A case series and a review of the literature. Anesthesiology 97:124, 2002.

68. Park KW, Darvish A, Lowenstein E: Airway management for adult patients with acute epiglottitis: A 12 year experience at an academic medical center (1984-1995). Anesthesiology 88:254, 1998.

69. Patil VU, Stehling LC, Zauder HL: Predicting the difficulty of intubation utilizing an intubating guide. Anesth Rev 10:32, 1983.

70. Pilkington S, Carli F, Dakin MJ, et al: Increase in Mallampati score during pregnancy. Br J Anaesth 74:638, 1995.

71. Piper JG: Perioperative management and surgical outcome of the acromegalic patient with sleep apnea. Neurosurgery 36:70, 1995.

72. Ralph SJ, Wareham CA: Rupture of the oesophagus during cricoid pressure. Anaesthesia 46:40, 1991.

73. Ramachandran K, Bhishma R: Unexpected difficult airway. Anesthesia 58:392, 2003.

74. Rashid J, Warltier B: Awake fibreoptic intubation for a rare cause of upper airway obstruction: An infected laryngocoel. Anaesthesia 44:834, 1989.

75. Redick LF: The temporomandibular joint and tracheal intubation. Anesth Analg 66:675, 1987.

76. Report on Confidential Enquiries into Maternal Deaths in England and Wales. 1982-1984, 1985-1987. London, Her Majesty's Stationery Office, 1989, 1991.

77. Riley R, Guilleminault C, Herran J, Powell N: Cephalometric analyses and flow-volume loops in obstructive sleep apnea patients. Sleep 6:303, 1983.

78. Roberts JT, Ali HH, Shorten GD: Using the bubble inclinometer to measure laryngeal tilt and predict difficulty of laryngoscopy. J Clin Anesth 5:306, 1993.

79. Roberts JT, Ali HH, Shorten GD: Using the laryngeal indices caliper to predict difficulty of intubation with a Macintosh #3 laryngoscope. J Clin Anesth 5:302, 1993.

80. Rochat RW, Koonin LM, Atrash HK, Jewett JF: Maternal mortality in the United States: Report from the Maternal Mortality Collaborative. Obstet Gynecol 72:91, 1988.

81. Rocke DA, Murray WB, Rout CC, Gouws E: Relative risk analysis of factors associated with difficult intubation in obstetric anesthesia. Anesthesiology 77:67, 1992.

82. Rose DDK, Cohen MM: The incidence of airway problems depends on the definition used. Can J Anaesth 43:30, 1996.

83. Samsoon GLT, Young JRB: Difficult tracheal intubation: A retrospective study. Anaesthesia 42:487, 1987.

84. Savva D: Prediction of difficult tracheal intubation. Br J Anaesth 73:149, 1994.

85. Sellick BA: Cricoid pressure to control regurgitation of stomach contents during induction of anaesthesia. Lancet 2:404, 1961.

86. Sellick BA: Rupture of the oesophagus following cricoid pressure? Anaesthesia 37:213, 1982.

87. Sethi DS, Stanley RE: Deep neck abscesses—Changing trends. J Laryngol Otol 108:138, 1994.

88. Task Force on Guidelines for Management of the Difficult Airway: Practice guidelines for management of the difficult airway. Anesthesiology 78:597, 1993.

89. Tham EJ, Gilldersleve CD, Sanders LD, et al: Effects of posture, phonation, and observer on Mallampati classification. Br J Anaesth 68:32, 1992.

90. Thompson B, Herndon DN, Trabor DL: Effect on mortality of inhalation injury. J Trauma 26:163, 1987.

91. Tokumine J, Sugahara K, Ura M, et al: Lingual tonsil hypertrophy with difficult airway and uncontrollable bleeding. Anaesthesia 58:390, 2003.

92. Tse JC, Rimm EB, Hussain A: Predicting difficult tracheal intubation in surgical patients scheduled for general anesthesia: A prospective blind study. Anesth Analg 81:254, 1995.

93. Turkan S, Ates Y, Cuhruk H, Tekdemir I: Should we reevaluate the variables for predicting the difficult airway in anesthesiology? Anesth Analg 94:1340, 2002.

94. Urakami Y, Takenaka I, Nakamura M, et al: The reliability of the Bellhouse test for evaluating extension capacity of the atlantoaxial complex. Anesth Analg 95:1437, 2002.

95. Vanner RG: Mini-symposium on the gastrointestinal tract and pulmonary aspiration: Mechanisms of regurgitation and its prevention with cricoid pressure. Int J Obstet Anesth 2:207, 1993.

96. Vetter TR: Acute airway obstruction due to arytenoiditis in a child with juvenile rheumatoid arthritis. Anesth Analg 79:1198, 1994.

97. Voyagis GS, Kyriakis KP, Dimitriou V, Vrettou I: Value of oropharyngeal Mallampati classification in predicting difficult laryngoscopy among obese patients. Eur J Anaesthesiol 15:330, 1998.

98. White A, Kander PL: Anatomic factors in difficult direct laryngoscopy. Br J Anaesth 47:468, 1975.

99. Whittington RM, Robinson JS, Thompson JM: Fatal aspiration (Mendelson's) syndrome despite antacids and cricoid pressure. Lancet 2:228, 1979.

100. Williamson JA, Webb RK, Szekely S, et al: The Australian Incident Monitoring Study. Difficult intubation: An analysis of 2000 incident reports. Anaesth Intensive Care 21:602, 1993.

101. Wilson ME, Spiegenhalter D, Roberston JA, et al: Predicting difficult intubation. Br J Anaesth 61:211, 1988.

102. Woods GM: Mandibular tori as a cause of inability to visualize the larynx. Anesth Analg 81:870, 1995.

103. Yentis SM: Predicting difficult intubation—Worthwhile exercise or pointless ritual? Anaesthesia 57:105, 2002.

9

THE AMERICAN SOCIETY OF ANESTHESIOLOGISTS' MANAGEMENT OF THE DIFFICULT AIRWAY ALGORITHM AND EXPLANATION-ANALYSIS OF THE ALGORITHM

Carin A. Hagberg
Jonathan L. Benumof

I. INTRODUCTION

The literature provides strong evidence that specific strategies facilitate management of the difficult airway. Specific strategies can be linked together to form more comprehensive treatment plans or algorithms. The purpose of the American Society of Anesthesiologists' (ASA) Algorithm on the Management of the Difficult Airway is to facilitate the management of the difficult airway and to reduce the likelihood of adverse outcomes. The principal adverse outcomes associated with the difficult airway include (but are not limited to) death, brain injury, cardiopulmonary arrest, unnecessary tracheostomy, airway trauma, and damage to teeth.

The original ASA Algorithm on the Management of the Difficult Airway was developed over a 2-year period by the ASA Task Force on Guidelines for Management of the Difficult Airway.[2] The task force consisted of Robert A. Caplan, M.D. (Chair); Jonathan L. Benumof, M.D.; Frederic A. Berry, M.D.; Casey D. Blitt, M.D.;

Robert H. Bode, M.D.; Frederick W. Cheney, M.D.; Richard T. Connis, Ph.D.; Orin F. Guidry, M.D.; and Andranik Ovassapian, M.D. and therein included academicians, private practitioners, airway experts, adult and pediatric anesthesia generalists, and a statistical methodologist. The algorithm was approved by the ASA House of Delegates, October 21, 1992, and became effective July 1, 1993. David Nickinovich, Ph.D. became an additional member of the task force in the revision of the practice guidelines, which were submitted and accepted for publication October 23, 2002.[47] This revised algorithm takes into account another 10 years of data and recommendations for a wider range of management techniques than was previously addressed.

This chapter presents and explains the ASA Algorithm on the Management of the Difficult Airway. The algorithm is concerned with the maintenance of airway patency at all times. Special emphasis is placed on an operating room setting (although the algorithm can be extrapolated to the intensive care unit and the ward). The algorithm is intended for use by anesthesiologists or by individuals who deliver anesthetic care and airway management under the direct supervision of an anesthesiologist. The guidelines themselves apply to airway management during all types of anesthetic care in different anesthetizing locations and are intended for all patients of all ages. Adherence to the principles of the difficult airway management algorithm and the widespread adoption of a precise plan for management of airway difficulties should result in reduction of respiratory catastrophes and a decrease in anesthesia morbidity and mortality.

II. THE ASA ALGORITHM ON THE MANAGEMENT OF THE DIFFICULT AIRWAY

A side-by-side comparison of the original (1993) and updated (2003) difficult airway management algorithm is depicted in Figure 9-1A and B. Differences between the two algorithms are listed in Box 9-1. The algorithm begins with the most basic question of whether or not the presence of a difficult airway is recognized (see Chapter 8). Obviously, if the potential for difficulty is recognized, one can make proper mental and physical preparation and the chance of a successful good outcome is increased, whereas failure to recognize the potential for difficulty means, by definition, that the actual difficulty will be unexpected, proper mental and physical preparation minimized, and the chance of a successful good outcome decreased.

When performing a proper airway evaluation, the practitioner should take into account any characteristics of the patient that could lead to difficulty in the performance of (1) bag-mask ventilation, (2) laryngoscopy, (3) intubation, and (4) a surgical airway. As mentioned earlier, the possibility of difficult mask ventilation (DMV) is now the first issue addressed in the revised algorithm.

Langeron and colleagues,[39] in a prospective study of 1502 patients, made the following observations: (1) the reported incidence of DMV was 5% in the general adult population, (2) DMV was reported more frequently when intubation was difficult, (3) anesthesiologists did not accurately predict DMV, and (4) five criteria (age older than 55 years, body mass index > 26 kg/m^2, lack of teeth, presence of mustache or beard, history of snoring) were independent risk factors for DMV and the presence of two of these risk factors indicated a high likelihood of DMV.

As perioperative physicians, anesthesiologists should keep these risk factors in mind in order to optimize the patient's condition, as some of them can be reversed. Thus, DMV may possibly be prevented by such simple precautions as shaving a mustache or beard, leaving dentures in place during bag-mask ventilation, and having the patient worked up for possible obstructive sleep apnea, if time permits. These points merit further investigation.

The following plan for routine evaluation of a patient's airway, assuming that the patient has no obvious pathologic airway problems, is a reasonable one (see Chapter 8 for a complete discussion of preoperative evaluation).

1. Before the initiation of anesthetic care and airway management in any patient, an airway history should be conducted, whenever feasible, to detect medical, surgical, and anesthetic factors that may indicate the presence of a difficult airway. Systemic diseases (e.g., respiratory failure and coronary artery disease) that might place limits on or require special attention during awake intubation, such as increased fraction of inspired oxygen (FiO_2) and prevention of sympathetic nervous system stimulation, respectively, should be noted. In addition, examination of previous anesthetic records, if available in a timely manner, may yield useful information about airway management.

2. Physical examination of the airway should also be conducted, whenever feasible, before the initiation of anesthetic care and airway management in all patients to detect physical characteristics that may indicate the presence of a difficult airway. Multiple airway features should be assessed (Table 9-1).
   a. Patients should be asked to open their mouths as widely as possible and extend their tongues. The mandibular opening (measured by ruler, if there is doubt about any limitation) and pharyngeal anatomy (e.g., uvula, tonsillar pillars) are observed.
   b. The length of the submental space (mandible to hyoid) and thyromental distance (mandible to thyroid notch) should be noted (measured by ruler, if there is any doubt).
   c. Patients should be viewed from the side to see their ability to assume the "sniffing" position (flexion of the neck on chest and extension of the head on the neck). The lateral view should also reveal any degree of maxillary overbite.

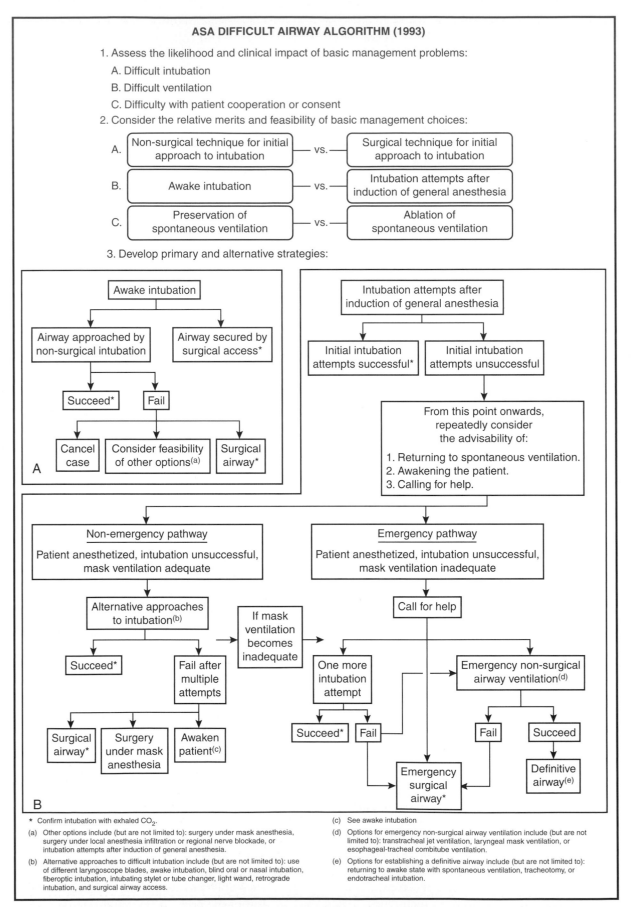

ASA DIFFICULT AIRWAY ALGORITHM (1993)

1. Assess the likelihood and clinical impact of basic management problems:
   A. Difficult intubation
   B. Difficult ventilation
   C. Difficulty with patient cooperation or consent

2. Consider the relative merits and feasibility of basic management choices:

   A. Non-surgical technique for initial approach to intubation — vs. — Surgical technique for initial approach to intubation

   B. Awake intubation — vs. — Intubation attempts after induction of general anesthesia

   C. Preservation of spontaneous ventilation — vs. — Ablation of spontaneous ventilation

3. Develop primary and alternative strategies:

A

Awake intubation
- Airway approached by non-surgical intubation
  - Succeed*
  - Fail
    - Cancel case
    - Consider feasibility of other options(a)
    - Surgical airway*
- Airway secured by surgical access*

Intubation attempts after induction of general anesthesia
- Initial intubation attempts successful*
- Initial intubation attempts unsuccessful
  - From this point onwards, repeatedly consider the advisability of:
    1. Returning to spontaneous ventilation.
    2. Awakening the patient.
    3. Calling for help.

B

Non-emergency pathway
Patient anesthetized, intubation unsuccessful, mask ventilation adequate
- Alternative approaches to intubation(b)
  - Succeed*
  - Fail after multiple attempts
    - Surgical airway*
    - Surgery under mask anesthesia
    - Awaken patient(c)

If mask ventilation becomes inadequate

Emergency pathway
Patient anesthetized, intubation unsuccessful, mask ventilation inadequate
- Call for help
  - One more intubation attempt
    - Succeed*
    - Fail
      - Emergency surgical airway*
  - Emergency non-surgical airway ventilation(d)
    - Fail
      - Emergency surgical airway*
    - Succeed
      - Definitive airway(e)

* Confirm intubation with exhaled CO₂.

(a) Other options include (but are not limited to): surgery under mask anesthesia, surgery under local anesthesia infiltration or regional nerve blockade, or intubation attempts after induction of general anesthesia.

(b) Alternative approaches to difficult intubation include (but are not limited to): use of different laryngoscope blades, awake intubation, blind oral or nasal intubation, fiberoptic intubation, intubating stylet or tube changer, light wand, retrograde intubation, and surgical airway access.

(c) See awake intubation

(d) Options for emergency non-surgical airway ventilation include (but are not limited to): transtracheal jet ventilation, laryngeal mask ventilation, or esophageal-tracheal combitube ventilation.

(e) Options for establishing a definitive airway include (but are not limited to): returning to awake state with spontaneous ventilation, tracheotomy, or endotracheal intubation.

Figure 9-1A The American Society of Anesthesiologists' (ASA) difficult airway algorithm. (From American Society of Anesthesiologists Task Force on Management of the Difficult Airway: Practice guidelines for management of the difficult airway: A report. Anesthesiology 78:597-602, 1993.)

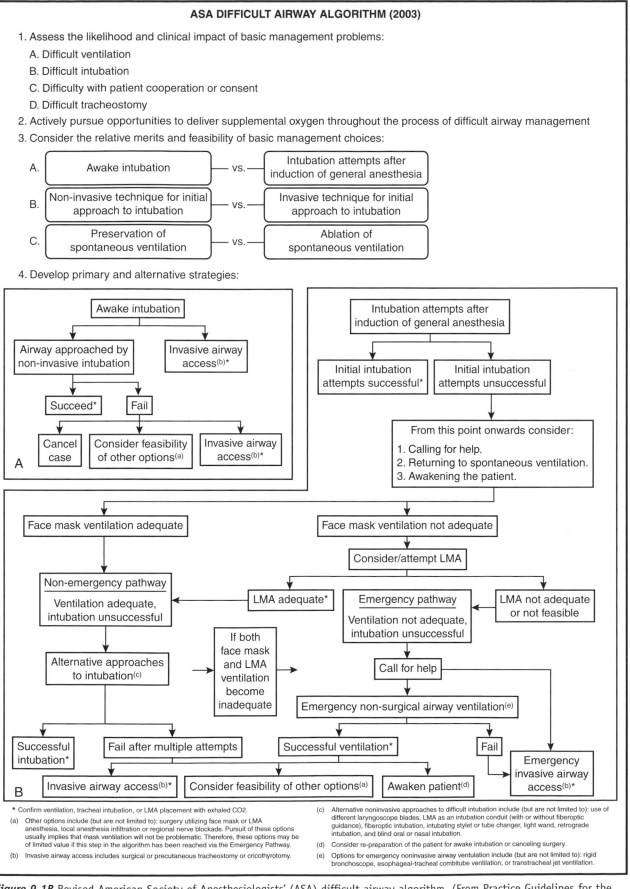

ASA DIFFICULT AIRWAY ALGORITHM (2003)

1. Assess the likelihood and clinical impact of basic management problems:

   A. Difficult ventilation

   B. Difficult intubation

   C. Difficulty with patient cooperation or consent

   D. Difficult tracheostomy

2. Actively pursue opportunities to deliver supplemental oxygen throughout the process of difficult airway management

3. Consider the relative merits and feasibility of basic management choices:

   A. Awake intubation — vs. — Intubation attempts after induction of general anesthesia

   B. Non-invasive technique for initial approach to intubation — vs. — Invasive technique for initial approach to intubation

   C. Preservation of spontaneous ventilation — vs. — Ablation of spontaneous ventilation

4. Develop primary and alternative strategies:

A

Awake intubation
- Airway approached by non-invasive intubation
  - Succeed*
    - Cancel case
  - Fail
    - Consider feasibility of other options(a)
    - Invasive airway access(b)*
- Invasive airway access(b)*

Intubation attempts after induction of general anesthesia
- Initial intubation attempts successful*
- Initial intubation attempts unsuccessful
  - From this point onwards consider:
    1. Calling for help.
    2. Returning to spontaneous ventilation.
    3. Awakening the patient.

B

Face mask ventilation adequate
- Non-emergency pathway
  Ventilation adequate, intubation unsuccessful
  - Alternative approaches to intubation(c)
    - Successful intubation*
    - Fail after multiple attempts
      - Invasive airway access(b)*
      - Consider feasibility of other options(a)

Face mask ventilation not adequate
- Consider/attempt LMA
  - LMA adequate*
  - LMA not adequate or not feasible
- Emergency pathway
  Ventilation not adequate, intubation unsuccessful
  - If both face mask and LMA ventilation become inadequate
  - Call for help
    - Emergency non-surgical airway ventilation(e)
      - Successful ventilation*
        - Awaken patient(d)
      - Fail
        - Emergency invasive airway access(b)*

* Confirm ventilation, tracheal intubation, or LMA placement with exhaled CO2.

(a) Other options include (but are not limited to): surgery utilizing face mask or LMA anesthesia, local anesthesia infiltration or regional nerve blockade. Pursuit of these options usually implies that mask ventilation will not be problematic. Therefore, these options may be of limited value if this step in the algorithm has been reached via the Emergency Pathway.

(b) Invasive airway access includes surgical or precutaneous tracheostomy or cricothyrotomy.

(c) Alternative noninvasive approaches to difficult intubation include (but are not limited to): use of different laryngoscope blades, LMA as an intubation conduit (with or without fiberoptic guidance), fiberoptic intubation, intubating stylet or tube changer, light wand, retrograde intubation, and blind oral or nasal intubation.

(d) Consider re-preparation of the patient for awake intubation or canceling surgery.

(e) Options for emergency noninvasive airway ventulation include (but are not limited to): rigid bronchoscope, esophageal-tracheal combitube ventilation, or transtracheal jet ventilation.

Figure 9-1B Revised American Society of Anesthesiologists' (ASA) difficult airway algorithm. (From Practice Guidelines for the Management of the Difficult Airway: An updated report by the American Society of Anesthesiologists Task Force on the Management of the Difficult Airway. Anesthesiology 98:1269-1277, 2003.)

Box 9-1 Differences between 1993 and 2003 ASA Management of the Difficult Airway Algorithms

1. Difficult ventilation is now listed first under assessment of the likelihood and clinical impact of basic management problems. Also, in the same category, difficult tracheostomy was added.
2. To pursue actively opportunities to deliver supplemental oxygen throughout the process of difficult airway management was added.
3. When considering the relative merits and feasibility of basic management choices, awake intubation versus intubation attempts after induction of anesthesia should now be considered first before nonsurgical techniques as the initial approach to intubation.
4. The use of the laryngeal mask airway (LMA) is incorporated into the algorithm in the awake limb and after induction of general anesthesia limb in both the nonemergency and emergency pathways (either as a ventilatory device or as a conduit for tracheal intubation).
5. Removed one more intubation attempt.
6. Added the rigid bronchoscope as an option for emergency noninvasive ventilation.

d. The patency of the nostrils.
e. The length and thickness of the neck.

Although each risk factor individually has a rather low positive predictive value for difficult intubation, when combined, the factors can provide a gestalt for difficult airway management.

3. Additional evaluation may be indicated in some patients to characterize the likelihood or nature of the anticipated airway difficulty. The findings of the airway history and physical examination may be useful in guiding the selection of specific diagnostic tests and consultation.[32]
4. In a few patients, an "awake look" using direct laryngoscopy (after adequate preparation) may be performed in order to assess intubation difficulty further. If an adequate view is obtained, endotracheal intubation may be performed, followed immediately by the administration of an intravenous induction agent.

If it is recognized that mask ventilation or the intubation is going to be difficult because of the presence of a pathologic factor or a combination of anatomic factors (large tongue size, small mandibular space, or restricted atlanto-occipital extension), airway patency should be secured and guaranteed (usually by intubation) while the patient remains awake.

A. AWAKE TRACHEAL INTUBATION

Although awake intubation is generally more time consuming for the anesthesiologist and a more unpleasant experience for the patient, there are several compelling reasons why intubation should be done while a patient with a recognized difficult airway is still awake. First, and most important, the natural airway is better maintained in most patients when they are awake ("no bridges are burned"). Second, in the awake patient, enough muscle

Table 9-1 Components of the Preoperative Airway Physical Examination

Airway Examination Component	Nonreassuring Findings
1. Length of upper incisors	Relatively long
2. Relation of maxillary and mandibular incisors during normal jaw closure	Prominent "overbite" (maxillary incisors anterior to mandibular incisors)
3. Relation of maxillary and mandibular incisors during voluntary protrusion of the jaw	Patient's mandibular incisors anterior to (in front of) maxillary incisors
4. Interincisor distance	< 3 cm
5. Visibility of uvula	Not visible when tongue is protruded with patient in sitting position (e.g., Mallampati class > II)
6. Shape of palate	Highly arched or very narrow
7. Compliance of mandibular space	Stiff, indurated, occupied by mass, or nonresilient
8. Thyromental distance	< 3 ordinary finger breadths
9. Length of neck	Short
10. Thickness of neck	Thick
11. Range of motion of head and neck	Patient cannot touch tip of chin to chest or cannot extend neck

tone is maintained to keep the relevant upper airway structures (the base of the tongue, vallecula, epiglottis, larynx, esophagus, and posterior pharyngeal wall) separated from one another and much easier to identify. In the anesthetized and paralyzed patient, loss of muscle tone tends to cause these structures to collapse toward one another (e.g., the tongue moves posteriorly), which distorts the anatomy.[30,48] Third, the larynx moves to a more anterior position with the induction of anesthesia and paralysis, which makes conventional intubation more difficult.[49] Thus, if a difficult intubation is anticipated, awake endotracheal intubation is indicated.

Crucial to the success of an awake endotracheal intubation is proper preparation of the patient (see Chapter 10). Most intubation techniques work well in patients when they are quiet and cooperative and have a larynx that is nonreactive to physical stimuli. The components of proper preparation for an awake intubation consist of psychological preparation (awake intubation proceeds more easily in the patient who knows and agrees with what is going to happen); appropriate monitoring (electrocardiogram, noninvasive blood pressure, pulse oximetry, and capnography); oxygen supplementation (nasal prongs, nasal cannula, suction channel of a fiberoptic bronchoscope [FOB], transtracheal catheter),[4,11,24,42] vasoconstriction of the nasal mucous membranes (if performing nasal intubation), administration of a drying agent, and topical anesthesia; judicious sedation (keeping the patient in meaningful contact with the environment); performance of laryngeal nerve blocks (e.g., block lingual branch of the glossopharyngeal nerve and the superior laryngeal nerve); aspiration prevention (see Chapter 11); and having the appropriate airway equipment available. Box 9-2 lists the suggested (ASA guidelines) contents of a portable airway management cart.[47]

There are numerous ways to intubate the trachea or ventilate a patient, or both (see Chapters 13 to 30). Box 9-3 shows a list of the techniques contained within the ASA guidelines. The techniques chosen depend, in part, upon the anticipated surgery, the condition of the patient, and the skills and preferences of the anesthesiologist.

Occasionally, awake intubation may fail owing to a lack of patient's cooperation, equipment, or operator limitations, or all of these. Depending on the precise cause of failure of awake intubation: (1) the surgery may be canceled (the patient needs further counseling, airway edema or trauma has resulted, or different equipment or personnel is necessary), (2) general anesthesia (GA) may be induced (the fundamental problem must be considered to be a lack of cooperation and mask ventilation considered to be nonproblematic), (3) regional anesthesia may be considered (requires careful clinical judgment balancing risks and benefits) (see Chapter 42), or (4) a surgical airway may be created (the surgery is essential and GA is considered inappropriate until intubation is accomplished). Occasionally, a surgical airway is the best choice for intubation (e.g., with laryngeal or tracheal

---

Box 9-2 Suggested Contents of the Portable Storage Unit for Difficult Airway Management

Important: The items listed in this box represent suggestions. The contents of the portable storage unit should be customized to meet the specific needs, preferences, and skills of the practitioner and health care facility.

1. Rigid laryngoscope blades of alternate design and size from those routinely used; this may include a rigid fiberoptic laryngoscope.
2. Endotracheal tubes of assorted sizes.
3. Endotracheal tube guides. Examples include (but are not limited to) semirigid stylets, ventilating tube changer, light wands, and forceps designed to manipulate the distal portion of the endotracheal tube.
4. Laryngeal mask airways of assorted sizes; this may include the intubation laryngeal mask airway (LMA-Fastrach) and the LMA-ProSeal (LMA North America, San Diego, CA).
5. Fiberoptic intubation equipment.
6. Retrograde intubation equipment.
7. At least one device suitable for emergency nonsurgical airway ventilation. Examples include (but are not limited to) the esophageal-tracheal Combitube (Tyco Healthcare, Mansfield, MA), a hollow jet ventilation stylet, and a transtracheal jet ventilator.
8. Equipment suitable for emergency surgical airway access (e.g., cricothyrotomy).
9. An exhaled CO_2 detector.
10. Rigid ventilating bronchoscope.

---

fracture or disruption, upper airway abscess, combined mandibular-maxillary fractures).

B. THE ANESTHETIZED PATIENT WHOSE TRACHEA IS DIFFICULT TO INTUBATE

There are three general situations in which an anesthesiologist is required to intubate the trachea of an unconscious or anesthetized patient whose airway is difficult to manage. First, the patient may already be unconscious (e.g., after trauma) or anesthetized (e.g., drug overdose). Second, the patient may absolutely refuse or not tolerate awake intubation (e.g., a child, a mentally retarded patient, or an intoxicated combative patient). Third, and perhaps most commonly, the anesthesiologist may fail to recognize intubation difficulty on the preoperative evaluation. Of course, even in the first and second situations, the preoperative airway evaluation is important because the findings may dictate the choice of intubation technique. In all three of these situations, the patient may, in addition, have a full stomach.

Box 9-3   Techniques for Difficult Airway Management

Important: This box displays commonly cited techniques. It is not a comprehensive list. The order of presentation is alphabetic and does not imply preference for a given technique or sequence of use. Combinations of techniques may be employed. The techniques chosen by the practitioner in a particular case depend upon specific needs, preferences, skills, and clinical constraints.

Techniques for Difficult Intubation

Alternative laryngoscope blades
Awake intubation
Blind intubation (oral or nasal)
Fiberoptic intubation
Intubating stylet or tube changer
Invasive airway access
Laryngeal mask airway as an intubating conduit
Light wand
Retrograde intubation

Techniques for Difficult Ventilation

Esophageal-tracheal Combitube
Intratracheal jet stylet
Invasive airway access
Laryngeal mask airway
Oral and nasopharyngeal airways
Rigid ventilating bronchoscope
Transtracheal jet ventilation
Two-person mask ventilation

All of the intubation techniques that are described for the awake patient[2,8] can be used in the unconscious or anesthetized patient without modification. However, direct and fiberoptic laryngoscopy may be slightly more difficult in the paralyzed, anesthetized patient compared with the awake patient because the larynx may become more anterior relative to other structures as a result of relaxation of oral and pharyngeal muscles.[49] In addition, and more important, the upper airway structures may coalesce into a horizontal plane instead of separating out in a vertical plane.[30,48]

In the anesthetized patient whose trachea has proved to be difficult to intubate, it is necessary to try to maintain gas exchange between intubation attempts by mask ventilation and also during intubation attempts, whenever possible. As depicted in the latest version of the difficult airway management algorithm, opportunities to deliver supplemental oxygen throughout whatever steps are taken to secure the airway should be pursued.[47] Positive-pressure ventilation may be continuously maintained during fiberoptic endoscopy–aided orotracheal intubation by using an anesthesia mask that has a special fiberoptic instrument port, which is covered by a self-sealing diaphragm (instead of standard mask), along with an airway intubator (instead of the standard oropharyngeal airway) (see Chapter 18)[45,48] or by using a laryngeal mask airway (LMA) as a conduit for the FOB (see Chapter 21).[7]

It is extremely important to realize that the amount of laryngeal edema and bleeding is likely to increase after every forceful intubation attempt. Although laryngeal edema and bleeding can occur with any intubation method, they are most common after use of a laryngoscope or retraction blade. Consequently, if there does not appear to be anything really new or different that can be atraumatically and quickly tried (e.g., better sniffing position, external laryngeal manipulation, new blade, new technique, much more experienced laryngoscopist) after a few failed intubation attempts and ventilation by mask can still be maintained, it is prudent to cease intubation attempts and consider the following options: (1) awaken the patient, (2) continue anesthesia by mask or LMA ventilation, or (3) perform a tracheostomy or cricothyrotomy before the ability to ventilate the lungs by mask is lost (see Fig. 9-1A and B). In fact, the most common scenario in the respiratory catastrophes in the ASA closed claims study was the development of progressive difficulty in ventilating by mask between persistent and prolonged failed intubation attempts; the final result was inability to ventilate by mask and provide gas exchange (see Chapter 53).[20] If the surgical procedure is not urgent, awakening the patient and doing the procedure another day will allow better planning. On the other hand, awakening the patient is often not possible in a failed airway situation, especially if the intubation is emergent. Many cases may be done (and may have to be done) by mask or LMA ventilation (e.g., cesarean section) if ventilation is reasonably easy. Finally, in some cases, the airway must be secured by a tracheostomy or cricothyrotomy (e.g., thoracotomy, intracranial-head-neck cases, and cases in the prone position).

If regurgitation or vomiting occurs at any time during attempts at endotracheal intubation in an anesthetized patient, there are a number of therapeutic steps that should be taken. First, the patient should be put in the Trendelenburg position and the head, and perhaps the body, turned to the left. Second, the mouth and pharynx should be suctioned with a large-bore suction device. Endotracheal intubation may then be tried with the patient in the lateral position; the advantage of this maneuver is that the tongue may be more out of the way, but the disadvantage is that this intubation position may be unfamiliar to most anesthesiologists. If the endotracheal tube (ET) has been passed into the esophagus, it may be left there; the advantage is that the ET may decompress the stomach and perhaps guide (by negative example) future intubation attempts. However, the disadvantage is that it may be more difficult to obtain a satisfactory mask seal between intubation attempts, even if the esophageal ET is sharply bent off to the side by the rim of the mask. Once the airway is secured and aspiration of gastric contents has been performed, standard treatment consists of suctioning, mechanical ventilation, positive end-expiratory pressure, fiberoptically guided saline lavage, and perhaps steroids and appropriate antibiotics after specific cultures and sensitivities are available (see Chapter 32).

C. THE PATIENT WHOSE LUNGS CANNOT BE VENTILATED BY MASK AND WHOSE TRACHEA CANNOT BE INTUBATED

In rare cases, it is impossible either to ventilate the lungs of a patient by mask or to intubate the trachea. Under these circumstances, unless there is an alternative ventilation method immediately available, death rapidly ensues. The LMA is a major advance in the management of both difficult intubation and difficult ventilation scenarios and was incorporated into the original ASA difficult airway management algorithm in five different places as either an airway (ventilation device) or a conduit for a flexible FOB in 1996.[9] In fact, it functions so well as a conduit that the LMA Fastrach (intubating LMA) was introduced into clinical practice in 1998.[7,14,42] Additional noninvasive options for emergency ventilation include the esophageal-tracheal Combitube (see Chapter 25), transtracheal jet ventilation (TTJV)[56] (see Chapter 26), and the rigid bronchoscope (see Chapters 27 and 35). It should be realized that both the Combitube and the LMA are supraglottic ventilatory devices and may not allow successful ventilation when airway obstruction occurs at or below the glottic opening. The same is true of TTJV. Thus, the rigid bronchoscope has now been introduced into the difficult airway management algorithm as a solution to maintain a patent airway and allow ventilation past an obstruction at these levels.

Although TTJV is easy to perform and can be lifesaving, time and the appropriate equipment are required to implement this technique, which precludes its use in many urgent emergency settings. Furthermore, the technique requires some patency of the glottis and upper airway. Severe subcutaneous emphysema may result if the needle or catheter is not entirely inside the tracheal lumen. In addition, barotrauma may result from over-anxious jet ventilation in the presence of a closed glottis or proximal airway obstruction.[54] Nonetheless, cricothyroid oxygen insufflation or jetting can convert an alarming situation into a controlled one, in which direct, fiberoptic, or retrograde intubation and other techniques become more practical.

The risks of an invasive rescue technique must be weighed against the risks of hypoxic brain injury or death.[50] Although most anesthesiologists think they should be able to perform a cricothyrotomy, less than 50% feel competent to perform one.[29] Failure of anesthesiologists to perform a cricothyrotomy expeditiously is often regarded as a criticism by plaintiff's experts in medicolegal actions. Therefore, when faced with a failed airway, preparations for a surgical airway must begin immediately, and once the decision is made, it is essential to use an effective technique (see Chapters 28 and 29). Invasive airway access, such as TTJV or cricothyrotomy (catheter or surgical), is a temporary measure to restore oxygenation. Definitive airway management will follow by either tracheal intubation[1,35] or formal tracheostomy.

D. TRACHEAL EXTUBATION OF A PATIENT WITH A DIFFICULT AIRWAY

Extubation of the patient with a difficult airway should be carefully assessed and performed, and the anesthesiologist should develop a strategy for safe extubation of these patients. The task force regards the concept of an extubation strategy as a logical extension of the intubation strategy. This strategy depends upon the surgery, the condition of the patient, and the skills and preferences of the anesthesiologist. The preformulated extubation strategy should include a consideration of the relative merits of awake extubation versus extubation before the return of consciousness; an evaluation for general clinical factors that may produce an adverse impact on ventilation after the patient has been extubated (e.g., abnormal mental status or gas exchange, airway edema, inability to clear secretions, inadequate return of neuromuscular functions); the formulation of an airway management plan that can be implemented if the patient is not able to maintain adequate ventilation after extubation; and consideration of the short-term use of a device that can serve as a guide for expedited reintubation. This type of device is usually inserted through the lumen of the tracheal tube and into the trachea before the tracheal tube is removed. The device may be rigid to facilitate intubation or hollow to facilitate ventilation, or both.

If tracheal extubation of a patient with a known difficult airway is followed by respiratory distress, reintubation and ventilation may be difficult or impossible. Thus, the ideal method of extubation is one that permits a withdrawal from the airway that is controlled, gradual, step by step, and reversible at any time. Extubation over a jet stylet closely approximates this ideal.

A jet stylet is a small inside diameter (ID), hollow, semirigid catheter that is inserted into an in situ ET prior to extubation. After the ET is withdrawn over the jet stylet, the small-ID hollow catheter may be used as a means of ventilation (i.e., the jet function) or as an intratracheal guide for reintubation (i.e., the stylet function), or both. The jet function may safely allow additional time to assess the need for the reintubation stylet function (see Chapter 47).

Miller and colleagues[45] formulated an algorithm for intubation of the difficult airway that incorporates the use of a ventilating tube exchanger and is suggested as one of several stepwise approaches to difficult airway management after extubation. The actual and optimal maneuvers involved in extubation may vary depending on patients' conditions and the skills of the practitioners delivering care. The necessary equipment that should be immediately available prior to extubating the difficult airway includes the same equipment that should be contained in a portable storage unit or cart for intubation of the difficult airway (see Chapter 47), as previously discussed.

E. FOLLOW-UP CARE OF A PATIENT WITH A DIFFICULT AIRWAY

The anesthesiologist should document the presence and nature of the airway difficulty in the medical record. The intent of this documentation is to guide and facilitate the delivery of future care. Aspects of documentation that may prove helpful include (but are not limited to):

1. A description of the airway difficulties that were encountered. If possible, the description should distinguish between difficulties encountered in mask ventilation and difficulties encountered in tracheal intubation, or both.
2. A description of the various airway management techniques that were employed. The description should indicate the extent to which each of the techniques played a beneficial or detrimental role in management of the difficult airway.

The anesthesiologist should inform the patient (or responsible person) of the airway difficulty that was encountered. The intent of this communication is to provide the patient (or responsible person) with information in guiding and facilitating the delivery of future care. The information conveyed may include (but is not limited to) the presence of a difficult airway, the apparent reasons for difficulty, and the implications for future care. Finally, the anesthesiologist should strongly consider dispensing or advising a Medic-Alert bracelet for the patient (see Chapter 52).

In addition, the anesthesiologist should evaluate and observe the patient for potential complications of difficult airway management. These complications include (but are not limited to) airway edema, bleeding, tracheal and esophageal perforation, pneumothorax, and aspiration.

III. SUMMARY OF THE ASA ALGORITHM

Difficulty in managing the airway is the single most important cause of major anesthesia-related morbidity and mortality. Successful management of a difficult airway begins with recognizing the potential problem. All patients should be examined for their ability to open the mouth widely and for the structures visible upon mouth opening, the size of the mandibular space, and ability to assume the sniffing position. If there is a good possibility that intubation or ventilation by mask, or both, will be difficult, the airway should be secured while

the patient is still awake rather than after induction of GA. For an awake intubation to be successful, it is absolutely essential that the patient be properly prepared; otherwise, the anesthesiologist will simply fulfill a self-defeating prophecy.

When the patient is properly prepared, any one of a number of intubation techniques is likely to be successful. If the patient is already anesthetized or paralyzed and intubation is found to be difficult, many repeated forceful attempts at intubation should be avoided because laryngeal edema and hemorrhage will develop progressively and the ability to ventilate the lungs by mask consequently may be lost. After several attempts at intubation, it may be best to awaken the patient, perform regional anesthesia (if appropriate; see Chapter 42), proceed with the case using mask or LMA ventilation, or do a semielective tracheostomy. In the event that the ability to ventilate by mask is lost and the patient's lungs still cannot be ventilated, LMA ventilation should be instituted immediately. If LMA ventilation does not provide adequate gas exchange, either TTJV or a surgical airway should be instituted immediately. Tracheal extubation of a patient with a difficult airway over a jet stylet permits a controlled, gradual, and reversible (in that ventilation and reintubation are possible at any time) withdrawal from the airway.

Four concepts emerge from the preceding discussion—four very important, take-home messages on the ASA difficult airway algorithm—as presented in Box 9-4.

Box 9-4 ASA Difficult Airway Algorithm Take-Home Messages

1. If suspicious of trouble → Secure the airway awake
2. If you get into trouble → Awaken the patient
3. Have a plan B, C, immediately available and in place = think ahead
4. Intubation choices → Do what you do best

IV. PROBLEMS WITH THE ASA ALGORITHM AND LIKELY FUTURE DIRECTIONS

The ASA difficult airway management algorithm has been before the anesthesia community, in one form or another, since 1991. This algorithm has undergone revisions as our knowledge and experience with managing the airway have grown and as new devices and techniques have become available. The strength of the ASA difficult airway management algorithm is twofold. First, it is very thorough and complete with respect to the options available when an anesthesiologist encounters a difficult airway. Second, it emphasizes the need for and importance of an organized approach to airway management.[40]

On the other hand, the algorithm has several deficiencies that diminish its application in clinical practice.

First, although it is intended to apply to all patients of all ages, there are certain populations of patients in which further considerations are necessary (e.g., pediatric and obstetric patients [see Chapters 33 and 34, respectively], nonfasted patients, or patients with obstruction at or below the vocal cords). Second, its clinical endpoint is successful intubation, but endotracheal intubation may not be necessary and successful ventilation may suffice. Third, the algorithm is fairly complex, allowing a wide choice of techniques at each stage, and its multiplicity of pathways may limit its clinical usefulness in guiding day-to-day practice.[33] It is not binary in nature, such as the algorithm used in advanced life support guidelines.[21] Fourth, somewhat vague terminology is used in its definitions of difficult tracheal intubation and difficult laryngoscopy. Definitions of optimal-best attempts at conventional laryngoscopy, mask ventilation, and difficult laryngoscopy or intubation are important because they provide an endpoint at which practitioners may quit a particular approach (limit risk) and move on to something that has a better chance of working (gain benefit). Fifth, the algorithm mentions ablation of spontaneous ventilation with muscle relaxants but does not discuss the great clinical management implications of muscle relaxants that have different durations of action. Sixth, although the algorithm advises confirmation of endotracheal intubation, the usefulness of capnography for this purpose is limited during cardiac arrest, which is not an uncommon consequence of the "cannot intubate, cannot ventilate" (CICV) scenario, whereas the esophageal detector device is not (see Chapter 30). Seventh, it does not provide a definitive flowchart for extubation of the difficult airway that incorporates the use of a device that can serve as a guide for expedited reintubation or ventilation, if necessary. Finally, the role of regional anesthesia in patients with a difficult airway requires further clarification (see Chapter 42).

A. DEFINITION OF DIFFICULT ENDOTRACHEAL INTUBATION

At present, the ASA difficult airway management algorithm defines difficult endotracheal intubation as "when tracheal intubation requires *multiple* attempts in the presence of tracheal pathology" and difficult laryngoscopy as "not being able to visualize any portion of the vocal cords after *multiple* attempts at conventional laryngoscopy." Because these definitions do not state a specific number of attempts, they can be interpreted differently by practitioners. Multiple may mean more than one, more than two, more than three, and so forth. Although this imprecise terminology may be deliberate, it may be more appropriate to provide a definitive number of attempts or not include a number at all and better define attempt (e.g., assuming best-optimal attempt is utilized and that an attempt is the physical placement and removal of the laryngoscope blade).

B. DEFINITION OF OPTIMAL-BEST ATTEMPT AT CONVENTIONAL LARYNGOSCOPY

Difficulty in performing endotracheal intubation is the end result of difficulty in performing laryngoscopy, which depends on the operator's level of expertise, patient's characteristics, and circumstances. The problem with multiple repeated attempts at conventional laryngoscopy is the creation of laryngeal edema and bleeding, which impair mask ventilation and subsequent endotracheal intubation attempts, thereby creating a CICV situation. Thus, it is imperative that the anesthesiologist make his or her optimal-best attempt at laryngoscopy as early as possible; if that fails, an alternative plan should be activated so that no further risk, without likely benefit, is incurred.

What is an optimal-best attempt at conventional laryngoscopy?[6] First, a reasonably experienced anesthesiologist who has had at least 3 full years of experience should perform the laryngoscopy. If an experienced anesthesiologist is having difficulty in visualizing the glottis, he or she should not ask or allow other anesthesiologists or ear, nose, and throat surgeons to attempt the *same* maneuver.

Second, the patient should always be in an optimal sniffing position (slight flexion of the neck on the head and severe extension of the head on the neck),[6] which aligns the oral, pharyngeal, and laryngeal axis into more of a straight line, unless contraindicated or unable to perform (cervical spine pathology). In some patients (such as the obese), obtaining an optimal sniffing position takes a great deal of work (Fig. 9-2), such as placing pillows and blankets under the scapula, shoulders, nape of the neck, and head, which is difficult when anesthesia and paralysis have made the patient a massive (dead) weight. Positioning the obese patient can be easily accomplished with a new positioning device, the Troop Elevation Pillow (Mercury Medical, Clearwater, FL) (Fig. 9-3). Thus, an endotracheal intubation attempt should not be wasted because of failure to have the patient in an optimal sniffing position before the induction of GA.

Third, if the laryngoscopic grade is II (arytenoids only), III (epiglottis only), or IV (soft palate only), optimal external laryngeal manipulation (OELM) or backward, upward, rightward pressure (BURP) should be used (Fig. 9-4).[6,10] Neither OELM nor BURP is cricoid pressure (see Fig. 9-4), and they can be achieved in 5 to 10 seconds.[10] Such maneuvers can frequently improve the laryngoscopic view by at least one entire grade and should be an inherent part of laryngoscopy and an instinctive reflex response to a poor laryngoscopic view.[10] Thus, an endotracheal intubation attempt should not be wasted because of failure to use these maneuvers.

Fourth, the proper function of both a Macintosh and a Miller blade is dependent on using an appropriate length of blade. In order to lift the epiglottis out of the line of sight, the Macintosh blade must be long enough to put tension on the glossoepiglottic ligament, and the Miller blade must be long enough to trap the epiglottis against the tongue. Thus, in some patients, it may be

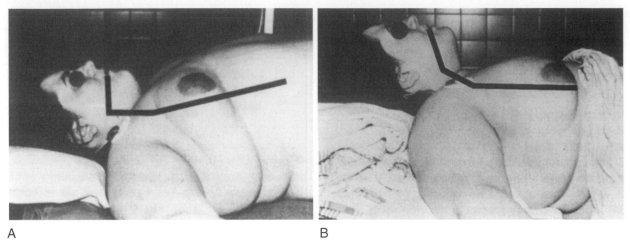

A   B

Figure 9-2 Getting the patient in an optimal sniffing position prior to the induction of general anesthesia occasionally (e.g., with very obese patients) takes a great deal of work. **A,** Just head on pillow. **B,** Scapula, shoulder, nape of neck, and head support results in the sniffing position. (Modified from Davis JM, Weeks S, Crone LA: Difficult intubation in the parturient. Can J Anesth 36:668-674, 1989.)

appropriate to change the length of the blade one time in order to obtain proper blade function.

Fifth, in some patients, a Macintosh blade may provide a superior view or intubating condition than a Miller blade, and vice versa. A Macintosh blade is generally regarded as a better blade whenever there is little upper airway room to pass the ET (e.g., small narrow mouth, palate, oropharynx), and a Miller blade is generally regarded as a better blade in patients who have a small mandibular space (anterior larynx), large incisors, or a long, floppy epiglottis.

In summary, an optimal-best attempt at laryngoscopy can be defined as involving (1) a reasonably experienced (at least 3 full recent years) laryngoscopist, (2) use of optimal sniffing position, (3) use of OLEM or BURP, and (4) change of length or type of blade one time. With this definition, and with no other confounding considerations, an optimal-best attempt at laryngoscopy may be achieved on the first attempt and should not take more than a maximum of three attempts. Thus, difficult endotracheal intubation may be readily apparent to a reasonably

experienced intubationist on the first attempt and therefore be independent of both number of attempts and time. A more logical definition would be based on optimal-best attempt laryngoscopic view and periglottic and subglottic pathology and retain number of attempts and time of attempt as maximal boundary airway conditions.

C. DEFINITION OF OPTIMAL-BEST ATTEMPT AT CONVENTIONAL MASK VENTILATION

If the patient cannot be intubated, gas exchange is dependent on mask ventilation. If the patient cannot be ventilated by mask, a CICV situation exists, and immediate

Determining optimal external laryngeal manipulation with free (right) hand

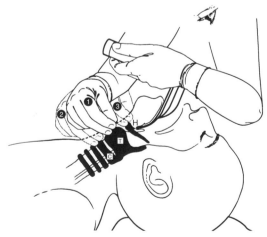

Figure 9-4 Determining optimal external manipulation (OELM) with free (right) hand. OELM should be an inherent part of laryngoscopy and is performed when laryngoscopic view is poor. Ninety percent of the time, the best view is obtained by pressing over the thyroid cartilage (1) or the cricoid cartilage (2); pressing over the hyoid bone (3) may also be effective.

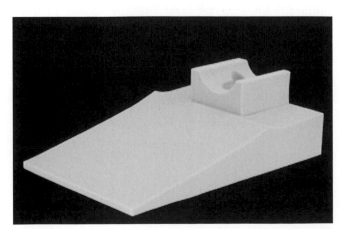

Figure 9-3 Troop Elevation Pillow with additional foam head rest. (Provided by Mercury Medical, Clearwater, FL.)

organ-lifesaving maneuvers must be instituted (see Section E following). Because each of the acceptable responses to a CICV situation has its own risks, the decision to abandon mask ventilation should be made after the anesthesiologist has made an optimal-best attempt at mask ventilation.

The first component of an optimal-best attempt at conventional mask ventilation is that it should be a two-person effort (Fig. 9-5) because far better mask seal, jaw thrust, and therefore tidal volume can be achieved with two people versus one person. The left-hand panel of Figure 9-5 shows a proper two-person mask ventilation effort when the second person knows how to perform a jaw thrust, and the right-hand panel of Figure 9-5 shows a proper two-person mask ventilation effort when the second person is capable only of squeezing the reservoir bag.

The second component of an optimal-best attempt at conventional mask ventilation is to use large oropharyngeal or nasopharyngeal airways, or both. If mask ventilation is very poor or nonexistent with a vigorous two-person effort in the presence of large artificial airways, it is time to move on to a potentially organ-lifesaving plan B (see Fig. 9-1 and Section E following).

D. DURATION OF ACTION OF MUSCLE RELAXANT

In patients presenting for elective surgery who end up in a CICV situation, the following is a common story. Preoperatively, the anesthesiologist does not recognize a difficult airway or feels the difficult airway is questionable; the anesthesiologist induces GA with an intravenous drug and paralyzes the patient with succinylcholine. Mask ventilation is initiated without difficulty, but endotracheal intubation with conventional laryngoscopy fails.

Appropriately, gas exchange is controlled by mask ventilation for a second time, and then, after some adjustment, endotracheal intubation with conventional laryngoscopy is attempted and fails for a second time. Mask ventilation controls gas exchange for a third time but is now perceptibly more difficult than before. After some adjustments, endotracheal intubation with conventional laryngoscopy

Two-person mask ventilation

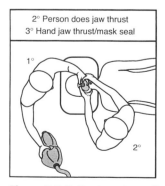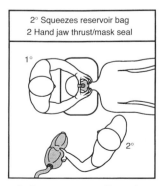

Figure 9-5 Optimal mask ventilation. *Left,* two-person effort when second person knows how to perform jaw thrust; *right,* two-person effort when second person can only squeeze the reservoir bag.

is attempted for the third time and fails. At this point, approximately 5 to 8 minutes have passed since the administration of succinylcholine. Although the anesthesiologist may want to exercise the awake option, the patient is not breathing spontaneously and mask ventilation is now attempted for a fourth time. However, mask ventilation is extremely difficult or impossible because the chest wall is rigid as a result of the patient sustaining a forceful exhalation mode and the presence of laryngospasm and edema related to the prior three laryngoscopies and intubation attempts. Now a race begins and the question arises whether the patient will resume adequate spontaneous ventilation (awaken) before experiencing severe hypoxemia, possibly resulting in organ or body damage. The answer is not certain and depends on many pharmacologic and physiologic variables. From this common story in patients who have ended up in a CICV situation, the advantages and disadvantages of muscle relaxants with different durations of action become obvious (Table 9-2). With the induction of GA in an uncooperative patient with a recognized difficult airway, the anesthesiologist should consider the relative merits of the preservation of spontaneous ventilation versus the use of muscle relaxants.

The use of succinylcholine in a patient with a recognized or questionable difficult airway may not be the best choice, particularly if it is thought that mask ventilation will be possible and a smooth transition to an alternative plan of action (e.g., fiberoptic bronchoscopy[48]) will be desirable. The key elements in the choice of a nondepolarizing muscle relaxant are the decision that mask ventilation will be adequate (see optimal attempt at mask ventilation) and the fact that rescue plans have been made.

Alternatively, endotracheal intubation can be successfully accomplished without the use of any muscle relaxant, and this option should be considered in certain situations.[55,57] Also, if a small dose of succinylcholine (0.5 to 0.75 mg/kg) is used, good intubating conditions can be achieved within 75 seconds for a duration of 60 seconds, allowing an early-awaken option. Another consideration is that in a large majority of patients, prior administration of a small dose of a nondepolarizing neuromuscular blocker may slightly diminish the duration of action of succinylcholine,[53] and thus the time to spontaneous recovery of airway reflexes may be shortened.

Lastly, whether to administer a second dose of succinylcholine following a cannot-intubate situation in which the patient resumes spontaneous ventilation is debatable, depending on the situation. If the chances of achieving successful endotracheal intubation are high (i.e., a fairly good laryngoscopic grade), yet it is difficult to accomplish intubation because of incomplete paralysis, the administration of a second dose of succinylcholine may be appropriate. It may also be considered appropriate in situations in which mask ventilation is possible, the laryngoscopist is highly skilled, and a simple change in either the patient's position or the type of

Table 9-2 **Advantages and Disadvantages of Muscle Relaxants with Different Durations of Action**

Muscle Relaxant	Advantages	Disadvantages
Succinylcholine	1. Permits the awaken option at the earliest time possible	1. A period of poor ventilation (either spontaneous or with positive pressure) may occur as the drug wears off 2. Does not permit a smooth transition to plan B (such as use of a fiberoptic bronchoscope[48]), etc.
Nondepolarizing	1. Permits a smooth transition to plan B, etc., provided mask ventilation is adequate	1. Does not allow awake option at an early time

laryngoscope is necessary. A small dose of glycopyrrolate (0.2 to 0.4 mg) should be administered in conjunction with the repeated dose of succinylcholine in order to prevent a bradycardic response.

E. APPROPRIATE OPTIONS FOR THE CANNOT INTUBATE, CANNOT VENTILATE SITUATION

Since 1992, most anesthesiologists in the United States have become very familiar with the LMA[13] and the Combitube[31] and have found that both work well in elective and emergency situations.[7,13,31] Although the algorithm does not dictate the order of preference of these devices in the CICV situation, the anesthesiologist must take the following considerations into account: (1) the anesthesiologist's own experience and level of comfort in the use of these methods, (2) the availability of these devices, (3) the type of airway obstruction (upper versus lower), and (4) the benefits and risks involved. Although the LMA-Classic is easily inserted, even by inexperienced personnel,[46] it does not provide an airtight seal around the larynx or protect the trachea from aspiration. Although there is increased complexity of insertion with the LMA-ProSeal, it forms a better seal[15,17-19,23,36,41] than the LMA-Classic and provides improved protection against aspiration.[16,27,28,37] Also, when properly positioned, the Combitube allows ventilation with a higher seal pressure than the LMA-Classic, protects against regurgitation,[5] and allows further attempts[52] at intubation while the esophageal cuff protects the airway. The Combitube has been successfully used in difficult intubation[3,5] and CICV situations,[12,26,38,51] including failure with an LMA.[43]

The decision to use the Combitube depends on availability, experience, and the clinical situation.[34] However, it must be remembered that both the LMA and the Combitube are supraglottic ventilatory devices (Fig. 9-6) and that is their inherent weakness. Thus, they cannot solve a truly glottic (e.g., spasm, massive edema, tumor, abscess) or subglottic problem.[31] If a truly glottic or subglottic problem exists, the only solution is to position the ventilatory mechanism below the level of the lesion

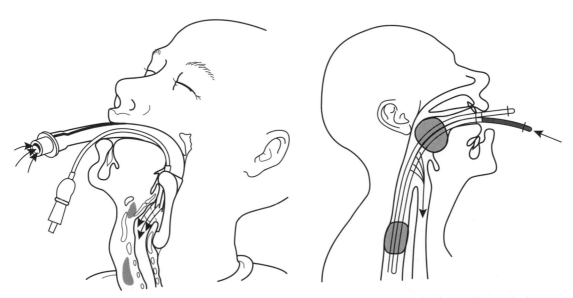

Figure 9-6 Both the laryngeal mask airway *(left)* and Combitube *(right)* are supraglottic ventilatory devices.

A

Respiratory system damaging
events by year of event

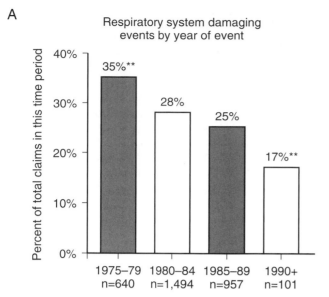

B

Claims for death and brain
damage by year of event

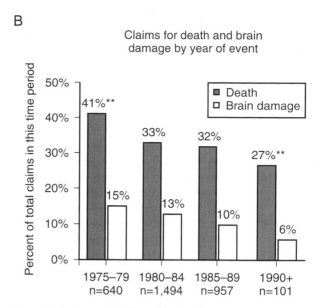

Figure 9-7 The incidence of respiratory system damaging events **(A)** and brain death and death **(B)** has significantly decreased. (From Cheney FW: Committee on Professional Liability—Overview. ASA Newsletter, 58:7-10, 1994.)

(e.g., ET, TTJV, rigid ventilating bronchoscope, surgical airway). One of the algorithm's inherent weaknesses is that it does not discriminate between the obstructed and the unobstructed airway in its guidelines.

V. CONCLUSION

In summary, the ASA difficult airway management algorithm has worked well over the past decade. In fact, there has been a very dramatic decrease (30% to 40%) in the number of respiratory-related malpractice lawsuits, brain damage, and deaths attributable to anesthesia since 1990 (Fig. 9-7).[22] However, a number of issues have emerged that indicate that the ASA difficult airway management algorithm can be improved, as discussed in this chapter. Consideration of these issues should make the algorithm still more clinically specific and functional. Nonetheless, the algorithm provides excellent guidelines for anesthesiologists

in their clinical decision-making for patients with difficult airways. Successful management of these patients is key for reducing the risk of anesthesia-related morbidity and mortality.

As the practice of airway management becomes more advanced, anesthesiologists must become both knowledgeable and proficient in the use of various airway devices and techniques. Although the algorithm cannot be practiced in its entirety on a regular basis, anesthesiologists need to incorporate these alternative devices and techniques into their daily practice so that they can develop the confidence and skill required for their successful use in the emergent setting. All of the equipment described should be available for regular practice, and a difficult airway cart or portable unit should be located near every anesthetizing location. Finally, appropriate follow-up and communication should be performed so that future caretakers will not unwittingly reproduce the same experience and risk.

REFERENCES

1. Ala-Kokko TI, Kyllonen M, Nuutinen L: Management of upper airway obstruction using a Seldinger minitracheotomy kit. Acta Anaesthesiol Scand 40:385-388, 1996.
2. American Society of Anesthesiologists Task Force on Management of the Difficult Airway: Practice guidelines for management of the difficult airway: A report. Anesthesiology 78:597-602, 1993.
3. Banyai M, Falger S, Roggla M, et al: Emergency intubation with the Combitube in a grossly obese patient with bull neck. Resuscitation 26:271-276, 1993.
4. Baraka A: Transtracheal jet ventilation during fiberoptic intubation under general anesthesia. Anesth Analg 65:1091-1092, 1986.

5. Baraka A, Salem R: The Combitube oesophageal-tracheal double lumen airway for difficult intubation. Can J Anaesth 40:1222-1223, 1993.

6. Benumof JL: Difficult laryngoscopy: Obtaining the best view. Can J Anaesth 41:361-365, 1994.

7. Benumof JL: Laryngeal mask airway: Indications and contraindications. Anesthesiology 77:843-846, 1992.

8. Benumof JL: Management of the difficult airway: With special emphasis on awake tracheal intubation. Anesthesiology 75:1087-1110, 1991.

9. Benumof JL: The laryngeal mask airway and the ASA difficult airway algorithm. Anesthesiology 84:686-699, 1996.

10. Benumof JL, Cooper SD: Quantitative improvement in laryngoscopic view by optimal external laryngeal manipulation. J Clin Anesth 8:136-140, 1996.

11. Benumof JL, Scheller MS: The importance of transtracheal jet ventilation in the management of the difficult airway. Anesthesiology 71:769-778, 1989.

12. Bigenzahn W, Pesau B, Frass M: Emergency ventilation using the Combitube in cases of difficult intubation. Eur Arch Otorhinolaryngol 248:129-131, 1991.

13. Brain AIJ, Ferson DZ: Laryngeal mask airway. In Hagberg CA (ed): Airway Management: Principles and Practice. 2nd ed. Philadelphia, Mosby, 2007.

14. Brain AI, Verghese C, Addy EV, Kapila A: The intubating laryngeal mask. I: Development of a new device for intubation of the trachea. Br J Anaesth 79:699-703, 1997.

15. Brain AI, Verghese C, Strube PJ: The LMA 'ProSeal'—A laryngeal mask with an oesophageal vent. Br J Anaesth 84:650-654, 2000.

16. Brimacombe J, Keller C: Airway protection with the ProSeal laryngeal mask airway. Anaesth Intensive Care 29:288-291, 2001.

17. Brimacombe J, Keller C: The ProSeal laryngeal mask airway: A randomized, crossover study with the standard laryngeal mask airway in paralyzed, anesthetized patients. Anesthesiology 93:104-109, 2000.

18. Brimacombe J, Keller C, Brimacombe L: A comparison of the laryngeal mask airway ProSeal and the laryngeal tube airway in paralyzed anesthetized adult patients undergoing pressure-controlled ventilation. Anesth Analg 95:770-776, 2002.

19. Brimacombe J, Keller C, Fullekrug B, et al: A multicenter study comparing the ProSeal and Classic laryngeal mask airway in anesthetized, nonparalyzed patients. Anesthesiology 96:289-295, 2002.

20. Caplan RA, Posner KL, Ward RJ, et al: Adverse respiratory events in anesthesia: A closed claims analysis. Anesthesiology 72:828-833, 1990.

21. Channing L, Cummins RO: ACLS Provider Manual. American Heart Association, Dallas TX, 2000.

22. Cheney FW: Committee on Professional Liability—Overview. ASA Newslett 58:7-10, 1994.

23. Cook TM, Nolan JP, Verghese C, et al: Randomized crossover comparison of the ProSeal with the Classic laryngeal mask airway in unparalysed anaesthetized patients. Br J Anaesth 88:527-533, 2002.

24. Dallen L, Wine R, Benumof JL: Spontaneous ventilation via transtracheal large bore intravenous catheter is possible. Anesthesiology 75:531-533, 1991.

25. Davies JM, Weeks S, Crone LA, Pavlin E: Difficult intubation in the parturient. Can J Anaesth 36:668-674, 1989.

26. Eichinger S, Schreiber W, Heinz T, et al: Airway management in a case of neck impalement: Use of the oesophageal tracheal Combitube airway. Br J Anaesth 68:534-535, 1992.

27. Evans NR, Gardner SV, James MF: ProSeal laryngeal mask protects against aspiration of fluid in the pharynx. Br J Anaesth 88:584-587, 2002.

28. Evans NR, Llewellyn RL, Gardner SV, James MF: Aspiration prevented by the ProSeal laryngeal mask airway: A case report. Can J Anaesth 49:413-416, 2002.

29. Ezri T, Szmuk P, Warters RD, et al: Difficult airway management practice patterns among anesthesiologists practicing in the United States: Have we made any progress? J Clin Anesth 15:418-422, 2003.

30. Fink RB: Respiration, the Human Larynx: A Functional Study. New York, Raven Press, 1975.

31. Frass M, Urtubia R, Hagberg C: The Combitube. In Hagberg CA (ed): Airway Management: Principles and Practice. 2nd ed. Philadelphia, Elsevier Science, 2006.

32. Hagberg CA, Ghatge S: Does the airway examination predict difficult intubation? In Fleisher L (ed): Evidence-Based Practice of Anesthesiology. Philadelphia, Elsevier Science, 2004, pp 34-46.

33. Heidegger T, Gerig HJ, Ulrich B, Kreienbühl G: Validation of a simple algorithm for tracheal intubation: Daily practice is the key to success in emergencies—An analysis of 13,248 intubations. Anesth Analg 92:517-522, 2001.

34. Henderson JJ, Popat MT, Pearce AC: Difficult Airway Society guidelines for management of the unanticipated difficult intubation. Anaesthesia 59:675-694, 2004.

35. Johnson C: Fiberoptic intubation prevents a tracheostomy in a trauma victim. AANA J 61:347-348, 1993.

36. Keller C, Brimacombe J: Mucosal pressure and oropharyngeal leak pressure with the ProSeal versus laryngeal mask airway in anaesthetized paralysed patients. Br J Anaesth 85:262-266, 2000.

37. Keller C, Brimacombe J, Kleinsasser A, Loeckinger A: Does the ProSeal laryngeal mask airway prevent aspiration of regurgitated fluid? Anesth Analg 91:1017-1020, 2000.

38. Klauser R, Roggla G, Pidlich J, et al: Massive upper airway bleeding after thrombolytic therapy: Successful airway management with the Combitube. Ann Emerg Med 21:431-433, 1992.

39. Langeron O, Masoo E, Huraux C, et al: Prediction of difficult mask ventilation. Anesthesiology 92:1229-1236, 2000.

40. Larson CP: A safe, effective, reliable modification of the ASA difficult airway algorithm for adult patients. Curr Rev Clin Anesth 23:1-12, 2002.

41. Lu PP, Brimacombe J, Yang C, Shyr M: ProSeal versus the Classic laryngeal mask airway for positive pressure ventilation during laparoscopic cholecystectomy. Br J Anaesth 88:824-827, 2002.

42. Mark L, Foley L, Michelson J: Effective dissemination of critical airway information: The Medical Alert National Difficult Airway/Intubation Registry. In Hagberg CA (ed): Airway Management: Principles and Practice. 2nd ed. Philadelphia, Elsevier Science, 2006.

43. McLellan I, Gordon P, Khawaja S, Thomas A: Percutaneous transtracheal high frequency jet ventilation as an aid to difficult intubation. Can J Anaesth 35:404-405, 1988.

44. Mercer M: Respiratory failure after tracheal extubation in a patient with halo frame cervical spine immobilization rescue therapy using the Combitube airway. Br J Anaesth 86:886-891, 2001.

45. Miller KA, Harkin CP, Bailey PL: Postoperative tracheal extubation. Anesth Analg 80:149-172, 1995.

46. Patil V, Stehling LC, Zauder HL, Koch JP: Mechanical aids for a fiberoptic endoscopy. Anesthesiology 57:69-70, 1982.

47. Penmant JH, Walker MB: Comparison of the endotracheal tube and laryngeal mask airway in airway management by paramedical personnel. Anesth Analg 74:531-534, 1992.

48. Practice Guidelines for the Management of the Difficult Airway: An updated report by the American Society of Anesthesiologists Task Force on the Management of the Difficult Airway. Anesthesiology 98:1269-1277, 2003.

49. Rogers S, Benumof JL: New and easy fiberoptic endoscopy aided tracheal intubation. Anesthesiology 59:569-572, 1983.

50. Salem R, Baraka A: Confirmation of tracheal intubation. In Hagberg CA (ed): Airway Management: Principles and Practice. 2nd ed. Philadelphia, Mosby, 2007.

51. Sivarajan M, Fink BR: The position and the state of the larynx during general anesthesia and muscle paralysis. Anesthesiology 72:439-442, 1990.

52. Tighe SQM: Failed tracheal intubation. Anaesthesia 47:356, 1992.

53. Tunstall ME, Geddes C: "Failed intubation" in obstetric anaesthesia. An indication for use of the "Esophageal Gastric Tube Airway." Br J Anaesth 56:659-661, 1984.

54. Urtubia RM, Aguila CM, Cumsille MA: Combitube: A study for proper use. Anesth Analg 90:958-962, 2000.

55. Walts P, Smith I: Clinical studies of the interaction between d-tubocurarine and succinylcholine. Anesthesiology 31:39-44, 1969.

56. Weymuller EA, Parlin EG, Paugh D, Cummings CU: Management of the difficult airway problems with percutaneous transtracheal ventilation. Ann Otol Rhinol Largyngol 96:34-37, 1987.

57. Wong AKH, Teco GS: Intubation without muscle relaxant: An alternative technique for rapid tracheal intubation. Anesth Intensive Care 24:224-230, 1996.

SECTION III

PREINTUBATION-VENTILATION PROCEDURES

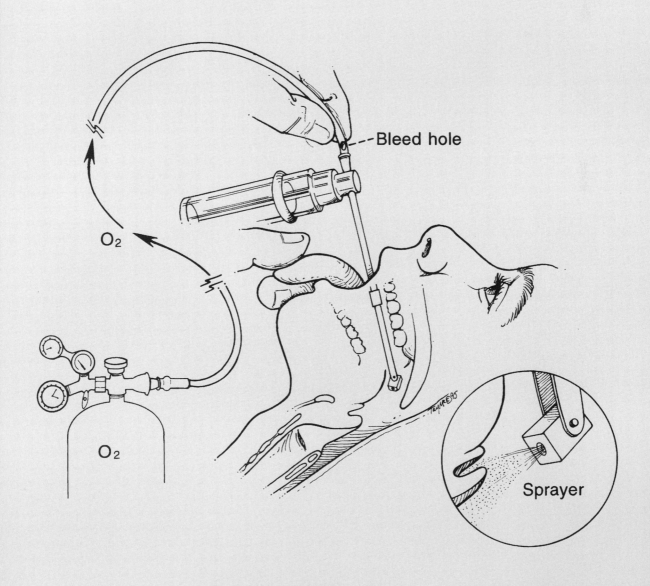

Bleed hole

O₂

O₂

Sprayer

10

PREPARATION OF THE PATIENT FOR AWAKE INTUBATION

Antonio Sanchez
Raj R. Iyer
Debra E. Morrison

I. BACKGROUND

A. HISTORY

"He sat in bed supporting himself with stiffened arms; his head was thrown forward, and he had the distressed anxiety so characteristic of impending suffocation depicted on his countenance. His inspirations were crowing and laboured.... He complained of intense pain...and begged that something should be done for his relief."

The preceding is from Dr. Macewend's 1880 account in the *British Medical Journal* of the first awake endotracheal intubation and describes a patient suffering from glottic edema. This patient underwent an *awake manual* endotracheal intubation using a *metallic* endotracheal tube (ET). This technique was performed without benefit of anesthesia and *without topical or regional blocks, sedatives, or analgesics*. The ET was kept in place with the patient in an awake state for 35 hours.[64] Although we may perceive this as brutal, Dr. Macewend was aware over 100 years ago that in spite of the patient's discomfort, the safest method for securing the airway was to perform an awake intubation (AI) rather than to provide comfort at the risk of compromising the airway totally.

There have been myriad subsequent reports of AI with favorable results,[32,59,66,68,73,95,97,103] yet many of us still hesitate to perform AI. It does appear that AI has been more readily accepted in the United States than in the European community.[62] In one large series from a single institution in the United States, 35% of all patients intubated and 21% of all patients anesthetized were intubated while awake.[59] The latter cannot, of course, be construed as indicative of the frequency of AI in the United States; this is unknown. AIs in Europe are performed only in specialized centers.

B. THE ASA ALGORITHM: A MILESTONE, "AWAKE INTUBATION"

In 1992, the American Society of Anesthesiologists (ASA) formed the Difficult Airway Task Force (DATF), which looked at closed claims malpractice suits and found that "inability to successfully manage very difficult airways has been responsible for as many as 30% of deaths totally attributable to anesthesia."[11] In the majority of these cases, patients did not display gross signs of airway difficulty, such as large tumors deviating the trachea of a patient in extremis, but had unrecognized difficult airways.[10] This implies that we are in need of more accurate predictors[42,65] of airway difficulty (fewer false positives and fewer false negatives within the predicted parameters) and that we must become better detectives. The DATF constructed an algorithm (see Chapter 9), which used as its cornerstone AI as the most prudent choice when an anesthesiologist is faced with a difficult airway. The difficult airway (DA) is defined as "the clinical situation in which a conventionally trained anesthesiologist experiences difficulty with mask ventilation, difficulty with endotracheal intubation, or both."[4,79]

C. PHYSICIAN RELUCTANCE TO PERFORM AWAKE INTUBATION

There seems to be an overall general hesitancy within the anesthesia community to perform AI.[62] At present there are no surveys to verify this statement,[63] but some of the reasons why there may be physician reluctance to perform AI are lack of a personal association with an airway disaster; the feeling that AI is too stressful emotionally and physically for the patient; that the physician may lack training; and fear of litigation or that the patient will refuse the procedure.

Although the majority of the reservations represented by these statements are addressed in other chapters of this textbook, we discuss patients' refusal in the section on the preoperative visit.

D. INDICATIONS AND CONTRAINDICATIONS FOR AWAKE INTUBATION

The ASA algorithm stresses the concept that formulation of a strategy for intubation should include the feasibility of three basic options: surgical versus nonsurgical techniques, preservation versus ablation of spontaneous ventilation, and AI versus intubation after induction of general anesthesia.[4] It is the opinion of most of the consultants of the DATF and expressed in the literature* that the safest method for a patient who requires endotracheal intubation and has a DA is for that individual to undergo AI for the following reasons:

1. The natural airway is preserved (patency of the airway is maintained through upper pharyngeal muscle tone).
2. Spontaneous breathing is maintained (maintaining oxygenation and ventilation).
3. A patient who is awake and well topicalized is easier to intubate (the larynx after induction of anesthesia moves to a more anterior position compared with the larynx in the awake patient).
4. The patient can still protect his or her airway from aspiration.
5. Patients are able to monitor their own neurologic symptoms (for example, the patient with potential cervical pathology).[11,59,103]

General indications for AI are compiled in Box 10-1.[30,59,67,85,103] There are no absolute contraindications to AI other than patient's refusal, a patient who is unable to cooperate (such as a child, a mentally retarded patient, or an intoxicated, combative patient), or a patient with a documented true allergy to all local anesthetics.[11]

---

*See references 4, 11, 30, 46, 50, 59, 66, 71, 84, 85, 93, 95, 97, 102.

Box 10-1   Indications for Awake Intubation[33,63,71,90,110]

1. Previous history of difficult intubation
2. Anticipated difficult airway (assessment on physical examination) as follows:
   Prominent protruding teeth
   Small mouth opening (scleroderma, temporomandibular joint pathology, anatomic variant)
   Narrow mandible
   Micrognathia
   Macroglossia
   Short muscular neck
   Very long neck
   Limited range of motion of the neck
   Congenital airway anomalies
   Obesity
   Pathology involving the airway (tracheomalacia)
   Malignancy involving the airway
   Upper airway obstruction
3. Trauma to the following:
   Face
   Upper airway
   Cervical spine
4. Anticipated difficult mask ventilation
5. Severe risk of aspiration
6. Respiratory failure
7. Severe hemodynamic instability

II. THE PREOPERATIVE VISIT

Because in the majority of the cases in the closed claims malpractice study the DA was unanticipated, we focus on elective patients, for whom there is time to evaluate the airway and communicate with the patient. In the setting of an emergency, which in itself should increase the probability of airway difficulty, especially with a patient in extremis,[70] the physician may not have time, nor can he or she be expected to be able to perform the detailed investigation of the airway described in this chapter.

A. THE DETECTIVE IN ALL OF US: REVIEWING OLD CHARTS

Whenever possible, previous anesthetic records (records, not just a record) should be examined because they may provide useful information.[4,7] Obviously, the most important are records involving intubation, especially the most recent ones. Other records documenting ease of mask ventilation and tolerance of drugs are also valuable. One should be alert for evidence of reactions to local anesthetics and of apnea with minimal doses of narcotics. Another reason for checking as many operating room (OR) records as possible, including noting the surgical procedure involved, is that the last intubation may have

been routine but the three previous ones may have been difficult, or the last intubation may have been routine but the operation then performed may have rendered the airway difficult.

When reading through a chart, one should focus on four important features.

1. Degree of difficulty of the endotracheal intubation (the difficulty encountered and the method used)
2. Positioning of the patient during laryngoscopy (sniffing position, other position)
3. Equipment used (even if the intubation was performed routinely in one attempt, a Bullard blade or a fiberoptic bronchoscope [FOB], neither of which requires the alignment of the three axes, may have been used)
4. Whether the technique that was used previously is familiar to you (one should not attempt to learn a new technique on a DA)

When the medical records have been reviewed, the preoperative interview should address the possibility of events having occurred since the last anesthetic (such as weight gain, laryngeal stenosis from previous airway intervention, suicide attempt with lye ingestion, motor vehicle accident, outpatient plastic surgery procedure such as chin implants, or worsening rheumatoid arthritis).

B. INTERVIEWING SKILLS

Dorland's Medical Dictionary defines empathy as the *intellectual* and *emotional* awareness and understanding of another person's thoughts, feelings, and behavior, even those that are distressing and disturbing. Although the anesthesiologist may participate in 1000 operations a year, few patients undergo more than five in a lifetime.[67] The patient's perception of empathy from the physician is the cornerstone of the patient's acceptance of an AI. Empathy helps the interviewer establish effective communication, which is important for accurate diagnosis and management of patients.[35] Two facets of medical education limit the clinician's development of empathy: the traditional format of interviewing training and the social ethos of medical training and medical practice, which stresses clinical detachment.[15,35] With empathy and the ability to communicate it, the physician can perform the interview in a more patient-oriented rather than disease-oriented fashion, resulting in better data gathering and patient's *compliance*.[38]

Plato recognized that "a life unexamined is not worth living." We as physicians must examine ourselves for biases[21] and unrecognized negative feelings toward an individual patient (such as the patient with morbid obesity, drug addiction, or simply the need to remain in control), which can be detrimental to effective communication and ultimately the patient's compliance.[21,99]

When we have determined that AI is in order, we should in a careful, unhurried manner describe to the patient the conventional intubation contrasted with AI. Focusing on the fact that the former is easier and less time consuming but that the latter is safer in light of the patient's own anatomy or condition, we must communicate to the patient that the knowledgeable, caring physician is willing to take extra measures to ensure the patient's safety. Recommendations should be presented to the patient with conviction but at the same time allowing the patient the option of the conventional method of intubation as a *last resort*.[85]

Complications of AI should also be presented, including local anesthetic toxicity, specific complications of the technique planned, discomfort, and recall. We should strive to develop sufficient skill in the techniques of AI in order to communicate honestly to the patient that he or she will experience a minimum of discomfort and unpleasantness, although he or she may or may not recall the intubation. Patients' recall after AI using different methods of sedation, analgesia, or local anesthetics has not been studied in a controlled fashion. Although episodes of explicit awareness during general anesthesia are rare (the incidence is 0.2% to 3%, depending on both depth of anesthesia and specific agents administered), it is anticipated that the incidence of recall of AI with minimal levels of sedation would be higher.[67] In reviewing 443 cases of AI (Table 10-1) in which various combinations of sedation and analgesia were utilized (11 patients had no sedation), 17% (mean of four studies) of the patients had partial recall and 6% (mean of four studies) had recall with unpleasant memories.[59,68,73,103]

If the patient refuses AI, the anesthesiologist may discuss the case with the primary care physician or the surgeon, or both, in order to recruit them in helping to convince the patient of the performance of an AI. If this, as well as subsequent discussion with the patient, is unsuccessful, the anesthesiologist should then document these data in the chart.

III. PREMEDICATION[27,32,73,117]

Once the patient is adequately prepared for AI, premedications are commonly employed to alleviate anxiety, provide a clear and dry airway, protect against the risk of aspiration, and enable adequate topicalization of the airway. Although adequate anxiolysis begins with the establishment of a good physician-patient relationship, a small percentage of patients requiring AI need pharmacologic agents to relieve anxiety and fear. In this section, we focus on the agents commonly utilized in the preoperative period, such as antisialogogues, sedatives/hypnotics, and analgesics.

A. SEDATIVES/HYPNOTICS[33,43,62,71,104]

Sedatives/hypnotics have an important role as they serve to provide anxiolysis, provide amnesia (anterograde > retrograde), sedate for patients' comfort, and improve patients' acceptance of securing the airway. Although they are beneficial, patients with significant airway compromise require conscious muscle tone to maintain airway patency. Thus, these agents should be used judiciously, if at all, in these situations. The following is a synopsis of some of the more commonly used agents.

1. Benzodiazepines

These are excellent anxiolytics, amnestics, sedatives, and hypnotics. Available agents include midazolam, diazepam, and lorazepam. Because of its ease in titration, *midazolam* is the more commonly used agent. Sedating doses average approximately 20 to 40 μg/kg (or 75 to 90 μg/kg intramuscularly [IM]), repeated every 5 minutes as needed to desired effect or up to 0.1 to 0.2 mg/kg. Onset of sedation is usually in 1 to 5 minutes, with a peak effect in 5 to 7 minutes and with a duration of 20 to 30 minutes. Although recovery is rapid, the half-life is about 1.7 to 3.6 hours, with increases noted with cirrhosis, congestive heart failure, obesity, elderly patients, and patients with renal failure. It is extensively metabolized by the liver (microsomal system) and renally eliminated as glucuronide conjugates. Comparative half-lives of diazepam and lorazepam are 20 to 50 hours and 11 to 22 hours, respectively.

Midazolam offers excellent anxiolysis and anterograde amnesia; doses should always be individualized, however, on the basis of the patient's age, underlying disease state, and concurrent medications. One should decrease the

Table 10-1 **Incidence of Recall in Patients Undergoing Awake Intubation**

Reference	No. of Awake Intubations	Complete Amnesia	Partial Recall	Unpleasant Memories
Thomas[104]	25	6	14	5
Kopman et al[59]	249	213	19	17
Mongan and Culling[68]	40	35	5	0
Ovassapian et al[74]	129	89	37	3
Total	443	343 (77%)	75 (17%)	25 (6%)

From Benumof JL: Airway Management: Principles and Practice. St. Louis, Mosby, 1996, p 162.

dose (~30%) if narcotics or other central nervous system depressants are administered concomitantly. A point of note is flumazenil. A specific benzodiazepine receptor antagonist, it is able to reverse the central nervous system depression (along with the amnestic, sedative/hypnotic, muscle relaxant, and psychomotor retardation effects) but not always the respiratory depression. Its half-life of 0.7 to 1.8 hours is shorter than that of the corresponding benzodiazepine agonists because of its rapid hepatic clearance. Thus, resedation can be a problem. Adult dosage for reversal of conscious sedation is initially 0.2 mg (or 3 μg/kg) over 15 seconds, then repeated as needed in 0.2-μg increments at 1-minute intervals. Maximum total cumulative dose is 1 mg (usually 0.6 to 1 mg). If resedation occurs, 0.2 to 0.5 mg is given every 20 minutes, with a maximum of 1 mg per dose or 3 mg/hr. Doses of 3 μg/kg are used, with a rapid onset of 1 to 3 minutes; duration after a 3-mg intravenous (IV) dose is about 45 to 90 minutes. For diagnostic and therapeutic reversal of a benzodiazepine agonist, 0.1 to 0.2 mg IV increments are given, up to 3 mg.

2. Opioids

These are effective sedatives and, with adequate plasma levels, offer important antitussive properties to depress laryngeal reflexes further. In addition, they alter the respiratory pattern to a slower and deeper rhythm. The attenuated airway reflexes then help prevent coughing and retching during airway instrumentation, and the slower respiratory pattern facilitates a better laryngeal view during an awake approach in securing the airway. However, in patients who are exquisitely sensitive and have decreased respiratory reserve, the risks of attendant hypoxemia and hypercarbia loom increasingly after administration of these agents. Thus, the doses of these agents must be highly individualized. Important aspects (although not all inclusive) of some of the opioids follow.

Fentanyl: IV doses (~1 to 2 μg/kg), onset in about 2 to 3 minutes, with a duration of 0.5 to 1 hour. Although it is commonly used intravenously, a transmucosal route is available. Transmucosally, the onset of effect is 5 to 15 minutes, with peak analgesia within 20 to 30 minutes. The transmucosal route (Actiq) allows rapid absorption (25% from the buccal mucosa and 75% swallowed with saliva and then slowly absorbed from the gastrointestinal [GI] tract). Actiq's bioavailability is about 50% (range 35% to 70%), with a half-life of 6.5 hours (range 5 to 15 hours). The transmucosal route is an attractive route when posed with a difficult pediatric airway as a bridge to alleviate separation anxiety and a smooth transfer to the OR.

Sufentanil: IV doses (up to 1 μg/kg), onset in 1 to 3 minutes, with duration being dose dependent. Especially with sufentanil, rapid IV dosing may result in skeletal muscle and chest wall rigidity, with subsequent impaired ventilation; thus, it should be used with caution as this effect could supercede any antitussive effect.

Alfentanil: When given slowly IV over 3 to 5 minutes (8 to 20 μg/kg) in a spontaneously breathing patient or when assisted ventilation is required, duration is less than 30 minutes. However, the same precautions regarding chest wall rigidity should be taken with this agent.

Remifentanil: This is an ultrashort-acting narcotic that is unique compared with the other short-acting agents in that it is metabolized by plasma and tissue esterases, with a half-life of 9 minutes. In a dose range 0.05 to 0.5 μg/kg/min (or higher), its onset is 1 minute, with a duration of 5 to 10 minutes. *Bolus doses are not recommended for sedation because of the risk of respiratory depression and muscle rigidity.* In addition, it is packaged as a powder to be reconstituted (for 50 μg/mL: 1 mg in 20 mL, 2 mg in 40 mL, or 5 mg in 100 mL; or for 25 μg/mL: 1 mg in 40 mL or 2 mg in 80 mL); this inherently could add to misuses and hazardous dosing. Therefore, it is extremely important to use these agents wisely lest their risks outweigh their benefits. Fentanyl seems to be the most useful regarding its risk/benefit profile.

3. Intravenous Hypnotics

Ketamine: Ketamine is a phencyclidine derivative producing dissociative anesthesia with electroencephalographic evidence of dissociation between the thalamus and limbic system. Clinically, patients present in a cataleptic state with eyes in a slow gaze and open. Intense analgesia (somatic > visceral) is present with anterograde amnesia. It is packaged as a racemic mixture (10, 50, and 100 mg/mL) in a slightly acidic solution (pH 3.5 to 5.5, pK_a 7.5, molecular weight 238); thus, ketamine is slightly basic. Intense analgesia results from selective inhibition of the medial thalamic nuclei and suppression of spinal cord activity necessary to transmit pain to higher centers. Usual doses for sedation range from 0.2 to 0.5 mg/kg IV (1 to 2 mg/kg IV is an induction dose), with peak plasma levels at less than 1 minute and a duration of 5 to 10 minutes. Analgesia continues much longer, requiring much lower plasma levels than those required for loss of consciousness. When used for the purpose of its respiratory axis effects, it does not cause significant respiratory depression. Ketamine maintains the minute ventilation response to CO_2; however, large doses can decrease the respiratory rate (decreasing for 2 to 3 minutes after administration, and apnea can occur if large doses are used, especially with opioids or other sedatives). A disadvantage is that it increases salivary and tracheobronchial secretions; thus, antisialogogues must be employed well in advance to prevent this effect if ketamine is to be used. Upper airway skeletal muscle tone is well maintained along with its bronchodilating effect; however, airway protection remains necessary in patients at risk for aspiration. In addition, emergence delirium can occur in 5% to 20% of the patients, with an increased incidence in patients older than 16 years, with doses greater than 2 mg/kg, and in those with prior personality disorders.

As a direct central sympathetic stimulant, it increases blood pressure (BP), heart rate (HR), cardiac output, and myocardial oxygen consumption; BP increases by about 20 to 40 mm Hg during the first 3 to 5 minutes after IV dosing and then decreases to prebaseline levels during the next 10 to 20 minutes. This sympathetic response can adversely augment the hemodynamic response to airway manipulation. In addition, ketamine is a potent cerebrovasodilator with a secondary increase in cerebral blood flow (~60% above baseline) and a secondary increase in intracranial pressure (ICP). Thus, although of some benefit, ketamine has significant disadvantages that have to be weighed before considering its use.

Propofol: Propofol is a sterically hindered phenol (2, 6-diisopropylphenol) with a pK$_a$ of 11.03 (it is highly alkaline). It exists as a sterile, nonpyrogenic, isotonic emulsion (pH 7 to 8.5) with 10% soybean oil, 2.25% glycerol, and 1.2% egg lecithin. It has rapid induction after IV induction doses in about 40 seconds with rapid emergence secondary to redistribution from vessel-rich groups to lean tissues. Its advantage is in greatly attenuating airway responses (unclear mechanism) with induction doses, with a smooth induction (less excitatory effects); emergence after a single dose is in about 4 minutes. Although it is typically an induction agent in doses of 2 to 2.5 mg/kg, a sedating dosage of about 0.25 mg/kg IV in incremental doses serves as an excellent sedative with a smooth plane achieved, good acceptance by patients (except for venoirritation, minimized with concomitant lidocaine, opioids, slower injection, or injection into larger venous access sites), amnesia, adequate anxiolysis, and beneficial antiemetic properties. As with any agent, doses need to be titrated judiciously to avoid overt apnea.

Dexmedetomidine: Dexmedetomidine is a highly specific α_2-adrenoreceptor agonist with sedative, analgesic, and anesthetic-sparing effects[3,12,36] that causes sedation without a change in ventilatory status. It stimulates α_2-adrenergic receptors in the locus ceruleus to provide sedation and in the spinal cord to enhance analgesia. It also causes sympatholysis through central and peripheral mechanisms. Dexmedetomidine binds α_2-receptors eight times more avidly than clonidine and is shorter acting.[29] In addition, it is a potent antisialogogue, which makes it desirable for cases involving airway instrumentation. Most of the clinical experience with dexmedetomidine has been with surgical patients undergoing cardiac and vascular procedures,[109] although there have been several reports of its use for sedation during AI.[96] Careful selection of patients and proper drug infusion are needed to avoid excessive deleterious hemodynamic changes, such as bradycardia and hypotension.[3,12] A loading dose of dexmedetomidine, 1 μg/kg IV over 10 minutes, followed by a continuous infusion of 0.2 to 0.7 μg/kg/hr can provide comfort and sedation throughout the procedure. In addition, it can be combined with ketamine for its cardio-stimulatory properties.[96] Unlike patients sedated with propofol, patients receiving dexmedetomidine are easily arousable and able to cooperate, thus able to take deep breaths and clear secretions during AI. Although lowering of bispectral index scores and partial amnesia have been reported with its use,[74] the true amnestic qualities of dexmedetomidine have yet to be defined. Further investigation with this sedative for use in AI is warranted.

4. Inhalational Anesthetics

Although not considered in the typical realm of sedative/hypnotics, these volatile anesthetics have a unique role in the pediatric DA, shorter recovery time, and patients with a DA who are uncooperative. Of the third-generation volatile anesthetics, desflurane and sevoflurane have clinical benefits.

Sevoflurane has a blood-gas partition coefficient of 0.63 to 0.69, brain-blood partition coefficient of 1.70, vapor pressure of 157 mm Hg (boiling point at 760 mm Hg of 58.5° C), and a minimum alveolar concentration (MAC) of 2.05 in 18- to 30-year-olds and 1.71 in 30- to 60-year-olds. Sevoflurane has a great advantage in enabling a smooth induction because of lack of pungency, minimizing coughing, breath holding, secretions, and laryngospasm. The purported benefits are great in the difficult pediatric (or adult) airway not possible to sedate adequately by conventional means. By achieving an appropriate depth of anesthesia while maintaining spontaneous ventilation, sevoflurane provides a bridge for maneuvers to secure the airway definitively.

Desflurane has a blood-gas partition coefficient of 0.42, brain-blood partition coefficient of 1.29, a vapor pressure of 670 mm Hg at 20° C and 798 mm Hg at 24° C (boiling point at 760 mm Hg of 22.5° C), and a MAC of 7.2 in 18- to 30-year-olds and 6.0 in 30- to 60-year-olds. Although desflurane has a clear disadvantage during inhalational induction because of pronounced coughing and breath holding, its lower brain-blood partition coefficient allows more rapid emergence. Thus, once an adequate anesthetic plane is established, one could theoretically change to desflurane to enable more rapid emergence without the inherent untoward effects experienced with induction sequence. The reader if referred to more selected texts for further details in this regard.

B. ASPIRATION PROPHYLAXIS

A small percentage of patients requiring AI may need prophylaxis against aspiration as they may have a full stomach (e.g., trauma victims) or be obese with DA, or both. Preoperative administration of nonparticulate antacids such as sodium citrate and citric acid (Bicitra) provides effective buffering of gastric acid pH.[37] Sodium citrate, potassium citrate, and citric acid (Polycitra) is a nonparticulate antacid with better buffering capacity than Bicitra.[25] A single dose of antacid increases gastric volume. This effect is offset by an increase in the pH of gastric fluid such that, if aspiration occurs, morbidity and mortality are significantly lower.[54]

H$_2$-receptor antagonists (cimetidine and ranitidine) are selective and competitive antagonists that block secretion of hydrogen ion (H^+) by gastric parietal cells and also decrease the secretion of gastric fluid. With IV administration of cimetidine (300 mg IV [150 mg/mL in 2 mL and 8 mL vials]) or ranitidine (50 mg), peak effects are achieved within 30 to 60 minutes, which increase gastric pH and decrease gastric volume.[39]

Metoclopramide is a dopamine antagonist that stimulates motility of the upper GI tract and increases lower esophageal sphincter tone. The net effect is accelerated gastric clearance of liquids and solids in the patent GI tract.[92] Doses are 0.15 to 0.3 mg/kg IV.

For complete aspiration prophylaxis, a combination of nonparticulate antacid, H_2-receptor blocking agent, and metoclopramide may be used.

C. ANTISIALOGOGUES[9,37,43,83]

Although innumerable combinations of medications can be employed successfully, there exists one important concept: *dry the airway.* Copious secretions present a twofold problem. Secretions obscure the view, whether it be by direct laryngoscopy or especially if flexible fiberoptic bronchoscopy is being used. In addition, an intervening layer of secretions prevents the local anesthetics from reaching intended areas, resulting in failed sensory blockade. Moreover, copious secretions could wash (and dilute) the local anesthetics away from a particular site, severely limiting their duration of action and potency. Thus, the first premedicant should be a drying agent.

The antisialogogues used in clinical practice are atropine, scopolamine, and glycopyrrolate. These agents prevent further liberation of secretions, but they do not eliminate secretions that have already accumulated. Consequently, antisialogogues are best administered approximately 1.5 hours prior to the application of local anesthetics. Pharmacodynamically, these are anticholinergic/antimuscarinic agents. They inhibit different muscarinic receptor subtypes at different plasma concentrations. In increasing concentrations, they inhibit salivary and bronchial secretions, myocardial and ophthalmic cholinergic receptors, and then GI and genitourinary receptors. Paradoxically, when given in small doses, these agents can be muscarinic agonists. The following are some salient details regarding the three agents used in clinical practice.

Atropine (0.4 to 0.6 mg IV, IM, subcutaneously [SC], or by mouth [PO]) has a rapid onset after IV administration (2 to 4 minutes); the onset after IM, SC, and PO dosing is delayed by 30 minutes to 2 hours (for PO dosing). It is well absorbed from all dosage forms, is widely distributed throughout the body, crosses the placenta, and crosses the blood-brain barrier. It is metabolized in the liver, with a half-life of 2 to 3 hours. The usual dosage varies with its use (as a drying agent, usually 7 to 10 μg/kg IV or 20 to 40 μg/kg IM). Although it can dry the airway (least of the three in its antisialogogic properties), a true disadvantage is that it is vagolytic even at doses that inhibit secretions. Therefore, undesired tachycardia usually results, which can be detrimental in patients with decreased cardiac

reserve. Considering the sympathetic stimulation usually encountered during securing the airway, this is an undesirable side effect. Also, as a tertiary amine, it crosses the blood-brain barrier and thus could lead to an anticholinergic syndrome with delirium, especially in elderly patients.

Glycopyrrolate (0.1 to 0.2 mg IV, IM, SC and 1 to 2 mg PO) has an onset after IV dosing in 1 to 2 minutes, after IM or SC dosing in 15 to 45 minutes, and after PO dosing in 50 minutes, with peak effect at 1 hour. Duration after IV dosing is 2 to 4 hours, after IM or SC dosing 2 to 3 hours for the vagolytic effect and 7 hours for the antisialogogic effects, and after PO dosing 6 hours. It is typically given in a dose of 7 to 10 μg/kg IV or 10 to 20 μg/IM. Its quaternary amine structure prevents its passage through the blood-brain barrier. In addition, if one administers it over at least 30 to 60 minutes, it is possible to prevent an untoward vagolytic effect, which is commonly seen with atropine (administered typically over 15 to 20 minutes).

Scopolamine (0.3 to 0.65 mg IV, IM, or SC) has an onset in 5 to 10 minutes after IV dosing and variably in 0.5 to 1 hour after IM or SC dosing. The duration of action is about 2 hours after IV dosing and 4 to 6 hours after IM or SC dosing. Although it is effective in drying (best of the three in its antisialogogic properties) secretions, its use is limited by its sedating effects (with amnesia) along with untoward delirium (peak effect occurs in 20 to 60 minutes, but it may take 3 to 7 days for full recovery). The authors' main drying agent is glycopyrrolate. Scopolamine is reserved for patients with high risk for cardiovascular compromise (as it is least vagolytic).

D. NASAL MUCOSAL VASOCONSTRICTORS

The nasal mucosa and nasopharynx are highly vascular. When a patient requires awake nasal intubation, adequate anesthesia of this area, along with vasoconstriction, is essential. Agents commonly used are 4% cocaine and 2% lidocaine with 1% phenylephrine.[47] When these agents are applied appropriately to the nasal area, adequate anesthesia and vasoconstriction can be achieved in 10 to 15 minutes, which facilitates awake nasal intubation (see "Nerve Blocks").

It is helpful to begin the process of vasoconstriction preoperatively by using nasal decongestants. When the patient is called to the OR, the floor nurse can be asked to apply 0.025% to 0.05% oxymetazoline hydrochloride nasal solution (Afrin spray), sprayed twice in each nostril, which vasoconstricts the anterior half of the nasal cavity. When the patient arrives in the holding area, the anesthesiologist repeats the process, allowing the solution to reach the posterior half of the nasal cavity.

IV. PREOPERATIVE PREPARATIONS

A. GENERAL PREOPERATIVE PREPARATIONS

The preparation of the patient for an AI begins, as discussed, with verbal communication to allay fear and appropriate premedication. The preparation for AI includes assembling necessary equipment, as discussed later, and arranging *in advance* for needed assistance. Patients' acuity must be considered when arranging transport to OR.

The decision must be made (1) to secure the airway at once (the patient in extremis who warrants a bedside emergency airway procedure), (2) to transport the patient to the OR with appropriate monitors (electrocardiogram [ECG], pulse oximeter, and automated BP cuff) and supplemental oxygen, accompanied by anesthesiologist or surgeon, or both, or (3) to call for routine transport to the OR. In the elective scenario, supplemental oxygen should be provided if appropriate (high-dose oxygen may be detrimental in some patients, such as those who rely on hypoxic respiratory drive),[67] and position should be considered (e.g., the morbidly obese patient may experience dramatic physiologic changes when supine and should be transported in a wheelchair or on a gurney in a semirecumbent position.).[76,105,107]

B. OPERATING ROOM PREPARATIONS

1. Staff

There should be "at least one additional individual who is immediately available to serve as an assistant in DA management."[4] Preferred whenever possible is a second anesthesiologist who can assist in the monitoring and ventilation of the patient (two-person ventilation and assistance in mask ventilation while the primary anesthesiologist performs fiberoptic intubation). In cases of the patient in extremis or a patient who refuses AI, a surgeon trained in performing a surgical airway should be at hand with a tracheostomy-cricothyrotomy tray, ready to perform an emergency surgical airway, if necessary.

2. Monitors

During AI the routine use of ECG, noninvasive BP monitor, pulse oximetry, capnography, and a precordial stethoscope is required as part of standard basic intraoperative monitoring. Depending on the complexity of the surgery and the patient's condition, monitoring may include more sophisticated and often invasive monitors.

ECG is a continuous display of the patient's cardiac activity during the intraoperative period and helps in diagnosis and necessary treatment of any changes seen in the HR or rhythm as well as heart blocks and ischemia. An audible indicator for each QRS complex allows the anesthesiologist to carry on with tasks in the OR while listening to cardiac rate and rhythm changes. ECG is usually monitored in lead II and lead V_5 for detection of dysrhythmias and myocardial ischemia, respectively.[13,98] Electrolyte changes, particularly those of potassium and calcium, can frequently be diagnosed with ECG.

BP is usually measured noninvasively by an oscillometric method during AI. Devices automatically measure BP at 1-, 2.5-, or 5-minute intervals and give accurate measurement of mean arterial pressure (MAP) even in hypotensive conditions.[77] The BP cuff width should be about 40% of the circumference of the arm. If the patient's general condition or the complexity of the operation demands, arterial BP may be recorded continuously by the "invasive" method by placement of an arterial catheter in the radial artery.

The precordial stethoscope is commonly placed on the suprasternal notch or over the left side of the chest under the clavicle area to monitor heart sounds and breath sounds continuously during the AI procedure. This device can help in detection of bronchospasm or obstructed airway.

Pulse oximetry is essential for detection of arterial oxygen saturation changes during AI, allowing early detection of hypoxemia so that the patient can be ventilated with 100% oxygen. Oxygen saturation values obtained by the pulse oximeter reading may not be accurate in the presence of hypotension, hypothermia, motion, OR lights, electrocautery interference, or peripheral vasoconstriction.[7]

Capnography measures carbon dioxide (CO_2) levels in inhaled and exhaled gases of the patient. Upon achievement of AI, the presence of three consecutive waveforms of end-tidal CO_2 confirms endotracheal intubation. The absence of an end-tidal CO_2 waveform on the monitoring device suggests esophageal intubation and alerts the anesthesiologist. Capnography also helps to diagnose other problems such as disconnection of anesthesia delivery system, obstruction in the airway, exhausted carbon dioxide absorber, and malfunctioning inspiratory or expiratory valve.[14]

3. Supplemental Oxygen

Administration of supplemental oxygen (O_2) should be considered during the entire process of DA management, which includes topicalization, intubation, and extubation.[4] Arterial hypoxemia has been well documented during bronchoscopy (an average decrease in arterial oxygen tension [PaO_2] of 20 to 30 mm Hg in patients breathing room air) and has been associated with cardiac dysrhythmias.[117] Daos and colleagues[28] have shown that the use of supplemental O_2 delayed circulatory arrest resulting from local anesthetic toxic effects in animals but did not show statistically significant improvement in the incidence of respiratory arrest. Considering the advantage of improving patients' safety, the use of supplemental O_2 must be encouraged in all patients undergoing AI.

In addition to the standard methods of supplementing O_2 (nasal prongs, face mask, and binasal airways), there are nonconventional methods for increasing the fractional concentration of O_2 in inspired gas (FIO_2): delivering O_2 through the suction port of the FOB,[11] delivering O_2 through the atomizer during topicalization,[18] or elective transtracheal jet ventilation (TTJV) in a patient in extremis.[9,11,18,83,105]

4. Airway Equipment

Consultants of the DATF agreed strongly that "preparatory efforts enhance success and minimize risk to the patient" (fewer adverse outcomes).[4] The concept of preassembled carts for emergency situations is not new ("crash carts" for cardiac arrest on every floor and malignant hyperthermia carts in every OR area). DATF recommendations are that *every anesthetizing location* should be equipped with a DA cart. (If the main OR is in a different location from the outpatient surgical center, two carts are necessary.) The DA cart should be a portable storage unit that contains specialized equipment for managing the DA. This cart should be customized to the individual *group* of anesthesiologists who use it (Box 10-2). For example, only one physician in the group may be familiar with a specific cricotome for establishing a surgical airway. The options are to train the rest of the staff in the mechanics of that particular instrument or to supply the cart with various equipment sufficient to satisfy all staff preferences and expertise. We have chosen the latter approach at our institution.

On top of our cart we have a dedicated capnograph and pulse oximeter because we are frequently asked to manage DAs outside the OR setting in locations such as the burn unit of the surgical intensive care unit. The top surface of the cart is used as a workstation for preparation of fiberoptic equipment and laying out equipment for topicalizing the airway and for nerve blocks (Fig. 10-1). The first drawer is for drugs (including flumazenil and naloxone) and ancillary fiberoptic equipment (Fig. 10-2). The FOBs themselves are suspended on the outside of the cart (Fig. 10-3), with tubes designated for clean or used bronchoscopes. The second drawer is for specialized blades, lighted stylets, and laryngeal mask airways (Fig. 10-4). Below the drawers, space is available for the fiberoptic light source, different sizes of ETs, and other ancillary equipment. On the outer wall of the airway cart we hang, on clips, emergency airway equipment such as cricotomes, retrograde kits, jet stylets, Combitubes and portable jet ventilator equipment (Fig. 10-5). Critical airway equipment can easily be obtained in a "pop-off" manner with one hand.

In addition to the equipment on the cart, on every OR anesthetic machine we have a designated Combitube, gum elastic bougie, and jet ventilator with a preassembled transtracheal kit. Multiple acceptable TTJV systems are available (see Chapter 26). We are currently using an injector (blowgun) powered by a regulated central wall O_2 pressure unit with a universal adapter to the O_2 wall outlet.[9] Taped to the jet ventilator is a kit containing a 14-gauge angiocatheter (for adult patients), an 18-gauge angiocatheter (for pediatric patients), and a 20-mL syringe. As part of our machine check, the jet ventilator is set at 40 to 50 psi[9,11,116] for adults and 5 psi for pediatric patients as starting pressures, to minimize the incidence of barotrauma.[10,11,35,77]

Box 10-2 Suggested Contents of the Portable Unit for Difficult Airway Management

1. Rigid laryngoscope blades of alternative designs and sizes from those routinely used.
2. Endotracheal tubes of assorted sizes.
3. Endotracheal tube guides. Examples include (but are not limited to) semirigid stylets with or without hollow core for jet ventilation, light wands, and forceps designed to manipulate the distal portion of the endotracheal tube.
4. Fiberoptic intubation equipment.
5. Retrograde intubation equipment.
6. At least one device for emergency nonsurgical airway ventilation. Examples include (but are not limited to) a transtracheal jet ventilation stylet, the laryngeal mask, and the esophageal-tracheal Combitube.
7. Equipment suitable for emergency surgical airway access (cricothyrotomy).
8. An exhaled CO_2 detector.
9. Pulse oximetry unit.
10. Portable O_2 tank.

Important: The items listed in this table represent suggestions. The contents of the portable storage unit should be customized to meet the specific needs, preferences, and skills of the practitioner and health care facility.

Modified from Practice guidelines for management of the difficult airway. Anesthesiology 78:597, 1993.

V. TOPICALIZATION

AI with airway instrumentation causes discomfort unless adequate topical anesthesia of the respiratory tract is performed, rendering the process painless. It is important to know the onset of action and mechanism of action, optimal concentration, and maximum amount of a drug that can be used safely.[2] The rate and amount of topical drug absorption usually vary depending on the site of application, amount of the drug applied locally, hemodynamic status of the patient, and patients' individual variations.[77] The rate at which the drug is absorbed from the respiratory tract is more rapid from the alveoli than from the tracheobronchial tree, which is more rapid than from the pharynx. It is still controversial whether the addition of vasoconstrictor to these drugs really prolongs the duration of action or slows the rate of absorption.[2] A second controversy exists with respect to topical anesthesia of the airway and risk of aspiration of gastric contents in any patients considered to have a full stomach. The authors were unable to find any reported cases in the literature of aspiration associated with topical anesthetic use in patients with a DA who underwent AIs. In addition, Keller and Brimacombe determined that resting gastroesophageal

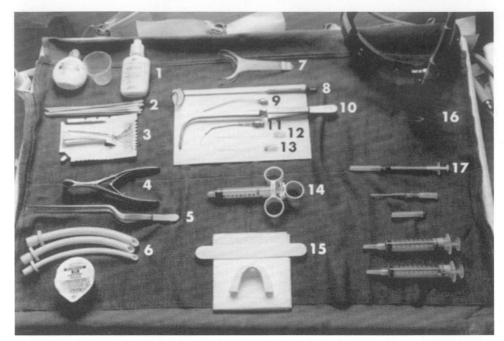

Figure 10-1 The top surface of our airway cart is used as a workstation for topicalization and nerve blocks. 1, Nasal vasoconstrictors and container for local anesthetics. 2, Long cotton-tipped applicators. 3, Neuropledgets. 4, Nasal speculum. 5, Bayonet forceps. 6, Nasal trumpets in various sizes with viscous lidocaine. 7, Cheek retractor. 8, Indirect mirror. 9, Modified Labat needle. 10, Krause's forceps. 11, Tonsillar needle. 12, Straight 25-gauge spinal needle for glossopharyngeal nerve block. 13, Angled 25-gauge spinal needle for sphenopalatine nerve block. 14, Three-ring syringe. 15, Tongue blade and mouth guard for glossopharyngeal nerve block. 16, Light source. 17, 25-gauge needle for superior laryngeal nerve block, 20-gauge angiocatheter for translaryngeal block, and syringes for local anesthetic. (From Benumof JL: Airway Management: Principles and Practice. St. Louis, Mosby, 1996, p 165.)

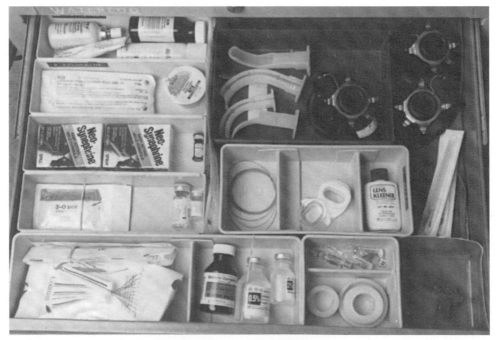

Figure 10-2 The first drawer of our airway cart contains drugs and ancillary equipment for fiberoptic bronchoscope (fiberoptic masks and oral airways). (From Benumof JL: Airway Management: Principles and Practice. St. Louis, Mosby, 1996, p 166.)

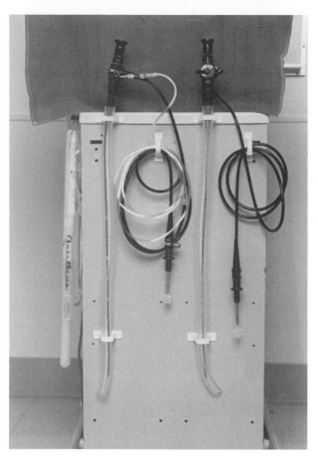

Figure 10-3 Fiberoptic bronchoscope suspended on the outside of the cart for easy access. Scope on the left has a triple stopcock and air hose to deliver oxygen as well as to administer local anesthetic through the suction port of the scope. (From Benumof JL: Airway Management: Principles and Practice. St. Louis, Mosby, 1996, p 166.)

pressure, upper esophageal sphincter pressure, and deglutition frequency were unaffected by oropharyngeal topical anesthesia.[57]

The most commonly used drugs for topical anesthesia are cocaine, benzocaine, lidocaine, and tetracaine.

A. COCAINE

Cocaine is a natural alkaloid that causes local anesthesia and vasoconstriction when applied topically; thus, cocaine is widely used in otolaryngologic surgical procedures.[91] The vasoconstrictive properties of cocaine result from interference with the reuptake of circulating norepinephrine by the adrenergic nerve endings.[6] Cocaine should be used with caution in patients with known hypersensitivity, coronary artery disease, hypertension, pseudocholinesterase deficiency, pregnancy with hypertension (preeclampsia), or hyperthyroidism as well as in children, elderly patients, and patients receiving monoamine oxidase inhibitors. After topical application of cocaine to the nasal mucosa, peak plasma levels are achieved within an hour and the drug persists in the plasma for 5 to 6 hours.[106] The metabolism of cocaine is mainly by plasma cholinesterase, with hepatic and renal excretion. The signs and symptoms of cocaine overdose include tachycardia, cardiac dysrhythmia, hypertension, and fever. It is important to remember that cocaine has addictive properties because of cortical stimulation resulting in euphoria, excitement, feeling "high," and increased muscle activity. Severe complications include convulsions, respiratory failure, coronary spasm, stroke, and death.

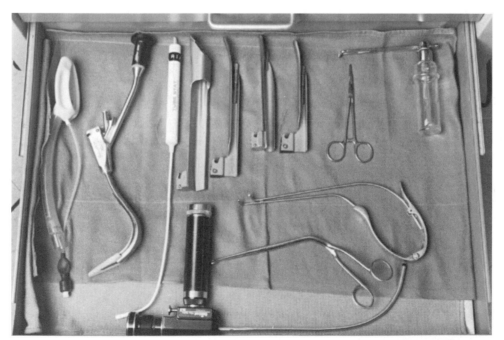

Figure 10-4 The second drawer of our airway cart contains assorted blades, lighted stylet, instruments to bend or manipulate endotracheal tubes, and laryngeal mask airways. (From Benumof JL: Airway Management: Principles and Practice. St. Louis, Mosby, 1996, p 167.)

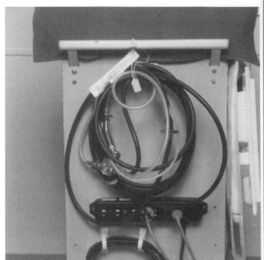
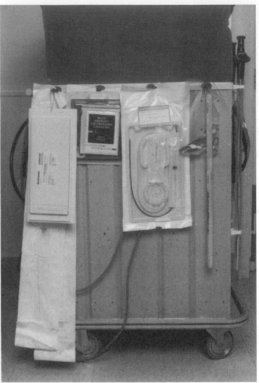

Figure 10-5 A and **B,** Suspended on outside of cart for easy access is emergency equipment (Combitube, jet stylet, cricotome, retrograde kit, and jet ventilator). (From Benumof JL: Airway Management: Principles and Practice. St. Louis, Mosby, 1996, p 167.)

Cocaine is available in two preparations, 4% and 10% solutions, for topical application. The 10% solution is not used because of a very high incidence of toxic effects. The dosage varies and depends on the area to be anesthetized, vascularity of the tissue, individual tolerance, and the technique of anesthesia. The dosage should be reduced in children and in elderly and debilitated patients. The maximum dose should not exceed 200 mg or 1 mg/kg.

B. BENZOCAINE

Benzocaine (ethyl aminobenzoate) is a water-insoluble ester-type local anesthetic agent that is mainly useful for topical application. The onset of action is rapid (<1 minute) with an effective duration of about 10 minutes. Benzocaine is available for use as 10%, 15%, and 20% solutions. To prolong its duration of action, it is usually mixed with 2% tetracaine. Topical application is usually nontoxic, although methemoglobinemia has been reported in adult patients taking sulfonamides and in pediatric patients.[58,69]

Benzocaine 20% spray (Hurricaine, Beutlich Pharmaceuticals, Waukegan, IL) contains 200 mg/mL; thus 0.5 mL is equal to the toxic dose, which is 100 mg. A half-second spray delivers approximately 0.15 mL, or 30 mg.

Cetacaine is a topical application spray containing benzocaine 14%, tetracaine 2%, butyl aminobenzoate 2%, benzalkonium chloride, and cetyldimethyl ethyl ammonium bromide, which has been shown to be effective for topicalizing the airway. Combining these agents

hastens onset of action and prolongs duration of action. Interestingly, there are case reports of methemoglobinemia occurring immediately after application of this spray. The risk of methemoglobinemia with the use of benzocaine led to an FDA warning in 2006, but there is no plan to remove the drug from the market at this time. (The Veterans Administration has halted the use of benzocaine spray in their hospital network.) Other drugs, including topical anesthetics, can cause methemoglobinemia (Table 10-2). In the patient who develops this complication, cyanosis appears first (at a methemoglobin level as low as 2.5%), and clinical symptoms (fatigue, weakness, headache, dizziness, and tachycardia) appear later (at methemoglobin levels of 20% to 50%). Treatment is with intravenous methylene blue (1 to 2 mg/kg [0.1 to 0.2 mL/kg of 1% solution] IV over 5 minutes, repeated in 1 hour as needed).[31,60,90]

C. LIDOCAINE

Lidocaine is an amide local anesthetic agent that is widely used. It is available in various preparations including aqueous (1%, 2%, and 4%) and viscous (1%) solutions, ointment (1%), and aerosol preparation. Xylocaine 10% metered-dose oral spray (Astra) delivers 10 mg per spray and rapidly anesthetizes the upper airway.

Once in the plasma, lidocaine is metabolized mainly by the hepatic microsomal system. In awake patients the toxic plasma level of lidocaine is 5 μg/mL.[14] In most of the

Table 10-2   **Methemoglobinemia**

I. Hereditary
  1. Patients with congenital M hemoglobins
  2. Patients with methemoglobin reductase deficiency
II. Acquired
  1. Nitrites and nitrates
    a. Amyl nitrite
    b. Butyl nitrite
    c. Nitric oxide
    d. Nitroglycerin
    e. Nitroprusside
    f. Silver nitrate
    g. Sodium nitrite
  2. Topical anesthetics
    a. Benzocaine
    b. Cetocaine
    c. Lidocaine
    d. Prilocaine
  3. Antimalarial agents
    a. Chloroquine
    b. Primaquine
  4. Others
    a. Acetanilide
    b. Aniline dyes

    c. Chlorates
    d. Dapsone
    e. Flutamide
    f. Menthol
    g. Metoclopramide
    h. Napthalene
    i. Phenacetin
    j. Phenazopyridine
    k. Phenols
    l. Phenytoin
    m. Pyridium
    n. Quinones
    o. Silver sulfadiazine
    p. Sulfonamides
III. Patient related (increased risk)
  1. Critically ill or febrile patients
  2. Patients with pulmonary disease (e.g., asthma, emphysema) and/or hypoxia
  3. Patients with coronary artery disease
  4. Geriatric population
  5. Pediatric population (<4 mo)

Modified from: Gupta PM, Lala DS, Arsura EL: Benzocaine-induced methemoglobinemia. South Med J 93:83, 2000.

clinical situations in which lidocaine is used as a local anesthetic agent for topicalization, the peak plasma level measured has been far below 5 or 6 µg/mL[60,88]; thus, severe toxic reactions secondary to lidocaine are uncommon in the context of airway management. Amitai and colleagues[5] reported the safety of topical lidocaine administered to nose, larynx, and bronchial tree in 15 children who underwent bronchoscopy (age 3 months to 9.5 years) and found that serum lidocaine concentrations were 1 to 3.5 µg/mL at doses up to 7 mg/kg given over a time range of 9 to 45 minutes. Symptoms of severe lidocaine toxicity include convulsions, respiratory failure, and circulatory collapse.

EMLA cream (eutectic mixture of local anesthetic) contains 2.5% lidocaine and 2.5% prilocaine and is considered a topical anesthetic for use on intact skin. Although the manufacturer does not recommend its use on mucosal surfaces because of faster systemic absorption, it has been employed as a topical anesthetic for AI. Larijani and coworkers described 20 adult patients who underwent awake fiberoptic intubation using 4 g of EMLA applied over the upper airway. The measured peak plasma concentrations of lidocaine or prilocaine did not reach toxic levels and methemoglobin levels did not exceed normal values (1.5%).[61]

D. TETRACAINE

Tetracaine is an amide local anesthetic agent with a longer duration of action than lidocaine and cocaine. It is available as 0.5%, 1%, and 2% solutions for local use. It is metabolized through hydrolysis by plasma cholinesterase. Tetracaine has been shown to have higher toxic effects when used as an aerosol with doses as small as 20 mg because absorption of the drug from the respiratory tract and GI tract is fast.[111] Severe toxic reactions following tetracaine overdose include convulsions, respiratory arrest, and circulatory collapse.[87] Fatalities have been reported with topical application of tetracaine 100 mg used to anesthetize mucous membrane.[1]

E. APPLICATION TECHNIQUES

1. Atomizers

Sprays and atomizers with long delivery systems are available to deliver local anesthesia to the larynx and trachea. Tetracaine (0.3% to 0.5% with epinephrine 1:200,000), maximum 4 to 7 mL, or lidocaine (4%), maximum 10 mL, is placed in an atomizer (Fig. 10-6), connected to the oxygen tank (flow, 8 to 10 L/min), and sprayed in the oropharynx for 10-second periods with 20-second rest intervals for about 20 minutes. Any residual agents from the oropharynx must be suctioned out to reduce absorption from the GI tract. This is a relatively safe and simple method to provide adequate anesthesia of the airway.

Alternatively, the Wolfe Tory Mucosal Atomization Device (MAD) is an inexpensive, disposable, latex-free device that when attached to a Luer fitted syringe

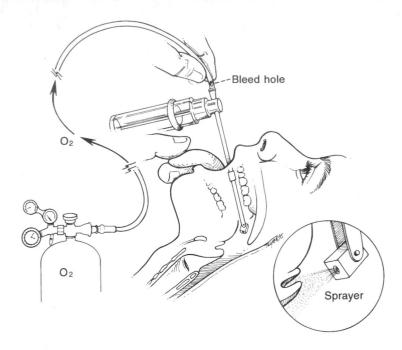

Figure 10-6 Atomizer hooked up to an oxygen (O_2) tank. A bleed hole is made close to the operator's hand, allowing intermittent spraying. Inset shows the tip of atomizer as it is angulated to spray toward the glottic opening. (From University of California, Irvine, Department of Anesthesia: D.A. Teaching Aids.)

containing an appropriate volume of local anesthetic can be used to quickly dispense an atomized solution orally or nasally. When time is not sufficient for a 20-minute preparation of the airway, quick atomization with a smaller volume of local anesthetic can allow the patient to accept an intubating oral airway treated with lidocaine jelly, or a series of graduated nasal trumpets treated with lidocaine jelly and the subsequent introduction of a fiberoptic bronchoscope. Topicalization of deeper structures can then be achieved by delivering the remaining volume of local anesthetic through the fiberoptic bronchoscope using the "spray as you go" techniques described in Section VI.

2. Nebulizers

The ultrasonic nebulizer utilizes 5 mL of 4% lidocaine to be nebulized with O_2 (6 to 8 L/min). The size of the droplet depends on the flow of O_2 and the type of nebulizer. With O_2 flow less than 6 L/min, droplet sizes of 30 to 60 μm can be achieved, coating the mucosa up to the trachea. The advantages of this technique include ease of application and safety. This is a difficult technique to use in small children and uncooperative patients. This approach is especially advantageous in patients with increased ICP, open eye injury, and severe coronary artery disease.[20] Foster and Hurewitz[41] reported the use of lidocaine with two different modalities (nebulizer-atomizer combination versus atomizer alone) in patients undergoing bronchoscopy. They found that the nebulizer-atomizer combination was more efficacious, resulting in a reduction of the dose required to anesthetize the upper airway.

Other less commonly used techniques for topical anesthesia include lozenges (amethocaine lozenges 60 mg) and gargle with 4% lidocaine gel,[19] which are not routinely used because they provide limited anesthesia.

VI. NERVE BLOCKS

Because of the multitude of nerves innervating the airway (see Chapter 1), there is no single anatomic site where a physician can perform a nerve block and anesthetize the entire airway. Even though topicalization of the mucosa serves, in the majority of patients, to anesthetize the entire airway adequately, some patients require supplementation to ablate sensation in the nerve endings running deep to the mucosal surface such as the periosteal nerve endings of the nasal turbinates and the stretch receptors at the base of the tongue, which are involved in gagging. The following nerve blocks are remarkable for their ease of performance, their minimal risk to the patient, the density of the block (complete ablation of sensory fibers), and the speed of onset.

A. NASAL CAVITY AND NASOPHARYNX[7,19,24,30,55,71,72,81,84-87]

1. Anatomy

The nasal cavity is innervated by a plethora of sensory fibers with multiple origins. The majority of the innervation is derived from two sources: the sphenopalatine ganglion and the anterior ethmoidal nerve.

The sphenopalatine ganglion (pterygopalatine, nasal, or Meckel's ganglion) is located in the pterygopalatine fossa (Fig. 10-7) posterior to the middle turbinate. It is covered by a 1- to 5-mm layer of connective tissue and mucous membrane. The ganglion is a 5-mm triangular or heart-shaped structure comprising branches primarily from the gasserian ganglion through the trigeminal nerve (V2). Although it sends out multiple branches, two nerves in particular, the greater and lesser palatine nerves, provide sensory innervation to the nasal turbinates

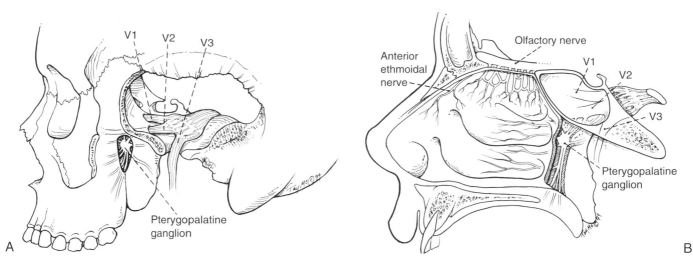

Figure 10-7 A, Left lateral view of the skull with temporal bone removed depicting the gasserian ganglion with the three branches (V1 to V3) of the trigeminal nerve. V2 is the major contributor to the pterygopalatine ganglion (shown as it sits in the pterygopalatine fossa). **B,** Left lateral view of the right nasal cavity depicting the anterior ethmoidal nerve, olfactory nerve, gasserian ganglion, and the trigeminal nerve (V1 to V3). The pterygopalatine ganglion lies just beneath the mucosal surface on the caudad surface of the sphenoid sinus (and forms the roof of the pterygopalatine fossa). (From University of California, Irvine, Department of Anesthesia, D.A. Teaching Aids.)

and to two thirds of the posterior nasal septum (including the periosteum).

The anterior ethmoidal nerve is one of the branches of the ciliary ganglion, which is located within the orbital cavity and inaccessible to nerve blocks. The anterior ethmoidal nerve (see Fig. 10-7B) gives sensory innervation to one third of the anterior portion of the nares.

2. Sphenopalatine Nerve Block: Oral Approach[7,24,30,55,71,81,87]

With the patient in the supine position, the physician stands facing the patient on the contralateral side of the nerve to be blocked. Using the left index finger, the greater palatine foramen (GPF) is identified. The GPF (Fig. 10-8) is located between the second and third maxillary molars

approximately 1 cm medial to the palatogingival margin and can usually be palpated as a small depression near the posterior edge of the hard palate. In approximately 15% of the population, the foramen is closed and inaccessible. A 25-gauge spinal needle, bent 2 to 3 cm proximal to the tip to an angle of 120 degrees, is used. Pain on insertion of the needle can be avoided by application of 2% viscous lidocaine with a cotton-tipped applicator for 1 to 2 minutes or digital pressure over the foramen. The 25-gauge spinal needle is then inserted into the GPF in a superior and slightly posterior direction (to a depth of 2 to 3 cm). An aspiration test is performed to ascertain that the sphenopalatine artery has not been cannulated, and 1 to 2 mL of 2% lidocaine with epinephrine 1:100,000 is injected. The epinephrine is used as a vasoconstrictor for the sphenopalatine artery, which runs

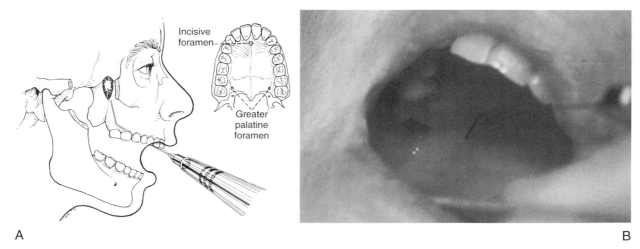

Figure 10-8 A, Inferior view of the hard palate showing location of the greater palatine foramen. Right lateral view of the head with zygomatic arch and coronoid process of the mandible removed exposing the pterygopalatine fossa (containing the pterygopalatine ganglion) with angulated spinal needle in place. **B,** Right sphenopalatine nerve block. (From University of California, Irvine, Department of Anesthesia, D.A. Teaching Aids.)

of 2% lidocaine with epinephrine 1:200,000 as the needle is withdrawn. The block is repeated on the opposite side.

b. External Approach: Cornu of the Thyroid

This is the same technique as stated previously but uses the cornu of the thyroid as the landmark. The benefit of this technique is that in many patients these structures are easier to palpate, and palpating them is less painful to the patient. A 4-cm, 25-gauge needle is walked off the cornu of the thyroid cartilage (see Fig. 10-16) in a superior-anterior direction aiming toward the lower third of the thyroid ligament; the same precautions as before are taken. The block is repeated on the opposite side.

c. External Approach: Thyroid Notch

The easiest landmark to identify in many of the patients, especially males, is the thyroid notch (Adam's apple). The thyroid notch is palpated, and the upper border of the thyroid cartilage is traced posteriorly for approximately 2 cm (see Fig. 10-16). Using a 2.5-cm, 25-gauge needle, the thyrohyoid ligament is directed posterior and cephalad and entered to a depth of 1.0 to 1.5 cm. This corresponds to the preepiglottic space, which normally contains the terminal branches of the SLN imbedded in a fat pad. The area is injected with the same solution, using precautions as previously described, but the entire volume is injected into the preepiglottic space before the needle is withdrawn. The block is repeated on the opposite side. An added benefit of this approach is the decreased likelihood of blocking the motor branch of the SLN.

d. Internal Approach: Pyriform Fossa

A noninvasive SLN block can be performed by applying local anesthetic to the pyriform fossa. (The internal branch of the SLN lies just superficial to the mucosa.) After local anesthetic is applied topically to the tongue and pharynx, the patient is placed in the *sitting* position with the physician standing on the *contralateral* side of the nerve to be blocked. The patient is asked to open the mouth wide with tongue protruded. The tongue is grasped with the left hand using a gauze pad (or depressed with a tongue blade) and gently pulled anteriorly. With the right hand a Jackson (Krause) forceps armed with cottonoids soaked in 4% cocaine is advanced (Fig. 10-17) over the lateral posterior curvature of the tongue (along the downward continuation of the tonsillar fossa). The tip of the forceps is advanced until it meets resistance (Fig. 10-18) and cannot be advanced any farther; at this point, the handle of the forceps should be in a horizontal position. The position of the tip of the forceps may be checked by palpating the neck lateral to the posterior-superior aspect of the thyroid cartilage. The forceps are kept in this position for at least 5 minutes, and the process is repeated on the opposite side.

4. Cautions, Complications, Contraindications

When performing the block from the external approaches, caution should be exercised in order not to insert

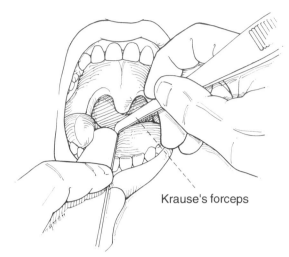

Figure 10-17 Superior laryngeal nerve block. External approach. Krause's forceps advanced over tongue toward pyriform sinus. (From University of California, Irvine, Department of Anesthesia, D.A. Teaching Aids.)

the needle into the thyroid cartilage because there is a possibility of injecting the solution at the level of the vocal cords, causing edema and airway obstruction. The carotid artery should be identified and displaced posteriorly to minimize the risk of intravascular injection; even small amounts of local anesthetics (0.25 to 0.5 mL) can induce seizures. On rare occasions (reported incidence of 2.7%), hypotension and bradycardia have been associated with SLN blocks. A number of possible causes of this reaction have been postulated: (1) apprehension and subsequent

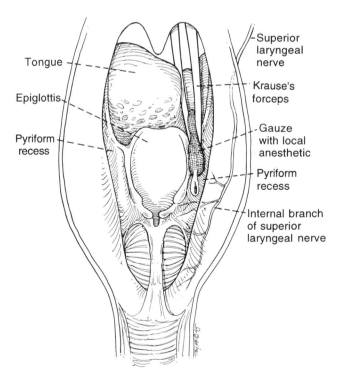

Figure 10-18 Superior laryngeal nerve block. External approach. Posterior view of the larynx showing tip of Krause's forceps at the level of the pyriform sinus. (From University of California, Irvine, Department of Anesthesia, D.A. Teaching Aids.)

vasovagal reaction related to painful stimulation, (2) digital pressure on the sensitive carotid sinus, (3) excessive manipulation of the larynx causing vasovagal reaction, (4) large doses of or accidental intravascular administration of local anesthetic drugs, and (5) direct neural stimulation of the branch of the vagus nerve by the needle. Therefore, it is recommended that anticholinergics be administered before the block is performed. The drying agent given before initiation of AI should suffice. Complications of the external approach also include hematoma (reported incidence of 1.4%), pharyngeal puncture, and rupture of the ET cuff in patients already intubated. Contraindications to the external approach are poor anatomic landmarks, local infections, local tumor growth, coagulopathy, and patients at risk for aspiration of gastric contents because of a depressed sensorium. The last is also a contraindication to the internal approach.

D. TRACHEA AND VOCAL CORDS*

1. Anatomy

The sensory innervation of the trachea and vocal cords is supplied by the vagus nerve through the recurrent laryngeal nerves (RLNs). The right RLN originates at the level of the right subclavian artery; the left originates at the level of the aortic arch (distal to the ligamentum arteriosum). Both ascend along the tracheoesophageal groove to supply sensory innervation to the tracheobronchial tree (up to and including the vocal cords) as well as supplying motor nerve fibers to the intrinsic muscles of the larynx (except the cricothyroid muscle). As both the sensory and motor fibers run together, nerve blocks cannot be performed because they would result in bilateral vocal cord paralysis and complete airway obstruction. The only alternative is topicalization of the mucosa. In addition to the use of nebulizers and atomizers to topicalize the trachea, there are three other techniques: translaryngeal anesthesia (transtracheal), "spray-as-you-go" technique through the FOB, and the Labat technique.

2. Translaryngeal (Transtracheal) Anesthesia: Positioning and Landmarks

The ideal position for translaryngeal anesthesia is the supine position with the neck hyperextended. In this position, the cervical vertebrae push the trachea and cricoid cartilage anteriorly and displace the strap muscles of the neck laterally. As a result, the cricoid cartilage and the structures above and below it are easier to palpate.

3. Translaryngeal (Transtracheal) Anesthesia: Technique

Using aseptic technique, a right hand–dominant person should stand on the left side of a supine patient. The patient

*See references 7, 11, 16, 22, 24, 40, 44, 45, 55, 67, 68, 70, 73, 75, 80, 84, 85, 100, 103, 110, 113, 117.

is asked not to talk, swallow, or cough until instructed. Using a tuberculin syringe, a small skin wheal is raised over the intended puncture site but not through the cricothyroid membrane (CTM). The left hand is then used to stabilize the trachea by placing the thumb and third digit on either side of the thyroid cartilage. The index finger of the left hand is used to identify the midline of the CTM and the upper border of the cricoid cartilage. The right hand then grasps the 20-gauge angiocatheter[7] and 10-mL syringe containing 4 to 5 mL of local anesthetic like a pencil; the fifth digit is used to brace the right hand on the patient's lower neck. The needle is aimed at a 45-degree angle (Fig. 10-19) in a caudad direction. As the needle passes through the CTM, resistance is felt, and at that point aspiration for air should be attempted to verify placement in the lumen of the airway. (The needle should not be advanced any further.) The sheath of the angiocatheter is advanced, the needle is removed and the syringe carefully reattached, and the aspiration test is again performed. The patient is asked to take a vital capacity breath, and at end of inspiration 4 mL of either 2% or 4% lidocaine is injected. We leave the sheath of the angiocatheter in place until the intubation is completed in case more local anesthetic is needed and to decrease the likelihood of subcutaneous emphysema (see Chapter 19). The coughing helps to nebulize the local anesthetic so that the inferior and superior surfaces of the vocal cords can be anesthetized.[81,86]

Whether the entry site is above or below the cricoid cartilage, a significant amount of local anesthetic bathes the tracheobronchial tree, false cords, true cords, epiglottis, vallecula, tongue, and posterior pharyngeal wall.[48] The success of translaryngeal anesthesia has been found to be as high as 95% and is attributed to both topicalization of the airway and systemic absorption.[17,23,48,53,85,108] After translaryngeal anesthesia using 5 mg/kg of a 10% lidocaine solution, therapeutic serum levels of lidocaine ($>1.4\ \mu g/mL$) were reached in a mean time of 5.1 minutes (±3.2 minutes).[17]

4. Translaryngeal (Transtracheal) Anesthesia: Cautions, Complications, Contraindications

The technique has been described using a 25-gauge needle, but we discourage this because of the possibility of breaking the needle as a result of the cricoid cartilage moving cephalad when the patient is coughing.[44] The tip of the needle should *not* be aimed in a cephalad direction because the tip of the angiocatheter sheath would then be advanced above the level of the vocal cords, resulting in local anesthetic above but not below the vocal cords. Coughing is a known factor in elevation of MAP, HR, ICP, and intraocular pressure (IOP). In a series of 186 AI patients using translaryngeal anesthesia, 34.8% coughed slightly, 47.5% coughed moderately severely, and 16.7% coughed severely (only 2 patients did not cough). The MAP and HR rose minimally during translaryngeal anesthesia; maximum increase in MAP (average 10 mm Hg

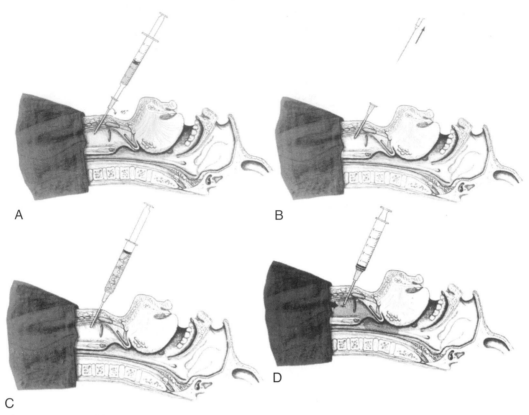

A B C D

Figure 10-19 A, Midsagittal view of the head and neck (translaryngeal anesthesia). Angiocatheter aimed at 45 degrees to the cricothyroid membrane. Aspiration test performed to verify position of tip of needle in tracheal lumen. **B,** Midsagittal view of the head and neck (translaryngeal anesthesia). Needle is removed from angiocatheter. **C,** Midsagittal view of the head and neck (translaryngeal anesthesia). Aspiration test repeated. **D,** Midsagittal view of the head and neck (translaryngeal anesthesia). Patient is asked to take a vital capacity breath and asked to cough. At end inspiration the local anesthetic is injected, resulting in coughing and nebulization of the local anesthetic *(stippled area)*. (From University of California, Irvine, Department of Anesthesia, The Retrograde Cookbook.)

above baseline) occurred during placement of the ET through the nares, and peak HR occurred as the ET entered the trachea.[73] In a study of 22 patients with brain tumors randomly assigned to either intravenous lidocaine or laryngotracheal lidocaine anesthesia, the laryngotracheal group showed higher ICP ("in excess of 40 torr") after laryngoscopy. Patients receiving laryngotracheal anesthesia, however, received the transtracheal lidocaine *after* laryngoscopy, suggesting that the elevation of ICP may have been due to laryngoscopy and not to the transtracheal administration of lidocaine. In another study, 20 patients (11 of whom had either cervical pathology or head and neck malignancy) were given translaryngeal anesthesia without undesirable side effects.[68]

Complications and contraindications are similar to those for retrograde intubation (see Chapter 19). Potential complications are bleeding (subcutaneous and intratracheal), infection, subcutaneous emphysema,[115] pneumomediastinum, pneumothorax, vocal cord damage, and esophageal perforation. These complications are rare, as illustrated by Gold and Buechael's study[44] of 17,500 cases of translaryngeal punctures with an incidence of complications of less than 0.01%.[44] Translaryngeal anesthesia is contraindicated in patients at risk for elevated ICP and

IOP; in those with severe cardiac disease, chronic cough, or unstable cervical fracture (unless adequate stabilization has been achieved); and in patients at risk for aspiration of gastric contents.

5. Spray as You Go[11,51,72,85]

In addition to using a nebulizer or an atomizer to anesthetize the vocal cords and trachea, a technique called *spray as you go* through the FOB can be performed. The technique is noninvasive and involves injecting local anesthetics through the suction port of the FOB. Two methods have been described. The *first* requires attaching a triple stopcock (Fig. 10-20) to the proximal portion of the suction port in order to connect oxygen tubing from a regulated oxygen tank set to flow at 2 to 4 L/min. Under direct vision through the bronchoscope, targeted areas are sprayed with aliquots of 0.2 to 1.0 mL of 2% to 4% lidocaine. The physician then waits 30 to 60 seconds before advancing to deeper structures and repeating the maneuver. The flow of oxygen allows higher F_{IO_2} delivery; keeps the FOB lens clean; disperses mucous secretions away from the lens, allowing a better view; and aids in nebulizing the local anesthetic. The *second* method involves

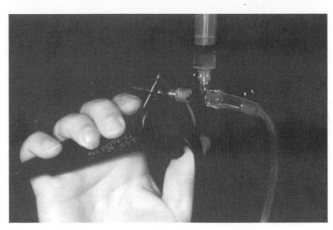

Figure 10-20 "Spray-as-you-go" technique. Oxygen hose and triple stopcock attached to the suction port of a fiberoptic bronchoscope with syringe attached containing local anesthetic; injected intermittently in aliquots of 0.2 to 1.0 mL. (From University of California, Irvine, Department of Anesthesia, D.A. Teaching Aids.)

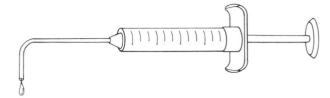

Figure 10-21 Labat needle for dripping local anesthetic over vocal cords. (From University of California, Irvine, Department of Anesthesia, D.A. Teaching Aids.)

passing a long angiographic or epidural catheter (internal diameter of 0.5 to 1.0 mm) through the suction port of an adult FOB. The catheter is cut short by 5 mm to prevent obstruction of the fiberoptic lens and allow more accurate placement of the local anesthetic (which flows as a stream instead of dribbling on the field). Shier[95] described a technique in which the successive placement of oral airways coated with viscous lidocaine is combined with the spray-as-you-go technique. The full time for successive intubation was 8 minutes. These techniques are especially useful in patients who are at risk for aspirating gastric contents because the topical anesthetic is applied only seconds before the intubation is accomplished and allows the patient to maintain his or her airway reflexes as long as possible.

6. Labat Technique[34,101,111]

The Labat technique is an antiquated method of anesthetizing the vocal cords and trachea. This technique requires a laryngeal mirror, a head lamp, and a Labat needle (Fig. 10-21). The patient is placed in the sitting position and asked to open the mouth wide. The tongue is pulled outward and an assistant is asked to hold the tongue with a gauze pad. In a right hand–dominant physician the left hand holds the laryngeal mirror over the oropharynx in order to identify the vocal cords. The right hand then holds the Labat needle and syringe (see Fig. 10-21) and drips local anesthetic (4 mL of 2% lidocaine) over the vocal cords. We use this technique only to illustrate to our residents that ear, nose, and throat

surgeons frequently make claim to an easy *direct* laryngoscopy because they were indeed able to visualize the vocal cords using the same method. This is misleading because it does not take into account the three-axis alignment required for direct laryngoscopy using a standard anesthesia laryngoscope.

VII. CONCLUSION

In the " Practice guidelines for management of the difficult airway: An updated report,"[79] if a DA is known or suspected, the anesthesiologist should inform the patient of the special risks and procedures pertaining to management of the DA and give consideration to the relative merits and feasibility of AI versus intubation after induction of general anesthesia. In our experience, we have only had one patient refuse an AI and would like to share this experience with the readers. The patient was a 22-year-old morbidly obese woman (BMI 42 kg/m^2) with a history of obstructive sleep apnea scheduled for an elective uvulopalatopharyngoplasty and tonsillectomy. On physical examination, she had a Mallampati III classification, "kissing tonsils," and a short thick neck in which the cricoid cartilage was located below the suprasternal notch. She refused an AI, saying "I would rather die." The surgeon was advised about the need for a chest cutter and sternal spreader for the emergency cricothyrotomy he would probably have to perform after induction of general anesthesia. The case was canceled by the surgeon. The patient's sister, seeing the logic of the strategy, convinced her to have an AI 3 days later, and we are all alive to tell the story.

ACKNOWLEDGMENTS

Dedicated to my wife, Vidya Iyer, whose unwavering support made this possible, and to parents, Lutgarda B. Sanchez and Andres Osvaldo Sanchez, M.D. With special thanks to Mrs. Debi Quilty, Mrs. Norma Claudio, and Elsie Vindiola for their research assistance and Tay McClellan for her outstanding medical illustrations.

REFERENCES

1. Adriani J, Campbell D: Fatalities following topical application of local anesthetic to the mucous membrane. JAMA 162:1527, 1956.
2. Adriani J, Zepernick R, Arens J, et al: The comparative potency and effectiveness of topical anesthetics in man. Clin Pharmacol Ther 5:49, 1964.
3. Aho M, Lehtinen AM, Erriola O, et al: The effect of intravenously administered dexmedetomidine on perioperative hemodynamics and isoflurane requirements in patients undergoing abdominal hysterectomy. Anesthesiology 74:997, 1991.

4. American Society of Anesthesiologists Task Force: Practice guidelines for management of the difficult airway. Anesthesiology 78:597, 1993.

5. Amitai Y, Zylber-Katz E, Avital A, et al: Serum lidocaine concentrations in children during bronchoscopy with topical anesthesia. Chest 98:1370, 1990.

6. Anderton JM, Nassar WY: Topical cocaine and general anesthesia: An investigation of the efficacy and side effects of cocaine on the nasal mucosa. Anaesthesia 30:809, 1975.

7. Barash PG, Cullen BF, Stoelting RK: Clinical Anesthesia. Philadelphia, Lippincott, 1989.

8. Bedder MD, Lindsay D: Glossopharyngeal nerve block using ultrasound guidance: A case report of a new technique. Reg Anesth 14:304, 1989.

9. Belleville JP, Ward DS, Bloor BC, Maze M: Effects of intravenous dexmedetomidine in humans: Sedation, ventilation, and metabolic rate. Anesthesiology 93:382, 2000.

10. Benumof JL, Scheller MS: The importance of transtracheal jet ventilation in the management of the difficult airway. Anesthesiology 71:769, 1989.

11. Benumof JL: Management of the difficult airway. Presented at the First International Symposium on the Difficult Airway, Newport Beach, Calif, Sept 16, 1993.

12. Benumof JL: Management of the difficult airway. Anesthesiology 75:1087, 1991.

13. Bertrand CA, Steiner NV, Jameson AG, et al: Disturbances of cardiac rhythm during anesthesia and surgery. JAMA 216:1615, 1971.

14. Bhavani-Shanker K, Mosely H, Kumar AY, et al: Capnometry and anesthesia. Can J Anaesth 39:617, 1992.

15. Block MR, Coulehan JL: Teaching the difficult interview in a required course on medical interviewing. J Med Educ 62:35, 1987.

16. Bonica JJ: Transtracheal anesthesia for endotracheal intubation. Anesthesiology 10:736, 1949.

17. Boster SR, Danzl DF, Madden RJ, et al: Translaryngeal absorption of lidocaine. Ann Emerg Med 11:461, 1982.

18. Boucek CD, Gunnerson HB, Tullock WC: Percutaneous transtracheal high-frequency jet ventilation as an aid to fiberoptic intubation. Anesthesiology 67:247, 1987.

19. Boudreaux AM: Simple technique for fiberoptic bronchoscopy. Am Soc Crit Care Anesthesiol 6(3):8, 1994.

20. Bourke DL, Katz J, Tonneson A: Nebulized anesthesia for awake endotracheal intubation. Anesthesiology 63:690, 1985.

21. Breytspraak LM, McGee J, Conger JC, et al: Sensitizing medical students to impression formation processes in the patient interview. J Med Educ 52:47, 1977.

22. Byron J, Bailey J: Head and Neck Surgery—Otolaryngology. Philadelphia, Lippincott, 1993.

23. Chu SS, Rah KH, Brannan MD, et al: Plasma concentration of lidocaine after endotracheal spray. Anesth Analg 54:438, 1975.

24. Clemente CD: Gray's Anatomy, 13th ed. Philadelphia, Lea & Febiger, 1985.

25. Conklin KA, Ziadlou-Rad F: Buffering capacity of citrate antacids. Anesthesiology 58:391, 1983.

26. Cooper M, Watson RL: An improved regional anesthetic technique for peroral endoscopy. Anesthesiology 43:372, 1975.

27. Coursin DB, Coursin DB, Maccioli GA: Dexmedetomidine. Curr Opin Crit Care 7:221, 2001.

28. Daos FG, Lopez L, Virtue RW: Local anesthetic toxicity modified by oxygen and by combination of the agents. Anesthesiology 23:755, 1962.

29. Demeester TR, Skinner DB, Evans RH, Benson DW: Local nerve block anesthesia for peroral endoscopy. Ann Thorac Surg 24:278, 1977.

30. Difficulties in tracheal intubation. In Latto IP, Rosen M (eds): Management of Difficult Intubation. London, Balliére Tindall, 1984, p 106.

31. Douglas WW, Fairbanks VF: Methemoglobinemia induced by a topical anesthetic spray (cetacaine). Chest 71:587, 1977.

32. Dundee JW, Haslett WHK: The benzodiazepines: A review of their actions and uses relative to anesthetic practice. Br J Anaesth 42:217, 1970.

33. Ebert TJ, Hall JE, Barney JA, et al: The effect of increasing plasma concentrations of dexmedetomidine in humans. Anesthesiology 93:382, 2000.

34. Egan TD, Lemmens HJM, Fiset P, et al: The pharmacokinetics of the new short-acting opioid remifentanil in healthy adult male volunteers. Anesthesiology 79:881, 1993.

35. Eriksson E: Illustrated Handbook in Local Anaesthesia. London, Lloyd Luke, 1979.

36. Evans BJ, Stanley RO, Burrows GD: Measuring medical students' empathy skills. Br J Med Psychol 66:121, 1993.

37. Eyler SW, Cullen BF, Murphy ME, et al: Antacid aspiration in rabbits: A comparison of Mylanta and Bicitra. Anesth Analg 61:288, 1982.

38. Farsad P, Galliguez P, Chamberlin R, et al: Teaching interviewing skills to pediatric house officers. Pediatrics 61:384, 1978.

39. Feldman M, Burton ME: Histamine receptor antagonists. N Engl J Med 323:1672, 1990.

40. Finucane TF, Santora HS: Principles of Airway Management. Philadelphia, Davis, 1988.

41. Foster WM, Hurewitz AN: Aerosolized lidocaine reduces dose of topical anesthetic for bronchoscopy. Am Rev Respir Dis 146:520, 1992.

42. Frerk CM: Predicting difficult intubation. Anaesthesia 56:1005, 1991.

43. Frumin MJ, Herekar VR, Jarvik ME: Amnestic actions of diazepam and scopolamine in man. Anesthesiology 45:406, 1976.

44. Gold MI, Buechael DR: Translaryngeal anesthesia: A review. Anesthesiology 20:181, 1959.

45. Gotta AW, Sullivan CA: Anaesthesia of the upper airway using topical anaesthetic and superior laryngeal nerve block. Br J Anaesth 53:1055, 1981.

46. Gotta AW, Sullivan CA: Superior laryngeal nerve block: An aid to intubating the patient with fractured mandible. J Trauma 24:83, 1984.

47. Gross JB, Hartigan ML, Schaffer DW: A suitable substitute for 4% cocaine before blind nasotracheal intubation: 3% lidocaine–0.25% phenylephrine nasal spray. Anesth Analg 63:915, 1984.

48. Hamill JF, Bedford RF, Weaver DC, Colohan AR: Lidocaine before endotracheal intubation: Intravenous or laryngotracheal? Anesthesiology 5:578, 1981.

49. Hast M: Otolaryngology. In English GM (ed): Anatomy of the Larynx, vol 3(14). Philadelphia, Harper & Row, 1987, p 46.

50. Hawkyard SJ, Morrison A, Doyle LA, et al: Attenuating the hypertensive response to laryngoscopy and endotracheal intubation using awake fibreoptic intubation. Acta Anaesthesiol Scand 36:1, 1992.

51. Hill AJ, Feneck RO, Underwood SM, et al: The hemodynamic effects of bronchoscopy: Comparison of propofol and thiopentone with and without alfentanil pretreatment. Anesthesia 46:266, 1991.

52. Hunt LA, Boyd GL: Superior laryngeal nerve block as a supplement to total intravenous anesthesia for rigid laser bronchoscopy in a patient with myasthenic syndrome. Anesth Analg 75:458, 1992.

53. Isaac PA, Barry JE, Vaughan RS, et al: A jet nebuliser for delivery of topical anesthesia to the respiratory tract. A comparison with cricothyroid puncture and direct spraying for fiberoptic bronchoscopy. Anaesthesia 45:46, 1990.

54. James CF, Modell JH, Gibbs CP, et al: Pulmonary aspiration effects of volume and pH in the rats. Anesth Analg 63:665, 1984.

55. Katz J: Atlas of Regional Anesthesia, 2nd ed. New York, Appleton & Lange, 1994.

56. Kazuhisa K, Norimasa S, Takanori M, et al: Glossopharyngeal nerve block for carotid sinus syndrome. Anesth Analg 75:1036, 1992.

57. Keller C, Brimacombe J: Resting esophageal sphincter pressures and deglutition frequency in awake subjects after oropharyngeal topical anesthesia and laryngeal mask device insertion. Anesth Analg 93:226, 2001.

58. Kern K, Langevin PB, Dunn BM: Methemoglobinemia after topical anesthesia with lidocaine and benzocaine for a difficult intubation. J Clin Anesth 12:167, 2000.

59. Kopman AF, Wollman SB, Ross K, et al: Awake endotracheal intubation: A review of 267 cases. Anesth Analg 54:323, 1975.

60. Kotler RL, Hansen-Flaschen J, Casey MP: Severe methemoglobinemia after flexible fibre optic bronchoscopy. Thorax 44:234, 1989.

61. Larijani GE, Cypel D, Gratz I, et al: The efficacy and safety of EMLA cream for awake fiberoptic endotracheal intubation. Anesth Analg 91:1024, 2000.

62. Latto IP: Awake intubation. Presented at the First International Symposium on the Difficult Airway, Newport Beach, Calif, Sept 16, 1993.

63. Le P, Ovassapian A, Benumof JL: Survey of university training programs: Residency training in airway management (unpublished data).

64. Macewend EM: Clinical observations on the introduction of tracheal tubes by the mouth instead of performing tracheostomy or laryngotomy. Br Med J July 24, 1880, p 122.

65. Mallampati SR, Gatt SP, Gugino LD, et al: A clinical sign to predict difficult tracheal intubation: A prospective study. Can J Anaesth 32:429, 1985.

66. Meschino A, Devitt JH, Koch P, et al: The safety of awake tracheal intubation in cervical spine injury. Can J Anaesth 39:114, 1992.

67. Miller DM: Anesthesia, 3rd ed. New York, Churchill Livingstone, 1990.

68. Mongan PD, Culling RD: Rapid oral anesthesia for awake intubation. J Clin Anesth 4:101, 1992.

69. Montero RF, Clark LD, Tolan MM, et al: The effects of small-dose ketamine on propofol sedation: Respiration, postoperative mood, perception, cognition, and pain. Anesth Analg 92:1465, 2001.

70. Murphy TM: Somatic blockade of head and neck. In Cousins MJ, Bridenbaugh PO (eds): Neural Blockade in Clinical Anaesthesia and Management of Pain, 2nd ed. Philadelphia, Lippincott, 1988, p 18.

71. Norton ML, Brown ACD: Atlas of the Difficult Airway. St. Louis, Mosby, 1991.

72. Ovassapian A: Fiberoptic Airway Endoscopy in Anesthesia and Critical Care. New York, Raven Press, 1990.

73. Ovassapian A, Krejcie TC, Yelich SJ, et al: Awake fibreoptic intubation in the patient at high risk of aspiration. Br J Anaesth 62:13, 1989.

74. Ovassapian A, Yelich SJ, Dykes MH, et al: Blood pressure and heart rate changes during awake fiberoptic nasotracheal intubation. Anesth Analg 62:951, 1983.

75. Paparella MM, Shumrick DA, Gluckman JL (eds): Otolaryngology. Philadelphia, WB Saunders, 1991.

76. Paul DR, Hoyt JL, Boutros AR: Cardiovascular and respiratory changes in response to change of posture in the very obese. Anesthesiology 45:73, 1976.

77. Perry LB: Topical anesthesia for bronchoscopy. Chest 73:691, 1978.

78. Platzer W: Atlas of Topographical Anatomy. Stuttgart, George Thieme Verlag, 1985.

79. Practice guidelines for management of the difficult airway: An updated report by the American Society of Anesthesiologists Task Force on Management of the Difficult Airway. Anesthesiology 98:1269, 2003.

80. Prakash UB: Bronchoscopy: A Text Atlas. New York, Raven Press, 1994.

81. Raj PP: Handbook of Regional Anesthesia. New York, Churchill Livingstone, 1985.

82. Ramsey M: Blood pressure monitoring: Automated oscillometric devices. J Clin Monit 7:56, 1991.

83. Ravussin P, Bayer-Berger M, Monnier P, et al: Percutaneous transtracheal ventilation for laser endoscopic procedures in infants and small children with laryngeal obstruction. Can J Anaesth 34:83, 1987.

84. Reed AF: Preparation for awake fiberoptic intubation. Presented at the ASA Refresher Course: Workshop on the Management of the Difficult Airway, Orlando, Fla, Nov 5, 1994.

85. Reed AF, Han DG: Preparation of the patient for awake intubation. Anesthesiol Clin North Am 9:69, 1991.

86. Reed AP: Preparation of the patient for awake flexible fiberoptic bronchoscopy. Chest 101:244, 1992.

87. Roberts JT: Anatomy and patient positioning for fiberoptic laryngoscopy. Anesthesiol Clin North Am 9:53, 1991.

88. Rosenberg PH, Heinonen J, Takasaki M: Lidocaine concentration in blood after topical anesthesia of the upper respiratory tract. Acta Anaesthesiol Scand 24:125, 1980.

89. Rovenstein EA, Papper EM: Glossopharyngeal nerve block. Am J Surg 75:713, 1948.

90. Sandza JG, Roberts RW, Shaw RC, Connors JP: Symptomatic methemoglobinemia with a commonly used topical anesthetic, cetacaine. Ann Thorac Surg 30:187, 1980.

91. Schenck NL: Local anesthesia in otolaryngology. Ann Otol Rhinol Laryngol 84:65, 1975.
92. Scher CS, Gitlin MC: Dexmedetomidine and low-dose ketamine provide adequate sedation for awake fiberoptic intubation. Can J Anaesth 50:607, 2003.
93. Shafer SL, Varvel JR: Pharmacokinetics, pharmacodynamics, and rational opioid selection. Anesthesiology 74:53, 1991.
94. Shibutani T, Hirota Y, Niwa H, et al: Cerebral arterial blood flow velocity during induction of general anesthesia: Rapid intravenous induction versus awake intubation. Anesth Prog 40:122, 1993.
95. Shier MEF: A simple technique for oral fiberoptic bronchoscopy. Anesth Analg 88:695, 1999.
96. Sidhu VS, Whitehead EM, Ainsworth QP, et al: A technique of awake fibreoptic intubation: Experience in patients with cervical spine disease. Anaesthesia 48:910, 1993.
97. Sinclair JR, Mason RA: Ankylosing spondylitis: The case for awake intubation. Anaesthesia 39:3, 1984.
98. Slogoff S, Keats AS, David Y, et al: Incidence of perioperative myocardial ischemia detected by different electrocardiographic systems. Anesthesiology 73:1074, 1990.
99. Smith RC: Teaching interviewing skills to medical students: The issue of "countertransference." J Med Educ 59:582, 1984.
100. Snell RS, Katz J: Clinical Anatomy for Anesthesiologists. New York, Appleton & Lange, 1989.
101. Snow JC: Anesthesia in Otolaryngology and Ophthalmology. London, Prentice-Hall International, 1982.
102. Sutherland AD, Williams RT: Cardiovascular responses and lidocaine absorption in fiberoptic-assisted awake intubation. Anesth Analg 65:389, 1986.
103. Talke P, Chen R, Thomas B, et al: The hemodynamic and adrenergic effects of perioperative dexmedetomidine infusion after vascular surgery. Anesth Analg 90:834, 2000.
104. Thomas JL: Awake intubation: Indications, techniques and a review of 25 patients. Anaesthesia 24:28, 1969.
105. Tornetta FJ: A comparison of droperidol, diazepam and hydroxyzine hydrochloride as premedication. Anesth Analg 56:496, 1977.
106. Tsueda K, Debrand M, Zeok SS, et al: Obesity supine death syndrome: Reports of two morbidly obese patients. Anesth Analg 58:4, 1979.
107. Van Dyke C, Barash PG, Jatlow P, et al: Cocaine: Plasma concentrations after intranasal application in man. Science 191:859, 1976.
108. Vaughan RW: Obesity: Implications in anesthetic management and toxicity. ASA Refresher Course in Anesthesiology, vol 9. Philadelphia, Lippincott, 1981.
109. Viegas O, Stoelting RK: Lidocaine in arterial blood after laryngotracheal administration. Anesthesiology 43:491, 1975.
110. Walts LF, Kassity KJ: Spread of local anesthesia after upper airway block. Arch Otolaryngol 81:77, 1965.
111. Weisel W, Tella RA: Reaction to tetracaine used as topical anesthetic in broncoscopy: A study of 1000 cases. JAMA 147:218, 1951.
112. White PF, Shafer A, Boyle WA, et al: Benzodiazepine antagonism does not provoke a stress response. Anesthesiology 70:636, 1989.
113. Wildsmith JAW, Armitage EN: Principles and Practices of Regional Anaesthesia. New York, Churchill Livingstone, 1987.
114. Wiles JR, Kelly J, Mostafa SM: Hypotension and bradycardia following superior laryngeal nerve block. Br J Anaesth 63:125, 1989.
115. Wong DT, McGuire GP: Subcutaneous emphysema following trans-cricothyroid membrane injection of local anesthetic. Can J Anaesth 47:165, 2000.
116. Yealy DM, Stewart RD, Kaplan RM: Myths and pitfalls in emergency translaryngeal ventilation: Correcting misimpressions. Ann Emerg Med 17:690, 1984.
117. Zupan J: Fiberoptic bronchoscopy in anesthesia and critical care. In Benumof JL (ed): Clinical Procedures in Anesthesia. Philadelphia, Lippincott, 1992.

SUGGESTED READINGS

Adriani J: Labat's Regional Anesthesia, 4th ed. St Louis, Warren HJ Green, 1985.

Benumof JL: Clinical considerations IV: Airway management. Annual Anesthesiology Refresher Course (UCSD), San Diego, Calif, May 19, 1989.

Efthimiou J, Higenbottam T, Holt D, Cochrane GM: Plasma concentration of lignocaine during fibre optic broncoscopy. Thorax 37:68, 1982.

McClure JM, Brown DT, Wildsmith JAW: Comparison of IV administration of midazolam and diazepam as sedation during spinal anesthesia. Br J Anaesth 55:1089, 1983.

Sanchez AS: The Retrograde Cookbook: First International Symposium on the Difficult Airway, Newport Beach, Calif, Sept 17, 1993.

Stoelting RK: Circulatory response to laryngoscopy and tracheal intubation with or without prior oropharyngeal viscous lidocaine. Anesth Analg 56:618, 1977.

11

ASPIRATION PREVENTION AND PROPHYLAXIS: PREOPERATIVE CONSIDERATIONS

Mark D. Tasch
Robert K. Stoelting

I. PERIOPERATIVE ASPIRATION

The pulmonary aspiration of gastric contents has generated a body of research and recrimination that might seem disproportionate to its reported incidence. Aspiration pneumonitis is an anesthetic complication whose consequences can be formidable but whose prevention would seem, at least in theory, to be readily attainable. Our desire to minimize risks led to rituals of fasting that have since been challenged, at least with respect to fluids. Any experience with aspiration and its dire sequelae may, however, inspire rigid adherence to conservative nil per os (NPO) standards and avid administration of prophylactic preoperative medications.

A. INCIDENCE

The statistical incidence of perioperative aspiration has been examined in long-term case reviews. Some authors have attempted to determine the incidence of silent aspiration, with or without clinical consequences. LoCicero[74] wrote that "between 16 and 27 percent of all anesthetized patients will have silent aspiration to some extent," often the result of either gastric inflation during ventilation by mask or intestinal manipulation during abdominal surgery. On the other hand, Hardy and colleagues[44] looked for gastroesophageal reflux (GER) by means of visual inspection of the pharynx and continuous measurement of upper esophageal pH and found no cases of GER during anesthetic induction in 100 patients.

A multicenter, prospective study of nearly 200,000 operations in France found the overall incidence of clinically apparent aspiration to be 1.4 per 10,000 anesthetics.[62] Leigh and Tytler's 5-year survey of nearly 110,000 anesthetics found six cases of aspiration requiring unplanned critical care.[71] Warner and colleagues,[161] retrospectively reviewing more than 215,000 general anesthetics, found an incidence of aspiration of 3.1 per 10,000 cases. Olsson and associates[103] examined the records of over 175,000 anesthetics administered at one hospital over 13 years and noted an incidence of aspiration of 4.7 per 10,000. Kallar and Everett's[62] multicenter survey of more than 500,000 outpatient anesthetics found the incidence of aspiration to be 1.7 per 10,000.

In their 1999 review of 133 Australian cases, Kluger and Short[68] reported that the incidence of passive regurgitation was three times that of active vomiting and that a majority of aspiration episodes accompanied anesthetics delivered by mask or by laryngeal mask airway (LMA). Thirty-eight percent of those who aspirated developed radiographic infiltrates, more often in the right lung than in the left. The authors also noted that "a recurring theme in many incidents was one of inadequate anaesthesia leading to coughing/straining and subsequent regurgitation/vomiting." In their 1999 survey of pediatric aspiration, Warner and coauthors[160] also wrote that "nearly all cases of pulmonary aspiration ... occurred in patients who gagged or coughed during airway manipulation or during induction of anesthesia."

Interestingly, several authors have noted that only about one half or fewer of the episodes of perioperative aspiration occur during anesthetic induction and intubation, perhaps because our concern is less heightened at other times.[62,68,71,90,103,153,161] These potentially catastrophic events also take place prior to induction (when the unguarded patient may be excessively sedated), during anesthetic maintenance, and during or after emergence and extubation.

B. CONSEQUENCES

When aspiration does occur, the subsequent clinical course can range from benign to fatal. Olsson and colleagues[103] reported that 18% of patients who aspirated perioperatively required mechanical ventilatory support and 5% died. All those who died were noted to have a poor preoperative physical status. Warner and coworkers[161] reported that 64% of patients did not manifest coughing, wheezing, radiographic abnormalities, or a 10% decrease in arterial oxygen saturation from preoperative room air values during the first 2 hours after aspiration. Such patients who remained asymptomatic for 2 hours developed no respiratory sequelae. Of the patients who did manifest signs or symptoms of pulmonary aspiration within 2 hours of the event, 54% required mechanical ventilatory support for at least 6 hours and 25% were ventilated for at least 24 hours. Unfortunately, half of those ventilated for at least 24 hours died, generating an overall mortality rate of under 5% of all aspirations.

Mortality rates resulting from perioperative pulmonary aspiration have ranged from less than 5% to greater than 80% in other reports.[22,27,50] In the studies of Warner[161] and Olsson[103] and their coworkers, there were no deaths in healthy patients undergoing elective surgery. Hickling and Howard[50] retrospectively studied patients in New Zealand who required mechanical ventilation for aspiration pneumonitis over a 5-year span. Of 38 such patients, 3 (8%) died of ventilatory failure or myocardial infarction. In their 1999 survey of 133 perioperative aspirations in Australia, Kluger and Short[68] wrote that "the deaths following aspiration events occurred in sicker patients ... although mortality can occur in healthy younger patients." Reviewing over 85,000 Scandinavian anesthetics, Mellin-Olsen and associates[90] noted that only 3 of 25 patients who aspirated developed serious morbidity, 2 of whom endured a prolonged course of illness but all of whom survived. In general, most healthy patients who aspirate only gastric fluid can expect to survive without residual respiratory impairment, albeit sometimes after a stormy postoperative course. Even in Mendelson's seminal report[91] of peripartum aspiration in 1946, the patients who were not promptly asphyxiated by solid material all survived, and "recovery was usually complete with an afebrile and uncomplicated course." On the other hand, as Gardner[33] wrote in 1958, "[a]spiration of vomit is ... often ... the *coup de grace* in an ill patient who might otherwise have a chance of survival."

C. RISK FACTORS

1. Demographic

Published surveys have determined some characteristics of patients or circumstances to be associated with cases of aspiration. Warner and colleagues[161] noted that the relative risk of aspiration was more than four times as high for emergency as for elective surgery. Higher American Society of Anesthesiologists (ASA) physical status classification was also associated with a higher risk of aspiration. The incidence of aspiration ranged from 1.1 per 10,000 elective anesthetics in ASA class I patients to 29.2 per 10,000 emergency anesthetics in ASA class IV and V patients. Contrary to conventional wisdom, "[a]ge, gender, pregnancy...concurrent administration of opioids, obesity...experience...of anesthesia provider, and types of surgical procedure were not independent risk factors for pulmonary aspiration .... The most common predisposing condition in all patients was gastrointestinal obstruction." Borland and coauthors[9] also wrote that "aspiration occurred significantly more often in patients with greater severity of underlying illness."

Olsson and colleagues[103] found that children and elderly persons were more likely than patients of intermediate ages to aspirate perioperatively. Statistically, the risk of aspiration was more than three times as high in emergency surgery as it was in elective operations. The incidence of aspiration was increased more than sixfold when surgery was performed at night rather than during daylight hours. In accordance with clinical intuition, the authors concluded that "[e]mergency cases anaesthetised in the middle of the night by an inexperienced anaesthetist constitute a high risk group for aspiration."[103] More recent studies[90,160] of both adult and pediatric cases have confirmed an impressively increased incidence of perioperative aspiration in emergency operations, but Borland and coauthors[9] found this increase to be only "marginally significant."

In Kallar and Everett's outpatient survey,[62] aspiration occurred most frequently in patients younger than 10 years. "In patients with no other identifiable risk factors, 67% of aspirations occurred after difficulties in airway management or intubation."[62] In the study of Olsson and colleagues[103] 15 of 83 aspirations were suffered by patients with no known risk factors. In 10 (67%) of these 15 cases, aspiration accompanied airway problems. In contrast to Kluger and Short's[68] findings, no patient aspirated while intubated.[103] Although regional techniques are often favored for the patient at increased risk for aspiration, elderly patients, in particular, have been reported to vomit and aspirate during subarachnoid anesthesia. Hypotension resulting from neuraxial sympathectomy can induce nausea and vomiting, and supplemental analgesics and sedatives given during lengthy operations can seriously obtund protective airway reflexes.[2,74,103]

Patients likely to have gastric contents of increased volume or acidity, elevated intragastric pressure, or decreased tone of the lower esophageal sphincter (LES) are traditionally considered to be at increased risk for perioperative pulmonary aspiration[22,44] (Boxes 11-1 and 11-2). As discussed later, pregnancy combines several of these likely risk factors. Although a lengthy NPO period before elective surgery is intended to minimize the volume of gastric contents, up to 90% of fasted patients have a gastric fluid pH less than 2.5.[27] Recent ethanol ingestion or hypoglycemic episodes stimulate gastric acid secretion,

---

Box 11-1 Risk Factors for Aspiration of Gastric Contents

Regurgitation or vomiting
  Hypotension in awake patient
  Opioids in awake patient
  Increased intragastric volume and pressure
  Decreased lower esophageal barrier pressure
Incompetent laryngeal protective reflexes
  Neurologic disease
  Neuromuscular disease
  Central nervous system depressants
  Advanced age or debility

Box 11-2 Factors That Increase Intragastric Volume and Pressure

Increased gastric filling
  Air inflation during mask ventilation
Increased gastric acid production
  Gastrin
  Histamine-2 receptor stimulation
  Recent ethanol ingestion
  Recent hypoglycemic episode
Decreased gastric emptying
  Intestinal obstruction
  Diabetic gastroparesis
  Opioids
  Anticholinergics
  Sympathetic stimulation (pain and anxiety)

---

and tobacco inhalation temporarily lowers LES tone. None of these effects are chronic.[27,44] LES tone has also been found to be reduced by gastric fluid acidity, caffeine, chocolate, and fatty foods.[27]

Surgical outpatients have traditionally been thought to arrive with gastric contents of expanded volume and reduced pH, possibly because of preoperative anxiety. Clinical studies, however, have not consistently confirmed this expectation.[62] Furthermore, Hardy and associates[44] contradicted several conventional notions by finding that neither gastric content volume nor pH correlated with preoperative anxiety, body mass index (BMI), ethanol or tobacco intake, or reflux history.

2. Obesity

Obese patients were traditionally thought to pose a relatively high risk for aspiration because of their greater gastric fluid volume and acidity, intragastric pressure, and incidence of GER.[47] This assumption has been challenged. In 1998, Harter and colleagues[47] studied 232 fasted, nondiabetic surgical patients who had received no relevant preoperative medication. Using conventional arbitrary criteria, they found that only 27% of obese patients, compared with 42% of the nonobese, had gastric contents of high volume and acidity. Grading obesity by BMI, they also found no association between degree of obesity and gastric fluid volume or pH.

The presumed sluggishness of gastric emptying in obese patients has also been denied. Verdich and coworkers[157] reported that obese and lean patients did not differ in their rates of gastric emptying in the first 3 hours after a test meal. Lower esophageal pressure has also been shown not to differ significantly between the obese and the nonobese.[47] On the other hand, the association between airway difficulties and aspiration episodes and the laryngoscopic challenges that arise with corpulence would appear to increase the risk of aspiration in these patients regardless of their gastrointestinal motility.

In a clinical review, Kadar and colleagues[61] reported their experiences with 50 obese patients who were administered a total of 660 electroconvulsive therapy (ECT) sessions without benefit of endotracheal intubation or pharmacologic aspiration prophylaxis. There were no cases of aspiration. This series included nine morbidly obese patients who received 97 ECT sessions.

3. Systemic Diseases

Patients with connective tissue, neurologic, metabolic, or neuromuscular diseases may be imperiled by esophageal dysfunction or laryngeal incompetence. Progressive systemic sclerosis and myotonia dystrophica have been specifically mentioned in case reports.[41,117,123] Hardoff and coworkers[42] found that "gastric emptying time in patients with Parkinson's disease was delayed compared with control volunteers ... [and] was even slower in patients treated with levodopa." Advanced age may be associated with attenuated cough or gag reflexes.

Long-standing diabetes mellitus is commonly considered to delay gastric emptying and may also compromise LES function.[122] Several authors have noted a high incidence of gastroparesis and prolonged mean gastric emptying times, at least for solid foods, when diabetic patients are compared with control subjects.[13,57,92,151] Impairment of gastric motility was usually found to correlate with findings of autonomic neuropathy but not with peripheral neuropathy or with indices of glycemic stability.

4. Pregnancy

Pregnancy imposes a constellation of potential risk factors. The enlarging uterus increases intragastric pressure by compressing the stomach, physically delays gastric emptying by pushing the pylorus cephalad and posteriorly, and promotes GER by altering the angle of the gastroesophageal junction. Progesterone decreases the tone of the LES, and excess gastrin, produced by the placenta, promotes gastric acid secretion.[32,54,122] The alterations in physique typical of late pregnancy can interfere with laryngoscopy and endotracheal intubation. Laryngeal and upper airway edema is also common in the parturient and can be exaggerated by preeclampsia.[95]

Studies of gastric emptying in pregnancy have produced somewhat inconsistent results. Wong and colleagues[163] found that water was readily cleared from the stomachs of nonobese, nonlaboring parturients at term and wrote that "recent studies of gastric emptying in nonlaboring term women ... suggest that gastric emptying is not delayed during pregnancy." Chiloiro and coworkers[16] found that gastric emptying time did not become slower with the progress of gestation but that total orocecal transit time did. A commoner clinical concern is the parturient in labor. Scrutton and associates[130] reported that laboring patients consuming a light solid meal had significantly greater gastric volumes than those allowed only water. Although pain, in any circumstance, is thought to delay gastric emptying, Porter and coauthors[110] stated that "pain does not appear to be the sole cause of gastric slowing in late labour since [there was] a similar delay in women in late labour who had received either epidural local anesthetic alone or no analgesia."

5. Pain and Analgesics

Pain and its treatment are considered risk factors for aspiration, notably in patients presenting with trauma. As noted by Crighton and colleagues,[24] "circulating catecholamines have an inhibitory effect on gastric emptying, and noradrenaline release in response to painful stimuli may cause inhibition of gastric tone and emptying." Reviews of pediatric emergency surgery found that the volume of gastric contents correlated with the severity of injury.[141] Carlin and associates[14] determined that gastric motility was significantly impaired for at least a week following trauma. Patients with either spinal cord or brain injuries have also been shown to manifest delayed gastric emptying of both liquid and solid contents.[63,64,75]

Administering opioids to alleviate pain is an essential act of kindness but may further impair gastrointestinal function. Opioid receptors can be found throughout the gastrointestinal tract; both human and animal studies suggest that there are both central and peripheral mechanisms by which these drugs retard gastric emptying.[98] Even modest intravenous doses of morphine demonstrably prolong gastric transit times in clinical studies.[24,40,97,166] On the other hand, tramadol, a parenteral analgesic with actions at opioid, noradrenergic, and serotonergic sites, appears to have little or no effect on gastrointestinal motility.[24,97]

Neuraxial opioids can also prolong gastric emptying. Guha and coauthors[38] reported that, in patients receiving thoracic epidural fentanyl and bupivacaine for postthoracotomy analgesia, gastric emptying was slower postoperatively than preoperatively. In this study, however, there was no control group of thoracotomy patients not given epidural analgesia, presumably for humanitarian reasons. In obstetric anesthesia, Kelly and associates[65] "conclude[d] that the administration of fentanyl 25 μg intrathecally delays gastric emptying in labor compared with both extradural fentanyl 50 μg with bupivacaine and extradural bupivacaine alone." Older reports indicated that epidural fentanyl boluses of 50 or 100 μg would retard gastric emptying. On the other hand, the addition of fentanyl (2 or 2.5 μg/mL) to dilute bupivacaine for epidural infusion during labor was not found to affect gastric motility.[110,167]

6. Positioning

Agnew and colleagues[1] continuously monitored esophageal and tracheal pH in thoracotomy patients "considered to be at low risk of GER." Twenty-eight percent of their patients not treated with an H_2-receptor antagonist were found to have acid reflux into the esophagus while in the lateral decubitus position, and nearly 8% had acid in the trachea. Although the authors did not correlate clinical outcomes with their findings, they did advise that patients undergoing thoracotomy be considered for routine preoperative aspiration chemoprophylaxis.

D. PATHOPHYSIOLOGY

When gastric contents enter the lungs, the resultant pulmonary pathology depends on the nature of the material aspirated (Box 11-3). Food particles small enough to enter the distal airways induce a foreign body reaction of inflammation and eventual granuloma formation. The aspiration of particulate antacids produces the same adverse response.[54,67] Acid aspiration induces an inflammatory response that begins within minutes and progresses over 24 to 36 hours.[25,67] In 1940, Irons and Apfelbach[56] wrote that the "characteristic microscopic changes are intense engorgement of the alveolar capillaries, … edema, and hemorrhage into the alveolar spaces …. Another outstanding characteristic is the extensive desquamation of the lining of the bronchial tree." Subsequent authors have also described hemorrhagic pulmonary edema, intense inflammation, and derangement of the pulmonary epithelium.[25,156] The membranous epithelial cells that produce surfactant are damaged or destroyed by the acid, to be replaced by granular epithelial cells.[74] As surfactant production fails, lung units progressively collapse. Fibrin and plasma leak from the capillaries into the pulmonary interstitium and alveoli, producing the noncardiogenic pulmonary edema often referred to as the adult or acute respiratory distress syndrome (ARDS).[25,74,108,137] Although most researchers have found that localized acid exposure leads to localized pathology, one animal study demonstrated that localized aspiration produced generalized pulmonary inflammation, presumably related to "inflammatory mediators" acting at sites distant from the original insult.[50] With effective supportive care, the acute inflammation can diminish, and epithelial regeneration begin, within 72 hours.

The clinical features of aspiration pneumonitis have been well described for over 6 decades. Even earlier, in 1887, Becker referred to bronchopneumonia as a postoperative complication related to the inhalation of gastric contents.[56] Hall, in 1940, published the first description of gastric fluid inhalation in obstetric patients. He distinguished between the aspiration of solid material, which could quickly kill by suffocation, and the aspiration syndrome produced by gastric fluid, for which he coined the term "chemical pneumonitis."[39] Mendelson,[91] in 1946, described the clinical features of 66 cases of peripartum aspiration observed from 1932 to 1945. Solid food produced airway obstruction, which was quickly fatal in two instances. Otherwise, wheezing, rales, rhonchi, tachypnea, and tachycardia were prominent. (Subsequent reports have not found wheezing to be so universal a manifestation, occurring in about one third of aspirations.) When present, wheezing is thought to result from bronchial mucosal edema and from a reflex response to acidic airway irritation.[25,27,53]

Refractory hypoxemia can ensue almost immediately as bronchospasm, airway edema or obstruction, and alveolar collapse or flooding increase the effective intrapulmonary shunt fraction (Box 11-4). The awake patient may experience intense dyspnea and cough up the pink, frothy sputum characteristic of pulmonary edema.[25,27,54] On the other hand, more modest aspirations may not become clinically evident for several hours.[35,54,134]

Hemodynamic derangements can also demand therapeutic attention. As the alveolar-capillary membrane loses its integrity, plasma leaks out of the pulmonary vasculature. If the leak becomes a flood, the loss of circulating fluid volume can produce hemoconcentration, hypotension, tachycardia, and even shock.[27,54] Pulmonary vasospasm may also contribute to right ventricular dysfunction.[27]

The radiographic evidence of pulmonary aspiration may become evident promptly, if aspiration is massive, or only after a delay of several hours. There is no pattern on the chest roentgenogram that is specific for aspiration. The distribution of infiltrates depends on the volume of material inhaled and on the patient's position at the time

---

Box 11-3 Pathophysiology of Aspiration

Particulate aspiration
   Airway obstruction
   Granulomatous inflammation
Acid aspiration
   Neutrophilic inflammation
   Hemorrhagic pulmonary edema
   Destruction of airway epithelium
   Loss of type I alveolar cells
   Loss of surfactant
      Alveolar instability and collapse
Disruption of alveolar-capillary membrane
Plasma leakage from pulmonary capillaries
   Noncardiogenic pulmonary edema
   Hypovolemia

Box 11-4 Aspiration and Hypoxemia

Upper airway obstruction
Increased lower airway resistance
   Obstruction by airway debris
   Airway edema
   Reflex bronchospasm
Alveolar collapse and flooding

of the event. Because of bronchial anatomy, aspiration occurring in the supine patient affects the right lower lobe most commonly, the left upper lobe least often.[27,54] If pulmonary aspiration is not complicated by secondary events, improvement in symptoms can be anticipated within 24 hours, but the radiographic picture may continue to worsen for another day.[54]

E. DETERMINANTS OF MORBIDITY

1. pH and Volume of Aspirate

In his 1946 report, Mendelson[91] also undertook to determine the relationship between gastric fluid acidity and pulmonary morbidity. When Mendelson instilled liquid containing hydrochloric acid (HCl) into rabbits' tracheas, the animals developed a syndrome "similar in many respects to that observed in the human following liquid aspiration," with cyanosis, dyspnea, and pink frothy sputum. On the other hand, when neutral liquid was instilled into their tracheas, the rabbits endured a brief symptomatic period, "but within a few hours they [were] apparently back to normal, able to carry on rabbit activities uninhibited."[91] (Mendelson maintained a discreet silence about the nature of these uninhibited rabbit activities.)

Since Mendelson's report, numerous attempts (and assumptions) have been made to define the "critical" volume and pH of gastric contents required to inflict significant damage on the lungs. Such neatly defined threshold values may be illusory objects of desire rather than features of clinical reality. Nonetheless, almost all researchers in the field of aspiration pneumonitis have made some use of such critical values to define the success or failure of drug therapies in the modification of gastric contents.

In 1952, Teabeaut[146] injected HCl solutions of different volumes and acidities into rabbits' tracheas. He found that solutions with a pH greater than 2.4 caused a relatively benign tissue response similar to that induced by the intratracheal injection of water. As the pH of the injectate was reduced from 2.4 to 1.5, a progressively more severe tissue reaction was elicited. At pH 1.5, the damage was maximal and equal to that found at lower pH values. From this study stemmed the popular concept of the pH value of 2.5 as a threshold for chemical pneumonitis. Other authors have advocated a higher standard, a pH of 3.5, for defining hazardous gastric content acidity. However, arguments for a "critical pH" value higher than 2.5 are generally based on case reports of severe pneumonitis caused by the aspiration of particulate gastric contents at higher pH values.[120]

The determination of a "critical volume" of gastric contents required to produce severe aspiration pneumonitis has been even more contentious than that of a critical pH. Two teams of investigators each found that, in dogs, pulmonary injury became independent of pH as the volume of aspirate was increased from 0.5 to 4.0 mL/kg.[27]

A preliminary experiment by Roberts and Shirley, involving gastric fluid instillation into the right main stem bronchus of a single monkey, long ago led to the acceptance, in some quarters, of 0.4 mL/kg as the volume of gastric fluid that placed the subject at risk for developing aspiration pneumonitis.[113,118,119] Subsequent researchers challenged this number. James and colleagues[59] demonstrated that aspirate volumes as low as 0.2 mL/kg could induce pulmonary injury if the aspirate pH was reduced to 1.09. On the other hand, Raidoo and coworkers,[113] also studying monkeys, found that the aspiration of 0.4 or 0.6 mL/kg of fluid with a pH of 1.0 produced mild or moderate pulmonary injury, and 0.8 or 1.0 mL/kg at pH 1.0 produced severe pneumonitis, with a 50% mortality rate (three of six) at 1.0 mL/kg. Clearly, the volume of aspirate that is considered hazardous depends on how much morbidity or pathology must be produced to be considered significant. Arguments have also been made concerning the experimental instillation of gastric fluid into one lung versus both lungs as well as the reliability of gastric fluid volume measurements. In addition, even if a critical volume for aspiration pneumonitis could be reliably determined, it cannot be known how much fluid must be present in the stomach in order to deposit this critical volume into the lung or lungs.[36,113] However, studies of therapeutic interventions must have criteria for defining success or failure, and threshold values for gastric fluid volume and pH will doubtless continue to be used, regardless of their validity.

2. Particulate Matter

Volume and acidity are not, of course, the only determinants of sequelae when gastric contents enter the lungs. Since the report of Bond and coworkers[8] in 1979, it has been appreciated that gastric fluid containing particulate antacids can produce severe aspiration pneumonitis, even at near-neutral pH, with wheezing, pulmonary edema, and hypoxemia requiring mechanical ventilatory support. Animal studies confirmed that nonparticulate gastric acid and particulate antacid solutions have similar potentials for pulmonary mischief if aspirated.[35] Although blood and digestive enzymes do not appear to induce chemical pneumonitis, feculent gastric contents with a high bacterial density readily produce pneumonitis and death in animals. (Acidic gastric contents are normally sterile.) Another study demonstrated that the mucus present in the gastric fluid of dogs with intestinal obstruction produced diffuse small airway obstruction and pulmonary injury when aspirated.[27]

II. PREVENTION OF ASPIRATION

The clinical challenges of perioperative pulmonary aspiration are prevention, prophylaxis, and treatment. Ideally, gastric contents can be physically prevented from entering the lungs in the first place. Should prevention fail, pharmacologic prophylaxis may modify the volume and character of gastric contents so that they inflict minimal damage on the lungs. Least desirably, aspiration pneumonitis can require intensive medical treatment and ventilatory support.

The nonpharmacologic means of keeping gastric contents out of the lungs are preoperative fasting, gastric decompression, and optimal airway management.

A. PREOPERATIVE FASTING

The commonest means of keeping gastric contents out of the lungs is to minimize the volume of such contents by way of preoperative fasting. In recent years, both the utility and the necessity of adhering to traditional NPO regimens for clear liquids have been challenged. As noted by Sethi and coauthors,[132] "the stomach can never be completely empty even after a midnight fast since it continues to secrete gastric juices." The issue has been studied in both pediatric and adult surgical patients and has become particularly contentious and emotional regarding obstetric anesthesia.

1. Pediatric

Conventional preoperative fasting can impose physical and emotional discomfort on children and their parents and may be difficult to enforce reliably in outpatients. Dehydration in infants and hypoglycemia in neonates may also result from prolonged NPO times.[22,62] The normal stomach can empty 80% of a clear liquid load within an hour of ingestion. While the stomach continues to secrete and reabsorb fluid throughout NPO time, ingested clear liquids are completely passed into the duodenum within 2.25 hours.[126] Several researchers have therefore sought to demonstrate that children may safely be allowed to drink clear liquids until just 2 to 3 hours before elective surgery.

Van der Walt and Carter[152] and other groups determined that healthy infants could drink limited volumes of clear liquids 3 to 4 hours before surgery with no effect on gastric content volumes. Splinter and colleagues[140] found that healthy infants could drink clear liquids ad libitum until 2 hours before anesthetic induction without altering gastric fluid volume or pH. (Gastric fluid pH was quite variable, and mean pH was less than 2.5 in all groups of patients studied, regardless of NPO time.) On the other hand, milk or formula intake on the morning of surgery (4 to 6 hours before induction) was associated with the presence of curds in many of the gastric aspirates. This was considered to represent an unacceptable risk of particulate aspiration. The authors thus concurred with previous recommendations that infants not be allowed milk or formula the morning of surgery.[140]

More recently, Cook-Sather and associates[21] studied 97 healthy infants undergoing elective surgery and found that gastric fluid volume was not increased when the fasting time for formula was reduced from 8 hours to either 6 or 4 hours. In their review of relevant studies, Splinter and Schreiner[141] concluded that the gastric emptying of breast milk is generally more rapid than that of commercial formulas but that both require more than 2 hours.

Schreiner and colleagues[128] compared the gastric contents of children subjected to conventional preoperative fasting (mean NPO time, 13.5 hours) with those of children permitted clear liquids until 2 hours before anesthetic induction (mean NPO time, 2.6 hours). Gastric fluid volumes actually tended to be somewhat smaller in the children allowed to drink clear liquids up to 2 hours preoperatively, and almost all children in both groups had gastric content pH values less than or equal to 2.5. Sandhar and coauthors,[126] studying children 1 to 14 years of age, also found that clear liquid ingestion 2 to 3 hours preoperatively did not significantly increase the mean volume of gastric contents and did not increase the number of patients with gastric contents more voluminous than 0.4 mL/kg. Reports by Splinter and Schaefer[139] and Moyao-Garcia,[96] Maekawa,[78] Ingebo,[55] and Gombar[34] and their colleagues all concluded that permitting children to drink nonparticulate fluids 2 or 3 hours before surgery had either no effect or even a small beneficial influence on the quantity and acidity of their gastric contents.

Clear liquids, alone, thus appear to pose no demonstrable hazard if taken at least 2 hours before anesthesia by children without gastrointestinal pathology. However, solid or semisolid foods are not cleared from the stomach as rapidly as clear liquids. Meakin and associates[88] found that a light breakfast of biscuits or orange juice with pulp, taken 2 to 4 hours before induction, did increase the volume of gastric aspirate in healthy children compared with those who had fasted for at least 4 hours. In all fasted children, and in almost all of those fed, the gastric content pH was less than or equal to 2.5. Hyperosmolar glucose solutions are also associated with delayed gastric emptying.[126]

In 1999, the ASA issued the report of its Task Force on Preoperative Fasting, which included practice guidelines. These guidelines were intended to apply to healthy patients, with no known relevant risk factors or injuries, scheduled for elective surgery. Noting these limitations, the ASA Task Force "support[ed] a fasting period for clear liquids of two hours for all patients ... [and] a fasting period for breast milk of four hours for both neonates and infants" while considering it "appropriate to fast from intake of infant formula for six or more hours."[111]

2. Adult

In adult surgical patients, too, considerable evidence demonstrates that clear liquid intake within 2 to 3 hours of anesthetic induction does not increase the risk of gastric acid aspiration. It is important to note that these studies typically involve healthy, nonpregnant, nonobese patients, free of known gastrointestinal pathology, not receiving opioids or other medications known to interfere with gastric emptying, undergoing elective surgery. The results of such studies cannot, therefore, be reliably applied to any groups of patients thus excluded.[73,93,109,144]

With adults, as with children, the basic arguments favoring relaxed NPO regimens for clear liquids involve their normally rapid gastric clearance. Over 90% of a 750-mL bolus of isotonic saline was found to pass from the normal stomach within 30 minutes.[81] Nygren and coauthors[100] reported that a 50-g liquid carbohydrate bolus is completely cleared from the stomach within 90 minutes. After 2 hours of fasting, the fluid in the stomach primarily represents the acid secreted by the stomach itself. Exogenous clear liquids thus tend to dilute endogenous gastric acid and may even accelerate gastric emptying.[36,109,128] Solids, lipids, and hyperosmotic liquids are thought to delay gastric emptying, and their intake would thus be considered ill advised prior to anesthetic induction.[36]

Several researchers have sought to correlate these theoretical considerations with clinical situations. Maltby and colleagues[81] studied outpatients who were either kept NPO from the previous midnight or given 150 mL of water 2.5 hours before anesthetic induction. Although the mean gastric pH did not differ significantly between the two groups, the mean gastric volume was significantly less in the patients who drank than in those who fasted. Read and Vaughan[116] similarly found that permitting patients to drink water ad libitum until 2 hours before surgery had no impact on gastric volume or pH but did decrease preanesthetic anxiety. Many patients had gastric pH values no greater than 2.5, regardless of the time elapsed since fluid intake.

Lewis and associates[72] divided healthy adult surgical inpatients into three groups, with NPO times for clear liquids being at least 3, 5, or more than 8 hours. (Clear liquids included Jell-O and black coffee or tea.) Neither gastric pH nor gastric volume differed significantly among these groups, but both values varied widely within each group. Phillips and colleagues[109] also determined that patients allowed to drink clear liquids until 2 hours preoperatively had gastric volume and pH values similar to those of patients fasted for 6 hours. Other studies have also confirmed that the ingestion of 150 mL of (pulp-free) orange juice, coffee, tea, or apple juice 2 to 3 hours before surgery has no detrimental effect on gastric pH or volume in surgical outpatients.[109] (Since the publication of these reports, one can only wonder how many hours of presurgical time have been consumed in contemplating the pulp content of orange juice that patients have admitted to consuming.)

The safety of clear liquid ingestion before surgery does not, of course, imply that solid food may also be taken with impunity. In an early study, Miller and coworkers[93] compared 22 adults kept NPO overnight before surgery with 23 adults permitted a light breakfast (one slice of buttered toast and tea or coffee with milk) the morning of surgery (mean NPO time, 3.8 hours). The two groups were found not to differ significantly in the mean volume or median pH of their gastric contents or in the percentage of patients with a gastric pH less than 3.0. Interestingly, in the subgroup of patients who were not given opioid premedication, seven of eight "fed" patients had a gastric pH less than 3.0 (median pH, 1.9), whereas only two of five fasted patients had a gastric pH less than 3.0 (median pH, 6.3). In addition, the authors remarked that "[i]t is likely that any large pieces of toast in the stomach would not be aspirated by the tube we used. Thus, the results of the study apply only to liquid in the stomach."[93] Soreide and coauthors[138] reported that the particulate elements of a light breakfast did not completely exit the stomach in less than 4 hours. Reflecting a consensus of clinical comfort, the aforementioned ASA task force recommended a 6-hour preoperative fast following a "light meal" and a fast of 8 hours or longer "for a meal that included fried or fatty foods or meat."[111]

3. Pregnant

As preoperative NPO standards became more relaxed, strenuous debate arose over the necessity of adhering to conventional NPO regimens for patients in labor. Obstetricians, nurse-midwifes, and psychologists joined the fray. On the one hand, anesthesiologists have long recognized that advanced gestation increases the risk of gastric content aspiration. On the other hand, proponents of liberalizing oral intake for parturients cited the infrequency of aspiration pneumonitis in modern practice, the futility of fasting in ensuring an empty stomach, and detrimental effects of fasting on maternal and fetal well-being. The fashionable battle cry of "patient autonomy" was also heard.

Elkington[29] cited a Washington state survey (1977 to 1981) in which none of 36 maternal deaths resulted from anesthetic complications and a North Carolina survey (1981 to 1985) in which only 1 of 40 maternal deaths resulted from aspiration. He did not advocate uninhibited feeding of patients in labor, however, but recommended that "[f]or otherwise uncomplicated parturients, a nonparticulate diet should be allowed as desired."

Ludka and Roberts[76] referred to a Michigan survey (1972 to 1984) showing that only 1 of 15 maternal deaths (0.82 per 100,000 live births) resulted from the aspiration of gastric contents, that no deaths were related to regional anesthesia, and that "failure to secure a patent airway was the primary cause of anesthesia-related maternal deaths." They cited other studies indicating that women who ate during labor were less ketotic, required less analgesic medication and oxytocin, and had more active fetuses and neonates with higher Apgar scores than women who fasted during labor. They also "found that laboring women self-regulated intake. Once active labor began, women usually preferred liquids."[76]

Regarding the inevitability of a full stomach in the parturient, Kallar and Everett[62] referred to an ultrasound study in which nearly two thirds of patients in labor had solid food in the stomach, regardless of how long they had fasted. Elkington[29] cited a report that about one fourth of parturients were "at risk" of aspiration pneumonitis, regardless of the duration of fasting, and that prolonged fasting was actually associated with increased gastric fluid volume at a lower pH. Broach and Newton[11] contended that "[a]dministration of narcotics, not labor itself, appears to be the major factor in delaying stomach emptying."

McKay and Mahan[87] wrote that "[a]mong many factors that can be linked to the occurrence of aspiration, the most important appears to be faulty administration of obstetric anesthesia." The authors further questioned "whether parturients should be kept … on restricted liquid intake to protect them from what appears to be the basic problem: inadequate anesthesia practices."[87] The apparent implication was that the parturient should eat, drink, and be merry, for if she should aspirate, only poor anesthetic care would be to blame.

On the other hand, Chestnut and Cohen[15] cited the Report on Confidential Enquiries into Maternal Deaths in England and Wales 1982-1984, which found that 7 of 19 anesthesia-associated maternal deaths resulted from the aspiration of gastric contents into the lungs, and an ASA review of closed malpractice claims in which "maternal aspiration was the primary reason for 8% of all claims against anesthesiologists for obstetric cases." The authors argued that "[t]hese data hardly suggest that the risk of maternal aspiration is remote"[15]

In his reply to McKay and Mahan, Crawford[23] noted that "[m]ost of the deaths from aspiration prior to the mid-1950s … were due to asphyxia, caused by respiratory obstruction with solid or semisolid material—since that time, with introduction of a firm dietary regimen for labor, only 2 of the 146 deaths noted have been in that category." Furthermore, he contended, "There is inevitably an incidence of cesarean section and of general anesthesia in every obstetric population … In an obstetric population the incidence of failed or difficult intubation is roughly one in 300."[23]

In the work of Scrutton and colleagues,[130] permitting parturients a "light diet" (as opposed to water only) had no effect on the course of labor or the neonatal Apgar scores but did increase the volume of gastric contents and of vomitus. They stated that "the presence of undigested food particles in the vomitus is probably of greater importance [than low pH] as a cause of mortality … [and] would not support the policy of encouraging women to eat any solid food once in labour particularly when isotonic drinks appear to offer an adequate calorific alternative."[130] In their review, Ng and Smith[99] concluded that "there is insufficient evidence to clarify changes in

risk in the first 24 hours of the postpartum period, when operative procedures are common."

Obviously, the pregnant patient with a difficult airway cannot always be avoided, nor can general anesthesia for cesarean section, no matter how aggressively regional analgesia is promoted. Regardless of gastric fluid volume or acidity, the presence of solid food imparts the immediate hazard of asphyxiation. Mendelson warned that "[m]isinformed friends and relatives often urge the patient to ingest a heavy meal early in labor before going to the hospital."[91] Crawford[23] concluded that "[g]rafting good anesthetic technique upon poor preparation of a patient for anesthesia is unjustifiable—there is an essential symbiosis between the two if safety is to be ensured."

B. PREINDUCTION GASTRIC EMPTYING

When a patient at increased risk for aspiration presents for surgery, the stomach can be emptied, at least in part, by an orogastric or a nasogastric (NG) tube. Many patients, of course, already have said tube placed for gastric decompression, particularly if intestinal obstruction has been diagnosed. In such cases, the anesthesiologist must decide whether to remove the gastric tube prior to induction. On the other hand, if gastric decompression has not been attempted, the anesthesiologist may wish to do so while the patient's protective airway reflexes remain intact.

It has long been argued that the presence of a gastric tube interferes with the sphincter function of the gastroesophageal junction and promotes GER by acting as a "wick."[143] The presence of a foreign body in the pharynx could also interfere with laryngoscopy. These considerations would favor removal of the gastric tube before induction. However, in an early study by Satiani and colleagues,[127] the incidence of "silent" GER was found to be 12% in anesthetized patients without an NG tube versus 6% in patients with an NG tube in place (a statistically insignificant difference). Hardy[43] wrote that "[a] nasogastric tube need not be withdrawn before induction of anesthesia. The tube can act as an overflow valve" and provide "a venting mechanism whereby pressure cannot build up in the stomach."

Dotson and associates[28] prospectively studied the effect of NG tube size on GER in normal subjects. Attempts were made to provoke GER with a device that elevated abdominal pressure stepwise to 100 mm Hg. In this report, GER "was not detected at any level of abdominal pressure regardless of the presence or size of a nasogastric tube."[28] Salem and colleagues[125] had previously demonstrated that "cricoid pressure is effective in sealing the esophagus around an esophageal tube against an intraesophageal pressure up to 100 cm H_2O." The authors also advocated the utility of an NG tube as a "blow-off valve" for increased intragastric pressure during induction. The presence of an NG tube, while allowing gastric decompression, may also hold open the LES.[27,66]

Manning and coworkers,[83] in a randomized study (of only 15 patients following elective abdominal surgery), concluded that the NG tube reduced LES barrier pressure, promoted the reflux of gastric contents, and impaired the clearance of fluid from the distal esophagus. The relevance of this report to the preinduction management of the emergency patient is clearly uncertain.

Vanner and Asai[153] advised that an NG tube already inserted "should be [suctioned and] left in place [for anesthetic induction], since its presence does not reduce the efficacy of cricoid pressure." On the other hand, Brock-Utne[12] contended that "the recommendation that a nasogastric tube should be left in situ during a rapid sequence technique induction is not supported by the evidence. Clinicians who have seen aspiration of gastric contents with an nasogastric tube in situ will, no doubt, remove the nasogastric tube before anesthetic induction." None of these writings address the usually surgical decision concerning which patients should have NG tubes placed before entering the operating room.

Some of the studies just cited would seem to indicate that an NG tube, already inserted, can be safely left in place during induction and may even have a protective benefit. Gastric decompression during surgery could also reduce the risk of regurgitation and aspiration in the postanesthetic period.[43] The necessity and utility of NG tube insertion just prior to induction are not so well defined. The benefits of awake gastric decompression depend, in part, on how completely the stomach can thereby be emptied. The primary drawback is patients' discomfort.

Several authors have studied the thoroughness of gastric emptying attainable by gastric tube suctioning, usually in the context of comparing different methods for estimating gastric residual volume. Ong and coauthors[104] reported as early as 1978 that the volume of fluid obtained by orogastric suctioning correlated poorly with the gastric residual volume calculated by a dilution method, "the volume aspirated being frequently much less than the volume calculated." The authors concluded that "[a]spiration through a gastric tube will not empty the stomach completely." Mechanical decompression of the stomach before induction might therefore be of limited reliability and thus provide a false sense of security.[104] Taylor and associates[145] studied 10 obese patients in whom gastric contents were first aspirated through a 16 F multiorificed Salem Sump tube, then "completely" removed by a gastroscope. "The blind aspirated volume underestimated true total gastric volume by an average of 14.7 mL, [which] was statistically significant … The residual content volume left in the stomach after blind aspiration varied from 4 mL to 23 mL," a maximal discrepancy far less than that found by Ong and coworkers[104] in 42 patients.

Hardy and colleagues[45] measured the volume of gastric fluid aspirated through an 18 F Salem Sump tube

in 24 patients, then directly inspected the stomach and measured the volume of fluid remaining. The residual volume that eluded orogastric suctioning ranged from 0 to 13 mL. The authors thus concluded "that the volume of aspirated gastric fluid … is a very good estimate of the volume present in the stomach at the time of induction" and that gastric tube suctioning "could also be suitable to empty the stomach of its liquid contents prior to anaesthesia."[45]

Alessi and Berci[3] first reported the results of a cinelaryngoscopic study of postoperative patients with NG tubes. They contended that the "[r]outine use of nasogastric tubes in major surgery is associated with unwarranted risks of aspiration through at least three mechanisms: hypersalivation—allowing pooling of secretions in the hypopharynx, a depressed cough reflex, … and various laryngeal and pharyngeal abnormalities … leading to an inability to handle secretions and protect the airway."[3] This study, however, involved patients subjected to prolonged nasogastric intubation after surgery and was not designed to address the immediate preoperative period.

It can be argued that any reduction in intragastric volume and pressure prior to anesthetic induction is desirable and should therefore be attempted. On the other hand, as Satiani and colleagues[127] conceded, "particulate matter … [is] impossible to evacuate through the lumen of an ordinary nasogastric tube." Salem and associates[125] concluded that "placement of a nasogastric tube before anesthetic induction seems to be indicated only in patients with overdistention of the stomach." Although obvious enteric obstruction is conventionally treated with gastric decompression prior to anesthetic induction, not every emergency or at-risk patient is subjected to NG tube insertion while awake. There is currently no consensus to dictate preinduction placement of a gastric tube in any set of patients without intestinal obstruction. In any case, gastric decompression in no way substitutes for proper perioperative management of the airway.

C. CRICOID PRESSURE

For the patient whose stomach is assumed to be full, the anesthesiologist must first decide whether to secure the airway before or after anesthetic induction. If anesthetic induction is to precede endotracheal intubation, the standard protective maneuver for more than four decades has been cricoid pressure. As described by Sellick[131] in 1961, "[t]he manoeuver consists in temporary occlusion of the upper end of the oesophagus by backward pressure of the cricoid cartilage against the bodies of the cervical vertebrae … Extension of the neck and application of pressure on the cricoid cartilage obliterates the oesophageal lumen at the level of the body of the fifth cervical vertebra … Pressure is maintained until intubation and inflation of the cuff of the endotracheal tube is completed."

Kopka[69] and Herman and colleagues[49] noted that cricoid pressure was used as early as 1774 to avert regurgitation related to gastric distention with air during resuscitation from drowning. In Sellick's original report[131] of 26 "high-risk" cases, 23 patients neither vomited nor regurgitated at any time near induction, and in the other 3 the "release of cricoid pressure after intubation was followed immediately by reflux into the pharynx of gastric or oesophageal contents, suggesting that in these three cases cricoid pressure had been effective."

Although the LES (as discussed later) has received considerable attention with regard to the pharmacology and pathophysiology of GER, there is also effective sphincter tone at the upper end of the esophagus. As described by Vanner and colleagues,[155] "[t]he upper oesophageal sphincter is formed mainly by the cricopharyngeus, a striated muscle situated behind the cricoid cartilage. The muscle tone of the cricopharyngeus creates a sphincter pressure which prevents regurgitation in the awake state." These authors found that general anesthesia with neuromuscular blockade reduced the upper esophageal sphincter pressure from 38 mm Hg (while awake) to 6 mm Hg, a pressure that would typically permit passive regurgitation. Although cricoid pressure could exceed the normal awake level of upper esophageal sphincter pressure, in only half of their study patients was it applied firmly enough to do so.[155]

Other authors have noted the inconsistency with which Sellick's maneuver is applied. As Stept and Safar[142] wrote in 1970, "[t]he attempt to close the esophagus by pressing the cricoid cartilage against the cervical vertebrae is rarely applied with proper timing, namely, starting with the onset of unconsciousness and continuing until the tracheal cuff is inflated." In their study of simulated cricoid pressure, Meek and coauthors[89] reported that target pressures could be sustained with a flexed arm for only 3.7 to 6.4 minutes (mean) and with an extended arm for 7.6 to 10.8 minutes (mean).

A rising chorus of skepticism concerning the efficacy of cricoid pressure has been heard. In their reviews, both Kluger and Short[68] and Thwaites and colleagues[147] cited reports of lethal aspiration occurring despite Sellick's maneuver. The former authors specifically questioned the "almost unerring faith in the efficacy of this manoeuvre."[68] In their prospective investigation of emergency intubations in critically ill patients, Schwartz and associates[129] reported that "twelve patients had an unexplained infiltrate that probably resulted from aspiration ... Nine of the twelve patients had cricoid pressure applied during airway management." Tournadre and coauthors[149] found that the application of cricoid pressure to awake subjects caused measurable decreases in LES barrier pressures. The relevance of these measurements to anesthetic induction is unknown. Specifically addressing medicolegal arguments, Jackson contended that "[t]here is no scientific validation for the commonly held belief

that 'improper application of cricoid pressure might explain any failures' to prevent aspiration."[58]

Although it is largely accepted that cricoid pressure limits the incidence of passive regurgitation, "it cannot be expected to prevent regurgitation during coughing, straining, or retching."[153] Sellick,[131] himself, warned against applying cricoid pressure to the patient actively vomiting lest the resulting increased pressure injure the esophagus. In addition, the maneuver itself can induce gagging and even vomiting in the awake patient.[153] Ralph and Wareham[114] reported a case in which "[r]upture of the oesophagus occurred during the application of cricoid pressure at induction of anaesthesia when the patient vomited." Fatal mediastinitis ensued.

It has also become more widely acknowledged that cricoid pressure can interfere with both pulmonary ventilation and endotracheal intubation. Hocking and associates[52] reported that "cricoid pressure produced a reduction in tidal volume and an increase in peak inspiratory pressure" in 50 female patients given mechanical ventilation by mask with an oral airway. Although the changes in pressure and volume were not large, "[c]omplete airway obstruction resulted on three occasions, all with cricoid pressure applied."[52] Saghaei and Masoodifar,[124] in their study of 80 healthy anesthetized adults, found that bimanual cricoid pressure induced decreases in tidal volume with significant increases in peak inspiratory pressure, blood pressure, and heart rate. Hartsilver and Vanner[48] reported similar findings, concluding that "the degree of airway obstruction is related to the force applied to the cricoid cartilage. Therefore, if it is difficult to ventilate via a facemask, the amount of cricoid pressure should be reduced."[48]

Cricoid pressure can also impede ventilation through an LMA. Asai and colleagues[4] reported that standardized cricoid pressure reduced the success rate of LMA ventilation from 100% (22 of 22) to 14% (3 of 22). Under fiberoptic visualization, the 18 LMAs that had been properly positioned became displaced when cricoid pressure was applied. Similarly, Harry and Nolan[46] stated that cricoid pressure reduced the success rate of endotracheal intubation through an intubating LMA from 84% to 52%. Using fiberoptic visualization by LMA, MacG Palmer and Ball[77] noted that cricoid pressure commonly caused cricoid deformation or occlusion, vocal cord closure, and impairment of ventilation, especially in women.

The application of cricoid pressure may either improve or impede conventional laryngoscopy. According to Vanner and coauthors,[154] standard cricoid pressure usually facilitated the exposure of the glottis, and "cricoid pressure in an upward (cephalad) and backward direction was more likely to give a better view at laryngoscopy than the standard technique." In a "substantial minority" of their patients, however, cricoid pressure had either no impact or a detrimental effect on laryngoscopy. Ho and associates[51] noted that "improperly applied" cricoid pressure could impede laryngoscopy and obstruct the airway. Other authors have contended that cricoid pressure tended to interfere with intubation with light wand or fiberoptic techniques.[5,135]

MacG Palmer and Ball[77] concluded that "[o]rthodox application of cricoid pressure may ... be directly implicated in the 'can't intubate, can't ventilate' scenario."[77] In their review of the current practice of rapid sequence induction, Thwaites and coworkers[147] sharpened the point of their critique by reminding us "that hypoxia can kill rapidly, while aspiration only might occur and only might kill." Although Sellick's maneuver remains a conventional element of aspiration prevention, many authors now assert that it should not be slavishly pursued to the detriment of gas exchange and airway securement.

III. MEDICAL PROPHYLAXIS OF ASPIRATION

A. GASTROESOPHAGEAL MOTILITY

Although preparation of the patient (rational NPO strategy and perhaps gastric suctioning) and airway management are the twin pillars of aspiration prevention, pharmacologic prophylaxis has been promoted as adjunctive to patients' safety. Because gastric contents must first pass through the esophagus before entering the pharynx and trachea, the LES has become a locus of attention. As described by Ciresi,[18] the LES "consists of functionally but not anatomically specialized smooth muscle, about 2-4 cm in length, just proximal to the stomach. The sphincteric muscle maintains closure of the distal esophagus through a mechanism of tonic contraction ... accompanied by a zone of intraluminal high pressure."[18] Normally, a cholinergic reflex loop acts to increase LES pressure when intragastric or intra-abdominal pressure rises.[103] The pressure gradient between the LES and the stomach is referred to as the barrier pressure and is responsible for preventing GER (Boxes 11-5 and 11-6).[2,101,112]

Box 11-5 Factors That Decrease Lower Esophageal Barrier Pressure

Gastric fluid components
  Increased acidity
  Lipids
  Hyperosmolar fluid
Progesterone
Pharmacologic agents
  Dopaminergic agonists
  β-Adrenergic agonists
  Theophylline and caffeine
  Anticholinergics
  Opioids

Box 11-6 Factors that Increase Lower Esophageal Barrier Pressure

Dopaminergic antagonists
  Metoclopramide
β-Adrenergic antagonists
Gastrointestinal cholinergic agonists
  Metoclopramide

LES function is modulated by neurohumoral influences. Cholinergic stimulation increases LES tone, and dopaminergic and adrenergic stimulations reduce it.[2,101,123] β-Adrenergic agents and theophylline reduce LES pressure and promote GER, often with symptomatic heartburn in awake patients. β-Adrenergic blockade elevates LES pressure.[6] Anticholinergics attenuate LES tone and impair the efficacy of medications given to increase LES barrier pressure.[35,62,86,115,122] Although prochlorperazine raises LES pressure (presumably by an antidopaminergic effect), promethazine lowers LES pressure because of its anticholinergic properties.[2] Among the wide variety of other drugs that may also reduce LES tone are benzodiazepines, opioids, barbiturates, dopamine, tricyclic antidepressants, calcium channel blockers, nitroglycerin, and nitroprusside.[62,122] Although succinylcholine-induced fasciculations can elevate intra-abdominal pressure, LES tone concurrently rises, and the barrier pressure is maintained or increased.[2,62] Apart from pharmacologic influences, Rabey and colleagues[112] demonstrated that "barrier pressure may be reduced after insertion of an LMA during anesthesia with spontaneous ventilation."

In many cases, agents that increase LES contractility also promote forward passage of gastric contents, and the factors that attenuate LES tone also retard gastric emptying. This correlation compounds our pharmacologic opportunities for either protection or mischief. Opioids and anticholinergics inhibit gastrointestinal motility, increasing the volume of gastric contents available for vomiting or regurgitation.[115,148] Although pain and anxiety delay gastric emptying through sympathetic stimulation, the administration of an opioid for analgesia can further retard the propulsion of gastric contents into the duodenum.[101,122]

1. Metoclopramide

Gastroprokinetic drugs are now available to promote gastric emptying while simultaneously enhancing LES barrier pressure. Metoclopramide is the prototypical agent in this category. The mechanisms of action proposed for metoclopramide include central antidopaminergic activity and prolactin stimulation as well as peripheral blockade of dopamine receptors and stimulation of cholinergic function in the upper gastrointestinal tract. Although metoclopramide retains its gastrokinetic effect in vagotomized subjects, atropine has been shown to interfere with this activity.[18,19] Metoclopramide both raises LES contractility and barrier pressure and accelerates gastric emptying. The latter effect is achieved by intensifying gastric longitudinal muscle contraction while relaxing the gastroduodenal sphincter and increasing the coordination of gastrointestinal peristalsis. Metoclopramide has no effect on gastric acid secretion.[18,35]

Metoclopramide has been extensively investigated as a chemoprophylactic agent for aspiration pneumonitis in children and in adults. Several original studies of patients given metoclopramide, in a dose of 10 or 20 mg, either orally (PO) or intravenously (IV), have demonstrated the drug's utility in reducing gastric residual volume.[35,82,133] Gonzalez and Kallar[35] wrote that "metoclopramide 10 mg PO or IV, in combination with Bicitra or an H_2-receptor antagonist, provides the most effective control of gastric volume and pH." Given PO, metoclopramide has an onset of action that reportedly varies from 30 to 60 minutes, with a duration of action of 2 to 3 hours.[35] Ciresi[18] found that metoclopramide at either 10 or 20 mg IV could reliably empty the stomach within 10 to 20 minutes. Manchikanti and coworkers reported that metoclopramide 10 mg IV reduced the increase in gastric volume that followed the ingestion of sodium citrate and citric acid (Bicitra) but did not interfere with Bicitra's antacid activity.[82] Metoclopramide was also found to reduce the volume of gastric contents in pediatric trauma patients.[141]

Other researchers found metoclopramide to be less uniformly effective, especially in the context of opioid coadministration or the recent ingestion of a solid meal.[86] Christensen and colleagues[17] demonstrated no influence of metoclopramide 0.1 mg/kg on the gastric pH or volume of healthy pediatric patients. As a perioperative antiemetic, metoclopramide was shown to be inconsistently useful.[86] Side effects attributed to metoclopramide have included somnolence, dizziness, and faintness. These problems may surface more frequently in elderly or severely ill patients.[18,35] Extrapyramidal reactions are a more serious problem but reportedly occur in only 1% of subjects.[18] Deehan and Dobb[26] reported a patient with traumatic brain injury in whom metoclopramide 10 mg IV twice induced a severe rise in intracranial pressure associated with increased cerebral blood flow.

Metoclopramide has also been investigated in obstetric anesthesia. The drug has been shown to increase LES tone in pregnant women and may thus be a useful prophylactic agent before cesarean section.[19,86] Studies of gastric emptying in the parturient have, however, provided less consistent results. Metoclopramide was shown to accelerate the gastric emptying of a test meal or of recently ingested food in patients undergoing scheduled or urgent cesarean section.[19,133] On the other hand, Cohen and associates[19] examined 58 healthy parturients after an overnight fast and found that metoclopramide, 10 mg IV, had no significant effect on mean gastric volume or pH or on the proportion of patients with a gastric content volume exceeding 25 mL. The authors suggested that

the drug might be more useful in the emergency setting characterized by active labor, recent food intake, pain, and anxiety.[19] Maternal metoclopramide administration does produce detectable and variable neonatal blood levels of the drug but without reported effects on Apgar scores or neurobehavioral test results.[19,106]

2. Erythromycin

Erythromycin is a macrolide antibiotic that has been in common use for more than 50 years. Given IV, it has been shown to improve gastric motility in patients with diabetic gastroparesis. Enteral feedings with erythromycin also pass more quickly through the stomach than control feedings. This action is thought to arise from the stimulation of motilin receptors in gastric smooth muscle. Berne and coworkers[7] demonstrated somewhat improved tolerance of gastric feedings in critically injured patients when erythromycin was given IV. The potential applicability of these findings to perioperative aspiration prophylaxis is interesting but unproved.

B. REDUCTION OF GASTRIC ACID CONTENT

Chemoprophylaxis of aspiration pneumonitis can also include the inhibition of gastric acid secretion or the neutralization of HCl already in the stomach. The former should eventually increase the pH and reduce the volume of gastric contents but has no effect on acidic fluid already in place. The latter should elevate gastric fluid pH but may also increase gastric fluid volume. The aspiration of particulate antacids can, as previously described, pose hazards equivalent to those of gastric acid inhalation. In 1982 Eyler and colleagues[31] demonstrated severe pulmonary pathology in rabbits resulting from the aspiration of a commercial particulate antacid. Oral antacid prophylaxis should therefore include only soluble, nonparticulate agents.

1. Neutralization of Gastric Acid

The clear antacid solutions most commonly studied are sodium citrate, 0.3 molar solution, and Bicitra. The pH of sodium citrate solutions typically exceeds 7.0, whereas that of Bicitra is 4.3.[82] Manchikanti and associates[82] compared surgical outpatients given Bicitra 15 or 30 mL PO with a matched control group. All patients studied were nonobese and NPO for at least 8 hours. Of the control patients, 88% had a gastric content pH less than or equal to 2.5, in contrast to 32% of those given Bicitra 15 mL and only 16% of those given Bicitra 30 mL. Among the Bicitra-treated patients, undesirably low pH values were typically found in those with lower gastric fluid volumes, confirming previous findings that the antacid effect was attenuated in patients with more rapid gastric emptying.[82]

Sodium citrate has been evaluated as a sole prophylactic agent in a variety of surgical settings, with inconsistent results. Kuster and colleagues[70] found that sodium citrate 30 mL, taken shortly before elective surgery, resulted in gastric fluid pH values greater than 3.5 in 95% of patients. Colman and coworkers[20] administered 15 or 30 mL of sodium citrate to 30 laboring parturients prior to emergency cesarean section. All 15 patients given 30 mL sodium citrate and 14 of 15 given 15 mL had gastric pH values of 2.5 or higher. In other reports, however, sodium citrate failed to alter gastric fluid pH in surgical patients. In a 0.3 molar solution, 30 mL may be more consistently effective than 15 mL but may still not have prolonged effects in patients with rapid gastric emptying.[2,60,105] Antacid prophylaxis may thus be adequate at the induction of anesthesia but inadequate at the time of awakening. Failure to neutralize gastric contents at the time of anesthetic induction may represent inadequate mixing of the sodium citrate with gastric fluid. Adequate mixing may require either adequate time for mixing or adequate movement of the patient.[27,70] Larger volumes of sodium citrate can induce nausea, vomiting, or diarrhea.[82]

2. Inhibition of Gastric Acid Secretion

a. H$_2$-Receptor Blockade

Gastric acid production is strongly modulated by the action of H$_2$ receptors. H$_2$-receptor blockade inhibits basal acid secretion as well as that stimulated by the presence of gastrin or food. Both H$_2$ antagonists and anticholinergic agents block the neural stimulation of gastric acid secretion.[18] However, this beneficial anticholinergic effect is overridden by the inhibition of gastrointestinal motility, so that gastric volume is not reduced and gastric pH is elevated only inconsistently.[35] Although H$_2$ antagonists do not delay gastric emptying, their inhibition of acid secretion tends to correlate inconsistently with both the timing and the magnitude of maximal drug concentration in the plasma.[99] Various H$_2$ antagonists have been evaluated in both surgical and obstetric settings, in different doses and routes of administration, with and without other prophylactic medications, to produce an expansive volume of findings.

i. Cimetidine   Given prior to elective surgery, a variety of cimetidine regimens can ensure that most patients have gastric fluid volume or pH values, or both, in the "safe" range, as defined by the investigators. These usually effective regimens include cimetidine 300 mg PO at bedtime followed by 300 mg PO or intramuscularly (IM) the morning of surgery, cimetidine 300 to 600 mg PO 1.5 to 2 hours preoperatively, or cimetidine 200 mg IV 1 hour before surgery. In one study cimetidine most reliably produced gastric content safety when combined with preoperative metoclopramide.[62] The reliability of oral cimetidine is generally improved if the drug is administered both the night before and the morning of anesthesia.[27]

A gastric fluid pH of 2.5 or less has been found in about 5% to 35% of patients treated with single 300-mg doses of cimetidine given PO, IM, or IV in different studies. Significant elevation of gastric pH requires 30 to 60 minutes to become evident after the intravenous administration of cimetidine and 60 to 90 minutes after intramuscular or oral dosing. Effective inhibition of gastric acid secretion persists for 4 to 6 hours.[35,86] Papadimitriou and colleagues[107] administered cimetidine 400 mg IV to 20 patients facing emergency surgery. Compared with 10 such patients given placebo treatment, those receiving cimetidine were found to have significantly lower mean gastric acidity, but the range of pH values was 1.6 to 7.2.

Cimetidine chemoprophylaxis has also been evaluated in obstetric anesthesia. In a study of women scheduled for elective cesarean section, the administration of cimetidine 400 mg PO the night before surgery, followed by 200 mg IM 90 minutes before induction, resulted in a mean gastric fluid pH of 6.2. However, 3 of the 16 patients studied had gastric fluid pH values less than 2.5.[20] In a study of 100 patients undergoing emergency cesarean section, cimetidine 200 mg IM was administered when surgical delivery was decided upon, followed by oral intake of a 0.3 molar solution of sodium citrate 30 mL just prior to induction. None of these patients had a gastric fluid pH less than 2.7, and only 1 of 100 had a gastric fluid pH less than 3.0.[87] Cimetidine administered in this fashion would most likely reduce gastric acidity by the time of extubation, whereas sodium citrate would be required to neutralize the acid already present.

To achieve both prompt neutralization of gastric HCl and subsequent inhibition of acid production, cimetidine (800 mg) and sodium citrate (1.8 g) have been combined in tablet form. (Alkalinization of gastric fluid has also been suggested to accelerate the systemic uptake of orally administered cimetidine.[27,105]) In healthy elective surgical patients, a single tablet of effervescent cimetidine provided both significant elevation of gastric content pH and significant reduction of gastric content volume when given 2 hours prior to induction, with no patient considered at risk for acid aspiration.[10] When given 10 to 50 minutes prior to elective or emergency cesarean section, one-half tablet of effervescent cimetidine achieved gastric pH values greater than 2.5 in 98% to 100% of patients at the times of both induction and extubation.[27,105] (Although this formulation is not available in the United States, commercial preparations of cimetidine and citrates can obviously be given together.)

Although cimetidine has a well-established record of safety when administered for perioperative aspiration prophylaxis, there are potential and observed side effects. The rapid intravenous infusion of large doses (e.g., 400 to 600 mg) has reportedly induced both hypotension and dangerous ventricular dysrhythmias.[86,101] Smith and colleagues[136] found that cimetidine 200 mg, given IV over 2 minutes to 20 critically ill patients, resulted in temporary and variable decreases in mean arterial pressure and systemic vascular resistance, not requiring treatment. Heart rate, cardiac output, and cardiac filling pressures were not altered. The authors advised that intravenous cimetidine be infused over at least a 10-minute period.[136] Other side effects sporadically associated with cimetidine include confusion, dizziness, headaches, and diarrhea, although these have not been reported to occur with single-dose preoperative administration.[18,86,101]

Cimetidine competitively inhibits the hepatic mixed-function oxidase system (cytochrome P450 enzyme) and also reduces hepatic perfusion.[6,86,101] As a result, cimetidine may elevate the blood concentrations of other drugs that are cleared by the liver, including warfarin, propranolol, diazepam, theophylline, phenytoin, meperidine, bupivacaine, and lidocaine. Clinically, this seems to be a greater concern with long-term than with one- or two-dose administration.[18,20,86]

ii. Ranitidine After cimetidine, ranitidine emerged as the next option for H_2 blockade. Ranitidine is considered to exert little or no inhibition of hepatic enzymes, has a longer duration of action (6 to 8 hours) than cimetidine, and has an efficacy greater than or equal to that of the original H_2 blocker. Effective onset times for the two drugs appear to be similar.[20,35,62,86,121] Smith and coauthors[136] reported that ranitidine 50 mg, given IV over 2 minutes to 20 critically ill patients, led to variable, transient reductions in mean arterial pressure and systemic vascular resistance. These hemodynamic effects occurred less frequently and were of lesser degree and duration than those resulting from cimetidine 200 mg, similarly administered. Previous sporadic case reports associated significant bradycardia with the intravenous administration of either cimetidine or ranitidine.[136]

In the study of adult surgical outpatients by Maltby and colleagues,[81] ranitidine 150 mg PO, given 2.5 hours prior to anesthetic induction, significantly decreased gastric residual volume and significantly increased gastric fluid pH when compared with placebo. In no patient was there the conventional (but arbitrary) at-risk combination of gastric pH less than 2.5 and gastric volume greater than 25 mL. Kuster and coworkers[70] administered ranitidine 300 mg PO the night before and 150 mg PO the morning of elective surgery. Gastric fluid pH was greater than 4.0 in all cases on both induction and extubation, "even after delayed or prolonged operations." McAllister and associates[84] treated adult patients with a single oral dose of ranitidine 300 mg 2 hours before surgery and found both a significant increase in mean gastric fluid pH and a significant decrease in mean gastric fluid volume compared with placebo treatment. Although some patients did have gastric fluid pH values below 2.5

despite the ranitidine regimen, the incidence of such low pH values was also significantly less than with placebo. The authors cautioned that "it is unsafe to assume that H_2 antagonists will always eliminate the risk of acid aspiration pneumonitis."[84]

In other studies, a single oral dose of ranitidine 150 mg, given 2 to 3 hours before anesthetic induction, has been found to produce gastric fluid pH values greater than 2.5 in most adult surgical patients. Another report indicated that ranitidine 150 mg PO, given both the night before and the morning of surgery, produced gastric fluid pH values greater than 2.5 in all such patients studied. Single-dose intravenous administration of ranitidine, 40 to 100 mg, has also been found to generate reliably gastric fluid pH values greater than 2.5 in adults, manifesting a greater efficacy than that of cimetidine 300 mg IV.[62]

Sandhar and coworkers[126] evaluated the efficacy of a single oral dose of ranitidine, 2 mg/kg, given 2 to 3 hours before surgery to patients aged 1 to 14 years. Although ranitidine significantly reduced both the volume and the acidity of gastric contents compared with placebo, 6 of 44 children receiving ranitidine did have gastric fluid pH values no greater than 2.5. These findings confirmed those of a similar study of Goudsouzian and Young,[37] although other authors have not demonstrated such a consistent reduction in gastric fluid volume.[62,81]

Papadimitriou and associates[107] compared ranitidine 150 mg IV with cimetidine 400 mg IV and with placebo given 1 hour before anesthetic induction to emergency surgical patients. Ranitidine and cimetidine caused similar reductions in gastric volume and acidity; only the reductions in acidity were statistically significant. Although the mean pH values in the cimetidine and ranitidine groups were similar, only ranitidine consistently produced safe gastric pH values (all of which were at least 5.0). Vila and colleagues,[158] evaluating H_2 antagonists in morbidly obese surgical patients, concluded that ranitidine was superior to cimetidine in elevating gastric fluid pH. When such patients were given ranitidine 150 mg PO the night before surgery and again 2 hours prior to induction, all pH values obtained were greater than 2.5. A literature review cited by Gonzalez and Kallar[35] also found that ranitidine more reliably ensured that gastric fluid pH would exceed 2.5 than did cimetidine, although neither agent consistently reduced gastric fluid volume into the range considered safe by given authors.

The effect of oral ranitidine (150 mg 2 to 3 hours before the scheduled time of surgery) with or without oral metoclopramide (10 mg 1 hour before surgery) and/or sodium citrate (30 mL on call to the operating room) on gastric fluid volume and pH was measured in 196 elective surgical inpatients.[80] Although no combination guaranteed a safe combination of fluid volume and pH, a single oral dose of ranitidine was statistically as effective as triple prophylaxis. In pediatric patients, both Gombar[34] and Maekawa[79] and their colleagues showed that oral ranitidine (either 2 mg/kg or 75 mg) effectively elevated gastric fluid pH with no appreciable effect on gastric volume.

Ranitidine has also been evaluated for prophylactic use in obstetric anesthesia. Ewart and associates[30] administered ranitidine 150 mg PO the night before and the morning of elective cesarean section. At both induction and extubation, all gastric aspirate volumes were less than 25 mL. However, 19% of patients had gastric fluid pH values less than 3.5, and 6% had values less than 2.5, either at induction or at extubation or both.[30] Colman and coworkers[20] administered ranitidine 150 mg PO 8 to 14 hours prior to elective cesarean section, then 50 mg IM 90 minutes before induction. All 20 patients in this study had gastric fluid volumes less than 25 mL and pH values greater than 2.5. A previous study by McAuley and others demonstrated that 79 of 80 parturients had gastric fluid pH values greater than 2.5 when given ranitidine 150 mg PO 2 to 6 hours prior to elective cesarean section.[85]

Rout and colleagues[121] evaluated the efficacy of ranitidine 50 mg IV given to laboring patients when cesarean section was decided upon. A control group received no H_2-antagonist therapy, but all patients were given 0.3 molar sodium citrate, 30 mL, shortly before induction. At the time of induction, 4% of those given only sodium citrate had a gastric fluid volume greater than 25 mL along with a pH less than 3.5, compared with 2.3% of those given both citrate and ranitidine ($P = .05$). At the time of extubation, 5.6% of those given only sodium citrate were considered at risk by the preceding criteria, compared with only 0.3% of those given both citrate and ranitidine ($P < .05$). There was no significant difference between the mean pH values of the two groups of patients. On the other hand, all gastric fluid pH values exceeded 3.5 in patients who received ranitidine more than 30 minutes prior to induction.

iii. Others A voluminous body of evidence thus documents the general safety and efficacy of preoperative cimetidine and ranitidine in ameliorating the acidity and volume of gastric contents. Newer agents, such as famotidine (10 mg PO) and nizatidine, have also been evaluated, with generally favorable results.[150,158] Wajima and colleagues[159] reported that nizatidine 300 mg PO was uniformly effective in maintaining gastric content pH above 2.5 and volume below 25 mL when given 2 hours prior to surgery.

On the basis of the presumably high ratio of benefit to risk, H_2-blocking agents are commonly recommended for surgical patients with an increased likelihood of inhaling gastric contents.[36,62] However, given the infrequency of perioperative aspiration pneumonitis, documentation of the actual clinical benefit of such practice has yet to be provided. In the review by Warner and coauthors[161] of more than 215,000 general anesthetics in adults, 35 patients with generally acknowledged risk factors did aspirate perioperatively. Of these 35, 17 had been given

prophylactic medication. In this small sample, aspiration prophylaxis produced no discernible difference in the incidence of pulmonary complications.[161] In general, the routine preoperative use of H_2 antagonists is not considered either essential or cost effective. As stated by Kallar and Everett,[62] "[I]t has yet to be proven that prophylaxis against acid aspiration changes morbidity or mortality in healthy patients having elective surgery."

b. Proton Pump Inhibition

Proton pump inhibitors (PPIs) constitute a newer class of agents for the suppression of gastric acid production. Acetylcholine, histamine, and gastrin all stimulate HCl secretion by the gastric parietal cell. Although these agonists stimulate different populations of receptors, their mechanisms of action all eventually result in the formation of cyclic adenosine monophosphate (cAMP). The cAMP activates the proton pump, H^+,K^+-adenosine triphosphatase (ATPase), which exchanges intraluminal potassium ions for intracellular hydrogen ions. Hydrogen ions are thereby secreted from the parietal cell into gastric fluids.[84,126] Omeprazole, the prototype PPI, is actually a prodrug, which is absorbed in the small intestine and is activated in the highly acidic milieu of the gastric parietal cell. Activated omeprazole then remains in the parietal cell for up to 48 hours, inhibiting the proton pump in a prolonged manner.[10,30,94,106] Inhibition of gastric acid secretion can be nearly complete, with no discernible side effects. A single dose of omeprazole, 20 to 40 mg, reduces gastric acidity for up to 48 hours. On the other hand, PPIs are characterized by variable first-pass metabolism with resulting inconsistencies in the plasma concentration after any given oral dose. As is the case with H_2 antagonists, there is also an unpredictable relationship between peak plasma concentration and peak inhibition of gastric acid production.[99]

Omeprazole has been evaluated as a preoperative agent for the chemoprophylaxis of aspiration pneumonitis. Bouly and colleagues[10] gave omeprazole 40 mg PO to healthy patients either the evening before or 2 hours prior to elective surgery. Although mean gastric fluid pH was significantly higher with omeprazole treatment than with placebo, gastric acidity was significantly greater with omeprazole than with effervescent cimetidine. Of 30 patients receiving omeprazole, 6 had gastric fluid pH values less than 2.5 at the time of induction. Omeprazole significantly reduced gastric fluid volume when compared with placebo. Wingtin and coworkers[162] administered either placebo or omeprazole 40 mg PO to healthy, nonobese adults the night before elective surgery. Patients receiving omeprazole had a significantly higher mean gastric fluid pH than those receiving placebo. The lowest gastric fluid pH observed with omeprazole was 2.4, in contrast to a minimal pH of 1.1 with placebo. Only 4.5% of omeprazole-treated patients had gastric fluid pH values less than 3.5, compared with 50% of those given a placebo. Yamanaka and coauthors[164] studied 13 patients given oral omeprazole 20 mg the night before surgery. The following morning, gastric content pH ranged from 2.5 to 7.0 and volume measurements were 0 to 30 mL.

Omeprazole has also been evaluated in obstetric anesthesia. Orr and associates[106] administered omeprazole 40 mg PO the night before and the morning of elective cesarean section. Only 1 of 30 patients had a gastric fluid pH less than 2.5 on induction, and all gastric fluid pH values exceeded 2.5 at the time of extubation. In no case did gastric fluid volume exceed 25 mL with a pH less than 2.5. Of 15 patients who also received metoclopramide 20 mg IM at least 20 minutes before elective cesarean section, all had gastric fluid pH values greater than 2.5, both on induction and at extubation. When omeprazole 80 mg PO was given only on the morning of elective cesarean section, 2 of 33 patients had a gastric fluid pH less than 2.5 at induction, 1 of whom also had a gastric fluid volume greater than 40 mL. All gastric fluid pH values were greater than 2.5 at extubation. Of 16 patients who also received metoclopramide 20 mg IM at least 20 minutes before elective cesarean section, 2 still had gastric fluid pH values less than 2.5 (with gastric fluid volumes less than 25 mL) on induction, but all gastric fluid pH values exceeded 2.5 at extubation.[106] Yau and coworkers[165] found that two doses of omeprazole 40 mg were superior to two doses of ranitidine 150 mg in producing gastric fluid pH values greater than 3.5 in nonlaboring patients undergoing elective cesarean section.

Ewart and colleagues[30] administered omeprazole 40 mg PO the night before and the morning of elective cesarean section. All gastric fluid pH values were at least 3.5, both on induction and at extubation, and all gastric fluid volumes were less than 25 mL. Moore and coworkers[94] administered omeprazole 80 mg PO the evening before elective cesarean section, with no subsequent morning dose, and noted somewhat less consistent antacid prophylaxis. Of 20 gastric fluid samples taken on induction, 1 met the authors' criteria for placing the patient at risk for aspiration pneumonitis. They concluded that this single-dose omeprazole regimen was not adequate to guarantee "acceptable gastric pH and volume 12-16 hours after administration."[94]

In general, the PPIs omeprazole, rabeprazole, and lansoprazole have been found most effective when given in two doses, the night before and the morning of surgery.[99] Given the dwindling proportion of patients hospitalized prior to elective surgery, two-dose regimens for chemoprophylaxis would seem somewhat impractical. Furthermore, Nishina and coauthors[102] reported that a single preoperative oral dose of ranitidine was more effective in reducing gastric acid content than two-dose regimens of rabeprazole or lansoprazole.

IV. CONCLUSION

It is clearly best to prevent gastric contents of any volume or pH from entering the trachea. Although this ideal may not always be attainable, even by the most skillful of clinicians, its likelihood would appear to be favored by optimal preparation of patients and a carefully executed, well-designed plan for anesthetic induction and airway management. The place of awake intubation and gastric emptying in high-risk cases is influenced by patients' characteristics and practitioner experience and confidence. Although cricoid pressure remains a standard prophylactic maneuver, it is now recognized that airway securement and effective ventilation may mandate its modification, or even discontinuation, in certain circumstances.

An impressive array of pharmacologic agents can now be employed to promote antegrade gastric emptying, inhibit GER, and reduce the acid content of gastric fluids. These drugs have been utilized with an established record of safety and offer us the reasonable expectation of rendering gastric fluid less threatening to the lungs. However, because of the limited incidence of clinically significant perioperative aspiration, it may not be possible to demonstrate statistically that the use of these agents actually improves patients' outcomes. In reference to gastric prokinetic drugs, antacids, and inhibitors of acid secretion, the ASA task force used the same phrasing, "the routine preoperative use of [such medications] ... in patients who have no apparent increased risk for pulmonary aspiration is not recommended." Chemoprophylaxis is only an adjunct to and not a substitute for otherwise sound clinical practice.

REFERENCES

1. Agnew NM, Kendall JB, Akrofi M, et al: Gastroesophageal reflux and tracheal aspiration in the thoracotomy position: Should ranitidine premedication be routine? Anesth Analg 95:1645-1649, 2002.
2. Aitkenhead AR: Anaesthesia and the gastro-intestinal system. Eur J Anaesthesiol 5:73-112, 1988.
3. Alessi DM, Berci G: Aspiration and nasogastric intubation. Otolaryngology 94:486-489, 1986.
4. Asai T, Barclay K, Power I, Vaughan RS: Cricoid pressure impedes placement of the laryngeal mask airway. Br J Anaesth 74:521-525, 1995.
5. Asai T, Murao K, Shingu K: Cricoid pressure applied after placement of laryngeal mask impedes subsequent fibreoptic tracheal intubation through mask. Br J Anaesth 85:256-261, 2000.

6. Barish CF, Wu WC, Castell DO: Respiratory complications of gastroesophageal reflux. Arch Intern Med 145:1882-1888, 1985.

7. Berne JD, Norwood SH, McAuley CE, et al: Erythromycin reduces delayed gastric emptying in critically ill trauma patients: A randomized, controlled trial. J Trauma 53:422-425, 2002.

8. Bond VK, Stoelting RK, Gupta CD: Pulmonary aspiration syndrome after inhalation of gastric fluid containing antacids. Anesthesiology 51:452-453, 1979.

9. Borland LM, Sereika SM, Woelfel SK, et al: Pulmonary aspiration in pediatric patients during general anesthesia: Incidence and outcome. J Clin Anesth 10:95-102, 1998.

10. Bouly A, Nathan N, Feiss P: Comparison of omeprazole with cimetidine for prophylaxis of acid aspiration in elective surgery. Eur J Anaesthesiol 10:209-213, 1993.

11. Broach J, Newton N: Food and beverages in labor. Part II. The effects of cessation of oral intake during labor. Birth 15:88-92, 1988.

12. Brock-Utne J: Gastroesophageal reflux and aspiration of gastric contents. Anesth Analg 94:762-763, 2002.

13. Caballero-Plasencia AM, Muros-Navarro MC, Martin-Ruiz JL, et al: Gastroparesis of digestible and indigestible solids in patients with insulin-dependent diabetes mellitus or functional dyspepsia. Dig Dis Sci 39:1409-1415, 1994.

14. Carlin CB, Scanlon PH, Wagner DA, et al: Gastric emptying in trauma patients. Dig Surg 16:192-196, 1999.

15. Chestnut DH, Cohen SE: At the water's edge: Where obstetrics and anesthesia meet. Obstet Gynecol 77:965-967, 1991.

16. Chiloiro M, Darconza G, Piccioli E, et al: Gastric emptying and orocecal transit time in pregnancy. J Gastroenterol 36:538-543, 2001.

17. Christensen S, Farrow-Gillespie A, Lerman J: Effects of ranitidine and metoclopramide on gastric fluid pH and volume in children. Br J Anaesth 65:456-460, 1990.

18. Ciresi SA: Gastrointestinal pharmacology review and anesthetic application to the combat casualty. Mil Med 154:555-559, 1989.

19. Cohen SE, Jasson J, Talafre M-L, et al: Does metoclopramide decrease the volume of gastric contents in patients undergoing cesarean section? Anesthesiology 61:604-607, 1984.

20. Colman RD, Frank M, Loughnan BA, et al: Use of i.m. ranitidine for the prophylaxis of aspiration pneumonitis in obstetrics. Br J Anaesth 61:720-729, 1988.

21. Cook-Sather SD, Harris KA, Chiavacci R, et al: A liberalized fasting guideline for formula-fed infants does not increase average gastric fluid volume before elective surgery. Anesth Analg 96:965-969, 2003.

22. Cotes CJ: NPO after midnight for children—A reappraisal. Anesthesiology 72:589-592, 1990.

23. Crawford JS: How can aspiration of vomitus in obstetrics best be prevented? Commentary: Setting the record straight. Birth 15:230-235, 1988.

24. Crighton IM, Martin PH, Hobbs GJ, et al: A comparison of the effects of intravenous tramadol, codeine, and morphine on gastric emptying in human volunteers. Anesth Analg 87:445-449, 1998.

25. Dal Santo G: Acid aspiration: Pathophysiological aspects, prevention, and therapy. Int Anesthesiol Clin 24:31-52, 1986.

26. Deehan S, Dobb GJ: Metoclopramide-induced raised intracranial pressure after head injury. J Neurosurg Anesthesiol 14:157-160, 2002.

27. DePaso WJ: Aspiration pneumonia. Clin Chest Med 12:269-284, 1991.

28. Dotson RG, Robinson RG, Pingleton SK: Gastroesophageal reflux with nasogastric tubes: Effect of nasogastric tube size. Am J Respir Crit Care Med 149:1659-1662, 1994.

29. Elkington KW: At the water's edge: Where obstetrics and anesthesia meet. Obstet Gynecol 77:304-308, 1991.

30. Ewart MC, Yau G, Gin T, et al: A comparison of the effects of omeprazole and ranitidine on gastric secretion in women undergoing elective caesarean section. Anaesthesia 45:527-530, 1990.

31. Eyler SW, Cullen BF, Murphy ME, Welch WD: Antacid aspiration in rabbits: A comparison of Mylanta and Bicitra. Anesth Analg 61:288-292, 1982.

32. Ezri T, Szmuk P, Stein A, et al: Peripartum general anaesthesia without tracheal intubation: Incidence of aspiration pneumonia. Anaesthesia 55:421-426, 2000.

33. Gardner AMN: Aspiration of food and vomit. Q J Med 27:227, 1958.

34. Gombar S, Dureja J, Kiran S, et al: The effect of pre-operative intake of oral water and ranitidine on gastric fluid volume and pH in children undergoing elective surgery. J Indian Med Assoc 95:166-168, 1997.

35. Gonzalez ER, Kallar SK: Reducing the risk of aspiration pneumonitis. DICP 23:203-208, 1989.

36. Goresky GV, Maltby JR: Fasting guidelines for elective surgical patients. Can J Anaesth 37:493-495, 1990.

37. Goudsouzian NG, Young ET: The efficacy of ranitidine in children. Acta Anaesthesiol Scand 31:387-390, 1987.

38. Guha A, Scawn ND, Rogers SA, et al: Gastric emptying in post-thoracotomy patients receiving a thoracic fentanyl-bupivacaine epidural infusion. Eur J Anaesthesiol 19:652-657, 2002.

39. Hall CC: Aspiration pneumonitis. JAMA 114:728, 1940.

40. Hammas B, Thorn SE, Wattwil M: Propofol and gastric effects of morphine. Acta Anaesthesiol Scand 45:1023–1027, 2001.

41. Hannon VM, Cunningham AJ, Hutchinson M, et al: Aspiration pneumonia and coma: An unusual presentation of dystrophica myotonia. Can Anaesth Soc J 33:803-806, 1986.

42. Hardoff R, Sula M, Tamir A, et al: Gastric emptying time and gastric motility in patients with Parkinson's disease. Mov Disord 16:1041-1047, 2001.

43. Hardy J-F: Large volume gastroesophageal reflux: A rationale for risk reduction in the perioperative period. Can J Anaesth 35:162-173, 1988.

44. Hardy J-F, Lepage Y, Bonneville-Chouinard N: Occurrence of gastroesophageal reflux on induction of anaesthesia does not correlate with the volume of gastric contents. Can J Anaesth 37:502-508, 1990.

45. Hardy J-F, Plourde G, Lebrun M, et al: Determining gastric contents during general anaesthesia: Evaluation of two methods. Can J Anaesth 34:474-477, 1987.

46. Harry RM, Nolan JP: The use of cricoid pressure with the intubating laryngeal mask. Anaesthesia 54:656-659, 1999.

47. Harter RL, Kelly WB, Kramer MG, et al: A comparison of the volume and pH of gastric contents of obese and lean surgical patients. Anesth Analg 86:147-152, 1998.

48. Hartsilver EL, Vanner RG: Airway obstruction with cricoid pressure. Anaesthesia 55:208-211, 2000.

49. Herman NL, Carter B, Van Decar TK: Cricoid pressure: Teaching the recommended level. Anesth Analg 83:859-863, 1996.

50. Hickling KG, Howard R: A retrospective survey of treatment and mortality in aspiration pneumonia. Intensive Care Med 14:617-622, 1988.

51. Ho AM, Wong W, Ling E, et al: Airway difficulties caused by improperly applied cricoid pressure. J Emerg Med 20:29-31, 2001.

52. Hocking G, Roberts FL, Thew ME: Airway obstruction with cricoid pressure and lateral tilt. Anaesthesia 56:825-828, 2001.

53. Hollingsworth HM: Wheezing and stridor. Clin Chest Med 8:231-240, 1987.

54. Hollingsworth HM, Irwin RS: Acute respiratory failure in pregnancy. Clin Chest Med 13:723-740, 1992.

55. Ingebo KR, Rayhorn NJ, Hecht RM, et al: Sedation in children: Adequacy of two-hour fasting. J Pediatr 131:155-158, 1997.

56. Irons EE, Apfelbach CW: Aspiration bronchopneumonia. JAMA 115:584, 1940.

57. Ishihara H, Singh H, Giesecke AH: Relationship between diabetic autonomic neuropathy and gastric contents. Anesth Analg 78:943-947, 1994.

58. Jackson SH: Efficacy and safety of cricoid pressure needs scientific validation. Anesthesiology 84:751-752, 1996.

59. James CF, Modell JH, Gibbs CP, et al: Pulmonary aspiration—Effects of volume and pH in the rat. Anesth Analg 63:655-658, 1984.

60. Joyce TH: Prophylaxis for pulmonary acid aspiration. Am J Med 83(Suppl 6A):46-52, 1987.

61. Kadar AG, Ing CH, White PF, et al: Anesthesia for electroconvulsive therapy in obese patients. Anesth Analg 94:360-361, 2002.

62. Kallar SK, Everett LL: Potential risks and preventive measures for pulmonary aspiration: New concepts in preoperative fasting guidelines. Anesth Analg 77:171-182, 1993.

63. Kao CH, ChangLai SP, Chieng PU, Yen TC: Gastric emptying in head-injured patients. Am J Gastroenterol 93:1108-1112, 1998.

64. Kao CH, ChangLai SP, Chieng PU, Yen TC: Gastric emptying in male neurologic trauma. J Nucl Med 39:1798-1801, 1998.

65. Kelly MC, Carabine UA, Hill DA, et al: A comparison of the effect of intrathecal and extradural fentanyl on gastric emptying in laboring women. Anesth Analg 85:834-838, 1997.

66. Khawaja IT, Buffa SD, Brandstetter RD: Aspiration pneumonia. Postgrad Med 92:165-168, 1992.

67. Kirsch CM, Sanders A: Aspiration pneumonia: Medical management. Otolaryngol Clin North Am 21:677-689, 1988.

68. Kluger MT, Short TG: Aspiration during anaesthesia: A review of 133 cases from the Australian Anaesthetic Incident Monitoring Study (AIMS). Anaesthesia 54:19-26, 1999.

69. Kopka A: The introduction of cricoid pressure. Anaesthesia 57:827, 2002.

70. Kuster M, Naji P, Gabi K, et al: Die intraoperative, direkte und kontinuirliche pH-Messung im Magen nach Vorbehandlung mit Ranitidin oder Natriumcitrat. Anaesthesist 38:59-64, 1989.

71. Leigh JM, Tytler JA: Admissions to the intensive care unit after complications of anaesthetic techniques over 10 years. Anaesthesia 45:814-820, 1990.

72. Lewis P, Maltby JR, Sutherland LR: Unrestricted oral fluid until three hours preoperatively: Effect on gastric fluid volume and pH. Can J Anaesth 37:S132, 1990.

73. Lindahl SG: Not only towards enhanced preoperative comfort. Anesth Analg 93:1091-1092, 2001.

74. LoCicero J: Bronchopulmonary aspiration. Surg Clin North Am 69:71-76, 1989.

75. Lockey DJ, Coats T, Parr MJ: Aspiration in severe trauma: A prospective study. Anaesthesia 54:1097-1098, 1999.

76. Ludka LM, Roberts CC: Eating and drinking in labor. J Nurse Midwifery 38:199-207, 1993.

77. MacG Palmer JH, Ball DR: The effect of cricoid pressure on the cricoid cartilage and vocal cords: An endoscopic study in anaesthetised patients. Anaesthesia 55:263-268, 2000.

78. Maekawa N, Mikawa K, Yahu H, et al: Effects of 2-, 4-, and 12-hour fasting intervals on preoperative gastric fluid pH and volume, and plasma glucose and lipid homeostasis in children. Acta Anaesthesiol Scand 37:783-787, 1993.

79. Maekawa N, Nishina K, Mikawa K, et al: Comparison of pirenzepine, ranitidine, and pirenzepine-ranitidine combination for reducing preoperative gastric fluid acidity and volume in children. Br J Anaesth 80:53-57, 1998.

80. Maltby JR, Elliott RH, Warnell I, et al: Gastric fluid volume and pH in elective surgical patients: Triple prophylaxis is not superior to ranitidine alone. Can J Anaesth 37:650-655, 1990.

81. Maltby JR, Sutherland AD, Sale JP, et al: Preoperative oral fluids: Is a five-hour fast justified prior to elective surgery? Anesth Analg 65:1112-1116, 1983.

82. Manchikanti L, Grow JB, Colliver JA, et al: Bicitra (sodium citrate) and metoclopramide in outpatient anesthesia for prophylaxis against aspiration pneumonitis. Anesthesiology 63:378-384, 1985.

83. Manning BJ, Winter DC, McGreatl G, et al: Nasogastric intubation causes gastroesophageal reflux in patients undergoing elective laparotomy. Surgery 130:788-791, 2001.

84. McAllister JD, Moote CA, Sharpe MD, et al: Random double-blind comparison of nizatidine, famotidine, ranitidine, and placebo. Can J Anaesth 37:S22, 1990.

85. McAuley DM, Moore J, McCaughey W, et al: Ranitidine as an antacid before elective Caesarean section. Anaesthesia 38:108-114, 1983.

86. McCammon RL: Prophylaxis for aspiration pneumonitis. Can Anaesth Soc J 33:S47-53, 1986.

87. McKay S, Mahan C: How can aspiration of vomitus in obstetrics best be prevented? Birth 15:222-235, 1988.

88. Meakin G, Dingwall AE, Addison GM: Effects of fasting and oral premedication on the pH and volume of gastric aspirate in children. Br J Anaesth 59:678-682, 1987.

89. Meek T, Vincent A, Duggen JE: Cricoid pressure: Can protective force be sustained? Br J Anaesth 80:672-674, 1998.

90. Mellin-Olsen J, Fasting S, Gisvold SE: Routine preoperative gastric emptying is seldom indicated. A study of 85,594 anaesthetics with special focus on aspiration pneumonia. Acta Anaesthesiol Scand 40: 1184-1188, 1996.

91. Mendelson CL: The aspiration of stomach contents into the lungs during obstetric anesthesia. Am J Obstet Gynecol 52:191, 1946.

92. Merio R, Festa A, Bergmann H, et al: Slow gastric emptying in type I diabetes: Relation to autonomic and peripheral neuropathy, blood glucose, and glycemic control. Diabetes Care 20:419-423, 1997.

93. Miller M, Wishart HY, Nimmo WS: Gastric contents at induction of anaesthesia: Is a 4-hour fast necessary? Br J Anaesth 55:1185-1188, 1983.

94. Moore J, Flynn RJ, Sampaio M, et al: Effect of single-dose omeprazole on intragastric acidity and volume during obstetric anaesthesia. Anaesthesia 44:559-562, 1989.

95. Morgan M: Anaesthetic contribution to maternal mortality. Br J Anaesth 59:842-855, 1987.

96. Moyao-Garcia D, Corrales-Fernandez MA, Blanco-Rodriguez G, et al: Benefits of oral administration of an electrolyte solution interrupting a prolonged preoperatory fasting period in pediatric patients. J Pediatr Surg 36:457-459, 2001.

97. Murphy DB, Sutton A, Prescott LF, Murphy MB: A comparison of the effects of tramadol and morphine on gastric emptying in man. Anaesthesia 52:1224-1229, 1997.

98. Murphy DB, Sutton JA, Prescott LF, Murphy MB: Opioid-induced delay in gastric emptying: A peripheral mechanism in humans. Anesthesiology 87:765-770, 1997.

99. Ng A, Smith G: Gastroesophageal reflux and aspiration of gastric contents in anesthetic practice. Anesth Analg 93:494-513, 2001.

100. Nygren J, Thorell A, Ljungqvist O: Preoperative oral carbohydrate nutrition: An update. Curr Opin Clin Nutr Metab Care 4:255-259, 2001.

101. Nimmo WS: Aspiration of gastric contents. Br J Hosp Med 34:176-179, 1985.

102. Nishina K, Mikawa K, Takao Y, et al: A comparison of rabeprazole, lansoprazole, and ranitidine for improving preoperative gastric fluid property in adults undergoing elective surgery. Anesth Analg 90:717-721, 2000.

103. Olsson GL, Hallen B, Hambraeus-Jonzon K: Aspiration during anaesthesia: A computer-aided study of 185,358 anaesthetics. Acta Anaesthesiol Scand 30:84-92, 1986.

104. Ong BY, Palahniuk RJ, Cumming M: Gastric volume and pH in out-patients. Can Anaesth Soc J 25:36-39, 1978.

105. Ormezzano X, Francois TP, Viaud J-Y, et al: Aspiration pneumonitis prophylaxis in obstetric anaesthesia: Comparison of effervescent cimetidine-sodium citrate mixture and sodium citrate. Br J Anaesth 64:503-506, 1990.

106. Orr DA, Bill KM, Gillon KRW, et al: Effects of omeprazole, with and without metoclopramide, in elective obstetric anaesthesia. Anaesthesia 48:114-119, 1993.

107. Papadimitriou L, Kandiloros A, Lakiotis K, et al: Protecting against the acid aspiration syndrome in adult patients undergoing emergency surgery. Hepatogastroenterology 39:560-561, 1992.

108. Pennza PT: Aspiration pneumonia, necrotizing pneumonia, and lung abscess. Emerg Med Clin North Am 7:279-307, 1989.

109. Phillips S, Hutchinson S, Davidson T: Preoperative drinking does not affect gastric contents. Br J Anaesth 70:6-9, 1993.

110. Porter JS, Bonello E, Reynolds F: The influence of epidural administration of fentanyl infusion on gastric emptying in labour. Anaesthesia 52:1151-1156, 1997.

111. Practice guidelines for preoperative fasting and the use of pharmacologic agents to reduce the risk of pulmonary aspiration: Application to healthy patients undergoing elective procedures: A report by the American Society of Anesthesiologists Task Force on Preoperative Fasting. Anesthesiology 90:896-905, 1999.

112. Rabey PG, Murphy PJ, Langton JA, et al: Effect of the laryngeal mask airway on lower oesophageal sphincter pressure in patients during general anaesthesia. Br J Anaesth 69:346-348, 1992.

113. Raidoo DM, Rocke DA, Brock-Utne JG, et al: Critical volume for pulmonary acid aspiration: Reappraisal in a primate model. Br J Anaesth 65:248-250, 1990.

114. Ralph SJ, Wareham CA: Rupture of the oesophagus during cricoid pressure. Anaesthesia 46:40-41, 1991.

115. Randell T, Saarvinaara L, Oikkonen M, et al: Oral atropine enhances the risk for acid aspiration in children. Acta Anaesthesiol Scand 35:651-653, 1991.

116. Read MS, Vaughan RS: Allowing pre-operative patients to drink: Effects on patients' safety and comfort of unlimited oral water until 2 hours before anaesthesia. Acta Anaesthesiol Scand 35:591-595, 1991.

117. Roberts JG, Sabar R, Gianoli JA, Kaye AD: Progressive systemic sclerosis: Clinical manifestations and anesthetic considerations. J Clin Anesth 14:474-477, 2002.

118. Roberts RB, Shirley MA: Antacid therapy in obstetrics. Anesthesiology 53:83, 1980.

119. Roberts RB, Shirley MA: Reducing the risk of acid aspiration during cesarean section. Anesth Analg 53:859-868, 1974.

120. Rocke DA, Brock-Utne JG, Rout CC: At risk for aspiration: New critical values of volume and pH? Anesth Analg 76:666, 1993.

121. Rout CC, Rocke DA, Gouws E: Intravenous ranitidine reduces the risk of acid aspiration of gastric contents at emergency cesarean section. Anesth Analg 76:156-161, 1993.

122. Ruffalo RL: Aspiration pneumonitis: Risk factors and management of the critically ill patient. DICP 24: S12-16, 1990.

123. Russin SJ, Adler AG: Pulmonary aspiration. Postgrad Med 85:155-161, 1989.

124. Saghaei M, Masoodifar M: The pressor response and airway effects of cricoid pressure during induction of general anesthesia. Anesth Analg 93:787-790, 2001.

125. Salem MR, Joseph NJ, Heyman HJ, et al: Cricoid compression is effective in obliterating the esophageal lumen in the presence of a nasogastric tube. Anesthesiology 63:443-446, 1985.

126. Sandhar BK, Goresky GV, Maltby JR, Shaffer EA: Effects of oral liquids and ranitidine on gastric fluid volume and pH in children undergoing outpatient surgery. Anesthesiology 71:327-330, 1989.

127. Satiani B, Bonner JT, Stone HH: Factors influencing intraoperative gastric regurgitation. Arch Surg 113: 721-723, 1978.

128. Schreiner MS, Triebwasser A, Keon TP: Ingestion of liquids compared with preoperative fasting in pediatric outpatients. Anesthesiology 72:593-597, 1990.

129. Schwartz DE, Matthay MA, Cohen NH: Death and other complications of emergency airway management in critically ill adults: A prospective investigation of 297 tracheal intubations. Anesthesiology 82:367-376, 1995.

130. Scrutton MJ, Metcalfe GA, Lowy C, et al: Eating in labour. A randomised controlled trial assessing the risks and benefits. Anaesthesia 54:329-334, 1999.

131. Sellick BA: Cricoid pressure to control regurgitation of stomach contents during induction of anaesthesia. Lancet 2:404, 1961.

132. Sethi AK, Chatterji C, Bhargava SK, et al: Safe pre-operative fasting times after milk or clear fluid in children. A preliminary study using real-time ultrasound. Anaesthesia 54:51-59, 1999.

133. Shaughnessy AF: Potential uses for metoclopramide. DICP 19:723-728, 1985.

134. Smith BE: Anesthetic emergencies. Clin Obstet Gynecol 28:391-404, 1985.

135. Smith CE, Boyer D: Cricoid pressure decreases ease of tracheal intubation using fibreoptic laryngoscopy (WuScope System). Can J Anaesth 49; 614-619, 2002.

136. Smith CL, Bardgett DM, Hunter JM: Haemodynamic effects of the i.v. administration of ranitidine in the critically ill patient. Br J Anaesth 59:1397-1402, 1987.

137. Sohma A, Brampton WJ, Dunnill MS, Sykes MK: Effect of ventilation with positive end-expiratory pressure on the development of lung damage in experimental acid aspiration pneumonia in the rabbit. Intensive Care Med 18:112-117, 1992.

138. Soreide E, Hausken T, Soreide JA, Steen PA: Gastric emptying of a light hospital breakfast. A study using real time ultrasonography. Acta Anaesthesiol Scand 40:549-553, 1996.

139. Splinter WM, Schaefer JD: Unlimited clear fluid ingestion two hours before surgery in children does not affect volume or pH of stomach contents. Anaesth Intensive Care 18:522-526, 1990.

140. Splinter WM, Schaefer JD, Bonn GE: Unlimited clear fluid ingestion by infants up to 2 hours before surgery is safe. Can J Anaesth 37:S95, 1990.

141. Splinter WM, Schreiner MS: Preoperative fasting in children. Anesth Analg 89:80-89, 1999.

142. Stept WJ, Safar P: Rapid induction/intubation for prevention of gastric-content aspiration. Anesth Analg 498:633, 1970.

143. Stone SB: Efficacy of cimetidine in decreasing the acidity and volume of gastric contents: Inadequacy of nasogastric suction and endotracheal intubation [letter]. J Trauma 21:996, 1981.

144. Strunin L: How long should patients fast before surgery? Time for new guidelines. Br J Anaesth 70:1,1993.

145. Taylor WJ, Champion MC, Barry AW, et al: Measuring gastric contents during general anaesthesia: Evaluation of blind gastric aspiration. Can J Anaesth 36:51-54, 1989.

146. Teabeaut JR: Aspiration of gastric contents. Am J Pathol 28:51, 1952.

147. Thwaites AJ, Rice CP, Smith I: Rapid sequence induction: A questionnaire survey of its routine conduct and continued management during a failed intubation. Anaesthesia 54:376-381, 1999.

148. Todd JG, Nimmo WS: Effect of premedication on drug absorption and gastric emptying. Br J Anaesth 55:1189-1193, 1983.

149. Tournadre JP, Chassard D, Berrada KR, Bouletreau P: Cricoid cartilage pressure decreases lower esophageal sphincter tone. Anesthesiology 86:7-9, 1997.

150. Trekova NA, Iavorovskii AG, Shmyrin MM, Grishin VV: Use of H2-receptor blocker famotidine in anesthesiology for cardiopulmonary bypass surgery. Anesteziol Reanimatol 1:16-19, 2002.

151. Vaisman N, Weintrob N, Blumenthal A, et al: Gastric emptying in patients with type I diabetes mellitus. Ann NY Acad Sci 873:506-511, 1999.

152. Van der Walt JH, Carter JA: The effect of different pre-operative feeding regimens on plasma glucose and gastric volume and pH in infancy. Anaesth Intensive Care 14:352-359, 1986.

153. Vanner RG, Asai T: Safe use of cricoid pressure. Anaesthesia 54:1-3, 1999.

154. Vanner RG, Clarke P, Moore WJ, Raftery S: The effect of cricoid pressure and neck support on the view at laryngoscopy. Anaesthesia 52:896-900, 1997.

155. Vanner RG, O'Dwyer JP, Pryle BJ, Reynolds F: Upper oesophageal sphincter pressure and the effect of cricoid pressure. Anaesthesia 47:95-100, 1992.

156. Veddeng OJ, Myhre ESP, Risoe C, Smiseth OA: Haemodynamic effects of selective positive end-expiratory pressure after unilateral pulmonary hydrochloric acid-aspiration in dogs. Intensive Care Med 18:356-361, 1992.

157. Verdich C, Madsen JL, Toubro S, et al: Effect of obesity and major weight reduction on gastric emptying. Int J Obes Relat Metab Disord 24:899-905, 2000.

158. Vila P, Valles J, Canet J, et al: Acid aspiration prophylaxis in morbidly obese patients: Famotidine vs. ranitidine. Anaesthesia 46:967-969, 1991.

159. Wajima Z, Shitara T, Inoue T, et al: The effect of previous administration of nizatidine on the neuromuscular effects of vecuronium and the effect of nizatidine on gastric secretion. Anaesth Intensive Care 28:46-48, 2000.

160. Warner MA, Warner ME, Warner DO, et al: Perioperative pulmonary aspiration in infants and children. Anesthesiology 90:66-71, 1999.

161. Warner MA, Warner ME, Weber JG: Clinical significance of pulmonary aspiration during the perioperative period. Anesthesiology 78:56-62, 1993.

162. Wingtin LN, Glomaud D, Hardy F, Phil S: Omeprazole for prophylaxis of acid aspiration in elective surgery. Anaesthesia 45:436-438, 1990.

163. Wong CA, Loffredi M, Ganchiff JN: Gastric emptying of water in term pregnancy. Anesthesiology 96:1395-1400, 2002.

164. Yamanaka Y, Mammoto T, Kita T, Kishi Y: A study of 13 patients with gastric tube in place after esophageal resection: Use of omeprazole to decrease gastric acidity and volume. J Clin Anesth 13:370-373, 2001.

165. Yau G, Kan AF, Gin T, et al: A comparison of omeprazole and ranitidine for prophylaxis against aspiration pneumonitis in emergency caesarean section. Anaesthesia 47:101-104, 1992.

166. Yuan CS, Foss JF, O'Connor M, et al: Effects of low-dose morphine on gastric emptying in healthy volunteers. J Clin Pharmacol 38:1017-1020, 1998.

167. Zimmermann DL, Breen TW, Fick G: Adding fentanyl 0.0002% to epidural bupivacaine 0.125% does not delay gastric emptying in laboring parturients. Anesth Analg 82:612-616, 1996.

12

PREOXYGENATION

Anis Baraka
M. Ramez Salem

I. HISTORICAL PERSPECTIVE

In 1948, Fowler and Comroe demonstrated that inhalation of 100% oxygen resulted in a very rapid increase of arterial oxyhemoglobin saturation (SaO_2) to 98% to 99%, but the attainment of the last 1% to 2% was a much slower process.[22] They also observed that the rate of increase is attenuated in patients with pulmonary emphysema or pulmonary artherosclerosis.[22] In 1955, Hamilton and Eastwood showed that "denitrogenation" was 95% complete within 2 to 3 minutes in subjects breathing normally from a circle anesthesia system with 5 L/min oxygen.[28] Dillon and Darsi, in the same year, observed significant arterial oxyhemoglobin desaturation during apnea following anesthetic induction with sodium thiopental and recommended that induction of anesthesia and endoscopy should be preceded by oxygen administration for 5 minutes.[17] Six years later, Heller and Watson found that 3 to 4 minutes of oxygen breathing was necessary in patients before anesthetic induction, whereas adequate oxygenation could be accomplished with the use of manual ventilation in 30 seconds.[31] With the introduction of the rapid sequence induction and intubation technique in the 1950s in patients who are at risk for aspiration of gastric contents, preoxygenation became an essential component of the technique.[46,59,63] Preoxygenation was also emphasized by Sellick when he introduced cricoid pressure in clinical practice in 1961.[57]

The administration of oxygen before anesthetic induction and intubation became a widely accepted maneuver designed to increase oxygen reserves and thereby delay the onset of arterial oxyhemoglobin desaturation during apnea. Various techniques and regimens have been advocated to ensure adequate preoxygenation. For many years, tidal volume breathing (TVB) of oxygen for 3 to 5 minutes has been commonly practiced.[17,28] Gold and colleagues challenged the need for 3 minutes of TVB by demonstrating that four deep breaths (DBs) within 0.5 minute and TVB for 5 minutes using a semiclosed circle absorber system were equally effective in increasing arterial oxygen tension (PaO_2).[26] Although some subsequent investigators corroborated their findings,[27,50] others showed that TVB for 3 minutes provided better preoxygenation and longer protection against hypoxemia during apnea than four DBs in 0.5 minute.[25,39,54,61] Later investigations suggested that the use of extended deep breathing to 8, 12, and

16 DBs in 1.0, 1.5, and 2.0 minutes, respectively, could produce maximal preoxygenation comparable to that achieved with TVB for 3 minutes and also delay the onset of apnea-induced oxyhemoglobin desaturation.[6,47]

Regardless of the technique used, preoxygenation has become an integral component of the rapid sequence induction technique and is particularly important if manual ventilation is not desirable, if there is difficulty with ventilation or endotracheal intubation is anticipated, and in patients with oxygen transport limitations. Because the "cannot ventilate, cannot intubate" situation is largely unpredictable, the desirability and need to preoxygenate maximally are theoretically present for all patients.[7] Along this line of thought, the original American Society of Anesthesiologists' (ASA) difficult airway algorithm made no mention of preoxygenation. In an updated report by the ASA Task Force on Management of the Difficult Airway (2003), "facemask preoxygenation before initiating management of the difficult airway" has been added.[53]

II. BODY OXYGEN STORES

Oxygen is carried in the blood in two forms: the greater portion is in reversible chemical combination with hemoglobin (HGB), and the smaller part is dissolved in plasma.[51] The ability to carry large amounts of oxygen in HGB is important because without it, the amount carried in the plasma would be so small that the cardiac output would need to be increased 20 times to yield an adequate oxygen flux.[51] The amount of chemically bound oxygen is directly related to the concentration of HGB and how saturated the HGB is with oxygen. Arterial oxygen content (CaO_2) can be calculated from the equation:

$$HGB \times 1.36 \times SaO_2 + PaO_2 \times 0.003$$

where 1.36 is the estimated mass volume of oxygen that can be bound by 1 g of normal HGB, SaO_2 is arterial oxyhemoglobin saturation (when fully saturated $SaO_2 = 100\%$), and 0.003 is the solubility coefficient of oxygen in human plasma. The CaO_2 of blood with an HGB concentration of 15 g/dL is about 20 mL of oxygen per 100 dL of blood. In addition, about 0.3 mL of oxygen per 100 dL of blood is in physical solution. This amount of dissolved oxygen normally accounts for only 1.5% of the total oxygen, but this contribution increases when PaO_2 is increased (dissolved oxygen is linearly related to PaO_2). The venous oxygen content ($C\bar{v}O_2$) of blood with a mixed venous oxygen tension ($P\bar{v}O_2$) of 40 mm Hg and mixed venous oxyhemoglobin saturation ($S\bar{v}O_2$) of 75% can be calculated accordingly.

Hemoglobin uptake and release of oxygen are regulated by a pattern demonstrated by the familiar oxyhemoglobin dissociation curve, which is a plot of SaO_2 as a function of PaO_2. The sigmoid shape of the curve reflects the fact that the four binding sites on a given HGB molecule interact with each other.[51] When the first site has bound a molecule of oxygen, the binding of the next site is facilitated, and so forth. The result is a curve that is steep up to a PO_2 of 60 mm Hg and becomes more shallow thereafter, approaching 100% saturation asymptotically. At a PO_2 of 100 mm Hg, the normal arterial value, 97% of the hemes have bound oxygen; at 40 mm Hg, a typical value for PO_2 in a resting person, the saturation declines to about 75%. The shape of the oxyhemoglobin dissociation curve has important physiologic implications. The flatness of the curve above a PO_2 of 80 mm Hg ensures a relatively constant SaO_2 despite wide variations in alveolar oxygen pressure. The steep portion of the curve between 20 and 60 mm Hg permits unloading of oxygen from HGB at relatively high PO_2 values, which favors the delivery of large amounts of oxygen into the tissue by diffusion.

The oxygen-binding properties of HGB are influenced by a number of factors, including pH, PCO_2, and temperature.[51] These factors cause shifts of the oxyhemoglobin dissociation curve to the right or left, without changing the slope of the curve. For example, an increase in temperature or a decrease in pH, such as may occur in active tissues, decreases the affinity of HGB for oxygen and shifts the oxyhemoglobin dissociation curve to the right. Thus, a higher PO_2 is required to achieve a given saturation, which facilitates unloading of oxygen at the tissue. To quantify the extent of a shift of the oxyhemoglobin dissociation curve, the so-called P50 is used, that is, the PO_2 required for 50% saturation. The P50 of normal adult HGB at 37° C and normal pH and PCO_2 is 26 to 27 mm Hg.

Despite its great importance, oxygen is a very difficult gas to store in a biologic system. In subjects breathing air, oxygen stores are small (Table 12-1).[15,51] The relatively steep oxyhemoglobin dissociation curve and the small oxygen stores imply that factors affecting PaO_2 produce

Table 12-1 **Body Oxygen Stores during Room Air and 100% Oxygen Breathing**

Store	Room Air	100% Oxygen
In the lungs (functional residual capacity)	450 mL	3000 mL
In the blood	850 mL	950 mL
Dissolved in tissue fluids	50 mL	100 mL
In combination with myoglobin	200 mL?	200 mL
Total	1550 mL	4250 mL

From Nunn JF (ed): Applied Respiratory Physiology, 4th ed. Oxford, Butterworth-Heinemann, 1995, p 288.

their full effects very quickly. This is in contrast to carbon dioxide (CO_2), for which the large size of the stores buffers the body against rapid changes. Thus, in a subject breathing air, a pulse oximeter probably gives an earlier indication of hypoventilation than CO_2 measurement. In contrast, in a subject breathing a high fraction of inspired oxygen (FIO_2), CO_2 measurement gives an earlier indication of hypoventilation.[51]

The principal stores of body oxygen while breathing air are significantly increased with breathing 100% oxygen (Fig. 12-1; see Table 12-1).[15,51] The maximal increase of oxygen stores occurs in the functional residual capacity (FRC). Storage of oxygen in the tissue is rather more difficult to assess, but assuming that Henry's law applies and the partition coefficient for gases approximates the gas-water coefficients, breathing oxygen for 3 minutes significantly increases tissue oxygen stores.[15]

III. APNEIC MASS-MOVEMENT OXYGENATION

Preoxygenation followed by oxygen insufflation during subsequent apnea maintains SaO_2 by apneic diffusion oxygenation.[23,24] In the apneic adult, total-body oxygen consumption ($\dot{V}O_2$) averages 230 mL/min while the output of CO_2 to the alveoli is limited to about 21 mL/min and the rest (about 90%) of CO_2 production is buffered within the body tissues. The lung volume initially decreases by the net gas exchange ratio of 209 mL/min. Thus, a pressure gradient is created between the upper airway and alveoli, resulting, if the airway is patent, in a subsequent mass movement of oxygen down the trachea into the alveoli. Conversely, CO_2 is not exhaled because of this mass movement of oxygen down the trachea and the alveolar carbon dioxide concentration ($PACO_2$) shows an initial rise of about 8 to 16 mm Hg in

the first minute and a subsequent fairly linear rise of about 3 mm Hg/min.[20] Fraioli and coauthors emphasized the importance of the FRC/body weight ratio during apneic diffusion and demonstrated that patients with a low FRC/body weight ratio could not tolerate apnea for more than 4 minutes, whereas those with a high FRC/body weight ratio (>53.3 ± 7 mL/kg) maintained PaO_2 at 90% of the control value.[23]

Apneic mass-movement oxygenation can easily be achieved by preoxygenation followed by insufflation of oxygen through a nasopharyngeal or oropharyngeal cannula or through a needle inserted in the cricothyroid or cricotracheal membrane. This provides at least 10 minutes of adequate oxygenation in healthy apneic patients whose airways are unobstructed and thus has many practical applications.[60] In patients who are difficult to intubate or ventilate, pharyngeal oxygen insufflation (or tracheal, in case of upper airway obstruction) may allow additional time for laryngoscopy and endotracheal intubation. This can be particularly advantageous in patients who also have decreased oxygen reserves secondary to decreased FRC and increased $\dot{V}O_2$, such as children, pregnant women, obese patients, and patients with adult respiratory distress syndrome (ARDS).[3] The combination of preoxygenation and apneic diffusion oxygenation can be used during bronchoscopy[33] and can provide the otolaryngologist with adequate time for glottic surgery unimpeded by the presence of the tracheal tube or by the patients' respiratory movements.

IV. EFFICACY AND EFFICIENCY OF PREOXYGENATION

Studies of preoxygenation have focused on measurements of indices reflecting its efficacy and efficiency.[7] Measurements of alveolar oxygen,[9,12,54] alveolar nitrogen,[16] or PaO_2[1,6,16,26] reflect the efficacy of preoxygenation, whereas the decline of SaO_2 during apnea is indicative of its efficiency.[7]

A. EFFICACY OF PREOXYGENATION

Preoxygenation increases the alveolar oxygen and decreases the alveolar nitrogen in a parallel fashion (Fig. 12-2). It is the washout of nitrogen from the lungs that is the key to achieving preoxygenation.[16] Preoxygenation and denitrogenation have been used synonymously to describe the same process, although a change in focus from preoxygenation to denitrogenation has been suggested.[16] Denitrogenation of the lungs is 95% complete within 3 minutes when the subject is breathing at a normal tidal volume from a circle absorber system with a 5-L fresh gas flow (FGF) of oxygen. With normal lung function, the oxygen washin and nitrogen washout are exponential functions and, thus, the rate of preoxygenation (or denitrogenation) is governed by the time constant (t) of the

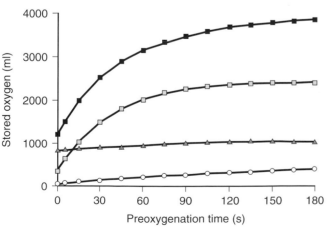

Figure 12-1 Variation in volume of oxygen stored in the functional residual capacity (□), the blood (▲), the tissue (○), and the whole body (■) with duration of preoxygenation. (From Campbell IT, Beatty PCW: Monitoring preoxygenation. Br J Anaesth 72:3-4, 1994.)

Figure 12-2 Comparison of mean end-tidal oxygen and nitrogen concentrations obtained at 30-second intervals during 5-minute periods of spontaneous tidal volume oxygenation using the circle absorber and NasOral systems in 20 volunteers. Data shown as mean ± SD. (From Nimmagadda U, Salem MR, Joseph NJ, et al: Efficacy of preoxygenation with tidal volume breathing. Comparison of breathing systems. Anesthesiology 93:693-698, 2000.)

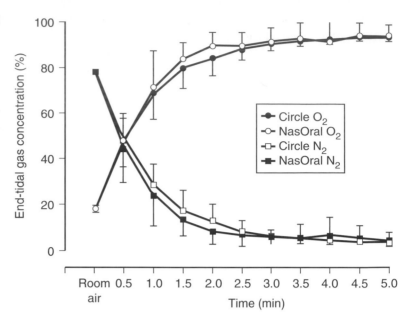

exponential curves. This t is the same for both washin and washout curves and is proportional to the ratio of alveolar ventilation to FRC ($\dot{V}_A$/FRC). The endpoints of maximal alveolar preoxygenation or denitrogenation have been defined as an end-tidal oxygen concentration (ET_{O_2}) of approximately 90% and an end-tidal nitrogen concentration (ET_{N_2}) of 5%.[9,12,61] Because of the obligatory presence of CO_2 and water vapor in the alveolar gas, an ET_{O_2} higher than 97% cannot be easily achieved. Factors affecting the efficacy of preoxygenation include F_{IO_2}, duration of breathing, and the $\dot{V}_A$/FRC ratio (Table 12-2).

1. Fraction of Inspired Oxygen

The main reasons for the failure to achieve an F_{IO_2} close to 1.0 are a leak under the face mask,[7,11,18,41,54] rebreathing exhaled gases, and the use of systems incapable of delivering a high oxygen concentration, such as resuscitation bags.[30] Even the presence of minor leaks may not be fully compensated for by increasing the FGF or by increasing the duration of preoxygenation. Bearded patients, edentulous patients, patients with sunken cheeks, the presence of nasogastric tubes, use of a wrong face mask size, improper use of head straps, and use of systems allowing air entrainment under the face mask are all common factors causing leaks between the face mask and the patient's head resulting in lower F_{IO_2}. Clinical endpoints indicative of a sealed system are movement of the reservoir bag in and out with each inhalation and exhalation, presence of a normal capnogram and ET_{CO_2}, and measurements of inspired and end-tidal oxygen values.[7,58]

There is reluctance among some anesthesiologists to use preoxygenation routinely because the mask presents discomfort to the patient and some patients find preoxygenation objectionable.[38] A study clearly found marked overestimation of the patient's discomfort by the anesthesiologist. In fact, patients' discomfort during preoxygenation is not more than the discomfort during other procedures such as the placement of intravenous lines.[38] It is the authors' experience that patients accept a tight-fitting mask if the procedure is explained beforehand and they are told that "it is important to fill the tank with oxygen."

Although anesthetic circuits can deliver 100% oxygen concentration, the F_{IO_2} can be influenced by the type of

Table 12-2 Factors Affecting the Efficacy and Efficiency of Preoxygenation

Factors Affecting Efficacy
Inspired oxygen concentration
Leak
System used
FGF, type of breathing (TVB or DB)
Duration of breathing
$\dot{V}_A$/FRC
Factors Affecting Efficiency
Capacity of oxygen loading
P_{AO_2} and FRC
Ca_{O_2} and CO
$\dot{V}_{O_2}$

Ca_{O_2} = arterial oxygen content; CO = cardiac output; DB = deep breathing; FGF = fresh gas flow; P_{AO_2} = alveolar oxygen concentration; TVB = tidal volume breathing; $\dot{V}_A$/FRC = alveolar ventilation to function residual capacity ratio; $\dot{V}_{O_2}$ = oxygen consumption.

breathing (TVB or DB), level of FGF, and the duration of breathing.[47] In a study involving volunteers comparing preoxygenation techniques using a semiclosed circle absorber with varying FGF in the same subjects, it was found that with TVB, inspired oxygen concentration was 95% with FGF of 5 L/min and increased to 98% with FGF of 7 and 10 L/min (Fig. 12-3).[47] However, with deep breathing, inspired oxygen concentration was only 88% at 5 L/min FGF, 91% at 7 L/min FGF, and 95% at 10 L/min FGF (see Fig. 12-3).[47] These findings imply that increasing the FGF from 5 to 10 L/min has little impact in increasing FIO_2 during TVB but has a noticeable effect during deep breathing.[47] Because of the breathing characteristics of the circle system, the minute ventilation during deep breathing may exceed the FGF, resulting in rebreathing of exhaled gases (N_2) and consequently decreasing the inspired oxygen concentration, whereas during TVB, rebreathing of exhaled gases is rather negligible and thus increasing the FGF (from 5 to 10 L/min) would have only a slight effect on the inspired oxygen concentration.[25,47]

2. Duration of Breathing and FRC and $\dot{V}_A$

Sufficient time is needed to accomplish maximal preoxygenation. With an FIO_2 close to 1, most healthy adult patients can reach the target level of ETO_2 greater than or equal to 90% (or $ETN_2 \leq 5\%$) in 3 to 5 minutes of TVB. The half-time for exponential change in alveolar oxygen fraction (FAO_2) with a step change in FIO_2 is given by the equation $0.693 \times VFRC/\dot{V}_A$ for a nonrebreathing system. With $V_{FRC} = 2.5$ L, the half-times are 26 and 13 seconds when $\dot{V}_A = 4$ and 8 L/min, respectively.[7] Thus, most of the oxygen that can be stored in the lungs can be brought in by hyperventilation with an $FIO_2 = 1.0$ for a shorter period of time than the oxygen that can be stored with TVB.[7] This is the basis for the deep breathing techniques, which have been introduced as an alternative to the traditional TVB.[8]

Changes in $\dot{V}_A$ and FRC can have a marked effect on the rate of rise in ETO_2 (and decrease in ETN_2) during preoxygenation. Because of the increase in $\dot{V}_A$ and decrease in FRC in pregnant women, ETO_2 rises faster than in nonpregnant women.[5,14,54] Similarly, preoxygenation can be accomplished faster in infants and children than in adults.[13,56]

B. EFFICIENCY OF PREOXYGENATION

The delay in arterial oxyhemoglobin desaturation during apnea depends on the efficacy of preoxygenation, capacity for oxygen loading, and $\dot{V}O_2$ (see Table 12-2). Patients with a decreased capacity for oxygen loading (decreased FRC, PAO_2, CaO_2, or cardiac output) or increased $\dot{V}O_2$, or both, desaturate much faster during apnea than healthy patients.[7,8,18,21,29,30] The main difference in the rate of apnea-induced oxyhemoglobin desaturation after different preoxygenation techniques is observed between SaO_2 of 100% and 99%.[7,8,21] This range represents the flat portion of the oxyhemoglobin dissociation curve. When oxygen reserves are depleted, rapid desaturation occurs regardless of the technique of preoxygenation and is similar to that observed in patients breathing air.

Farmery and Roe developed an intriguing computer model describing the rate of oxyhemoglobin desaturation during apnea.[21] This model was found to agree reasonably well with actual data from patients whose weight and degree of normalcy and preoxygenation were reliably known (Fig. 12-4).[8,21] Because it would be dangerous to obtain time to marked oxyhemoglobin desaturation data in humans, this model is uniquely useful for analysis of oxyhemoglobin saturation using pulse oximetry (SpO_2)

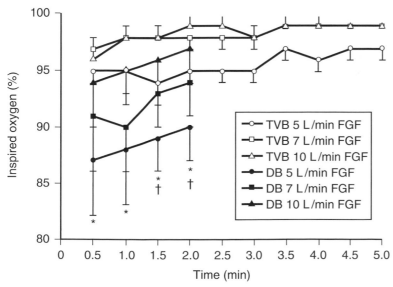

Figure 12-3 Comparison of tidal volume breathing (TVB) and deep breathing (DB) preoxygenation techniques on inspired oxygen using 5, 7, and 10 L/min fresh gas flow (FGF). *Significant difference between 5, 7, and 10 L/min FGF; †significant difference from DB at 0.5 and 1.0 minute. Statistical difference accepted when $P < .05$. (From Nimmagadda U, Chiravuri SD, Salem MR, et al: Preoxygenation with tidal volume and deep breathing techniques: The impact of duration of breathing and fresh gas flow. Anesth Analg 92:1337-1341, 2001.)

Figure 12-4 Arterial oxyhemoglobin saturation (Sa_{O_2}) versus time of apnea in the obese patient, in a 10-kg child (low functional residual capacity and high O_2), and in a moderately ill adult versus a healthy adult. (From Benumof JL, Dagg R, Benumof R: Critical hemoglobin desaturation will occur before return to unparalyzed state from 1mg/kg succinylcholine. Anesthesiology 87:979-982, 1997.)

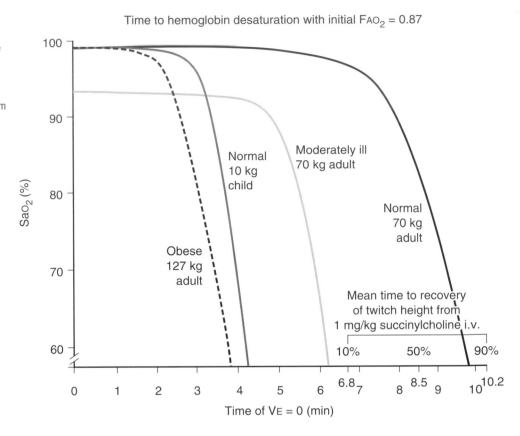

below 90%.[8,21] When preapnea FA_{O_2} is progressively decreased from 0.87 to 0.8, 0.7, 0.6, 0.5, 0.4, 0.3, and 0.13 (air) for a healthy 70-kg patient, apnea times to $Sa_{O_2} = 60\%$ are progressively decreased from 9.9 to 9.31, 8.38, 7.30, 6.37, 5.40, 4.40, 3.55, and 2.8 minutes, respectively.[8,21] Figure 12-4 shows that for a healthy 70-kg adult, a moderately ill 70-kg adult, a healthy 10-kg child, and an obese 127-kg adult, $Sa_{O_2} = 80\%$ is reached after 8.7, 5.5, 3.7, and 3.1 minutes, respectively, whereas $Sa_{O_2} = 60\%$ is reached at 9.9, 6.2, 4.23, and 3.8 minutes, respectively.[8] Critical oxyhemoglobin desaturation is defined as Sp_{O_2} less than or equal to 80% and decreasing; for the patients shown in the figure at Sp_{O_2} less than or equal to 80%, the range in rate of decrease is 20% to 4% per minute.

V. TECHNIQUES OF PREOXYGENATION

Two main techniques are used: TVB and deep breathing (Table 12-3).

A. TIDAL VOLUME BREATHING

The traditional TVB of oxygen has been undoubtedly proved to be an effective preoxygenation technique. To ensure maximal preoxygenation, the duration of TVB should be 3 minutes or longer in most adults and

an FI_{O_2} near 1 should be maintained (see Table 12-3 and Fig. 12-2). Various anesthetic systems (circle absorber,[25-27,50] Mapleson A,[10,54] Mapleson D,[39,54,61] and nonrebreathing systems[28,39,41]) and FGFs ranging from 5 to 35 L/min have been used successfully.[27,61] However, the semiclosed circle absorber system (the commonest system used in the operating room) at an FGF as low as 5 L/min is just as effective.[47] Increasing the FGF from 5 to 10 L/min has little effect in enhancing preoxygenation during TVB (Fig. 12-5).[47]

Table 12-3 Techniques of Preoxygenation

Tidal Volume Breathing
Traditional tidal volume breathing (3-5 min)
One vital capacity breath followed by tidal volume breathing
Deep Breathing
Single vital capacity breath
4 deep breaths (4 inspiratory capacity breaths)
8 deep breaths (8 inspiratory capacity breaths)
Extended deep breathing (12-16 inspiratory capacity breaths)
One vital capacity breath followed by deep breathing

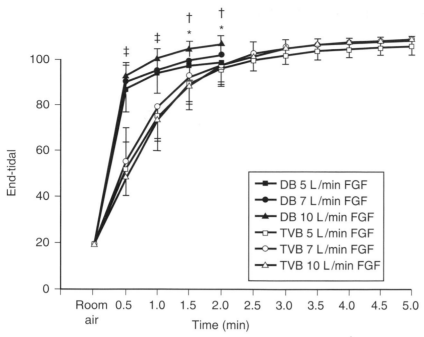

Figure 12-5 Comparison of tidal volume breathing (TVB) and deep breathing (DB) preoxygenation techniques on end-tidal oxygen using 5, 7, and 10 L/min fresh gas flow (FGF). *Significant difference from DB at 5 and 7 L/min FGF; †significant difference from DB at 0.5 and 1.0 minute; ‡significant difference from TVB. Statistical difference accepted when $P < .05$. (From Nimmagadda U, Chiravuri SD, Salem MR, et al: Preoxygenation with tidal volume and deep breathing techniques: The impact of duration of breathing and fresh gas flow. Anesth Analg 92:1337-1341, 2001.)

B. DEEP BREATHING TECHNIQUES

On the basis of the assumption that alveolar denitrogenation can be achieved rapidly by deep breathing, Gold and colleagues introduced the 4 DBs in 0.5 minute (4 DB/0.5 min) method of preoxygenation.[26] They showed that PaO_2 after 4 DB/0.5 min was not different from PaO_2 after TVB for 3 minutes (TVB/3 min). Although a few studies corroborated their findings,[27,50] other investigations showed that TVB/3 min provided more effective preoxygenation (see Fig. 12-5) and longer protection against hypoxemia during apnea than the 4 DB/0.5 min method, particularly in pregnant women, morbidly obese patients, and elderly patients.[25,39,54,61]

There are two main reasons why the 4 DB/0.5 min method is inferior to TVB. First, if the ventilation in 0.5 minute is much greater than the oxygen inflow rate, rebreathing of exhaled nitrogen must occur, which decreases FIO_2. Nimmagadda and coworkers confirmed that 4 DB/0.5 min provided suboptimal preoxygenation in volunteers (no subject achieved an ETO_2 value $\geq 90\%$) (see Fig. 12-5).[47] Another possible reason why patients preoxygenated with 4 DB/0.5 min desaturate faster is that the tissue and venous compartments need more than 0.5 minute to fill with oxygen.[15] Probably, these compartments have the capability of storing additional oxygen above that contained while breathing room air.[47] Such stored oxygen increases in an exponential fashion. Thus, it is possible that the 4 DB/0.5 min technique results in rapid arterial oxygenation without substantial increase in the tissue oxygen stores and hence results in more rapid desaturation during subsequent apnea than would a longer period of preoxygenation with TVB.[6] Because the 4 DB/0.5 min technique yields submaximal

preoxygenation, it should be reserved for emergency situations only when time is limited.[47]

To optimize the deep breathing method of preoxygenation, investigators focused on (1) extending the duration of deep breathing to 1, 1.5, and 2 minutes to allow 8, 12, and 16 DB, respectively,[6,47] and (2) the use of high FGF greater than or equal to 10 L/min.[6,47] These maneuvers result in maximal preoxygenation (evidenced by higher ETO_2, PaO_2, and lower ETN_2) and improved efficiency (delayed onset of oxyhemoglobin desaturation during apnea) than the original 4 DB/0.5 min.[6,47] An investigation suggested that preoxygenation using 8 DB/1.0 min at an FGF of 10 L/min is associated with slower oxyhemoglobin desaturation than that following 4 DB/0.5 min and TVB/3 min (Fig. 12-6).[6] Several explanations were given for this surprising finding, including leftward shift of the oxyhemoglobin dissociation curve secondary to hyperventilation-induced reduction in $PaCO_2$ (Fig. 12-7) and the occurrence of several extra DBs during anesthetic induction.[7,55]

The use of maximal exhalation before any preoxygenation maneuver has been suggested.[4,40] In a healthy subject with an FRC of 3 L, forced exhalation to the residual volume decreases the lung volume to about 1.5 L. A 50% reduction of the FRC leads to 50% reduction in the t (time constant) of the oxygen washin (nitrogen washout) curve. This maneuver of maximal exhalation can improve the efficacy of preoxygenation with either 4 DB/0.5 min or TVB (Fig. 12-8).[4,40]

It has also been demonstrated that preoxygenation using the single vital capacity breath (SVCB) technique can provide within 30 seconds a PaO_2 comparable to that achieved by TVB/min (Fig. 12-9). This technique

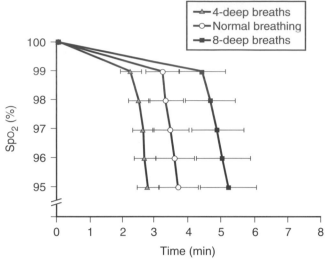

Figure 12-6 Mean times to reach percentage decrease in hemoglobin saturation during apnea after three different preoxygenation techniques. Spo₂, oxygen saturation from pulse oximetry. (From Baraka AS, Taha SK Aouad MT, et al: Preoxygenation. Comparison of maximal breathing and tidal volume breathing techniques. Anesthesiology 91:612-616, 1999.)

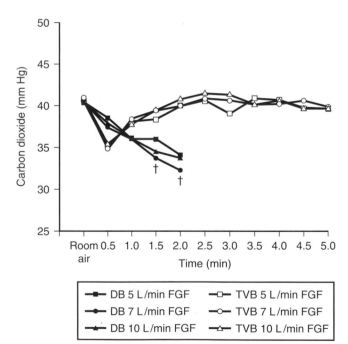

Figure 12-7 Effect of the deep breathing (DB) technique on end-tidal carbon dioxide using 5, 7, and 10 L/min fresh gas flow (FGF). TVB, tidal volume breathing. †Significant difference from DB at 0.5 and 1.0 minute. Statistical difference accepted when $P < .05$. (From Nimmagadda U, Chiravuri SD, Salem MR, et al: Preoxygenation with tidal volume and deep breathing techniques: The impact of duration of breathing and fresh gas flow. Anesth Analg 92:1337-1341, 2001.)

is basically a triphasic process. The first phase consists of forced exhalation to the residual volume. This minimizes lung nitrogen content and the subsequent dilution of incoming oxygen. The second phase is deep inspiration to expand the lungs to their total capacity, with a consequent maximal increase of the P_{AO_2}. The third phase consists of holding the chest in full inspiratory position, which may increase the alveolar-capillary oxygen diffusion. The breath-hold also allows gas movement from the compliant alveoli to the less compliant alveoli (pendelluft maximization) because the time constants of filling between alveoli are not uniform. The SVCB technique can optimize preoxygenation, especially when it is used for fast induction of inhalation anesthesia.

VI. BREATHING SYSTEMS FOR PREOXYGENATION

All anesthetic circuits (the standard semiclosed circle absorber, Mapleson's classified systems) used in the operating room are capable of delivering high F_{IO_2} and thus can provide maximal preoxygenation. A relatively new system designed specifically for preoxygenation has gained some popularity in Europe (NasOral, LogoMed GambH, Windhagen, Germany).[42,43] The NasOral system is a nonrebreathing system that delivers oxygen from a 3.3-L reservoir bag to a small nasal mask, with exhalation occurring by the oral route by means of a mouthpiece.[42,43] One-way valves in the nasal mask and the mouthpiece ensure unidirectional flow (Fig. 12-10). The FGF is adjusted to the individual ventilation to maintain an inflated reservoir bag.[42,43] Investigations showed that the circle absorber and NasOral systems are equally effective in achieving alveolar oxygenation despite their different characteristics (see Fig. 12-2).[49] Accordingly, there is little justification for the additional cost of this device for use in the operating room, where the circle absorber system can be used for preoxygenation, administration of anesthesia, and positive-pressure ventilation.[49]

In the critical care setting, resuscitation bags are commonly used for preoxygenation. However, the effectiveness of various resuscitation bags differs markedly during spontaneous respiration.[49] Some, because of their design, cannot deliver high F_{IO_2} despite an FGF of 15 L/min or greater (Fig. 12-11).[49] Resuscitation bags can be categorized into two groups depending on the type of valve mechanism. Disk-type valve systems use single or multiple disks to allow fresh gas to flow to the subject (and seal the exhalation port) during inspiration. The disk returns to its former position and opens the exhalation port during exhalation (Fig. 12-12). Because this disk valve function is not dependent on compression of the reservoir bag, this type of resuscitation bag functions equally well during manual and spontaneous ventilation. Consequently, this type of resuscitation bag can be used

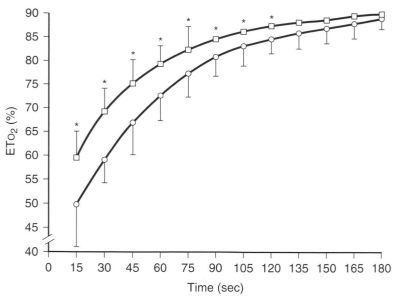

Figure 12-8 Comparison of end-tidal oxygen values over a 3-minute period during preoxygenation by the tidal volume breathing technique following maximal exhalation (□) versus tidal volume breathing (○). (From Baraka A, Taha SK, El-Khatib MF, et al: Oxygenation using tidal volume breathing after maximal exhalation. Anesth Analg 97:1533-1535, 2003.)

effectively for preoxygenation in the critical care setting.[32,44,49]

Resuscitation bags using duckbill inspiratory valves function differently during manual and spontaneous ventilation.[44,49] During manual ventilation, gas is forced through the valve base, opening the duckbill valve and delivering fresh gas to the patient's lungs. This force also seals the valve base to the exhalation port. During exhalation, the valve base returns to its former position, and exhaled gases are vented to the exhalation port (Fig. 12-13). The efficacy of the duckbill-type resuscitation bags in delivering high F_{IO_2} during spontaneous breathing has been studied by Mills and associates.[44] They found that duckbill-type resuscitation bags, without one-way exhalation valves to prevent air entrainment, showed variability in delivered oxygen concentration during spontaneous breathing.[44] These findings have been

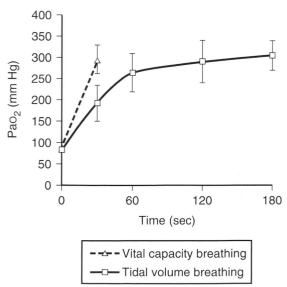

Figure 12-9 The mean arterial oxygen tension (Pa_{O_2}) achieved after preoxygenation by the single vital capacity breath technique (△) compared with that achieved by the traditional preoxygenation technique (○). (From Baraka A, Haroun-Bizri S, Khoury S, et al: Single vital capacity breath for preoxygenation. Can J Anaesth 47:1144-1146, 2000.)

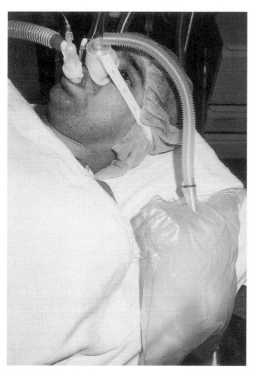

Figure 12-10 The NasOral system uses a small nasal mask for inspiration of oxygen from a reservoir bag. Exhalation occurs through a mouthpiece. One-way valves in the nasal mask and the mouthpiece ensure unidirectional flow. (From Nimmagadda U, Salem MR, Joseph NJ, et al: Efficacy of preoxygenation with tidal volume breathing. Comparison of breathing systems. Anesthesiology 93:693-698, 2000.)

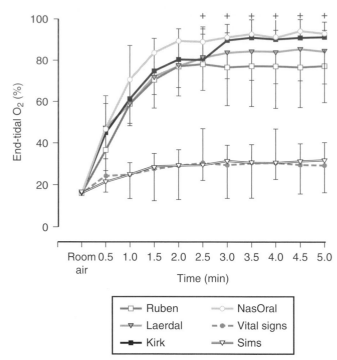

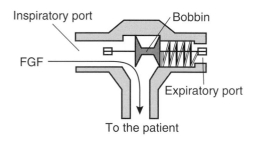

Figure 12-11 Comparison of mean end-tidal oxygen concentrations obtained at 30-second intervals during 5-minute periods of spontaneous tidal volume oxygenation using the NasOral system and five resuscitation bags in 20 volunteers. Data shown as mean ± SD. +Significant difference between systems. (From Nimmagadda U, Salem MR, Joseph NJ, et al: Efficacy of preoxygenation with tidal volume breathing. Comparison of breathing systems. Anesthesiology 93:693-698, 2000.)

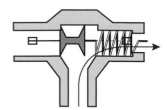

Figure 12-12 Diagram of a typical disk valve in a disk-type resuscitation bag. During inhalation (*top*), the piston seals the exhalation port and allows fresh gas to flow to the patient. During exhalation (*bottom*), the fresh gas port is sealed by the piston while gas is allowed to flow to the exhalation port. FGF, fresh gas flow. (From Moyle JTB, Davey A [eds]: Ward's Anaesthetic Equipment. London, WB Saunders, 1998, p 190.)

confirmed by Nimmagadda and colleagues,[49] who showed that some duckbill resuscitation bags cannot deliver a high F_{IO_2} during spontaneous ventilation even if a high FGF is used. In the absence of a one-way valve on the exhalation port, generation of sufficient negative pressure to open the duckbill valve becomes impossible.[49] During inspiration, the unsealed valve base allows room air to enter through the exhalation port and mix with oxygen from a partially open duckbill valve (see Fig. 12-13).[49] The addition of a one-way valve on the exhalation port, duckbill-type resuscitation bags (Laerdal and Kirk) can reliably deliver an F_{IO_2} greater than 0.9 with an FGF of 15 L/min.[49] This valve seals the exhalation port during inspiration and allows the patient to generate sufficient negative pressure to open the duckbill valve, permitting oxygen to flow without dilution (see Fig. 12-13).[49]

The NasOral system has advantages over resuscitation bags when used for preoxygenation. (1) It provides better preoxygenation than all available resuscitation bags because of a higher F_{IO_2} and reduced apparatus dead space (see Fig. 12-11). (2) It is economical when oxygen tanks are used because it requires an FGF comparable to the subject's minute ventilation.[48] (3) It can provide apneic oxygenation through the nasal mask during laryngoscopy and orotracheal intubation, if needed. Disadvantages of the NasOral system are that it requires patients' cooperation to use the mouthpiece and the system cannot be used for positive-pressure ventilation.[49]

The inability of a resuscitation bag to deliver a high F_{IO_2} may have serious consequences during rapid sequence induction and intubation in the critical care setting or during transport of the spontaneously breathing, critically ill patient.[49] Clinicians should ascertain that the resuscitation bags used in their institution are capable of delivering a high F_{IO_2} during spontaneous ventilation.[49]

VII. SPECIAL SITUATIONS

A. PREGNANCY

Because pregnant women are at high risk for pulmonary aspiration, rapid sequence induction or intubation is desirable whenever general anesthesia is administered to them. Maximal preoxygenation can be achieved faster in pregnant than in nonpregnant women because of the increased $\dot{V}_A$ and decreased FRC.[14,50,54] However, during apnea, pregnant women become hypoxemic more rapidly because of the limited oxygen stores in their small FRC and the increased $\dot{V}_{O_2}$.[5] From the fifth month of pregnancy, the FRC decreases to 80% of that in the nonpregnant state, while the $\dot{V}_{O_2}$ increases by 30% to 40%. In pregnant women, preoxygenation can be accomplished by TVB for 3 minutes or by deep breathing for 1 minute or longer before anesthetic induction. A combination of both techniques may also be used. Because the 4 DB/0.5 min technique provides suboptimal oxygenation, it should be

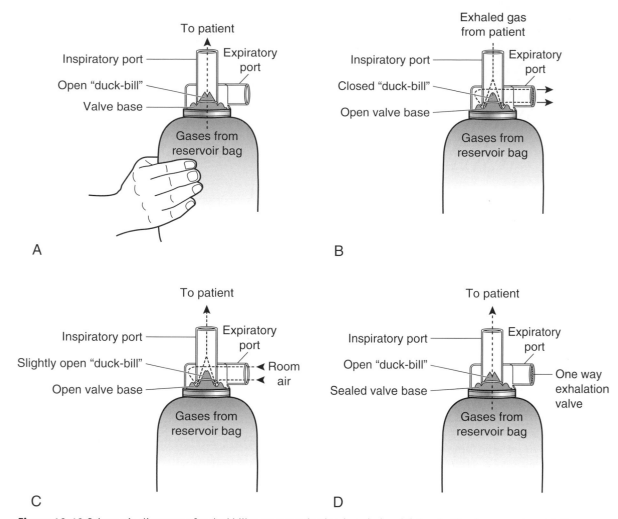

To patient

Inspiratory port

Open "duck-bill"

Valve base

Expiratory port

Gases from reservoir bag

A

Exhaled gas from patient

Inspiratory port

Closed "duck-bill"

Open valve base

Expiratory port

Gases from reservoir bag

B

To patient

Inspiratory port

Slightly open "duck-bill"

Open valve base

Expiratory port

Room air

Gases from reservoir bag

C

To patient

Inspiratory port

Open "duck-bill"

Sealed valve base

Expiratory port

One way exhalation valve

Gases from reservoir bag

D

Figure 12-13 Schematic diagrams of a duckbill-type resuscitation bag during (**A**) inspiration by manual ventilation, (**B**) exhalation by manual or spontaneous ventilation, (**C**) spontaneous inspiration without a one-way exhalation valve, and (**D**) spontaneous inspiration with a one-way exhalation valve.

used only in emergency situations when time is limited. The influence of preoxygenation in the supine position versus 45-degree head-up position on the duration of apnea leading to a decrease in SaO_2 to 95% has been investigated.[5] The average time to 95% arterial oxyhemoglobin desaturation was shorter in pregnant than nonpregnant patients (173 versus 243 seconds) in the supine position.[5] Using the head-up position resulted in an increase in the oxyhemoglobin desaturation time in nonpregnant patients but no effect in pregnant patients.[5]

B. MORBIDLY OBESE PATIENTS

Because of their relatively small FRC (limited oxygen reservoir) and their higher than normal $\dot{V}O_2$, apnea in morbidly obese patients can result in progressive oxyhemoglobin desaturation[10,27,34] (Fig. 12-14). Accordingly, it is imperative to achieve maximal preoxygenation in these patients before the onset of apnea by either TVB/3 min

or deep breathing for 1 minute or longer of oxygen. There appears to be little difference between preoxygenation performed in the head-up or lateral position compared with the supine position in morbidly obese patients.[48] In these patients, oxygen insufflation through a nasopharyngeal or oropharyngeal catheter during laryngoscopy and intubation may further delay the onset of arterial oxyhemoglobin desaturation during apnea.

C. ELDERLY PATIENTS

Several changes that occur during the aging process may influence the period of preoxygenation that is needed in elderly patients and the subsequent time of oxyhemoglobin desaturation to a given level.[12,39,61] On one hand, the basal $\dot{V}O_2$ declines with age (from 143 mL/min · m² in a male aged 20 years to 124 mL/min · m² in a male aged 60 years) so that the demand for oxygen is less; on the other hand, changes in the lung function make oxygen

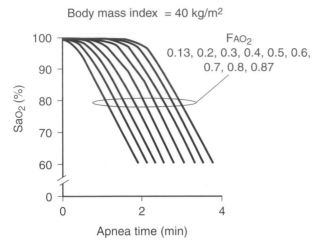

Figure 12-14 Diagram comparing the mean time to apnea-induced oxyhemoglobin desaturation during apnea in a morbidly obese patient. F_{AO_2}, alveolar oxygen fraction ; Sa_{O_2}, arterial oxyhemoglobin saturation. (From Benumof JL: ASA Refresher Course Lectures, 2002.)

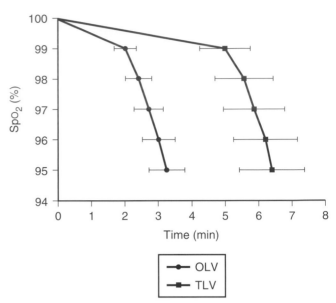

Figure 12-15 Diagram comparing the mean time to apnea-induced oxyhemoglobin desaturation from pulse oximetry oxygen saturation (Sp_{O_2}) of 100% down to 95% following two-lung ventilation (TLV) versus one-lung ventilation (OLV). (From Baraka A, Aouad M, Taha S, et al: Apnea-induced hemoglobin desaturation during one-lung vs two-lung ventilation. Can J Anaesth 47:58-61, 2000.)

uptake less efficient. In particular, the closing volume increases with age, leading to less efficient denitrogenation; this could mean that longer periods of preoxygenation are required in elderly patients. The reduction of oxygen demand in elderly patients does not compensate fully for less efficient oxygen uptake because the mean times to 93% preoxygenation in elderly patients are approximately one half those reported for equivalent preoxygenation periods in young patients. Reliable preoxygenation can be achieved with extended TVB or deep breathing for longer than 3 minutes or 1 minute, respectively.

D. LUNG DISEASE

Patients with ARDS have decreased FRC, increased intrapulmonary shunting, and increased $\dot{V}_{O_2}$, and hence interruption of ventilation or suctioning can result in rapid oxyhemoglobin desaturation. It has been shown that in patients undergoing thoracic surgery the rate of oxyhemoglobin desaturation during apnea is faster after one-lung ventilation that after two-lung ventilation. The time of oxyhemoglobin desaturation after one-lung ventilation is nearly one half the time after two-lung ventilation (Fig. 12-15).[2] This fast rate of oxyhemoglobin desaturation during one-lung ventilation can be attributed to collapse of the nonventilated lung with a consequent decrease of the FRC oxygen store; the rate of oxyhemoglobin desaturation may be further exaggerated by the associated right-to-left intrapulmonary shunt.[2] A similar decrease of the safety margin may occur in patients with lung disease characterized by decreased FRC or increased intrapulmonary shunting, or both. In these patients, maximal preoxygenation should precede interruption of ventilation or tracheobronchial suction.

E. PEDIATRIC PATIENTS

Because of their smaller FRC and increased metabolic requirements, pediatric patients are at increased risk for developing faster oxyhemoglobin desaturation than adults whenever there is an interruption of their oxygen delivery.[13,19,35-37,45,52,62] The younger the child, the faster is the onset of hypoxemia.[20,37,38] With a satisfactory mask fit, the efficacy of preoxygenation depends on the age of the child and the duration and type of breathing.[13,45,56] Studies in pediatric patients demonstrated that maximal preoxygenation can be reached faster than in adults.[13,56] With TVB, an ET_{O_2} of 90% or greater is reached within 60 to 100 seconds in almost all children.[13,45,56] In the first year of life, it is reached in 36 seconds (range 20 to 60 seconds); between 3 and 5 years in 50 seconds (range 30 to 90 seconds), and above 5 years in 68 seconds (range 30 to 100 seconds).[45] It has been shown that deep breathing in children results in faster preoxygenation than TVB in the same children and also faster than deep breathing in adults (Fig. 12-16).[56] Thus, contrary to that in adults, optimal preoxygenation can be accomplished in children using deep breathing for 30 seconds.[56]

Several factors affect the onset of apnea-induced oxyhemoglobin desaturation after preoxygenation in children. These include the efficacy of preoxygenation (duration, alveolar ventilation), age (or weight), the presence of disease, and the composition of gases in the lungs. Some studies examined the time for Sp_{O_2} to decrease from 100% to 95%,[35,36] although others targeted a level as low as 90%.[19,62,64] In a comparison of three groups of children

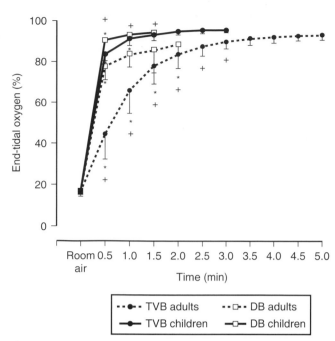

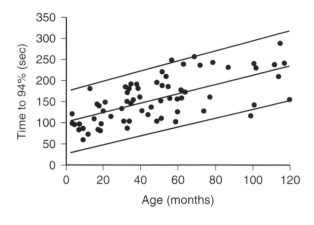

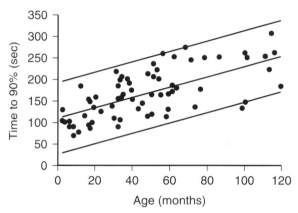

Figure 12-16 Comparison of tidal volume breathing (TVB) and deep breathing (DB) preoxygenation techniques on end-tidal oxygen. *Significant difference from all other time periods; +significant difference between adults and children. (From Salem MR, Joseph NJ, Villa EM, et al. Preoxygenation in children: Comparison of tidal volume and deep breathing techniques [abstract]. Anesthesiology 97:A1247, 2001.)

Figure 12-17 Relationship between desaturation times to 94% (*top*) and to 90% (*bottom*) and age with a prediction interval of 95% (*P* < .001). (From Dupeyrat A, Dubreuil M, Ecoffey C: Preoxygenation in children [letter]. Anesth Analg 79:1027, 1994.)

who breathed 100% O_2 at TVB for 1, 2, and 3 minutes before apnea, times for SpO_2 to decrease from 100% to 98%, 95%, and 90% were shorter in those who breathed O_2 for 1 minute.[64] On the basis of these findings, 2 minutes of preoxygenation with TVB in children seems to provide maximum benefit and allows 2 minutes or longer of safe apnea.[64] The time for SpO_2 to decrease from 100% to 95% and 90% is shorter in young children than in older children.[19] Most infants reach an SpO_2 of 90% in 70 to 90 seconds (Fig. 12-17). This duration is shortened in the presence of upper respiratory infection.[36]

Although the time for oxyhemoglobin desaturation is mainly dependent on the oxygen content of the lung at the start of apnea, other gas components may play a role. If 60% nitrous oxide in O_2 is used, the time for SpO_2 to decrease to 95% is shortened to approximately one third.[35] However, this duration is still longer than that following air-O_2 breathing while maintaining the same delivered oxygen concentration.[35] This can be explained by the second-gas effect. Nitrous oxide continues to dissolve into the blood and is carried away from the lungs, resulting in an increase in the PaO_2 and hence delaying the onset of oxyhemoglobin desaturation.[35]

It should be emphasized that the apnea-desaturation studies were performed in essentially healthy children who had a patent airway (open tracheal tube). It is conceivable that the presence of cardiac or respiratory disease or airway obstruction would lead to faster oxyhemoglobin

desaturation during apnea in infants and children.[35] Premature infants are usually given a low FIO_2 using an air-O_2 mixture because of fear of retinopathy of prematurity. Oxyhemoglobin desaturation occurs very quickly in these infants even after a short period of apnea. Transient increase in FIO_2, limiting apnea to very short periods, and close monitoring are important considerations.

VIII. SUMMARY

Oxygenation prior to anesthetic induction and endotracheal intubation has become an accepted maneuver designed to increase oxygen reserves and, thereby, delay the onset of arterial oxyhemoglobin desaturation during apnea. It is particularly important when manual mask ventilation is undesirable and when difficulty with ventilation or endotracheal intubation is anticipated. Because the cannot ventilate, cannot intubate situation is largely unpredictable, maximal preoxygenation is desirable in all patients. It is also essential in patients with a decreased capacity for oxygen loading (decreased FRC, PaO_2, or cardiac output) or increased $\dot{V}O_2$ or both. Preoxygenation should be considered when maneuvers that deplete the oxygen reserves such as suctioning, one-lung ventilation, or apneic oxygenation are performed.

In the operating room, maximal preoxygenation can be accomplished in most patients with the commonly used anesthetic systems with either tidal volume breathing for 3 to 5 minutes or deep breathing for 1.0 to 1.5 minutes. Elderly patients and patients with pulmonary disease may require longer periods of preoxygenation, whereas pediatric patients may need a shorter time. Except in children, the 4 DB/0.5 min technique provides submaximal preoxygenation and therefore should be reserved for emergency situations when time is limited. When deep breathing is used, an FGF of 10 L/min or greater is necessary; otherwise, rebreathing of exhaled gases occurs, leading to decreased inspired oxygen concentration. During preoxygenation, it is important that a tight-fitting mask is used to avoid air entrainment and that the reservoir bag is fully inflated. Almost all patients gladly accept mask preoxygenation if the procedure and its importance are explained to them beforehand.

Clinical endpoints indicative of maximal preoxygenation are movement of the reservoir bag in and out with each inspiration and exhalation, presence of a normal capnographic tracing, and a near-normal $ETCO_2$ throughout the period of preoxygenation. Monitoring O_2 or N_2, or both, by means of oxygraphy or mass spectrometry to ensure a target level of ETO_2 greater than or equal to 90% or an ETN_2 less than or equal to 5% is desirable if available.

We predict that in the near future there will be universal use and teaching of preoxygenation techniques in anesthetic practice and in the critical care setting. There will also be extensive research into means to maximize the efficacy and efficiency of preoxygenation. Examples include use of extended deep breathing, use of maximal exhalation before preoxygenation, enhancing the storage of O_2 in the tissue and venous compartments, and utilization of apneic diffusion oxygenation in a variety of clinical settings.

REFERENCES

1. Archer GW, Marx GF: Arterial oxygen tension during apnoea in parturient women. Br J Anaesth 46:358-360, 1974.
2. Baraka A, Aouad M, Taha S, et al: Apnea-induced hemoglobin desaturation during one-lung vs two-lung ventilation. Can J Anaesth 47:58-61, 2000.
3. Baraka A, Haroun-Bizri S, Khoury S, Chehab IR: Single vital capacity breath for preoxygenation. Can J Anaesth 47:1144-1146, 2000.
4. Baraka A, Salem MR, Joseph NJ: Critical hemoglobin desaturation can be delayed by apneic diffusion oxygenation. Anesthesiology 90:332-333, 1999.
5. Baraka AS, Hanna MT, Jabbour SI, et al: Preoxygenation of pregnant and nonpregnant women in head-up versus supine position. Anesth Analg 46:824-827, 1991.
6. Baraka AS, Taha SK, Aouad MT, et al: Preoxygenation. Comparison of maximal breathing and tidal volume breathing techniques. Anesthesiology 91:612-615, 1999.
7. Benumof JL: Preoxygenation: Best method for both efficacy and efficiency [editorial]. Anesthesiology 91:603-605, 1999.
8. Benumof JL, Dagg R, Benumof R: Critical hemoglobin desaturation will occur before return to unparalyzed state from 1mg/kg succinylcholine. Anesthesiology 87:979-982, 1997.
9. Berry CB, Miles PS: Preoxygenation in healthy volunteers: A graph of oxygen "washin" using end-tidal oxygraphy. Br J Anaesth 72:116-118, 1994.
10. Berthoud MC, Peacock JE, Reilly CS: Effectiveness of preoxygenation in morbidly obese patients. Br J Anaesth 67:464-466, 1991.
11. Berthoud M, Read DH, Norman J: Pre-oxygenation—How long? Anaesthesia 38:96-102, 1983.
12. Bhatia PK, Bhandari SC, Tulsioni KL, Kumar Y: End-tidal oxygraphy and safe duration of apnea in young adults and elderly patients. Anaesthesia 52:175-178, 1997.
13. Butler PJ, Munro HM, Kenny MB: Preoxygenation in children using expired oxygraphy. Br J Anaesth 77:333-334, 1996.
14. Byrne F, Oduro-Dominah A, Kipling R: The effect of pregnancy on pulmonary nitrogen washout. A study of pre-oxygenation. Anaesthesia 42:148-150, 1987.
15. Campbell IT, Beatty PCW: Monitoring preoxygenation. Br J Anaesth 72:3-4, 1994.
16. Carmichael FJ, Cruise CJE, Crago RR, Paluck S: Preoxygenation: A study of denitrogenation. Anesth Analg 68:406-409, 1989:
17. Dillon JB, Darsi ML: Oxygen for acute respiratory depression due to administration of thiopental sodium. JAMA 159:1114-1116, 1955.
18. Drummond GB, Park GR: Arterial oxygen saturation before intubation of the trachea. Br J Anaesth 54:987-992, 1984.
19. Dupeyrat A, Dubreuil M, Ecoffey C: Preoxygenation in children [letter]. Anesth Analg 79:1027, 1994.
20. Eger EJ II, Severinghaus JW: The rate of rise of $PACO_2$ in the apneic anesthetized patient. Anesthesiology 22:419-425, 1961.
21. Farmery AD, Roe PG: A model to describe the rate of oxyhemoglobin desaturation during apnoea. Br J Anaesth 76:284-291, 1996.
22. Fowler WS, Comroe JH: Lung function studies. 1: The rate of increase of arterial oxygen saturation during the inhalation of 100% oxygen. J Clin Invest 27:327-334, 1948.

23. Fraioli RL, Sheffer LA, Steffenson JL: Pulmonary and cardiovascular effects of apneic oxygenation in man. Anesthesiology 39:588, 1973.

24. Fruman MJ, Epstein RM, Cohen G: Apneic oxygenation in man. Anesthesiology 20:789-798, 1959.

25. Gambee AM, Hertzka RE, Fisher DM: Preoxygenation techniques: Comparison of three minutes and four breaths. Anesth Analg 66:468-470, 1987.

26. Gold MI, Duarte I, Muravchik S: Arterial oxygenation in conscious patients after 5 minutes and after 30 seconds of oxygen breathing. Anesth Analg 60:313-315, 1981.

27. Goldberg ME, Norris MC. Larijani GE, et al: Preoxygenation in the morbidly obese: A comparison of two techniques. Anesth Analg 68:520-522, 1989.

28. Hamilton WK, Eastwood DW: A study of denitrogenation with some inhalation anesthetic systems. Anesthesiology 16:861-867, 1955.

29. Hayes AH, Breslin DS, Mirakhur RK, et al: Frequency of haemoglobin desaturation with the use of succinylcholine during rapid sequence induction of anesthesia. Acta Anaesthesiol Scand 45:746-749, 2001.

30. Heier T, Feiner JR, Lin J, et al: Hemoglobin desaturation after succinylcholine-induced apnea. A study of the recovery of spontaneous ventilation in healthy volunteers. Anesthesiology 94:754-759, 2001.

31. Heller ML, Watson TR Jr: Polarographic study of arterial oxygenation during apnea in man. N Engl J Med 264:326-330, 1961.

32. Hess D, Hirsch C, Marquis-D'Amico C, Macmarek RM: Imposed work and oxygen delivery during spontaneous breathing with adult disposable manual ventilators. Anesthesiology 81:1256-1263, 1994.

33. Holmdahl MH: Pulmonary uptake of oxygen, acid-base metabolism, and circulation during prolonged apnoea. Acta Chir Scand 212(Suppl):1-128, 1956.

34. Jense HG, Dubin SA, Silverstein PJ, O'Leary-Escolas U: Effect of obesity on safe duration of apnea in anesthetized humans. Anesth Analg 72:89-93, 1991.

35. Kinouchi K, Fukumitsu K, Tashiro C, et al: Duration of apnoea in anaesthetized children required for desaturation of haemoglobin to 95%: Comparison of three different breathing gases. Paediatr Anaesth 5:115-119, 1995.

36. Kinouchi K, Tanigami H, Tashiro C, et al: Duration of apnea in anesthetized infants and children required for desaturation of hemoglobin to 95%. Influence of upper respiratory infection. Anesthesiology 77:1105-1107, 1992.

37. Laycock GJA, McNicol LR: Hypoxemia during induction of anesthesia—An audit of children who underwent general anaesthesia for routine elective surgery. Anaesthesia 43:981-984, 1988.

38. Machlin HA, Myles PS, Berry CB, et al: End-tidal oxygen measurement compared with patient factor assessment for determining preoxygenation time. Anaesth Intensive Care 21:409-412, 1993.

39. McCarthy G, Elliott P, Mirakhur RK, McLoughlin C: A comparison of different pre-oxygenation techniques in the elderly. Anaesthesia 46:824-827, 1991.

40. McCrory JW, Matthews JNS: Comparison of four methods of preoxygenation. Br J Anaesth 64:571-574, 1990.

41. McGowan P, Skinner A: Preoxygenation—The importance of a good face mask seal. Br J Anaesth 75:777-778, 1995.

42. Mertzlufft F, Zander R: Intrapulmonary O_2 storage with the NasOral system. Anasthesiol Intensivmed Notfallmed Schmerzther 29:235-237, 1994.

43. Mertzlufft F, Zander R: Optimal preoxygenation: The NasOral system. Adv Exp Med Biol 345:45-50, 1994.

44. Mills PJ, Baptiste J, Preston J, Barnas GM: Manual resuscitators and spontaneous ventilation—An evaluation. Crit Care Med 19:1425-1431, 1991.

45. Morrison JE, Collier E, Friesen RH, Logan L: Preoxygenation before laryngoscopy in children: How long is enough? Paediatr Anaesth 8:293-298, 1998.

46. Morton HJV, Wylie WD: Anaesthetic deaths due to regurgitation or vomiting. Anaesthesia 6:190, 1951.

47. Nimmagadda U, Chiravuri SD, Salem MR, et al: Preoxygenation with tidal volume and deep breathing techniques: The impact of duration of breathing and fresh gas flow. Anesth Analg 92:1337-1341, 2001.

48. Nimmagadda U, Joseph NJ, Ugboma S, Salem MR: Does positioning affect the efficacy of preoxygenation in the morbidly obese [abstract]? Anesthesiology 97:A1088, 2002.

49. Nimmagadda U, Salem MR, Joseph NJ, et al: Efficacy of preoxygenation with tidal volume breathing. Comparison of breathing systems. Anesthesiology 93:1-7, 2000.

50. Norris MC, Dewan DM: Preoxygenation for cesarean section: A comparison of the two techniques. Anesthesiology 62:827-829, 1985.

51. Nunn JF: Oxygen stores and the steady state. In Nunn JF (ed): Applied Respiratory Physiology, 4th ed. Oxford, Butterworth-Heinemann, 1995, p 288.

52. Patel R, Lenczyck M, Hannallah RS, McGill WA: Age and onset of desaturation in apnoeic children. Can J Anaesth 41:771-774, 1994.

53. Practice guidelines for management of difficult airway. An updated report by the American Society of Anesthesiologists Task Force on Management of the Difficult Airway. Anesthesiology 98:1269-1277, 2003.

54. Russell GN, Smith CL, Snowdon SL, Bryson THL: Pre-oxygenation and the parturient patient. Anaesthesia 42:346-351, 1987.

55. Salem MR, Joseph NJ, Crystal GJ, Nimmagadda U: Preoxygenation: Comparison of maximal breathing and tidal volume techniques [letter]. Anesthesiology 92:1845-1847, 2000.

56. Salem MR, Joseph NJ, Villa EM, et al: Preoxygenation in children: Comparison of tidal volume and deep breathing techniques [abstract]. Anesthesiology 95:A1247, 2001.

57. Sellick BA: Cricoid pressure to control regurgitation of stomach contents during induction of anesthesia. Lancet 2:404-406, 1961.

58. Schlack W, Heck Z, Lorenz C: Mask tolerance and preoxygenation: A problem for anesthesiologists but not for patients [letter]. Anesthesiology 94:546, 2001.

59. Snow RG, Nunn JF: Induction of anaesthesia in the foot down-position for patients with a full stomach. Br J Anaesth 31:493-497, 1959.

60. Teller LE, Alexander GM, Fruman MJ, Gross JB: Pharyngeal insufflation of oxygen prevents arterial desaturation during apnea. Anesthesiology 69:980-982, 1988.

61. Valentine SJ, Marjot R, Monk CR: Preoxygenation in the elderly: A comparison of the four-maximal-breath and the three-minute techniques. Anesth Analg 71:516-519, 1990.

62. Videira RLR, Neto PPR, Gomide RV, et al: Preoxygenation in children: For how long? Acta Anaesthesiol Scand 36:109-111, 1992.

63. Wylie WD: The use of muscle relaxants at the induction of anaesthesia of patients with a full stomach. Br J Anaesth 35:168, 1963.

64. Xue F-S, Tong S-Y, Wang X-L, et al: Study of the optimal duration of preoxygenation in children. J Clin Anesth 7:93-96, 1995.

THE AIRWAY TECHNIQUES

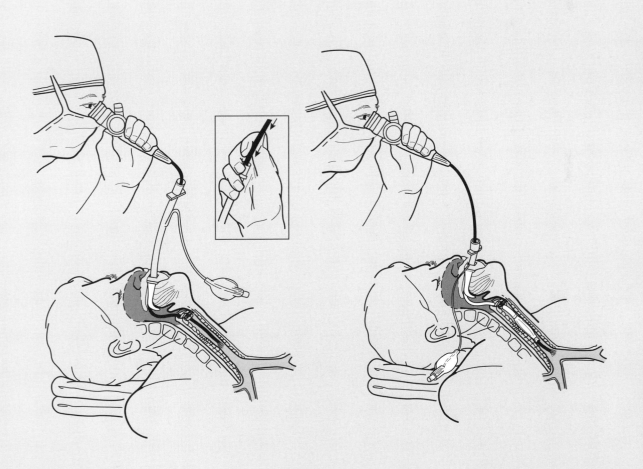

13

OXYGEN DELIVERY SYSTEMS, INHALATION THERAPY, AND RESPIRATORY THERAPY*

Jeffrey S. Vender
Joseph W. Szokol

I. INTRODUCTION

Many patients suffer from acute and chronic dysfunction of the cardiopulmonary system. Appropriate management of the surgical and critical care patient necessitates an understanding of both prophylactic and therapeutic techniques to support gas exchange and pulmonary function. Oxygen therapy is one of the most commonly employed medical interventions. An understanding of oxygen delivery systems and devices is essential for optimal care. Bronchial hygiene is now a cornerstone in prophylactic care of the perioperative surgical patient. The bronchial hygiene techniques employed are supportive of the natural cough mechanism. Finally, any medications that are specifically intended to treat pulmonary pathophysiology can

*Portions of the text from Vender JS, Clemency MV: Oxygen delivery systems, inhalation therapy, respiratory care. In Benumof JL (ed): Clinical Procedures in Anesthesia and Intensive Care. Philadelphia, JB Lippincott, 1992, pp 63-87.

be delivered by inhalation therapy with both greater efficiency and less toxicity than oral or parenteral methods. This chapter is an overview of the various procedures and techniques employed in the respiratory care of our patients.

II. OXYGEN THERAPY

A. INDICATIONS

Oxygen (O_2) is one of the most common therapeutic substances used in the practice of critical care medicine. Oxygen therapy has been shown to improve outcomes in patients undergoing surgery. The use of higher concentrations of oxygen (80% fraction of inspired oxygen [FIO_2]) intraoperatively and for 2 hours postoperatively through a face mask reduces the incidence of wound infections and postoperative nausea and vomiting in patients undergoing colorectal surgery.[14,15] This section reviews some of the indications, goals, and modes of O_2 therapy in the adult patient.

Treatment or prevention of hypoxemia is the most common indication for O_2 therapy, and the final goal of effective treatment is the avoidance or resolution of tissue hypoxia. Tissue hypoxia exists when delivery of O_2 is inadequate to meet the metabolic demands of the tissues. O_2 content (Box 13-1) depends on the arterial partial pressure of O_2 (PaO_2), the hemoglobin concentration of arterial blood, and the saturation of hemoglobin with O_2. O_2 delivery (DO_2) is calculated by multiplying cardiac output (liters per minute) by the arterial O_2 content. DO_2 is measured in milliliters of O_2 per minute and, for a 70-kg healthy patient, is approximately 1000 mL/min (Box 13-2).

Hypoxia may result from a decrement of any of the determinants of DO_2, including anemia, low cardiac output, hypoxemia, or abnormal hemoglobin affinity (e.g., carbon monoxide toxicity). Hypoxia may also arise from a failure of O_2 utilization at the tissue level (e.g., the microvascular perfusion defect of shock) or even at the cell itself (e.g., cyanide poisoning).

Aerobic metabolism requires a balance between DO_2 and O_2 consumption. Breathing enriched inspired

---

Box 13-1   Calculation of Arterial Oxygen Content (CaO_2)

$$CaO_2 = SaO_2 \times Hg \times 1.34 + PaO_2 \times 0.0031$$

CaO_2 = arterial oxygen content (vol%)
Hg = hemoglobin (g%)
1.34 = oxygen-carrying capacity of hemoglobin
PaO_2 = arterial partial pressure of oxygen (torr)
0.0031 = solubility coefficient of oxygen in plasma

From Benumof JL (ed): Airway Management: Principles and Practice. St. Louis, Mosby, 1996, p 206.

Box 13-2   Calculation of Oxygen Delivery (DO_2)

$$DO_2 = CaO_2 \times CO \times 10$$

CaO_2 = arterial oxygen content in cm^3 per 100 cm^3 blood (vol%). This value is approximately 20 in the normal adult with a hemoglobin of 15 g%.
CO = cardiac output in liters per minute. This value is approximately 5 in the healthy 70-kg adult.
DO_2 = oxygen delivery in cm^3 per minute. This value is approximately 1000 mL/min in the healthy 70-kg adult.

From Benumof JL (ed): Airway Management: Principles and Practice. St. Louis, Mosby, 1996, p 206.

---

concentrations of O_2 may increase the PaO_2, the percentage of saturation of hemoglobin, and O_2 content, thereby augmenting DO_2 until the underlying cause of the hypoxia can be corrected (e.g., transfusing the anemic patient). The clinical situation in which O_2 therapy is most effective, however, is in the treatment of hypoxemia.

Hypoxemia may be defined as a relative deficiency of O_2 tension in the arterial blood. The most common causes of hypoxemia include true shunt, ventilation-perfusion inequalities, and decreased mixed venous O_2 content ($\bar{C}O_2$).

True intrapulmonary shunting is defined as the condition in which deoxygenated blood from the right heart enters the left heart without the benefit of alveolar gas exchange. True intrapulmonary shunts cause hypoxemia that is poorly responsive to O_2 therapy. The greater the percentage of the cardiac output shunted, the less responsive to O_2 the hypoxemia. Therapy for this "oxygen-refractory" hypoxemia is aimed at reducing the shunt. Respiratory therapy such as tracheobronchial toilet to remove mucous plugging of a lobar bronchus or adjusting an endotracheal tube (ET) that has advanced into a main stem bronchus may be effective. Positive airway pressure therapy can reduce intrapulmonary shunting in certain disease states associated with a diffuse reduction in functional residual capacity.

Mismatch of ventilation and perfusion ($\dot{V}/\dot{Q}$; shunt effect) causes hypoxemia when mixed venous blood flowing past the alveolar-capillary membrane (ACM) takes away O_2 molecules faster than ventilation to the alveolus can replace them. The alveolus receives perfusion in excess of ventilation and is considered an area of low $\dot{V}/\dot{Q}$. The resultant partial pressure of O_2 in the alveolus (PAO_2) is too low to oxygenate fully the blood flowing past it. When a significant number of the lungs' gas-exchanging units are affected, hypoxemia results.

The easiest way to understand the hypoxemic effect of low PAO_2 is to consider the effect of breathing gas with a subnormal O_2 tension (e.g., 100% nitrous oxide). In time, there would be a washout of the O_2 in the alveoli. The PAO_2 would drop and hypoxemia would ensue.

Although the critical care clinician is unlikely to encounter this situation, a similar drop in PaO_2 is seen in many other circumstances.

Hypoventilation causes hypoxemia when an increase in alveolar carbon dioxide (CO_2) "crowds out" the oxygen molecules and decreases PAO_2. Clinical entities associated with low PAO_2 include chronic obstructive pulmonary disease (COPD), asthma, retained secretions, sedative or narcotic administration, acute lung injury syndrome, and early or mild pulmonary edema. Breathing enriched inspired concentrations of O_2 under these circumstances increases PAO_2, which increases the O_2 gradient across the ACM, resulting in faster equilibration of mixed venous blood exposed to the ACM and a higher pulmonary venous, left atrial, left ventricular, and arterial PO_2.

Even small increases in inspired O_2 tension can correct hypoxemia when low PAO_2 is the cause. Indeed, drug-induced alveolar hypoventilation resulting in hypoxemia on room air is exquisitely sensitive to increases in inspired O_2 concentration. Appropriate initial management of patients with alteration in mental status includes the use of O_2 therapy as long as ventilatory needs are also monitored.

Cases of hypoxemia caused by either true shunt or $\dot{V}/\dot{Q}$ mismatch share a common phenomenon. Both pathophysiologic mechanisms are enhanced by a decreased mixed venous hemoglobin saturation (low $\overline{S}O_2$). Decreased $\overline{S}O_2$ results in a decreased O_2 content of the mixed venous blood. Low $\overline{C}O_2$ causes hypoxemia by worsening the hypoxemic effect of any existing shunt or areas of low $\dot{V}/\dot{Q}$ by presenting more desaturated blood to the left atrium and lowering PaO_2 by binding dissolved O_2 to the desaturated hemoglobin. Decreased $\overline{C}O_2$ arises from low O_2 delivery (e.g., low cardiac output, anemia, or hypoxemia) or increased O_2 consumption (e.g., high fever or increased minute ventilation and work of breathing).

The consequences of untreated hypoxemia include tachycardia and increased myocardial O_2 demand as well as increased minute volume and work of breathing. By treating hypoxemia, supplemental O_2 restores homeostasis and greatly decreases the stress response and its attendant cardiopulmonary sequelae.

B. OXYGEN DELIVERY SYSTEMS

With the exception of anesthetic breathing circuits, virtually all O_2 delivery systems are nonrebreathing. In nonrebreathing circuits, the inspiratory gas is not made up in any part by the exhaled tidal volume (V_T), and the only CO_2 inhaled is that which exists in any entrained room air (RA). To avoid rebreathing, exhaled gases must be sequestered by one-way valves and inspired gases must be presented in sufficient volume and flow to allow the high peak flow rates and minute ventilation demonstrated in critically ill patients. Inspiratory entrainment of RA or the use of inspiratory reservoirs (including the

anatomic dead space of the nasopharynx, oropharynx, and non–gas-exchanging portion of the bronchial tree) and one-way valves typifies nonrebreathing systems and defines them into two groups.[20,23,32] Low-flow systems depend on inspiration of RA to meet inspiratory flow and volume demands. High-flow systems provide the entire inspiratory atmosphere. High-flow systems use reservoirs or very high flow rates to meet both the large peak inspiratory flow demands and the exaggerated minute volumes found in many critically ill patients.

1. Low-Flow Oxygen Systems

A low-flow, variable-performance system depends on RA entrainment to meet the patient's peak inspiratory and minute ventilatory demands that are not met by the inspiratory gas flow or oxygen reservoir alone. Low-flow devices include nasal cannulas, simple face masks, partial rebreathing masks, nonrebreathing masks, and tracheostomy collars. Low-flow systems are characterized by the ability to deliver high and low FIO_2. The FIO_2 becomes unpredictable and inconsistent when these devices are used for patients with abnormal or changing ventilatory patterns. Low-flow systems produce FIO_2 values ranging from 21% to 80%. The FIO_2 may vary with the size of the oxygen reservoir, oxygen flow, and the patient's ventilatory pattern (e.g., V_T, peak inspiratory flow, respiratory rate, and minute ventilation). With a normal ventilation pattern, these devices can deliver a relatively predictable and consistent FIO_2.

It is imperative to understand and appreciate the fact that low-flow systems do not mean low FIO_2 values. As stated, with changes in V_T, respiratory rate, oxygen reservoir size, and so on, the FIO_2 can vary dramatically at comparable oxygen flow rates. The following two examples are theoretical mathematical estimates of an FIO_2 produced by a low-flow system (e.g., nasal cannula) in two different clinical conditions.

The following example for estimation of FIO_2 from a low-flow system is based on the textbook "normal" patient and ventilatory pattern. The following assumptions are used for the FIO_2 calculation: the anatomic reservoir for a nasal cannula consists of nose, nasopharynx, and oropharynx and is approximately one third of the entire normal anatomic dead space (including trachea)—for example, $1/3 \times 150$ mL = 50 mL; a nasal cannula oxygen flow rate of 6 L/min (100 mL/sec); a V_T of 500 mL; a respiratory rate of 20 breaths per minute; inspiratory time (I) of 1 second; and expiratory time (E) of 2 seconds. If the terminal 0.5 second of the 2-second expiratory time has negligible gas flow, the anatomic reservoir (50 mL) completely fills with 100% oxygen, assuming an oxygen flow rate of 100 mL/sec. Using the preceding normal variables, the FIO_2 is calculated for a patient with a 500-mL and a 250-mL V_T.

The preceding 50% variability in FIO_2 at 6 L/min of oxygen flow clearly demonstrates the effects of a variable

Example 1

Cannula	6 L/min	V_T, 500 mL	
Mechanical reservoir	None	I/E ratio, 1:2	
Anatomic reservoir	50 mL	Rate, 20 breaths per min	
100% O_2 provided/sec	100 mL	Inspiratory time, 1 sec	
Volume inspired O_2			
Anatomic reservoir	50 mL		
Flow/sec	100 mL		
Inspired room air	0.2 × 350 mL = 70 mL		
O_2 inspired	220 mL		

$$\text{FiO}_2 = \frac{220 \text{ mL } O_2}{500 \text{ mL } V_T} = 0.44$$

ventilatory pattern. In general, the larger the V_T or faster the respiratory rate, the lower the FiO_2. The smaller the V_T or lower the respiratory rate, the higher the FiO_2.

Low-flow oxygen devices are the most commonly employed oxygen delivery systems because of simplicity, ease of use, familiarity, economics, availability, and acceptance by patients. In most clinical situations (see "High-Flow Oxygen Systems" Section II. B. 2 and "High-Flow Devices" Section II. C. 2 in this chapter) these systems should be initially employed.

2. High-Flow Oxygen Systems

High-flow, fixed-performance systems are nonrebreathing systems that provide the entire inspiratory atmosphere needed to meet the peak inspiratory flow and minute

Example 2

If V_T is decreased to 250 mL:

Volume inspired O_2

Anatomic reservoir	50 mL
Flow/sec	100 mL
Inspired room air (0.20 × 100 cm³)	0.2 × 100 mL = 20 mL
O_2 inspired	170 mL

$$\text{FiO}_2 = \frac{170 \text{ mL } O_2}{250 \text{ mL } V_T} = 0.68$$

ventilatory demands of the patient. To meet the patient's peak inspiratory flow, the flow rate and reservoir are very important. Flows in excess of 30 to 40 L/min (or four times the measured minute volume) are often necessary. High-flow devices include aerosol masks and T pieces that are powered by air-entrainment nebulizers or air-oxygen blenders and Venturi masks (see "Oxygen Delivery Devices" Section II. C.). The advantage of high-flow systems is the ability to deliver predictable, consistent, and measurable high and low FiO_2s, despite the patient's ventilatory pattern, and to control the humidity and temperature of the delivered gases. The primary limitations of these systems are cost, bulkiness, and patients' tolerance.

There are two primary indications for high-flow oxygen devices:

1. Patients who require a consistent, predictable, minimal FiO_2 to reverse hypoxemia yet prevent hypoventilation because of a dependence on hypoxic ventilatory drive.
2. The patient with increased minute ventilation and abnormal respiratory pattern who needs predictable and consistent high FiO_2s.

C. OXYGEN DELIVERY DEVICES

1. Low-Flow Devices

a. Nasal Cannulas

Because of their simplicity and the ease with which patients tolerate them, nasal cannulas are the most frequently used oxygen delivery devices. The nasal cannula consists of two prongs, one inserted into each naris, that deliver 100% oxygen. To be effective, the nasal passages must be patent, but the patient need not breathe through the nose. The flow rate settings range from 0.25 to 6 L/min. The nasopharynx serves as the oxygen reservoir (Fig. 13-1). Gases should be humidified to prevent mucosal drying if the oxygen flow exceeds 4 L/min. For each 1 L/min increase in flow, the FiO_2 is assumed to increase 4% (Table 13-1).

Thus, an FiO_2 of 0.24 to 0.44 can be delivered predictably if the patient breathes at a normal minute ventilation rate with a normal respiratory pattern. Increasing flows to greater than 6 L/min does not significantly increase the FiO_2 above 0.44 and is often poorly tolerated by the patient.

The components needed for nasal cannula assembly include nasal cannula prongs, delivery tubing, adjustable restraining headband, and oxygen flowmeter to provide a controlled gas delivery from a wall outlet; a humidification system increases patients' comfort at higher flows (4 L/min or more).

Procedurally, the initiation of any oxygen therapy should be preceded by a review of the chart and documentation of the oxygen concentration and device ordered. If a humidifier (typically prefilled, single-use, disposable)

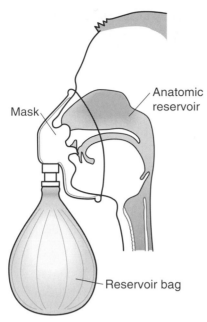

Figure 13-1 The three reservoirs of low-flow oxygen therapy. (From Vender JS, Clemency MV: Oxygen delivery systems, inhalation therapy, and respiratory care. In Benumof JL [ed]: Clinical Procedures in Anesthesia and Intensive Care. Philadelphia, JB Lippincott, 1992, pp 63-87.)

is used, it should be filled to the appropriate level with sterile water and connected to the flowmeter.

The nasal prong should be secured in the patient's naris and the cannula secured around the patient's head by a restraining strap.

Avoidance of undue cutaneous pressure is essential. Gauze may be needed to pad pressure points around the cheeks and ears during prolonged use. The flowmeter should be adjusted to the prescribed liter flow to attain the desired FIO_2 (see Table 13-1).

Although nasal cannulas are simple and safe, several potential hazards and complications exist. Oxygen supports

combustion, and any type of oxygen therapy is a fire hazard. Nasal trauma from prolonged use of or pressure from the nasal prongs can cause tissue damage. With poorly humidified, high gas flows, dehydration of the airway mucosal surface can occur. This mucosal dehydration can result in mucosal irritation, nosebleeds, laryngitis, earache, substernal chest pain, and bronchospasm.[4,20,32] Finally, because this is a low-flow system, it is imperative to remember the FIO_2 can be inaccurate and inconsistent, leading to the potential for underoxygenation or overoxygenation. This problem is of special concern with overoxygenation in patients with COPD with increased hypoxic drive to breathe. Underoxygenation potentiates any problems associated with hypoxemia.

b. Simple Face Mask

To provide a higher FIO_2 than that provided by nasal cannula with low-flow systems, the size of the oxygen reservoir must increase (see Fig. 13-1). A simple face mask consists of a mask with two side ports. The mask serves as an additional 100 to 200 mL oxygen reservoir. The side ports allow RA entrainment and exit for exhaled gases. The mask has no valves. An FIO_2 of 0.40 to 0.60 can be achieved predictably when patients exhibit normal respiratory patterns. Gas flows greater than 8 L/min do not significantly increase the FIO_2 above 0.60 because the oxygen reservoir is filled. A minimum flow of 5 L/min is necessary to prevent CO_2 accumulation and rebreathing. The actual delivered oxygen is dependent on the ventilatory pattern of the patient, similar to the situation with nasal cannulas.

The equipment needed is identical to that used for nasal cannula oxygen administration. The only difference is the use of a face mask. The predicted FIO_2 can be estimated from the oxygen flow rate (Table 13-2). Appropriate mask application is needed with all masks to maximize the FIO_2 and the patient's comfort. The mask should be positioned over the nasal bridge and the face, restricting oxygen escape into the patient's eye, which can cause ocular drying and irritation. The use of face masks has the added risk of aspiration because of concealed vomitus. If FIO_2 values above 0.60 are required, a partial rebreathing

Table 13-1 Approximate FIO_2 Delivered by Nasal Cannula*

Flow Rate (L/min)	Approximate FIO_2
1	0.24
2	0.28
3	0.32
4	0.36
5	0.40
6	0.44

*Based on normal ventilatory patterns.
FIO_2, fraction of inspired oxygen.
From Benumof JL: Airway Management: Principles and Practice. St. Louis, Mosby, 1996, p 209.

Table 13-2 Approximate FIO_2 Delivered by Simple Face Mask*

Flow Rate (L/min)	FIO_2
5-6	0.4
6-7	0.5
7-8	0.6

*Based on normal ventilatory patterns.
FIO_2, fraction of inspired oxygen.
From Benumof JL: Airway Management: Principles and Practice. St. Louis, Mosby, 1996, p 209.

mask, nonrebreathing mask, or high-flow system should be employed. All oxygen devices that deliver higher FIO_2 increase the potential of oxygen toxicity (see "Complications," Section II.F).

c. Partial Rebreathing Mask

To deliver an FIO_2 above 60% with a low-flow system, the oxygen reservoir system must be increased (see Fig. 13-1).[32] A partial rebreathing mask adds a reservoir bag with a 600- to 1000-mL capacity. Side ports allow entrainment of RA and the exit of exhaled gases. The distinctive feature of this mask is that the first 33% of the patient's exhaled volume fills the reservoir bag. This volume is from the anatomic dead space and contains little carbon dioxide. During inspiration, the bag should not completely collapse. A deflated reservoir bag results in a decreased FIO_2 because of entrained RA. With the next breath, the first exhaled gas (which is in the reservoir bag) and fresh gas are inhaled—thus the name partial rebreather. Fresh gas flows should equal or exceed 8 L/min, and the reservoir bag must remain inflated during the entire ventilatory cycle to ensure the highest FIO_2 and adequate carbon dioxide evacuation. An FIO_2 of 0.60 to 0.80+ can be delivered with this device if the mask is applied appropriately and the ventilatory pattern is normal (Table 13-3). This mask's rebreathing capacity allows oxygen conservation and thus may be useful during transportation, when oxygen supply may be limited. Complications with partial rebreathing oxygen delivery systems are similar to those with other mask devices with low-flow systems.

d. Nonrebreathing Mask

A nonrebreathing mask (Fig. 13-2) is similar to a partial rebreathing mask but adds three unidirectional valves.

Table 13-3   Approximate FIO_2 Delivered by Mask with Reservoir Bag*

Flow Rate (L/min)	FIO_2
6	0.6
7	0.7
8	0.8
9	0.8+
10	0.8+

*Based on normal ventilatory patterns.
FIO_2, fraction of inspired oxygen.
From Benumof JL: Airway Management: Principles and Practice. St. Louis, Mosby, 1996, p 210.

One valve is located on each side of the mask to permit the venting of exhaled gases and prevent RA entrainment. The third unidirectional valve is situated between the mask and the reservoir bag and prevents exhaled gases from entering the bag.

The bag must be inflated throughout the ventilatory cycle to ensure the highest FIO_2 and adequate carbon dioxide evacuation. Typically, the FIO_2 is 0.80 to 0.90. Fresh gas flow is usually 15 L/min (range, 10 to 15 L/min). If RA is not entrained, an FIO_2 approaching 1.0 can be achieved. If fresh gas flows do not meet ventilatory needs, many masks have a spring-loaded tension valve that permits RA entrainment if the reservoir is evacuated. This is often needed to meet the increased inspiratory drive of critically ill patients. This spring valve is often called a safety valve. The spring valve tension should be checked periodically. If such a valve is not present, one of the unidirectional

Nonrebreathing oxygen mask

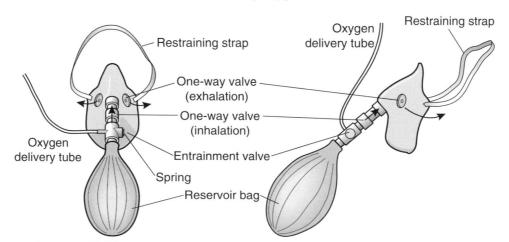

Figure 13-2 A nonrebreathing oxygen mask. In addition to the exhalation valve, the mask has a one-way inhalation valve. (From Vender JS, Clemency MV: Oxygen delivery systems, inhalation therapy, and respiratory care. In Benumof JL [ed]: Clinical Procedures in Anesthesia and Intensive Care. Philadelphia, JB Lippincott, 1992.)

valves on the mask should be removed to allow RA entrainment if needed to meet ventilatory demands. If the total ventilatory needs are met without RA entrainment, the rebreathing mask performs like a high-flow system. The operational application of a nonrebreathing mask is similar to that of other mask devices. To optimize the system, the mask should fit snugly (without excessive pressure) to avoid air entrainment around the mask, which would dilute the delivered gas and lower the FIO_2. If the mask fit is appropriate, the reservoir bag responds to the patient's inspiratory efforts. The high flows often employed increase the potential for several problems. Gastric distention, cutaneous irritation, and distention of the venting valves in the open position allowing RA entrainment can all occur with excessive gas flows.

e. Tracheostomy Collars

Tracheostomy collars are used primarily to deliver humidity to patients with artificial airways. Oxygen may be delivered with these devices, but, as with the nasal cannula, the FIO_2 is unpredictable, inconsistent, and dependent on ventilatory pattern.

2. High-Flow Devices

a. Venturi Masks

As discussed earlier, high-flow systems have flow rates and reservoirs large enough to provide the total inspired gases reliably. Most high-flow systems use gas entrainment to provide the flow and FIO_2 needs. Venturi masks entrain air by the Bernoulli principle and constant pressure-jet mixing.[30] This physical phenomenon is based on a rapid velocity of gas (e.g., oxygen) moving through a restricted orifice. This produces viscous shearing forces, which create a decreased pressure gradient (subatmospheric) downstream relative to the surrounding gases. This pressure gradient causes RA to be entrained until the pressures are equalized. Figure 13-3 illustrates the Venturi principle.

Venturi principle

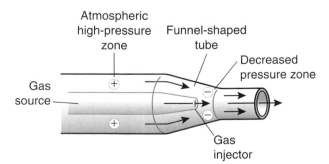

Figure 13-3 Illustration of the Venturi principle. (From Vender JS, Clemency MV: Oxygen delivery systems, inhalation therapy, and respiratory care. In Benumof JL [ed]: Clinical Procedures in Anesthesia and Intensive Care. Philadelphia, JB Lippincott, 1992.)

Altering the gas orifice or entrainment port size causes the FIO_2 to vary. The oxygen flow rate determines the total volume of gas provided by the device. It provides predictable and reliable FIO_2 values of 0.24 to 0.50 that are independent of the patient's respiratory pattern.

These masks come in the following varieties:

1. A fixed FIO_2 model, which requires specific inspiratory attachments that are color coded and have labeled jets that produce a known FIO_2 with a given flow.
2. A variable FIO_2 model (Fig. 13-4), which has a graded adjustment of the air entrainment port that can be set to allow variation in delivered FIO_2.

To use any air entrainment device properly to control the FIO_2, the standard air-oxygen entrainment ratios and minimum recommended flows for a given FIO_2 must be used (Table 13-4). The minimum total flow requirement should result from entrained RA added to the fresh oxygen flow and equal three to four times the minute ventilation. This minimal flow is required to meet the patient's peak inspiratory flow demands. As the desired FIO_2 increases, the air-oxygen entrainment ratio decreases with a net reduction in total gas flow. Therefore, the higher the desired FIO_2, the greater the probability of the patient's needs exceeding the total flow capabilities of the device.

Venturi masks are often useful when treating patients with COPD who depend on hypoxic ventilatory drive and accurate FIO_2s.[13] The Venturi mask's ability to deliver a high flow with no particulate H_2O makes it beneficial in treating asthmatics, in whom bronchospasm may be precipitated or exacerbated by aerosolized H_2O administration.

Several specific concerns regarding the application of a Venturi mask must be recognized to provide appropriate function. Obstructions distal to the jet orifice can produce back pressure and an effect referred to as "Venturi stall." When this occurs, RA entrainment is compromised, causing a decreased total gas flow and an increased FIO_2. Occlusion or alteration of the exhalation ports can also produce this situation. Aerosol devices should not be used with these devices. Water droplets can occlude the oxygen injector. If humidity is needed, a vapor-type humidity adapter collar should be used.

b. Aerosol Masks and T Pieces with Nebulizers or Air-Oxygen Blenders

FIO_2s greater than 0.40 with a high-flow system are best provided by large-volume nebulizers and wide-bore tubing. Aerosol masks, in conjunction with air entrainment nebulizers or air-oxygen blenders, deliver consistent and predictable FIO_2s, regardless of the patient's ventilatory pattern. A T piece is used in place of an aerosol mask for patients with an artificial airway.

Air entrainment nebulizers can deliver FIO_2s of 0.35 to 1.00 and produce an aerosol. The maximum gas flow through the nebulizer is 14 to 16 L/min. As with the Venturi masks, less RA is entrained with higher FIO_2s.

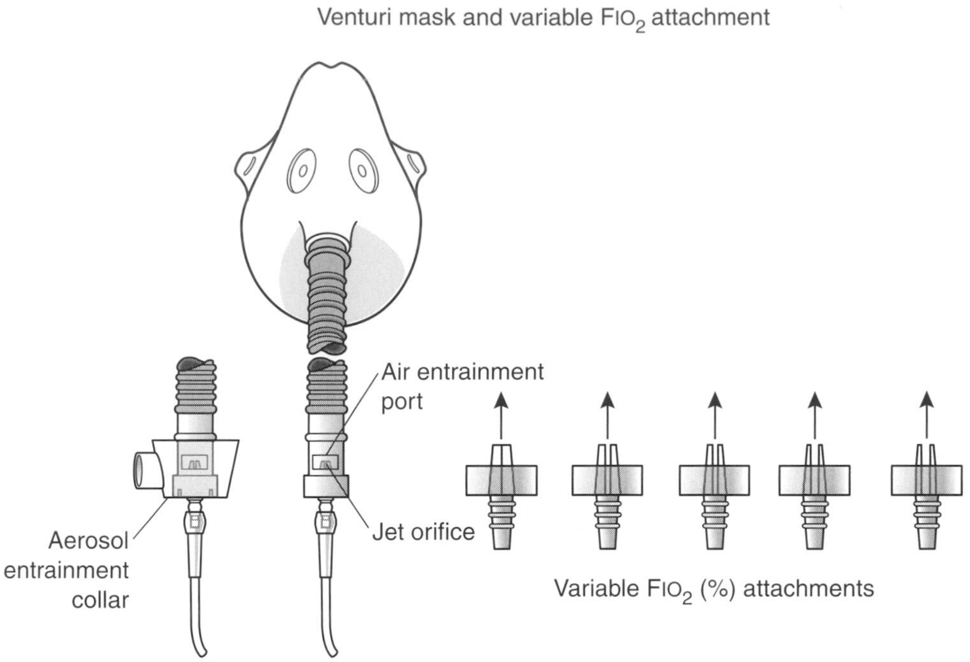

Venturi mask and variable F_{IO₂} attachment

Figure 13-4 Air entrainment Ventimask. Specific F$_{IO_2}$ levels are provided by the various jet orifices. (From Vender JS, Clemency MV: Oxygen delivery systems, inhalation therapy, and respiratory care. In Benumof JL [ed]: Clinical Procedures in Anesthesia and Intensive Care. Philadelphia, JB Lippincott, 1992.)

As a result, total flow at high F$_{IO_2}$s is decreased. To meet ventilatory demands, two nebulizers may feed a single mask to increase the total flow, and a short length of corrugated tubing may be added to the aerosol mask side ports to increase the reservoir capacity (Fig. 13-5). If the aerosol mist exiting the mask side ports disappears during inspiration, RA is probably being entrained and flow should be increased.

Table 13-4 **Approximate Air Entrainment Ratio and Gas Flow (F$_{IO_2}$)***

F$_{IO_2}$ (%)	Ratio	Recommended O$_2$ Flow (L/min)	Total Gas Flow (to Port) (L/min)
24	25.3:1	3	79
26	14.8:1	3	47
28	10.3:1	6	68
30	7.8:1	6	53
35	4.6:1	9	50
40	3.2:1	12	50
50	1.7:1	15	41

*Varies with manufacturer.
F$_{IO_2}$, fraction of inspired oxygen.
From Benumof JL: Airway Management: Principles and Practice. St. Louis, Mosby, 1996, p 212.

Circuit resistance can increase as a result of water accumulation or kinking of the aerosol tubing. The increased pressure at the Venturi device decreases RA entrainment, increases F$_{IO_2}$, and decreases total gas flow. Thus, if a predictable F$_{IO_2}$ above 0.40 is desired, an air-oxygen blender should be used. Air-oxygen blenders can deliver consistent and accurate F$_{IO_2}$s from 0.21 to 1.0 and flows of up to 100 L/min. The higher flows tend to produce excessive noise through the long-bore tubing. They are usually used in conjunction with humidifiers. Air-oxygen blenders are recommended for patients with increased minute ventilation who require a high F$_{IO_2}$ and in whom bronchospasm may be precipitated or worsened by a nebulized H$_2$O aerosol.

With an artificial airway, a 15- to 20-inch reservoir tube should be added to the Briggs T piece (Hudson, RCI, Temecula, CA) to prevent the potential of entraining air into the system.

D. HUMIDIFIERS

Humidity is the water vapor in a gas. When air is 100% saturated at 37° C, it contains 43.8 mg H$_2$O/L. The amount of water vapor a volume of gas contains depends on the temperature and water availability. The vapor pressure exerted by the water vapor is equal to 47 mm Hg. Alveolar gases are 100% saturated at 37° C. When the inspired atmosphere contains less than 43.8 mg H$_2$O/L or has a vapor pressure below 47 mm Hg, a gradient exists between the respiratory mucosa and the inhaled gas. This gradient

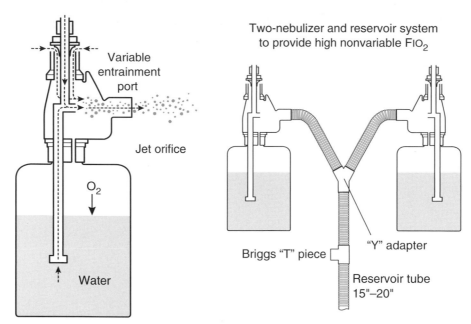

Figure 13-5 Single-unit and double (tandem)-unit mechanical aerosol systems. (From Vender JS, Clemency MV: Oxygen delivery systems, inhalation therapy, and respiratory care. In Benumof JL [ed]: Clinical Procedures in Anesthesia and Intensive Care. Philadelphia, JB Lippincott, 1992.)

causes water to leave the mucosa and to humidify the inhaled gas.

RA that has a relative humidity of 50% at 21° C has a relative humidity of 21% at 37° C. Under normal conditions, the lungs contribute approximately 250 mL/H$_2$O per day to saturate inspired air 100%.[32]

The administration of dry oxygen lowers the water content of the inspired air. The upper respiratory tract filters, humidifies, and warms inspired gases. Nasal breathing is more efficient than oral breathing for conditioning inspired gases. The use of an artificial airway bypasses the nasopharynx and oropharynx, where a significant amount of warming and humidification of inspired gases are accomplished. As a result, oxygen administration and the use of artificial airways increase the demand on the lungs to humidify the inspired gases.

This increased demand ultimately leads to mucosal drying, inspissated secretions, and decreased mucociliary clearance. This can eventually result in bacterial infections, atelectasis, and pneumonia. To prevent these complications, a humidifier or nebulizer should be used to increase the water content of the inspired gases.

Indications for humidity therapy include high-flow therapeutic gas delivery to nonintubated patients, delivery of gases through artificial airways, and reduction of airway resistance in asthma. It is generally accepted that low flows (1 to 4 L/min) do not need humidification except in specific individuals and that all O$_2$ delivered to infants should be humidified.

A humidifier increases the water vapor, either heated or unheated, in a gas. This can be accomplished by passing gas over heated water (heated passover humidifier);

by fractionating gas into tiny bubbles as gas passes through water (bubble diffusion or jet humidifiers); by allowing gas to pass through a chamber that contains a heated, water-saturated wick (heated wick humidifier); and by vaporizing water and selectively allowing the vapor to mix with the inspired gases (vapor-phase humidifier). Other variations of humidification systems exist but are beyond the scope of this chapter.[19]

Bubble humidifiers can be used with nasal cannulas, simple face masks, partial and nonbreathing masks, and air-oxygen blenders. They increase the relative humidity of gas from 0% to 70% at 25° C, which is approximately equal to 34% at 37° C.[16,21] Large-volume bubble-through humidifiers are available for use with ventilator circuits or high-gas-flow delivery systems.

A heated humidifier should be used when delivering dry gases to patients with ETs because it allows delivery of gases with an increased water content and relative humidity exceeding 65% at 37° C. When heated humidifiers are used, proximal airway temperature should be monitored to ensure a gas temperature that allows maximum moisture-carrying capacity yet prevents mucosal burns.

Heat and moisture exchangers (HMEs) are simple, small humidifier systems designed to be attached to an artificial airway. The HMEs are often referred to as an "artificial nose." The efficiency of these devices is quite variable, depending on the HME design, V$_T$, and atmospheric conditions. HMEs are typically used for short-term ventilatory support and for humidification during anesthesia. Several noted contraindications include neonatal and small pediatric patients; copious secretions; significant spontaneous breathing, in which the patient's V_T exceeds the HME specifications; and large-volume losses through a bronchopleural fistula or leakage around the ET.[19]

A nebulizer increases the water content of the inspired gas by generating aerosols (small droplets of particulate water) that become incorporated into the delivered gas stream and then evaporate into the inspired gas as it is warmed in the respiratory tract. There are two basic kinds of nebulizers, pneumatic and electric. Pneumatic nebulizers operate from a pressured gas source and are either jet or hydrodynamic. Electric nebulizers are powered by an electrical source and are referred to as "ultrasonic." There are several varieties of both types of nebulizers, and they depend more on design differences than on the power source. A more in-depth discussion of nebulizers is available elsewhere.[4,32] The resultant humidity ranges from 50% to 100% at 37° C, depending on the device used. If heated, the relative humidity of the gas can exceed 100% at 37° C. Air entrainment nebulizers are used in conjunction with aerosol masks and T pieces.

There are three general purposes for aerosol therapy. First, aerosol therapy increases the particulate and molecular water content of the inspired gases. The aerosol increases the water content of desiccated and retained secretions, enhancing bronchial hygiene. This does not alleviate the need for systemic hydration. Second, delivery of medications is a primary indication for aerosol therapy, for example, α_2-agonists, corticosteroids, anticholinergics, and antiviral-bacterial agents (see "Inhalation Therapy," Section IV). Third, aerosol therapy has also been employed for sputum inductions. The success of aerosol therapy depends on proper technique of administration and an appropriate indication for use.

The aerosol generated by the nebulizer can precipitate bronchospasm of hyperactive airways.[20,32] Prophylactic bronchodilator therapy should be entertained prior to or during the aerosol treatment. Fluid accumulation and overload have been reported. These are more common in pediatrics and with continuous ultrasonic rather than intermittent or jet therapy. Dry secretions are hydrophilic and can swell because of the absorbed water content. If secretions swell, they can obstruct airways. Mobilization of secretions limits this problem. Aerosol therapy for drug delivery has been reported to precipitate the same side effects as systemic drug delivery. Therapeutic aerosols have been implicated in nosocomial infections.[8] Cross-contamination between patients must be avoided.

E. MANUAL RESUSCITATION BAGS

Manual resuscitation bags are used primarily for resuscitation and manual ventilation of ventilator-dependent patients. These bags can deliver an FIO_2 above 0.90 and V_Ts up to 800 mL when oxygen flows to the bag are 10 to 15 mL/min. Factors that promote the highest FIO_2s include the use of an oxygen reservoir, connection to an oxygen source, and slow rates of ventilation that allow the bag to refill completely. Positive end-expiratory pressure (PEEP) valves should be used for patients who require more than 5 cm H_2O PEEP. One should be aware of different capabilities among various resuscitation bags in delivery of maximum FIO_2.[1,2,5]

F. COMPLICATIONS

Complications related to oxygen delivery can be divided into two groups: complications related to the oxygen delivery systems (see sections that discuss the specific devices) and pathophysiologic complications related to oxygen therapy.

Pathophysiologic complications related to oxygen therapy can lead to serious consequences. The three major complications encountered in adults are hypoventilation, absorption atelectasis, and oxygen toxicity.

Oxygen therapy must be used appropriately in patients with COPD who rely on hypoxic ventilatory drive for breathing. They typically have a chronically elevated arterial carbon dioxide tension ($PaCO_2$), a normal pH, and a PaO_2 usually below 60 mm Hg. Because the increased $PaCO_2$ is compensated by an increased bicarbonate ion concentration in the arterial blood and the cerebral spinal fluid, the patient may become desensitized to ventilatory stimulation from changes in the $PaCO_2$. Instead, the chemoreceptors in the aortic and carotid bodies control ventilation. They are sensitive to PaO_2s below 60 mm Hg. When worsening hypoxemia is treated with supplemental oxygen, the goal is to raise the PaO_2 just to the patient's chronic level. Thus, the minimum FIO_2 needed to accomplish this goal should be delivered. If oxygen administration raises the PaO_2 above this level, the patient's hypoxic drive is blunted and hypoventilation can result. If hypoventilation is not reversed rapidly, respiratory failure necessitating mechanical ventilation ensues.

Absorption atelectasis occurs when high alveolar oxygen concentrations cause alveolar collapse. Nitrogen, already at equilibrium, remains within the alveoli and "splints" alveoli open. When high FIO_2s are administered, nitrogen is washed out of the alveoli, which are then filled primarily with oxygen. In areas of the lungs with reduced ventilation-perfusion ratios, oxygen is absorbed into the blood faster than ventilation can replace it. The affected alveoli become smaller and smaller until surface tension becomes so great as to cause their collapse. Progressively higher fractions of inspired oxygen above 0.50 cause absorption atelectasis in healthy individuals. Fractions of inspired oxygen of 0.50 or more may precipitate this phenomenon in patients with decreased ventilation-perfusion ratios.

The third pathophysiologic complication of oxygen therapy, oxygen toxicity, becomes clinically important after 8 to 12 hours of exposure to a high FIO_2. Oxygen toxicity probably results from direct exposure of the alveoli to a high FIO_2. Healthy lungs appear to tolerate FIO_2s of less than 0.6. In damaged lungs, FIO_2s greater than 0.50 can result in a toxic alveolar oxygen concentration. Because most oxygen therapy is delivered at 1 atm barometric pressure, the F_{IO_2} and the duration of exposure become the determining factors in the development of most clinically significant oxygen toxicity.

The mechanism of oxygen toxicity is related to the significantly higher production of oxygen free radicals including superoxide anions (O_2^-), hydroxyl radicals (OH^-), hydrogen peroxide (H_2O_2), and single oxygen. These radicals affect cell function by inactivating sulfhydryl enzymes, disrupting DNA synthesis, and disrupting cell membranes' integrity. Vitamin E, superoxide dismutase, and sulfhydryl compounds promote normal, protective free radical scavenging within the lung. During periods of lung tissue hyperoxia, these protective mechanisms are overwhelmed and toxicity results.[11]

The classical clinical manifestations of oxygen toxicity include cough, substernal chest pain, dyspnea, rales, pulmonary edema, progressive arterial hypoxemia, bilateral pulmonary infiltrates, decreasing lung compliance, and atelectasis. These signs and symptoms are nonspecific; thus, oxygen toxicity is frequently difficult to distinguish from severe underlying pulmonary disease. Often, only subtle progression of arterial hypoxemia heralds the onset of pulmonary oxygen toxicity.

On pathologic study, there are two distinct phases of classical oxygen toxicity. The early or exudative phase, observed during the first 24 to 48 hours, is characterized by the destruction of type I pneumocytes and the development of interstitial and intra-alveolar hemorrhage and edema. The late or proliferative phase, which begins after 72 hours, is characterized by resorption of early infiltrates, hyperplasia, and proliferation of type II pneumocytes and increased collagen synthesis. When oxygen toxicity progresses to the proliferative stage, permanent lung damage may result from scarring and fibrosis.

The treatment for oxygen toxicity is prevention. Oxygen therapy should be directed at improving oxygenation with the minimum F_{IO_2} needed to obtain an Sao_2 greater than 90%. Inhalation treatments and raised expiratory airway pressure may be useful adjuncts in improving pulmonary toilet, decreasing V/Q mismatch, and improving arterial oxygenation and may be used to maintain adequate oxygenation at an F_{IO_2} of 0.50 or less.

III. TECHNIQUES OF RESPIRATORY CARE

The provision of adequate pulmonary gas exchange is implicit in our teaching and management of respiratory care. For optimal gas exchange to occur, the airways must be maintained clear of foreign material (secretions). The various therapeutic techniques available are aimed at the mobilization and removal of pulmonary secretions. In addition, various therapies are intended to optimize breathing efficiency. Respiratory therapy aimed at the patient with impaired pulmonary function can improve

several outcome measures. Using common physiotherapy techniques such as postural drainage, vibration, percussion, and suction on critically ill patients leads to decreases in intrapulmonary shunt by a mean of 20% and significant improvements in lung compliance.[22] The lining of the lungs secretes a mucous layer that usually moves toward the larynx at a rate of 1 to 2 cm/min by ciliary motion. This mucous layer is responsible for transporting foreign particles from the lungs to the larynx. Critically ill patients have multiple factors contributing to the presence of increased secretions. Alterations in the mucociliary escalator system related to smoking, stress, high F_{IO_2}s, anesthesia, foreign bodies in the trachea (e.g., ET), various tracheobronchial diseases, and abnormalities in mucus production are all recognized contributors to retention of airway secretions. To help compensate for these deficiencies, the patient must be able to promote an adequate cough. In the critically ill patient or the individual with an artificial airway, an adequate cough is often absent. If any of these problems is present, there is an increased tendency to retain secretions.

Retained secretions promote several potential complications. Occlusion of the airway promotes ventilation-perfusion inequalities and eventually absorption atelectasis. This produces a progressively worse hypoxemia that is less responsive to oxygen therapy (see indications in "Oxygen Delivery Systems," Section II.B). Retained secretions and distal airway occlusion promote an increased incidence of stasis pneumonia. In addition, retained secretions increase the patient's work of breathing because of an increased airway resistance associated with the airway inflammation and partial airway occlusion and result in a reduced pulmonary compliance because of the atelectasis and reduced lung volumes.

Many of the fundamental practices of respiratory care are aimed at the provision of optimal airway care, tracheobronchial toilet, and the prevention and management of retained secretions. Because dehydration is a common cause of retained secretions, adequate hydration and humidification of gas delivery are essential. Humidity and aerosol therapy were discussed in the oxygen (gas) delivery section of this chapter. The remainder of this section addresses other techniques commonly employed in respiratory care. These include airway suctioning, chest physical therapy, and incentive spirometry. Intermittent positive-pressure breathing (IPPB) is discussed separately because it is used for both the promotion of tracheobronchial toilet and the delivery of medication (see "Inhalation Therapy," Section IV).

A. SUCTIONING

Airway suctioning is commonly employed in respiratory care to promote optimal tracheobronchial toilet and airway patency in critically ill patients. Because of the perceived simplicity and limited complications, airway suctioning is frequently employed. If proper indications and technique are not appreciated, however, the potential for significant complications exists.

1. Indications

Suctioning of the airway should not be done without appropriate clinical indications. The audible (auscultatory) or visible presence of airway secretions is the most common indication. Increasing peak inspiratory pressures in mechanically ventilated patients are often indicative of retained secretions. Routine prophylactic suctioning is unwarranted except in neonates, in whom the small airway diameters can be acutely obstructed by a small accumulation of secretions.

In addition to removal of secretions, suction catheters are employed as aids in evaluating airway patency. If an artificial airway appears to be occluded, an attempt to pass a suction catheter can help assess airway patency. Several causes of artificial airway occlusion are mucous plugging, foreign body obstructions, kinking, and cuff herniations. If the suction catheter cannot be passed and ventilation is obstructed, several successive maneuvers are advisable. The cuff should be deflated and the airway repositioned; if improvement is inadequate, the artificial airway should be replaced.

The actual provision of airway suctioning depends on an appreciation of the available equipment, the appropriate techniques, and the potential complications.

2. Equipment

Numerous commercial suction catheters exist.[6,20,32] The ideal catheter is one that optimizes secretion removal and minimizes tissue trauma. Specific features of the catheters include the material of construction, frictional resistance, size (length and diameter), shape, and position of the aspirating holes. An opening at the proximal end of the catheter to allow the entrance of RA, neutralizing the vacuum without disconnecting the vacuum apparatus, is ideal. The proximal hole should be larger than the catheter lumen. Tracheal suctioning can occur only with occlusion of this proximal opening. The conventional suction catheter has both side holes and end holes (Fig. 13-6).

The Argyle Aero-Flo (Sherwood Medical, St. Louis) catheter provides a distal orifice, multiple side holes, and a flared end. Reportedly, this catheter is not as efficacious as the conventional one for removing secretions. The flared tip is to minimize tissue trauma, but it increases the overall catheter diameter, potentially making insertion more difficult and traumatic. Other catheters are designed with special anatomic or physiologic needs in mind. The Coudé angle-tipped catheter (Bard, Covington, GA) is shaped to increase the selective cannulation of the left main stem bronchus. This is facilitated by turning the head to the right during suctioning. Newer systems have been developed to provide a "closed system" for suctioning. These self-contained catheters allow suctioning of

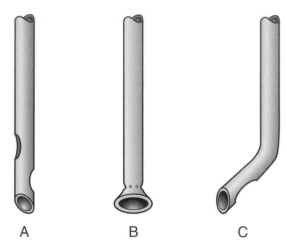

Side and end holes of suction catheters

Figure 13-6 Three suction catheters with side and end holes. **A,** Conventional catheter. **B,** Argyle Aero-Flow catheter (distal orifice and multiple side holes; flared end decreases tissue trauma but increases insertion difficulty). **C,** Coudé angle tipped catheter (increases cannulation of left main stem bronchus). (From Vender JS, Clemency MV: Oxygen delivery systems, inhalation therapy, and respiratory care. In Benumof JL [ed]: Clinical Procedures in Anesthesia and Intensive Care. Philadelphia, JB Lippincott, 1992.)

the patient without discontinuation of mechanical ventilation. This can limit some of the complications associated with suctioning and ventilatory disconnection.

The length of the typical catheter should pass beyond the distal tip of the artificial airway. The diameter of the suction catheter is very important. The optimal catheter diameter should not exceed one half the internal diameter of the artificial airway. Too large a catheter can produce an excessive vacuum and evacuation of gases distal to the tip of the airway, promoting atelectasis because of inadequate space for entrainment of air around the suction catheter. If too small a catheter is employed, removal of secretions can be compromised.

3. Technique

The technique of suctioning is important for the optimal removal of secretions and limitation of complications. This is a sterile procedure necessitating appropriate care in handling the catheter. Gloves and hand washing are necessary unless a closed system is employed. Other necessary equipment includes a vacuum source, sterile rinsing solution, AMBU oxygen system, and lavage solution. The optimal vacuum pressure should be adjusted for the patient's age.

Prior to suctioning, the patient should be preoxygenated by increasing the FIO_2 or by manual resuscitator ventilatory assistance. Preoxygenation minimizes the hypoxemia induced by FIO_2 disconnection and application of the suction vacuum. After preoxygenation, the sterile catheter is advanced past the distal tip of the artificial airway without the vacuum. When the catheter can no longer easily advance, it should be slightly withdrawn and intermittent vacuum pressure applied while the catheter is removed in a rotating fashion. This technique reportedly reduces mucosal trauma and enhances secretion clearance. The vacuum (suction) time should be limited to 10 to 15 seconds, and discontinuation of ventilation and oxygenation should not exceed 20 seconds. After removal of the catheter, reoxygenation and ventilation are essential. Throughout the procedure, the patient's stability and tolerance should be monitored. If signs of distress or dysrhythmias develop, the procedure should be immediately discontinued and oxygenation and ventilation reestablished. Suctioning is repeated until secretions have been adequately removed. After airway suctioning, oropharyngeal secretions should be suctioned and the catheter should be disposed.

Optimization of secretion removal necessitates adequate hydration and humidification of delivered gases. Occasionally, secretions can become quite viscous. Instillation of 5 to 10 mL of sterile normal saline can aid removal.

In critically ill patients, using a closed-system or swivel adapter to allow simultaneous suctioning and ventilation limits the consequences of airway disconnection and enhances sterility. These disposable systems are usually more costly but are used for 24 hours.

When an artificial airway is absent, nasotracheal suctioning techniques are employed. These techniques are technically less effective and more difficult than oral suctioning without an artificial airway and have the potential for additional complications. After appropriate lubrication, the catheter is inserted into a patient's nasal passage (often through a previously placed nasopharyngeal airway). The catheter is advanced into the larynx. Breath sounds from the proximal end of the catheter are often used as an audible guide. Upon the catheter's entry into the larynx, the patient often coughs. The vacuum is connected, and suctioning of the trachea is accomplished as previously described.

4. Complications

Complications of suctioning can be significant.[10,32] Although the suction vacuum is used to remove secretions, it also removes oxygen-enriched gases from the airway. If inappropriately applied and monitored, suctioning can produce significant hypoxemia. The use of arterial oxygen monitors (e.g., pulse oximetry) can often help detect alterations in arterial oxygenation (SaO_2) and heart rate and the presence of dysrhythmias.

Cardiovascular alterations are common. Dysrhythmias and hypotension are the most frequent cardiac complications. Arterial hypoxemia (and eventually myocardial hypoxia) and vagal stimulation secondary to tracheal suctioning are two recognized precipitory etiologies for cardiovascular complications. In addition, coughing induced by stimulation of the airway can reduce venous return and ventricular preload. Avoidance of hypoxemia, prolonged suctioning (greater than 10 seconds), and appropriate monitoring and sedation help reduce the incidence and significance of these complications.[7]

As discussed earlier, inappropriate suction catheter size can produce an excessive evacuation of gas distal to the artificial airway because of inadequate space for proximal air entrainment. This leads to hypoxemia and atelectasis. It is best avoided by reducing the catheter size to less than one half the internal diameter of the airway. Presuctioning and postsuctioning auscultation of the lungs helps detect significant atelectasis. After suctioning, several hyperinflations of the lungs can help reinflate atelectatic lung segments.

Mucosal irritations and trauma are common with frequent suctioning. The incidence and severity of trauma depend on the frequency of suctioning; technique; catheter design; absence of secretions, allowing more direct mucosal contact; and amount of vacuum pressure applied. Blood in the secretions is usually the first sign of tissue trauma. Meticulous technique is essential to limit this common complication. Airway reflexes can be irritated by direct mechanical stimulation. Wheezing resulting from bronchoconstriction can necessitate bronchodilator therapy. Nasotracheal suctioning can induce several additional complications. Nasal irritation, epistaxis, and laryngospasm are all noted complications. Laryngospasm can be life threatening if it is not recognized and appropriately managed.

B. CHEST PHYSICAL THERAPY

Chest physical therapy techniques are an integral part of respiratory care. Chest physical therapy plays an important role in the provision of bronchial hygiene and optimization of ventilation. The mucociliary escalator systems and cough can be aided by adjunctive techniques. This section discusses postural drainage techniques, percussion and vibration therapy, and incentive spirometry. Other breathing exercises and coughing techniques are covered in more extensive reviews of respiratory care.

1. Postural Drainage and Positional Changes

The fundamental goal of postural drainage is to move loosened secretions toward the proximal airway for eventual removal. Pulmonary drainage takes advantage of the fact that liquids flow in the direction of gravity. Flow of secretions is optimized by liquefaction (see "Humidifiers" Section II. D. in this chapter).

The primary indications for pulmonary drainage are malfunctioning of normal bronchial hygiene mechanisms and excessive or retained secretions.[4,17,32,36] In patients with ineffective lung volumes and cough, pulmonary drainage can be used prophylactically to prevent accumulation of secretions. Several clinical conditions typically benefiting from pulmonary drainage are bronchiectasis, cystic fibrosis, COPD, asthma, lung abscess, spinal cord injuries, atelectasis, pneumonia, and healing after thoracic and abdominal surgery.

To administer postural drainage appropriately, the practitioner must be able to visualize the location of the involved lung segments and the proper position to optimize drainage into the proximal airway. The lungs are divided into lobes, segments, and subsegments (Table 13-5).

Precise anatomic descriptions of the various pulmonary subsegments and positions are beyond the scope of this section. The large posterior and superior basal segments of the lower lobe are commonly involved in hospital patients with atelectasis and pneumonia. In the typical hospital patient these segments are most gravity dependent, causing stasis of secretions (Fig. 13-7).

Appropriate positioning of the patient can enhance gravitational flow. This therapy also includes turning or rotating the body around its longitudinal axis. Newer critical care beds have this feature incorporated into their design and function. Commonly employed positions for postural drainage are demonstrated in Figure 13-8.

Postural drainage should be done several times per day. For optimal results, postural drainage should follow humidity treatments and other bronchial hygiene therapies. Postural drainage should precede meals by 30 to 60 minutes, and the duration of treatment continues as long as the patient tolerates the therapy and may last up to 1 hour in certain populations of patients (cystic fibrosis patients).

Dependent lung segments

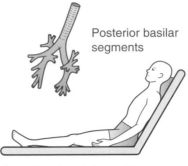

Posterior basilar segments

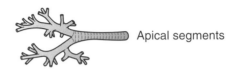

A Semi-upright position

Apical segments

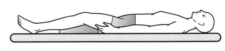

B Supine position

Figure 13-7 Lung segments typically at risk for retained secretions, atelectasis, and pneumonia that are due to body position during convalescence. **A**, Posterior basilar segment of the lower lobe. **B**, Apical segment of the lower lobe. (From Vender JS, Clemency MV: Oxygen delivery systems, inhalation therapy, and respiratory care. In Benumof JL [ed]: Clinical Procedures in Anesthesia and Intensive Care. Philadelphia, JB Lippincott, 1992.)

Table 13-5 Lung Segments

Right Side	Left Side
Upper lobe	*Upper lobe*
Apical	Apical-posterior
Posterior	Anterior
Anterior	
Middle lobe	*Lingula*
Lateral	Superior
Medial	Inferior
Lower lobe	*Lower lobe*
Superior	Superior
Medial basal	Anterior basal
Anterior basal	Lateral basal
Lateral basal	Posterior basal
Posterior basal	

From Benumof JL: Airway Management: Principles and Practice. St. Louis, Mosby, 1996, p 218.

Postural drainage can produce physiologic and anatomic stresses that are potentially detrimental to specific patients.[34] Alterations in the cardiovascular system from abrupt changes in position are well recognized. Hypotension or congestive heart failure that is due to changes in preload can be induced by positional change. Ventilation-perfusion relationships are altered by changes in position. Ideally, if the diseased pulmonary drainage is in the uppermost position, blood preferentially flows to the gravity-dependent, nondiseased segments, improving the ventilation-perfusion relationships. The head-down position, which is commonly used, is best avoided in patients with intracranial disease. The decreased venous return from the head could increase intracranial pressure.

The prone position has been demonstrated to improve oxygenation in patients with acute respiratory distress syndrome. The placement of critically ill patients in the prone position can be done without significant morbidity despite the presence of multiple sites of vascular access and intubation. The improvement in oxygenation is thought to be due to recruitment of collapse alveoli, more evenly distributed pleural pressure gradients, and caudad movement of the diaphragm.[18]

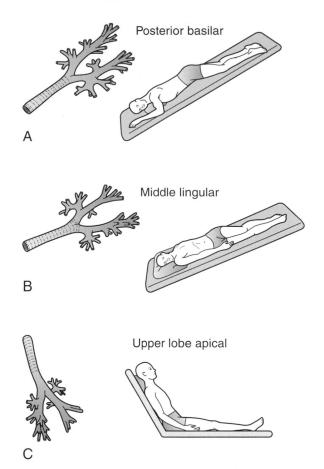

Figure 13-8 Common position for optimizing postural drainage of **(A)** the posterior basilar, **(B)** middle lingular, and **(C)** upper lobe apical segments. (From Vender JS, Clemency MV: Oxygen delivery systems, inhalation therapy, and respiratory care. In Benumof JL [ed]: Clinical Procedures in Anesthesia and Intensive Care. Philadelphia, JB Lippincott, 1992.)

Continuous rotational therapy employs dedicated intensive care unit beds that slowly and continuously rotate the patient along a longitudinal axis. The theory is that rotation of patients prevents gravity-dependent airway closure or collapse, worsening of pulmonary compliance and atelectasis, and pooling of secretions and possible subsequent pulmonary infection caused by long-term immobilization.[33] The use of rotational therapy may lead to a significantly lower incidence of patients diagnosed with pneumonia compared with patients cared for on conventional beds.[9]

Continual assessment of patients' tolerance during the procedure is necessary. Vital signs, oxygenation monitoring, general appearance, level of consciousness, and subjective comments by the patient are all part of the appraisal process.

2. Percussion and Vibration Therapy

Percussion and vibration therapy are used in conjunction with postural drainage to loosen and mobilize secretions that are adherent to the bronchial walls.[29,32]

Percussion involves a manually produced, rhythmic vibration of varying intensity and frequency. In a "clapping" (cupped hands) motion, a blow is delivered during inspiration and expiration over the affected area while the patient is in the appropriate position for postural drainage (Fig. 13-9).

Mechanical energy is produced by compression of the air between the cupped hand and the chest wall. Proper percussion should produce a popping sound (similar to striking the bottom of a ketchup bottle). Proper force and rhythm can be accomplished by placing the hands not farther than 5 inches from the chest and then alternating a flexing and extending of the wrists (similar to a waving motion). The procedure should last 5 to 7 minutes per affected area.

Like all respiratory care, percussion therapy should not be performed without a medical order. Therapy should not be performed over bare skin, surgical incisions, bone prominences, kidneys, and female breasts or with hard objects. If a stinging sensation or reddening of the skin develops, the technique should be reevaluated.

Special care must be given to the fragile patient. Fractured ribs, localized pain, coagulation abnormalities, bone metastases, hemoptysis, and empyemas are relative contraindications to percussion therapy.

Vibration therapy is used to promote bronchial hygiene in a fashion similar to chest percussion. Manually or mechanically (Fig. 13-10) gentle vibrations are transmitted through the chest wall to the affected area during exhalation. Vibration frequencies in excess of 200 per minute can be achieved if the procedure is done correctly. In patients receiving IPPB, all chest physical therapy procedures should be performed during the IPPB.

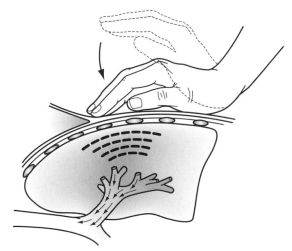

Figure 13-9 Typical hand position for chest percussion therapy. The hand is cupped and positioned about 5 inches from the chest, and the wrist is flexed. The hand strikes the chest in a waving motion. (From Vender JS, Clemency MV: Oxygen delivery systems, inhalation therapy, and respiratory care. In Benumof JL [ed]: Clinical Procedures in Anesthesia and Intensive Care. Philadelphia, JB Lippincott, 1992.)

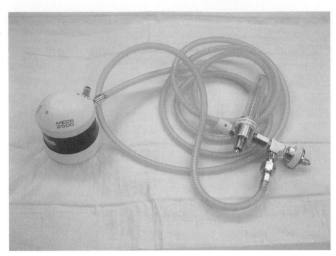

Figure 13-10 Image of a pneumatic chest percussion device. It uses Newton's third law of motion to assist the respiratory therapist in controlling percussion intensity. Therapists control the pulse intensity by how firmly they press the device. This device provides percussion without the need for clapping. It is less fatiguing for the therapist and may be more comfortable for the patient than manual percussion.

3. Incentive Spirometry

In the 1970s, alternative methods for prophylactic bronchial hygiene were developed to replace the more costly and controversial use of IPPB. Incentive spirometry (IS) was developed after several techniques utilizing expiratory maneuvers (e.g., blow and glove bottles) and carbon dioxide–induced hyperventilation were found either to be clinically ineffective or to cause other risks.[4,20,32]

IS was developed with an emphasis on sustained maximal inspiration (SMI). IS provides a visual goal or incentive for the patient to achieve SMI. Normal spontaneous breathing patterns have periodic hyperinflations that prevent the alveolar collapse associated with shallow tidal ventilation breathing patterns. Narcotics, sedative drugs, general anesthesia, cerebral trauma, and abdominal or thoracic surgery can all promote shallow tidal ventilation breathing patterns. Complications from this breathing pattern include atelectasis, retained secretions, and pneumonia.

The physiologic principle of SMI is to produce a maximal transpulmonary pressure gradient by generating a more negative intrapleural pressure. This pressure gradient produces alveolar hyperinflation with maximal airflow during the inspiratory phase.[37]

The indications for IS and SMI are primarily related to bronchial hygiene. These techniques should be employed perioperatively in surgical patients at an increased risk for pulmonary complications. IS involves the patient in his or her care and recovery, which can be psychologically beneficial while also being cost advantageous relative to the equipment and personal costs associated with other forms of respiratory care (e.g., IPPB).

The goals of IS and SMI therapy are to optimize lung inflation to prevent atelectasis, to optimize the cough mechanism by providing larger lung volumes, and to provide a baseline standard to assess the effectiveness of therapy or detect the onset of acute pulmonary disease (as noted by a deteriorating performance). To achieve these goals optimally necessitates instruction and supervision of the patient. It is now well recognized that preoperative education enhances the effectiveness of postoperative bronchial hygiene therapy (e.g., IS and SMI). The purpose of IS and SMI is not to replace an adequate cough and deep-breathing regimen but to provide the tool to support the patient who for various reasons is ineffective in spontaneous ability to provide bronchial hygiene. Appropriate instruction for proper breathing techniques can help produce an effective cough mechanism.

Various clinical models of incentive spirometers are available.[4] The devices vary in how they function, guide the therapy, or recognize the achievements. Each manufacturer provides instructions for use that should be followed. The devices are aimed at generating the largest inspiratory volumes during 5 to 15 seconds. The actual device used or rate of flow is not as important as the frequency of use and the attainment of maximal inspiratory volumes and sustained inspiration. Maximal benefit with most devices can be achieved only with user education.

The administration of IS and SMI therapy necessitates a physiologically and emotionally stable patient. The patient's cooperation and motivation are very important. For the therapy to be optimally effective, the patient should be free of acute pulmonary disease and have a forced vital capacity of more than 15 mL/kg and a spontaneous respiratory rate of less than 25 beats per minute. Ideally, the patient should not require a high F_{IO_2}. Therapy should be done hourly while the patient is awake. Typically, the patient should do four to five SMIs at a 30- to 60-second interval. The patient should be coached to inspire slowly while attaining maximal inspiratory volumes.

Although the use of IS is widespread throughout the United States, a review cast doubts on the superiority of IS over other methods of postoperative respiratory care. Overend and colleagues[28] examined all studies utilizing IS. They determined that most studies showed no benefit of IS and only one well-conducted study demonstrated an improvement in postoperative respiratory care but found no advantage of IS over IPPB or the encouragement of deep breathing exercises. There are no significant complications associated with IS and SMI therapy. The only contraindications are patients who are uncooperative, physically disabled with acute pulmonary disease, or unable to generate minimum volumes for lung inflation (e.g., 12 to 15 mL/kg).

C. INTERMITTENT POSITIVE-PRESSURE BREATHING

In the past four decades, few respiratory care therapies have been as controversial as IPPB.[4,20,26,32] Objective data assessing therapeutic benefit relative to cost and alternative therapies have been less than confirmatory.[26,37] Numerous conferences have been sponsored by medical organizations to evaluate literature supporting and opposing IPPB. The inconclusive result of these efforts has significantly reduced (and in some situations eliminated) the use of IPPB. Alternative techniques (previously discussed) have been substituted. This section is intended to define IPPB, recognize its indications, and describe the technique of administration and potential side effects and complications. An extensive historical and in-depth analysis of IPPB controversies is beyond the scope of this section.

1. Indications

IPPB is the therapeutic application of inspiratory positive pressure to the airway and is distinctly different from intermittent positive-pressure ventilation (PPV) or other means of prolonged, continuous ventilation.

The clinical indications for IPPB are subjective and unproved. It is easier to assess IPPB if the indications are described as clinical goals. The fundamental basis and singular goal of IPPB is to provide a larger V_T to the spontaneously breathing patient in a physiologically tolerable manner. If this goal is achieved, IPPB could be employed (1) to improve and promote the cough mechanism, (2) to improve distribution of ventilation, and (3) to enhance delivery of inhaled medications.

Bronchial hygiene can be compromised in patients with a reduced or inadequate cough mechanism. An adequate vital capacity (15 mL/kg) is necessary to generate the volume and expiratory flow needed to produce an effective cough. Although IPPB can increase V_T significantly, effectiveness still depends on the pressure and flow patterns generated as well as on an understanding of cough technique. Therefore, if cough is improved, one can indirectly see the benefit of IPPB for removal of secretions and for limiting complications associated with this problem.

The increased V_T produced by IPPB can be used to improve the distribution of ventilation. As in most respiratory care therapies, the efficacy depends on the patient's underlying condition, selection of patients, optimal technique, and frequency of application. Continual assessment of the therapy is mandatory. Theoretically, if ventilation increases, atelectasis can be prevented or treated.

In patients who are unable to provide an adequate inspiratory volume, IPPB can enhance drug delivery and distribution. When the patient is capable of an adequate cough and spontaneous deep breath, a hand nebulizer is as efficacious as IPPB. IPPB is rarely used solely for delivery of medication.

2. Administration

The effectiveness of IPPB depends on the individual administering the therapy.[4] It is incumbent for that individual (1) to understand the appropriate operation, maintenance and clinical application of the mechanical device employed; (2) to select the appropriate patient; (3) to provide the necessary education to the patient to optimize the effort; (4) to assess the effectiveness relative to goals and indications; and (5) to identify complications or side effects associated with the therapy.

The generic device uses a gas pressure source, a main control valve, a breathing circuit, and an automatic cycling control. Typically, IPPB is delivered by a pressure-cycled ventilator. Positive pressure (e.g., 20 to 30 cm H_2O) is used to expand the lungs. To be effective, the increase in V_T from the IPPB treatment must exceed the patient's limited spontaneous vital capacity by 100%. A prolonged inspiratory effort to the preset pressure limit should be emphasized. Therapy is typically 6 to 8 breaths per minute, lasting 10 minutes.

Keys to successful therapy include (1) machine sensitivity to the patient's inspiratory effort, (2) a tight seal between the machine and patient because these are pressure-limited devices, (3) a progressive increase in the inspiratory pressure as tolerated by the patient in an effort to achieve a desired exhaled volume, and (4) a cooperative, relaxed, and well-educated patient.

The physiologic side effects and complications associated with IPPB are well described in the literature.[4] Both hyperventilation and variable oxygenation can result from IPPB therapy. Hypocarbia that is due to an increased V_T and respiratory frequency can produce altered electrolytes (K^+), dizziness, muscle tremors, and tingling and numbness of the extremities. Proper instruction to the patient and a 5- to 10-minute rest period after therapy can minimize this problem. Hypoxemia and hyperoxia that are due to inaccurate FIO_2 values can be a concern in patients who are dependent on hypoxic respiratory drive (carbon dioxide retainers).

The use of IPPB can increase mean intrathoracic pressure, resulting in a decreased venous return. As with other forms of PPV, a decreased venous return (preload) can produce a decreased cardiac output and subsequent vital sign changes (hypotension or tachycardia). In addition to cardiovascular changes, IPPB can impede venous drainage from the head. This is a potential but limited concern in patients with increased intracranial pressure if IPPB is appropriately administered in the sitting position.

Barotrauma is a concern with all forms of PPV. The exact etiologic mechanism of PPV in the development of pneumothorax and ruptured lobes is unclear. Clearly, PPV results in increased intrapulmonary volume and pressure, but the same conditions tend to promote a better cough mechanism that causes sudden marked changes in pressure and lobe rupture. Before proceeding with an IPPB treatment, any chest pain complaints must be evaluated to rule out barotrauma.

Other reported complications include, but are not limited to, gastric insufflation and secondary nausea and vomiting, psychological dependency, nosocomial infections, altered airway resistance, and adverse reactions to administered medications. The incidence and significance of these adverse effects are often the result of inappropriate administration, noncompliance by the patient, selection of patients, and simple lack of attention to detail. Asthmatics reportedly tolerate IPPB poorly and have an increased airway resistance and a higher incidence of barotrauma.

There are few definite contraindications to IPPB. Relative contraindications to IPPB are focused on its lack of documented efficacy. Untreated pneumothorax is a definite contraindication to IPPB. Good clinical contraindications are lack of a definite indication for IPPB or an available, less expensive alternative therapy.

IV. INHALATION THERAPY

Inhalation therapy is often used synonymously with the term *respiratory care*. In a general context, inhalation therapy can be thought of as the delivery of gases for ventilation and oxygenation, as aerosol therapy, or as a means of delivering therapeutic medications.

Therapeutic aerosols have been employed in the treatment of pulmonary patients with bronchospastic airway disease, COPD, and pulmonary infection. The basic goals of aerosol therapy are to improve bronchial hygiene, humidify gases delivered through artificial airways, and deliver medications. The first two goals were discussed earlier in this chapter.

The advantages of delivering drugs by inhalation are multiple. Easier access, rapid onset of action, reduced extrapulmonary side effects, reduced dosage, coincidental application with aerosol therapy for humidification, and psychological benefits have all been cited.[4,20,32] In the nonintubated patient, aerosol therapy necessitates the patient's cooperation and skilled help. The equipment is a potential source of nosocomial infections.[8] Aerosol therapy has many of the same disadvantages noted with humidification. Although drug usage is often reduced, precise titration and dosages are difficult to ascertain because of variable degrees of drug deposition in the airway.

This section provides an overview of inhalation pharmacology. The basic principles, devices for medication delivery, and specific pharmacologic agents that are employed are discussed. For a more comprehensive topic review and specific drug information, one should refer to available reference texts.

A. BASIC PHARMACOLOGIC PRINCIPLES

The basic pharmacology of inhalation therapy necessitates a brief pharmacologic review. A medication is a drug that is given to elicit a physiologic response and is used for therapeutic purposes. Undesired responses (side effects) are also produced. The medication can interact with receptors by direct application (topical effect) or absorption into the bloodstream.

Various routes of pharmacologic administration are used for respiratory care. Subcutaneous, parenteral, gastrointestinal, and inhalation administrations are all commonly employed in the management of pulmonary diseases. Inhalation therapy employs the increased surface area of the lung parenchyma as a route of medication administration. This necessitates the drug reaching the alveolar and tracheobronchial mucosal surfaces for systemic capillary absorption.

Although inhaled medications can have topical effects, the primary reasons for the inhalation of medications are convenience, a safe method for self-administration, and maximal pulmonary benefit with reduced side effects. If the drug depends on systemic absorption, the drug's distribution and blood concentration are important. Blood concentration is altered by several mechanisms, such as dosage, route of administration, absorption, metabolism, and excretion. Alteration in liver and kidney function can produce unexpected drug levels and side effects.

If multiple drugs are employed for respiratory care, various drug interactions can occur. *Potentiation* is the result of one drug with limited activity changing the response of another drug; *synergism* results when two drugs with similar action produce a greater response than the sum of the individual responses. If the response to the two drugs is the sum of the responses to the individual medications, they are *additive*. *Tolerance* necessitates increasing drug levels to elicit a response, and *tachyphylaxis* results in the inability of larger doses to produce the expected response. Finally, the nomenclature for drug dosages should be understood. Two common methods for expressing drug dosage are *ratio strength* (drug dilutions) and *percentage strength* (percentage solutions). The following facts are necessary to understand this often confusing topic. A *solution* is a homogeneous mixture of two substances. A *solute* is the dissolved drug, and a *solvent* is the fluid in which the drug is dissolved. A gram of water equals 1 mL of water, and 1 g equals 1000 mg. *Ratio strength* is expressed in terms of parts of solute in relation to the total parts of solvent (or grams of solute per grams of solvent). A 1:1000 solution is 1 g of a drug in 1000 g of solvent (or 1000 mg/1000 mL—1 mg/1 mL). *Percentage strength* is expressed as the number of parts of solute in 100 parts of solvent (or grams of solute per 100 g of solvent). A 1% solution is 1 g of drug in 100 g of solvent.

B. AEROSOLIZED DRUG DELIVERY SYSTEMS

Therapeutic aerosols are commonly employed in respiratory care. As stated earlier, inhalation delivery of drugs can often produce therapeutic drug effects with reduced toxicity. The effectiveness of aerosols is related to the amount of drug delivered to the lungs. Actual pulmonary deposition of aerosolized drugs is a result of drug sedimentation that is due to gravity, inertial impact that is due to airway size, and directional change of airflow and kinetic energy.[32] Aerosol delivery also depends on particle size, pattern of inhalation, and degree of airway obstruction. Particle size should be smaller than 5 µm; otherwise, the particles may become trapped in the upper airway and never reach the site of action in the lungs. Aerosol particles that can traverse artificial airways (e.g., ET) are usually less than 2 µm in diameter. Also, particles smaller than 2 µm are deposited in peripheral airways. Particles less than 0.6 µm in diameter are often exhaled before reaching their site of action.

The ideal pattern of inhalation should be large volume, slow inspiration (5 to 6 seconds), and accentuated by an inspiratory hold (10 seconds). This breath holding enhances sedimentation and diffusion. Faster inspiratory inflows increase deposition of particles on oropharyngeal and upper airway surfaces. If airway obstruction is significant, adequate deposition of drugs can be limited. If the obstruction is not relieved, larger dosages or increased frequency of administration may be necessary. Application of the aerosol early in inspiration allows deeper penetration into the lungs, whereas delivery of medications at the back end of the breath enhances application to slower filling lung units. Concerns are raised in areas of the lung with poor ventilation related to airflow obstruction or low compliance. There are several methods for delivering aerosolized medications to the patient: jet nebulizers, pressurized metered-dose inhalers (MDIs), dry powder inhalers, ultrasonic nebulizers, and IPPB (discussed earlier).

Dry powder inhalers and pressurized MDIs are the most common delivery systems because of their low cost and ease of use. The MDI is a convenient, self-contained, and commonly employed method of aerosolized drug delivery (Figs. 13-11 and 13-12).[4,20] These prefilled drug canisters are activated by manual compression and deliver a predetermined unit (metered) of medication. Appropriate instruction is necessary for optimal use.[31] With the canister in the upside-down position, the device should be compressed only once per inhalation. A slow

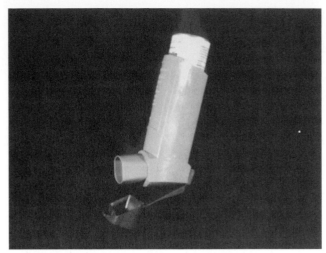

Figure 13-12 Metered-dose inhaler for handheld use. (From Benumof JL [ed]: Airway Management: Principles and Practice. St. Louis, Mosby, 1996, p 223.)

maximal inspiration with a breath-hold is typically recommended. It is imperative that the tongue not obstruct flow, but it is controversial whether the device should be placed in the mouth or held several centimeters from the lips with the mouth wide open. Concerns about excessive oral deposition of large particles must be offset against consistency of administration when the device is held away from the mouth. Other issues regarding use of MDIs include ideal lung volume for actuation, time of inspiratory hold, and inspiratory flow rate. If multiple doses are prescribed, an interval of several minutes between puffs is advisable.

Several problems with MDI drug delivery have been recognized. Manual coordination is necessary to activate the canister. Arthritis can cause difficulty, as can misaiming the aerosol. Pharyngeal deposition can lead to local abnormalities (e.g., oral candidiasis secondary to aerosolized corticosteroids). Systemic effects that are due to swallowing the drug can be reduced if the pharynx is rinsed after inhalation to reduce pharyngeal deposition.[20] The new MDI devices have been designed to reduce some of these problems. In addition, several spacing devices are available as extensions to MDIs. Spacers are designed to eliminate the need for hand-breath coordination and reduction of large-particle deposition in the upper airway.

The gas-powered nebulizers can be handheld or placed in line with the ventilatory circuit (Fig. 13-13).[4,20] The handheld devices are typically employed for more acutely ill individuals and as an alternative to an MDI. The full handheld system uses a nebulizer, a pressurized gas source, and a mouthpiece or face mask. Patients' cooperation is not required, and high doses of drugs can be delivered. Disadvantages include expense and less ease of use.

These systems are more expensive, cumbersome, and often less efficient than MDIs. Supervision is usually necessary for appropriate drug preparation and administration. Typically, the drug is diluted in saline. The drug is usually

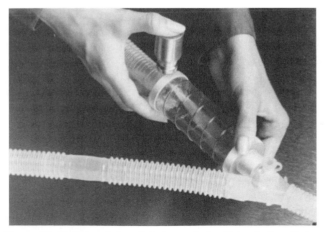

Figure 13-11 Metered-dose inhaler and circuit inspiratory limb spacer. (Aero Vent-Monaghan Medical, Plattsburgh, NY)

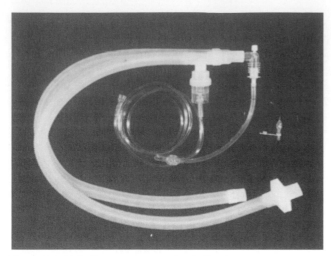

Figure 13-13 In-line, gas-powered nebulization system. (From Benumof JL [ed]: Airway Management: Principles and Practice. St. Louis, Mosby, 1996, p 223.)

more concentrated because a majority of the drug is never aerosolized or is lost during exhalation. Only the drug that is inspired can reach the lung.

The total volume to be nebulized is usually 3 mL (see "Pharmacologic Agents" Section IV. C. in this chapter) at gas flows of 6 to 8 L/min (device dependent). The treatment time is usually 5 to 10 minutes. During the course of treatment, the patient's vital signs and subjective tolerance must be monitored. Aerosolization of medication for drug delivery is different from aerosol therapy for humidification (see "Humidifiers" Section II. D.).

Both the MDI and the gas-powered nebulizers can be used in line with an artificial airway or ventilator circuit, or both (see Figs. 13-11 and 13-13). The drug delivery system is positioned in the inspiratory limb, as proximal to the artificial airway as possible. In-line drug delivery is usually less efficient in ventilated patients than in spontaneously breathing, nonintubated patients because of the breathing pattern, drug deposition on the ET, and airway disease.

C. PHARMACOLOGIC AGENTS

Numerous drugs are used in the management of pulmonary diseases. Inhaled medications offer advantages over intravenous or oral administration. These include more specific targeting to the site of action and resulting lower doses limiting systemic side effects. Nebulized (aerosolized) drug delivery is commonly employed to improve mucociliary clearance (mucokinetics) and relieve bronchospastic airway disease. The major drugs employed for inhalation therapy can be categorized by their ability to affect these two issues. In addition, certain anti-inflammatory, antiasthmatic, antifungal, antiviral, and antibacterial drugs are given by aerosol. The following reviews some of the commonly employed *aerosolized* drugs and is not meant to be a comprehensive review of respiratory pharmacology. All listed dosages are meant to

be representative for adult patients (if needed, specific product literature should be referred to prior to use).

1. Mucokinetic Drugs

Mucokinetic drugs are employed to enhance mucociliary clearance. These agents can be classified according to their mechanism of action. Hypoviscosity agents are the most commonly employed mucokinetic agents. Saline, sodium bicarbonate, and alcohol are the specific agents most commonly used. The mechanism of action for each drug varies but tends to affect mucus viscosity by disrupting the mucopolysaccharide chains that are the primary components of mucus. The other category of mucokinetic aerosol agents is made up of the mucolytics. The following is a brief synopsis of the various drugs in these two groups.[3]

a. Hypoviscosity Agents

Saline is the most commonly employed mucokinetic agent. It can be used as a primary drug or a solvent. The mechanism of action is reduction of viscosity by dilution of the mucopolysaccharide strands. The indication for use is thick, tenacious mucous secretions. The typical concentration is 0.45% to 0.9% sodium chloride (NaCl). The two major side effects associated with aerosolized saline are overhydration and the promotion of bronchospasm in patients with hyperactive airway disease (especially in newborns).

Alcohol (ethyl alcohol and ethanol) decreases the surface tension of pulmonary fluid. The typical concentration is 30%, and the dosage is 4 to 10 mL. The primary indication is pulmonary edema. This agent should be administered by side-arm nebulization or IPPB but not as a heated aerosol. The contraindication is a hypersensitivity to alcohol or its derivative. Side effects include airway irritation, bronchospasm, and local dehydration.

b. Mucolytic Agents

Acetylcysteine 10% (Mucomyst) is an effective mucolytic. The mechanism of action is lysis of the disulfide bonds in mucopolysaccharide chains, reducing the viscosity of the mucus. The indication is for management of viscous, inspissated, mucopurulent secretions. The actual effectiveness in the treatment of mucostasis is inconclusive, and each individual must be monitored to determine the benefit of therapy. The usual dosage is 2 to 5 mL every 6 hours. Hypersensitivity is a contraindication. In general, acetylcysteine is relatively nontoxic. Side effects include unpleasant taste and odor, local irritation, inhibition of ciliary activity, and bronchospasm. For these reasons, pretreatment with a bronchodilator is recommended. Other reported side effects include nausea, vomiting, stomatitis, rhinorrhea, and generalized urticaria. Acetylcysteine is incompatible with several antibodies. The drug should be avoided or used with extreme caution in patients with bronchospastic airway disease.

Other special concerns are a need for refrigeration, reactivity with rubber, and limited use after opening (96 hours).[12]

2. Bronchodilators and Antiasthmatic Drugs

Acute and chronic bronchospastic airway diseases afflict many individuals. Many drugs, varying primarily by their mechanism of action and route of delivery, are available to manage this problem. This section deals only with aerosolized drugs that are commonly employed in the therapy of bronchospastic airway disease (Table 13-6).[19,24,35] The drug groups are divided by their mechanism of action: sympathomimetics, anticholinergics, corticosteroids, and cromolyn. A comprehensive review of these drugs, the various mechanisms for bronchodilation, and the management of specific pathophysiologic problems is beyond the scope of this chapter.

a. Sympathomimetics

Sympathomimetics include the β-adrenergic agonists and methylxanthines (not available in aerosol). β-Adrenergic agents couple to the β_2-adrenoreceptor through the G protein α subunit to adenylate cyclase, which results in an increase in intracellular cyclic adenosine monophosphate (cAMP), which then leads to activation of protein kinase A. Activated protein kinase A inhibits phosphorylation of certain muscle proteins that regulate smooth muscle tone and also inhibits release of calcium ion from intracellular stores. In general, the responses of sympathomimetic drugs are classified according to whether the effects are α, β_1, or β_2. The β_2 receptors are responsible for bronchial smooth muscle relaxation. The common side effects associated with β-adrenergic agonists are due to their additional β_1 and α effects. β_1 effects cause an increase in heart rate, dysrhythmias, and cardiac contractility; α effects increase vascular tone. Potent β_2 stimulants can produce unwanted symptoms: anxiety, headache, nausea, tremors, and sleeplessness. Prolonged utilization can lead to receptor down-regulation and reduced drug response. Ideally, the more pure the β_2 response, the better the therapeutic benefit relative to side effects. The following sympathomimetics are commonly employed in clinical practice.[12,20,32,37]

Isoetharine hydrochloride 1% (Bronkosol) is available in a 1% solution. Its primary action is β_2 with weak β_1 (therapeutic doses) and no α effects. The nebulized dosage is usually 0.1 to 0.2 mg/kg/dose in 4.0 mL of normal saline. The bronchodilatory effects are weaker than those of isoproterenol and last 1 to 3 hours. The drug is available in an MDI. Typical dosage of the MDI is two puffs (340 μg per puff) four times a day.

Metaproterenol sulfate 5% (Alupent) is very similar to isoetharine, but the duration of action is approximately 5 hours. The dosage is 0.3 mL (5%) in 2.5 mL of normal saline. Metaproterenol is available in an MDI.

Albuterol (Ventolin, Proventil) is a sympathomimetic agent available in an MDI. It has a strong β_2 effect with limited β_1 properties. Its β_2 duration of action is approximately 6 hours.

Racemic epinephrine 2.25% (Vaponephrine) is a mixture of levo and dextro isomers of epinephrine. It is a weak β and mild α drug. The α effects provide mucosal constriction. In the aerosol form, this drug acts as a good mucosal decongestant. The drug has minimal bronchodilatory action. Cardiovascular side effects are limited. Typical dosage is 0.5 mL (2.25%) in 3.5 mL of saline, given as frequently as every hour in adult patients. Racemic epinephrine is commonly mixed with 0.25 mL (1 mg) of dexamethasone for the management of postextubation swelling and croup.

Isoproterenol (Isuprel) is the prototype pure β-adrenergic bronchodilator. Bronchodilation depends on adequate blood levels. In addition, isoproterenol is a pulmonary and mucosal vascular dilator. This causes an increased rate of absorption, higher blood levels, and increased β_1 side effects. The side effects can be quite significant and often reduce the utilization of this agent in patients with cardiac disease; dysrhythmias, myocardial ischemia, and palpitations can all occur. If the pulmonary vasculature vasodilates to areas of low ventilation, the potential to augment ventilation-perfusion mismatch and increase intrapulmonary shunt exists. Typical dosage is 0.25 to 0.5 mL (0.5%) in 3.5 mL of saline. The effect lasts 1 to 2 hours. Isoproterenol is also available as an MDI.

Newer inhaled β-adrenergic drugs include salmeterol, pirbuterol, and bitolterol (a catecholamine). Salmeterol can be administered by either a pressurized MDI (21 μg) or a dry powered inhaler (50 μg). Pirbuterol acetate is usually administered through a pressurized MDI (200 μg). Bitolterol can be provided as either a pressurized MDI or a solution. Salmeterol was the first long-acting adrenergic bronchodilator approved for use in the United States. Its duration of action is approximately 12 hours, with an onset of about 20 minutes and a peak effect occurring in 3 to 5 hours. It is particularly useful in patients with nocturnal asthma because of its longer duration of action. The prolonged effect of some of the newer bronchodilators is due to their increased lipophilicity (Table 13-7).

b. Anticholinergic Agents and Antibiotics

Anticholinergic drugs play an increasing role in the management of bronchospastic pulmonary disease but generally have been found more effective as maintenance treatment of bronchoconstriction in COPD. These drugs inhibit acetylcholine at the cholinergic receptor site, reducing vagal nerve activity. This produces bronchodilation (preferentially in large airways) and a reduction in mucus secretion. Major side effects include dry mouth, blurred vision, headache, tremor, nervousness, and palpitations.

Ipratropium bromide (Atrovent) is a commonly used anticholinergic. Its effects are primarily β_2. It is available as an MDI. The standard dosage is 36 μg four times a day (18 μg per puff). Hypersensitivity to the drug is

Table 13-6　Aerosolized Bronchodilators and Antiasthmatic Drugs

Type of Drug	Method	Dose*	Mechanism
Sympathomimetics			*β₂ agonist increase in cyclic AMP*
Short-acting beta agonists			
Albuterol (Ventolin, Proventil)	MDI/Neb	2 puffs (90 µg/puff) q4 hr prn	
Levalbuterol hydrochloride (Xopenex)	Neb	0.63-1.25 mg nebulized solution q 6-8 hr	
Pirbuterol acetate (Maxair)	MDI	2 puffs (200 µg/puff) 4 hr prn	
Racemic epinephrine	Neb	0.25 mL in 3.5 mL	
Long-acting beta agonists			
Salmeterol xinafoate (Serevent)	DPI	1 puff (50 µg) bid	
Formoterol fumarate (Foradil)	DPI	1 capsule (12 µg) via Aerolizer inhaler bid	
Anticholinergics			*Cholinergic blocker increasing β stimulation*
Ipratropium bromide (Atrovent)	MDI/Neb	2 puffs (18 µg/puff) qid 17 µg (0.02%) qid	
Tiotropium bromide (Spiriva)	DPI	1 capsule inhaled (18 µg) via HandiHaler qd	
Anti-inflammatory			
Inhaled corticosteroids			*Anti-inflammatory Inhibit leukocyte migration Potentiate β-agonists*
Beclomethasone acetate (Vanceril, Beclovent)	MDI	2 puffs (42 µg/puff) qid	
Flunisolide (AeroBid)	MDI	2-4 puffs (250 µg/puff) bid	
Triamcinolone acetonide (Azmacort)	MDI	2-8 puffs (100 µg/puff) bid	
Budesonide (Pulmicort)	DPI/Neb	1-4 puffs (200 µg/puff) bid 0.25 mg/2 mL bid 0.5 mg/2 mL bid	

Fluticasone propionate (Flovent)
  44 µg
  110 µg
  220 µg
	MDI	Up to a maximum of 880 µg/day	

Mometasone furoate (Asmanex)	DPI	1-2 puffs (220 µg/puff) qd	
Nonsteroidal anti-inflammatory agents			*Mast cell suppression*
Cromolyn sodium 1% (Intal)	MDI/Neb	2 puffs (800 µg/puff) qid 20 mg in 2-4 mL qid	
Nedocromil (Tilade)	MDI	2 puffs (1.75 mg/puff) qid	
Combination Products			
Albuterol sulfate/ipratropium bromide (Combivent)	MDI/Neb	2 puffs (0.09 mg/0.018 mg per puff) qid 1 vial (3 mg/0.5 mg) qid	

Fluticasone propionate/salmeterol Xinafoate (Advair)
  100 µg/50 µg
  250 µg/50 µg
  500 µg/50 µg
	DPI	1 puff bid	

*Dosages may vary; references to specific drug inserts are recommended.
MDI, metered-dose inhaler; Neb, nebulizer; DPI, dry-powder inhaler; bid, twice a day; qid, four times a day; qd, once a day.
Modified from Benumof JL: Airway Management: Principles and Practice. St. Louis, Mosby, 1996.

Table 13-7 **Onset and Duration of Commonly Used Bronchodilators**

Drug	Onset (min)	Peak (min)	Duration (hr)
Isoproterenol*	2-5	5-30	1-2
Isoetharine*	2-5	15-60	1-3
Bitolterol*	3-5	30-60	5-8
Metaproterenol	2-5	60	2-6
Albuterol	15	30-60	3-8
Pirbuterol	5	30	5
Salmeterol	20	180-300	12

*A catecholamine.

From Benumof JL: Airway Management: Principles and Practice. St. Louis, Mosby, 1996.

a contraindication. Caution should be exercised in patients with narrow-angle glaucoma.

Antibiotics are also delivered by an inhalational route. Aerosolized tobramycin is used in patients with cystic fibrosis, and ribavirin is employed in children against respiratory syncytial virus. Pentamidine can be employed as prophylaxis against *Pneumocystis carinii*.

c. Antiallergy and Asthmatic Agents

The two main groups of aerosolized agents in this category are cromolyn and corticosteroids. These drugs are often used in concert with other medications.

Cromolyn sodium 1% and nedocromil are rarely used to prevent bronchospasm in exercise-induced asthma. They have been replaced by inhaled corticosteroids. These drugs are not effective in the management of acute bronchospasm. The mechanism of action is suppression of mast cell response to antigen-antibody reactions. Cromolyn sodium is available in a powder (spinhaler), liquid, and MDI for inhalation therapy. The typical dosages are 20 mg four times a day by nebulizer or two puffs four times a day (800 µg per puff) with the MDI. The MDI appears to be tolerated best. Hypersensitivity is a contraindication. Side effects include local irritation, allergic symptoms (rash and urticaria), and airway hyperactivity (most common with the powder).

Newer mediator antagonists are now available. These include zafirlukast, montelukast, and zileuton. Zafirlukast

and montelukast work as leukotriene receptor antagonists and selectively inhibit leukotriene receptors LTD_4 and LTE_4. Leukotrienes are produced by 5-lipoxygenase from arachidonic acid and stimulate leukotriene receptors to cause bronchoconstrictions and chemotaxis of inflammatory cells. As with cromolyn sodium, these agents are not to be used for acute asthmatic attacks but rather for long-term prevention of bronchoconstriction.[35]

Corticosteroids are commonly used for maintenance therapy in patients with chronic asthma.[25,27] The mechanism of action is attributed to their anti-inflammatory properties, reducing leakage of fluids, inhibiting migration of macrophages and leukocytes, and possibly blocking the response to various mediators of inflammation. Corticosteroids have been reported to potentiate the effects of the sympathomimetic drugs.[4] Both systemic and topical side effects can occur with inhaled corticosteroids. These effects include adrenal insufficiency, acute asthma episodes, possible growth retardation, and osteoporosis. Local effects include oropharyngeal fungal infections and dysphonia. Adrenal suppression is usually not a concern with doses below 800 µg/day.

Dexamethasone sodium phosphate (Decadron) is the prototypic steroid for respiratory care. It is used most often for its anti-inflammatory action and after extubation with racemic epinephrine. The typical dosage is 0.25 mL (1 mg) in 2.5 mL of saline. The side effects of corticosteroids are related to their chronicity of use and degree of systemic absorption. Because of its systemic effects, dexamethasone is used on a limited basis as an aerosol.

Beclomethasone dipropionate (Vanceril, Beclovent) is an aerosolized corticosteroid that is highly active topically and that has limited systemic absorption or activity. The typical dosage is two puffs (42 µg per puff) three or four times a day. Hoarseness, sore throat, and oral candidiasis are reported side effects. The candidiasis can be managed with topical antifungal drugs. Mild adrenal suppression is reported with high doses, and caution is advised when switching from oral to inhaled corticosteroids.

The preceding pharmacologic agents are representative of those commonly employed by aerosol in respiratory care. Appropriate pharmacologic management necessitates assessing response to therapy. Objective and subjective relief of symptoms and improvement in pulmonary function while minimizing side effects of these drugs are the endpoints of good inhalation therapy.

REFERENCES

1. Barnes TA, Watson ME: Oxygen delivery performance of four adult resuscitation bags. Respir Care 27:139, 1982.
2. Barnes TA, Watson ME: Oxygen delivery performance of old and new designs of the Laerdal, Vitalograph and AMBU adult manual resuscitators. Respir Care 28:1121, 1983.
3. Barton AD: Aerosolized detergents and mucolytic agents in the treatment of stable chronic obstructive pulmonary disease. Am Rev Respir Dis 110:104, 1974.
4. Burton GL, Hodgkin JE (eds): Respiratory Care, 2nd ed. Philadelphia, JB Lippincott, 1984.
5. Carden E, Friedman D: Further studies of manually operated self-inflating resuscitation bag. Anesth Analg 56:202, 1977.
6. Chapman GA, Kim CS, Frankel J, et al: Evaluation of the safety and efficiency of new suction catheter design. Respir Care 31:889, 1986.

7. Cohen D, Horiuchi K, Kemper M, et al: Modulating effects of propofol on metabolic and cardiopulmonary responses to stressful intensive care procedures. Crit Care Med 24:612, 1996.
8. Craven DE, Goulartet A, Maki BJ: Contaminated condensate in mechanical ventilator circuits: A risk factor for nosocomial pneumonia? Am Rev Respir Dis 129:625, 1984.
9. deBoisblanc BP, Castro M, Everret B, et al: Effect of air-supported, continuous, postural oscillation on the risk of early ICU pneumonia in nontraumatic critical illness. Chest 103:1543, 1993.
10. Demers RR: Complications of endotracheal suctioning procedures. Respir Care 27:453, 1982.
11. Deneke SM, Fanburg BL: Normobaric oxygen toxicity of the lung. N Engl J Med 303:76, 1980.
12. Eubanks DH, Bone RC: Comprehensive Respiratory Care. St Louis, Mosby, 1985.
13. Gibson RL, Comer PB, Beckham RW et al: Actual tracheal oxygen concentrations with commonly used oxygen equipment. Anesthesiology 44:71, 1976.
14. Greif R, Akca O, Horn E, et al: Supplemental perioperative oxygen to reduce the incidence of surgical-wound infection. N Engl J Med 342:161, 2000.
15. Greif R, Laciny S, Rapf B, et al: Supplemental oxygen reduces the incidence of postoperative nausea and vomiting. N Engl J Med 91:1246, 1999.
16. Hall TO: Aerosol generators and humidifiers. In Barnes TA (ed): Respiratory Care Practice. Chicago, Year Book, 1988, pp 356-405.
17. Harris JA, Jerry BA: Indications and procedures for segmental bronchial drainage. Respir Care 20:1164, 1975.
18. Jolliett P, Bulpa P, Chevrolet RC: Effects of prone position on gas exchange and hemodynamics in severe respiratory distress syndrome. Crit Care Med 12:1977, 1998.
19. Kacmarek RM: Humidity and aerosol therapy. In Pierson DJ, Kacmarek RM (eds): Foundations of Respiratory Care. New York, Churchill Livingstone, 1992, pp 793-824.
20. Kacmarek RM, Stoller JK (eds): Current Respiratory Care. Toronto, BC Decker, 1988.
21. Klein EF, Shah DA, Shah NJ, et al: Performance characteristics of conventional and prototype humidifiers and nebulizers. Chest 64:690, 1973.
22. Mackenzie CF, Shin B: Cardiorespiratory function before and after chest physiotherapy in mechanically ventilated patients with post-traumatic respiratory failure. Crit Care Med 13:483, 1985.
23. Marini JJ: Postoperative atelectasis: Pathophysiology, clinical importance, and principles of management. Respir Care 29:516, 1984.
24. McFadden RR: Aerosolized bronchodilators and steroids in the treatment of airway obstruction in adults. Am Rev Respir Dis 122:89, 1980.
25. Morse HG: Mechanisms of action and therapeutic role of corticosteroids and asthma. J Allergy Clin Immunol 75:1, 1985.
26. Murray JF: Review of the state of the art of intermittent positive pressure breathing therapy. Am Rev Respir Dis 110:193, 1974.
27. Newhouse MT, Dolovich MB: Control of asthma by aerosols. N Engl J Med 315:870, 1986.
28. Overend TJ, Anderson CM, Lucy SD, et al: The effect of incentive spirometry on postoperative pulmonary complications: A systematic review. Chest 120:971, 2001.
29. Radford R: Rational basis for percussion: Augmented mucociliary clearance. Respir Care 27:556, 1982.
30. Scacci R: Air entrainment masks: jet mixing is how they work; the Bernoulli and Venturi principles are how they don't. Respir Care 24:928, 1979.
31. Self TH, Brooks JB: Necessity of teaching patients correct bronchodilator inhalation technique. Immunol Allergy Pract 4:40, 1982.
32. Shapiro BA, Kacmarek RM, Cane RD, et al: Clinical Application of Respiratory Care, 4th ed. St Louis, Mosby, 1991.
33. Stiller K: Physiotherapy in intensive care: Towards an evidence-based practice. Chest 118:1801, 2000.
34. Tyler ML: Complications of positioning and chest physiotherapy. Respir Care 27:458, 1982.
35. Weinberger M, Hendeles L, Ahrens R: Pharmacologic management of reversible obstructive airway disease. Med Clin North Am 65:529, 1981.
36. Zadai CL: Physical therapy for the acutely ill medical patient. Phys Ther 61:1746, 1981.
37. Ziment I: Why are they saying bad things about IPPB? Respir Care 18:677, 1973.

SUGGESTED READINGS

American College of Chest Physicians-Heart, Lung and Blood Institute: National Conference on Oxygen Therapy. Chest 85:234, 1984.

Fisher AB: Oxygen therapy: Side effects and toxicity. Am Rev Respir Dis 122:61, 1980.

Grabovac MT, Kim KK, Quinn TE, et al: Respiratory care. In Miller RD (ed): Anesthesia, 6th ed. Philadelphia, Churchill Livingstone, 2005, pp 2811-2830.

Vender JS, Clemency MV: Oxygen delivery systems, inhalation therapy, and respiratory care. In Benumof JL (ed): Clinical Procedures in Anesthesia and Intensive Care. Philadelphia, JB Lippincott, 1992, pp 63-87.

14

NONINTUBATION MANAGEMENT OF THE AIRWAY: MASK VENTILATION*

John P. McGee II
Jeffrey S. Vender

I. OVERVIEW

Maintaining a patent airway is the first principle of resuscitation and life support. It is an essential skill for those caring for anesthetized or critically ill patients. Clinicians working in a hospital setting (respiratory care, nursing, intensive care, and emergency room physicians) should all be competent in the basic essentials of airway care.

Too frequently, inexperienced personnel believe airway management necessitates intubation of the trachea. The focus of this chapter is twofold: a review of tools and skills of nonintubation airway management and a discussion of potential airway management techniques. Other chapters focus on techniques of endotracheal intubation and pharyngeal intubation (laryngeal mask airway). Airway management can be divided into the establishment and maintenance of a patent airway and respiratory support. Establishing and maintaining a patent airway are achieved by manipulating the head and neck in ways that maximize the anatomic airway or by using artificial airway devices. Respiratory support techniques control the atmosphere the patient breathes and allow manual ventilatory assistance.

A. AIRWAY ANATOMY

The airway is the passageway that air or respiratory gases must traverse. Nonintubation airway management seeks to produce patency to gas flow through the oropharynx, nasopharynx, and larynx without the use of artificial airway devices that extend into the trachea or laryngopharynx.

---

*Figures and portions of the text from McGee JP, Vender S: Nonintubation management of the airway. In Benumof JL (ed): Clinical Procedures in Anesthesia and Intensive Care. Philadelphia, JB Lippincott, 1992, pp 89-114.

A thorough understanding of airway anatomy is necessary to appreciate the therapeutic maneuvers and devices employed in airway management (Fig. 14-1). Very detailed reviews of airway anatomy can be found in Chapters 1 and 2 of this book and various atlases and texts.[5,6,38,41]

Gas passes from outside the body through the nose or mouth. If through the nares, it passes through the choanae, nasopharynx (where it is warmed and humidified), oropharynx, hypopharynx or laryngopharynx, and glottis. If through the mouth, the oropharynx and hypopharynx are traversed. Nasal passages can be obstructed by choanal atresia, septal deviation, mucosal swelling, or foreign material (e.g., mucus, blood). The entry to the oropharynx can be blocked by the soft palate lying against the posterior pharyngeal wall. The pathway of gas by either route can be restricted by the tongue in the oropharynx or the epiglottis in the hypopharynx. These are sites of pharyngeal collapse.[9,13,17,27] Airway manipulation and devices can treat these causes of obstruction fairly efficaciously in most cases.[18,24,25,28] Laryngeal obstruction related to spasm must be treated by positive airway pressure, deeper anesthesia, muscle relaxants, or endotracheal intubation.[4]

Laryngeal closure can occur from intrinsic or extrinsic muscles of the larynx. Tight airway closure (laryngospasm or effort closure) results from contraction of the external laryngeal muscles, which force the mucosal folds of the quadrangular membrane into apposition (Fig. 14-2). Muscle groups also extend from the thyroid cartilage to the hyoid and cricoid. When they contract, the interior mucosa and soft tissue (ventricular and vocal folds) are forced into the center of the airway and the thyroid shield is deformed (compressed inward), providing a spring to open the airway rapidly once these muscles relax.[6] The larynx closes at the level of the true cords by action of the intrinsic muscles of the larynx (especially interarytenoid and cricothyroid) during phonation, but this closure is not as tight as the laryngeal spasm described earlier.

Opening of the pharynx and larynx is achieved by elongating and unfolding the airway from the hyoid to the cricoid cartilage.[1,5,6,20] Muscles tether the hyoid bone and the tongue to the chin or anterior mandible (geniohyoid, digastric, hyoglossus, and genioglossus). Other muscles tether the cricoid and thyroid cartilages to the sternum and first rib (sternothyroid). The "strap muscles" tether the hyoid bone to the sternum and rib (sternohyoid

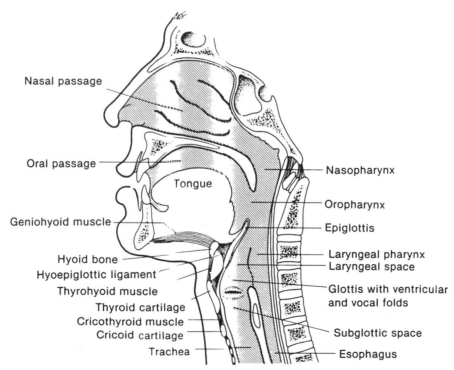

Figure 14-1 Normal airway anatomy: lateral view of head and neck in neutral position. The various components of the airway and surrounding structures are labeled. Note that (1) the tongue and soft palate could easily obliterate the airway at the oropharynx by falling backward (the likelihood of the epiglottis sealing against the posterior pharyngeal wall is better seen in the xerograms [see Figs. 14-3 and 14-4]) and that (2) the muscular line from the mentum to hyoid bone (geniohyoid muscle) to thyroid cartilage (thyrohyoid muscle and membrane) to cricoid (cricothyroid muscle) has a folded and right-angle character. This line can be straightened by extending the head and pulling the jaw forward (anteriorly), thus pulling the epiglottis and tongue away from the posterior wall. (From Benumof JL [ed]: Airway Management: Principles and Practice. St. Louis, Mosby, 1996, p 229.)

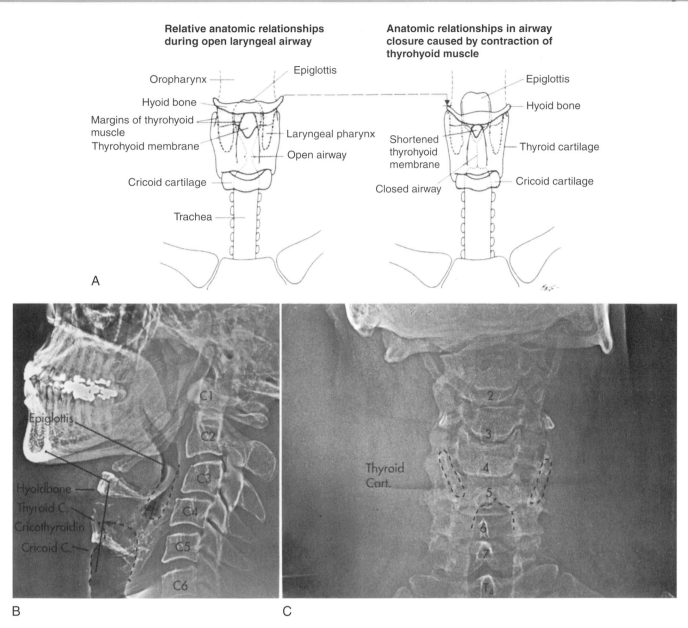

Figure 14-2 Laryngeal closure. **A,** Both panels are schematic frontal views of the airway at the larynx. The left panel shows an open airway with an air column visible centrally and the hyoid bone clearly above the thyroid shield. The right panel shows obliteration of the air column (caused by apposition of the ventricular and vocal folds) and approximation of the hyoid bone to the thyroid cartilage, caused by contraction of the thyrohyoid muscle. **B** and **C,** Lateral and frontal xerograms during Valsalva-induced laryngeal closure. In the lateral view, note the marked thyrohyoid approximation, and in the frontal view, the abrupt airway cutoff and lack of air column within the thyroid shield, which is at the level of C4-C5. (From Benumof JL [ed]: Airway Management: Principles and Practice. St. Louis, Mosby, 1996, p 230.)

and omohyoid). When the head is tilted, the chin and the mandible are displaced forward on the temporomandibular sliding joint (a jaw-thrust maneuver); maximum stretch occurs at the hyoid-thyroid-cricoid area. The hyoid bone is pulled in an anterior direction along with the epiglottis and root of the tongue, opening up the oropharynx. The ventricular and vocal folds flatten against the sides of the thyroid cartilage, opening the laryngeal airway.[6]

The inferior and middle constrictors close the superior part of the esophagus (cervical sphincter) to prevent regurgitation. Muscle relaxants open the airway by relaxing the intrinsic and extrinsic laryngeal muscles that close the airway. They can also relax the pharyngeal constrictors,

potentially permitting regurgitation (and aspiration). These two problems, airway patency versus airway protection, represent the major dilemma of airway management without an endotracheal tube (ET).

B. UPPER AIRWAY OBSTRUCTION

1. Pharyngeal Collapse—Lessons from Studies of Obstructive Sleep Apnea

Upper airway obstruction encountered in anesthetizing patients with "normal" airways has long been attributed to a relaxed tongue (treated with chin lift and an oral airway) or laryngospasm (crowing) treated with positive pressure or succinylcholine, or both.[1,4,19,30] With the emergence of obstructive sleep apnea (OSA) as a syndrome treatable with nasal continuous positive airway pressure (nCPAP),[36] the concept of the airway collapsing like a flexible tube has replaced the concept of a cylinder being obstructed by a specific tissue mass. The investigation of pharyngeal collapse during the respiratory cycle and during sleep has exploded.[2,9,10,14-17,23,27,31,32] Although these investigations are done primarily during sleep, they give insight into problems and frustrations known to those who have practiced mask anesthesia. Anesthesiologists have encountered patients who, despite a nasal and oral airway or a triple airway maneuver, still did not have a patent airway, even in the absence of specific pathology.

During the awake state the pharynx is patent, in part because of its tubular structure and in part because of the tonic activity in pharyngeal dilator muscles. The tongue electromyogram (EMG) is the most easily recorded.[10,27] If breathing through the nose is made more difficult, the tongue EMG increases to keep the airway patent.[11,12,23] During sleep, the tonic and phasic EMG decreases and the pharyngeal resistance rises.[40] In certain instances, the airway can collapse and become obstructed. This most commonly occurs at the level of the soft palate.[10,16] In fewer instances, the obstruction is at the level of the epiglottis (hypopharynx).[27] In patients susceptible to OSA, the geometry of the pharynx can be altered during normal sleep.[10] It is usually oval with the long axis in the transverse plane; in OSA, it is round or oval with the long axis in the anterior-posterior plane (the lateral walls are thickened).[31,32] This obstruction can often be treated effectively with nCPAP. Alternatively, intraoral devices (mandibular advancement device) that advance the mandible to a similar extent as the jaw-thrust maneuver can be employed.[18,25,28]

If nCPAP is used, the pressure is increased until a critical pressure is reached and some airflow begins. The airflow is limited in inspiration until a higher level of CPAP is reached at which snoring stops, inspiratory velocity increases, and ventilation is unobstructed.[34] This effective level of CPAP is abbreviated nCPAP$_{eff}$ as opposed to the critical pressure, P$_{crit}$. In patients with symptomatic sleep disturbance, the P$_{crit}$ is about 5 cm H$_2$O and nCPAP$_{eff}$ is 10 to 15 cm H$_2$O. An nCPAP of 20 cm H$_2$O is rarely required. In healthy patients who do not snore, negative pressure applied at the nose can cause pharyngeal collapse, snoring, and airway obstruction.[33] This requires −10 to −20 cm H$_2$O, so the basic physiologic concepts seem to apply to the whole population. Finally, CPAP applied through a face mask (to both nose and mouth) is not as effective as nCPAP alone.[35] However, oral airway devices were not used in this situation. It is probable, although unproved, that general anesthesia makes the pharyngeal airway less stable and shifts these nasal pressures needed to open the airway in a positive direction.

Hypopharyngeal obstruction has been investigated by placing a nasal fiberscope at the level of the soft palate in anesthetized patients.[20] The epiglottis and the glottic opening can be seen, recorded digitally, and analyzed. The percentage of glottic opening (POGO) seen from this view can be determined. In general, airflow increases and snoring decreases as POGO increases. However, a POGO of 100% has been documented with airway occlusion, and a POGO of 0% has been documented with no stridor and obvious ventilation, so this score is only an index. These evaluations do support the potential of airflow restriction at the hypopharynx and are consistent with this being related to the epiglottis obstructing the airway.

2. Clinical Airway Collapse

Upper airway obstruction is a common airway emergency necessitating nonintubation airway manipulation and airway devices. Soft tissue obstructions of the pharynx and larynx are the usual causes of upper airway obstruction.

Recognition of upper airway obstruction is essential and is dependent on observation, suspicion, and clinical data. The causes of soft tissue upper airway obstruction at the pharynx include loss of pharyngeal muscle tone resulting from a central nervous system abnormality (anesthesia, trauma, coma, stroke) [11,14,23,27]; expanding, space-occupying lesions (tumor, mucosal edema, abscess, and hematoma); and foreign substances (such as teeth, vomitus, or foreign body). Laryngeal obstruction is most often related to increased muscle activity from attempted vocalization or a reaction from foreign substances (secretions, foreign bodies, or tumors). The presentation of airway obstruction can be partial or complete. *Partial* airway obstruction is recognized by noisy inspiratory sounds. Depending on the magnitude, cause, and location of the obstruction, the tone of the sounds can vary. Snoring is the typical sound of partial airway obstruction in the nasopharynx and oropharynx and generally is most audible during expiration. Stridor or crowing suggests glottic (laryngeal) obstruction or laryngospasm and is heard most often in inspiration. In addition, signs and symptoms of hypoxemia or hypocarbia, or both, should make one suspicious of an airway obstruction.

Complete airway obstruction is a medical emergency. Signs of complete obstruction in the spontaneously breathing individual are inaudible breath sounds or the inability to perceive air movement; use of accessory neck muscles; sternal, intercostal, and epigastric retraction with inspiratory effort and absence of chest expansion on inspiration; and agitation.

Prevention and relief of airway obstruction are the focus of this chapter. Rapid, simple maneuvers should take precedence in the management of this problem.

II. MANAGEMENT OF THE AIRWAY WITHOUT INTUBATION

A. SIMPLE (NONINSTRUMENTAL) AIRWAY MANEUVERS: HEAD TILT, CHIN LIFT, JAW THRUST

The sections on airway anatomy and airway obstruction in this chapter, as well as Chapter 1, constitute essential background to the understanding of airway maneuvers. When muscles of the floor of the mouth and tongue relax, the tongue lies close to or on the back wall of the oropharynx, causing soft tissue obstruction.[27,30] It is also possible for the epiglottis to overlie and obstruct the glottic opening or to seal against the posterior pharyngeal wall.[1,9,27] This is exaggerated by flexing the head and neck or opening the mouth, or both (Fig. 14-3). The distance between the chin and the thyroid notch is relatively short in the flexed position. Any maneuver that increases the distance straightens out the mentum-geniohyoid-hyoid-thyroid line, thus elevating the hyoid bone farther from the pharynx. The hyoid elevates the epiglottis through the hyoepiglottic ligament. There are two maneuvers to lengthen this anterior neck distance.

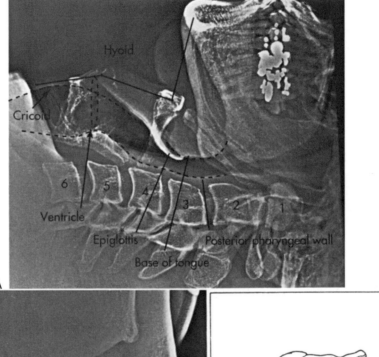

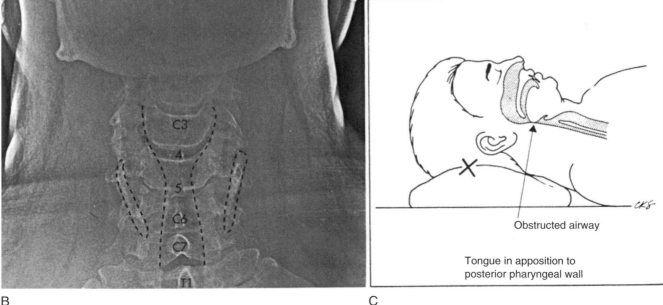

Figure 14-3 **A,** Lateral xerogram of the head and neck in neutral position. Patient is awake and supine. Mentum overlies the hyoid bone, the temporomandibular joint is in place, the base of the tongue and the epiglottis are close to the posterior pharyngeal wall, and the thyroid shield and cricoid cartilage are at the level of C5-C6. Note that an oral airway could easily touch the tip of the epiglottis, pushing it down. **B,** Frontal view, demonstrating the air column within the thyroid shield with its narrowest site at the level of the vocal cords (C5-6). **C,** Diagram of flexed head with tongue in apposition to posterior pharyngeal wall. (From Benumof JL [ed]: Airway Management: Principles and Practice. St. Louis, Mosby, 1996, p 232.)

The first maneuver (head tilt) is to tilt the head back on the atlanto-occipital joint while keeping the mouth closed (teeth approximated). This distance may be further augmented by elevating the occiput 1 to 4 inches above the level of the shoulders (sniffing position), as long as the larynx and posterior pharynx stay in their original position.

In some patients the cervical spine is stiff enough that elevating the head also elevates the C4-5 laryngeal area, leaving the airway unchanged. In children younger than 5 years the upper cervical spine is more flexible and can bow upward, forcing the posterior pharyngeal wall upward against the tongue and epiglottis, thereby exacerbating the obstruction. Therefore, a child's airway is usually best maintained by leaving the head in a more neutral position than that described for an adult. The head tilt is the simplest and first airway maneuver in resuscitation (Fig. 14-4). Head tilt may be accomplished by a chin lift or neck-occipital pivot. Extreme caution should be exercised in patients with suspected neck injuries or cerebrovascular disease. The head tilt by chin lift is reportedly more effective than the head tilt by neck-occipital pivot. In the latter, the mouth opens, the geniohyoid is slack, and the hyoid bone (and epiglottis) may remain close to the pharyngeal wall.[21]

The second maneuver more directly lifts the hyoid bone and tongue away from the posterior pharyngeal wall by subluxating the mandible forward onto the sliding part of the temporomandibular joint (mandibular advancement). The occluded teeth prevent the movement of the mandible, so the thumbs depress the mentum while the fingers grip the rami of the mandible and lift it upward to protrude the mandibular teeth in front of the maxillary teeth after the mouth opens slightly. (The insertion of a small airway sometimes makes this procedure easier because it separates the teeth, allowing the mandible to slide forward.) This is called the jaw-thrust maneuver and reliably opens the airway (Fig. 14-5). In most people the mandible is readily drawn back into the joint by elasticity of the joint capsule and masseter muscle; consequently, this position is difficult to maintain with one hand.

Some 20% of patients occlude the nasopharynx with the soft palate during exhalation, when the muscles are relaxed. If the mouth and lips are closed, exhalation is impeded. In these cases, an airway device is required to allow free exhalation. Without an airway device, the mouth must be opened slightly to ensure that the lips are parted. These three maneuvers (head tilt, jaw thrust, and open mouth), done together, are known as the triple airway maneuver (Box 14-1; see Fig. 14-5). The triple airway maneuver is the most reliable manual method to achieve upper airway patency.

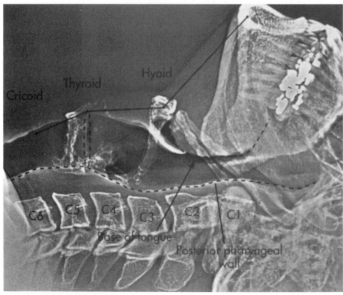

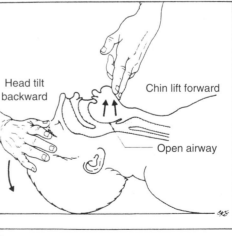

Head tilt and chin lift to obtain extended position

A

B

Figure 14-4 **A,** Head and neck in extended position (head tilt). Lateral xerogram with labeling as in Figure 14-3. Mentum is now superior to the hyoid bone, the temporomandibular joint is still in place (reduced position), the base of the tongue and epiglottis are farther off the posterior pharyngeal wall, and the thyroid and cricoid shield are at the level of C4-C5. The hyoid bone has been raised and elevated from C3-C4 to C2-C3. **B,** The drawing shows the head tilted back and the chin lifted forward, both of which contribute to opening the airway. (From Benumof JL [ed]: Airway Management: Principles and Practice. St. Louis, Mosby, 1996, p 233.)

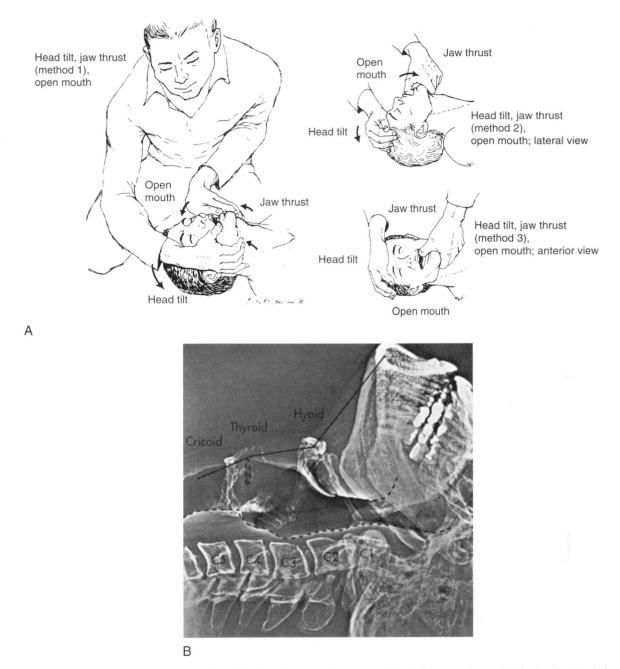

Figure 14-5 Triple airway maneuver (head tilt, jaw thrust, and open mouth). **A,** Diagram shows (1) the head extended on the atlanto-occipital joint, (2) the mouth opened to get the teeth out of occlusion as well as to open the oral fissure, and (3) the mandible forced upward, forcing the mandibular condyles to slide anteriorly at the temporomandibular joint. **B,** Lateral xerogram of jaw protrusion (patient awake). In addition to the extended position, the mandibular incisors protrude beyond the maxillary incisors, the teeth are not in occlusion, and the condyles of the mandible are forward, out of the hollow of the temporomandibular joint and onto the sliding portion (subluxated). (From Benumof JL [ed]: Airway Management: Principles and Practice. St. Louis, Mosby, 1996, p 234.)

B. HEIMLICH MANEUVER

As previously discussed, airway maneuvers can help obtain airway patency but do not relieve airway obstruction that is due to foreign material lodged in the upper airway. A foreign body obstruction should be suspected with a witnessed aspiration and when the patient cannot talk, when ventilation is absent, or when positive-pressure ventilation meets resistance after routine airway maneuvers have been done. Prior to the insertion of artificial airway devices, a manual effort (finger sweep) should be made to evacuate any foreign material present in the oropharynx. A Heimlich maneuver is indicated when coughing or traditional means are unable to relieve *complete* airway obstruction that is due to foreign material.

Box 14-1   Simple (Noninstrumental) Airway Maneuvers

Head Tilt
PROCEDURE

1. With the patient supine and operator at the patient's side, place one hand under the neck and the heel of the other hand on the forehead.
2. Extend the head by displacing the forehead back and lifting the occiput up (neck lift).

INDICATION:	Soft tissue upper airway obstruction
CONTRAINDICATIONS:	Fractured neck
	Basilar artery syndrome
	Infants
COMPLICATIONS:	Sore neck
	Pinched nerve

Chin Lift
PROCEDURE:

1. With the patient supine and operator at the head of the patient, place one hand on the forehead, with the first two fingers of the other hand over the underside of the chin.
2. Simultaneously tilt the forehead and exert upward traction on the chin.

INDICATION:	Alternative to neck lift for head tilt
CONTRAINDICATIONS:	Same as head tilt
COMPLICATIONS:	Same as head tilt

Jaw Thrust
PROCEDURE:

1. From above the patient's head, place thumbs on the maxilla and fingers behind the angle of the mandible (bilaterally), opening, lifting, and displacing the jaw forward.
2. Retract the lower lip with thumbs.
3. Tilt the head backward (unless contraindicated).

INDICATION:	Head tilt contraindicated (e.g., fractured neck) or ineffective
CONTRAINDICATIONS:	Fractured jaw
	Dislocated jaw
	Awake patient
COMPLICATIONS:	Dislocated jaw
	Damaged teeth

Open Mouth
PROCEDURE:

1. Open lips with thumbs after subluxating jaw as part of triple airway maneuver.

INDICATION:	Expiratory obstruction after head tilt
CONTRAINDICATIONS:	Worsening of inspiratory airway
COMPLICATIONS:	None

The intent is to increase intrathoracic pressure sufficiently to stimulate a cough. The Heimlich maneuver (subdiaphragmatic abdominal thrusts) is a recently recommended alternative to back blows (Fig. 14-6; Box 14-2). Alternatively, a forceful chest compression in the manner of a rapidly executed bear hug if the patient is upright or a sternal compression if supine is equally effective. In emergency situations, one technique should not exclude the other alternatives. The Heimlich maneuver is not advocated by all authorities.[29]

C. ARTIFICIAL AIRWAY DEVICES

When airway maneuvers are inadequate to establish airway patency, it is often necessary to employ artificial airway devices. The following addresses the various available

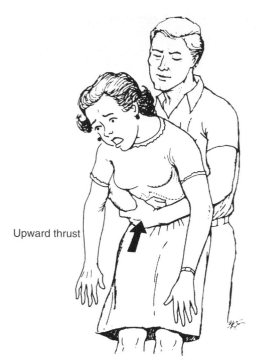

Upward thrust

Figure 14-6 Heimlich maneuver. Opening an airway obstructed by a laryngeal foreign body by compressing the lungs through external pressure on the abdominal viscera, forcing the diaphragm cephalad. An alternative method to create this "external cough" is by compressing the thorax directly. (From Benumof JL [ed]: Airway Management: Principles and Practice. St. Louis, Mosby, 1996, p 236.)

devices and discusses techniques of insertion and maintenance as well as indications, contraindications, and complications.

1. Oropharyngeal Airways

An oral airway can be used as a bite block to prevent occlusion of the teeth, but more often it is used to

Box 14-2	The Heimlich Maneuver

PROCEDURE
In the upright patient, wrap both arms around the chest with the right hand in a closed fist in the low sternal-xiphoid area and the left hand on top of the fist. With a rapid forceful thrust, compress upward, increasing subdiaphragmatic pressure and creating an artificial cough.

INDICATION:	Complete upper airway obstruction by a foreign body threatening asphyxia
CONTRAINDICATIONS:	Fractured ribs (relative) Cardiac contusion (relative) Partial airway obstruction
COMPLICATIONS:	Fractured ribs, sternum Liver or spleen trauma

provide a patent airway. The oral airways range in size from 0 for neonates to 4 for adults. The airways are usually made of plastic, metal, or rubber. They should be wide enough to make contact with two or three teeth on the mandible and maxilla and be slightly compressible so that the pressure of a clenched jaw is distributed over all the teeth in contact while the lumen remains patent. The airway is designed with a straight bite section to touch the teeth, a flange at the buccal (proximal) end to prevent swallowing or overinsertion of the airway, and a distal semicircular section to follow the curvature of the mouth, tongue, and posterior pharynx so that the tongue is displaced anteriorly (concave side against the tongue) (Fig. 14-7). In addition, an air channel is often provided to facilitate oropharyngeal suctioning.

There are several types of oral airways; all the ones described in the following list have a flange, straight section, and pharyngeal curve (see Fig. 14-7).

1. The Guedel airway has a plastic elliptic tube with a central lumen reinforced by a harder inner plastic tube at the level of the teeth and by plastic ridges along the pharyngeal section. Because the airway is completely enclosed, redundant oral and pharyngeal mucosae cannot occlude or narrow the lumen from the side. Because it is oval, the four central incisors usually make contact with it with great force during masseter spasm.

2. The Berman airway consists of two horizontal plates joined by a median ridge. The plates are usually flat and make contact with more of the teeth than the Guedel airway. The Berman airway has been designed with movable upper and lower plates and a hinged lower section meant to lift the base of the tongue (see Fig. 14-7). Such airways frequently penetrate deeper into the pharynx, touch the epiglottis, and cause airway reactivity (laryngospasm) in a lightly anesthetized patient (see later).

3. The Ovassapian airway has a large anterior flange to control the tongue and a large opening at the level of the teeth, open posteriorly, to allow a fiberscope and ET to be passed through it and later disengaged from the airway.

The use of an oral airway seems deceptively simple, but it is essential to do it correctly. The patient's pharyngeal and laryngeal reflexes should be depressed to avoid worsening the airway because of the reaction to a foreign body. The mouth is opened and a tongue blade placed at the base of the tongue and drawn upward, lifting the tongue off the posterior pharyngeal wall (Fig. 14-8A). The airway is placed so that the oropharyngeal tube is just off the posterior wall of the oropharynx with 1 to 2 cm protruding above the incisors (Fig. 14-8B). (If the flange is at the teeth when the tip is just at the base of the tongue, the airway is too small.) A jaw-thrust maneuver is done with the fingers of both hands to lift

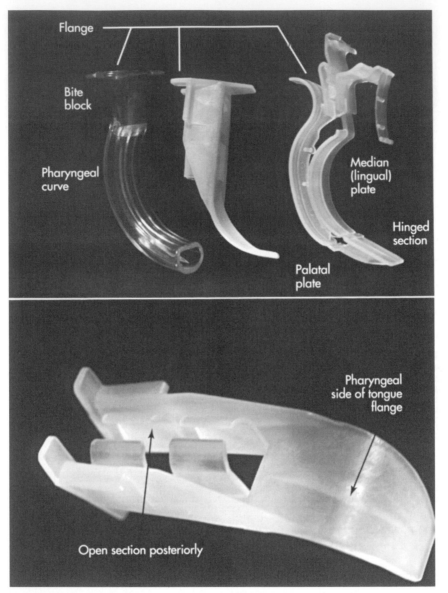

Figure 14-7 Types of oropharyngeal airways. All oral airways have a flange to prevent overinsertion, a straight bite-block portion, and a pharyngeal curve section. The Guedel airway is a bent cylinder, enclosed at the sides so that soft tissue cannot restrict the central airway. A small suction catheter (less than 14 gauge) can usually be inserted through the Guedel airway into the lower oropharynx, but the oral cavity must still be suctioned around it to remove oral secretions. The Ovassapian airway has a large anterior flange to control the tongue. The airway is open posteriorly so that an endotracheal tube can be inserted through the airway with the fiberoptic technique and the assembly later separated. The absence of a posterior flange allows easier manipulation of the fiberoptic bronchoscope. The Berman airway has anterior and posterior flanges and a central ridge. The open sides of the airway allow secretions to pool toward the center, where a suction catheter inserted down the airway can reach them. The flanges are usually sufficiently close together that soft tissue does not bulge in from the sides. The type shown has a hinged lower plate and a sliding mechanism allowing the lingual flange to slip upward, tilting the lower plate up to elevate the root of the tongue off the pharyngeal wall. Posterior view of Ovassapian airway showing open posterior section. (From Benumof JL [ed]: Airway Management: Principles and Practice. St. Louis, Mosby, 1996, p 237.)

the tongue off the pharyngeal wall; the thumbs then tap the airway down the last 2 cm so that the curve of the pharyngeal airway lies behind the base of the tongue (Fig. 14-8C). The condyles of the mandible are then allowed to reduce back into the temporomandibular joint. The mouth should be inspected so that neither tongue nor lips are caught between teeth and airway.

An alternative method of insertion is to insert the airway backward (convex side toward the tongue) until the tip is close to the pharyngeal wall of the oropharynx and then to rotate it 180 degrees (Fig. 14-8D). Rather than pushing the tongue straight downward, the tip rotates and sweeps under from the side. This method is not as reliable as the tongue-blade-assisted method mentioned earlier and has the added risk that the twisting motion can catch gapped teeth and loosen them in patients with poor dentition. If the airway is not patent after the placement of an oral airway, the following situations must be considered.

A short airway with a pronounced curve may impinge on the base of the tongue or the tongue may obstruct the pharyngeal airway below the plastic oral airway (POA). The solution is to try a longer airway or make the existing airway more flexible. If a longer plastic oral airway still results in obstruction, the curve of the airway may carry it into the vallecula or the airway may have pushed the epiglottis into the glottis or posterior wall of the pharynx. In the lightly anesthetized or awake patient, this stimulation causes coughing or laryngeal spasm. The best treatment for this problem is to withdraw the airway 1 to 2 cm. A topical anesthetic spray of the pharynx (tetracaine [Cetacaine] 0.5%, lidocaine 4%) or a water-soluble, local anesthetic lubricant on the airway, or both, reduces the chance of laryngeal activity but should be used judiciously or avoided in the patient thought to be at risk for aspiration. Another approach is to modify the plastic airway to make it more flexible and to give its leading edge a wedge shape (Fig. 14-9). If the obstruction is not relieved, one should then employ an alternative airway technique.

Indications for use of an oropharyngeal airway (OPA) consist of an obstructed upper airway (complete or partial) in the unconscious patient and a need for a bite block in the unconscious patient.

There are three major complications with the use of oral airways: trauma, airway hyperactivity, and airway obstruction. Minor trauma, including pinching of the lips and tongue, is common. Potential ulceration and necrosis of oropharyngeal structures from pressure and long-term (days) contact have been reported.[5] These problems necessitate intermittent surveillance during use. Dental injury can result from twisting of the airway, involuntary clenching of the jaw, or direct axial pressure. Dental damage is most common in patients with periodontal disease, dental caries, pronounced degrees of dental proclination, and isolated teeth.[24]

Airway hyperactivity is potentially lethal. Oropharyngeal and laryngeal reflexes can be stimulated by the placement of an artificial airway. Coughing, retching, emesis, laryngospasm, and bronchospasm are common reflex responses. Any OPA that touches the epiglottis or vocal cords can cause these responses, but the problem is more common with larger OPAs. The initial management is to withdraw the OPA partially. If an anesthetic is being administered, the level is deepened with an intravenous agent. In cases of laryngospasm, it might be necessary to apply mild positive airway pressure and, in trained hands, to administer cautiously small doses of succinylcholine for prompt cessation. A variant of the oral airway is the cuffed oropharyngeal airway (COPA) in which a cuff is inflated in the oropharynx or hypopharynx behind the base of the tongue. The COPA has a 14-mm adapter and is meant to connect directly to a breathing circuit.

2. Nasopharyngeal Airways

The nasopharyngeal airway (NPA) is an alternative airway device for treating soft tissue upper airway obstruction. Once in place, an NPA is less stimulating than an OPA and therefore better tolerated in the awake, semicomatose, or lightly anesthetized patient. In oropharyngeal trauma, the nasal airway is often preferable. NPAs are pliable bent cylinders made of plastic or soft rubber in variable lengths and widths (Fig. 14-10). A flange or movable disk prevents the outside end from passing beyond the nares and controlling the depth of insertion. The concavity is meant to follow the superior side of the hard palate and posterior wall of the naso-oropharynx. The airway is beveled on the left side to aid in following the airway and minimizing mucosal trauma as it advances. A narrow nasopharyngeal tube is often desired to minimize nasal trauma but may be too short to reach behind the tongue. An ET of the same diameter may be cut to a longer length and softened in hot water to provide a longer airway. A safety pin or 15-mm adapter should be inserted in the cut ET to prevent its migration into the nasopharynx (see Fig. 14-10A). A variant of this airway is known as a cuffed nasopharyngeal tube. It is cut shorter than the ET tube but retains the inflatable cuff. The cuff is blown up in the oropharynx or laryngopharynx and the tube pulled back so that the cuff lies against the soft palate and displaces the base of the tongue forward. This inflatable airway is more stimulating to the patient and the airway than the uncuffed type but is readily managed in an anesthetized patient.[26]

The nose should be inspected to determine its size and patency and the presence of nasal polyps or marked septal deviation. Vasoconstriction of the mucous membranes can be accomplished with cocaine or phenylephrine (Neo-Synephrine) drops or spray. Cotton swabs can be saturated in the solution and gently passed parallel to the palate into the nasopharynx. If three cotton swabs can be

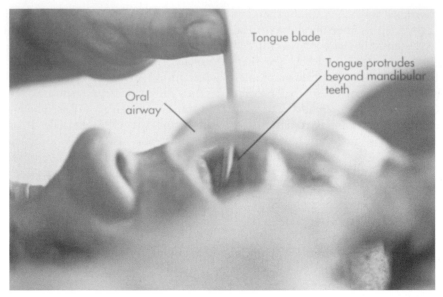

A

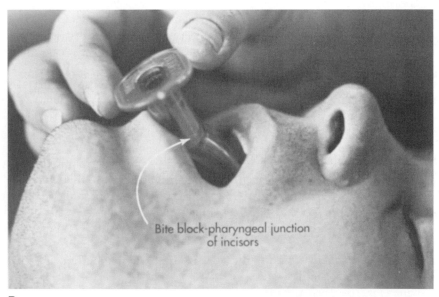

B

Figure 14-8 Oropharyngeal airway insertion technique. **A** to **C**, standard technique; **D**, an alternative when no tongue blade is available. **A**, The tongue blade is placed deep into the mouth and depresses the tongue at its posterior half. The tongue is then pulled forward by the tongue blade in an attempt to pull it off the back wall of the pharynx. The airway is inserted with the concave side toward the tongue until the incisors are at the junction of the pharyngeal curve and the bite-block sections. The tongue blade is removed. **B**, The oral airway has been placed by the right hand and the tongue blade removed.

Continued

accommodated in the nasal passage, a size 7.5 airway usually passes. The airway is generously lubricated with a water-soluble anesthetic ointment. The swabs are removed, and the airway is gently passed with the concave side against the hard palate (Fig. 14-11) through the nasal passage parallel to the palate until resistance is felt in the posterior nasopharynx (anterior wall of the retropharyngeal space).

Sometimes it is helpful to rotate the NPA 90 degrees counterclockwise, bringing the open part of the bevel against the posterior nasopharyngeal mucosae, and to resume gentle pressure. As the tube makes the bend (indicated by a relative loss of resistance to passage), it should be rotated back to the original position. If the tube does not pass with moderate pressure, there are three management options: a narrower tube, redilation

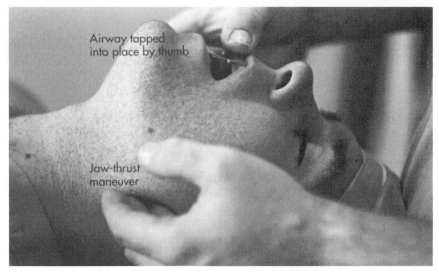

C   Alternative method of oropharyngeal airway insertion

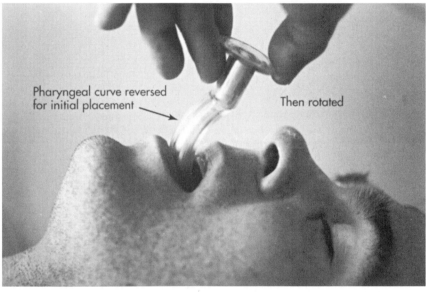

D

Figure 14-8, cont'd. **C,** A jaw-thrust maneuver is done with the fingers at the angle of the jaws (to elevate the posterior tongue) while the thumb taps the airway into place (behind the tongue). When the jaw is allowed to relax, inspect the lips to ensure that they are not caught between the teeth and airway. **D,** In an alternative technique the airway is placed in reverse manner (concave toward palate) and then spun into place so that the lower section of the airway rotates between the tongue and posterior pharyngeal wall. The junction of the bite-block section and the pharyngeal curve should be near the incisors before the spin move is done.

of the naris, and attempting passage in the other naris. If the tube does not pass into the oropharynx, one should withdraw the tube 2 cm, pass a suction catheter through the nasal airway as a guide, and push the airway forward over the suction tube. If the patient coughs or reacts as the nasal tube is inserted to its full extent, it should be withdrawn 1 to 2 cm. (The tip has probably touched the epiglottis or vocal cords.) If the patient's airway is still obstructed after insertion, the airway should be checked for obstruction by passing a small suction catheter. If the obstruction persists, it is possible that the NPA is too short and the base of the tongue lies at its tip. A size 6.0 ET can be cut at 18 cm to provide a longer airway. If laryngospasm is suspected, one should withdraw the NPA 1 to 2 cm and manage further as previously described.

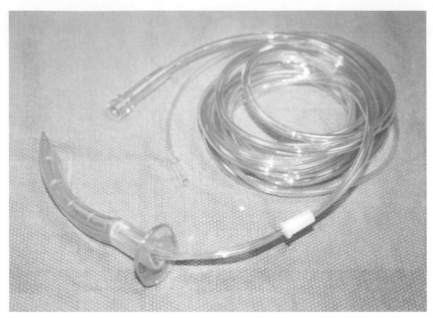

Figure 14-9 A Guedel airway modified to increase flexibility and minimize pushing the epiglottis down. It is also modified to allow oxygenation and capnography by the insertion of small tubes to supply O_2 and aspirate gas to a side-stream capnograph. A small suction catheter (10 or 14 Fr) can also be inserted. Used for moderate to deep intravenous sedation techniques; can be used under a mask.

The indications for an NPA consist of relief of upper airway obstruction in awake, semicomatose, or lightly anesthetized patients; in patients who are not adequately treated with OPAs; in patients with dental indications or oropharyngeal trauma; and in patients in whom there is a need to facilitate oropharyngeal and laryngopharyngeal suctioning.

The contraindications (absolute or relative) consist of nasal airway occlusion, nasal fractures, marked deviated septum, coagulopathy (risk of epistaxis), prior transsphenoidal hypophysectomy or Caldwell-Luc procedures (nose packed), cerebrospinal fluid rhinorrhea, and adenoid hypertrophy (relative, usually in pediatrics).

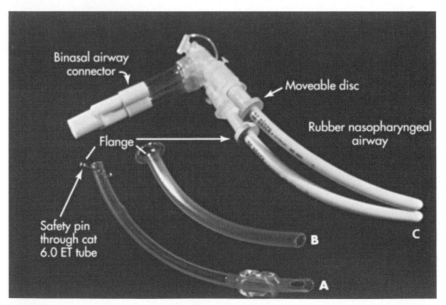

Figure 14-10 Nasopharyngeal airways. **A,** A size 6.0 endotracheal tube cut at 18 cm with a safety pin through the proximal end to prevent overinsertion. Added length allows tube to go behind the tongue or epiglottis. **B,** Clear nasal airway with flange at proximal end. **C,** Binasal airway. Two standard airways (these have movable disks to prevent overinsertion) connected to a double-lumen tube adapter. (From Benumof JL [ed]: Airway Management: Principles and Practice. St. Louis, Mosby, 1996, p 240.)

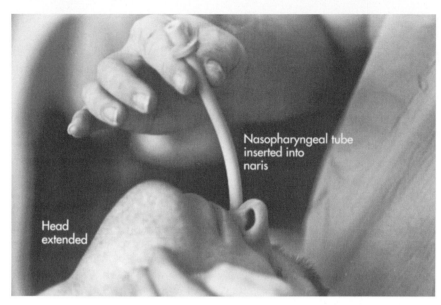

Figure 14-11 Insertion of nasopharyngeal airway. The airway is oriented concave to the hard palate and inserted straight back. Gripping the airway near the top allows the tube to bend if resistance to passage is extreme. If it is gripped close to the naris, sufficient force can be transmitted to shear off a turbinate. (From Benumof JL [ed]: Airway Management: Principles and Practice. St. Louis, Mosby, 1996, p 241.)

The complications of NPAs consist of failure of passage of the airway, epistaxis (mucosal tears or avulsion of the turbinate), submucosal tunneling, and pressure sores. Epistaxis is usually self-limiting and resolves spontaneously. The problem usually arises when the nasal tube is removed, removing the tamponade. Anterior plexus bleeding is treated by applying pressure to the nostrils. If the posterior plexus is bleeding, one should leave the airway in, suction the pharynx, ventilate the patient, and consider intubating the trachea if the bleeding does not stop rapidly. The patient should be positioned on his or her side to avoid aspiration of blood. A nasal pack or otolaryngology consultation may be necessary. The management of submucosal tunneling in the retropharyngeal space is to withdraw the airway. When this occurs, it is unlikely that an NPA can be successfully passed by this route. Passage through the other nostril may be attempted or an OPA used. The patient should be observed periodically for pressure sores of the ala nasi or for evidence of sinusitis. Upon extubation, some mucosal ulceration may be observed.

3. Binasal Airways

The use of two NPAs joined together by an adapter (see Fig. 14-10C) has been previously described.[26,39] This technique allows spontaneous and potentially low positive-pressure ventilation if the mouth is occluded. To allow assisted ventilation in the usual fashion, the nasal tubes must be inserted past the collapsed section of the pharynx (usually at least to the lower oropharynx), and the flexible pharynx usually provides some seal. The use of two tubes provides enough bulk to seal and enough cross-sectional area to minimize airway resistance. (Two 6-mm NPAs have a cross-sectional area exceeding that of an 8-mm airway.) If the nasal airways are shortened or inserted only 2 to 4 cm into the nares, the device can be used to produce CPAP to open the airway. Under these circumstances, the positive pressure stents the airway open. A sufficient seal to allow circuit pressures of 15 cm H_2O is usually needed to stent the airway open. It is helpful to have an anesthesia machine with a pressure relief valve calibrated in cm H_2O (e.g., North American Drager Fabius). Commercially available nasal CPAP masks can be adapted to an anesthesia circuit (see Fig 14-16). These devices are dedicated for one patient and cannot be readily sterilized for use in multiple patients. In any technique that requires positive pressure and assisted ventilation that may further augment inspiratory pressure, gastric inflation is possible.[22] The laryngeal mask airway (LMA) is likely to be a better management option in any circumstance in which prolonged positive pressure is required, although a greater level of anesthesia is probably needed for the LMA insertion (see Chapter 21).

D. NONINTUBATION VENTILATION

Despite a patent airway, ventilation can be inadequate. Ventilatory assistance can be achieved through several alternatives other than intubation. Standard cardiopulmonary resuscitation courses have long taught the effectiveness of mouth-to-mouth and mouth-to-nose ventilation.

Mouth-to-artificial-airway ventilation using a disposable face mask or an S tube (two Guedel airways with the flanges bonded together) overcomes many of the aesthetic objections to the previous techniques. More sophisticated approaches to ventilatory assistance (as in anesthesia) typically include the use of bag-mask-valve systems. Ventilation of a patient generally requires a sealed interface between the patient and a delivery system that supplies airway gases and can be pressurized. For nonintubation ventilation, this seal is either on the skin of the face (face mask techniques) or in the hypopharynx (LMA). A partial seal can be obtained in the oropharynx or nasopharynx by the binasal airway, the cuffed NPA, or the COPA, but the effectiveness of the seal is limited. The most reliable seal, allowing high positive pressures, is in the trachea, through endotracheal intubation.

1. Face Masks

The face mask is typically the starting point for linking a positive-pressure generating device to a patient's airway. Nasal masks can be used in limited circumstances, but achieving a sufficient seal to ventilate a patient promptly is problematic. Face masks differ in material, shape, type of seal, and transparency. The mask is composed of three parts: the body, seal (or cushion), and connector (or collar). The body is the main structure of the mask. Because the body rises above the face, all face masks increase dead space. A more malleable body allows a better fit to the face and a reduced dead space. The added dead space is usually not significant when ventilation is spontaneous, and it is never significant if ventilation is controlled. Respiratory gas analysis (capnography) can verify ventilation. The seal is the actual rim of the mask that comes in contact with the face. The two types of seals are a cushion rim that is often inflatable and a rubber or plastic edge that is noninflatable. The connector is at the top of the body and provides a 22-mm female adapter for a breathing circuit or air-mask-bag unit (Ambu)-bag elbow. A collar with hooks allows a mask-retaining strap to be attached to help hold the mask to the face. The precise application of the straps (e.g., crossed [ipsilateral strap to contralateral hook] or uncrossed) is a matter of individual preference and is usually the result of a trial-and-error process to find the best seal and airway patency for the individual patient.

The Ohio anatomic face mask has a body contoured to the face, with a sharp notch for the nose, a double curve to fit the malar eminence of the cheek, and a curved chin section (Fig. 14-12). It is made of conductive rubber, is slightly malleable, and has a high-pressure, low-volume cushion. For those whom it fits, it allows the chin to be lifted high into the mask while sealing the sides and maintaining maxillary pressure, providing the best compromise between adequacy of seal and patency of airway. Its disadvantages include poor fit on a face with a broad, flat bridge of the nose and poor malleability to different-sized faces.

The correct size is important, and several sizes should be readily available. It is opaque, so vomitus cannot be readily seen, and it requires extensive aeration with the seal cushion collapsed after ethylene oxide sterilization because the ethylene oxide absorbed in the rubber can cause a chemical burn on the skin. Disposable transparent plastic masks have been made with high-volume, low-pressure cushions that seal to the face much more easily. They have little or no chin curve, and obtaining a patent airway is slightly more difficult. The base of the body of these transparent masks is flat; the large, flexible cushion fits a wide variety of faces. The cushion may be factory sealed or have a nipple for the injection of air. A progression of this style is the "easy-seal" mask having a reinforced flexible disk for a body and a large, floppy cushion constituting the entire undersurface of the disk except for the 22-mm adapter air passage. This mask is used in arrest situations but has not been commonly used to administer anesthesia.

The proper use of a face mask depends on obtaining a good seal between the mask and the patient's face; successfully doing this is fundamental to administering adequate ventilation and inhalation anesthesia. The mask should comfortably fit both the hand of the user and the face of the patient. If the mask is too long, the face can be elongated 1 to 2 cm by placing an oral airway. If the mask is too short with the OPA placed, the OPA can be removed and an NPA placed. The mask can also be moved 1 to 2 cm along the bridge of the nose to make a small mask fit at the chin.

Several methods are described for holding the mask. Regardless of the precise method, close monitoring for leaks is necessary. The left hand grips the mask with the thumb and index finger around the collar (Figs. 14-13 and 14-14). The left side of the mask fits into the palm. The hypothenar eminence of the left hand should extend below the left side of the mask. If it does not, the mask is too big for the user's hand and a smaller mask should be tried. The problem with a large mask is that the left hypothenar eminence cannot pull the patient's cheek against the left side of the mask to maintain a seal if pronation is necessary to seal the right side (see later).

The patient may, of course, require a large mask, in which case retaining straps are usually necessary to get a satisfactory seal in all quadrants. The middle finger can be on the mask or chin, depending on the span of the user's hand, the size of the mask and face, and the ease of fit. The proximal interphalangeal joints of the fingers and the distal interphalangeal joint of the thumb should be at the midline of the mask, allowing the pads of the fingers to put pressure on the right side of the mask. To seal the mask at the bridge of the nose, one should spread the sides of the mask and place it on the bridge of the nose so that the mask does not put pressure on the eyes. The nose is subsequently sealed by downward pressure of the thumb. One lowers the mask onto the face and notes where the lower edge of the mask touches the patient's face. If it touches at the teeth, a larger mask should be

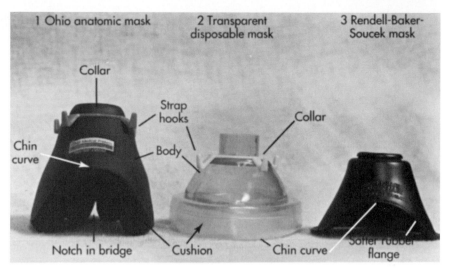

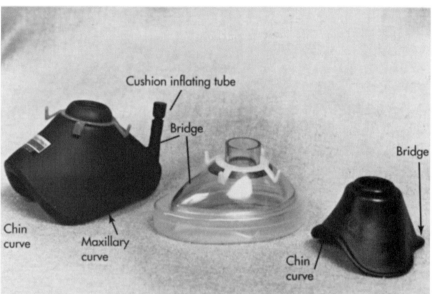

Figure 14-12 Face masks, front **(top)** and side **(bottom)** views. 1, Ohio anatomic mask. 2, Transparent disposable mask. 3, Rendell-Baker-Soucek mask. The various parts of the masks and different cushions and contours are evident; strap hooks can also be put on the Rendell-Baker-Soucek mask if desired. The use of high-volume, low-pressure cuffs has eliminated the need for an anatomically formed body of the mask to achieve an adequate seal to the face and has reduced the chances of pressure points over the face. However, this type of mask does little to aid the maintenance of a patent airway, making the use of artificial airways more important. (From Benumof JL [ed]: Airway Management: Principles and Practice. St. Louis, Mosby, 1996, p 243.)

used or the current one slid down the nose 1 to 2 cm. If the chin curve hits the mentum instead of the alveolar ridge, the sides of the mask may not seal to the face. To seal the chin section, the mandible is gripped with the fingers and the wrist rotated so as to pull the mandible up into the mask with the fingers while pushing the bridge of the mask down with the thumb. To seal the left side of the mask, skin of the cheek is gathered against the side of the mask with the hypothenar eminence. To seal the right side, the left forearm is pronated while pressing the ends of the thumb, index finger, and possibly middle finger onto the right side of the mask.

The sides of the mask are malleable to adjust to wide or narrow faces. In edentulous patients, the cheeks are often too hollow to allow an adequate fit. Edentulous patients also lose vertical dimension to their face that can be restored by an oral airway. In rare situations, dentures are left in place to allow a better mask fit, but the dentures can be lost, broken, or dislodged with consequent obstruction. Alternatively, one can use a large mask so that the

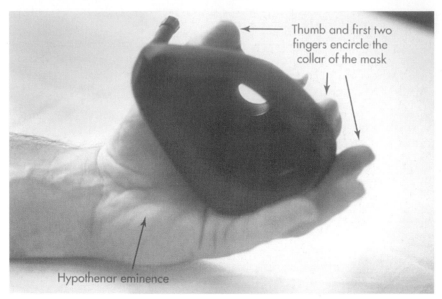

Thumb and first two fingers encircle the collar of the mask

Hypothenar eminence

Figure 14-13 Proper hand grip of face mask. Hypothenar eminence extends down from mask while thumb and two fingers encircle collar. (From Benumof JL [ed]: Airway Management: Principles and Practice. St. Louis, Mosby, 1996, p 244.)

chin fits entirely inside the mask with the seal on the caudal surface of the chin, the cheeks fit within the mask, and the sides of the mask seal along the lateral maxilla and mandible. These maneuvers to make a difficult mask fit possible are often best sidestepped by endotracheal intubation or use of an LMA, but clinical judgment must determine when this is the case (Box 14-3). Mask-retaining straps can be placed at the occiput and connected to the mask collar to put pressure at various angles to assist the seal. The tension on the straps should be no more than necessary to achieve a seal. External gauze sponges may be used to protect the skin from excessive pressure by a strap. When straps or gauze sponges are employed, extreme care must be taken to avoid ocular trauma.[30] An additional maneuver to compensate for mask leaks is to increase fresh gas flow.

Masks with high-volume, low-pressure cuffs deform to seal more easily and make contact with a larger surface area of skin, minimizing the chance of pressure ischemia. The chin and cheek areas seal more easily, but the size of the cushion occasionally results in pressure on the globe of the eye if the mask is high on the bridge of the nose. The thumb can pull the mask caudad to roll the cushion away from the eye. The cushions may be factory sealed or inflatable. The latter should be filled sufficiently that the edge of the body of the mask does not touch the face. Some masks do not have cushions (Rendell-Baker-Soucek masks), but the rubber or plastic edge is usually tapered and flexible so that it deforms along the face to give a larger area of contact than just the edge.

A face mask is indicated to seal a patient's airway to allow application of a mixture of gases to either ventilate, oxygenate, or anesthetize. Mask ventilation is relatively contraindicated in situations requiring general anesthesia with a large likelihood of gastric contents soiling the trachea, such as a full stomach, hiatus hernia, esophageal motility disorders, and pharyngeal diverticula. In addition, whenever there is a likelihood of gas inflating the stomach (such as with a weakened cricopharyngeal sphincter, a need for high airway pressures, known or suspected sleep apnea, marked kyphoscoliosis), an adverse position, or inability to reach the head of the patient easily, use of a mask for positive-pressure ventilation must be done cautiously. Mask ventilation is also relatively contraindicated whenever there is a need to avoid the head and neck manipulation that may be necessary to maintain the airway or whenever there is a need to avoid touching the neck or an inability to seal the mask. Lack of integrity of the dermis, resulting in marked bullae from friction (e.g., epidermolysis bullosa), is a contraindication to the use of a face mask. Finally, inability to sustain adequate assisted or spontaneous ventilation is a relative contraindication to further use of a face mask.

2. Respiratory (Resuscitator) Bags

The air-mask-bag unit (Ambu) was developed in 1955 by Rubin. The Ambu has provided an alternative means of artificial ventilation to the standard anesthesia bag and circuit. The bag can be used with a mask or ET. Its advantage is in being self-inflating, thus avoiding the need for compressed gas. The disadvantages are that the "feel" of the airway (compliance and resistance) is poor and the delivery of high concentrations of oxygen more complex. Various types of hand resuscitator units exist. They use various valve systems to ensure nonrebreathing, and the

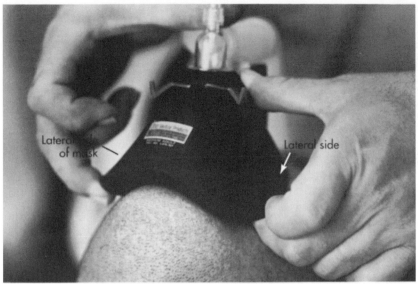

A   Application of mask to face

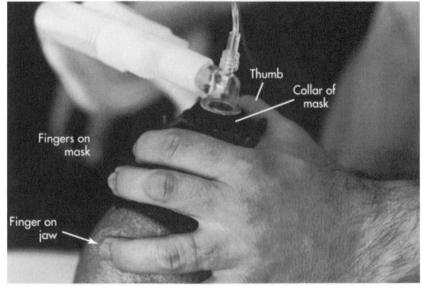

B   Standard one handed grip of mask to face

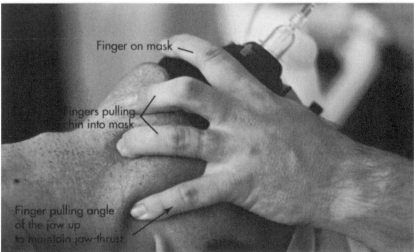

C   One handed mask grip with jaw-thrust

Figure 14-14 Sealing and holding the mask to the face. **A,** Application of mask to face. Fingers spread the bridge and lateral sides of the mask as it is lowered onto face. **B,** Side view of standard one-handed grip of mask to face. The thumb and first two fingers encircle the collar of the mask while the last two fingers pull mandible up into the mask and extend the head. **C,** One-handed mask grip: maintaining jaw thrust. Caudad view of hand grip shows little finger at the angle of the jaw maintaining backward and upward pull to maintain jaw thrust. Because of the increased span required of the hand, only the first finger is now on the mask, while the second and third fingers pull the mandible into the face and extend the head. (The exact position of each of the four fingers depends slightly on the size of the left hand.) To prevent teeth from grating on one another, this technique usually requires the prior insertion of an oral airway. The jaw-thrust position is initiated with the usual two-handed maneuver; this one-handed grip can at best only maintain the position. The strong pull on the mandible resulting in friction of the incisors on the bite-block portion of the oral airway does as much to maintain the position as does the little finger at the angle of the jaw. (From Benumof JL [ed]: Airway Management: Principles and Practice. St. Louis, Mosby, 1996, p 245.)

Box 14-3 **Airway Management Choices**

Nasal Continuous Positive Airway Pressure (CPAP) Mask

INDICATIONS	Obstructed airway with minimal sedation
	Known obstructive sleep apnea
ADVANTAGES	Minimal increase in sedation needed for tolerance
	Can be used to administer volatile anesthetic
DISADVANTAGES	Nasal airway seal can be difficult
	Requires constant monitoring, variable CPAP
	High gas flows needed. Scavenging difficult
CONTRAINDICATIONS	Marked obesity
	More than limited surgery
	Inability to have ready access to head to alter technique
	Gastroesophageal reflux disease
COMPLICATIONS	Gastric insufflation

Mask with Oropharyngeal Airway

INDICATIONS:	Ventilation preceding endotracheal intubation
	Failed endotracheal intubation
	Awake patient requires high levels of inspired O_2
ADVANTAGES:	Can be done in awake patient without airway
	Does not require relaxants
	Minimal response of patient
DISADVANTAGES:	Requires constant attention (left hand is constantly on patient's face or mask; skill required throughout)
	Gastric inflation and inadequate ventilation if positive pressure consistently over 20 torr
CONTRAINDICATIONS:	Known increased risk of vomiting or regurgitation
	Known significant airway obstruction
COMPLICATIONS:	Lip or dental trauma on airway
	Inadequate airway patency (laryngospasm, pharyngeal obstruction)
	Facial pressure injury (skin, supraorbital, or infraorbital nerves, mental nerves from fingers or mask straps)
	Aspiration risk highest of the three techniques

Laryngeal Mask Airway

INDICATIONS:	Failed intubation
	Difficult face mask fit
ADVANTAGES:	Minimal response of patient, but does require anesthetic
	Does not require relaxant
	Smooth emergence
	Once placed, hands are free; requires intermediate level of monitoring
	Regurgitation and laryngospasm less likely than with mask
DISADVANTAGES:	Cannot generate airway pressures >20 torr reliably
	Requires anesthetic level; can be misplaced
	Laryngospasm possible
	Regurgitation more likely than with endotracheal tube
CONTRAINDICATIONS:	Known increased risk of vomiting, regurgitation
	High airway pressures required
COMPLICATIONS:	Regurgitation/aspiration
	Inadequate placement and inadequate ventilation
	Hypoglossal nerve palsy
	Pharyngeal trauma

Continued

Box 14-3 **Airway Management Choices—cont'd**

Endotracheal Tube Airway

INDICATIONS:	Increased risk of vomiting, regurgitation
	High airway pressures anticipated (obese patient)
	Inaccessibility of airway
ADVANTAGES:	Most secure airway, once placed and confirmed
	Skill requirement low after initial placement
	Seals trachea from gastrointestinal tract; high pressure possible
DISADVANTAGES:	Nociceptive response to tracheal foreign body
	Coughing during and after extubation
	Postextubation laryngospasm, noncardiac pulmonary edema
	Usually requires relaxant to place
	Can result in death if esophageal placement unrecognized
CONTRAINDICATIONS:	No capnography available (relative)
	Chance of minor voice changes unacceptable (professional singer—relative)
COMPLICATIONS:	Cough, straining on endotracheal tube or at extubation (suture lines compromised)
	Noncardiac pulmonary edema, croup
	Hypertension, tachycardia
	Bronchospasm in susceptible individual
	Undiscovered esophageal intubation (if no capnograph)
	Hoarseness (usually 24 hours; can be 6 months)

---

units vary in size, weight, percentage of oxygen delivery, volume, reinflation time, cycling rate, and number of parts.

Criteria for selection of an AMBU should include easy, foolproof assembly; a nonsticking valve system to prevent rebreathing while allowing exhalation; a closable pressure pop-off valve with standard 15- to 22-mm connection; capability to deliver 95% oxygen and 0 to 12 cm H_2O positive end-expiratory pressure (PEEP); airway pressure monitor; capability to be sterilized; and performance under varying common environmental conditions. Limited complications have been associated with the use of Ambu equipment.

3. Determining the Effectiveness of Nonintubation Ventilation and Use of Supplemental Airway Maintenance Techniques

The mask seal should be sufficient to permit a positive pressure of 20 cm H_2O with a minimal leak. It is important to limit positive airway pressure to 25 cm H_2O to avoid inflating the stomach, which increases the chance of regurgitation.[7,22,30] The effectiveness of ventilation should be judged by exhaled tidal volume, movement of the chest, good bilateral breath sounds, vital signs, and available monitors of oxygenation and ventilation. Pulse oximetry and capnography should be used if available. If the patient cannot be ventilated with 25 cm H_2O positive pressure, either the upper airway is obstructed, the patient has sufficient muscle tone to prevent chest expansion, or there is a decrease in pulmonary compliance or increased airway resistance. The oral airway, triple airway maneuver, or CPAP corrects the first; a small dose of

succinylcholine decreases laryngeal spasm and muscle tone; and definitive treatment of the compliance and resistance issues depends on the etiologic factors. Tracheal tug or paradoxical movement of the chest suggests airway obstruction. An NPA or OPA may open the pharyngeal airway. The known presence of anatomic airway obstruction (tumor or polyp) precludes the use of muscle relaxants because loss of muscle tone may cause nearly untreatable airway obstruction.

The difficulty in maintaining a mask fit and a patent airway with one hand is occasionally so great that the patient's safety is best served if the mask fit and airway are controlled by two hands while a second person ventilates the patient's lungs by squeezing the bag.[7] The two-handed airway technique uses the fingers to perform a jaw-thrust maneuver while the thumbs hold the mask in place by pressure on the lateral sides of the mask (Fig. 14-15). This maneuver can be done from the side of the patient, facing the patient's mandible, as well as from behind. This is not a stable situation. Either the airway improves within 5 minutes, or an alternative airway technique (LMA or endotracheal intubation) should be chosen.

III. SPECIFIC CLINICAL SITUATIONS

Airway maintenance without endotracheal intubation is a necessity of the practice of anesthesia, respiratory care, emergency medicine, and critical care. Occasionally, nonintubation techniques are desirable because they avoid the foreign body responses to endotracheal intubation

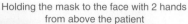

Holding the mask to the face with 2 hands
from above the patient

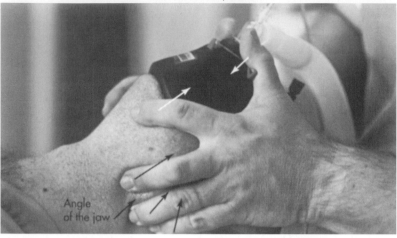

A

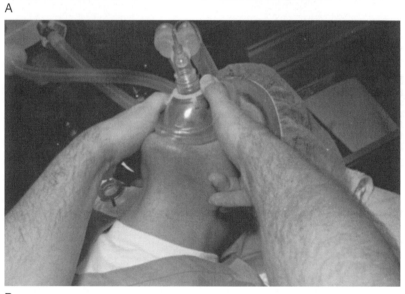

B

Figure 14-15 Holding the mask to the face with two hands. **A,** Thumbs are hooked over collar of the mask, with lower fingers maintaining jaw thrust (if needed) and upper fingers pulling mandible into the mask and extending the head. (*Arrows* indicate direction of force.) A second individual must ventilate the patient. In this figure the airway is maintained from above the head. **B,** The airway and mask fit is maintained from the side of the patient, allowing the person ventilating the patient improved access to the patient. The thumbs maintain downward pressure from the collar of the mask, the thenar eminence maintains lateral pressure on the mask, and the first and second fingers maintain jaw thrust from the angle of the jaw. This position is helpful if the person ventilating the patient is preparing to intubate the patient's trachea under direct vision using a laryngoscope or by fiberoptic bronchoscopy. (From Benumof JL [ed]: Airway Management: Principles and Practice. St. Louis, Mosby, 1996, p 249.)

(tachycardia, hypertension, and coughing). The risks of nonintubation of the airway have been previously discussed. This technique is not well suited to prolonged positive-pressure ventilation. Airway maintenance during a prolonged steady state (30 minutes to 3 hours) presents a different set of problems and vigilance requirements from those of airway maintenance in a transitional period between a natural airway and the placement or removal of an ET tube. Three situations requiring airway

maintenance without endotracheal intubation that deserve special mention are sedation, transitional periods surrounding endotracheal intubation, and induction and maintenance of a general anesthetic.

A. DURING SEDATION

Sedation is used to allay patients' anxiety or minimize discomfort associated with position or duration of the procedure when the stimuli of surgery have been largely ablated by a regional anesthetic block or local anesthetic infiltration. Mild sedation during which the patient can converse typically requires no special airway management, although supplemental oxygen per nasal cannulas or clear plastic oxygen insufflation mask should be used. Sedation to the point of somnolence or stertor requires some intervention to ensure adequacy of ventilation and oxygenation. Chin lift or jaw thrust usually results in increased patient's awareness and clearing of the stertor, reassuring the anesthetist that the patient is not overly sedated. If stertor returns, turning the head 45 degrees to one side or the other may help. In patients whom a mask does not fit at all closely (edentulous patients being the most common), sedation can be temporarily deepened, the nares anesthetized, and a small NPA inserted, into which a 15-mm adapter (which goes to an oxygen source) has been inserted. A more complete seal and wider airway can be achieved by using two nasal airways (see "Binasal Airways" Section II. C. 3) or a nasal mask with CPAP (Fig. 14-16). These techniques produce less hemodynamic disturbances than do endotracheal intubation, but they require monitoring and the ability to revise techniques as determined by the level of sedation. Because of field avoidance, mask techniques are usually not feasible during monitored anesthesia care for cataract surgery or facial plastic surgery. An oral airway is usually not successful because it is more stimulating than the nasal airway and may induce retching with this level of sedation.

The trend to moderate and deep sedation in situations in which anesthesiologists are involved is apparent in our practice. These techniques routinely require airway support (either airway maneuvers or the use of airway devices). A convenient system that is easily constructed consists of a Guedel airway that is made more flexible by making relaxing cuts in the anterior curve and inserting small lines to deliver O_2 from one and aspirate pharyngeal gas to a capnometer from the other (see Fig 14-8).

B. TRANSITIONAL AIRWAY TECHNIQUES

Before intubation of the trachea, the patient usually has received a neuromuscular blocker or, in the case of cardiopulmonary arrest, has no muscle tone. The larynx is open, and laryngeal spasm is not a consideration. The previously discussed techniques of airway maintenance are usually sufficient to permit ventilating the patient. Airway maintenance from extubation to smooth, spontaneous ventilation can be complicated by the presence of a reactive larynx capable of spasm. Therefore, the timing of extubation is an important consideration. Extubation can be either at a deep stage of anesthesia with minimal airway reactivity or during very light anesthesia (nearly or fully awake) so that there is full control of reflex activity. The patient extubated during the middle ground of moderate anesthetic depth is at increased risk for laryngospasm.

The correct timing is estimated as follows. The patient should be breathing spontaneously and considered to have an empty stomach. The oropharynx is suctioned (with a flexible suction catheter) to remove pooled secretions. If smooth, spontaneous breathing continues, the cuff

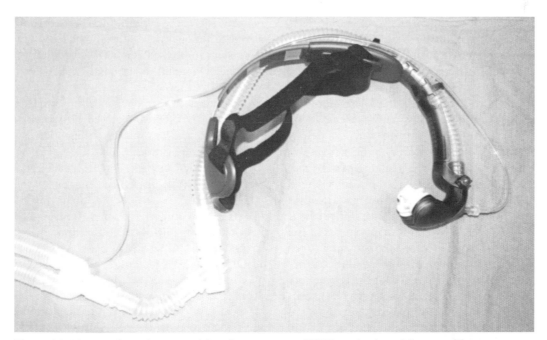

Figure 14-16 A nasal continuous positive airway pressure (CPAP) mask adapted for use with an anesthesia machine and breathing circuit. Note the ability for capnography. A compliant reservoir bag is necessary for this technique to generate CPAP.

is deflated. If the patient continues to breathe smoothly, the trachea is extubated during inspiration with pressure on the reservoir bag. If, on the other hand, coughing and straining ensue, extubation must be delayed until the patient again breathes smoothly for two or three cycles. In either event, an inspiratory breath is augmented maximally and the ET is withdrawn at end inspiration, allowing rapid expiratory airflow or a cough to clear retained secretions from around the vocal cords. A triple airway maneuver is done immediately.[8,20] Spontaneous ventilation is confirmed, and a mask with oxygen is applied to the face. If secretions are copious or intraoral blood is expected, the patient should be put into a position to optimize drainage.

C. INDUCTION AND MAINTENANCE OF ANESTHESIA WITHOUT MUSCLE RELAXATION

The major difference between airway management during inhalation anesthesia without muscle relaxation and with muscle relaxation is that the larynx is responsive to irritation. Spasm can occur in response to irritation of the epiglottis and laryngeal introitus from OPAs or NPAs, pungent anesthetics, secretions, and surgical stimulation if the anesthetic level is inadequate.[4] The most important feature of mask airway management during the maintenance of anesthesia is monitoring the progress of the operation and the state of the airway. Increasing levels of stimuli must be anticipated and the anesthetic deepened prior to their occurrence, usually by increased concentration of inhaled volatile anesthetic. The smooth conduct of an inhalation anesthetic by mask requires more vigilance, anticipation, and knowledge of the individual surgeon than does one by an ET tube or an LMA.

Fatigue is a common problem if the operation lasts more than 1 hour and the airway is difficult to manage. There are many ways to minimize fatigue. The patient's head should be at a level between the anesthetist's waist and shoulders. The anesthetist should stand or sit on a variable-height chair to accomplish this. The elbow of the anesthetist's left arm should be kept tucked against his or her left side to minimize shoulder strain, and weight can be substituted for muscle power if the left arm is allowed to extend and the anesthetist leans backward. Resting the elbow on the table next to the patient's head also relaxes the shoulder. The right hand may hold the mask temporarily to give the left hand a rest if the patient is breathing spontaneously. A head strap can assist the anesthetist's forearm muscles. Strapping the mask does not free the left hand for other than the briefest of times (15 to 30 seconds) because the pads of the fingers are irreplaceable monitors. The left hand still provides extension of the head, sometimes required to maintain a patent airway even with artificial airways in place.

There are times when both hands must be used to open the airway (jaw-thrust maneuver) and to seal the mask to the face. If a second person is not available to ventilate, judicious use of PEEP or CPAP of 5 to 10 torr may allow adequate tidal volumes with spontaneous ventilation. This is a common procedure immediately following removal of an ET as a transitional state to full spontaneous ventilation as the airway rapidly improves and stabilizes. It is possible to use positive pressure to ventilate a patient whose airway is opened by this maneuver. One must realize that positive pressure greater than 20 cm H_2O, especially if delivered out of phase with the patient's spontaneous attempts to ventilate, is more likely to distend the stomach than ventilate the lungs, thereby increasing the risk of regurgitation. It is best to have a second person with an "educated hand" to augment the patient's spontaneous attempts to breathe. It is possible to use standard circle system ventilation instead of a second person in healthy patients undergoing routine surgical procedures, but its usefulness has not been determined in the hypoxic or hypercarbic patient requiring immediate airway management.[37] If possible, a pressure-limited setting of 20 to 25 cm H_2O should be used with a rate of 8 to 20 breaths per minute, adjusted to best results determined by pulse oximetry or capnography if available. This is not a stable situation. If the airway does not improve rapidly, the alternative plan next in line in the difficult airway algorithm (including surgical airway) should be executed.

IV. DECIDING WHICH AIRWAY TECHNIQUE TO USE

Choosing the airway technique is every bit as important a medical decision as choosing the drugs used (see Box 14-3). It is based on a risk-benefit analysis and is individualized for each patient-anesthetist combination. The airway techniques that allow a semiclosed or closed breathing system to be used and allow some degree of assisted or controlled ventilation are nasal CPAP, face mask, COPA, laryngeal tube airway (LTA), LMA (classical and ProSeal), and endotracheal intubation. These techniques vary in the ability to seal the airway, maintain airway patency, free the hands, evoke the patient's response, and potential complications.

The airway can be sealed to a delivery system at the face (nasal CPAP mask, face mask), in the oropharynx (COPA, LTA), in the laryngopharynx or hypopharynx (LMA), or within the trachea (endotracheal). The ET tube cuff is capable of the highest pressure seal; the LMA ProSeal, LTA, and LMA classical less (15 to 30 cm H_2O); the COPA less; and the face mask the most variable level of seal depending on facial anatomy and operator skill. The face mask, nCPAP mask, COPA, and classical LMA are best suited to a spontaneously breathing patient with assisted ventilations. The LMA ProSeal and the LTA have increased protection against regurgitation[22] and a cuff pattern to allow higher airway pressures[3] and so are better for periods of controlled ventilation or muscle relaxation. Patients requiring controlled ventilation, especially if muscle relaxation or high ventilatory pressures are needed, are best served by endotracheal intubation. Patency of the airway is best ensured by an ET tube followed by either type of LMA.

Nonintubation management of the airway remains a critically important topic and skill in patients' care for sedation, anesthesia, and critical care management. The trend to moderate or deep sedation for a variety of procedures and diagnostic tests requires knowledge and skill in this arena, yet it is imperative to understand the limitations and the alternatives to airway management that have become available in the last 10 years. Nonintubation management of the airway is an essential part of every other airway management technique, either as a transitional phase during induction and emergence or as a backup alternative plan. The increasing use of moderate or deep sedation frequently requires it as a major adjunct or rescue technique from an unintended deeper level of sedation. However, two trends in the past 10 years have decreased the advisability of nonintubation airway management during general anesthesia. One is the proliferation of oral pharyngeal invasive devices of various sizes (LMAs of various styles and COPA). The other is the improved ability to eliminate the transitional period before endotracheal intubation with improved drugs and application techniques for sedation, topical anesthesia, and fiberoptic intubation. The ability to intubate asleep patients reliably has been improved using fiberoptic-assisted intubation with fast track LMA and Wu-Scope or Bullard intubating laryngoscopes. Understanding the advantages, disadvantages, and limitations of any airway management technique remains a cornerstone of judgment in selecting the optimal management path.

REFERENCES

1. Boidin MP: Airway patency in the unconscious patient. Br J Anaesth 57:306, 1985.
2. Dempsey JA, Skatrud JB, Jacques AJ, et al: Anatomic determinants of sleep-disordered breathing across the spectrum of clinical and nonclinical male subjects. Chest 122:840, 2002.
3. Figueredo E, Martinez M, Pintanel T: A comparison of the ProSeal laryngeal mask and the laryngeal tube in spontaneously breathing anesthetized patients. Anesth Analg 96:600, 2003.
4. Fink BR: Etiology and treatment of laryngeal spasm. Anesthesiology 17:569, 1956.
5. Fink BR: The Human Larynx. New York, Raven Press, 1975.
6. Fink BR, Demerest RJ: Laryngeal Biomechanics. Cambridge, Mass, Harvard University Press, 1978.
7. Finucane BT, Santori AH: Principles of Airway Management. Philadelphia, FA Davis, 1988.
8. Gleeson K, Swillich C, Bendrick T: Effect of inspiratory nasal loading on pharyngeal resistance. J Appl Physiol 60:1882, 1986.
9. Haponik EF, Smith PL, Bohlman ME, et al: Computerized tomography in obstructive sleep apnea: Correlation of airway size with physiology during sleep and wakefulness. Am Rev Respir Dis 127:221, 1983.
10. Horner RL, Shea SA, McIvor J, et al: Pharyngeal size and shape during wakefulness and sleep in patients with obstructive sleep apnoea. Q J Med 268:719, 1989.
11. Hudgel D, Mulholland M, Hendricks C: Neuromuscular and mechanical responses to inspiratory resistive loading during sleep. J Appl Physiol 63:603, 1987.
12. Issa FG, Edwards P, Szeto E, et al: Genioglossus and breathing responses to airway occlusion: Effect of sleep and route of occlusion. J Appl Physiol 64:543, 1988.
13. Issa FG, Sullivan CE: Upper airway closing pressures in snorers. J Appl Physiol 57:528, 1984.
14. Macey PM, Henderson A, Macey KE, et al: Brain morphology associated with obstructive sleep apnea. Am J Respir Crit Care Med 166:1382, 2002.
15. Malhotra A, Huang Y, Fogel R, et al: The male predisposition to pharyngeal collapse: Importance of airway length. Am J Respir Crit Care Med 166:1388, 2002.
16. Malhotra A, Pillar G, Fogel R, et al: Upper airway collapsibility: Measurements and sleep effects. Chest 120:156, 2001.
17. Malhotra A, White DP: Obstructive sleep apnea. Lancet 360:237, 2002.
18. Marklund M, Sahlin C, Stenlund H: Mandibular advancement device in patients with obstructive sleep apnea: Long term effects on apnea and sleep. Chest 120:162, 2001.
19. McGee JP, Vender JS: Nonintubation management of the airway. In Benumof JL (ed): Clinical Procedures in Anesthesia and Intensive Care. New York, JB Lippincott, 1992, pp 89-114.
20. Meier S, Geiduschek J, Paganoni R, et al: The effect of chin lift, jaw thrust, and continuous positive airway pressure on the size of the glottic opening and on the stridor score in anesthetized, spontaneously breathing children. Anesth Analg 94:494, 2002.
21. Meurice J-C, Marc I, Carrier G, et al: Effects of mouth opening on airway collapsibility in normal sleep subjects. Am J Respir Crit Care Med 153:255, 1996.
22. Ng A, Smith G: Gastroesophageal reflux and aspiration of gastric contents in anesthetic practice. Anesth Analg 93:494, 2001.
23. Onal E, Burrows DL, Hart RH, et al: Induction of periodic breathing during sleep causes upper airway obstruction in humans. J Appl Physiol 61:1438, 1986.
24. Petit FX, Pepin JL, Bettega G, et al: Mandibular advancement devices: Rate of contraindications in 100 consecutive obstructive sleep apnea patients. Am J Respir Crit Care Med 166:274, 2002.
25. Pitsis AJ, Darendeliler MA, Gotsopoulos H: Effect of vertical dimension on efficacy of oral appliance therapy in obstructive sleep apnea. Am J Respir Crit Care Med 166:860, 2002.

26. Ralston SJ, Charters P: Cuffed nasopharyngeal tube as "dedicated airway" in difficult intubation. Anaesthesia 49:133, 1994.

27. Rama A, Tekwani S, Kushida C: Sites of obstruction in obstructive sleep apnea. Chest 122:1139, 2002.

28. Randerath WJ, Heise M, Hinz R, et al: An individually adjustable oral appliance vs continuous positive airway pressure in mild-to-moderate obstructive sleep apnea syndrome. Chest 122:569, 2002.

29. Redding JS: The choking controversy: Critique of evidence on the Heimlich maneuver. Crit Care Med 7:745, 1979.

30. Safar P, Bircher NG: Cardiopulmonary Cerebral Resuscitation. Philadelphia, WB Saunders, 1988.

31. Schwab RJ, Gefter WB, Hoffman EA: Dynamic upper airway imaging during awake respiration in normal subjects and patients with sleep disordered breathing. Am Rev Respir Dis 148:1385, 1993.

32. Schwab RJ, Gupta KB, Gefter WB, et al: Upper airway and soft tissue anatomy in normal subjects and patients with sleep disordered breathing: Significance of the lateral pharyngeal walls. Am J Respir Crit Care Med 152:1673, 1995.

33. Schwartz AR, Smith PL, Wise RA, et al: Induction of upper airway occlusion in sleeping individuals with subatmospheric nasal pressure. J Appl Physiol 64:535, 1988.

34. Sforza E, Petiau C, Weiss T, et al: Pharyngeal critical pressure in patients with obstructive sleep apnea syndrome: Clinical implications. Am J Respir Crit Care Med 159:149, 1999.

35. Smith PL, Wise RA, Gold AR, et al: Upper airway pressure-flow relationships in obstructive sleep apnea. J Appl Physiol 64:789, 1988.

36. Sullivan CE, Issa FG, Berthon-Jones M, et al: Reversal of obstructive sleep apnea by continuous positive airway pressure applied through the nares. Lancet 1:862, 1981.

37. von Goedecke A, Voelckel WG, Wenzel V, et al.: Mechanical versus manual ventilation via a face mask during the induction of anesthesia: A prospective, randomized, crossover study. Anesth Analg 98:260, 2004.

38. Weiglein AH, Putz R, Pabst R: Sobotta Atlas of Human Anatomy, vol 1, 21st ed. Philadelphia, Lippincott Williams & Wilkins, 2000.

39. Weisman H, Bauer RO, Huddy RA, et al: An improved binasopharyngeal airway system for anesthesia. Anesth Analg 51:11, 1972.

40. Wiegand L, Zwillich CW, White DP: Collapsibility of the human upper airway during normal sleep. J Appl Physiol 66:1800, 1989.

41. Williams PL, Warwick R, Dyson M, et al: Gray's Anatomy, 37th ed. Edinburgh, Churchill Livingstone, 1989.

15

INDICATIONS FOR TRACHEAL INTUBATION

Tiberiu Ezri
R. David Warters

I. INTRODUCTION

Tracheal intubation may be indicated for several purposes as shown in Box 15-1. Tracheal intubation provides a patent airway, thus preventing obstruction as a result of either loss of consciousness or edema or compression (e.g., tumors, hematoma). Endotracheal tube (ET) placement also protects the airway against the aspiration of gastric contents, blood, secretions, and foreign bodies (e.g., dislodged teeth in facial trauma). The propensity for aspiration is greatly increased by loss of consciousness related to head injury or other neurologic insults or to general anesthesia. Although the presence of an ET should decrease the incidence of gastric inflation with the inherent risk of aspiration of gastric contents, silent aspiration around a partially inflated cuff may still occur.[28] An ET also allows effective positive-pressure ventilation, although this can also be accomplished with supraglottic airway devices, such as the laryngeal mask airway (LMA) and the esophageal tracheal Combitube. Removal of tracheobronchial secretions and blood is also eased by the presence of an ET. This is especially crucial in patients who are unable to cough effectively (e.g., comatose patients, those with chest trauma). In addition, an ET

decreases the upper airway dead space by approximately 75%,[23] which may be critical for preserving normocarbia, especially in patients suffering from increased intracranial pressure. Lastly, an ET may serve as a route for emergency drug administration during cardiac arrest when intravenous access is not available.[1] Tracheal intubation may be required to achieve one or any combination of these goals.

This chapter begins with a brief history of endotracheal intubation and then discusses the preceding indications for tracheal intubation according to degree of urgency.

II. HISTORICAL INDICATIONS FOR TRACHEAL INTUBATION

Historically, the earliest known reference to tracheostomy is made in Rig Veda, a Hindu book dating back to around 2000 BC.[8] The legend says that Alexander the Great in about 400 BC cut open with his sword the trachea of a suffocating soldier.[8] The Greek Asculapiades (Aesculapius) possibly performed tracheostomy routinely around the year 100 BC.[10] Vesalius in 1543 performed a tracheostomy in a living animal.[18] The first tracheostomies

---

Box 15-1   Purposes of Tracheal Intubation

1. Provides a patent airway
2. Protects the airway against aspiration of secretions, blood, and gastric contents
3. Allows positive-pressure ventilation
4. Allows removal of tracheobronchial secretions
5. Decreases the anatomic dead space
6. Oxygenation—provides a controlled concentration of oxygen up to 100%
7. Serves as a route for emergency drug administration during cardiac arrest

---

and endotracheal intubations were for resuscitation of drowned persons and for those suffering from laryngeal diphtheria. In 1760, Buchan described the first use of an opening in the patients' "windpipe" during resuscitation, and Cullen suggested the use of tracheal intubation and ventilation with bellows for reviving the apparently dead.[8] Subsequently, Curry and Fine developed intralaryngeal cannulas for resuscitation.[8]

At the end of the 18th century, Cogan and Harves founded a society for drowned persons in London, emphasizing that tracheal intubation was more efficient than mouth-to-mouth ventilation.[19] At about the same time, John Snow resuscitated a baby with a tracheal catheter.[19]

In 1833, Trousseau saved the lives of 200 persons suffering from diphtheria.[8]

By reproducing the technique of tracheostomy developed by John Snow in animals, the German Trendelenburg administered the first endotracheal anesthesia in humans in the early 1870s.[19]

The first elective use of endotracheal intubation for an anesthetic was reported by William Macewan, a surgeon, in 1878.[18,19] The patient was intubated awake for the resection of an oral tumor. He performed an awake, digital, "blind" intubation for a tongue surgery using chloroform anesthesia.[18] His apparent goals were to provide an uninterrupted, smooth anesthesia and avoid aspiration of blood into the airways.[18,19] Most of the early reported endotracheal anesthesias were performed in patients undergoing surgery on the upper airway. Beside the previously mentioned advantages in these cases, endotracheal anesthesia would move the anesthetist away from the surgical field and ease the surgeon's tasks.

In 1885, after witnessing the mutilating effect of hasty tracheostomies, Joseph O'Dwyer, an American surgeon, developed a series of metal tracheal tubes that he inserted orally between the vocal cords in diphtheric patients.[18] In 1888, he successfully intubated and artificially ventilated patients undergoing thoracic surgery.[25] At the end of the 19th century, the German Franz Kuhn constructed metal tubes, which he inserted orally with the digital, blind technique.[18] Kuhn described the use of a curved tube introducer. He preferred packing the hypopharynx

with gauze instead of using cuffed tubes for prevention of aspiration.[18] Kuhn also published the first paper on nasal intubation.[18] Eisenmenger, Dorrance, Guedel, and Waters were the first to attach an inflatable cuff to the tracheal tubes.[4] The "cocainization" of the airway to decrease the reflex reaction to awake intubation was pioneered by Rosenberg and Kuhn in Germany and further developed by Magill in England.[18,19]

During World War I, Magill and Rowbotham performed several intubations for patients suffering from severe facial injuries who underwent reconstructive surgeries in England.[9,33] They also developed a forceps useful for nasal intubation (the Magill forceps) and introduced the term blind intubation by performing nasal intubation with rubber tubes following cocainization of the airway.[18,19] One-lung intubation for thoracic surgery was first used by Ralph Waters, and in the beginning it was performed with double-cuffed, single-lumen tubes developed by Gale, Waters, and Guedel.[12,18] In 1939 Gebauer[13] and in 1949 Eric Carlens[6] from Sweden reported on a similar double-lumen bronchial tube for separation of the lungs. The first modern double-lumen tubes were developed by Robertshaw[29] in 1962.

Indirect laryngoscopy was first described in the 19th century by Garcia in England,[19] and the German Kirstein in 1895 was the first to perform direct laryngoscopy.[19] In 1913 Jackson[18] designed a laryngoscope that was later modified by Magill, Miller, and Macintosh.[3,19]

In 1942, Harold Griffith, a Canadian anesthetist, used curare for the first time in anesthesia. He intubated the trachea in 25 patients, providing abdominal relaxation for surgery.[14] The use of endotracheal intubation became routine after the introduction of muscle relaxants into anesthesia practice.

III. CLINICAL INDICATIONS FOR TRACHEAL INTUBATION ACCORDING TO DEGREE OF URGENCY

Tracheal intubation may be required for emergent, urgent, or elective reasons. A list of major clinical indications for tracheal intubation according to urgency is presented in Table 15-1. Indications may also be categorized according to the perioperative period as in Table 15-2.

A. EMERGENT INTUBATION

Intubation is always indicated during cardiopulmonary resuscitation (CPR). ET placement during CPR provides effective ventilation and oxygenation, frees the operator's hands from mask ventilation, improves the conditions for chest compression, avoids gastric distention and aspiration of gastric contents into the lungs, and allows accurate measurement of end-tidal CO_2, which may be critical for assessment of the effectiveness of resuscitation.[15]

Table 15-1 **Classification of Clinical Indications for Tracheal Intubation according to Degree of Urgency**

Condition	Emergent	Urgent	Elective
CPR	Cardiac arrest of any origin		
Trauma	Loss of spontaneous ventilation Loss of airway patency Facial burns with respiratory distress	Facial burns with risk of airway loss Partial airway obstruction with upper airway/facial trauma Loss of consciousness High aspiration risk Respiratory failure Shock syndrome	Anesthesia for uncooperative trauma patients for diagnostic procedures Anesthesia for trauma surgery
Medical conditions	Loss of spontaneous ventilation Total airway obstruction	Partial airway obstruction Loss of consciousness Respiratory failure of any origin Shock syndrome of any origin	Special diagnostic procedures
Perioperative indications	Loss of airway patency that is unrelieved by other airway devices CPR during anesthesia	Partial airway obstruction unrelieved by other airway devices Hypoxemia/hypercarbia under mask ventilation Unstable hemodynamics Unexpected anesthetic complication	Risk of aspiration Surgery in the proximity of the airway Special surgeries (cardiac, chest, head) Prolonged surgeries Special patient's positioning

CPR, cardiopulmonary resuscitation.

Supraglottic devices (e.g., LMA, esophageal tracheal Combitube) have been successfully used as temporary means of ventilation during CPR,[11] but they do not provide the same degree of protection from aspiration or the same reliability of gas exchange. A tracheal tube may also serve as a route for medication administration (epinephrine, atropine, lidocaine) when intravenous access is not established.[1]

Emergent intubation is indicated in any situation leading to apnea or total airway obstruction. Pathophysiologically, a condition requiring emergent intubation may arise as "drive" failure (head injury), "pump" failure (severe chest trauma), airway obstruction, or a combination of these. Emergency intubation in facial burn or facial trauma cases is indicated if the patient is unconscious (e.g., carbon monoxide intoxication) with respiratory distress and with total loss of the airway (such as major upper airway disruption). Emergent intubation may be needed in severe face and neck trauma (Le Fort III fracture or upper airway compression by hematoma).

Table 15-2 **Perioperative Indications for Endotracheal Intubation**

Preoperative	Intraoperative	Postoperative
Unstable patients scheduled for emergency surgery	Risk of aspiration Any surgery requiring muscle relaxation Any cardiac, thoracic, upper abdominal, or neurosurgery Patients in unusual positions for surgery Surgery in the vicinity of the airway Risk of loss of the airway Need for avoidance of hypercarbia Major surgery Loss of the airway during anesthesia in unintubated patients Intraoperative complications	Continuation of artificial ventilation for multiple reasons Unstable (bleeding) patients Opioid overdose Partial curarization Pulmonary edema Pneumothorax

B. URGENT INTUBATION

Urgent indications for endotracheal intubation present the biggest challenge in airway management. Whereas most emergent indications are readily recognized, urgent situations can be more difficult to identify and manage expeditiously. Urgent indications may include shock states of any origin (increased work of breathing with excessive oxygen consumption), partial airway obstruction (e.g., tumors involving the airway or neck), and respiratory failure of any origin (e.g., neuromuscular diseases, brain tumors, chronic obstructive lung disease). Pulmonary edema (cardiogenic and hyperpermeability) and pulmonary embolism are other reasons for acute respiratory failure.

In the absence of frank cardiopulmonary arrest, the diagnosis of impending or actual respiratory failure in awake patients is based on objective quantitative criteria or subjective qualitative criteria, or both. There are many causes of respiratory failure, and detailing them is beyond the scope of this book. The treatment for respiratory failure is mechanical ventilation. The following discussion of indications for tracheal intubation of the awake patient in respiratory failure emphasizes this primary goal of tracheal intubation.

1. Objective Quantitative Criteria for Tracheal Intubation

The three right-hand columns of Table 15-3 describe a deterioration in the results of respiratory function testing from an acceptable range to an unstable, possible intubation status requiring close monitoring and intensive nontracheal intubation support (see Chapters 13 and 14) to probable intubation and mechanical ventilation necessary status.[26] Respiratory function testing can be divided into mechanical, oxygenation, and ventilation categories. In practice, arterial partial pressures of oxygen (PaO_2) and carbon dioxide ($PaCO_2$) are used most often as indicators of proper tracheal intubation, and vital capacity, peak inspiratory force, and respiratory rate are most often used as variables to determine the appropriateness of tracheal extubation.

The trend of the data in Table 15-3 is as important as the data themselves. For example, progressively increasing $PaCO_2$ from a normal $PaCO_2$ in a patient without previous lung disease is more important than an already high $PaCO_2$ in a patient with emphysema. Thus, a PaO_2 of 50 mm Hg and a $PaCO_2$ of 65 mm Hg might be considered normal for a patient with chronic obstructive pulmonary disease (COPD), but the same values would indicate a marked degree of respiratory embarrassment for a patient with no lung disease. Knowledge of the patient's usual state of health is very helpful in making the decision to intubate the trachea.

2. Subjective Qualitative Criteria for Tracheal Intubation

Because the degree of respiratory failure in awake patients is amenable to quantification, the most important indications for tracheal intubation in most of these patients are the objective tests of respiratory function. However, in some situations objective criteria are not available and the gross appearance of the patient alone is sufficient indication (Box 15-2).

Preoperative preventive or urgent intubation in awake patients may sometimes be required in the emergency room for safer transportation of the patient to the operating theater for emergency surgery (e.g., major trauma).

Table 15-3 Objective Quantitative Criteria for Tracheal Intubation

Respiratory Function		Acceptable Range	Chest PT, Oxygen, Drugs, Close Monitoring	Possible Intubation, Probable Intubation and Ventilation
Category	**Variable**			
Mechanics	Vital capacity (mL/kg)	67-75	65-15	<15
	Inspiratory force (mL H₂O)	100-50	50-25	<25
Oxygenation	A-aDO₂ (mm Hg) room air	<38	38-55	>55
	FIO₂ = 1.0	<100	100-450	>450
	PaO₂ (mm Hg) room air	<72	72-55	<55
	FIO₂ = 1.0	>400	400-200	<200
Ventilation	Respiratory rate (breaths/min)	10-25	25-40 or <8	>40 or <6
	PaCO₂ (mm Hg)	35-45	45-60	>60

Adapted from Pontpoppidan H, Geffin B, Lowenstein E: Acute respiratory failure in the adult (second of three parts). N Engl J Med 287:743, 1972.
A-aDO₂, alveolar-arterial partial pressure of oxygen difference; FIO₂, inspired concentration of oxygen; PaO₂ and PaCO₂, arterial partial pressure of oxygen and carbon dioxide, respectively; PT, physical therapy.

This may be the case in patients who still have a stable airway but may unexpectedly deteriorate during transportation.

The postoperative patient emerging from anesthesia often has a significant element of several of these objective and subjective indications for continued tracheal intubation and mechanical ventilation. These elements include residual anesthesia or paralysis (mental state obtunded, weak breathing muscles, and no swallowing), objective deterioration in lung function, and need for a smooth transition into a postoperative period that will include many other intensive therapies for other major organs.

C. ELECTIVE INTUBATION

Indications for elective intubation involve anticipation of the need for controlled ventilation or airway protection. Patients who undergo diagnostic or surgical procedures often require tracheal intubation. Elective intubation may be necessary in trauma patients for performance of special investigations (e.g., computed tomography scans) in uncooperative, combative patients or those with painful injuries.[32]

Endotracheal intubation during general anesthesia may reflect a primary or a secondary need for a guaranteed airway. Patients who have a primary need for a guaranteed airway (e.g., patients who undergo neurosurgical, cardiothoracic, ear, nose, mouth, and throat procedures and major intra-abdominal procedures) or patients who develop a secondary need (which may become urgent) for a guaranteed airway (e.g., if ventilation by mask or supraglottic ventilatory devices [SVDs] becomes inadequate, the procedure is changed after induction of anesthesia, or a major complication occurs) require tracheal intubation (see last section in this chapter). In both groups of patients, the usual purposes of tracheal intubation, in descending order of importance, are to provide airway patency, mechanical ventilation, airway protection, and the ability to remove secretions. Airway protection is relatively more important in patients considered at risk for aspiration of gastric contents (i.e., full stomachs) and in patients undergoing intra-abdominal procedures. A severely poisoned patient is equivalent to a generally anesthetized patient with a full stomach and requires tracheal intubation for airway protection, patency, and mechanical ventilation. Preoperative knowledge of the surgical procedure is crucial in determining the importance of securing the airway with an ET during the procedure. In anesthetized, unintubated patients (e.g., patients ventilated by mask or SVD, patients undergoing regional anesthesia, or sedated patients with local anesthesia), intraoperative signs of airway obstruction may be most important.

1. Primary Need for a Guaranteed Airway

Box 15-3 summarizes the primary needs for a guaranteed airway during general anesthesia. Many surgical procedures require that the patient be tracheally intubated (see Box 15-3). Surgical procedures (performed with the patient under general anesthesia) that prevent the anesthesiologist from having access to or control over the patient's natural airway, or both, require tracheal intubation. *This still remains the commonsense approach and the basis for a safe practice.* These procedures consist of all neurosurgical, ear, nose, mouth, and tracheal procedures. Although surgeries in the vicinity of the airway usually demand endotracheal intubation, the LMA instead of an ET has been used successfully during tonsillectomy and awake craniotomy in both adults and children.[16,17] The risks of loss of airway during the procedure should be weighed against the possible benefits.

Also, all procedures performed with the patient in the prone position, most procedures performed with the patient in the lateral decubitus position, and any procedure that involves turning the patient so that the anesthesiologist is not at the patient's head should include endotracheal intubation. Intrathoracic and intra-abdominal procedures require tracheal intubation because of both mechanical and physiologic impediments to adequate gas exchange. Surgical procedures of very long duration usually require tracheal intubation because the ability of the anesthesiologist[1] to maintain an adequate airway decreases with time. Procedures that require a great deal of the anesthesiologist's attention and time for nonrespiratory matters (e.g., those involving massive blood loss or extensive monitoring) require tracheal intubation so that the anesthesiologist's hands and attention are not tied to maintaining a guaranteed airway. As noted earlier, the patient emerging from anesthesia for a major surgical procedure often requires continued tracheal intubation and mechanical ventilation for multiple reasons.

For patients requiring muscle relaxation for surgery, endotracheal intubation may be safer than supraglottic devices in terms of less risk of aspiration, less air leak, and less propensity for dislodgement of the airway. However, prolonged surgery and use of muscle relaxants do not preclude the use of an LMA instead of an ET.[34] Special attention is required for patients with decreased chest-lung compliance (COPD, obesity), who may need high inflation pressures for effective ventilation with SVD, with the inherent risk of gastric distention. See Chapter 42 regarding further detail of the proper use of regional anesthesia in patients who may be at high risk for intubation difficulties.

The American Society of Anesthesiologists Practice Guidelines for Management of the Difficult Airway[27] strongly recommend elective, awake intubation in patients with previous or predicted difficult intubation, although this has been challenged in obstetric anesthesia, with regional anesthesia performed in at-risk patients scheduled for cesarean section.[2]

2. Secondary Need for a Guaranteed Airway

When a secondary need for a guaranteed airway arises, it is usually unexpected and may not be planned. For example, ventilation by mask or SVD may become inadequate, the surgical procedure may be changed, or a major surgical or anesthetic complication may occur (Box 15-4). The difficulty of tracheal intubation under these circumstances may be increased.

Box 15-4   Secondary Need for a Guaranteed Airway

1. Mask ventilation is inadequate.
2. Surgical procedure is changed after anesthesia is induced.
3. A major anesthetic or surgical complication occurs.

---

a. Inadequate Ventilation

Airway obstruction is the most common serious cause of inadequate ventilation by a mask, and major airway obstruction unrelieved by such maneuvers as anterior jaw dislocation and insertion of a nasopharyngeal or oropharyngeal airway is a strong indication for tracheal intubation; other options less certain to succeed include insertion of an LMA (Chapter 21) and a Combitube (Chapter 25). Nonetheless, airway obstruction may also occur with the use of any of the SVDs. The obstruction can be at any level in the airway and may cause preferential ventilation of the esophagus (pathway of least resistance), resulting in distention of the stomach. Stomach distention, in turn, further impairs ventilation of the lungs. Patients under general anesthesia who are breathing through an anesthesia mask make up the largest group with this indication for tracheal intubation. However, patients in respiratory failure who are narcotized by carbon dioxide retention, patients who are excessively intravenously sedated or narcotized while under regional anesthesia, patients who are poisoned or have taken or been given (iatrogenically) a drug overdose, and head-injured patients are also in this category.

Total airway obstruction is characterized by lack of breath sounds, which may be coupled with continuing, sometimes strenuous but ineffectual efforts at breathing. Excessive diaphragmatic activity may cause abdominal movements and chest retraction yet not necessarily movement of air. The diagnosis is made by the absence of breath sounds, failure to observe movement of the breathing bag or failure to feel the movement and warmth of air at the airway outlet, and absence of a carbon dioxide excretion waveform.

Partial upper airway obstruction is characterized by restriction of air movement with inspiration that prolongs the inspiratory phase, diminished tidal exchange and breath sounds, excessive diaphragmatic activity, retraction of the upper chest, discrepancy between the movements of the breathing bag and the chest wall, and various characteristic sounds. Partial obstruction caused by the tongue causes a rough, irregular, stuttery noise frequently associated with stertorous respiration. Preoperatively, one's index of suspicion for partial obstruction of the upper airway by a large tongue falling against the pharynx can be increased by a history of heavy snoring and sleep apnea, and the size of the tongue relative to the oropharynx can be determined by having the patient open his or her mouth widely. If the uvula and tonsillar pillars are obscured by the tongue, the tongue is very large in relation to the oropharynx.[22,30] Partial laryngospasm usually causes a high-pitched whistle or squeak. On the other hand, partial obstruction by the lips is most noticeable during expiration and is accompanied by a low-pitched, rough, fluttery sound. Pharyngeal secretions cause a gurgling, bubbling noise. Partial obstruction at the trachea related to foreign materials and secretions produces a rattly or sloshy noise.

Lower airway obstruction is characterized by diminished tidal exchange, excessive intercostal and diaphragmatic activity, active inspiration and expiration during spontaneous respiration, and, most important, adventitious breath sounds consisting of rales, rhonchi, or wheezing. Bronchiolar secretions cause rhonchi, and bronchiolar constriction causes wheezing. Alveolar obstruction may be associated with all types of adventitious sounds, but rales are most common. With lower airway obstruction the breathing bag classically empties and refills slowly, and moderate changes in compliance can be felt by squeezing the reservoir bag.

Langeron and colleagues[21] observed a 5% incidence of difficult mask ventilation, defined as inability of an unassisted anesthesiologist to maintain oxygen saturation greater than 92% or to prevent or reverse signs of inadequate ventilation under general anesthesia. In their study of 1502 patients that excluded ear, nose and throat; obstetric; and emergency patients, they found five criteria (age >55 years, body mass index >26 kg/m^2, lack of teeth, presence of a beard, history of snoring) to be independent risk factors for difficult mask ventilation, with two of these criteria indicating a high likelihood of difficult mask ventilation (sensitivity of 72%, specificity of 73%).

Very obese patients may be predictably difficult to ventilate by mask because of the difficulty in raising the heavy chest wall and displacing the massive abdominal wall. Patients with dentures may be difficult to ventilate by mask because of large air leaks between the sunken cheeks and the mask, and it may be advisable to leave a patient's dentures in place during the performance of bag-mask ventilation but remove them prior to endotracheal intubation. Although such maneuvers as changing the size of the mask, pressing the mask closer to the face, and changing the contour of the patient's face (e.g., placing saline-soaked gauze rolls in the buccal pouches to round out the cheeks) may sometimes diminish or eliminate the air leak, tracheal intubation is often necessary.

b. Change in Intended Surgical Procedure
Change in the planned surgical procedure most frequently follows diagnostic procedures such as conversion of a breast biopsy into a mastectomy, conversion of a cesarean section to a hysterectomy, and conversion of a bronchoscopy or mediastinoscopy to a lung resection.

c. Anesthetic or Surgical Complications
The occurrence of a major anesthetic or surgical complication, such as a high or total spinal anesthetic, massive blood loss, malignant hyperthermia, or wearing off of a regional anesthetic (patient experiences undue pain), often requires tracheal intubation (along with other important treatments).

IV. SUMMARY

Both awake and anesthetized patients may require tracheal intubation. Tracheal intubation provides airway patency, protects the airway from aspiration, allows mechanical ventilation, and allows airway suctioning. In awake patients, the decision to intubate is based on objective quantitative and subjective qualitative criteria and trends in all available data. In anesthetized patients, the need for tracheal intubation is usually identified preoperatively but may occasionally arise unexpectedly after the induction of anesthesia. Thus, tracheal intubation may be either an expected, elective, planned procedure or an unexpected, nonelective, emergency procedure. Chapters 15 through 30 describe the techniques one may use to accomplish this very important procedure.

REFERENCES

1. A.H.A.- A.C.L.S. Guidelines. Circulation 102-I 129-I 135(Suppl), Part 6 ACLS, Section 6, Pharmacology II, 2000.
2. Benumof JL: ASA difficult airway algorithm: New thoughts and considerations. In Hagberg C (ed): Handbook of Difficult Airway Management. Philadelphia, Churchill Livingstone, 1996, p 31.
3. Boulton TB: Classical files. Surv Anesthesiol 27:396, 1983.
4. Calverley RK: Classical file. Surv Anesthesiol 28:70, 1984.
5. Campbell EJM, Agostini E, Davis EN: The Respiratory Muscles: Mechanics and Neural Control, 2nd ed. London, Lloyd Luke, 1970.
6. Carlens E: New flexible double-lumen catheter for bronchospirometry. J Thorac Surg 18:742, 1949.
7. Cohen BM: The interrelationship of the respiratory functions of the nasal and lower airways. Bull Physiopathol Respir 7:895, 1971.
8. Colice GL: Historical background. In: Tobin MJ (ed): Principles and Practice of Mechanical Ventilation. New York, McGraw-Hill, 1994, p 1.
9. Condon HA, Gilchrist E: Stanley Rowbotham, twentieth century pioneer anaesthetist. Anaesthesia 41:46, 1986.
10. Frost E: Tracing the tracheostomy. Ann Otol 85:618, 1974.
11. Gabrielli A, Layon AJ, Wenzel V, et al: Alternative ventilation strategies in cardiopulmonary resuscitation. Curr Opin Crit Care 8:199, 2000.
12. Gale JW, Waters RM: Closed endotracheal anesthesia in thoracic surgery: Preliminary report. Curr Res Anesth Analg 11:283, 1932.
13. Gebauer PW: A catheter for bronchospirometry. J Thorac Surg 8:674, 1939.
14. Grifith HR, Johnson GE: The use of curare in general anesthesia. Anesthesiology 3:418, 1942.
15. Grmec S, Klemen P: Does the end-tidal carbon dioxide (EtCO$_2$) concentration have prognostic value during out-of-hospital cardiac arrest? Eur J Emerg Med 8:263, 2001.
16. Hagberg CA, Gollas A, Berry JM: The laryngeal mask airway for awake craniotomy in the pediatric patient: Report of three cases. J Clin Anesth 16:43, 2004.

17. Hatcher IS, Stack CG: Postal survey of the anaesthetic techniques used for paediatric tonsillectomy surgery. Paediatr Anaesth 9:311, 1999.

18. History of endotracheal anaesthesia. In Gillespie NA: Endotracheal Anaesthesia, 2nd ed. Madison, University of Wisconsin Press, 1948.

19. Intubation of the trachea. In Rushman GB, Davies NJH, Atkinson RS: A Short History of Anaesthesia: The First 150 Years. Oxford, Butterworth-Heinemann, 1996, p 92.

20. Knelson JH, Howatt WF, Demuth GR: The physiologic significance of grunting respiration. Pediatrics 44:393, 1969.

21. Langeron O, Mazzo E, Huraux C, et al: Prediction of difficult mask ventilation. Anesthesiology 92:1229, 2000.

22. Mallampati RS, Gatt SP, Gugino LD, et al: A clinical sign to predict difficult tracheal intubation: A prospective study. Can Anaesth Soc J 32:429, 1985.

23. Mecca RS: Postoperative recovery. In Barash PG, Cullen BF, Stoelting RK (eds): Clinical Anesthesia, 3rd ed. Philadelphia, Lippincott-Raven, 1997, p 1290.

24. Mueller RE, Petty TL, Filley GF: Ventilation and arterial blood-gas changes induced by pursed-lips breathing. J Appl Physiol 28:784, 1970.

25. Mushin WW, Rendell-Baker L: Thoracic Anesthesia. Past and Present (reprinted by the Wood Library Museum, 1991). Springfield, Ill, Charles C Thomas, 1953, p 44.

26. Pontpoppidan H, Geffin B, Lowenstein E: Acute respiratory failure in the adult (second of three parts). N Engl J Med 287:743, 1972.

27. Practice guidelines for management of the difficult airway: A report by the American Society of Anesthesiologists Task Force on Management of the Difficult Airway. Anesthesiology 78:597, 1993.

28. Rello J, Sonora R, Jubert P, et al: Pneumonia in intubated patients: Role of respiratory airway care. Am J Respir Crit Care Med 154:111, 1996.

29. Robertshaw FL: Low resistance double-lumen endotracheal tubes. Br J Anaesth 34:576, 1962.

30. Samsoon GLT, Young JRB: Difficult tracheal intubation: A retrospective study, Anaesthesia 42:487, 1987.

31. Schmidt RW, Wasserman K, Lillington GA: The effect of air flow and oral pressure on the mechanics of breathing in patients with asthma and emphysema. Am Rev Respir Dis 90:564, 1964.

32. Stene JK, Grande CM: Anesthesia for trauma. In Miller RD (ed): Anesthesia, 5th ed. Philadelphia, Churchill Livingstone, 2000, p 2157.

33. Thomas KB: Sir Ivan Whiteside Magill. A review of his publications and other references to his life and work. Anaesthesia 33:628, 1978.

34. Verghese C, Brimacombe JR: Survey of laryngeal mask airway usage in 11,910 patients: Safety and efficacy for conventional and nonconventional usage. Anesth Analg 82:129, 1996.

16

CONVENTIONAL (LARYNGOSCOPIC) OROTRACHEAL AND NASOTRACHEAL INTUBATION (SINGLE LUMEN TUBE)

James M. Berry

I. A SHORT HISTORY OF TRACHEAL INTUBATION

As we participate in the 21st century practice of medicine, it is useful to recollect the origin and development of some of the techniques commonly used today for airway management. It is remarkable that modern airway techniques are less than 50 years old but derive from physiologic experiments done primarily in the 18th and 19th centuries. However, skilled airway management is one of the central pillars of the practice of anesthesiology, resuscitation, and critical care, and an appreciation of the evolution and development of airway techniques can improve our understanding and application of these essential skills.

Cannulation of the trachea, or *aspera arteria*, as it was called by Robert Hooke, was initially described as a technique for positive-pressure ventilation:

> ...the Dog being kept alive by the Reciprocal blowing up of his Lungs with Bellowes, and they suffered to subside, for the space of an hour or more, after his Thorax had been so display'd, and his Aspera Arteria cut off just below the Epiglotis, and bound on upon the nose of the Bellows.[10]

However, the use of tracheal cannulation for the administration of anesthetics (as well as the provision of a patent airway) was first reported in 1858 by John Snow in *On Chloroform and Other Anaesthetics*,[21] wherein he described a tracheotomy and cannulation for the administration of chloroform in a spontaneously breathing rabbit. The first human use of tracheostomy for anesthesia and protection against aspiration was reported by Trendelenburg in 1869, again accompanied by spontaneous ventilation.[23] In the next 10 years, numerous investigators developed nonsurgical techniques and apparatus for cannulation of the trachea, for either surgical (ear, nose, throat) or medical (diphtheria) indications. Matas was among the first to advocate the use of positive-pressure ventilation through a tracheal cannula to avoid the catastrophic consequences of pneumothorax for a spontaneously ventilating patient during thoracotomy.[17]

Endotracheal anesthesia came into its own during and immediately after World War I owing to the volume of facial and mandibular injuries treated in England, especially at the hospital at Sidcup. Soon thereafter was published one of many descriptive treatises on intubation in anesthesia:

> The maintenance of a free airway has long been recognized as a first principle in general anesthesia and the danger of complete laryngeal obstruction has always been obvious. On the other hand, the cumulative effects of partial respiratory obstruction have, in the past, been frequently

overlooked and it is not improbable that many of the surgical difficulties, postoperative complications, and even fatalities attributed to the anesthetic agent have been primarily due to an imperfect airway. It may be said without exaggeration that in remedying this defect endotracheal anesthesia has proved as great a factor in the advances of anesthesia as the discovery of new drugs or the development of improved apparatus. I.W. Magill, Am J Surg, 1936.

However, immediately thereafter he inserts a caveat:

...owing to the ease of control it affords, there is a tendency towards its employment in every operation, regardless of other considerations. This tendency is to be deprecated, especially in the teaching of students. The novice should learn airway control by simple methods in the first instance, for he may be called to administer an anesthetic in circumstances in which artificial devices are not available. Moreover, as the method involves instrumentation, which is not devoid of the risk of trauma, even though it may be slight, intubation should only be attempted when the necessity for it has been considered carefully.

The historical lesson here is that, no matter how routine tracheal intubation becomes, it is still an invasive procedure with nontrivial risks and significant complications. It should be used for specific indications and only after careful consideration of the balance of risks to and benefits for the patient.

II. CONVENTIONAL (LARYNGOSCOPIC) OROTRACHEAL INTUBATION

The orotracheal route is the simplest and most direct approach to tracheal cannulation. Done under direct laryngoscopic vision, this technique is the most straightforward, simple, and direct for the purposes of administering general anesthesia, ventilation of critically ill patients, and cardiopulmonary resuscitation. The vocal cords are visualized with the aid of a handheld laryngoscope, and the endotracheal tube (ET) is then introduced and positioned in the trachea under continuous direct observation. After confirmation of correct placement, the tube is then fixed in place and ventilation assisted or controlled as indicated.

A. PREPARATION AND POSITIONING

Box 16-1 lists the basic materials required for conventional orotracheal intubation. The materials are grouped according to the temporal sequence of events. All items are required for either routine intubation, dealing with common difficulties, or preventing complications. Redundancy is the key in preparing for a critical event such as tracheal intubation. All essential equipment (laryngoscope handles, tubes) should have a readily available backup in case of unexpected failure. An assortment of laryngoscope blades, both straight (Miller) and curved (Macintosh), should be available.

Box 16-1   Basic Equipment for Tracheal Intubation

Preoxygenation and Ventilation
1. Oxygen source
2. Ventilation bag or anesthesia circuit (for positive-pressure ventilation)
3. Appropriately sized face mask
4. Appropriately sized oropharyngeal and nasopharyngeal airways
5. Tongue blade

Endotracheal Tubes
6. Appropriately sized tracheal tubes (at least two)
7. Malleable stylet
8. Syringe for tube cuff, 10 mL
9. Jelly and/or ointment, 4% lidocaine (Xylocaine)

Drugs
10. Intravenous anesthetics and muscle relaxants (ready to administer)
11. Reliable, free-flowing intravenous infusion (some pediatric exceptions)
12. Topical anesthetics and vasoconstrictors (for nasal intubation)

Laryngoscopy
13. Working suction apparatus with "tonsil tip"
14. Assortment of Miller blades with functioning battery handle
15. Assortment of Macintosh blades with functioning battery handle
16. Bolsters (folded sheets, towels) for positioning of head and shoulders

Fixation of the Endotracheal Tube
17. Tincture of benzoin
18. Appropriate tape or tie
19. Stethoscope
20. End-tidal CO_2 monitor
21. Pulse oximeter

The proper sequence of events prior to laryngoscopy includes:

1. Adequate access to the head of the bed or table. Removal of side rails and headboard (if outside the surgical suite) ensures freedom of movement; ensuring that the bed/table is locked in position prevents unnecessary and stress-inducing pursuit of the patient around the room. The height of the surface should be adjusted to the level of the operator's chest. An experienced aide should be in constant attendance to provide items such as suction lines, airways, tubes, and drugs to the primary operator as well as to apply laryngeal pressure as needed.
2. Proper positioning of the patient prior to laryngoscopy. Patients who are uncooperative, agitated, or otherwise mobile may require rapid and efficient positioning after sedation; thus, pads or rolls should be prepared in advance and be readily at hand.

The earliest attempts at laryngoscopy used the "classical" positioning of full extension. Described by Jackson in 1913, this position required full extension of the head and neck on a flat surface. Twenty years later, he amended his view to one that supported the contemporary "sniffing" position of flexion at the neck and extension at the head.[11,12] This was accomplished by supporting the head on a pillow of at least 10 cm thickness. Numerous authors have examined radiographs of subjects to determine the optimal positioning for orotracheal access. Simultaneously, various theoretical models of positioning for intubation have been proposed. For the past 60 years, the three-axis theory has proposed that the oral, pharyngeal, and laryngeal axes should be brought into approximate alignment in order to best facilitate orotracheal visualization and intubation (Fig. 16-1). Proposed by Bannister and MacBeth in 1944, this model presumes that laryngoscopy is done in the midline (two-dimensional model) and that laryngeal axis alignment is necessary for proper intubation.[4] This has been challenged by the work of Adnet and colleagues in both imaging studies and clinical comparisons.[1-3] In general, no advantage of the sniffing position (flexion at C6-C7 and extension at occiput-C1) over simple neck extension could be demonstrated. However, in patients with limited extension at the occiput, the sniffing position was found to be beneficial.

Along with extension of the upper cervical spine-occipital junction, either a neutral to extended or a flexed position of the lower cervical spine may prove optimal for intubation. The reasonable option in view of conflicting evidence (and patients' variability) is to position the patient with the occiput on a pad (traditional sniffing position) and be prepared to remove the pad (convert to simple extension) should initial laryngoscopy be inadequate (Fig. 16-2). Obese patients may often require more extensive padding (planking) starting at the midpoint of the back to the head in order to assume an optimal position for laryngoscopy.

Occasionally, in obese patients it is necessary to also place towels and blankets under the scapula, shoulders, and nape of the neck, as well as the head, in order to flex the neck on the chest (see Figs. 16-1B and 16-2) and extend the head on the neck (see Figs. 16-1C and 16-2); in this instance, the purpose of the scapula, shoulder, and neck support is to give the head room so that it may be extended on the neck. When in doubt, the final assessment of the position should be from a lateral view of the

Head and neck position and the axes of the head and neck upper airway

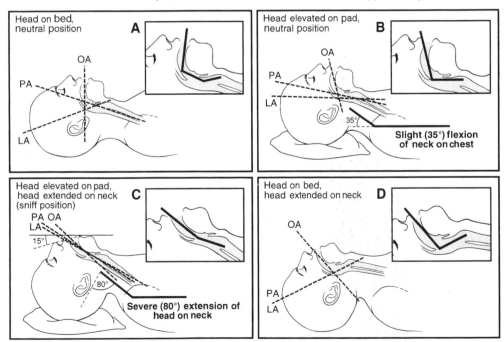

Figure 16-1 Schematic diagram showing the alignment of the oral axis (OA), pharyngeal axis (PA), and laryngeal axis (LA) in four different head positions. Each head position is accompanied by an inset that magnifies the upper airway (the oral cavity, pharynx, and larynx) and superimposes, as a variously bent bold line, the continuity of these three axes within the upper airway. **A,** The head is in the neutral position with a marked degree of nonalignment of the LA, PA, and OA. **B,** The head is resting on a large pad that flexes the neck on the chest and aligns the LA with the PA. **C,** The head is resting on a pad (which flexes the neck on the chest): concomitant extension of the head on the neck, which brings all three axes into alignment (sniffing position), is shown. **D,** Extension of the head on the neck without concomitant elevation of the head on a pad, which results in nonalignment of the PA and LA with the OA. (From Benumof JL [ed]: Airway Management: Principles and Practice. St. Louis, Mosby, 1996, p 263.)

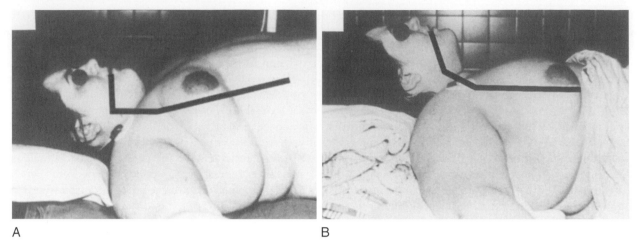

A   B

Figure 16-2 **A,** In some obese patients, simply placing the head on a pillow does not result in the sniffing position; in the obese patient shown, and as illustrated by the overlying heavy bold black line, the oral and laryngeal axes are perpendicular to one another, the neck is not flexed on the chest, and the head is not extended on the neck at the atlanto-occipital joint. **B,** In the same patient, placing support (blankets, towels, and the like) under the scapula, shoulders, nape of the neck, and head results in a much better sniffing position: the oral, pharyngeal, and laryngeal axes form only a slightly bent curve, the neck is flexed on the chest, and the head is extended on the neck at the atlanto-occipital joint. (From Benumof JL [ed]: Airway Management: Principles and Practice. St. Louis, Mosby, 1996, p 264.)

patient because only a lateral view enables precise assessment of the chest, neck, face, and head axes (see Figs. 16-1C and 16-2).

B. PREOXYGENATION

Instrumentation of the airway may be done on an awake, spontaneously breathing patient; and, at times, this may be the safest and most prudent approach. However, most commonly, laryngoscopy and intubation are performed on an anesthetized and (usually) apneic patient. Because this requires some finite period of time, the patient is at risk for arterial desaturation and hypoxic injury. Preoxygenation is done prior to laryngoscopy to minimize this risk.

The administration of 100% oxygen through a tight-fitting mask may occur either by way of the patient's spontaneous respirations or by positive-pressure bag-mask ventilation. In either case, adequate ventilation must occur in order to "wash out" alveolar nitrogen and fill the lungs with oxygen. The goal is to fill not only the alveoli used in normal tidal breathing but also the remaining alveoli and airways constituting the functional residual capacity (FRC). This additional oxygen serves as a reservoir to delay the onset of arterial hypoxia for as long as 5 minutes. A number of guidelines have been proposed to accomplish this potentially lifesaving goal.

Depending on the minute ventilation of the patient (either spontaneous or assisted), the time to complete effective preoxygenation varies from 1 to 5 minutes; although, in an awake and cooperative patient, this may be mostly accomplished with three or four full, vital capacity breaths.[7-8] Work has documented the increased efficacy of eight full breaths in approximately 60 seconds, with times to desaturation approaching those of the more traditional 3- to 5-minute preoxygenation.[5] Obviously, a higher minute ventilation leads to more rapid and complete preoxygenation. Measures of the adequacy of preoxygenation include (1) real-time gas analysis of expired oxygen concentration (goal of 95%) and (2) analysis of expired nitrogen (goal of < 5%). Essential to either of these measurements is the presence of a capnograph waveform with a plateau reflecting the expected alveolar carbon dioxide concentration. This documents the presence of an effective seal of circuit-bag to the patient's airway and the effective delivery of 100% oxygen. The use of an Ambu-type bag-valve-mask without an expiratory valve may not provide optimal preoxygenation.[19]

The effectiveness of preoxygenation in preventing hypoxia during laryngoscopy is significantly reduced in the morbidly obese patient. Even with the most careful preoxygenation, the duration of apnea before the onset of hypoxia is half the duration seen in patients with normal body weight. This is hypothesized to be due to the considerable reduction in FRC and vital capacity in the obese patient and to the additional reduction attributable to the cephalad diaphragmatic shift related to supine positioning.[13] This places morbidly obese patients at significantly increased risk for injury should any difficulty with ventilation or intubation be encountered.

Pharyngeal insufflation of oxygen can significantly prolong the safe duration of apnea. In a typical adult, approximately 250 mL/min of oxygen is transferred from the lungs into the bloodstream, while only 200 mL/min of CO_2 enters the lungs from the bloodstream (respiratory quotient of 0.8). This alveolar gas deficit causes alveolar pressures to become slightly subatmospheric. Thus, if the airway is patent, there is a net flow of gas from the pharynx into the alveoli (apneic oxygenation). If, following adequate preoxygenation, the pharynx is filled with oxygen, the onset of hypoxia is delayed because oxygen, rather than air, would be drawn into the lungs by this mechanism. Pharyngeal insufflation may be conveniently achieved by passing a catheter into the pharynx through a nasopharyngeal airway and attaching an oxygen source at 2 to 3 L/min. Alternatively, some laryngoscopes have a sideport suitable for attachment of oxygen tubing. When preoxygenation is followed by pharyngeal insufflation as previously described, in normal but apneic patients, the oxygen saturation from pulse oximetry [SpO_2] remains equal to 98% for a minimum of 10 minutes (although at the end of 10 minutes the arterial carbon dioxide tension [$PaCO_2$] may be expected to be ~80 mm Hg).[22]

C. LARYNGOSCOPY

The purpose of direct laryngoscopy is to provide adequate visualization of the glottis to allow correct placement of the ET with the minimum effort, elapsed time, and potential for injury to the patient. Considerable effort has been expended to develop laryngoscopic techniques and equipment to facilitate this important procedure. Although this volume outlines numerous techniques for tracheal cannulation, the facilitative use of direct laryngoscopy is by far the most common technique.

There are two basic types of laryngoscope blades: the curved blade (Macintosh) and the straight blade with curved tip (Miller).[16,18] They are designed for right hand-dominant use; the laryngoscope is held in the left hand while the right hand manipulates the ET. Historically, either (or both) hands could be initially used, shifting the laryngoscope to the left hand while the right hand manipulated the tube. Both of these blade styles include a flange on the left side of the blade for lateral retraction of the tongue and also contain a light-emitting area (bulb or fiberoptic tip). Each blade has a channel with an open right side for visualization of the larynx and for insertion of the ET (Figs. 16-3 to 16-10). There are numerous modifications and variations of these two themes, but, fundamentally, they are all lighted, handheld retractors for oropharyngeal soft tissues.

Although contact with the upper incisors from the laryngoscope blade is to be avoided, some patients with limited mouth opening, front caps, or obvious decay are at risk for damage by even the most innocuous, transient trauma. It seems prudent, if the possibility of incisor trauma exists, to provide some protection for the upper teeth. A number of materials have been used in the past to guard the upper teeth: a folded strip of lead (introduced by Magill and now obsolete), folded tape, cardboard or alcohol wipe, or a purpose-built mouth guard (as used in contact sports). The disadvantage of any of these is that they occupy a few millimeters of the available mouth opening, thus reducing the available aperture for laryngoscopy.

There are two methods to open the mouth and facilitate the introduction of the blade. First, extension of the head on the neck (by pressure from the right hand at the vertex) causes the lips to part and the mouth to open (see Fig. 16-4). Alternatively, the thumb of the right hand can press down on the right lower molar teeth, and the index finger of the right hand can simultaneously press up on the right upper molar teeth (scissors maneuver) (see Fig. 16-5).

The laryngoscope blade is then inserted into the right side of the mouth (see Fig. 16-3A). During the insertion of the laryngoscope, the patient's lower lip should be pulled away from the lower incisors (with the right hand or by an assistant) to prevent injury to the lower lip by entrapment of the lower lip between the laryngoscope blade and the lower incisor teeth. The blade is simultaneously advanced forward toward the base of the tongue and the tip directed centrally toward the midline so that the tongue is completely displaced to the left side of the mouth by the flange of the laryngoscope blade (see Fig. 16-3B). After the blade has been applied to the base of the tongue, the laryngoscope is lifted to expose the epiglottis (see Fig. 16-3C). During this process, the left wrist should remain straight, all lifting being done by the left shoulder and arm. If the operator follows a natural inclination to radial-flex the wrist further, thereby using the laryngoscope like a lever whose fulcrum is the upper incisor or gum, injury is likely to result. With the patient properly positioned, the direction of force necessary to lift the mandible and tongue and thereby expose the glottis is along an approximately 45-degree straight line above the long axis of the patient. It has been proposed that the best aid to inexperienced operators learning laryngoscopy would be a 10-pin bowler's wrist brace, which would immobilize the wrist.

Once the epiglottis is visualized, the next step depends on the type of laryngoscope blade being used. If the blade is curved (Macintosh), the tip should be placed in the vallecula (space between the base of the tongue and the pharyngeal surface of the epiglottis) (see Fig. 16-3D). Subsequent forward and upward movement of the blade tenses the hyoepiglottic ligament, causing the epiglottis to move upward like a trapdoor, first exposing the arytenoid cartilages and then allowing more and more of the glottic opening and vocal cords to come into view (see Fig. 16-3D).

The ability to identify the epiglottis and then lift anteriorly to reveal progressively more of the glottic aperture has led to a convenient system for grading the laryngoscopic view of any given patient.[6,24] A grade I laryngoscopic view consists of visualization of the vocal cords in their entirety. A grade II laryngoscopic view is visualization of the posterior portion of the laryngeal aperture (the arytenoid cartilages) but not any portion of the vocal cords. A grade III laryngoscopic view is visualization of just the epiglottis

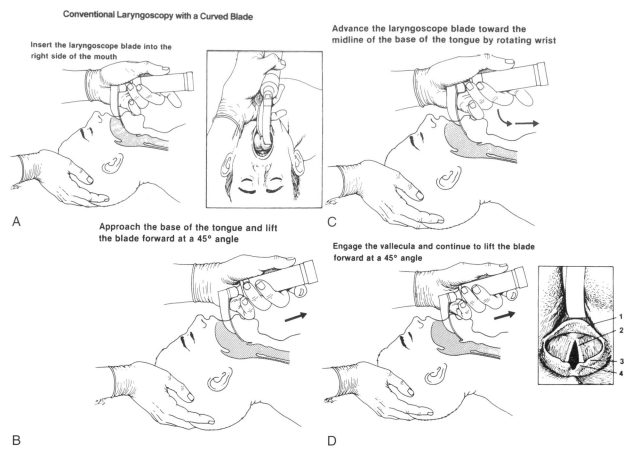

Conventional Laryngoscopy with a Curved Blade

Insert the laryngoscope blade into the right side of the mouth

A

Approach the base of the tongue and lift the blade forward at a 45° angle

B

Advance the laryngoscope blade toward the midline of the base of the tongue by rotating wrist

C

Engage the vallecula and continue to lift the blade forward at a 45° angle

D

Figure 16-3 The four-part schematic diagram shows how to perform laryngoscopy with a Macintosh blade (curved blade). **A** and **D**, Both lateral and frontal views are shown. **B** and **C**, Lateral views. **A**, The laryngoscope blade is inserted into the right side of the mouth so that the tongue is to the left of the flange. **B**, The blade is advanced around the base of the tongue, in part by rotating the wrist so that the handle of the blade becomes more vertical (*arrows,* C). **C**, The handle of the laryngoscope is lifted at a 45-degree angle (*arrow*) as the tip of the blade is placed in the vallecula **(D)** with continued lifting of the laryngoscope handle at a 45-degree angle, resulting in exposure of the laryngeal aperture. 1, Epiglottis; 2, vocal cords; 3, cuneiform part of arytenoid cartilage; and 4, corniculate part of arytenoid cartilage. (From Benumof JL [ed]: Airway Management: Principles and Practice. St. Louis, Mosby, 1996, p 267.)

but not the posterior portion of the laryngeal aperture, and a grade IV laryngoscopic view is visualization of just the soft palate but not the epiglottis. This grading system is necessarily subjective and skill dependent, but it does correlate somewhat with difficult intubation.

If the blade is straight (Jackson, Wisconsin, or Miller), however, the tip should extend just behind (posterior to) or beneath the laryngeal surface of the epiglottis (see Fig. 16-6). As with a curved laryngoscope blade, subsequent forward and upward movement of the straight blade (exerted along the axis of the handle, not by pulling back on the handle) exposes the glottic opening (see Fig. 16-6).

The use of a curved blade is thought to be less stimulating to the patient and possibly less traumatic to the epiglottis for two reasons. First, the tip of a curved blade does not normally touch the epiglottis. Second, the pharyngeal surface of the epiglottis is innervated by the glossopharyngeal nerve, whereas the superior laryngeal nerve supplies the laryngeal surface of the epiglottis.

Stimulation of the laryngeal surface of the epiglottis is thought to predispose to laryngospasm and bronchospasm more than stimulation of the pharyngeal surface of the epiglottis. Curved blades are also thought to be less traumatic to the teeth and to provide more room for passage of the tracheal tube through the oropharynx. On the other hand, straight blades provide a better view of the glottis in a patient with a long, floppy epiglottis or an anterior larynx. Therefore, straight blades are preferred in infants, pediatric patients, and patients with an anterior larynx. Use of a longer blade (curved or straight) is more appropriate in very large patients and patients with a very long thyromental distance.

Four major common problems are encountered in performing laryngoscopy. First, with either laryngoscope blade, inserting the blade too deeply into the pharynx may elevate the entire larynx so that the opening of the esophagus is visualized rather than the glottic aperture (see Fig. 16-7). Insertion of a curved blade too far into

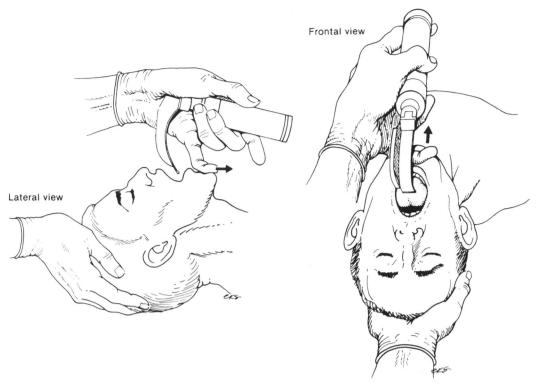

Figure 16-4 The mouth can be opened wide by concomitantly extending the head on the neck with the right hand while the small finger and medial border of the left hand push the anterior aspect of the mandible in a caudad direction (extraoral technique). As the blade approaches the mouth, it should be directed toward the right side of the mouth. Gloves should be worn during laryngoscopy because the hands may come in contact with patient's secretions. (From Benumof JL [ed]: Airway Management: Principles and Practice. St. Louis, Mosby, 1996, p 265.)

the vallecula, as well as continued rotation of the handle to the vertical, may push the epiglottis down over the glottic opening, resulting in limited exposure of the larynx (see Fig. 16-8).

The tracheal and esophageal openings are usually easily distinguished: the esophagus is located just to the right of the midline and more posterior, and the esophageal opening is round and puckered, with no structures around it. The glottis is located in the midline, has a triangular shape, and contains the prominent knobs of the arytenoids posteriorly and the pale white true vocal cords bilaterally.

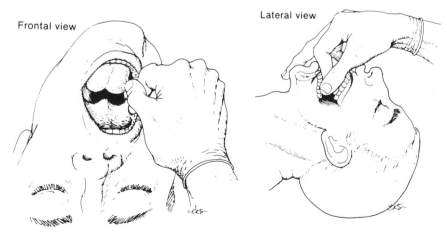

Figure 16-5 The mouth can be opened wide by pressing the thumb of the right hand on the right lower posterior molar teeth in a caudad direction while the index finger of the right hand simultaneously presses on the right upper posterior molar teeth in a cephalad direction (intraoral technique). Gloves should be worn during laryngoscopy because the hands may come into contact with patient's secretions. (From Benumof JL [ed]: Airway Management: Principles and Practice. St. Louis, Mosby, 1996, p 266.)

Conventional Laryngoscopy with a Straight Blade

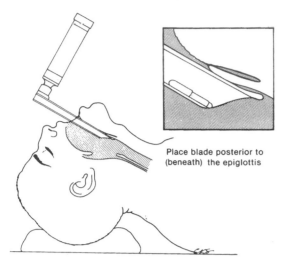

Place blade posterior to (beneath) the epiglottis

Figure 16-6 Conventional laryngoscopy with a straight blade. A straight laryngoscope blade (Miller) should be passed underneath the laryngeal surface of the epiglottis; then the handle of the laryngoscope should be elevated at a 45-degree angle, similar to the lifting that takes place in the use of a curved laryngoscope blade. (From Benumof JL [ed]: Airway Management: Principles and Practice. St. Louis, Mosby, 1996, p 268.)

Second, it is important to keep the tongue completely to the left side of the mouth with the flange of the laryngoscope blade. Many unsuccessful or difficult intubations result from the tongue protruding over the flange of the blade toward the right side of the mouth, thus obstructing a clear path through which the vocal cords

Insertion of the Laryngoscope Blade Too Deeply into the Pharynx Elevates the Larynx and Exposes the Esphagus

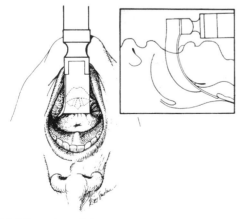

Figure 16-7 Insertion of the laryngoscope blade too deeply into the pharynx may result in elevation of the entire larynx so that the opening of the esophagus rather than the glottic aperture is visualized. The esophagus is located just to the right of the midline and posteriorly, and the esophageal opening is round and puckered with no structure around it. (From Benumof JL [ed]: Airway Management: Principles and Practice. St. Louis, Mosby, 1996, p 268.)

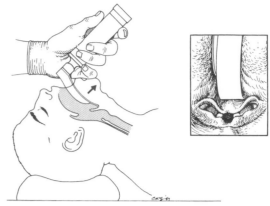

Figure 16-8 Insertion of the laryngoscope blade too deeply into the vallecula may push the epiglottis down over the laryngeal aperture, diminishing exposure of the vocal cords. (From Benumof JL [ed]: Airway Management: Principles and Practice. St. Louis, Mosby, 1996, p 267.)

must be visualized and the ET passed (see Fig. 16-9B). Vision is obscured further when the ET occupies part of the view. Thus, with a partially obstructed or "tunnel" view the endoscopist can partially visualize, but not instrument, the larynx. Therefore, all of the tongue must be to the left of the blade (Fig. 16-9A).

A third common error in performing laryngoscopy is, in an effort to keep the tongue to the left, displacement of the blade tip to the right of the midline. This position obscures the view of the epiglottis and may precipitate trauma and bleeding from friable tissue in the tonsillar bed. Especially with the use of the straight blade, the shaft of the blade can be to the right of midline (over the right molars), but the tip must reside exactly in the midline of the hypopharynx. An assistant may be useful to retract the right cheek and enlarge the space to the right of the blade, thus facilitating visualization of the larynx and introduction of the ET.

Fourth, in barrel-chested, obese, or large-breasted patients, it may be difficult initially to insert the blade of a laryngoscope correctly into the mouth and avoid obstruction to movement of the handle of the laryngoscope by the chest wall. In these patients, further initial neck extension or a 45-degree rotation of the laryngoscope handle to the right permits easier introduction of the blade of the laryngoscope into the mouth. Alternatively, a short laryngoscope handle (designed for this situation) may be used instead of the full-length handle.

The use of optimal external laryngeal pressure can significantly improve the laryngoscopic view. For example, routine use of external laryngeal pressure may reduce the incidence of a grade III view from 9% to a range from 5.4% to 1.3%.[14] Optimal external laryngeal pressure is usually backward, upward, and to the right (BURP) on the thyroid cartilage, but the best way to determine optimal external laryngeal manipulation (OELM) is for the operator to determine this with his or her own free right hand

**The Tongue should be to the Left of
the Laryngoscope Blade**

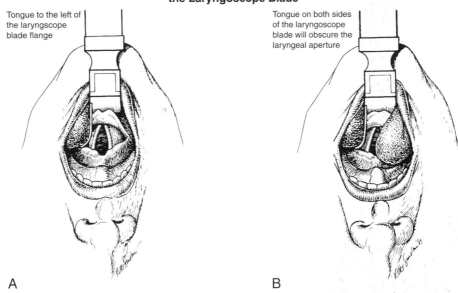

A

B

Figure 16-9 The tongue should be to the left of the laryngoscope blade. **A,** The flange on the laryngoscope blade should keep the tongue completely to the left side of the mouth. If this is accomplished, the tongue does not obstruct the view of the vocal cords. The tracheal rings on the anterior aspect of the trachea are evident. **B,** If the tongue slips over the laryngoscope blade and occupies part of the right side of the mouth, the view of the vocal cords is obscured by the part of the tongue that is on the right side of the mouth. (From Benumof JL [ed]: Airway Management: Principles and Practice. St. Louis, Mosby, 1996, p 269.)

Determining optimal external layngeal manipulation with free (right) hand

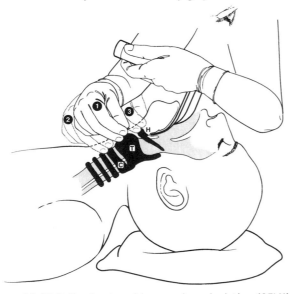

Figure 16-10 Optimal external laryngeal manipulation (OELM) to improve the laryngoscopic view is determined by the laryngoscopist by quickly pressing in both the cephalad and posterior direction with the right hand over (1) the thyroid (T) (most common), (2) cricoid (C), and (3) hyoid cartilages (H). If the laryngoscopic view is critically improved by this maneuver, the laryngoscopist can use an assistant's hands or fingers as an extension of his or her own right hand to reproduce the OELM. (From Benumof JL [ed]: Airway Management: Principles and Practice. St. Louis, Mosby, 1996, p 268.)

(see Fig. 16-10) after it is free from the duties of head extension and mouth opening.

D. TRACHEAL INTUBATION

The actual insertion of the ET is frequently easy once the vocal cords are exposed (and the tongue out of the way) (see Fig. 16-9A). However, it is not uncommon that the vocal cords can be visualized but endotracheal placement of the tube is problematic. Adult tracheas readily accept tracheal tubes with internal diameters of 7 to 9 (or even 10) mm (see Chapter 33 for pediatric sizes). If it is thought that fiberoptic bronchoscopy will be necessary subsequently for either diagnosis or therapy, at least an 8-mm size should be used. If it is thought that the space between the upper and lower teeth will be small and the cuff of the tube may come in contact with the teeth, the distal tube and cuff should be lubricated to facilitate the cuff sliding by the teeth. Also, in the case of limited mouth opening, all air should be evacuated from the cuff in order to allow as low a cuff profile as possible. The tip of the ET should be introduced into the far right corner of the mouth and passed along an axis that intersects the line of the laryngoscope blade at the glottis. In this manner, the tube does not interrupt the view of the vocal cords down the channel of the blade. The common error of trying to use the laryngoscope blade as a midline guide, through which the tube is passed, violates this principle, obscures vision, and is a significant source of difficulty for the inexperienced operator. The tube tip is passed through the cords, stopping 2 cm after the tube cuff completely passes the vocal cords; alternatively, when the external tube markings of 22 to 24 cm are at the lower incisors, the tip of the tube is at the midtrachea.[11] It is of paramount importance that the operator not take his or her eyes off the laryngeal aperture until the cuff disappears just beyond the vocal cords. The most common cause of inadvertent esophageal intubation is failure to see clearly the tube pass through the cords (and inspect it in situ after placement). The arytenoid cartilages frequently displace the tube tip posteriorly into the esophagus unless care is taken to pass the tip anteriorly and squarely into the tracheal lumen.

The use of a stylet may be valuable in controlling the direction of passage of an ET. By providing increased rigidity and malleability, it allows more control of the tube. However, the ET cannot be readily reshaped after it is introduced past the teeth. The insertion of an ET through the mouth allows only two degrees of free movement: depth of insertion and rotation of the tip. It is important to understand that the direction of the tube tip can be changed only by rotation; thus, the ET should be inserted as far to the right lateral aspect of the mouth as possible to facilitate the motion of the tip through torque applied to the connector end of the ET. In general, when speed of intubation is important (as in a patient with a full stomach), an ET should always be equipped with a stylet. A stylet should be easily malleable and well lubricated (although plastic-coated stylets may be adequately slippery) and not extend beyond the tip of the tube. Occasionally, a curved, styleted ET impinges on the anterior tracheal wall as it is being inserted and after passage through the vocal cords. Under these circumstances, after the ET tip is through the vocal cords, the stylet should be withdrawn, which returns the tip of the ET to its inherent flexibility and permits further passage distally.

After placement of the ET, the laryngoscope is removed from the mouth and the cuff of the tube is inflated to a cuff pressure of 22 to 32 cm H_2O. If a cuff pressure gauge is unavailable, the tube is inflated until moderate tension is felt in the pilot balloon to the cuff. The tube should then be connected to a source of positive-pressure ventilation and held in place by one hand. The hand holding the ET in place should be securely resting against the cheek (as a temporary fixation) until the ET is finally secured to prevent any sudden movement from dislodging the ET.

E. VERIFICATION OF CORRECT PLACEMENT

The next, most important task is to determine definitively that the tube has been inserted into the trachea rather than the esophagus (Box 16-2). This issue is extensively discussed in Chapter 15, and only a brief summary of the signs of tracheal intubation is given here. Helpful, but not absolute, signs of tracheal intubation consist of breath sounds in the axillary chest wall, lack of breath sounds

---

Box 16-2   Signs of Tracheal Intubation
Less Reliable Signs
1. Breath sounds in axillary chest wall
2. No breath sounds over stomach
3. No gastric distention
4. Chest rise and fall
5. Large spontaneous exhaled tidal volumes
6. Hearing air exit from the endotracheal tube when the chest is compressed
7. Reservoir bag having the appropriate compliance
8. Maintenance of arterial saturation by pulse oximetry
More Reliable Signs
1. Carbon dioxide excretion waveform
2. Rapid expansion of a tracheal indicator bulb
Most Reliable Signs
1. Endotracheal tube visualized between vocal cords (laryngoscopy)
2. Fiberoptic visualization of cartilaginous rings of the trachea and tracheal carina

---

over the stomach, lack of gastric distention, chest rise with inspiration, large exhaled tidal volumes, the sound of air exiting from the ET when the chest is compressed, and appropriate compliance of a reservoir bag during hand ventilation. A progressive decrease in SpO_2 may indicate failure to intubate the trachea, but it is a very late sign of esophageal intubation (especially on 100% oxygen), and it may also indicate bronchospasm, endobronchial intubation, aspiration, kinking of the tube, machine or equipment malfunction, or merely the normal response delay inherent in pulse oximetry.

More reliable signs of tracheal intubation are the presence of a normal CO_2 waveform (capnogram) and rapid expansion of a large rubber tracheal indicator bulb (see Chapter 15). Cardiac arrest (when no CO_2 is excreted), severe bronchospasm, or kinking or plugging of the ET may prevent the appearance of CO_2 in the exhaled gas (a false-negative finding), and CO_2 may appear if the tip of the tube is proximal to but near the larynx (a false-positive finding). The self-inflating bulb has high sensitivity and specificity in normal patients, but it has a significant false-negative rate in obese patients.[15]

The only absolutely reliable methods of definitively determining tracheal intubation are direct observation of the ET going through the vocal cords and the use of a fiberoptic bronchoscope. Direct visualization of the tube lying in the glottic opening may be enhanced by displacing the tube posteriorly, which may pull the glottic opening posteriorly and into a better view. The fiberoptic bronchoscope allows visualization of the cartilaginous rings of the trachea and the tracheal carina but is not an accepted practice for routine determination of correct tube placement.

If there is no CO_2 waveform, breath sounds cannot be heard, or no chest movement occurs, one should remove the ET, ventilate the patient with a mask and bag system several times with 100% O_2, and attempt tracheal intubation again after inspecting the used tube for defects or plugs in the lumen. Changes in the shape or curvature of the ET and in the position of the head and neck, as well as the need for anterior tracheal pressure, should be considered and coordinated during the period of mask ventilation.

The next task is to ascertain that the tip of the ET is above the carina. This is done by observing equal expansion of both hemithoraces and by stethoscopic examination for breath sounds throughout both peripheral lung fields. However, hearing uniform breath sounds throughout all lung fields does not guarantee correct tube position. If there is any question about a possible main stem bronchus intubation, one should retract the tube about 1 cm at a time and reexamine the breath sounds (stopping prior to complete withdrawal above the vocal cords). In one study, an insertion depth of 21 cm in adult women and 23 cm in adult men resulted in no incidence of main stem bronchial intubation.[20] Simultaneous palpation of pulsed pressures in the cuff in the suprasternal notch and the pilot balloon of the cuff is another simple way of determining the location of the tube in the trachea. Fiberoptic bronchoscopy is another, but complex, way of determining the location of the tube in the trachea. Outside the operating room, it is always advisable to confirm ET position by chest radiography. Ideally, the tip of the tube should be 2 to 4 cm above the carina at the clavicular (midtracheal) level.

When the tracheal tube is placed and during taping of the ET, the marking of the ET at the level of the teeth should be noted for reference should the tube become displaced.

F. FIXATION OF THE TUBE

After the mark of the tube at the teeth level has been noted, the tube should be tightly secured in place. This is important not only to prevent accidental extubation but also to minimize tube movement within the airway. Taping the tube to the facial skin with adhesive tape is the most common method of securing the tube.

The skin of the maxilla should be considered the primary source of fixation for an orotracheal tube because it is less mobile and thus less apt to allow excessive motion of the tube within the airway. As well, the tube then lies along the palate and is less likely to be displaced by the tongue of a conscious patient. The fixation of the tube in place can be improved by having the lateral ends of the tape completely encircle the neck; however, the risk of restriction of venous return from the head (especially in intracranial pathology) requires careful consideration. Application of tincture of benzoin to the skin before the tape is applied helps provide a stronger bond between the tape and skin. In case of prolonged intubation, changing the tape and reapplying it to a new area on the face every 2 days helps prevent maceration of the skin.

In patients with beards or in whom the adhesive tape fails to stick to the skin, the tube can be tied into the place with a length of umbilical tape that is knotted around the tube and then encircles the neck. Adhesive tape may be used over the umbilical tape for added security. As well, a surgical face mask, reversed so that the ties are in front and the mask at the occiput, can serve as a reasonable, temporary means of fixation. Another reliable method of securing an orotracheal tube is to wire the tube to a tooth. One or two layers of adhesive tape are wrapped around the tube at the level of the upper incisor teeth. Stainless steel wire (25 to 28 gauge) is passed around an upper incisor tooth and twisted around the tape on the tube. In anesthetized patients a suture may be passed through the gum and then either around a ring of adhesive tape on the ET (as with wire) or through the wall of the ET and then tied to the tube. A bite block, rolled gauze, or an oral airway (used in the vast majority of tracheal intubations for general anesthesia) should be placed between the teeth to prevent the patient from biting down and occluding the lumen of an oral tube. Numerous commercial products are available to attempt to improve the stability, patient's comfort, and convenience of stabilizing and immobilizing an orotracheal tube.

III. CONVENTIONAL (LARYNGOSCOPIC) NASOTRACHEAL INTUBATION

Intubation by the nasal route is generally a more difficult procedure than oral intubation. On the other hand, nasal tubes are thought to be better tolerated than oral tubes. Therefore, nasal tubes have been considered the tube of choice for medium-term mechanical ventilation. The issue of nasotracheal tubes contributing to the development of sinusitis and pneumonia has been investigated, and existing evidence has not demonstrated an association.[9] Nonetheless, the use of nasotracheal intubation for longer term ventilation has been declining in favor of orotracheal intubation or early tracheostomy. The use of nasotracheal tubes is currently confined to surgical procedures requiring free access to the oropharynx (e.g., dental procedures, mandibular fixation) and to some pediatric procedures in which stability and security of the tube are of overwhelming concern (usually because of its proximity to the surgical field).

The tracheal tube is inserted into a nostril (preferably the right) and then passed through the nasal cavity and nasopharynx to the oropharynx. Once the tube has been passed into the oropharynx, it can be guided into the glottis under conventional direct laryngoscopic vision, or it can be grasped by a Magill forceps and thus directed into the glottis. Nasal intubation is accompanied by a transient bacteremia, and endocarditis prophylaxis should be used in susceptible patients.

A. PREPARATION

Prior to insertion of the nasotracheal tube, the nasal mucosa should be sprayed with a vasoconstrictor drug. Vasoconstriction of blood vessels in the nasal mucosa minimizes bleeding related to the unavoidable trauma, and it increases the diameter of the nasal passages by constricting (shrinking) the nasal mucosa. In addition, softening the tip of the nasotracheal tube by soaking it in a warm saline solution may decrease the incidence of mucosal damage and bleeding. The naris selected should be the one that the patient thinks is the most patent (because of the significant incidence of septal deviation in patients). However, if both nares offer equal resistance, the right-sided naris should be chosen because the bevel of the nasotracheal tube, when introduced through the right naris, more easily passes the vocal cords (Fig. 16-11).

The question of potential trauma to the turbinates by the open bevel of the tube and the best orientation of the bevel in passing the turbinates has not been completely resolved. There is a risk that the tube tip, in passing the inferior turbinate, may strike and damage or avulse the turbinate. In the worst case, the turbinate may be dislodged and occlude the lumen of the tube, causing both epistaxis and complete tube obstruction. Therefore, care must be taken to pass the tube along the floor of the nose below the inferior turbinate and to avoid any excessive force in advancing the tube. Other measures might include preliminary vasoconstriction, lubrication of the tube, gentle rotation as the tube is advanced, and evacuation of all air from the cuff to minimize its effective diameter. Efforts to rationalize the direction of the bevel as it passes the turbinate have not been demonstrated to change the incidence of this complication.

In the vast majority of adults, tubes with an internal diameter of 7.0 to 7.5 mm pass easily through the nares. The other prelaryngoscopy maneuvers described under direct-vision orotracheal intubation (positioning of the head, suctioning, and preoxygenation) should be performed for direct-vision nasal intubation. The nasotracheal tube should be lubricated and passed through the nose in one smooth posterior, caudad, medially directed movement until resistance to forward movement significantly decreases as the tube enters the oropharynx (usually at a distance of 15 to 16 cm). Significant resistance should be overcome not by force but by withdrawal, rotation, and reinsertion of the tube. Difficult passage should prompt the selection of the opposite nostril or of a smaller tube.

The pathway that the nasotracheal tube takes should be visualized as lying on its side. The curve of the tracheal tube should be aligned to facilitate passage along this curved course. As the tube passes through the nose into the nasopharynx, it must turn downward to pass through the pharynx. In making this turn, it may strike against

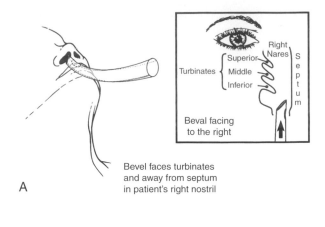

Bevel faces turbinates and away from septum in patient's right nostril

A

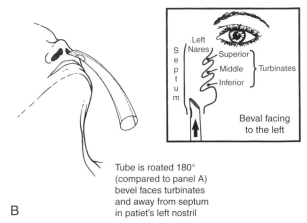

Tube is roated 180° (compared to panel A) bevel faces turbinates and away from septum in patiet's left nostril

B

Figure 16-11 Insertion of a nasotracheal tube into the nares. **A,** When the nasotracheal tube is passed into the right naris, the bevel should be facing to the right toward the turbinates (see inset). In this way, the tip of the tube is against the septum and the risks of catching the tip of the tube on a turbinate and tearing or dislocating it are minimized. In this orientation the concavity of the tube is pointing anteriorly. **B,** When the nasotracheal tube is passed into the left naris, the bevel should be facing to the left toward the turbinates (see inset). In this way, the tip of the tube is against the septum and the risks of catching the tip of the tube on a turbinate and tearing or dislocating it are minimized. In this orientation the concavity of the tube is pointing posteriorly. (From Benumof JL [ed]: Airway Management: Principles and Practice. St. Louis, Mosby, 1996, p 273.)

the posterior nasopharyngeal wall and resist any attempt to push it further. The tube should be pulled back a short distance, and the patient's head should be extended further to facilitate attempts to pass this point smoothly and atraumatically. If this is not performed and the tube is forced, the mucosal covering of the posterior nasopharyngeal wall may be torn open and the tube may be passed into the submucous tissues. This false passage is accompanied by a "boggy" feeling and the complete obstruction of the tube lumen.

B. LARYNGOSCOPY

The laryngoscopy for nasal intubation is identical to that described for oral intubation.

C. TRACHEAL INTUBATION

Once the tube is in the oropharynx, the tip of the tube must be aligned with the glottic opening. This requires that the tip of the tube be visible in the hypopharynx. The tube should be advanced or withdrawn until this is the case. It is possible that a combination of tube rotation and repositioning of the head will allow clear passage of the tube tip into the trachea; however, it is likely that the tube will require guidance from Magill forceps held in the operator's right hand.

The advantage of the design of these forceps is that when the grasping ends are parallel to the long axis of the tracheal tube, the handle is outside the right side of the mouth and at a right angle to the long axis of the tube. Because the handle is outside the right side of the mouth, it is away from the line of sight. As the forceps are grasped parallel to the long axis of the tube, a backhand motion of the right hand passes the tube toward the glottic opening (Fig. 16-12). Thus, the operator can

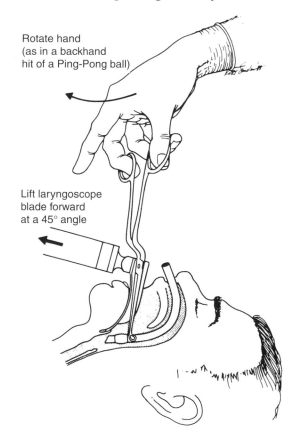

Guiding a Nasotracheal Tube into the Larynx Using a Magil Forceps

Rotate hand (as in a backhand hit of a Ping-Pong ball)

Lift laryngoscope blade forward at a 45° angle

Figure 16-12 A nasotracheal tube can be guided under direct vision (laryngoscopic control) through the laryngeal aperture with a Magill forceps by simply rotating the hand as one would do when using a backhand motion in hitting a Ping-Pong ball. The Magill forceps should grab the nasotracheal tube proximal to the cuff of the endotracheal tube. (From Benumof JL [ed]: Airway Management: Principles and Practice. St. Louis, Mosby, 1996, p 275.)

have the larynx exposed by the laryngoscope held in the left hand, the tube in full view, a means (the forceps) of manipulating the alignment of the tube, and a means of advancing the tube. However, it is often desirable to have an assistant advance the proximal end of the tube so that the operator is free simply to guide the tube into the larynx without having to pull it with the Magill forceps. The tip of the tube should be grasped to guide it into the trachea; grasping the cuff area is likely to lead to cuff trauma and possible damage. Also, the addition of a small amount of air into the ET cuff should center the ET within the glottis, and as the ET is advanced, the cuff deflates.

In some patients, as the tube enters the trachea, the tube's anterior curvature may direct it against the anterior tracheal wall and interfere with passage past this point. To resolve this difficulty, the head must be lifted (flexed) slowly as the tube is advanced. A nasotracheal tube should be advanced until the cuff is 2 cm below the vocal cords or until the external markings are 24 to 25 cm for women and 26 to 27 cm for men (3 cm more than for oral tubes) at the nares. The tube's correct placement must be verified as in any intubation (see orotracheal intubation), but this is particularly critical with nasal intubations because the relationship to external tube markings and the location of the tube tip is not as firmly established as it is for orotracheal tubes. If nasal bleeding occurs, it is probably wise to leave the ET in place to provide tamponade. If the bleeding is severe, the ET can be retracted and the cuff inflated to provide better tamponade.

D. FIXATION OF THE TUBE

The nasotracheal tube can be secured with adhesive tape as described for orotracheal tubes. In addition, a nasotracheal tube can be secured by a suture through the nasal septum and then tied, after being tightly wound around an adhesive band on the tube or passed through the wall of the tube by a needle and then tied.

IV. CONCLUSION

The art of laryngoscopic tracheal intubation is one of infinite variety and unpredictability. We face a diverse population of patients with a variety of disease processes. When their pathology includes airway abnormalities, gaining control of the airway can be a life-threatening as well as a lifesaving process. Ongoing study and practice in a variety of airway techniques are the only protection we have in the intrinsically hazardous field of airway management. Mastery of the art begins with a mastery of the fundamentals. Although practiced by a wide variety of health professionals, laryngoscopic intubation is an extraordinarily complex and continually evolving branch of anesthesiology and critical care.

REFERENCES

1. Adnet F, Baillard C, Borron SW, et al: Randomized study comparing the "sniffing position" with simple head extension for laryngoscopic view in elective surgery patients. Anesthesiology 95:836, 2001.
2. Adnet F, Borron SW, Dumas JL, et al: Study of the "sniffing position" by magnetic resonance imaging. Anesthesiology 94:83, 2001.
3. Adnet F, Borron SW, Lapostolle F, et al: The three axis alignment theory and the "sniffing position": Perpetuation of an anatomic myth? Anesthesiology 91:1964, 1999.
4. Bannister FB, MacBeth RG: Direct laryngoscopy and tracheal intubation. Lancet 2:651, 1944.
5. Baraka AS, Taha SK, Aouad MT, et al: Preoxygenation: Comparison of maximal breathing and tidal volume breathing techniques. Anesthesiology 91:612, 1999.
6. Cormack RS, Lehane J: Difficult tracheal intubation in obstetrics. Anaesthesia 39:1105, 1984.
7. Gambee AM, Hertzka RE, Fisher DM: Preoxygenation techniques: Comparison of three minutes and four breaths. Anesth Analg 66:468, 1987.
8. Gold MI, Durate I, Muravchick S: Arterial oxygenation in conscious patients after 5 minutes and after 30 seconds of oxygen breathing. Anesth Analg 60:313, 1981.
9. Holzapfel L, Chevret S, Madinier G, et al: Influence of long-term oro- or nasotracheal intubation on nosocomial maxillary sinusitis and pneumonia: Results of a prospective, randomized clinical trial. Crit Care Med 21:1132, 1993.
10. Hooke R: The technique of insertion of intratracheal insufflation tubes. Philos Trans R Soc 2:539, 1667.
11. Jackson C: An account of an experiment made by M. Hook of preserving animals alive by blowing through their lungs with bellows. Surg Gynaecol Obstet 17:507, 1913.
12. Jackson C: Bronchoscopy, Oesophagoscopy, and Gastroscopy, 3rd ed. Philadelphia, WB Saunders, 1934, p 85.
13. Jense HG, Dubin SA, Silverstein PI, et al: Effect of obesity on safe duration of apnea in anesthetized humans. Anesth Analg 72:89, 1991.
14. Knill RL: Difficult laryngoscopy made easy with a "BURP." Can J Anaesth 40:279, 1993.
15. Lang DJ, Wafai Y, Salem R, et al: Efficacy of the self-inflating bulb in confirming tracheal intubation in the morbidly obese. Anesthesiology 85:246, 1996.
16. Macintosh RR: An aid to oral intubation. Br Med J 1:28, 1949.
17. Matas, R: On the management of acute traumatic pneumothorax. Ann. Surg 29:409, 1899.
18. Miller RA: A new laryngoscope. Anesthesiology 2:317, 1941.
19. Nimmagada U, Salem MR, Joseph NJ, et al: Efficacy of preoxygenation with tidal volume breathing: Comparison of breathing systems. Anesthesiology 93:693, 2000.
20. Owen RL, Cheney FW: Endobronchial intubation: A preventable complication. Anesthesiology 67:255, 1987.
21. Snow J: On Chloroform and Other Anaesthetics. London, John Churchill, New Burlington Street, 1858, p 117.
22. Teller LE, Alexander CM, Frumin MJ, et al: Pharyngeal insufflation of oxygen prevents arterial desaturation during apnea. Anesthesiology 69:980, 1988.
23. Trendelenburg F: Beiträge zur den Operationen an den Luftwegen. 2. Tamponnade der Trachea. Arch Klin Chir 12:121, 1871.
24. Wilson ME, Spiegelhalter D, Robertson JA, et al: Predicting difficult intubation. Br J Anaesth 61:211, 1988.

17

BLIND DIGITAL INTUBATION

Chris C. Christodoulou

Michael F. Murphy

Orlando R. Hung

I. HISTORY

Although probably first described by Herholdt and Rafn[8] in 1796 for the management of drowning victims, blind digital orotracheal intubation had received scant attention in the medical literature until the mid-1980s, when revived by Stewart[14,15] in emergency medicine and prehospital care. Notable publications on the topic over the years have portrayed the technique as an acceptable, if not preferable, alternative to standard laryngoscopic endotracheal intubation, particularly when the standard technique is contraindicated, has failed, or is not possible because of a lack of equipment.

In 1880, MacEwen[12] described the technique utilizing a curved metal tube in awake patients, and Sykes[16] recommended the routine use of the digital technique in anesthetic practice in the 1930s. Siddall[13] and Lanham[11] relegated the technique to last-ditch efforts following the failure of conventional intubation methods.[14] The technique has been described in neonatal resuscitation[17,18] and as an adjunct in blind nasotracheal intubation.[10]

Currently, there is widespread variation in awareness, expertise, and application of the technique in anesthesia, emergency medicine,[6,7] and prehospital care. Although advances in airway management equipment and expertise have made obsolete the routine use of blind digital orotracheal intubation, it remains a valuable skill in some patients, especially in the emergency setting[14] or under circumstances in which the intubator cannot be positioned at the head of the patient, rendering laryngoscopic intubation impossible.

II. INDICATIONS

The use of the digital technique is neither aesthetically pleasing, easily accomplished, nor entirely safe. As one might imagine, placing one's fingers far enough down a patient's throat to elevate the epiglottis and guide an endotracheal tube into the trachea has implications related to selection of patients and the manual dexterity and anatomic features of the intubator.

The technique has found some popularity in the prehospital care environment where difficult position of the patient, poor lighting conditions, disrupted anatomy, potential cervical spine instability, and unknown status regarding infectious disease are the norm. Digital intubation is ordinarily used when other maneuvers have failed or are likely to fail or when alternative equipment is unavailable or inoperative.

Successful digital intubation demands that the patient be unconscious to tolerate the intense oropharyngeal stimulus and prevent bite injuries to the intubator. Neuromuscular blockade facilitates the technique, although it is relatively contraindicated in patients with anatomically difficult or disrupted airways. Digital intubation may be indicated as follows:

1. When equipment required to undertake alternative techniques is unavailable or inoperative.
2. When positioning of the patient or the intubator prevents conventional intubation.
3. When other methods have failed or are likely to fail and the skill and experience of the intubator make the digital technique the one of choice.
4. In the presence of potential or actual cervical spine instability, when the intubator selects the digital technique on the basis of the risk-benefit analysis. Although there is no evidence to suggest that the technique of digital intubation will alter the neurologic outcome of a patient, we believe that there is less cervical spine motion during intubation with the digital technique as compared with the conventional laryngoscopic orotracheal intubation without in-line stabilization.
5. When adequate visualization of the airway to allow conventional intubation is not possible because of the absence of adequate suction to clear secretions, blood, or vomitus in the oropharynx or because of traumatic disruption of the upper airway anatomy.

III. TECHNIQUE OF DIGITAL INTUBATION

A. PREPARATION

As with any intubation technique, preparation involves assembling the necessary equipment and personnel, including emergency drugs and adequate suction, to optimize success and preserve ventilation and oxygenation. An appropriate size of endotracheal tube (ET) is selected. The use of a stiff but malleable stylet improves maneuverability during the intubation. Lubrication of the stylet with a water-soluble lubricant ensures easy retraction following the placement of the tip of the ET in the glottic opening. The stylet is inserted into the ET so that the distal end of the stylet is at the level of the Murphy eye. With the stylet in place, the distal half of the ET and the stylet (ET-ST) unit is bent to a configuration as seen in Figure 17-1. The proximal half of the ET is then bent approximately 90 degrees to the dominant side of the intubator to allow manipulation of the ET-ST by the dominant hand during intubation (Figs. 17-2 and 17-3). The degree of bend should be individualized and depends on the intubator's experience. The tip of the ET should be well lubricated with a water-soluble lubricant. In the uncommon event that the intubation is performed in an awake patient, especially an uncooperative patient, a bite block should be placed between the patient's molars on one side to minimize the risk of injury to the intubator's fingers.

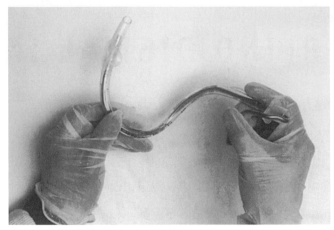

Figure 17-1 With the stylet in place, the distal half of the tube is bent in a U shape.

B. POSITIONING

The patient should be supine with the head in a slight sniffing position as for laryngoscopic intubation. The intubator stands (or kneels if the patient is on the ground) beside the patient so that the nondominant side of the intubator is closest to the patient. An assistant can help to facilitate the intubating procedure.

C. TECHNIQUE

It is our experience that pulling the tongue forward by an assistant facilitates palpation of the epiglottis, thus improving the success rate for digital intubation. The patient's mouth is opened and the tongue grasped gently by the assistant with a gauze sponge (Fig. 17-4). Traction on the tongue moves the epiglottis slightly cephalad, enhancing its palpability and facilitating the placement of the tip of the ET into the glottic opening. One then inserts the index and middle fingers of the nondominant

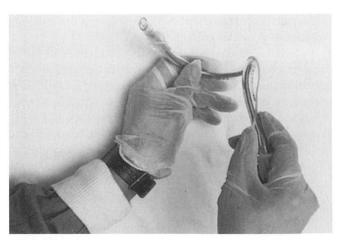

Figure 17-2 The proximal half of the endotracheal tube is bent 90 degrees toward the dominant side of the intubator.

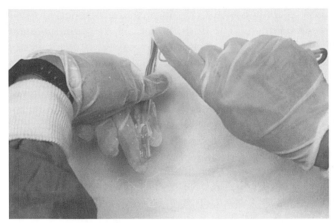

Figure 17-3 Final configuration allows improved control of the endotracheal tube with both hands. During the intubation, the index finger of the dominant hand can help advance the endotracheal tube while the index and middle fingers of the nondominant hand guide the tip of the tube into the glottis.

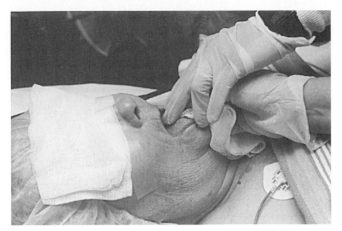

Figure 17-5 The index and middle fingers of the nondominant hand are inserted into the mouth palm down.

hand into the oral cavity and slides the palm down along the surface of the tongue (Fig. 17-5). The tip of the middle finger touches the tip of the epiglottis, which is then directed anteriorly (Fig. 17-6). The ease of palpating and lifting the epiglottis depends on the length of the intubator's fingers, the height of the patient, the anatomy of the oropharynx, and the presence or absence of teeth.

Once the epiglottis is identified and directed anteriorly, the ET-ST is inserted through the corner of the mouth (Fig. 17-7). The ET-ST glides along the groove between the middle and index fingers on the palmar surface of the nondominant hand. While firm anterior pressure is maintained against the epiglottis with the middle finger, the ET-ST is advanced slowly into the glottic opening by the dominant hand (Fig. 17-8). The index finger may be used to guide the tip of the ET-ST into the glottic opening. Stabilize the ET while withdrawing the stylet (Fig. 17-9), and advance the ET slowly

into the trachea. During the intubation, the ET-ST should never be advanced forcefully against resistance. Accurate placement is confirmed by conventional techniques, such as auscultation and carbon dioxide detection. Occasionally, the tip of the epiglottis cannot be palpated. An upward (cephalad) and backward (posterior) pressure applied anteriorly to the larynx by an assistant may be helpful. As an alternative, the index and middle fingers of the nondominant hand may be used to keep the ET-ST in the midline, while observing tissue movement in the anterior neck during gentle rocking of the ET-ST back and forth in an attempt to locate the glottic opening.

An alternative technique described by Cook begins with placement of the index and middle finger tips of the nondominant hand in the hypopharynx, posterior to the larynx.[2] The ET held in the dominant hand is then passed into the pharynx. The volar surfaces of the fingers serve as a "basketball backstop" to guide the ET held in the dominant hand through the glottic opening. If required,

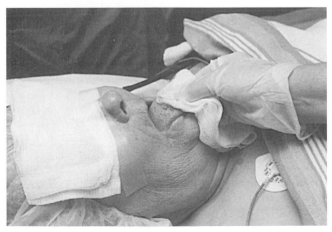

Figure 17-4 An assistant retracts the tongue using a piece of gauze.

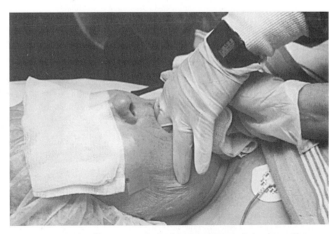

Figure 17-6 The fingers are advanced to the point where the middle finger is able to palpate the tip of the epiglottis and push it anteriorly.

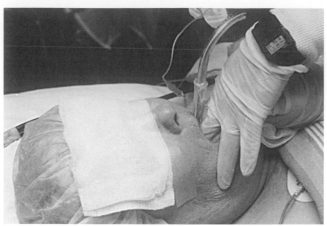

Figure 17-7 The endotracheal tube and stylet unit (ET-ST) is advanced along the groove between the index and middle fingers, over the top of the tongue.

the index finger of the nondominant hand may be flexed to help guide the tube through the glottis.

D. NEONATAL DIGITAL INTUBATION

Blind digital intubation in neonates has not gained widespread acceptance as a primary technique of intubation. It has been used in several third-world countries where experience with and access to standard laryngoscopes are limited.[17] Hancock and Peterson have employed the blind digital intubation technique in neonatal resuscitation and accidental extubation situations.[5] The intubator uses the gloved index finger of the nondominant hand to identify the epiglottis and glottic opening. The index finger is then used to guide the ET through the glottic opening. The thumb of the nondominant hand can be used to apply external cricoid pressure. A styletted ET is recommended. The fifth finger of the nondominant hand can be used in very small neonates. Advantages of the blind digital technique in neonates include reduced lip and gum trauma, controlled palpation of anatomic landmarks, and easy access to the airway in various transport scenarios, without the need to adjust lines and monitoring equipment leads in unstable patients. The technique can also be used to confirm accidental extubation of the trachea. Caution should be exercised when airway pathology is suspected. Blind digital intubation of neonates and infants can be considered in situations in which other direct visualization techniques have failed.

E. COMBINED TECHNIQUES

The technique of blind digital intubation has been combined with the BAAM Whistle (Beck Airway Airflow Monitor, Great Plains Ballistics, Lubbock, TX) and Endotrol (Mallinckrodt Medical, Argyle, NY) tube to facilitate endotracheal intubation in several situations where direct laryngoscopy has failed.[3,4] The BAAM device was initially developed to facilitate the teaching of nasotracheal intubation techniques under spontaneous ventilation. The BAAM produces a whistling sound of slightly different pitches during inspiration and expiration if the ET is positioned within the air column leaving or entering the trachea. The device has also been shown to be effective in guiding nasotracheal tube placement in situations in which external cardiac massage is being applied.[4]

The Endotrol tube's unique design allows the intubator to adjust the distal tip anteriorly by pulling on a plastic wire that runs along the concave curvature of the ET. This motion allows better alignment of the distal tip of the tube with the glottic opening.

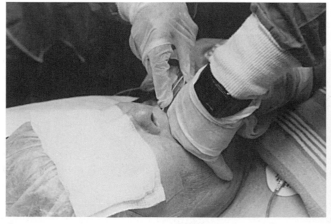

A

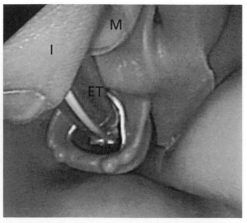

B

Figure 17-8 A, The endotracheal tube and stylet unit (ET-ST) is guided into the glottis, directed by the index fingertip if necessary. **B,** View of the larynx (of a mannequin) demonstrating the guidance of the endotracheal tube into the glottic opening by the tip of the index finger of the nondominant hand. ET, endotracheal tube; I, index finger; M, middle finger. Note: gloves should be worn at all times when performing the technique on patients.

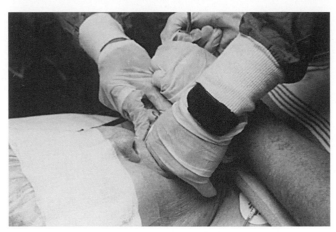

Figure 17-9 The endotracheal tube is stabilized while the stylet is removed.

In fiberscope-guided endotracheal intubation, it can be difficult to advance the ET into the trachea. Asai and colleagues reported the use of the digital technique to help guide a 39 Fr double-lumen tube off the fiberscope into the trachea of a patient undergoing an anterior thoracic laminectomy procedure.[1] The anatomy of the patient's airway and that of the intubator's hand are key determinants in deciding which technique should be utilized in a given situation.

Light-guided tracheal intubation using the Trachlight (Laerdal Medical, Wappingers Falls, NY) can be difficult in patients with a long and floppy epiglottis.[9] This difficulty can be overcome by using the combined light-guided digital intubating technique. During the intubation, the middle finger of the nondominant hand can be used to lift the epiglottis off the posterior wall of the pharynx to allow the ET with the Trachlight to go underneath the epiglottis into the glottic opening. The light glow from the anterior neck can be used to confirm the correct placement of the ET tip into the glottis. During the past several years, we have performed more than 20 intubations using this combined light-guided digital intubating technique.

IV. CASE HISTORY

Blind digital intubation is a relatively simple technique that can be learned easily. The following case history serves to illustrate the role of digital intubation in the emergency airway management of a patient who could not be intubated by the conventional method.

A call was received by the 911 center of a large, urban emergency medical services (EMS) system reporting a "man not breathing" at a downtown hotel. A mobile intensive care unit from the nearest ambulance station was dispatched within 40 seconds of the call having been received.

On arrival 3 minutes later, the EMS team was directed to the top floor of the hotel, where a wedding reception was in progress. On the floor of a small washroom, the 120-kg patient was found in cardiac arrest, pulseless, and not breathing. According to the history given by relatives, the patient had chest pain while dancing after a large meal. He went into the washroom and collapsed.

Cardiopulmonary resuscitation (CPR) with bag-mask ventilation was begun immediately. Vomiting ensued, obscuring the view of the paramedic who was attempting orotracheal intubation using a laryngoscope. Suctioning was attempted using a portable suction unit, but so much vomitus was present that the collecting bottle of the suction unit filled rapidly and further suctioning was not successful in clearing the upper airway. "Quick-look" paddles revealed asystole.

While chest compressions and bag-mask ventilation continued, attempts at intravenous access were successful. Second and third attempts at direct-vision tracheal intubation resulted in esophageal placement, readily recognized by the paramedic team.

It became clear that attempts at direct visualization of the airway would not be successful because of the large amount of vomitus in the oropharynx. Because of this, the decision was made to place the ET using the tactile (digital) method. Using a 7.5-mm ET, a physician carried out a digital intubation through the vomitus and secretions and was successful on the first attempt. Ventilation and suctioning were begun through the in-place ET, and the patient's color improved. CPR continued during transport to a local hospital.

V. LIMITATIONS

The more alert the patient is, the less likely that digital intubation will be tolerated or successful. The very setting, by itself, of a patient who is already the victim of multiple failed intubation attempts places limitations on the likelihood of success of the digital technique. Patients with limited mouth opening, carious or prominent dentition, small mouths, and large tongues as well as very tall patients can be predictably difficult to intubate, no matter what method is employed, including the digital method. With practice, however, digital intubation has been shown to be an effective, alternative method of intubation.[4]

The risk of injury to the intubator by the patient's teeth and body fluids is real. This risk can be minimized by selecting unconscious or paralyzed patients or by placing a bite block between the patient's molars. In our experience, double gloving provides a measure of protection against barrier interruption, injury from teeth, and the potential for disease transmission.

As with other techniques of intubation, complications such as trauma to the upper airway can occur during the digital intubation. However, trauma can be minimized by advancing the ET gently during the intubation. Other potential complications of digital intubation, including esophageal intubation, can be avoided by a good technique, gentle manipulation, and by employing tracheal placement confirmation techniques such as carbon dioxide detection.

Digital intubation is a "blind" technique and therefore relatively contraindicated in patients with upper airway compromise resulting from such disorders as infectious diseases, neoplasms, foreign bodies, caustic and thermal burns, and anaphylaxis.

VI. CONCLUSION

Digital intubation is seldom the method of first choice in securing a definitive airway. However, it offers an alternative that, in the event of failure of conventional techniques, may prove lifesaving. Successful digital intubation depends largely on the intubator's preparation, experience, and skill.

REFERENCES

1. Asai T, Matsumoto S, Shingu K: Use of the McCoy laryngoscope or fingers to facilitate fiberscope-aided tracheal intubation. Anaesthesia 53:903, 1998.
2. Cook RT: Digital endotracheal intubation [letter]. Am J Emerg Med 10:396, 1992.
3. Cook RT Jr, Polson DL: Use of BAAM with a digital intubation technique in a trauma patient. Prehosp Disaster Med 8:357, 1993.
4. Cook RT Jr, Stene JK, Marcolina B Jr: Use of a Beck Airway Airflow Monitor and controllable-tip endotracheal tube in two cases of nonlaryngoscopic oral intubation. Am J Emerg Med 13:180, 1995.
5. Hancock PJ, Peterson G: Finger intubation of the trachea in newborns. Pediatrics 89:325, 1992.
6. Hardwick WC, Bluhm D: Digital intubation. J Emerg Med 1:317, 1984.
7. Hartmannsgruber MW, Gabrielli A, Layon AJ, et al: The traumatic airway: The anesthesiologist's role in the emergency room. Int Anesthesiol Clin 38:87, 2000.
8. Herholdt JD, Rafn CG: Life-Saving Measures for Drowning Persons. Copenhagen, H Tikiob, 1796.
9. Hung OR, Pytka S, Morris I, et al: Clinical trial of a new lightwand (Trachlight) to intubate the trachea. Anesthesiology 83:509, 1995.
10. Korber TE, Henneman PL: Digital nasotracheal intubation. J Emerg Med 7:275, 1989.
11. Lanham HG: Tactile orotracheal intubation [letter]. JAMA 236:2288, 1976.
12. MacEwen W: Clinical observations on the introduction of tracheal tubes by the mouth instead of performing tracheotomy or laryngotomy. Br Med J 1:163, 1880.
13. Siddall WJW: Tactile orotracheal intubation. Anaesthesia 21:221, 1966.
14. Stewart RD: Digital intubation. In Dailey RH, Simon B, Stewart RD, et al (eds): The Airway: Emergency Management. St Louis, Mosby, 1992, pp 111-114.
15. Stewart RD: Tactile orotracheal intubation. Ann Emerg Med 13:175, 1984.
16. Sykes WS: Oral endotracheal intubation without laryngoscopy: A plea for simplicity. Curr Res Anesth Analg 16:133, 1937.
17. Wijesundera CD: Digital intubation of the trachea. Ceylon Med J 35:81, 1990.
18. Woody NC, Woody HG: Direct digital intratracheal intubation for neonatal resuscitation. J Pediatr 73:903, 1968.

18

FIBEROPTIC ENDOSCOPY–AIDED TECHNIQUES

Melissa Wheeler
Andranik Ovassapian

I. HISTORICAL BACKGROUND

The first recorded fiberoptic nasotracheal intubation was performed in 1967 on a patient with Still's disease, using a flexible fiberoptic choledochoscope.[128] Five years later, a fiberoptic bronchoscope (FOB) was used for nasotracheal intubation in patients with severe rheumatoid arthritis in whom conventional endotracheal intubation techniques were not possible.[49,194] The first series of 100 fiberoptic endotracheal intubations was reported by Stiles and colleagues[189] in 1972. Intubations were performed both orally and nasally; four intubations failed because of copious secretions. Stiles and colleagues indicated that with experience, fiberoptic intubation could be performed in less than 1 minute.

In 1973 Davis[55] mentioned the use of the FOB to check endotracheal tube (ET) position in relation to the carina. Reports of fiberoptic evaluation of ET position and fiberoptic repositioning of ET intraoperatively soon followed.[126,198,208] Fiberoptic evaluation of ET position was demonstrated to be as good as chest radiographic evaluation in both adults and children.[57,132]

Raj and associates in 1974 were the first to report the use of the FOB to assist placement and positioning of a left-sided double-lumen endobronchial ET.[162] Other reports of the use of the FOB for positioning single-lumen and double-lumen endobronchial ETs followed.[6,178] Ovassapian and Schrader[145] described a new fiberoptic technique for positioning of right-sided double-lumen ETs in 1987. Benumof and coworkers[23] published their findings on evaluation of the left and right main stem bronchi in 1987, demonstrating the high safety margin of the left-sided double-lumen ET and further demonstrating why placement of a right-sided double-lumen ET is not possible in some patients.

During this time period, the FOB was also being used in critically ill patients, both pediatric and adult, to evaluate the upper and lower airway.[63,64,68,109,110,134,179,214] Early adopters of flexible fiberoptic bronchoscopy cited several advantages. Diagnostic and therapeutic procedures could be performed at the bedside without general anesthesia and without interruption of ongoing mechanical ventilation. It could be performed orally, nasally, or through an in situ ET or tracheostomy. The main disadvantage of its use through airway devices is the increased airway resistance encountered particularly in pediatric patients because the FOB may occupy a significant portion of the lumen.

The FOB was not originally developed for the management of the difficult intubation.[92] The value of the FOB, however, in this area was recognized by anesthesiologists from the beginning, and they played an important role in expanding its use in the management of the difficult airway (DA).[49,128,139,189,194] The FOB was used for patients with Ludwig's angina,[175] rheumatoid arthritis,[122,165] trauma,[127,170] unstable cervical spine,[181] cut throat (disruption) injuries,[53] acromegaly,[138] Pierre Robin syndrome,[104,173] and many other DA conditions.[3,61,100,123,130,143,148,202]

The significant role of the FOB in securing the airway in the conscious patient, especially when associated with an increased risk of aspiration, has been demonstrated by several investigators.[61,100,130,143,148,202] Ovassapian and colleagues[142] reported the first series of patients ($n = 129$) at increased risk for aspiration who had awake fiberoptic intubation. None had evidence of aspiration after successful completion of the technique.

The relative ease of exploring the upper and lower airway with or without the benefit of general anesthesia has expanded the role of the anesthesiologist as a diagnostician in the perioperative period.[146] Uses of the FOB include evaluation of preoperative or postextubation stridor; diagnosis of acute atelectasis or unintentional endobronchial intubation causing unexpected hypoxemia; ET blockage by secretions, kinking, or cuff herniation; and incidental discoveries of laryngeal polyps or other airway lesions.

The continuous improvement and refinement of technique, the development of new FOBs and related ancillary equipment, and recognition of the value of the FOB in airway management have led to the enormous popularity that the FOB enjoys today. Increased publication of papers related to fiberoptic airway management and books and monographs entirely devoted to fiberoptic use in anesthesia attest to the widespread interest of clinicians in this area.[140,146]

The teaching of fiberoptic airway endoscopy is part of most anesthesia resident training programs. One of the first graduate-level training programs was developed by Ovassapian and colleagues.[149] This program was later incorporated into a workshop format for training clinicians in practice.[59] Since then, a number of new ideas have been introduced for the step-by-step, progressive training of the art of fiberoptic intubation.[45,47,169,172,186]

II. FIBEROPTIC BRONCHOSCOPE

The first FOB was designed and produced on the basis of specifications provided by Ikeda[92] in 1966. Since then, FOBs in various sizes and lengths have been introduced for use in patients ranging in age and size from the preterm infant to the adult (Table 18-1).[149] Knowledge of the physical principles used in construction of an FOB is essential to understanding its function and its frailties. Frequent damage to the instrument not only is costly but also means that the FOB is unavailable and therefore underutilized.

A. ANATOMY AND PHYSICS

Fiberoptic laryngoscopes and bronchoscopes are manufactured by various companies using the same basic principles and design (Fig. 18-1). The handle contains the eyepiece for viewing or an integrated camera that connects to a video screen. The eyepiece contains a diopter adjustment ring to focus and adjust the eyepiece to fit each

Table 18-1 **Characteristics of Fiberoptic and Video Bronchoscopes**

Instrument	Insertion Cord Diameter (mm)	Insertion Cord Length (mm)	Working Channel (mm)	Tip Bending (degrees)	Field of View (degrees)
Olympus					
LF-2*	4.0	600	1.5	Up 120 Down 120	90
LF-P*†	2.2	600	None	Up 120 Down 120	75
LF-TP*§	5.2	600	2.6	Up 180 Down 130	75
LF-GP*§	4.1	600	1.5	Up 120 Down 120	90
LF-DP*§	3.1	600	1.2	Up 120 Down 120	90
BF-3C160‡	3.8	600	1.2	Up 180 Down 130	120
BF-P160‡	4.9	600	2.0	Up 180 Down 130	120
BF-160‡	5.3	600	2.0	Up 180 Down 130	120
Pentax					
FB-8V	2.8	600	1.2	Up 180 Down 130	100
FB-10V	3.4	600	1.2	Up 180 Down 130	120
FB-15V	4.9	600	2.2	Up 180 Down 130	120
EB-1570‡	5.1	600	2.0	Up 180 Down 130	120
Karl Storz					
11301-ABN1‡	2.8	500	1.2	Up 140 Down 140	90
11301-AB1	2.8	500	1.2	Up 140 Down 140	90
11302-BDN1‡	3.7	650	1.5	Up 140 Down 140	90
11302-BD1	3.7	650	1.5	Up 140 Down 140	90
1131-BNN1‡	5.2	650	2.3	Up 140 Down 140	90
1131-BN1	5.2	650	2.3	Up 140 Down 140	90

*Intubation fiberscopes.
†Smallest with directable tip.
‡Video bronchoscope.
§Integrated miniature light source.

viewer's vision. Karl Storz Company (Tuttlingen, Germany) has developed a different visualization system that integrates a Micro-Video-Module into the FOB. With this system, only focusing of the FOB (not both the camera and the FOB) is required. For all types of FOB, other components of the handle are the lever for controlling the bending section of the tip, the suction button, and the access port to the suction channel. The bending lever is located on the back of the handle and controls movement of the insertion cord tip in one plane of motion. Handles are designed to be held comfortably by either hand and to allow maneuvering of the bending lever by the thumb and activation of the suction by the index finger. This one-handed operation allows the operator's other hand to be free to advance, withdraw, or manipulate the insertion cord or ET.

The insertion cord is the portion of the FOB that is inserted into the patient and over which the ET is passed during fiberoptic intubation. The insertion cord contains the light and image transmission bundles, the suction channel, and the tip bending control wires. These components are held together with a stainless steel mesh and are wrapped with a water-impermeable plastic coating. The outside diameter of the insertion cord is what determines the size of the smallest ET that can be used. The insertion cord is flexible and tolerates gentle bending to accommodate the curves of the airway. Keep in mind, however, that the only portion of the insertion cord that is designed for maximum bending is the distal tip. Vigorous bending of other areas of the insertion cord results in breakage of fiberoptic fibers.

Light is transmitted within the insertion cord through one or two light transmission bundles to the tip of the FOB. The glass fibers of the light transmission bundles extend to the light guide bundle of the universal cord, which is connected to the external light source or to the light source integrated into the handle of portable FOBs. The viewing portion of the FOB incorporates part of the handle (the eyepiece or camera) and parts of the insertion cord (the image transmission bundle and objective lens). All FOBs are frontal view instruments; that is, the objective lens is perpendicular to the longitudinal axis of the instrument; the image viewed through the lens is in the same orientation as the actual object. The FOB also has fixed focus at the distal tip. Light reflected off the object is focused by the objective lens onto the distal end of the image transmission bundle. This image is then transmitted to the proximal end of the image transmission bundle near the eyepiece or camera. The glass fibers in the image transmission bundle are placed so that each fiber is in the same relative location on both ends of the bundle to represent the true nature of the object (coherent bundle).

The suction or working channel extends from the handle of the FOB to the tip of the insertion cord and can be used to suction secretions, spray local anesthetics, pass various biopsy and brush instruments, or insufflate oxygen. Movement of the bending lever located on the handle manipulates the distal section of the insertion cord.

Two wires originating from the bending lever and ending at the tip of the FOB provide the mechanism (Fig. 18-2). When the lever is moved downward, the wire that controls the anterior deflection of the tip is tightened and the tip of the FOB bends upward or anteriorly. When the lever is moved upward, the tip of the FOB bends downward or posteriorly. Substantial usage and improper handling, such as applying excessive pressure on the lever while the tip of FOB is inside the ET lumen, result in breakage of the delicate wire and loss of bending control.

The universal cord is the portion of the FOB that contains the light transmission fiber bundle and electrical wiring for the automatic exposure system. It ends in a light guide connector that contains the light guide, a venting connector, and electrical contacts for photography. It is plugged into the light source before use of the FOB. The venting connector is where the ethylene oxide (ETO) sterilization-venting cap and leakage tester are placed (Fig. 18-3). When the ETO cap is attached, it vents the interior of the FOB to equalize internal and external pressures. The ETO cap must be installed when FOB is subjected to gas sterilization and aeration and during airfreight transportation. The ETO cap must be removed before immersion of the FOB into water or disinfectant solution or when the FOB is in use.

The light source is an integral part of the fiberoptic endoscope system. Various light sources are available, which provide adequate illumination not only for viewing but also for taking photographs or videotapes. An intense light is generated and is focused on the proximal end of the light guide cable by a source lens or a spherical reflecting mirror. A heat filter or reflecting mirror is used to reduce the amount of heat focused on the light guide cable. FOBs with the light source incorporated into the body of the scope are available. These increase the portability of the instrument, making its use both outside and inside the operating room more simple and convenient (Olympus Optical Co. [Europa] GmbH, Hamburg, Germany).

B. CLEANING AND DISINFECTING

Universal precautions are now mandatory in every health care institution to minimize the risk of transmission of infectious diseases. Cleaning and disinfecting the FOB following each use are a must for safe practice of bronchoscopy.[83,84]

After each use the FOB should be cleaned and disinfected to prevent damage to the FOB and to prevent transmission of disease from patient to patient. Specific recommendations for sterilization or disinfection made by the manufacturer and by each health care facility should be followed. Most modern FOBs are constructed to withstand complete immersion in disinfectant solution.

The FOB should be washed immediately after each use, and the working channel should be flushed with water to remove secretions before they dry. The use of a cleaning brush may be needed for complete removal of secretions from the working channel. The brush should be inserted

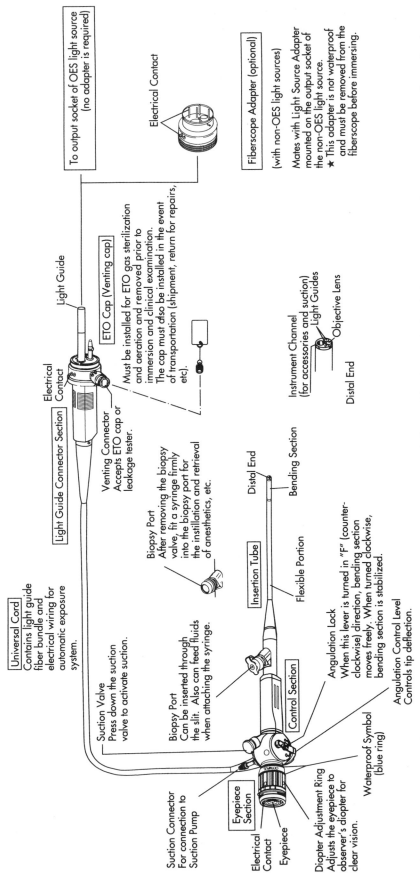

Figure 18-1 Components of a fiberoptic bronchoscope. Olympus BF-20D series. ETO, ethylene oxide; OES, optical emission spectroscopy. (From Ovassapian A: Fiberoptic Airway Endoscopy in Anesthesia and Critical Care. New York, Raven Press, 1990.)

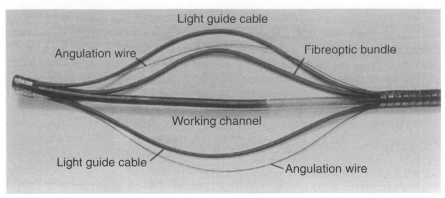

Figure 18-2 Inside a fiberoptic bronchoscope (FOB) insertion cord. Two angulation wires control the bending of the tip of the fiberoptic. Two light guide cables contain fiberoptic bundles (incoherent), which bring light to the tip of the FOB. The fiberoptic bundle contains the coherent bundle, which transmits images from the objective lens at the tip of the FOB to the eyepiece of the FOB. The working channel is used for suctioning of secretions, instillation of local anesthetics, and insufflation of oxygen. (From Ovassapian A: Fiberoptic Airway Endoscopy in Anesthesia and Critical Care. New York, Raven Press, 1990.)

through the suction port at the handle downward toward the tip of the insertion cord to avoid FOB damage. Retrograde insertion of a wire through the working channel is not recommended because it increases the risk of damage to the internal lining of the suction channel of the FOB. Before being soaked in disinfecting solution, the FOB should be inspected for defects that might allow liquids to penetrate the scope. The rubber covering of the distal portion of the insertion cord should be carefully examined because frequent use may cause tears and defects in this covering. The FOB should be tested for leaks using a leakage tester supplied by the manufacturer. If an air leak is detected, the instrument should be sent promptly to the manufacturer for appropriate repair.

After initial inspection, the suction and biopsy port assembly should be removed and the FOB placed in disinfectant solution. A syringe of disinfecting solution is used to fill the working channel of the FOB. One such solution is 2% alkaline glutaraldehyde. Recommended immersion times after use in noninfected patients vary from

10 minutes for glutaraldehyde to 20 minutes for the iodine-containing solutions. Each solution is potentially caustic to the materials in the FOB; thus, the manufacturers' recommendations for disinfectant concentration and maximum soaking time should be carefully observed. The FOB should be washed and the working channel suctioned with water to remove all traces of the disinfectant solution. Suctioning air for 10 to 15 seconds dries the inside of the suction channel.

If the patient has tuberculosis or another transmissible illness, the FOB should be sterilized. Sterilization of the bronchoscope is also critical before use in patients with immune deficiencies. Complete sterilization of the FOB can be accomplished with ETO gas. The ETO cap must be securely attached to the venting connector and must remain in place throughout the sterilization and aeration process. The gas sterilization procedure is lengthy; it may take as long as 24 hours before the FOB is ready for use. The ideal container allows the insertion cord to remain straight. Carrying cases or small sterilization trays, in which

Figure 18-3 Air leak tester. The cap is attached to the fiberscope venting connector. The adapter is attached to the light source. The air pumped by the light source pressurizes the fiberscope. Any air leak from the fiberscope indicates that the waterproof system is damaged and needs to be repaired before it can be soaked in solution. (From Ovassapian A: Fiberoptic Airway Endoscopy in Anesthesia and Critical Care. New York, Raven Press, 1990.)

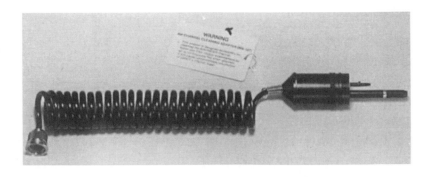

the insertion cord is bent, are less desirable for storage because the bending ultimately changes the shape and integrity of the insertion cord. The storage location must be clean, dry, well ventilated, and maintained at room temperature. Direct sunlight, high temperature, high humidity, and x-ray exposure may cause damage to the FOB.

III. FIBEROPTIC INTUBATION OF THE ADULT TRACHEA

The value of the FOB in difficult endotracheal intubation is well established.* However, the use of an FOB should not be limited to patients in whom endotracheal intubation may be difficult (Box 18-1). Many patients who might be denied general anesthesia or might receive tracheostomy can be safely intubated with the help of the FOB. Fiberoptic intubation is accomplished simply, quickly, and easily when certain preparatory steps are taken.

A. PREPARATION OF EQUIPMENT

1. Fiberoptic Bronchoscope and Cart

Anesthesiologists must be prepared to manage any kind of airway at any time. The ability to transport rapidly fiberoptic equipment and supplies is critical for effective use of this instrument, especially when emergency conditions exist. Whether these emergencies arise in the ward, the intensive care unit, the emergency room, or the operating room, a readily available mobile bronchoscopy cart is invaluable (Fig. 18-4). The cart should have large wheels for stability and easy transport and be equipped with

---

*References 1, 3, 21, 53, 61, 104, 122, 123, 127, 130, 138, 139, 143, 148, 165, 170, 173, 175, 181, 202.

Box 18-1	**Indications for Fiberoptic Intubation**

  I. Routine intubation
 II. Difficult intubation
     A. Known or anticipated
     B. Unanticipated failed intubation
III. Compromised airway
     A. Upper airway
     B. Lower airway (tracheal compression)
 IV. Intubation of the conscious patient preferred
     A. High risk of aspiration
     B. Movement of neck not desirable
     C. Known difficult mask ventilation
     D. Morbid obesity
     E. Self-positioning
  V. High risk of dental damage
 VI. Previous tracheostomy or prolonged intubation

FOBs, a light source, drugs for application of topical anesthesia, and various other airway supplies such as gauzes, tongue blades, intubating and nasal airways, cotton-tipped swabs, bronchoscopy swivel adapter, lubricant (K-Y jelly or silicone lubricant), and endoscopy masks, which may be needed for fiberoptic intubation. Integration of this cart with a DA cart is reasonable as the FOB is one of the first-line tools to approach the patient with a DA.

All equipment and supplies for administration of anesthesia, resuscitation, and monitoring should be available in the operating room and should be checked following a standard protocol before beginning a nonemergent fiberoptic intubation. In the operating room, the fiberoptic cart is placed at the left side of the endoscopist. The FOB is connected to the light source, the light is turned on, and the focus is adjusted by looking at written material until a clear view is obtained. The light is then turned off until the time of intubation. The insertion cord of the FOB and the ET (cut to an appropriate length with the cuff checked) are placed in warm water; the insertion cord is warmed to prevent fogging and the ET is warmed to soften and to improve its pliability. Alternatively, a commercial defogging solution may be applied to the optical tip of the FOB. The necessary supplies are laid out on top of the fiberoptic cart, and suction is prepared and at hand.

2. Ancillary Equipment

Various intubating airway devices, nasopharyngeal airways, endoscopy masks, and bronchoscopy swivel adapters have been used to facilitate fiberoptic ET intubation.[24,54,73,93,116,136,151,212,213] Some are reviewed in the following.

a. Intubating Airways

The Berman II intubating airway is disposable and is tubular along its entire length (Fig. 18-5).[24] It was originally designed for blind orotracheal intubation. It has also been used for fiberoptic intubation.[146] It has a longitudinal opening on its side, which can be opened wide to disengage it from the ET and remove it from the patient's mouth. The airway is available in different sizes. Because of its length and tubular shape, the FOB cannot be maneuvered by bending its tip once it is placed through the airway. Therefore, if the distal end of the airway is not in line with the glottic opening, exposure of the cords can be accomplished only by partial withdrawal of the airway.

The Ovassapian fiberoptic intubating airway is designed to provide an open air space in the oropharynx, to protect the FOB from being bitten by the patient, and to be removed from the mouth without disconnecting the ET adapter (Fig. 18-6).[136] It is available in only one size. The airway has a flat lingual surface on the proximal half, which minimizes its movement. The wide distal half of the airway curves to prevent the tongue and soft tissues of the anterior pharyngeal wall from falling back and obstructing

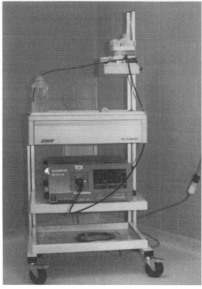

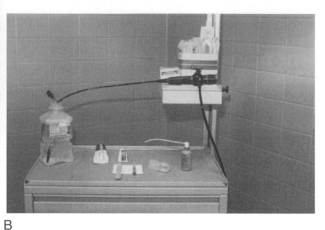

A   B

Figure 18-4 **A,** A simple fiberoptic cart arrangement. Fiberoptic bronchoscope, after being cleaned and disinfected after each use, is stored on the top of cart covered with towels. All necessary supplies are in drawer. **B,** Close view of the top of the fiberoptic cart showing the equipment and drugs prepared for an awake intubation (warm water bottle with endotracheal tube and fiberoptic bronchoscope placed inside, lubricant, local anesthetic jelly, tongue blade, local anesthetic solution for transtracheal injection, intubating airway, and lidocaine spray).

the view of the glottis. This feature also maintains an open space for maneuvering the tip of the FOB. This airway accommodates an ET up to 8.5 mm in inner diameter (ID).

The Patil fiberoptic airway is available in only one size and is made of aluminum.[151] A groove at the middle portion of the distal part of the airway provides room for anterior-posterior maneuvering of the FOB. However, an ET does not pass through the airway, and it should be removed before advancement of the ET.

The Williams airway intubator was designed for "blind" orotracheal intubation, but its use in fiberoptic intubation has been described.[212] The proximal half is cylindrical; the distal half has an open lingual surface. The airway is

made in two sizes, 90 and 100 mm, which admit ETs up to 8 and 8.5 mm ID, respectively (Fig. 18-7). Because of its design, the tip of the FOB cannot be maneuvered in an anteroposterior or a lateral direction. If the distal end of the airway is not in line with the glottic opening, the exposure of the cords becomes difficult, necessitating partial withdrawal of the airway. The ET adapter should be removed before intubation to allow removal of the airway.

b. Endoscopy Masks and Adaptors
A face mask with an endoscopy port to assist fiberoptic intubation in anesthetized patients was first described by Mallios[116] in 1980 and later by Patil and coauthors[151]

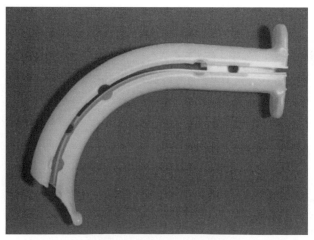

Figure 18-5 Berman airway.

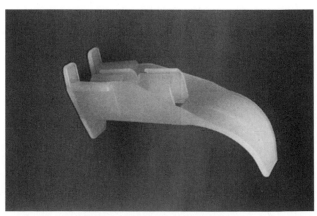

Figure 18-6 Ovassapian airway.

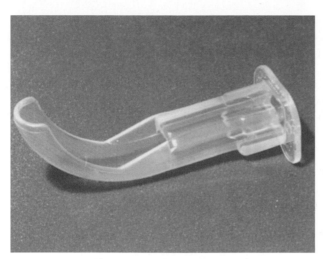

Figure 18-7 Williams airway.

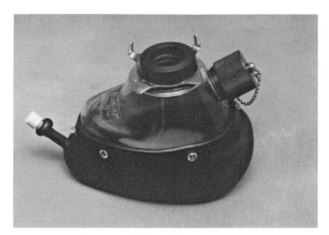

Figure 18-8 Patil-Syracuse mask.

(Fig. 18-8). Modification of oropharyngeal airways and pediatric anesthesia masks to facilitate pediatric fiberoptic intubation is also described.[73,213] The endoscopy mask permits passage of an FOB through the port into the oropharynx in an anesthetized patient being ventilated by face mask. Because a rubber diaphragm covers the port, an air leak is not developed and mask ventilation can be continued throughout the procedure.

A face mask adapter for fiberoptic intubation of the anesthetized patient has been described (bronchoscopy swivel adapter). This adapter consists of two parts: a rotating elbow, which possesses a port, and the body of the adapter, which attaches to the face mask.[93]

B. FIBEROPTIC INTUBATION OF THE CONSCIOUS PATIENT

When the airway is compromised or difficult intubation is expected, awake intubation (AI) with or without conscious sedation is indicated (see Box 18-1).[21,146] AI should also be considered in the following circumstances: for patients

at high risk for gastric aspiration, for those who have an unstable cervical spine, for the morbidly obese, and for patients in ventilatory failure or who are otherwise seriously ill. Patients with tracheal stenosis or with extrinsic compression of the trachea secondary to thoracic aortic aneurysm, substernal thyroid, or mediastinal mass may also benefit from AI. The advantages of fiberoptic intubation for these patients are the maintenance of spontaneous ventilation and the ability to position the tip of the ET precisely beyond the compression site. Fiberoptic intubation is easiest in the awake patient because the tongue does not fall back in the pharynx, and spontaneous ventilation tends to keep the airway open. In addition, by deep breathing the patient can assist the operator in locating the glottis when the airway anatomy is distorted.

There are several factors that are critical for successful completion of an awake fiberoptic endotracheal intubation. These are psychological preparation of the patient, pharmacologic preparation of the patient, appropriate monitoring and delivery of oxygen during preparation of the patient and the procedure, an expert endoscopist, and a well-functioning FOB (Box 18-2).

1. Preparation of the Patient

Psychological preparation of the patient starts with an informative, reassuring preoperative visit to the patient. A detailed explanation of the technique is provided, and

---

Box 18-2   Keys to Successful Awake Intubation

I. Preparation of the patient
 A. Psychological preparation: informative, reassuring preoperative visit
 B. Pharmacologic preparation
  1. Premedication
   a. Light or no sedation for calm patients
   b. Heavy sedation for anxious patients
   c. Narcotics when pain is present
   d. Specific drugs for habitual drug users
   e. Antisialagogue unless contraindicated
  2. Intravenous sedation
   a. No sedation for patients with severely compromised airway
   b. Conscious sedation for most patients
   c. Heavy sedation for uncooperative patients
  3. Topical anesthesia
   a. Oral intubation: oropharynx, laryngotracheal
   b. Nasal intubation: nasal mucosa, laryngotracheal
  C. Monitoring and oxygen
II. Expert endoscopist
III. Functional fiberoptic bronchoscope and supplies

questions are answered. If intubation is to be performed with no sedation, the reason should be explained to the patient, emphasizing that this is done for the patient's safety. The patient's active participation in the process of intubation is asked for. The patient is informed of what he or she can do to assist in a smooth intubation, for example, maintaining the head position, taking deep breaths, or swallowing secretions when requested. A well-informed patient who knows that the technique is chosen to maximize his or her safety appreciates the efforts and helps the physician in the process of intubation. When minimal or no sedation is used, the patient should also be informed that recall of the procedure is expected. With the patient thus prepared, any negative psychological impact is minimized. If the patient's condition permits providing conscious sedation, the patient should be further assured that it is most likely he or she will not remember the intubation. When the visit is successful, the patient's apprehension is relieved and therefore the need for sedation is lessened and the patient's cooperation is maximized.

Pharmacologic preparation of the patient consists of premedication, conscious sedation at the time of intubation, and application of topical anesthesia. The goal of premedication is twofold. One goal is to provide sedation that complements the psychological preparation of the patient. The second is to provide an antisialagogue to reduce secretions. Benzodiazepines are the most commonly prescribed drugs for premedication and sedation. Diazepam (Valium) 5 to 10 mg by mouth or midazolam 1 to 3 mg intramuscularly or 10 to 20 mg by mouth provides adequate sedation in most patients. Opioids should be considered if the patient is in pain or is a habitual user. However, if the patient's airway or physical condition is compromised, no sedative or opioid should be given prior to the patient's arrival at a monitored setting where the anesthesiologist is in attendance.

Standard monitoring is applied to all patients receiving airway endoscopy, whether the procedure is performed in the operating room suite, intensive care unit, or any other location. Anesthesia, intravenous sedation, or application of topical anesthesia is started on the basis of the needs of the patient and the urgency of the airway intervention. Oxygen is provided by nasal cannula at a flow rate of 3 L/min to all adult patients undergoing AI in whom this therapy is not contraindicated.

An antisialagogue agent is used to reduce secretions. This is essential for establishing good topical anesthesia and to optimize conditions for fiberoptic visualization of the glottis.[21,83,146] Glycopyrrolate and atropine are given intramuscularly as a premedicant or intravenously before sedation begins. Because glycopyrrolate does not cross the blood-brain barrier and causes less tachycardia, it is considered the anticholinergic agent of choice.

The next phase of pharmacologic preparation is conscious sedation administered intravenously in immediate preparation for intubation. Conscious sedation is desirable to minimize awareness of the procedure and to increase the patient's acceptance, provided that safety is not compromised. The goal of conscious sedation is to have a calm and cooperative patient who can follow verbal commands and maintain adequate oxygenation and ventilation. Depending on the patient's condition and the indication for AI, an opioid, a sedative, or a combination is used. Opioids produce profound analgesia, are strong depressants of the airway reflexes, and facilitate airway instrumentation while the patient is still capable of following verbal commands. However, patients become more susceptible to aspiration of gastric contents if regurgitation or vomiting occurs. Airway protective reflexes remain more active when a sedative such as diazepam or midazolam is used, but the patient may be less cooperative and react more vigorously to instrumentation of the airway. A combination of fentanyl and midazolam (1.5 μg/kg and 30 μg/kg, respectively) has been used successfully for conscious sedation. Remifentanil infusion has also been used successfully for sedation for fiberoptic intubation.[160,161,164]

The last phase of pharmacologic preparation is application of topical anesthesia. Instrumentation of the airway without adequate topical anesthesia is uncomfortable and distressing to a conscious patient and may make successful completion of intubation more difficult or impossible. Awake airway instrumentation must be made painless and nonstressful, especially in those who may need repeated operations. Good topical anesthesia of the respiratory tract mucous membranes eliminates pharyngeal, laryngeal, and tracheobronchial reflexes. Judicious use of topical anesthetics requires a sound knowledge of their pharmacology and skills in the techniques for their effective application. Reduction of secretions to provide a dry mucosa is essential to good topical anesthesia. Excess secretions dilute the local anesthetic solution, create a barrier between agent and mucosa, and carry the local anesthetic away from the site of action.[146,163]

The principles and guidelines for the safe use of topical anesthetics have been summarized by Adriani and coauthors.[1] It is essential to know the optimum effective concentration of each drug, the rapidity of onset of action, the recommended maximum safe dose, and the appropriate techniques for application. As a rule, the onset time shortens and the duration of anesthesia lengthens as the concentration of drug is increased. However, the maximum effective concentration is not necessarily either safe or recommended. For example, cocaine is maximally effective at 20% concentration, far in excess of the 4% to 10% recommended for clinical use. Combining two local anesthetics at their maximum effective concentrations neither improves nor prolongs the duration of topical anesthesia. However, systemic effects of the two drugs are additive and increase the possibility of systemic toxicity.[35] In a mixture of short- and long-acting drugs, the duration of anesthesia is that of the longer acting drug. For example, benzocaine, with its rapid onset, and tetracaine, with its prolonged action, complement each other.

The rate and amount of topical anesthetic absorbed vary according to the site of application, the dose of the drug, and general condition of the patient.[26,43,44,153] Absorption is more rapid from alveoli than from the tracheobronchial tree and more rapid from the tracheobronchial tree than from the pharynx. Vasoconstrictor added to solutions of topical anesthetics neither slows their absorption nor prolongs their duration.[1] Plasma levels rise more rapidly after topical application to the respiratory tract than after injection into tissue; therefore, recommended doses of topical anesthetics for use within the respiratory tract are approximately half of the doses of the same drug injected into tissue.

2. Orotracheal Intubation of the Conscious Patient

a. Topical Anesthesia

Application of topical anesthesia should wait until after sedation has been given to minimize the patient's discomfort. For the oropharynx, application of a 4% solution or a 10% aerosol preparation of lidocaine spray provides excellent topical anesthesia by abolishing pain sensation and obtunding gag and swallowing reflexes.

For topical anesthesia of the larynx and trachea, 4% lidocaine can be injected across the cricothyroid membrane (translaryngeal injection technique) or sprayed through the FOB. Translaryngeal injection using a 20-gauge catheter or a 22-gauge needle provides good topical anesthesia of the trachea and larynx. Most patients cough, often for period of 8 to 20 seconds. The main advantage of this technique is that the topical anesthesia is established prior to endoscopy. This feature prevents the severe cough and laryngeal spasm that can be seen with advancement of the FOB. In addition, it provides better, more solid topical anesthesia than the "spray-as-you-go" technique.[204] A local anesthetic jelly, lidocaine 5% or benzocaine 20% (Americaine), is applied to the base of the tongue and to the anterior tonsillar pillars with a tongue blade at approximately 60 to 90 seconds after translaryngeal injection. This maneuver checks the adequacy of the oropharyngeal topical anesthesia by the lidocaine spray and supplements the block if it is not adequate.

The spray-as-you-go application of topical anesthesia involves spraying the anesthetic through the suction channel of an advancing FOB.[204] The epiglottis and vocal cords are visualized through the FOB and sprayed directly. After 30 to 45 seconds, the FOB is advanced into the trachea, the anterior wall is sprayed, and as the FOB is advanced toward the carina, incremental doses are sprayed on the walls of the tracheobronchial tree. The size of the FOB channel is important with this technique. A small suction channel (0.5 to 1.0 mm) enables the operator to use 0.2 mL of solution at a time and produces a fine stream that reaches the targeted area. Most adult FOBs have larger suction channels (2 to 2.5 mm) for suctioning, brushing, and using biopsy forceps. With this larger channel, spray of small volumes of local anesthetic becomes difficult, and

spread of the solution is less uniform. This problem can be overcome by passing an epidural catheter (internal diameter 0.5 to 1 mm cut to the length of the insertion cord) through the suction channel and using it for spraying the local anesthetic.[146] A three-way stopcock placed at the hub of the epidural catheter allows suctioning to alternate with spraying without losing the anesthetic solution during suctioning; the three-way stopcock is closed during suctioning and open during spraying. The spray-as-you-go technique provides flexibility for the operator to anesthetize part or all of the respiratory passages. It is useful for most awake endotracheal intubations but particularly for patients at high risk for aspirating gastric contents because the topical anesthetic is applied only *after* the vocal cords are exposed and intubation is achieved without the lower airway being anesthetized.

Anesthesia of the airway may be supplemented with bilateral superior laryngeal and lingual nerve blocks.[21,163] The sensory innervation of the larynx above the level of the vocal cords is supplied by the superior laryngeal nerve. This branch of the vagus nerve is easily blocked bilaterally by injecting 2 to 3 mL of 1% lidocaine by an anterior neck approach. The lingual branch of the glossopharyngeal nerve carries the sensory innervation of the pharynx, tonsils, and posterior third of the tongue. The block of the lingual nerve bilaterally depresses the gag reflex during endotracheal intubation in the conscious patient. In most patients, the local anesthetic applied topically to the back of the tongue and throat is sufficient. If this does not produce satisfactory anesthesia, injection of local anesthetic (2 mL of 1% lidocaine) bilaterally at the palatolingual arches (anterior tonsillar pillars) blocks the lingual branch of the glossopharyngeal nerve.

b. Procedure

After topical anesthesia has been established, the patient's head is put into a neutral position for intubation, an airway intubator is placed in the mouth, the oropharynx is suctioned, and the lubricated ET is placed 4 to 5 cm inside the intubating airway. The fourth and fifth fingers of the right hand hold the ET to prevent premature advancement of the ET, while the index finger and thumb advance the FOB through the ET (Fig. 18-9). As the FOB is advanced toward the oropharynx, the white pharyngeal surface of the airway and the patient's soft palate and uvula come into view (Fig. 18-10). As the FOB is advanced, its tip is deflected anteriorly to expose the epiglottis and vocal cords. In the presence of a large, floppy epiglottis, the tip of the FOB must be manipulated underneath the epiglottis to visualize the vocal cords. Extending the head at the atlanto-occipital joint and keeping the mouth closed keeps the epiglottis away from posterior pharyngeal wall. On rare occasions during an AI, an assistant must perform a jaw thrust or must pull the tongue forward to facilitate glottic exposure. These maneuvers increase the pharyngeal space by elevation of the tongue and epiglottis away from the

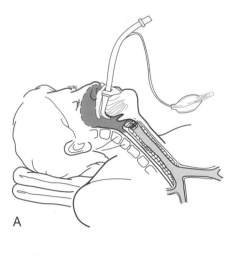

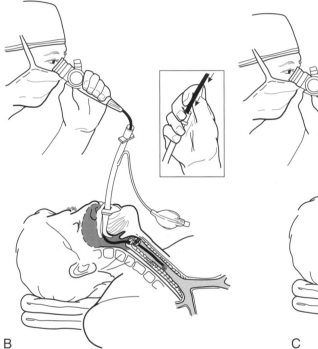

Figure 18-9 Fiberoptic orotracheal intubation in a conscious patient. **A,** Ovassapian intubating airway and endotracheal tube (ET) position. **B,** The bronchoscope is advanced through ET into midtrachea. Inset illustrates position of hand for holding tracheal ET and advancing the bronchoscope. **C,** The ET is advanced over the bronchoscope into the trachea. (From Ovassapian A: Fiberoptic Airway Endoscopy in Anesthesia and Critical Care. New York, Raven Press, 1990.)

posterior pharyngeal wall. This improves visualization of the larynx and provides more room to maneuver the FOB tip.

After the vocal cords are visualized, they are maintained in *the center of the field of view* by fine rotation of the body of the FOB and manipulations of the tip control lever as the FOB is being advanced. Without such maneuvering, the tip of the FOB often ends up in the anterior commissure or against the anterior laryngeal wall. If this occurs, pulling the FOB back and flexing the tip of the FOB posteriorly brings the laryngeal inlet and tracheal lumen into view. The FOB is then advanced into the midtrachea, and the ET is slipped over the firmly held stationary FOB into the trachea. The FOB is kept stationary to ensure that it is neither advanced farther down into the tracheobronchial tree nor pulled out of the trachea during

advancement of the ET. Ideally, the tip of the ET is positioned 3 to 4 cm above the carina by direct visualization through the FOB.

The oral approach can be somewhat more difficult than the nasal approach because of the sharp curve leading from the oral cavity into the larynx. In many patients, even though the FOB has entered the trachea, the ET impinges on the epiglottis or lodges in the pyriform sinus and cannot be advanced into the trachea.[31,146] Orientation of the leading edge bevel is the most important determinant of successful passage of the ET. The bevel-down orientation appears to improve the success of oral fiberoptic endotracheal intubation by allowing the ET to slip past the potentially obstructing right arytenoid cartilage.[99,174] Advancing the ET while instructing the patient to take a deep breath also improves successful passage.

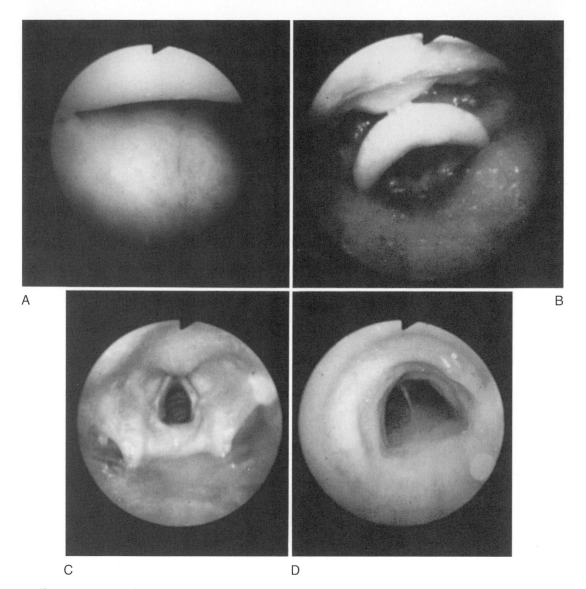

Figure 18-10 Bronchoscopic views during fiberoptic orotracheal intubation. **A,** Pharyngeal surface of the Ovassapian airway is seen in white in the upper half of the picture. Soft palate is seen in the lower half of the picture. **B,** The tip of bronchoscope is in oropharynx. Distal end of Ovassapian airway covering the base of the tongue. Epiglottis is in view. **C,** The tip of bronchoscope passed beneath the tip of epiglottis. Glottis is in view. **D,** The tip of the bronchoscope in lower third of the trachea. Carina is in view. (From Ovassapian A: Fiberoptic Airway Endoscopy in Anesthesia and Critical Care. New York, Raven Press, 1990.)

In some patients this maneuver may have to be repeated two to three times, particularly when a small-size FOB is used for placement of a large-size ET. Whenever feasible, the size of the FOB and the ID of the ET should be matched as closely as possible to minimize "play" between the two but still allow smooth passage of the ET over the FOB. The larger a gap is between the FOB and ET, the more chance there is that the ET may not have slipped into the trachea.[146] An ET made more pliable by placement in warm water may also minimize this occurrence. The passage of a spiral-wound (anode) ET may be less likely to be impeded by glottic structures,[31] although this has been disputed by other investigators.[48,103] Other specialized ETs have also been suggested for use to improve ET passage.[80,105] It is our experience that meticulous attention to the orientation of the bevel solves most problems with ET passage, and thus special ETs that may be more expensive or difficult to find are not needed.[206] Laryngospasm resulting from poor topical anesthesia may also prevent ET advancement. In this circumstance, additional topical anesthesia applied through the FOB improves conditions for intubation.

3. Nasotracheal Intubation of the Conscious Patient

a. Topical Anesthesia

To anesthetize the mucous membrane of the nose, the more patent nostril is selected and filled with 2% lidocaine gel. Then cotton-tipped applicators soaked in 4% to 5% cocaine or a mixture of lidocaine with phenylephrine (Neo-Synephrine)[106] or oxymetazoline (Afrin) (3 mL 4% lidocaine plus 1 mL 1% phenylephrine or 0.05% oxymetazoline) can be placed in the nose with minimal reaction by the patient. These agents provide topical anesthesia and shrinkage of the nasal mucosa. Allow 4 minutes for maximal anesthetic and vasoconstrictive effect. Two milliliters of agent is adequate for anesthetizing one nostril. Using cotton-tipped applicators is also helpful in evaluating the patency of nasal passages and in predicting the angle for ET insertion.

Laryngotracheal anesthesia is achieved by translaryngeal injection or by spraying through the FOB during the process of intubation. There is no need for application of topical anesthesia to the oropharynx because the gag reflex is not stimulated by the nasal route.[146,148]

b. Procedure

Fiberoptic nasotracheal intubation is often easier than the oral approach because the FOB is usually pointed straight at the glottis as it enters the oropharynx, there is no sharp turn to negotiate, and the vocal cords are usually visible from a distance.[146,148] For nasotracheal intubation in conscious patients, either the ET is placed in the nostril first and the FOB is passed through it or the ET is mounted over the FOB, which is then passed through the nostril. Placing the ET first avoids the possibility of nasal secretions covering the objective lens and obscuring the view, and a tight nasal passage can be recognized when the FOB is being advanced. Once the FOB has been passed through the ET into the trachea, advancement of the ET over the FOB is easily accomplished. There are two disadvantages to placing the ET into the nostril first. One is the increased possibility of causing nasal bleeding and thus rendering the FOB virtually useless. The other disadvantage is that, in some patients, the direction established by the ET prevents manipulation of the FOB into the glottis. The main disadvantage of passing the FOB first is that the adequacy of the nasal passage cannot be judged. Insertion of a 4- or 5-mm outside diameter FOB through the nose does not guarantee the subsequent passage of a 7- or 8-mm ID ET. In the case of a tight nasal passage, if the ET is advanced over the FOB by force, removal of the FOB may be impossible, necessitating removal of the ET and FOB together.

If the plan is to place the ET in the nose first, it should be softened in warm water and generously lubricated. It is introduced gently through the anesthetized nostril until it just enters the posterior oropharynx. If it does not make the bend, it is pulled back, rotated 90 degrees to the right or left, and reintroduced. If this maneuver is unsuccessful, the FOB may be used to direct the ET tip into the oropharynx. After the ET tip is placed in the oropharynx, secretions are suctioned through the ET. Then the lubricated FOB is advanced through it into the oropharynx (Fig. 18-11). In 80% to 85% of patients the epiglottis and vocal cords are seen with minimal or no manipulation of the tip of the FOB.[148] In heavily sedated patients or in elderly, edentulous patients, the tongue and pharyngeal tissue may fall back and block the exposure of the larynx and vocal cords. As described for oral intubation, extending the head, applying jaw thrust, or pulling the tongue forward often helps in visualizing the vocal cords. The FOB is advanced into the midtrachea, followed by the ET. With nasotracheal intubation the incidence of the ET meeting resistance and not entering the trachea is relatively low. However, to improve successful ET passage the ET should be turned *90 degrees clockwise* from its usual orientation so that the *bevel is facing up*, thus avoiding the epiglottis.[99] This is the opposite of the ET orientation recommended for oral fiberoptic intubation.

C. FIBEROPTIC INTUBATION IN THE ANESTHETIZED PATIENT

Fiberoptic intubation with the patient under general anesthesia is accomplished with the patient either breathing spontaneously or paralyzed and receiving controlled ventilation. The main disadvantage of intubation under general anesthesia is that the tongue and pharyngeal tissues lose their tonicity and close down the pharyngeal space, blocking visualization of the larynx. To minimize apnea time when the patient is paralyzed and to facilitate laryngeal exposure, an assistant is needed. The assistant is directed to do the following tasks: first, to mount the ET on the lubricated FOB and have it ready to hand to the anesthesiologist as soon as the anesthesia mask is removed; second, to apply jaw thrust to maintain an open oropharynx; and third, to observe the apnea time and monitor the patient. The endoscopy cart is placed at the head of the table on the left side of the patient while the assistant stands on the patient's left side facing the anesthesiologist.

If the patient is breathing spontaneously, supplemental oxygen should be administered. This may be provided by nasal cannula, by blow-by from the anesthesia circuit, by use of an insufflation catheter, by standard face mask used over only the oropharynx[86] or nasopharynx, or by endoscopy mask or nasopharyngeal airways. For the apneic patient with a DA, ventilation may be performed with an endoscopy mask or a small standard face mask applied over the oropharynx[86] or nasopharynx. If mask ventilation is difficult or impossible, jet ventilation by a modified Fogarty embolectomy catheter or transtracheal catheter has been described.[12] It is important to note that low-flow tracheal oxygen can help maintain oxygenation.[114,115] Even delivery of 5 L of O_2 by nasal cannula to provide apneic oxygenation has been shown to slow the rise in arterial carbon dioxide tension ($Paco_2$) and decline in Pao_2.[108]

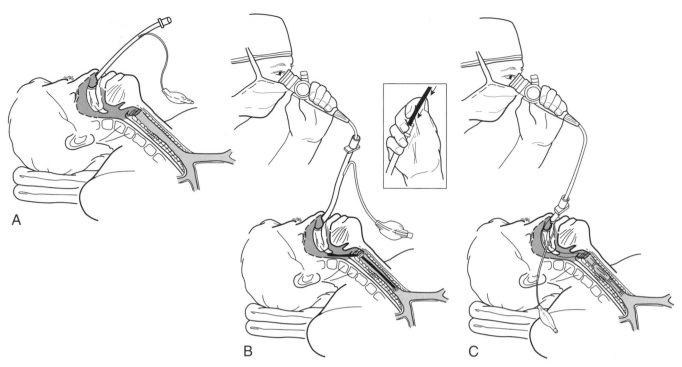

Figure 18-11 Fiberoptic nasotracheal intubation in conscious patient. **A,** The position of the tip of the nasotracheal endotracheal tube (ET) making the bend into oropharynx. **B,** The fiberscope advanced through the nasotracheal ET into the midtrachea. Inset illustrates position of hand for holding tracheal ET and advancing the fiberscope. **C,** The tracheal ET threaded over the fiberscope into the trachea. (From Ovassapian A: Fiberoptic Airway Endoscopy in Anesthesia and Critical Care. New York, Raven Press, 1990.)

1. Orotracheal Intubation

After general anesthesia and muscle relaxation are established, the anesthesia mask is removed, the intubating airway is placed inside the mouth, and the oropharynx is suctioned. Ventilation is resumed by mask and continued for 30 to 60 seconds. The assistant has the FOB ready, with the ET mounted on its insertion cord. The anesthesia mask is removed, and the anesthesiologist grasps the body of the FOB with the left hand and the tip of the insertion cord with the right hand. The tip of the insertion cord is placed inside the intubating airway and advanced into the oropharynx. The assistant applies a jaw thrust after handing the FOB to the endoscopist. This maneuver is vital and constitutes the most important step in fiberoptic intubation under general anesthesia.

If an intubating airway is not available, the assistant may pull the patient's tongue forward away from the palate and posterior pharyngeal wall. This maneuver also moves the epiglottis away from the posterior pharyngeal wall, thus assisting exposure of the vocal cords. Care must be taken because forceful stretch of the tongue over the lower teeth may cause trauma and laceration of the tongue. Lung forceps and mouth gag with tongue holder have also been applied to keep the tongue forward.[139,154] The assistant may also use both hands to apply jaw thrust, while simultaneously opening the mouth by downward pressure on the chin. Without the intubating airway, the FOB is more likely to move from the midline position and make exposure of the vocal cords more difficult.[139]

After placement of the FOB in the midtrachea, the ET is advanced with a rotating motion into the trachea; the tip of the ET is placed 3 cm above the carina. As previously discussed, orientation of the leading edge bevel is the most important determinant of successful passage of the ET. The bevel-down orientation (Murphy eye up for a straight polyvinyl chloride ET) should be assured for oral fiberoptic intubation to facilitate entry into the trachea by slipping past the potentially obstructing right arytenoid cartilage. If the ET faces resistance and does not enter the trachea, it is pulled back, rotated 180 degrees to the right or left, and then advanced while the assistant continues to apply jaw thrust. The FOB is then removed, and the breathing system is attached to the ET. In case of a prolonged intubation time, the position of the ET should be checked only after ventilation has been resumed.

2. Nasotracheal Intubation

The general preparation for and the technique of intubation are as described for orotracheal intubation, and the assistant performs the same duties. An oropharyngeal airway or an intubating airway is used to retract the tongue from the posterior pharyngeal wall. Application of a vasoconstrictor to the nostril prior to intubation either before or after induction of anesthesia is recommended to decrease the incidence of bleeding. To minimize apnea time, the lubricated ET is mounted on the insertion cord of the FOB before the anesthesia mask is removed rather than being placed into the nostril after the mask is removed. As soon as the mask is removed from the patient's face, the operator grasps the FOB as described earlier and inserts its tip into the selected nostril; while looking through the FOB, the operator advances it toward the larynx and trachea. The assistant applies jaw thrust to keep the posterior pharyngeal space open. After the FOB is placed in the midtrachea, the ET is threaded over the FOB into the trachea. To ensure adequate nasopharyngeal patency and to reduce nasal trauma, sequential introduction of increasing sizes of small flexible nasopharyngeal airways can be used to dilate the nasal passages gently. This maneuver ensures that the ET easily threads over the FOB and into the trachea. The patient may also be ventilated between each placement of a nasopharyngeal airway.

3. Rapid Sequence Induction and Intubation

The combination of a difficult intubation and full stomach in patients receiving emergency operation presents a special problem. If the patient is uncooperative, is intoxicated, or is a child, AI to secure the airway before induction of general anesthesia may not be a viable option. Under these conditions, general anesthesia using the rapid sequence induction and intubation technique is commonly used. Compression of the cricoid cartilage to block passive regurgitation of gastric contents into the oropharynx is applied with this induction technique. Failure of endotracheal intubation with rigid laryngoscopy during a rapid sequence induction leaves the patient's airway vulnerable to aspiration. Fiberoptic intubation while cricoid pressure is maintained is a possibility that should be considered. Advanced experience and confidence in the use of FOB are necessary for successful use of FOB under these circumstances.[141]

The ability to perform rapid fiberoptic intubation in patients at high risk for aspiration may play an important role in diminishing major airway-related catastrophes. Repeated attempts at blind nasal or rigid laryngoscopy for endotracheal intubation traumatize the airway and may change a manageable airway into an unmanageable one. Air may be introduced into the stomach if ventilation is required during repeated intubation attempts, even if cricoid pressure is maintained, and this may increase the risk of aspiration of stomach contents.[121,190] The application of a rapid fiberoptic intubation, before either of these scenarios occurs, may be a lifesaving measure.

4. Intubation Using an Endoscopy Mask

An anesthesia mask with endoscopy port can be used during the course of fiberoptic intubation to provide oxygen to the spontaneously breathing patient or to allow positive-pressure ventilation of the anesthetized and paralyzed patient.[14,72,102,165] An assistant who is capable of administering anesthesia and maintaining mask ventilation is essential. Anesthesia is induced and maintained with an endoscopy mask. The use of an intubating airway is mandatory for success with this technique. After placement of this airway, the oropharynx is suctioned and mask ventilation is resumed. The FOB, loaded with an ET that has its 15-mm adapter removed, is advanced through the rubber diaphragm of the endoscopy port into the intubating airway and through the vocal cords into the trachea (Fig. 18-12).[165] The ET is threaded over the FOB through the endoscopy port and intubating airway into the trachea. After the FOB is removed, the endoscopy mask is disengaged from the ET and removed. The ET 15-mm adapter is now replaced and connected to the anesthesia circuit. Caution should be exercised to avoid accidental injury of face or eyes during placement of the ET adapter, which must be pushed into the ET securely.

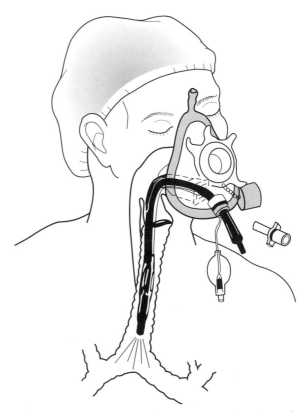

Figure 18-12 Intubation through endoscopy mask. Schematic diagram showing fiberoptic orotracheal intubation through endoscopy mask in an anesthetized and paralyzed patient. The fiberoptic bronchoscope and endotracheal tube (ET) have been introduced through the diaphragm in the endoscopy mask. After intubation, the fiberoptic bronchoscope is removed from within the ET and the endoscopy mask is removed over the ET. ET adapter is replaced and connected to anesthesia machine breathing system. (From Rogers SN, Benumof JL: New and easy techniques for fiberoptic endoscopy-aided tracheal intubation. Anesthesiology 59:569-572, 1983.)

It is also possible to use the endoscopy mask for nasotracheal intubation.[116] However, the length of an uncut ET threaded over the FOB may prevent placement of the tip of the FOB in the midtrachea without advancing the ET through the diaphragm of the endoscopy port. As soon as the ET is passed through the diaphragm, it opens the system and positive-pressure ventilation cannot be continued. Cutting the ET or using an FOB with an insertion cord length of 60 cm, such as the Olympus LF-2, allows the FOB tip to reach the midtrachea before the nasotracheal ET enters the endoscopy port, avoiding the problem with ventilation.

A modified endoscopy mask technique is another alternative to avoid this problem. This technique also protects the insertion cord of the FOB from damage that may be caused by the port of the mask and therefore may be used for oral intubations as well. For this modified method, the ET is prepared with its 15-mm adapter loosely attached to the ET for later easy disconnection. A bronchoscopy swivel adapter (SIMS Portex, Keene, NH) is mounted on the ET 15-mm adapter. The 15-mm side arm of the swivel adapter is blocked with tape. The prepared ET is lubricated and is passed through the diaphragm of the endoscopy mask port to a depth of approximately 10 cm (Fig. 18-13). Additional lubrication is applied to the distal end of the ET after it has passed through the diaphragm. Anesthesia is induced using a regular anesthesia mask. After achieving surgical depth of anesthesia and complete relaxation, the anesthesia mask is removed, an intubating airway is placed, and the oropharynx is suctioned. The endoscopy mask mounted with the ET is now placed over the face with the tip of the ET entering the airway. The anesthesia is continued with the endoscopy mask in place. The FOB is now advanced through the bronchoscopic port of the swivel adapter, through the ET into the oropharyngeal airway and into the trachea. The ET is advanced over the FOB into the trachea. The FOB

and both adapters are removed together, leaving the ET in place. The endoscopy mask is then disengaged from the ET and removed. The ET 15-mm adapter is reattached to the ET, completing the intubation process. For nasotracheal intubation, if the ET is placed into the endoscopy mask first, it may be impossible to manipulate the FOB tip into the nose; therefore, the ET with loosely attached adapters is mounted over the FOB before intubation. The breathing circuit remains closed when the ET passes through the endoscopy port.

5. Intubation Using a Nasal Airway

In the anesthetized and spontaneously breathing patient, anesthesia may be maintained through a nasopharyngeal airway to allow time for unhurried endotracheal intubation. For orotracheal intubation, a binasal airway is placed in the nostrils and connected to the anesthesia breathing system. An intubating airway is placed, and the FOB mounted with the ET is inserted through the airway to perform the intubation.[123] For nasotracheal intubation, a nasopharyngeal airway mounted with an ET adapter is inserted in one nostril.[112,203] The breathing circuit of the anesthesia machine is attached to the nasopharyngeal airway. The FOB mounted with the ET is passed through the other nostril to perform endotracheal intubation. With both the oral and the nasal approach, because the patient is breathing spontaneously and the level of anesthesia is maintained, more time is provided for intubation.

D. COMBINING FIBEROPTIC INTUBATION WITH OTHER INTUBATION OR AIRWAY MANAGEMENT TECHNIQUES

The FOB can be used in combination with other intubation or airway management techniques to overcome many difficult and seemingly impossible airways. The FOB can be used in combination with a rigid laryngoscope, laryngeal mask airway, or a Combitube. It can be used to improve the technique of a retrograde wire intubation or of a blind nasal intubation. Also, the principles of light wand intubation can be applied with an FOB.

1. Fiberoptic Intubation Aided by Rigid Laryngoscopy

In patients with an oropharyngeal mass, upper airway edema, or a posteriorly displaced epiglottis (because of a supraglottic mass or because the epiglottis is large and floppy), the passage of an FOB beneath the epiglottis to expose the glottic opening may be extremely difficult. Combining rigid laryngoscopy with fiberoptic intubation is helpful under these circumstances.[51,94,146,171]

The epiglottis is exposed using a rigid laryngoscope by a second anesthesiologist. By looking directly inside the mouth (not through the FOB), the first anesthesiologist passes the tip of the FOB under the epiglottis.[146] The tip

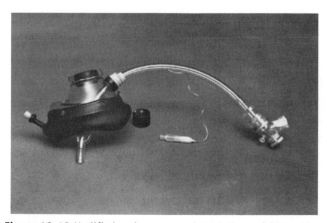

Figure 18-13 Modified endoscopy mask technique of fiberoptic intubation. Endoscopy mask mounted with endotracheal tube (ET) with loosely attached tracheal ET and bronchoscopy swivel adapters. (From Ovassapian A: Fiberoptic Airway Endoscopy in Anesthesia and Critical Care. New York, Raven Press, 1990.)

of the FOB can also be guided toward the glottis by the anesthesiologist who performs the rigid laryngoscopy while the first one is looking through the FOB.[51] If successful, this allows easy exposure of the vocal cords and advancement of the FOB into the trachea to complete the intubation.

The combined use of rigid and fiberoptic laryngoscopes is also helpful in changing an existing ET in a patient with a history of difficult intubation. Excessive pharyngeal soft tissue, edema of the airway, and a large volume of secretions are common in these patients and interfere with fiberoptic visualization of the larynx. Rigid laryngoscopy helps in exposing the supraglottic area and allows complete suctioning of secretions. In addition, a curved blade lifts the epiglottis, which may be embracing the ET, and allows passage of the FOB beneath the epiglottis. This is crucial for exposure of the anterior commissure and passage of the FOB into the trachea alongside an existing ET.[146]

2. Fiberoptic Intubation through the Laryngeal Mask Airway

The laryngeal mask airway (LMA) has become a routine airway management tool for the administration of general anesthesia.[27,155] Its ease and speed of insertion without the use of rigid laryngoscopy or muscle relaxants has prompted the anesthesiologist to use the laryngeal mask for management of the DA and failed intubation.* A number of case reports attest to the value of the LMA in failed intubation and in restoring artificial ventilation when it otherwise could not be achieved by bag and face mask.[5,10,28,34,39,131] The revised practice guidelines for management of the difficult airway recommend placement of the LMA when intubation and face mask ventilation have both failed.[156] Endotracheal intubation through the LMA has been successfully carried out in awake and anesthetized patients, using blind or fiberoptic-aided techniques.[22,29,30,38,52,56,58,96,120] Fiberoptic-aided techniques have the advantage of providing direct visualization of the larynx and therefore improve the success rate of intubation through the LMA (Fig. 18-14).

The LMA is placed, and breathing through the LMA is confirmed. An appropriate-sized ET and FOB are selected. A well-lubricated FOB loaded with an ET is advanced through the LMA.[22] The larynx is exposed, and the FOB is advanced into the trachea. The ET is threaded over the FOB into the trachea, and the cuff of the ET is inflated. The FOB is removed, and ventilation is carried out through the ET. At the conclusion of anesthesia the ET is removed first, allowing the patient to breath through the LMA until protective airway reflexes return. Then the LMA can be removed.

There are shortcomings of the LMA used as a guide for intubation. One is the limitation imposed on the size of the ET that can be placed. Another potential problem is the length of the ET and the possibility of intralaryngeal placement of the ET cuff. For example, the 6-mm cuffed ET is 28 cm in length. The length of a size 4 LMA is 19 cm, and the distance from the LMA grille to the vocal cords is 3.5 cm. This allows only 5 cm of the ET to go beyond the vocal cords.[11] As a result, the cuff of the ET may be inflated in the larynx rather than the trachea, and this may cause recurrent laryngeal nerve palsy. Removing the adapter of the LMA before intubation shortens the length of the LMA by 18 mm, which leads to deeper placement of the ET inside the trachea and may prevent this problem. This, however, eliminates the advantage of using the LMA to provide ventilation during fiberoptic intubation. A nasal Ring-Adair-Elwyn (RAE) tube has a greater length than a conventional ET by approximately 5 to 6 cm, and the use of this ET placed by FOB and by a ventilating bronchoscopic swivel adapter has been described to overcome these problems.[19,20,168] Occasionally, the added length may be too great and the proximal 2 cm may need to be trimmed before the ET can be safely and successfully placed.[19]

If removal of the LMA is desired, a "tube-in-tube" method has been suggested as another way to add sufficient length that the LMA can be safely removed without dislodging the ET.[40] This involves the placement of either one full size larger ET over the end of the ET used for intubation or one full size smaller ET inside the ET used for intubation. The 15-mm adapter is removed for both ETs. The LMA is withdrawn over the combined ET after successful fiberoptic intubation. The ET used for lengthening is removed and the 15-mm adapter replaced. An alternative is to place and exchange catheter or guidewire through the ET placed for intubation. The 15-mm adapter and LMA are removed while maintaining the position of the ET in the trachea. The 15-mm adapter is then replaced.

If an ET with a larger ID is desired, it may be changed to a larger size of ET with the help of an ET changer or the FOB. An alternative described by Hasham and colleagues[85] is to use the FOB to place a smaller ET through the LMA into the trachea to be used as a final intubation guide. An 8.5-mm ET is then railroaded over the "guide" ET and into the trachea.

The FOB has also been used through the LMA to place a guidewire into the trachea.[8,200] In one technique, the guidewire was used to place a ureteral catheter.[200] Correct placement was confirmed by detection of CO_2, and the LMA was then removed and the ureteral catheter used as a guide to pass the appropriately sized ET.[200] In the other report, a wire was placed with an FOB that was too large for the appropriately sized ET.[8] The LMA was left in place and the wire used as a guide for intubation.

---

*References 22, 28-30, 34, 38, 85, 87, 94, 96, 120, 131, 155.

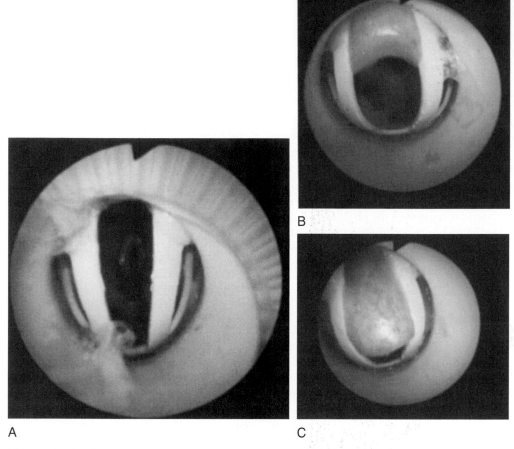

Figure 18-14 Endoscopic view through laryngeal mask airway (LMA). The fiberoptic bronchoscope is placed inside the LMA with the tip 2 cm away from the inside bars of the LMA. **A,** Perfect positioning of LMA. The epiglottis is out of view. Blind intubation through LMA is highly likely but still may fail, depending on the position of the tip of the endotracheal tube in relation to glottic anatomy. Fiberoptic intubation would be successful. **B,** The tip of epiglottis blocking half of the LMA distal opening. Blind endotracheal intubation may be successful; however, the chance of failure is great. Fiberoptic intubation would be successful. **C,** The epiglottis blocking more than 90% of the distal opening of the LMA. Blind endotracheal intubation through LMA not possible. Fiberoptic intubation is likely.

A Cook Retrograde Intubation Kit and FOB have also been used together to change the LMA to a larger conventional ET than could otherwise be placed.[7] This technique uses the FOB to place an exchange stylet through the LMA and into the trachea. The exchange stylet is superior to a conventional guidewire because of the added diameter and rigidity. This method allows the airway to be maintained until the LMA is exchanged with an ET. Anesthesia may be maintained and the airway instrumented without difficulty using this technique.[7]

Another approach to the ET size limitation of endotracheal intubation through the LMA is to split an LMA longitudinally. The cuff of the split LMA is sealed with silicone and the LMA shaft bound with micropore tape. The split, taped LMA is inserted and its cuff fully inflated.

Through this LMA a larger size of ET can be advanced into the trachea over the FOB.[52] The FOB mounted with the ET is passed through the LMA into the trachea. The LMA is then deflated. The tape is removed from the LMA and the ET threaded over the FOB through the LMA into the trachea.

The LMA-Fastrach was designed to overcome the limitations described for the classical LMA and to facilitate endotracheal intubation with larger ETs.[41,74] Differences from the classical LMA are a larger, shorter, more rigid barrel; a mobile rather than a fixed epiglottic bar; and a rigid handle to facilitate one-handed manipulation. Either a blind or a fiberoptic-assisted technique may be used to complete intubation. A purpose-specific ET and intubation guide come with each LMA-Fastrach. It is available only in sizes 3, 4, and 5, so it cannot be used for children smaller than 30 kg.

3. Fiberoptic Endotracheal Intubation with a Combitube in Place

When endotracheal intubation has failed and mask ventilation is impossible, other approaches may be taken to establish ventilation to avoid anoxic brain damage. The esophageal-tracheal double-lumen ET (Combitube) is one such device that is recommended for rapid establishment of ventilation.[70] The Combitube provides ventilation whether it is placed in the esophagus (common) or in the trachea (uncommon). The Combitube is placed blindly, and more than 90% of the time it enters the esophagus. Ventilation is achieved through the pharyngeal lumen of the airway while the esophageal cuff blocks the air entry into the esophagus and the pharyngeal cuff seals the upper airway. With the Combitube in the esophagus, suctioning of the trachea is not possible. The Combitube is also not recommended for prolonged mechanical ventilation. Replacement of the Combitube with an ET is necessary to avoid possible complications, to provide a more secure airway, and to have access to the trachea for suctioning.

In a series of 14 patients, fiberoptic intubation of the trachea was attempted in the presence of a Combitube.[144] Endotracheal intubation was successful in 12 patients. In one patient the fiberoptic intubation failed because of poor relaxation, and in the other the Combitube was removed before intubation was completed. The Combitube often elevates the epiglottis, making fiberoptic exposure of the vocal cords easy. However, because of the large diameter of the Combitube, manipulation of the FOB can be difficult. Combination of blind placement of the Combitube followed by fiberoptic endotracheal intubation has been described for management of the DA.[76]

4. Fiberoptic-Assisted "Blind Nasal" Intubation

The FOB can be used in two different ways to assist in completion of a difficult or failed blind nasotracheal intubation. When the size of the nasal passage prohibits passage of the FOB through the nasotracheal ET, the FOB may be introduced through the contralateral nostril to visualize the position of the tip of the ET and assist in its passage through the vocal cords.[3] Under visual observation, the nasotracheal ET and the patient's head are manipulated to direct the nasotracheal ET toward the larynx.

In some patients with a distorted and compromised airway, blind nasotracheal intubation and fiberoptic exposure of the glottis may fail independently. A combination of blind nasal and fiberoptic intubation techniques may prove successful. The nasotracheal ET is advanced blindly, gently, and slowly while the practitioner is listening to the breath sounds of the spontaneously breathing patient. The advancement of the ET is stopped when the breath sounds are loudest. At this position the tip of the ET is

a short distance from the glottic opening, and the ET has passed beyond the distorted obstructed airway. Passage of a lubricated FOB through the nasotracheal ET brings the tip of the FOB close to the glottis. The epiglottis and the glottic opening are easily identified. The FOB is advanced into the trachea and followed by the nasotracheal ET to complete intubation.

5. Fiberoptic-Assisted Retrograde Guidewire Intubation

A guidewire introduced through the cricothyroid membrane may be used to direct the FOB toward the glottis and trachea when attempts at conventional retrograde technique of intubation have failed. Two different principles have been applied for completion of retrograde intubation with the FOB. First, the ET that cannot be advanced over the guidewire into the larynx is left in place. The FOB is inserted into the ET and is advanced alongside the guidewire past the end of the ET and beyond the entrance of the guidewire into the trachea. When the position of the FOB is assured in the lower trachea, the guidewire is removed and the ET is threaded over the FOB into the trachea.[18] The second approach is to pass the guidewire in a retrograde fashion through the suction channel of an FOB that is mounted with an ET. The FOB is guided and advanced over the guidewire into the trachea. The wire is removed, and the ET is threaded over the FOB into the trachea.[107]

6. Use of the Fiberscope as a Light Wand

The light wand is a lighted stylet with a bright light on its tip and is applied for blind endotracheal intubation. The light wand is loaded with the ET and is advanced blindly toward the trachea. Strong transillumination of the anterior neck confirms its entrance into the trachea, at which time the ET is railroaded over the stylet into the trachea. If the light wand is not advanced enough to reach the larynx or if it enters the esophagus, the light is not transmitted through the anterior neck. When the light wand is off center, the light is detected on the lateral aspect of the larynx in the lateral neck.

The FOB has a strong light and can be used as a light wand to enter the trachea by observing the distribution of the light on the anterior neck. This approach may prevent failure of fiberoptic intubation when copious secretions or blood interferes with visualization of the airway anatomy. We have used this approach on a few occasions, and it has also been described by others.[209] The FOB loaded with the ET is passed through the intubating airway toward the larynx. While jaw thrust is applied, the FOB is advanced, first keeping its distal tip straight to facilitate its passage beneath the epiglottis and then deflecting it anteriorly to enter the larynx. The position of the transilluminated light on the neck dictates the maneuvers necessary to enter the trachea.

IV. FIBEROPTIC INTUBATION IN CHILDREN AND INFANTS

The technique of fiberoptic endoscopy for airway management in the adult patient is well established. Less frequently discussed are the uses of fiberoptic endoscopy for the management of the pediatric airway. This is unfortunate because the difficult pediatric airway can be a frightening and challenging experience for any anesthesiologist, and any technique that can be added to our airway management skills should be understood and used. In particular, with the introduction of ultrathin fiberoptic endoscopes that have directable tips (LF-P, Olympus Optical Co. [Europa] GmbH, Hamburg, Germany), even preterm neonates requiring ETs as small as 2.5 mm ID are not excluded from the option of a fiberoptic approach to airway management.

Other FOBs for use in older patients are also available. A pediatric FOB with the light source incorporated into the body of the scope, the LF-DP, is larger than the LF-P (3.1 mm outer diameter) and has a working channel (1.2 mm ID). It can accommodate an ET as small as 3.5 mm ID. Karl Storz Company (Tuttlingen, Germany) has developed an FOB for pediatric endotracheal intubation that integrates a Micro-Video-Module into the fiberoptic scope (11301 AAN). This is similar to their adult FOB. An FOB that is identical except that it incorporates an eyepiece is also available. These scopes have working channels (1.2 mm internal diameter) and have a 2.8 mm external diameter so that they can accommodate an ET as small as 3.5 mm ID.

All indications for fiberoptic endoscopic airway management in adult patients can also be applied to pediatric patients. However, conditions that are more frequently or are exclusively found in the pediatric population warrant special mention. Conditions that are unique to or more common in children and are associated with DA fall into the following broad categories: (1) acquired pathology and (2) congenital syndromes and hereditary diseases (Boxes 18-3 and 18-4). Fiberoptic endoscopic airway management for some of these conditions has been described in the literature.*

Although airway management is potentially adversely affected in any of these syndromes, some generalizations can be made about the type of problem each may present. Many conditions that predispose to a DA in children (airway obstruction or difficult laryngoscopy) are best managed by fiberoptic intubation. For example, because this technique does not require extensive head or neck manipulation, it is useful for patients who have either cervical inflexibility (Klippel-Feil syndrome) or instability (Down syndrome, achondroplastic dwarfism, trauma).

---

*References 3, 9, 13, 16, 25, 33, 66, 79, 104, 123, 124, 167, 170, 173, 193, 205, 210.

> **Box 18-3   Acquired Pathology Associated with Difficult Airway**
>
> Infection: epiglottitis, upper airway abscess
> Obesity
> Trauma and burns
> Tumors and masses: upper and lower airways

Patients with micrognathia (Pierre Robin sequence, Treacher Collins syndrome, Goldenhar syndrome) may be impossible to intubate by rigid laryngoscopy because the tongue cannot be compressed into the small mandibular space. Fiberoptic intubation does not depend on this displacement and therefore can be successfully performed in these patients. Also, fiberoptic intubation is well tolerated by the awake, sedated, and spontaneously breathing patient; therefore, it is a useful technique for patients who may be difficult or impossible to ventilate by mask (mucopolysaccharidoses).[146] These pathologies and others that are associated with a DA in children are reviewed extensively elsewhere.[33,97,205]

A. SEDATION OF CHILDREN FOR FIBEROPTIC INTUBATION

Traditionally, the approach to the anticipated DA in adults is to place the ET and secure the airway while the patient is awake but with topical anesthesia and conscious sedation. Commonly applied in adults, a benzodiazepine and narcotic combination is also quite effective for adolescents and mature preteens. For pediatric usage, dosing is based on weight but also guided by clinical parameters, including preexisting medical conditions that may affect sensitivity to these medications. An advantage of opioids and benzodiazepines is that each class has a reversal agent. However, for an already frightened young child or older child or adolescent who is intellectually impaired, benzodiazepine-opioid sedation may be difficult; enough sedation to ensure compliance with securing the airway may be too much to preserve adequate spontaneous ventilation. There are, however, safe and effective alternatives to the benzodiazepine-narcotic combinations (Box 18-5). Remifentanil has been described both for sedation for painful procedures in children[111] and as an adjunct to fiberoptic intubation.[160,161,164] Experience using this drug for sedation should be gained in patients with normal airways prior to attempting this technique in patients with potentially DAs. The advantages and disadvantages of this medication as an adjunct to fiberoptic intubation have yet to be examined in a controlled clinical trial.

Ketamine is a potent hypnotic and analgesic agent that produces a "dissociative" anesthetic.[81] In most circumstances, ketamine preserves adequate spontaneous ventilation while providing sufficient anesthesia to prevent

Box 18-4   Congenital Syndromes and Hereditary Diseases Associated with Difficult Airway

Micrognathia and Mandibular Hypoplasia
Achondrogenesis, types I and II
Branchio-oculo-facial syndrome
Campomelic dysplasia
Carpenter's syndrome
Cat-eye syndrome
Catel-Manzke syndrome
Cerebrocostomandibular syndrome
Cerebro-ocular-facio-skeletal (COFS) syndrome
Cheney's syndrome
Christ-Siemens-Touraine syndrome
Cri du chat syndrome
Cornelia de Lange syndrome
DiGeorge's syndrome
Dubowitz syndrome
Edwards' syndrome (trisomy 18)
Escobar syndrome
Frontometaphyseal dysplasia
Fryns syndrome
Goldenhar's syndrome
Hallermann-Streiff syndrome
King-Denborough syndrome
Langer-Giedion syndrome
Langer mesomelic dysplasia
Lenz-Majewski hyperostosis syndrome
Letterer-Siwe disease
Marshall-Smith syndrome
Marden-Walker syndrome
Meckel-Gruber syndrome
Melnick-Needles syndrome
Miller syndrome
Möbius' syndrome
Nager syndrome
Noonan syndrome
Oculo-auricular-vertebral spectrum
Opitz syndrome
Oral-facial-digital syndrome
Oto-palatal-digital syndrome, type I
Osteochondrodystrophies (dwarfism)
Patau syndrome (trisomy 13)
Pierre Robin sequence
Roberts-SC phocomelia
Robinow syndrome
Rubinstein-Taybi syndrome
Russell-Silver syndrome
Schwartz-Jampel syndrome
Seckel syndrome
Smith-Lemli-Opitz syndrome
Stickler syndrome
Treacher Collins syndrome
Turner syndrome
Yunis-Varon syndrome

Macroglossia
Alpha-thalassemia
Beckwith-Wiedemann syndrome
Down syndrome (trisomy 21)
Farber's disease
Hurler's syndrome (mucopolysaccharidosis, type I)
Pompe's disease (glycogen storage disease, type II)
Cervical Instability or Limited Cervical Mobility
Aarskog syndrome
Achondroplasia
Acrodysostosis
Aicardi syndrome
Arnold-Chiari malformation
Atelosteogenesis
Baller-Gerold syndrome
Cervico-oculo-acoustic syndrome
Down syndrome (see macroglossia)
Frontometaphyseal dysplasia
Hurler's syndrome (see macroglossia)
Klippel-Feil sequence
Larsen syndrome
Marfan syndrome
Maroteaux-Lamy syndrome (mucopolysaccharidosis, type VI)
Morquio's syndrome (mucopolysaccharidosis, type IV)
Osteochondrodystrophies (dwarfism)
Oto-palatal-digital syndrome, type II
Pallister-Hall syndrome
Peters-plus syndrome
Syndromes Affecting Temporomandibular Joint and/or Limited Mouth Opening
Arthrogryposis
Behçet's syndrome
Cockayne-Touraine syndrome (dystrophic epidermolysis bullae)
CREST syndrome
Epidermolysis bullosum
Freeman-Sheldon syndrome (whistling face)
Hecht syndrome
Juvenile rheumatoid arthritis (Still's disease)
Myositis ossificans
Nager syndrome
Rapp-Hodgkin ectodermal dysplasia
Scleroderma
Treacher Collins syndrome
Xeroderma pigmentosa
Midface Hypoplasia and Prominent or Abnormal Mandible
Andersen's syndrome
Antley-Bixler syndrome
Apert's syndrome
Crouzon syndrome

Box 18-4   Congenital Syndromes and Hereditary Diseases Associated with Difficult Airway—cont'd

Midface Hypoplasia and Prominent or Abnormal Mandible—cont'd
Frontonasal dysplasia sequence
Hallermann-Streiff syndrome
Oral-facial-digital syndrome
Oto-palatal-digital syndrome, type I
Pfeiffer's syndrome
Rieger's syndrome
Schinzel-Giedion syndrome
Obstructing Mass
Cherubism (tumors)
Encephalocele
Farber's disease (tumors of larynx; see macroglossia)
Kasabach-Merritt syndrome (hemangioma)
Letterer-Siwe disease (laryngeal fibrosis; see micrognathia)
Neurofibromatosis (fibroma)

Stevens-Johnson syndrome (bullae)
Sturge-Weber syndrome (hemangioma)
Enlarged Mandible or Distortion of Facial Features
Fragile X syndrome
Gaucher disease
Hunter's syndrome
Hurler's syndrome
Hurler-Scheie syndrome
Hypomelanosis of Ito
Maroteaux-Lamy syndrome
Morquio's syndrome
Pyle's disease
Saethre-Chotzen syndrome
Sanfilippo's syndrome (mucopolysaccharidosis, type III)
Scheie syndrome
Sotos' syndrome (cerebral gigantism)

CREST, calcinosis cutis, Raynaud's phenomenon, esophageal dysfunction, sclerodactyly, and telangiectasia.

---

reaction to airway manipulation. These characteristics make it a reasonable choice for sedation of the infant, the young child, or the mentally delayed older child or adolescent. It may be used alone or in conjunction with midazolam. However, careful titration of the dose is essential because ketamine has been documented to cause apnea in a healthy pediatric patient[184] and there are no reversal agents. An attractive feature of ketamine is that it has many routes for administration. If an intravenous line is difficult or impossible to obtain, a small intramuscular, intranasal, oral, or rectal dose can be effectively used for heavy sedation. However, caution is required with the use of any sedative provided before securing intravenous access in a patient with a potential DA. As soon as possible, an intravenous line should be secured, and further sedation, if necessary, may be given intravenously.

Ketamine has not been widely used in adult anesthesia because of the associated high incidence of psychomimetic emergence reactions.[81] However, these reactions are less common in children,[88] particularly if ketamine is combined with midazolam.[37] Ketamine can produce increased upper airway secretions, which might interfere with fiberoptic airway management; therefore, a preoperative antisialagogue in conjunction with preendoscopy suctioning of the airway is strongly recommended. There are anecdotal reports of "hyperreactive" airway reflexes when ketamine is used. However, adequate ketamine or ketamine-midazolam doses combined with good suctioning and skilled endoscopy techniques are the best defense against airway reactivity. In fact, ketamine is a commonly described anesthetic agent for fiberoptic airway management in children with DAs, and no problems with increased airway reactivity have been noted.[4,50,89,159]

Propofol infusion titrated to provide a more profound degree of sedation but to maintain spontaneous ventilation is another anesthetic option.[117] The technique is tricky, however, and advanced experience is required because of the risk of oversedation and apnea. Propofol has the advantage of quick awakening after the infusion is discontinued, unlike titrated doses of ketamine. A disadvantage shared with ketamine is the lack of a specific reversal agent.

General anesthesia with maintenance of spontaneous ventilation is an alternative when abnormal airway anatomy is present and difficulty with the patient's cooperation is anticipated. However, the risks of apnea, laryngospasm, and loss of the airway must be carefully considered before general anesthesia is attempted. Both inhalational and intravenous induction and maintenance techniques have been described.[15,113,196] A slow and careful inhalation induction with halothane may provide better intubating conditions than sevoflurane,[133] although sevoflurane has been advocated and used successfully in this setting.[65,98,125,183,196,201] Controlled ventilation is gradually assumed, and this ensures that the child's airway can be managed by mask. If mask ventilation is easily

---

Box 18-5   Sedation for Fiberoptic Intubation in Pediatrics

Ketamine 0.5 mg/kg, intravenous (IV) in incremental doses
Midazolam 10-20 µg/kg, IV in incremental doses
Fentanyl 0.5 µg/kg, IV in incremental doses
Remifentanil 0.1 µg/kg/min, IV infusion
Propofol 0.5-2 mg/kg, IV bolus; 150-300 µg/kg/min, IV infusion

performed, a muscle relaxant can be given and fiberoptic intubation begun. This approach obviates any risk of laryngospasm or of sudden movement of the patient, which can occur with sedation or light anesthesia, with preserved spontaneous ventilation. However, time for each fiberoptic attempt for intubation is decreased because of the patient's apnea. Muscle relaxation also changes upper airway dynamics and patency, and thus mask ventilation may be adversely affected or may become impossible. If the use of a muscle relaxant is inadvisable and maintaining spontaneous ventilation increases the patient's safety, 4% lidocaine should be sprayed on the vocal cords to prevent or minimize the incidence and severity of laryngospasm before the FOB is advanced into the trachea.

B. TOPICAL ANESTHESIA: SPECIAL CONSIDERATIONS

For endotracheal intubation under sedation, topical anesthesia of the airway improves patients' acceptance, prevents laryngospasm, and increases the success rate by decreasing airway reflexes. For fiberoptic intubation under general anesthesia with spontaneous ventilation preserved, topical anesthesia is also important to minimize airway reflexes.

In general, all techniques for application of local anesthetic that are used in adults may be used in children, with a few caveats. One should keep in mind the smaller size of the patient and the subsequent restrictions on the volumes and amount of local anesthetic that can be used. Also, Cetacaine spray and Americaine ointment, because they contain the ingredient benzocaine, may cause methemoglobinemia in infants; it is best to avoid using them in children who are smaller than 40 kg.[91] Translaryngeal injection is technically difficult in infants younger than 6 months and therefore should be avoided in these children.

Nebulized lidocaine has been used successfully in adults and children.[26,77] Many children have used nebulizers in the treatment of asthma or bronchospastic disease and therefore readily accept the lidocaine nebulizer. A suggested dosing schedule for nebulized lidocaine is presented in Table 18-2.

C. PEDIATRIC FIBEROPTIC INTUBATION

Any fiberoptic technique is more successful if a preoperative antisialagogue is administered either intramuscularly or intravenously before proceeding with the fiberoptic intubation. Except for intubation of the older child or adolescent under conscious sedation, an assistant is necessary to aid in the safe monitoring of the patient and to provide jaw thrust. Jaw thrust is necessary to elevate the tongue off the posterior pharynx and facilitate visualization of the vocal cords.

Endoscopy masks can be used to provide oxygen to the spontaneously breathing patient and to ventilate the paralyzed patient during fiberoptic laryngoscopy. The Frei endoscopy mask (VBM Medizintechnik GmbH, Sulz,

Table 18-2 Lidocaine Nebulizer: Suggested Doses for Children

Patient Weight (kg)	4% Lidocaine (mL)	Normal Saline (%)
10-14	0.5	2
15-19	1.0	2
20-24	1.5	3
25-29	2.0	4
30-34	2.5	—
35-39	3.0	—
40-44	3.5	—
45 and up	4.0	—

Germany) and the Patil-Syracuse endoscopy masks (Anesthesia Associates, San Marcos, CA) are commercially available. The Patil-Syracuse masks are available in a size for children but are too large for most children younger than 4 years. Masks similar to the commercially available endoscopic mask designed by Frei can also be made using a disposable face mask. A hole is drilled in the back of the disposable mask and a piece of corrugated tubing that has a 15-mm adapter at its proximal end is affixed to the mask at the site of the hole. This tubing can then be attached to the anesthesia circuit. A silicon diaphragm is attached to the mask over the usual site for circuit attachment. A slit is made in this diaphragm to allow passage of the FOB. Once the FOB has been successfully positioned in the airway, the diaphragm is removed to allow passage of the ET. This mask configuration allows the FOB to be placed in a central position, overlying the nose and mouth, which is more favorable for intubation.[71,72]

Another pediatric anesthesia mask suitable for fiberoptic intubation has been described.[102] This mask is made by modifying a commercially available disposable mask that has a ventilation port (Vent port) on its side. The authors added a large fiberoptic port (22 mm ID) in the middle of the mask to allow the passage of all sizes of pediatric ETs. This fiberoptic port was covered with an elastic rubber membrane to allow fiberscopic manipulation under continuous manual ventilation through Vent port connected to the breathing circuit. Fiberoptic intubation, mainly nasotracheal, was performed safely through the port in several infants and children with DA.[102] Another alternative is to combine a disposable face mask with a bronchoscopic swivel adapter.[213] The FOB can then be passed through the diaphragm of the adapter while ventilation is maintained by the anesthesia circuit. It should be noted that intubation through a face mask may be more difficult than direct intubation without the face mask. The face mask may impede full range of motion of the FOB or mandate angles of approach that may be more difficult to negotiate.

As with adults, the LMA can be useful as a guide for fiberoptic intubation.[5,96,150] Several of the techniques previously described were developed for intubation of children with a DA.[8,200] The use of the FOB for intubation through the LMA rather than attempts at blind intubation is supported by several studies that found that in children (especially neonates with a size 1 LMA placed) the epiglottis is frequently overlying the glottis even when there is no evidence of airway obstruction.[58,78,199] The incidence of overlying epiglottis is also particularly high in children with mucopolysaccharidoses.[199] This overlying epiglottis can impede the blind placement of an ET.[96] Because of this problem, the FOB has been used for direct ET placement,[62] for guidewire placement,[8,200] and to ensure correct placement of the LMA prior to blind placement of an ET.[176]

Commercial oral airways are available for use in pediatric patients (VBM Medizintechnik GmbH, Sulz, Germany); however, there are only three sizes (infant, child, and adult) and no studies have evaluated their usefulness in assisting fiberoptic intubation in children. Guedel airways can also be modified for use as an oral intubation guide.[213] A strip is cut from the convex surface of the airway to create a channel for placement of the FOB. This modified airway may be used to maintain a midline approach to the glottis, but it is ineffective as a bite block.

1. Single-Stage Intubation

The single-stage intubation or routine technique is the traditional adult technique as described previously in this chapter. This is the method of choice if a small, directable-tip FOB is available. For example, the Olympus LF-P directable-tip FOB, which has an external diameter of 1.8 mm, may be used in ETs as small as 2.5 mm ID.

Preparation for fiberoptic intubation should include checking the FOB, light source, and related supplies as well as preparation of rigid laryngoscopy equipment, masks, circuit, appropriate drugs, ETs, and stylets. Some small FOBs have no suction channel, and the regular suction catheter is used to clear the oropharyngeal secretions. The suction control port of the catheter is blocked by tape to make it suitable for one-hand operation.

As discussed for adults, a method for delivering supplemental oxygen should also be available. The patient should be positioned in an appropriate fashion to ensure the greatest possibility of success. The body should be positioned with the arms tucked on either side. A strap should be placed over the legs. For infants, a "papoosing" technique is useful. A small blanket or towel is folded so that it is the width of the patient's body and approximately three times the length. The infant is placed on the blanket and the length of the blanket is tucked over each arm and then under the body. This technique keeps arms restrained but maintains free excursion of the chest and abdomen. Head position should be neutral or extended rather than sniffing because the neutral or extended position ensures

a better angle for visualization of the larynx with the FOB.[180]

To begin fiberoptic laryngoscopy, thread an ET that is sized appropriately for the patient's age onto the FOB. Stand at the head of the patient as one would for rigid laryngoscopy. Hold the FOB with the left hand as one would a rigid laryngoscope. Use the right hand to guide the insertion cord. To facilitate fiberoptic laryngoscopy, an assistant should perform a jaw thrust to open the posterior pharyngeal space. Alternatively, a bite block or intubating airway may be used to keep the tongue away from the pharyngeal wall and create a space in which to direct the FOB. Direct forward traction on the tongue, which optimally opens the posterior pharyngeal space, may be required in some patients. The tongue may be pulled forward by grasping it firmly with disposable sponge forceps or gauze pad. In some cases, a tongue suture may be required so that adequate traction can be applied.

In contrast to the approach in adults, the FOB is usually passed into the airway before passing the ET through the nose or oropharynx. This prevents interference with motion of the FOB and the directable tip and, in the case of nasal intubation, decreases the likelihood of epistaxis prior to visualization of the vocal cords. The tip of the FOB should be introduced behind the tongue, in the midline, and gradually advanced under direct vision until a recognizable anatomic structure is observed. To maintain midline position during an oral approach, the right hand is rested on the patient's face to keep the insertion cord of the FOB at the midpoint of the mouth. Particularly in neonates and small infants, the fingers of the right hand may need to be placed inside the mouth to hold the FOB in the midline position.

Because the pediatric vocal cords are angled and the trachea is directed posteriorly,[60] it may be difficult to pass the FOB tip through the cords and into the trachea unless the glottis is approached directly. To achieve this direct approach, it is vital that the FOB be passed in the midline and that the insertion cord be kept straight to minimize looping. Keeping the insertion cord straight is also important to maintain orientation in the airways. Using this method, when the FOB is rotated, the tip should rotate in the same direction. The right hand, which is guiding the insertion cord, should not grip too tightly or rotation of the cord will be impossible. Because the airway distances in children are shorter than in adults, the most common initial error for those with experience in adult fiberoptic intubation is to advance the FOB too deeply and into the esophagus. To avoid this pitfall, the FOB should not be advanced until identifiable airway structures are seen. The depth of anesthesia or sedation as well as oxygen saturation must be carefully monitored throughout the procedure.

The narrowest portion of the airway in children is the circular cricoid cartilage, in contrast to the elliptical glottic opening in adults. The circular shape of the cricoid cartilage allows uncuffed ETs to fit without excessive leak.

When an uncuffed ET is used, a larger ID tube, which has reduced resistance, can be placed. Thus, uncuffed tubes are commonly chosen for intubation of children. However, the use of uncuffed ETs creates a problem unique to children: inability to ventilate or protect the airway effectively after ET placement because the inserted ET is too small. One solution is to use an ET changer to switch to an ET a half-size larger. The FOB can then be used to confirm the correct placement of the new ET. As an alternative, the FOB can be loaded with the new ET and the tip directed to the larynx to the side of the previously placed ET. An assistant can then withdraw the old ET as the FOB is directed through the glottis. The new ET is then advanced into the trachea and the FOB removed as usual. If appropriate, the problem may be avoided altogether by using a small cuffed ET for the first attempt.

The single-stage or routine technique of fiberoptic intubation may also be used with a nasal rather than an oral approach, but one must be aware of the possibility of sheared adenoid tissue and subsequent bleeding. This is of particular concern in children between 2 and 6 years of age, when adenoid tissue is often hypertrophied. In general, there is no clear advantage to the nasal approach, although some practitioners believe that the midline approach is more easily maintained and the view of the larynx more direct with the nasal approach. The oral approach with good jaw thrust is easily performed, and the potential problems of shearing adenoid tissue and of creating a nasal bleed are avoided. If a nasal approach is used in young children, phenylephrine or oxymetazoline drops may be used to vasoconstrict the nasal passages. This may ease placement and decrease the possibility of bleeding. Another method to reduce nasal trauma is sequential introduction of increasing sizes of small flexible nasopharyngeal airways to dilate the nasal passages gently. Softening the ET in warm water also decreases nasal trauma.

2. Two-Stage Intubation

The two-stage intubation technique is used in infants and small children when the FOBs that are available are too large to pass through the appropriately sized ET. In the original technique described by Stiles,[188] a standard cardiac catheter and guidewire with the proximal connector removed were used. An FOB with a working channel is required for this technique. The cardiac catheter guidewire is passed through the working channel of the FOB to within 1 inch of its distal portion. The FOB is then introduced into the mouth and positioned at the top of the vocal cords. The guidewire is then advanced under direct observation through the glottis into the trachea. The FOB is removed, leaving the guidewire in place. The patient then receives mask ventilation while an assistant passes the cardiac catheter over the guidewire. The cardiac catheter is used to stiffen the guidewire, facilitating passage of the ET over the guidewire and into the trachea. The catheter

guidewire combination is then removed, leaving the ET in the trachea. This technique has been used for the intubation of an infant with Pierre Robin syndrome.[173] However, those authors found that threading of the cardiac catheter over the guidewire was an unnecessary step and that the 3.5-mm ID ET could be passed directly over the guidewire into the trachea without difficulty.

A modification for a spontaneously breathing patient utilized an ET as a nasopharyngeal airway through which oxygen was delivered.[8] If the FOB has no working channel, an 8 Fr red rubber catheter can be attached by waterproof tape to the insertion cord of the FOB.[69] The larynx is visualized in the usual fashion, and then a cardiac catheter guidewire is threaded through the rubber catheter into the trachea. With the guidewire in position, the FOB is withdrawn and an ET passed into the trachea over the guidewire.

3. Three-Stage Intubation

A three-stage fiberoptic intubation technique for infants has been described.[52] This approach is another alternative that can be used when the FOB is too large and lacks a working channel. For this technique, an ET that is larger than the larynx of the infant is advanced over the FOB and positioned on top of the vocal cords. The FOB is then removed, and an ET changer or catheter is advanced into the trachea through the ET. The larger ET is then removed and the appropriate-sized ET is threaded over the ET changer or catheter into the trachea. This technique was used successfully in a 6-month-old infant whose operation had been previously canceled because of failure to intubate.[25]

4. Intubation under Fiberoptic Observation

This technique is an alternative that can be used for nasotracheal intubation when the available FOB is too large to pass through the appropriate-sized ET. In this technique the FOB is introduced through one naris while the ET is passed through the second naris. The ET is manipulated into the glottis while the glottis and the tip of the ET are observed through the FOB.[3] As an alternative, if the observed ET is not easily passed into the glottis, a small catheter may be more easily manipulated into the glottic entry and then used as a guide over which the ET can be passed.[79] A disadvantage of these techniques is that a minimum of two people and ideally a third person are needed. One person would perform the fiberoptic laryngoscopy to expose the larynx and ET, a second person would hold and manipulate the head of the patient, and the third person would manipulate the ET or catheter into the larynx. These techniques were used successfully in two neonates; one had congenital fusion of the jaws, and the other had Dandy-Walker syndrome associated with Klippel-Feil syndrome, micrognathia, hypoplasia of the soft palate, and anteversion of the uvula.[3,79]

V. FIBEROPTIC ENDOTRACHEAL TUBE EXCHANGE

It may be necessary to replace an ET for a variety of reasons (Box 18-6).[2] Before changing an ET, four basic steps should be followed. First, the patient should be evaluated to verify the necessity of changing the ET. Second, the route of intubation should be decided, either oral or nasal. Third, the technique for ET changing should be decided. Fourth, all necessary equipment should be secured and an assistant enlisted before beginning the procedure (Box 18-7). The route of intubation (oral or nasal) is often optional but may be mandated by the patient's condition and the reason for ET change.[2]

Several techniques may be used for changing an ET: an airway exchange catheter, rigid laryngoscopy, and fiberoptic laryngoscopy (see Chapter 47).[2,146] The airway exchange catheter may be used when the route of intubation remains the same. Both the rigid laryngoscope and the FOB can be used for ET changing that maintains the same route or when the route of intubation is changed. The most common technique is direct rigid laryngoscopy because all anesthesiologists are familiar and experienced with it.[2]

When the use of a rigid laryngoscope is technically difficult or may be hazardous, fiberoptic ET change may be advantageous. Patients with acute ventilatory failure who

---

Box 18-6   Indications for Changing an Endotracheal Tube

I. Problems with ventilation
   A. Blockade of the endotracheal tube by secretions, blood, foreign material
   B. Endotracheal tube kink
   C. Broken cuff
   D. Cuff leak from too short an endotracheal tube (laryngeal placement)
   E. Endotracheal tube too small (pediatric uncuffed tube)
II. Patient-related indications
   A. Sinusitis complicating nasal intubation
   B. Endotracheal tube too short (laryngeal placement with potential trauma)
   C. Change orotracheal to nasotracheal endotracheal tube for patient's comfort
III. Procedure-related indications
   A. Endotracheal tube too small for bronchoscopy or major surgery
   B. Change single-lumen to double-lumen endotracheal tube for thoracotomy
   C. Change double-lumen to single-lumen endotracheal tube for postoperative ventilatory support

---

Box 18-7   Steps and Techniques for Changing an Endotracheal Tube

1. Evaluation and verification of the need for endotracheal tube change
   Immediate (emergent)
   Urgent
   Nonurgent
2. Determination of the route of intubation
   Unchanged
   Change from oral to nasal route
   Change from nasal to oral route
3. Determination of the technique for endotracheal tube changing
   Direct rigid laryngoscopy
   Airway exchange catheter
   Fiberoptic laryngoscopy

---

require high positive end-expiratory pressure (PEEP) (10 to 20 cm H_2O) to maintain a minimum acceptable PaO_2 decompensate very quickly when mechanical ventilation and high PEEP are disrupted. Mask ventilation with 100% oxygen is usually ineffective to maintain or improve the PaO_2 in these patients. The removal of the existing ET, followed by a failure to reintubate immediately, may be extremely dangerous. In this type of patient, the FOB can be positioned through the vocal cords and beside the ET prior to its removal. This ensures rapid ET replacement, minimizing the chance of airway loss and ventilatory failure.

Fiberoptic ET change may also be preferred when accidental esophageal intubation must be avoided. For example, in patients who have undergone esophagectomy with a gastric pull-up, esophageal intubation must be avoided to prevent potential trauma at the site of the anastomosis. Although use of the FOB does not guarantee avoidance of inadvertent esophageal intubation, it minimizes the incidence of such occurrences. Two other groups of patients who may benefit from fiberoptic ET change are patients with a known difficult intubation and patients with an unstable cervical spine.

A. CHANGE OF AN ORAL TO A NASAL ENDOTRACHEAL TUBE

The first use of FOB to change an ET was reported in 1981.[166] If the patient is conscious, the procedure is explained and the patient's cooperation is secured. An antisialagogue is administered intravenously or intramuscularly 15 to 30 minutes before ET change to minimize secretions. A narcotic is included with intravenous sedation to assist in suppression of the pharyngeal and laryngeal reflexes. The nasal mucosa is anesthetized and a vasoconstrictor applied. An ET, softened by placement in warm water, is lubricated with a clear, water-soluble lubricant.

It is then inserted into the nose and advanced into the oropharynx. The tracheal ET cuff is rechecked to ensure that it is intact. The pharynx is thoroughly suctioned, and the FOB is advanced through the nasal ET into the pharynx. All secretions are suctioned, and 4 to 5 mL of 4% lidocaine is sprayed over the larynx to provide topical anesthesia. After 2 to 3 minutes, the airway is suctioned. An assistant applies jaw thrust or helps pull the tongue forward. The goals are to advance the FOB alongside the existing ET into the trachea and position the tip of the FOB just above the carina. Positioning the tip of the FOB just above the carina prevents accidental extubation of the FOB during removal of the existing ET.

An orally placed ET occupies the posterior half of the larynx and lies against the arytenoids and interarytenoid muscle, leaving the anterior portion of the glottis open. The FOB is maneuvered so that its tip will be placed anterior to the existing ET to bring the anterior commissure of the larynx into view (Fig. 18-15).[146] The FOB is advanced into the larynx and trachea until the ET cuff is identified. The cuff is deflated, and the FOB is advanced beyond it to 2 to 3 cm above the carina. The tape is removed from the existing ET and, while the operator is looking through the FOB to ensure that the FOB tip stays close to the carina, the assistant pulls out the existing ET. As soon as the oral ET is out of the larynx, the new nasal ET is threaded over the FOB into the trachea. The FOB is removed, and ventilation is resumed.

If the FOB cannot be advanced into the trachea beside the ET, a second approach to ET changing is to position the FOB on top of the vocal cords and to advance into the trachea after the ET is withdrawn.[146] For complete clearance of secretions, the cuff of the existing orotracheal ET is deflated and one or two positive-pressure ventilation breaths are given to move secretions accumulated above the cuff into the oropharynx. The cuff is reinflated,

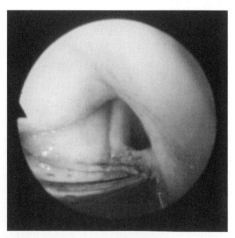

Figure 18-15 Endoscopic view of the existing orotracheal endotracheal tube (ET). The anterior commissure is free. The tip of the fiberoptic bronchoscope, which is rotated to the left 90 degrees, is positioned above the orotracheal ET and is ready to enter the larynx.

and all secretions are suctioned again. The FOB is positioned above the cords and the cuff of the ET is then deflated again. This ET is pulled out while jaw thrust is maintained. The FOB is immediately advanced into the trachea and the new ET is threaded into place. The shortcoming of this approach is that after extubation secretions and soft tissue may block the laryngeal view and delay or cause failure of endotracheal intubation. This necessitates mask ventilation before a second attempt at intubation. The failure rate with this technique is relatively high.[82,146,166] Combining rigid laryngoscopy with fiberoptic intubation may increase the success rate of ET changing under difficult conditions.

B. CHANGE OF A NASAL TO AN ORAL ENDOTRACHEAL TUBE

Most of the considerations described earlier for change from an oral to a nasal ET also apply to fiberoptic change of a nasal to an oral ET. The nasal ET lies against the posterior pharyngeal wall and therefore interferes less with advancement and manipulation of the FOB. There is less restriction in selection of the size of an oral ET, and there is a lesser possibility of accidental damage to the ET cuff. The technique for advancement of the FOB alongside the existing nasotracheal ET, removal of the existing ET, and advancement of the orotracheal ET is similar to the technique described for fiberoptic change of an oral to a nasal ET.

VI. ADVANTAGES OF FIBEROPTIC INTUBATION

The primary advantage of fiberoptic intubation is its effectiveness in the management of both difficult and failed conventional endotracheal intubation (Box 18-8). The FOB is flexible and thus can conform to a variety of anatomic variations that can occur in patients with a DA. It can be used orally or nasally and for all age groups. Whenever movement of the head and neck is not possible or is undesirable and the opening of the mouth is restricted, the FOB provides the most successful and easy approach for securing the airway.

Another advantage of fiberoptic intubation is placement of the ET under visual observation and therefore avoidance of esophageal or endobronchial intubation. However, in a patient with abnormal airway anatomy and in the presence of secretions, it is possible that the FOB may still be advanced into the esophagus instead of the trachea. The lumen of the esophagus is usually flat, but on occasion the lumen of the esophagus is open and tubular and may be mistaken for the trachea, especially in the presence of secretions and poor visualization. When tracheal rings are not satisfactorily identified, the FOB should be advanced farther to expose the carina. The presence of tracheal bifurcation excludes the possibility of esophageal intubation.

Box 18-8   Advantages of Fiberoptic Intubation

Related to the Fiberoptic Bronchoscope
Flexible instrument adaptable to airway anatomy
Applicable for oral or nasal intubations
Applicable to all age groups
Excellent visualization of the airway
Ability to apply topical anesthesia and insufflate oxygen during intubation
Ability to integrate a video system
Related to the Intubation Technique
High success rate in difficult intubation
Prevention of unrecognized esophageal and endobronchial intubation
Definitive check of endotracheal tube position
Allows evaluation of the airway before intubation
Less traumatic than rigid laryngoscopic intubation
Less cardiovascular response during awake intubation (AI) than with rigid laryngoscopic intubation
Excellent acceptance of AI by patients

This technique also permits excellent visualization of the airway, which allows evaluation of the larynx and trachea before intubation. This may provide key information in patients with compromised airway. The FOB makes precise placement of the ET beyond the tracheal compression possible in patients with an anterior mediastinal mass.[157] This is a critical factor in avoiding airway disasters such as those reported during anesthetic management of patients with an anterior mediastinal mass.[75,101,157,158,177]

Fiberoptic intubation of the trachea in conscious patients is well tolerated, less stressful, and associated with a lesser degree of hypertension and tachycardia than with rigid laryngoscopy.[147,192] However, cardiovascular response to fiberoptic intubation under general anesthesia has not been shown to be more favorable when compared with rigid laryngoscopy.[185,187]

Fiberoptic intubation can easily be performed with the patient in the supine, sitting, lateral, or even prone position. The FOB provides the only hope for securing the airway and providing general anesthesia to patients in whom access to the anterior neck is not possible because of severe cervical flexion deformity.[143] Other advantages include less trauma and avoidance of tooth damage, which is a common complication and the most common cause of malpractice suits against anesthesiologists.[32,215] The ability to apply topical anesthesia and insufflate oxygen through the working channel of the FOB and the option of using a video camera system are additional advantages of this technique.

After completion of intubation, the distance from the tip of the ET to the carina is measured and the length of the ET at teeth level is recorded. This information is useful for subsequent repositioning or retaping of the ET in critically ill patients to avoid bronchial intubation and to obviate the need for chest radiographic confirmation of the ET position.

VII. DISADVANTAGES AND COMPLICATIONS OF FIBEROPTIC INTUBATION

Two major disadvantages of the FOB itself are the expense of the instrument and its size (Box 18-9). Bronchoscopes are delicate instruments and most need a separate light source for proper illumination during endoscopy; therefore, they occupy a larger space and need their own cart and setup. Cleaning, sterilization, and storage consume more time and resources. Another disadvantage of the FOB is that a small amount of secretions or blood may completely obscure the view and interfere with airway evaluation and endotracheal intubation. As the FOB is advanced through the tracheal ET, the effective lumen left for air exchange is compromised and airway resistance increases greatly when compared with the rigid bronchoscope, which provides a large lumen for air exchange.

With fiberoptic intubation, the passage of the ET through the vocal cords is done blindly, and the depth of tracheal ET cuff placement inside the trachea is unknown. Blind passage of the ET through the vocal cords may result in intralaryngeal placement of the ET cuff with the potential of causing recurrent laryngeal nerve injury and vocal cord palsy. Forceful advancement of the ET should be avoided because it may traumatize the larynx.

A poorly lubricated FOB with a tight fit may cause intussusception of the outer cover of the FOB, complete obstruction of the ET, and failure to withdraw the FOB.[18,182] Passing the FOB through the Murphy eye, or side opening, of the ET can cause failure of intubation

---

Box 18-9   Disadvantages of Fiberoptic Intubation

Related to the Fiberoptic Bronchoscope
Fragile
Expensive
Separate light source may be required
Time consuming to clean and disinfect
Vision is obscured easily by secretions or blood
Related to the Intubation Technique
Different skill is required than in rigid laryngoscopy
Lack of expertise is a disadvantage if the practitioner is not taught during training. Most of the lumen of the endotracheal tube is blocked by the fiberoptic bronchoscope
Passage of the endotracheal tube through the vocal cords is blind
Advancement of the endotracheal tube into the trachea may pull the fiberoptic bronchoscope out of trachea
Resistance during advancement of endotracheal tube into the trachea is more common

and inability to remove the FOB.[137] Foreign body aspiration of part of the endoscopy mask during fiberoptic intubation has been reported.[152,211,216]

Positioning of the insertion cord of the FOB into the trachea also does not guarantee tracheal placement of the ET. While the FOB is in the trachea, the ET may enter the esophagus, pulling the FOB out of the trachea. This is most likely to happen when a small FOB is used for passage of a large ET.[146] In addition, a correctly placed ET may inadvertently be withdrawn from the trachea during taping of the ET and positioning of the patient. Checking ET position with the FOB after completion of intubation and taping ensures the correct placement of the ET.

The hemodynamic response to endotracheal intubation during awake fiberoptic intubation has been shown to be less severe than the response to rigid laryngoscopic intubation.[147,192] This advantage of fiberoptic intubation has not been shown to be true when intubation has been performed in anesthetized adult patients[67,185,187] or in anesthetized pediatric patients.[167] In one such study the fiberoptic intubation was associated with a greater increase in systolic blood pressure (BP) and heart rate than with rigid laryngoscopic intubation. Fiberoptic intubations were performed by holding the tongue and pulling it forward, which could be painful. Prolonged intubation time and retraction of the tongue may have contributed to this exaggerated response.[185] In another study no differences were demonstrated in systolic BP; however, the increase in pulse rate was higher in the fiberoptic group than in the rigid laryngoscopy group.[67] Schaefer and colleagues[172] demonstrated no difference in hemodynamic response to endotracheal intubation with fiberoptic bronchoscopic or rigid laryngoscopic techniques in adults. Roth and coworkers[167] also demonstrated no difference in infants younger than 24 months. More studies are needed to clarify the differences reported by various investigators. Both Roth[167] and Schaefer[172] and their colleagues reported that the incidence of postoperative sore throat, dysphagia, and hoarseness after fiberoptic intubation was similar to that with rigid laryngoscopic intubation, despite a longer period of airway manipulation and lack of visual control of tracheal ET insertion in the fiberoptic group.

Among 111 pediatric fiberoptic intubations in 15 reports, six complications were noted.* Of 20 patients who required fiberoptic intubation for a variety of illnesses, 2 patients had oxygen saturation levels of 86% and 89%.[13] However, no supplemental oxygen was being used in these patients, and saturation levels rapidly returned to normal with administration of supplemental oxygen. In another study of 20 patients intubated by FOB, 2 patients were noted by the parents to have a barky cough 24 hours after intubation. These coughs resolved without consequence.[167] It should be noted that in a control group of

children who had traditional intubation, 2 of 20 also had a barky cough at 24 hours after surgery and in these children the cough also resolved without consequence.[167] In a report of 20 intubations in four children with gangrenous stomatitis, one episode of epistaxis was reported.[193]

The most dramatic complication associated with the fiberoptic intubation is a case report of postobstructive pulmonary edema in a 12-year-old child with Hurler's syndrome.[210] Hurler's syndrome is a mucopolysaccharidase deficiency that results in deposition of mucopolysaccharides in tissues, causing facial and airway deformities. Postobstructive pulmonary edema has been described in normal children because of acute airway obstruction associated with forceful respiratory attempts after extubation.[135] Thus, it is not the technique of intubation but rather airway obstruction and the subsequent relief of that obstruction that contributes to the development of this complication.

VIII. CAUSES OF FAILURE OF FIBEROPTIC INTUBATION

The single most common cause of failure of fiberoptic intubation is lack of training and experience.

A large, floppy epiglottis or the presence of secretions or blood contributes to a difficult fiberoptic intubation. The objective lens at the tip of the FOB is easily covered with secretions and blood, which interfere with the visualization of laryngeal structures (Box 18-10).[146] Administration of an adequate dose of an antisialagogue and proper suctioning of secretions before intubation are important preliminary steps in avoiding this problem. The conscious patient can be asked to swallow or breathe deeply to clear secretions. Secretions can also be suctioned through the working channel of the FOB. Insufflation of oxygen through the suction channel helps keep secretions away and improves exposure, but one should be aware of the possibility of barotrauma to lungs if the FOB is advanced through a narrowed airway, limiting the oxygen escape

---

*References 3, 9, 13, 16, 25, 66, 79, 90, 104, 123, 124, 167, 170, 173, 191, 193, 210.

> **Box 18-10   Causes of Failure of Fiberoptic Intubation**
>
> Lack of expertise
> Presence of secretions and blood
> Fogging of the objective and focusing lenses
> Poor topical anesthesia
> Decreased space between epiglottis and the posterior pharyngeal wall
> Distorted airway anatomy
> Passage of fiberoptic bronchoscope through the Murphy eye
> Inadequate lubrication of a tightly fitting fiberoptic bronchoscope

from the lungs. In case of unexpected difficult rigid laryngoscopy and endotracheal intubation, fiberoptic intubation should be instituted as soon as possible and before causing trauma and bleeding.

Fogging of objective and ocular lenses also interferes with exposure of the laryngeal structures. Exit of exhaled air from the upper border of the operator's protective face mask causes fogging of the ocular lens in a cold operating room. Insertion of the tip of the insertion cord in warm water or application of a commercially available defogging solution solves the problem of objective lens fogging.

In case of inadequate topical anesthesia, instrumentation of the oropharynx increases secretions and may cause coughing, choking, or vomiting. Excessive swallowing or coughing may move the laryngeal structures out of the visual field. Laryngospasm is likely if poorly anesthetized vocal cords are touched with the FOB. Even if the FOB can be passed through the vocal cords, it may be impossible to pass the ET.

In many patients, the tip of the epiglottis may be next to the posterior pharyngeal wall, which interferes with navigating the FOB to the larynx. In the presence of a large, floppy epiglottis, application of jaw thrust or pulling the tongue moves the epiglottis away from the posterior pharyngeal wall and corrects the problem (Fig. 18-16). If difficulty is experienced because of a supraepiglottic mass or inflammation and edema of the upper airway, simple jaw thrust may not solve the problem. Under these circumstances, even if the FOB is advanced into the trachea, threading the ET over the FOB into the trachea may fail (Fig. 18-17). Anterior displacement of the base of the tongue with a rigid laryngoscope may be necessary to assist

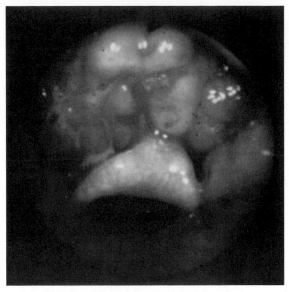

Figure 18-17 A large, benign lymphoid mass at the base of the tongue compressing the epiglottis. This condition makes fiberoptic exposure of the glottis opening difficult and may interfere with smooth passage of the endotracheal tube over the fiberoptic bronchoscope into the trachea.

the passage of the ET. With severe flexion deformity of the cervical spine the entire larynx is pushed backward against the posterior pharyngeal wall, making fiberoptic intubation quite difficult (Fig. 18-18).[146]

Distorted anatomy that is due to previous surgery, a mass, edema, or soft tissue contracture may contribute to the difficult vocal cord exposure (Fig. 18-19). A deviated nasal septum may direct a nasotracheal ET away from the glottis, and in severe cases, even though the FOB may enter the trachea, the ET may not follow it. Selecting the nostril toward which the larynx is deviated reduces this possibility and makes exposure of the glottis simpler.

Difficulty in advancing the ET into the trachea is a common phenomenon during orotracheal intubation. Advancement of the tracheal ET may also be difficult when the FOB is passed through the Murphy eye rather than the distal opening of the ET.[137] When the FOB is passed through the Murphy eye of the endotracheal ET, withdrawal of the FOB may be difficult or impossible without damaging the instrument. In this instance, the FOB and ET should be withdrawn together as a unit, the FOB disengaged, and the procedure repeated. It may also be difficult to remove an unlubricated FOB that has a tight fit. If the FOB has a loose plastic cover and the ET is a tight fit, intussusception can result, leading to difficulty in removing the instrument from the ET.[182]

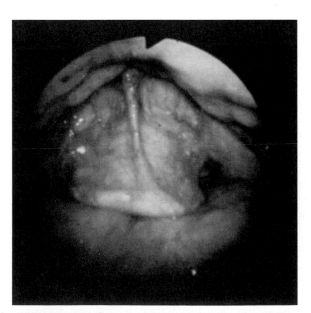

Figure 18-16 Large, floppy epiglottis blocks the view of the glottis. Jaw thrust or pulling the tongue forward moves the tip of the epiglottis away from the posterior pharyngeal wall, making exposure of the glottis possible. (From Ovassapian A: Fiberoptic Airway Endoscopy in Anesthesia and Critical Care. New York, Raven Press, 1990.)

IX. LEARNING FIBEROPTIC INTUBATION

The flexible fiberoptic choledochoscope was the first of the new generation of flexible instruments to be used for difficult endotracheal intubation.[128] Shortly after the

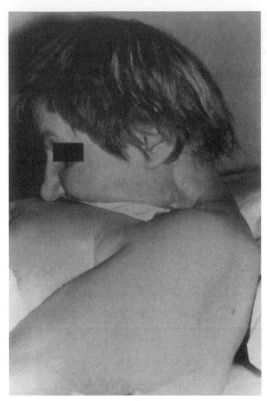

Figure 18-18 Lateral view of a patient with severe degree of cervical spine flexion deformity resulting from advanced rheumatoid arthritis and pathologic fracture of cervical vertebrae related to fall. Fiberoptic exposure of the vocal cords was extremely difficult because posterior displacement of the entire larynx was pushing the tip of epiglottis against posterior pharyngeal wall. (From Ovassapian A: Fiberoptic Airway Endoscopy in Anesthesia and Critical Care. New York, Raven Press, 1990.)

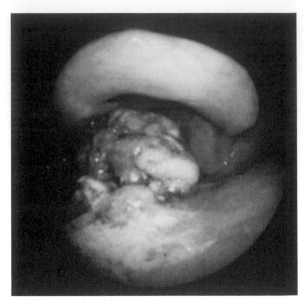

Figure 18-19 Large malignant mass of larynx originating from left piriform sinus. The tip of epiglottis is in view with large fungating mass beneath it. The glottic opening cannot be seen. A 6-mm internal diameter endotracheal tube was passed atraumatically into the trachea using Olympus LF-1 fiberoptic intubation scope. The fiberoptic scope was passed from the 1 o'clock position to the back of the mass where glottic opening with normal vocal cords could be seen. Moderately difficult fiberoptic intubation.

introduction of the FOB into clinical bronchology practice, its use was applied to difficult endotracheal intubation by anesthesiologists.[49,92,128,189,194] Despite the early recognition by some anesthesiologists of the value of flexible fiberoptic instruments in airway management and their early introduction into clinical anesthesia practice, widespread introduction of the instrument into clinical practice has been slow. This has remained so despite newer, modern instrument design and equipment and their efficacy in a wide range of clinical circumstances of importance to the anesthesiologist.

In recent years there has been significant interest in and increase in learning this valuable skill by many disciplines of medicine involved in airway management, especially by anesthesiologists. This view is supported by the large number of regional and national scientific meetings devoted entirely or in part to the role of the FOB in airway management and by the increased number of publications about fiberoptic airway management.

Our "hands-on" workshop teaching the use of the FOB in airway management was started in 1984. Over the past 5 years the number of workshops devoted to airway management and fiberoptic intubation has escalated.

This is in keeping with the findings of a 1985 survey of academic department chairpersons, members of the Society for Education in Anesthesia, and private-practice anesthesiologists, who were asked which procedural skills should be learned by anesthesia residents; fiberoptic intubation received one of the highest priorities.[146]

Fiberoptic endotracheal intubation is a psychomotor skill completely different from conventional techniques. There are three components to learning the art of fiberoptic intubation. First, one must understand the instrument, its application, and the skills required (cognitive); second, one must learn to perform the skills (psychomotor); and third, one must be able to apply the new skills in clinical practice.

A. UNDERSTANDING THE FIBEROPTIC BRONCHOSCOPE

Understanding the physical characteristics of the bronchoscope, the manner in which it functions, and how to avoid damaging it are critical for its successful use. Demonstration of the FOB and in-service training for the physicians, nurses, and technicians who use and take care of the bronchoscope are essential to avoid unnecessary breakage, which contributes to underuse of the instrument.

The endoscopist should have a clear understanding of what the instrument can do, its limitations, and how it can be used most beneficially. Viewing of various videotapes that demonstrate the clinical application of the instrument, its characteristics, and its handling is a basic step in learning its use.[140]

B. HANDLING THE FIBEROPTIC BRONCHOSCOPE

The handling and maneuvering of the FOB can be learned by working on models, patients, or both. It seems logical that the early phase of exercise for becoming acquainted with the instrument and developing the dexterity that is essential for successful use of this instrument be done on models. Working on the model is easy and avoids the stress of the operating room. Exercise can be done at any time, and valuable operating room time is not consumed for this purpose. The most important advantage is becoming dexterous and learning what to do when the technique is applied to the patient.

The selection of patients for the first few fiberoptic intubations is also critical. Patients with normal airway anatomy provide the opportunity to train the eye to the airway anatomy, manage problems created by secretions, and learn to keep the larynx in the visual field during patients' movement and swallowing. Only after gaining skill and confidence with use of the FOB in patients with normal airways does the management of a complicated airway become both practical and likely to succeed. The following steps are suggested for learning proper maneuvering of the FOB.

1. Practice on the Tracheobronchial Tree Model or Dexterity Model

Hands-on work is necessary to educate the trainee to maneuver the FOB and develop the eye-motor coordination and optic recognition essential to its use. Manipulation of the instrument should be natural and spontaneous and can easily be achieved by working on a tracheobronchial or dexterity model (e.g., Dexter, Replicant Medical Simulators, Wellington, New Zealand).[17,59,118,140,149,186,195] Naik and colleagues demonstrated that training on a simple model is more effective than conventional didactic instruction for resident acquisition of fiberoptic intubation skills.[129]

The practitioner should have access to the FOB and a model for unlimited practice. Practice on a model is critical for learning effective and proper manipulation of the FOB. Practice should continue until the operator can quickly and predictably maneuver the FOB in a given direction to expose various segments of the lung model. An acceptable level of dexterity is achieved with 3 to 4 hours of practice.

2. Practice on the Intubation Mannequin

An intubation mannequin simulates normal airway anatomy and is used to demonstrate the steps of fiberoptic intubation that are performed in awake and anesthetized patients. ET position is checked by measuring the distance between the tip of the ET and carina. Fiberoptic ET changing techniques, double-lumen tube positioning, and intubation through an LMA are also practiced. Each procedure is practiced several times to become familiar with the steps of these fiberoptic intubation techniques.[45,59,140,149,172,186]

3. Practice on Patients

The final stage of learning flexible fiberoptic intubation involves performing intubations orally or nasally with the patient either sedated or anesthetized and paralyzed.[45,46,59,95,140,149,172,186] This approach is practical and justified because fiberoptic intubation is now considered a routine procedure and has been shown to be safe in adults and children.[46,167] However, even after practice with mannequins or training aids, the first fiberoptic intubation of a patient may be challenging. Recognition and management of the problems created by secretions, blood, fogging, and inadequate topical anesthesia with airway reactivity and movement and identification of the epiglottis and the glottic opening from this new perspective are key.

A sedated patient in stable condition with good topical anesthesia provides an unhurried opportunity for the inexperienced endoscopist to try his or her first fiberoptic intubation. The endoscopist gains confidence in handling managing the airway with the FOB with each successful routine intubation. Because patients' overall acceptance of awake or sedated fiberoptic intubations is excellent, more liberal use of AIs should be encouraged.

Teaching fiberoptic orotracheal intubation with the patient under general anesthesia is an alternative method with its own advantages (see Chapter 51). The number of patients available for teaching is not limited, and the anxiety about performing a new technique in a conscious patient is avoided.[172] Fiberoptic orotracheal intubations are performed routinely in less than 60 seconds; therefore, time is not usually a factor.

Initial intubations by the inexperienced endoscopist should be limited to patients with normal upper airway anatomy who are scheduled for routine surgical procedures.[45,59,140,149,172,186] The instructor who is teaching the technique should emphasize the role of an assistant in performing the maneuvers that support the relaxed oropharyngeal structures in the anesthetized patient. With experience, intubation of patients with abnormal airway anatomy and patients in whom rigid laryngoscopy has failed becomes an easier task to perform.

C. VIDEO SYSTEM AS A LEARNING AND TEACHING TOOL

In addition to the tracheobronchial model and intubation mannequin, other equipment is helpful in teaching fiberoptic intubation. The fiberoptic teaching attachment makes it possible for the instructor and trainee simultaneously to observe and demonstrate the intubation procedure. A video camera and television screen can be used to demonstrate the techniques for endotracheal intubation, airway evaluation, or the positioning of endobronchial ETs.

Smith and colleagues[186] for intubation of adults and Wheeler and associates[207] for intubation of children have demonstrated that the use of a video system was more effective in teaching the step-by-step technique of fiberoptic intubation than other methods.

D. ASSESSING PROFICIENCY

Proficiency in fiberoptic intubation technique cannot simply be based on the number of performances attempted. Trainees who have learned the use and proper manipulation of the FOB by practicing on a tracheobronchial tree model and have used the FOB to expose laryngeal structures can be successful in more than 85% of their first six attempts at nasotracheal intubation in patients with normal airway anatomy.[149]

Johnson and Roberts[95] reported that an acceptable level of technical expertise in fiberoptic intubation can be obtained by performing 10 intubations in anesthetized patients. This finding is based on the performance of four anesthesia residents with at least 8 months of training and with no previous experience in fiberoptic intubation. Each resident had a 15-minute practice session on a teaching mannequin with an instructor before attempting orotracheal intubation in anesthetized patients.

If intubation was not achieved within 3 minutes, ventilation in the patient was performed before a second attempt was made. The duration of the intubation procedure was measured from the last mask ventilation to the first breath through the ET, minus the time during which a second mask ventilation was performed. In the first five intubations, the success rate for the first attempt at fiberoptic intubation was 50%; the rate improved to 90% in the next five patients and to 100% in the following five patients.[95]

The authors concluded that an acceptable level of technical expertise in fiberoptic intubation is achieved within 10 intubations and that the time needed for intubation remains stable after the 10th intubation at an average level of 1.2 to 1.5 minutes. Their findings were similar to the experience of Delaney and Hessler,[56] who reported their clinical experiences in the use of the FOB in emergency room nasotracheal intubations; they found a significant decrease in the time needed for intubation after their 9th to 10th cases.

Although the level of proficiency cannot be based only on the number of intubations performed by the individual, in our experience most trainees, after practicing on tracheobronchial and intubation models, learn to use the FOB effectively in awake patients with normal airway anatomy after 15 to 20 such intubations. The same number of intubations with patients under general anesthesia seems to be adequate to give the trainee the necessary skill and experience for independent use of the FOB. However, the amount of training or experience necessary for safe, effective use of the FOB in patients with compromised airways is not known and needs to be studied.

On the basis of the observations of a few of our anesthesia fellows and staff who have used the FOB for considerable lengths of time, expert mastery of the FOB requires significant experience of 100 cases or more. A varied exposure to multiple airway evaluations, endotracheal intubations, ET changes, and double-lumen ET placement may be needed to gain the necessary experience for independent, successful use of the FOB in patients with compromised airways.

Minimal competence standards for cognitive and technical skills to perform fiberoptic endotracheal intubation, placement, and positioning of double-lumen ETs and limited bronchoscopy should be established. A selected minimum number of fiberoptic intubation performances should be only one of the criteria used to judge competence. Each trainee must be evaluated individually regarding overall performance.

If instruction in flexible fiberoptic laryngoscopy is initiated early in the anesthesia training program, there will be ample time and opportunity for every trainee to become proficient in the use of the FOB. Successful teaching of a psychomotor skill requires an instructor who is knowledgeable and proficient in the skill and displays a positive attitude toward the clinical applications and effectiveness of the technique.[59]

E. INTRODUCING FIBEROPTIC INTUBATION INTO ONE'S OWN PRACTICE

Anesthesiologists who have not been trained to perform fiberoptic intubation during their residency training program face a special challenge in introducing this new technique into their daily practice. The following steps are suggested to assist with the smooth introduction of the technique.

The first step requires gaining the necessary cognitive skills concerning the instrument and its clinical application by referring to the published literature. The second step requires organizing a fiberoptic cart that is reliably maintained with all necessary required equipment and supplies, along with a system for the routine care and cleaning of the FOB. The learning of basic technique by participating in fiberoptic workshops, along with practice on tracheobronchial and intubation models, is the third step before fiberoptic intubation in patients is attempted.[59]

When the basic knowledge and handling of the FOB are learned and an organized, well-functioning fiberoptic cart is assembled, an assistant should be enlisted. A colleague, nurse, or technician can provide the necessary assistance for performing intubation with the patient under general anesthesia.

Attempts at laryngeal exposure in the anesthetized patient tend to proceed smoothly and to have a relatively high success rate. The well-prepared anesthesiologist does not appear to be clumsy or leave a negative impression on the surgeon or other personnel in the operating room. Initial failure of a technique, particularly when it is new, is an acceptable and familiar circumstance to most individuals who work in the operating room environment. However, attempting a technique without any preparation is unacceptable and leaves a bad impression.

The goal of the first few attempts at fiberoptic intubation should be limited to laryngeal exposure only. The importance of jaw thrust in the anesthetized patient, the role of the assistant, and difficulties created by secretions will all be appreciated. Very soon, laryngeal exposure time is minimized and time is available to complete the process of intubation.

F. SKILL RETENTION

Marsland and colleagues have highlighted the problem of skill retention.[118] They point out that "dexterity deficit and dexterity decay" undermine the psychomotor component of fiberoptic intubation and contribute to the underutilization of this recommended technique. The psychomotor skill of endoscopic airway management has been reported to be difficult to maintain.[119] It is the authors' perception, gained from teaching fiberoptic intubation at numerous conferences, that many practitioners believe pressures for efficiency in the operating room prevent the frequent use of the FOB that is required to maintain skills. In response to this problem, Marsland and colleagues have developed an endoscopic dexterity training system, Dexter. The system components include a mannequin, an image chart, a series of maps, and a structured training manual. The objective is to explore the mannequin endoscopically and find the images placed inside it. These are identified from the image chart, and a letter corresponding to the image is written in the correct location on the appropriate map. The developers hope that Dexter will foster the skilled use of FOBs in airway management, thus improving patients' care and operating room efficiency when FOBs are used in the clinical setting. However, no formal clinical trials using this device have been published thus far.

Even if basic psychomotor skills can be retained through model practice, there is no substitute for the step-by-step use of the FOB in patients. Skills in sedation and application of topical anesthesia are no less important to the successful completion of fiberoptic intubation and are best acquired in the clinical setting.

X. CONCLUSION

The maintenance of a patent airway is one of the fundamental responsibilities of every anesthesiologist. Unexpected difficult intubations associated with difficult mask ventilation are responsible for a large proportion of anesthetic-related complications that result in permanent disability or death.[36,42] When an airway problem is encountered, one should use the technique that one is most familiar or experienced with to gain control of the situation. However, this should not be used as an excuse to avoid learning new techniques that may be superior or more successful under those difficult circumstances. Two editorials have emphasized the value of fiberoptic intubation technique and the importance of developing training programs to teach every anesthesia trainee.[119,197]

Fiberoptic intubation has proved itself to be the technique of choice for the management of securing the DA. The appropriate selection and use of the FOB minimize disastrous outcomes and increase the safety of airway management. Fiberoptic endotracheal intubation is critical in airway management and should be mastered by all physicians involved in airway management.

REFERENCES

1. Adriani J, Zepernick R, Arens J, Authement E: The comparative potency and effectiveness of topical anesthetics in man. Clin Pharmacol Ther 5:49-62, 1964.
2. Alfery DD: Changing an endotracheal tube. In Benumof JL (ed): Procedures in Anesthesia and Intensive Care. Philadelphia, Lippincott, 1991.
3. Alfery DD, Ward CF, Harwood IR, Mannino FL: Airway management for a neonate with congenital fusion of the jaws. Anesthesiology 51:340-342, 1979.
4. Antila H, Laitio T, Aantaa R, et al: Difficult airway in a patient with Marshall-Smith syndrome. Paediatr Anaesth 8:429-432, 1998.
5. Appleby JN, Bingham RM: Craniodiaphyseal dysplasia; another cause of difficult intubation. Paediatr Anaesth 6:225-229, 1996.
6. Aps C, Towey RM: Experiences with fibre-optic bronchoscopic positioning of single-lumen endobronchial tubes. Anaesthesia 36:415-418, 1981.
7. Arndt GA, Topp J, Hannah J, et al: Intubation via the LMA using a Cook retrograde intubation kit. Can J Anaesth 45:257-260, 1998.
8. Arul A, Jacob R: A different under vision approach to a difficult intubation. Paediatr Anaesth 9:260-261, 1999.
9. Asada A, Tatekawa S, Terai T, et al: The anesthetic implications of a patient with Farber's lipogranulomatosis. Anesthesiology 80:206-209, 1994.
10. Asai T: Use of the laryngeal mask for fibrescope-aided tracheal intubation in an awake patient with a deviated larynx. Acta Anaesthesiol Scand 38:615-616, 1994.
11. Asai T, Latto IP, Vaughan RS: The distance between the grille of the laryngeal mask airway and the vocal cords. Is conventional intubation through the laryngeal mask safe? Anaesthesia 48:667-669, 1993.
12. Auden SM: Additional techniques for managing the difficult pediatric airway. Anesth Analg 90:878-880, 2000.

13. Audenaert SM, Montgomery CL, Stone B, et al: Retrograde-assisted fiberoptic tracheal intubation in children with difficult airways. Anesth Analg 73:660-664, 1991.

14. aWengen DF, Probst RR, Frei FJ: Flexible laryngoscopy in neonates and infants: Insertion through a median opening in the face mask. Int J Pediatr Otorhinolaryngol 21:183-187, 1991.

15. Bahk JH, Han SM, Kim SD: Management of difficult airways with a laryngeal mask airway under propofol anaesthesia. Paediatr Anaesth 9:163-166, 1999.

16. Baines DB, Goodrick MA, Beckenham EJ, Overton JH: Fibreoptically guided endotracheal intubation in a child. Anaesth Intensive Care 17:354-356, 1989.

17. Bainton CR: Models to facilitate the learning of fiberoptic technique. Int Anesthesiol Clin 32:47-55, 1994.

18. Barriot P, Riou B: Retrograde technique for tracheal intubation in trauma patients. Crit Care Med 16: 712-713, 1988.

19. Benumof JL: A new technique of fiberoptic intubation through a standard LMA. Anesthesiology 95:1541, 2001.

20. Benumof JL: Laryngeal mask airway and the ASA difficult airway algorithm. Anesthesiology 84:686-699, 1996.

21. Benumof JL: Management of the difficult adult airway with special emphasis on awake tracheal intubation. Anesthesiology 75:1087-1110, 1991.

22. Benumof JL: Use of the laryngeal mask airway to facilitate fiberscope-aided tracheal intubation. Anesth Analg 74:313-315, 1992.

23. Benumof JL, Partridge BL, Salvatierra C, Keating J: Margin of safety in positioning modern double-lumen endotracheal tubes. Anesthesiology 67:729-738, 1987.

24. Berman RA: A method for blind oral intubation of the trachea or esophagus. Anesth Analg 56:866-867, 1977.

25. Berthelsen P, Prytz S, Jacobsen E: Two-stage fiberoptic nasotracheal intubation in infants: A new approach to difficult pediatric intubation. Anesthesiology 63: 457-458, 1985.

26. Bourke DL, Katz J, Tonneson A: Nebulized anesthesia for awake endotracheal intubation. Anesthesiology 63:690-692, 1985.

27. Brain AI: The laryngeal mask—A new concept in airway management. Br J Anaesth 55:801-805, 1983.

28. Brain AI: Three cases of difficult intubation overcome by the laryngeal mask airway. Anaesthesia 40:353-355, 1985.

29. Brimacombe J, Berry A: Placement of a Cook airway exchange catheter via the laryngeal mask airway. Anaesthesia 48:351-352, 1993.

30. Brimacombe J, Newell S, Swainston R, Thompson J: A potential new technique for awake fibreoptic bronchoscopy—Use of the laryngeal mask airway. Med J Aust 156:876-877, 1992.

31. Brull SJ, Wiklund R, Ferris C, et al: Facilitation of fiberoptic orotracheal intubation with a flexible tracheal tube. Anesth Analg 78:746-748, 1994.

32. Burton JF, Baker AB: Dental damage during anaesthesia and surgery. Anaesth Intensive Care 15:262-268, 1987.

33. Butler MG, Hayes BG, Hathaway MM, Begleiter ML: Specific genetic diseases at risk for sedation/anesthesia complications. Anesth Analg 91:837-855, 2000.

34. Calder I, Ordman AJ, Jackowski A, Crockard HA: The Brain laryngeal mask airway. An alternative to emergency tracheal intubation. Anaesthesia 45:137-139, 1990.

35. Campbell D, Adriani J: Absorption of local anesthetics. JAMA 168:873, 1958.

36. Caplan RA, Posner KL, Ward RJ, Cheney FW: Adverse respiratory events in anesthesia: A closed claims analysis. Anesthesiology 72:828-833, 1990.

37. Cartwright PD, Pingel SM: Midazolam and diazepam in ketamine anaesthesia. Anaesthesia 39:439-442, 1984.

38. Chadd GD, Ackers JW, Bailey PM: Difficult intubation aided by the laryngeal mask airway. Anaesthesia 44:1015, 1989.

39. Chadd GD, Crane DL, Phillips RM, Tunell WP: Extubation and reintubation guided by the laryngeal mask airway in a child with the Pierre-Robin syndrome. Anesthesiology 76:640-641, 1992.

40. Chadd GD, Walford AJ, Crane DL: The 3.5/4.5 modification for fiberscope-guided tracheal intubation using the laryngeal mask airway. Anesth Analg 75: 307-308, 1992.

41. Chan YW, Kong CF, Kong CS, et al: The intubating laryngeal mask airway (ILMA): Initial experience in Singapore. Br J Anaesth 81:610-611, 1998.

42. Cheney FW, Posner KL, Caplan RA: Adverse respiratory events infrequently leading to malpractice suits. A closed claims analysis. Anesthesiology 75:932-939, 1991.

43. Chinn WM, Zavala DC, Ambre J: Plasma levels of lidocaine following nebulized aerosol administration. Chest 71:346-348, 1977.

44. Chu SS, Rah KH, Brannan MD, Cohen JL: Plasma concentration of lidocaine after endotracheal spray. Anesth Analg 54:438-441, 1975.

45. Coe PA, King TA, Towey RM: Teaching guided fibreoptic nasotracheal intubation. An assessment of an anaesthetic technique to aid training. Anaesthesia 43:410-413, 1988.

46. Cole AF, Mallon JS, Rolbin SH, Ananthanarayan C: Fiberoptic intubation using anesthetized, paralyzed, apneic patients. Results of a resident training program. Anesthesiology 84:1101-1106, 1996.

47. Colt HG, Crawford SW, Galbraith O III: Virtual reality bronchoscopy simulation: A revolution in procedural training. Chest 120:1333-1339, 2001.

48. Connelly NR, Kyle R, Gotta J, et al: Comparison of wire reinforced tubes with warmed standard tubes to facilitate fiberoptic intubation. J Clin Anesth 13:3-5, 2001.

49. Conyers AB, Wallace DH, Mulder DS: Use of the fiber optic bronchoscope for nasotracheal intubation: Case report. Can Anaesth Soc J 19:654-656, 1972.

50. Cormack RS: Anaesthesia with the difficult airway. Anaesthesia 52:710, 1997.

51. Couture P, Perreault C, Girard D: Fibreoptic bronchoscopic intubation after induction of general anaesthesia: Another approach. Can J Anaesth 39:99, 1992.

52. Darling JR, Keohane M, Murray JM: A split laryngeal mask as an aid to training in fibreoptic tracheal intubation. A comparison with the Berman II intubating airway. Anaesthesia 48:1079-1082, 1993.

53. Davies JR: The fibreoptic laryngoscope in the management of cut throat injuries. Br J Anaesth 50: 511-514, 1978.

54. Davis K: Alterations to the Patil-Syracuse mask for fiberoptic intubation. Anesth Analg 74:472-473, 1992.

55. Davis NJ: A new fiberoptic laryngoscope for nasal intubation. Anesth Analg 52:807-808, 1973.

56. Delaney KA, Hessler R: Emergency flexible fiberoptic nasotracheal intubation: A report of 60 cases. Ann Emerg Med 17:919-926, 1988.

57. Dietrich KA, Strauss RH, Cabalka AK, et al: Use of flexible fiberoptic endoscopy for determination of endotracheal tube position in the pediatric patient. Crit Care Med 16:884-887, 1988.

58. Dubreuil M, Laffon M, Plaud B, et al: Complications and fiberoptic assessment of size 1 laryngeal mask airway. Anesth Analg 76:527-529, 1993.

59. Dykes MH, Ovassapian A: Dissemination of fibreoptic airway endoscopy skills by means of a workshop utilizing models. Br J Anaesth 63:595-597, 1989.

60. Eckenhoff JE: Some anatomic considerations of the infant larynx influencing endotracheal anesthesia. Anesthesiology 12:401-410, 1951.

61. Edens ET, Sia RL: Flexible fiberoptic endoscopy in difficult intubations. Ann Otol Rhinol Laryngol 90:307-309, 1981.

62. Ellis DS, Potluri PK, O'Flaherty JE, Baum VC: Difficult airway management in the neonate: A simple method of intubating through a laryngeal mask airway. Paediatr Anaesth 9:460-462, 1999.

63. Fan LL, Flynn JW: Laryngoscopy in neonates and infants: Experience with the flexible fiberoptic bronchoscope. Laryngoscope 91:451-456, 1981.

64. Fan LL, Sparks LM, Dulinski JP: Applications of an ultrathin flexible bronchoscope for neonatal and pediatric airway problems. Chest 89:673-676, 1986.

65. Fenlon S, Pearce A: Sevoflurane induction and difficult airway management. Anaesthesia 52:285-286, 1997.

66. Finer NN, Muzyka D: Flexible endoscopic intubation of the neonate. Pediatr Pulmonol 12:48-51, 1992.

67. Finfer SR, MacKenzie SI, Saddler JM, Watkins TG: Cardiovascular responses to tracheal intubation: A comparison of direct laryngoscopy and fibreoptic intubation. Anaesth Intensive Care 17:44-48, 1989.

68. Fitzpatrick SB, Marsh B, Stokes D, Wang KP: Indications for flexible fiberoptic bronchoscopy in pediatric patients. Am J Dis Child 137:595-597, 1983.

69. Ford RW: Adaptation of the fiberoptic laryngoscope for tracheal intubation with small diameter tubes. Can Anaesth Soc J 28:479-480, 1981.

70. Frass M, Frenzer R, Rauscha F, et al: Evaluation of esophageal tracheal Combitube in cardiopulmonary resuscitation. Crit Care Med 15:609-611, 1987.

71. Frei FJ, aWengen DF, Rutishauser M, Ummenhofer W: The airway endoscopy mask: Useful device for fibreoptic evaluation and intubation of the paediatric airway. Paediatr Anaesth 5:319-324, 1995.

72. Frei FJ, Ummenhofer W: A special mask for teaching fiber-optic intubation in pediatric patients. Anesth Analg 76:458, 1993.

73. Frei FJ, Ummenhofer W: Difficult intubation in paediatrics. Paediatr Anaesth 6:251-263, 1996.

74. Fukutome T, Amaha K, Nakazawa K, et al: Tracheal intubation through the intubating laryngeal mask airway (LMA-Fastrach) in patients with difficult airways. Anaesth Intensive Care 26:387-391, 1998.

75. Furst SR, Burrows PE, Holzman RS: General anesthesia in a child with a dynamic, vascular anterior mediastinal mass. Anesthesiology 84:976-979, 1996.

76. Gaitini LA, Vaida SJ, Fradis M, et al: Replacing the Combitube by an endotracheal tube using a fibre-optic bronchoscope during spontaneous ventilation. J Laryngol Otol 112:786-787, 1998.

77. Gjonaj ST, Lowenthal DB, Dozor AJ: Nebulized lidocaine administered to infants and children undergoing flexible bronchoscopy. Chest 112:1665-1669, 1997.

78. Goudsouzian NG, Denman W, Cleveland R, Shorten G: Radiologic localization of the laryngeal mask airway in children. Anesthesiology 77:1085-1089, 1992.

79. Gouverneur JM, Veyckemans F, Licker M, et al: Using an ureteral catheter as a guide in difficult neonatal fiberoptic intubation. Anesthesiology 66:436-437, 1987.

80. Greer JR, Smith SP, Strang T: A comparison of tracheal tube tip designs on the passage of an endotracheal tube during oral fiberoptic intubation. Anesthesiology 94:729-731, 2001.

81. Haas DA, Harper DG: Ketamine: A review of its pharmacologic properties and use in ambulatory anesthesia. Anesth Prog 39:61-68, 1992.

82. Halebian P, Shires GT: A method for replacement of the endotracheal tube with continuous control of the airway. Surg Gynecol Obstet 161:285-286, 1985.

83. Hanson PJ, Collins JV: AIDS and the lung. 1—AIDS, aprons, and elbow grease: Preventing the nosocomial spread of human immunodeficiency virus and associated organisms. Thorax 44:778-783, 1989.

84. Hanson PJ, Meah S, Tipler D, Collins JV: Costs of infection control in endoscopy units. BMJ 298:866-867, 1989.

85. Hasham F, Kumar CM, Lawler PG: The use of the laryngeal mask airway to assist fibreoptic orotracheal intubation. Anaesthesia 46:891, 1991.

86. Heard CM, Gunnarsson B, Fletcher JE: Teaching fiberoptic intubation in the pediatric patient. Anesth Analg 91:1044, 2000.

87. Heath ML, Allagain J: Intubation through the laryngeal mask. A technique for unexpected difficult intubation. Anaesthesia 46:545-548, 1991.

88. Hollister GR, Burn JM: Side effects of ketamine in pediatric anesthesia. Anesth Analg 53:264-267, 1974.

89. Hostetler MA, Barnard JA: Removal of esophageal foreign bodies in the pediatric ED: Is ketamine an option? Am J Emerg Med 20:96-98, 2002.

90. Howardy-Hansen P, Berthelsen P: Fibreoptic bronchoscopic nasotracheal intubation of a neonate with Pierre Robin syndrome. Anaesthesia 43:121-122, 1988.

91. Hughes JR: Infantile methemoglobinemia due to benzocaine suppository. J Pediatr 67:509-510, 1965.

92. Ikeda S: Atlas of Flexible Bronchofiberoscopy. Baltimore, University Park, 1974.

93. Imai M, Kemmotsu O: A new adapter for fiberoptic endotracheal intubation for anesthetized patients. Anesthesiology 70:374-375, 1989.

94. Johnson C, Hunter J, Ho E, Bruff C: Fiberoptic intubation facilitated by a rigid laryngoscope. Anesth Analg 72:714, 1991.

95. Johnson C, Roberts JT: Clinical competence in the performance of fiberoptic laryngoscopy and endotracheal intubation: A study of resident instruction. J Clin Anesth 1:344-349, 1989.

96. Johnson CM, Sims C: Awake fibreoptic intubation via a laryngeal mask in an infant with Goldenhar's syndrome. Anaesth Intensive Care 22:194-197, 1994.

97. Jones KL: Smith's Recognizable Patterns of Human Malformation, 5th ed. Philadelphia, WB Saunders, 1997.

98. Kandasamy R, Sivalingam P: Use of sevoflurane in difficult airways. Acta Anaesthesiol Scand 44:627-629, 2000.

99. Katsnelson T, Frost EA, Farcon E, Goldiner PL: When the endotracheal tube will not pass over the flexible fiberoptic bronchoscope. Anesthesiology 76:151-152, 1992.

100. Keenan MA, Stiles CM, Kaufman RL: Acquired laryngeal deviation associated with cervical spine disease in erosive polyarticular arthritis. Use of the fiberoptic bronchoscope in rheumatoid disease. Anesthesiology 58:441-449, 1983.

101. Keon TP: Death on induction of anesthesia for cervical node biopsy. Anesthesiology 55:471-472, 1981.

102. Kitamura S, Fukumitsu K, Kinouchi K, et al: A new modification of anaesthesia mask for fibreoptic intubation in children. Paediatr Anaesth 9:119-122, 1999.

103. Klafta JM: Flexible tracheal tubes facilitate fiberoptic intubation. Anesth Analg 79:1211-1212, 1994.

104. Kleeman PP, Jantzen JP, Bonfils P: The ultra-thin bronchoscope in management of the difficult paediatric airway. Can J Anaesth 34:606-608, 1987.

105. Kristensen MS: The Parker Flex-Tip tube versus a standard tube for fiberoptic orotracheal intubation: A randomized double-blind study. Anesthesiology 98:354-358, 2003.

106. Latorre F, Otter W, Kleemann PP, et al: Cocaine or phenylephrine/lignocaine for nasal fibreoptic intubation? Eur J Anaesthesiol 13:577-581, 1996.

107. Lechman MJ, Donahoo JS, MacVaugh H III: Endotracheal intubation using percutaneous retrograde guidewire insertion followed by antegrade fiberoptic bronchoscopy. Crit Care Med 14:589-590, 1986.

108. Lee SC: Improvement of gas exchange by apneic oxygenation with nasal prong during fiberoptic intubation in fully relaxed patients. J Korean Med Sci 13:582-586, 1998.

109. Lindholm CE, Ollman B, Snyder J, et al: Flexible fiberoptic bronchoscopy in critical care medicine. Diagnosis, therapy and complications. Crit Care Med 2:250-261, 1974.

110. Lindholm CE, Ollman B, Snyder JV, et al: Cardio-respiratory effects of flexible fiberoptic bronchoscopy in critically ill patients. Chest 74:362-368, 1978.

111. Litman RS: Conscious sedation with remifentanil and midazolam during brief painful procedures in children. Arch Pediatr Adolesc Med 153:1085-1088, 1999.

112. Lu GP, Frost EA, Goldiner PL: Another approach to the problem airway. Anesthesiology 65:101-102, 1986.

113. MacIntyre PA, Ansari KA: Sevoflurane for predicted difficult tracheal intubation. Eur J Anaesthesiol 15:462-466, 1998.

114. Mackenzie CF, Barnas G, Nesbitt S: Tracheal insufflation of oxygen at low flow: Capabilities and limitations. Anesth Analg 71:684-690, 1990.

115. Mackenzie CF, Barnas GM, Smalley J, et al: Low-flow endobronchial insufflation with air for 2 hours of apnea provides ventilation adequate for survival. Anesth Analg 71:279-284, 1990.

116. Mallios C: A modification of the Laerdal anaesthesia mask for nasotracheal intubation with the fiberoptic laryngoscope. Anaesthesia 35:599-600, 1980.

117. Marsh B, White M, Morton N, Kenny GN: Pharmacokinetic model driven infusion of propofol in children. Br J Anaesth 67:41-48, 1991.

118. Marsland CP, Robinson BJ, Chitty CH, Guy BJ: Acquisition and maintenance of endoscopic skills: Developing an endoscopic dexterity training system for anesthesiologists. J Clin Anesth 14:615-619, 2002.

119. Mason RA: Learning fibreoptic intubation: Fundamental problems. Anaesthesia 47:729-731, 1992.

120. McCrirrick A, Pracilio JA: Awake intubation: A new technique. Anaesthesia 46:661-663, 1991.

121. Melker RJ: Alternative methods of ventilation during respiratory and cardiac arrest. Circulation 74:IV63-IV65, 1986.

122. Messeter KH, Pettersson KI: Endotracheal intubation with the fibre-optic bronchoscope. Anaesthesia 35:294-298, 1980.

123. Monrigal JP, Granry JC, Le Rolle T, et al: Difficult intubation in newborns and infants using an ultra thin fiberoptic bronchoscope. Anesthesiology 75(3A):A1044, 1991.

124. Montgomery G, Dueringer J, Johnson C: Nasal endotracheal tube change with an intubating stylette after fiberoptic intubation. Anesth Analg 72:713, 1991.

125. Mostafa SM, Atherton AM: Sevoflurane for difficult tracheal intubation. Br J Anaesth 79:392-393, 1997.

126. Moyers J, Gregory GA: Use of fiberoptic bronchoscopy to reposition an endotracheal tube intraoperatively. Anesthesiology 43:685, 1975.

127. Mulder DS, Wallace DH, Woolhouse FM: The use of the fiberoptic bronchoscope to facilitate endotracheal intubation following head and neck trauma. J Trauma 15:638-640, 1975.

128. Murphy P: A fibre-optic endoscope used for nasal intubation. Anaesthesia 22:489-491, 1967.

129. Naik VN, Matsumoto ED, Houston PL, et al: Fiberoptic orotracheal intubation on anesthetized patients: Do manipulation skills learned on a simple model transfer into the operating room? Anesthesiology 95:343-348, 2001.

130. Nakayama M, Kataoka N, Usui Y, et al: Techniques of nasotracheal intubation with the fiberoptic bronchoscope. J Emerg Med 10:729-734, 1992.

131. Nath G, Major V: The laryngeal mask in the management of a paediatric difficult airway. Anaesth Intensive Care 20:518-520, 1992.

132. O'Brien D, Curran J, Conroy J, Bouchier-Hayes D: Fibre-optic assessment of tracheal tube position. A comparison of tracheal tube position as estimated by fibre-optic bronchoscopy and by chest X-ray. Anaesthesia 40:73-76, 1985.

133. O'Brien K, Kumar R, Morton NS: Sevoflurane compared with halothane for tracheal intubation in children. Br J Anaesth 80:452-455, 1998.

134. Olopade CO, Prakash UB: Bronchoscopy in the critical-care unit. Mayo Clin Proc 64:1255-1263, 1989.

135. Oudjhane K, Bowen A, Oh KS, Young LW: Pulmonary edema complicating upper airway obstruction in infants and children. Can Assoc Radiol J 43:278-282, 1992.

136. Ovassapian, A: A new fiberoptic intubating airway. Anesth Analg 66:S132, 1987.

137. Ovassapian A: Failure to withdraw flexible fiberoptic laryngoscope after nasotracheal intubation. Anesthesiology 63:124-125, 1985.

138. Ovassapian A, Doka JC, Romsa DE: Acromegaly—Use of fiberoptic laryngoscopy to avoid tracheostomy. Anesthesiology 54:429-430, 1981.

139. Ovassapian A, Dykes MHM: The role of fiberoptic endoscopy in airway management. Semin Anesth 6:93, 1987.

140. Ovassapian A, Dykes MH, Golmon ME: A training programme for fibreoptic nasotracheal intubation. Use of model and live patients. Anaesthesia 38:795-798, 1983.

141. Ovassapian A, Krejcie TC, Joshi CW: Fiberoptic vs. rigid laryngoscopy for rapid sequence intubation of the trachea. Anesthesiology 74:S229, 1992.

142. Ovassapian A, Krejcie TC, Yelich SJ, Dykes MH: Awake fibreoptic intubation in the patient at high risk of aspiration. Br J Anaesth 62:13-16, 1989.

143. Ovassapian A, Land P, Schafer MF, et al: Anesthetic management for surgical corrections of severe flexion deformity of the cervical spine. Anesthesiology 58:370-372, 1983.

144. Ovassapian A, Liu SS, Krejcie TC. Fiberoptic tracheal intubation with Combitube in place. Anesth Analg 75:S315, 1993.

145. Ovassapian A, Schrader SC: Fiber-optic aided bronchial intubation. Semin Anesth 6:133, 1987.

146. Ovassapian A, Wheeler M: Fiberoptic endoscopy-aided techniques. In Benumof JL (ed): Airway Management: Principles and Practice. St. Louis, Mosby, 1996, pp 282-319.

147. Ovassapian A, Yelich SJ, Dykes MH, Brunner EE: Blood pressure and heart rate changes during awake fiberoptic nasotracheal intubation. Anesth Analg 62:951-954, 1983.

148. Ovassapian A, Yelich SJ, Dykes MH, Brunner EE: Fiberoptic nasotracheal intubation—Incidence and causes of failure. Anesth Analg 62:692-695, 1983.

149. Ovassapian A, Yelich SJ, Dykes MH, Golman ME: Learning fibreoptic intubation: Use of simulators v. traditional teaching. Br J Anaesth 61:217-220, 1988.

150. Patel A, Venn PJ, Barham CJ: Fibreoptic intubation through a laryngeal mask airway in an infant with Robin sequence. Eur J Anaesthesiol 15:237-239, 1998.

151. Patil V, Stehling LC, Zauder HL, Koch JP: Mechanical aids for fiberoptic endoscopy. Anesthesiology 57:69-70, 1982.

152. Patil VU: Concerning the complications of the Patil-Syracuse mask. Anesth Analg 76:1165-1166, 1993.

153. Patterson JR, Blaschke TF, Hunt KK, Meffin PJ: Lidocaine blood concentrations during fiberoptic bronchoscopy. Am Rev Respir Dis 112:53-57, 1975.

154. Pelimon A, Simunovic Z: Mouth gag and tongue holder for fibre-optic laryngoscopy. Anaesthesia 40:386, 1985.

155. Pennant JH, White PF: The laryngeal mask airway. Its uses in anesthesiology. Anesthesiology 79:144-163, 1993.

156. Practice guidelines for management of the difficult airway: An updated report by the American Society of Anesthesiologists Task Force on Management of the Difficult Airway. Anesthesiology 98:1269-1277, 2003.

157. Prakash UB, Abel MD, Hubmayr RD: Mediastinal mass and tracheal obstruction during general anesthesia. Mayo Clin Proc 63:1004-1011, 1988.

158. Price SL, Hecker BR: Pulmonary oedema following airway obstruction in a patient with Hodgkin's disease. Br J Anaesth 59:518-521, 1987.

159. Przybylo HJ, Stevenson GW, Vicari FA, et al: Retrograde fibreoptic intubation in a child with Nager's syndrome. Can J Anaesth 43:697-699, 1996.

160. Puchner W, Egger P, Puhringer F, et al: Evaluation of remifentanil as single drug for awake fiberoptic intubation. Acta Anaesthesiol Scand 46:350-354, 2002.

161. Puchner W, Obwegeser J, Puhringer FK: Use of remifentanil for awake fiberoptic intubation in a morbidly obese patient with severe inflammation of the neck. Acta Anaesthesiol Scand 46:473-476, 2002.

162. Raj PP, Forestner J, Watson TD, et al: Technics for fiberoptic laryngoscopy in anesthesia. Anesth Analg 53:708-714, 1974.

163. Reed AP, Han DG: Preparation of the patient for awake fiberoptic intubation. Anesth Clin North Am 9:69, 1991.

164. Reusche MD, Egan TD: Remifentanil for conscious sedation and analgesia during awake fiberoptic tracheal intubation: A case report with pharmacokinetic simulations. J Clin Anesth 11:64-68, 1999.

165. Rogers SN, Benumof JL: New and easy techniques for fiberoptic endoscopy-aided tracheal intubation. Anesthesiology 59:569-572, 1983.

166. Rosenbaum SH, Rosenbaum LM, Cole RP, et al: Use of the flexible fiberoptic bronchoscope to change endotracheal tubes in critically ill patients. Anesthesiology 54:169-170, 1981.

167. Roth AG, Wheeler M, Stevenson GW, Hall SC: Comparison of a rigid laryngoscope with the ultrathin fibreoptic laryngoscope for tracheal intubation in infants. Can J Anaesth 41:1069-1073, 1994.

168. Roth DM, Benumof JL: Intubation through a laryngeal mask airway with a nasal RAE tube: Stabilization of the proximal end of the tube. Anesthesiology 85:1220, 1996.

169. Rowe R, Cohen RA: An evaluation of a virtual reality airway simulator. Anesth Analg 95:62-66, table, 2002.

170. Rucker RW, Silva WJ, Worcester CC: Fiberoptic bronchoscopic nasotracheal intubation in children. Chest 76:56-58, 1979.

171. Russell SH, Hirsch NP: Simultaneous use of two laryngoscopes. Anaesthesia 48:918, 1993.

172. Schaefer HG, Marsch SC, Keller HL, et al: Teaching fibreoptic intubation in anaesthetised patients. Anaesthesia 49:331-334, 1994.

173. Scheller JG, Schulman SR: Fiber-optic bronchoscopic guidance for intubating a neonate with Pierre-Robin syndrome. J Clin Anesth 3:45-47, 1991.

174. Schwartz D, Johnson C, Roberts J: A maneuver to facilitate flexible fiberoptic intubation. Anesthesiology 71:470-471, 1989.

175. Schwartz HC, Bauer RA, Davis NJ, Guralnick WC: Ludwig's angina: Use of fiberoptic laryngoscopy to avoid tracheostomy. J Oral Surg 32:608-611, 1974.

176. Selim M, Mowafi H, Al Ghamdi A, Adu-Gyamfi Y: Intubation via LMA in pediatric patients with difficult airways. Can J Anaesth 46:891-893, 1999.

177. Shamberger RC, Holzman RS, Griscom NT, et al: Prospective evaluation by computed tomography and pulmonary function tests of children with mediastinal masses. Surgery 118:468-471, 1995.

178. Shinnick JP, Freedman AP: Bronchofiberscopic placement of a double-lumen endotracheal tube. Crit Care Med 10:544-545, 1982.

179. Shinwell ES, Higgins RD, Auten RL, Shapiro DL: Fiberoptic bronchoscopy in the treatment of intubated neonates. Am J Dis Child 143:1064-1065, 1989.

180. Shorten GD, Ali HH, Roberts JT: Assessment of patient position for fiberoptic intubation using videolaryngoscopy. J Clin Anesth 7:31-34, 1995.

181. Sidhu VS, Whitehead EM, Ainsworth QP, et al: A technique of awake fibreoptic intubation. Experience in patients with cervical spine disease. Anaesthesia 48:910-913, 1993.

182. Siegel M, Coleprate P: Complication of fiberoptic bronchoscope. Anesthesiology 61:214-215, 1984.

183. Smith CE, Fallon WF Jr: Sevoflurane mask anesthesia for urgent tracheostomy in an uncooperative trauma patient with a difficult airway. Can J Anaesth 47:242-245, 2000.

184. Smith JA, Santer LJ: Respiratory arrest following intramuscular ketamine injection in a 4-year-old child. Ann Emerg Med 22:613-615, 1993.

185. Smith JE: Heart rate and arterial pressure changes during fibreoptic tracheal intubation under general anaesthesia. Anaesthesia 43:629-632, 1988.

186. Smith JE, Fenner SG, King MJ: Teaching fibreoptic nasotracheal intubation with and without closed circuit television. Br J Anaesth 71:206-211, 1993.

187. Smith M, Calder I, Crockard A, et al: Oxygen saturation and cardiovascular changes during fibreoptic intubation under general anaesthesia. Anaesthesia 47:158-161, 1992.

188. Stiles CM: A flexible fiberoptic bronchoscope for endotracheal intubation of infants. Anesth Analg 53:1017-1019, 1974.

189. Stiles CM, Stiles QR, Denson JS: A flexible fiber optic laryngoscope. JAMA 221:1246-1247, 1972.

190. Stone BJ, Chantler PJ, Baskett PJ: The incidence of regurgitation during cardiopulmonary resuscitation: A comparison between the bag valve mask and laryngeal mask airway. Resuscitation 38:3-6, 1998.

191. Suriani RJ, Kayne RD: Fiberoptic bronchoscopic guidance for intubating a child with Pierre-Robin syndrome. J Clin Anesth 4:258-259, 1992.

192. Sutherland AD, Sale JP: Fibreoptic awake intubation— A method of topical anaesthesia and orotracheal intubation. Can Anaesth Soc J 33:502-504, 1986.

193. Tassonyi E, Lehmann C, Gunning K, et al: Fiberoptically guided intubation in children with gangrenous stomatitis (noma). Anesthesiology 73:348-349, 1990.

194. Taylor PA, Towey RM: The broncho-fiberscope as an aid to endotracheal intubation. Br J Anaesth 44:611-612, 1972.

195. Thomas DI, Bosch O: Training box for fibreoptics. Anaesthesia 55:815-816, 2000.

196. Thurlow JA, Madden AP: Sevoflurane for intubation of an infant with croup. Br J Anaesth 80:699-700, 1998.

197. Vaughan RS: Training in fibreoptic laryngoscopy. Br J Anaesth 66:538-540, 1991.

198. Vigneswaran R, Whitfield JM: The use of a new ultra-thin fiberoptic bronchoscope to determine endotracheal tube position in the sick newborn infant. Chest 80:174-177, 1981.

199. Walker RW: The laryngeal mask airway in the difficult paediatric airway: An assessment of positioning and use in fibreoptic intubation. Paediatr Anaesth 10:53-58, 2000.

200. Walker RW, Allen DL, Rothera MR: A fibreoptic intubation technique for children with mucopolysaccha-ridoses using the laryngeal mask airway. Paediatr Anaesth 7:421-426, 1997.

201. Wang CY, Chiu CL, Delilkan AE: Sevoflurane for difficult intubation in children. Br J Anaesth 80:408, 1998.

202. Wang JF, Reves JG, Corssen G: Use of the fiberoptic laryngoscope for difficult tracheal intubation. Ala J Med Sci 13:247-251, 1976.

203. Wangler MA, Weaver JM: A method to facilitate fiberoptic laryngoscopy. Anesthesiology 61:111, 1984.

204. Webb AR, Fernando SS, Dalton HR, et al: Local anaesthesia for fiberoptic bronchoscopy: Transcricoid injection or the "spray as you go" technique? Thorax 45:474-477, 1990.

205. Wheeler M, Coté CJ, Todres ID: In Coté CJ, Todres ID, Goudsouzian NG, Ryan JF (eds): The Pediatric Airway, a Practice of Anesthesia for Infants and Children, 3rd ed. Philadelphia, WB Saunders, 2001, pp 79-120.

206. Wheeler M, Dsida RM: Fiberoptic intubation: Troubles with the "Tube"? Anesthesiology 99:1236-1237, 2003.

207. Wheeler M, Roth AG, Heffner CL, Coté CJ: Teaching flexible fiberoptic intubation of infants and children: Does a videoscope system improve skill acquisition? Anesthesiology A-1112, 2002.

208. Whitehouse AC, Klock LE: Letter: Evaluation of endotracheal tube position with the fiberoptic intubation laryngoscope. Chest 68:848, 1975.

209. Whitlock JE, Calder I: Transillumination in fibreoptic intubation. Anaesthesia 42:570, 1987.

210. Wilder RT, Belani KG: Fiberoptic intubation complicated by pulmonary edema in a 12- year-old child with Hurler syndrome. Anesthesiology 72:205-207, 1990.

211. Williams L, Teague PD, Nagia AH: Foreign body from a Patil-Syracuse mask. Anesth Analg 73:359-360, 1991.

212. Williams RT, Harrison RE: Prone tracheal intubation simplified using an airway intubator. Can Anaesth Soc J 28:288-289, 1981.

213. Wilton NC: Aids for fiberoptically guided intubation in children. Anesthesiology 75:549-550, 1991.

214. Wood RE: Spelunking in the pediatric airways: Explorations with the flexible fiberoptic bronchoscope. Pediatr Clin North Am 31:785-799, 1984.

215. Wright RB, Manfield FF: Damage to teeth during the administration of general anaesthesia. Anesth Analg 53:405-408, 1974.

216. Zornow MH, Mitchell MM: Foreign body aspiration during fiberoptic-assisted intubation. Anesthesiology 64:303, 1986.

19

RETROGRADE INTUBATION TECHNIQUE

Antonio Sanchez

I. HISTORY

The first reported case of retrograde intubation (RI) was by Butler and Cirillo in 1960.[22] The technique involved passing a red rubber catheter cephalad through the patient's previously existing tracheostomy. When the catheter exited the oral cavity, it was tied to the endotracheal tube (ET), allowing it to be pulled into the trachea.

The first person to perform RI as presently practiced was Waters, a British anesthesiologist in Nigeria.[155] In 1963, he reported treating patients who had cancrum oris, an invasive gangrene that deforms the oral cavity, severely limiting mouth opening. His technique involved passing a standard Tuohy needle through the cricothyroid membrane (CTM) and feeding an epidural catheter cephalad into the nasopharynx. He "fished" the catheter out of the nasopharynx through the nares, using a hook he devised. The epidural catheter was then used as a stylet to guide the ET through the nares and into the trachea.

Over the ensuing years, RI did not gain clinical acceptance because of its invasiveness and the potential for complications from the CTM puncture. After 1964, when fiberoptic technology became available, RI was irregularly but occasionally discussed in the literature.[1-165] In 1993, RI was designated as part of the anesthesiologist's armamentarium by the American Society of Anesthesiologists Difficult Airway Task Force.[9]

The name "retrograde intubation," used by Butler and Cirillo, is a misnomer.[77] The technique is actually a

Box 19-1   Number of Retrograde Intubations in the Literature (539 Patients and 137 Cadavers)

Oral Cavity
Cancrum oris, 27
Mandibular or maxillary fracture, 31
Mandibular prognathia, 1
Perimandibular abscess, 1
Ankylosis of temporomandibular joint, 8
Microstomia, 1
Macroglossia, 1
Cancer of tongue, 8
Oral myxoma, 1
Lingual tonsil, 1
Hypopharyngeal tumors, 2
Cervical
Spinal cord injury, 98
Ankylosing spondylitis, 19
Rheumatoid arthritis, 32

Pharynx and Larynx
Laryngeal cancer, 163
Pharyngeal abscess, 1
Epiglottitis, 1
Pharyngeal edema, 1
Laryngeal edema after burn, 3
Others
Pediatric anomalies, 27
Obesity, 13
Coronary artery bypass grafting (failure to intubate), 28
Tracheostomy stoma, 16
Trauma (failure to intubate), 34
Disease not specified (failure to intubate), 21
Cadaver studies, 137

From University of California–Irvine Department of Anesthesia: Teaching Aids.

translaryngeal guided intubation, but for historical reasons we continue using the name retrograde intubation.

II. INDICATIONS

The RI technique has been used both in the hospital setting and in prehospital mobile units (in the field).[12,95] It has been employed with the anticipated[4,5,12,26,155] and unanticipated* difficult airway, following failure to intubate using conventional means (direct laryngoscopy,[26,95,29] blind nasal intubation,[19,29] bougie,[35,47] laryngeal mask airway [LMA], and fiberoptic laryngoscopy[18,62,65,126]). It has been employed in both humans and animals.[30,131] In the literature, as well as in the author's experience, there have been approximately 807 cases using RI (670 patients and 137 cadavers) as a means of securing the airway. Although in the majority of cases RI has been used to place a single-lumen ET, one case report described placement of a double-lumen ET through RI.[4]

Airway disease necessitating RI has been of a wide variety (Box 19-1). RI has been most frequently associated with limited range of motion of the neck (153 trauma victims with potential cervical spine injury), and its use has been reported in facial trauma. It has been employed in both adults and pediatric patients with success (Box 19-2).

Not all reports have described the amount of time required to perform the technique, but in one study involving emergency medical service personnel (paramedics and registered nurses) using training mannequins, the average time was 71 seconds (range, 42 to 129 seconds).[152] Barriot and Riou[12] described 13 patients with maxillofacial trauma who could not be intubated in the field using direct laryngoscopy (six attempts: average time, 18 minutes). Intubation was subsequently performed in the patients on the first RI attempt in an average time of less than 5 minutes. An additional six patients were intubated in less than 5 minutes when RI was used as the initial method of choice. Slots and colleagues reported a modified technique using a Mini-Trach II set on 20 cadavers with an average time for intubation of 6.7 seconds (range 3 to 10 seconds); it was subsequently used on a an emergency basis on three patients with an average time of 10 seconds. The investigators concluded that the RI technique was a rapid, efficacious method for intratracheal intubation of trauma patients, especially patients with maxillofacial trauma.[141]

Historical indications for RI are the following:

1. Failed attempts at laryngoscopy, LMA, or fiberoptic intubation
2. Urgent establishment of an airway where visualization of the vocal cords is prevented by blood, secretions, or anatomic derangement in scenarios in which ventilation is still possible
3. Elective use when deemed necessary in clinical situations such as unstable cervical spine, maxillofacial trauma, or anatomic anomaly

Box 19-2   Characteristics of Retrograde Intubations (RIs) in the Literature

1. Number of adult patients (RI): 509
2. Number of pediatric patients (RI): 30
3. Age range: 1 day old (weight, 2.9 kg) to 84 years
4. Average time for technique: 0.2 minute (range, 0.5 to 15 minutes)
5. Elective cases: 249 patients
6. Failed attempts using RI: 12 patients.

From University of California–Irvine Department of Anesthesia: Teaching Aids.

*References 12, 19, 29, 42, 47, 57, 83, 95, 96, 111, 126, 148, 153, 155.

III. CONTRAINDICATIONS

Contraindications to RI have been cited, often anecdotally (Box 19-3). Most are relative contraindications and can be divided into four categories: unfavorable anatomy, laryngotracheal disease, coagulopathy, and infection.

A. UNFAVORABLE ANATOMY

Because in most cases RI is performed above or below the cricoid cartilage, absolute lack of access to this region, as in severe flexion deformity of the neck, is a contraindication if not an impossibility.[107,108] For the same reason, the patient with nonpalpable landmarks,[55,100,144] obesity,[132] overlying malignancy,[100] or large thyroid goiter[100] should be approached cautiously. Shantha[138] reported a case of RI in a patient with a large thyroid goiter. After failure of conventional intubating methods (including fiberoptic), the surgeons dissected down to the CTM and subsequently passed the catheter cephalad. Thirteen cases of RI have been reported in obese patients without major complications.[42,126,129,132]

B. LARYNGOTRACHEAL DISEASE

Theoretically, laryngotracheal stenosis[55,155] may contraindicate RI because narrowing of the trachea or larynx could be made worse by either the needle puncture or the catheter.[55,155] However, RI has been used in patients with laryngeal cancer,[56] epiglottitis,[64] and laryngeal edema resulting from burn injuries.[65,96] It should not be used when there is laryngeal tracheal stenosis directly under the intended puncture site.

C. COAGULOPATHY[1,2,55,68,100,112,120,149]

Preexisting bleeding diathesis should be considered a relative contraindication. Although there is a potential for bleeding, the CTM is considered a relatively avascular plane (see "Anatomy" in Section IV). A small, self-limited hematoma[26] was reported in a patient who underwent a coronary artery bypass graft with intraoperative heparin and postoperative disseminated intravascular coagulation.

D. INFECTION

RI in the presence of preexisting infection over the puncture site or in the path of the puncture, as in pretracheal abscess or Ludwig's angina, could result in transmittal of bacterial flora into the trachea and should be avoided. This, again, should be considered a relative contraindication because transtracheal aspiration is performed for a sputum sample in patients with pneumonia despite the possibility of pretracheal abscess (see "Complications" Section VIII in this chapter).[36,53,55,100,120,165]

IV. ANATOMY

The performance of RI requires basic anatomic knowledge of the cricoid cartilage (Fig. 19-1) and the structures above and below it, to minimize complications and failure. Indeed, regardless of the intubation technique planned, the cricoid cartilage and CTM should be identified preoperatively in every patient.[128] Cartilage and membrane, vascular structures, and the thyroid gland are relevant anatomy.

A. CARTILAGE AND MEMBRANE

The cricoid cartilage is in the shape of signet ring (see Fig. 19-1). It consists of a broad, flat, posterior plate called the lamina and a narrow, convex, anterior structure called the arch.[23,27] In most cases the cartilage can be easily palpated by identifying the thyroid notch and running a

---

Box 19-3 Contraindications to Retrograde Intubation and Examples

Unfavorable Anatomy
Lack of access to cricothyroid muscle (severe flexion deformity of the neck)
Poor anatomic landmarks (obesity)
Pretracheal mass (thyroid goiter)
Laryngotracheal Disease
Malignancy
Stenosis
Coagulopathy
Infection (Pretracheal Abscess)

From University of California–Irvine Department of Anesthesia: Teaching Aids.

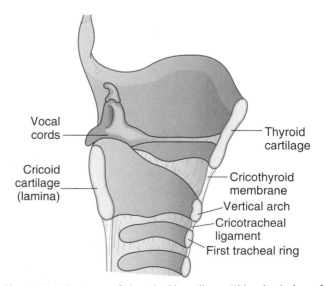

Figure 19-1 Anatomy of the cricoid cartilage. Midsagittal view of the larynx and trachea. (From Sanchez AF: *The Retrograde Cookbook.* Irvine, University of California–Irvine Department of Anesthesia, 1993.)

finger down the midline in a caudad direction until a rigid rounded structure is encountered. The vertical height (Fig. 19-2) of the arch is 0.5 to 0.7 cm.[27] The CTM connects the superior border of the arch to the inferior border of the thyroid cartilage and measures approximately 1 cm in height[23] and 2 cm in width.[78] The lateral borders are the paired cricothyroid muscles.[36] The cricotracheal ligament connects the inferior border of the arch to the upper border of the first tracheal ring and measures 0.3 to 0.6 cm in height.[139] The distance between the inferior border of the thyroid cartilage and the vocal cords varies with gender but is approximately 0.9 cm.[105]

B. VASCULAR STRUCTURES

There are paired major blood vessels above and below the cricoid cartilage: the cricothyroid artery and the superior thyroid artery (Fig. 19-3).

The cricothyroid artery,[6,16,27,78,105] a branch of the superior thyroid artery, runs along the anterior surface of the CTM, usually close to the inferior border of the thyroid cartilage. In some cases, the cricothyroid arteries anastomose in the midline and give rise to a descending branch that feeds the middle lobe of the thyroid gland when present. On the basis of dissections on cadavers performed by the author, the cricothyroid artery becomes insignificant in size as it approaches the midline. No major venous plexus could be found mentioned in the literature or found in dissections by the author.

The anterior branch of the superior thyroid artery[6,16,27,105] runs along the upper border of the thyroid

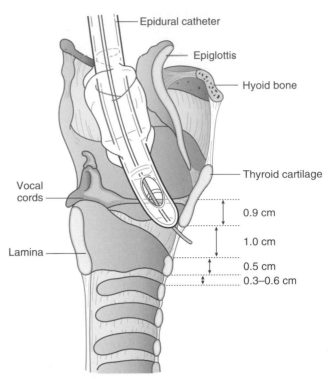

Figure 19-2 Midsagittal view of the larynx and trachea showing the distance between the vocal cords and the upper border of the first tracheal ring. Only a small portion of the endotracheal tube Murphy eye is below the vocal cords. (From Sanchez AF: The Retrograde Cookbook. Irvine, University of California–Irvine Department of Anesthesia, 1993.)

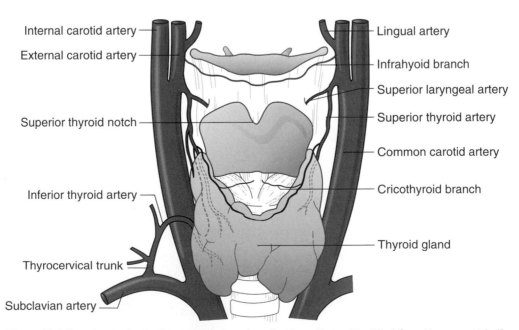

Figure 19-3 Vascular anatomy above and below the cricoid cartilage. (Modified from Naumann H [ed]: Head and Neck Surgery. Philadelphia, WB Saunders, 1984.)

isthmus to anastomose with its counterpart from the opposite side. The inferior thyroid artery also anastomoses with the superior thyroid artery at the level of the isthmus. The arteries are remarkable for their large size and frequent anastomoses. In less than 10% of the population, an unpaired thyroid ima artery ascends ventral to the trachea (from either the aortic arch or brachiocephalic artery) to anastomose at the level of the isthmus. It is usually small but may be very large. A rich venous plexus is formed in and around the isthmus.

C. THYROID GLAND (ISTHMUS, PYRAMIDAL LOBE)

The isthmus of the thyroid gland (see Fig. 19-3) is rarely absent and generally lies anterior to the trachea between the first and fourth tracheal rings (usually between the second and third), although there are many variations. Its size and vertical height vary; the average vertical height and depth are 1.25 cm. Extending from the isthmus, the highly vascular pyramidal lobe (Fig. 19-4) is well developed in one third of the population. It is found more frequently on the left of the midline and may extend up to the hyoid bone (the upper continuation is usually thyromuscular[6,16,23,27,30]).

V. PHYSIOLOGY

Sympathetic stress responses (increased heart rate, blood pressure, intraocular pressure, and intracranial pressure and elevated catecholamine levels) have been reported with laryngoscopy, endotracheal intubation, coughing, translaryngeal local anesthesia, laryngotracheal anesthesia, and fiberoptic intubation. Therefore, concern is appropriate when performing RI in patients with coronary artery disease, elevated intraocular pressure, and elevated intracranial pressure.[11,33,69,101,107,108,140,145,156] It is reasonable to argue, however, that RI, performed skillfully, is not more stimulating than any other technique for managing the airway.

No apparent significant changes in hemodynamics were reported in multiple case reports of patients with cardiac disease (congenital anomalies, ischemic coronary artery disease, valvular disease, pericarditis, and congestive heart failure) who underwent RI, both awake with topical anesthesia and under general anesthesia.* Casthely and colleagues[26] reported 25 patients with difficult airway because of rheumatoid arthritis who came for open heart surgery (coronary artery bypass graft and valve replacement). The patients had invasive monitors placed (Swan-Ganz catheters and peripheral arterial lines) preoperatively. The initial 24 patients underwent a cardiac induction of anesthesia (diazepam 10 mg, fentanyl 25 to 30 μg/kg, and pancuronium 0.1 mg/kg) before rigid laryngoscopy, followed by RI. Comparison of hemodynamic responses to rigid laryngoscopy (Macintosh and Miller blades) versus RI demonstrated that the former was more stressful (Table 19-1). Patient 25 underwent RI before induction of anesthesia after application of topical anesthesia with no significant hemodynamic response.

Two case reports[5,57] documented patients with a previous history of difficult airway and intracranial pathology (pseudotumor cerebri and intracranial tumor with elevated intracranial pressure) who underwent elective, awake RI after topical anesthesia with no evidence of further increase in intracranial pressure.

The author, unmedicated except for topical lidocaine, underwent awake RI with no significant hemodynamic changes.[128]

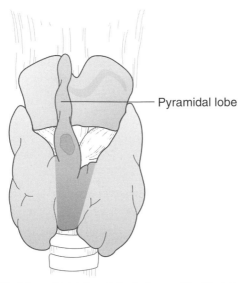

Figure 19-4 Pyramidal lobe of the isthmus. (Modified from Naumann H [ed]: Head and Neck Surgery, vol 4. Philadelphia, WB Saunders, 1984.)

— Pyramidal lobe

VI. TECHNIQUES

A. PREPARATION

1. Positioning

The ideal position for RI is the supine sniffing position with the neck hyperextended.[46,54] In this position, the cervical vertebrae push the trachea and cricoid cartilage anteriorly and displace the strap muscles of the neck laterally. As a result, the cricoid cartilage and the structures above and below it are easier to palpate. RI can also be performed with the patient in a sitting position,[128] which may be the only position in which some patients can breathe comfortably. Potential cervical spine injury or limited range of motion of the cervical spine may necessitate RI with the neck in a neutral position, which is a well-documented practice (see Box 19-1).

---

*References 24, 26, 28, 29, 64, 83, 84, 93, 111, 118, 134.

Table 19-1   **Hemodynamic Effects of Retrograde Intubation**

	Laryngoscopy	Retrograde Intubation
HR	Increase	No change from baseline
MAP	Increase	No change from baseline
CI	Decrease	No change from baseline
PCWP	Increase	No change from baseline
ECG	3-mm ST depression	No change from baseline

HR, heart rate; MAP, mean arterial pressure; CI, cardiac index; PCWP, pulmonary capillary wedge pressure; ECG, electrocardiogram (ST segment changes in lead V_5)
Modified from Casthely PA, Landesman S, Fynaman PN: Retrograde intubation in patients undergoing open heart surgery. Can Anaesth Soc J 32:661, 1985.

2. Skin Preparation

Although most documented RIs have not been elective, every effort should be made to perform RI using aseptic technique. Recommendations have been made for prophylactic antibiotics in diabetic or immunocompromised patients, who may be more susceptible to infection.[13]

3. Anesthesia

If time permits, the airway should be anesthetized to prevent sympathetic stimulation, laryngospasm, and discomfort. In the literature, many different combinations of techniques have been described:

1. Translaryngeal anesthesia during intravenous sedation or general anesthesia[5,19,26,75,96,126,155]
2. Translaryngeal anesthesia with superior laryngeal nerve block[10,12,95]
3. Translaryngeal anesthesia with topicalization of the pharynx (aerosolized or sprayed)[4,34,57,60]
4. Glossopharyngeal nerve block and superior laryngeal nerve block with nebulized local anesthetic[111]

(Refer to Chapter 10 for a detailed description of neural blockade of the airway.)

In the author's experience,[128] an awake RI can be performed with translaryngeal anesthesia (4 mL 2% lidocaine) supplemented with topicalization (nebulized or sprayed local anesthetics) of the pharynx and hypopharynx. Special caution should be exercised when performing the translaryngeal anesthesia because coughing, grunting, sneezing, or swallowing causes the cricoid cartilage to travel cephalad with the potential for breaking the needle in the trachea.[106,160] To avoid this, one can insert a 20-gauge angiocatheter and remove the needle before injecting the local anesthetic.

4. Entry Site

The transtracheal puncture for RI can be made either above or below the cricoid cartilage. The CTM is relatively avascular and has less potential for bleeding (see "Anatomy" in Section IV). The disadvantage of the CTM is that initially only 1 cm of ET is actually placed below the vocal cords and the angle of entry of the ET into the trachea is more acute. An initial puncture performed at the cricotracheal ligament or lower affords the added advantage of the ET traveling in a straighter path as well as allowing a longer initial length of ET below the vocal cords. The disadvantage is that this site (below the cricoid cartilage) has more potential for bleeding (although none has been reported). Both entry sites have been used successfully. In cadaver studies[89,90] the success rate for RI was higher with less vocal cord trauma when the cricotracheal ligament rather than the CTM was used. Vocal cord trauma has not been reported in living patients.

B. CLASSICAL TECHNIQUE

The classical technique of RI is performed percutaneously using a standard 17-gauge Tuohy needle and epidural catheter.

After positioning (Fig. 19-5), skin preparation, and anesthesia, a right hand–dominant person should stand on the right side of a supine patient. The left hand is used to stabilize the trachea by placing the thumb and third digit on either side of the thyroid cartilage. The index

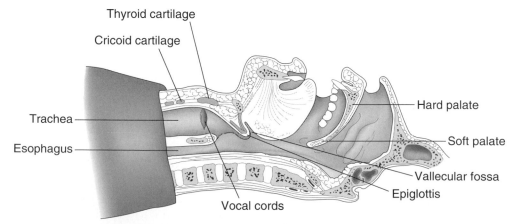

Figure 19-5 Midsagittal view of the head and neck. (From Sanchez AF: The Retrograde Cookbook. Irvine, University of California–Irvine Department of Anesthesia, 1993.)

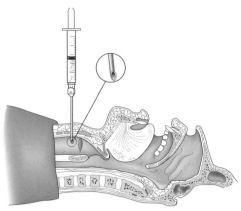

Figure 19-6 Standard No. 17 Tuohy needle (with saline-filled syringe) is advanced (with bevel pointing cephalad) through the cricothyroid membrane at a 90-degree angle (trying to stay as close as possible to the upper border of the cricoid cartilage). Entrance into the trachea is verified by aspiration of air. (From Sanchez AF: The Retrograde Cookbook. Irvine, University of California–Irvine Department of Anesthesia, 1993.)

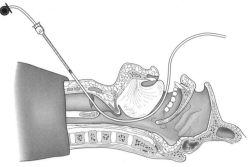

Figure 19-8 Epidural catheter is advanced through the vocal cords and into the pharynx. During this time the patient is asked to stick tongue out, or tongue can be pulled out manually. Most of the time the epidural catheter comes out of the mouth on its own. Tuohy needle is then withdrawn to the caudal end of epidural catheter. (From Sanchez AF: The Retrograde Cookbook. Irvine, University of California–Irvine Department of Anesthesia, 1993.)

finger of the left hand is used to identify the midline of the CTM and the upper border of the cricoid cartilage.

Because the Tuohy needle is blunt, a small incision through the skin and subcutaneous tissue with a No. 11 scalpel blade is recommended. Because of the significant force required to perforate the skin and the CTM, there is a risk of perforating the posterior tracheal wall as well. This has been verified in cadaver studies using a fiberoptic bronchoscope (FOB).[132]

The right hand then grasps the Tuohy needle and saline syringe like a pencil (using the fifth digit to brace the right hand on the patient's lower neck) and performs the puncture, aspirating to confirm placement in the lumen of the airway (Figs. 19-6 and 19-7).

Once the Tuohy needle is in place, the epidural catheter is advanced into the trachea (Fig. 19-8). When advancing the epidural catheter, it is important to have the tongue pulled anteriorly to prevent the catheter from coiling up in the oropharynx. The catheter usually exits on its own

from either the oral (Fig. 19-9) or nasal cavity. A hemostat should be clamped to the catheter at the neck skin line to prevent further movement of the epidural catheter. If the catheter has to be retrieved from the oropharynx, the author's preferred instrument is a nerve hook (V. Mueller NL2490, Baxter, Deerfield, IL). Magill forceps have been used, but these were designed to grasp large structures such as an ET and may not grip the relatively small catheter (the distal tips of the forceps do not completely occlude) and, in addition, may traumatize the pharynx. Arya and associates described an innovative atraumatic method of retrieving catheters from the oral pharynx in patients with limited mouth opening. They used a "pharyngeal loop" that they devised using a ureteral guidewire that was threaded through a 3-mm uncuffed polyvinyl chloride ET and doubled up to form a loop. The pharyngeal loop allowed them to retrieve the catheter from the oropharynx in a patient who had limited mouth opening.[8]

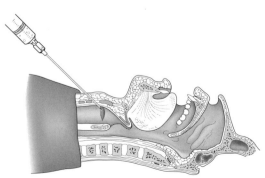

Figure 19-7 Angle of Tuohy needle is changed to 45 degrees with bevel pointing cephalad (again verifying position by aspirating air). (From Sanchez AF: The Retrograde Cookbook. Irvine, University of California–Irvine Department of Anesthesia, 1993.)

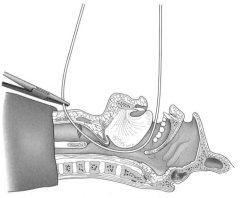

Figure 19-9 Pull epidural catheter out of the mouth to an appropriate length; then clamp a hemostat flush with the skin. (From Sanchez AF: The Retrograde Cookbook. Irvine, University of California–Irvine Department of Anesthesia, 1993.)

Figure 19-10 Cross section of larynx and trachea with endotracheal tube (ET) and catheter guide passing through the cricothyroid membrane. **A**, Catheter passes through end of ET, and 1 cm of ET passes the cords. **B**, The catheter exits the side hole, allowing 2 cm of ET to pass beyond the vocal cords.

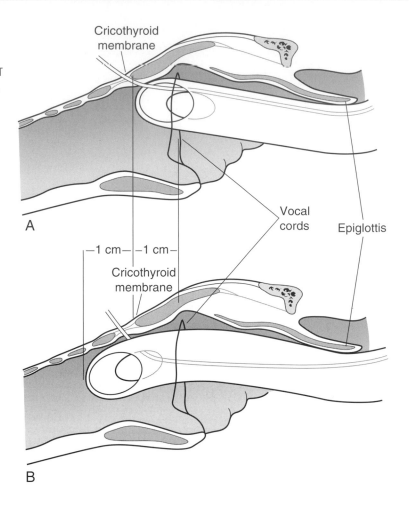

Originally, the catheter was threaded through the main distal lumen (beveled portion) of the ET. Bourke and Levesque[20] modified the technique by threading the catheter through the Murphy eye (Fig. 19-10), reasoning that this would allow an additional 1 cm of ET to pass through the cords. Lleu and coworkers,[89,90] in cadaver studies, showed that using the cricotracheal ligament as the puncture site in combination with threading the epidural catheter through the Murphy eye enhanced success compared with the original technique.

When the ET is being advanced over the epidural catheter (Figs. 19-11 to 19-13), a moderate amount of tension should be employed.[2,47] Excessive tension pulls the ET anteriorly, making it more likely to be caught up against the epiglottis, vallecula, or anterior commissure of the vocal cords. If there is difficulty in passing the opening of the glottis, the ET can be rotated 90 degrees counterclockwise[47,62,132] or exchanged for a smaller tube.[132]

Ideally, one would like to verify that the ET is below the vocal cords *before* removing the epidural catheter (Fig. 19-14; see Fig. 19-13). The methods are the following:

1. By direct vision, using the FOB (see "Fiberoptic Technique" Section VI. D)
2. If the patient is breathing spontaneously, by listening to breath sounds through the ET

3. By capnography, using a fiberoptic elbow adapter connected to a capnograph [14]
4. By luminescent techniques using a light wand[66]

C. GUIDEWIRE TECHNIQUE

The modified technique using a guidewire* was developed because the flexible epidural catheter is prone to kinking.[30,47,62] Equipment consists of an 18-gauge angiocatheter, a J-tip guidewire (0.038-inch outer diameter and 110 to 120 cm in length), and a guide catheter (Fig. 19-15).

Use of a guidewire offers the following advantages:

1. The J tip tends to be less traumatic to the airway.[1,34,49,65]
2. Retrieval of the guidewire from the oral or nasal cavity is easier.[34,49,144]
3. The guidewire is less prone to kinking.[114]
4. The guidewire can be used with the FOB (see "Fiberoptic Technique" Section VI. D).
5. The guidewire is easy to handle.[10,49,100]
6. The technique takes less time to perform than the classical technique.[144,152]

---

*References 1, 4, 10, 24, 30, 32, 34, 38, 47-49, 55, 57, 62, 64, 65, 72, 75-77, 83, 100, 101, 124, 140, 144, 145, 148, 156, 162.

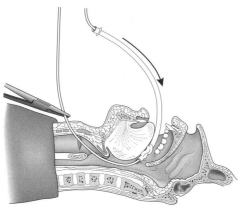

Figure 19-11 Thread a well-lubricated endotracheal tube (ET) over the epidural catheter. Maintain a moderate amount of tension on the epidural catheter as you advance the ET *(arrow)* forward; you will feel a small click as ET travels through the vocal cords. (From Sanchez AF: The Retrograde Cookbook. Irvine, University of California–Irvine Department of Anesthesia, 1993.)

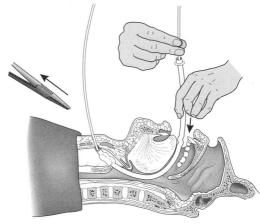

Figure 19-13 Have an assistant remove hemostat *(large arrow)* while pressure is maintained *(small arrow)* to push the endotracheal tube up against the cricothyroid membrane. (The epidural catheter may be cut flush with the hemostat before hemostat is removed.) (From Sanchez AF: The Retrograde Cookbook. Irvine, University of California–Irvine Department of Anesthesia, 1993.)

Discrepancy between the external diameter of the guidewire and the internal diameter of the ET allows a "railroading" effect to occur, with the tip of the ET catching peripherally on the arytenoids or vocal cords instead of going straight through the cords. Sliding the guide catheter over the guidewire from above (antegrade) when it has exited the mouth or nose increases the external diameter of the guidewire,[14] and use of the guide catheter in combination with a smaller diameter ET allows the ET to enter the glottis in a more centralized position with respect to the glottic opening.

Various types of antegrade guide catheters have been used: FOBs (see next section), nasogastric tubes,[92,132] suction catheters,[59,132] plastic sheaths from Swan-Ganz catheters,[72] Eschmann stylets,[47] and tube changers.[65,76]

The Cook Critical Care retrograde guidewire kit (Cook Incorporated, Bloomington, IN) contains a tapered antegrade guide catheter, which is the author's choice of antegrade guide catheter (see Fig. 19-15), and is used to describe the basic guidewire and antegrade guide catheter technique.

The guidewire and antegrade guide catheter technique is as follows. Identify the trachea in Figures 19-16 to 19-18 with the syringe and 18-gauge angiocatheter. The J wire is then fed through the intratracheal catheter (Fig. 19-19) until it passes out the mouth (Fig. 19-20). The guidewire is then clamped at the neck skin line, and the tapered antegrade guide catheter is fed over the guidewire (Fig. 19-21) until the antegrade guide catheter reaches the CTM (Fig. 19-22). The ET is then fed over the

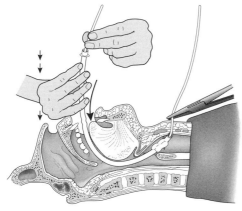

Figure 19-12 When the endotracheal tube (ET) reaches the cricothyroid membrane (CTM), it is important to maintain pressure *(small arrows)*, forcing the ET into the oropharynx *(large arrow)* to cause continuing pressure against the CTM with the tip of the ET. (Note: moderate tension is still maintained on the epidural catheter.) (From Sanchez AF: The Retrograde Cookbook. Irvine, University of California–Irvine Department of Anesthesia, 1993.)

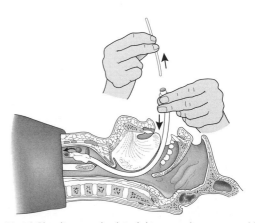

Figure 19-14 Simultaneously *(straight arrows)* remove epidural catheter as you advance the endotracheal tube (ET). The tip of the ET will drop from its position up against the CTM to mid-trachea *(curved arrow)*. Advance ET to desired depth. (From Sanchez AF: The Retrograde Cookbook. Irvine, University of California–Irvine Department of Anesthesia, 1993.)

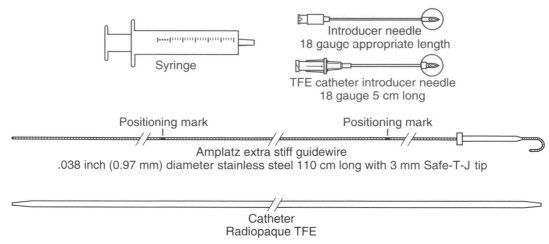

Figure 19-15 Retrograde kit TFE (Teflon guide catheter). (From Cook Inc., Bloomington, IN)

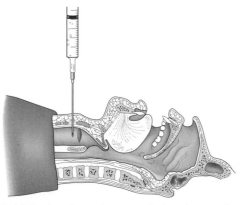

Figure 19-16 Angiocatheter (18-gauge) placed at 90-degree angle to the cricothyroid membrane, aspirating for air to confirm position. (From Sanchez AF: The Retrograde Cookbook. Irvine, University of California–Irvine Department of Anesthesia, 1993.)

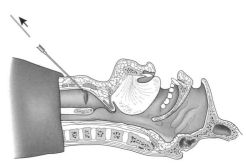

Figure 19-18 Advance sheath of angiocatheter cephalad, and remove needle. (From Sanchez AF: The Retrograde Cookbook. Irvine, University of California–Irvine Department of Anesthesia, 1993.)

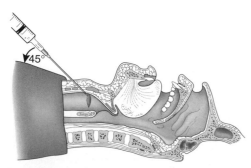

Figure 19-17 Angle is changed to 45 degrees (again aspirating air to confirm position). (From Sanchez AF: The Retrograde Cookbook. Irvine, University of California–Irvine Department of Anesthesia, 1993.)

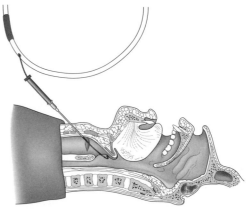

Figure 19-19 Advance J-tip guidewire through angiocatheter sheath. (From Sanchez AF: The Retrograde Cookbook. Irvine, University of California–Irvine Department of Anesthesia, 1993.)

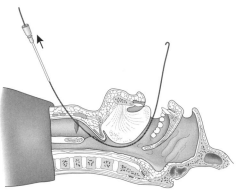

Figure 19-20 Retrieve end of guidewire from mouth as in classical technique. Remove angiocatheter *(small arrow)*. (From Sanchez AF: The Retrograde Cookbook. Irvine, University of California–Irvine Department of Anesthesia, 1993.)

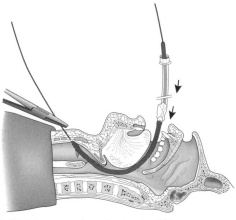

Figure 19-23 Advance endotracheal tube (ET) over entire structure *(arrows)*. Use an ET that has 6.0 to 7.0 mm internal diameter. Size of the ET is dictated by the external diameter of the guide catheter. (From Sanchez AF: The Retrograde Cookbook. Irvine, University of California–Irvine Department of Anesthesia, 1993.)

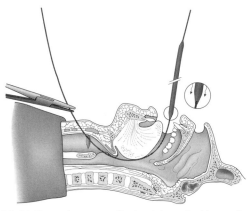

Figure 19-21 Clamp hemostat flush with neck skin, and advance tapered tip of guide catheter *(inset)* over guidewire into mouth. (From Sanchez AF: The Retrograde Cookbook. Irvine, University of California–Irvine Department of Anesthesia, 1993.)

antegrade guide catheter (Figs. 19-23 and 19-24) and the antegrade guide catheter is removed (Fig. 19-25). The standard Cook RI set has been modified to include a tapered antegrade guide catheter with distal sideports and Rapi-Fit adapters (Arndt Airway Exchange Catheter) in order to allow oxygenation and ventilation of the patient as well as facilitate placement of an ET.

Three other modifications have been reported using guide catheters. First, the guidewire is removed when the guide catheter abuts against the CTM (see Fig. 19-21). The guide catheter alone is then advanced farther into the trachea and used as a stylet for the ET.[72,75,76] Second, an RI is performed with the bare guidewire (or epidural catheter) alone. When the ET abuts the CTM, the guide catheter is advanced through the ET from above (antegrade), passing distally to the carina.[29] The guidewire is then removed and the guide catheter is again used as a stylet for the ET. In the author's opinion, the best results

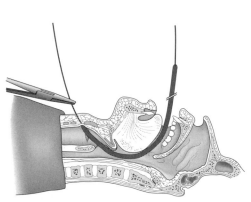

Figure 19-22 Advance guide catheter to cricothyroid membrane. (From Sanchez AF: The Retrograde Cookbook. Irvine, University of California–Irvine Department of Anesthesia, 1993.)

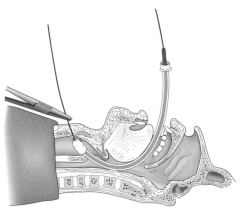

Figure 19-24 Advance endotracheal tube through vocal cords and up against the cricothyroid membrane. (From Sanchez AF: The Retrograde Cookbook. Irvine, University of California–Irvine Department of Anesthesia, 1993.)

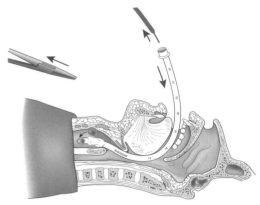

Figure 19-25 Removal of wire and catheter as in classical technique, except that the guidewire and guide catheter are removed simultaneously. (From Sanchez AF: The Retrograde Cookbook. Irvine, University of California–Irvine Department of Anesthesia, 1993.)

from a blind RI would be obtained by using the cricotracheal ligament as a puncture site and the guide catheter over the guidewire technique. Third, an LMA has been used as conduit for the exit of the guidewire; a jet stylet is then placed over the guidewire and both the LMA and guidewire are then removed leaving the jet stylet as a guide catheter for the ET. Benefits of this technique include a longer time for ventilation and the ability to place a larger ET than the LMA would have accommodated.[7]

D. FIBEROPTIC TECHNIQUE

The FOB is a versatile tool for the anesthesiologist,[6] but the FOB, like RI, has its limitations. In some cases, the combination of two techniques when previously either technique alone has failed[10,14,24,57,64,83,132,148] allows achievement of tracheal intubation. The combination of RI with direct laryngoscopy[64] and RI using FOB[10,24,57,83,148] can improve the chance of successful intubation. The advantages of passing an FOB antegrade over a guidewire placed by RI are as follows:

1. The outer diameter of the guidewire and the internal diameter of the suction port of the FOB form a tight fit that prevents railroading between both cylinders, allowing the FOB to follow a straight path through the vocal cords without being caught on anatomic structures.
2. The FOB acts as a large antegrade guide catheter (see "Guidewire Technique" Section VI. C) and prevents railroading of the ET.
3. When the FOB has passed over the wire through the vocal cords, it can be advanced freely beyond the puncture site to the carina, which eliminates the problem of distance between vocal cords and puncture site.
4. Use of the FOB allows placement of the ET under direct vision.

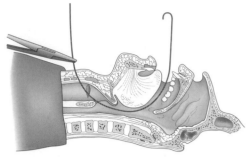

Figure 19-26 Guidewire placed as in guidewire technique and pulled out to appropriate length to accommodate fiberoptic bronchoscope (hemostat in place). (From Sanchez AF: The Retrograde Cookbook. Irvine, University of California–Irvine Department of Anesthesia, 1993.)

5. The FOB can be used by the less experienced operator.
6. Oxygen can be delivered continuously through the FOB with the guidewire still in place (see "Pediatrics" Section VII).

Preparation of the FOB should be completed before RI is initiated. The rubber casing from the proximal portion of the suction port must be removed (to allow the guidewire to exit from the FOB handle), and the FOB should be armed with the appropriate-sized ET (6.5 to 7.0 mm inner diameter). The RI is performed using the guidewire technique (Fig. 19-26) and the FOB then passed antegrade over the guidewire like a guide catheter (Figs. 19-27 to 19-30). Once the tip of the FOB abuts the CTM (Fig. 19-31), there are the following options:

1. Remove the guidewire distally (Fig. 19-32) or proximally (through the fiberoptic handle) and, after advancing under direct vision to the carina, intubate (Figs. 19-33 and 19-34). Removal of the guidewire distally is less likely to dislodge the FOB

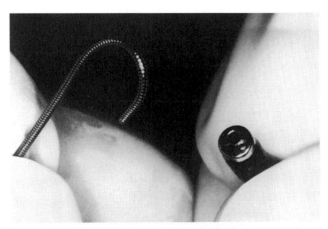

Figure 19-27 Close-up view of J tip of guidewire and distal tip of fiberoptic bronchoscope. (From Sanchez AF: The Retrograde Cookbook. Irvine, University of California–Irvine Department of Anesthesia, 1993.)

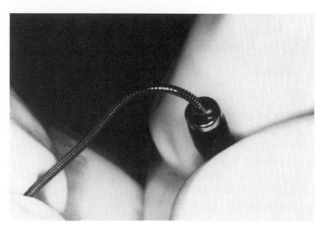

Figure 19-28 Close-up view of J tip being fed into suction port of fiberoptic bronchoscope. (From Sanchez AF: The Retrograde Cookbook. Irvine, University of California–Irvine Department of Anesthesia, 1993.)

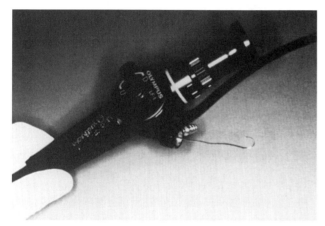

Figure 19-29 J tip exiting from fiberoptic bronchoscope handle. (From Sanchez AF: The Retrograde Cookbook. Irvine, University of California–Irvine Department of Anesthesia, 1993.)

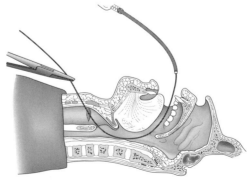

Figure 19-30 Begin advancing the fiberoptic bronchoscope (armed with the endotracheal tube) over the guidewire. (From Sanchez AF: The Retrograde Cookbook. Irvine, University of California–Irvine Department of Anesthesia, 1993.)

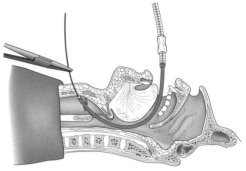

Figure 19-31 Advance fiberoptic bronchoscope to the cricothyroid membrane. (From Sanchez AF: The Retrograde Cookbook. Irvine, University of California–Irvine Department of Anesthesia, 1993.)

from the trachea, but anecdote suggests that removal proximally should decrease the incidence of infection resulting from oral contaminants.[13,122]

2. Instead of removing the guidewire, allow it to relax caudad into the trachea, advance the FOB below the cricoid cartilage, and then remove the guidewire. This allows a greater length of the FOB in the trachea before the guidewire is removed.

3. Remove the guidewire proximally only until it is seen through the FOB to have popped out of the CTM and into the trachea; then advance the guidewire through the FOB to the carina. The FOB can then be advanced antegrade over the guidewire to the carina. (Caution: Be sure both ends of the guidewire are floppy.)

4. Tobias[148] used a fiberoptic technique that did not make use of the suction port of the FOB. He performed a standard RI, feeding the guidewire or epidural catheter, first, through the main lumen (bevel) of the ET and immediately exiting out of the Murphy eye. The ET was then advanced to the level of the CTM (Fig. 19-35). At this time, the FOB was advanced proximally through the ET to the level of the carina. The retrograde guidewire was then removed, and a standard fiberoptic intubation was performed.

(The author prefers the third option.)

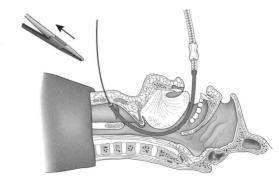

Figure 19-32 Have assistant remove hemostat *(arrow)*. (From Sanchez AF: The Retrograde Cookbook. Irvine, University of California–Irvine Department of Anesthesia, 1993.)

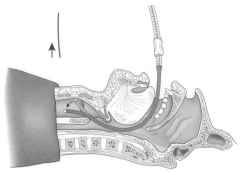

Figure 19-33 Remove guidewire from the cricothyroid membrane *(straight arrow)*. The tip of the fiberoptic bronchoscope then drops into midtracheal position *(curved arrow)*. (From Sanchez AF: The Retrograde Cookbook. Irvine, University of California–Irvine Department of Anesthesia, 1993.)

The combination of FOB and RI is the easiest to perform of all the RI techniques. The disadvantages are that it requires more equipment (not readily available in cases of emergency) and more preparation time and may not be suitable in certain conditions (airway with large amounts of blood or secretions).

E. SILK PULL-THROUGH TECHNIQUE

Various pull-through techniques have been described using epidural catheters,[1,79] central venous pressure catheters,[118] monofilament sutures,[60] and Fogarty catheters[25]; the silk technique is also a pull-through technique.[128,129,132] The basic principle involves advancing the epidural catheter retrograde as in the classical technique, attaching it to a length of silk, attaching the length of silk to the tip of the ET, and then using the catheter-silk combination to pull the ET into the trachea. The silk technique offers the following advantages:

1. Equipment is readily available in the operating room.
2. The silk is intimately attached to the ET, eliminating railroading.

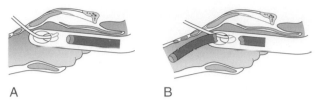

Figure 19-35 A, Midsagittal view of the larynx with the endotracheal tube (ET) tip at the level of the cricothyroid membrane. The fiberoptic bronchoscope (FOB) is advanced through the main lumen of the ET. **B,** The FOB is advanced to the level of the carina, *before* the guidewire is removed. (Modified from Tobias R: Increased success with retrograde guide for endotracheal intubation [letter]. Anesth Analg 62:366, 1983.)

3. Multiple attempts at intubation are allowed without having to repeat the procedure (CTM puncture) if it fails initially.
4. Oxygen can be delivered through the ET using a standard anesthesia circle system, and in-line capnography can be used to verify placement of the ET.
5. If necessary, postoperative reintubation can be accomplished using the silk, which is left in place until the time of discharge from the recovery room.

The silk technique employs the principles and equipment of the classical technique, with the addition of a length of silk suture (3-0 nylon monofilament may also be used). Once the epidural catheter (which is used only to place the silk) is out of either the oral or nasal cavity (Fig. 19-36), the silk suture is tied to the cephalad end of the catheter (see Fig. 19-36) and the silk is pulled antegrade through the CTM (Fig. 19-37). The epidural catheter is cut off and discarded (see Fig. 19-37), and the cephalad end of the silk is tied to the Murphy eye (Fig. 19-38). The silk suture is then used to pull the ET gently into the trachea (Fig. 19-39; see Fig. 19-38). When a floppy epiglottis causes obstruction, one can deliberately intubate the esophagus; as the ET is being gently withdrawn from the esophagus, tension applied simultaneously

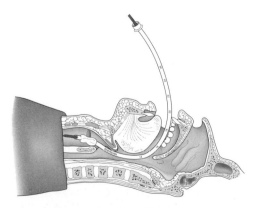

Figure 19-34 Continue as you would in a standard fiberoptic intubation. (From Sanchez AF: The Retrograde Cookbook. Irvine, University of California–Irvine Department of Anesthesia, 1993.)

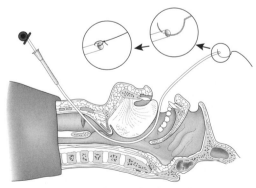

Figure 19-36 After proceeding as in classical technique, when the epidural catheter has exited the oral cavity, it is tied to a 3-0 noncutting silk suture (30-inch length), as shown in the insets. (From Sanchez AF: The Retrograde Cookbook. Irvine, University of California–Irvine Department of Anesthesia, 1993.)

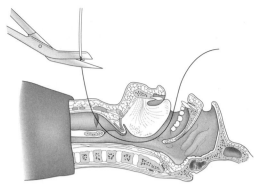

Figure 19-37 Pull the epidural catheter caudad until the silk suture exits the skin above the cricothyroid membrane; then cut off the epidural catheter. (From Sanchez AF: The Retrograde Cookbook. Irvine, University of California–Irvine Department of Anesthesia, 1993.)

to the distal end of the silk pops the tip of the ET anteriorly, lifts up the epiglottis, and allows the ET to enter the larynx. When the ET abuts up against the CTM, the tension on the silk suture is released (Fig. 19-40) and the ET is passed further to enter the trachea (see Fig. 19-40). If a nasal intubation is required, a urologic catheter can be used to cause the epidural catheter to exit the nasal rather than the oral cavity (Figs. 19-41 to 19-44).

In practice, it may be difficult to suture the silk onto the epidural catheter. A small learning curve is required not to allow any slack on the silk until the CTM is reached and to gauge properly the fine balance between pulling on the silk and simultaneously advancing the ET. The technique is easy, and because the silk can be left in place with no discomfort for the duration of the anesthetic and after extubation, emergent reintubation can be accomplished. The author has had two occasions to reintubate in the recovery room using this technique; both patients had

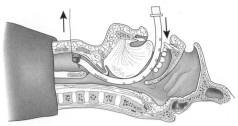

Figure 19-39 Simultaneously pull the silk caudad *(arrow)* as you advance the endotracheal tube (ET) *(arrow)* with the opposite hand. Advance ET to the cricothyroid membrane. (From Sanchez AF: The Retrograde Cookbook. Irvine, University of California–Irvine Department of Anesthesia, 1993.)

suffered maxillofacial trauma, had initially been intubated awake using the retrograde silk technique, and had arch bars placed in the operating room.

VII. PEDIATRICS

In pediatric patients, the physician is faced with the formidable problems of small anatomic structures that are difficult to palpate, immature anatomic structures such as anterior larynx and narrow cricoid cartilage, congenital anomalies, and pathologic disorders that intimately affect the airway (e.g., acute epiglottitis). Because the pediatric airway is different, concerns have been raised about whether RI is indicated or contraindicated in infants.[34,46,54,85] Some have claimed that RI is dangerous[85] without citing any clinical supportive evidence. The number of articles and case reports in the medical literature on the subject of RI in the pediatric population is limited.*

---

*References 2, 10, 19, 20, 29, 34, 46, 54, 64, 85, 96, 132, 153, 155.

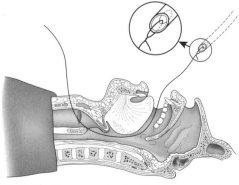

Figure 19-38 Tie the suture to the Murphy eye as shown. Have assistant pull patient's tongue forward. Begin pulling the suture with one hand while the opposite hand holds the endotracheal tube (ET) steady and in midline. At all times maintain tension on the suture while advancing the ET. (From Sanchez AF: The Retrograde Cookbook. Irvine, University of California–Irvine Department of Anesthesia, 1993.)

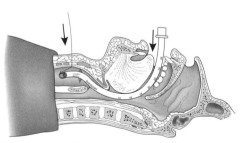

Figure 19-40 Release the suture, and with the opposite hand advance the endotracheal tube (ET) to desired depth. The suture partially retracts *(arrow)* into the trachea as the ET is advanced *(arrow)* past the cricothyroid membrane. The remaining suture is secured to the neck with transparent dressing. On extubation the silk is left in place as a precaution, should reintubation be required. The suture is removed in the recovery room upon patient's discharge by cutting it flush with the skin and pulling it out of the oral cavity. (From Sanchez AF: The Retrograde Cookbook. Irvine, University of California–Irvine Department of Anesthesia, 1993.)

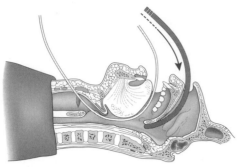

Figure 19-41 With the epidural catheter already in place, a 16-Fr red rubber urologic catheter is advanced *(arrow)* through the nose. (From Sanchez AF: The Retrograde Cookbook. Irvine, University of California–Irvine Department of Anesthesia, 1993.)

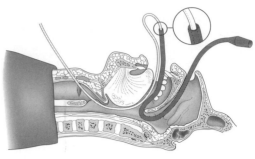

Figure 19-43 The epidural catheter is fed into the urologic catheter *(inset)* and may be tied together. (From Sanchez AF: The Retrograde Cookbook. Irvine, University of California–Irvine Department of Anesthesia, 1993.)

RI has been used in the anticipated and the unanticipated difficult pediatric airway, primarily after failure of conventional intubating techniques (blind nasal intubation, direct laryngoscopy, or fiberoptic intubation). The technique used is the same as in the adult, but a higher incidence of difficulties has been reported, including problems in cannulating the ET and inability to pass the ET through the glottic opening.[3,10,29]

In some cases, combined techniques have offered more success than blind RI. In one case report of a 16-year-old with acute epiglottitis, intubation was accomplished only by RI combined with rigid laryngoscopy; the retrograde catheter marked a path through an otherwise completely distorted anatomy.[64] The largest pediatric series with the highest success rate was reported by Audenaert and colleagues[10]; in that series RI was performed in 20 pediatric patients, aged 1 day to 17 years, with difficult airways primarily resulting from congenital anomalies (Table 19-2). The authors' preferred approach, a combination of fiberoptic with retrograde guidewire intubation, offers the following:

1. Higher success rate
2. Faster intubation
3. Ability to insufflate oxygen through the suction port of the FOB with the guidewire in place (Table 19-3)
4. No hanging up of the ET in the glottis

5. No need to rely on anatomic landmarks to guide the FOB into the trachea
6. Less requirement for experience to manage the FOB

No major complications were reported, and the technique was considered a valuable addition to pediatric airway management.

Przybylo and Stevenson described a unique method of managing the airway in a pediatric patient for closure of a tracheocutaneous fistula. The patient was a 4-year-old female with severe micrognathia and limited temporomandibular joint motion and mouth opening requiring a tracheostomy in the neonatal period for upper airway obstruction. Attempts at oral-nasal fiberoptic intubation were unsuccessful; the FOB was passed through the existing tracheocutaneous fistula in a cephalad direction, into the nasal cavity, and the FOB was then used as a stylet for nasal intubation.[115]

VIII. COMPLICATIONS AND CAUTIONS

Although it has been demonstrated that transtracheal needle puncture is safe and associated with only minor complications (Box 19-4), numerous potential

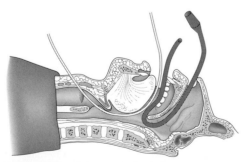

Figure 19-42 The tip of the urologic catheter is retrieved from the oral cavity. (From Sanchez AF: The Retrograde Cookbook. Irvine, University of California–Irvine Department of Anesthesia, 1993.)

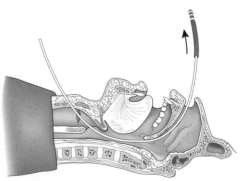

Figure 19-44 Urologic catheter is removed *(arrow)*, with the epidural catheter now exiting the nose. The epidural catheter can now be used as a nasotracheal guide. (From Sanchez AF: The Retrograde Cookbook. Irvine, University of California–Irvine Department of Anesthesia, 1993.)

Table 19-2 **Summary of Clinical Approaches to Pediatric Patients with Airways Difficult to Manage Clinically**

Case No.	Age	Weight (kg)	Primary/Surgical Diagnosis	Airway Problems	Scope	Tube	Rationale or Failed Means of Tracheal Intubation
1	1 day	2.9	Congenital anomalies/ omphalocele	Micrognathia, nonvisualization	AUR-8	3.0	A, D
2	6 mo	4.5	Congenital anomalies/ bilateral radial club hand	Nonvisualization	AUR-8	3.0	D
3	7 mo	5.7	Amyoplasia/congenital hip dislocation	Micrognathia, nonvisualization, limited mouth opening	AUR-8	4.0	A, D, F*
4	8 mo	6.8	Amyoplasia/clubfoot	Micrognathia, limited mouth opening, nonvisualization	AUR-8	4.0	A, D
5	10 mo	4.9	Pierre Robin syndrome/ cleft palate	Micrognathia, nonvisualization	AUR-8	3.5	A, D
6	11 mo	7.8	Arthrogryposis/clubfoot	Klippel-Feil, micrognathia	AUR-8	4.0	A
7	15 mo	8.0	Undiagnosed congenital anomalies/congenital hip dislocation	Nonvisualization	AUR-8	4.0	D
8	24 mo	13.2	Hurler's syndrome/bone marrow transplant	Short neck, large tongue, limited neck motion, nonvisualization	AUR-8	4.0	A, D
9	26 mo	11.4	Camptomelic dysplasia/ cervical fusion	Cervical spine abnormalities and instability, limited motion of neck, mouth	AUR-8	3.0	A, C
10	3 yr	11.2	Hallermann-Streiff syndrome/ophthalmologic procedures	Narrowed trachea, micrognathia, malar hypoplasia, microstomia, nonvisualization	AUR-8	4.5	A, D
11	5 yr (6 yr)	15.1 (16.9)	Escobar syndrome (multiple pterygium)/ orthopedic and plastic procedures	Klippel-Feil, brevicollis, limited mouth and neck motion, nonvisualization	LF-1	5.0	A, D
12	6 yr	11.3	Multiple congenital anomalies/infantile scoliosis	Micrognathia, cervical hemivertebra, limited mouth opening, nonvisualization	LF-1	5.0	H, A, D, R, F*
13	7 yr	17.1	Spondyloepiphyseal dysplasia congenital/ C1-2 subluxation	C-spine abnormalities	LF-1	5.5	C

Continued

Table 19-2   **Summary of Clinical Approaches to Pediatric Patients with Airways Difficult to Manage Clinically—cont'd**

Case No.	Age	Weight (kg)	Primary/Surgical Diagnosis	Airway Problems	Scope	Tube	Rationale or Failed Means of Tracheal Intubation
14	7 yr (7 yr)	15.9 (17.1)	Schwartz-Jampel syndrome/ C2-3 subluxation	Microstomia, limited neck and mouth motion, C-spine abnormalities	LF-1	5.0	A, C
15	9 yr	14	Cerebral palsy/ congenital hip dislocation	Nonvisualization	AUR-8	5.5	D
16	12 yr	22	Escobar syndrome (multiple pterygium)/ scoliosis	Klippel-Feil, brevicollis, limited mouth, neck motion, micrognathia nonvisualization	LF-1	5.5	A, D, L
q17	12 yr	15.2	Undiagnosed congenital progressive neuromuscular disease/extreme cervicothoracolumbar fixed lordosis for release and fusion	Extreme fixed cervicothoracic lordosis, micrognathia nonvisualization	AUR-8	5.0	A, D
q18	14 yr	51	Juvenile rheumatoid arthritis/joint fusion	Limited motion, neck and mouth	LF-1	5.5	H, A
q19	15 yr	71	Juvenile rheumatoid arthritis/phalangeal replacements	Limited motion, neck and mouth	LF-1	6.0	H, A
20	17 yr	74	Trauma/cervical spine and facial fractures	Facial fractures, in cervical traction, unstable cervical spine	LF-1	7.5	C

*Use of a Bullard rigid fiberoptic laryngoscope afforded an excellent view of the vocal cords, but owing to limited mouth opening the endotracheal tube could not be properly positioned.

Case numbers have been assigned for reference and convenience only. The tracheas of patients 11 and 14 have each been intubated twice with retrograde-assisted fiberoptic technique. Under "airway problems," nonvisualization refers to failure to expose the cords or arytenoid cartilages with direct laryngoscopy. On all occasions on which the AUR-8 scope was used, the 22-gauge catheter and 0.018-inch wire (see text) were also used. Likewise, where the LF-1 scope was used, the 20-gauge catheter and 0.025-inch wire (see text) were used. "Tube" refers to the endotracheal tube's internal diameter in millimeters. The "rationale or failed means of tracheal intubation" column reveals a few patients in whom this technique was used primarily, usually for cervical spine consideration (C) or when the airway was known to be extremely difficult by history or previous experience (H) or by preoperative assessment (A). Direct laryngoscopy (D), fiberoptic laryngoscopy (F), light wand (L), and retrograde alone (R) techniques were attempted unsuccessfully where so noted.

From Audenaert SM, Montgomery CL, Stone B: Retrograde-assisted fiberoptic tracheal intubation in children with difficult airways. Anesth Analg 73:660, 1991.

complications of RI have been cited in the literature (Box 19-5). Documented complications of RI are relatively few, and most were self-limited (Box 19-6). The most common complications were bleeding[1,2,12,26,55,56,95,114] and subcutaneous emphysema.[95,114,153]

A. BLEEDING

Insignificant bleeding (four to five drops of blood) has been observed with CTM puncture during RI.[2,114] Even a patient who had received heparin intraoperatively and had postoperative disseminated intravascular coagulation had only a small, self-limited hematoma following the procedure.[26] Controversy exists with respect to making the puncture below the cricoid cartilage because of a greater potential for bleeding.[1,90,155] Three studies[1,95,153] involving 57 patients who underwent RI with punctures at the cricotracheal ligament or between the second and third tracheal rings showed no evidence of major bleeding. There are, however, scattered reports of severe

Table 19-3 **Flow Measurement of Various Fiberscopes**

Scope (Mfg)	Outer Scope Diameter (mm)	Inner Lumen Diameter (mm)	Working Length (cm)	Maximum Tip Flexion (degrees)	Scope Configuration	Maximum O₂ Flow (L/min)
AUR-8 (Circon ACMI)	2.7	0.8	37	140	Straight	9.4 ± 0.1
					90-degree curve and 90-degree tip flexion	9.4 ± 0.0
					90-degree curve with 0.018-inch wire in place	4.37 ± 0.01
LF-1 (Olympus)	3.8	1.2	60	120	Straight	18.1 ± 0.2
					90-degree curve and 90-degree tip flexion	17.9 ± 0.1
					90-degree curve with 0.025-inch wire in place	12.4 ± 0.1
BF-1 (Olympus)	5.9	2.8	55	100	Straight	159 ± 5
					90-degree curve and 90-degree tip flexion	152 ± 1
					90-degree curve with 0.035-inch wire in place	145 ± 1

Flow measurements represent mean ± SD.
Mfg, manufacturer.
From Audenaert SM, Montgomery CL, Stone B: Retrograde-assisted fiberoptic tracheal intubation in children with difficult airways. Anesth Analg 73:660, 1991.

hemoptysis after transtracheal needle puncture with resultant hypoxia, cardiorespiratory arrest, dysrhythmias, and death.[63,68,133,142,149] Two patients had epistaxis[2,30] after nasal intubation (no vasoconstricting agent was used). The following measures have been suggested to decrease the potential for bleeding:

1. Avoid RI in patients with bleeding diathesis.
2. Apply pressure to the puncture site for 5 minutes.
3. Apply pressure dressing to the puncture site for 24 hours.
4. Maintain patient in the supine position for 3 to 4 hours after puncture.

B. SUBCUTANEOUS EMPHYSEMA*

Subcutaneous emphysema localized to the area of a transtracheal needle puncture site is common but self-limited. In severe cases, air may track through the fascial

---

*References 14, 58, 63, 95, 97, 106-108, 112, 116, 133, 142, 153, 161.

Box 19-4 **Translaryngeal Anesthesia (Complications)**

17,500 Reported Cases
2 broken needles
2 laryngospasms
4 soft tissue infections

Modified from Gold MI, Buechel DR: Translaryngeal Anesthesia: A review. Anesthesiology 20:181, 1959.

planes of the neck, leading to tracheal compression with airway compromise, pneumomediastinum, and pneumothorax.[97,107,108,112,149,150,160,161] Accumulation of air occurs gradually[97,112] (1 to 6 hours) after a transtracheal puncture. Severe subcutaneous emphysema has been attributed to use of a large-bore needle, multiple CTM punctures, and exposure of the puncture site to persistent elevated intratracheal pressure (coughing, grunting, or sneezing). In addition, pneumomediastinum has been reported in patients who underwent transtracheal puncture with a needle and was attributed to elevated endotracheal pressure (paroxysmal coughing and sneezing).[68,112,120] When the patient has been intubated by the retrograde technique, elevated peak inspiratory and end-expiratory

---

Box 19-5 **Potential Complications of Retrograde Intubation**

Esophageal perforation
Hemoptysis
Intratracheal submucosal hematoma with distal obstruction
Laryngeal edema
Laryngospasm
Pretracheal infection
Tracheal fistula
Tracheitis
Vocal cord damage

From University of California–Irvine Department of Anesthesia: Teaching Aids.

Box 19-6   Reported Complications of Retrograde Intubation

Self-Limited
Bleeding
   Puncture site, 8
   Peritracheal hematoma, 1
   Epistaxis, 2
Subcutaneous emphysema, 4
Pneumomediastinum, 2
Breath holding, 1
Catheter traveling caudad,* 4
Not Self-Limited
Trigeminal nerve trauma, 1
Incorrect placement (pharyngeal), 1
Pretracheal abscess, 1
Pneumothorax, 1
Loss of hook,† 2

*Refers to catheter traveling in a caudad direction toward the lungs instead of cephalad toward the oral cavity.
†Refers to Dr. Waters' technique of retrieving catheter from nasopharynx using a self-made hook. From Waters DJ: Guided blind endotracheal intubation: For patients with deformities of the upper airway. Anaesthesia 18:158, 1963.
From University of California–Irvine Department of Anesthesia: Teaching Aids.

pressures (PIP and PEEP, respectively) should not increase the likelihood of these complications intraoperatively because the puncture site is located above the ET cuff. The result is that the area of the initial puncture site would not be exposed to high pressure. Lee and co-authors[84] reported a patient (history of noncardiogenic pulmonary edema and atelectasis) who, after RI, received 7.5 cm of water with PEEP (PIP values were not reported) with no complications.

C. OTHER COMPLICATIONS

Other reported self-limited complications were breath holding[2] and the catheter (a straight, flexible guidewire) traveling caudally.[32,153]

   Complications that were not self-limited were as follows:

1. Trigeminal nerve trauma,[42] which the author suspects was due to multiple laryngoscopies

2. Guidewire fracture, in which wire had to be surgically removed[28]
3. Loss of hook (the type that was originally used by Waters and is no longer used)[2,3,155]
4. Pneumothorax, which necessitated a chest tube[112]
5. Pretracheal abscess in diabetic patients after multiple punctures at the CTM requiring incision and drainage[13]

IX. CONCLUSION

The anesthesia care provider is charged with the responsibility for securing the airway. In the vast majority of cases this can be accomplished using conventional techniques, but in a small number of cases these techniques cannot be successfully applied to the clinical problem at hand. No method, including RI, offers 100% success; therefore, it is wise to have multiple available options and to be facile with alternative techniques for intubation.

   RI has been a particularly useful alternative in difficult intubations after multiple manipulations have caused bleeding, in facial injuries where bleeding is already present, and in patients with limited neck movement and mouth opening. The technique is easy to learn, requires little equipment, and in practiced hands is a rapid, safe, and effective method for intubating the trachea.

   International awareness (in multiple specialties) of the value of RI in selected clinical settings has increased.[86,104] In the author's opinion, RI is a valuable additional airway management technique and should be included as part of the armamentarium of health care providers involved in the care of seriously injured or ill patients.

ACKNOWLEDGMENTS

Dedicated to my daughter, Danielle. With special thanks to Mrs. Debi Quilty, Mrs. Norma Claudio, and Elsie Vindiola for their research assistance and Tay McClellan for her outstanding medical illustrations.

REFERENCES

1. Abou-Madi MN, Trop D: Pulling versus guiding: A modification of retrograde guided intubation. Can J Anaesth 36:336, 1989.
2. Akinyemi OO: Complications of guided blind endotracheal intubation. Anaesthesia 34:590, 1979.
3. Akinyemi OO, John A: A complication of guided blind intubation. Anaesthesia 29:733, 1974.
4. Alfery DD: Double-lumen endobronchial tube intubation using retrograde wire technique [letter]. Anesth Analg 76:1374, 1993.
5. Amanor-Boadu SD: Translaryngeal guided intubation in a patient with raised intracranial pressure. Afr J Med Med Sci 21:65, 1992.
6. Anson BJ: Morris Human Anatomy: A Complete System Treatise, 12th ed. New York, McGraw-Hill, 1966.

7. Arndt GA, Topp J, Hannah J, et al: Intubation via the LMA using a Cook retrograde intubation kit. Can J Anaesth 45:257, 1998.

8. Arya VK, Dutta A, Chari P, et al: Difficult retrograde endotracheal intubation: The utility of a pharyngeal loop. Anesth Analg 92:470, 2002.

9. ASA Difficult Airway Task Force: Practice guidelines for management of the difficult airway. Anesthesiology 78:597, 1993.

10. Audenaert SM, Montgomery CL, Stone B: Retrograde-assisted fiberoptic tracheal intubation in children with difficult airways. Anesth Analg 73:660, 1991.

11. Barash PG, Cullen BF, Stoelting RK (eds): Clinical Anesthesia. Philadelphia, JB Lippincott, 1989.

12. Barriot P, Riou B: Retrograde technique for tracheal intubation in trauma patients. Crit Care Med 16:712, 1988.

13. Beebe DS, Tran P, Belani KG, Adams GL: Pretracheal abscess following retrograde tracheal intubation. Anaesthesia 50:470, 1995.

14. Benumof JL: Management of the difficult adult airway. Anesthesiology 75:1087, 1991.

15. Benumof JL: Retrograde intubation [letter]. Anesthesiology 76:1060, 1992.

16. Bergman R, Thompson S, Afifi AK, et al: Compendium of Human Anatomic Variation: Text, Atlas, and World Literature. Baltimore, Urban & Schwarzenberg, 1988.

17. Bissinger U, Guggenberger H, Lenz G: Retrograde-guided fiberoptic intubation in patients with laryngeal carcinoma. Anesth Analg 81:408, 1995.

18. Bissinger U, Guggenberger H, Lenz G: A safer approach to retrograde-guided fiberoptic intubation. Anesth Analg 82:1108, 1996.

19. Borland LM, Swan DV: Difficult pediatric endotracheal intubation: A new approach to the retrograde technique. Anesthesiology 55:577, 1981.

20. Bourke D, Levesque PR: Modification of retrograde guide for endotracheal intubation. Anesth Analg 53:1013, 1974.

21. Bowes WA 3rd, Johnson JO: Pneumomediastinum after planned retrograde fiberoptic intubation. Anesth Analg 78:795, 1994.

22. Butler FS, Cirillo AA: Retrograde tracheal intubation. Anesth Analg 39:333, 1960.

23. Caparosa RJ, Zavatsky AR: Practical aspects of the cricothyroid space. Laryngoscope 67:577, 1957.

24. Carlson CA, Perkins HM: Solving a difficult intubation. Anesthesiology 64:537, 1986.

25. Carlson RR, Sadove MS: Guided non-visualized nasal endotracheal intubation using a transtracheal Fogarty catheter. Ill Med J 143:364, 1973.

26. Casthely PA, Landesman S, Fynaman PN: Retrograde intubation in patients undergoing open heart surgery. Can Anaesth Soc J 32:661, 1985.

27. Clemente C (ed): Gray's Anatomy, 13th ed. Philadelphia, Lea & Febiger, 1985.

28. Contrucci RB, Gottlieb JS: A complication of retrograde endotracheal intubation. Ear Nose Throat J 69:776, 1989.

29. Cooper CMS, Murray-Wilson A: Retrograde intubation: Management of a 4.8 kg. 5-month infant. Anaesthesia 42:1197, 1988.

30. Corleta O, Habazettl H, Kreimeier U: Modified retrograde orotracheal intubation technique for airway access in rabbits. Eur Surg Res 24:129, 1992.

31. Cossham PS: Difficult intubation. Br J Anaesth 57:239, 1985.

32. Criado A, Planas A: Intubacion orotraqueal retrograda (Cartas al director). Rev Esp Anestesiol Reanim 35:344, 1988.

33. Cuchiara RF, Black S, Steinkeler JA: Anesthesia for intracranial procedures. In Barash PG, Cullen BF, Stoelting RK (eds): Clinical Anesthesia. Philadelphia, JB Lippincott, 1989, p 652.

34. Dailey RD, Simon B: Retrograde tracheal intubation. In Purcell T (ed): The Airway Emergency Management. St Louis, Mosby, 1992, p 84.

35. Dennison PH: Four experiences in intubation of one patient with Still's disease. Br J Anaesth 50:636, 1978.

36. Deresinski SC, Stevens DA: Anterior cervical infections: Complications of transtracheal aspirations. Am Rev Respir Dis 110:354, 1974.

37. Dhara SS: Guided blind endotracheal intubation [letter]. Anaesthesia 35:81, 1980.

38. Dhara SS: Retrograde intubation: A facilitated approach. Br J Anaesth 69:631, 1992.

39. Diaz J: The difficult intubation kit. Anesth Rev 17:49, 1990.

40. Dubey PK, Kumar A: A device for cricothyrotomy and retrograde intubation. Anaesthesia 55:702, 2000.

41. Eidelman L, Pizov R: A safer approach to retrograde-guided fiberoptic intubation. Anesth Analg 82:1108, 1996.

42. Faithfull NS: Injury to terminal branches of the trigeminal nerve following tracheal intubation. Br J Anaesth 57:535, 1985.

43. Faithfull NS: Retrograde intubation. Summary of papers presented at the sixth European Congress. Anaesthesia 1(Suppl 22):458, 1982.

44. Faithfull NS, Erdmann W, Groenland THN: Alternatieve intubatie routes. Ned Tijdschr Anaesth Medewerkers 25:8, 1985.

45. Finucane BT, Santora AH: Principles of Airway Management. Philadelphia, FA Davis, 1988.

46. France NK, Beste DJ: Anesthesia for pediatric ear, nose and throat surgery. In Gregory GA (ed): Pediatric Anesthesia, 2nd ed. New York, Churchill Livingstone, 1989, p 169.

47. Freund PR, Rooke A, Schwid H: Retrograde intubation with a modified Eschmann stylet [letter]. Anesth Analg 67:596, 1988.

48. Gerenstein RI: J-wire facilitates translaryngeal guided intubation [letter]. Anesthesiology 76:1059, 1992.

49. Gerenstein RI, Arria-Devoe G: J-wire and translaryngeal guided intubation [letter]. Crit Care Med 17:486, 1989.

50. Gordon RA: Anesthetic management of patients with airway problems. Int Anesthesiol Clin 10:37, 1972.

51. Graham WP III, Kilgore ES III: Endotracheal intubation in complicated cases. Hosp Physicians 3:60, 1987.

52. Greaves JD: Endotracheal intubation in Still's disease. Br J Anaesth 51:75, 1979.

53. Green DC, Strait GB: A complication of transtracheal anesthesia: Nocardia cellulitis. Ann Thorac Surg 8:561, 1969.

54. Gregory GA: Induction of anesthesia. In Gregory GA (ed): Pediatric Anesthesia, 2nd ed. New York, Churchill Livingstone, 1989.

55. Guggenberger H, Lenz G: Training in retrograde intubation [letter]. Anesthesiology 69:292, 1980.

56. Guggenberger H, Lenz G, Heumann H: Success rate and complications of a modified guided blind technique for intubation in 36 patients. Anaesthesist 36:703, 1987.

57. Gupta B, McDonald JS, Brooks HJ: Oral fiberoptic intubation over a retrograde guidewire. Anesth Analg 68:517, 1989.

58. Hahn HH, Beaty HN: Transtracheal aspiration in the evaluation of patients with pneumonia. Ann Intern Med 72:183, 1970.

59. Harmer M, Vaughan R: Guided blind oral intubation [letter]. Anaesthesia 35:921, 1986.

60. Harrison CA, Wise CC: Retrograde intubation [letter]. Anaesthesia 43:609, 1988.

61. Harvey SC, Fishman RL, Edwards SM: Retrograde intubation through a laryngeal mask airway. Anesthesiology 85:1503, 1996.

62. Heller EM, Schneider K, Saven B: Percutaneous retrograde intubation. Laryngoscope 99:555, 1989.

63. Hemley SD, Arida EJ, Diggs AM, et al: Percutaneous cricothyroid membrane bronchography. Radiology 76:763, 1961.

64. Heslet L, Christensen KS, Sanchez R, et al: Facilitated blind intubation using a transtracheal guide wire. Dan Med Bull 32:275, 1985.

65. Hines MH, Meredith JW: Modified retrograde intubation technique for rapid airway access. Am J Surg 159:597, 1990.

66. Hung OR, al-Qatari M: Light-guided retrograde intubation. Can J Anaesth 44:877, 1997.

67. Jagtap SR, Malde AD, Pantvaidya SH: Anaesthetic considerations in a patient with Fraser syndrome. Anaesthesia 50:39, 1995.

68. Kalinske RW, Parker RH, Brandt D: Diagnostic usefulness and safety of transtracheal aspiration. N Engl J Med 276:604, 1967.

69. Kaplan JA: Postoperative respiratory care. In Kaplan JA (ed): Thoracic Anesthesia. New York, Churchill Livingstone, 1983.

70. King HK: Translaryngeal guided intubation [letter]. Anesth Analg 64:650, 1985.

71. King HK: Translaryngeal guided intubation: A lifesaving technique. A review and case report. Anesth Sin 22:279, 1984.

72. King HK: Translaryngeal guided intubation using a sheath stylet. Anesthesiology 63:567, 1985.

73. King HK, Khan AK, Wooten DJ: Translaryngeal guided intubation solved a critical airway problem. J Clin Anesth 1:112, 1988.

74. King KH, Wang LF, Khan AK: Soft and firm introducers for translaryngeal guided intubation [letter]. Anesth Analg 68:826, 1989.

75. King HK, Wang LF, Khan AK: Translaryngeal guided intubation for difficult intubation. Crit Care Med 15:869, 1987.

76. King KK, Wang LF, Khan AK, Wooten DJ: Antegrade vs retrograde insertion introducer for guided intubation in needle laryngostomized patient. Can J Anaesth 36:252, 1989.

77. King HK, Wang LF, Wooten DJ: Endotracheal intubation using translaryngeal guided intubation vs percutaneous retrograde guidewire insertion [letter]. Crit Care Med 15:183, 1987.

78. Kress TD, Balasubramaniam S: Cricothyroidotomy. Ann Emerg Med 11:197, 1982.

79. Kubo K, Takahashi S, Oka M: A modified technique of guided blind intubation in oral surgery. J Maxillofac Surg 8:135, 1980.

80. Latto IP, Rosen M: Management of difficult intubation. In Latto IP, Rosen M (eds): Difficulties in Tracheal Intubation. Philadelphia, Baillière Tindall, 1984.

81. Lau HP, Yip KM, Liu CC: Rapid airway access by modified retrograde intubation. J Formos Med Assoc 95:347, 1996.

82. Layman PR: An alternative to blind intubation. Anaesthesia 38:165, 1983.

83. Lechman MJ, Donahoo JS, Macvaugh H: Endotracheal intubation using percutaneous retrograde guidewire insertion followed by antegrade fiberoptic bronchoscopy. Crit Care Med 14:589, 1986.

84. Lee YW, Lee YS, Kim JR: Retrograde tracheal intubation. Yonsei Med J 28:228, 1987.

85. Levin RM: Anesthesia for cleft lip and cleft palate. Anesthesiol Rev 6:25, 1979.

86. Levitan RM, Kush S, Hollander JE: Devices for difficult airway management in academic emergency departments: Results of a national survey. Ann Emerg Med 33:694, 1999.

87. Lin BC, Chen IH: Anesthesia for ankylosing spondylitis patients undergoing transpedicle vertebrectomy. Acta Anaesthesiol Sin 37:73, 1999.

88. Linscott MS, Horton WC: Management of upper airway obstruction. Otolaryngol Clin North Am 12:351, 1979.

89. Lleu JC, Forrler M, Forrler C, et al: L'intubation oro-trachéale par void rétrograde. Ann Fr Anesth Reanim 8:632, 1989.

90. Lleu JC, Forrler M, Pottecher T: Retrograde intubation using the subcricoid region [letter]. Br J Anaesth 55:855, 1983.

91. Lopez G, James NR: Mechanical problems of the airway. J Clin Anesth 36:118, 1984.

92. Luhrs R, Fuller E: A case study: The use of trans-tracheal guide for a patient with a large protruding oral myxoma. J Am Assoc Nurse Anesth 55:81, 1987.

93. Maestro CM, Andujar MJJ, Sancho CJ, et al: Intubacion retrograda en un paciente con una malformacion epiglotica (Cartas al director). Rev Esp Anestesiol Reanim 35:344, 1988.

94. Mahajan R, Sandhya X, Chari P: An alternative technique for retrograde intubation. Anaesthesia 56, 2001.

95. Mahiou P, Bouvet FR, Korach JM: Intubation retrograde [abstract R26]. Proceedings of the Thirty-First Congress de Intubation Tracheal, Paris, July 14, 1983.

96. Manchester GH, Mani MM, Master FW: A simple method for emergency orotracheal intubation. Plast Reconstr Surg 49:312, 1972.

97. Massey JY: Complications of transtracheal aspiration: A case report. J Ark Med Soc 67:254, 1971.

98. Matot I, Hevron I, Katzenelson R: Dental mirror for difficult nasotracheal intubation. Anaesthesia 52:780, 1997.

99. Mclean D: Guided blind oral intubation [letter]. Anaesthesia 37:605, 1982.

100. McNamara RM: Retrograde intubation of the trachea. Ann Emerg Med 16:680, 1987.

101. Miller RD: Anesthesia, vol 2, 2nd ed. New York, Churchill Livingstone, 1990.

102. Miller RD: Endotracheal intubation. In Anesthesia, 3rd ed. New York, Churchill Livingstone, 1986.

103. Morais RJ, Kotsev SN, Hana SJ: Modified retrograde intubation in a patient with difficult airway. Saudi Med J 21:490, 2000.

104. Morton T, Brady S, Clancy M: Difficult airway equipment in English emergency departments. Anaesthesia 55:485, 2000.

105. Naumann H: Head and Neck Surgery. Philadelphia, WB Saunders, 1984.

106. Newman J, Schultz S, Langevin RE: Bronchography by cricothyroid catheterization. Laryngoscope 75:774, 1965.

107. Ovassapian A: Fiberoptic tracheal intubation. In Ovassapian A (ed): Fiberoptic Airway Endoscopy in Anesthesia and Critical Care, 3rd ed. New York, Raven Press, 1990.

108. Ovassapian A: Topical anesthesia. In Ovassapian A (ed): Fiberoptic Airway Endoscopy in Anesthesia and Critical Care. New York, Raven Press, 1990.

109. Parmet JL, Colonna-Romano P, Horrow JC, et al: The laryngeal mask airway reliably provides rescue ventilation in cases of unanticipated difficult tracheal intubation along with difficult mask ventilation. Anesth Analg 87:661, 1998.

110. Payne KA: Difficult tracheal intubation. Anaesth Intensive Care 8:84, 1980.

111. Pintanel T, Font M, Aguilar JL, et al: Intubation orotracheal retrograde (Cartas al director). Rev Esp Anestesiol Reanim 35:344, 1988.

112. Poon YK: Case history number 89: A life-threatening complication of cricothyroid membrane puncture. Anesth Analg 55:298, 1976.

113. Poradowska-Jeszke M, Falkiewicz H: Intubation rétrograde chez un nourrisson atteint de maladie de Pierre Robin. Cah Anesthesiol 37:605, 1989.

114. Powell WF, Ozdil T: A translaryngeal guide for tracheal intubation. Anesth Analg 46:231, 1967.

115. Przybylo HJ, Stevenson GW: Retrograde fibreoptic intubation in a child with Nager's syndrome. Can J Anaesth 43:697, 1996.

116. Radigan LR, King RD: A technique for the prevention of postoperative atelectasis. Surgery 47:184, 1960.

117. Ramsay MAE, Salyer KE: The management of a child with a major airway abnormality. Plast Reconstr Surg 67:668, 1981.

118. Raza S, Levinsky L, Lajos TZ: Transtracheal intubation: Useful adjunct in cardiac surgical anesthesia. J Thorac Cardiovasc Surg 76:721, 1978.

119. Reynaud J, Lacour M, Diop L, et al: Intubation tracheale guidée a bouche fermée (technic de D.J. Waters). Bull Soc Med Afr Noire Lang Fr 12:774, 1967.

120. Ries K, Levison ME, Kaye D, et al: Transtracheal aspiration in pulmonary infection. Arch Intern Med 133:453, 1974.

121. Riou B: Intubation difficile. In Conference d'actualisation, 1990, Société Francaise d'Anesthésie Réanimation, Paris, July 3, 1990, Masson.

122. Rizzi F, Ambroselli V, Mezzetti MG: Sull'impiego dell'intubazione retrograda in emergenza. Minerva Anestesiol 57:1705, 1991.

123. Roberts JR: Clinical Procedures in Emergency Medicine. Philadelphia, WB Saunders, 1985.

124. Roberts KW: New use for Swan-Ganz introducer wire [letter]. Anesth Analg 60:67, 1981.

125. Roberts KW, Solgonick RM: A modification of retrograde wire-guided, fiberoptic-assisted endotracheal intubation in a patient with ankylosing spondylitis. Anesth Analg 82:1290, 1996.

126. Rossini L: The tunneling technique: An approach to difficult intubations. J Am Assoc Nurse Anesth 52:189, 1984.

127. Salem MR, Mathrubhutham M, Bennett EJ, et al: Difficult intubation. N Engl J Med 295:879, 1976.

128. Sanchez AF: ASA airway safety video. II. Cricothyroid membrane, 1992.

129. Sanchez AF: Preventing the difficult from becoming the impossible airway: Retrograde intubation. Presented at the annual meeting of the American Society of Anesthesiologist, Las Vegas, Oct 16, 1990.

130. Sanchez, AF: Retrograde intubation. Anesthesiol Clin North Am 13:439, 1995.

131. Sanchez AF: Retrograde intubation in the llama. Presented at the American Association of Zoological Veterinarians, annual meeting, St. Louis, Nov 3, 1993.

132. Sanchez AF: The retrograde cookbook. Presented at the first international symposium on the difficult airway, Newport Beach, Calif, June 6, 1993.

133. Schillaci RF, Iacovoni VE, Conte RS, et al: Transtracheal aspiration complicated by fatal endotracheal hemorrhage. N Engl J Med 295:488, 1976.

134. Schmidt SI, Hasewinkel JV: Retrograde catheter-guided direct laryngoscopy. Anesthesiol Rev 16:6, 1989.

135. Scurr C: A complication of guided blind intubation [letter]. Anaesthesia 30:411, 1975.

136. Seavello J, Hammer GB: Tracheal intubation in a child with trismus pseudocamptodactyly (Hecht) syndrome. J Clin Anesth 11:254, 1999.

137. Sellers W: Finding a use for the lumen in the Portex Tracheal Tube Guide. Anaesthesia 58:190, 2003.

138. Shantha TR: Retrograde intubation [letter]. Br J Anaesth 55:855, 1983.

139. Shantha TR: Retrograde intubation using the subcricoid region. Br J Anaesth 68:109, 1992.

140. Shapiro HM, Drummond JC: Neurosurgical anesthesia and intracranial hypertension. In Miller RD (ed): Anesthesia, vol 2, 3rd ed. New York, Churchill Livingstone, 1990, p 854.

141. Slots P, Vegger P, Bettger H, et al: Retrograde intubation with a Mini-Trach II kit. Acta Anaesth Scand 47:274, 2003.

142. Spencer CD, Beaty HN: Complications of transtracheal aspiration. N Engl J Med 286:304, 1972.

143. Stehling SC: Management of the airway. In Barash PG, Cullen BF, Stoelting RK (eds): Clinical Anesthesia. Philadelphia, JB Lippincott, 1989, p 652.

144. Stern Y, Spitzer T: Retrograde intubation of the trachea. J Laryngol Otol 105:746, 1991.

145. Stone DJ, Gal TJ: Airway management. In Miller RD (ed): Anesthesia, vol 2, 3rd ed. New York, Churchill Livingstone, 1990, p 1105.

146. Stordahl A, Syrovy G: Blind endotracheal intubation over retrograde. Tidsskr Nor Laegeforen 106:1590, 1986.

147. Talyshkhanov KK: Retrograde intubation of the trachea. Anesteziol Reanimatol 5-6:58, 1992.

148. Tobias R: Increased success with retrograde guide for endotracheal intubation [letter]. Anesth Analg 62:366, 1983.

149. Unger KM, Moser KM: Fatal complication of transtracheal aspiration: A report of two cases. Arch Intern Med 132:437, 1973.

150. van der Laan KT, Ballast B, Wouters B, van Overbeek JJ: Retrograde endotracheale intubatie met behulp van een catheter. Ned Tijdschr Geneeskd 131:2324, 1987.

151. Van Stralen D, Perkin RM: Retrograde intubation difficulty in an 18-year-old muscular dystrophy patient. Am J Emerg Med 13:100, 1995.

152. Van Stralen DW, Rogers M, Perkin RM, et al: Retrograde intubation training using mannequin. Am J Emerg Med 13:50, 1995.

153. VanNiekerk JV, Smalhout B: Retrograde endotracheal intubation using a catheter. Ned Tijdschr Geneeskd 131:1663, 1987.

154. Ward CF, Salvatierra A: Special intubation techniques for the adult patient. In Benumof JL (ed): Clinical Procedures in Anesthesia and Intensive Care. Philadelphia, JB Lippincott, 1992, p 156.

155. Waters DJ: Guided blind endotracheal intubation: For patients with deformities of the upper airway. Anaesthesia 18:158, 1963.

156. Wedel DJ, Brown DL: Nerve blocks. In Miller RD (ed): Anesthesia, vol 2, 3rd ed. New York, Churchill Livingstone, 1990, p 235.

157. Wijesinghe HS, Gough JE: Complications of a retrograde intubation in a trauma patient. Acad Emerg Med 7:1267, 2000.

158. Williams JB, Sahni R: Performance of retrograde intubation in a multiple-trauma patient. Prehosp Emerg Care 5:49, 2001.

159. Williamson R: Pediatric intubation: Retrograde or blind [letter]? Anaesthesia 42:802, 1988.

160. Willson JKV: Cricothyroid bronchography with a polyethylene catheter: Description of a new technique. Am J Roentgenol 81:305, 1959.

161. Won KH, Rowland DW, Croteau JR, et al: Massive subcutaneous emphysema complicating transcricothyroid bronchography. Am J Roentgenol Radium Ther Nucl Med 101:953, 1967.

162. Yealy DM, Paris PM: Recent advances in airway management. Emerg Med Clin North Am 7:83, 1989.

163. Yoneda I, Nakamura M, Satoh T: A simple method of retrograde intubation. Masui (Jpn J Anesthesiol) 40:124, 1991.

164. Yonfa AE, Waite PD, Ballard JB, et al: Retrograde approach to nasotracheal in a child with severe Pierre Robin syndrome. Anesthesiol Rev 10:28, 1983.

165. Yoshikawa TT, Chow AW, Montgomerie JZ, et al: Paratracheal abscess: An unusual complication of transtracheal aspiration. Chest 65:105, 1974.

20

INTUBATING STYLETS

Orlando R. Hung
Ronald D. Stewart

I. INTRODUCTION

The procedure of placing an endotracheal tube (ET) in the trachea for ventilation and oxygenation is more than 1000 years old. It was first performed on pigs by the Arab Avicenna between 980 and 1037.[17,42] But it was not until 1796 that Herholdt and Rafn described the method of "blind" tactile digital intubation in a resuscitation protocol for drowning victims.[21] MacEwen in 1880 reported the placement of a curved metal tube into the trachea orally by tactile means in awake patients.[37] However, modern methods of endotracheal intubation did not emerge until early in the 20th century following the introduction of a flexible metal tube by Kuhn and the laryngoscope by Jackson.[31]

Over the years, laryngoscopic intubation has been shown to be an effective, safe, and relatively easy technique. In fact, it has become the standard method of endotracheal intubation in the operating room, intensive care unit, and emergency department. Unfortunately, even in the hands of experienced laryngoscopists, accurate and prompt placement of the ET remains a significant challenge in some patients. This is particularly true in "unprepared" patients or patients requiring emergency intubation. Direct visualization of the glottis can be difficult in the presence of an anatomic abnormality such as a receding mandible, prominent upper incisors, a restricted mouth opening, or limited movement of the cervical spine. It has been estimated that 1% to 3% of surgical patients have "difficult" airways, making laryngoscopic intubation difficult and sometimes impossible.[35] In the obstetric population, the incidence of failed laryngoscopic intubation has been reported to be between 0.05% and 0.35%.[11]

Many predictors of difficult laryngoscopic intubation have been suggested in the literature.[40,58] However, no single predictor is reliable in predicting difficult laryngoscopic intubation.[12,32,50] Because of these several factors, alternative intubation techniques, such as fiberoptic intubation, have been developed. Although effective and reliable, this technique requires expensive equipment as well as special skill and training. In addition, fiberoptic intubation is difficult in emergency situations in which unprepared or uncooperative patients may have copious secretions or blood in the oropharynx.

Because of the difficulties posed by direct-vision laryngoscopic intubation, particularly under emergency conditions, the search for other techniques has led to the development of blind techniques using a variety of devices. During the past few decades, intubating guides and light-guided intubation using the principle of transillumination have proved to be effective, safe, and simple. This chapter briefly reviews the principles and techniques of these alternative intubation procedures.

Although many types of intubating guides and lighted stylets have been commercially available for many years, our discussion focuses only on devices proved effective and safe in the medical literature. It should be emphasized, however, that the concepts and techniques of intubation are applicable to other similar devices.

II. INTUBATING STYLETS OR GUIDES

A. HISTORY

Intubation using an introducer or guide was first reported by MacIntosh in 1949.[39] The guide used in his report was a 60-cm-long, 15 Fr gauge elastic catheter (Eschmann Tracheal Tube Introducer, Portex Limited, Hythe, UK) with a J (coudé) tip (a 40-degree angle bend) at the distal end (Fig. 20-1). This "bougie" is most suitable for patients whose laryngeal aperture cannot be seen under direct vision using a laryngoscope (e.g., grade III laryngoscopic view as described by Cormack and Lehane[10]). Under these circumstances, the bougie is "hooked" underneath the epiglottis and is advanced into the trachea. If it is accurately placed, a tactile clicking sensation may be felt as the tip of the bougie slides over the tracheal rings while advancing into the trachea. Furthermore, if the bougie enters the trachea correctly, the bougie is lodged in a distal airway and cannot advance beyond the 30- to 35-cm mark. In contrast, if it is placed in the esophagus, the entire bougie can be advanced without encountering any resistance. After the bougie is placed in the trachea, the ET is advanced distally over the bougie and is guided into the trachea. A jaw lift or jaw thrust by the nondominant hand of the clinician or by a laryngoscope facilitates the advancement of the ET over the bougie by elevating the tongue and epiglottis. If difficulty persists while advancing the ET, rotating the ET 90 degrees counterclockwise turns the ET bevel posteriorly and minimizes the risk of catching on the structures of the glottic opening.[20]

Following intubation, the position of the ET is confirmed using conventional methods, such as end-tidal CO_2 and auscultation.

B. ADDITIONAL INTUBATING GUIDES

In the several decades since the introduction of the bougie, many intubating guides of different sizes, shapes, lengths, and materials have been developed. All of the designs serve a function similar to that of the gum elastic bougie, but many have some additional features.

1. The Flex-Guide Endotracheal Tube Introducer (GreenField Medical Sourcing, Northborough, MA) is a flexible plastic introducer with a curved distal tip.[43]
2. The Cook Airway Exchange Catheter (Cook Inc., Bloomington, IN) is a hollow flexible straight tube designed as a tube exchanger for patients with difficult airways (DAs) (Figs. 20-2 and 20-3). With an adaptor at the proximal end, the device can be used to ventilate patients under difficult circumstances through the inner lumen and the distal ports. However, it does not have a curved tip at the distal end similar to that of the gum elastic bougie.
3. The Sheridan Tube Exchanger (Sheridan Catheter Corp., Oregon, NY) serves a function similar to that of the Cook Airway Exchange Catheter with a hollow flexible straight tube.
4. An intubating catheter with a curved tip at the distal end has been introduced (Frova Intubation Introducer, Cook Inc.) (see Figs. 20-2 and 20-3). It has two side ports and a hollow lumen. The introducer has two side ports, a hollow lumen, and a rigid removable internal cannula to increase its stiffness to facilitate tracheal placement. The Frova

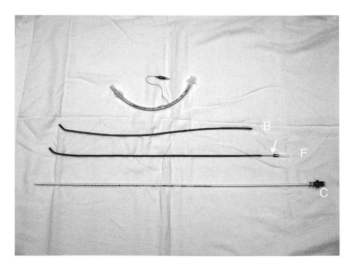

Figure 20-2 The gum elastic bougie (B), the Cook Airway Exchange Catheter (C), and the Frova Intubation Introducer (F), which has a rigid removable internal cannula *(arrow)* to facilitate tracheal placement.

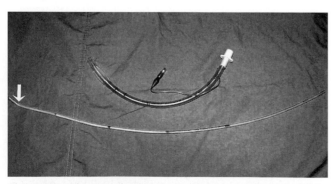

Figure 20-1 The gum elastic bougie (Eschmann catheter) with a J (coudé) tip *(arrow)*.

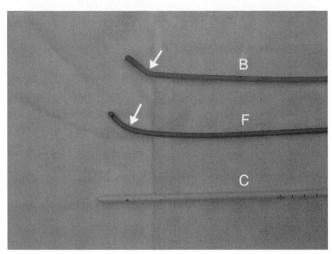

Figure 20-3 Both the Cook Airway Exchange Catheter (C) and the Frova Intubation Introducer (F) have a hollow inner lumen and distal ports to permit ventilation. However, the Frova Intubation Introducer but not the Cook Airway Exchange Catheter has a J (coudé) tip *(arrow)* similar to that of the gum elastic bougie (B).

introducer has two sizes: the adult version for ET with greater than 5.5 mm inner diameter and the pediatric version for ETs 3.0 to 5.0 mm in inner diameter.

5. The Schroeder (Parker Flex-It Directional Stylet) Oral/Nasal Directional Stylet (Parker Medical, Englewood, CO) is a disposable articulating stylet that requires no bending prior to intubation. Inserting the stylet into an ET allows the clinician to elevate the tip of the ET by wrapping all four fingers around the proximal ET and using the thumb to depress the proximal end of the stylet (Fig. 20-4).

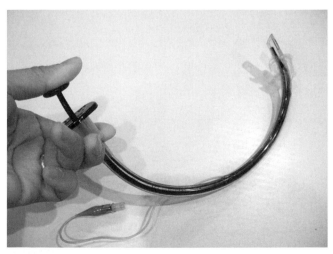

Figure 20-4 The Schroeder Directional Stylet can be used to elevate the tip of the endotracheal tube by wrapping all four fingers around the proximal tracheal tube and using the thumb to depress the proximal end of the stylet.

Although the stylet is suitable for both oral and nasal intubation, it has been reported to be somewhat awkward to use and the curvature created is not at the tip but rather over the distal half of the tube.[36] However, it has been reported to be effective for difficult as well as for blind intubations.[57]

A number of studies have reported the effectiveness of these intubating guides in patients with a DA.[33,47-49] Most of these studies, however, used the gum elastic bougie. With only a few exceptions, there are currently few data to support the use of the newer devices for endotracheal intubation, particularly in patients with a history of DA. It should be emphasized that most of these new intubating guides and stylets are disposable and designed for a single use. In contrast, the gum elastic bougie is more cost effective because it is reusable.

IV. LIGHTED STYLETS (LIGHT WANDS)

A. HISTORY OF LIGHT WANDS

In 1957, MacIntosh and Richards reported the use of a lighted introducer to assist the placement of an ET in the trachea under direct vision using a laryngoscope.[38] However, they did not describe the technique of transillumination of the soft tissues of the neck. The technique of transillumination was probably first described by Yamamura and colleagues in 1959 when they reported the use of a lighted stylet for nasotracheal intubation.[59]

A lighted stylet uses the principle of transillumination of the soft tissues of the anterior neck to guide the tip of the ET into the trachea. It also takes advantage of the anterior (superficial) location of the trachea relative to the esophagus. When the tip of the lighted ET enters the glottic opening, a well-defined circumscribed glow can be readily seen slightly below the thyroid prominence (Fig. 20-5). However, if the tip of the tube is in the esophagus, the transmitted glow is diffuse and cannot be readily detected easily under ambient lighting conditions (Fig. 20-6). If the tip of the ET is placed in the vallecula, the light glow is diffuse and appears slightly above the thyroid prominence. Using these landmarks and principles, the clinician can guide the tip of the ET easily and safely into the trachea without the use of a laryngoscope.

Despite its potential clinical advantages, intubation using a lighted stylet (light wand) did not receive widespread popularity until a commercial intubating device became available. During the past decade, several versions of the lighted stylet have been introduced, including the Flexilum (Concept Corporation, Clearwater, FL), Tubestat (Concept Corporation), and Fiberoptic Lighted-Intubation Stilette (Benson Medical Industries, Markham, Ontario, Canada) (Fig. 20-7). After more than a decade of experience, these devices have proved to be effective and safe in placing the ET both orally and nasally.[4,13,55]

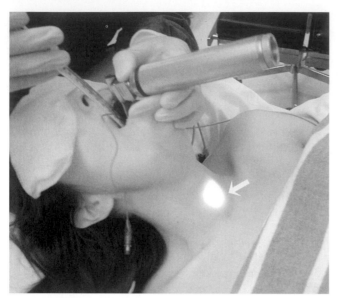

Figure 20-5 When the tip of the endotracheal tube with the light wand is placed at the glottic opening under direct laryngoscopy, a well-defined circumscribed glow *(arrow)* in the anterior neck just below the thyroid prominence can be readily seen.

In 1985, Vollmer and colleagues reported an 88% success rate in 24 field intubations using the Flexilum with three failures.[55] The average time of intubation was 20 seconds. In 1986, Ellis and associates reported successful intubations in 50 elective surgical patients using the Tubestat with an average time to intubate of 37 seconds.[13]

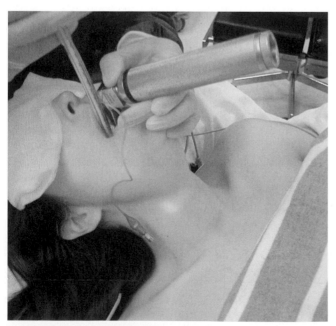

Figure 20-6 When the tip of the endotracheal tube is placed in the esophagus under direct laryngoscopy, transillumination is poor and the transmitted glow is diffuse in the anterior neck and cannot be seen easily under ambient lighting conditions.

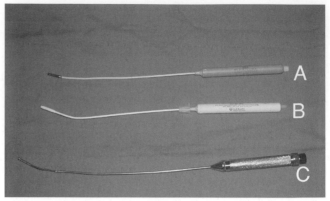

Figure 20-7 Commercially available lighted-stylets: (**A**) Flexilum, (**B**) Tubestat, and (**C**) Fiberoptic Lighted-Intubation Stilette.

Most of the patients were intubated following one attempt (72%), with 22% requiring two attempts and 6% three attempts. In a larger study with 200 patients, Ainsworth and Howell successfully intubated all patients using the Tubestat within 60 seconds.[4] However, the authors commented that "satisfactory conditions are met only when a darkened environment can be obtained and that transillumination in daylight may not be a reliable indicator of successful intubation." Weis and Hatton also reported successful intubations of 250 patients using the lighted stylet with three failures in patients who were grossly obese.[56]

Despite these favorable results, the growing experience with the technique of light-guided intubation revealed some limitations with the available lighted-stylet devices. These included (1) light intensity; (2) short length, limiting the use of the lighted-stylet device to short or cut ETs; (3) absence of a connector to secure the ET to the lighted-stylet device; (4) rigidity of the lighted stylet, which hampered use of the devices for other intubating techniques, including light-guided nasal intubation; and (5) the fact that most lighted stylets were designed for single use, thus increasing the cost of intubation.

To address the shortcomings of these existing devices, a lighted stylet was designed specifically for intubation and introduced in 1995 (Trachlight, Laerdal Medical Corp., Wappingers Falls, NY).[25] It incorporated an improved light source and a more flexible wand portion of the device. This added flexibility broadened the utility of the device for both oral and nasal intubation, made intubation easier, and permitted the evaluation of the position of the tip of the ET after intubation.

The Trachlight consists of three parts: a reusable handle, a flexible wand, and a stiff retractable stylet (Fig. 20-8). The power control circuitry and batteries are encased within the handle. The Trachlight requires three triple-A alkaline batteries, which are readily changed as needed. A locking clamp located on the front of the handle accepts and secures a standard ET connector. The stylet or wand

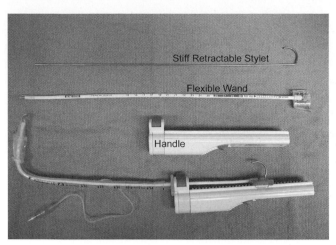

Figure 20-8 The Trachlight (TL) consists of three parts: a handle, a flexible wand, and a stiff retractable stylet wire. With the TL placed inside the endotracheal tube (ET), the ET-TL unit is bent at a 90-degree angle just proximal to the cuff of the tube in the shape of a field-hockey stick.

consists of a durable, flexible plastic shaft with a bright light bulb affixed at the distal end. Because of improved bulb technology, the light emitted by the Trachlight is extremely bright with minimal heat production (a maximum surface temperature of approximately 60° C). The bulb of the Trachlight, in addition to projecting the light forward as in most lighted stylets, projects the light laterally at a much wider angle. This additional feature further improves transillumination of the soft tissues of the neck. The improved light source of the Trachlight permits intubation to be performed under ambient lighting conditions, and in most cases it is unnecessary to dim the room light. After 30 seconds of illumination, the light bulb blinks to minimize heat production and provide a convenient reminder of elapsed time. Because the tip of the stylet is encased within the ET and because of the efficient heat exchange capacity of the upper airway mucosa, it is extremely unlikely that heat from the bulb would cause any thermal injury during intubation. An animal study confirmed that there are no histopathologic changes following the use of the Trachlight.[45]

A rigid plastic connector with a release arm at the proximal end of the Trachlight allows adjustment of the wand along the handle when the release arm is depressed. Enclosed within the wand is a stiff but malleable, retractable wire stylet. When the wire stylet is retracted, the wand becomes pliable, permitting the ET to advance easily into the trachea. This may well be the most important feature of this lighted-stylet device because it significantly improves its ease of use.

The retractable wire stylet stiffens the wand sufficiently that it can be shaped in the form of a field-hockey stick (see Fig. 20-8). This configuration directs the bright light of the bulb against the anterior wall of the larynx and trachea. In addition, the hockey stick configuration enhances maneuverability during intubation and facilitates the placement of the ET through the glottic opening. However, once through the glottis, the field-hockey stick configuration can impede further advancement of the tube into the trachea. Retraction of the wire stylet produces a pliable ET-Trachlight unit (ET-TL), facilitating its advancement into the trachea. This flexibility also allows accurate placement of the tip of the ET. Once the internal wire stylet is retracted, the pliable ET-TL can be advanced into the trachea until the tip reaches the sternal notch. At the sternal notch, the tip of the endotracheal tip is located about halfway between the vocal cords and the carina.[51]

B. TECHNIQUE OF LIGHT WAND INTUBATION:

The authors have had significant involvement in the development of the Trachlight, and the following intubation technique is a reflection of their experience and therefore bias using the Trachlight. However, the concept of intubation using the principle of transillumination is applicable to other types of lighted stylets. Undoubtedly, successful intubation using a lighted stylet, including the Trachlight, depends somewhat on the clinician's experience and skill. In other words, as with any intubation technique, regular use of a Trachlight improves the clinician's performance and may also reduce the likelihood of complications.

1. Preparation

Lubrication of the wire internal stylet of the wand using silicon fluid (Endoscopic Instrument Lubricant AE-1, ACMI, Southborough, MA) ensures its easy retraction during intubation. With the wire internal stylet in place, the clinician attaches the wand to the handle. The internal wall of the ET should be well lubricated with a water-soluble lubricant to facilitate retraction of the wand following the ET placement. The wand is inserted into the ET, and the tube is firmly attached to the handle. The length of the wand is adjusted by sliding the wand along the handle, and the light bulb is placed close to, but not protruding beyond, the tip of the ET.

With the Trachlight in place, the ET-TL unit is bent at a 90-degree angle just proximal to the cuff of the tube in the shape of a field-hockey stick (see Fig. 20-8). Even though the degree of bend should be individualized to the patient, the 90-degree angle bend generally makes the intubation considerably easier. When the tip of the ET is in the glottic opening, the 90-degree angle bend projects the maximum light intensity toward the surface of the skin, producing a well-defined exterior circumscribed glow. If the Trachlight is bent to 45 degrees, the maximum light intensity is directed down the trachea, whereas a 90-degree bend generally provides better transillumination by directing the light through the soft tissues of the neck, making the light-guided intubation considerably easier. Even though the wider angle of light projection from the light bulb of the Trachlight enhances transillumination substantially, it is the authors' preference to keep a "tight" 90-degree bend for most intubations. For obese patients or patients with short necks, a more acute bend (>90-degree bend) provides better transillumination.

Although it is our experience that the recommended bent length of the Trachlight (6.5 to 8.5 cm) is generally suitable for most patients, some investigators suggested that the bent length of the Trachlight should be approximated to the patient's thyroid prominence–to–mandibular angle distance (TMD).[9] Chen and colleagues[9] found that a shorter bent length (6.5 cm) is more suitable with a shorter TMD (<5.5 cm). Perhaps this study serves to remind us that the bent length should be individualized; that is, a longer bent length (the higher limit of the bent length, such as 8.5 cm) would be more appropriate for patients with a longer TMD and a lower limit (e.g., 6.5 cm) for patients with a shorter TMD. To facilitate slipping the tip of the ET into trachea during intubation, the tip should be coated with a water-soluble lubricant.

2. Positioning

In the hospital setting, the clinician usually stands at the head of the table or bed. It is also possible to use the device from the front or side of the patient, enhancing its utility in the prehospital environment. Depending on the clinician's height, it may be advisable to lower the table or to use a footstool to allow maximal visualization of the anterior neck of the patient during intubation. In contrast to the technique for laryngoscopic intubation, the patient's head and neck should be in a neutral or relatively extended and not a sniffing position. The epiglottis is in close contact with the posterior pharyngeal wall when the head is in the sniffing position, making it more difficult for the Trachlight to pass posterior to the epiglottis. However, the epiglottis is lifted off the posterior pharyngeal wall when the head is extended. This position facilitates the entrance of the ET into the glottic opening.

3. Control of Ambient Light

With improved bulb technology, the light emitted by the Trachlight is extremely bright with a directed beam that enhances soft tissue transillumination of the neck. In most cases, patients can be intubated easily under ambient lighting conditions. In fact, in a large clinical study, we were able to perform endotracheal intubation using the Trachlight under ambient light in 85% of the cases.[26] In very thin patients, the light bulb is so bright that it is possible to misinterpret an esophageal intubation as an intratracheal placement, although the glow from an intra-esophageal intubation is much more diffuse in character. It is therefore recommended that all intubations using the Trachlight be carried out under ambient light. Dimming room lights should be used only when absolutely necessary, such as in the case of obese patients or patients with

thick necks. In the emergency department or prehospital setting when controlling the ambient lighting is not possible, it may be helpful to shade the neck with a towel or hand.

4. Technique of Intubation

a. Oral Intubation

As with other intubation techniques, proper oxygenation of the patient should precede light-guided intubation. Under anesthesia and with the patient supine, the tongue falls posteriorly, pushing the epiglottis against the posterior pharyngeal wall (Fig. 20-9). In order to have a clear passage to the glottic opening during intubation, it is necessary for the clinician to grasp the jaw and lift upward using the thumb and index finger of the nondominant hand. (Fig. 20-10). This lifts the tongue and epiglottis away from the posterior pharyngeal wall to facilitate placement of the tip of the ET posterior to the epiglottis and into the glottic opening (see Fig. 20-10). The nondominant hand should be kept close to the corner of the mouth to ensure an unobstructed path in the midline for the lighted stylet. The Trachlight is grasped in the dominant hand, switched on, and the ET-TL inserted into the midline of the oropharynx. The midline position of the ET-TL is maintained while the device is advanced gently in a rocking motion along an imaginary arc. The ET-TL should always be advanced gently. When resistance is felt, the ET-TL should be rocked backward (cephalad) and the tip redirected toward the laryngeal prominence using the glow of the light as a guide.

A faint glow seen above the laryngeal prominence indicates that the tip of the ET-TL is located in the vallecula.

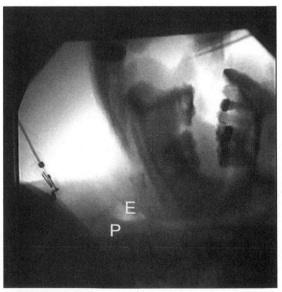

Figure 20-9 This lateral radiographic view of the upper airway of an anesthetized patient shows that the tongue falls posteriorly, pushing the epiglottis (E) against the posterior pharyngeal wall (P).

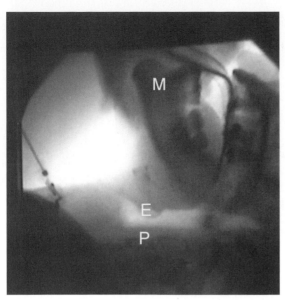

Figure 20-10 This lateral radiographic view of the upper airway of an anesthetized patient shows that a jaw (or mandible [M]) lift can elevate the tongue and the epiglottis (E) off the posterior pharyngeal wall (P) with an open passage for the endotracheal tube–Trachlight to enter the glottic opening.

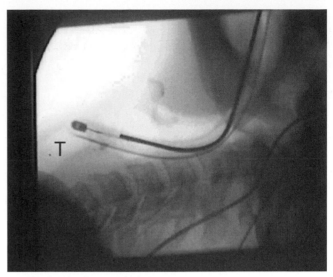

Figure 20-12 This lateral radiographic view of the upper airway of an anesthetized patient shows that when the tip of the endotracheal tube–Trachlight is placed at the glottic opening, the endotracheal tube cannot be advanced readily into the trachea (T) because of the hockey stick configuration of the Trachlight.

A jaw lift helps to elevate the epiglottis and enhance the passage of the ET-TL under the epiglottis. When the tip of ET-TL enters the glottic opening, a well-defined circumscribed glow can be seen in the anterior neck slightly below the laryngeal prominence (Fig. 20-11). However, the ET-TL cannot be advanced into the trachea because of the hockey stick configuration of the Trachlight (Fig. 20-12). Retracting the wire inner stylet approximately 10 cm makes the ET-TL more pliable, allowing advancement into the trachea with reduced risk of trauma (Fig. 20-13). The ET-TL is then advanced until the glow begins to disappear at the sternal notch

(Fig. 20-14), indicating that the tip of the ET is approximately 5 cm above the carina in the average adult.[51] Following release of the locking clamp, the Trachlight wand can be removed from the ET.

Occasionally, the circumscribed glow cannot be readily seen in the anterior neck because of anatomic features such as morbid obesity or a short neck. Neck extension as described previously may be helpful. Retraction of the breast or chest wall tissues together with indentation of the tissues around the trachea by an assistant enhances

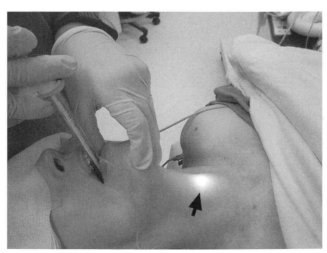

Figure 20-11 When the tip of the endotracheal tube with the light wand is placed at the glottic opening, a well-defined glow *(arrow)* can be readily seen in the anterior neck just below the thyroid prominence.

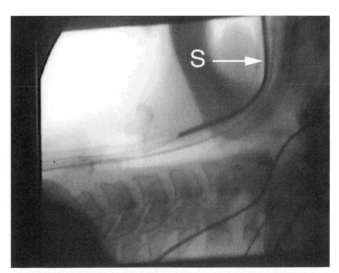

Figure 20-13 This lateral radiographic view of the upper airway of an anesthetized patient shows that with the stiff internal stylet wire (S) retracted approximately 10 cm, the distal endotracheal tube–Trachlight becomes more pliable, allowing easy advancement of the endotracheal tube into the trachea.

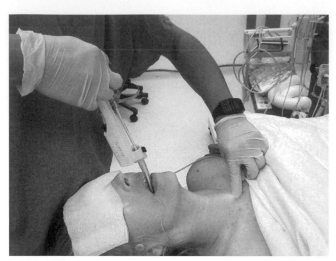

Figure 20-14 Following retraction of the stiff internal stylet wire, the endotracheal tube–Trachlight becomes pliable, permitting the endotracheal tube to be advanced further into the trachea. The endotracheal tube is advanced until the glow is at the sternal notch.

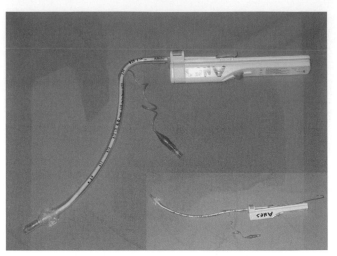

Figure 20-15 If a nasal RAE tracheal tube is used, the stiff internal stylet wire of the Trachlight can be retracted halfway (about 15 cm) to allow unbending of the proximal curvature of the nasal RAE tube *(inset)*.

transillumination of the soft tissues in the anterior neck, but dimming the ambient light is required only on rare occasions.

Following the retraction of the wire stylet, the tip of the tube and lighted stylet can sometimes be caught at the vestibular folds of the cords or tracheal ring (hung up) and cannot be advanced into the trachea readily because the tip of the ET is pointing toward the anterior wall of the larynx or trachea. While maintaining the tube tip in contact with the laryngeal or tracheal wall, the clinician should rotate the ET-TL sideways 90 degrees or more to the right or left side of the head. The tip of the ET then points sideways or downward, and this repositioning enhances the entrance of the ET into the trachea. Alternatively, grasping the anterior larynx with the nondominant hand with an upward lift helps the tip of the ET to come off the vestibular folds or tracheal ring.

b. Nasal Intubation

Although nasotracheal intubation is used infrequently by anesthesiologists in oral procedures, it remains a useful alternative technique for many situations, particularly in emergency medicine. Light-guided nasotracheal intubation using the Trachlight is particularly useful when guided or blind nasal intubation is indicated, such as in emergency airways for patients with a limited mouth opening and cervical spine instability.

Removal of the internal wire stylet of the lighted stylet prior to the insertion of the Trachlight into the ET makes the ET-TL pliable enough for nasotracheal intubation. If a nasal Ring-Adair-Elwyn (RAE) ET is used, the inner wire stylet of the Trachlight can be retracted halfway (about 15 cm) to allow unbending of the proximal curvature of the nasal RAE tube (Fig. 20-15). This facilitates light-guided nasotracheal intubation using the nasal

RAE tube. Application of a vasoconstrictor nasal spray to the nasal mucosa prior to intubation minimizes bleeding. The ET-TL should be immersed in a bottle of warm sterile water or saline to soften the ET and further reduce the risk of mucosal damage during nasal intubation. Water-soluble lubricant is applied to the nostril to facilitate entry of the ET-TL through the nose. As with oral intubation, a jaw lift during intubation elevates the tongue and epiglottis away from the posterior wall of the pharynx, facilitating the placement of the tip of the ET behind the epiglottis and into the glottic opening.

The Trachlight is switched on once the tip of the ET-TL has advanced into the oropharynx, positioned in the midline, and advanced *gently* using the light glow as a guide. When resistance is felt, the ET-TL should be withdrawn slightly and the tip redirected toward the laryngeal prominence using the glow of the light as a guide. A faint glow seen above the laryngeal prominence indicates that the tip of the ET-TL is located in the vallecula. A jaw lift and slight withdrawal of the ET-TL help to elevate the epiglottis and enhance the passage of the ET-TL under it. When the ET-TL enters the glottic opening, a well-defined circumscribed glow is seen in the anterior neck just below the thyroid prominence (Fig. 20-16). To ensure that the tip of the ET-TL is located at the optimal position within the trachea, the tip of the ET is advanced until the glow begins to disappear at the sternal notch. Following the release of the locking clamp, the Trachlight is withdrawn from the ET. Correct tube placement should be confirmed using end-tidal CO_2 or auscultation, or both.

Because of the natural curvature of the ET, the tip of the ET commonly goes posteriorly into the esophagus during blind or light-guided nasal intubation. To bring the tip of the ET anteriorly during intubation, it is sometimes necessary to flex the neck of the patient while

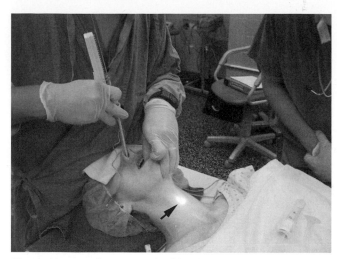

Figure 20-16 During nasotracheal intubation using the Trachlight, the jaw is grasped and lifted upward by the nondominant hand. This elevates the tongue and epiglottis away from the posterior wall of the pharynx to facilitate the placement of the tip of the endotracheal tube into the glottic opening. When the endotracheal tube–Trachlight enters the glottic opening, a well-defined circumscribed glow *(arrow)* is seen in the anterior neck just below the thyroid prominence.

advancing the ET-TL slowly. In the event that flexing the neck of the patient is contraindicated, inflating the ET cuff completely with 20 cm³ of air helps to elevate the ET tip and align it with the glottis during intubation.[23] Alternatively, the use of a directional-tip tube (Endotrol tube, Mallinckrodt, St Louis, MO) also facilitates the lifting of the tip of the ET during nasal intubation.[6] In some difficult circumstances, nasotracheal intubation can be performed effectively and safely with the internal stiff stylet in place.[3] Although there may be an increased risk of nasal trauma with the stylet in place, this technique may be associated with fewer head-neck manipulations and perhaps better control of the tip of the ET.

C. CLINICAL APPLICATIONS

We conducted a large study involving 950 elective surgical patients to determine the effectiveness and safety of oral intubation with either light-guided intubation using the Trachlight or direct-vision placement using a laryngoscope.[26] There was a statistically significant difference in the total intubation time between the groups (15.7 ± 10.8 seconds for Trachlight versus 19.6 ± 23.7 seconds for laryngoscopy). However, such a small difference is probably of little clinical importance. The Trachlight also appears to compare favorably with the conventional laryngoscopic technique with regard to its effectiveness and failure rate. There was a 1% failure rate with the Trachlight and 92% of intubations were successful on the first attempt, compared with a 3% failure rate and an 89% success rate on the first attempt using the laryngoscope. There were significantly fewer traumatic

events and sore throats in the Trachlight group compared with laryngoscopy patients. Tsutsui and Setoyama reported similar findings in a study with 511 patients.[54] Trachlight intubation appears to be highly effective (99%) with the majority of the intubations successful (93%) after one attempt. Unsuccessful intubation even at the third attempt occurred in three patients (1%).

Fewer failures and complications compared with the conventional technique using laryngoscopy and the ease of intubation irrespective of patients' upper airway anatomy led to speculation that the Trachlight might be potentially useful in intubating patients with DAs.[26] During the development of the device, we demonstrated the effectiveness of Trachlight intubation in patients with a DA.[27] Two hundred and sixty-five patients were studied with 206 patients in group 1 (patients with a documented history of difficult intubation or anticipated DAs) and 59 in group 2 (anesthetized patients with an unanticipated failed laryngoscopic intubation). In group 1, intubation was successful in all but two of the patients with a mean (±SD) time to intubation of 25.7 ± 20.1 seconds. The tracheas of these two patients (a morbidly obese patient weighing 220 kg and a patient with severe flexion deformity of the cervical spine) were intubated successfully using a fiberoptic bronchoscope. Orotracheal intubation was successful in all patients in group 2 using the Trachlight with a mean (±SD) time to intubation of 19.7 ± 13.5 seconds. Apart from minor mucosal bleeding (mostly from nasal intubation), no serious complications were observed in any of the study patients. The results of this study indicate that Trachlight is a useful and effective technique for placement of ETs both nasally and orally for patients with an anticipated as well as an unanticipated DA.

Other investigators have also reported successful use of the Trachlight for tracheal placement in patients with a DA. These include patients with a history of limited mouth opening,[15] cervical spine abnormality,[29] Pierre Robin syndrome,[30] and cardiac patients with a DA.[18]

Although many studies have reported the comparative hemodynamic changes associated with Trachlight intubation and laryngoscopic intubation, the results were inconsistent. Several studies involving only a small number of patients ($n = 40$ to 60) showed that there was no statistical difference in the hemodynamic changes following endotracheal intubation using either the lighted stylet or the laryngoscope.[16,22,53] However, none of these studies performed a power analysis to determine the appropriate sample size for the study, thus running the risk of having a type II error. Furthermore, one of these studies did not include a standardized general anesthetic technique.[16] These findings were not consistent with the results of other studies with lower hemodynamic responses following endotracheal intubation using a lighted stylet compared with a laryngoscope.[28,34,44,54]

In a small study ($n = 40$), Nishikawa and colleagues[44] showed that the lighted-stylet technique significantly attenuates hemodynamic changes after intubation in comparison with the laryngoscopic technique in normotensive patients. However, they did not find any significant difference in hemodynamic changes between the two techniques in patients with hypertension. These results were in direct contrast to the findings of another comparative study of the hemodynamic changes between three intubating techniques using either a Macintosh laryngoscope, a Trachlight, or an intubating laryngeal mask airway (LMA) (Fastrach) ($n = 75$).[34] The investigators reported that both the Fastrach and the Trachlight lighted stylet attenuate the hemodynamic stress response to endotracheal intubation compared with the Macintosh laryngoscope in hypertensive but not in normotensive patients.

In a large study ($n = 511$), Tsutsui and Setoyama reported that the Trachlight intubation was associated with less elevation of the blood pressure during intubation than with laryngoscopic intubation.[54] During the development of the Trachlight, we also conducted a study involving 450 elective surgical patients and showed that the increase in mean arterial pressure and heart rate following intubation was significantly less with the Trachlight than with laryngoscopy.[28] Unfortunately, in our study, the anesthetic technique employed was not standardized. Clearly, future studies involving a large number of patients are necessary to clarify these conflicting data regarding the hemodynamic stimulation associated with light-guided endotracheal intubation.

D. OTHER POTENTIAL USES

Tracheal intubation can fail with Trachlight as well as with the laryngoscope. However, in our study with 950 patients, we showed that all Trachlight failures were resolved with direct laryngoscopy. Similarly, all failures of direct laryngoscopy were resolved with Trachlight. These results suggest that a success rate approaching 100% can be achieved in endotracheal intubation with the use of a technique combining the two methods. The combined technique could be particularly useful for unanticipated difficult laryngoscopic intubation (e.g., patients with Cormack's grade 3 laryngoscopic view). Instead of using an ET-stylet with a 90-degree bend, the ET can be used together with the Trachlight (ET-TL) with a 90-degree bend. Under direct laryngoscopy, the tip of the ET-TL can be hooked under the epiglottis. If the tip of the ET is placed at the glottic opening, a well-defined circumscribed glow can be seen in the anterior neck slightly below the laryngeal prominence. If a glow is not seen, the ET-TL should be repositioned until a glow can be seen in the anterior neck. Since the development of the Trachlight, the authors have recorded more than a dozen failed intubations using either the Trachlight or laryngoscope. In each of these failures, endotracheal intubation was successful using the laryngoscope with the Trachlight. Other investigators have also reported successful use of this combined technique.[2] In this study, the investigators successfully performed endotracheal intubation in 350 surgical patients with a simulated DA using the laryngoscope together with the Trachlight.

In addition to its use with the laryngoscope, the Trachlight has been combined successfully with other intubating techniques. These include intubation through the LMA-Classic,[7,8] use in conjunction with the Fastrach,[14] use with the Bullard laryngoscope,[19,41] and use with a retrograde intubating technique.[24]

The Trachlight has also been shown to be useful in identifying the ET tip intratracheal position during percutaneous tracheostomy.[1] This simple technique can help to avoid puncturing the ET or cuff, thus ensuring adequate ventilation and oxygenation during the percutaneous tracheostomy. The technique is also inexpensive and minimizes the risk of damaging equipment such as the fiberoptic bronchoscope. If it is used properly, it is possible that this simple light-guided technique can also be used to determine accurately when the tip of the ET is above the surgical tracheostomy site as the tube is pulled back during surgical tracheostomy.

It should be emphasized that the distinct advantages of the Trachlight (flexibility of the wand and the retractable wire internal stylet) have been clearly shown in managing patients with a variety of airway challenges. These additional uses clearly demonstrate the versatility of the Trachlight device.

E. LIMITATIONS

Although the Trachlight and other lighted stylets have been demonstrated to be effective and safe devices for intubation, the technique requires transillumination of the soft tissues of the anterior neck without visualization of the laryngeal structure. Therefore, Trachlight should not be used in patients with known abnormalities of the upper airway, such as tumors, polyps, infection (e.g., epiglottitis and retropharyngeal abscess), and trauma of the upper airway or if there is a foreign body in the upper airway. In these cases, other alternatives using direct vision, such as fiberoptic intubation, should be considered. Trachlight should also be used with caution in patients in whom transillumination of the anterior neck may not be adequate, such as patients who are grossly obese or patients with limited neck extension. However, these contraindications and precautions must be weighed in light of the urgency of achieving a patent airway in any patient whose ventilation may be compromised in whom urgent intubation is indicated. Intuitively, this light-guided technique should not be attempted with an awake uncooperative patient unless a bite block is used to prevent damage to the device or injury to the clinician.

Since its introduction in 1995, the Trachlight has been used extensively in many countries. Although there are potential risks of damaging the glottic opening during endotracheal intubation using a "nonvisualizing" intubating technique, there have been no reported serious complications of the use of the device to date. However, Aoyama and coworkers reported that the epiglottis of a patient was partially pushed into the laryngeal inlet along with the ET following Trachlight intubation.[5] To investigate the potential risk of laryngeal damage during Trachlight intubation, the investigators used a nasally placed fiberoptic bronchoscope. They reported that during the placement of the ET using the Trachlight, structures around the glottic opening, including the epiglottis and the arytenoids, can be transiently displaced. In some instances, the epiglottis was pushed into the glottic opening. Fortunately, the epiglottis usually spontaneously returned to the correct position. The investigators suggested that there are potential risks of laryngeal damage in addition to the downfolding of the epiglottis during ET placement using the Trachlight. But such occurrences have not been observed to cause permanent damage, and the reduction in the incidence of sore throat in patients intubated using the Trachlight compared with laryngoscopic intubation would suggest that such reports are of little clinical significance.[26]

Intubation using a lighted stylet has some risks. Stone and other investigators reported disconnection of the light bulb from a lighted stylet requiring retrieval from a major bronchus.[52] However, the lighted-stylet device (Flexilum) was not designed or recommended for endotracheal intubation. A later version of the same design solved the problem of bulb loss into the trachea by encasing stylet and bulb in a tough plastic sheath (Tubestat). It is extremely unlikely that the light bulb would be detached from the Trachlight because the light bulb is firmly attached to the durable plastic sheath of Trachlight, in contrast to the older devices. In fact, since its introduction in 1995, there has been no reported case of a light bulb detached from the Trachlight. Although rare, subluxation of the cricoarytenoid cartilage has also been reported by a study using an older version of a lighted stylet (Tubestat). However, with the retractable stylet, the risk of damaging the arytenoid cartilage during Trachlight intubation is low.

Noguchi and associates reported that the application of an 8% lidocaine (Xylocaine) pump spray as a lubricant for the Trachlight had resulted in disappearance of the print markings of the wand.[46] However, the lidocaine jelly and glycerin showed no effect on the print mark. The investigators suggested that lidocaine pump spray should not be used as a lubricant on the Trachlight wand.

Although the Trachlight has been shown to be an effective and safe intubating device, its potential risks and complications, as well as its indications, must be kept in mind.

IV. SUMMARY

Occasional difficult laryngoscopic intubation has led to the development of many alternative techniques for placing an ET. An intubating guide, such as the gum elastic bougie, has been shown to be effective in guiding the ET into the trachea when the laryngeal aperture cannot be seen under direct vision using a laryngoscope. Transillumination of the soft tissues of the neck using a lighted stylet has been shown to be an effective intubation technique for decades. Although many versions of lighted stylets are available, the Trachlight has incorporated many design modifications to facilitate both oral and nasal intubation in both awake and anesthetized patients. It has been demonstrated to be an effective and safe intubating device in a large number of surgical patients and patients with documented DAs. However, it should not be used in patients with anatomic abnormalities of the upper airways. As with any intubation technique, regular use and practice with these intubating devices improve performance and may also reduce the likelihood of complications.

REFERENCES

1. Addas BM, Howes WJ, Hung OR: Light-guided tracheal puncture for percutaneous tracheostomy. Can J Anaesth 47:919-922, 2000.
2. Agro F, Benumof JL, Carassiti M, et al: Efficacy of a combined technique using the Trachlight together with direct laryngoscopy under simulated difficult airway conditions in 350 anesthetized patients. Can J Anaesth 49:525-526, 2002.
3. Agro F, Brimacombe J, Marchionni L, et al: Nasal intubation with the Trachlight. Can J Anaesth 46:907-908, 1999.
4. Ainsworth QP, Howell TH: Transilluminated tracheal intubation. Br J Anaesth 62:494-497, 1989.
5. Aoyama K, Takenaka I, Nagaoka E, et al: Potential damage to the larynx associated with light-guided intubation: A case and series of fiberoptic examinations. Anesthesiology 94:165-167, 2001.
6. Asai T: Endotrol tube for blind nasotracheal intubation [letter]. Anaesthesia 50:507, 1996.
7. Asai T, Latto IP: Unexpected difficulty in the lighted stylet–aided tracheal intubation via the laryngeal mask. Br J Anaesth 76:111-112, 1996.
8. Asai T, Latto IP: Use of the lighted stylet for tracheal intubation via the laryngeal mask airway. Br J Anaesth 75:503-504, 1995.
9. Chen TH, Tsai SK, Lin CJ, et al: Does the suggested lightwand bent length fit every patient? The relation between bent length and patient's thyroid prominence–to–mandibular angle distance. Anesthesiology 98:1070-1076, 2003.
10. Cormack RS, Lehane J: Difficult tracheal intubation in obstetrics. Anaesthesia 39:1105-1111, 1984.
11. Davies JM, Weeks S, Crone LA, et al: Difficult intubation in the parturient. Can J Anaesth 36:668-674, 1989.
12. El-Ganzouri AR, McCarthy RJ, Tuman KJ, et al: Preoperative airway assessment: Predictive value of a

multivariate risk index. Anesth Analg 82:1197-1204, 1996.

13. Ellis DG, Jakymec A, Kaplan RM, et al: Guided orotracheal intubation in the operating room using a lighted stylet: A comparison with direct laryngoscopic technique. Anesthesiology 64:823-826, 1986.

14. Fan KH, Hung OR, Agro F: A comparative study of tracheal intubation using an intubating laryngeal mask (Fastrach) alone, or together with a lightwand (Trachlight). J Clin Anesth 12:581-585, 2000.

15. Favaro R, Tordiglione P, Di Lascio F, et al: Effective nasotracheal intubation using a modified transillumination technique. Can J Anaesth 49:91-95, 2002.

16. Friedman PG, Rosenberg MK, Lebonbom-Mansour M: A comparison of light wand and suspension laryngoscopic intubation techniques in outpatients. Anesth Analg 85:578-582, 1997.

17. Frostad AB, Ronning-Amesen A: Tracheostomy in acute obstructive laryngitis. J Laryngol Otol 87:1101-1106, 1973.

18. Gille A, Komar K, Schmidt E, Alexander T: Transillumination technique in difficult intubations in heart surgery. Anasthesiol Intensivmed Notfallmed Schmerzther 37:604-608, 2002.

19. Gutstein HB: Use of the Bullard laryngoscope and light-wand in pediatric patients. Anesthesiol Clin North Am 16:795-812, 1998.

20. Hagberg CA: Special devices and techniques. Anesthesiol Clin North Am 20:907-932, 2002.

21. Herholdt JD, Rafn CG: Life-Saving Measures for Drowning Persons. Copenhagen, H Tikiob, 1796, pp 52-53.

22. Hirabayashi Y, Hiruta M, Kawakami T, et al: Effects of lightwand (Trachlight) compared with direct laryngoscopy on circulatory responses to tracheal intubation. Br J Anaesth 81:253-255, 1998.

23. Hung OR: Nasal intubation with the Trachlight. Can J Anaesth 46:907-908, 1999.

24. Hung OR, Al-Qatari M: Light-guided retrograde intubation. Can J Anaesth 44:877-882, 1997.

25. Hung OR, Stewart RD: Lightwand intubation: I—A new lightwand device. Can J Anaesth 42:820-825, 1995.

26. Hung OR, Pytka S, Morris I, et al: Clinical trial of a new lightwand device (Trachlight) to intubate the trachea. Anesthesiology 83:509-514, 1995.

27. Hung OR, Pytka S, Morris I, et al: Lightwand intubation: II—Clinical trial of a new lightwand for tracheal intubation in patients with difficult airways. Can J Anaesth 42:826-830, 1995.

28. Hung OR, Pytka S, Murphy MF, et al: Comparative hemodynamic changes following laryngoscopic or lightwand intubation. Anesthesiology 79(3A):A497, 1993.

29. Inoue Y, Koga K, Shigematsu A: A comparison of two tracheal intubation techniques with Trachlight and Fastrach in patients with cervical spine disorders. Anesth Analg 94:667-671, 2002.

30. Iseki K, Watanabe K, Iwama H: Use of the Trachlight for intubation in the Pierre-Robin syndrome. Anaesthesia 52:801-802, 1997.

31. Jackson C: The technique of insertion of intratracheal insufflation tubes. Surg Gynecol Obstet 17:507, 1913.

32. Karkouti K, Rose DK, Wigglesworth D, Cohen MM: Predicting difficult intubation: A multivariable analysis. Can J Anaesth 47:730-739, 2000.

33. Kidd JF, Dyson A, Latto IP: Successful difficult intubation. Use of the gum elastic bougie. Anaesthesia 43:437-438, 1988.

34. Kihara S, Brimacombe J, Yaguchi Y, et al: Hemodynamic responses among three tracheal intubation devices in normotensive and hypertensive patients. Anesth Analg 96:890-895, table of contents, 2003.

35. Latto IP: Management of difficult intubation. In Latto IP, Rosen M (eds): Difficulties in Tracheal Intubation. London, Baillière Tindall, 1987, pp 99-141.

36. Levitan R, Ochroch EA: Airway management and direct laryngoscopy: A review and update. Crit Care Clin 16:373-388, 2000.

37. MacEwen W: Clinical observations on the introduction of tracheal tubes by the mouth instead of performing tracheostomy or laryngotomy. Br Med J 122:163, 1880.

38. MacIntosh R, Richards H: Illuminated introducer for endotracheal tubes. Anaesthesia 12:223-225, 1957.

39. MacIntosh RR: An aid to oral intubation. Br Med J 1:28, 1949.

40. Mallampati SR, Gugino LD, Desai SP, et al: A clinical sign to predict difficult tracheal intubation: A prospective study. Can Anesth Soc J 32:429-434, 1985.

41. McGuire G, Krestow M: Bullard assisted trachlight technique. Can J Anaesth 46:907, 1999.

42. Mihic D, Binkert E, Novoselac M: The first endotracheal intubation [letter]. Anesthesiology 52:523, 1980.

43. Moscati R, Jehle D, Christiansen G, et al: Endotracheal tube introducer for failed intubations: A variant of the gum elastic bougie. Ann Emerg Med 36:52-56, 2000.

44. Nishikawa K, Omote K, Kawana S, Namiki A: A comparison of hemodynamic changes after endotracheal intubation by using the lightwand device and the laryngoscope in normotensive and hypertensive patients. Anesth Analg 90:1203-1207, 2000.

45. Nishiyama T, Matsukawa T, Hanaoka K: Safety of a new lightwand device (Trachlight): Temperature and histopathological study. Anesth Analg 87:717-718, 1998.

46. Noguchi T, Koga K, Shiga Y, Shigematsu A: Preliminary report: Dissolving effect of 8% lidocaine pump spray on the print mark of the Trachlight wand. Masui 51:503-504, 2002.

47. Nolan JP, Wilson ME: Evaluation of the gum elastic bougie. Anaesthesia 47:878-881, 1992.

48. Nolan JP, Wilson ME: Orotracheal intubation patients with potential cervical spine injury. Anaesthesia 48:630-633, 1993.

49. Rao TL, Mathru M, Gorski DW, Salem MR: Experience with a new intubation guide for difficult tracheal intubation. Crit Care Med 10:882-883, 1982.

50. Rose DK, Cohen MM: The airway: Problems and predictions in 18,500 patients. Can J Anaesth 41:372-383, 1994.

51. Stewart RD, LaRosee A, Kaplan RM, Ilkhanipour K: Correct positioning of an endotracheal tube using a flexible lighted stylet. Crit Care Med 18:97-99, 1990.

52. Stone DJ, Stirt JA, Kaplan MJ, McLean WC: A complication of lightwand-guided nasotracheal intubation. Anesthesiology 61:780-781, 1984.

53. Takahashi S, Mizutani T, Miyabe M, Toyooka H: Hemodynamic responses to tracheal intubation with laryngoscope versus lightwand intubating device (Trachlight) in adults with normal airway. Anesth Analg 95:480-484, 2002.

54. Tsutsui T, Setoyama K: A clinical evaluation of blind orotracheal intubation using Trachlight in 511 patients. Masui 50:854-858, 2001.

55. Vollmer TP, Stewart RD, Paris PM, et al: Use of a lighted stylet for guided orotracheal intubation in the prehospital setting. Ann Emerg Med 14:324-328, 1985.

56. Weis FR, Hatton MN: Intubation by use of the light-wand: Experience in 253 patients. J Oral Maxillofac Surg 47:577-560, 1989.

57. Weiss M: Management of difficult tracheal intubation with a video-optically modified Schroeder intubation stylet. Anesth Analg 85:1181-1182, 1997.

58. Wilson ME, Speiglhalter D, Robertson JA, Lesser P: Predicting difficult intubation. Br J Anaesth 61:211-216, 1988.

59. Yamamura H, Yamamoto T, Kamiyama M: Device for blind nasal intubation. Anesthesiology 20:221, 1959.

21

LARYNGEAL MASK AIRWAY

David Z. Ferson
Archie I. J. Brain

FOREWORD

The laryngeal mask airway (LMA; LMA Company, Henley, England) is a supraglottic airway device developed by Archie Brain, M.D. (Honorary Consultant Anesthetist, Royal Berkshire Hospital, Reading, England) and introduced into clinical practice in 1988. In the first paper on the LMA, published in the *British Journal of Anaesthesia* in 1983,[21] Dr. Brain described the device as "an alternative to either the endotracheal tube or the face-mask with either spontaneous or positive pressure ventilation." Twenty years and more than 150 million safe uses later, the LMA has significantly improved the comfort and safety of airway management worldwide. Many authorities in anesthesia consider the LMA to be the most important development in airway management in the past 50 years. It would be too simplistic, therefore, in an evaluation of the quality of anesthesia patients' care, to view the LMA as just another airway device. In fact, while experimenting with different shapes and materials as he developed the LMA, Dr. Brain recognized the importance of studying, understanding, and incorporating into the LMA design the anatomic and physiologic principles that govern the oro-pharyngo-laryngeal complex. This effort resulted in an airway device that is not only very effective but also minimally intrusive. Realizing that one LMA model could not fulfill all clinical needs, Dr. Brain introduced three additional models from 1993 to 2003: the LMA-Flexible, the intubating LMA-Fastrach, and the LMA-ProSeal. These models represent only a fraction of the potentially useful clinical designs that have originated from Dr. Brain's research.—David Ferson, M.D.

I. INTRODUCTION

The LMA is a minimally invasive device designed for the management of the airway in the unconscious patient. It consists of an inflatable mask fitted with a tube that exits the mouth to permit ventilation of the lungs. The mask fits against the periglottic tissues, occupying the hypopharyngeal space and forming a seal above the glottis instead of within the trachea (Fig. 21-1). The LMA is

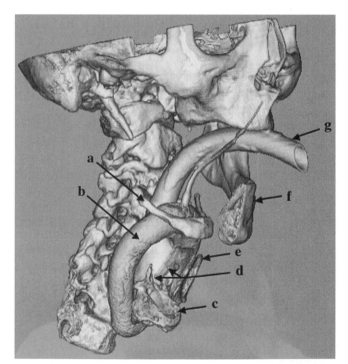

Figure 21-1 Three-dimensional radiologic reconstruction of the human airway with the laryngeal mask airway (LMA) in situ: (a) hyoid bone; (b) LMA's cuff; (c) cricoid ring; (d) arytenoid cartilages; (e) thyroid cartilage (digitally partially removed to demonstrate the position of the LMA); (f) mandible (digitally partially removed to demonstrate the position of the LMA); (g) LMA's shaft. The LMA's cuff forms a seal with the periglottic tissues and provides a continuous connection between the natural airway and the device.

thus a *supraglottic* airway management device. Originally produced as a single general-purpose design in a range of sizes, it is currently made in various forms to satisfy different requirements. The LMA's inventor (AB, one of the present authors) originally set out to design a device that would provide greater control than the face mask without the invasive disadvantages of the endotracheal tube (ETT). Now, more than 20 years later, a substantial worldwide body of literature, while supporting the wisdom of exercising caution when learning to use the supraglottic approach, provides ample evidence of a wide range of uses that go beyond those originally postulated.[7] For example, the LMA is becoming increasingly popular outside the operating room (OR), as evidenced by its endorsement by the European Resuscitation Council and, more recently, the American Heart Association.[76] Its more exotic uses include the adoption of the LMA-Fastrach, the intubating form of the LMA, by the National Aeronautics and Space Administration (NASA) as part of its emergency medical kit for space travel. There is also evidence from the literature that the later varieties of the LMA, including the LMA-Flexible, LMA-Fastrach,[13] and LMA-ProSeal,[19] may be more appropriate tools for specific uses than the original LMA. Well over 2000 scientific articles have been written about the LMA; therefore, describing the full impact of this device on modern anesthetic practice is beyond the scope of a single chapter. Our aim instead is to provide an up-to-date overview of the LMA's current uses worldwide. After a historical review and comments regarding the correct LMA insertion technique, we explore the principal uses of each of the LMA models, as indicated by published research, and discuss possible problems as well as offer suggestions for getting the best results from each device. Also, we describe the evolution of the LMA's use in patients with difficult-to-manage airways and include the current recommendations for LMA use from the American Society of Anesthesiologists (ASA) difficult airway algorithm.[116]

II. HISTORY AND DEVELOPMENT

In 1988, the definitive device now referred to as the "Classic" LMA was released commercially in the United Kingdom (UK). Although the LMA was rapidly adopted in the UK, it was not until 1991 that the Food and Drug Administration permitted the release of the device in the United States and then only with the stricture that "the LMA is not a replacement for the endotracheal tube." In the presence of what at that time was a very unconventional way of managing the airway, this caution was understandable. Nevertheless, it resulted in a somewhat slower acceptance of the concept of "masking the larynx" in the United States than in the UK, where the LMA was purchased by every health authority within 2 years of its launch, resulting almost immediately in a reduction in ETT use (Fig. 21-2).

Harold Wood Hospital:
Percentage of Cases Managed with an Endotracheal Tube and the
Laryngeal Mask Airway From June 1986 to November 1991

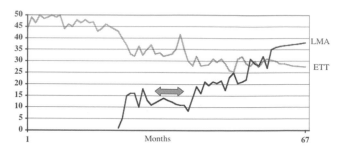

Endotracheal Tube (ETT): Dotted Line
Laryngeal Mask Airway (LMA): Solid Line
Horizontal Arrow: Period of LMA Shortage

Figure 21-2 Harold Wood Hospital (England) data on laryngeal mask airway (LMA) and endotracheal tube (ETT) utilization from June 1986 through November 1991. The use of the ETT has significantly declined in favor of the LMA. This illustrates the rapid growth of LMA use in the United Kingdom.

A. FROM IDEA TO FIRST PROTOTYPE

The inventor (AB) is often asked why and how the idea of the LMA first arose. Like many before him, he believed that a supraglottic approach would be less traumatic than intubation and thus more desirable, provided the method could be easier to control and more reliable than the face mask. Other inventors had mainly explored the oral and pharyngeal spaces above the larynx,[64,75,78,90,113,123] but the LMA was the first device actually to encircle the periglottic tissues in the hypopharynx with a mask. As to the question of how the LMA came about, the inventor conceived his idea in early 1981. Later that year, he began providing dental anesthesia at the outpatient clinic of the Royal London Hospital. At that time, a device known as the Goldman Dental Nose Piece was being used for airway maintenance during dental extractions in anesthetized patients. This was a reusable vulcanized rubber mask that could be detached from its rigid base for cleaning (Fig. 21-3). The mask was designed to fit over the nose, leaving the mouth free for surgical access. Noting a certain similarity between the contours around the nose and those around the glottis, the inventor wondered if the Goldman mask could be modified to fit over the larynx. Placing a device over the larynx would short-circuit the upper airway passages, perhaps eliminating some of the problems associated with maintaining their patency under anesthesia.

Because the Goldman mask was scheduled to be discontinued in favor of a disposable version, the author was able to obtain samples for experimentation. Using an acrylic adhesive, he glued a diagonally cut Portex 10-mm ETT to the rubber mask's attachment flange, which he had to draw across the mask aperture into the midline to form a base (Fig. 21-4). Figure 21-5 is a 1981 photograph

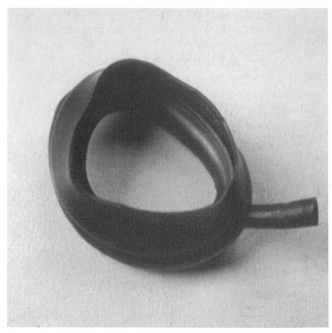

Figure 21-3 Goldman dental mask nose piece, which was used to develop the early cuffs for the laryngeal mask airway prototypes. The central portion of the mask was cut out to allow attachment of the tube.

taken of the inventor as he is about to insert one of the resulting prototypes into his anesthetized pharynx to test the validity of his hypothesis. In his diary, he recorded an absence of any complications, despite having repeated the experiment four times. This observation, combined with broadly worded institutional review board approval, provided the justification for subsequent extensive clinical investigation, which was to occupy the author for the next 7 years. During this time, he built many prototypes, which he used in approximately 7000 patients.[20] He also took extensive notes in private diaries to record his progress but published only a small number of cases;

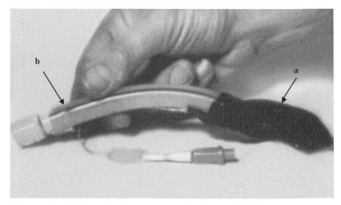

Figure 21-4 The early laryngeal mask airway (LMA) prototype made of a modified Goldman dental nose piece, which formed a cuff (a) and a diagonally cut endotracheal tube (b). The two pieces were glued together to form the first LMA to be tested clinically.

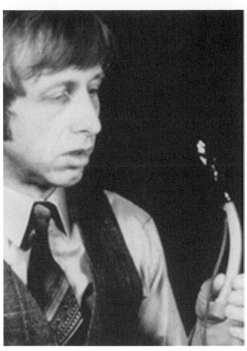

Figure 21-5 Archie Brain, M.D. (1981), the inventor of the laryngeal mask airway (LMA), as he is about to insert one of the LMA prototypes into his anesthetized pharynx to test his hypothesis that a supraglottic device is effective, safe, and much less invasive than the endotracheal tube.

he believed there was little point in presenting data concerning an invention that was not yet ready for production.

B. EARLY PUBLICATIONS

The first article about the LMA, published in the *British Journal of Anaesthesia* in 1983, presented data from only 23 patients and received little attention.[21] A second description 2 years later in *Anaesthesia* was subtitled "development and trials of a new type of airway" and detailed the LMA's use in 118 patients, although it also reported that the author had by this time gained experience in more than 500 cases.[25] On the basis of this experience and a case report published the previous year in *Archives of Emergency Medicine*,[18] which described the successful use of modified versions of the initial prototype in cases of difficult intubation, Brain and colleagues[25] felt justified in concluding that "the laryngeal mask may have a valuable role to play in all types of inhalational anesthesia, while its proven value in some cases of difficult intubation indicates that it may contribute to the safety of general anesthesia."

In the same issue, the author presented further evidence of the potential usefulness of the device in cases of difficult intubation, but there was still no response to these claims from the profession, perhaps because no product was yet available for independent assessment.[23] However, the author had given one of his prototypes to a visiting American anesthesiologist, Ronald Katz, M.D., chairman of the anesthesiology department at the University of California-Los Angeles. Dr. Katz provided the first independent description of the LMA based on his experience with this prototype, writing in Wellcome Trends in Anesthesiology in October 1985[145] and again in February 1986.[146] This second article provided the first published image—reproduced from one of the inventor's transparencies—of the glottis seen fiberoptically through the LMA prototype and noted the potential of the device to overcome intubation problems. American awareness of the LMA thus preceded its availability in the United States by 6 years.

C. FROM HANDMADE MODELS TO CLINICAL USE

It may be asked why it took so long for the LMA to become clinically available. There were three reasons: the initial lack of commercial interest, which meant there were no models available for others to use; the solitary nature of the LMA's development, which was carried out virtually single-handedly by a clinician with a substantial clinical commitment who continued to work with largely homemade equipment until the first commercial prototypes were made in early 1988; and perhaps most important, the complexity of the airway anatomy, which made it hard to design a device that was both safe and effective. One advantage of the long development process was that the considerable clinical history that the inventor accumulated between 1981 and 1988 guided the development of the LMA, so the first factory-made models required little modification. These were produced in Gary, Indiana, tested by the author, and then demonstrated to colleagues in the Royal East Sussex Hospital, Hastings (UK), in April 1988. The chairman of the anesthesiology department at the Royal East Sussex Hospital, Colin Alexander, M.D., immediately authorized the LMA's use in his department, publishing his experience in a letter entitled "Use your Brain" in *Anaesthesia* that year.[2] He concluded that the device "should be considered whenever the indication for tracheal intubation does not include protection of the airway from gastric contents." Meanwhile, a few colleagues who had been given prototypes by the author (or, in one case, had built their own) continued to explore the LMA's use in known cases of difficult intubation, with encouraging results.[20]

Arguably the most influential clinical study using the author's hand-built prototypes was not published until 1989, after the commercial form of the device had already become available. Brodrick and colleagues[36] studied 100 cases in which the patients breathed spontaneously. Eighteen anesthesiologists took part in the study and recorded a "clear and unobstructed airway in 98% of cases," but obstruction on initial placement of the LMA occurred in 10 cases and "appeared to be as a result of downfolding of the epiglottis." A stainless steel introducer tool with a handle similar to that of the LMA-Fastrach and a blade fitting into a slot in the distal anterior end of the LMA's mask had been designed to overcome this problem. An aperture in the blade into which the epiglottis fit caused the epiglottis to be drawn upward as the tool was removed from the patient's pharynx. This insertion tool was in fact used successfully in these cases, but fears that it could cause trauma led to it being abandoned in the commercial form of the LMA. Brodrick's paper is often quoted in support of limiting the use of the LMA to spontaneously breathing patients. However, because the LMAs used by Nunn's group were prototypes, only a size 3 device was available for use in 72 men as well as in 28 women (weight not recorded). Given the possibility that the LMA's size was less than optimal, it is not surprising that eight patients could not be ventilated using positive pressure without unacceptable leaks and that the mean leak pressure was 17 cm H_2O, similar to that recorded by the author 6 years earlier.[20]

In addition to the information accumulated in his clinical work, study of the anatomy and physiology of the larynx and pharynx guided the author throughout the development of the LMA. As the work progressed, the author found himself struggling to achieve a balance between simplicity, efficacy, and safety. The essential problem was that in designing a device that fits into the lower pharynx, measures favoring efficacy tended to counteract those favoring simplicity. Improving the seal, for example, required more complex construction to avoid potential trauma related to high mucosal pressures. Likewise, an effort to make the device easier to insert led to the development of an insertion tool, which was determined (by the author) to be potentially unsafe and therefore abandoned, in spite of the efficacy it demonstrated.[20] Ultimately, the solutions chosen were compromises. Regarding the seal, the author realized that seals with a leak pressure much higher than 20 cm H_2O were rarely necessary in practice and that an inadequate seal often could be overcome by using a more appropriately sized device, using a better fixation technique, or giving a more appropriate anesthetic. To make insertion of the LMA maximally reliable and minimally traumatic, a technique gradually evolved that is based on the swallowing mechanism. Unfortunately, the author underestimated the difficulty of teaching others to understand and master such a subtle technique. Indeed, the technique is virtually impossible to learn without direct, hands-on demonstration and guidance.[59] As a result, a considerable portion of the articles in the LMA literature suggest variant insertion methods, most of which had already been tried and rejected by the author for being unreliable or traumatic.

In spite of these difficulties, the history of the LMA since its first commercial launch is essentially a story of steady expansion in use around the world. Availability, cost, and user education have governed the speed at which the various forms of the LMA have been accepted. Figure 21-2 shows data collected by the anesthesiology department of Harold Wood Hospital, a typical general hospital near London, on the influence of the Classic LMA, in the first 3 years of its availability, on the use of the ETT and the face mask. The dip in the curve representing LMA use indicates a period of commercial nonavailability. These data show clearly that use of the ETT almost immediately declined in favor of the new method of airway management and illustrate the rapid growth of LMA use in the UK. They also cast some doubt on the widely held view that the popularity of the LMA in the UK has been due to the more frequent use of the face mask there than in the United States.

As new models of the LMA have become available, countries with different anesthetic traditions have responded to them with varying degrees of enthusiasm. In all cases, however, use of the LMA has steadily increased (personal communication, March 2004, LMA International SA).

III. THE LARYNGEAL MASK AIRWAY INSERTION TECHNIQUE

The LMA occupies a potential space that is shared by the respiratory and alimentary tracts, which are subject to the control and coordination of several complex reflexes. Although one does not need a detailed knowledge of the specific reflexes to use the LMA, one does need to understand the basic concept behind the recommended insertion technique, which not only ensures the greatest success but also results in the fewest complications. Physiologically, the alimentary tract is capable of either accepting (swallowing) or rejecting (vomiting) liquids or solids in the form of food. In contrast, the respiratory tract mobilizes defensive responses (coughing, laryngospasm, bronchospasm) only when invaded by liquids or solids (e.g., an ETT). When inserted correctly, the LMA does not stimulate the respiratory tract defenses because the device forms an end-to-end seal against the periglottic tissues.

Investigations using magnetic resonance imaging (MRI) to assess the effect of the LMA on the anatomy of the airway may help to explain the reliability of the device. A study by Shorten and coworkers of 46 adults requiring sagittal MRI views of the head and neck compared the anatomic differences between awake, sedated, and anesthetized patients.[124] With an LMA in place, the epiglottic angle was more than twice as great with respect to the posterior pharyngeal wall in the anesthetized group as it was in either the sedated or awake group. This had no apparent effect on ventilatory function in most patients. This is probably due to the depth of the LMA bowl, which the inventor found to be a critical dimension when experimenting with different design ideas during the 1980s. The recommended standard insertion technique evolved slowly as the inventor gained experience, and it was not until he had been inserting LMAs for almost 10 years that he realized that his technique was becoming more and more similar to the physiologic act of swallowing food. Once he realized this, it was a simple matter to study this mechanism more closely and make allowances for the fact that in the anesthetized patient, this reflex is partially or completely abolished. The following key points emerged:

1. *Correct mask deflation is important.* The purpose of chewing food is to form a soft, atraumatic paste that can easily be passed through the pharynx and esophagus. At the onset of the act of swallowing, this paste, the so-called food bolus, is pressed by the tongue into the hard palate. The pressure generated is distributed widely over the palatal surface, so there is no localized high-pressure point, which would give the sensation of a sharp object and lead to rejection instead of swallowing. The inventor realized that to imitate this sensation of a soft food bolus, he needed to deflate the mask so that it presented an elastic, hollow shape. When this shape was pressed into the dome of the palate, the hollow form would need to be inverted. The pressure required by the inserting finger to achieve this would cause the outer rim of the mask to act like a gentle spring, producing the desired effect of spreading pressure smoothly over the entire posterior surface of the mask. This spring effect cannot be achieved without deflating the mask to a vacuum pressure of about −40 cm H_2O. Only in this way was it possible to prevent the pointed distal end of the mask bowl from transmitting an irritating localized pressure point as it was pressed into the oropharyngeal curve. Partial mask inflation could not achieve this aim, however, because the soft distal end of the mask simply rolled backward, allowing the pointed tip of the mask bowl to scratch the palatal surface. Deflating the mask such that it followed the curvature of the palate had the same disadvantage, as this made the pointed end even more prominent. Finally, inserting a fully inflated mask introduced excessive bulk, which created the possibility of tearing the cuff against the teeth and was physiologically equivalent to swallowing too large a bolus of food, which again could lead to the rejection reflex.

2. *The deflated mask must be lubricated if the oral cavity is not already wet.* Again, there is a parallel with swallowing because lubrication is a key part of deglutition. Because the mask is to be slid against the palate, it makes sense to apply a bolus of lubricant to the distal hollowed posterior surface of the mask immediately prior to insertion. Water-soluble jelly is a good substitute for oral secretions. It is not necessary or desirable to spread the lubricant over the whole surface of the mask prior to insertion.

3. *Flatten the mask against the hard palate.* Initially during swallowing, the tongue flattens the softened food bolus against the hard palate; thus, during the first step in LMA insertion, the mask, correctly prepared to impart a sensation similar to that of a soft food bolus, is flattened by pressing it against the hard palate. Placing the index finger on the airway tube at its junction with the mask under the deflated proximal rim of the cuff is the best way to impart the necessary force.

4. *Cranioposterior movement of the index finger.* In swallowing, the bolus of food is advanced into the pharynx, esophagus, and ultimately the stomach through the precise coordination of several muscle groups, beginning with the tongue. During LMA insertion, the clinician must use her or his index finger to advance the mask in the cranioposterior direction, thus imitating the action of the tongue. This allows a completely deflated tip to slide smoothly along the hard palate, soft palate, and posterior pharyngeal wall, while minimizing the contact of the mask with anterior structures such as the base of the tongue, the epiglottis, and the laryngeal inlet. It is important to realize that the finger must continue to push in a cranioposterior direction even though the anatomy forces the mask and, with it the finger, to move caudally. The finger must never consciously be directed caudally and should be inserted to its fullest extent until resistance is felt as the mask tip enters the upper esophageal sphincter (UES). It is anatomically impossible to perform this action correctly without *extending* the proximal metacarpopharyngeal joint of the index finger and *flexing* the wrist.

5. *Widening the oropharyngeal angle—first role of the nondominant hand.* Cadaveric work demonstrates that if the head of the supine subject is pushed by the supinated hand in a caudal direction, head extension, neck flexion, and mouth opening are simultaneously achieved. This maneuver widens the oropharyngeal angle to greater than 90 degrees in the normal subject and draws the larynx away from the posterior pharyngeal wall. Both of these effects facilitate LMA insertion. The nondominant hand should therefore maintain firm caudal pressure on the occiput from the start of insertion until the mask has passed behind the tongue.

6. *Removal of the index finger—second role of the nondominant hand.* To prevent the mask sliding out of position once fully inserted, the nondominant hand should move from behind the head to grasp the proximal end of the LMA before the index finger is removed. As the index finger is removed, the mask is held steady or, if it has not been fully inserted, can be pressed further into position by the nondominant hand.

7. *Mask inflation.* As the mask is inflated, its increased bulk and the relatively large radius of the airway tube cause it to slide cranially. It can be shown anatomically that this results in loss of contact between the mask tip and the UES. However, the LMA should not be held in place during inflation because this could result in the

distal end of the mask stretching the UES. All LMAs should be inflated to a pressure of less than 60 cm H_2O (pressures above this have been found to cause discomfort in awake volunteers).

8. *Device fixation—restoring the seal against the UES.* Finally, the distal end of the tube is again pressed into the curve of the hard palate to reestablish firm contact between the proximal end of the device and the UES. While this pressure is maintained, adhesive tape is applied to the maxilla on one side of the patient's face and passed over and under the tube in a single loop before fixing to the opposite maxilla. This form of fixation ensures stability of the device and is likely to afford maximum protection in the event of unexpected regurgitation as well as reduce the incidence of gastric insufflation during positive-pressure ventilation.*

The basic insertion technique is identical for all LMA models. Unfortunately, misunderstanding of and a lack of commitment to mastering this technique are extremely widespread, as reflected in the multiplicity of insertion methods advocated in the literature and the common belief that a failure rate of 10% is acceptable. When variant insertion techniques are used, the failure rate is about five-fold higher than it is with the standard insertion technique. The risk of complications, such as laryngeal or pharyngeal trauma and pulmonary aspiration, probably increases even more than the failure rate when the standard insertion technique is not used. In addition, the use of variant insertion techniques may hinder or prevent the user from acquiring the skills necessary for advanced clinical applications of the LMA. As shown in several reports, use of the standard insertion technique results in a reliable airway, a minimal stress response, and an extremely low risk of complications. This is probably because the LMA's position in relation to the respiratory and alimentary tracts is optimal when the standard insertion technique is used. We refer the reader to instruction manuals for the LMA Classic, the LMA-Flexible, the LMA-Fastrach, and the LMA-ProSeal for detailed, step-by-step instructions on the recommended insertion technique.[94]

IV. LMA CLASSIC

A. BASIC USES

1. Indications for Use

A common question put to the inventor is "What are the indications for LMA use?" This is not easy to answer because although it has long been accepted that success

rates for establishing an airway with the LMA tend to be high, even in relatively unskilled hands, it is equally clear that there is more to the art of using the LMA than simply getting it into place. The evidence for this is the steady expansion in indications as the device's popularity has spread. Just as complications tend to diminish with increasing user experience, so the more confident and more adept user seems to find applications for the LMA that might previously have seemed inappropriate. Using the LMA for airway maintenance during atrial septal defect repair in children, for example, would no doubt strike many American anesthesiologists as highly unconventional, just as it would have alarmed the inventor had it been suggested he try this in 1988.[152] The problem of defining indications for the LMA is perhaps best resolved by recommending that, as with any skill, it is best to start at a simple level and progress gradually to more complex uses. What then are appropriate basic uses for the LMA? Broadly speaking, any nonemergency case requiring general anesthesia in a patient in the supine position who has an ASA classification of I (ASA I) or II and in whom the surgeon is performing a routine, short procedure that does not involve the alimentary or respiratory tract would constitute an appropriate basic use. In practice, such cases are likely to be found in the ambulatory setting and would include simple orthopedic, urologic, superficial, or gynecologic procedures. Although it involves external manipulation of the bowel, inguinal canal surgery would also fall within this category.

2. Inherent Teaching Difficulties—A Vicious Circle

The learning curve for correct LMA insertion extends beyond the often-quoted 10 to 15 uses by one or even two orders of magnitude.[97] For the anesthesiologist who is just starting to get used to the LMA, an important advantage of confining its use to simple cases is that, in many locations, they represent the greater part of the surgical caseload; thus, there are many opportunities for learning and practice. Most anesthesiology residents, however, start out in a teaching hospital, where the caseload tends to be weighted more heavily toward long and complex procedures for which LMA use would be inappropriate in any but the most experienced hands. For this reason, perhaps, it is common in the UK and in the United States to hear experienced consultant anesthesiologists complain that newly appointed colleagues, who have spent the greater part of their training years within teaching hospitals, appear to have only the most rudimentary concept of LMA use. It is, unfortunately, the same academic colleagues who carry out many of the studies that make up the core of evidence-based knowledge related to the LMA. This represents a vicious circle that is not easy to break, particularly at a time when there is increasing pressure on the medical profession to justify all clinical activity by reference to "proven" techniques. A suggested way out of this impasse is outlined subsequently.

---

*One study involving 108 patients showed that a malpositioned LMA was 26 times more likely to be associated with gastric insufflation.[89]

3. Graduating from Simple to Specialized Uses of the LMA

Clearly, the safety of the patient must be the guiding principle when deciding whether someone is qualified to perform specialized uses of the LMA. As a simple rule, a clinician whose first-time insertion success rate is 90% or less should not be considered adequately trained to progress beyond the simplest procedures in ASA I patients. (Davies and colleagues reported a success rate of 94% in the first 10 cases in which naval medical trainees used the LMA for the first time in ASA I anesthetized patients.[48]) Obviously, the insertion success rate depends on the types of cases routinely encountered, and the preceding generalization applies to clinicians in an average peripheral hospital that performs a broad range of common procedures. Those who wish to gain greater expertise in the use of the LMA, but whose practice is based in specialized centers that lack suitable simple cases, might consider the practice of inserting an LMA routinely at the start of a case and then switching to the preferred airway technique before the surgery. The inventor has found this to be a useful strategy within the teaching hospital environment. Its justification is that the skills acquired could be lifesaving in the event of an airway emergency. In addition, if the LMA has been inserted successfully and the patient subsequently proves impossible to intubate, the clinician has an already proven way of at least maintaining oxygenation while other strategies are considered. Alternatively, if the clinician has been unable to use the LMA successfully in a certain patient, time is not wasted in trying to use it after a subsequent failed intubation in this patient.

B. SPECIALIZED USES

1. Procedures outside the Operating Room

a. Radiology and Magnetic Resonance Imaging

The potential advantages of the LMA in investigative imaging were first noted in a letter to *Anaesthesia* from Glasgow, Scotland, in 1990.[118] The authors pointed out that the LMA permitted hands-free control of the airway in patients who needed to be kept immobile for prolonged periods, a situation often necessitating general anesthesia in restless or young patients. Later, to improve its performance and durability, the LMA's valve was fitted with a small, stainless steel spring, which unfortunately interfered with MRI of the head and neck. However, LMAs equipped with valves made of nonferrous material were subsequently made available for use in this situation. Stevens and Burden, in a letter to *Anaesthesia* in 1994, commented that they had used the LMA Classic with the modified, nonmetallic valve in more than 500 small children undergoing MRI and that it had proved safe and reliable.[131] They presented an MRI image demonstrating that, by contrast, the LMA-Flexible cannot be used for investigations involving the head and neck because the tube contains a wire, which obliterates the image of the surrounding area.

Goudsouzian and associates were the first authors in America to note the efficacy of the LMA during MRI, using the images obtained during investigations in 28 children to comment on the position of the device when inserted by residents in training.[71] They noted that in spite of poor user skills (21% of attempts resulted in a failure to insert, 21% of the cases required more than one insertion attempt, 82% had a downward deflection of the epiglottis, and 7% had oropharyngeal misplacement), satisfactory ventilatory parameters were maintained in all the children. The safety of the LMA, even in less than fully skilled hands, is a powerful argument for its use in areas remote from the OR. Van Obbergh and colleagues, working in Brussels, Belgium, presented results from somewhat more experienced users.[137] The LMA was used during MRI in 100 consecutive procedures in children that were carried out using propofol. The position of the LMA was not recorded, but only 16% of the cases required more than one insertion attempt, there were no failures to insert, and oxygen saturation values of 99.1% or above were maintained in all the children. Ventilation was manually assisted using an Ayre T-piece.

b. Radiation Therapy

Grebenik and coworkers were the first to describe the use of the LMA in pediatric radiation therapy, studying 25 children who underwent a total of 312 courses of radiation therapy under anesthesia.[73] The children were between 3 weeks and 3 years old, and eight of them were anesthetized once a day for 20 or more consecutive days. In each case, the LMA was left in place until the protective reflexes returned. The absence of complications suggests that the LMA might be appropriate for procedures requiring frequent, repeated anesthetics in children.

A major advantage of the LMA over the ETT in children receiving radiation therapy on a daily basis during a 4- to 6-week course of treatment is that the LMA does not invade the trachea. Therefore, the risk of tracheal ulcerations, granulation tissue, and subsequent tracheal stenosis associated with repeated intubations with an ETT is eliminated. Also, the LMA causes much less stimulation than does an ETT; thus, anesthetic requirements for the LMA are significantly lower. For example, at the University of Texas M. D. Anderson Cancer Center in Houston, all children undergoing radiation therapy receive an intravenous infusion of propofol as the sole anesthetic agent during their treatment. The LMA is frequently used for airway management, and spontaneous respiration is preserved (Fig. 21-6). This allows more rapid turnover of patients and more efficient use of the radiation therapy suite.

c. Diagnostic and Short Therapeutic Procedures in Children

The LMA can be very useful during short diagnostic, therapeutic, and minor surgical procedures performed in children either in the hospital's procedure room or

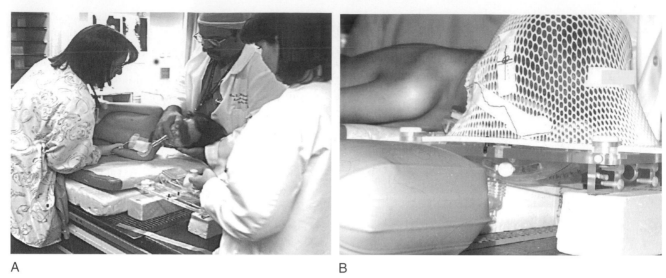

Figure 21-6 Use of the laryngeal mask airway (LMA) in a child undergoing a series of radiation treatments at the University of Texas M. D. Anderson Cancer Center in Houston. **A,** Propofol is used to induce general anesthesia, and after the LMA is inserted, the child is placed in a prone position. **B,** Continuous intravenous infusion of propofol is used as the sole anesthetic agent during radiation treatment, while the child is breathing spontaneously through the LMA. This allows more rapid turnover of patients and more efficient use of the radiation therapy suite.

in the OR. These procedures include, but are not limited to, spinal puncture with or without intrathecal therapy, bone marrow aspirations, insertion or removal of a central line or a Port-a-Cath, and minor biopsies (Fig. 21-7). Most children tolerate these procedures well under deep intravenous sedation with propofol and local anesthesia with maintenance of spontaneous respiration. However, some children develop respiratory depression or airway obstruction during deep sedation. In those children,

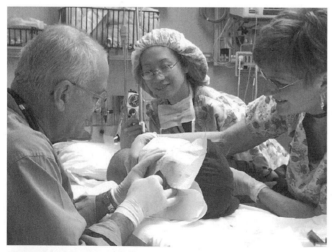

Figure 21-7 Lumbar spinal tap and intrathecal therapy performed on a small child at the University of Texas M. D. Anderson Cancer Center in Houston. Continuous infusion of propofol is used to achieve deep sedation. The laryngeal mask airway (LMA) is used to maintain the open airway and the child is allowed to breathe spontaneously. The LMA is less invasive than the tracheal tube, and less medication is required to tolerate the device.

the LMA can be an excellent and much less invasive alternative to endotracheal intubation, resulting in a clear airway without resorting to general anesthesia and muscle relaxation.

d. Cardiology

The LMA can also be useful in patients undergoing transesophageal echocardiography (TEE). TEE is an invasive procedure, and many patients experience significant discomfort or are unable to tolerate TEE under topical anesthesia. In the cardiology clinic setting, TEE is usually performed with topical anesthesia consisting of spraying the oropharynx with a local anesthetic (e.g., 4% lidocaine or 20% benzocaine), with or without sedation.[49,86] However, a significant number of patients experience discomfort during the procedure, and many patients cannot tolerate the insertion of the probe, even after sedation.[39,46] Because topical anesthesia and light sedation do not completely abolish the gag reflex, deep sedation or even general anesthesia may be necessary for patients with highly sensitive reflexes in the upper airway and pharynx. One possible solution for patients who cannot tolerate the insertion of the TEE probe with topical anesthesia and light sedation is deep sedation with propofol. The LMA can be used to maintain the airway in patients undergoing TEE examination during deep sedation with propofol.[52] The LMA can easily be inserted with the TEE probe in place, and the presence of the LMA does not interfere with the manipulation of the TEE probe (Fig. 21-8).

The LMA can also be a better alternative than endotracheal intubation in patients undergoing cardioversion in whom face mask ventilation is difficult or inadequate.

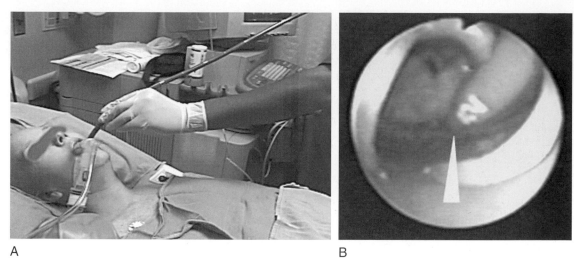

A   B

Figure 21-8 Use of the laryngeal mask airway (LMA) during transesophageal echocardiography (TEE) at the University of Texas M. D. Anderson Cancer Center in Houston. The LMA is inserted subsequent to TEE placement. **A,** The presence of the LMA does not interfere with TEE examination. **B,** Fiberoptic view through the LMA shows the TEE probe *(arrowhead)* inside the LMA bowl.

The minimal hemodynamic stimulation associated with insertion of the LMA, which contrasts with a significant hemodynamic response during endotracheal intubation, offers a great advantage in patients with cardiovascular disease.[79]

2. Head and Neck Surgery

Most of the applications of the LMA in procedures involving the head and neck are discussed in the section about the LMA-Flexible. However, one of the unique advantages of the Classic LMA in these patients is the access to the larynx that the device allows (Fig. 21-9). This is particularly useful for diagnostic evaluation of the larynx and trachea and during neodymium:yttrium-aluminum-garnet (Nd:YAG) laser surgery. It is difficult to manage the airway using an ETT in patients who require Nd:YAG laser treatment of lesions located in the vocal cords or the proximal part of the trachea because the presence of the ETT limits access to these lesions. Also, there is a high risk of a laser-induced airway fire when an ETT is used. In contrast, the LMA provides an unobstructed view of the surgical field and virtually eliminates the risk of airway fire (Fig. 21-10).

Head and neck surgery is associated with the risk of bruising or otherwise traumatizing nerves that control the motor functions of the larynx. The LMA can be very useful in evaluating the function of the vocal cords at the

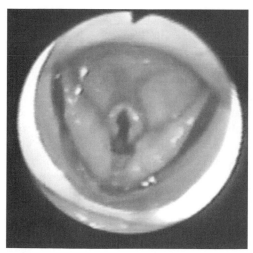

Figure 21-9 View of the larynx through a fiberscope placed coaxially through the optimally positioned laryngeal mask airway. The epiglottis is not downfolded and the tip of the mask lies behind the larynx, occluding the upper esophageal sphincter.

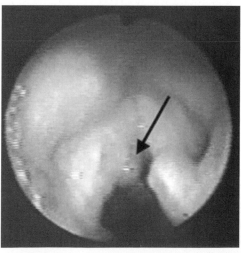

Figure 21-10 Fiberoptic view through the LMA of the left vocal cord lesion *(arrow)*. This type of lesion would be very difficult to handle with the Nd:YAG laser if an endotracheal tube were used.

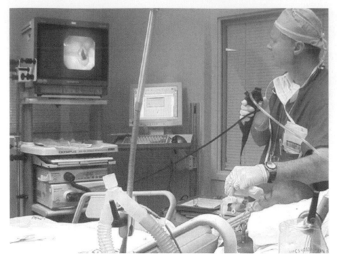

Figure 21-11 A child admitted to the intensive care unit after brain stem surgery at the University of Texas M. D. Anderson Cancer Center in Houston. Using deep sedation with propofol, the laryngeal mask airway (LMA) was inserted behind the endotracheal tube (ETT). After successful LMA insertion, the ETT is removed to allow visualization of the vocal cords and evaluation of their function in a spontaneously breathing child. This helps the intensivist and the surgeon determine whether the patient will be able to maintain her or his airway postoperatively.

conclusion of neck dissection and thyroid and parathyroid surgery.[55] While the patient is still under general anesthesia, the LMA is inserted behind the ETT and inflated. The anesthesiologist then removes the ETT, and the patient is allowed to breathe spontaneously. As the patient emerges from general anesthesia, a fiberoptic bronchoscope (FOB) is inserted through the lumen of the LMA to observe the function of the vocal cords. At M. D. Anderson Cancer Center this technique has become a very important diagnostic tool to detect the functional status of the nerves providing motor function to the larynx and has allowed the anesthesiologists and surgeons to make more informed decisions about the postoperative airway management of their patients. Similarly, patients undergoing brain stem surgery in the area that involves the lower cranial nerves, which control the pharynx and larynx, can be evaluated fiberoptically through the LMA in the intensive care unit. This helps the intensivist and the surgeon determine whether the patient will be able to maintain her or his airway postoperatively (Fig. 21-11).

3. Pulmonary Medicine and Thoracic Surgery

a. Bronchoscopy in Children and Adults

Physicians in the fields of thoracic surgery and pulmonary medicine have shown interest in the LMA because of the unique access it provides to the larynx and respiratory tree. Diagnostic fiberoptic laryngoscopy and

FOB can be performed readily through the LMA in patients under general anesthesia or under topical anesthesia with sedation.[35,51,60] Maekawa and colleagues in a 1991 letter to *Anesthesiology* describing the use of a size 1 LMA as a conduit for FOB with a 3.6-mm flexible endoscope in two children, ages 2 and 8 months, listed the following advantages: (1) The LMA tube is much larger (5 mm internal diameter) than the corresponding ETT, permitting the use of a larger bronchoscope, which gives a better view than that obtained through the 2- to 2.5-mm bronchoscope normally required to fit through the ETT in this age group; (2) use of the LMA permitted examination of the larynx, including vocal cord movement and the part of the trachea normally occupied by the ETT; (3) the larger diameter LMA airway tube permits easy ventilation, which in turn permits uninterrupted observation; and (4) not using an ETT may be valuable in cases of laryngeal or tracheal stenosis that might be made worse by the passage of the ETT.[98]

Theroux and associates, in another letter to *Anesthesiology*, described the use of the size 1 LMA as a conduit for intubation in a 2.5-kg baby with Schwarz-Jampel syndrome who could not be intubated by other means.[132] The uncuffed ETT was advanced over a 2.2-mm bronchoscope, which was easily passed into the trachea through the LMA. In 1997, Mizikov and coauthors reported their experience of using FOB through the LMA in 45 children: 15 diagnostic cases, 22 cases of lavage, 7 cases of foreign body removal, and 1 case of electrocoagulation of an adenoma.[108] Total intravenous anesthesia and positive-pressure ventilation were used in all cases. Patients' ages ranged from neonatal to 15 years. With the size 1 LMA, they used the Olympus BF3C20 bronchoscope (diameter, 3.6 mm), and with the size 2 LMA, the Olympus BFP30 (diameter, 5 mm) was used. The epiglottis was within the mask in 96.5% of cases but was not associated with significant airway obstruction in any case.

b. Laser Surgery of the Trachea

In 1992, Slinger and colleagues provided a detailed account of a difficult case of palliative laser resection of a severely obstructing distal tracheal mass.[128] The airway was initially managed using a size 4 LMA, through which a 6-mm Olympus FOB was passed by a swivel connector to apply the laser. Spontaneous ventilation with propofol-isoflurane anesthesia was used. After 120 minutes, 50% of the tracheal lumen had been restored, at which point it was decided to convert to rigid bronchoscopy so that the surgeon could remove larger pieces of tissue by forceps, thereby speeding the procedure. The authors repeated this approach in two other, less severe, cases without complications. They pointed out that the laser is not likely to burn the silicone LMA tube if it is switched on only when in the trachea. However, the authors stressed that use of the rigid bronchoscope remained the "gold standard" for such cases.

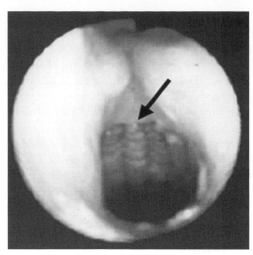

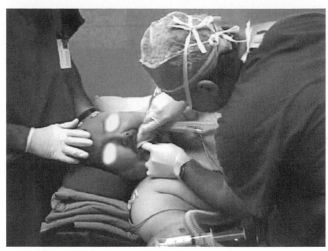

Figure 21-12 Fiberoptic view of the tracheal stent *(arrow)* placed high in the trachea (1.5 cm below the vocal cords) through the laryngeal mask airway (LMA). The LMA's shaft permits use of a 6-mm fiberoptic bronchoscope and provides a bigger cross-sectional area than a 9-mm endotracheal tube (ETT), thus allowing better ventilation during stent placement than the ETT in patients who already have compromised respiratory functions.

Figure 21-13 Insertion of the laryngeal mask airway (LMA-ProSeal) into a patient undergoing craniotomy with awake intraoperative speech mapping. The anesthesiologist is facing the patient and uses his thumb to insert the LMA-ProSeal into the patient.

c. Tracheobronchial Stent Placement

Another advantage of using the LMA in patients with pathology involving the tracheobronchial tree is evident during stent placement using fiberoptic guidance.[43] The LMA's shaft permits use of a 6-mm FOB and provides a larger cross-sectional area than does a 9-mm ETT, which is usually employed during stent placement. Thus, the LMA allows better ventilation during stent placement than does an ETT in patients who already have compromised respiratory function. Also, in patients who have an obstruction high in the trachea, the LMA is much better than an ETT because it allows placement of the stent without the risk of extubating the patient (Fig. 21-12).

4. Neurosurgery

The hemodynamic stability associated with LMA use may be beneficial during induction in patients undergoing neurosurgical repair of an intracranial aneurysm and in patients with increased intracranial pressure. Also, Silva and Brimacombe reported that hypertension, coughing, and bucking, all of which are common during emergence from general anesthesia with an ETT, were prevented in neurosurgical patients by simply replacing the ETT with the LMA at the end of the procedure.[127] The insertion and use of the LMA in patients under general anesthesia have been associated with minimal changes in intracranial pressure.[58] This characteristic might be particularly useful during ventriculoperitoneal shunt placement in children, adults, and patients who have suffered a traumatic brain injury.

Other uses for the LMA in neurosurgical patients include awake craniotomy and stereotactic procedures in children and adults. In an awake craniotomy, eloquent areas of the brain are mapped and monitored intraoperatively by stimulating the cerebral cortex with an electrical current. This direct electrical stimulation of the cerebral cortex greatly increases the risk of focal or generalized seizures. Airway management using a face mask and endotracheal intubation during generalized seizures can be very difficult for two reasons: (1) the patient is usually lying on her or his side, giving the anesthesiologist limited access to the airway; and (2) the patient's head is fixed by metal pins and a frame to provide a stable surgical field and allow the use of modern intraoperative image guidance. However, an experienced and skilled anesthesiologist can easily insert the LMA into such patients, thus allowing ventilation and oxygenation in this potentially difficult clinical situation (Fig. 21-13).[122]

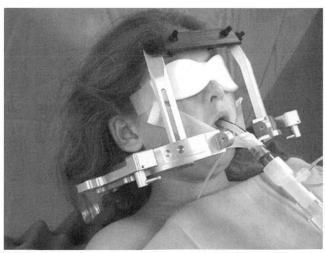

Figure 21-14 A young child undergoing stereotactic biopsy at the University of Texas M. D. Anderson Cancer Center in Houston. Anesthesia is induced with propofol in the radiology suite, and the laryngeal mask is inserted.

Stereotactic biopsies can also be performed in children using the LMA. Anesthesia is induced with propofol in the radiology suite, and the LMA is inserted (Fig. 21-14). Local anesthetic is then injected to anesthetize the skin before pins for the stereotactic frame are applied. During continuous infusion of propofol, an MRI is obtained while the child breathes spontaneously through the LMA. While asleep, the child is transported to the OR for the stereotactic biopsy. This technique provides optimal comfort for the children and excellent operating conditions for the radiologists and surgeons.

V. LMA-FLEXIBLE

Many surgeries, particularly procedures performed on the head and neck, require the anesthesiologist and surgeon to share access to the airway. Traditionally, special ETTs that have a spiral coil built into them to increase the flexibility of the tube and to prevent kinking have been used to allow the surgeon to manipulate the ETT during surgery to gain access to the operating field. To make an LMA specifically for head and neck procedures, a similar spiral coil was incorporated into the LMA's shaft, creating the LMA-Flexible (FLMA) (Fig. 21-15), which was introduced into clinical practice in 1994. The FLMA has since been used successfully in patients undergoing a variety of head and neck surgeries.

A. TONSILLECTOMY AND ADENOIDECTOMY

Several authors have reported the successful use of the FLMA during tonsillectomies and adenoidectomies. The main advantages of using the FLMA for these procedures are better tolerance of the FLMA by the patients,

fewer adverse airway events during emergence and upon extubation, and less blood soiling of the airway owing to the shielding of the larynx by the LMA's cuff. Williams and Bailey[147,148] reported that when the FLMA was used in children during adenotonsillectomies, there was little soiling of the trachea with blood. In contrast, when an uncuffed ETT was used, blood was almost always present in the trachea, causing coughing on emergence. At the end of surgery, there were also fewer episodes of airway obstruction in the FLMA group than in the ETT patients. This is probably because the FLMA was better tolerated by the patients, allowing extubation when the airway reflexes were less obtunded and the patients were able to maintain an open airway. Also, Fiani and coworkers demonstrated in a randomized study of patients undergoing elective tonsillectomies that fewer complications such as laryngospasm, bleeding, bronchospasm, and desaturation occurred in the FLMA group than in the ETT group.[62]

The FLMA is also useful during ear and nose surgery, such as tympanoplasty, myringoplasty, rhinoplasty, septoplasty, and nasal polypectomy.[16,45,47,53,119,147,149] As reported by Watcha and coauthors, the LMA provided better oxygen saturation and better surgical conditions in pediatric patients undergoing myringoplasties than did the face mask.[144] Although in other studies the FLMA and the ETT were equally effective in adult patients undergoing nasal surgery, there was less blood in the trachea and fewer airway events during emergence in the FLMA group.[45,144]

B. DENTAL AND ORAL SURGERY

The FLMA has also been found to be useful during dental procedures and oral surgery in children and adults (Fig. 21-16).[70,117] For example, George and Sanders,[67] in a comparison of the FLMA with the nasal mask during

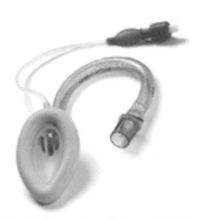

Figure 21-15 Flexible laryngeal mask airway (FLMA), which was introduced into clinical practice in 1994, has a spiral coil built into the shaft to increase the flexibility of the tube and to prevent kinking. This allows the surgeon to manipulate the FLMA's shaft during the surgery and to have good access to the operating field. The FLMA has been used successfully in patients undergoing a variety of head and neck, eye, and oral surgeries.

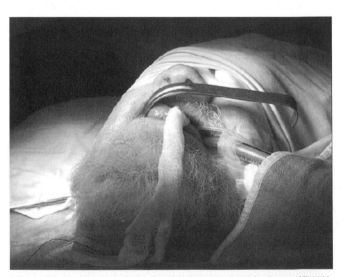

Figure 21-16 The use of the flexible laryngeal mask airway (FLMA) in a patient undergoing oral surgery. The FLMA causes less hemodynamic stimulation than the endotracheal tube and thus is safer to use in patients with severe atherosclerotic heart disease.

dental procedures in children, reported significantly fewer instances of airway obstruction, oxygen desaturation, and cardiac dysrhythmias in children in the FLMA group. Other oral surgeries in which the FLMA has been used successfully include repair of a cleft palate,[15,101,151] glossopexy,[106] removal of a tongue tumor,[82] and fixation of mandibular fractures after failed endotracheal intubation.[3]

C. OPHTHALMOLOGIC PROCEDURES

Patients with increased intraocular pressure who are undergoing intraocular procedures are frequently at higher risk for injury from sudden changes in intraocular pressure during laryngoscopy and endotracheal intubation.[12] Also, coughing and bucking on the ETT during emergence from general anesthesia can be detrimental and may even lead to suture rupture.[134] The benefits of using the FLMA for eye surgery include less change in the intraocular pressure during induction and emergence from general anesthesia and less hemodynamic stimulation.[88,110] The FLMA has been shown to be particularly useful during cataract surgery, trabeculectomy, and vitroretinal surgery.[142] The use of the device has also benefited children undergoing strabismus repair, gonioscopy, nasolacrimal duct probing, eyelid repair, scleral and conjunctival procedures, and foreign body removal.[10]

IV. LARYNGEAL MASK AIRWAY USE IN PATIENTS WITH DIFFICULT-TO-MANAGE AIRWAYS

One of the most important tasks of an anesthesiologist is to provide ventilation and oxygenation for the patient during surgery. This requires establishing and maintaining a patent airway during the course of anesthesia. As reported in 1990 in a closed claims study published by the ASA, airway-related problems were among the leading causes of major morbidity and mortality directly related to anesthesia.[38] This study laid the groundwork for the development of the ASA difficult airway algorithm, which established pathways for the care of patients with difficult-to-manage airways.[37] Although the algorithm provides an organized approach to airway management based on preoperative findings, it does not constitute a foolproof system. Many patients still prove difficult to intubate by means of conventional laryngoscopy, even when the preoperative interview and physical examination do not yield any signs of potential difficulty. Also, it is well known that airway swelling may ensue quickly after multiple intubation attempts. Although face mask ventilation in these patients might have been adequate initially, it may soon become difficult, thus creating the very dangerous and potentially life-threatening situation of inadequate oxygenation.

During the past 10 years, the LMA has received a great deal of attention because it can be effective in patients who are difficult to intubate by conventional laryngoscopy and difficult to ventilate with a face mask. The success of the LMA in these patients is due to its design. The LMA fits into the potential space of the pharynx much like a hand fits into a glove. Also, in contrast to rigid laryngoscopy, insertion of the LMA does not rely upon direct visualization of the larynx. Therefore, many factors that are associated with difficult rigid laryngoscopy (e.g., Mallampati class III and IV and Cormack-Lehane grade 3 and 4 views) do not affect the insertion of and ventilation through the LMA.[44,99]

A. LMA CLASSIC

The potential of the LMA for the emergency and nonemergency management of patients with difficult airways was appreciated shortly after its invention. In February 1983, an early prototype was used successfully by Dr. Brain in a 114-kg male undergoing laparotomy who could not be intubated. However, the first publication describing the LMA as a possible solution to airway management problems in emergency situations did not appear in the scientific literature until 1984.[22] By 1985, the LMA had been used successfully in five adults in whom difficult intubation was anticipated, and in October 1987 it was used, for the first time, in cases of failed pediatric intubation.[20] In 1989, Allison and McCrory[4] used fiberoptic guidance for endotracheal intubations, and in 1991, McCrirrick and Pracilio first reported an awake intubation through the LMA.[104] Numerous case reports appeared describing airway management with the LMA in several clinical situations including, but not limited to, adult and pediatric patients with (1) cervical spine pathology, including cervical spine instability[6,96,104,123,129]; (2) morbid obesity[68]; (3) micrognathia and macrognathia[9,133]; (4) Klippel-Feil syndrome[1]; (5) Treacher Collins syndrome[65]; (6) Pierre Robin syndrome[11]; (7) Goldenhar's syndrome[81]; (8) Hurler's syndrome[69]; (9) Down syndrome[74]; and (10) unexpected failed intubation associated with difficult face mask ventilation.[103,126]

A major step in recognizing the LMA's potential in the management of airway emergencies took place in 1993, when the LMA was incorporated into the "Practice guidelines for management of the difficult airway" by the ASA Task Force on Management of the Difficult Airway.[37] Not enough data were available then to appreciate fully the LMA's role in difficult airway situations. By 1996, the reported experience with the LMA had substantially increased, and Jonathan Benumof, M.D. (who participated in the development of the ASA algorithm), assessed the LMA's potential in a difficult airway scenario.[14] His recommendations were that the LMA should be considered not only as originally recommended in the emergency pathway of the algorithm but also in four additional situations: (1) during awake intubation as an aid to endotracheal intubation, (2) as a definite airway in nonemergency situations, (3) as an aid to tracheal intubation in anesthetized patients, and (4) as an aid to tracheal intubation after the airway is established in emergency situations. In his review, Benumof concluded, "With multiple uses and multiple places of use, the LMA is an important option within the ASA difficult airway algorithm. More importantly, the clinical record of LMA use in 'cannot intubate, cannot ventilate' situations has been excellent, and in patients whose lungs cannot be ventilated because of the supraglottic obstruction and whose trachea cannot be intubated due to unfavorable anatomy (but not periglottic pathology), the LMA should be immediately available and considered as the first treatment of choice." In 2003, Benumof's recommendations fully materialized in the new "Practice guidelines for management of the difficult airway," updated by the ASA Task Force on Management of the Difficult Airway.[116] Essentially, depending on the user's level of expertise, the LMA can now be used in any place in the algorithm.

B. LMA-FASTRACH

In 1983, while developing the LMA, Dr. Brain conducted a fiberoptic investigation that revealed the LMA's potential as a guide for endotracheal intubation. The same year, he developed a prototype LMA and used it to intubate blindly three patients using a 9-mm ETT (Fig. 21-17). However, the development of an intubating LMA was not revisited by Dr. Brain until 1994. In response to clinicians' growing demands for a device that had the same ventilatory properties as the LMA Classic but would serve as a better conduit for intubation, he designed the intubating LMA-Fastrach (ILMA; LMA North America, San Diego, CA), which was introduced in 1997 (Fig. 21-18).

The ILMA is designed to facilitate blind or fiberoptically guided endotracheal intubations without the need to move the cervical spine during intubation. Available only in adult sizes, the ILMA consists of an anatomically

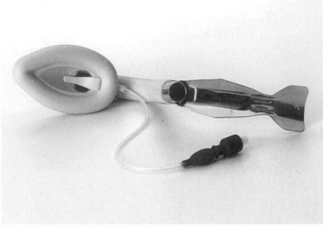

Figure 21-18 The intubating laryngeal mask (LMA-Fastrach), which was introduced in 1997, consists of the mask, which has the same shape as the LMA Classic, and the 13-mm internal diameter stainless steel shaft, which can accommodate an endotracheal tube up to 8.5 mm in internal diameter.

curved stainless steel tube 13 mm in internal diameter that is connected firmly at its distal end to the laryngeal mask. The angle of the metal shaft was carefully designed, using measurements from sagittal MRI images, to fit well into the oral and pharyngeal space while keeping the head and neck in a neutral position. Proximally, the metal shaft forms a standard 15-mm connector for the anesthesia circuit, and a rigid guiding handle serves both to insert the device, eliminating the need to insert fingers into the mouth, and to stabilize and direct the device during intubation attempts. In addition, the two bars at the aperture of the LMA Classic have been replaced in the ILMA by a single, movable epiglottic elevating bar that pushes the epiglottis out of the way and allows smooth and unobstructed passage of the ETT as it emerges from the distal end of the ILMA's metal shaft (Fig. 21-19). This shaft can accommodate an ETT up to 8.5 mm in diameter. In addition, the shaft of the ILMA is shorter than that of the LMA Classic, eliminating the need for longer ETTs in patients with long necks.

The ILMA was first described by Brain and coworkers[27] in 1997 in the *British Journal of Anaesthesia*. In the same issue, there were also two separate reports, by Brain[26] and Kapila[84] and their colleagues, of early clinical experience with the ILMA. Unfortunately, Kapila's report described results obtained 3 years earlier using a more primitive prototype of the ILMA and thus created some confusion regarding the technique of intubation through the device. At the same time, early versions of the ILMA instruction manual included recommendations for use based on these early prototypes. Subsequently, however, the results from a large study[61] that evaluated the effectiveness of the ILMA in patients with different types of difficult-to-manage airways rendered most of these earlier recommendations irrelevant by showing that the only technique that

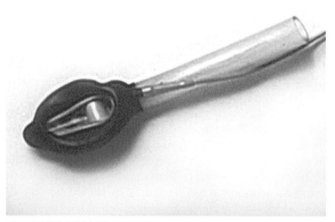

Figure 21-17 A prototype of the intubating laryngeal mask built and used by Dr. Archie Brain in 1983, which was used to intubate blindly three patients who had a history of difficult intubation with a 9-mm internal diameter tracheal tube.

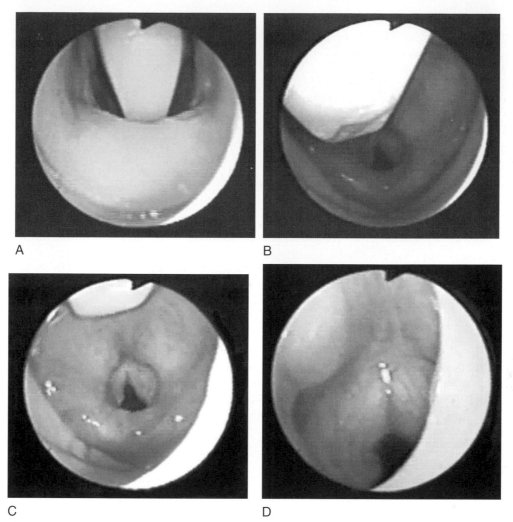

Figure 21-19 Fiberoptic view of intubation through the LMA-Fastrach. **A,** Epiglottic elevating bar (EEB), as seen from inside the shaft. **B,** The tip of the endotracheal tube, as it advances through the LMA-Fastrach, pushes the EEB upward. **C,** This movement of the EEB lifts the epiglottis out of the way and **(D)** provides a clear passage for the ETT through the vocal cords.

improved the rate of blind intubation through the ILMA was Chandy's maneuver (Chandy Verghese, M.D., consultant in anaesthesia and intensive care, Royal Berkshire Hospital, Reading, England, verbal communication, January 1998).

Chandy's maneuver consists of two steps, which are performed sequentially. The first step, which is important for establishing optimal ventilation, is to rotate the ILMA slightly in the sagittal plane using the metal handle until the least resistance to bag ventilation is achieved. The second step of Chandy's maneuver is performed just before blind intubation and consists of using the metal handle to lift slightly (but not tilt) the ILMA away from the posterior pharyngeal wall. This facilitates the smooth passage of the ETT into the trachea (Fig. 21-20). The same study assessed the effectiveness of the ILMA in 254 patients, including patients with Cormack-Lehane grade 4 views, immobilized cervical spines, and airways distorted by tumors, surgery, or radiation therapy and patients wearing stereotactic frames.[61] Insertion of the ILMA was accomplished in three attempts or fewer in all patients. The overall success rates for blind and fiberoptically guided intubations were 97% and 100%, respectively. This represents the largest analysis to date examining the use of the ILMA in patients with difficult-to-manage airways and demonstrates that the ILMA may be a particularly valuable tool in the emergency or elective airway management of patients in whom other techniques have failed and in the treatment of patients with immobilized cervical spines.

The ILMA can also be used as an intubating tool in patients with normal airways. In fact, in a study conducted by Brain and colleagues, the hemodynamic response to the ILMA was similar to the response to the LMA Classic; thus, in patients with compromised cardiovascular systems the ILMA could be a less stimulating alternative to rigid

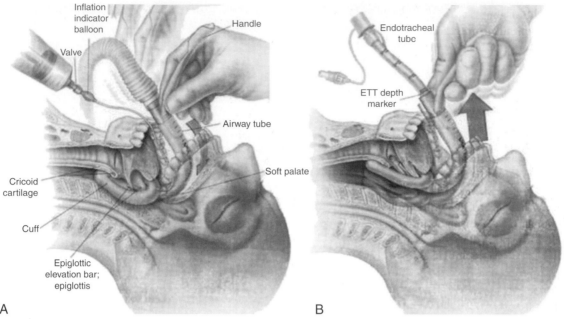

A   **B**

Figure 21-20 Chandy's maneuver consists of two steps, which are performed sequentially. **A**, The first step, which is important for establishing optimal ventilation, is to rotate the ILMA slightly in the sagittal plane using the metal handle until the least resistance to bag ventilation is achieved. **B**, The second step of Chandy's maneuver is performed just before blind intubation and consists of using the metal handle to lift slightly (but not tilt) the ILMA away from the posterior pharyngeal wall. This facilitates the smooth passage of the ETT into the trachea.

laryngoscopy for intubation of the trachea.[26,83] Also, using the ILMA in patients with normal airways allows clinicians to develop good skills and familiarity with the device before using it in emergency situations.

VII. LMA-PROSEAL

The LMA-ProSeal (LMA North America) (Fig. 21-21) was designed by the author (AB) with the principal objective of providing a separate conduit to permit gastric fluids to bypass the glottis. The inventor believed such a device was needed because even in fasted patients one can never be completely certain that the stomach is empty. The LMA-ProSeal also permits access to the stomach using standard gastric tubes, provides a more reliable seal around the glottis, reduces the leakage of inspired gases into the stomach, provides a more comfortable fit within the pharynx, facilitates the use of mechanical ventilation, and permits the diagnosis of incorrect LMA placement.

The LMA Classic may or may not block the esophagus, depending on how precisely it is positioned in the hypopharynx. The inventor, realizing this, developed an insertion and fixation technique that would ensure correct positioning, but these recommendations are widely ignored or unknown to the majority of users, who continue to choose their own favored insertion techniques and methods of fixation. It comes as no surprise, therefore, that there are cases of aspiration in the LMA literature, although they are

rare.[111] In the LMA-ProSeal, the drain tube opening at the distal tip of the mask ensures that if the tip is not correctly placed against the UES, inflation of the reservoir bag causes some of the gas to be diverted back up the drain tube, providing measurable evidence of inadequate device placement. The reader is referred to the LMA-ProSeal instruction manual for further details of the diagnostic functions made possible by the drain tube.[95]

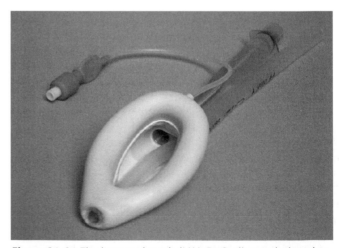

Figure 21-21 The laryngeal mask (LMA-ProSeal) was designed to achieve two objectives: (1) to separate the respiratory and gastrointestinal tracts and (2) to provide a better seal around the glottis and allow positive-pressure ventilation in a more reliable manner than the LMA Classic.

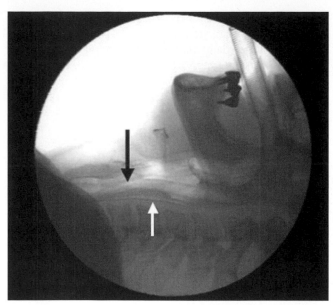

Figure 21-22 Lateral neck radiograph with the LMA-ProSeal in place. When inflated correctly with up to 60 cm of water pressure, the posterior cuff of the mask expands only slightly *(white arrow)*. This ensures the patency of the gastric drain tube *(black arrow)*.

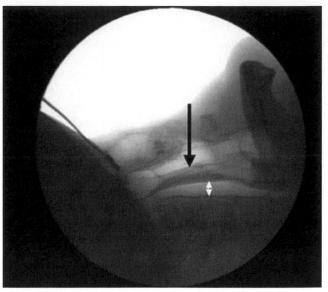

Figure 21-23 Lateral neck radiograph with the LMA-ProSeal in place. If the cuff is inflated with excessive volume, exceeding 60 cm of water pressure, the gastric drain tube can be partially or completely occluded *(black arrow)* by the bowl of the mask pushed toward the glottis by the overinflated cuff *(white double arrow)*.

LMA-ProSeal, which will soon be available in the same range of sizes as the LMA Classic (excluding size 6), has a number of important differences. The adult sizes are fitted with a posterior extension to the cuff that expands to a relatively small degree when inflated within the confined space of the pharynx, as demonstrated radiologically (Fig. 21-22). Similar images in which the cuff is inflated excessively demonstrate that the presence of the posterior cuff, while probably increasing the seal pressure by about 10%, introduces two dangers that must be guarded against. One danger is the possibility of herniating the cuff bowl forward toward the glottis, thereby causing partial or complete blockage of the delicate drain tube and compromising the airway (Fig. 21-23). Second, overinflation may cause the mask to slide proximally, thus reducing the efficacy of its seal against the UES. It is important to understand the consequences of these two effects: if the drain tube is blocked and its opening is simultaneously moved away from contact with the UES, the major advantages of the device are lost because, although the seal may appear to be excellent, there is no longer any guarantee that a seal even exists against the UES. The LMA-ProSeal is therefore a more sophisticated device than the LMA Classic, and instructions for its use must be followed carefully.

Pediatric sizes of the LMA-ProSeal feature the drain tube but no posterior cuff. The relatively larger airway and drain tube configuration required for optimal functioning in the pediatric anatomy result in a wider device angle when viewed laterally. If a posterior cuff were added, this angle would become critically large, causing the device to slide proximally out of the pharynx as it is inflated.

VIII. DISPOSABLE LARYNGEAL MASK AIRWAYS

A. RATIONALE

Recent events have served to remind us that infection is a perennial risk to health care workers and patients. The risk of infection in hospitals seems to be about as intractable a problem as iatrogenic disease. New antimicrobial agents encourage the emergence of resistant organisms just as more powerful therapeutic tools offer new opportunities for human error in their application. Although laryngeal masks have never been proved to be a source of infection transmission, the continuing uncertainty surrounding the size of the population of Creutzfeldt-Jakob disease carriers and the risk of transmission of the infectious agent through the tonsillar bed, together with the difficulties in ensuring effective device sterilization against small virus-like particles, have led to increased interest in disposable airway equipment, particularly in some European countries. In the UK, the Department of Health (DOH) required surgeons and anesthetists to use disposable equipment for tonsillectomies but reversed this decision when the use of poorly designed disposable surgical instruments was implicated in the death of a patient. In London's main otolaryngologic hospital, the Royal Throat, Nose, and Ear Hospital, the reusable flexible LMA had for some years been used in approximately 90% of tonsillectomies (Paul Bailey, M.D., personal communication, March 2004), and substitution with the disposable ETT was believed to be a retrospective step. Accordingly, the DOH agreed to fund the cost of treating the reusable flexible LMA as a single-use item, pending the availability of a disposable version of the device.

The lessons learned from this experience were that we should be wary of rushing to embrace disposable forms of an established device until we are sure that their function is equivalent and that the avoidance of a theoretical risk of low probability (transmission of prion infection associated with tonsillectomy) should not take precedence over the avoidance of known risks (the imposition of untried and unfamiliar equipment for an operation, the safety of which is highly dependent on skill and training using well-established techniques).

Accordingly, all pediatric and adult sizes of the disposable LMA (LMA Unique; LMA North America) have been subjected to a rigorous series of tests to ensure that, as much as possible, their function is equivalent to that of the reusable silicone device.[138,140] This has not been easy to accomplish because vinyl plastic materials lack the elasticity of silicone, and this tends to affect the insertion and seal characteristics of the LMA. It is likely that the plastic disposable LMAs will be found to be less appropriate for positive-pressure ventilation than the Classic LMA. However, this limitation may be regarded as academic because the LMA ProSeal is specifically designed for use with positive pressure.

IX. PROBLEMS AND CONTROVERSIES

Several reports have addressed problems and complications associated with the use of the LMA. The occurrence of such problems and complications, however, appears to be inversely proportional to the experience and skill level of the operator. Most adverse events associated with LMA are probably the result of incorrect use of the device or inappropriate selection of patients. Also, some of the advanced clinical applications of the device (e.g., use of positive-pressure ventilation with the LMA) have been considered controversial. However, as their experience and skill with the LMA advance, many clinicians find it to be a very useful airway tool in situations that they had previously considered to be controversial. Thus, it is the skill level and experience of the clinician and not the type of clinical application that should guide the use of the LMA. In this section, we discuss some of the reported problems and complications and ways to manage them when they occur. We also address controversies regarding the LMA's use.

A. ORO-PHARYNGO-LARYNGEAL MORBIDITY

Any foreign body that comes into contact with airway structures can potentially cause complications. The LMA passes through and occupies anatomic areas from the oral cavity to the hypopharynx. Structures that are at high risk for injury from supraglottic airways, including the LMA, are mucous membranes, soft tissues of the pharynx and larynx, salivary glands, nerves and blood vessels of the neck, laryngeal cartilages, and bones of the neck. When injury occurs, it usually manifests itself in minor complaints such as a dry mouth or sore throat.[105] These usually resolve quickly and have no long-term sequelae. However, more serious complications, such as hypoglossal and lingual nerve palsy, trauma to the epiglottis and larynx, dysarthria, dysphonia, and tongue cyanosis related to vascular compression, have been reported.[8,63,80,93,109,121,150]

1. Sore Throat

Sore throat, dry throat, pharyngeal erythema, and minor pharyngeal abrasions have been reported with the LMA, and the published incidence of sore throat varies between 0% and 70%.[105,121] Initially, it was not clear why the incidence of sore throat varied so much. Factors that may affect the incidence of sore throat include the insertion technique, duration of the procedure, type of lubricant, type of ventilation (spontaneous or controlled), and intracuff pressure.[30,33,72,85] Of these, the only variable that has been shown to reduce the incidence of sore throat reliably is lowering the intracuff pressure.[32] Overinflation of the LMA's cuff is a common practice when the size of the device is too small for a given patient and the practitioner encounters a significant leak while attempting assisted or positive-pressure ventilation. The overinflated cuff becomes stiff and exerts high local pressure on tissues, especially those surrounding bony structures such as the hyoid bone and cervical spine. Also, nitrous oxide diffuses through the silicone walls of the LMA, increasing the pressure inside the cuff.[115] This can be remedied by monitoring the intracuff pressure and periodically withdrawing the gas from the LMA's cuff. Based on unpublished research by the inventor in awake volunteers, the maximum pressure inside the LMA's cuff should not exceed 60 cm H_2O because higher pressure causes discomfort, presumably owing to stretching of the constrictor muscles. Appropriate LMA size selection combined with a good insertion technique and low intracuff pressure reduces significantly the incidence of postoperative sore throat.

2. Vascular Compression and Nerve Damage

Although rare, compression of the blood vessels of the tongue, leading to tongue cyanosis, has been observed after LMA insertion.[93] This complication is likely to occur when the LMA is not inserted deeply enough or when the LMA's cuff is overinflated. Also, the blood vessels of the tongue or the lingual nerve can be compressed by malpositioning of the LMA's shaft on the lateral side of the tongue (based on cadaveric research by the authors). Similarly, if during LMA insertion the cuff is partially or fully inflated, the device frequently lies higher than when the correct insertion technique is used. This malpositioning of the LMA can lead to the compression of the lingual or hypoglossal nerve, resulting in transient or prolonged nerve palsy. The hypoglossal nerve, which supplies all of the intrinsic and all but one of the extrinsic muscles of the tongue, is particularly vulnerable to injury at the point where the nerve loops anteriorly, close to the greater cornu of hyoid bone, and then runs along the lateral surface of the hyoglossal muscle and above the posterior border of the mylohyoid muscle before dividing into several branches that supply tongue muscles. To best avoid these complications, one should select the appropriate LMA size, use the standard insertion technique, and ensure that the intracuff pressure is no higher than 60 cm H_2O.

B. RISK OF ASPIRATION

Aspiration during general anesthesia has an overall incidence that ranges between 1.4 and 6.5 per 10,000 cases and a mortality rate of 5%.[41,91,114,135] In a study of 215,488 anesthetic cases, Warner and coauthors[143] reported that the incidence of aspiration was 2.6 per 10,000 in patients undergoing elective surgery and 11 per 10,000 in patients undergoing emergency procedures. A mortality rate of 0.14 per 10,000 in ASA III-V patients was also reported. Warner's study did not include patients whose airways were managed using the LMA.

The LMA does not protect reliably against aspiration and therefore should not be used electively in patients who are at high risk for this complication. However, as stated earlier, the majority of users do not adhere to the recommended insertion or fixation techniques when using the LMA, which, as explained earlier, is designed to optimize the seal of the distal end of the device against the UES. Even so, a meta-analysis of published literature on the LMA by Brimacombe and Berry[31] revealed that the overall incidence of pulmonary aspiration with the LMA is around 2 per 10,000. In fact, 18 cases of suspected pulmonary aspiration during LMA use have been found by meta-analysis, and only 10 of these were confirmed radiographically. In only three patients did the aspiration warrant ventilatory support, which lasted from 1 to 7 days. None of the patients who aspirated through the LMA suffered any long-term effects. Of particular interest is that most of these patients had one or more factors predisposing them to aspiration. These included emergency surgery in a patient who had not fasted, a difficult airway, obesity, steep Trendelenburg's position with intra-abdominal insufflation, and previous gastric surgery. Although the meta-analysis study contained only reports published through September 1993, a subsequent analysis of 11,910 LMA anesthetic cases by Verghese and Brimacombe[139] yielded an even smaller incidence of aspiration (0.84 per 10,000). Even allowing for the fact that critical events in anesthesia are frequently underreported, the absence of admissions to intensive care units for ventilatory support indicates that aspiration with the LMA is rare. Nevertheless, one must

always be meticulous about selecting patients appropriately, using the correct insertion technique to obtain the optimal LMA position, paying attention to the appropriate depth of anesthesia, and maintaining constant vigilance during surgery. If, despite all of these measures, regurgitation or aspiration occurs, the following plan of action should be implemented:

1. Do not attempt to remove the LMA because a significant amount of regurgitant fluid may be trapped behind the LMA's cuff. One should consider that the cuff shields and protects the larynx from the trapped fluid, and removing the LMA may worsen the situation.
2. Temporarily disconnect the circuit to allow drainage of the fluid while tilting the patient's head down and to the side.
3. Suction the LMA and administer 100% oxygen to the patient.
4. Ventilate the patient manually using low gas flows and small tidal volumes to minimize the risk of forcing any fluid from the trachea into the small bronchi.
5. Use a large FOB to evaluate the tracheobronchial tree, and suction any remaining fluid.
6. If aspiration below the vocal cords is confirmed, consider intubating the patient with an ETT and institute appropriate treatment protocols.

The risk of aspiration with the LMA is likely to be significantly reduced in the new LMA-ProSeal, which incorporates a drainage tube into the LMA design, warns of an inadequate UES seal, and permits more reliable positive-pressure ventilation than does the LMA Classic.

C. POSITIVE-PRESSURE VENTILATION

When the first independent trial of the LMA was carried out, only a size 3 was available, and the correct fixation technique ensuring an adequate seal against the UES had not been developed.[24] Thus, when used in large patients, the device was not very reliable when applying positive-pressure ventilation. Also, because the LMA concept was very new, it was prudent for clinicians initially to limit the use of the LMA to patients who were breathing spontaneously. Even now, positive-pressure ventilation should be considered an advanced use of the LMA, and clinicians should practice and gain experience using the LMA in patients who are breathing spontaneously before attempting controlled ventilation. However, after the LMA was introduced commercially in a range of sizes, first for adults and then for children, many LMA users found that when they became experienced, the LMA could be very effective during positive-pressure ventilation.[142] Devitt and colleagues[50] compared the effectiveness of the LMA with that of the ETT in 48 patients and showed that positive-pressure ventilation (range, 15 to 30 cm H_2O) through the LMA was adequate and comparable to that achieved through the ETT. Epstein and associates[56] studied the effectiveness of the LMA with controlled ventilation in children 3 months to 17 years old and concluded that the device performed effectively and reliably. In another study, Epstein and coauthors established that the airway seal pressures (25.9 to 31.2 cm H_2O) were well maintained with the LMA in children.[57]

Two separate large clinical studies of more than 7000 patients led by Verghese and Van Damme established that the LMA is as effective as the ETT for controlled ventilation.[136,140] Van Damme's study also assessed the airway seal pressures and demonstrated that at 15 cm H_2O or less, leaks occurred with the LMA in only 2.7% of patients. Subsequently, Verghese reported his experience of using the LMA successfully in 5236 patients undergoing a variety of surgical procedures under general anesthesia and positive-pressure ventilation.[139]

The following basic principles should be considered when using the LMA with positive-pressure ventilation:

1. *Selection of patients*: Most patients with normal lung compliance who have fasted can be mechanically ventilated effectively with the LMA.
2. *Size selection*: Select the largest LMA size appropriate for the patient. This prevents a tendency to compensate for inadequate seal pressure by overinflating the cuff.
3. *Insertion technique*: Carefully follow the correct insertion technique to ensure the optimal positioning of the LMA in the airway.
4. *Fixation technique*: Use the correct method of taping the LMA. This ensures proper contact between the LMA's tip and the esophagus and prevents gastric insufflation.
5. *Auscultation*: Always auscultate over the stomach to ensure that gastric insufflation is not taking place.
6. *Ventilatory parameters*: Limit tidal volumes to 8 mL/kg and control the end-tidal CO_2 by adjusting the respiratory rate.
7. *Treatment of inadequate tidal volume*: Maintain an adequate level of anesthesia for the particular surgical procedure.

If leaking does occur when using the LMA for positive-pressure ventilation, one should investigate the cause and try to correct the situation. If the device has been correctly fixed in place and remains correctly inflated, the problem is usually due to the need for more relaxant or deeper anesthesia.

D. USE FOR PROLONGED PROCEDURES

The maximum duration for which the LMA can be safely used is not well established. However, a limit of 2 hours was suggested soon after the LMA became available for wide clinical use.[6] This recommendation was based on the possible increased risk of aspiration or pharyngeal morbidity. Subsequent reports, however, demonstrated

that in the hands of experienced users the LMA can be safely used during procedures lasting up to 8 hours.[29,34] In fact, in rare circumstances the LMA has been used in the intensive care arena to provide effective respiratory support for 10 to 24 hours with no evidence of any adverse effects to the patients.[5] The LMA-ProSeal, which is designed for positive-pressure ventilation and has a gastric drainage tube to minimize the risk of aspiration, may be best suited for prolonged procedures.[28] However, regardless of the model used, clinicians must always remain vigilant and provide adequate anesthesia to their patients, thus minimizing the risks of any complications. Also, if nitrous oxide is administered to the patient, one needs to remember that this gas diffuses into the LMA's cuff, increasing intracuff pressure. Thus, during prolonged LMA use, close monitoring of the intracuff pressure is recommended. Also, in order to minimize the risk of mucosal ischemia associated with high intracuff pressures, hourly removal of a few milliliters of air from the cuff is considered a prudent practice.[77]

E. USE IN NONSUPINE POSITIONS

Use of the LMA in patients in other than the supine position should be considered an advanced use.[40,54,92,107,112,125] Also, one needs to have an alternative plan in case the device dislodges from its original position during the procedure. Because of the risk of LMA dislodgment in patients in nonsupine positions, one should consider inducing general anesthesia and inserting the LMA into the patient after the patient has been positioned for the procedure. This would allow the clinician to ensure the feasibility of inserting the LMA into the patient at any time during procedure. Also, if the insertion cannot be performed successfully, one should reconsider whether the LMA should be used in that particular patient at all. The LMA insertion technique in patients in the lateral or prone position differs significantly from the insertion technique in supine patients. Using one's thumb to insert the LMA might be the most useful method in patients positioned either prone or laterally.[17] One of the quoted advantages of using the LMA in patients in the prone position is that the patients are able to position themselves comfortably before induction of general anesthesia, thus potentially reducing the incidence of back problems.[102]

F. DEVICE PROBLEMS

As with any medical device, prior to its clinical release the LMA was subjected to rigorous testing to ensure compliance with the medical industry standards. However, a number of device complications have been reported. These include, but are not limited to, separation of the LMA cuff from the shaft,[87,141] fragmentation of the device inside the patient,[130] kinking of the LMA's shaft,[100] and failure to inflate or deflate the cuff.[66,120] Most of these complications are related to the use of the device beyond the manufacturer's recommendations and to the use of the wrong chemicals for sterilization as well as coating the device with silicone lubricants, which are not recommended for the LMA. Strict adherence to the manufacturer's instructions for cleaning, sterilization, and use should always be followed. These include not exceeding the recommended 40 uses per device. If a malfunction occurs, one needs to follow the instructions from the manufacturer's manual. Perhaps with the introduction of the disposable LMA models, the number of device problems linked to overuse and wrong sterilization techniques will be eliminated. However, all LMAs should always be inspected and tested prior to use to ensure optimal performance and safety.

X. CONCLUSION

When the LMA was first introduced, it was considered to be an alternative to the face mask. However, today its clinical applications exceed the original recommendations and benefit patients undergoing operations in all surgical and anesthetic subspecialties. Also, many modern surgical techniques are much less invasive than traditional operations, and a large number of patients undergo procedures in day surgical centers. As described, the LMA is much less stimulating to patients than the ETT and is now considered the first choice for diagnostic and minimally invasive surgical procedures. The LMA has been shown to be very effective, and frequently lifesaving, in patients with different types of difficult-to-manage airways. A study by Combes and colleagues[42] demonstrated that the ILMA and gum elastic bougie were the most frequently used and most successful techniques in patients with unexpected difficult intubation in the OR.

Most important, the LMA has unequivocally established the precedence that the supraglottic approach to airway management is not only feasible but also preferred in many clinical situations. This has created an interest on the part of the medical industry in developing other supraglottic airways. Although this represents a healthy exploration of different clinical approaches to airway management, clinicians should be careful when inserting these new devices into their patients because there are no separate standards or regulations guiding the safety and efficacy of supraglottic airways. This means that the responsibility for any complications from the use of these devices rests with the clinicians using them. The good news is that recently the American Society for Testing and Materials and the Food and Drug Administration developed standards and regulations for this new category of airway devices—the supralaryngeal airways. The new standards will aim to guide the development of airway devices, which we hope will have the same record of safety as the LMA.

REFERENCES

1. Adejumo SWA, Davies MW: The laryngeal mask airway—Another trick. Anaesthesia 51:604, 1996.
2. Alexander CA, Leach AB, Thompson AR, Lister JB: Use your Brain! Anaesthesia 43:893-894, 1988.
3. Allen JG, Flower EA: The Brain laryngeal mask. An alternative to difficult intubation. Br Dent J 168: 202-204, 1990.
4. Allison A, McCrory J: Tracheal placement of a gum elastic bougie using the laryngeal mask airway. Anaesthesia 45:419-420, 1990.
5. Arosio EM, Conci F: Use of the laryngeal mask airway for respiratory distress in the intensive care unit. Anaesthesia 50:635-636, 1995.
6. Asai T: Fiberoptic tracheal intubation through the laryngeal mask airway in an awake patient with cervical spine instability. Anesth Analg 77:404, 1993.
7. Asai T, Morris S: The laryngeal mask airway: Its features, effects, and role. Can J Anaesth 41:930-960, 1994.
8. Asai T, Murao K, Yukawa H, Shingu K: Re-evaluation of appropriate size of the laryngeal mask airway. Br J Anaesth 83:478-479, 1999.
9. Aye T, Milne B: Use of the laryngeal mask prior to definitive intubation in a difficult airway: A case report. J Emerg Med 13:711-714, 1995.
10. Balog CC, Bogetz MS, Good WH, et al: The laryngeal mask is an ideal airway for many outpatient pediatric ophthalmologic procedures. Anesth Analg 78:S17, 1994.
11. Baraka A: Laryngeal mask airway for resuscitation of a newborn with Pierre Robin syndrome. Anesthesiology 83:645-646, 1995.
12. Barclay K, Wall T, Wareham K, Asai T: Intra-ocular pressure changes in patients with glaucoma—Comparison between laryngeal mask airway and tracheal tube. Anaesthesia 49:159-162, 1994.
13. Baskett PJF, Parr MJA, Nolan JP: The intubating laryngeal mask: Results of a multicentre trial with experience of 500 cases. Anaesthesia 53:1174-1179, 1998.
14. Benumof J: The laryngeal mask airway and the ASA difficult airway algorithm. Anesthesiology 84: 686-699, 1996.
15. Beveridge ME: Laryngeal mask anaesthesia for repair of cleft palate. Anaesthesia 44:656-657, 1989.
16. Bing J: Masque larynge pour réduction de fractura du nez. Ann Fr Anesth Reanim 10:494, 1991.
17. Brain A: Thumb insertion technique. In Brimacombe JR, Brain AIJ, Berry AM (eds): The Laryngeal Mask Airway—A Review and Practical Guide. Philadelphia, WB Saunders, 1997, p 287.
18. Brain AI: The laryngeal mask airway—A possible new solution to airway problems in the emergency situation. Arch Emerg Med 4:229-232, 1984.
19. Brain AI, Verghese C, Strube PJ: The LMA ProSeal—A laryngeal mask with an esophageal vent. Br J Anaesth 84:650-654, 2000.

20. Brain AIJ: The development of the laryngeal mask— A brief history of the invention, early clinical studies and experimental work from which the laryngeal mask evolved. Eur J Anaesthesiol 4:5-17, 1991.

21. Brain AIJ: The laryngeal mask—A new concept in airway management. Br J Anaesth 55:801-805, 1983.

22. Brain AIJ: The laryngeal mask airway—A possible new solution to airway problems in the emergency situation. Arch Emerg Med 1:229-232, 1984.

23. Brain AIJ: Three cases of difficult intubation overcome by use of the laryngeal mask. Anaesthesia 40:353-355, 1985.

24. Brain AIJ, Brimacombe JR: Alternative insertion techniques. In Brimacombe JR, Brain AIJ, Berry AM (eds): The Laryngeal Mask Airway—A Review and Practical Guide. Philadelphia, WB Saunders, 1997, pp 83-85.

25. Brain AIJ, McGhee TD, McAteer EJ, et al: The laryngeal mask airway. Development and preliminary trials of a new type of airway. Anaesthesia 40:356-361, 1985.

26. Brain AIJ, Verghese C, Addy EV, et al: The intubating laryngeal mask II: A preliminary clinical report of a new means of intubating the trachea. Br J Anaesth 79: 704-709, 1997.

27. Brain AIJ, Verghese C, Kapila A, Brimacombe J: The intubating laryngeal mask I: Development of a new device for intubation of the trachea. Br J Anaesth 79:699-703, 1997.

28. Braun U, Zerbst M, Fullekrug B, et al: A comparison of the Proseal laryngeal mask to the standard laryngeal mask on anesthesized, non-relaxed patients. Anasthesiol Intensivmed Notfallmed Schmerzther 37:727-733, 2002.

29. Brimacombe J, Archdeacon J: The laryngeal mask airway for unplanned prolonged procedures. Can J Anaesth 42:1176, 1995.

30. Brimacombe J, Berry A: Laryngeal mask airway cuff pressure and position during anaesthesia lasting one to two hours. Can J Anaesth 41:589-593, 1994.

31. Brimacombe J, Berry A: The incidence of aspiration associated with the laryngeal mask airway—A meta-analysis of published literature. J Clin Anesth 7:297-305, 1995.

32. Brimacombe J, Holyoake L, Keller C, et al: Emergence characteristics and postoperative laryngopharyngeal morbidity with the laryngeal mask airway: A comparison of high versus low initial cuff volume. Anaesthesia 55:338-343, 2000.

33. Brimacombe J, Holyoake L, Keller C, et al: Pharyngolaryngeal, neck, and jaw discomfort after anesthesia with the face mask and laryngeal mask airway at high and low cuff volumes in males and females. Anesthesiology 93:26-31, 2000.

34. Brimacombe J, Shorney N: The laryngeal mask airway and prolonged balanced anesthesia. Can J Anaesth 40:360-364, 1993.

35. Brimacombe J, Tucker P, Simmons S: The laryngeal mask airway for awake diagnostic bronchoscopy: A retrospective study of 200 consecutive patients. Eur J Anaesthesiol 12:1017-1023, 1995.

36. Brodrick PM, Webster NR, Nunn JF: The laryngeal mask airway—A study of 100 patients during spontaneous breathing. Anaesthesia 44:238-241, 1989.

37. Caplan RA, Benumoff JL, Berry FA, et al: Practice guidelines for management of the difficult airway: A report by the ASA Task Force on Management of the Difficult Airway. Anesthesiology 78:597-602, 1993.

38. Caplan RA, Posner KL, Ward RJ, Cheney FW: Adverse respiratory events in anesthesia: A closed claims analysis. Anesthesiology 72:828-833, 1990.

39. Chan KL, Cohen GI, Sochowski RA, Baird MG: Complications of transesophageal echocardiography in ambulatory adult patients: Analysis of 1500 consecutive examinations. J Am Soc Echocardiogr 4:577-582, 1991.

40. Chen CH, Lin CC, Tan PP: Clinical experience of laryngeal mask airway in lateral position during anesthesia. Acta Anaesthesiol Sin 33:31-34, 1995.

41. Cohen MM, Duncan PG, Pope WDB, Wolkenstein C: A survey of 112000 anaesthetics at one teaching hospital. Can Anaesth Soc J 33:22-31, 1986.

42. Combes X, Le Roux B, Suen P, et al: Unanticipated difficult airway in anesthetized patients: Prospective validation of a management algorithm. Anesthesiology 5:1146-1150, 2004.

43. Conacher ID: Anaesthesia and tracheobronchial stenting for central airway obstruction in adults. Br J Anaesth 90:367-374, 2003.

44. Cormack RS, Lehane J: Difficult tracheal intubation in obstetrics. Anesthesia 39:1105-1111, 1984.

45. Dain SL, Webster AC, Morley-Foster P, et al: Propofol for insertion of the laryngeal mask airway for short ENT procedures in children. Anesth Analg 82:S83, 1996.

46. Daniel WG, Erbel R, Kasper W, et al: Safety of transesophageal echocardiography: A multicenter survey of 10,419 examinations. Circulation 83:817-821, 1991.

47. Daum RE, O'Reilly BJ: The laryngeal mask airway in ENT surgery. J Laryngol Otol 106:28-30, 1992.

48. Davies PR, Tighe SQ, Greenslade GL, Evans GH: Laryngeal mask airway and tracheal tube insertion by unskilled personnel. Lancet 336:977-979, 1990.

49. De Belder MA, Leech G, Camm AJ: Transesophageal echocardiography in unsedated outpatients: Technique and patients' tolerance. J Am Soc Echocardiogr 2: 375-379, 1989.

50. Devitt JH, Wenstone R, Noel AG, O'Donnell RRT: The laryngeal mask airway and positive-pressure ventilation. Anesthesiology 80:550-555, 1994.

51. Du Plessis M, Barr AM, Verghese C, Lyall JR: Fiberoptic bronchoscopy under general anesthesia using the laryngeal mask airway. Eur J Anaesthesiol 10:363-365, 1993.

52. Ferson D, Thakar D, Swafford J, et al: Use of deep intravenous sedation with propofol and the laryngeal mask airway during transesophageal echocardiography. J Cardiothorac Vasc Anesth 17:443-446, 2003.

53. Ebata T, Nishiki S, Masuda A, Amaha K: Anaesthesia for Treacher Collins syndrome using a laryngeal mask airway. Can J Anaesth 38:1043-1045, 1991.

54. Elias M: Laryngeal mask airway for radiotherapy in the prone position. Anaesthesia 47:1005, 1992.

55. Eltzschig HK, Posner M, Moore FD Jr: The use of readily available equipment in a simple method for intraoperative monitoring of recurrent laryngeal nerve function during thyroid surgery: Initial experience with more than 300 cases. Arch Surg 137:452-456, 2002.

56. Epstein RH, Ferouz F, Jenkins MA: Airway sealing pressures of the laryngeal mask airway in children. Anesthesiology 81:A1322, 1994.

57. Epstein RH, Ferouz F, Jenkins MA: Airway sealing pressures of the laryngeal mask in pediatric patients. J Clin Anesth 8:93-98, 1996.

58. Ferson DZ: The effect of the laryngeal mask insertion on intracranial pressure in a patient with posterior fossa tumor. Internet J Anesthesiol 3, 1997.

59. Ferson DZ, Bui TP, Arens JF: Evaluation of the effectiveness of two methods of training for the insertion of the laryngeal mask airway. Anesthesiology 95:A558, 2001.

60. Ferson DZ, Nesbitt JC, Nesbitt K, et al: The laryngeal mask airway: A new standard for airway evaluation in thoracic surgery. Ann Thorac Surg 63:768-772, 1997.

61. Ferson DZ, Rosenblatt WH, Johansen MJ, et al: Use of the intubating LMA-Fastrach in 254 patients with difficult-to-manage airways. Anesthesiology 95:1175-1181, 2000.

62. Fiani N, Scandella C, Giolitto N, et al: Comparison of reinforced laryngeal mask airway vs endotracheal intubation in tonsillectomy. Anesthesiology 81:A491, 1994.

63. Figueredo E, Vivar-Diago M, Munoz-Blanco F: Laryngo-pharyngeal complaints after use of the laryngeal mask airway. Can J Anaesth 46:220-225, 1999.

64. Fink BR: Roentgen ray studies of airway problems. I. The oropharyngeal airway. Anesthesiology 18:162-163, 1957.

65. Fuchs K, Kukule I, Knoch M, Wiegand W: Larynxmske versus Intubation bei erschwerten Intubationsbedingungen beim Franceschetti-Zwahlen-Klein-Syndrom (Treacher-Collins-Syndrom). Anasthesiol Intensivmed Noftalmed Schmerzther 28:190-192, 1993.

66. George A: Failed cuff inflation of a laryngeal mask. Anaesthesia 49:80, 1994.

67. George JM, Sanders GM: The reinforced laryngeal mask airway in paediatric outpatient dental surgery. 11th World Congress of Anesthesiology, Sydney, April 14-20, 1996, Abstract Handbook, p 477.

68. Godley M, Ramachandra AR: Use of LMA for awake intubation for caesarian section. Can J Anaesth 43:299-302, 1996.

69. Goldie AS, Hudson I: Fiberoptic tracheal intubation through a modified laryngeal mask. Paediatr Anaesth 2:344, 1992.

70. Goodwin A, Ogg TW, Lamb W, Adlam D: The reinforced laryngeal mask airway in dental day surgery. Ambulatory Surg 1:31-35, 1993.

71. Goudsouzian NG, Denman W, Cleveland R, Shorten G: Radiologic localization of the laryngeal mask in children. Anesthesiology 77:1085-1089, 1992.

72. Grady DM, McHardy F, Wong J, et al: Pharyngolaryngeal morbidity with the laryngeal mask airway in spontaneously breathing patients: Does size matter? Anesthesiology 94:760-766, 2001.

73. Grebenik CR, Ferguson C, White A: The laryngeal mask airway in pediatric radiotherapy. Anaesthesiology 72:474-477, 1990.

74. Gronert BJ: Laryngeal mask airway for management of airway and extracorporeal shock wave lithotripsy. Paediatr Anaesth 6:147-150, 1996.

75. Guedel AE: A nontraumatic pharyngeal airway. J Am Med Assoc 100:1862, 1933.

76. Guidelines 2000 for Cardiopulmonary Resuscitation and Emergency Cardiovascular Care. An International Consensus on Science. The American Heart Association in collaboration with the International Liaison Committee on Resuscitation. Circulation 102(Suppl), 2000.

77. Hamakawa T: Sore throat after the use of the LM. J Clin Anesth 17:245-246, 1993.

78. Hewitt F: Clinical observation upon respiration during anesthesia. Proc R Med Chir Soc 3:31-38, 1981.

79. Imai M, Matsamura C, Hanaoka Y, et al: Comparison of cardiovascular responses to airway management: Fiberoptic intubation using a new adapter, laryngeal mask insertion, or conventional laryngoscopic intubation. J Clin Anesth 7:14-18, 1995.

80. Inomata S, Nishikiwa T, Suga A, Yamashita S: Transient bilateral vocal cord paralysis after insertion of a laryngeal mask airway. Anesthesiology 82:787-788, 1995.

81. Johnson CM, Sims C: Awake fiberoptic intubation via a laryngeal mask in an infant with Goldenhar's syndrome. Anaesth Intensive Care 22:194-197, 1994.

82. Kadota Y, Oda T, Yoshimura N: Applications of a laryngeal mask to a fiberoptic bronchoscope–aided tracheal intubation. J Clin Anesth 4:503-504, 1992.

83. Kahl M, Eberhart LHJ, Behnke H, et al: Stress response to tracheal intubation in patients undergoing coronary artery surgery: Direct laryngoscopy versus an intubating laryngeal mask airway. J Cardiothorac Vasc Anesth 18(3):275-280, 2004.

84. Kapila A, Addy EV, Verghese C, Brain AIJ: The intubating laryngeal mask airway: An initial assessment of performance. Br J Anaesth 79:710-713, 1997.

85. Keller C, Sparr HJ, Brimacombe JR: Laryngeal mask lubrication. A comparative study of saline versus 2% lignocaine gel with cuff pressure control. Anaesthesia 52:592-597, 1997.

86. Khandheria BK: The transesophageal echocardiographic examination: Is it safe? Echocardiography 11:55-63, 1994.

87. Khoo ST: The laryngeal mask airway—An unusual complication. Anaesth Intensive Care 21:249-250, 1993.

88. Lamb K, James MFM, Janicki PK: The laryngeal mask airway for intraocular surgery: Effects on intraocular pressure and stress responses. Br J Anaesth 69:143-144, 1992.

89. Latorre F, Mienert R, Eberle B, et al: Laryngeal mask airway position and gastric insufflation [abstract]. 18th Annual Meeting of the European Academy of Anaesthesiology, Copenhagen, Denmark, Aug 29–Sept 1, 1996.

90. Leech BC: The pharyngeal bulb gasway: A new aid in cyclopropane anesthesia. Anesth Analg 16:22-25, 1937.

91. Leigh JM, Tytler JA: Admissions to the intensive care unit after complications of anaesthetic techniques over 10 years. Anaesthesia 45:814-820, 1990.

92. Lim W, Cone AM: Laryngeal mask and the prone position. Anaesthesia 49:542, 1994.

93. Lloyd Jones FR, Hegab A: Recurrent laryngeal nerve palsy after laryngeal mask insertion. Anaesthesia 51:171-172, 1996.

94. LMA Instruction Manual, LMA North America, Inc, San Diego.

95. LMA ProSeal Instruction Manual, LMA North America, Inc, San Diego.

96. Logan A: Use of the laryngeal mask in a patient with an unstable fracture of the cervical spine. Anaesthesia 46:987, 1991.

97. Lopez-Gil M, Brimacombe J, Cebrian J, Arranz J: The laryngeal mask airway in pediatric practice—A prospective study of skill acquisition by resident anesthesiologists. Anesthesiology 84:807-811, 1996.

98. Maekawa N, Mikawa K, Tanaka O, et al: The laryngeal mask may be a useful device for fiberoptic airway endoscopy in pediatric anesthesia. Anesthesiology 75:169-170, 1991.

99. Mallampati SR, Gatt SP, Gugino LD: A clinical study to predict difficult tracheal intubation. A prospective study. Can J Aneasth 32:429-434, 1985.

100. Martin DW: Kinking of the laryngeal mask airway in two children. Anaesthesia 45:488, 1990.

101. Mason DG, Bingham RM: The laryngeal mask airway in children. Anaesthesia 45:760-763, 1990.

102. McCaughey W, Bhanumurthy S: Laryngeal mask placement in the prone position. Anaesthesia 48:1104-1105, 1993.

103. McClune S, Regain M, Moore J: Laryngeal mask airway for caesarean section. Anaesthesia 45:227-228, 1990.

104. McCrirrick A, Pracilio JA: Awake intubation: A new technique. Anaesthesia 46:661-663, 1991.

105. McHardy FE, Chung F: Postoperative sore throat: Cause, prevention and treatment. Anaesthesia 54:444-453, 1999.

106. Mecklem D, Brimacombe J, Yarker J: Glossopexy in Pierre Robin sequence using the laryngeal mask airway. J Clin Anesth 7:267-269, 1995.

107. Milligan KA: Laryngeal mask in the prone position. Anaesthesia 49:449, 1994.

108. Mizikov VM, Variushina TV, Kirimov I: Fiberoptic bronchoscopy via laryngeal mask in children. Anesteziol Reanimatol 5:78-80, 1997.

109. Morikawa M: Vocal paralysis after use of the LM. J Clin Anesth 16:1194, 1992.

110. Myint Y, Singh AK, Peacock JE, Padfield A: Changes in intra-ocular pressure during general anaesthesia. A comparison of spontaneous breathing through a laryngeal mask with positive pressure ventilation through a tracheal tube. Anaesthesia 50:126-129, 1995.

111. Nanji GM, Maltby JR: Vomiting and aspiration pneumonitis with the laryngeal mask airway. Can J Anaesth 39:69-70, 1992.

112. Ngan Kee WD: Laryngeal mask airway for radiotherapy in the prone position. Anaesthesia 47:446-447, 1992.

113. Northrup WP: Apparatus for artificial prolonged forcible respiration. Br Med J ii:697, 1984.

114. Olsson GL, Hallen B, Hambraeus Jonzon K: Aspiration during anesthesia: A computer-aided study of 185,358 anaesthetics. Acta Anaesthesiol Scand 84-92, 1986.

115. Ouellette RG: The effect of nitrous oxide on laryngeal mask cuff pressure. AANA J 68:411-414, 2000.

116. Practice guidelines for management of the difficult airway: An updated report by the American Society of Anesthesiologists Task Force on Management of the Difficult Airway. Anesthesiology 98:1269-1277, 2003.

117. Quinn AC, Samaan A, McAteer EM, et al: The reinforced laryngeal mask for dento-alveolar surgery. Br J Anaesth 77:185-188, 1996.

118. Rafferty C, Burke AM, Cossar DF, Farling PA: Laryngeal mask and magnetic resonance imaging. Anaesthesia 45:590-591, 1990.

119. Rheineck Leyssius AT, Vos RJ, Blommesteijn R, Kalkman CJ: Use of the laryngeal mask airway versus orotracheal intubation to secure a patient airway in rhinoplastic surgery. Anesthesiology 81:A1293, 1994.

120. Richards JT: Pilot tube of the laryngeal mask airway. Anaesthesia 49:450-451, 1994.

121. Rieger A, Brunne B, Hass I, et al: Laryngo-pharyngeal complaints following laryngeal mask airway and endo-tracheal intubation. J Clin Anesth 9:42-47, 1997.

122. Sarang A, Dinsmore J: Anaesthesia for awake craniotomy—Evolution of a technique that facilitates awake neurological testing. Br J Anaesth 90:161-165, 2003.

123. Shipway F: Airway for intranasal operations. Br Med J (Apt 13): 767, 1935.

124. Shorten GD, Opie NJ, Graziotti P, et al: Assessment of upper airway anatomy in awake, sedated, and anesthetised patients using magnetic resonance imaging. Anaesth Intensive Care 22:165-169, 1994.

125. Sidhu VS: Laryngeal mask airway for anesthesia in the prone position. Anaesth Intensive Care 20:119, 1992.

126. Silk JM, Hill HM, Calder I: Difficult intubation and the laryngeal mask. Eur J Anaesthesiol 4:47-51, 1991.

127. Silva L, Brimacombe JR: Tracheal tube/laryngeal mask exchange for emergence. Anesthesiology 85:218, 1996.

128. Slinger P, Robinson R, Shennib H, et al: Alternative technique for laser resection of a carinal obstruction. J Cardiothorac Vasc Anesth 6:749-755, 1992.

129. Smith BL: Brain airway in anesthesia for patients with juvenile chronic arthritis. Anaesthesia 43:421-422, 1988.

130. Squires SJ, Woods K: Fragmented laryngeal mask airway. Anaesthesia 47:274, 1992.

131. Stevens JE, Burden G: Reinforced laryngeal mask airway and magnetic resonance imaging. Anaesthesia 49:79-80, 1994.

132. Theroux MC, Kettrick RG, Khine HH: Laryngeal mask airway and fiberoptic endoscopy in an infant with Schwartz-Jampel syndrome. Anesthesiology 82:605, 1995.

133. Thomson KD: A blind nasal intubation using a laryngeal mask airway. Anaesthesia 48:785-787, 1993.

134. Thomson KD: The effect of the laryngeal mask airway on coughing after eye surgery under general anaesthetic. Ophthalmic Surg 23:630-631, 1992.

135. Tiret L, Desmonts JM, Hatton F, Vourc'h G: Complications associated with anaesthesia: A prospective survey in France. Can Anaesth Soc J 33:336-344, 1986.

136. Van Damme E: Die Kehlkopfmaske in der ambulanten Anasthesia—Eine Antwertung vom 5000 ambulanten Narkosen. Anasthesiol Intensivmed Notfallmed Schmerzther 29:284-286, 1994.

137. Van Obbergh LJ, Muller G, Zeippen B, Dooms G: Propofol infusion and laryngeal mask for magnetic resonance imaging in children. Anesthesiology 77:A1177, 1992.

138. Verghese C, Berlet J, Kapila A, Pollard R: Clinical assessment of the single use laryngeal mask airway—The LMA-Unique. Br J Anaesth 80:677-679, 1998.

139. Verghese C, Brimacombe J: Survey of laryngeal mask usage in 11910 patients—Safety and efficacy for conventional and nonconventional usage. Anesth Analg 82:129-133, 1996.

140. Verghese C, Smith TCG, Young E: Prospective survey of the use of the laryngeal mask airway in 2359 patients. Anaesthesia 48:58-60, 1993.

141. Vickers R, Springer A, Hindmarsh J: Problem with the laryngeal mask airway. Anaesthesia 45:892, 1994.

142. Wainwright AC: Positive pressure ventilation and the laryngeal mask airway in ophthalmic anaesthesia. Br J Anaesth 75:249-250, 1995.

143. Warner MA, Warner WE, Webber JG: Clinical significance of pulmonary aspirations during the perioperative period. Anesthesiology 78:56-56, 1993.

144. Watcha MF, Garner FT, White PF, Lusk R: Laryngeal mask airway vs face mask and Guedel airway during pediatric myringotomy. Arch Otolaryngol Head Neck Surg 120:877-880, 1994.

145. Wellcome Trends in Anesthesiology, October 1985.

146. Wellcome Trends in Anesthesiology, February 1986 (Katz R: Clinical update: The laryngeal mask airway. Wellcome Trends Anaesthesiol Feb 1986).

147. Williams PJ, Bailey PM: Comparison of reinforced laryngeal mask airway and tracheal intubation for adenotonsillectomy. Br J Anaesth 70:30-33, 1993.

148. Williams PJ, Bailey PM: The reinforced laryngeal mask for adenotonsillectomy. Br J Anaesth 72:729, 1994.

149. Williams PJ, Thompsett C, Bailey PM: Comparison of reinforced laryngeal mask airway and tracheal intubation for nasal surgery. Anaesthesia 50:987-989, 1995.

150. Wynn JM, Jones KL: Tongue cyanosis after laryngeal mask insertion. Anesthesiology 80:1403-1404, 1994.

151. Zagnoev M, McCloskey J, Martin T: Fiberoptic intubation via the laryngeal mask airway. Anesth Analg 78:813-814, 1994.

152. Zerafa M, Baulch S, Elliott MJ, Petros AJ: Use of the laryngeal mask airway during repair of atrial septal defect in children. Paediatr Anaesth 9:257-259, 1999.

NEW GENERATION SUPRAGLOTTIC VENTILATORY DEVICES

Carin A. Hagberg
Felice E. Agro
Tim M. Cook
Allan P. Reed

I. INTRODUCTION

In the past, the choice of an airway device essentially was limited to the face mask or the endotracheal tube (ET).[1] Tracheal intubation is the overall accepted "gold standard" for securing the airway and providing adequate ventilation. However, training in tracheal intubation requires time, appropriate instruments, and adequate circumstances with respect to space and illumination. Furthermore, tracheal intubation requires continued practice and carries with it its own set of complications.

The practice of airway management has become more advanced. This advancement is demonstrated by the introduction of many new airway devices, several of which have been included in the American Society of Anesthesiologists (ASA) difficult airway algorithm.[64] The standard laryngeal mask airway, LMA Classic (cLMA; LMA North America, San Diego, CA) was introduced into clinical practice in 1988 and rapidly transformed airway management. Since that time, and particularly in the past 5 years, there has been an explosion of new supraglottic airway devices designed to compete with the cLMA, particularly single-use devices. There are several driving forces for the introduction of single-use devices, including the concern over sterility of cleaned, reusable devices (e.g., elimination of proteinaceous material and the risk of transmission of prion disease) and the inability to recycle the device enough to be cost effective. There are more than a dozen manufacturers of the single-use LMA (LMA Unique or uLMA), yet only those manufactured by Intavent or LMA North America have epiglottic bars at the distal end of the airway tube because of patent reasons.

Supraglottic airway (SGA) is a general term that includes airways with and without sealing characteristics. In an editorial, Brimacombe[18] recommended that the term "extraglottic" airway be used instead because many of these devices have components that are infraglottic (hypopharynx and upper esophagus). Nonetheless, this book describes all airway devices that have a ventilation orifice or orifices above the glottis as "supraglottic" and those that deliver anesthetic gases or oxygen below the vocal cords (e.g., transtracheal jet ventilation, cricothyrotomy) as "infraglottic."

Both Brimacombe (Table 22-1) and Miller (Table 22-2) suggested there be a classification system for this increasing complex family of devices. According to Miller,[56] there are three main sealing mechanisms: cuffed perilaryngeal sealers, cuffed pharyngeal sealers, and cuffless anatomically preshaped sealers. The explanation for each provides reasons for the differences observed in the sealing pressures achieved with each of the different types of devices. Further subdivision can be made by considering whether the device is single use or reusable and whether protection from aspiration of gastric contents is offered. Figure 22-1 illustrates the three sealing mechanisms, the force vector being determined by the airway pressure in the pharynx proximal to the sealing site.

Table 22-1 **Classification of Extraglottic Airway Devices by Presence or Absence of a Cuff, Oral or Nasal Route of Insertion, and Anatomic Location of the Distal Portion**

Cuffed, orally inserted laryngopharyngeal airways
  Williams airway intubator*
  Patil oral airway*
  Ovassapian fiberoptic intubating airway*
  Combined oropharyngeal airway and dental pack
  Modified Connell airway

Cuffed, orally inserted laryngopharyngeal airways
  Mehta's cuffed oropharyngeal airway†
  Cuffed oropharyngeal airway†

Uncuffed, nasally inserted laryngopharyngeal airways
  Variable flange nasopharyngeal airway
  Linder nasopharyngeal airway

Cuffed, nasally inserted laryngopharyngeal airways   Boheimer's cuffed nasopharyngeal airway†

Cuffed, orally inserted hypopharyngeal airways
  Classic LMA‡
  Flexible LMA‡
  Intubating LMA*
  Disposable LMA‡
  ProSeal LMA‡
  Glottic aperture seal airway‡
  Streamlined pharynx airway liner‡
  SoftSeal laryngeal mask‡
  Laryngeal Tube airway†
  Laryngeal Tube suction†
  Airway management device†
  Pharyngeal airway express†
  Cobra pharyngeal lumen airway†

Uncuffed, orally inserted esophageal airways   Tracheoesophageal airway

Cuffed, orally inserted esophageal airways
  Pharyngeal tracheal lumen airway†
  Esophageal tracheal Combitube

Many of the names of extraglottic airway devices do not fit this classification system. For example, the distal ends of the "Patil oral airway" and the "Linder nasopharyngeal airway" are in the laryngopharynx and not in the oral cavity and nasopharynx, respectively. There are no extraglottic airway devices whose distal portion is intended to sit in the oral cavity, nasal cavity, or nasopharynx.
*Primary function as an airway intubator
†proximal pharyngeal cuff
‡periglottic cuff
LMA, laryngeal mask airway.
From Brimacombe J: A proposed classification system for extraglottic airway devices [letter]. Anesthesiology 101:559, 2004.

Table 22-2 Miller's Supraglottic Classifications

	Cuffed Perilaryngeal Sealers		Cuffed Pharyngeal Sealers		
	Without Directional Sealing	**With Directional Sealing**	**Without Esophageal Sealing Cuffs**	**With Esophageal Sealing Cuffs**	**Cuffless Preshaped Sealers**
Devices	Laryngeal mask airway Intubating laryngeal mask airway SoftSeal laryngeal mask Ambu AuraOnce Intubating Laryngeal Airway	ProSeal laryngeal mask airway	Cobra PLA	Laryngeal Tube Laryngeal Tube—suction Esophageal—tracheal Combitube	Streamlined Liner of the Pharynx Airway
Sealing mechanism	Relies on simple opposition of the cuff that surrounds the larynx	Sealing site is at or around the entrance of the larynx.	Pharyngeal cuff seals at the base of the tongue.		Anatomically preshaped hollow airway that seals the outlet from the pharynx at the base of the tongue to the entrance to the esophagus, as a result of the resilience of the walls of the shaped airway
Advantages	Minimal risk of precipitating laryngospasm Well tolerated at lower anesthetic levels	Higher seal pressures Decreased risk of regurgitated fluid entering airway channel	Better sealing pressures Pressure exerted perpendicular to airway channel	Minimizes aspiration risk Most provide access to esophagus.	Hollow structure provides aspiration protection by storage of regurgitation liquid. Safe to suction regurgitated liquid without risk of laryngospasm Preshaped airway provides specific positioning and a stable airway. Easier to use No NO_2 influence Able to insert through limited mouth opening

	Cuffed Perilaryngeal Sealers		Cuffed Pharyngeal Sealers		Cuffless Preshaped Sealers
	Without Directional Sealing	*With Directional Sealing*	*Without Esophageal Sealing Cuffs*	*With Esophageal Sealing Cuffs*	
Disadvantages	Low seal pressures Little storage space for regurgitated liquid Increased risk of gastroesophageal insufflation No protection from aspiration Backward-slanting profile can become caught in back of mouth.	Harder to insert More easily rotated out of position Folding of tip can occur upon insertion, occluding the drainage tube.	No sealing of the downward outlet increasing risk of gastroesophageal insufflation Reliance based on tone of gastroesophageal sphincter No protection from aspiration Increased need for repositioning	Increased potential for mucosal trauma due to stiffer tube Congestion of tongue with excessive increases in cuff pressure and potential lingual nerve damage Increased need for repositioning	Difficult to select proper size Less flexibility in positioning Not for use in abnormal or distorted upper airway anatomy

PLA, perilaryngeal airway.

Adapted from Miller DM: A proposed classification and scoring system for supraglottic sealing airways: A brief review. Anesth Analg 99:1553-1559, 2004.

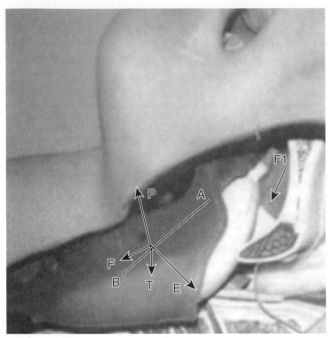

Figure 22-1 The laryngeal mask (LM) airway is inserted into an Ambu Manikin Trainer. AB represents the side view of the axis of the bowl of the LM, which comprises the area over which the sealing force is exerted. The expulsive force E is exerted at right angles to this plane (AB). To prevent the airway from being expelled at the peak inflation pressure, equal and opposite forces need to be exerted. These comprise a force vector P from the posterior pharyngeal wall and T from the base of the tongue with resultant frictional force F that resists expulsion. If F is insufficient, strapping or tying of the silicone tube at the mouth may be necessary to provide an additional force F1 that is transmitted through the tube to increase the total force vector F. Notice that the LM tends to kink in the middle of its perilaryngeal cuff. This may alter the direction of the vector E in a more expulsive direction, necessitating a larger value for F. (From Miller DM: A proposed classification and scoring system for supraglottic sealing airways: A brief review. Anesth Analg 99:1553-1559, 2004.)

Only the devices currently used in clinical practice in both the United Kingdom and the United States, with the exception of the Streamlined Liner of the Pharynx Airway, are discussed in this chapter. See Chapters 21 and 25 for extensive reviews of the LMA and Combitube.

II. CLASSIFICATION OF SUPRAGLOTTIC VENTILATORY DEVICES

A. CUFFED PERIPHARYNGEAL SEALERS

1. Ambu AuraOnce

a. History

In the fall of 2002, the Danish medical device manufacturer Ambu A/S (Ambu, Glen Burnie, MD), primarily known for the invention of the manual resuscitator some 50 years ago, was looking for new clinical areas in which

the company could utilize its experience in airway management and unique production capabilities.

After a series of visits to anesthesiology departments and interviews with experienced users of laryngeal mask concepts currently on the market, Ambu and a group of internationally renowned anesthesiologists designed a laryngeal mask to be used under routine anesthesia that offered new benefits to its users. The result, the Ambu AuraOnce (formerly called the Ambu laryngeal mask), was commercially launched globally in February 2004.

b. Device Description

The Ambu AuraOnce (AAO) is a sterile, single-use product made of polyvinyl chloride (PVC), molded in one piece, featuring a special built-in curve that carefully replicates natural human anatomy (Fig. 22-2). The curve ensures that the patient's head remains in a natural, supine position when the mask is in use. Together with the reinforced tip, the curve also facilitates insertion of the mask without extra stress on the upper jaw. In addition, internal ribs built into the curve give the airway tube the flexibility needed to adapt to individual anatomic variances and a wide range of head positions.

It is molded in one piece with an integrated inflation line and no epiglottic bars on the anterior surface of the cuff. The cuff is elliptical and is shaped to reside in the hypopharynx at the base of the tongue. Its curved shape and design without epiglottic bars allow easy access for flexible fiberoptic devices. The product is sterile and latex free and is available in both adult and pediatric sizes 1 to 5. The proper size is based on the weight and size of the patient (Table 22-3).

The Ambu Aura40 is the reusable, silicon version of the AAO. It is the first reusable laryngeal mask to feature a built-in curve that carefully replicates the natural human anatomy. It can be steam autoclaved up to 40 times. The Aura40 offers all the same features as the AAO.

c. Insertion Technique and Device Removal

It is important that the individual who inserts or ventilates through the AAO is familiar with the warnings, precautions, indications, and contraindications in the use

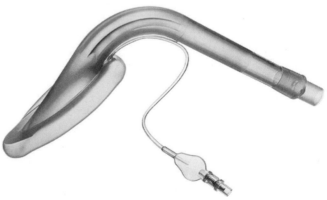

Figure 22-2 Ambu AuraOnce. (Courtesy of Ambu A/S.)

Table 22-3   **Ambu AuraOnce Size and Cuff Volume**

Mask Size	Patient Weight (kg)	Tube Outer Diameter(mm)	Maximum Cuff Volume (mL)	Maximum Cuff Pressure (cm H$_2$O)
No. 3	30-50	158	20	60
No. 4	50-70	177	30	60
No. 5	70	198.5	40	60

Courtesy of Ambu A/S.

of this device. Before insertion, the following points are of the highest importance:

- The size of the AAO must be appropriate for the patient. Use the guidelines from Table 22-3 combined with clinical judgment to select the correct size. Consideration should also be given to the patient's experience with the device and the size used.
- Check for correct cuff deflation and lubricate the posterior surface of the device with a water-soluble lubricant.
- Always have a spare AAO ready for use.
- Excess force must be avoided at all times.
- Preoxygenate and implement standard monitoring procedures.
- Ensure an adequate level of anesthesia (or unconsciousness) before attempting insertion. Resistance or swallowing may indicate inadequate anesthesia or inappropriate technique, or both. Inexperienced users should choose a deeper level of anesthesia.
- Insert AAO in a fashion similar to that described for the traditional LMAs in Chapter 21. When the mask is fully inserted, resistance is felt.
- If the cuff fails to flatten or curls over as it is advanced, it is necessary to withdraw the mask and reinsert it. In case of tonsillar obstruction, a diagonal shift of the mask is often successful.

d. Indications and Advantages

The AAO is intended for use as an alternative to the face mask for achieving and maintaining control of the airway during routine and critical anesthetic procedures in fasted patients. It may be used where unexpected difficulties arise with airway management and even preferred in some critical airway situations. The AAO may also be used to establish a clear airway during resuscitation in the profoundly unconscious patient with absent glossopharyngeal and laryngeal reflexes who may need artificial ventilation. The device is not intended for use as a replacement for the ET and is best suited for use in fasted surgical procedures where tracheal intubation is not deemed necessary.

The AAO features an extra soft cuff. The cuff is flexible and the tip is reinforced. These features facilitate insertion and also prevent the tip from folding during insertion. The cuff, mask, and airway tube of the AAO are not glued together but molded in a single unit, thus preventing the mask from separating during use. The one-piece molding process also ensures that the product is free from ridges that can scratch the walls of the patient's airways during placement.

e. Disadvantages

Given that airway pressures should be limited to no greater than 20 to 25 cm H$_2$O, the AAO may not be appropriate for patients with reduced lung compliance or increased airway resistance. The major disadvantage of the device is that it does not protect against aspiration and does not secure the airway as effectively as the tracheal tube. In addition, the AAO cannot prevent or treat airway obstruction at or beyond the larynx.

f. Comparison with Face Mask Ventilation and Endotracheal Intubation

In contrast to the face mask, the AAO is associated with less dead space ventilation and no gastric inflation if reasonable airway pressures are used. Furthermore, it allows the anesthesiologist to have the hands free for other important tasks. Compression of eyes and facial and infraorbital nerves is avoided, and operating room pollution from vapors and anesthetic gas is less likely.

Compared with the ET, the AAO is easier to place, avoids laryngoscopy and its associated problems, and is less invasive. Furthermore, the insertion of this device does not require the use of muscle relaxants.

g. Guide to Endotracheal Intubation

The AAO may be used as an intubation conduit. This may be performed by loading an Aintree airway exchange catheter (Cook Critical Care, Bloomington, IN) onto a fiberoptic bronchoscope (FOB) and then passing it into the lumen of the AAO. This can be performed either with or without the use of a Bodai adapter (Sontek Medical, Lexington, MA). The use of the Bodai adapter allows oxygen and gas administration through the attached breathing circuit during the exchange of the AAO to an ET. When the device is correctly positioned and the mask opening is opposite the vocal cords, the device directs the FOB directly toward the larynx. When the FOB has passed through the vocal cords, the Aintree catheter can be advanced into the trachea until the carina is visualized.

The FOB should then be removed. If oxygenation is necessary at this point, either one of the Rapi-Fit adapters packaged with the device can be utilized to administer oxygen. The cuff of the AAO is then deflated and removed over the catheter. Using direct laryngoscopy, an appropriately sized ET should be passed over the catheter and into the trachea. Once successfully placed, the catheter can be removed. Confirmation of tracheal placement should be performed by capnography and chest auscultation. Blind intubation through the AAO by simply advancing an ET through it or by using a bougie guide may be successful, but passage into the trachea is not consistently obtained, and the preceding technique is far preferable.

h. Medical Literature

A multicenter study of the clinical performance of the AAO was conducted by Hagberg and colleagues[41] to evaluate the ease of insertion, insertion success, airway seal, and ventilation. Device placement was successful in all 118 nonparalyzed, anesthetized patients on the first or second attempt (92.4% and 7.6%, respectively). Adequate ventilation was achieved in all patients, and the vocal cords could be visualized by fiberoptic endoscopy in 91.5% of patients. Complications and patients' complaints were minor and were quickly resolved. They found that the curvature of the tube facilitates insertion and the large, soft cuff allows a higher oropharyngeal leak pressure than is commonly found in other laryngeal masks; thus, it can be used more safely for controlled ventilation. In addition, the tip of the AAO is reinforced to avoid folding that can lead to air leakage, a common problem with other LMAs.

In one study center, ventilation using the AAO in different head positions was evaluated. Gentzwuerker and coauthors[37] evaluated the stability of the device in 30 patients in five different head positions: (1) head on a standard pillow, (2) head rotated 90 degrees to the left side, (3) head rotated 90 degrees to the right side, (4) head with chin lift on a standard pillow, and (5) head flat on a table without a pillow. No changes in the performance of the device in terms of ventilatory criteria were documented with any position changes. Thus, the AAO may be a useful SGA for cases in which head movement may be necessary for surgery.

Francksen and coworkers[30] compared the performance of the uLMA and the AAO in 80 patients undergoing minor routine gynecologic surgery. They demonstrated that the time of insertion and failure rate were comparable. In addition, blood gas samples and ventilation variables revealed sufficient ventilation and oxygenation with either device. Again, airway leak pressures were higher with the AAO compared with the uLMA (18 versus 16 cm H_2O median and 12 to 38 versus 5 to 28 cm H_2O range; $P < .013$). No gastric inflation was found to occur with either device, nor was postoperative airway morbidity comparable.

Gernoth and colleagues[39] compared the performance of the cLMA and the AAO for airway management in 60 patients with immobilization of the cervical spine scheduled for elective ambulatory interventions. An AAO or cLMA was inserted after cervical immobilization with an extrication collar. In this study, insertion time, number of insertion attempts, and airway leak pressures were comparable (AAO 25.6 ± 5.3 cm H_2O and cLMA 26.5 ± 6.5 cm H_2O). Thus, they concluded that both devices are suitable for rapid and reliable airway management in patients with cervical immobilization.

2. SoftSeal Laryngeal Mask

a. History

The SoftSeal laryngeal mask (SSLM) is another new disposable SGA device (Smiths Medical ASD, Keene, NH; Smiths Medical, Hythe, Kent, England) that was developed through the Smiths Internal Research and Development group and is covered by several patents.

The project development for this mask began in November 1998. At that time, it was planned to use an extruded tube portion attached to a molded shoe with a blow-molded cuff, similar to the existing disposable uLMA. The first prototype added a "ski tip" form at the nose that was intended to help guide the tube around the oropharynx and into position. A new method of blow molding the cuff of the device became necessary in order to embed the inflation line for the cuff into the wall of the tubing. The development of this aspect took a considerable period of time.

The second prototype of the SSLM was developed in September 2000. The ski tip had to be removed as it actually increased the impact of forces on the rear of the oropharynx. The heel at the back of the cuff was raised to retain the inflation line, which was also intended to provide a natural position for the finger when used to insert the device using the finger technique, as described by Brain.[50]

The third prototype of the SSLM appeared in January 2001. The connector of the device had evolved to include a knurled edge to provide an improved grip for clinicians when connecting and disconnecting the device. Further detail changes around the tip were also incorporated that utilized ultraviolet-activated glue. An artificial oropharynx was developed in order to test the device prior to any clinical use, which allowed measurement of the forces applied on the hard and soft palates, on the rear pharyngeal wall, and against the laryngeal inlet. Following testing of this prototype in the model oropharynx, further design modifications were made, including smoothing the joint between the tube and the shoe and reducing the heel height. A subsequent prototype of this new design was used to perform cadaver studies in Belgium and the United States during March 2001. Following these trials, future modifications were developed, including lowering the tip of the shoe below the upper edge of the cuff and

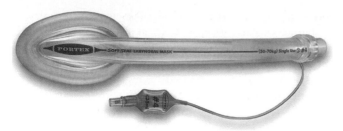

Figure 22-3 SoftSeal laryngeal mask. (Courtesy of Smiths Medical.)

Table 22-5 **SoftSeal Maximum Recommended Air Volume**

Mask Size	Maximum Cuff Volume (mL)
No. 3	25
No. 4	35
No. 5	55

Courtesy of Smiths Medical, Inc.

eliminating the thickened step in the wall. The shoe and tube were also made as one piece.

The last prototype of the SSLM has a lower lip that allows enhanced flexibility, resulting in measured insertion forces similar to those achieved with the cLMA. The connector has a more scalloped design. All of these aspects were combined in the preproduction prototypes used for evaluation trials in Australia, Sweden, South Africa, and Canada and continued into the product launch. The final product was commercially launched in Australia in May 2002. It was launched in January 2003 in the United States.

b. Device Description

The SSLM is a tubular oropharyngeal airway with a mask and an inflatable peripheral cuff attached to the distal end (Fig. 22-3). It is designed to produce an airtight seal around the laryngeal inlet and so provide a secure airway suitable for spontaneous or controlled ventilation during general anesthesia. It can be inserted without laryngoscopy and paralysis in most cases. Once in place, it provides more secure airway control than with a face mask and there is no need to support the patient's chin, allowing "hands-free" airway management.

The device is available in seven sizes. The proper size is based on the weight and size of the patient. In general, the size indications for adults are shown in Table 22-4. No. 3 for small females, a No. 4 for most males and females, and a No. 5 for larger male patients.

c. Insertion Technique and Device Removal

Prior to insertion, the valve depressor should be removed from the inflation valve and the integrity of the cuff and inflation system should be checked by deflating

Table 22-4 **SoftSeal Size Chart**

Mask Size	Patient Weight (kg)
No. 3	30-50
No. 4	50-70
No. 5	70+

Courtesy of Smiths Medical, Inc.

the cuff with a syringe and reinflating with the maximum recommended volume of air (Table 22-5). The tube and cuff should be examined for any signs of damage and the lumen should be free of any blockage.

Although there are currently many insertion techniques in use, insertion of the SSLM with the partially inflated cuff technique (approximately 30 mL of ambient air) is recommended to provide optimal results. The valve depressor should be replaced onto the inflation valve to allow the cuff to return to atmospheric pressure.

A sterile water-based gel lubricant should be used to lubricate the posterior surface of the laryngeal mask just before insertion. Application of lubricant to the anterior surface of the mask should be avoided as it may cause aspiration of excess lubricant or tube blockage. Also, lidocaine is not recommended as a lubricant as it may lead to an increase in some postoperative complications[47] and toxicity in pediatric patients.

Just before insertion, the valve depressor should be removed to ensure that the cuff has retained an inflated appearance with no wrinkles or depressions. If not contraindicated, the patient's head should be placed in the "sniffing" position (neck flexed and head extended). If a muscle relaxant was administered prior to insertion, use of a triple airway maneuver (mouth opening, head extension, jaw thrust) should decrease the incidence of epiglottic downfolding.[11]

The device should be held between the fingers and thumb of the dominant hand with the blue line on the tube aligned midline with the nasal septum and upper lip to confirm direct orientation. The top should be directed against the hard palate, as during traditional LMA insertion, while performing a jaw lift with the nondominant hand. The mask should be advanced into the oropharynx with a slight twisting motion to negotiate the tongue and tonsils. The nondominant hand should then hold the 15-mm connector and push the mask into the hypopharynx until resistance is encountered. Force should never be utilized.

The cuff should be inflated with air until a "just-seal" pressure is obtained. A maximum intracuff pressure of 60 cm H_2O is recommended to ensure an adequate seal and minimize trauma. The tube usually moves out of the mouth up to 15 mm and tissues in the neck bulge slightly when the cuff is inflated, confirming correct placement.

The device should not be held or secured prior to cuff inflation.

The tube should then be connected to the breathing system, and adequacy of ventilation should be assessed. A bite block should be inserted to prevent occlusion upon emergence and the tube securely taped in position to the patient's face.

d. Indications and Advantages

The SSLM may be used for airway management in any patient in whom anesthesia can be safely maintained through a face mask (with the exception of patients with oropharyngeal pathology or abnormal anatomy). The device can also be used as a "rescue airway" in either the cannot intubate, cannot ventilate (CICV) or cannot intubate, difficult to ventilate (CIDV) scenario. Because the SSLM does not provide airway protection, it is advisable to facilitate endotracheal intubation in order to secure the airway if the patient is considered at risk for aspiration. The wider ventilation orifice (can accommodate up to a size 7.5 mm ET) and absence of aperture bars could possibly facilitate this procedure.

Use of the SSLM may be considered in an unconscious patient at risk for airway obstruction who may require artificial respiration when endotracheal intubation is unavailable. The clinician must balance the risk of pulmonary aspiration against the benefits of obtaining an adequate airway or oxygenation of the patient.

e. Disadvantages

Given that airway pressures should be limited to no greater than 20 to 25 cm H_2O, the SSLM may not be appropriate for patients with reduced lung compliance or increased airway resistance. The major disadvantage of the device is that it does not protect against aspiration and does not secure the airway as effectively as the tracheal tube. In addition, the SSLM cannot prevent or treat airway obstruction at or beyond the laryngeal inlet.

f. Comparison with Face Mask Ventilation and Endotracheal Intubation

As with the AAO, the use of the SSLM should be associated with less dead space ventilation and no gastric inflation, if reasonable airway pressures are used, as compared with face mask ventilation. Furthermore, it allows the anesthesiologist to be hands free for other important tasks. Compression of eyes and facial and infraorbital nerves is avoided, and operating room pollution from vapors and anesthetic gas is less likely.

Compared with the ET, the SSLM is easier to place, avoids laryngoscopy and its associated problems, and is less invasive. Furthermore, the insertion of this device does not require the use of muscle relaxants.

g. Guide to Endotracheal Intubation

The SSLM may be used as an intubation conduit. This may be done by either directly passing an ET through the shaft of the SSLM or loading an Aintree airway exchange catheter (Cook Critical Care) onto an FOB and then passing it into the lumen of the SSLM. When the device is correctly positioned and the mask opening is opposite the vocal cords, the device directs the FOB directly toward the larynx. When the FOB has passed through the vocal cords, the Aintree catheter can be advanced into the trachea until the carina is visualized and then the FOB removed. If oxygenation is necessary at this point, either one of the Rapi-Fit adapters can be utilized to administer oxygen. The cuff of the SSLM is then deflated and removed over the catheter. Using direct laryngoscopy, an appropriately sized ET (≥ 7.0 mm) should be passed over the catheter and into the trachea. When it is successfully placed, the catheter can be removed. Confirmation of tracheal placement should be performed by capnography and chest auscultation. Blind intubation through the SSLM by simply advancing an ET through it or by using a bougie guide may be successful, but passage into the trachea is not consistently obtained, and the preceding technique is far preferable.

h. Medical Literature

Several studies have been performed comparing the performance of the SSLM with the uLMA during both spontaneous and positive-pressure ventilation. Brimacombe and colleagues[23] studied 90 healthy, paralyzed, anesthetized patients undergoing routine superficial or peripheral surgery in a crossover fashion, in which both devices were utilized for positive-pressure ventilation in each patient. They found that the uLMA is superior to the SSLM in terms of ease of insertion, fiberoptic position, and mucosal trauma but similar in terms of oropharyngeal leak pressure and ease of ventilation.

In another randomized, crossover study comparing the SSLM and the uLMA in 168 anesthetized, spontaneously breathing patients, Paech and associates[63] determined that although both devices performed equivalently with respect to first-time placement, the SSLM was often rated more difficult to insert and more likely to show mucosal trauma. On the other hand, the fiberoptic view of the larynx was better through the SSLM and it more frequently provided a ventilation seal at 20 cm H_2O. Also, in contrast to the uLMA, its cuff pressure did not increase during nitrous oxide anesthesia. In this study there was a larger proportion of females, a smaller mask size was used for both males and females, and the SSLM was inserted with a partially inflated cuff.

When the SSLM was compared with the cLMA, Van Zundert and coworkers[71] found that in spontaneously breathing adult patients requiring a size 4 LMA, the new disposable SSLM is an acceptable alternative to the cLMA, resulting in a good laryngeal seal and similar clinical performance. They also determined that the cuff pressures substantially increased with the cLMA and that there was less trauma to patients using the SSLM, as assessed by the incidence of sore throat in the early postoperative period. This decreased incidence of both trauma and sore throat may be due to partial inflation of the cuff with ambient room air at 10 mm Hg (15 cm H_2O) above atmospheric pressure. Hagberg and colleagues[42,43] also demonstrated that partial cuff inflation (30 cm³ of ambient air) enhances ease of insertion and minimizes mucosal trauma, as previously recommended.

3. Intubating Laryngeal Airway

a. History
The Intubating Laryngeal Airway (ILA, Cookgas L.L.C., St. Louis, MO) distributed by Mercury Medical (Clearwater, FL) is a new, Food and Drug Administration (FDA)-approved, reusable hypercurved intubating laryngeal airway invented by Dr. Daniel Cook, who spent over 8 years in its development. The ILA was introduced into clinical practice in December 2004 for airway management as an SGA or as a conduit for endotracheal intubation.

b. Device Description
The ILA is manufactured of medical grade silicon and is 100% latex free. There are ridges located in both the airway tube and the mask. The ridges below the airway connector were designed to improve the tube seal. They also allow easy removal of the connector during intubation through the device. The airway tube of the ILA is hypercurved to approximate the anatomy of the oral-pharyngeal passage, designed to eliminate the tendency to overbend and kink the airway tube (Fig. 22-4).

The large oval mask cavity allows intubation using standard ETs (sizes 5.0 to 8.5 mm). There is a keyhole-shaped airway outlet designed to direct the ETs toward the laryngeal inlet. It also creates ample space for other medical instruments used for intubation. There are three internal ridges located in the distal portion of the mask that approximate the anatomic shape of the posterior pharynx, which are designed to create increased airway stability, smooth insertion, and improved airway alignment.

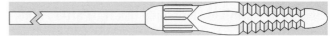

Figure 22-5 ILA Removal Stylet. (Courtesy of Dr. Daniel Cook.)

When the ILA cuff is inflated, these ridges move against the posterior larynx and improve the anterior mask seal, thus helping to isolate the esophagus and reduce the potential for aspiration.

Three ILA sizes are available (2.5, 3.5, and 4.5). Generally, the 2.5 is used in children and adolescents 20 to 50 kg (smallest size ET 5.0 mm), the 3.5 is used in small adults (50 to 70 kg), and the 4.5 is used in large adults (70 to 100 kg). They are available in half sizes because these fit a broader range of patients.

The removal following intubation is accomplished with the Cookgas ILA Removal Stylet (Fig. 22-5). This stylet was specifically designed to be used in conjunction with the ILA. The stylet stabilizes the previously inserted ET and allows controlled removal of the ILA without dislodging the ET from the trachea. It is manufactured with polypropylene and can be used up to 10 times. It must be cleansed in a detergent solution; it is not autoclavable, as is the ILA. The ILA Removal Stylet consists of an adapter connected to a rod. The adapter is tapered from bottom to top and has horizontal ridges and vertical grooves. The taper allows the stylet to accommodate standard ETs in multiple sizes (5.0 to 8.5 mm). It is designed with ridges and grooves, each serving a purpose. The ridges engage the ET in a firm, secure grip, giving the user control of the ET during the ILA removal process. The grooves allow spontaneously breathing patients unimpeded air passage within the ET during the removal of the ILA.

c. Insertion Technique and Device Removal
Before use, the integrity of the cuff and inflation system should be checked by completely deflating and reinflating the cuff with the maximum recommended volume of air (Tables 22-6 and 22-7). All air should then be removed

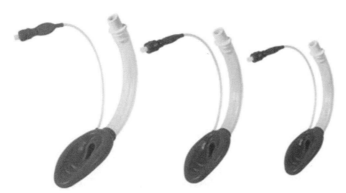

Figure 22-4 Intubating laryngeal airway. (Courtesy of Dr. Daniel Cook.)

Table 22-6 ILA Sizing Chart

Mask Size	Patient Weight (kg)
2.5	20-50
3.5	50-70
4.5	70-100

Courtesy of Tyco Healthcare.

Table 22-7   **LMA Cuff Pressures (cm H$_2$O) after Filling Completely Emptied Cuff with Recommended Volume of Air**

LMA/Size	1	1.5	2	2.5	3
Classic	71 ± 2	>120	>120	85 ± 5	97 ± 5
Unique	83 ± 1	>120	>120	>120	>120
ProSeal	NA	78 ± 3	70 ± 3	42 ± 2	18 ± 2
SoftSeal	62 ± 1	53 ± 3	34 ± 3	70 ± 2	55 ± 2
Marshall	48 ± 1	91 ± 5	107 ± 2	97 ± 2	>120
LaryngoSeal	>120	>120	>120	>120	>120

LMA, laryngeal mask airway.
Maino P: Eur J Anaesthesiol 22:A-572, 2005.

from the cuff by active aspiration with a syringe while pressing the anterior portion of the mask onto a sterile flat surface. The posterior portion of the device should be lubricated with a sterile, water-based lubricant just prior to insertion.

Although it is not necessary, insertion of the ILA is best accomplished with the patient's head and neck in the sniffing position (neck flexed and head extended). The use of a jaw lift is recommended during insertion. This maneuver elevates the epiglottis off the posterior pharyngeal wall, thereby enhancing passage and seating of the device. The ILA should be inserted using a technique similar to that used with the LMA, gently applying inward and downward pressure, using the curvature of the ILA mask and airway tube as a guide. Minimal manipulation may be necessary to turn the corner into the upper pharynx. The device should be passed into the hypopharynx until resistance is met. The cuff should then be inflated with air (10 to 20 cm^3) until a proper seal is obtained or up to an intracuff pressure of 60 cm H$_2$O. Usually, cuff inflation with 10 cm^3 of air is sufficient to achieve a seal. The breathing system is then connected to the 15-mm connector and adequacy of ventilation is assessed. If adequate ventilation is not obtained, an "up-down" movement may clear a downfolding epiglottis and remedy the situation. The ILA may now be utilized for airway management as a SGA. A bite block should be inserted alongside the tube and taped in place in the usual fashion.

If tracheal intubation is necessary or desired, ILA positioning should be assessed for optimal ventilation (i.e., easy airflow, higher tidal volumes). Before intubation, the laryngeal musculature and vocal cords must be relaxed by administration of either a local anesthetic or a muscle relaxant. The patient should be preoxygenated with 100% oxygen for 3 to 5 minutes. An appropriately sized ET (5.0 to 8.5 mm) should be prepared by completely deflating the ET cuff and lubricating the external surface. It is important to deflate the ET cuff completely to allow the ET to slide easily within the ILA.

The ILA connector should then be removed (but not discarded). The previously deflated and lubricated ET should be inserted through the ILA to a depth of approximately 12 to 15 cm, depending on the ILA size. This places the distal tip of the ET at or just proximal to the opening of the ILA airway tube within the mask cavity. There are several acceptable methods that can now be employed to advance the ET further into the trachea.

Fiberoptic Technique. A fiberoptic bronchoscope can be directly passed through the ET and into the trachea by indirect visualization. When the carina is visualized, the ET can be passed through the laryngeal inlet and into the proximal trachea, using the scope as a guide. The ET cuff can then be inflated, the scope removed, and the ET connector replaced. Adequacy of ventilation should be checked by capnography, adequate chest excursion, and auscultation of bilateral breath sounds.

Stylet Technique. An intubation stylet (Eschmann tracheal tube introducer or Frova intubation catheter) can be passed through the ET and into the trachea. By gently placing the fingers of the left hand over the cricoid cartilage, the stylet may be felt as it passes through the cricoid ring. When the stylet passes into the trachea, the ET is simply advanced over the stylet, through the laryngeal inlet, and into the trachea, using the intubation stylet as a guide. The ET cuff can then be inflated, the stylet removed, and the 15-mm ET connector replaced. Adequate ventilation should then be assessed, as described previously.

Blind Technique. The ET should be slowly advanced through the ILA in the direction of the laryngeal inlet. For spontaneously breathing patients, the circuit can be attached to the ET connector and capnography may be used as a guide to successful tracheal placement. The Beck Airway Airflow Monitor (Great Plains Ballistics, Lubbock, TX) can also be used to facilitate blind tracheal intubation. If resistance to further advancement is encountered, repositioning of the ILA should be performed. When successful tracheal intubation has been achieved, the ET cuff should be inflated and adequate ventilation should be assessed, as noted previously.

When proper position of the ET is confirmed, the 15-mm connector of the ET should be removed and the ILA Removal Stylet (tapered end first) should be placed into the proximal end of the ET until the adapter fits snugly within the ET. With firm inward pressure, the stylet adapter is rotated in a clockwise direction until the adapter firmly engages the ET. The cuff of the ILA should be deflated to allow easier removal of the device. While exerting an inward stabilizing force on the stylet, the ILA is slowly withdrawn outward over the ET-ILA stylet and out of the patient's mouth. The ILA stylet is unscrewed from the ET in the counterclockwise direction using outward tension on the ILA stylet in order to disengage it from the ET. The 15-mm connector can then be replaced on the ET and proper position of the ET in the trachea reconfirmed.

d. Indications and Advantages

As previously mentioned, the ILA was designed for airway management as a routine airway or as a conduit for either blind, stylet-guided, or fiberoptically guided endotracheal intubation. It should be used only in unconscious or adequately topically anesthetized patients. It incorporates design features that facilitate ease and reliability of insertion. Its larger bowl enhances entry into the mouth and passage along the oropharyngeal curve. The natural curve of its leading edge facilitates passage behind the epiglottis and arytenoid cartilages and into the upper esophageal inlet without the need for special deflation techniques or insertion devices. Each ILA accepts routinely used PVC ETs (2.5 can accommodate a 5.0- to 6.5-mm ET, 3.5 up to a 7.5-mm ET, and 4.5 up to an 8.5-mm ET).

Unlike the intubating LMA (ILMA), the ILA does not necessarily require removal when it has been used as a conduit. It can remain in place and later be used as a bridge to extubation during emergence. In addition, 10 cm^3 of air is usually sufficient to inflate the cuff of the ILA, and thus the same 10 cm^3 syringe routinely used for the ET cuff inflation can also be used for the ILA cuff inflation. Lastly, the ILA Removal Stylet is designed with grooves that allow spontaneous ventilation within the ET during ILA removal, thus facilitating the performance of awake or asleep intubation during spontaneous ventilation with this device.

e. Disadvantages

The ILA is nonsterile when delivered. It should be washed thoroughly and autoclaved prior to its use. The ILA Removal Stylet is also delivered nonsterile and should be washed with soap and water and rinsed with alcohol before its use. As with the ILMA, the ILA is available only in sizes that do not allow intubation of infants and young children. In addition, when simply used as a SAG SGA, it should not be used in anesthetized patients at increased risk for pulmonary aspiration of gastric contents, with poor lung compliance or increased airway resistance, or with lesions of the oropharynx or epiglottis. Its use as an emergency airway device has not been studied.

f. Comparison with Face Mask Ventilation and Endotracheal Intubation

In theory, the use of the ILA (when utilized as a SGA) should result in less dead space ventilation and minimal gastric inflation if reasonable airway pressures are used. It allows anesthesiologists to have their hands free to perform other tasks. Compression of the eyes and facial and infraorbital nerves is avoided, and operating room pollution from vapors and anesthetic is less likely.

g. Guide to Endotracheal Intubation

See "Insertion Technique and Device Removal."

h. Medical Literature

Thus far, there is little reported in the literature regarding the ILA. An observational study was performed by Klein and Jones[48] that involved 28 patients scheduled for gynecologic surgery. The ILA was used for endotracheal intubation in 22 patients. A FOB was passed down the lumen of the ILA following placement to evaluate its relationship to airway structures in the first 20 patients and to facilitate endotracheal intubation in selected patients. Blind passage of an ET was attempted in 6 of the first 20 patients and in all of the final 8 patients. They determined that the ILA is effective as a device for airway management and as a conduit for endotracheal intubation. The ILA was successfully placed on the first attempt in 27 of 28 (96.4%) patients. They found that leaks during manual ventilation could be corrected with slight withdrawal of the device. Although the glottis was visualized in all patients with the FOB, some degree of epiglottic downfolding was observed on fiberoptic examination on most cases. The "Klein maneuver" describes the correction of epiglottic downfolding by jaw lift and withdrawal of the ILA, followed by reinsertion. Intubation using the ILA as a conduit was 100% successful using fiberoptic guidance. Successful blind intubation was enhanced with the flexible reinforced tracheal tube (Mallinckrodt). Optimal techniques for blind intubation, as well as the utility of the device in difficult airways, require further investigation.

B. CUFFED PHARYNGEAL SEALERS

1. Laryngeal Tube

a. History

The Laryngeal Tube (LT) (VBM Medizintechnik, Sulz am Neckar, Germany) and King Laryngeal Tube (King Systems, Noblesville, IN) are SGA devices that were introduced to the European market in 1999[7] and to the United States in February 2003.

b. Device Description

The LT consists of a silicon reusable airway tube provided with two cuffs (pharyngeal and esophageal), a single balloon for pressure control,[7,35] and a 15-mm

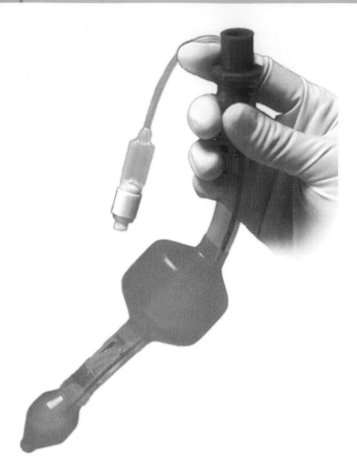

Figure 22-6 King Laryngeal Tube. (Courtesy of King Systems.)

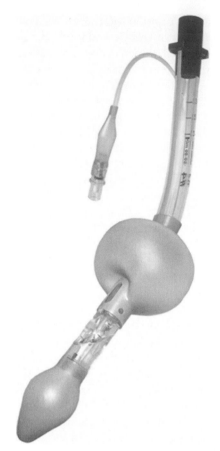

Figure 22-7 King Laryngeal Tube—disposable (Courtesy of King Systems.)

standard male adapter (Fig. 22-6), which is designed to be reused up to 50 times. The airway tube is short and J shaped; it has an average diameter of 11.5 mm and a blind tip. Six sizes, suitable for neonates up to large adults, are available[7,35] (Table 22-8). LT size selection must be based on the patient's weight from size 0 to 2 and on height from size 3 to 5. The disposable version (King LTD) is currently being sold in sizes 3 to 5 worldwide (Fig. 22-7). Pediatric sizes will become available in the near future.

Table 22-8   Laryngeal Tube Size Recommendations

Size	Use	Color
0	Infants < 5 kg	Transparent
1	Children 5-12 kg	White
2	Children 12-25 kg	Green
3	Adults with height < 155 cm	Yellow
4	Adults with height 155–180 cm	Red
5	Adults with height > 180 cm	Violet

Courtesy of King Systems.

After device insertion, the proximal cuff lies in the hypopharynx and the distal in the upper esophagus. Both cuffs are high volume and low pressure to avoid ischemic damage and permit a good seal. The original version of the LT was designed with a single ventilation opening between the two cuffs in the ventral part of the tube. This version also had two separate inflation lines for the two cuffs. Changes in the design of this device before its launch in the United States included two ventilation outlets rather than the one located between the two cuffs. The proximal cuff is protected by a bend located in a V dent of the pharyngeal cuff. With cuff inflation, soft tissue is deflected from this opening, helping to maintain a patent airway.[20] A wedge-shaped block closes the tip of the tube, diverting the inflated mixture to the trachea. The cuffs should be inflated, with the aid of the laryngeal cuff pressure gauge, to 60 cm H_2O. Because there is a single inflation line, both cuffs inflate simultaneously.

In addition, there are two side eyelets (one on either side of the main ventilation orifices). The latest version of the LTD has three side eyelets on each side to allow improved collateral ventilation should the epiglottis obstruct the main ventilation orifice. This version has also been manufactured 1.0 cm longer to facilitate deeper placement of the device, thus ensuring proper

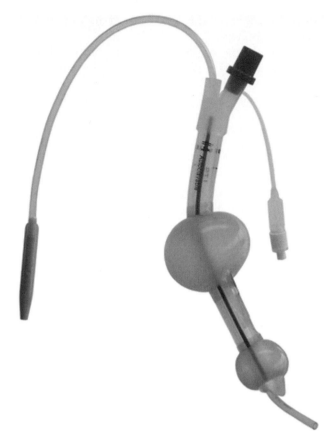

Figure 22-8 King Laryngeal Tube—Suction. (Courtesy of King Systems.)

positioning of the two main ventilation orifices and location of the proximal cuff beneath the tongue so that the epiglottis is more likely to be raised with cuff inflation in much the same manner as with a Macintosh laryngoscope blade.

The Laryngeal Tube Suction (LTS) is a double-lumen silicon LT that incorporates a second esophageal lumen placed behind the ventilatory lumen (Fig. 22-8). This second lumen represents a relief valve for increases in gastric pressure that permits gastric suctioning and egress of gastric contents.[28] Although this version of the LT is FDA 510(k) approved in the United States, the LTS is currently available only in Europe. Clinical trials involving a disposable version that differs in design from the silicon or reusable LT are to be conducted in the United States.

c. Insertion Technique and Device Removal

Before each use, the nondisposable LT must be cleaned and sterilized. The LT must first be washed in warm water using a mild soap or a diluent with 8% to 10% sodium bicarbonate solution. The LT must not be exposed to any chemicals, disinfectants, or cleaning agents not recommended for use with silicon. The LT should then be carefully inspected to ensure that all visible foreign matter has been removed. All air should be removed from the cuffs with a syringe prior to its sterilization.

When the cuffs are tightly deflated, the device may be placed in an appropriate autoclave-proof bag before autoclaving. Steam autoclaving is the only method recommended for the sterilization of this device. The maximum autoclave set-point temperature should not exceed 134° C at 2.4 bar for 10 minutes. After autoclaving and before each use, the cuffs of the LT should be checked for any leakage.

The LT should be placed after induction of anesthesia when the patient is apneic and loses the eyelash reflex and there is no resistance to manipulation of the lower jaw. If no muscle relaxing agent is used, anesthesia should be deep enough to obtund the airway reflexes. An appropriately sized LT should be chosen according to the selection criteria described previously. Before insertion, the cuffs must be fully and correctly deflated and lubricated. A neutral head position is ideal, although the sniffing position with jaw lift makes it easier to go around the corner in the posterior pharynx. The device characteristics ensure the placement of the tube for any given position of the head and of the operator. The LT should be held in the dominant hand and inserted blindly along the midline of the tongue with the tip against the hard palate in the caudal direction. Then it should be passed smoothly along the palate into the hypopharynx until resistance is felt.

The proximal and distal cuffs should then be inflated with the aid of the cuff pressure gauge (King Systems) to 60 cm H_2O. If it is not available or time is of the essence, the cuffs can be inflated with the aid of a dedicated syringe (Table 22-9). Because of the specially designed inflation line, the proximal cuff is first filled, stabilizing the tube. When the proximal cuff adjusts to the anatomy of the patient, the distal cuff automatically inflates. The LT can be now connected to the breathing system. Indicators of correct LT placement are auscultation of bilateral lung sounds, bilateral chest excursion, absence of gastric insufflation, and capnography. When the LT is correctly positioned, the bite block can be attached to the tube.

Correct placement of the LT may be verified using a test with a light wand (Trachlight) without the metallic stylet. The light wand can be inserted into the LT and advanced through it until a faint glow can be seen above

Table 22-9 **Maximum Laryngeal Tube Cuff Volumes**

Mask Size	Maximum Cuff Volume (mL)
0	10
1	20
2	35
3	60
4	80
5	90

Courtesy of King Systems.

the thyroid prominence. It indicates that the tip of the light wand is just in front of the laryngeal inlet. The light wand can be advanced still further until a well-defined circumscribed glow is seen in the anterior neck slightly below the thyroid prominence. When the LT is correctly positioned, the light wand tip easily enters into the glottic opening, showing a well-defined circumscribed glow. The Trachlight test must be considered negative when transillumination shows a glow with a halo near the thyroid prominence. This could be due to the Trachlight tip lying against the epiglottis or the glossoepiglottic fold. The visualization of a lateral glow indicates that the hole for ventilation is not in front of the laryngeal inlet even though ventilation may be effective.

After LT placement, respiration is initially supported by manual ventilation and the patient is allowed to resume spontaneous ventilation. Even when spontaneous ventilation is planned, it is suitable to use positive-pressure ventilation initially, thus ensuring good ventilation in addition to providing information about correct LT placement.

The LT is well tolerated until the return of the protective reflexes. Slight cuff deflation at this point allows better toleration of the oropharyngeal cuff. The device should be removed with the patient either deeply anesthetized or totally awake; otherwise, laryngospasm, coughing, or gagging may occur. Before removal of the device, the cuffs should be completely deflated. Inadequate cuff deflation can make removal difficult, risking cuff damage and discomfort for the patient.

d. Indications and Advantages

The LT is designed for use during spontaneous or controlled ventilation. The slim profile of the LT allows easy insertion with little mouth opening; thus, it can be considered for airway management in patients with restricted mouth opening. The insertion is relatively easy and guarantees a clear airway in most patients on the first attempt, and extensive training is not necessary.

Because of the form and length of the tube, an inadvertent endotracheal intubation should not occur. The LT is associated with an extremely low incidence of trauma with respect to sore throat, hoarseness, or blood compared to other SGA devices. This is due to the soft tip, soft cuff material, and low cuff pressures. High-volume, low-pressure cuffs provide a good seal and protect against ischemic damage; the presence of only one pilot balloon allows quick cuff inflation; and it is useful in emergency situations.

As a supraglottic device, the LT can be used to detect laryngopharyngeal activity and can provide information about the depth of anesthesia in nonparalyzed patients. Inactivity of the vocal cords is considered an important indicator of depth of anesthesia in nonparalyzed patients. As with any SGA, surgical stimulation can cause laryngospasm. Vocal cord activity may be detected by alteration of capnography and airway resistance. If vocal cord activity is present, the flow-volume monitoring shows alterations of the loop related to the laryngeal resistor component.

In addition, the ventilation can be controlled by the LT during attempts at fiberoptic nasotracheal intubation. Both the FOB and the ET can be advanced through the nose into the oral cavity without deflating the cuffs of the LT. When endotracheal intubation is determined to be successful, the cuffs of the LT can be deflated and the device removed.

e. Disadvantages

At present, it is not prudent to use the LT in anesthetized patients at increased risk for pulmonary aspiration of gastric contents. Also, the LT may not be appropriate in patients with poor lung compliance or increased airway resistance or patients with lesions of the oropharynx or epiglottis. Lastly, the LT cannot prevent or treat airway obstruction at or beyond the glottis.

f. Comparison with Face Mask Ventilation and Endotracheal Intubation

Because of the presence of the ventilation holes and the interval wedge-shaped block, three maneuvers are possible: (1) aspiration of blood and secretions, (2) passage of an FOB, and (3) passage of a tube exchanger. Compared with the face mask, the LT allows better access to the airway, resulting in minimal dead space and gastric inflation. Furthermore, the LT allows anesthesiologists to have their hands free and reduces environmental pollution from vapors and anesthetic gas.

g. Guide to Endotracheal Intubation

The trachea can be intubated using small ETs (up to 6.5 mm), which can be passed blindly through the LT. The ET connector must be removed and the tube must be well lubricated. The tip of the ET is gently advanced forward until it passes through the glottic opening. Resistance can be due to incorrect positioning of the LT, epiglottis obstruction of ET passage, or inadequate lubrication of the ET. This procedure can be visualized by video laryngoscopy using the DCI Video Intubation System (Karl Storz Endoscopy, Culver City, CA). When the ET is positioned, the cuffs of the LT must be deflated and the device can then be removed. The shorter tube shaft on the LT, compared with the LMA, allows the ET to be inserted far enough so that the cuff can be placed as desired in the trachea without removal of the LT. Unless indicated otherwise, the LT should remain in place with both cuffs deflated after tracheal intubation has been performed. The disadvantage of this procedure is that the diameter of the ET is limited by the LT size. Because removal of the LT over the ET can be problematic, exchanging the ET and LT using a tube exchanger and then passing a larger ET, if desired and appropriate, is recommended.

To overcome this problem, a tube exchanger may be used. Tracheal intubation through the LT can be performed also with fiberoptic placement of the Aintree airway exchange catheter (Cook Critical Care) (see Chapter 47). Throughout the procedure, oxygen administration can continue through the LT until its removal using a Bodai adapter (Sontek Medical, Lexington, MA).[38]

h. Medical Literature

Most available trials have used earlier revisions of the LT rather than the currently available device. Nonetheless, the results of these trials are mostly positive. Doerges, Asai, and their colleagues determined that after blind insertion, the device provides a patent airway in the majority of patients at the first attempt.[17,28] The LT tube can be inserted quickly without extensive training; it is considered a suitable airway management device with a high rate of successful insertion, requiring a mouth opening as limited as 23 mm.[34,36] LT placement is easy,[34] and its acceptance among physicians, nurses, and paramedics is high.[4,5] Simple handling and aspiration protection are its substantial advantages.[28] Correct LT positioning may require more adjustments in patients with an increased body mass index.[9]

Insertion time is comparable to that with the LMA.[28] Asai and colleagues[16] reported successful use of the LT in three patients in whom insertion of the LMA had failed. These authors hypothesized that the success and failure might have been related to a difference in the width of these two devices. The pharyngeal space was narrowed by swollen tonsils, goiter, and redundant oropharyngeal tissue; thus, they recommended that when LMA insertion is difficult or impossible because of a narrowed pharynx, insertion of the LT may be attempted before considering endotracheal intubation.

Halothane, enflurane, isoflurane, sevoflurane, desflurane, and total intravenous anesthesia may be used for maintenance of anesthesia with the LT. Nitrous oxide may be used to maintain anesthesia, although cuff pressures should be monitored with its use.[13,32] A rise of 15 cm H_2O in the intracuff pressure 30 minutes after its insertion caused by diffusion of nitrous oxide into the cuff has been demonstrated.[13,32]

Ventilation achieved with the LT is comparable to that obtained with other SGAs. In fact, its seal pressure has been found to be better than that of the standard LMA.[61] It provides a good airway seal to 30 cm H_2O of airway pressure[15,17] and has been shown to be efficacious during mechanical ventilation in adult and pediatric patients undergoing elective surgery.[7,17,65]

Because of the ease of insertion and a good airtight seal, the LT may have a potential role in airway management during cardiopulmonary resuscitation.[65] It was reported that 28 Fire Defense Academy students who had experience with the LMA could insert the LT on the first attempt in mannequins; the majority of participants stated that its insertion was easier than insertion of the LMA.[12] Doerges and coauthors[28] confirmed that the LT allows immediate ventilation of the patient, possibly decreasing the evidence of further oxygen desaturation in difficult conditions such as cardiopulmonary resuscitation without the possibility of preoxygenation.

Numerous studies have shown the King LT to be effective during mechanical ventilation,[22,25,28,32] but there are some studies, most notably that of Miller and colleagues,[60] which found the King LT to be unsatisfactory for spontaneous ventilation. The findings of Miller and colleagues were based on a frequent failure rate (7 of 17 patients) secondary to loss of airway control during surgery. These findings were based on a first-generation model of the LT manufactured by VBM (Sulz am Neckar, Germany) that did not feature a second large ventilation aperture and two lateral ventilatory openings that were present in the first-generation King LT (King Systems).

In a study by Hagberg and coworkers,[40] the King LT was demonstrated to be a reliable SGA for airway management during elective surgery with spontaneous ventilation. In this study the mean depth of insertion was higher than expected for each size of the King LT; thus, the company now manufactures this device 1 cm larger in the silicon version and 2 cm larger in the disposable version. The first-time placement success rate was 86%, consistent with the first-time placement rates of 85% to 95% found in previous studies.[17,22,36] The King LT provided a good airtight seal in most patients and often there was no gas leak around the cuff at an airway pressure of 25 cm H_2O, which is comparable to findings in studies conducted by Asai and others.[14,15,62] However, in unfasted patients and in some elective procedures (e.g., positioning in the prone position), endotracheal intubation is still required to protect the patient from aspiration.[27,66] Although the design of the LT or King LT is such that it should minimize the risk of aspiration, as with the Combitube, further study is warranted in a large number of patients at high risk for aspiration and regurgitation.

2. Cobra PLA

a. History

The Cobra perilaryngeal airway (Cobra PLA, Engineered Medical Systems, Indianapolis, IN) (Fig. 22-9) was introduced into the anesthetic community in 1997 when Dr. David Alfery modified a well-known instrument helpful in airway management, the Guedel oral airway. The initial idea was to modify the Guedel airway in order to accomplish mask ventilation in the most difficult airways encountered. The first changes consisted of lengthening and widening the distal end of the Guedel airway and placing a slot in the widened end to accommodate the epiglottis. This modification of the airway functioned quite well to hold soft tissues away from the laryngeal inlet, but a decision was soon made to convert it into an SGA device.

Thus, the proximal portion of the airway was attached to a breathing tube, adding a circumferential cuff proximal to the distal breathing hole, modifying the shape of

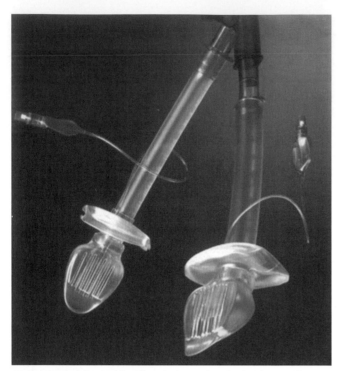

Figure 22-9 Cobra perilaryngeal airway (PLA). (Courtesy of Engineered Medical Systems.)

the distal "cobra head" portion, putting a 15-mm adapter on the proximal end, and adding a grill to the distal anterior surface. Later refinements to the product included a distal flexible tongue, an internal ramp inside the Cobra head to help guide an ET into the glottis, a temperature monitor to be able to measure core temperature, and a distal gas-sampling port on the pediatric models, the Cobra PLUS.

b. Device Description

The Cobra PLA consists of a breathing tube with a circumferential inflatable cuff proximal to the ventilation outlet portion, a 15-mm standard adapter, and a distal widened Cobra head that holds soft tissues apart and allows ventilation of the trachea. When in proper position, the Cobra head lies in front of the laryngeal inlet and seals the hypopharynx. In this respect, it differs from many other SGAs as the distal tip lies proximal to the esophageal inlet. Internal to the Cobra head, there is a ramp to direct the breathing gas (or an ET) into the trachea. Over the distal anteriorly placed breathing hole of the Cobra head, there is a soft grill. This feature helps deflect the epiglottis off the Cobra head, preventing the epiglottis from obstructing the breathing hole. The bars of the grill are flexible enough to allow passage of an ET when that maneuver is performed. The cuff is circumferential and is shaped to reside in the hypopharynx at the base of the tongue. When inflated, it raises the base of the tongue, exposing the laryngeal inlet, as well as affecting an airway seal, thus allowing positive-pressure ventilation to be carried out.

The device is named Cobra because of the shape of the distal part of the airway; when turned over and looked at on end, it appears similar to the head of a cobra snake. This special shape allows the device to pass more easily along the hard palate during the insertion procedure and holds soft tissues widely away from the laryngeal inlet, once in place. "Perilaryngeal" refers to the fact that the widened distal Cobra end pushes soft tissues away from the laryngeal inlet and describes its anatomic location.

The Cobra PLA is available in eight sizes according to the weight and size of the patient (Table 22-10). The proper size is that which comfortably fits through the patient's mouth. Generally, the size indication is a No. 3 for most female patients, a No. 4 for most men, and a No. 5 for larger men. When unsure of the appropriate size, especially when learning placement technique, it is advisable to pick the smaller of any two sizes under consideration. When a practitioner is comfortable with insertion technique, and especially when a muscle relaxant has been administered (providing maximal jaw relaxation, which aids passage of the Cobra PLA), it is possible to choose the larger of two sizes under consideration. Again, the most important consideration is to choose a size that fits through the patient's mouth without undue difficulty. There is a range of potential weights of patients for any given Cobra PLA size because of body habitus differences in patients with mouths of equivalent size. In fact, the size 3 Cobra PLA has been successfully used in patients smaller than 40 to 130 kg (Dr. David Affrey, personal communication). The manufacturer's suggested range for each size is indicated in Table 22-10. It can be noted that for most weights two or more sizes are considered and that there is no suggested upper limit for any given size. The reason is that a patient with a relatively high weight may have a very small mouth in relation to his or her weight.

Agro and colleagues[2] suggested the following range for choosing the Cobra PLA size: size 3 less than 60 kg, size 4 between 60 and 80 kg, and size 5 greater than

Table 22-10   Cobra PLA Sizes

Size	Weight (kg)
½	2.5-7.5
1	5-15
1½	10-35
2	20-60
3	40-100
4	70-130
5	100-160
6	>130

PLA, perilaryngeal airway.

Table 22-11 **Range for Choosing the Cobra Size Suggested by Agrò et al**

Size	Weight (kg)
3	<60
4	60-80
5	>80

From Agrò F, Barzoi G, Gallì B: The Cobra PLA in 110 anaesthetized and paralysed patients: What size to choose? [letter]. Br J Anaesth 92: 777-778, 2004.

80 kg (Table 22-11). In this study, relatively large Cobra PLAs were used because the author was skilled in the insertion technique, scissoring the mouth open and performing jaw lift (Agro maneuver), and patients were given muscle relaxants. When using Agro's range, the cuff inflation volume can be reduced from the maximum recommended by the manufacturer (Table 22-12). In this fashion, the cuffs can function similarly to the cuffs on ETs, as high-volume, low-pressure cuffs. In addition, use of these larger sizes allows considerably higher cuff sealing pressures to be obtained (if desired) than those that result from choosing lower sizes.

A newly patented Cobra PLUS is to be released in the near future. It combines the advancement of the Cobra PLA plus monitoring of core temperature on all adult sizes. For pediatric sizes, the Cobra PLUS combines both core temperature and distal CO_2 monitoring.[67]

c. Insertion Technique and Device Removal

The Cobra PLA is easily inserted in most cases, with the insertion technique simple to carry out. First, the cuff is fully deflated and folded back against the breathing tube. A lubricant is liberally applied to the front and the back of the Cobra head and to the cuff, with care taken to avoid obstructing the anterior situated grill. The patient's head and neck are positioned in the sniffing position and the mouth is opened with a scissor maneuver by one's nondominant hand, gently pulling the mandible upward. The Cobra PLA tip should not be directed against the

Table 22-12 **Cobra PLA Cuff Inflation Volumes Suggested by Manufacturer and by Agrò et al***

Size	Volume (mL) (Manufacturer)	Volume (mL) (Agrò et al)
3	<65	26.5 ± 2.1
4	<70	31.9 ± 4.0
5	<85	40.0 ± 4.1

PLA, perilaryngeal airway.
*Agro F, Barzoi G, Galli B: The Cobra PLA in 110 anaesthetized and paralysed patients: What size to choose? [letter]. Br J Anaesth 92: 777-778, 2004.

hard palate, as is often done when inserting an LMA.[19] This maneuver could make insertion more difficult by increasing the curve that the device tip must take at the back of the mouth. Rather, the distal end of the Cobra PLA is directed straight back between the tongue and hard palate. When the Cobra head is inserted into the mouth, an anteriorly directed jaw lift maneuver should be effected with the nondominant hand while inserting the device with the dominant hand. Conversely, pushing the jaw downward makes insertion more difficult. In addition, modest neck extension (without jaw lift maneuver) may aid passage of the device as it turns toward the glottis at the back of the mouth.

When the Cobra PLA is advanced to the back of the mouth, it often turns caudally toward the larynx with minimal resistance, as the flexible distal tip (or tongue) guides the device downward. Alternatively, in some situations a gentle push past posterior resistance is required to orient the Cobra PLA toward moving to its final position. The Cobra PLA is correctly seated when modest resistance to further distal passage is encountered as the device tip reaches the glottis. When positioning is correct, the flexible tip lies under the arytenoids, the ramp-grill lifts the epiglottis, and the cuff lies in the hypopharynx at the base of the tongue.

The smallest Cobra PLAs have a unique feature in that the distal gas-sampling port is located in the head of the Cobra, directly adjacent to where exhaled gas leaves the trachea. This is especially useful in newborns and infants, in whom very rapid respiratory rates and low tidal volumes result in inaccurate gas-sampling values when obtained from the Y-circuit connector to a supraglottic device. Distal gas sampling from the Cobra head removes much of the dead space from the gas sampling in the smallest patients, resulting in more accurate end-tidal gas-sampling levels.

Following proper positioning of the Cobra PLA, the cuff can be inflated. Initial cuff inflation should be done with less than the maximum volume recommended until there is no leak with positive-pressure ventilation (minimal leakage technique). When an adequate depth of anesthesia is achieved, the cardiovascular response to the Cobra PLA insertion appears be similar to that following placement of other SGA devices and less than that with laryngoscopy and endotracheal intubation.

Manual ventilation is performed to confirm correct placement and to measure the pressure at which an audible leak occurs. Indicators of correct placement are auscultation of neck, bilateral lung sounds and chest excursion, absence of gastric insufflation, and positive capnometry. It is not advisable to ventilate with more than 25 cm H_2O of airway pressure, even when testing for ventilation and cuff seal, because gastric insufflation may occur at pressures over this level.

As previously mentioned, it is recommended to inflate the cuff with only enough air to achieve a good seal. The cuff should never be overinflated. If possible, a cuff pressure gauge should be utilized to monitor intracuff pressure (60 cm H_2O approximately). If positive-pressure ventilation is carried out, ventilation pressures should be limited to approximately 20 to 25 cm H_2O. This is accomplished by setting a low inspiratory flow rate and then adjusting the tidal volume. If adequate ventilation is not achieved, it is possible that the Cobra PLA is inserted too far; in that case, it must be pulled back 1 to 2 cm. Halothane, enflurane, isoflurane, sevoflurane, desflurane, and total intravenous anesthesia are all acceptable for maintenance of anesthesia with the Cobra PLA. Patients may be allowed to breathe spontaneously or may be mechanically ventilated according to the desires of the anesthesiologist.

With respect to insertion of the Cobra PLA, some practical points should be borne in mind. First, an adequate depth of anesthesia should be achieved before insertion is attempted. Laryngospasm may occur and has been attributed to attempting to insert the device at too light a level of anesthesia. Second, if the size of the Cobra PLA is unsuitable for the patient, it can be removed and a new size reinserted with minimal trauma to the oropharynx. Third, if the Cobra PLA is not inserted far enough, inflation of the cuff may cause the tongue to protrude from the patient's mouth and an adequate seal may not be achieved. In this case, it should be advanced further or a smaller Cobra PLA chosen for use when properly positioned. The cuff should not be visible at the base of the tongue when the mouth is opened. Fourth, it is possible to advance the Cobra PLA past the laryngeal inlet, in which case ventilation is not possible. This is most often encountered on initial insertions (as one is learning insertion technique) and when a smaller Cobra PLA is used. The solution to this problem is merely to pull back the airway 1 to 2 cm and reattempt ventilation. This step can be repeated as necessary. Overall, proper insertion technique of the Cobra PLA can be easily mastered within 5 to 10 insertions and often on the first attempt.[2]

When the patient responds to simple commands such as "open your mouth," the cuff may be partially deflated and the Cobra PLA gently withdrawn from the patient. The partial deflation of the cuff allows it to squeeze secretions up out of the mouth as the Cobra PLA is removed.

d. Indications and Advantages

The precise indications for use of the Cobra PLA have not been fully established, but they should be similar to those for other SGAs. However, it is fundamental to emphasize that this device cannot be relied on to protect the upper airway from aspiration in anesthetized patients. Thus, elective use should be confined to patients not at risk for regurgitation or vomiting of gastric contents.

The Cobra PLA is designed for spontaneous and controlled ventilation. It can be used as a rescue airway in either CICV or CIDV scenarios. Because the Cobra PLA does not provide airway protection, it is advisable

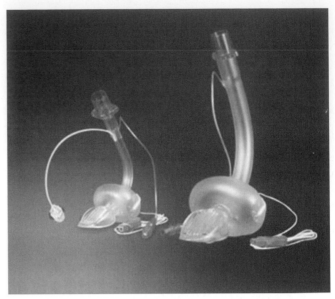

Figure 22-10 Cobra PLUS. (Courtesy of Engineered Medical Systems.)

to facilitate endotracheal intubation in order to secure the airway if the patient is considered a risk for aspiration.

Another important advantage of the Cobra PLA that is particularly useful in the management of emergency airway problems is that the insertion technique is very simple, and even when it is used by personnel with little or no experience in supraglottic devices (as evidenced by physicians' experience when beginning their residency training), success is often achieved.[2] Thus, it could be useful for those who undertake airway management infrequently. A large clinical study is under way evaluating the use of the Cobra PLA in the out-of-hospital emergency airway situation when difficulty in establishing an adequate airway is encountered.

There are additional advantages afforded by the Cobra PLUS (Fig. 22-10), which involves monitoring of core body temperature as well as distal CO_2 monitoring in the pediatric-sized devices.

e. Disadvantages

Because airway pressures should be limited to no greater than 20 to 25 cm H_2O, the Cobra PLA may not be appropriate for patients with reduced lung compliance or increased airway resistance. The major disadvantage of the device is that it does not protect against aspiration and does not secure the airway as effectively as the tracheal tube. In addition, the Cobra PLA cannot prevent or treat airway obstruction at or beyond the larynx.

f. Comparison with Face Mask Ventilation and Endotracheal Intubation

In contrast to the face mask, the Cobra PLA is associated with less dead space ventilation and no gastric inflation if reasonable airway pressures are used. Furthermore, it allows the anesthesiologist to have hands free for other important tasks (such as administration of drugs). Compression of eyes and facial and infraorbital nerves is avoided, and operating room pollution from vapors and anesthetic gas is less likely.

Compared with an ET, the Cobra PLA is easier to place, avoids laryngoscopy and its associated problems, and is less invasive. Furthermore, the insertion of this device does not require the use of muscle relaxant drugs.

g. Guide to Endotracheal Intubation

The Cobra PLA may be used as a intubation conduit. This may be done by loading a standard ET onto an FOB and then passing it into the lumen of the Cobra PLA. When the device is correctly positioned and the distal breathing hole is opposite the vocal cords, the internal ramp directs the FOB directly toward the larynx. When the FOB has passed through the vocal cords, the ET can be advanced into the trachea and the FOB removed. The large diameter of the Cobra PLA permits the passage of an adequately sized ET, as indicated in Table 22-13. The Cobra PLA can be left in place with its cuff deflated while ventilation is carried out by the ET.

When an FOB is not available and the Trachlight (TL) is available, it is also possible to execute a semiblind technique for airway rescue.[3,4,29] Once the Cobra PLA has been inserted and an emergency airway successfully achieved, the TL, with the rigid internal stylet removed and, with a standard ET tube loaded onto it is inserted into the lumen of the Cobra PLA. When a bright halo of the TL is transilluminated in the anterior part of the neck underneath the proximal trachea, it indicates that the breathing hole of the Cobra PLA is directly in front of the vocal cords and the TL is correctly positioned in the trachea.[8] The ET can then be passed over the TL and the TL removed. Blind intubation through the Cobra PLA by simply advancing an ET through it or by using a bougie guide may be successful, but passage into the trachea is not consistently obtained, and the preceding techniques are far preferable in the emergency situation.

Table 22-13 **Passage of Endotracheal Tube into the Cobra PLA**

Cobra Size	ET Size (mm)
½	3.0
1	4.5
1½	4.5
2	6.5
3	6.5
4	8.0
5	8.0
6	8.0

ET, endotracheal tube; PLA, perilaryngeal airway.

Unlike other supraglottic devices, it has been made short enough to allow a standard ET to be passed through it far enough that the cuff resides below the vocal cords. Thus, when it is used in this manner, it is not necessary to use an especially long ET (such as a nasal Ring-Adair-Elwyn or microlaryngoscopy tube) to remove the Cobra PLA or to do additional maneuvers to accomplish this goal.

h. Medical Literature

There is limited medical literature related to the use of the Cobra PLA because it is such a new medical product. The first report of use of the Cobra PLA in a peer-reviewed journal was that of Agro and colleagues[1] in 2003, which involved 28 anesthetized and mechanically ventilated patients. Although the investigating team had experienced only insertion of the Cobra PLA in mannequins when the study commenced, they still reported successful insertion in 100% of patients within 10 ± 3 seconds. Immediate ventilation was achieved in 57% of patients, and 43% required a positioning maneuver (e.g., pulling back) to achieve success. The need for adjusting the position of the Cobra PLA was related to an increased body mass index. Oxygen saturation always remained greater than 98%, and there were no complications. In a later study, Agro and others studied a series of 110 patients.[2] Successful insertion was observed in every patient (no failures) in 6.8 ± 2 seconds. Again, there were no adverse airway events or significant complications. They were able to achieve mean cuff leak pressures of 34 cm H_2O using very low cuff inflation volumes by choosing relatively large Cobra PLAs.

Akca and coauthors[10] compared the uLMA with the Cobra PLA in a randomized series of 81 patients. They reported that insertion times, airway adequacy, number of repositioning episodes, and minor complications were similar in both groups of patients. However, the cuff sealing pressure of the Cobra PLA was significantly greater than that of the uLMA (23 ± 6 versus 18 ± 5 cm H_2O). They also found cuff sealing pressures to be lower than those found by Agro, most likely because Akca and associates used smaller Cobra PLAs. Finally, Gaitini and coworkers[31] presented a study that compared the uLMA, the Cobra PLA, and the Pharyngeal Airway Xpress (PAXpress). In this study, which comprised 25 patients in each group, the authors found that the three devices were equivalent in providing safe and effective airways, with the Cobra PLA having significantly higher cuff leak pressures (33 ± 6 cm H_2O for the Cobra PLA, 24 ± 5 cm H_2O for the PAXpress, and 20 ± 5 cm H_2O for the uLMA) and a better fiberoptic score (i.e., better positioning in front of the vocal cords) than with the other two devices.

Szmuk and others[68] have described the use of the Cobra PLA in an elective case with a known difficult airway. They reported use in a 2.3-kg, 3-week-old infant undergoing G-button placement for feeding access. This infant suffered from Desbuquois syndrome, a rare condition characterized by multiple congenital anomalies including hypoplastic midfacies, subluxation of C5-6, and thoracic abnormalities. This constellation of findings results in an airway that is known to be difficult to intubate, and the authors successfully managed the airway using a size 1/2 Cobra PLA.

To date, there are three reports of an airway rescue using the Cobra PLA. In the first, Agro and colleagues[5] describe a patient who experienced sudden airway obstruction following extubation after undergoing a total thyroidectomy. As the initial intubation in this patient had been difficult, the airway was emergently secured using a Cobra PLA. Following this maneuver, an ET was advanced into the trachea using bronchoscopic guidance. In the second report, Szmuk and coauthors[68] discuss a patient undergoing a cadaver kidney transplant in whom orotracheal intubation proved impossible to achieve and bag and mask ventilation was carried out only with difficulty. A Cobra PLA was inserted, ventilation easily achieved, and an ET was passed into the trachea under fiberoptic guidance. The operation was then carried out with the Cobra PLA left in place, and the Cobra PLA and ET were removed as a unit at the end of the case.

In the third report, Agro and colleagues[6] used the Cobra PLA in a 71-year-old male patient with respiratory failure during the performance of a cricothyrotomy following the Griggs technique. The FOB, through the Cobra PLA, permitted an internal view of the tracheostomy site so that the anesthesiologist could observe the needle and guidewire entering the trachea by ensuring the proper placement of the introducer and dilator while having continuous airway control.

From these initial reports, it appears that the Cobra PLA functions quite well as an SGA, with some unique advantages (e.g., ability to pass a standard ET fully into the trachea) for both elective and emergency situations. The final place for the Cobra PLA in airway management will be determined after additional experience with its use and additional studies are reported.

C. CUFFLESS PRESHAPED SEALERS

1. Streamlined Liner of the Pharynx Airway

a. History

The SLIPA (Hudson Respiratory Care, Temecula, CA) airway is named as such because it is an acronym for Streamlined Liner of the Pharynx Airway and because it looks like a slipper.[57] The SLIPA was developed by Dr. Donald Miller, whose motivation for developing the device was his personal experience with three inconsequential aspirations in elective fasted children, who regurgitated and aspirated small quantities of bile-stained fluid during the emergent phase of anesthesia (personal communication). This triggered the idea of an airway that lined the pharynx to provide an enlarged cavity for trapping regurgitated liquids before pulmonary aspiration occurs. This idea made a cuff inflation mechanism for sealing to achieve positive-pressure ventilation not only

less necessary but also less desirable, as any cuff inflating mechanism occupies space, thus decreasing storage capacity. In addition, a device without a cuff inflating mechanism decreases manufacturer's costs, thus achieving a less expensive single-use airway device.

Although the SLIPA was launched and has been commercially available in Europe since June 2004, production stopped when there was a change in the manufacturer of the device (Hudson to Teleflex). At that time 510(k) or FDA approval was not necessary. The product should be available for sale again soon, and FDA approval is now pending.

b. Device Description

The SLIPA is a new type of SGA, fabricated from soft plastic with an anatomically preformed shape that lines the pharynx. Thus, positive-pressure ventilation may be achieved without a cuff inflating mechanism that is required in other SGAs, such as the LMA. It comprises a hollow, blow-molded chamber shaped like a boot with a toe (T), bridge (B) that seals at the base of the tongue, and a heel (H) (Fig. 22-11), which anchors the device in a stable position between the esophagus and nasopharynx.[58]

Toward the tow side of the lateral bulges of the bridge are smaller secondary lateral bulges leaving an indentation (I in Fig. 22-11), the positions of which were extrapolated from a study on cadavers to coincide with the tips of the hyoid bone. The design aims at relieving pressure at this vulnerable anatomic site[59] and should thereby prevent damage to the hypoglossal nerve and perhaps also the recurrent laryngeal nerve from pressure effects that may occur with cuff inflating devices.[21,49,51,69]

As the device is hollow, a limited volume of pharyngeal secretions or regurgitated liquids can pass through the anterior hole and be trapped within the airway, thereby providing some protection from aspiration. The chamber provides a large capacity (50 mL in the equivalent SLIPA [size 53] compared with 3.5 mL in the LMA [size 4]) for providing maximum but limited storage of regurgitated liquids should they arise from the stomach, thus preventing their inadvertent overflow into the trachea.[58] The safety advantages of simplicity and minimization of aspiration risk of a device without a cuff inflating mechanism necessitate double the number of sizes in order to obtain a good-quality seal for positive-pressure ventilation.

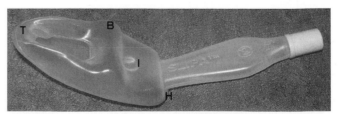

Figure 22-11 Streamlined Liner of the Pharynx Airway. (Courtesy of Dr. Donald Miller.)

There are currently six adult sizes: 47, 49, 51, 53, 55, and 57. Sizes 47, 49, and 51 are suitable for small, medium, and large females and sizes 53, 55, and 57 are suitable for small, medium, and large males. The numbers refer to the widest transverse diameter (in mm) at the level of the bridge. Matching this dimension to the distance between left and right cornua of the thyroid cartilage is a useful and possibly even more precise method of choosing the correct size.

c. Insertion Technique and Device Removal

Insertion technique differs from that of the LMA because it passes the oropharyngeal curve with greater ease and it is not helpful to try pushing it up against the hard palate. Insertion simply requires extension of the head and advancement of the device toward the esophagus until the heel of the device spontaneously locates itself in the nasopharynx. As with most other SGAs, it is helpful if an assistant lifts the jaw forward during insertion. Alternatively, the anesthesiologist can lift the jaw forward with the thumb and finger.

The crescent shape of the tow lowers the risk of obstructing the airway, whether caused by folding the epiglottis down or by invoking laryngospasm. The toe of the chamber slips easily into the entrance to the esophagus, where it seals against the cricopharyngeus sphincter. The bridge in the center of the chamber with its two lateral bulges fits into the pyriform fossa at the base of the tongue, which it displaces away from the posterior pharyngeal wall, thus helping to prevent the epiglottis from closing on the glottis. The anterior opening in the SLIPA achieves the same effect by means of the narrowed lower portion that keeps a particularly long epiglottis from closing completely on the glottis. The heel of the chamber anchors the SLIPA in position by sliding over the soft palate and nasopharyngeal opening. Once positioned, it provides a reliable airway with no need for further manipulation.

It is usually not necessary for the SLIPA to be tied or strapped into position. The hollow chamber is able to flatten to facilitate insertion, and once in position, it reverts spontaneously to its preinsertion shape. In addition, because there is no cuff to deflate, the SLIPA can be removed when there is return of protective airway reflexes.

d. Indications and Advantages

The SLIPA is a simple, inexpensive disposable device designed to minimize the risk of aspiration during controlled ventilation. The SLIPA consists of a hollow blow-molded soft plastic airway shaped to form a seal in the pharynx rather than an inflatable cuff. This design feature of being hollow allows liquid entrapment, thus possibly providing protection against aspiration. Although the SLIPA may provide this protection, its use is still recommended only in types of cases similar to those in which other SGAs are recommended.

As with the use of other SGAs, use of the SLIPA does not require paralysis or laryngoscopy with its inherent risks and disadvantages; thus, there is less cardiovascular stress than with tracheal intubation as well as a decreased incidence of sore throats. Also, it is designed without a cuff. Because no cuff is necessary for the device to seal in the pharynx, the cost of production of the SLIPA, compared with other SGAs, is decreased. Furthermore, because of its unique design, once it is in place, a need to manipulate and manage the airway is unlikely.

e. Disadvantages

Appropriate sizing of the SLIPA to the patient is necessary because the dimensions of the airway need to match for this device to form a seal; thus, many sizes need to be available and there is a greater possibility that the wrong size may be chosen. Indeed, the literature reflects that when difficulty was encountered, it appeared to be associated with incorrect size selection. Matching of the width of the thyroid cartilage to the SLIPA's dimension aids in the appropriate choice of device size. Several studies have been conducted on the function of this device in laboratory models only. Randomized clinical trials may be required to establish the role of the SLIPA in relation to other airway devices.

f. Comparison with Face Mask Ventilation and Endotracheal Intubation

As previously mentioned, the SLIPA should be used only in types of cases similar to those in which other SGAs are recommended. Further study is necessary to determine its usefulness in patients with poor lung compliance or increased airway resistance. Its use should be avoided in patients with lesions of the oropharynx or epiglottis and patients with an obstruction at or beyond the level of the glottis. Compared with endotracheal intubation, the use of this device may be associated with less cardiovascular stress and fewer sore throats. The use of muscle relaxants is not necessary, unless desired for the operative procedure. Despite the irregular shape of the SLIPA, it does not pose a greater resistance to airflow than other SGAs or an oral ET.

g. Guide to Endotracheal Intubation

The use of the SLIPA as an intubation conduit has yet to be evaluated.

h. Medical Literature

Most of the studies on the SLIPA have been led by the inventor, with only two independent reports. The initial pilot study on 22 patients using only one size of the SLIPA demonstrated a remarkable 91% success rate.[57] In a study involving 120 patients, the SLIPA was compared with the LMA with three sizes to choose from. In all the basic requirements for performance in an SGA, namely ease of use, success rate, sealing for positive-pressure ventilation, stress response to placement, and postoperative

Table 22-14 **Capacity of the Various Sizes of SLIPA to Retain Fluid in the Horizontal and 10-Degree Head-Down Positions (*n* = 6)**

Size (mm)	Horizontal (mL)	Head-Down (mL)
47	29 ± 0.3	45 ± 0.3
49	30 ± 1.0	48 ± 0.7
51	32 ± 1.3	54 ± 0.7
53	36 ± 1.0	62 ± 0.6
55	45 ± 1.2	68 ± 1.1
57	54 ± 0.8	72 ± 1.2

Values are mean ± SD.
SLIPA, Streamlined Liner of the Pharynx Airway.
Courtesy of Dr. Donald Miller.

trauma and sore throat, both devices were comparable. The success rate for both the SLIPA and cLMA was 59 of 60 patients. The oropharyngeal leak pressure was found to be greater than with the LMA, but this finding was not significant.[58]

In the same report,[58] a laboratory study using a lung model was performed in which aspiration into the lungs could be quantified in relation to regurgitation volumes during positive-pressure ventilation. The SLIPA, cLMA, and ProSeal LMA (pLMA) were compared. Both the SLIPA and pLMA compared favorably with the cLMA. The effectiveness of the pLMA was limited by volume capacity in the laboratory study.[58] The cLMA proved to be vulnerable to aspiration, occurring if the volume exceeded 3.5 mL, whereas the SLIPA volumes at which aspiration began were approximately 50 mL. Table 22-14 shows the relation of SLIPA size to volume where aspiration may occur.

Although the storage volumes of the SLIPA are probably more than adequate to prevent aspiration for more than 99% of fasted patients, they may not be adequate for nonfasted patients. Nevertheless, for resuscitation, it would appear to have some major theoretical advantages over the cLMA. Not only is the SLIPA storage capacity 10 times greater than that of the LMA, suction into the SLIPA chamber is much less likely to pass into the trachea, possibly stimulating laryngospasm. Also, large particles of food may easily pass into the chamber (they could obstruct the drainage tube of the pLMA). In the desperate situation in which vomiting is occurring, the chamber can be removed, its contents shaken out, and the SLIPA reinserted again (theoretically, it may even provide a quicker means initially of removing vomitus than with a suction apparatus).

In a study of its application in gynecologic laparoscopies involving 150 patients (50 in each group), the SLIPA was compared with the pLMA and the use of tracheal tubes. The SLIPA was comparable to the pLMA

regarding ease of insertion, oropharyngeal leak or pressure, seal quality, systolic pressure response to insertion, and operating room time saving when compared with endotracheal intubation. There were fewer sore throats with the pLMA than with use of an ET ($P < .05$) and SLIPA airway. The oropharyngeal leak pressure of 30 cm H_2O was not significantly different from that of the pLMA of 31 cm H_2O.

An independent study of new users of the SLIPA resulted in a success rate for the first attempted insertion of 17 of 20 for a single user and of 36 of 40 for multiple users with no discernible learning curve.[45] In this study, most users found the SLIPA to be easy or very easy to use as an effective airway for spontaneous or assisted ventilation. A further study comparing the SLIPA with the SSLM showed the former to have a higher first-time insertion success rate, and it was easier to use.[46] Fluid dynamic studies of various SGAs revealed that there was less resistance to gas flow in the SLIPA than other devices.[24]

III. DESIRABLE FEATURES AND OPTIMAL METHODS FOR TESTING

A. ISSUES

Until the late 1980s, the options for maintaining the airway during anesthesia were largely limited to the ET or the face mask combined with an oropharyngeal airway. The initial response was skeptical, but despite this, many tried it and it was soon firmly established in anesthetic practice. Since then, the LMA (now called the LMA Classic, cLMA) has been used in approximately 150 million anesthesias and there are over 2400 studies published on the use of the device.

The market for SGAs is extensive. Surveys in three European countries have reported that the cLMA is used in approximately 65% of general anesthesias. In the United Kingdom this represents 3.5 million uses each year. At approximately $3 per use, this market costs in excess of $12 million per year in the United Kingdom. Of course, the United Kingdom represents only a fraction of the global market.

There are five variations of the laryngeal mask (classic, flexible, intubating, double-lumen, and disposable) and at least 10 other distinct SGAs currently on the market. Two more are in final development (AMD, glossopharyngeal tube [GPT]). Three were introduced and have now been abandoned: cuffed oropharyngeal airway (COPA), the Pharyngeal airway express (PAXpress), and the Laryngoseal. The glottic aperture airway (GO₂, Eden Prairie, MN) actually never made it into clinical use.

The market for single-use devices is increasing. There are 5 different manufacturers of single-use cLMAs (Ambu, Intavent Orthofix [probably LMA company for

North America], Intersurgical, Marshalls, and Portex) at the time of writing, and this is expected to increase to 12 within a year. There are important design differences between all five single-use cLMAs. If all variants are included, there are 19 SGAs available for nonintubated patients and 9 more soon to be released. All but three of these devices have been introduced in Europe in the past 3 years.

B. TESTING OF NEW GENERATION AIRWAY DEVICES

A small survey of SGA device manufacturers[26] showed that for several recently introduced devices, the number of patients in whom the device had been used before marketing was less than 150 in all cases but one. The number of trials published in peer-reviewed journals at the time of launching the product has varied from 0 to 12. One device launched in 2001 remained without published data 18 months later. Only two of seven devices underwent comparison with the cLMA in randomized controlled trials before marketing, and the largest of these involved only 60 patients.

How does an anesthesiologist start to use a new airway device? Typically, a company representative may provide a few anesthesiologists with samples of the new device and provide education in its use. These anesthesiologists try the device on a few patients and form an opinion. Many hundreds of anesthesiologists may go through this process, exposing perhaps thousands of patients to relatively untested devices, before a consensus is slowly reached. The quality of each evaluation varies with the individual's practice and experience. Companies may use informal comments from one user to encourage other users. Individual uptake may therefore be swayed considerably by limited personal experiences and new devices can be introduced without adequate evaluation of clinical efficacy or safety, or, conversely, the devices may be rejected without due cause. In contrast, some companies restrict the distribution of new devices to a few hospitals or to experts in the field. Some attempt to collect an assessment of the device's performance each time it is used. Some perform extensive laboratory, model, and clinical evaluations before marketing. However, these practices are far from universal.

Is it still acceptable to evaluate new devices in such an ad hoc manner? This process should be contrasted with the introduction of a new drug, which must go through laboratory and preclinical studies even before clinical trials are considered. Three phases of clinical trials are reviewed before release to the market. Postmarketing surveillance is mandatory and extensive.

What regulations govern the introduction of new medical devices, particularly airway devices? In the United Kingdom, the use of medical devices is controlled by three European Directives as part of European law.[54] Within these there are specific directives applicable to airway devices. Adherence to these directives is overseen by a statutory (regulatory) body. This statutory body has responsibility for ensuring that medical devices do not threaten patients' health and safety. Statutory requirements are largely harmonized throughout Europe, and compliance with one country's requirements allows distribution and marketing of a device throughout the European Union. In addition to the statutory body, there are other agencies that might have an interest in monitoring the release of new anesthetic equipment. In the United Kingdom, the National Institute for Clinical Excellence (NICE) and the Commission for Health Assessment and Improvement (CHAI) might be expected to be interested in this area. However, their specific remits are for the evaluation of new devices, which are used as part of a new procedure. Thus, the new SGAs fall outside this remit.

The statutory requirements (of safety and quality) do include a statement to the effect that the device should function as intended by the manufacturer. However, in practice, the statutory assessments focus on production quality control and manufacturing standards. A mixture of self-assessment and external assessment is obtained, depending on the risk that the device is considered to pose to patients. These assessments must be passed to allow continued marketing of a device. Airway devices are considered to be of low or intermediate risk and are primarily subject to manufacturers' self-assessment. They may be marketed before completion of external assessment. Performance of the desired function, efficacy, and cost-effectiveness are not a focus of these assessments. Passing statutory requirements and obtaining a CE mark (a mark to indicate this, which allows marketing of such a device throughout Europe) imply that the device is "fit for its intended purpose," but assessment of performance, efficacy, and cost-effectiveness appears to be left to the manufacturers, distributors, and end users in the postmarketing phase.

Once a device is marketed, clinical trials are not required to demonstrate efficacy or quality of performance. Manufacturers are legally bound to report "serious or potentially serious" adverse incidents.[3] The statutory body requires reporting of incidences in which "malfunction of or deterioration in the characteristics and performance of a device" leads to "actual or potential patient harm."[3] There is also a mechanism for voluntary reporting of incidents by users. Whether these mechanisms lead to reliable reporting of such incidents and whether these schemes identify devices that are simply poorly designed or underperform is not clear. Formal assessment of performance may come from postmarketing cohort or comparative studies. However, these are infrequent and are published a long time after a device has been marketed.

This creates a further problem. New devices are often redesigned after initial release to the market, in the light of clinical experience and customer feedback. These new "improved" devices go through a similar process before being marketed. Second-generation (or even third- and fourth-generation) devices are then marketed, often under the same name as the original. As an example, one SGA device was modified three times (four versions, all named identically) in the 18 months after it was initially marketed. Publication delay leads to considerable confusion, as the unsuspecting reader of journals may not realize that a newly published paper relates to a device that has subsequently been modified. The performance of the old version may be very different from that of the current version. There have been five published studies on the device referred to previously, but none evaluated the currently available version. Although this does not make trials of the previous version of each device completely redundant, it does make interpretation of the limited data even more difficult.

It would be better to determine the desirable features of a new airway device and use these to assess the design and function of a new device before and after it is marketed.

C. DESIRABLE FEATURES OF SUPRAGLOTTIC AIRWAYS

There are certain questions that influence the anesthesiologist's choice of an airway for an individual patient. For instance, does the anesthesiologist use a single-use device, a device that can be reused most often, the cheapest device, or the device that causes least trauma? Do all devices maintain the airway reliably? Do any of them protect the airway from regurgitation and pulmonary aspiration? Which devices enable safe and effective positive-pressure ventilation? Will the device enable access to the airway if required? Other questions relate to how well these devices function in large cohorts. Are there differences in ease of insertion and airway seal pressure between the various devices? How often are manipulations needed to maintain a clear airway during anesthesia? Which devices are tolerated best during emergence? What are the relative incidences of airway trauma and postoperative pharyngolaryngeal morbidity? Unfortunately, in the majority of cases, remarkably few data are available. The manner in which new medical devices are regulated contributes to this.

The desirable features of an ideal supraglottic device relate to efficacy, versatility, safety, reusability, and cost. Manufacturing a quality product is important. The device should be made of good-quality nonharmful materials. A long shelf life is desirable. Devices designed to be reusable should be robust enough to allow multiple uses without deterioration of performance. Similarly, design should enable appropriate cleaning without damage or deterioration. Most of these factors are overseen during the statutory evaluations. Desirable features may be viewed from the patient's or anesthesiologist's perspective.

The anesthesiologist wants a device that is inserted reliably on the first attempt, producing a clear airway for both spontaneous and controlled ventilation. It must enable the anesthesiologist to maintain hands-free anesthesia. Emergence should be without complications.

The incidence of airway trauma and postoperative sore throat should be acceptably low. Design features or clinical evidence of protection against aspiration is desirable, as is the ability to reach the trachea through the device. From the patient's perspective, the ideal device should not cause intraoperative complications, device-associated trauma, or pharyngolaryngeal morbidity. We first consider the anesthesiologist's requirements.

The device should enable insertion with minimal mouth opening (most require 2 to 3 cm mouth opening) and with a light depth of anesthesia (the dose range for different airways varies approximately twofold). Supraglottic devices requiring a muscle relaxant for insertion are of limited use.

All SGA devices may cause airway obstruction from epiglottic downfolding. This is reduced by ensuring correct insertion technique and by designing devices with a slim leading edge. The slim profile of the deflated LT and the deflation device and tip flattener that are provided with the cLMA and pLMA are examples of such design. The epiglottis may also cause obstruction by entering the orifice of the airway device, and a variety of design features are aimed at avoiding this. These include epiglottic bars (cLMA and flexible FLMA), a large orifice too big to obstruct (pLMA), multiple holes (Combitube, LT), and a hooded orifice with protective fins (PAXpress).

First-time insertion success should be high and require a minimum of manipulations. With current devices, first-time insertion success ranges from below 70% to above 95%. The average number of manipulations required to enable insertion ranges widely, from less than one manipulation in 25 cases to more than one per case.

The anesthesiologist requires an airway that, once inserted, does not require airway manipulations or repositioning during anesthesia, enabling hands-free anesthesia. The most functional devices require an intervention in less than 1 in 25 cases, but others require intervention in two thirds of cases.

The airway should be stable when head and neck position varies, such as during rotation to improve surgical access, or when the head and neck are repositioned for further procedures. Limited evidence suggests that the stability of different SGA devices under these circumstances is variable.

Intraoperative complications (e.g., airway obstruction, loss of airway, regurgitation, laryngospasm) should be infrequent. The published incidence of minor complications with existing devices ranges sixfold, from less than 10% to 60%. Serious and minor repetitive complications or the need to perform repeated or continuous manipulations to maintain the airway may force early removal of the airway. This is the ultimate failure of the airway device, and it occurs with an incidence of less than 1 in 50 cases to more than 1 in 5 cases.

The ideal SGA is reliable for both spontaneous and controlled ventilation. Of the existing devices, several versions of one device function poorly during spontaneous ventilation and another is designed specifically to facilitate controlled rather than spontaneous ventilation. Several devices that produce a low-pressure seal with the airway may be unsuitable during controlled ventilation because of the risk of gastric inflation and regurgitation risk.

Protection of the airway from aspiration is critically important. SGAs are increasingly used in more obese patients, in those with minor gastroesophageal reflux, and during controlled ventilation. Several of the newer devices have features that lessen the likelihood of gastric inflation and enable access to the esophagus or stomach to drain the stomach or enable venting of regurgitated matter. For some of these devices, there is experimental and clinical evidence to support the function of these innovations, but for other similar devices there is none. Regurgitation and aspiration are infrequent events. Evidence proving better safety of one device compared with another could come only from studies of several million patients. Such studies are impractical. Instead, safety data have to be acquired by analyzing the design features, surrogate measures of airway safety, and bench models. SGAs are also used for nasal and oropharyngeal surgery, yet only a few have been demonstrated to protect of the airway from pharyngeal secretions. It remains unclear which of the newer devices are safe for such operations.

The ideal airway device causes no trauma to the airway. With existing devices the incidence of trauma to the airway, as evidenced by blood visible on the device, ranges from almost 0% to more than 50%. SGAs commonly cause sore throat, dysphonia, and dysphagia, but these symptoms are usually minor and transient. The possibility of nerve injuries is of greater concern. The ideal airway minimizes or eliminates both of these problems. However, the intracuff and mucosal pressures vary in intensity and location with different SGAs. The incidence of sore throat varies with different devices from below 10% to above 40%. Clinically significant nerve injury is rare with all SGAs, and the relative risks of each device are not known.

In addition to its role in maintaining the airway during anesthesia, an SGA may usefully enable access to the airway. This may help with the treatment of some intraoperative complications and may help in the management of the difficult airway. The ILMA is designed specifically for these roles. There are several techniques for its use. An ET can be passed blindly through a cLMA, but it requires a long, narrow tube and some luck. Light-guided, fiberscope-guided, and catheter exchange techniques are better but they require a short SGA that is wide enough throughout its length. The larynx must be reliably visible from the airway orifice. SGA devices vary in length and diameter. The proximal orifice of some accept tubes and fiberscopes of only 5.0 mm external diameter whereas others accommodate ETs of 8.5 mm internal diameter. At their distal end, grills, bars, small orifices, and difficult angles may impede or prevent access to the trachea. The ability to view the laryngeal inlet from the airway orifice ranges between devices from above 90% to below 40%.

Although most devices are used by experienced anesthesiologists, SGAs may be used by the inexperienced for anesthesia, out-of-hospital rescue, or resuscitation. The ideal airway should therefore be intuitive to use, have a high success rate for the naive user, and have a short learning curve. For most devices, these data are not available, but what little there is suggests that insertion and airway maintenance by nonanesthesiologists and by naive users vary considerably among devices.

Finally, there is an implicit assumption that reusable devices may be replaced by cheaper, single-use devices, and some believe that single-use devices are intrinsically preferable. However, many single-use devices differ from the reusable devices they seek to replace, both in design and in the materials used. Some of these modifications appear minor, but the implications for performance have not been evaluated. Work on single-use laryngoscopes[70] and intubation stylets[52] provides evidence that changes in product material may alter performance considerably. Data on the current versions of the single-use cLMAs and comparisons between these and the reusable LMA are not yet available.

No single device meets all the criteria for the ideal SGA. Indeed, some of these criteria are mutually exclusive. For instance, a device that is large enough to accommodate an adequately sized ET is unlikely to be as easily inserted as a smaller device. Epiglottic bars reduce airway obstruction but hinder instrumental access to the trachea. A single-use device is less likely than a more expensive reusable device to be made of the best materials to optimize handling characteristics and minimize pharyngolaryngeal trauma. Therefore, it is likely that several different airways will always be needed for use in different clinical situations.

D. SUGGESTED NEW METHODS OF ASSESSMENT

New airway devices, indeed all new equipment, should undergo mandatory assessment of manufacturing quality *and* clinical performance before marketing. The function of SGAs should be evaluated in bench models and in vivo. The characteristics of the ideal SGA, outlined earlier, provide a checklist against which function can be assessed. A three-stage performance evaluation of new devices would be best.

Stage 1. Bench evaluation using mannequins or models designed to test function and safety.
Stage 2.* A rigorous cohort study to determine whether the device is effective and safe.
Stage 3.* A randomized controlled trial against the current gold standard for the procedure for which the new device is expected to be used (cLMA, pLMA, ILMA).

---

*Stages 2 and 3 require ethical approval and written consent by the patient.

1. Stage 1: Bench Evaluation

Bench models include airway mannequins and others such as those specifically designed to test aspiration risk.[58] The problem with all these nonclinical models is determining whether function in models mimics that in patients. The existing mannequins are not designed for this role, and the performance of SGAs in them is not representative of their performance in patients. With the increasing use of SGAs during resuscitation, during out-of-hospital rescue, and by nonanesthesiologists, there is an urgent need for realistic mannequins to be developed for testing and training. Several companies are developing these mannequins, which should enable reliable bench testing of SGA devices. Functions that can be tested with these mannequins include ease of insertion, laryngeal seal, airway resistance, stability of the device in different head and neck positions, ease of passage of a gastric tube, positioning of the airway over the larynx, and suitability for fiberscopic or catheter exchange techniques. Learning curves and use by nonanesthesiologists can be examined. Comparisons can be made between new and existing devices. Suitable models may be constructed to assess airway protection and protection from aspiration. Bench testing might lead to further development of a device before starting clinical studies.

2. Stage 2: Cohort Study

A cohort study might be used for the first assessment of clinical performance in patients. A cohort study enables full clinical evaluation of the new device under routine clinical conditions. Such a study enables examination of all the functions that can be tested with bench tests (with perhaps the exception of aspiration protection). It also enables assessment of function during spontaneous respiration and determination of any airway trauma or pharyngolaryngeal morbidity. The cohort must be large enough to enable identification of common problems, but unless it is very large it will not detect uncommon or rare problems. For instance, for an event that does not occur in a cohort study of n cases, the 95% confidence interval for frequency of that event is approximately 1 in $3/n$.[44] For example, if no nerve injuries occur in a cohort study of 100 cases, the upper limit of the 95% confidence interval for risk of nerve injury is 1 in 33. A cohort of more than 100 would be a reasonable compromise between being large enough to identify important uncommon events and still remain a practical size.

3. Stage 3: Randomized Control Trial

After successful completion of bench and cohort evaluation, the need for further modifications of the device should be considered. Significant modifications necessitate repetition of the early evaluations. On successful completion of the early evaluations, the new device should be compared with its best existing competitor. In most cases this would be the cLMA. Such an evaluation should be a randomized controlled trial of adequate size to identify clinically important differences in function. The previous evaluations would have indicated any important differences in function between the new and standard device (e.g., significant differences in airway seal pressure) and enabled power calculations to determine appropriate study size. However, trials of at least 100 patients would provide more comprehensive and clinically useful comparisons. Economic evaluation of cost-effectiveness of the new device might also take place at this stage.

Data from the three phases of evaluation might then be used to determine what role the new airway device has in the market. It might be licensed for only one aspect of airway care (e.g., for spontaneous breathing only, for controlled ventilation in patients with good pulmonary compliance, or for airway maintenance when tracheal access is likely to be necessary). License extensions might be granted in the light of further research.

The use of this methodology would still result in only 200 to 300 uses of the device in patients before release to market. This number would not be enough to identify uncommon and perhaps unexpected problems, complications, or advantages. Therefore, the proposed method of evaluation does not obviate the need for postmarketing surveillance or reporting of adverse incidents. A formal method of such evaluation could be developed. For instance, the first 5000 devices used after marketing might have evaluation cards attached, to be returned after use. Alternatively, the manufacturer might be required to seek reports of all adverse incidents for the first 2 years after release (similar to the Yellow Card system for new drugs that applies in the United Kingdom).

The structured nature of the evaluation would have advantages for manufacturer, clinician, and patient. For successful devices, the manufacturer would have robust data to support performance claims and a clearer vision of the likely advantages and roles of the new device. This would enhance marketing and raise credibility. For devices that performed poorly, the manufacturer could avoid the expense of large-scale production and marketing of devices that would ultimately fail to achieve market share. The clinician would have better evidence on which to base personal evaluation. Researchers would have clearer ideas of how a new device might be evaluated to define function further and investigate wider indications for use. Finally, the patient would be less likely to be exposed to unnecessary risk during the use of a new device.

IV. CONCLUSION

Anesthesiologists and patients rely on equipment to be safe during anesthesia. The relationship between manufacturer and clinician, acting for the patient, is symbiotic. Care of patients can improve only through a sustained effort by clinicians and manufacturers to improve the medical devices used during anesthesia. In this respect, much has been achieved in airway care in the past 15 years and the practice of anesthesia has been transformed. Innovation does not come cheap, and much of the cost of advances or improvements comes during research and development. This cost is borne entirely by the manufacturer. A more open relationship between interested parties and the early involvement of objective structured evaluation of new airway equipment is recommended. Such an approach should prevent undertested or underdeveloped products coming to market and so protect patients. Although this is the essential aim, an evaluation program should encourage and support equipment manufacturers and needs careful balance to achieve both these goals.

REFERENCES

1. Agro F, Barzoi G, Carassiti M, Gallì B: Getting the tube in the oesophagus and oxygen in the trachea: Preliminary results with the new supraglottic device (Cobra) in 28 anaesthetised patients. Anaesthesia 58:920-921, 2003.
2. Agro F, Barzoi G, Gallì B: The Cobra PLA in 110 anaesthetized and paralysed patients: What size to choose? [letter]. Br J Anaesth 92:777-778, 2004.
3. Agro F, Brimacombe J, Carassiti M, et al: Lighted stylet as an aid to blind tracheal intubation via the LMA [letter]. J Clin Anesth 10:263-264, 1998.
4. Agro F, Brimacombe J, Carassiti M, et al: Use of a lighted stylet for intubation via the laryngeal mask airway. Can J Anaesth 45:556-560, 1998.
5. Agro F, Carassiti M, Barzoi G, et al: A first report of the diagnosis and treatment of acute postoperative airway obstruction with CobraPLA. Can J Anaesth 51:640-641, 2004.
6. Agro F, Carassiti M, Magnani C: Percutaneous dilatational cricothyroidotomy: Airway control via CobraPLA. Anesth Analg 99:628, 2004.
7. Agro F, Cataldo R, Alfano A, Gallì B: A new prototype for airway management in an emergency: The laryngeal tube. Resuscitation 41:284-286, 1999.
8. Agro F, Hung OR, Cataldo R, et al: Lightwand intubation using the Trachlight: A brief review of current knowledge. Can J Anaesth 48:592-599, 2001.
9. Agro FE, Galli B, Cataldo R, et al: Relationship between body mass index and ventilation with the Laryngeal Tube in 228 anesthetized paralyzed patients: A pilot study. Can J Anaesth 49:641-642, 2002.
10. Akca O, Wadhwa A, Sengupta P, et al: The perilaryngeal airway (Cobra-PLA) provides better airway sealing pressures than the laryngeal mask airway (LMA). Anesthesiology 99:A566, 2003.
11. Aoyama K, Takenaka I, Sata T, Shigematsu A: The triple airway manoeuvre for insertion of the laryngeal mask airway in paralyzed patients. Can J Anaesth 42:1010-1016, 1995.
12. Asai T, Hidaka I, Kawachi S: Efficacy of the laryngeal tube by inexperienced personnel. Resuscitation 55:171-175, 2002.
13. Asai T, Kawachi S: Pressure exerted by cuff of laryngeal tube on the oropharynx. Anaesthesia 56:912, 2001.
14. Asai T, Kawashima A, Hidaka I, Kawachi S: Laryngeal tube: Its use for controlled ventilation. Masui 50:1340-1341, 2001.
15. Asai T, Kawashima A, Hidaka I, Kawadri S: The laryngeal tube compared with the laryngeal mask: Insertion, gas leak pressure and gastric insufflation. Br J Anaesth 89:729-732, 2002.
16. Asai T, Matsumoto S, Shingu K, et al: Use of the laryngeal tube after failed insertion of a laryngeal mask airway. Anaesthesia 60:625-626, 2005.
17. Asai T, Murao K, Shingu K: Efficacy of the laryngeal tube during intermittent positive-pressure ventilation. Anaesthesia 55:1099-1102, 2000.
18. Brimacombe J: A proposed classification system for extraglottic airway devices [letter]. Anesthesiology 101:559, 2004.
19. Brimacombe JR, Berry A: Insertion of the laryngeal mask airway—A prospective study of four techniques. Anaesth Intensive Care 21:89-92, 1993.
20. Brimacombe JR, Brain AIJ: The Laryngeal Mask Airway. A Review and Practical Guide. Philadelphia, WB Saunders, 1997.
21. Brimacombe J, Clarke G, Keller C: Lingual nerve injury associated with the ProSeal laryngeal mask airway: A case report and review of the literature. Br J Anaesth 95:720-723, 2005.
22. Brimacombe J, Keller C, Brimacombe L: A comparison of the laryngeal mask airway ProSeal and the laryngeal tube airway in paralyzed anesthetized adult patients undergoing pressure-controlled ventilation. Anesth Analg 96:1535, 2003.
23. Brimacombe J, von Goedecke A, Keller C, et al: The laryngeal mask airway Unique versus the Soft Seal laryngeal mask: A randomized, crossover study in paralyzed, anesthetized patients. Anesth Analg 99:1560-1563, 2004.
24. Coetzee GH: Flow through disposable alternatives to the laryngeal mask. Anaesthesia 58:280-281, 2003.
25. Cook TM, McCormick B, Asai T: Randomized comparison of the laryngeal tube with classical laryngeal mask airway for anaesthesia with controlled ventilation. Br J Anaesth 91:373-378, 2003.
26. Cook TM: Spoilt for choice? New supraglottic airways. Anaesthesia 58:107-110, 2003.
27. Coppolo DP, May JJ: Self-extubations. A 12-month experience. Chest 98:165-169, 1990.
28. Doerges V, Ocker H, Wenzel V, Schmucker P: The laryngeal tube: A new simple airway device. Anesth Analg 90:1220-1222, 2000.
29. Fan KH, Hung OR, Agro F: A comparative study of tracheal intubation using an intubating laryngeal mask (Fastrach) alone or together with a lightwand (Trachlight). J Clin Anesth 12:581-585, 2000.
30. Francksen H, Bein B, Obermoeller T, et al: Ambu laryngeal mask vs. Laryngeal mask Unique: Evaluation of two modified disposable ventilatory devices. Anesthesiology 103:A1440, 2005.

31. Gaitini LA, Somri MJ, Kersh K, et al: A comparison of the Laryngeal Mask Airway Unique, Pharyngeal Airway X press and Perilaryngeal Airway Cobra in paralysed anesthetized adult patients. Anesthesiology 99:A1495, 2003.

32. Gaitini L, Vaida SJ, Somri M, et al: An evaluation of the laryngeal tube during general anesthesia using mechanical ventilation. Anesth Analg 96:1750-1755, 2003.

33. Gaitini LA, Vaida SJ, Mostafa S, Janovski B: The effect of nitrous oxide on the cuff pressure of the laryngeal tube. Anaesthesia 57:506, 2002.

34. Galli B, Mattei A, Antonelli S, et al: A new adjunct for airway management: The laryngeal tube, preliminary data. Eur J Anaesthesiol 18:124, 2001.

35. Genzwuerker H, Hilker T, Hohner E, Kuhnert-Frey B: Der Larynxtubus: Eine Alternative für die vorübergehende Oxygenierung bei schwieriger Intubation? [abstract]. Anaesthesiol Intensivmed 40:40, 1999.

36. Genzwuerker HV, Hilker T, Hohner E, Kuhnert-Frey B: The laryngeal tube: A new adjunct for airway management. Prehosp Emerg Care 4:168-172, 2000.

37. Gentzwuerker H, Hinklebein J, Krivosic-Hober R, et al: Performance of the new single-use Ambu laryngeal mask in different head positions. Anesthesiology 101:A1590, 2004.

38. Genzwuerker HV, Vollmer T, Ellinger K: Fibreoptic tracheal intubation after placement of the laryngeal tube. Br J Anaesth 89:733-738, 2002.

39. Gernoth C, Jandewerth O, Contzen M, et al: Comparison of two different laryngeal mask models for airway management in patients with immobilization of the cervical spine. [German] Anaesthesist 55:263-269, 2006.

40. Hagberg CA, Bogomolny Y, Gilmore C, et al: An evaluation of the insertion and function of a new supra-glottic airway device, the King LT, during spontaneous ventilation. Anesth Analg 102:621-625, 2006.

41. Hagberg CA, Jensen FS, Genzwuerker HV, et al: International, multi-center study of the Ambu laryngeal mask in nonparalyzed, anesthetized patients. Anesth Analg 101:1862-1866, 2005.

42. Hagberg C, Sciard D, Bogomolny Y, et al: A clinical comparison of the SoftSeal laryngeal mask and the Unique single-use laryngeal mask in adults. Anesthesiology 103:A1441, 2005.

43. Hagberg C, Sciard D, Bogomolny Y, et al: Optimal insertion method of the SoftSeal laryngeal mask in adult patients. Anesthesiology 103:A1442, 2005.

44. Hanley JA, Lippman-Hand A: If nothing goes wrong, is everything all right? Interpreting zero numerators. JAMA 249:1743-1745, 1983.

45. Hein C, Owen H, Plummer J: The SLIPA-A disposable supraglottic airway device that is easy to use. Anesthesiology 101:A1534, 2004.

46. Hein C, Owen H, Plummer J: Randomised comparison of the SLIPA and SoftSeal laryngeal mask airway by health professional trainees. Personal communication.

47. Keller C, Sparr HJ, Brimacombe JR: Laryngeal mask lubrication. A comparative study of saline versus 2% lignocaine gel with cuff pressure control. Anaesthesia 52:592-597, 1997.

48. Klein MT, Jones J: Utility of the intubating laryngeal airway: Report of an observational study. Anesthesiology 103:A846, 2005.

49. Laffon M, Ferrandiere M, Mercier C, Fusciardi J: Transient lingual and glossopharyngeal nerve injury: A complication of cuffed oropharyngeal airway. Anesthesiology 94:719-720, 2001.

50. LMA Instruction Manual. San Diego, LMA North America.

51. Lowinger D, Benjamin B, Gadd L: Recurrent laryngeal nerve injury caused by a laryngeal mask airway. Anaesth Intensive Care 27:202-205, 1999.

52. Marfin AG, Pandit JJ, Hames KC, et al: Use of the bougie in simulated difficult intubation. Comparison of single-use with multiple-use bougie. Anaesthesia 58:852-855, 2003.

53. Medical Devices Agency Directives Bulletin No 3. The Vigilance System. Medical Devices Agency, 2002.

54. Medical Devices Agency Directives Bulletin No 8. Information about the EC Medical Devices Directives. Medical Devices Agency, 2002.

55. Miller DM: Advantages of the ProSeal and SLIPA airways compared to using tracheal tubes in day case laparoscopic gynaecological procedures. Eur J Anaesthesiol 12:S-21, 2004.

56. Miller DM: A proposed classification and scoring system for supraglottic sealing airways: A brief review. Anesth Analg 99:1553-1559, 2004.

57. Miller DM, Lavelle M: A streamlined pharynx airway liner: Pilot study in 22 patients in controlled and spontaneous ventilation. Anesth Analg 94:759-761, 2002.

58. Miller DM, Light D: Laboratory and clinical comparisons of the Streamlined Liner of the Pharynx Airway (SLIPA) with the laryngeal mask airway. Anaesthesia 58:136-142, 2003.

59. Miller DM, Newton NI: Risk of hypoglossal nerve injury and supraglottic airways: A magnetic resonance image study. Anesthesiology 101:A1531, 2004.

60. Miller DM, Youkhana I, Pearce AC: The laryngeal mask and VBM laryngeal tube compared during spontaneous ventilation. A pilot study. Eur J Anaesthesiol 18:593-598, 2001.

61. Ocker H, Doerges V, Heringslake M, Schmucker P: Der neue Larynxtubus vs. Larynxmaske-suffiziente Beatmung mit Aspirationsschutz? [abstract]. Anaesthesiol Intensivmed 41:376, 2000.

62. Ocker H, Wenzel V, Schmucher P, et al: A comparison of the laryngeal tube with the laryngeal mask airway during routine surgical procedures. Anesth Analg 95:1094-1097, 2002.

63. Paech MJ, Lain S, Garrett WR, et al: Randomised evaluation of the single-use SoftSeal and the re-usable LMA Classic laryngeal mask. Anaesth Intensive Care 32:66-72, 2004.

64. Practice guidelines for management of the difficult airway: An updated report by the American Society of Anesthesiologists Task Force on Management of the Difficult Airway. Anesthesiology 98:1269-1277, 2003.

65. Richebe P, Semjen F, El Hammar F, et al: Clinical evaluation of the laryngeal tube (LT) in pediatric anesthesia. Anesthesiology 93:A1268, 2000.

66. Robertson C, Steen P, Adgey J, et al: The 1998 European Resuscitation Council guidelines for adult advanced life support: A statement from the Working Group on Advanced Life Support, and approved by the executive committee. Resuscitation 37:81-90, 1998.

67. Szmuk P, Ghelber O, Matuszczak M, et al: CobraPLA with an end tidal CO_2 sampling site: Differences between proximal and distal sampling sites. Anesthesiology 103:A1389, 2005.

68. Szmuk P, Matuszczeak M, Carlson RF, et al: Use of CobraPLA for airway management in a neonate with Desbuquois syndrome. Case report and anaesthetic implications. Paediatr Anaesth 15:602-605, 2005.

69. Trumpelmann P, Cook T: Unilateral hypoglossal nerve injury following the use of a ProSeal laryngeal mask. Anaesthesia 60:101-102, 2005.

70. Twigg S, McCormick B, Cook TM: A randomised evaluation of the performance of single use laryngoscopes in simulated easy and difficult intubation. Br J Anaesth 90:8-13, 2003.

71. Van Zundert AAJ, Fonck K, Al-Shaikh B, Mortier E: Comparison of the LMA-Classic with the new disposable soft seal laryngeal mask in spontaneously breathing adult patients. Anesthesiology 99:1066-1071, 2003.

THE EVOLUTION OF UPPER AIRWAY RETRACTION: NEW AND OLD LARYNGOSCOPE BLADES

J. Adam Law
Carin A. Hagberg

I. INTRODUCTION

Historically, most laryngoscopy performed for the purpose of endotracheal intubation has been *direct* in that laryngoscopy has afforded the operator a direct line-of-sight view of the laryngeal inlet. However, the introduction of the flexible fiberoptic bronchoscope (FOB) in the 1970s introduced the ability to visualize the glottis *indirectly* through an image transmitted by a fiberoptic bundle (i.e., endoscopically). Subsequently, various rigid fiberoptic and video-aided laryngoscopes joined the indirect laryngoscope family. As instruments that help overcome many of the anatomic determinants of difficult direct laryngoscopy, the latter tools can be useful. However, direct laryngoscopy is still performed for most intubations. This chapter reviews blades used for direct laryngoscopy as well as the rigid and semirigid fiberoptic and video-aided devices. Emphasis is placed on blades that have evolved into common usage, although passing mention may also be made of instruments of historical interest.

II. HISTORY

Many techniques of endotracheal intubation have been described since MacEwen's 1880 publication[106] of his successful digital intubation of four patients. This fascinating report most likely describes the first use of endotracheal

intubation for elective surgery as well as documenting the short-term intubation of two patients for life-threatening inflammatory conditions of the laryngeal inlet. Although mirror-based indirect laryngoscopy had been described for the first time by the singer Garcia in 1855[54] and later refined by Türck and Czermak,[163] not until 1895 was the first report of direct laryngoscopy published by Alfred Kirstein. Kirstein's interest in developing a direct laryngoscope in turn stemmed from a colleague's observation to him of the accidental tracheal placement of an esophagoscope. Initially, Kirstein was able to visualize the larynx directly with a shorter esophagoscope. Subsequently, he attached the esophagoscope to an electric hand lamp to create his "autoscope" for laryngoscopy; light from the source in the handle was deflected down the esophagoscope lumen by a prism.[79] Concern about excess levering force on the teeth and extreme head extension led Kirstein to refine his scope by redesigning the blade from an enclosed "O" shape to an open crescent shape, with two variations differing in distal width and thickness for direct or indirect lifting of the epiglottis (Fig. 23-1). While recognizing the laryngoscope's potential, Kirstein himself never used his instruments for intubation or bronchoscopy. Rather, his student Gustav Killian in 1897 went on to use the original Kirstein autoscope to extract a foreign body from a bronchus. This and subsequent work with bronchoscopy earned Killian the title of "father of bronchoscopy."[186]

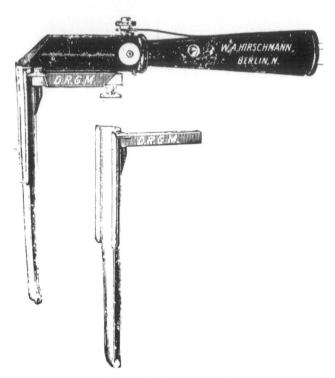

Figure 23-1 Kirstein's modified autoscope. Standard blade is attached to handle. Intralaryngeal blade is shown separately **(bottom).** (From Hirsch NP, Smith GB, Hirsch PO: Alfred Kirstein—Pioneer of direct laryngoscopy. Anaesthesia 41:42, 1986.)

Meanwhile, recognizing the benefits of endotracheal delivery of inhalational anesthesia as well as the potential for difficulty in intubating the trachea, Janeway in 1913 described a smaller and more portable laryngoscope powered by batteries located in the handle. It featured a straight blade with a slight distal curve and, as introduced by Chevalier Jackson in 1907, a light bulb located distally on the blade (Fig. 23-2).[83] The Jackson laryngoscope was U shaped with the handle used for lifting

parallel to the blade. Jackson emphasized, as did earlier authors, the importance of head extension to help expose the glottis. The Jackson laryngoscope had an O-profiled blade with a removable portion, leaving it with a C-shaped profile, in common with many other straight blades (e.g., Magill, Flagg) used over the succeeding three decades.[57,111] Indeed, blades and laryngoscopic technique used for intubation underwent little apparent evolution until the early 1940s, at which time Macintosh described his blade and technique for indirect elevation of the epiglottis. The Macintosh blade and the Miller version of the straight blade evolved into common usage, becoming benchmarks with which other direct laryngoscope blades are compared. Many attempts at improving upon the original design of these blades have been described since then. Some have come to commercial production, and some have not. Only in the 1970s did the flexible FOB introduce another option for use in difficult situations, and rigid fiberoptic devices such as the Bullard laryngoscope were first introduced in the late 1980s. The 1990s in turn saw the introduction of additional rigid fiberoptic laryngoscopes as well as commercially available fiberoptic stylets. Most recently, video-assisted devices have become increasingly represented on the market.

III. DIRECT LARYNGOSCOPE DESIGN

A. COMPONENTS OF A DIRECT LARYNGOSCOPE

A laryngoscope consists of a handle, a blade, and a light source. The main shaft of the blade is called the *spatula* or *tongue* (Fig. 23-3). The blade is used to compress and displace the tongue and soft tissues to help obtain a direct line-of-sight view from the operator's eye past the upper teeth to the laryngeal inlet. It may be straight or

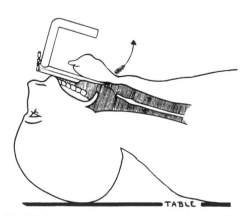

Figure 23-2 Jackson laryngoscope positioned in oropharynx. *Arrow* illustrates direction of motion that should be imparted on laryngoscope blade to assist in exposure of the larynx and insertion of endotracheal tube. (From Jackson C: The technique of insertion of intratracheal insufflation tubes. Surg Gynecol Obstet 17:507, 1913.)

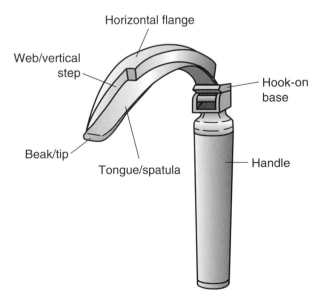

Figure 23-3 The components of a Macintosh bladed direct laryngoscope. (Courtesy of Anne Law.)

curved in all or part of its length. The upward projection on the blade toward the roof of the mouth is called the *web* or *vertical step*. The lateral projection from the vertical step is called the *flange*, although some authorities also refer to the vertical component as the flange.

Differences in laryngoscope blade design are predicated upon variations in blade shape (curved or straight in all or part), the tip, and the step/flange configuration. The last varies from almost none, wherein the blade is little different from a tongue depressor with a variable amount of curve, to that of a Macintosh blade, with its reverse-Z configuration, to a complete O in the case of a totally enclosed (e.g., Bainton) blade. Functionally, the spatula of the blade is used to compress the tongue; the vertical step helps displace the tongue and soft tissues, usually to the left; and the flange also aids in controlling the tongue. The *beak* is the tip of the blade and is usually thickened and blunt to avoid tissue trauma. In close proximity to the beak is a light source, supplied directly from a bulb or transmitted down a fiberoptic bundle from a more proximally located bulb. At the base (or *heel*) of the blade is the block, housing an electrical contact that serves to turn on the light. Most blades are designed to detach from the handle by a hook on the blade and slot on the handle.

B. DIRECT LARYNGOSCOPE LIGHTING CONSIDERATIONS

Visualization of the laryngeal inlet during direct laryngoscopy depends on adequate illumination of airway structures by the laryngoscope.[45] Illumination is a function of both the intensity and color of the supplied light and the area over which it falls. This in turn is dependent on the nature of the laryngoscope blade's light source and the potential of the power source applied to it.[45] Light can be measured at a number of points, including its source (e.g., *luminous flux*, measured in *lumens*) and the surface receiving the light, that is, being illuminated (*illuminance*, measured in *lux*) (Fig. 23-4), or by looking at the amount of light reemitted from a surface in a given direction (*luminance*, measured in *candela per square meter [cd/m²]*).[152] During direct laryngoscopy, perception of the surface brightness of the larynx depends on light transmitted back to the laryngoscopist's eyes from the surface of the larynx; this is the luminance. The luminance of the larynx is dependent, in turn, on both the illuminance and the light reflected from the tissues. Skilton and colleagues[152] determined the minimum required luminance for effective laryngoscopy to be 100 cd/m².

A direct laryngoscope blade emits light close to its distal end from an incandescent bulb or through a fiberoptic bundle. In the latter, a bulb located in the laryngoscope handle (or occasionally in the base of the blade) transmits light down a fiberoptic bundle to the light source tip. Generally, power is supplied from batteries located in the laryngoscope handle, although use of a separate power supply has been described.[9] Investigators have

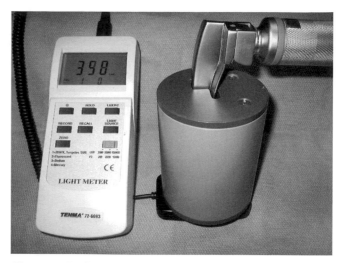

Figure 23-4 A lux meter for measuring laryngoscope illuminance. The jig into which the blade is inserted ensures standardized distance and orientation of blade light source to light meter. (Courtesy of Paul Brousseau.)

demonstrated that illumination[28,165] and luminance[45] are affected by factors such as the type of light source (bulb or fiberoptic bundle), handle type, manufacturer, and sterilization history of the blade. The studies have shown that, in general, better illumination[152,165] and luminance[45] are supplied by distal bulbs, not fiberoptic blades. Bulbs on blades also tend to supply a larger area of illumination.[165] Conversely, fiberoptic blades have the advantage of a cool (and secure) light source, with easier cleaning considerations.[165] Incandescent but not fiberoptic light appears to be affected by handle type, with short handles compromising supplied illumination.[165] In addition, illumination supplied by different manufacturers' versions of the same blade varies over a wide range.[23,28,165] Blade design may also affect light delivery to the target area, particularly if the light tip can be occluded by the tongue—in some straight blades, the light tip's location on the blade's left edge may render it susceptible to partial occlusion by the tongue, pharyngeal, or paraepiglottic tissues as the blade displaces the tongue to the left (Fig. 23-5).[21] Remedies to this have included directing the bulb or bundle tip to the right and locating the bulb or bundle tip to the right of the vertical step proximal to its end. Miller, in the original report of his blade, also illustrated the need to place the light source close to the tip of the blade (Fig. 23-6).[122]

Other sources of lighting compromise, particularly in fiberoptic blades, include cleaning and thermal sterilization cycles and possibly trauma to the blade. Bucx and coworkers[28] have demonstrated that after 200 to 300 steam sterilization cycles at 134° C, light output from fiberoptic blades degraded significantly although they withstood washing and 90° C disinfection reasonably well.[23] A suboptimal connection between the handle and fiberoptic blade may also compromise illumination by allowing light to escape between the bulb source in the

Figure 23-15 Schematic of Gubuya-Orkin blade: **A**, side view; **B**, fitting view; **C**, end view of tip section; **D**, top view. (From Gabuya R, Orkin LR: Design and utility of a new curved laryngoscope blade. Anesth Analg 38:364, 1959.)

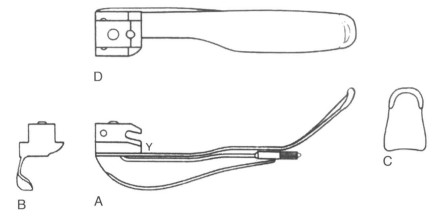

7. Curved Blades with Exaggerated Distal Curvature

A number of blades have been described with a more acute curvature of the distal spatula than the Macintosh. Of historical interest, the *Gubuya-Orkin* blade, described in 1959, was unique in having an S-shaped blade with its distal 3 cm malleable. The authors described bending it through a range from 15 to 45 degrees, with optimal position thought to be 35 degrees from the horizontal for indirect lifting of the epiglottis (Fig. 23-15).[63] Found to be effective in some cases in which Macintosh laryngoscopy had failed, the blade may have been the forerunner of other blades with a marked fixed or variable distal curvature. The *Blechman* blade also differs from the Macintosh in having an accentuated curve toward the blade tip. In addition, the reverse-Z vertical step and flange begin distal to the block/heel of the blade and extend only to within 5 cm of blade tip. The curved *Fink* blade similarly has a sharper curve at the distal spatula and reduced vertical step proximally as compared with the Macintosh. The *Upsher ULX* (Mercury Medical, Clearwater, FL) blade has a more pronounced curve throughout the entire blade length than the standard Macintosh. The *Wiemers* or *Freiburg* blade, marketed in Europe, with less initial curvature than a Macintosh, has a fairly acutely curved tip (Fig. 23-16).[112] As a group, these blades may have utility in patients with limitations of mouth opening, impaired head and neck mobility, or prominent upper incisors, in whom the tip of a Macintosh blade may otherwise fail to engage the glossoepiglottic fold at the appropriate angle. More specific indications for these blades await scientific evaluation.

B. MILLER AND RELATED STRAIGHT BLADES

1. Miller Laryngoscope Blade

Straight blade use, with entrapment and direct lifting of the epiglottis, was already the common laryngoscopic technique when Robert Miller introduced his modification of the straight laryngoscope blade in 1941. The blade he described was longer than medium-sized blades available at the time, narrower at the tip, and featured a gradual curve

starting 2 inches (5 cm) from the distal end. The vertical step was also substantially less (see Fig. 23-6). Miller contended that the shallower step would allow less mouth opening (thus permitting freer anterior movement of the mandible) and less potential for damage to the teeth. With the lesser degree of mouth opening, Miller conceded that available room for ET manipulation would be less and that a stylet would be desirable.[122] Cassels in 1942 echoed Miller's contention that a greater distal curvature of the straight blade would facilitate exposure of the laryngeal inlet, accompanying his report with an elegant diagram to help illustrate his theory.[32] Figure 23-17 demonstrates that especially in the presence of limited mouth opening, for a given position of the base of a straight blade between the teeth, a curved distal tip should enable the laryngoscopist to visualize a more anterior aspect of the laryngeal inlet. The Miller laryngoscope blade continues to be a commonly used straight blade.

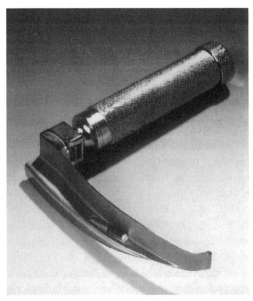

Figure 23-16 The Wiemers blade, with its reduced initial curvature and sharply curved tip. (From Maleck WH, Koetter KP, Lentz M, et al: A randomized comparison of three laryngoscopes with the Macintosh. Resuscitation 42:241-245, 1999.)

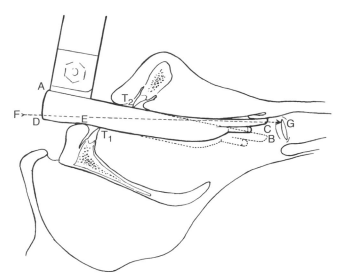

Figure 23-17 Cassels' 1942 diagram illustrates the advantages of a distal curve to an otherwise straight blade. With compromised interincisor opening (T1 to T2), limited upward angulation of a straight blade (A-B) may afford only a view of the posterior laryngeal inlet. Curving the distal blade (A-C) permits a more anterior view from point D looking along line F-G. (From Cassels WH: Advantages of a curved laryngoscope. Anesthesiology 3:580, 1942.)

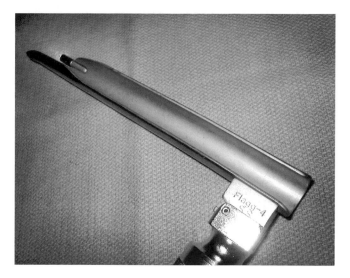

Figure 23-18 The Flagg blade.

2. Historical Straight Blades

Three older straight blades that warrant mention are the Magill, Flagg, and Guedel blades, which all predate the Miller. Indeed, Miller developed his blade at least partly in response to perceived shortcomings of these blades. Nonetheless, all three blades continue to be marketed in adult and pediatric sizes, attesting to their ongoing popularity. The *Magill* blade, dating to 1921, is mainly straight, with a U-shaped step and flange concave to the right. The step and flange continue to within an inch of the end of the blade. The *Flagg* blade is straight with a very slight curve at the distal tip and was originally designed for use with Flagg catheters and tubes. With a light source placed quite distally, the C-shaped cross section tapers gradually from its proximal to distal end (Fig. 23-18).[51] The *Guedel* is similar to the Flagg blade, but the distal tip has slightly more curve and the blade is angled on its base to result in a 72-degree angle with the handle to help promote a lifting action instead of using the teeth as a fulcrum.

3. Soper Blade

The Soper is a straight blade described originally in 1947. Wing-Commander Soper developed the blade in response to the Macintosh's occasional failure to elevate a long "flabby" epiglottis.[158] Although described as a modification of the Macintosh blade, it is largely straight save for a slight distal curvature. It retains the reverse Z-shaped vertical step and flange of the Macintosh blade. A small transverse slot cut into the blade a few millimeters from

the tip is designed to help prevent the epiglottis from slipping off the blade (Fig. 23-19). The Soper is still commercially available in both adult and pediatric lengths.

4. Gould Blade

Gould, in 1954, modified a Soper blade by (1) lining the flange with rubber and reducing the proximal vertical step and (2) lengthening and blunting the distal end of the blade (Fig. 23-20). He made a similar modification to a Macintosh blade, although neither version attained widespread use.[69]

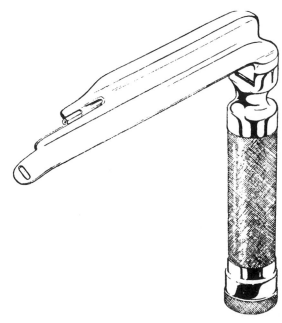

Figure 23-19 The Soper laryngoscope. (From Soper RI: A new laryngoscope for anaesthetists. Br Med J 1:265, 1947.)

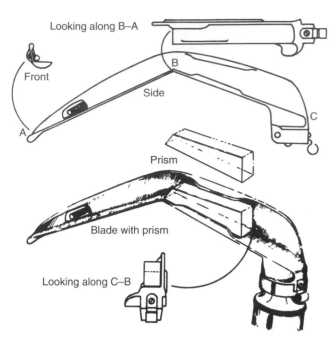

Figure 23-25 The Belscope angulated laryngoscope. The top diagram illustrates the view obtained from the blade angle along the distal blade (line B-A). Failing this, indirect visualization can occur with prism (through line C-B). (From Bellhouse CP: An angulated laryngoscope for routine and difficult tracheal intubation. Anesthesiology 69:126, 1988.)

Often a styletted ET curved anteriorly is necessary for advancement through the glottis.[13]

c. Clinical Experience

Bellhouse[13] reported his experience of 3500 intubations in which he used the Belscope without failure. The report included a subseries of 12 patients in whom the Belscope successfully exposed the glottis where the Macintosh

Figure 23-26 Use of the Belscope by the right paraglossal route **(left)**, with view assisted by retraction of the lip. Occasionally, use of the prism may be required for indirect visualization of the larynx **(right)**. (From Bellhouse CP: An angulated laryngoscope for routine and difficult tracheal intubation. Anesthesiology 69:126, 1988.)

had failed. Bellhouse emphasized the need for practice in the use of the blade, as its feel is different from that of other blades.[13] Separately, Mayall reported a second series of 12 patients with Cormack grade 3 laryngoscopies with the Macintosh blade, all of whom were converted to a "good view of the cords" with the Belscope without use of the prism.[115] In a crossover study by Sultana and colleagues comparing Macintosh and Belscope laryngoscopy, of 22 grade 3 views obtained, 19 were with the Macintosh blade. ET passage using the Belscope required lip retraction by an assistant more frequently than with the Macintosh.[162]

Gajraj and coworkers[64] looked at cervical spine movement using the Belscope (with prism) compared with the Macintosh blade. They detected no difference in cervical spine movement between the blades as assessed by cross-table cervical spine radiographs.

2. Choi Double-Angle Laryngoscope

Choi in 1990 described a double-angled blade with the spatula incorporating two incremental angles—the proximal (20 degrees) and the distal (30 degrees) (Fig. 23-27). The spatula and beak are wide and flat for tongue or epiglottis control, and there is no vertical step or flange. The light source lies along the left edge of the blade, between the two angles, with the bulb pointing toward the center of the glottis. The blade can be used with either direct or indirect lifting of the epiglottis. It is commercially available in one adult and one pediatric size.[35]

3. Orr Laryngoscope

The Orr blade was developed to help eliminate contact with the upper teeth. Two right-angle bends (Fig. 23-28)

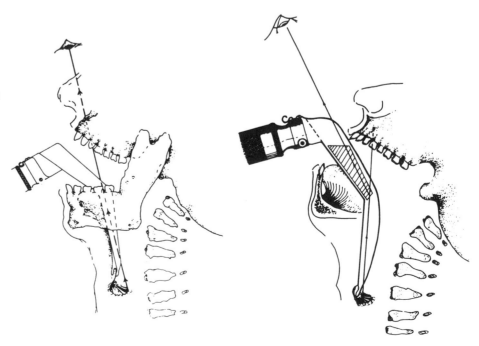

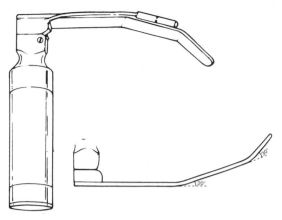

Figure 23-27 The Choi double-angle laryngoscope, with incremental 20-degree and 30-degree angles on its blade. (From Choi JJ: A new double-angle blade for direct laryngoscopy. Anesthesiology 72:576, 1990.)

are designed to enable the blade to sit down inside the mouth, shifting the fulcrum into the pharynx and away from the teeth. It is generally used to elevate the epiglottis directly, and ET advancement is from the right side of the mouth. Rarely used now, the Orr blade was available in two lengths.[126]

4. Levering Tip Laryngoscope

a. Description

The levering tip or articulating laryngoscope (McCoy, Corazzelli-London-McCoy or CLM blade, Mercury Medical, Clearwater, FL) is a modification of standard curved (and straight) laryngoscope blades. First described applied to a curved blade in 1993 and now marketed by a number of manufacturers (e.g., the Flipper [Rüsch Inc, Duluth, GA] and Heine Flex Tip [Heine Optotechnik,

Herrsching, Germany]), these laryngoscope blades have a hinged distal tip activated by a lever that lies adjacent to the handle of the laryngoscope. Depressing the lever toward the handle elevates the tip, located 25 mm from the end of the blade, by approximately 70 degrees (Fig. 23-29).[117] The lever acts on the tip through a spring-loaded drum on the proximal end of the blade, which in turn pushes a shaft linking with the distal hinge. In the resting position, the blade looks and acts like a standard blade, with the vertical step of the distal adjustable tip locking with that of the rest of the blade. The blade-lever assembly can be used with any compatible standard handle. When activated, the levering tip laryngoscope may have the advantage of having a fulcrum at a point lower in the pharynx, helping to provide an optimal tip angle and contact with the hyoepiglottic ligament in situations such as limited mouth opening, large tongue, or prominent or overriding upper teeth. It is available in different curved blade sizes (e.g., Macintosh 3 and 4) as well as straight blade sizes.[51]

b. Blade Use

The curved levering tip blade is most often used by placing the tip in the vallecula, although the tip can also be placed beneath the epiglottis. In the presence of poor glottic visualization, the lever can be depressed, activating the distal tip upward. This in turn may help the blade tip make contact with the hyoepiglottic ligament, in turn helping to lift the epiglottis and improve glottic visualization. Endotracheal intubation is then performed in a standard fashion. The lever is released and the blade is removed with the tip in the neutral position.

c. Clinical Experience

Since the introduction of the CLM, a number of case reports have attested to its value in difficult situations.[33,86,168] Subsequent prospective series have

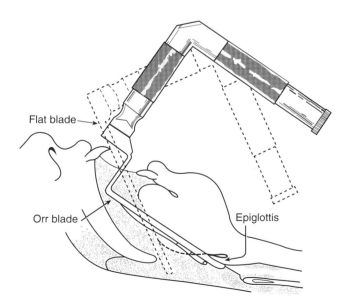

Figure 23-28 The Orr laryngoscope blade. (From Orr RB: A new laryngoscopy blade designed to facilitate difficult endotracheal intubation. Anesthesiology 31:377, 1969.)

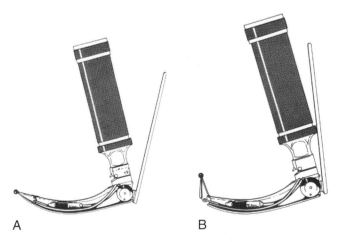

Figure 23-29 The Corazzelli-London-McCoy (CLM) blade in the default **(A)** and activated with tip elevated **(B)** positions. (From McCoy ED, Mirakhur RK: The levering laryngoscope, Anaesthesia 48:516, 1993.)

confirmed the CLM's utility in some difficult situations as well as confirming clinical suspicions that its use in otherwise easy situations may in fact worsen the view. Studies have been consistent in their findings that without cervical spine precautions, improvement with use of blade tip activation from Cormack[44] grade 3 views to grade 2 or better is significant, occurring 44% to 91% of the time.[34,40,74,137,166] In this population presenting with a grade 3 view, the view rarely worsens with blade tip activation.[34,40,74,166] In most[34,137,166] but not all[74] studies, the CLM blade has failed to meaningfully improve Cormack grade 4 views.

The levering tip blade is less useful in otherwise easy laryngoscopies. Although one report documented a 66% improvement in laryngoscopic view in 38 Cormack grade 2 (arytenoids only) patients, the same report revealed a 22% overall incidence of worsening of the view obtained with tip activation, all in patients in Cormack grades 1 and 2.[166] One explanation for this effect may be that in easy laryngoscopy situations, the blade tip easily engages and can lift the hyoepiglottic ligament and hyoid bone at the appropriate angle. With no potential for further upward travel, blade tip activation instead forces the midportion of the blade downward and into the direct line of sight, thus potentially obscuring the view (Fig. 23-30).[104] The better the view before tip activation, the more likely this phenomenon appears to be.[40,74,137,166]

Two studies have documented that the improvement in laryngoscopic view obtained with tip activation of the CLM is less than that obtained simply with external laryngeal pressure,[74,137] although application of both external laryngeal pressure and tip activation has an additive effect.[74]

McCoy and colleagues[119] found that force incurred when using the levering tip blade was significantly less than that needed to visualize the larynx with the Macintosh blade. There was no increase in heart rate, mean arterial pressure, or plasma norepinephrine levels with use of the levering tip blade,[118] possibly because of the lesser need to provide forward displacement of attached structures while elevating the epiglottis.

The CLM blade may be useful in patients in whom cervical spine precautions are in effect. In three separate studies simulating cervical spine precautions with use of either manual in-line stabilization or application of a cervical collar, activation of the levering tip improved the Cormack laryngeal view by at least one grade in 45% to 74% of patients, and in the patients with a grade 3 view, conversion to a grade 2 or better view occurred in 83% to 92% of cases.[61,102,167] Interestingly, in the 319 patients enrolled in these three studies, the view was worsened by use of the activated CLM blade in only one case. A separate study looking at head extension using external anatomic markers during CLM laryngoscopy demonstrated that 6 to 8 degrees less head extension was necessary for both arytenoid-only and full glottic exposure compared with Macintosh blade use.[161] MacIntyre and coauthors[109] however, using lateral radiographs to look at cervical spine movement with Macintosh and CLM blade use, could not demonstrate a significant difference in the degree of extension occurring between C0 and C3. Finally, in a cadaver series with surgically induced lesions at C5-6, Miller, Macintosh, and McCoy blade laryngoscopy use was assessed fluoroscopically. The Miller was superior to the Macintosh or the CLM blade at minimizing axial

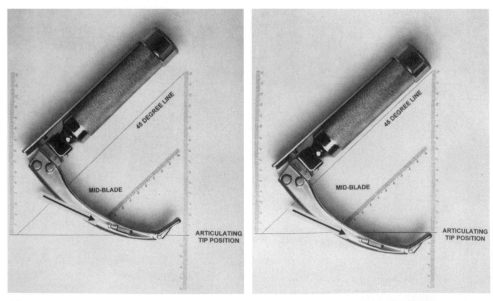

Figure 23-30 When the Corazzelli-London-McCoy (CLM) blade improves the view **(left),** the tip elevates base of tongue and vallecula. However, if these structures are already maximally elevated, tip activation forces the blade posteriorly into the line of sight **(right),** possibly worsening the view. (From Levitan RM, Ochroch EA: Explaining the variable effect on laryngeal view obtained with the McCoy laryngoscope [letter]. Anaesthesia 54:599-601, 1999.)

distraction, but no significant difference in anteroposterior displacement or angular rotation at the level of the lesion was otherwise demonstrated between blades.[66]

The CLM has been well studied since its introduction and, in summary, appears to be potentially useful in some difficult situations while not helping or in fact worsening the view in already easy direct laryngoscopy situations. Published evidence suggests that it may be particularly useful in situations in which Cormack grade 3 views have been induced by cervical spine precautions.

5. Flexiblade

a. Description

The Flexiblade (Arco Medic, Omer, Israel) is a second device incorporating a flexible component into a rigid blade. This direct laryngoscope is flexible in the intermediate portion of the blade. Activation of the trigger, which, unlike that in the CLM, lies along the front of the handle, results in variable flexion of six intermediate segments located 3.5 to 10 cm from the blade's tip. This adjusts the blade's curvature through a 20-degree arc, going from a shape similar to that of a Miller to that of a Macintosh blade (Fig. 23-31).[182] The Flexiblade can be attached to a standard laryngoscope handle or a remote light source by a fiberoptic cable and is available in three sizes, corresponding roughly to Macintosh 2, 3, and 4 blades.

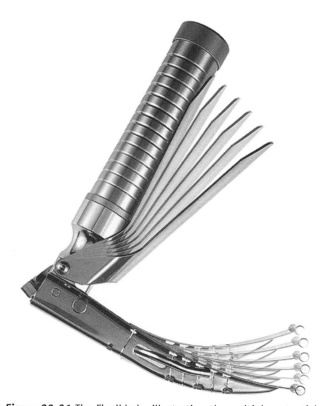

Figure 23-31 The Flexiblade, illustrating the multiple potential positions of its variably flexing blade. (Courtesy of Arco Medic Ltd.)

b. Blade Use

Use of the Flexiblade is similar to the technique used with the CLM blade. With the tip of the blade located in the vallecula, activation of the trigger increases the amount of blade flexion, which may in turn help with glottic visualization. ET passage follows in the usual fashion.

c. Clinical Experience

Perera and coauthors[130] evaluated the Flexiblade in 200 patients. In patients initially Cormack grade 3 with the Flexiblade in the neutral position, blade activation converted the view to Cormack grade 2 or 1 in 84% of cases. In the series, blade activation worsened the view in only four patients, and, as with the CLM blade, all of those patients were grade 1 or 2 before blade flexion. Yardeni and colleagues[183] performed an in vitro technical analysis of the blade after the technique described by Marks and associates and confirmed that the Flexiblade behaves in similar fashion to a Miller or Macintosh blade at the neutral and fully elevated positions, respectively.

D. BLADES DESIGNED FOR OTHER SPECIFIC ANATOMIC VARIANTS

1. Blades with Reduced Vertical Step

A number of blades have been designed with a reduced vertical step. In theory, this should help with blade insertion in patients with limited mouth opening and lower risk to the upper teeth. The latter risk is obviously increased if the laryngoscopist levers on the teeth, but studies have also demonstrated that the horizontal flanges of well-used Macintosh blades show significant signs of wear at the level of the upper teeth, suggesting frequent contact with the blade, and other studies have demonstrated that even experienced clinicians generate significant axial force on the upper incisors.[26,27] Although these findings may suggest that one of the functions of the vertical step is in fact to maintain mouth opening through contact with the upper teeth, most clinicians prefer at least to attempt to minimize contact with the upper teeth. To address the issue of step/flange contact with the upper teeth, a number of modifications to blades have been described.

a. Bizzarri-Giuffrida Blade

The Bizzarri-Giuffrida blade was developed in response to the problem of the Macintosh blade's vertical step and flange proximally touching the upper teeth, causing (particularly with limited mandibular mobility) difficulty in rotation of the blade into the hypopharynx and full insertion into the valleculae. The blade is curved in similar fashion to the Macintosh blade and simply omits the vertical step with the exception of a minimal amount midblade, where needed to protect the light carrier (Fig. 23-32). The inventors' experience in several hundred patients was one of "complete satisfaction," particularly in patients with "buck" teeth, receding jaw, "bull neck," and anterior larynx. They also noted successful use of the blade during

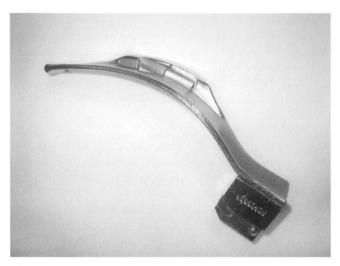

Figure 23-32 The Bizzarri blade, with its almost total absence of vertical step.

awake direct laryngoscopy.[17] Other studies, however, have not confirmed this opinion. When compared with the Macintosh in a mannequin study, the blade took longer to achieve intubation and was rated subjectively lower.[112] The blade may be useful in certain difficult situations but requires further study.

b. Callander-Thomas blade

Callander and Thomas in 1987 described a blade incorporating a reduction in the proximal portion of the vertical step and flange of the Macintosh blade (Fig. 23-33). The reduction in the step height was postulated to improve the blade's potential utility in patients with limited mouth opening as well as decrease the risk of dental damage.[29]

c. Bucx blade

A modification similar to the Callander-Thomas blade was made by Bucx after technical analysis suggested it to

be a good model.[25] This blade, with a Macintosh-style curve, has a vertical step and flange reduced to a minimum from blade base to 8 cm from the blade tip (Fig. 23-34). Bucx and coworkers[25] followed up with a clinical evaluation of the blade, randomly assigning 46 patients into two groups for laryngoscopy and intubation with either a regular Macintosh or the modified blade. Although the mean force exerted on the maxillary incisors was significantly reduced in the modified blade group, there was a decided tendency toward anteflexion of the head during laryngoscopy with the modified blade and an increased need for the assistant to retract the upper lip to aid with intubation. These findings were confirmed in a second mannequin study.[24] Although the accepted purpose of the vertical step of laryngoscope blades is stated to be soft tissue, especially tongue, control, this study suggests the possibility that the vertical step and flange at the level of the upper teeth may in fact help to maintain mouth opening and counteract the tendency of the head to anteflex during laryngoscopy.

d. Onkst Blade

Onkst in 1961 modified a Macintosh 3 blade to help avoid undue pressure on the upper incisors. The proximal portions of the blade's vertical step and flange are hinged and, although normally kept in the upright position by a weak spring, allow the vertical step/flange to fold down in response to pressure on the teeth, thus theoretically avoiding dental damage (Fig. 23-35).[125]

e. Racz-Allen Hinged-Step Blade

Racz and Allen introduced another blade with hinged step and flange. This modified straight blade has its vertical step hinged and maintained in position by a spring. During laryngoscopy, any pressure on the vertical step from the upper teeth causes an upward and lateral deflection of

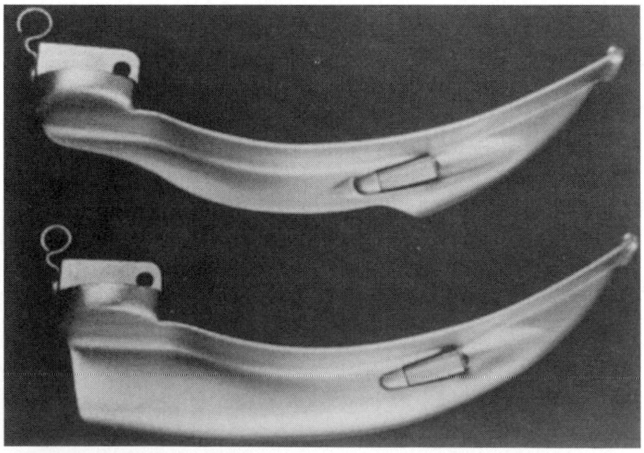

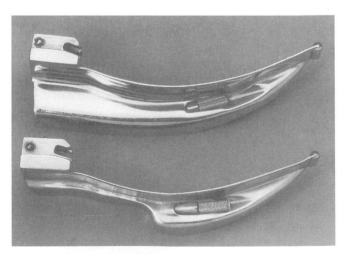

Figure 23-33 The Callander-Thomas blade **(top),** with reduced vertical step proximally, compared with the Macintosh **(bottom).** (From Callander CC, Thomas J: Modification of Macintosh laryngoscope for difficult intubation [letter]. Anaesthesia 42:671, 1987.)

Figure 23-34 The Bucx blade **(bottom),** with reduced proximal vertical step, compared with the Macintosh **(top).** (From Bucx MJL, Snijders CJ, van der Vegt MH, et al: Reshaping the Macintosh blade using biomechanical modeling. Anaesthesia 52:662-667, 1997.)

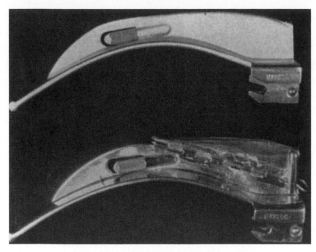

Figure 23-35 The Onkst blade **(bottom),** with its hinged vertical component, compared with standard Macintosh blade **(top).** (From Onkst R: Modified laryngoscope blade. Anesthesiology 22:846, 1961.)

the hinged portion. The main blade is convex in cross section to a greater extent than the Miller to help maintain vision when the concave hinged portion is displaced. A threaded shaft is removable, allowing disassembly of the two portions of the blade for cleaning (Fig. 23-36).[136] The blade is intermediate in length between a Miller 2 and 3. Racz and Allen reported over 2000 successful intubations at their institution with the blade.

2. Blades and Devices That Avoid Chest Impingement

A number of adaptations have been reported to help avoid unwanted impingement of a laryngoscope's handle during laryngoscopy. This is particularly important in morbidly obese patients, parturients with mammomegaly,

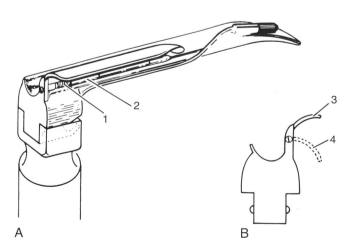

Figure 23-36 Side **(A)** and fitting **(B)** views of the Racz-Allen hinged blade. 1, spring; 2, threaded screw; 3, normal position; 4, full displacement of the hinged component of the blade. (From Racz GB, Allen FB: A new pressure-sensitive laryngoscope. Anesthesiology 62:356, 1985.)

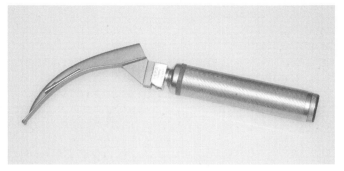

Figure 23-37 The Polio blade is a standard Macintosh blade that fits onto a standard handle at a very obtuse angle.

patients in an "iron lung," and during the application of cricoid pressure, when an assistant's hand is present. Equipment solutions have included shortened handles as well as making the angle between the laryngoscope handle and blade more obtuse by means of modifications to the blade itself, the handle, or insertion of adapters. It should be emphasized, however, that appropriate positioning of the patient often renders these devices unnecessary.

a. Modified Blades

The *Polio* blade was introduced by Foregger in 1954, designed for use during intubation of patients in iron lung respirators. It features a Macintosh-style blade that attaches to a battery handle at an obtuse angle of 170 degrees (Fig. 23-37).[170] It may still have application in situations where a regular handle attachment setup may encounter forward impingement (e.g., obesity, kyphosis with barrel chest deformity, mammary gland hypertrophy, or a short neck),[100] although the extremely obtuse angle of blade to handle may make it difficult to generate an adequate lifting force. The *Kessel* modification involved remaking a Macintosh blade's block so that the blade comes off the handle at an angle of 110 degrees instead of the usual 90 degrees. No other modifications were made (Fig. 23-38).[92] Beaver described a straight

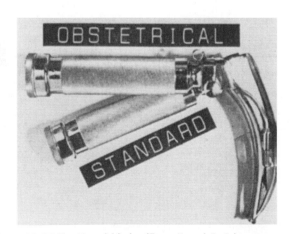

Figure 23-38 The Kessel blade. (From Kessel J: A laryngoscope for obstetrical use: An obstetrical laryngoscope. Anaesth Intensive Care 5:265, 1977.)

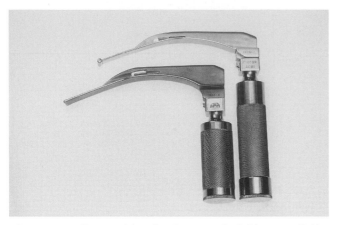

Figure 23-39 Shortened handles (e.g., on the left) are available to help avoid chest impingement during laryngoscopy.

blade with a handle set at 25 degrees to facilitate intubation of patients in "box" respirators.[12]

b. Modified Handles

Short handles at half the length of regular laryngoscope handles have been described to help avoid chest or breast impingement (Fig. 23-39).[47] In addition, some handles (e.g., the Heine fiberoptic angled handle [Heine USA Ltd., Dover, NH]) are available with a blade hook attachment configuration that results in more obtuse angulation of any attached laryngoscope blade (Fig. 23-40). Patil and colleagues have described a shortened, adjustable angle laryngoscope handle incorporating a blade lock device that allows positioning of the blade at 180, 135, 90, or 45 degrees to the handle (Fig. 23-41). When there is potential impingement of a laryngoscope handle on a patient's chest, the instrument can be inserted at 180 degrees; then the angle of the blade to handle can be reduced to a more regular 135 or 90 degrees, allowing laryngoscopy to be performed.[128]

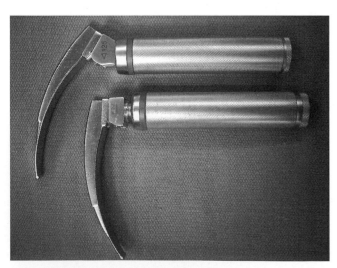

Figure 23-40 The Heine handle with an angled hook configuration allowing more obtuse angulation of any type of Greenline specification fiberoptic blade.

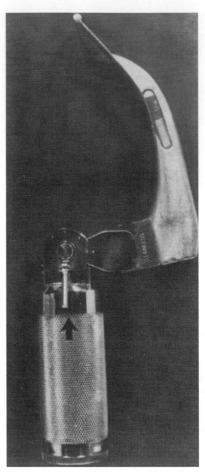

Figure 23-41 The Patil handle allows positioning of the laryngoscope blade at an angle of 45, 90, 135, or 180 degrees to the (shortened) handle. (From Patil VU, Stehling LC, Zauder HL: An adjustable laryngoscope handle for difficult intubations [letter]. Anesthesiology 60:609, 1984.)

c. Adapters

The *Jellicoe* adapter was described to overcome the reality of the true angle between Macintosh blade tip and handle being 58 degrees. The adapter simply increases this angle to 90 degrees (Fig. 23-42), potentially facilitating blade entry into patients' oral cavities in some situations.[84] Dhara and Cheong in 1991 described a multiple angle laryngoscope adapter that fits between handle and blade and makes available working angles of 65, 90, 110, 130, 150, and 180 degrees between blade and handle (Fig. 23-43).[48] Finally, the *Yentis* adapter is a 2.5-cm cube block that fits between a standard handle and laryngoscope blade (Fig. 23-44). It allows insertion of the blade into the patient's mouth with the handle swung 90 degrees to the right. When the blade is inserted, the handle can be swung back to the normal position for laryngoscopy.[184]

3. Blades for Small Infraoral Cavity

a. Bainton Blade

The Bainton blade is unique in this collection of blades in that it is designed specifically for pathologic conditions

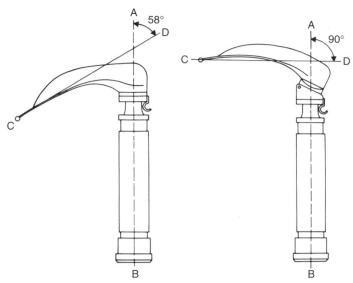

Figure 23-42 Diagram illustrating the 58-degree functional angle between the standard Macintosh blade tip and handle **(left)** and 90-degree angle with interposed Jellicoe adaptor **(right)**. (From Jellicoe JA, Harris NR: A modification of a standard laryngoscope for difficult tracheal intubation in obstetric cases. Anaesthesia 39:800-802, 1984.)

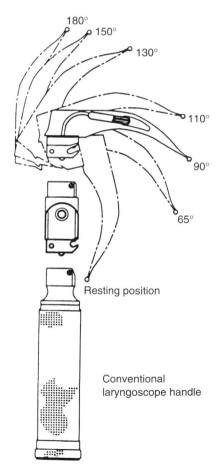

Figure 23-43 The Dhara adapter makes available multiple angles between laryngoscope blade and handle. (From Dhara SF, Cheong TW: An adjustable multiple angle laryngoscope adaptor. Anaesth Intensive Care 10:243, 1991.)

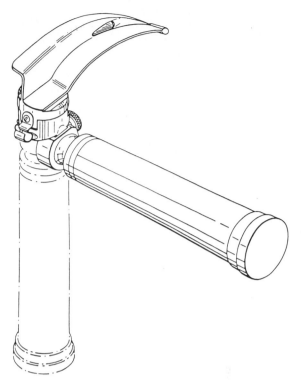

Figure 23-44 The Yentis adapter allows lateral pivoting of the laryngoscope handle to aid blade insertion. (From Yentis SM: A laryngoscope adaptor for difficult intubation. Anaesthesia 42: 764, 1987.)

creating obliteration of the hypopharynx. It is essentially a straight blade, compatible with regular laryngoscope handles, the distal 7 cm of which has a tubular design to help create a pharyngeal space where there may be none (Fig. 23-45). The lumen accepts up to a size 8.0 ET, and an intraluminal light source ensures that lighting is not compromised by tissues crowding the bulb. Bainton tested his prototype on dogs with artificially induced hypopharyngeal swelling and also in a small series of 12 patients with edematous conditions of the pharynx (one with a friable bleeding tumor), with complete success.[11] The blade has gone on to commercial production.

b. Diaz Pediatric Tubular Laryngoscope

This laryngoscope features a U-shaped handle and blade assembly. With a gradual distal curve, the blade is composed of two halves that are held together with a removable screw. A tubular scope of straight blade design results when the two halves are attached (Fig. 23-46). The enclosed channel houses two light sources, one on each side, which are powered from an external fiberoptic light source. Endotracheal intubation is accomplished through the lumen of the scope, which must be disassembled by removal of the screw prior to the scope's removal from the patient.[50]

E. PEDIATRIC LARYNGOSCOPES

Both Macintosh and Miller blades are available in pediatric sizes. A size 1 in both blades is generally appropriate

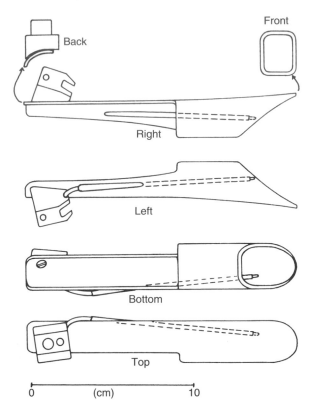

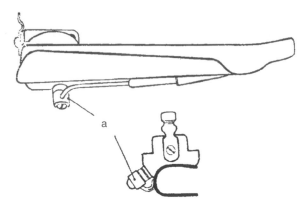

Figure 23-47 The Oxford pediatric blade as described by Bryce-Smith. Letter "a" represents the light carrier. (From Bryce-Smith R: A laryngoscope blade for infants. Br Med J 1:217, 1952.)

Figure 23-45 The Bainton laryngoscope blade is tubular distally to help overcome pharyngeal obstruction. (From Bainton CR: A new laryngoscope blade to overcome pharyngeal obstruction. Anesthesiology 67:767, 1987.)

for an infant and a size 2 for a child. Additional Miller sizes 0 and 00 are available for the premature and small premature infant, respectively. Other pediatric blades are available commercially; descriptions of them follow.

1. Oxford (Bryce-Smith) Blade

The Oxford, or Bryce-Smith blade, was intended for neonates but is applicable to infants up to age 3. Primarily a straight blade, it tapers gradually from its proximal width of 1.8 cm to 1 cm distally. The step and flange are U shaped,

and although the distal 2.5 cm is open, a slight distal step remains for tongue control. The horizontal flange is quite broad proximally, helping prevent the upper lip from obscuring the view and also potentially helping in difficult cleft-palate situations (Fig. 23-47).[22]

2. Seward Blade

The Seward blade was created for use in the neonate, although is also compatible with children up to age 5. The primarily straight blade is 10.5 cm in length, with a mild distal angulation and sharply tapering width, ending in a thickened beak. The adult bulb is protected from the tongue on the inside of the reverse Z-shaped step and flange (Fig. 23-48).[143]

3. Robertshaw Blade

Robertshaw originally modified a baby Soper straight blade by slightly curving the distal end while also modifying the step and flange from the Soper's reverse Z to a slight C. The light source was well protected from the

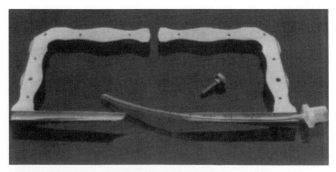

Figure 23-46 Two-piece tubular pediatric laryngoscope as described by Diaz and colleagues. (From Diaz JH, Guarisco JL, LeJeune FE: A modified tubular pharyngolaryngoscope for difficult pediatric laryngoscopy. Anesthesiology 73:357, 1990.)

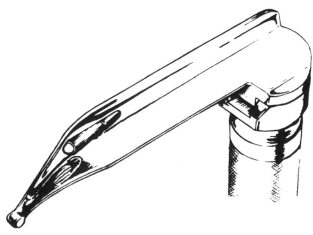

Figure 23-48 The Seward newborn laryngoscope blade. (From Seward EH: Laryngoscope for resuscitation of the newborn. Lancet 2:1041, 1957.)

tongue inside the vertical step. A subsequent modification, the Mark 2, exhibited additional leftward bending of the vertical step, creating a wider channel for visualization (Fig. 23-49).[138]

4. Others

The *Propper* or *Heine* blade is straight with a slightly curved tip. The horizontal flange is in the reverse-Z configuration, curving away from the blade.[51] A number of other modifications have been described for pediatric use. Matsuki[114] described a widened thin blade attached to the handle at a slightly obtuse angle to aid in control of the infant tongue. Rokowski and Gurmarnik[139] described a modification of the standard Miller 0 blade in which the distal portion of the blade was widened into a triangular configuration for neonates or circular configuration for infants. In addition, the width of the flange was reduced by 2 mm without modifying the height of the step, to improve the area available for ET manipulation and laryngeal visualization. Diaz[49] combined a number of described improvements in pediatric blades into one unit by modifying a Miller 1 blade to include an attached oxygen insufflation port, a corrugated lingual surface, and outward bending of the C-shaped flange to widen the cross-sectional area. No formal evaluation has been published.

F. LARYNGOSCOPE BLADES WITH ACCESSORY DEVICES

1. Blades with Integrated Oxygen Delivery Channel

A number of blades, mainly in pediatric sizes, are available with integrated channels designed for the insufflation of oxygen during direct laryngoscopy. The concept has evolved from earlier reports of oxygen insufflation through feeding tubes taped to blades during laryngoscopy of neonates and infants.[43,180] Hencz subsequently described permanently affixing a wide-bore aspirating needle for the same purpose.[76] Todres and Crone[164] formally described the *Oxyscope* laryngoscope incorporating a built-in oxygen insufflation channel. It was originally made available in Miller 0 and 1 blades and subsequently in Macintosh blades. Studies during laryngoscopy in spontaneously breathing anesthetized infants have demonstrated higher oxygen tensions with oxygen administration through these blades.[103,164] They continue to be marketed under various brand names, mainly in the Miller configuration.

2. Blades with Integrated Suction Channel

Adult[62,93] and pediatric[55] blades with an integrated suction channel or blades that allow suction through an oxygen administration port have been described. The modified blades could potentially be useful in patients with copious secretions or emesis or situations such as bleeding after tonsillectomy, by allowing suctioning during ongoing laryngoscopy.[105] The *Khan* blade consisted of a 1.75 mm ID tube welded to a straight blade with a proximal hub angled so that the laryngoscopist's thumb could occlude a port to control the amount of suction applied.[93] *Tull* suction blades, available in Miller and Macintosh versions, have a finger-controlled valve lying next to the laryngoscope handle to enable the laryngoscopist to apply suction at will.[51]

V. RIGID INDIRECT LARYNGOSCOPES AND STYLETS

Rigid indirect laryngoscopes enable a view of the laryngeal inlet indirectly through a fiberoptic bundle, video camera, or other optical aid. Examples of optically aided laryngoscopes include the Siker blade with its built-in mirror; blades using attachable prisms (e.g., the Huffman and Belscope), and the Viewmax laryngoscope (which refracts a distal image through the use of a series of lenses). Other indirect laryngoscopes deliver an image endoscopically through a fiberoptic bundle or using video technology. These laryngoscopes have the advantage of enabling vision "around the corner" of the tongue, thus potentially bypassing some of the problems inherent in direct laryngoscopy. Indirect laryngoscopes in each of the optical, fiberoptic, and video categories vary in shape from those using classically shaped Macintosh blades to instruments of entirely different design. The ensuing discussion is limited to rigid and semirigid indirect devices, as flexible fiberoptic and rigid direct bronchoscopes are covered elsewhere in this text.

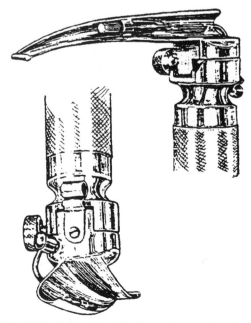

Figure 23-49 The Robertshaw blade, Mark 2 version. (From Robertshaw FL: A new laryngoscope for infants and children. Lancet 2:1034, 1962.)

A. RIGID INDIRECT LARYNGOSCOPES WITH OPTICALLY ASSISTED VIEW

1. Siker Laryngoscope

Siker in 1956 described an angled laryngoscope with an incorporated reflecting surface. The portion of the blade distal to the mirror is angulated at 135 degrees from the proximal section (Fig. 23-50). The stainless steel mirror is attached to the blade by means of a copper jacket to facilitate conduction of heat from the patient, thereby minimizing fogging of the mirror.[151] After blade insertion, if the laryngeal inlet cannot be directly visualized, the mirror can be used to indirectly identify first epiglottis and then cords. Facility with the use of this blade takes some experience, as the mirror inverts the reflected image. A styletted tube is essential; as the tube enters the larynx, it appears to move in a posteroinferior direction. Siker in his original publication described the blade's use in 100 "unselected" patients. Laryngoscopy failed in just one patient because of excessive blade length. In three other patients with failed laryngoscopy and intubation with standard blades, the Siker succeeded. The author has emphasized the need for practice in the use of the blade.[151]

2. McMorrow-Mirakhur Mirrored Laryngoscope

McMorrow and Mirakhur described a modification of the levering tip laryngoscope that incorporates an adjustable mirror. Looking like a regular CLM laryngoscope in resting position (Fig. 23-51), it can be operated as both a regular Macintosh blade or levering tip blade, as previously described. The difference is that it has a mirror lying posteriorly on the blade. As the levering tip is activated by

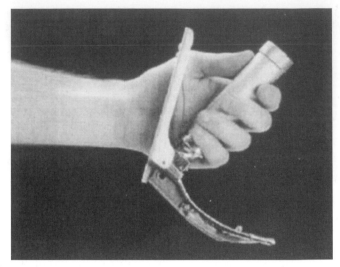

Figure 23-51 The McMorrow-Mirakhur laryngoscope in the resting position. (From McMorrow RCN, Mirakhur RK: A new mirrored laryngoscope. Anaesthesia 58:998-1002, 2003.)

moving the control lever toward the laryngoscope handle, (Fig. 23-52) the mirror is deployed posteriorly and inferiorly with respect to the blade. If necessary, further depression of the control lever toward the handle changes the mirror pitch to a usable angle (Fig. 23-53), ultimately providing an additional 60-degree field of view compared with the Macintosh alone. If intubation is performed between the blade and the mirror, the scope has to be removed in its activated state. The blade should be heated or the mirror defogged prior to each use.

McMorrow and Mirakhur tested the laryngoscope in 15 patients presenting for elective surgery, comparing it

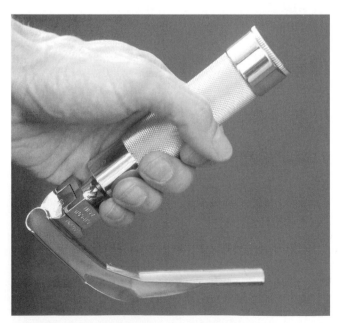

Figure 23-50 The Siker blade, with its reflecting mirror located inferiorly, midblade.

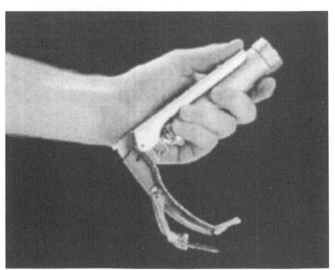

Figure 23-52 The McMorrow-Mirakhur laryngoscope in the half-deployed positions; the levering tip is activated and the mirror is ignored. (From McMorrow RCN, Mirakhur RK: A new mirrored laryngoscope. Anaesthesia 58:998-1002, 2003.)

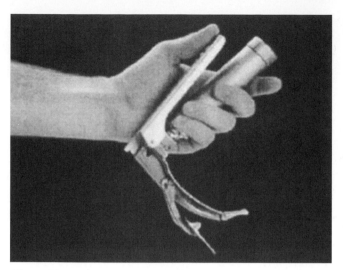

Figure 23-53 The McMorrow-Mirakhur laryngoscope in the fully deployed position with the distal mirror providing an additional 6 degrees of visual field. (From McMorrow RCN, Mirakhur RK: A new mirrored laryngoscope. Anaesthesia 58:998-1002, 2003.)

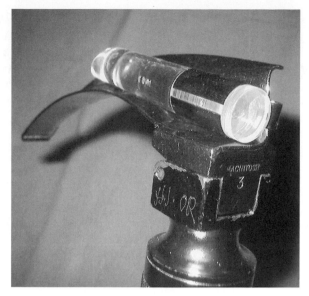

Figure 23-54 A Huffman prism attached to a Macintosh 3 blade.

with both the Macintosh and McCoy blades. Manual in-line neck stabilization was used to create difficult conditions for laryngoscopy, and all patients were reported as Cormack[44] grade 3 views with the Macintosh blade. Using the McMorrow-Mirakhur blade with mirror deployment, an improvement from a grade 3 to a grade 1 view occurred in 50% of patients and to grade 2 in 21%. The view was considered worse in 7%, and no change was noted in 21% of patients.[121]

3. Huffman Prism

Although a prism had been described by Janeway in 1913, Huffman revisited the concept in 1968, attaching a Plexiglas prism to a Macintosh 3 blade by means of a steel clip. Because the image of the cords is deflected by approximately 30 degrees, Huffman theorized that less force on tongue and hypopharynx would be needed to achieve laryngeal inlet visualization (Fig. 23-54).[81] Subsequently, he affixed a second prism distal to the first to achieve a total refraction of 80 degrees. He used the resulting instrument as a tool to inspect the larynx at light planes of anesthesia but also speculated that it may be a useful tool for the difficult laryngoscopy situation.[82] Huffman prisms continue to be available in various sizes for Macintosh blades.

4. Rüsch Viewmax Laryngoscope

The Viewmax (Rüsch Inc, Duluth, GA) laryngoscope blade is similar in shape to a Macintosh but incorporates a removable lens system (the Viewscope) ending in a proximal eyepiece, which can refract the distal image 20 degrees from the horizontal (Fig. 23-55). This has the potential to improve laryngeal inlet visualization compared with

that obtainable by direct vision. The blade of the Viewmax is wider than that of a standard Macintosh, and although the lens system provides some vertical component, the blade otherwise has little formal vertical step. With the resultant lessened ability to sweep the tongue to the left, the blade can be used midline in the patient's mouth. The Viewmax is available in an adult and a pediatric size, corresponding to Macintosh size $3\frac{1}{2}$ and 2 blades, respectively. (It should be noted that at the time of writing the name Viewmax is also applied to another company's [Timesco, London, England] version of the improved view Macintosh blade.)

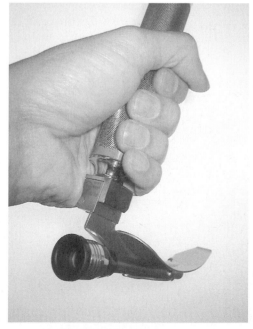

Figure 23-55 The Rüsch Viewmax blade. A lens system refracts the distal image by 20 degrees. (Courtesy of Rüsch Canada.)

B. RIGID INDIRECT FIBEROPTIC LARYNGOSCOPES

Rigid indirect laryngoscopes were first introduced into anesthetic practice in the late 1980s, with more widespread use occurring throughout the 1990s. Initially, most of these devices made use of fiberoptic technology for image transmission; primary video imaging has since been introduced.

1. Bullard Laryngoscope

a. Description

The Bullard laryngoscope (BL; ACMI Corporation, Southborough, MA) is an indirect rigid fiberoptic laryngoscope. Available in adult and pediatric versions, it has been used to facilitate intubations in awake and anesthetized patients by the oral and nasal[91,144,145] routes with standard, armored,[1] Ring-Adair-Elwyn (RAE),[91] Endotrol,[19,42] and double-lumen[68,149] ETs. The BL's anatomically shaped blade permits indirect laryngoscopy without aligning the oral, pharyngeal, and laryngeal axes, making the device potentially useful for patients with limitation of cervical spine mobility or mouth opening and those with prominent upper incisors.

Introduced in the late 1980s, the BL features a rigid L-shaped blade incorporating fiberoptic bundles that transmit an image to a proximal eyepiece (Fig. 23-56). The fiberoptic bundle, located on the posterior aspect of the blade, comes to within 26 mm of the distal tip of the blade and affords a 55-degree field of view at the level of the larynx. The eyepiece can accept a video camera attachment and on more recent versions allows adjustable diopter correction. Power is supplied from a standard battery handle or with use of an adapter, through a flexible fiberoptic cable connected to a high-intensity (e.g., halogen or xenon) light source. A 3.7-mm hollow working channel also lies posteriorly on the blade, with a proximal Luer-lock connection. This channel can be used for suction, oxygen insufflation, or the administration of local anesthetics during laryngoscopy.

The BL is the only indirect fiberoptic laryngoscope to offer two styles of attachable metal stylets designed to facilitate ET advancement, although its use has also been described with a styletted ET used freehand.[19,110] Intubating forceps used early in the scope's history have been largely abandoned in favor of the stylets. The original attached nonmalleable wire stylet (Fig. 23-57) has an external diameter of 3.3 mm, anchors to a port on the BL blade, and follows the contour of the blade to its tip. The more recently introduced multifunctional intubating stylet (MFIS) (Fig. 23-58) features a hollow lumen allowing prior passage of a flexible catheter or an 11 Fr airway exchange catheter (Cook Inc, Bloomington, IN)[38] over which an ET can be advanced. Available in adult and pediatric sizes, the MFIS attaches to either the eyepiece shaft or the same port as the original wire stylet, according to the model. The BL's blade is only 6.4 mm thick, allowing its use in patients with minimal interincisor opening. However, when it is used with one of the loaded attached stylets, the greatest limitation to insertion of the BL is the external diameter of the ET, as the entire blade-stylet-tube unit is inserted simultaneously (Fig. 23-59).

A disposable plastic blade tip extender has been made available to extend the length of the BL blade tip (see Fig. 23-56). Designed to aid in picking up the epiglottis in larger patients, this device clicks firmly to the metal blade tip and requires significant effort or a tool to remove, making its inadvertent loss in the patient's hypopharynx unlikely if it is properly applied. If the extender is used, however, the blade should be inspected for its presence after withdrawal from the patient's mouth.

Two pediatric versions of the scope are available, the neonatal (newborn to 2 years) and the pediatric (newborn

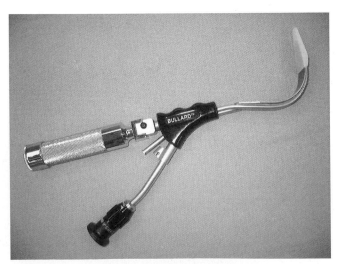

Figure 23-56 The adult Bullard laryngoscope. Note presence of the plastic tip extender.

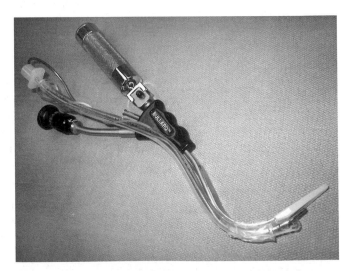

Figure 23-57 The adult Bullard laryngoscope with loaded attached wire stylet and blade tip extender. Note that distal tip of stylet is placed through Murphy eye of endotracheal tube.

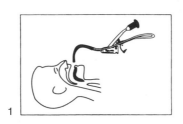

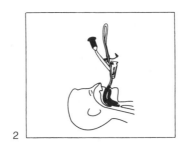

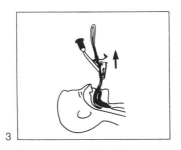

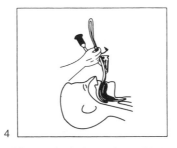

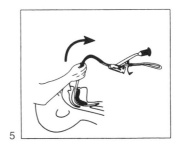

Figure 23-58 Bullard laryngoscope use with attached wire stylet. With head and neck in the neutral position, the scope-stylet-tube assembly is inserted into the patient's mouth **(1)**. As the handle is rotated from a horizontal to a vertical plane **(2)** the blade slides down and around the tongue. Once vertical, the blade is allowed to drop gently against posterior pharyngeal wall, moved caudad, then lifted vertically **(3)**, directly lifting epiglottis and exposing cords when the image is sought through the eyepiece. With the stylet tip aimed at the glottic opening, the endotracheal tube is advanced off the stylet through the cords **(4)**. Following intubation, the unit is rotated forward to the horizontal and out of the patient's mouth **(5)**. (From Cooper SD, Benumof JL, Ozaki GT: Evaluation of the Bullard laryngoscope using the new intubating stylet: Comparison with conventional laryngoscopy. Anesth Analg 79:965, 1994.)

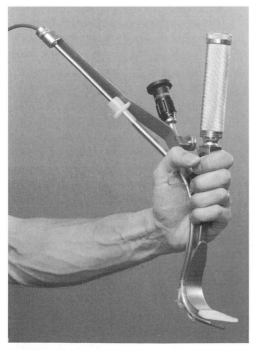

Figure 23-59 The Bullard laryngoscope with attached multifunctional intubating stylet (in this case attached to the viewing arm). Endotracheal intubation can be preceded by passage of a flexible guiding catheter, seen here protruding from the distal end of the stylet.

to 10 years) (Fig. 23-60). Both blades are narrower with a width of 1.3 cm, in contrast to the adult blade's 2.5-cm width, and have a decreased internal curvature radius.[150]

b. Instrument Use

Before use, the BL must be defogged, as with any indirect fiberoptic laryngoscope. This can be achieved with a commercial defogging or silicon solution, warming of the scope (e.g., in a forced air warmer[53] or between warm blankets), or insufflation of oxygen at 6 to 8 L/min.[46] If an attached stylet is used, it should be attached to the BL in the appropriate location, lubricated, and loaded with an ET. Removal of the 15-mm connector may aid ET loading and unloading. If the original wire stylet is used, the tube is loaded with the distal stylet tip placed just through the Murphy eye (see Fig. 23-57). Alternatively, if a freehand technique is used, the tube and stylet *must* be bent appropriately, conforming approximately to the shape of the blade. For light source activation, the battery handle or fiberoptic adapter is engaged by pushing distally on a safety lock button located on the proximal laryngoscope blade.

Insertion of the scope begins with the handle parallel to the patient's chest (see Fig. 23-58). With the patient's mouth opened, the blade is inserted into the mouth in the midline, with the tube and attached stylet held snugly to the undersurface of the blade. As the blade is advanced,

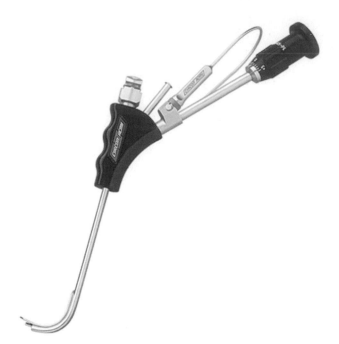

Figure 23-60 Pediatric Bullard laryngoscope with wire stylet attached. (Courtesy of ACMI Corporation.)

it is rotated down into the hypopharynx, in the midline, until the handle is vertical. At that point, the entire assembly is allowed to drop gently against the posterior pharyngeal wall, moved caudad, then lifted vertically. This "scooping" maneuver aids in picking up the epiglottis. The image of the laryngeal inlet is then sought through the eyepiece. The stylet and tube are lined up with the glottic opening, whereupon the ET is advanced off the stylet through the glottis. If the multifunctional stylet is used, tube passage can be preceded by passing the intubation catheter. Proper endotracheal placement can be confirmed under endoscopic visualization through the eyepiece as the tube is advanced. Following ET placement, while holding the ET, the BL or BL-stylet assembly is removed by rotating forward and toward the patient's chest.

As with any of the scopes in this category of device, the ET advances from the right side rather than in the midline position. This may occasionally result in difficulty with tube passage into the trachea despite good vocal cord visualization because of the leading edge of the ET's bevel striking the right arytenoid cartilages, aryepiglottic fold, or vocal cord. Various responses have been described for this dilemma, including aiming the wire stylet at the middle third of the left vocal fold,[89] moving the BL tip 2 to 3 mm to the left and reattempting tube passage,[90] loading the tube (on the original wire stylet) reversed with bevel directed to the right,[88,90] permanently lessening the terminal angulation of the attached wire stylet from 20 to 15 degrees, or moving the scope slightly cephalad before another attempt.[46] In addition, it should be appreciated that positioning the blade-tube-stylet assembly too

close to the glottis can be detrimental to easy tube passage. Finally, in spite of visualization of the tube tip passing successfully through the cords, occasionally ET passage beyond the cricoid cartilage is impeded; one solution may be to angulate the BL slightly forward to help align the stylet's axis with that of the trachea.[90]

c. Clinical Experience

Following the BL's introduction, many case reports detailed its successful use in awake and anesthetized patients with difficult airways (DAs).[37-39,67,68] Where the BL enables the clinician to "see around the corner," generally an excellent view of the glottis is obtained, even when direct laryngoscopy has failed. Indeed, Cooper and colleagues reported in a series of 50 patients that the view, time to intubation, and ease of intubation with the BL were independent of Cormack views obtained at direct laryngoscopy.[42] When compared with the flexible FOB in both awake and anesthetized patients, the BL has been found to require less time to obtain a view and achieve intubation than the flexible FOB, with an equal success rate even with manual in-line neck stabilization.[36,37,148] Most studies have found BL use to be unaffected by cricoid pressure application, in contrast to the flexible FOB.[148] No differences have been demonstrated in the hemodynamic (diastolic blood pressure or heart rate) response to intubation when comparing BL with Macintosh direct laryngoscopy.[8]

The Bullard is easily used with the head and neck in the neutral position and may be a good instrument to use in the patient with limitation to head and cervical spine mobility. Hastings and colleagues studied head and neck movement during laryngoscopy and intubation with the BL, Macintosh, and Miller blades and found that significantly less head extension occurred with use of the BL. Radiographically determined upper cervical spine extension was also significantly less using the BL compared with the Macintosh, and glottic visualization was significantly better with the BL.[75] A second study similarly found cervical spine extension to be significantly less with the BL compared with Macintosh direct laryngoscopy both with and without manual in-line neck stabilization.[169]

The BL has been used to facilitate nasal intubations. Used orally to help guide intubation with an ET passed nasally, the blade can be used with minimal mouth opening. Shigematsu and colleagues have described Bullard-aided nasal intubation with an Endotrol (Mallinckrodt Inc, St. Louis, MO) tube to be a useful technique,[144,145] and Katsnelson and coworkers described use of an epidural catheter passed distally through the Murphy eye of a nasal RAE tube and looped proximally to aid tip control during BL-aided nasal intubation.[91]

BL use in the pediatric setting has been studied using the adult scope. In one series of 50 pediatric patients, all but 4 patients were successfully intubated with the adult BL, with all the failures occurring in patients younger than 38 months.[150] When use of the adult BL was compared with the Wis-Hipple 1½ blade in pediatric patients, no significant difference was found in terms of total time to intubation, and a similar number of failed intubations occurred with each blade.[147] The only series reporting use of the pediatric Bullard described successful laryngoscopy (although not intubation) in 90 of 93 pediatric patients, 31% of whom had predictors or a history of difficult laryngoscopy.[19]

Finally, a single series has been published describing the use of the BL for double-lumen tube placement. Using the original wire intubating stylet with the terminal angulation decreased to 15 degrees,[46] the double-lumen tube was successfully placed in the trachea in 28 of 29 patients, including two with a history of known difficult direct laryngoscopy, in an average of 28 seconds. The bronchial lumen was found to be correctly located in the left main stem in only 9 of the 28 patients.[149]

The BL is a useful instrument for use in the DA and in the patient with cervical spine precautions. Dr. Roger Bullard, a now-retired obstetric anesthesiologist, continues to be a tireless advocate of the instrument. To the practitioner who takes the time to become familiar with its use in the elective patient, the BL can become an invaluable tool in the anticipated or unanticipated difficult situation.

2. UpsherScope

a. Description

Simplest in design of the rigid fiberoptic laryngoscopes is the UpsherScope (Mercury Medical, Clearwater, FL). Similar in design to the BL, it consists of a rigid curved blade that can also attach to either a battery-powered handle or a high-intensity light source through a fiberoptic cable. It differs from the BL in having a J- rather than L-shaped blade, which is narrower and more rounded in profile (Fig. 23-61). Located on the posterior surface of the blade is a C-shaped tube-guiding channel, which ends 2 cm from the distal end of the blade. It is designed to guide passage of an ET up to 7.5 mm ID in size to the glottic opening, and an open slot in the tube guide allows the ET to be disengaged from the device following intubation. The light channel and viewing fibers also run posteriorly, to the left of the tube guide. The device does not have any extra ports, and any suctioning, insufflation of oxygen, or local anesthetic instillation is performed directly through the lumen of the ET. The UpsherScope Ultra (Mercury Medical) has been introduced and features improved optics, a flatter blade tip for improved epiglottis control, and, most important, an elongated lower flange that helps direct the ET anteriorly, in turn potentially decreasing the amount of vertical lift needed when using the scope. The scope is presently available in only a single adult size.

b. Instrument Use

The laryngoscope is prepared for use by lubricating the posterior delivery channel with a water-soluble lubricant

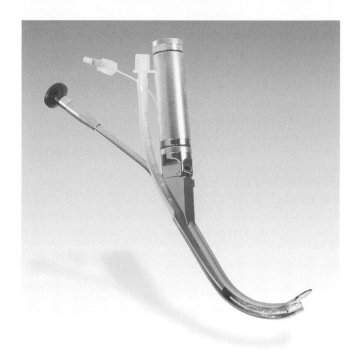

Figure 23-61 The UpsherScope Ultra with endotracheal tube loaded in tube delivery channel. Note the extended lower flange designed to help direct the endotracheal tube anteriorly. (Courtesy of Mercury Medical.)

and performing an antifog maneuver. As with all fiberoptic scopes, secretions can interfere with the view, and the oropharynx should be suctioned prior to the insertion of the device. An ET is loaded into the delivery channel, with its distal tip positioned just proximal to the optical bundle so as not to obscure the view of the cords. The eyepiece should be focused (UpsherScope only) and the light source activated.

Insertion of the scope into the patient should be started with the scope handle parallel to the patient, with the head and neck in the neutral position. Only 15 mm of mouth opening is needed for scope and tube insertion. The laryngoscope is rotated into the patient until the handle is perpendicular to the patient, and, as with the Bullard, the scope is allowed to drop gently against the posterior pharynx, then lifted prior to attempting visualization through the eyepiece. Once upright, some additional gentle vertical movement of the scope (or additional jaw lift) aids in increasing the working space in the hypopharynx and also helps align the ET with the glottic opening. With the newer UpsherScope Ultra, lining up the lower flange with the arytenoid cartilages ensures good vertical placement for tube passage. Once the cords are visualized, the ET can be advanced through the tube guide under endoscopic visualization. Following ET passage, the UpsherScope is withdrawn while the tube is stabilized in place and pinched to facilitate its disengagement from the guiding channel.

Failure to visualize the glottic opening may be the result of the scope being off midline. Reorientation to patient and scope midline helps, as may further jaw lift to create additional working room for minor left-right corrections. In addition, failure to pick up the epiglottis may compromise glottic visualization; increasing flexion of head and neck may help if this is a persistent problem. Difficulty with ET passage has been described especially with the original version of the UpsherScope, possibly because the ET tended to be directed posteriorly and slightly to the right when delivered from the channel guide.[185] Further vertical lifting of the scope or additional jaw lift may help align the ET with the glottic opening, as may slight leftward movement if the leading edge of the ET bevel strikes a right-sided structure. Prior passage of a gum elastic bougie through the ET into the laryngeal aperture has been reported to greatly improve successful use of the scope.[185]

c. Clinical Experience

In a series of 200 patients with normal airways, Pearce and associates[129] reported that 191 were successfully intubated with the UpsherScope in a median time of 38 seconds. Apart from secretions and fogging, the main problems identified with scope use were difficulty in picking up the epiglottis and ET passage. Fridrich and colleagues[60] compared use of the UpsherScope with direct Macintosh laryngoscopy in a randomized prospective trial. In the UpsherScope group, 87% of patients were successfully intubated in a mean time of 50 seconds, compared with a 97% success rate for direct laryngoscopy with a mean time to intubation of 23 seconds. This study also documented some occurrences of poor control of the epiglottis and misdirection of the ET. Scientific evaluation may reveal that the UpsherScope Ultra version has improved the utility of this laryngoscope.

3. WuScope

a. Description

The WuScope (Achi Corporation, Fremont, CA) is a tubular, curved, bivalved laryngoscope that was first described in 1994 by Wu and Chou.[178] As a rigid fiberoptic device, it is conceptually similar to the Bullard laryngoscope and the UpsherScopes. The instrument has two main components—a removable flexible fiberoptic endoscope that provides light and image transmission and the blade assembly (Fig. 23-62). The blade is a tubular assembly in turn composed of three stainless steel parts that fit together: the handle, the main blade, and the bivalve element (Fig. 23-63). The handle houses the removable endoscope body and attaches to the main blade at an angle of 110 degrees. When the components are assembled, the main blade and bivalve elements create two channels: one is the passageway through which the ET is advanced, and the other houses the fiberoptic endoscope. Alongside the endoscope passage runs an oxygen channel. The resulting blade is 16 to 18 mm in vertical height and is tubular in nature, helping to maintain space in the hypopharynx in the presence of pathology or

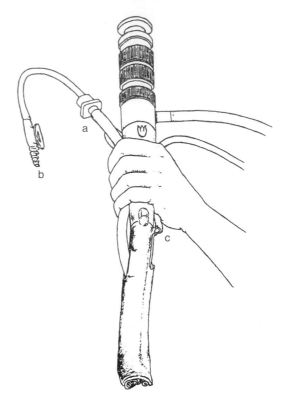

Figure 23-62 Drawing of assembled WuScope with loaded endotracheal tube (a), suction catheter guide within the ET lumen (b), and oxygen tubing attached to the oxygen port (c). (From Wu T, Chou H: A new laryngoscope: The combination intubating device. Anesthesiology 81:1085, 1994.)

redundant tissue and also offering some protection to the endoscope tip from blood and secretions. The fiberoptic endoscope (e.g., the Achi FA-10WUBS, Achi Corporation) is similar to a rhinopharyngoscope without the distal angulation control and is now available in a battery-powered version[179] to create a self-contained and portable unit (Fig. 23-64). The WuScope is available in two sizes: the large adult, accommodating ETs up to 9.5 mm ID, and the adult, suitable for adults less than 70 kg, and accepting up to 8.5 mm ID tubes. For double-lumen tubes, the large adult blade accommodates left 35 and 37 Fr sizes, and the smaller adult blade is limited to a 35 Fr tube.[154] Both detachable blades are interchangeable with the same handle, although an extender must be used when using the adult blade—this enables the same fiberscope to be used with both lengths of blade.

b. Instrument Use

The WuScope has been used to facilitate intubations in awake and anesthetized patients by the oral and nasal routes. The device is prepared by assembling the three handle-blade components and inserting the defogged fiberscope. The bivalve element can be attached or released easily at the main blade and the handle by separate interlocking mechanisms.[178] A lubricated ET, with its cuff completely deflated, is loaded into the ET passageway,

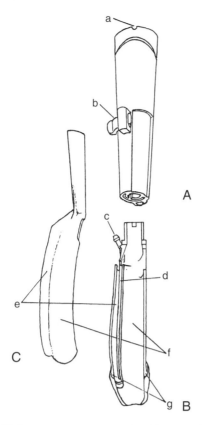

Figure 23-63 WuScope components: **A,** handle; **B,** main blade; and **C,** bivalve element. (a) Locator on the handle that aligns with a locator on the fiberscope, (b) a latch for the proximal interlocking mechanism, (c) the oxygen port, (d) the oxygen channel, (e) the fibercord passageway, (f) the endotracheal tube passageway, and (g) slits for the distal interlocking mechanism. (From Wu T, Chou H: A new laryngoscope: The combination intubating device. Anesthesiology 81:1085, 1994.)

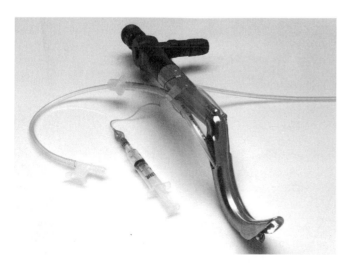

Figure 23-64 A battery-powered version of the WuScope, with loaded endotracheal tube and suction catheter. (Courtesy of Dr. Hsiu-Chin Chou.)

and a suction catheter, also well lubricated, may be positioned in the ET. The Murphy eye of the tube is positioned just distal to the end of the bivalve element. With the patient's head and neck in the neutral position, holding the metal handle, the scope-tube-catheter assembly is inserted into the mouth in the midline. A minimum of 20 mm of mouth opening is required for scope insertion. As the blade tip passes the uvula, an image is sought through the endoscope eyepiece and the scope is rotated farther down into the hypopharynx (Fig. 23-65). Most often the tip of the main blade is located in the vallecula, although occasionally it may be necessary to pick up the epiglottis. When the laryngeal inlet is visualized, the scope tip is positioned as needed to align the suction catheter or ET, or both, with the glottis; sideways, forward, upward, or backward (cephalad) adjustments of the scope tip may be needed to attain this. The suction catheter can then be advanced through the glottis, followed by endotracheal intubation over the suction catheter. Visual confirmation of tube passage can be obtained by ongoing viewing through the eyepiece. The bivalve element is then disengaged and removed, followed by the main blade-handle-endoscope assembly as one unit while the ET is held in situ.

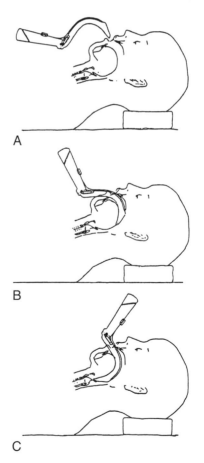

Figure 23-65 WuScope insertion. With head and neck in neutral position **(A),** the blade is slid down and around the tongue **(B),** with the blade tip most often entering the vallecula **(C).** (From Wu T, Chou H: A new laryngoscope: The combination intubating device. Anesthesiology 81:1085, 1994.)

To facilitate nasotracheal intubations, the WuScope is used without the bivalve blade. After the ET is passed through the nares into the oropharynx, the WuScope main blade is inserted and the concave undersurface of the blade allowed to straddle the ET. The blade can then be used for lateral adjustment of the tube as it is advanced toward the glottis.

As with other rigid fiberoptic devices, as the ET is advanced, posterior displacement occasionally occurs. Appropriate responses include (1) vertically lifting the scope, (2) cephalad movement of the scope prior to reattempting passage of the suction catheter, and (3) advancing the ET 5 to 10 mm, then readvancing the suction catheter through the cords.

c. Clinical Experience

The Wu Scope was evaluated in more than 300 endotracheal intubations over a 12-month period by the inventor, including intubations in 48 patients with Mallampati classification III and IV, without any complications.[178] Smith and coworkers[156] also reported their initial experience using the scope. Of 69 patients, 24 with predictors of difficult intubation, all but 2 were successfully intubated with the WuScope, all with a grade 1 view and a maximum of two attempts. Of the patients with predictors of difficulty, 71% were intubated easily on the first attempt.

Case reports have documented the successful use of the WuScope in cases in which impaired space in the hypopharynx was present (e.g., related to lingual tonsil hyperplasia[6] and expanding neck hematoma[159]). The WuScope may have a unique advantage among the rigid fiberoptic endoscopes in conditions such as these because of its rigid "exoskeleton" protecting the fiberoptic endoscope from redundant soft tissue, blood, and secretions. Other case reports have described WuScope use as an aid to ET change in patients with DAs; the device was used to deliver either a suction catheter[7] or a second small ET[159,160] through the cords prior to removal of the defective ET. As with other devices, application of cricoid pressure has been shown to impede and even prevent intubation in some patients during use of the WuScope.[153]

The WuScope was compared with conventional Macintosh laryngoscopy in patients with and without manual in-line neck stabilization by Sandhu and coauthors.[141] They found that in the unstabilized neck, WuScope use required less head extension, and with applied manual in-line neck stabilization the laryngeal view obtained using the WuScope was much superior to that with the Macintosh blade with no change in atlanto-occipital angle. WuScope intubation was successful in all patients. Smith and colleagues[155] made a similar comparison in patients with manual in-line neck stabilization and reported that successful intubation occurred in 95% of the WuScope group and 93% of the conventional direct laryngoscopy group. Although intubation took slightly longer with the WuScope in this study, 79% in the WuScope group had an Intubation Difficulty Scale

(IDS) score of 0 as described by Adnet and colleagues,[2] representing a straightforward intubation, as distinct from only 18% in the conventional group.

4. Augustine Scope and Augustine Guide

a. Augustine Scope

The Augustine Scope is another rigid fiberoptic L-shaped device that evolved from the Augustine Guide. Following a report[101] of the use of the Augustine Guide (AG) as a guide for fiberoptic oral intubation, a purpose-made battery-powered fiberoptic scope was proposed. The scope consists of an L-shaped blade, fiberoptic viewing bundle, built-in light source, and a tube delivery channel similar to that of the UpsherScope (Fig. 23-66). The leading edge of the blade, located superiorly when the scope is positioned in the patient, has a midline indentation and two lateral bulbous protrusions (Fig. 23-67) and is designed to sit in the valleculae. When in position and lifted, the blade places tension on the hyoepiglottic ligament to help raise the epiglottis. A second device to help raise the epiglottis is a small metallic flap hinged superiorly on the scope, overlying

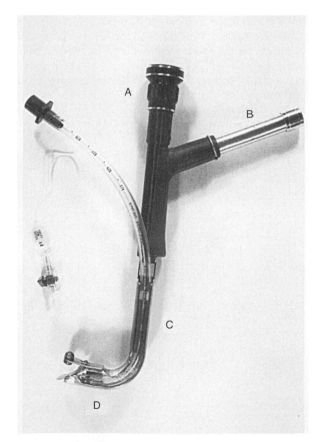

Figure 23-66 The Augustine Scope: (A) the eyepiece, (B) a battery pack, (C) the endotracheal tube channel, and (D) the viewing tip. (From Krafft P, Krenn CG, Fitzgerald RD, et al: Clinical trial of a new device for fiberoptic orotracheal intubation [Augustine Scope]. Anesth Analg 84:606-610, 1997.)

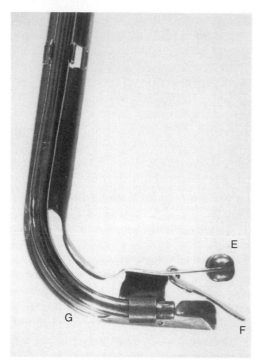

Figure 23-67 The Augustine Scope: close-up of distal viewing tip. (E) The paired bulbous protrusions designed to sit in the recesses of the valleculae, (F) the epiglottis elevator, and (G) the fiberoptic bundle. (From Krafft P, Krenn CG, Fitzgerald RD, et al: Clinical trial of a new device for fiberoptic orotracheal intubation [Augustine Scope]. Anesth Analg 84:606-620, 1997.)

laryngoscopy in a series of 200 patients. No significant difference was noted between the instruments in terms of first-attempt success or time to intubation. To date, the Augustine Scope has not been commercially marketed.

b. Augustine Guide

i. Description The AG is a plastic device designed to assist blind oral intubation and as a nonlaryngoscope is described in this section only for completeness. The guide has an L-shaped blade with a central channel for an esophageal detector–guiding stylet and ET passage. The guide blade is designed to sit down and around the tongue and distally has a midline indentation with two lateral protrusions, designed to sit on either side of the glosso-epiglottic fold (Fig. 23-68). When it is properly placed, vertical elevation of the AG tenses the hyoepiglottic ligament and lifts the epiglottis, facilitating access to the underlying vocal cords for ET passage.[98]

ii. Instrument Use For use, the patient's head and neck are placed in the neutral position and the mouth opened. The tongue can be gently withdrawn, although if this is done care must be taken to not lacerate its undersurface on the lower teeth. A bite block may be placed. The AG, with channel well lubricated, is then rotated down into the hypopharynx, remaining in close proximity to the tongue to help achieve correct placement in the vallecula. External palpation of the neck helps to confirm correct device positioning. As the correctly placed guide is gently rotated to left and right, the hyoid bone may be felt to move correspondingly in the neck (Fig. 23-69).[30] The AG is then gently elevated, and the esophageal detector-stylet is blindly advanced. Free aspiration of air from the stylet by pulling back on an attached 30-cm³ syringe confirms tracheal placement of the catheter, whereupon the ET can be advanced off the stylet into the trachea (Fig. 23-70).[97]

the tube channel (see Fig. 23-67). With advancement of the ET, the lifter is elevated, possibly helping to lift the epiglottis. The tube delivery channel runs alongside the fiberoptic bundle and helps to orient the tip of the ET directly in front of the glottis. Krafft and coworkers[99] compared the Augustine Scope with direct Macintosh blade

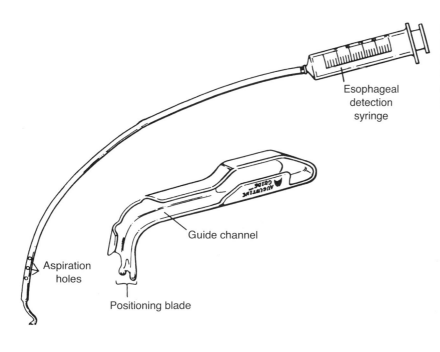

Esophageal detection syringe

Guide channel

Aspiration holes

Positioning blade

Figure 23-68 Component parts of the Augustine Guide: stylet **(top)** and intubation guide **(bottom).** (From Carr RJ, Belani KGB: Clinical assessment of the Augustine Guide for endotracheal intubation. Anesth Analg 78:983, 1994.)

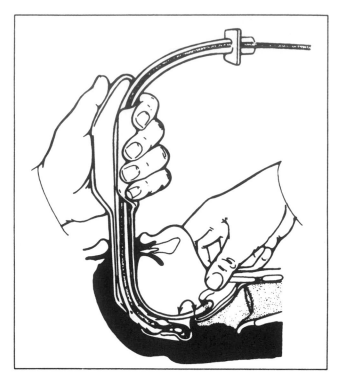

Figure 23-69 The Augustine Guide positioned in the vallecula—location being confirmed with external palpation of the hyoid bone. (Courtesy of Augustine Medical Inc from Kovac AL: The Augustine Guide: A new device for blind orotracheal intubation. Anesthesiol Rev 20:25, 1993.)

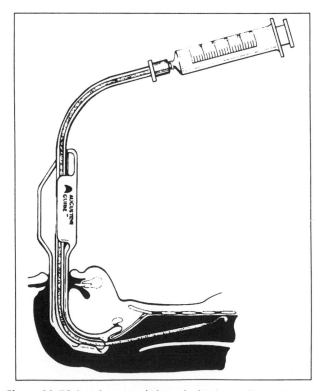

Figure 23-70 A stylet passed through the Augustine Guide. If correctly located in the trachea, free aspiration of air by the esophageal detecting syringe occurs. (Courtesy of Augustine Medical Inc from Kovac AL: The Augustine Guide: A new device for blind orotracheal intubation. Anesthesiol Rev 20:25, 1993.)

iii. Clinical Experience Clinical evaluation of the AG in a number of studies revealed a first-attempt intubation success rate of 68% to 92%, with an overall success rate (i.e., up to three attempts) of 94% to 100%.[5,30,31,98] In one large series of patients, Ambesh and Kaushik[5] reported that intubation success using the AG was unrelated to either the Mallampati or Cormack score. Carr and colleagues[30] published a series of 44 patients with DAs either predicted or discovered after induction. All patients were successfully intubated using the AG, 36 on the first attempt. Similarly, in the series published by Krafft and coauthors,[98] seven of eight patients with Mallampati scores of 3 or 4 were successfully intubated with the AG, four on the first attempt. The sole Mallampati 4 patient, successfully intubated with the AG, had experienced multiple failed attempts at direct laryngoscopy.

The stress response to intubation with the AG was looked at by Pernerstorfer and colleagues, who detected a significant rise in both systolic and mean arterial pressure after intubation using direct laryngoscopy; any increase with AG intubation was less, although failing to achieve statistical significance. Serum noradrenalin and prolactin responses were significantly less in the AG group.[131] Finally, in a study assessing upper cervical (occiput to C3) movement radiologically, the AG was associated with a median of 17 degrees less extension compared with direct laryngoscopy.[56] The AG is no longer marketed.

C. RIGID AND SEMIRIGID FIBEROPTIC STYLETS

Endotracheal intubation using a fiberoptic stylet was first described in 1969 by Murphy, when he published a report of his use of a flexible choledochoscope through a nasally introduced ET.[123] In 1979, Berci and Katz[14] published a description of the use of a straight endoscope as an ET stylet with many of the features of present-day units—a proximal viewing element and a sliding ET adapter with a Luer-lock inlet through which oxygen or air could be insufflated. The authors advocated its use with an external light source in conjunction with direct laryngoscopy. A curved distal tip was added to this format of scope with the introduction of the Bonfils stylet. These and other fiberoptic stylets described subsequently can be used on their own with the proximal eyepiece or can be used in conjunction with an integrated or attachable camera to obtain a video image on a monitor.

1. Seeing Optical Stylet System (Shikani Stylet)

a. Description

One example of a fiberoptic stylet is the Seeing Optical Stylet (SOS) (Clarus Medical, Minneapolis, MN). It is considered a semirigid device as the distal shaft of the stainless steel instrument is somewhat malleable and can be bent by hand or a bending tool to conform to the patient's anatomy. The stylet attaches by a threaded connector to a proximal eyepiece called a SITEcoupler, which has no focus adjustment and is compatible with most video camera adapters. An adjustable plastic tube stop fits over the shaft of the stylet and retains an ET in the desired position. The tube stop incorporates an oxygen port connector enabling the insufflation of oxygen down the ET during intubation. The image is transmitted proximally to the eyepiece through a high-resolution (30,000 pixel) fiberoptic bundle, and light is carried distally by several illumination bundles. Light can be supplied from one of three types of light source. The SITElite handle, to which the stylet is easily attached, is a bright halogen light source powered by four AA batteries (Fig. 23-71). Alternatively, an adapter is available enabling stylet use with a standard green-specification fiberoptic laryngoscope handle. Third, the SOS can be used with most remote light sources using a compatible fiberoptic cable. The SOS is currently available in two sizes; the adult version accepts ETs of 5.5 mm or greater ID and a pediatric version accepts ETs of 3.0 to 5.0 mm ID. As a modular system, the stylet component of the SOS can be completely detached from the SITEcoupler eyepiece for cleaning, disinfection, or sterilization.

b. Instrument Use

An ET is loaded onto the lubricated stylet with placement of the distal lens tip just proximal to the ET bevel. This position is maintained by inserting the ET's 15-mm connector into the adjustable tube stop, which is in turn affixed to the stylet's shaft with a tightening screw. The lens tip must be defogged by heating or application of an antifog solution. Although the SOS is supplied with a J-shaped distal bend, if desired a more acute bend (up to 120 degrees) can be introduced before use. The SOS-ET tube assembly can be used as a stand-alone device or in conjunction with direct laryngoscopy. In the former situation, good tongue control by use of a concomitant jaw lift facilitates orientation as the scope is advanced under endoscopic control. Alternatively, if used in conjunction with direct laryngoscopy, the stylet-scope assembly can

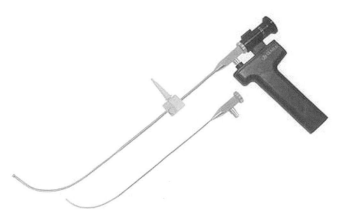

Figure 23-71 The adult and pediatric Shikani Seeing Optical Stylets, with battery-powered SiteLite light source handle. (Courtesy of Clarus Medical.)

be inserted beneath the epiglottis under direct vision, at which time it can be advanced under endoscopic control toward the glottis. With either technique the distal ET-stylet is passed through the cords into the trachea; then the SOS is withdrawn as the ET is advanced further into the trachea.

c. Clinical Experience

Shikani originally described the SOS in 1999 and reported its use for the intubation of 120 patients, 74 of them children, including 7 patients with Cormack grade 3 or 4 airways. In this initial report, the scope was used with video monitoring. All patients were successfully intubated without complications, 88% on the first attempt. In some of the more difficult cases, concomitant use of a laryngoscope was made.[146] Agro and colleagues[4] reported their initial experience with the device in 20 patients after only mannequin experience. Fifty-five percent were intubated on the first attempt in a mean time of 8.6 seconds. Another report described use of the SOS in a series of seven pediatric patients, six with Cormack grade 3 views at direct laryngoscopy. All but one were successfully intubated with the SOS.[132]

Additional versions of the original SOS have been developed. The Foley Flexible Airway Scope Tool (FAST) (Clarus Medical, Minneapolis, MN) is similar in design to the SOS, but the stylet is fully passively flexible. It can be used as a quick objective way to confirm ET placement or to help with ET placement through an intubating laryngeal mask airway. This device is currently being modified with a new tip, the FAST Plus, that will allow it to be used to aid nasal intubation.

2. Bonfils Retromolar Intubation Fiberscope (Bonfils Stylet)

a. Description

The Bonfils Retromolar Intubation Fiberscope (Karl Storz GmbH, Tuttlingen, Germany) is a rigid fiberoptic stylet with a fixed 40-degree distal anterior curvature. It is 5 mm in diameter and is available with and without a 1.2-mm working channel. The proximal eyepiece, with adjustable diopter correction, can be angled up or down relative to the stylet shaft (Fig. 23-72). An adapter provides for ET fixation on the stylet shaft and oxygen insufflation. Power is supplied through a cable from a remote xenon light source or by an attachable lithium battery–powered xenon light source. The scope is also available in a version with an integrated microvideo module to allow image display on a monitor without the use of a separate camera head.

b. Instrument Use

In an early paper, Bonfils described a retromolar approach to laryngoscopy and intubation,[18] and this method is also espoused when using the Bonfils stylet, as the fixed 40-degree curvature may be inadequate to negotiate the orotracheal angle when using a midline approach.

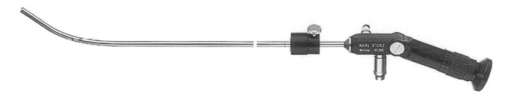

Figure 23-72 The Bonfils retromolar intubating Stylet. (Courtesy of Karl Storz.)

Before use, the optical system should be defogged by pre-heating or applying antifogging agents and the oropharynx should be suctioned. Using the retromolar approach, the scope is advanced from the corner of the mouth, over or behind the molars, while a concomitant jaw lift or thrust is performed to create working space in the hypopharynx. With the stylet positioned just proximal to the ET bevel, the stylet-tube assembly is passed beneath the epiglottis and the ET tip placed through the glottis, whereupon the ET is advanced off the stylet. Additional tongue and soft tissue control can be afforded with concomitant laryngoscopy.

c. Clinical Experience

Rudolph and Schlender in a prospective study successfully intubated 103 of 107 patients with the Bonfils scope, 95% on the first attempt. Seventeen patients with Cormack grade 3 or 4 views at direct laryngoscopy were all successfully intubated with the Bonfils. Concomitant use of Macintosh direct laryngoscopy was made in 21% of the series cases.[140]

3. StyletScope

a. Description

The fiberoptic StyletScope (FSS, Nihon Koden Corporation, Tokyo, Japan) is a lightweight stylet incorporating a plastic fiberoptic system for lighting and visualization, together with a flexible distal tip and built-in light source. The image guide is 3500 pixels with attached lens, which in turn gives a 50-degree field of view. A viewing eyepiece is mounted on the proximal end of the scope handle, and the distal end of the handle fits the standard 15-mm connector of an ET. Depressing a lever originating on the upper surface of the scope handle causes the distal end of the stylet, with loaded ET, to flex up to 75 degrees anteriorly (Fig. 23-73A). The scope is battery powered by two 1.5-volt batteries located in the handle. The FSS is reusable and can be sterilized in ethylene oxide.[96]

b. Instrument Use

The FSS is introduced into a size 7.0 or larger ET and locked into place. The distal tip of the stylet is adjusted to sit just proximal to the bevel of the tube by sliding the ET connector within the handle housing. An antifog agent should be applied to the distal lens tip. If used in conjunction with standard laryngoscopy, the stylet-tube assembly is placed beneath the epiglottis under direct vision, whereupon an image of the glottic opening can be sought through the FSS eyepiece and the tube-scope assembly passed through the glottis (Fig. 23-73B). Stand-alone use of the scope using a jaw lift has also been described.[95,181] If needed, during use the distal stylet-tube assembly can be bent anteriorly by depressing the lever of the FSS.

c. Clinical Experience

Kitamura and colleagues reported a prospective series of sequential patients in whom the device was used in conjunction with direct laryngoscopy. After induction, using manual in-line neck stabilization and electively revealing only Cormack[44] grade 3 views, intubation was successful on the first attempt in 94% of patients in an average of 29 seconds.[96] Yamada and coauthors subsequently described use of the scope without concomitant laryngoscopy by successfully intubating 10 of 11 patients on the first attempt in a mean time of 22 seconds.[181] In addition, case reports have documented successful use of the scope in patients with limited mouth opening[124] and C-spine precautions.[73]

In terms of hemodynamic effects, comparing routine direct laryngoscopic with laryngoscope-facilitated FSS intubation, the FSS intubation caused significantly less blood pressure increase at 1 minute in normotensive and hypertensive patients.[94] When use of the FSS on its own was compared with direct laryngoscopic intubation, less increase in heart rate was demonstrated with no significant difference in blood pressure change.[95] Stand-alone[95] and laryngoscope-facilitated FSS[94] intubations have also resulted in a lower incidence of sore throat compared with direct laryngoscopy alone.

D. VIDEO-ASSISTED RIGID AND SEMIRIGID DEVICES

Perhaps inevitably, many new airway devices take advantage of video technology, and video adaptation of existing equipment is also taking place. The newly minted acronym VAAMa (video-assisted airway management)[172] can be applied to (1) the use of video transmission of the view from the tip of conventional devices such as laryngoscope blades and ETs, (2) the video display of an image obtained through fiberoptic bundles, or (3) video use as

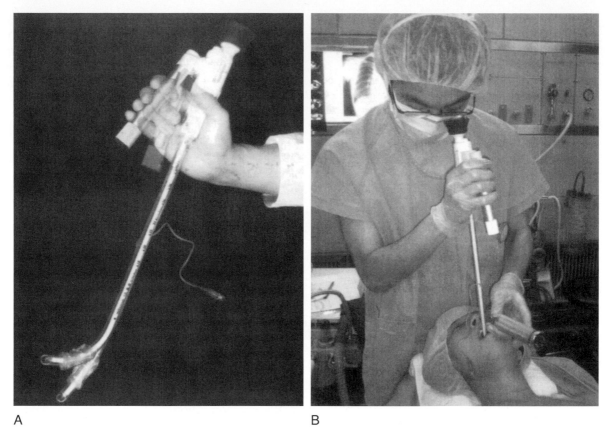

A   B

Figure 23-73 The StyletScope: photographs illustrating the maneuverable nature of the scope's tip **(A)** and the scope being used in conjunction with direct laryngoscopy **(B).** (From Kimura A, Yamakage M, Chen X, et al: Use of the fiberoptic stylet scope (StyletScope) reduces the hemodynamic response to intubation in normotensive and hypertensive patients. Can J Anaesth 48:919-923, 2001.)

the primary visualization system. A number of potential benefits accrue from use of video-assisted airway devices. First, having laryngoscopy and intubation displayed on a video monitor in the operating room can be an excellent teaching tool, providing a large image of laryngeal anatomy while allowing the supervising clinician to monitor the progress of endotracheal intubation.[87] Second, an assistant may better appreciate the effect of manipulations such as applied external laryngeal pressure. Third, these devices may aid either nasotracheal or orotracheal intubation and they have potential for use in reintubation procedures. Finally, immediate recognition of an esophageal intubation and appropriate positioning of the ET above the carina[177] are additional benefits, as may be the recognition of subglottic pathology or anatomic variants.[174] Use of video-assisted equipment in the patient with a DA is still sporadic, but increasing scientific evaluation of this final potential benefit can be anticipated over the coming years.

1. Visualized Endotracheal Tube

First described by Frass and colleagues[59] in 1997, the Visualized Endotracheal Tube (VETT) (Pulmonx Inc, Palo Alto, CA) was first used in a series of intubated intensive care unit (ICU) patients with the described advantages of being able to monitor tube position and visualize the state of tracheobronchial secretions. It consists of a polyvinyl chloride tube with embedded illumination fibers that transmit light from a standard light source to the tip of the tube while image fibers transmit an image to a video monitoring system (Fig. 23-74). An airflow lumen located next to the distal image lens enables lens rinsing with normal saline. The VETT was originally available in a size of 7.0 mm ID. The device was evaluated in a group of 40 ICU patients with randomization to VETT or regular ET. VETT patients all had their tubes positioned 5 cm above the carina primarily, whereas in the regular group two patients needed to have tubes withdrawn when evaluated by chest radiography. During the course of the ICU stay, VETT patients required less suctioning on the basis of direct visualization of tracheobronchial tree secretions.[59]

2. Video-Assisted Semirigid Stylets

a. Weiss Video-Optical Intubation Stylet

i. Description The evolution of Weiss' video-optical intubation stylet (VOIS) has been described in a number of

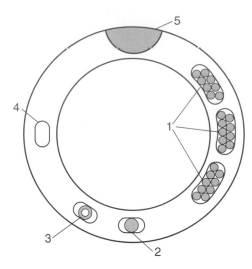

Figure 23-74 The Visualized Endotracheal Tube (VETT) cross section. Illumination fibers (1), image fibers (2), airflow lumen (3), inflation lumen (4), and radiopaque stripe (5). (From Frass M, Kofler J, Thalhammer F, et al: Clinical evaluation of a new visualized endotracheal tube (VETT). Anesthesiology 87:1262-1263, 1997.)

published reports. Initially, he simply placed an ultra-thin fiberoptic endoscope into an ET with a Schroeder directional stylet.[171] Thereafter, the fiberscope was bound with a thin metallic element by a plastic tube,[173] and still later the endoscope was placed in the lumen of a hollow malleable intubation stylet.[16] Now commercially marketed in Europe, the VOIS (Acutronic Medical Systems AG, Baar, Switzerland) is a semirigid fiberoptic stylet, malleable distally to 90 degrees, with an adapter proximally to fit the 15-mm connector of an ET (Fig. 23-75). A 2-m-long cable carrying image and light transmission fibers exits the proximal end of the stylet for insertion into a camera–light source unit. The VOIS is reusable and can be sterilized in ethylene oxide.

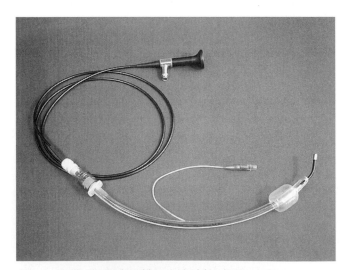

Figure 23-75 The Weiss video-optical intubation stylet. (Courtesy of Dr. Markus Weiss.)

ii. Instrument Use For use, the VOIS is lubricated, defogged, inserted into an ET, locked proximally to the ET connector with its sliding adapter, and bent into the desired shape. Conventional laryngoscopy and intubation can be performed and the procedure monitored with the VOIS. In the presence of difficult direct laryngoscopy, the tip of the ET can be advanced under direct vision beneath the epiglottis, at which point further guidance of the ET toward and through the glottis occurs while watching the monitor image of the view transmitted from stylet tip.[15] Unlike some other fiberoptic stylets, the Weiss VOIS has generally been used in conjunction with direct laryngoscopy.

ii. Clinical Experience In a mannequin study, with only a Cormack grade 3 view exposed by direct laryngoscopy, intubation using the VOIS was compared with that using a conventional malleable stylet. Forty-five clinicians attempted five intubations with each technique. At an average of 20 seconds, the VOIS took twice as long to achieve intubation; however, it was associated with no ET malpositioning, compared with a 20% incidence of both esophageal and endobronchial intubations with the blind technique.[16] In a study of 100 pediatric patients using the VOIS in conjunction with straight-blade direct laryngoscopy, all intubations were successful on the first attempt, without oxygen desaturation. Endobronchial intubations were detected and corrected in 12 patients, and one esophageal intubation was detected and immediately corrected. The series included six patients with a Cormack[44] grade 3 view at direct laryngoscopy who were all successfully intubated with the stylet.[177] In a second operating room study, 50 pediatric patients had only a grade 3 view exposed at direct laryngoscopy. Endotracheal intubation using the VOIS was successful in 92% of the patients in a median time of 15 seconds.[17]

b. Gravenstein Nanoscope

The Nanoscope (Nanoptics, Inc, Gainesville, FL) is a semirigid fiberoptic stylet that incorporates proprietary plastic optical bundles. An oral version of the scope incorporates a stiffening stylet; the nasal version remains fully flexible. Both bundles are embedded in a 37-cm-long malleable intubating stylet with an outer diameter of 6 mm. Fibers extending from the proximal end of the stylet connect to a charge-coupled device and light source. The image is then displayed on a video monitor. In assessing the efficacy of this device, Gravenstein and coworkers[70] compared intubation with Macintosh or Miller direct laryngoscopy with the Nanoscope or the flexible FOB in a group of 81 patients. Total time to intubation was shortest for direct laryngoscopy, followed by use of the Nanoscope, with the FOB taking the longest. The quality of the view obtained with the Nanoscope was inferior to that obtained with direct laryngoscopy or the flexible FOB, but this did not interfere with the ability to intubate.

3. Video-Assisted Laryngoscopes

a. Angulated Video-Intubation Laryngoscope

i. Description The angulated video-intubation laryngoscope (AVIL) is an endoscopic device consisting of a cast plastic laryngoscope blade with an integrated channel permitting insertion of a thin fiberoptic endoscope to a point 3 cm from the blade tip. The blade has a flattened vertical step as well as a fixed distal angulation, in similar fashion to an activated CLM blade (Fig. 23-76). The 2.8 mm outer diameter endoscope carries bundles for both illumination and image transmission.

Proximally, the viewfinder of the endoscope is attached to a conventional video-endoscope camera system, transmitting in turn to a bedside video monitor.[52]

ii. Instrument Use The scope should be prepared for use by employing an antifog maneuver to the distal lens tip. The scope is inserted and is designed to expose cords merely by gently elevating the tongue. If needed, the blade can elevate the epiglottis to visualize cords. Once cords are visualized, a styletted ET (bent to 45 degrees distally) can be introduced from the side of the mouth, advanced initially under direct vision along the blade's vertical step, and then advanced under videoscopic control to and through cords.[175] Final ET positioning can be achieved by observing ET depth markings or cuff position on the monitor.

iii. Clinical Experience Weiss and associates[175] evaluated the AVIL in a series of 100 consecutive pediatric patients, comparing it with the Macintosh blade. In this population of patients, with applied manual in-line neck stabilization, use of the AVIL provided better glottic visualization than direct Macintosh laryngoscopy. Endotracheal intubation was successfully performed in all patients. Transient difficulties from lens misting were reported in 12 patients, underscoring the need for good defogging maneuvers. Weiss also compared the AVIL with the VOIS in a mannequin study in which the head was immobilized to permit only a grade 3 view. The two devices were judged to be equally easy to use, although the intubation time with the VOIS was slightly less.[15]

b. Direct Couple Interface (DCI) Video Laryngoscope System

i. Description The video laryngoscope (Karl Storz GmbH, Tuttlingen, Germany) was designed using a regular Macintosh blade and laryngoscope handle. The batteries in the handle are replaced with a small video camera (DCI camera). A combined image–light bundle issues from the handle and inserts into a small metal guide on the Macintosh blade. A camera and light cable lead from the handle to a control unit and light source (Fig. 23-77). A universal cart can accommodate all components of the system, with recording capability, including a video monitor. Other devices (e.g., flexible FOBs) can also be plugged into the same camera control and light source.[87]

ii. Instrument Use For use of the DCI Video Laryngoscope System, components are assembled and an antifog solution is applied to the tip of the

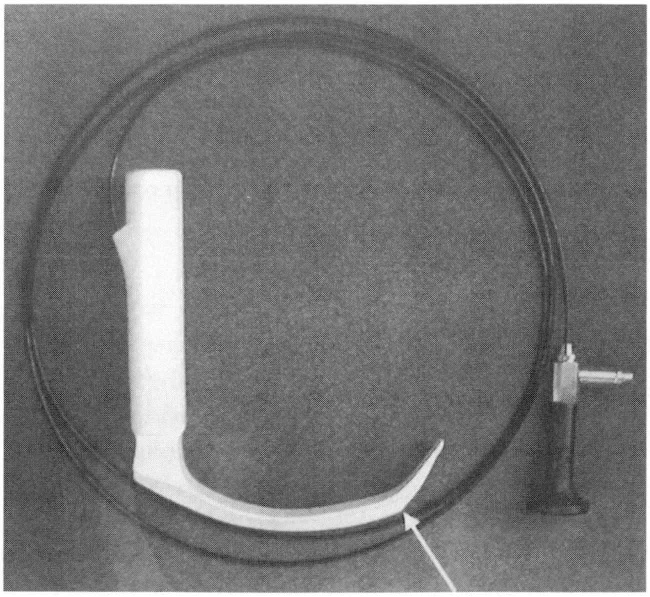

Figure 23-76 The angulated video-intubation laryngoscope. The fiberoptic lens tip is located at the site of the distal angulation of the blade *(arrow)*. (From Dullenkopf A, Holzmann D, Feurer R, et al: Tracheal intubation in children with Morquio syndrome using the angulated video-intubation laryngoscope. Can J Anaesth 49:198-202, 2002.)

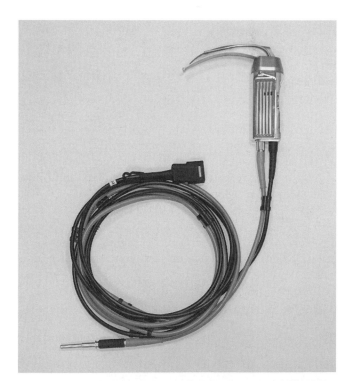

Figure 23-77 The DCI Video Laryngoscope System with the DCI camera incorporated in its handle (Courtesy of Karl Storz Endoscopy.)

image–light bundle. The laryngoscope is then used as a regular Macintosh blade, but upon insertion of the scope into the patient's mouth, the image can be viewed on the video monitor. Although the familiar Macintosh blade technique is used with this device, the presence of a distal viewing bundle may necessitate less anterior lift on the blade and may also permit a view of part or all of the glottic opening in otherwise difficult laryngoscopies.

iii. Clinical Experience Kaplan and associates[87] reported a series of 235 patients in whom they used the DCI Video Laryngoscope System. Of these, 217 were predicted to be straightforward, and in all but one the DCI Video Laryngoscope System was successfully used, with 10% requiring external laryngeal manipulation. A second group of 18 patients had anatomic predictors of difficult laryngoscopy; this group all required external laryngeal manipulation but were all successfully intubated with the DCI Video Laryngoscope System. Hagberg and colleagues[71] compared the view obtained using the DCI Video Laryngoscope System by direct vision with that obtained on the monitor and found that the image on the monitor was the same as or better than the direct line-of-sight view in 98% of patients undergoing routine anesthesia. In patients with predictors of possible difficult laryngoscopy, the same group reported a pilot study that also suggested a significant improvement in laryngoscopic view using the projected image as opposed to direct view. In this latter series of 33 patients, 39% were Cormack grade 3 or 4 by direct view, yet all were converted to grade 2 or better with the projected view.[72] A portable unit, the Medipack, as well as the DCI Video Laryngoscope System will become available that allows interchange of difference sizes and types of laryngoscope blades.

c. GlideScope

i. Description The GlideScope (Saturn Biomedical Systems, Burnaby, British Columbia) is a video camera–based laryngoscope that displays an image of the laryngeal inlet on an accompanying monitor. Made of medical-grade plastic, the laryngoscope has a miniature video camera embedded posteriorly midway along the blade, resulting in a vertical profile of 18 mm. An angulation of 60 degrees at midblade is designed to permit laryngeal inlet visualization with little tissue manipulation (Fig. 23-78). An antifogging mechanism effectively prevents fogging of the view. Lighting is supplied by two light-emitting diodes, one blue, one red. The black-and-white image is transmitted to a 7-inch liquid crystal display high-resolution monitor through a video cable. The monitor, with an integrated cradle for the laryngoscope storage when not in use (Fig. 23-79), can be affixed to a mobile, height-adjustable stand or an intravenous pole. The video cable is easily detached from the GlideScope, and the connecting terminal can be capped to permit complete submersion for disinfection. The laryngoscope should not be autoclaved, although the video cable can be.

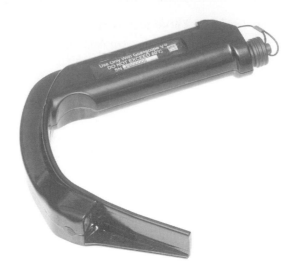

Figure 23-78 The GlideScope blade with integrated video camera.

ii. Instrument Use Preparation for use of the GlideScope is limited to ensuring that the power is connected and turned on. When the instrument has been turned on for a few minutes, no additional defogging maneuver is needed. A styletted ET is needed with distal curvature of 45 to 60 degrees to aid access to the glottic opening. Blade insertion is as for a Macintosh blade, although in this indirect technique the blade tip need not be advanced to the vallecula, nor need a lift be performed to the same extent as with the Macintosh blade. When the best view of the glottis is achieved on the video monitor with or without external laryngeal manipulation, the ET is advanced alongside and posterior to the blade. Intubation can be achieved by positioning the ET at the glottic opening, then advancing it off the stylet through the cords. If difficulty with tube passage is encountered, relaxation of any upward tongue lift should be attempted; alternatively, backing away slightly from the laryngeal inlet with the scope may help. Good visualization of the process should be available throughout on the monitor.

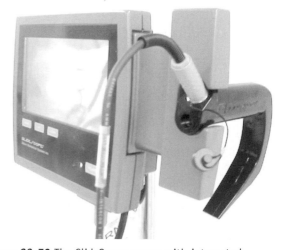

Figure 23-79 The GlideScope screen with integrated laryngoscope cradle.

iii. Clinical Experience In a small series of 15 patients wearing cervical collars, Agro and colleagues compared the Cormack[44] views obtained with the Macintosh laryngoscope and the GlideScope. In 14 of 15 patients, the view with the GlideScope improved one full grade compared with that obtained with the Macintosh blade. In particular, of the nine patients with grade 3 views during direct laryngoscopy, eight improved to a grade 2 view with use of the GlideScope. Average time to intubation was 38 seconds.[3] An additional case report documents the successful use of the GlideScope in a patient with a previously documented grade 3 to 4 laryngoscopy. With use of the GlideScope, a grade 1 view of the glottis was obtained and intubation was accomplished within 15 seconds.[41] Further research may prove the GlideScope to be a useful instrument for the DA in addition to its role as a teaching device.

VI. SUMMARY AND CONCLUSIONS

Direct laryngoscopy for intubation confers the known advantages of familiarity, direct glottic visualization, cost effectiveness, equipment availability, and a steep learning curve. The time interval between this and the last version of this chapter has seen the addition of more evidence in the literature on some direct laryngoscopes (e.g., the levering tip laryngoscope), a few new blades, and a resurgence of interest in straight blade laryngoscopy. However, the prevalence of grade 3 views at direct laryngoscopy is stubbornly persistent. Adjunctive maneuvers such as external laryngeal manipulation and head lift, together with adjuncts such as ET introducers (bougies), remain crucial to the success of difficult direct laryngoscopy. Alternative intubation techniques introduced in a timely fashion are also essential to achieving success in the latter situation, including the very effective lighted stylet (e.g., Trachlight), intubating laryngeal mask airway (Fastrach), and flexible fiberoptic bronchoscopy. However, indirect laryngoscopic techniques using rigid fiberoptic and video-based instruments or fiberoptic stylets can also be considered. As a group, these devices are relatively expensive and can fall victim to blood and secretions in the airway, yet they confer the advantage of (indirect) laryngeal inlet visualization, in contrast to the Trachlight and Fastrach. Thus, they may have additional utility in situations in which blind techniques are contraindicated (e.g., in the presence of anatomic abnormalities of the airway). Ongoing research is needed to further delineate the role of these devices in the management of the DA.

As an increasing array of fiberoptic and video-aided devices become available, it will be incumbent on the individual clinician to become familiar with the use of some of these instruments in elective cases in order to expect them to be useful in the difficult situation. Conversely, it will also be important for teaching programs to ensure that excellent skills in direct laryngoscopy are still taught, obtained, and maintained and that competence with different direct laryngoscopy blades (e.g., curved, straight, and levering tip) is attained.

REFERENCES

1. Adamo AK, Katsnelson T, Rodriquez ED, Karasik E: Intraoperative airway management with pan-facial fractures: Alternative approaches. J Craniomaxillofac Trauma 2: 30-35, 1996.
2. Adnet F, Borron SW, Racine SX, et al: The intubation difficulty scale (IDS): Proposal and evaluation of a new score characterizing the complexity of endotracheal intubation. Anesthesiology 87:1290-1297, 1997.
3. Agro F, Barzoi G, Montecchia F: Tracheal intubation using a Macintosh laryngoscope or a GlideScope in 15 patients with cervical spine immobilization [letter]. Br J Anaesth 90:705-706, 2003.
4. Agro F, Cataldo R, Carassiti M, et al: The Seeing Stylet: A new device for tracheal intubation. Resuscitation 44:177-180, 2000.
5. Ambesh SP, Kaushik S: Blind orotracheal intubation with the Augustine Guide: A prospective study. Anesth Analg 86:435-437, 1998.
6. Andrews SR, Mabey MF: Tubular fiberoptic laryngoscope (WuScope) and lingual tonsil airway obstruction. Anesthesiology 93:904-905, 2000.
7. Andrews SR, Norcross SD, Mabey MF, et al: The WuScope technique for endotracheal tube exchange [letter]. Anesthesiology 90:929-930, 1999.
8. Araki K, Nomura R, Tsuchiya N, et al: Cardiovascular responses to endotracheal intubation with the Bullard and the Macintosh laryngoscopes [letter]. Can J Anaesth 49:526, 2002.
9. Arthurs GJ: Fibre-optically lit laryngoscope. Anaesthesia 54:873-874, 1999.
10. Asai T, Matsumoto S, Fujise K, et al: Comparison of two Macintosh laryngoscope blades in 300 patients. Br J Anaesth 90:457-460, 2003.
11. Bainton CR: A new laryngoscope blade to overcome pharyngeal obstruction. Anesthesiology 67:767-70, 1987.
12. Beaver RA: Special laryngoscopes. Anaesthesia 10:83-84, 1955.
13. Bellhouse CP: An angulated laryngoscope for routine and difficult tracheal intubation. Anesthesiology 69: 126-129, 1988.
14. Berci G, Katz R: Optical stylet: An aid to intubation and teaching. Ann Otol 88:828-831, 1979.
15. Biro P, Weiss M: Comparison of two video-assisted techniques for the difficult intubation. Acta Anaesthesiol Scand 45:761-765, 2001.
16. Biro P, Weiss M, Gerber A, et al: Comparison of a new video-optical intubation stylet versus the conventional

malleable stylet in simulated difficult tracheal intubation. Anaesthesia 55:886-889, 2000.

17. Bizzarri DV, Giuffrida JG: Improved laryngoscope blade designed for ease of manipulation and reduction of trauma. Anesth Analg 37:231-232, 1958.

18. Bonfils P: Schwierge Intubation bei Pierre-Robin-Kindern, eine neue Methode: Der retromolare Weg. Anaesthetist 32:363-367, 1983.

19. Borland LM, Casselbrant M: The Bullard laryngoscope—A new indirect oral laryngoscope (pediatric version). Anesth Analg 70:105-108, 1990.

20. Bowen RA, Jackson I: A new laryngoscope. Anaesthesia 7:254-256, 1952.

21. Bruin G: The Miller blade and the disappearing light source [letter]. Anesth Analg 83:888, 1996.

22. Bryce-Smith R: A laryngoscope blade for infants. Br Med J 1:217, 1952.

23. Bucx MJ, De Gast HM, Veldhuis J, et al: The effect of mechanical cleaning and thermal disinfection on light intensity provided by fibrelight Macintosh laryngoscopes. Anaesthesia 58:461-465, 2003.

24. Bucx MJL, Snijders CJ, van der Vegt MH, et al: An evaluation of a modified Macintosh laryngoscope in a manikin. Can J Anaesth 45:483-487, 1998.

25. Bucx MJ, Snijders CJ, van der Vegt MH, et al: Reshaping the Macintosh blade using biomechanical modelling. Anaesthesia 52:662-667, 1997.

26. Bucx MJ, Snijders CJ, van Geel RT, et al: Forces acting on the maxillary incisor teeth during laryngoscopy using the Macintosh laryngoscope. Anaesthesia 49:1064-1070, 1994.

27. Bucx MJ, van Geel RT, Wegener JT, et al: Does experience influence the forces exerted on maxillary incisors during laryngoscopy? A manikin study using the Macintosh laryngoscope. Can J Anaesth 42:144-149, 1995.

28. Bucx MJ, Veldman DJ, Beenhakker MM, et al: The effect of steam sterilisation at 134 degrees C on light intensity provided by fibrelight Macintosh laryngoscopes. Anaesthesia 54:875-878, 1999.

29. Callander CC, Thomas J: Modification of Macintosh laryngoscope for difficult intubation [letter]. Anaesthesia 42:671-672, 1987.

30. Carr R, Reyford H, Belani K, et al: Evaluation of the Augustine Guide for difficult tracheal intubation. Can J Anaesth 42:1171-1175, 1995.

31. Carr RJ, Belani KG: Clinical assessment of the Augustine Guide for endotracheal intubation. Anesth Analg 78:983-987, 1994.

32. Cassels WH: Advantages of a curved laryngoscope. Anesthesiology 3:580-581, 1942.

33. Chadwick IS, McCluskey A: Another trachea intubated with the McCoy laryngoscope [letter]. Anaesthesia 50:571, 1995.

34. Chisholm DG, Calder I: Experience with the McCoy laryngoscope in difficult laryngoscopy. Anaesthesia 52:896-913, 1997.

35. Choi JJ: A new double-angle blade for direct laryngoscopy [letter]. Anesthesiology 72:576, 1990.

36. Cohn AI, Zornow MH: Awake endotracheal intubation in patients with cervical spine disease: A comparison of the Bullard laryngoscope and the fiberoptic bronchoscope. Anesth Analg 81:1283-1286, 1995.

37. Cohn AI, Hart RT, McGraw SR, et al: The Bullard laryngoscope for emergency airway management in a morbidly obese patient. Anesth Analg 81:872-873, 1995.

38. Cohn AI, Isaac P, Ramakrishnan U, et al: Bullard laryngoscope: Preliminary experience with the new multifunctional stylet [letter]. J Clin Anesth 10:681-682, 1998.

39. Cohn AI, McGraw SR, King WH: Awake intubation of the adult trachea using the Bullard laryngoscope. Can J Anaesth 42:246-248, 1995.

40. Cook TM, Tuckey JP: A comparison between the Macintosh and the McCoy laryngoscope blades. Anaesthesia 51:977-980, 1996.

41. Cooper RM: Use of a new videolaryngoscope (Glidescope) in the management of a difficult airway. Can J Anaesth 50:611-613, 2003.

42. Cooper SD, Benumof JL, Ozaki GT: Evaluation of the Bullard laryngoscope using the new intubating stylet: Comparison with conventional laryngoscopy. Anesth Analg 79:965-970, 1994.

43. Cork RC, Woods W, Vaughan RW, et al: Oxygen supplementation during endotracheal intubation of infants [letter]. Anesthesiology 51:186, 1979.

44. Cormack RS, Lehane J: Difficult tracheal intubation in obstetrics. Anaesthesia 39:1105-1111, 1984.

45. Crosby E, Cleland M: An assessment of the luminance and light field characteristics of used direct laryngoscopes. Can J Anaesth 46:792-796, 1999.

46. Crosby ET: Techniques using the Bullard laryngoscope [letter]. Anesth Analg 81:1314-1315, 1995.

47. Datta S: Modified laryngoscope for endotracheal intubation of obese patients [letter]. Anesth Analg 60:120-121, 1981.

48. Dhara SS, Cheong TW: An adjustable multiple angle laryngoscope adaptor. Anaesth Intensive Care 19:243-245, 1991.

49. Diaz JH: Further modifications of the Miller blade for difficult pediatric laryngoscope [letter]. Anesthesiology 60:612-613, 1984.

50. Diaz JH, Guarisco JL, LeJeune FE: A modified tubular pharyngolaryngoscope for difficult pediatric laryngoscopy [letter]. Anesthesiology 73:357-358, 1990.

51. Dorsch JA, Dorsch SE: Understanding Anesthesia Equipment, 4th ed. Baltimore, Williams & Wilkins, 1999.

52. Dullenkopf A, Holzmann D, Feurer R, et al: Tracheal intubation in children with Morquio syndrome using the angulated video-intubation laryngoscope. Can J Anaesth 49:198-202, 2002.

53. Dunn SM, Pulai I: Forced air warming can facilitate fiberoptic intubations [letter]. Anesthesiology 88:282, 1998.

54. Fink BR: The Human Larynx: A Functional Study. New York, Raven Press, 1975.

55. Fishelev W, Vatashsky E, Aronson HB: Suction catheter attached to laryngoscope [letter]. Anaesthesia 39:188-189, 1984.

56. Fitzgerald RD, Krafft P, Skrbensky G, et al: Excursions of the cervical spine during tracheal intubation: Blind oral intubation compared with direct laryngoscopy. Anaesthesia 49:111-115, 1994.

57. Flagg PJ: Intratracheal inhalation anesthesia in practice. Arch Otolaryngol 15:844-859, 1932.

58. Fletcher J: Laryngoscope light intensity [letter]. Can J Anaesth 42:259-260, 1995.

59. Frass M, Kofler J, Thalhammer F, et al: Clinical evaluation of a new visualized endotracheal tube (VETT) [letter]. Anesthesiology 87:1262-1263, 1997.

60. Fridrich P, Frass M, Krenn CG, et al: The UpsherScope in routine and difficult airway management: A randomized, controlled clinical trial. Anesth Analg 85:1377-1381, 1997.

61. Gabbott DA: Laryngoscopy using the McCoy laryngoscope after application of a cervical collar. Anaesthesia 51:812-814, 1996.

62. Gabrielczyk MR: A new integrated suction laryngoscope [letter]. Anaesthesia 41:970-971, 1986.

63. Gabuya R, Orkin LR: Design and utility of a new curved laryngoscope blade. Anesth Analg 38:364-369, 1959.

64. Gajraj NM, Chason DP, Shearer VE: Cervical spine movement during orotracheal intubation: Comparison of the Belscope and Macintosh blades. Anaesthesia 49:772-774, 1994.

65. Gerlach K, Wenzel V, von Knobelsdorff G, et al: A new universal laryngoscope blade: A preliminary comparison with Macintosh laryngoscope blades. Resuscitation 57:63-67, 2003.

66. Gerling MC, Davis DP, Hamilton RS, et al: Effects of cervical spine immobilization technique and laryngoscope blade selection on an unstable cervical spine in a cadaver model of intubation. Ann Emerg Med 36:293-300, 2000.

67. Ghouri AF, Bernstein CA: Use of the Bullard laryngoscope blade in patients with maxillofacial injuries [letter]. Anesthesiology 84:490, 1996.

68. Gorback MS: Management of the challenging airway with the Bullard laryngoscope. J Clin Anesth 3:473-477, 1991.

69. Gould RB: Modified laryngoscope blade. Anaesthesia 9:125, 1954.

70. Gravenstein D, Melker R, Lampotang S: Clinical assessment of a plastic optical fiber stylet for human tracheal intubation. Anesthesiology 91:648-656, 1999.

71. Hagberg CA, Iannucci DG, Goodrich AL: A comparison of the glottic view obtained with the Macintosh Video Laryngoscope in anesthetized, paralyzed, apneic patients: Direct view vs. video monitor. Anesthesiology 99:A1501, 2003.

72. Hagberg CA, Iannucci DG, Goodrich AL: An evaluation of the Macintosh Video Laryngoscope in the intubation of potential difficult to intubate patients: A pilot study. Anesthesiology 99:A1500, 2003.

73. Hamada T, Morokura N, Suzuki Y, et al: Orotracheal intubation using a Styletscope in a patient to avoid neck recurvation. Masui 50:519-520, 2001.

74. Harioka T, Nomura K, Mukaida K, et al: The McCoy laryngoscope, external laryngeal pressure, and their combined use. Anaesth Intensive Care 28:537-539, 2000.

75. Hastings RH, Vigil AC, Hanna R, et al: Cervical spine movement during laryngoscopy with the Bullard, Macintosh, and Miller laryngoscopes. Anesthesiology 82:859-869, 1995.

76. Hencz P: Modified laryngoscope for endotracheal intubation of neonates [letter]. Anesthesiology 53:84, 1980.

77. Henderson JJ: Laryngeal view and ease of endotracheal intubation achieved with a new straight laryngoscope (Henderson laryngoscope). Anesthesiology 91:A563, 1999.

78. Henderson JJ: The use of paraglossal straight blade laryngoscopy in difficult tracheal intubation. Anaesthesia 52:552-560, 1997.

79. Hirsch NP, Smith GB, Hirsch PO: Alfred Kirstein—Pioneer of direct laryngoscopy. Anaesthesia 41:42-45, 1986.

80. Horton WA, Fahy L, Charters P: Disposition of cervical vertebrae, atlanto-axial joint, hyoid and mandible during x-ray laryngoscopy. Br J Anaesth 63:435-438, 1989.

81. Huffman JP: The application of prisms to curved laryngoscopes: A preliminary study. J Am Assoc Nurse Anesth 36:138-139, 1968.

82. Huffman JP, Elam JO: Prisms and fiber optics for laryngoscopy. Anesth Analg 50:64-67, 1971.

83. Janeway HH: Intratracheal anesthesia from the standpoint of the nose, throat and oral surgeon with a description of a new instrument for catheterizing the trachea. Laryngoscope 23:1082-1090, 1913.

84. Jellicoe JA, Harris NR: A modification of a standard laryngoscope for difficult tracheal intubation in obstetric cases. Anaesthesia 39:800-802, 1984.

85. Jephcott A: The Macintosh laryngoscope—A historical note on its clinical and commercial development. Anaesthesia 39:474-479, 1984.

86. Johnston HM, Rao U: The McCoy levering laryngoscope blade [letter]. Anaesthesia 49:358, 1994.

87. Kaplan MB, Ward DS, Berci G: A new video laryngoscope—An aid to intubation and teaching. J Clin Anesth 14:620-626, 2002.

88. Katoh H, Nishiyama J, Takiguchi M, et al: A better method to attach an endotracheal tube to the stylet of the Bullard laryngoscope. Masui 42:237-241, 1993.

89. Katsnelson T, Farcon E, Cosio M, et al: The Bullard laryngoscope and size of the endotracheal tube [letter]. Anesthesiology 81:261-262, 1994.

90. Katsnelson T, Farcon E, Schwalbe SS, et al: The Bullard laryngoscope and the right arytenoid [letter]. Can J Anaesth 41:552-553, 1994.

91. Katsnelson T, Straker T, Farcon E, et al: The Bullard laryngoscope and a "directional tip" RAE tube [letter]. J Clin Anesth 8:80-81, 1996.

92. Kessell J: A laryngoscope for obstetrical use—An obstetrical laryngoscope. Anaesth Intensive Care 5:265-266, 1977.

93. Khan AK: A controllable suctioning laryngoscope [letter]. Anesth Analg 71:200, 1990.

94. Kimura A, Yamakage M, Chen X, et al: Use of the fibreoptic stylet scope (StyletScope) reduces the hemodynamic response to intubation in normotensive and hypertensive patients. Can J Anaesth 48:919-923, 2001.

95. Kitamura T, Yamada Y, Chinzei M, et al: Attenuation of haemodynamic responses to tracheal intubation by the StyletScope. Br J Anaesth 86:275-277, 2001.

96. Kitamura T, Yamada Y, Du H-L, et al: Efficiency of a new fiberoptic Stylet Scope in tracheal intubation. Anesthesiology 91:1628-1632, 1999.

97. Kovac A: Learning to intubate with the Augustine Guide. Anesth Analg 78:S219, 1994.

98. Krafft P, Fitzgerald R, Pernerstorfer T, et al: A new device for blind oral intubation in routine and difficult airway management. Eur J Anaesth 11:207-212, 1994.

99. Krafft P, Krenn CG, Fitzgerald RD, et al: Clinical trial of a new device for fiberoptic orotracheal intubation (Augustine Scope). Anesth Analg 84:606-610, 1997.

100. Lagade MRG, Poppers PJ: Revival of the Polio laryngoscope blade [letter]. Anesthesiology 57:545, 1982.

101. LaTourette P, Patil VU: The Augustine Guide as a fiberoptic bronchoscope guide [letter]. Anesth Analg 76:1164-1165, 1993.

102. Laurent SC, de Melo AE, Alexander-Williams JM: The use of the McCoy laryngoscope in patients with simulated cervical spine injuries. Anaesthesia 51:74-75, 1996.

103. Ledbetter JL, Rasch DK, Pollard TG, et al: Reducing the risks of laryngoscopy in anaesthetised infants. Anaesthesia 43:151-153, 1988.

104. Levitan RM, Ochroch EA: Explaining the variable effect on laryngeal view obtained with the McCoy laryngoscope [letter]. Anaesthesia 54:599-601, 1999.

105. Loeser EA: Oxygen- and suction-equipped laryngoscope blade [letter]. Anesthesiology 62:376, 1985.

106. MacEwen W: Introduction of tracheal tubes by the mouth instead of performing tracheotomy or laryngotomy. Br Med J 2:122-124, 163-165, 1880.

107. Macintosh RR: A new laryngoscope. Lancet 1:205, 1943.

108. Macintosh RR: Laryngoscope blades [letter]. Lancet 485, 1944.

109. MacIntyre PA, McLeod ADM, Hurley R, et al: Cervical spine movements during laryngoscopy. Anaesthesia 54:413-418, 1999.

110. MacQuarrie K, Hung OR, Law JA: Tracheal intubation using a Bullard laryngoscope for patients with a simulated difficult airway. Can J Anaesth 46:760-765, 1999.

111. Magill IW: Technique in endotracheal anaesthesia. Br Med J 2:817-819, 1930.

112. Maleck WH, Koetter KP, Lentz M, et al: A randomized comparison of three laryngoscopes with the Macintosh. Resuscitation 42:241-245, 1999.

113. Marks RD, Hancock R, Charters P: An analysis of laryngoscope blade shape and design: New criteria for laryngoscope evaluation. Can J Anaesth 40:262-270, 1993.

114. Matsuki A: New pediatric laryngoscope [letter]. Anesthesiology 57:556, 1982.

115. Mayall RM: The Belscope for management of the difficult airway [letter]. Anesthesiology 76:1059-10, 1992.

116. McComish PB: Left sided laryngoscopes [letter]. Anaesthesia 15:326, 1960.

117. McCoy EP, Mirakhur RK: The levering laryngoscope. Anaesthesia 48:516-519, 1993.

118. McCoy EP, Mirakhur RK, McCloskey BV: A comparison of the stress response to laryngoscopy. Anaesthesia 50:943-946, 1995.

119. McCoy EP, Mirakhur RK, Rafferty C, et al: A comparison of the forces exerted during laryngoscopy. Anaesthesia 51:912-915, 1996.

120. McIntyre JWR: Laryngoscope design and the difficult adult tracheal intubation. Can J Anaesth 36:94-98, 1989.

121. McMorrow RC, Mirakhur RK: A new mirrored laryngoscope. Anaesthesia 58:998-1002, 2003.

122. Miller RA: A new laryngoscope. Anesthesiology 2:317-320, 1941.

123. Murphy P: A fibre-optic endoscope used for nasal intubation. Anaesthesia 22:489-491, 1967.

124. Nagashima M, Saito T, Takahata O, et al: Orotracheal intubation using a StyletScope in a patient with restricted opening of the mouth. Masui 51:775-776, 2002.

125. Onkst HR: Modified laryngoscope blade. Anesthesiology 22:846-848, 1961.

126. Orr RB: A new laryngoscope blade designed to facilitate difficult endotracheal intubation. Anesthesiology 31:377-378, 1960.

127. Parrott CM: Modification of Macintosh's curved laryngoscope [letter]. Br Med J 2:1031, 1951.

128. Patil VU, Stehling LC, Zauder HL: An adjustable laryngoscope handle for difficult intubations [letter]. Anesthesiology 60:609, 1984.

129. Pearce AC, Shaw S, Macklin S: Evaluation of the Upsherscope. Anaesthesia 51:561-564, 1996.

130. Perera CN, Wiener PC, Harmer M, et al: Evaluation of the use of the Flexiblade. Anaesthesia 55:890-893, 2000.

131. Pernerstorfer T, Krafft P, Fitzgerald RD, et al: Stress response to tracheal intubation: Direct laryngoscopy compared with blind oral intubation. Anaesthesia 50:17-22, 1995.

132. Pfitzner L, Cooper MG: The Shikani Seeing Stylet for difficult intubation in children: Initial experience. Anaesth Intensive Care 30:462-466, 2002.

133. Phillips OC, Duerksen RL: Endotracheal intubation: A new blade for direct laryngoscopy. Anesth Analg 52:691-7, 1973.

134. Pope ES: Left handed laryngoscope. Anaesthesia 15:326-328, 1960.

135. Racz GB: Improved vision modification of the Macintosh laryngoscope [letter]. Anaesthesia 39:1249-1250, 1984.

136. Racz GB, Allen FB: A new pressure-sensitive laryngoscope [letter]. Anesthesiology 62:356-358, 1985.

137. Randell T, Maattanen M, Kytta J: The best view at laryngoscopy using the McCoy laryngoscope with and without cricoid pressure. Anaesthesia 53:536-539, 1998.

138. Robertshaw FL: A new laryngoscope for infants and children. Lancet 2:1034, 1962.

139. Rokowski WJ, Gurmarnik S: Laryngoscope blades modified for neonates and infants [letter]. Anesth Analg 62:241-242, 1983.

140. Rudolph C, Schlender M: Clinical experiences with fiber optic intubation using the Bonfils intubation fiber scope. Anaesthesiol Reanim 21:127-130, 1996.

141. Sandhu NS, Schaffer S, Capan LM, et al: Comparison of the Wuscope and Macintosh #3 blade in normal and cervical spine stabilized patients. Anesthesiology 91:A480, 1999.

142. Schapira M: A modified straight laryngoscope blade designed to facilitate endotracheal intubation. Anesth Analg 52:553-554, 1973.

143. Seward EH: Laryngoscope for resuscitation of the newborn. Lancet 2:1041, 1957.

144. Shigematsu T, Miyazawa N, Kobayashi M, et al: Nasal intubation with Bullard laryngoscope: A useful approach for difficult airways. Anesth Analg 79:132-135, 1994.

145. Shigematsu T, Miyazawa N, Yorozu T: Nasotracheal intubation using Bullard laryngoscope [letter]. Can J Anaesth 38:798, 1991.

146. Shikani AH: New "seeing" stylet-scope and method for the management of the difficult airway. Otolaryngol Head Neck Surg 120:113-116, 1999.

147. Shulman B, Connelly NR: The adult Bullard laryngoscope as an alternative to the Wis-Hipple 1½ in paediatric patients. Paediatr Anaesth 10:41-45, 2000.

148. Shulman GB, Connelly NR: A comparison of the Bullard laryngoscope versus the flexible fiberoptic bronchoscope during intubation in patients afforded inline stabilization. J Clin Anesth 13:182-185, 2001.

149. Shulman GB, Connelly NR: Double lumen tube placement with the Bullard laryngoscope. Can J Anaesth 46:232-234, 1999.

150. Shulman GB, Connelly NR, Gibson C: The adult Bullard laryngoscope in paediatric patients. Can J Anaesth 44:969-972, 1997.

151. Siker ES: A mirror laryngoscope. Anesthesiology 17: 38-42, 1956.

152. Skilton RW, Parry D, Arthurs GJ, et al: A study of the brightness of laryngoscope light. Anaesthesia 51:667-672, 1996.

153. Smith CE, Boyer D: Cricoid pressure decreases ease of tracheal intubation using fiberoptic laryngoscopy (WuScope system). Can J Anaesth 49:614-619, 2002.

154. Smith CE, Kareti M: Fiberoptic laryngoscopy (WuScope) For double-lumen endobronchial tube placement in two difficult-intubation patients [letter]. Anesthesiology 93:906-907, 2000.

155. Smith CE, Pinchak AB, Sidhu TS, et al: Evaluation of tracheal intubation difficulty in patients with cervical spine immobilization—Fiberoptic (WuScope) versus conventional laryngoscopy. Anesthesiology 91:1253-1259, 1999.

156. Smith CE, Sidhu TS, Lever J, et al: The complexity of tracheal intubation using rigid fiberoptic laryngoscopy (WuScope). Anesth Analg 89:236-239, 1999.

157. Snow J: Modification of laryngoscope blade. Anesthesiology 23:394, 1962.

158. Soper RL: A new laryngoscope for anaesthetists. Br Med J 1:265, 1947.

159. Sprung J, Weingarten T, Dilger J: The use of WuScope fiberoptic laryngoscopy for tracheal intubation in complex clinical situations. Anesthesiology 98:263-265, 2003.

160. Sprung J, Wright LC, Dilger J: Use of WuScope for exchange of endotracheal tube in a patient with difficult airway. Laryngoscope 113:1082-1084, 2003.

161. Sugiyama K, Yokoyama K: Head extension angle required for direct larynygoscopy with the McCoy laryngoscope blade [letter]. Anesthesiology 94:939-940, 2001.

162. Sultana A, Simmons M, Gatt S: The Belscope—A new angulated laryngoscope: Randomised, prospective, controlled comparison with the Macintosh laryngoscope. Anaesth Intensive Care 22:98, 1994.

163. Sykes WS: The cheerful centenarian, or the founder of laryngoscopy. In Essays on the First Hundred Years of Anaesthesia. Edinburgh, E & S Livingstone, 1961, pp 95-113.

164. Todres ID, Crone RK: Experience with a modified laryngoscope in sick infants. Crit Care Med 9:544-545, 1981.

165. Tousignant G, Tessler MJ: Light intensity and area of illumination provided by various laryngoscope blades. Can J Anaesth 41:865-869, 1994.

166. Tuckey JP, Cook TM, Render CA: An evaluation of the levering laryngoscope. Anaesthesia 51:71-73, 1996.

167. Uchida T, Yoshio H, Saito Y, et al: The McCoy levering laryngoscope in patients with limited neck extension. Can J Anaesth 44:674-676, 1997.

168. Ward M: The McCoy levering laryngoscope blade [letter]. Anaesthesia 49:357-358, 1994.

169. Watts ADJ, Gelb AW, Bach DB, et al: Comparison of the Bullard and Macintosh laryngoscopes for endotracheal intubation of patients with a potential cervical spine injury. Anesthesiology 87:1335-1342, 1997.

170. Weeks DB: A new use for an old blade. Anesthesiology 40:200-201, 1974.

171. Weiss M: Management of difficult tracheal intubation with a video-optically modified Schroeder intubation stylet. Anesth Analg 85:1181-1182, 1997.

172. Weiss M: Video-assisted airway management. Internet J Anesthesiol 3: http://www.ispub.com/journals/IJA/Vol3N1/vaam.htm, 1999. Accessed 6/30/2003.

173. Weiss M: Video-intuboscopy: A new aid to routine and difficult tracheal intubation. Br J Anaesth 80:525-527, 1998.

174. Weiss M, Villiger C: Subglottic video-airway imaging. Internet J Anesthesiol 2: http://www.ispub.com/journals/IJA/vol2n3/svai.xml, 1998. Accessed 6/30/2003.

175. Weiss M, Hartmann K, Fischer JE, et al: Use of angulated video-intubation laryngoscope in children undergoing manual in-line neck stabilization. Br J Anaesth 87:453-458, 2001.

176. Weiss M, Hartmann K, Fischer J, et al: Video-intuboscopic assistance is a useful aid to tracheal intubation in pediatric patients. Can J Anaesth 48:691-696, 2001.

177. Weiss M, Schwarz U, Dillier CM, et al: Video-intuboscopic monitoring of tracheal intubation in pediatric patients. Can J Anaesth 47:1202-1206, 2000.

178. Wu T, Chou H: A new laryngoscope: The combination intubating device [letter]. Anesthesiology 81:1085-1087, 1994.

179. Wu T, Chou H: WuScope versus conventional laryngoscope in cervical spine immobilization [letter]. Anesthesiology 93:588, 2000.

180. Wung J, Stark R, Indyk L: Oxygen supplement during endotracheal intubation of the infant. Pediatrics 59:1046-1048, 1977.

181. Yamada Y, Takayuki K, Du H-L, et al: An efficient technique for tracheal intubation using the StyletScope alone [letter]. Anesthesiology 92:1210, 2000.

182. Yardeni IZ, Abramowitz A, Zelman V: A new laryngoscope with flexible adjustable rigid blade. Br J Anaesth 83:537-539, 1999.

183. Yardeni IZ, Gefen A, Smolyarenko V, et al: Design evaluation of commonly used rigid and levering laryngoscope blades. Acta Anaesthesiol Scand 46: 1003-1009, 2002.

184. Yentis SM: A laryngoscope adaptor for difficult intubation. Anaesthesia 42:764-766, 1987.

185. Yeo V, Chung DC, Hin LY: A bougie improves the utility of the UpsherScope. J Clin Anesth 11:471-476, 1999.

186. Zollner F: Gustav Killian: Father of bronchoscopy. Arch Otolaryngol 82:656-659, 1965.

24

SEPARATION OF THE TWO LUNGS (DOUBLE-LUMEN TUBES, BRONCHIAL BLOCKERS, AND ENDOBRONCHIAL SINGLE-LUMEN TUBES)

Roy Sheinbaum
Gregory B. Hammer
Jonathan L. Benumof

I. INTRODUCTION

This chapter deals with the physiology, indications, and techniques of single-lung ventilation (SLV). Although lung isolation is most commonly utilized during thoracic and cardiovascular procedures, it can often be of great assistance in other procedures and in some cases lifesaving. It is therefore important to have a good understanding of the physiology and techniques of SLV.

The advent of better designed double-lumen tubes (DLTs), single-lumen tubes (SLTs) with built-in blockers, and new blocking devices and the improvement in fiberoptic technology are making SLV easier and safer to perform.

II. PHYSIOLOGY

The most common physiologic problem with SLV is the creation of a large intrapulmonary shunt. This shunt, if severe and left uncorrected, can result in hypoxia with severe irreversible end-organ damage. Most anesthesiologists aim to maintain arterial saturation above 90%, as the oxygen saturation curve drops sharply below this value.

The physiologic goal is to promote blood flow to the dependent lung. This is performed by making the pulmonary vascular resistance (PVR) of the dependent lung as low as possible. Excess positive end-expiratory pressure (PEEP), tidal volumes, and hypovolemia all contribute to increasing PVR of the dependent lung and therefore increase shunt fraction. Correction of the shunt can be accomplished by either decreasing blood flow or supplying oxygen to the nondependent lung.

Hypoxic pulmonary vasoconstriction is a powerful reflex that increases PVR of the hypoxic lung and therefore shunts blood to the better oxygenated lung. It is therefore useful to limit agents that inhibit hypoxic pulmonary vasoconstriction (nitrates, high concentrations of volatile agents, and hypercapnia).

Supplementation of oxygen to the nondependent lung can also alleviate hypoxia. The goal is to allow enough oxygen to the nondependent lung to reverse hypoxia but not so much flow as to inflate the lung and obscure the surgical field. This can be accomplished by the application of an external continuous positive airway pressure (CPAP) circuit to the nondependent lung or ever more simply by two or three partial inflations of the nondependent lung.

III. INDICATIONS FOR LUNG SEPARATION

There are both absolute and relative indications for SLV.

A. ABSOLUTE

Absolute indications for lung separation (Box 24-1) include prevention of spillage of blood or pus from a bleeding or infected lung into the normal lung, establishment of adequate gas exchange when there is a change in pulmonary compliance or lung pathology, and bronchopulmonary lavage. Accumulation of blood or pus in the noninvolved lung can lead to severe atelectasis, pneumonia, sepsis, and death. Bleeding of the lung from trauma or a pulmonary lesion can lead to drowning of the nonaffected lung. Lung isolation in these scenarios is often lifesaving.

Several unilateral lung problems can lead to inadequate ventilation. A large bronchopleural or bronchocutaneous fistula can lead to little or no ventilation of the normal lung. In this situation, the increased compliance to gas flow of the diseased lung results in most of the positive-pressure ventilation being directed toward the diseased lung, thus bypassing the normal lung and

---

Box 24-1   Indications for Separation of the Two Lungs (Double-Lumen Tube Intubation) or One-Lung Ventilation

I. Absolute
  A. Isolation of one lung from the other to avoid spillage or contamination
    1. Infection
    2. Massive hemorrhage
  B. Control of the distribution of ventilation
    1. Bronchopleural fistula
    2. Bronchopleural cutaneous fistula
    3. Surgical opening of a major conducting airway
    4. Giant unilateral lung cyst or bulla
    5. Tracheobronchial tree disruption
    6. Life-threatening hypoxemia related to unilateral lung disease
  C. Unilateral bronchopulmonary lavage
    1. Pulmonary alveolar proteinosis

II. Relative
  A. Surgical exposure—high priority
    1. Thoracic aortic aneurysm
    2. Pneumonectomy
    3. Thoracoscopy
    4. Upper lobectomy
    5. Mediastinal exposure
  B. Surgical exposure—medium (lower) priority
    1. Middle and lower lobectomies and subsegmental resections
    2. Esophageal resection
    3. Procedures on the thoracic spine
  C. Postcardiopulmonary bypass pulmonary edema/ hemorrhage after removal of totally occluding unilateral chronic pulmonary emboli
  D. Severe hypoxemia related to unilateral lung disease

producing inadequate gas exchange. In a similar manner, a relatively noncompliant transplanted lung cannot compete with the better compliance of the native lung and thus the transplanted lung can be severely underventilated. Another scenario involves a lung with bullous or cystic disease or a lung with tracheobronchial disruption.[35] Exposure of this lung to elevated airway pressures could result in lung rupture with tension pneumothorax or mediastinum.

Patients with alveolar proteinosis may require bronchopulmonary lavage. Bronchpulmonary lavage involves multiple instillations of large fluid volumes into the target lung with subsequent drainage of the effluent fluid. Lung separation is mandatory because of the large volume of fluid required to perform the lavage and to avoid cross-lung contamination and drowning.

B. RELATIVE

Relative indications for lung isolation involve facilitating surgical exposure, avoiding lung trauma related to lung retraction or instrumentation, and improving gas exchange.

Examples include surgery for repair of thoracic aneurysms, lung lobectomies (especially upper lobe), thoracoscopies, esophageal and spinal surgeries, and unilateral lung trauma.

IV. TECHNIQUES

A. DOUBLE-LUMEN TUBES

1. Anatomy

DLTs are in essence two tubes bonded together, allowing each tube segment to ventilate a specified lung. DLTs are designed as right- and left-sided tubes. Left-sided DLTs have a bronchial port that extends into the left main stem bronchus, and the tracheal port is designed to sit above the carina (Fig. 24-1). Right-sided DLTs are designed with the bronchial port extending into the right main stem bronchus, also with the tracheal port designed to sit above the carina (see Fig. 24-1). In addition, the cuff of the right-sided DLT is often at an oblique angle, allowing the Murphy eye to be in position to ventilate the right upper lobe bronchus (see Fig. 24-1).

The original DLTs were reusable red rubber tubes with high-pressure cuffs. Over time the tubes became stiff and brittle, making placement more difficult and traumatic. The new DLTs are made of nontoxic plastic (the Z-79 marking) and are disposable. As the plastic heats up to the surrounding body temperature, the DLT better conforms to the anatomy of the patient. The increased malleability, however, makes it more difficult to reposition the same tube. The DLTs employ high-volume, low-pressure, color-coded cuffs. The bronchial cuff, pilot balloon, and connector are blue. The tracheal cuff, pilot balloon, and connector are white. Cuff inflation pressure goals are to attain a balance between an adequate seal and maintaining mucosal blood flow. In general, cuff pressures between 15 to 30 mm Hg achieve these goals.[9,16,40,47] For those who still use nitrous oxide, cuff pressures should be checked periodically. Tubes are sized by gauge (French).[26,28,35,37,39,42] In most adult applications a 39 Fr fits well. A black radiopaque line is placed at the end of each lumen, allowing placement recognition by radiography.

A Y-type adapter allows ventilation of both lumens through a single circuit. DLTs are curved at the distal end, allowing placement into the larynx and positioning into the main stem bronchus. Once the bronchial portion is past the cords, the tubes must be rotated toward the side of the bronchial lumen in order to sit properly. The rotation and advancement of the DLT should be

Double-Lumen Tubes

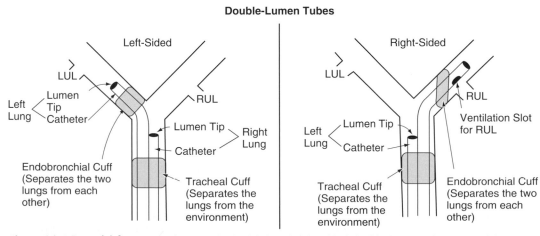

Figure 24-1 Essential features and parts of left-sided and right-sided double lumen tubes. RUL, right upper lobe; LUL, left upper lobe. (From Benumof JL: Anesthesia for Thoracic Surgery. Philadelphia, WB Saunders, 1987.)

performed after removal of the stylet in order to minimize potential laryngeal trauma. If resistance is encountered upon rotating or advancing the tube, the use of a smaller tube needs to be considered. Confirmation of placement by fiberoptic bronchoscopy is mandatory. The DLTs from different manufacturers (Mallinckrodt, Sheridan, Rusch, Portex) have their own characteristic feel. One should use the device that best suits both the anesthesiologist's and the patient's needs.

2. Advantages

Despite the advent of new lung isolation devices, the DLT still has inherent advantages. When properly positioned, the DLT allows independent ventilation of either lung. This can be of great advantage in cases in which each lung needs to be ventilated using different modalities. Because DLTs have a relatively large luminal access into each main stem bronchus, suctioning is better. Preventing desaturation is easier with DLTs because CPAP or partial lung inflation is easy to perform.

3. Disadvantages

Intubation with a DLT is more difficult than with an SLT.[16] Intubation is even more complex in patients with difficult airway anatomy.[52] In cases of a distorted or compressed tracheobronchial tree, the placement of DLTs can be impossible. DLTs are larger than SLTs and can contribute to airway damage if left in place for long periods of time. The process of exchanging a DLT to an SLT can also be dangerous, especially after procedures in which airway edema occurs. It is also more difficult to wean intensive care unit (ICU) patients from a DLT than from an SLT.

4. Choice

a. Right versus Left Double-Lumen Tube

It has been recommended that in order to minimize tube displacement, the nonoperated bronchus be intubated (i.e., for right lung surgery use a left-sided DLT) (Fig. 24-2). Controversy exists, however, when performing left lung procedures. Anatomic anomalies of the right upper lobe occur commonly, and the bronchial port of a right-sided tube may not be positioned to allow adequate ventilation of the right upper lobe bronchus. This can result in severe hypoxia during isolated right lung ventilation.[41]

For this reason, many anesthesiologists prefer to use left-sided DLTs for all lung surgery (see Fig. 24-2). If manipulation of the left main stem bronchus is required, the left DLT is then withdrawn and positioned with the bronchial port above the carina. Our preference for left main stem surgery and left lung collapse is to use a right-sided DLT and position it to visualize the right upper lobe bronchus orifice (Fig. 24-3).

Contraindications for use of left-sided tubes include anatomic barriers that make positioning improbable or dangerous (i.e., left-sided carinal or bronchial lesions,

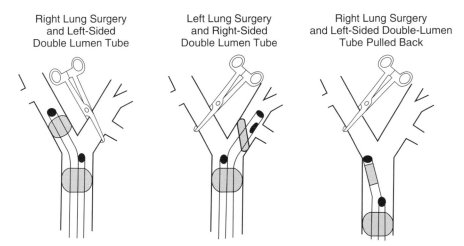

| Right Lung Surgery and Left-Sided Double Lumen Tube | Left Lung Surgery and Right-Sided Double Lumen Tube | Right Lung Surgery and Left-Sided Double-Lumen Tube Pulled Back |

Figure 24-2 Use of left-sided and right-sided double-lumen tubes for left and right lung surgery (as indicated by clamp). When surgery is going to be performed on the right lung, a left-sided double-lumen tube should be used (**A**). When surgery is going to be performed on the left lung, a right-sided double-lumen tube may be used (**B**). However, because of uncertainty about the alignment of right upper lobe ventilation slot to the right upper lobe orifice, a left-sided double-lumen tube can also be used for left lung surgery (**C**). If left lung surgery requires a clamp to be placed high on left main stem bronchus, the left endobronchial cuff should be deflated, the left-sided double-lumen tube pulled back into the trachea, and the right lung ventilated through both lumens (use double-lumen tube as a single-lumen tube). (From Benumof JL: Anesthesia for Thoracic Surgery. Philadelphia, WB Saunders, 1987.)

**Use of Fibreoptic Bronchoscope to Determine
Precise Right-Sided Double-Lumen Tube Position**

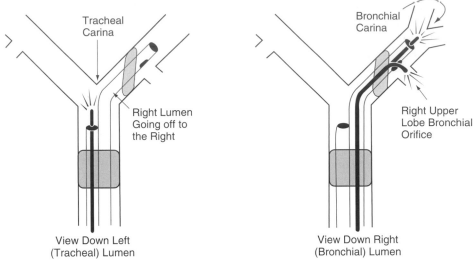

Figure 24-3 This schematic diagram portrays use of a fiberoptic bronchoscope to determine precise position of right-sided double-lumen tube. **A**, When fiberoptic bronchoscope is passed down left (tracheal) lumen, endoscopist should see a clear, straight-ahead view of the tracheal carina and right lumen going off into right main stem bronchus. **B**, When fiberoptic bronchoscope is passed down right (bronchial) lumen, endoscopist should see bronchial carina in the distance; when fiberoptic bronchoscope is flexed laterally and cephalad and passed through the ventilation slot of the right upper lobe, the bronchial orifice of the right upper lobe should be visualized. (From Benumof JL: Anesthesia for Thoracic Surgery. Philadelphia, WB Saunders, 1987.)

strictures, and vascular compression by aortic aneurysm).[10,16] To date, however, in over 1000 cases of thoracoabdominal aortic aneurysm, we have never encountered an aneurysm that ruptured because of placement of a left DLT. We have, on the other hand, had to place right-sided DLTs because of tortuosity and compression of the trachea or left main stem bronchus, which made placement of a left-sided DLT impossible. Sleeve resection of the left main stem bronchus is also a relative contraindication for the use of a left-sided DLT.

b. Size of Double-Lumen Tube

The ideal size of a DLT is one that results in a near seal of the bronchial lumen. The high inflation pressures of a small tube can cause as much mucosal damage as forcing too large a tube into a small bronchus (square peg–round hole scenario).[27] Unfortunately, even when using height- and weight-based estimates, it is impossible to choose the correct size of tube all the time.[7,10] It is important never to force a DLT into position. A good practice is to place a fiberoptic bronchoscope (FOB) through the bronchial lumen after the bronchial port is placed past the cords. The FOB is then guided down the trachea, identifying the carina and visualizing the main stem bronchus. One can then better gauge the size of the main stem opening. If the main stem opening is deemed appropriate for the size of DLT, the FOB is advanced into the main stem bronchus and the bronchial

port of the DLT can be guided over the FOB into position (Table 24-1).

5. Positioning

Malposition of the DLT can lead to life-threatening consequences. Gas exchange can be severely impaired, leading to hypoxia, gas trapping, tension pneumothorax, cross-contamination of lung contents, and interference with surgical procedure. Multiple studies have shown that DLTs are often malpositioned.[7,10] On the basis of these studies and personal experience, it is our opinion that the only reliable method for confirmation of placement of DLTs is a visualization technique such as FOB. Different techniques utilizing FOB are discussed here.

a. Placement of Double-Lumen Tube

In general, DLTs are placed similarly to SLTs but with some additional maneuvers and considerations. DLTs are larger in diameter and longer than SLTs, which makes them more difficult to place. For laryngoscopy, the shoulder of a Macintosh blade provides better tongue displacement and more space from which to insert the tube. The bronchial extension of the DLT is placed through the cords and the stylet is then removed (to prevent tissue trauma). The tube can then be rotated 90 degrees and advanced in the direction of the bronchial lumen. The average depth of insertion is

Table 24-1   **Relationship of FOB* size to DLT* size**

FOB Size, Outside Diameter (mm)	DLT Size (French)	Fit of FOB inside DLT
5.6	All sizes	Does not fit
	41	Easy passage
	39	Moderately easy passage
4.9	37	Tight fit, needs lubricant,† hand push
	35	Does not fit
3.6-4.2	All sizes	Easy passage
Approximately 2.0	All sizes	Most operating rooms need special arrangements to obtain this size FOB

*DLT, double-lumen tube; FOB, fiberoptic bronchoscope.
†Lubricant recommended is a silicon-based fluid made by the American Cystoscope Co.

29 cm for a 170-cm individual. For each 10-cm change in height, the tube depth is increased or decreased 1 cm.[10] When the tube depth is reached, the tracheal cuff is inflated and the patient connected to the ventilator. Care must be taken not to tear or puncture the tracheal cuff during intubation. Placing an unopened alcohol swab over the front teeth can minimized endotracheal tube (ET) cuff damage. Confirmation of CO_2 is critical. When the tube is confirmed to be in the airway, an FOB is placed through the tracheal lumen (Fig. 24-4). The FOB is advanced and the carina identified. The bronchial lumen of the tube must be visualized entering the appropriate main stem (i.e., for a right-sided DLT, the bronchial lumen should be in the right main stem bronchus).

Use of Fiberoptic Bronchoscope Down the Right Lumen to Determine Precise Left-Sided Double-Lumen Tube Position

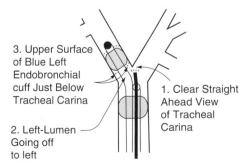

3. Upper Surface of Blue Left Endobronchial cuff Just Below Tracheal Carina

1. Clear Straight Ahead View of Tracheal Carina

2. Left-Lumen Going off to left

Figure 24-4 Use of fiberoptic bronchoscope down the right lumen to determine precise position of left-sided double-lumen tube. The endoscopist should see a clear straight-ahead view of the tracheal carina, the left lumen going off into the left main stem bronchus, and, most important (in bold print), the upper surface of the blue left endobronchial cuff just below the tracheal carina. (From Benumof JL: Anesthesia for Thoracic Surgery. Philadelphia, WB Saunders, 1987.)

The balloon of the bronchial lumen should be inflated under direct vision and lie just distal to the carina. The tube may have to be repositioned in order to visualize the balloon. Direct visualization of the balloon inflation helps to confirm tube position and size. Direct visualization is also necessary to ensure that the bronchial balloon does not herniate over the carina or that the tracheal portion of the DLT does not encroach on the carina (Fig. 24-5).

Determination and orientation of right versus left main stem bronchus are done by determination of the anterior and posterior aspects of the trachea. The anterior of the trachea is identified by the tracheal rings, which extend the anterior two thirds of the trachea. Posteriorly, the trachea consists of the membranous component, with longitudinal striations. When the anterior and posterior of the trachea are identified, right and left orientation is possible. It is often necessary to suction the DLT prior to insertion of the FOB. Lubrication and antifogging agents applied to the FOB can facilitate manipulation and visualization. Use of antisialagogues can also be useful in limiting secretions before DLT placement. These agents should be used with caution in patients with coronary artery disease, as they can produce undesirable tachycardias.

An alternative method of DLT placement is to use the FOB as a stylet and guide the bronchial lumen of the DLT directly into the correct main stem bronchus. This is accomplished by inserting the FOB through the bronchial port of the DLT after the bronchial port is past the cords. The FOB is then advanced down the trachea, identifying anterior-posterior and right-left orientation. The FOB is advanced further, identifying the carina and right and left main stem bronchi. The FOB is advanced into the appropriate main stem bronchus and the DLT advanced over the FOB. It is then necessary to remove the FOB and place it down the tracheal lumen in order to confirm the position of the bronchial cuff and also to

**Use of Fiberoptic Bronchoscope to Determine
Precise Left-Sided Double-Lumen Tube Position**

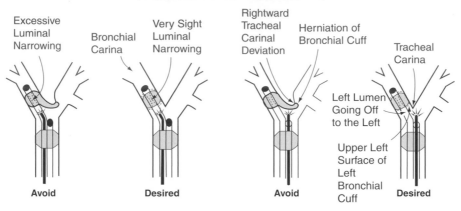

View Down Left (Bronchial) Lumen   **View Down Right (Tracheal) Lumen**

Figure 24-5 Complete fiberoptic bronchoscopy picture of left-sided double-lumen tubes (both desired view and view to be avoided from both lumens). When bronchoscope is passed down the right lumen of the left-sided tube, the endoscopist should see a clear, straight-ahead view of the tracheal carina, the left lumen going off into the main stem bronchus, and the upper surface of the blue left endotracheal cuff just below the tracheal carina. Excessive pressure in the endobronchial cuff, as manifested by tracheal carinal deviation to right and herniation of endobronchial cuff over carina, should be avoided. When bronchoscope is passed down left lumen of left-sided tube, endoscopist should see a very slight left luminal narrowing and a clear, straight-ahead view of bronchial carina in the distance. Excessive left luminal narrowing should be avoided. (From Benumof JL: Anesthesia for Thoracic Surgery. Philadelphia, WB Saunders, 1987.)

ensure that the tracheal lumen is not encroaching on the carina. This technique allows better assessment of the carina and tracheal rings than the "blind" advancement approach and allows placement in tortuous airways. The technique, however, takes more time to perform, and in some patients with poor pulmonary reserve this extra time can lead to oxygen desaturation.

Once proper position is confirmed, the DLT is secured in position and the patient positioned. It is imperative to recheck DLT position when the patient is repositioned as movement of the tube is common.

b. Confirmation of Placement

Many maneuvers have been described to assess the proper position of DLTs.[13,14] These include visualization of chest excursion while alternately clamping and unclamping the tracheal and bronchial ports, auscultation of lung fields while alternately clamping and unclamping the tracheal and bronchial ports, and radiographic confirmation.[5,15] After many years of performing these maneuvers, we are convinced that the only practical and reliable method of confirming DLT placement is by direct FOB (Fig. 24-6). All else is a waste of time and energy and does not provide direct assessment of bronchial cuff and tracheal lumen position.[1,29,37] The periodic use of an FOB in patients intubated with an SLT as a tool to maintain the skills required for FOB is recommended.

6. Complications

As previously stated, the most common complication of DLTs is malpositioning (Fig. 24-7).[44,55] Other complications include traumatic laryngeal injury, tracheobronchial tree disruption, inadvertent suturing of the DLT to thoracic structures, and direct vocal cord injury.[49] Although most complications (except malpositioning) have been reported in the older style DLTs (Carlens and Robertshaw), the newer designs can also pose a risk.[19,22,48]

7. Changing the Double-Lumen Tube to a Single-Lumen Tube

a. Procedure

Although the DLT has great advantages for lung isolation, it has some drawbacks. Because of the relatively large outer diameter of DLTs, they are more likely to produce laryngeal trauma the longer they remain in place. It is also more difficult to wean patients from a DLT in the ICU. It is therefore desirable to replace the DLT with an SLT at the end of the surgical procedure if the patient is to remain intubated postoperatively.

There is often some pressure by a surgeon or ICU attending to replace the DLT with an SLT. Replacing a DLT with an SLT can be life threatening and must be performed with great caution. Prior to changing out a DLT, one must ensure that the patient is well preoxygenated and paralyzed. An SLT with stylet, face mask,

**Use of Fiberoptic Bronchoscope to
Insert Left-Sided Double-Lumen Tube**

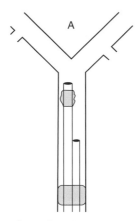 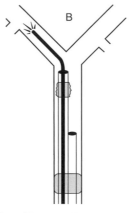 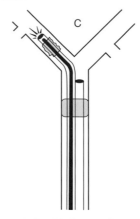

| Insert Double-Lumen Tube Into Trachea in Conventional Manner and Ventilate Both Lungs | Pass Fiberoptic Bronchoscope Down Left Lumen Into Left Main Stem Bronchus | Push Double-Lumen Tube in Over Fiberoptic Bronchoscope Until Left Lumen is in Left Main Stem Bronchus |

Figure 24-6 Double-lumen tube can be put into trachea in a conventional manner, and both lungs can be ventilated by both lumens (**A**). Fiberoptic bronchoscope may be inserted into left lumen of double-lumen tube through a self-sealing diaphragm in the elbow connector to the left lumen; this allows continued positive-pressure ventilation of both lungs through right lumen without creating a leak. After fiberoptic bronchoscope has been passed into the left main stem bronchus (**B**), it is used as a stylet for left lumen (**C**); fiberoptic broncho-scope is then withdrawn. Final precise positioning of double-lumen tube is performed with fiberoptic bronchoscope in right lumen (see Figs. 24-9 and 24-10). (From Benumof JL: Anesthesia for Thoracic Surgery. Philadelphia, WB Saunders, 1987.)

Double-Lumen Tube Malpositions

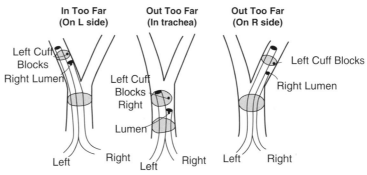

Procedure	Breath Sounds Heard		
Clamp Right Lumen Both Cuffs Inflated	Left	Left and Right	Right
Clamp Left Lumen Both Cuffs Inflated	None or Very ↓	None or Very ↓	None or Very ↓
Clamp Left Lumen Deflaft Left Cuff	Left	Left and Right	Right

Figure 24-7 There are three major (involving a whole lung) malpositions of a left-sided double-lumen endotracheal tube. The tube can be in too far on the left (both lumens are in the left main stem bronchus), out too far (both lumens are in the trachea), or down the right main stem bronchus (at least the left lumen is in the right main stem bronchus). In each of these three malpositions, the left cuff, when fully inflated, can completely block the right lumen. Inflation and deflation of the left cuff while the left lumen is clamped create a breath sound differential diagnosis of tube malposition. See text for full explanation. L, left; R, right; ↓, decreased. (From Benumof JL: Anesthesia for Thoracic Surgery. Philadelphia, WB Saunders, 1987.)

and suction needs to be readily available. When all is ready, the bronchial cuff is deflated and the oropharynx is suctioned. Direct laryngoscopy is then performed, preferably with a Miller blade. If the DLT and larynx can be visualized well, the blade can be passed into the larynx just past the vocal cords. When the laryngoscope is positioned as such, an assistant deflates the tracheal cuff of the DLT upon instruction, and the DLT is retracted under constant direct vision. When the DLT is removed, the assistant hands the SLT, which is placed directly into the larynx. It is vital not to lose sight of the larynx and not to reposition the laryngoscope blade. When the SLT is past the cords, the cuff is inflated, the patient is ventilated, and CO_2 confirmation is obtained. If, upon laryngoscopic inspection of the airway, the vocal cords are too edematous, bloody, or difficult to visualize, the tube exchange should be aborted. "It is better to be a live coward than have a dead patient."

b. Use of Airway Exchange Catheters

Alternative techniques of tube exchange involve the use of tube exchangers. Of the available tube exchangers, it is our preference to use the Cook tube exchangers because they are easy to use, hollow, and allow ventilation if the need arises. The technique involves placing a tube exchanger through the existing DLT (either the tracheal or bronchial port may be used, although the bronchial port may provide more stability) and then removing the DLT. Care must be taken to keep the tube exchanger in place as the DLT is removed. Once the DLT is removed, the SLT is "railroaded" over the tube exchanger into the trachea. The tube exchanger is removed (keeping the SLT in place) and the cuff inflated. Confirmation of CO_2 is then obtained.

The tube exchangers are not, however, foolproof. It is easy to dislodge a tube exchanger at any point during the attempted exchange. Also, often the fit between the exchanger and SLT is such that the SLT becomes caught up at the level of the cords. Rotating the SLT clockwise, the corkscrew maneuver, can overcome the obstruction, but it can also cause dislodgement of the tube and tube exchanger.

A combination technique of using a tube exchanger under direct vision may be a safer approach. With this technique, the larynx and DLT are visualized while a tube exchanger is inserted through the DLT. The yellow color of the Cook exchanger is seen passing into the distal airway. Under direct vision, the DLT is withdrawn and the tube exchanger position is confirmed. The SLT (without stylet) is advanced over the tube exchanger while visualizing the larynx. The tube is guided under direct vision into the larynx and the exchanger removed. Proper placement is determined by CO_2 confirmation.

8. Contraindications

Not all patients requiring lung separation are candidates for DLTs. Contraindication to placing DLTs can be

separated into the following categories: (1) known or anticipated technical difficulty in DLT placement, (2) dangerous anatomy (dangerous curves ahead), (3) small airways or patients, and (4) unstable patients. For these patients, alternative means of lung separation will be discussed.

B. SINGLE-LUMEN TUBES

There exist several situations in which lung isolation is required but the use of a DLT is not practical. In these instances, the use of a modified SLT with integrated blockers or the use of blockers in conjunction with an SLT is appropriate.

1. Difficult Airway

Patients presenting with difficult airway anatomy can be a particular challenge for lung isolation, as the placement of conventional DLTs can be impossible in these patients.[30] In these cases the use of an SLT or Univent tube is advised, as these devices are more easily placed than DLTs.

In patients who have an SLT in place and have developed significant airway edema or are in the prone or lateral position and then require lung isolation, a blocker device is the safest technique to invoke lung isolation. Similarly, in patients who have an SLT and develop traumatized or bloodied airways, the insertion of a DLT is very difficult because of the inability to visualize airway anatomy properly with the FOB. The use of an SLT or Univent allows better airway suctioning and improved safety for lung isolation.

There are cases in which postoperative airway edema is inevitable and the prospect of changing a DLT to an SLT postoperatively would pose too great a risk to the patient. In these cases, it is worth considering the use of an SLT with blocker or a Univent tube. The blockers can be withdrawn when no longer required, without removal of the ET, and the patient transported to the ICU and then weaned from the ventilator.

a. Small Airway

In patients with small airway anatomy, it is not possible to place a DLT. In these cases, the use of an SLT (with or without a blocker) or Univent tube is the only method of isolating the lung without surgical compression of the lung. ETs as small as 5.0 mm can accommodate blockers. In ETs smaller than 5.0 mm it is not possible to pass both blocker and FOB through the tube. In cases requiring a very small ET (less than 5.0 mm), the technique of "main stemming" the ET in order to achieve lung isolation can be utilized.

b. Desire for Segmental Lobe Isolation

There are some instances when selectively blocking lung segments is desired. In these cases, a blocker device can be advanced into the desired lung segment. It is not possible to isolate lung segments with a DLT. For example, a patient with a left lung pneumonia and right lower lobe (RLL) and right middle lobe (RML) bronchocutaneous fistulas underwent a trial of right lung isolation, yet this method failed because of profound desaturation. An SLT with a blocker isolating the RLL and RML allowed adequate saturation while the patient recovered from the pneumonia and the bronchocutaneous fistula sealed.

2. Disadvantages

a. Lung Deflation
When bronchial blockers are used to isolate the lung, the deflation of the blocked lung is slow. This is because the gas trapped in the isolated lung cannot escape and must be resorbed. Deflation of the lung with the Univent tube is somewhat faster because of the small lumen extending through the blocker. It is also possible to administer suction to the blocker lumen of the Univent tube and facilitate lung deflation. In order to accelerate lung deflation, the patient should be ventilated with 100% oxygen for several minutes prior to bronchial cuff inflation. This accelerates deflation because oxygen is reabsorbed more rapidly than air. Alternatively, if the patient's pulmonary function permits, the patient can be temporarily disconnected from the ventilator circuit and both lungs allowed to deflate spontaneously. The blocker cuff is then inflated and the patient reconnected to the ventilator.

b. Secretion Removal
The relatively large lumens of DLTs allow passage of small suction catheters and good removal of blood or secretions. The same is not the case for SLTs with blockers or Univent tubes.

c. Bronchial Mucosal Damage
Unlike DLTs, which utilize high-volume, low-pressure cuffs in both the tracheal and bronchial cuffs, bronchial blockers and Univent tubes have low-volume, higher-pressure cuffs. Prolonged inflation of the bronchial balloons may result in mucosal ischemia and irreversible damage. For this reason, it is prudent to deflate the bronchial cuff at the earliest opportunity after lung isolation is no longer required.

Some authors advocate techniques of "just seal" bronchial cuff inflation volumes in order to minimize mucosal ischemia and damage.[9,47] These techniques tend to be of little or no value, as most of those described are cumbersome and require specialized connectors between the ET, the blocking device, and the circuit. In addition, the cuff pressure required for the blocker can change because of compliance changes of the ventilated lung.

d. Treatment of Desaturation
In all cases of one-lung ventilation and desaturation, one must use a checklist. It is necessary to ensure that the patient is receiving 100% oxygen, ensure adequate ventilation, and verify tube or blocker position, or both. Once these issues are resolved, desaturation can be further treated. With DLTs, desaturation with one-lung ventilation can be treated by several maneuvers. The nondependent lung can have CPAP applied, the nondependent lung can be partially expanded, PEEP to the dependent lung can be altered, and finally both lungs can be ventilated. Similar options are as readily available for SLT and Univent tubes.

C. UNIVENT TUBES

The Univent tube is a Silastic SLT that has a built-in internal chamber allowing the advancement of the integrated blocker (Fig. 24-8).[30,31,39] The integrated blocker has a small lumen along the entire length to facilitate lung deflation and limited suctioning. At the distal tip of the blocker is a small balloon. The proximal end of the blocker section contains a cap. This cap needs to be engaged when the blocker balloon is deflated. Failure to engage the cap when the blocker balloon is deflated results in a circuit leak. Univent tubes are available in multiple sizes (Table 24-2), all designated by internal lumen size. It is important to note that because of the thickness of the tube wall and the integrated blocker chamber, the outer size of these devices is much larger

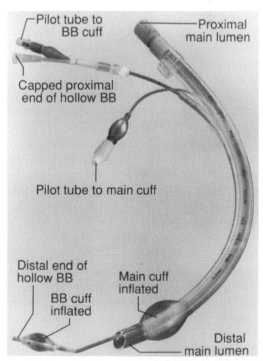

Figure 24-8 Univent single-lumen tube and bronchial blocker system.

Table 24-2   **Comparative Tube Sizes**

Univent ID, mm	Univent FG of Single Main Lumen (Marked on Tube)	Univent OD, mm Lateral/AP	Equivalent SLT OD, mm	Equivalent DLT, FG
7.5	31	11.0/12.0	9.6	35
8.0	33	11.5/13.0	10.9	37
8.5	35	12.0/13.5	11.6	39
9.0	37	12.5/14.0	12.2	41

AP, anteroposterior; DLT, double-lumen tube, Bronchocath; FG, French gauge; ID, internal diameter; OD, outside diameter; SLT, single-lumen tube, Shiley. FG = OD in mm × 3. The AP diameter is greater than the lateral diameter because of the presence of bronchial blocker lumen.
Data from MacGillvray RG: Evaluation of a new tracheal tube with a moveable bronchus blocker. Anaesthesia 43:687, 1988 and Slinger P: Con: The Univent tube is not the best method of providing one-lung ventilation. J Cardiothorac Vasc Anesth 7:108-112, 1993.

than that of a similarly designated SLT. For example a 7.5-mm Univent tube has an outer diameter size of 11.2 mm versus a 7.5-mm SLT, which has an outer diameter of 10.2 mm. Sizing aside, these tubes are very useful.

Prior to placing the Univent tube, it must be prepared. Preparation involves removing the distal and proximal tension wires, which help keep the Univent's shape during storage. The cuffs of the blocker and main tube need to be checked and deflated. The blocker needs to be retracted into the blocker chamber so that the distal tip of the blocker is flush with the main tube. The tube is then inserted into the larynx and trachea. It is best not to advance the main balloon much past the cords. The main tube cuff is then inflated. A distance of at least 2 to 3 cm is required between the distal tip of the main tube and the carina in order to maintain and manipulate the "hockey stick" curve of the blocker as it is advanced past the tip of the main tube. Failure to provide this adequate distance between the tip of the main tube and the carina in effect straightens the hockey stick shape of the blocker and makes directional control of the blocker very difficult.

The Silastic material of the Univent tube makes passage of a nonlubricated FOB difficult, and the FOB should be well lubricated prior to insertion into the main segment of the tube. It is often helpful to attach some type of self-sealing diaphragm device between the Univent tube and the elbow connection of circuit. This allows continuous ventilation while the blocker is being positioned. The FOB is advanced past the distal tip of the tube and the anterior tracheal rings are identified. This allows proper orientation of the right and left main stem bronchi. With the FOB past the main tube opening and above the carina, the main stem bronchi are identified. The blocker portion of the tube is advanced under FOB vision and while securing the main tube (Fig. 24-9).

Placement of the blocker into the desired main stem bronchus is achieved by advancing the blocker with either a clockwise or counterclockwise rotation. If this maneuver is not sufficient to align the blocker into the desired main stem bronchus, the entire Univent tube may also be rotated in the desired direction in order to assist the blocker orientation. The blocker is advanced into the desired location, and the locking cuff at the proximal end of the blocker is secured. It is useful to note the distance marker on the blocker. One needs to ensure that the proximal cap of the blocker is engaged, or a tube leak will be present. When lung isolation is desired, the blocker cuff is inflated (best performed under direct FOB visualization) and the proximal cap of the blocker may be disengaged in order to assist egress of gas from the lung and enhance lung deflation (see Fig. 24-9). Blind placement of the blocker is unsuccessful, especially if the left main stem bronchus is the target. Also, blind placement may result in trauma to the tracheobronchial tree, resulting in bleeding or even tension pneumothorax.

D. BRONCHIAL BLOCKERS

It is also possible to perform lung isolation without the use of specialized tubes. In these cases a blocking device is inserted either through the lumen of an SLT or outside the SLT, between the tracheal cuff and the trachea. Placement is confirmed by fiberoptic bronchoscopy.

1. Para-Axial Endotracheal Blockers (Fig. 24-10)

The advantage of placing the blocker device outside the SLT is that this method allows blocker placement with smaller ETs because the blocker does not share the ET lumen. It is often easier to position the blocker, as the blocker and FOB do not become caught up with one another in the ET lumen. Disadvantages of this paratube technique include (1) the need to perform laryngoscopy in order to place the blocker into the trachea, (2) the need

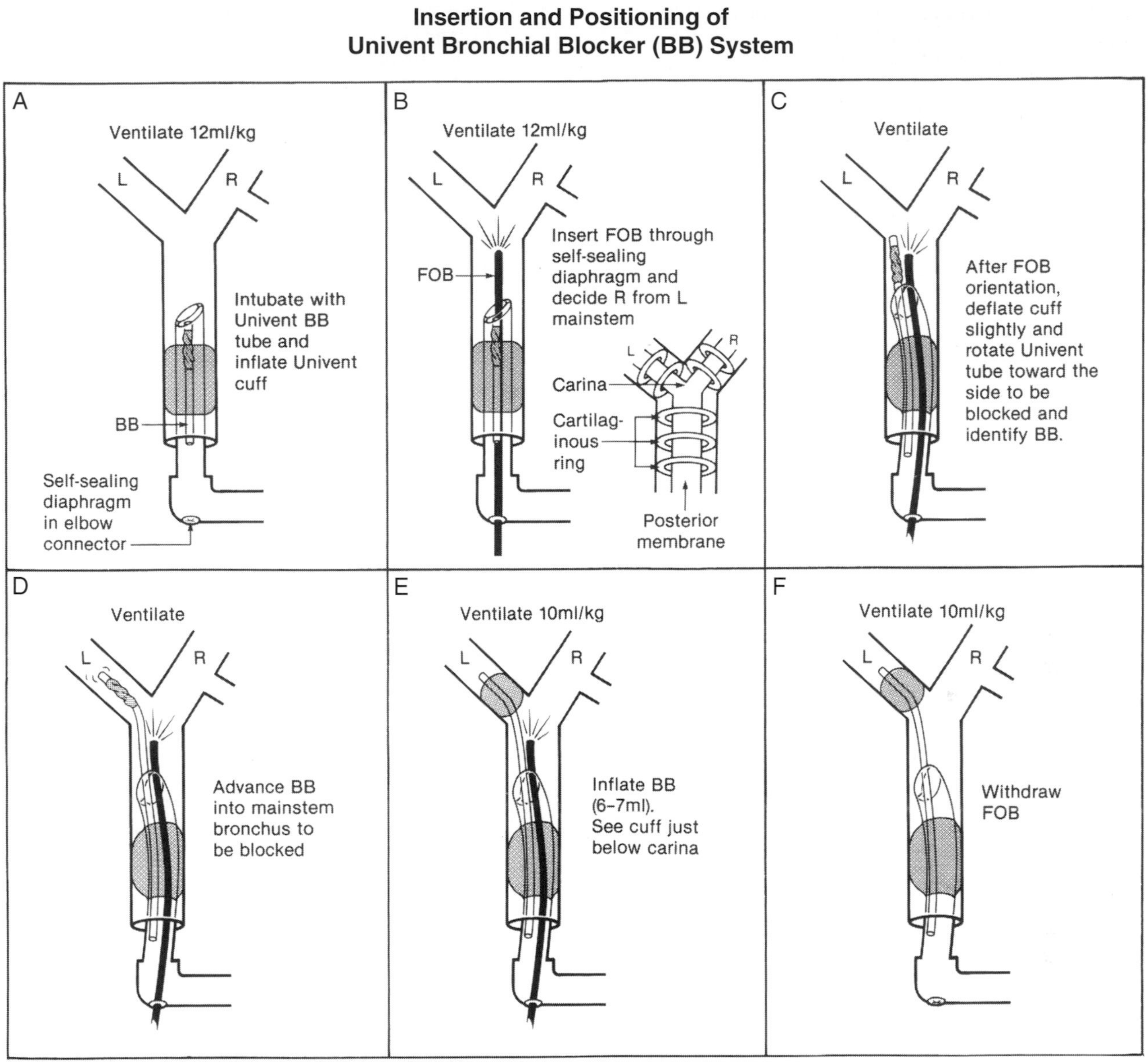

Insertion and Positioning of
Univent Bronchial Blocker (BB) System

Figure 24-9 The sequential steps of the fiberoptic-aided method of inserting and positioning the Univent bronchial blocker in the left main stem bronchus. See text for full explanation. One- and two-lung ventilation is achieved by simply inflating and deflating, respectively, the bronchial blocker balloon. FOB, fiberoptic bronchoscope; L, left; R, right. (From Benumof JL: Anesthesia for thoracic surgery. Philadelphia, WB Saunders, 1987.)

to deflate the tracheal cuff while positioning the blocker, and (3) the potential to rupture the ET cuff while manipulating the blocker. It is because of these disadvantages that we prefer to use a "through the tube" blocker technique.

2. Coaxial Stand-Alone Endotracheal Blockers
(Fig. 24-11)

Any device that has a balloon-tipped catheter can be used as a blocker.[21] The most common devices used are Fogarty embolectomy catheters and the Cook bronchial blockers.[58]

a. Fogarty Catheters

The Fogarty catheters come with a rigid wire stylet in place. This allows the creation of a hockey stick curve at the end of the catheter, which allows better directional control of the blocker. Once the blocker is positioned (by FOB), the stylet is removed and a stopcock is placed over the balloon port. Under FOB vision, the balloon is inflated until the desired lumen is occluded. The Fogarty is then secured to the ET. The main disadvantage of this device is the inability to suction or insufflate distal to the occluded bronchial lumen. Another disadvantage is that the balloon utilizes a high-pressure, low-volume cuff.

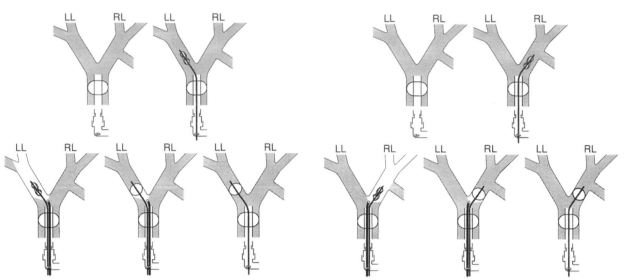

A. Lung Separation With Single Lumen Tube and Left Lung Bronchial Blocker Inside of Single Lumen Tube

B. Lung Separation With Single Lumen Tube and Right Lung Bronchial Blocker Inside of Single Lumen Tube

Figure 24-10 Sequence for lung separation with single-lumen tube and bronchial blocker within the single-lumen tube. **A**, Left lung bronchial blocker. **B**, Right lung bronchial blocker. The bronchial blocker (Fogarty embolectomy catheter) is placed in the correct main stem bronchus under fiberoptic vision. (From Benumof JL: Anesthesia for Thoracic Surgery. Philadelphia, WB Saunders, 1987.)

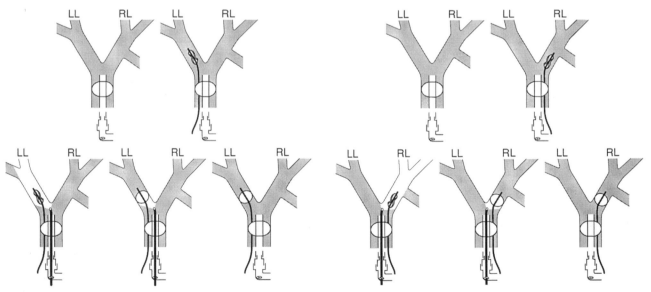

A. Lung Separation With Single Lumen Tube and Left Lung Bronchial Blocker Outside of Single Lumen Tube

B. Lung Separation With Single Lumen Tube and Right Lung Bronchial Blocker Outside of Single Lumen Tube

Figure 24-11 How to separate two lungs with a single-lumen tube, fiberoptic bronchoscope, and a left lung **(A)** and a right lung **(B)** bronchial blocker that is outside the single-lumen tube. Sequence of events is as follows. Single-lumen tube is inserted, and patient is ventilated (upper left diagram, **A** and **B**). Bronchial blocker is passed alongside the indwelling endotracheal tube (upper right diagram, **A** and **B**). Fiberoptic bronchoscope is passed through a self-sealing diaphragm in elbow connector to the endotracheal tube and is used to place bronchial blocker into the appropriate main stem bronchus under direct vision (lower left diagram, **A** and **B**). Balloon on the bronchial blocker is also inflated under direct vision and is positioned just below the tracheal carina (lower middle diagram, **A** and **B**). During the lower panel sequence (insertion and use of fiberoptic bronchoscope), the self-sealing diaphragm allows patient to continue to be ventilated with positive-pressure ventilation (around the fiberoptic bronchoscope but within the lumens of the endotracheal tube). LL, left lung; RR, right lung. (From Benumof JL: Anesthesia for Thoracic Surgery. Philadelphia, WB Saunders, 1987.)

b. Arndt and Cohen Bronchial Blockers

The Cook corporation has produced two specialized blockers. These are the Arndt and Cohen blockers. Each blocker utilizes a high-volume, low-pressure cuff and is introduced through a multiport airway adapter. This adapter has an ingenious sealing diaphragm that allows passage of blockers of different sizes. It also incorporates a separate port for the introduction of the FOB. The multiport adapter can be used with any stand-alone blocker. The Arndt blocker comes in various sizes. It has a small central lumen to allow minimal insufflation and suctioning. It is to be directed by snaring the monofilament guide loop through an FOB and upon placement in the desired position, release of the snare, which is often easier said than done. The Cohen blocker also comes in various sizes and employs a directional tip, which makes placing this device easier than placing the Arndt blocker.

The main disadvantages of these commercial blockers are that their outer diameters are greater than those of the Fogarty catheters, which makes placing them in ETs smaller than 6.0 difficult to impossible. For cases in which a small ET (less than 6 mm) is used, a Cook multiport adapter with a small Fogarty catheter may be preferred.

V. PEDIATRIC LUNG ISOLATION

A. VENTILATION-PERFUSION DURING THORACIC SURGERY

Ventilation is normally distributed preferentially to dependent regions of the lung so that there is a gradient of increasing ventilation from the most nondependent to the most dependent lung segments. Because of gravitational effects, perfusion normally follows a similar distribution, with increased blood flow to dependent lung segments. Therefore, ventilation and perfusion are normally well matched. During thoracic surgery, several factors act to increase ventilation-perfusion ($\dot{V}/\dot{Q}$) mismatch. General anesthesia, neuromuscular blockade, and mechanical ventilation cause a decrease in functional residual capacity of both lungs. Compression of the dependent lung in the lateral decubitus position may cause atelectasis. Surgical retraction or SLV or both result in collapse of the operative lung. Hypoxic pulmonary vasoconstriction, which acts to divert blood flow away from underventilated lung, thereby minimizing ($\dot{V}/\dot{Q}$) mismatch, may be diminished by inhalational anesthetic agents and other vasodilating drugs. These factors apply equally to infants, children, and adults. The overall effect of the lateral decubitus position on ($\dot{V}/\dot{Q}$) mismatch, however, is different in infants compared with older children and adults.

In adults with unilateral lung disease, oxygenation is optimal when the patient is placed in the lateral decubitus position with the healthy lung dependent ("down") and the diseased lung nondependent ("up").[50] Presumably, this is related to an increase in blood flow to the dependent, healthy lung and a decrease in blood flow to the nondependent, diseased lung related to the hydrostatic pressure (or gravitational) gradient between the two lungs. This phenomenon promotes ($\dot{V}/\dot{Q}$) matching in the adult patient undergoing thoracic surgery in the lateral decubitus position.

In infants with unilateral lung disease, however, oxygenation is improved with the healthy lung up.[28] Several factors account for this discrepancy between adults and infants. Infants have a soft, easily compressible rib cage that cannot fully support the underlying lung. Therefore, functional residual capacity is closer to residual volume, making airway closure likely to occur in the dependent lung even during tidal breathing.[42] When the adult is placed in the lateral decubitus position, the dependent diaphragm has a mechanical advantage because it is "loaded" by the abdominal hydrostatic pressure gradient. This pressure gradient is reduced in infants, thereby reducing the functional advantage of the dependent diaphragm. The infant's small size also results in a reduced hydrostatic pressure gradient between the nondependent and dependent lungs. Consequently, the favorable increase in perfusion to the dependent, ventilated lung is reduced in infants.

Finally, the infant's increased oxygen requirement, coupled with a small functional residual capacity, predisposes to hypoxemia. Infants normally consume 6 to 8 mL of O_2/kg/min, compared with a normal O_2 consumption in adults of 2 to 3 mL/kg/min.[18] For these reasons, infants are at increased risk for significant oxygen desaturation during surgery in the lateral decubitus position.

B. INDICATIONS AND TECHNIQUES FOR SINGLE-LUNG VENTILATION IN INFANTS AND CHILDREN

Prior to 1995, nearly all thoracic surgery in children was performed by thoracotomy. In the majority of cases, anesthesiologists ventilated both lungs with a conventional ET and the surgeons retracted the operative lung in order to gain exposure to the surgical field. During the past decade, the use of video-assisted thoracoscopic surgery (VATS) has dramatically increased in both adults and children. Reported advantages of thoracoscopy include smaller chest incisions, reduced postoperative pain, and more rapid postoperative recovery compared with thoracotomy.[2,46,60] Advances in surgical technique as well as technology, including high-resolution microchip cameras and smaller endoscopic instruments, have facilitated the application of VATS in smaller patients.

VATS is being used extensively for pleural débridement in patients with empyema, lung biopsy, and wedge resections for interstitial lung disease, mediastinal masses, and metastatic lesions. More extensive pulmonary resections, including segmentectomy and lobectomy, have been performed for lung abscess, bullous disease, sequestrations, lobar emphysema, CAM, and neoplasms. In selected centers, more advanced procedures have been reported, including closure of patent ductus arteriosus, repair of hiatal hernias, and anterior spinal fusion.

VATS can be performed while both lungs are being ventilated using CO_2 insufflation and placement of a retractor to displace lung tissue in the operative field. However, SLV is extremely desirable during VATS because lung deflation improves visualization of thoracic contents and may reduce lung injury caused by the use of retractors.[4] There are several different techniques that can be used for SLV in children.

C. SINGLE-LUMEN TUBE

The simplest means of providing SLV is to intubate the ipsilateral main stem bronchus with a conventional single-lumen ET.[51] When the left bronchus is to be intubated, the bevel of the ET is rotated 180 degrees and the head turned to the right.[34] The ET is advanced into the bronchus until breath sounds on the operative side disappear. An FOB may be passed through or alongside the ET to confirm or guide placement. When a cuffed ET is used, the distance from the tip of the tube to the distal cuff must be shorter than the length of the bronchus so that the cuff is not entirely in the bronchus.[36] This technique is simple and requires no special equipment other than an FOB. This may be the preferred technique of SLV in emergency situations such as airway hemorrhage or contralateral tension pneumothorax.

Problems can occur when using a single-lumen ET for SLV. If a smaller, uncuffed ET is used, it may be difficult to provide an adequate seal of the intended bronchus. This may prevent the operative lung from adequately collapsing or fail to protect the healthy, ventilated lung from contamination by purulent material from the contralateral lung. One is unable to suction the operative lung using this technique. Hypoxemia may occur because of obstruction of the upper lobe bronchus, especially when the short right main stem bronchus is intubated.

Variations of this technique have been described, including intubation of both bronchi independently with small ETs.[17,45,59,61] One main stem bronchus is initially intubated with an ET, after which another ET is advanced over an FOB into the opposite bronchus.

D. BALLOON-TIPPED BRONCHIAL BLOCKERS

A Fogarty embolectomy catheter or an end-hole, balloon wedge catheter may be used for bronchial blockade to provide SLV.[21,26,38,57] Placement of a Fogarty catheter is facilitated by bending the tip of its stylet toward the bronchus on the operative side. An FOB may be used to reposition the catheter and confirm appropriate placement. When an end-hole catheter is placed outside the ET, the bronchus on the operative side is initially intubated with an ET. A guidewire is then advanced into that bronchus through the ET. The ET is

removed and the blocker is advanced over the guidewire into the bronchus. An ET is then reinserted into the trachea alongside the blocker catheter. The catheter balloon is positioned in the proximal main stem bronchus under fiberoptic visual guidance. With an inflated blocker balloon the airway is completely sealed, providing more predictable lung collapse and better operating conditions than with an ET in the bronchus.

A potential problem with this technique is dislodgement of the blocker balloon into the trachea. The inflated balloon then blocks ventilation to both lungs or prevents collapse of the operated lung, or both. The balloons of most catheters currently used for bronchial blockade have low-volume, high-pressure properties and overdistention can damage or even rupture the airway.[8] One study, however, reported that bronchial blocker cuffs produced lower "cuff-to-tracheal" pressures than DLTs.[23] When closed-tip bronchial blockers are used, the operative lung cannot be suctioned and CPAP cannot be provided to the operative lung if needed.

Adapters have been used that facilitate ventilation during placement of a bronchial blocker through an indwelling ET.[3,56] A new 5 Fr endobronchial blocker that is suitable for use in children with a multiport adapter and FOB has been described (Cook, Bloomington, IN).[25] The risk of hypoxemia during blocker placement is diminished, and repositioning of the blocker may be performed with fiberoptic guidance during surgery. Even with use of an FOB with a diameter of 2.2 mm, however, the indwelling ET must be at least 5.0 mm ID to allow passage of the catheter and FOB. This technique, therefore, is generally limited to children older than 18 months to 2 years.

E. UNIVENT TUBE

The Univent tube (Fuji Systems, Tokyo, Japan) is a conventional ET with a second lumen containing a small tube that can be advanced into a bronchus.[20,31,32] A balloon located at the distal end of this small tube serves as a blocker. Univent tubes require an FOB for successful placement. Univent tubes are now available in sizes as small as a 3.5 and 4.5 mm inner diameter for use in children older than 6 years.[24] Because the blocker tube is firmly attached to the main ET, displacement of the Univent blocker balloon is less likely than when other blocker techniques are used. The blocker tube has a small lumen, which allows egress of gas and can be used to insufflate oxygen or suction the operated lung.

A disadvantage of the Univent tube is the large amount of cross-sectional area occupied by the blocker channel, especially in the smaller tubes. Smaller Univent tubes have a disproportionately high resistance to gas flow.[54] The Univent tube's blocker balloon has low-volume, high-pressure characteristics, and mucosal injury can occur during normal inflation.[6,33]

F. DOUBLE-LUMEN TUBES

All DLTs are essentially two tubes of unequal length molded together. The shorter tube ends in the trachea and the longer tube in the bronchus. Marraro described a bilumen tube for infants.[43] This tube consists of two separate uncuffed ETs of different length attached longitudinally. This tube is not available in the United States. DLTs for older children and adults have cuffs located on the tracheal and bronchial lumens. The tracheal cuff, when inflated, allows positive-pressure ventilation. The inflated bronchial cuff allows ventilation to be diverted to either or both lungs and protects each lung from contamination from the contralateral side.

Conventional plastic DLTs, once available only in adult sizes (35, 37, 39, and 41 Fr), are now available in smaller sizes. The smallest cuffed DLT is 26 Fr (Rusch, Duluth, GA)

Table 24-3   Limitations to the Use of the Univent Bronchial Blocker Tube and Solutions to the Limitations

Limitation	Solution
1. Slow inflation time	1. (a) Deflate bronchial blocker cuff and administer a positive-pressure breath through the main single lumen; (b) carefully administer one short high-pressure (20-30 psi) jet ventilation.
2. Slow deflation time	2. (a) Deflate bronchial blocker cuff and compress and evacuate the lung through the main single lumen; (b) apply suction to bronchial blocker lumen.
3. Blockage of bronchial blocker lumen by blood or pus	3. Suction, wire stylet, and then suction.
4. High-pressure cuff	4. Use just-seal volume of air.
5. Intraoperative leak in bronchial blocker cuff	5. Make sure bronchial blocker cuff is subcarinal, increase inflation volume, and rearrange surgical field.

and may be used in children as young as 8 years. DLTs are also available in sizes 28 and 32 Fr (Mallinckrodt Medical, St. Louis, MO) suitable for children 10 years of age and older.

DLTs are inserted in children using the same technique as in adults.[12] The tip of the tube is inserted just past the vocal cords and the stylet is withdrawn. The DLT is rotated 90 degrees to the appropriate side and then advanced into the bronchus. In the adult population the depth of insertion is directly related to the height of the patient.[11] No equivalent measurements are yet available in children. If fiberoptic bronchoscopy is to be used to confirm tube placement, an FOB with a small diameter and sufficient length must be available.[53]

A DLT offers the advantage of ease of insertion as well as the ability to suction and oxygenate the operative lung with CPAP. Left DLTs are preferred to right DLTs because of the shorter length of the right main bronchus.[7] Right DLTs are more difficult to position accurately because of the greater risk of right upper lobe obstruction.

DLTs are safe and easy to use. There are very few reports of airway damage from DLTs in adults and none in children. Their high-volume, low-pressure cuffs should not damage the airway if they are not overinflated with air or distended with nitrous oxide while in place.

Guidelines for selecting appropriate tubes (or catheters) for SLV in children are shown in Table 24-3. There is significant variability in overall size and airway dimensions in children, particularly in teenagers. The recommendation shown in Table 24-3 are based on average values for airway dimensions. Larger DLTs may be safely used in large teenagers.

VI. CONCLUSION

The anesthesiologist caring for patients requiring SLV faces many challenges. An understanding of the primary underlying lesion as well as associated anomalies that may affect perioperative management is paramount. A working knowledge of respiratory physiology and anatomy is required for the planning and execution of appropriate intraoperative care. Familiarity with a variety of techniques for SLV suited to the patient's size and needs allows maximal surgical exposure while minimizing trauma to the lungs and airways.

REFERENCES

1. Alliaume B, Coddens J, Deloof T: Reliability of auscultation in positioning of double-lumen endobronchial tubes. Can J Anaesth 39:687, 1992.
2. Angelillo Mackinlay TA, Lyons GA, Chimondeguy DJ, et al: VATS debridement versus thoracotomy in the treatment of loculated postpneumonia empyema. Ann Thorac Surg 61:1626-1630, 1996.
3. Arndt GA, De Lessio ST, Kranner PW, et al: One-lung ventilation when intubation is difficult—Presentation of a new endobronchial blocker. Acta Anaesthesiol Scand 43:356-358, 1999.
4. Benumof JL: Anesthesia for Thoracic Surgery, 2nd ed. Philadelphia, WB Saunders, 1995.

5. Benumof JL: The position of a double-lumen tube should be routinely determined by fiberoptic bronchoscopy [editorial]. J Cardiothorac Vasc Anesth 7:513, 1993.

6. Benumof JL, Gaughan SD, Ozaki GT: The relationship among bronchial blocker cuff inflation volume, proximal airway pressure, and seal of the bronchial blocker cuff. J Cardiothorac Vasc Anesth 6:404-408, 1992.

7. Benumof JL, Partridge BL, Salvatierra C, Keating J: Margin of safety in positioning modern double-lumen endotracheal tubes. Anesthesiology 67:729-738, 1987.

8. Borchardt RA, LaQuaglia MP, McDowall, Wilson RS: Bronchial injury during lung isolation in a pediatric patient. Anesth Analg 87:324-325, 1998.

9. Brodsky JB, Adkins MO, Gaba DM: Bronchial cuff pressures of double-lumen tubes. Anesth Analg 69:608, 1989.

10. Brodsky JB, Benumof JL, Ehrenwerth J, et al: Depth of placement of left double-lumen endobronchial tubes. Anesth Analg 73:570, 1991.

11. Brodsky JB, Macario A, Mark JBD: Tracheal diameter predicts double-lumen tube size: A method for selecting left double-lumen tubes. Anesth Analg 82:861-864, 1996.

12. Brodsky JB, Mark JBD: A simple technique for accurate placement of double-lumen endobronchial tubes. Anesth Rev 10:26-30, 1983.

13. Brodsky JB, Shulman MS, Mark JBD: Malposition of left-sided double-lumen endobronchial tubes. Anesthesiology 62:667, 1985.

14. Burk WJ III: Should a fiberoptic bronchoscope be routinely used to position a double-lumen tube? Anesthesiology 68:826, 1988.

15. Cohen E, Goldofsky S, Neustein S, et al: Fiberoptic evaluation of endobronchial tube position: Red rubber vs polyvinylchloride. Anesth Analg 68(Suppl):54, 1989.

16. Cohen JA, Denisco RA, Richards TS et al: Hazardous placement of a Robertshaw-type endobronchial tube. Anesth Analg 65:100, 1986.

17. Cullum AR, English CW, Branthwaite MA: Endobronchial intubation in infancy. Anaesthesia 28:66-70, 1973.

18. Dawes GS: Fetal and Neonatal Physiology. Chicago, Yearbook Medical, 1973.

19. Dryden GE: Circulatory collapse after pneumonectomy (an unusual complication from the use of a Carlens catheter): Case report. Anesth Analg 56:451, 1977.

20. Gayes JM: The Univent tube is the best technique for providing one-lung ventilation. Pro: One-lung ventilation is best accomplished with the Univent endotracheal tube. J Cardiothorac Vasc Anesth 7:103-105, 1993.

21. Ginsberg RJ: New technique for one-lung anesthesia using a bronchial blocker. J Thorac Cardiovasc Surg 82:542-546, 1981.

22. Guernelli N, Bragaglia RB, Briccoli A et al: Tracheobronchial ruptures due to cuffed Carlens tubes. Ann Thorac Surg 28:66, 1979.

23. Guyton DC, Besselievre TR, Devidas M, et al: A comparison of two different bronchial cuff designs and four different bronchial cuff inflation methods. J Cardiothorac Vasc Anesth 11:599-603, 1997.

24. Hammer GB, Brodsky JB, Redpath J, Cannon WB: The Univent tube for single lung ventilation in children. Paediatr Anaesth 8:55-57, 1998.

25. Hammer GB, Harrison TK, Vricella LA, et al: Single lung ventilation using a new pediatric bronchial blocker. Paediatr Anaesth 12:69-72, 2001.

26. Hammer GB, Manos SJ, Smith BM, et al: Single lung ventilation in pediatric patients. Anesthesiology 84:1503-1506, 1996.

27. Hansen TB, Watson CB: Tracheobronchial trauma secondary to a Carlens tube [abstract]. Presented at the Society of Cardiovascular Anesthesiologists fifth annual meeting, 1983.

28. Heaf DP, Helms P, Gordon MB, Turner HM: Postural effects on gas exchange in infants. N Engl J Med 28:1505-1508, 1983.

29. Hurford WE, Alfille PH: A quality improvement study of the placement and complications of double-lumen endobronchial tubes. J Cardiothorac Vasc Anesth 7:517-520, 1993.

30. Inoue H, Shohtsu A, Ogawa J, et al: New device for one lung anesthesia: Endotracheal tube with moveable blocker. J Thorac Cardiovasc Surg 83:940, 1982.

31. Kamaya H, Krishna PR: New endotracheal tube (Univent tube) for selective blockade of one lung. Anesthesiology 63:342-343, 1985.

32. Karwande SV: A new tube for single lung ventilation. Chest 92:761-763, 1987.

33. Kelley JG, Gaba DM, Brodsky JB: Bronchial cuff pressures of two tubes used in thoracic surgery. J Cardiothorac Vasc Anesth 6:190-194, 1992.

34. Kubota H, Kubota Y, Toshiro T, et al: Selective blind endobronchial intubation in children and adults. Anesthesiology 67:587-589, 1987.

35. Kvetan V, Carlon GC, Howland WS: Acute pulmonary failure in asymmetric lung disease: Approach to management. Crit Care Med 10:114, 1982.

36. Lammers CR, Hammer GB, Brodsky JB, Cannon WB: Failure to isolate the lungs with an endotracheal tube positioned in the bronchus. Anesth Analg 85:944, 1997.

37. Lewis JW, Serwin JP, Gabriel FS, et al: The utility of a double-lumen tube for one-lung ventilation in a variety of noncardiac thoracic surgical procedures. J Cardiothorac Vasc Anesth 5:705, 1992.

38. Lin YC, Hackel A: Paediatric selective bronchial blocker. Paediatr Anaesth 4:391-392, 1994.

39. MacGillvray RG: Evaluation of a new tracheal tube with a moveable bronchus blocker. Anaesthesia 43:687, 1988.

40. Magee PT: Endobronchial cuff pressures of double-lumen tubes. Anesth Analg 72:265, 1991.

41. Maguire DP, Spiro AW: Bronchial obstruction and hypoxia during one-lung ventilation. Anesthesiology 66:830, 1987.

42. Mansell A, Bryan C, Levison H: Airway closure in children. J Appl Physiol 33:711-714, 1972.

43. Marraro G: Selective bronchial intubation in paediatrics: The Marraro paediatric bilumen tube. Paediatric Anaesthesia 4:255-258, 1994.

44. McKenna MJ, Wilson RS, Botelho RJ: Right upper lobe obstruction with right-sided double-lumen endobronchial tubes: A comparison of two types. J Cardiothorac Vasc Anesth 2:734, 1988.

45. McLellan I: Endobronchial intubation in children. Anaesthesia 29:757-758, 1974.

46. Mouroux J, Clary-Meinesz C, Padovani B, et al: Efficacy and safety of videothoracoscopic lung biopsy in the diagnosis of interstitial lung disease. Eur J Cardiothorac Surg 11:22-26, 1997.

47. Neto PPR: Bronchial cuff pressure of endobronchial double-lumen tubes. Anesth Analg 71:209, 1990.

48. Newman RW, Finer GE, Downs JE: Routine use of the Carlens double-lumen endobronchial catheter: An experimental and clinical study. J Thorac Cardiovasc Surg 42:327, 1961.

49. Read RC, Friday CD, Eason CN: Prospective study of the Robertshaw endobronchial catheter in thoracic surgery. Ann Thorac Surg 24:156, 1977.

50. Remolina C, Khan AU, Santiago TV, Edelman NH: Positional hypoxemia in unilateral lung disease. N Engl J Med 304:523-525, 1981.

51. Rowe R, Andropoulos D, Heard M, et al: Anesthetic management of pediatric patients undergoing thoracoscopy. J Cardiothorac Vasc Anesth 8:563, 1994.

52. Saito S, Dohi S, Tajima K: Failure of double-lumen endobronchial tube placement: Congenital tracheal stenosis in an adult. Anesthesiology 66:83, 1987.

53. Slinger PD: Fiberoptic bronchoscopic positioning of double-lumen tubes. J Cardiothorac Anesth 3:486-496, 1989.

54. Slinger PD, Lesiuk L: Flow resistances of disposable double-lumen, single-lumen, and Univent tubes. J Cardiothorac Vasc Anesth 12:142-144, 1998.

55. Smith GB, Hirsch NP, Ehrenwerth J: Placement of double-lumen endobronchial tubes. Br J Anaesth 58:1317, 1986.

56. Takahashi M, Horinouchi T, Kato M, et al: Double-access-port endotracheal tube for selective lung ventilation in pediatric patients. Anesthesiology 93:308-309, 2000.

57. Turner MWH, Buchanon CCR, Brown SW: Paediatric one lung ventilation in the prone position. Paediatr Anaesth 7:427-429, 1997.

58. Veil R: Selective bronchial blocking in a small child. Br J Anaesth 41:453, 1969.

59. Watson CB, Bowe EA, Burk W: One-lung anesthesia for pediatric thoracic surgery: A new use for the fiberoptic bronchoscope. Anesthesiology 56:314-315, 1982.

60. Weatherford DA, Stephenson JE, Taylor SM, et al: Thoracoscopy versus thoracotomy: Indications and advantages. Ann Surg 61:83-86, 1995.

61. Yeh TF, Pildes RS, Salem MR: Treatment of persistent tension pneumothorax in a neonate by selective bronchial intubation. Anesthesiology 49:37-38, 1978.

25

THE COMBITUBE: ESOPHAGEAL-TRACHEAL DOUBLE-LUMEN AIRWAY

Michael Frass
Ricardo M. Urtubia
Carin A. Hagberg

I. HISTORY AND DEVELOPMENT OF THE COMBITUBE

A. ROLE OF THE ENDOTRACHEAL TUBE FOR INTUBATION AND VENTILATION

Rapid establishment of a patent airway to facilitate adequate ventilation during cardiopulmonary resuscitation (CPR) is the primary task of the rescuer. Mouth-to-mouth ventilation carries the disadvantages of possible gastric insufflation and a danger of aspiration. Endotracheal intubation remains the gold standard in airway maintenance. However, this skill is only acquired after intensive training and requires constant practice. Often the people performing resuscitation procedures are untrained in intubation. In addition, endotracheal intubation is difficult[9] or impossible even for skilled personnel on many occasions, since endotracheal intubation requires good exposure of the patient's airway, a skilled endoscopist, and equipment or facilities for intubation. Therefore, as the main objectives of airway management are ventilation and oxygenation, the need arises for a simple and efficient alternative to endotracheal intubation.

B. DEVELOPMENT AND DESCRIPTION OF THE ESOPHAGEAL OBTURATOR AIRWAY AS AN ALTERNATIVE AIRWAY ADJUNCT

The esophageal obturator airway was constructed by Don Michael and Gordon as an alternative to the endotracheal tube during emergency intubation.[20] The esophageal obturator airway is a 34-cm-long tube with a balloon at its distal tip (Fig. 25-1). The balloon should lie below the level of the tracheal bifurcation after insertion. The distal end is blocked. Proximal to the balloon there are 16 holes, which are positioned in the region of the hypopharynx after positioning of the airway. At the proximal end, a facemask is connected to the airway, sealing mouth and nose during ventilation.

The esophageal obturator airway is inserted by first grasping the back of the patient's tongue and the lower jaw with thumb and index finger and then guiding the airway gently into the esophagus. The distal balloon is inflated to occlude the esophagus while the mask is pressed against the patient's face. Air enters the proximal end and then enters the hypopharynx through perforations, since the distal end is blocked. From there, air is forced over the opened glottis into the trachea, since the mouth and nose are sealed by the mask and the esophagus by the balloon (Fig. 25-1).

C. STUDIES WITH THE ESOPHAGEAL OBTURATOR AIRWAY

Subsequent physiologic testing and field trials of the esophageal obturator airway have been performed.

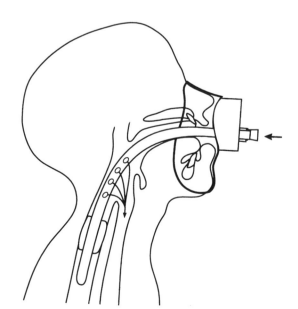

Figure 25-1 Esophageal obturator airway. Air is blown through proximal port and travels through perforations into hypopharynx (small arrows) and trachea, since mouth and nose are sealed by the mask and esophagus by the balloon.

Schofferman et al.[79] evaluated the airway in 18 patients suffering from cardiac arrest, in which resuscitation was performed by paramedics. Arterial blood-gas analysis was obtained during ventilation with the esophageal obturator airway and subsequently with the endotracheal tube (ET). There was little or no improvement in oxygenation after endotracheal intubation, implying that failure to oxygenate some patients was not due to the esophageal obturator airway. Shea et al.[82] compared two similar groups of patients during cardiopulmonary arrest with ventricular fibrillation: 296 patients were intubated with either the ET or the esophageal obturator airway. Survival rates and neurologic sequelae of survivors showed no statistically significant difference between the two groups. Hammargren et al.[42] compared both devices after standardizing the method of oxygen delivery and assuring true sampling of arterial blood. In 48 victims of prehospital cardiac arrest, blood gases were drawn during ventilation with the esophageal obturator airway and subsequent ventilation with the ET. There was no statistically significant difference in the PaO_2 or $PaCO_2$ between the two devices. The authors concluded that the esophageal obturator airway was an effective means of airway management, with the ventilation achieved equal to that of an ET.

Nevertheless, it soon became apparent from studies in the controlled environment of the operating room that considerable technical difficulties were associated with the esophageal obturator airway.[13]

D. DISADVANTAGES OF THE ESOPHAGEAL OBTURATOR AIRWAY

The esophageal obturator airway is discussed controversially in the literature because of the following possible complications:

1. There are significant difficulties in obtaining a tight face-mask seal and maintaining the seal during transportation. Effective use requires at least two hands to seal the mask. Complaints are related to significant difficulty obtaining an adequate mask fit particularly in edentulous or bearded patients.[13,42]
2. Inadvertent or unrecognized tracheal intubation.[38] In this case, the patient's airway is completely obstructed, and attempts at repositioning are usually unsuccessful.
3. Esophageal or gastric ruptures.[16,49,80] Ruptures of the esophagus or the stomach may be due to the length of the esophageal obturator airway. Since many cardiac arrest patients exhibit left atrial dilatation with subsequent lateral deviation of the lower half of the esophagus, the esophageal obturator airway may be forced into the left lateral direction in addition to the sagittal curved direction, which might lead to ruptures.

E. DEVELOPMENT OF THE COMBITUBE ESOPHAGEAL/TRACHEAL DOUBLE-LUMEN AIRWAY

The above disadvantages and the idea that both tracheal and esophageal intubation allow ventilation and oxygenation, led to the development of the Combitube. It was devised by Michael Frass in cooperation with Reinhard Frenzer and Jonas Zahler, Moedling and Vienna, Austria.[24-26,30]

The intent of the Combitube design was to deal effectively with the problem of managing the airway with the highest level of success possible. In fact, studies in large populations[36,72,78,85] demonstrate that the Combitube provides a much better chance of ventilation and oxygenation than other devices, isolating and protecting the airway from digestive regurgitation and aspiration, at the same time. Thus, the Combitube can be used in cases in which airway management is difficult independent of the cause: anatomic factors, patient's position with respect to the operator, space and illumination, presence of a full stomach. In addition, the Combitube does not need special equipment, energy or complex techniques to be properly used. Finally, as the Combitube is available in only two sizes (37 and 41 French), no time is lost in selecting the proper size among many alternatives.

II. DESCRIPTION OF THE COMBITUBE

A. TECHNICAL DESCRIPTION

The Esophageal Tracheal Combitube (Combitube; Tyco Healthcare, Mansfield, MA) is a device for emergency intubation that combines the functions of an esophageal obturator airway and a conventional ET (Fig. 25-2). The Combitube is a double-cuff and double-lumen tube (Fig. 25-3). The so-called oropharyngeal balloon is located at the middle portion of the tube and the so-called tracheoesophageal cuff is located at the distal end.[90] The lumens are separated by a partition wall. Proximally, both lumens are opened and linked by short tubes with universal connectors. Distally, the so-called pharyngeal lumen is blocked and has 8 perforations at the level between the cuffs, and the so-called tracheoesophageal lumen is open. This design allows ventilation both when the Combitube is positioned in the esophagus through the perforations of the pharyngeal lumen, and in the trachea, through the opened distal end of the tracheoesophageal lumen. The pharyngeal balloon seals the oral and nasal cavity after inflation. Printed ring marks proximal to the oropharyngeal balloon indicate the limit of insertion.

The Combitube is produced in two sizes: the 37 Fr SA (Small Adult) model may be used in patients with a height from 4 up to 6 ½ feet[36,93,99] while the 41 Fr model is used in patients taller than 6 feet with some overlap. The preferred model for most patients is the 37 Fr SA because it has been reported to work well in patients up to 6 feet or taller.

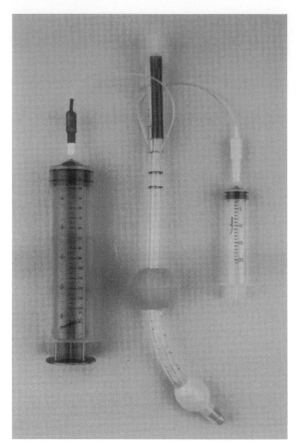

Figure 25-2 Combitube, with large syringe for inflation of oropharyngeal balloon and small syringe for inflation of distal cuff.

B. INSERTION TECHNIQUES

As previously mentioned, the Combitube can be successfully inserted independently of the patient's position with regard to the operator. The patient's head is preferably in neutral position, or a small cushion may be used. Sniffing position may actually impede Combitube insertion.

1. Conventional Technique

With the operator behind the patient's head, the lower jaw and tongue are lifted by the thumb and index finger. The tongue is pressed forward by the thumb and the tube is inserted in a downward curved movement until the printed ring marks lie between the teeth, or the alveolar ridges in edentulous patients (Fig. 25-4A). Insertion should be performed along the tongue to avoid potential damage of the posterior pharyngeal mucosa. Sometimes, a rocking motion may alleviate insertion. Next, the oropharyngeal balloon is inflated with up to 85 mL of air with the 37 Fr SA Combitube (or up to 100 mL with the 41 Fr Combitube through port No. 1 with the blue pilot balloon using the large syringe with blue color code (Fig. 25-4B). The minimal volume technique may be used in which enough air is inflated to obtain a seal (discussed later in "General Anesthesia") or a cuff pressure gauge may be

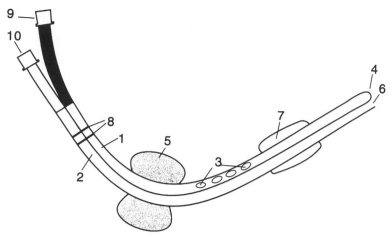

Figure 25-3 Cross-sectional view of Combitube. 1, "Pharyngeal" lumen (longer tube with blocked distal end); 2, "tracheoesophageal" lumen (shorter tube with open distal end); 3, perforations of esophageal lumen 1 at pharyngeal section; 4, blocked distal end of esophageal lumen 1; 5, oropharyngeal balloon; 6, open distal end of tracheal lumen 2; 7, distal cuff for obturating either esophagus or trachea; 8, printed ring marks for indicating depth of insertion between the teeth or alveolar ridges; 9, connector for (blue) tube leading to esophageal lumen 1; 10, connector for (transparent) tube leading to tracheal lumen 2.

utilized to achieve a seal of 60 mm Hg. If sufficient sealing of the mouth and nose cannot be accomplished, the oropharyngeal balloon may be filled with an additional 50 mL of air up to a total amount of 150 mL.[31]

During inflation, the tube may move slightly out of the patient's mouth because of the self-positioning properties of the balloon. In addition, a useful sign indicating malposition due to insufficient insertion is that the inflated pharyngeal balloon can be seen when looking into the patient's mouth (Fig. 25-5). If this occurs, the pharyngeal balloon should be deflated and the tip's position should be reevaluated. The Combitube may have kinked upon insertion and reinsertion may be necessary. The anatomic relationships of the oropharyngeal balloon were shown with the help of x-rays.[31] It was demonstrated that the balloon protruded in an oral direction after overinflation so it did not close the epiglottis.

Figure 25-6 shows an MRI image with a cross-sectional view of the Combitube in the esophageal position. It displays an anterior movement of the larynx, a situation that can often be observed clinically. Knowledge of this may facilitate subsequent location of the larynx for endotracheal intubation.

Then, the distal balloon is inflated with 10 ± 1 mL of air[43] through port No. 2 with the white pilot balloon using the small syringe. With blind insertion, there is a high probability that the tube will be placed into the esophagus. Therefore, test ventilation is recommended through the longer blue tube No. 1 leading to the esophageal lumen (see Fig. 25-4C). Air passes into the pharynx and then through the glottis into the trachea, since the mouth, nose, and esophagus are blocked by the balloons. Auscultation of

breath sounds in the absence of gastric insufflation confirms adequate ventilation when the Combitube is in the esophagus. Ventilation is then continued through this lumen. In this position, the Combitube allows for active decompression of the stomach.[2] In addition, gastric contents can be suctioned through the other unused tracheoesophageal lumen with the help of a small suction catheter (10 or 12 Fr) included in the kit.

The most common cause for failed ventilation through the blue connector is tracheal position of the distal tip (see Fig. 25-4D). Without changing the position of the Combitube, ventilation is changed to the shorter transparent tube No. 2, leading to the tracheoesophageal lumen, and position is again confirmed by auscultation. Now, air flows directly into the trachea. The oropharyngeal balloon may now be deflated in case of regurgitation to allow suction with a conventional catheter. Otherwise, the balloon should remain inflated to stabilize the Combitube.

While ventilating through the blue connector, if no breath sounds are heard over the lungs or a capnographic curve is absent, the second most common cause is that the Combitube has been inserted too deeply, in which the oropharyngeal balloon lies just opposite the laryngeal aperture and occludes the airway.[39] In this situation, both balloons should be deflated and the Combitube pulled back for about 2 to 3 cm out of the patient's mouth and then fixed in this position. The third most common cause is a phenomenon leading to high airway pressure (e.g., laryngo- or bronchospasm, pulmonary edema). In this situation, the phenomenon should be identified and treated. Contrary to other airway devices, the Combitube allows ventilation against high airway pressure and administration

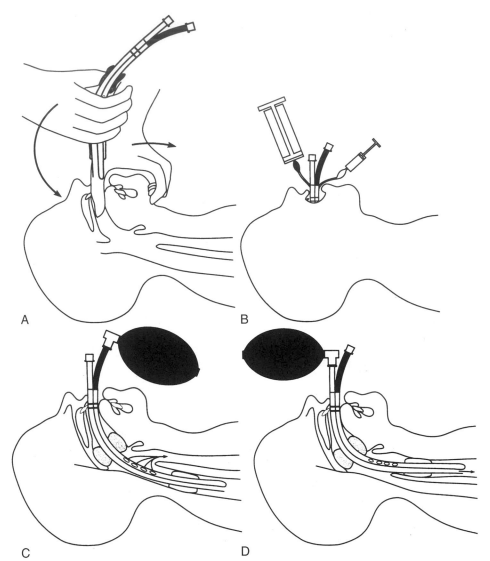

Figure 25-4 Guidelines for introduction of the Combitube. **A,** Insertion of Combitube: Lifting of chin and lower jaw, introducing of Combitube in downward curved movement. **B,** Inflation of oropharyngeal balloon with 100 mL of air, then distal cuff with 5 to 15 mL of air. **C,** Combitube in esophageal position: Ventilation is performed via longer blue tube No. 1. Air flows through holes into pharynx and from there into trachea. **D,** Combitube in tracheal position: Ventilation is performed via shorter transparent tube No. 2. Air flows directly into trachea.

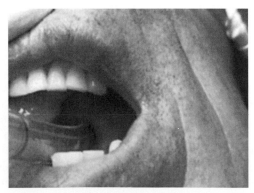

Figure 25-5 The possibility of seeing the inflated oropharyngeal balloon in the patient's mouth indicates malposition of the Combitube.

of inhaled bronchodilators,[1,2] so proper treatment of the spastic phenomenon can be started immediately after full inflation of the balloons in order to ensure high-pressure ventilation.

2. Alternative Insertion Technique

Another way of inserting the Combitube has been described by Urtubia et al.[95] The new insertion technique (Fig. 25-7A and B) consists in grasping the upper teeth or the upper alveolar ridge with the index finger while pushing the chin with the middle finger.

For patients in sitting and prone position, or when the operator is facing the patient, a similar technique would be useful. The index finger grasps the lower teeth or alveolar ridge while the middle finger pushes the cheek (Fig. 25-7C).

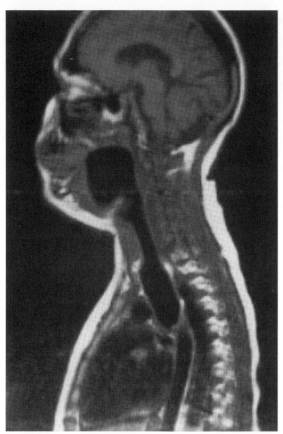

Figure 25-6 MRI imaging: Cross-sectional view of a patient intubated with Combitube in esophageal position. (Courtesy of Dr. B. Panning, Department of Anesthesiology II, and Dr. C. Ehrenheim, Department of Nuclear Medicine and Special Biophysics, Hannover School of Medicine, Hannover, Germany.)

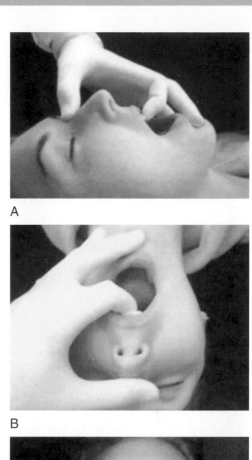

A

B

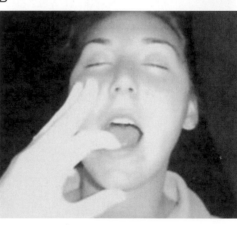

C

Figure 25-7 New insertion technique, as described in Urtubia and coauthors.[88] (**A and B**). Alternative insertion technique (**C**).(Courtesy of Dr. Carin Hagberg.)

The enlarged interincisor distance would allow easier insertion of the Combitube especially in partially edentulous patients and in patients with limited oral opening (Fig. 25-8A and B). In addition, as the original technique, it does not require any cervical movement, which would make it also suitable for cervical spine trauma patients.

The Combitube may be inserted blindly or with the aid of a laryngoscope. The laryngoscope is recommended during the initial training period, when endotracheal intubation using laryngoscopy fails (i.e., insert Combitube with the laryngoscope still in place), and when blind insertion of the Combitube fails.[2]

III. INDICATIONS FOR USE OF THE COMBITUBE

A. EMERGENCY INTUBATION OUT-OF-HOSPITAL

The Combitube is especially suitable for emergency intubation in and out of the hospital whenever endotracheal intubation is not immediately possible. It may be used in the following situations: (1) in patients with difficult anatomy (e.g., bull neck, lockjaw, small mouth opening; the Combitube can be inserted in patients with an interincisor distance [oral aperture] as small as 15 mm[52]; see Box 25-1); (2) under difficult circumstances with respect to space (e.g., difficult access to a patient's head when the patient lies on the floor in a small room, when the patient is lying with his head close to the wall in the general ward or in the intensive care unit [ICU] with many lines at the side impeding quick access to the head, or with patients trapped in a car after an accident); and (3) under difficult illumination (e.g., bright light, massive bleeding, or regurgitation that might inhibit direct laryngoscopy). The Combitube prevents aspiration, which might occur with repeated suction maneuvers.[41,58,93]

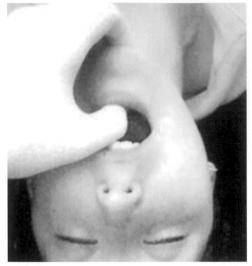

A

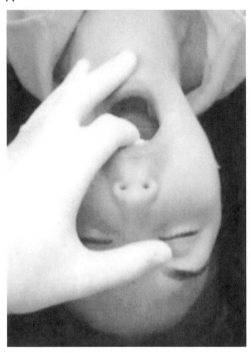

B

Figure 25-8 **A** and **B,** Comparison of oral aperture between the two insertion techniques. Observe the larger interincisor distance in **B.** (Courtesy of Dr. Carin Hagberg)

B. ELECTIVE AND EMERGENCY SURGERY

1. General Anesthesia

Use of the Combitube is indicated in routine surgery in patients for whom conventional intubation is not mandatory, such as singers and actors, who may be afraid of damage to the vocal cords by endotracheal intubation, or patients with rheumatoid arthritis with atlantoaxial subluxation. The main advantages of the Combitube in elective and emergency surgery are a higher insertion or ventilation rate, reliable protection of the airway against

regurgitation and aspiration of gastric contents (patients with a full stomach, gynecologic laparoscopy), and ventilation and oxygenation against high airway pressures (obesity, laryngo- or bronchospasm). As with emergency intubation, it is especially suitable in patients with difficult anatomic conditions. Whenever endotracheal intubation cannot be performed immediately, the Combitube should be considered (see Box 25-1). The main advantage in the failed intubation or ventilation setting is immediate esophageal insertion of the Combitube under direct vision without removing the laryngoscope.

There are some special considerations for the use of the Combitube by anesthesiologists who are expert in endotracheal intubation.

1. The patient's head does not have to be placed in the traditional "sniffing position" as recommended for conventional endotracheal intubation. The patient's head should remain in a neutral position that allows free movement of the lower jaw. Depending on the situation, the chin may be lifted toward the patient's chest. Some clinicians prefer to extend the head or to

use a small cushion. In patients with cervical spine injury, the Combitube allows airway management avoiding mobilization of the neck.

2. The position of the operator (Fig. 25-9) may be behind the patient, especially when a laryngoscope is used (Fig. 25-9A); to the side of the patient's head (Fig. 25-9B); or face to face—the operator may stand beside the patient's thorax facing the patient (Fig. 25-9C). In all three positions, it is necessary to insert the Combitube with a curved downward-caudal movement.

3. During elective surgery, it is always necessary to achieve an adequate depth of anesthesia, with or without additional relaxation. Half of intubation dose of a neuromuscular blocking agent might be enough to assure a smooth insertion.[36] Gaitini et al. have used the Combitube in patients with controlled mechanical ventilation with, and in spontaneously breathing patients without, relaxation.[36] However, grasping and elevating the epiglottis with the fingers during insertion might reduce the need for relaxation. Recommended induction agents are propofol or sevoflurane with or without opioids. In a study of 50 female patients undergoing gynecologic laparoscopy, Urtubia et al. successfully inserted the Combitube in 100% of the cases using inhalational induction with sevoflurane as sole agent, without opioids or neuromuscular blockade.[92]

4. It is recommended that a laryngoscope be used to avoid any potential damage to the oral and pharyngeal mucosa. Nevertheless, with a well-performed blind insertion technique and an adequate level of anesthesia, the risk of damage is comparable to that with the laryngeal mask airway (LMA) or the ET, in terms of postoperative sore throat (16% to 25%).[36,43,93] With the laryngoscope, the Combitube is then intentionally introduced into the esophagus. In emergencies, the situation could be as follows: failed endotracheal intubation occurs and, with the laryngoscope still in the patient's mouth, a Combitube is placed under direct visualization.

5. Another method that may facilitate Combitube insertion and minimize insertion trauma is warming the Combitube in a bottle of warm saline or water, similar to the procedure performed with an ET for nasal intubation. This technique also allows Combitube insertion without additional application of lubricant.

6. The minimal volume technique should be applied in elective cases as well as in emergencies after stabilization of the patient. Studies have shown[36,43,93] that adequate sealing of the oropharyngeal balloon can be achieved with 40 to 85 mL of air with the SA Combitube. Therefore, the balloon should be initially filled with 40 mL of air only. If a tight seal can be achieved as evaluated by auscultation, comparable to inspiratory and expiratory tidal volume and flow-volume curve, the

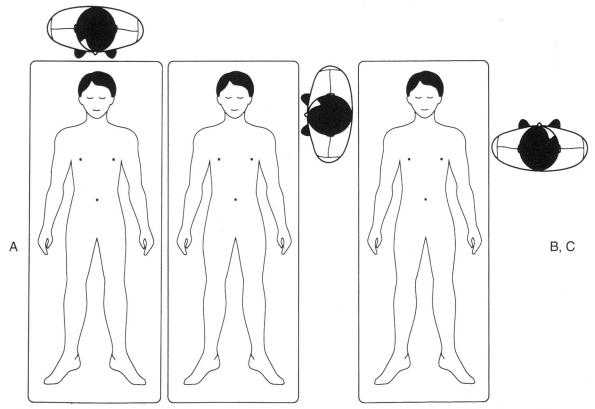

Figure 25-9 Position of operator during insertion of Combitube. **A**, Behind the patient, especially with use of a laryngoscope. **B**, Operator standing to side of patient's head. **C**, Face to face, operator standing beside patient's thorax.

volume is not increased. If a leak is observed, then additional increments of 10 mL of air each are added into the balloon until a tight seal is reached. The volumes of the oropharyngeal balloon also need to be adjusted with use of nitrous oxide and volatile anesthetics.

2. Awake Intubation

Panning has shown in a self-experiment that the Combitube can be inserted with local pharyngeal anesthesia (personal communication). Keller et al. have inserted the Combitube in four awake volunteers with topical anesthesia.[50] Nevertheless, unless an urgent insertion is required, the Combitube should always be inserted when gag reflexes are suppressed due to the risk of mucosal damage or vomiting.

3. Replacement of the Combitube

The Combitube may be left in place for up to 8 hours.[27] While emergency and routine surgical procedures may be successfully carried out in this time period, the Combitube is not intended for long-term ventilation, since the pressure on the pharyngeal mucosa may be harmful. Therefore, we recommend replacing the Combitube after a maximum duration of 8 hours.

Replacement of the Combitube in the esophageal position by an ET can be performed in several ways with no danger of aspiration:

1. While the distal cuff remains inflated, deflate the oropharyngeal balloon completely, with the Combitube remaining in the esophagus. Displace the Combitube to the left corner of the mouth and insert an ET by laryngoscopy or by fiberoptic intubation.[68] After successful placement of the ET, insert a suction catheter through the tracheoesophageal lumen into the esophagus and during continuous suctioning, deflate the distal cuff and remove the Combitube. If insertion of the ET is not possible, push the Combitube back into its original midline position, re-inflate the oropharyngeal balloon and continue ventilating via the longer blue No. 1 lumen of the Combitube until the next endotracheal intubation attempt or until a surgical airway is established.

2. Another method has been described by Gaitini et al.[37] The oropharyngeal balloon is partly deflated according to the "minimal volume technique" so that the least amount of air allows adequate sealing of the oral and nasal cavities. Then, during continued ventilation through the longer blue No. 1 lumen, a fiberoptic bronchoscope mounted with an ET is introduced through the patient's mouth. Without time limit, the bronchoscope may be advanced into the trachea. The unique feature of this method is that ventilation is not interrupted during the entire replacement procedure.

All the patients in this study had Mallampati class III or IV.

3. In addition, the Combitube may be replaced by surgical means, such as cricothyrotomy or tracheostomy.[100] In fact, these were the first surgical procedures performed with the Combitube. An advantage of this method is that the trachea is not occupied by an ET, thus ventilation may be continued while the surgical airway is established. As a disadvantage, the trachea is not protected against aspiration of blood generated during the surgical procedure.

4. Replacement of the Combitube in the tracheal position by an ET can be performed as follows: After lubrication, a pediatric (8 Fr) Tracheal Tube Exchanger (Cook Critical Care, Bloomington, IN) is introduced into the tracheoesophageal lumen via the shorter transparent No. 2 lumen into the trachea, the Combitube is removed and an ET advanced using the tube exchanger as a guide.[74,75] Laryngoscopy should be performed, if not contraindicated, in order to facilitate advancement of the ET through the glottis.

4. Extubation

Extubation after surgery in the awake patient is possible, and the patient will not show signs of significant distress. As a first step, the oropharyngeal balloon is deflated. Now, communication with the patient is possible. Deflation of the distal cuff and final extubation during continuous suctioning via the shorter transparent No. 2 lumen should only be performed after recovery of protective reflexes.

After deflation of the oropharyngeal balloon, the pharyngeal structures could occlude the ventilating perforations of the Combitube. Thus, it would be advisable to deflate the balloon up to the point at which breathing is normal. Once the patient fully resumes spontaneous ventilation, the Combitube can be withdrawn with a curved movement out of the patient's mouth in a similar fashion as insertion.

C. ADVANTAGES

The Combitube has a wide range of applications and advantages (Box 25-2). Those benefiting from its use include physicians working in anesthesia and/or emergency departments,[36,72,93] paramedics and emergency medical technicians,[6,12,21,44,47,54,74,82] combat medics,[72] parkmedics,[58] and physicians in private practice (e.g., when faced with anaphylactic reactions).[1,2] Cardiac arrests usually do not occur under ideal circumstances, and often CPR is performed in awkward locations, poorly lit areas, and with limited access to the patient's head. Since the Combitube can be inserted without a laryngoscope, establishment of a patent airway is not hampered by either adverse environmental factors or staff unskilled in endotracheal intubation.[47] It is safe against aspiration, and high ventilatory pressures may be applied.

> **Box 25-2   Advantages of the Combitube**
>
> Noninvasive as compared to cricothyrotomy
> Universal size (Combitube 37 Fr SA fits patients with a height from 4 up to 6½ feet)[36,92,96]
> Universal model (one type only)
> Easy to learn even by untrained personnel (P. Knacke, personal communication, 2003)[51-53]
> No preparations necessary; tube and syringes are ready to use
> Helpful under difficult circumstances with respect to space and illumination
> Blind insertion technique
> Neck extension unnecessary
> Simultaneous fixation after inflation of oropharyngeal balloon
> Works in either tracheal or esophageal position
> Active decompression of esophagus and stomach
> Minimized risk of aspiration[41,45,54,92]
> Use of controlled mechanical ventilation possible at high ventilation pressures (up to 50 cm H_2O)[33,52,69]
> Independent of power supply (e.g., batteries of laryngoscope)
> Well suited for obese patients[7,18]
> May be used in paralyzed patients who cannot be intubated or mask ventilated

There is no need for additional fixation of the Combitube after inflation of the oropharyngeal balloon, because the anterior upper wall of the oropharyngeal balloon lies just behind the posterior end of the hard palate, thereby guaranteeing strong anchoring during ventilation and transportation. This is a very attractive advantage of the Combitube, as compared to other devices during transportation of emergency patients, providing a more secure airway. Studies have shown that the Combitube is easy to learn.[54]

D. DISADVANTAGES

A potential disadvantage of the Combitube is that suctioning of tracheal secretions is impossible in the esophageal position. However, studies of use of the esophageal obturator airway in cardiac arrest patients[42,82] have shown that the outcome of those cases is not statistically different when compared with cases in which endotracheal intubation is used. The Combitube is designed to bridge the relatively short gap between the prehospital setting and admission of the patient to the emergency department. If prolonged ventilation is required, the administration of glycopyrronium bromide may be used to suppress tracheal secretions (e.g., during surgery). Krafft et al.[55] have described a redesigned Combitube in which two proximal anterior holes are replaced by one large hole allowing a bronchoscope to pass for inspection and suctioning of the trachea as well as a means for replacing the Combitube using a guide wire.

E. CONTRAINDICATIONS

The Combitube is contraindicated in patients with the following: intact gag reflexes (irrespective of their level of consciousness); height less than 6 ft (41Fr Combitube) and less than 4 ft (37 Fr SA Combitube); central-airway obstruction; ingestion of caustic substances; and known upper esophageal pathology (Zencker's diverticulum).

F. COMPLICATIONS

Ovassapian[78] (personal communication) observed livid discoloration of the tongue during ventilation with the Combitube in a few patients without further sequelae. In an out-of-hospital study with paramedics as rescuers, two lacerations of the esophagus could be found in autopsies of cardiac arrest patients ventilated with the Combitube.[98] However, the authors state that the distal cuff was overfilled with 20 to 40 mL of air (instead of 10 ± 1 mL). As outlined in the instructions, the Combitube should not be advanced with use of force. Klein[51] has reported an esophageal rupture after insertion of a Combitube, stiff suctioning catheter, LMA, laryngoscope and ET. Most probably a traumatic procedure with one or more of these devices was the cause of the complication.

Oczenski et al.[67] have reported a very high number of complications in elective surgery. When compared to the studies of Gaitini, Hartmann, and Urtubia,[36,43,93] the total complication rate found by Oczenski is four-fold. This unexpectedly high rate of complications was probably due to traumatic maneuvers during airway management, which is in accordance with the occurrence of 8% of pharyngeal hematoma with the LMA. The study of Oczenski clearly demonstrates that all precautions should be considered when there are obvious handling problems. Recommendation is that when facing difficulties during insertion, a laryngoscope is immediately used to insert the Combitube intentionally into the esophagus under direct vision.

IV. STUDIES

A. COMBITUBE IN CARDIAC ARREST PATIENTS

1. In-Hospital Studies

The application of the Combitube during CPR has been investigated.[26-28,85] The first paper[26] described a study consisting of two parts: in the first part, blood-gas analyses of 19 patients after 15 minutes of ventilation with the Combitube were shown. In the second part, a sample of blood-gas analyses were taken of 12 patients during ventilation with the Combitube and compared to subsequent ventilation with a conventional ET. Blood-gas analyses showed higher arterial oxygen pressures (124 ± 33 mm Hg with the Combitube vs. 103 ± 30 mm Hg with an ET, P <.001). Carbon dioxide pressure was not significantly different. The second paper[29] reported the use of the Combitube during in-hospital CPR. In randomized sequence, either the Combitube or a conventional ET was used in 43 patients. After stabilization of the patients, each tube was replaced with the other type of tube. Blood-gas analyses again showed the phenomenon of increased oxygen tensions during Combitube ventilation. Additionally, it was found that intubation time was significantly shorter with the Combitube.

Another study evaluated the safety and effectiveness of the 41 Fr Combitube as used by ICU nurses under medical supervision compared with an ET established by ICU physicians during CPR.[83] Again, intubation time was shorter for the Combitube and blood gases for each device were comparable, although arterial oxygen tension was slightly higher during ventilation with the Combitube. The study suggests that the Combitube, as used by ICU nurses, is as effective as the ET as used by ICU physicians during CPR.

2. Out-of-Hospital Studies

Atherton and Johnson investigated the ability of paramedics in a non-urban emergency medical setting to use the 41 Fr Combitube in prehospital cardiac arrest patients.[6] Fifty-two cases of prehospital Combitube insertion by paramedics were examined, and 11 paramedics were evaluated for skill retention. Combitube insertion was attempted in 52 prehospital cardiac arrest patients, 69% of whom were intubated successfully. Paramedics recognized esophageal versus tracheal placement in 100% of the cases. The Combitube was inserted successfully in 64% of the patients who could not be intubated by the conventional visualized method. The Combitube was inserted successfully 71% of the time when used as a first-line airway adjunct. Fifteen months later, a follow-up study in 9 of 11 randomly selected paramedics demonstrated inadequate skill retention (improper insertion angle resulting in resistance and inability to insert the tube, inappropriate inflation of the balloons, insertion too deep or not deep enough). Following this reevaluation and retraining, the success rate rose to almost 100%.[48] These results demonstrate that as with every device, there is a necessity of reevaluation of skills a short time after the first training and that skills need to be maintained.

In a prehospital study,[78] three alternative airway devices and the oral airway were compared in a modified randomized crossover design study by non-advanced life support emergency medical assistants (EMAs). The Pharyngeal Tracheal Lumen Airway (PTL), the Laryngeal Mask Airway (LMA), and the 41 Fr Combitube were compared objectively for success of insertion, ventilation, and arterial blood gas and spirometry measurements performed upon hospital arrival. Subjective assessment was carried out by EMAs and receiving physicians. Operating room training was performed with the LMA only. Autopsy findings and survival to hospital discharge were analyzed. The study took place in four non-ALS communities over $4\frac{1}{2}$ yrs and involved 470 patients in cardiac and/or respiratory arrest. EMAs had automatic external defibrillator training but no endotracheal intubation skills. Successful insertion and ventilation was highest for the Combitube (86% vs. 82% PTL, and 73% with LMA, $P = 0.048$). Significant comparative differences in subjective evaluation were found. The Combitube was associated with the least problems with ventilation and was most preferred by the majority of EMAs. Unlike LMA use, no aspirations were found with the use of the Combitube in autopsies.

A retrospective study[85] was designed to determine the choice of airway devices used for non-traumatic, out-of-hospital cardiac arrest patients and to evaluate the success and failure of insertion and airway control/ventilation by three airway adjuncts, the 41 Fr Combitube, the esophageal gastric tube airway (EGTA), and the LMA, which were used in conjunction with the bag-valve-mask (BVM) by emergency life-saving technicians (ELSTs) in Japan. A survey of 1079 ELSTs was performed to identify the type of airway devices, the success rates of airway insertion, the effectiveness of airway control/ventilation, and associated complications in 12,020 cases of cardiac arrest. The choice of airway devices included: BVM, 7180 cases; EGTA, 545 cases; Combitube, 1594 cases; and LMA, 2701 cases. Successful insertion rates on the first attempt were: EGTA, 82.7%; Combitube, 82.4%; and LMA, 72.5% ($P < 0.0001$). Failed insertions: EGTA, 8.2%; Combitube, 6.9%; and LMA, 10.5% ($P < 0.0001$). Successful ventilation rates were: EGTA, 71.0%; Combitube, 78.9%; and LMA, 71.5% ($P < 0.0004$). Six cases of aspiration were reported in the LMA group, whereas nine cases of soft-tissue injuries, including one esophageal perforation, were reported in the 41 Fr Combitube group; 17.8% had vomited either prior or during airway placement. The Combitube appears to be the most appropriate choice among the airway devices examined.

The ability to train emergency medical technicians-defibrillation (EMT-Ds) to effectively use the 41 Fr Combitube for intubations in the prehospital environment was evaluated in this prospective field study lasting for 18 months.[66] Indications for use of the Combitube included unconsciousness without a purposeful response, absence of the gag reflex, apnea or respiratory rate < 6 breaths/min, age > 16 years, and height at least 5 feet tall. Twenty-two EMT-D provider agencies, involving approximately 500 EMT-Ds, were included as study participants. Combitube insertions were attempted in 195 prehospital patients in cardiorespiratory arrest. An overall successful intubation rate of 79% was observed with identical success rates for medical and trauma patients. The device was placed in the esophagus 91% of the time. Resistance during insertion was the major reason for unsuccessful Combitube intubations. An overall hospital admission rate of 19% was observed. No complications were reported. In conclusion, EMT-Ds can be trained to use the Combitube as a means of establishing an airway in the prehospital setting.

Rural EMTs were educated in selected advanced skills, and then the safety and effectiveness of practice were evaluated.[44] After a minimum of 72 hours of training, EMTs employed three skills (Combitube, glucometry, automated external defibrillation) and seven medications (albuterol, nitroglycerin, naloxone, epinephrine, glucagon, activated charcoal, and aspirin). Congruence between prehospital assessment and emergency department (ED) diagnosis was assessed, along with correct use of airway skills (18 of 36 months). The Combitube worked well in 15 out of 19 cases (79%), and EMTs always correctly found the respective lumen to ventilate.

The purpose of another study was to assess the feasibility, safety and effectiveness of the Combitube when used by EMT-Ds in cardiorespiratory arrest patients of all etiologies.[57] The EMTs had automatic external defibrillator (AED) training but no prior advanced airway technique skills. The prehospital intervention was reviewed using the EMTs cardiac arrest report, the AED tape recording of the event and the assessment of the receiving emergency physician. The patients' hospital records and autopsy report were reviewed in search of complications. Eight hundred and thirty-one adult cardiac arrest patients were studied. Placement was successful in 725 (95.4%) of the 760 patients where Combitube insertion was attempted and ventilation was successful in 695 (91.4%) patients. An autopsy was performed in 133 patients and no esophageal lesions or significant injuries to the airway structures were observed. Results suggest that EMT-Ds can use the Combitube for control of the airway and ventilation in cardiorespiratory arrest patients safely and effectively.

In another field study investigating time for post shock analysis after out-of-hospital defibrillation with automated external defibrillators,[12,17] 86 (93.7%) out of 96 patients were successfully intubated with the Combitube.

3. Case Reports

A case of successful Combitube treatment of an acute respiratory arrest secondary to an acute asthma exacerbation was reported by Liao et al.[58] An advanced EMT-II (National Park Service Parkmedic) utilized this device. The female patient was successfully intubated and ventilated and was flown by helicopter for more than 2 hours. Despite repeated episodes of vomiting, no aspiration occurred in this patient. The Combitube was replaced by an ET and the patient was extubated 2 days later and discharged on day 3 after the event.

The Combitube was helpful in a bullnecked patient when movement of the neck and opening of the mouth were impossible[7,62]; and in the case of rapidly enlarging cervical hematoma, which caused upper airway obstruction and thus required immediate intubation after endotracheal

intubation had failed because the epiglottis could not be visualized with a laryngoscope.[10]

In Chile, a 65-year-old female patient with chronic renal insufficiency and atrial fibrillation experienced sudden respiratory arrest during the dialysis procedure at an out-of-hospital dialysis center. Ventilation with a facemask was not possible. As rapid deterioration of her condition was noted, successful blind insertion of a Combitube by a non-skilled nurse reestablished patient's oxygenation.[91]

B. COMBITUBE IN TRAUMA PATIENTS

1. Studies

Blostein et al. have prospectively studied the use of the Combitube in trauma patients in whom orotracheal rapid sequence intubation (RSI) failed.[11] Flight nurses were trained in the use of the Combitube by mannequin simulation, videotape review, and didactic sessions. Combitube insertion was attempted after failure of two or more attempts at orotracheal RSI. Over a 12-month period, 12 patients had successful Combitube insertion, and 10 cases qualified for review. Injuries, number of failed orotracheal RSI attempts, definitive airway, initial arterial blood gas results, and outcome were recorded. Combitube insertion was successful in all 10 patients in whom placement was attempted. Definitive airway control was achieved by conversion to orotracheal intubation in 7 patients, emergency department cricothyroidotomy in 1 patient, and operative room tracheostomy in 2 patients. No patient died because of failure to control the airway. Seven patients requiring Combitube had mandible fractures, 4 had traumatic brain injuries, 2 had facial fractures, and 1 had hemopneumothorax. Data suggest that Combitube insertion is an effective method of airway control in trauma patients who fail orotracheal RSI. It may be particularly useful in the patient with maxillofacial trauma and offers a practical alternative to surgical cricothyroidotomy in difficult airway situations.

In Davis's study,[17] the ability of paramedic RSI to facilitate intubation of patients with severe head injuries in an urban out-of-hospital system was evaluated. Adult patients with head injuries were prospectively enrolled over a 1-year period by using the following inclusion criteria: Glasgow Coma Scale score of 3 to 8, transport time of greater than 10 minutes, and inability to intubate without RSI. Midazolam and succinylcholine were administered before laryngoscopy, and rocuronium was given after tube placement was confirmed by means of capnometry, syringe aspiration, and pulse oximetry. The Combitube was used as a salvage airway device. Outcome measures included intubation success rates, preintubation and postintubation oxygen saturation values, arrival arterial blood gas values, and total out-of-hospital times for patients intubated en route versus on scene. Of 114 enrolled patients, 96 (84.2%) underwent successful endotracheal intubation, and 17 (14.9%) underwent Combitube intubation, with only 1 (0.9%) airway failure. There were no unrecognized esophageal intubations. On arrival at the trauma center, median oxygen saturation was 99%, mean arrival PaO_2 was 307 mm Hg, and mean arrival $PaCO_2$ was 35.8 mm Hg.

A Combitube was inserted into 40 patients undergoing general anesthesia.[62] A rigid cervical collar was then used to immobilize the neck of each patient. In all 40 subjects, adequate ventilation of the lungs was possible in this position as assessed by chest movement and auscultation, measurement of expired tidal volume and maintenance of satisfactory arterial oxygen saturation. In 18 out of 40 patients (45%), small traces of blood were present on the Combitube after removal. Reducing the volume of air injected into the proximal balloon of the ETC appeared to reduce the incidence of airway trauma during insertion.

In another study, a rigid cervical collar was used to immobilize the neck in 15 ASA 1 and 2 patients under general anesthesia.[63] Insertion of the Combitube airway was then attempted. In 10 out of 15 (66%) patients, blind insertion was not possible. In 5 out of 15 (33%) successful blind insertions the Combitube entered the esophagus on each occasion. In 8 out of 10 of the failures, re-insertion of the Combitube was attempted with the aid of a Macintosh laryngoscope. In 6 out of 8 cases (75%) satisfactory placement was then possible with the Combitube again entering the esophagus on each occasion. Ventilation was satisfactory in all patients when insertion was successful. Blood staining of the Combitube was present in 7 out of 15 (47%) patients. The authors state that the Combitube cannot be recommended for use in patients whose necks are immobilized in rigid cervical collars. The alternative insertion technique might improve the rate of successful insertion in this group of patients, because it provides a larger oral aperture than the classic maneuver. However, in cases of suspected or evident cervical spine injury, manual in-line traction prior to intubation and application of a cervical collar is recommended.

2. CASE REPORTS

A 14-year-old boy had been hit by a motorcycle while riding his bicycle. He suffered severe oronasal bleeding associated with craniofacial injury.[64] Computed tomographic (CT) scanning at admission indicated multiple craniofacial fractures (left frontal bone, maxilla, mandible, sphenoidal bone, zygomatic bone, nasal bone, and ethmoidal bone) with epidural hematoma of the frontal lobe. His face was depressed about the nose. To keep the airway from oronasal bleeding, emergency tracheostomy was performed after endotracheal intubation. Nasal and oral packing using Foley balloon catheters was performed but failed to control oronasal bleeding. Bradycardia appeared with ventricular fibrillation during the course owing to marked hypovolemia. To get tighter packing, we inserted

a Combitube. When the pharyngeal cuff of the Combitube was inflated, blood pressure (BP) rose from 105/60 mm Hg to 140/90 mm Hg, and the heart rate immediately decreased from 145 to 95 beats per minute. Stable circulation was realized by this method during angiography. Embolization was performed with consequent hemostasis. The Combitube was removed the next day. Surgery for facial fracture was conducted on the 16th hospital day, and the patient was discharged on the 70th hospital day.

The Combitube was utilized in this case to control severe oronasal bleeding before performing angiography. This method was effective in controlling oronasal bleeding and was easy to perform. The authors thus recommend the Combitube for oronasal bleeding before embolization.

In another case, an 18-year-old man was driving and lost control over his car crashing into trees standing aside the street.[53] Upon arrival of the ambulance, the patient required immediate intubation; however, he was trapped in the car. The car stuck in a tree and the windshield was broken. Therefore, intubation was performed with the Combitube through the windshield with one hand only, and ventilation was performed successfully. The patient could then be extracted and was intubated by an endotracheal airway. The patient survived and passed examinations of high school soon after the accident.

A similar situation occurred in a 24-year-old patient who was trapped in his jeep following a motor vehicle collision.[61] During his rescue, immediate intubation became mandatory. Since access to the patient's head was limited, a Combitube was inserted standing in front of the patient, and ventilation was easily accomplished. The patient was admitted to the hospital and was weaned from the ventilator 3 days later. After 4 weeks, he was discharged from the hospital without having suffered any neurologic sequelae. In conclusion, the Combitube appeared to be a valid alternative to endotracheal intubation in cases of difficult access to the patient's head.

In several unusual cases, the Combitube has proven superior to conventional endotracheal intubation. The Combitube proved to be useful in the case of neck impalement with a large wooden splinter entering at the left angle of the mandible, traversing the pharynx and soft palate and entering the right maxillary cavity below the floor of the orbit.[22]

C. ANESTHESIOLOGIC STUDIES

1. General Anesthesia

Function and effectiveness of the Combitube were first tested in animal experiments[26] and subsequently in humans.[24] The effectiveness of ventilation with the Combitube was compared to ventilation with an ET during routine surgery in a crossover study.[30] Twenty-three patients were ventilated first with the Combitube and then with an ET (group 1). In group 2, application of the tubes was performed in a reversed order in eight patients. After 20 minutes of ventilation with each airway, arterial blood samples were analyzed. In all cases, patients were ventilated with the Combitube without problems comparable to ventilation with an ET. In addition, arterial oxygen pressure was higher during ventilation with the Combitube (142 ± 43 mm Hg with the Combitube vs. 119 ± 40 mm Hg with the ET in group 1, $P < .001$; 117 ± 16 mm Hg with the endotracheal airway vs. 146 ± 13 mm Hg with the Combitube in group 2, $P < .001$), whereas the differences in arterial carbon dioxide tension and pH were not significant.

The reasons for increased oxygen tension during ventilation with the Combitube were investigated in another study.[33] In 12 patients undergoing general anesthesia during routine surgery, a thin catheter was placed with its tip 10 cm below the vocal cords. Patients were then ventilated by mask, by the Combitube in esophageal position, and by an ET in randomized sequence. Pressures were recorded in the trachea and at the airway openings. Blood gases again showed a higher arterial oxygen tension with the Combitube when compared to ET (151 ± 37 mm Hg vs. 125 ± 32 mm Hg, $P < .05$) and a higher arterial carbon dioxide tension (36 ± 4 mm Hg vs. 33 ± 4 mm Hg, $P < .05$). This slightly higher carbon dioxide tension with the Combitube might be partly due to the integration of the hypopharynx into the physiologic dead space. Compared to mask ventilation, carbon dioxide tension was lower with the Combitube.

The following differences in intratracheal pressures were found. The rising pressure during inspiration was highest with the ET (19 ± 6 mm Hg/second with the ET vs. 14 ± 6 mm Hg/second with the Combitube, $P < .05$). The smaller rising pressure with the Combitube may lead to a more favorable distribution of ventilation. Expiratory flow time was prolonged during ventilation with the Combitube (2.0 ± 1.0 sec vs. 1.3 ± 0.6 sec with the ET). This effect is probably due to an increase in expiratory resistance because of the double-lumen design and might favor the formation of a small positive end-expiratory pressure (PEEP). Auto-PEEP might also be caused by integration of the vocal cords into the airway with the Combitube, while they are bypassed by the ET. The auto-PEEP does not exceed 2 mm Hg and therefore does not influence cerebral perfusion during CPR. The smaller rising pressure, prolonged expiratory-flow time, and auto-PEEP together seem to be responsible for the improved conditions for alveolar-arterial gas exchange.

While peak pressures at the airway openings may be high due to the resistance of the double-lumen airway, intratracheal pressures were comparable between the two tubes (peak endotracheal pressure: 10 ± 4 mm Hg with a Combitube vs. 12 ± 6 mm Hg with an ET, $P =$ ns; endotracheal-plateau pressure: 8 ± 2 mm Hg with the Combitube vs. 8 ± 4 mm Hg with the ET, $P =$ ns).[33]

The Combitube may also be used for prolonged ventilation.[27] In seven patients in the intensive care unit, the Combitube was used over a period of 2 to 8 hours during mechanical ventilation. Results showed adequate ventilation compared with subsequent endotracheal ventilation. Lipp et al.[60] have used the Combitube with an average time for insertion of 12 to 23 seconds. In 3 out of 50 patients, the Combitube had to be withdrawn for 1 to 2 cm.

Urtubia et al. have studied the proper use of the Combitube.[93] While the manufacturer recommends that the SA Combitube be used in patients with a height between 122 and 152 cm, the aim of this study was to evaluate whether ventilation is effective and reliable in patients taller than 152 cm with the Combitube in the esophageal position. Also, it was evaluated whether the airway protection is adequate and whether direct intubation of the trachea with the Combitube inserted in the esophagus is possible. Urtubia et al. studied 25 anesthetized, paralyzed adult patients, 150 to 180 cm in height. Methylene blue was given orally to all patients before anesthesia induction. Under direct vision, a SA Combitube was inserted in the esophagus of all patients. The pharyngeal balloon inflation volume was titrated to air leak and cuff pressures were measured. During surgery, a laryngoscope was inserted into the pharynx with the pharyngeal balloon deflated and the laryngoscopic view was evaluated by using the Cormack-Lehane scale. The presence of methylene blue in the hypopharynx was investigated by direct laryngoscopy. Ventilation was effective and reliable in all 25 patients who were 150 to 180 cm in height (average $169 +/- 7$ cm). In addition, a direct relationship between the pharyngeal balloon volume and patient height was established ($P < 0.05$), by using linear regression models, suggesting that the 37 Fr SA Combitube can be used in patients up to 6 feet (185 cm) of height, implying also that the SA Combitube is the preferred size for most patients. The laryngoscopic view of the glottis was adequate to allow direct tracheal intubation. No trace of methylene blue was detected in the hypopharynx. The authors concluded that the SA Combitube may be used in patients from 122 to 185 cm in height. The trachea could be directly intubated with the Combitube in the esophageal position in patients with normal airways. The airway protection appears to be adequate.

In a study of Gaitini and colleagues the effectiveness of the Combitube in elective surgery during both mechanical and spontaneous ventilation was investigated.[36] Two hundred ASA physical status I and II patients, with normal airways, scheduled for elective surgery were randomly allocated into two groups: nonparalyzed, spontaneously breathing ($n = 100$); or paralyzed, mechanically ventilated ($n = 100$). After induction of general anesthesia and insertion of the Combitube, SpO_2, $EtCO_2$ and isoflurane concentration, systolic and diastolic BP and heart rate, as well as breath-by-breath spirometry data were obtained every 5 minutes. In 97% of patients, it was possible to maintain oxygenation, ventilation, and respiratory mechanics, as well as hemodynamic stability during either mechanical or spontaneous ventilation for the entire duration of surgery. The duration of surgery was between 15 and 155 min. The results of this study suggest that the Combitube is an effective and safe airway device for continued management of the airway in 97% of elective surgery cases.

Walz et al. decided to test the smaller SA Combitube in patients exceeding 5 feet in height.[99] They reported 104 patients (66 male, 38 female; 3.93–6.5 feet [120–198 cm]) who received the SA Combitube during general anesthesia, most often during automatic implantable cardioverter defibrillator implantation. The duration of the procedures ranged from 45 to 360 min. In each case, they were able to document with the use of pulse oximetry, capnometry, and ventilation parameters that the patients could be oxygenated and ventilated adequately. The oropharyngeal cuff volume of 85 mL, recommended by the manufacturer, was sufficient in 71 patients (68%). The remaining 33 patients required an additional insufflation volume of 25 to 50 mL in the oropharyngeal balloon to prevent air leakage. They concluded that the SA Combitube can be instituted without restriction in patients exceeding 5 feet in height. Due to its smaller size, the SA Combitube is easier to use and seems to be less traumatic to soft tissues. The authors preferred to use a laryngoscope during insertion of the SA Combitube, which not only resulted in less trauma but also reduced the number of intubation failures.

Evaluation of safety, efficacy, and maximum ventilatory pressures during routine surgery was investigated in another study.[32] Five hundred patients receiving general anesthesia were enrolled into the study. Type of surgery, duration of surgery, ease of insertion, and potential complications were recorded. In addition, maximum ventilatory pressures and leaks were evaluated in this study. The Combitube worked well in all but two patients. Duration of surgery varied between 30 and 360 minutes. The Combitube happened to be placed into the esophagus in 97% of the patients. More than 95% of the blind Combitube insertions were successful at the first attempt with an average intubation time of less than 15 seconds. Efficacy of oxygenation and ventilation of the Combitube, as evaluated by pulse oximetry and $EtCO_2$, showed an SpO_2 greater than 95% in all cases and an $EtCO_2$ of 35 to 45 mm Hg. Leak, expressed as a fraction of the inspired volume, did not increase more than 5% up to a ventilation pressure of 50 cm H_2O. Data suggest that the Combitube appears to be a safe and easy device, which may be used whenever ET is not immediately possible. In addition, this study demonstrated its usefulness during routine surgery.

Schreier et al. studied the 37 Fr SA Combitube in 20 children.[81] The age was 9.3 ± 2.4 years, height 137.3 ± 10.5 cm, and weight 35 ± 10.8 kg. The Combitube worked well in all cases. This study shows that the 37 Fr SA Combitube could be used in cases of "cannot intubate-cannot-ventilate" in children taller than 122 cm.

A 46-year-old obese white female with a short neck was scheduled for excision of a thyroid goiter.[52] One hour following extubation, a hematoma of the right anterior neck was noted. Immediate intubation was mandatory. While fiberoptics failed, a blind attempt at inserting an ET resulted in an esophageal intubation. An interincisor distance of 13 mm prevented insertion of a No. 3 LMA. An SA Combitube was then inserted blindly. Oxygen saturation rapidly improved and could be maintained at 97% with an FiO_2 of 1.0. General anesthesia was completed and the hematoma was evacuated. Following evacuation of the hematoma, ventilation improved as peak airway pressures declined. The superiority of the Combitube in this case is due to its slim design thereby surpassing the LMA. The Combitube should be considered as an additional tool for managing patient airways under difficult circumstances.

A similar case was reported by Hagberg and colleagues[40] in which the Combitube was successfully used in a 50-year-old patient status post previous burn injury to the face, resulting in severe contracture formation of the mouth and significant tracheal stenosis following prolonged intubation. His airway evaluation revealed a Mallampati class IV airway, one fingerbreadth mouth opening and full range of neck mobility.

Because of the patient's airway exam and the concern for endotracheal intubation causing further subglottic tracheal stenosis, a Combitube was chosen for airway management. ENT surgeons were present in the room with the patient's neck prepared and draped, along with equipment set-up for the performance of a tracheostomy, if necessary. Additionally, a fiberoptic bronchoscope was present and prepared for use. The authors found the Combitube to be a very advantageous airway device in establishing an airway in this case and can be considered for elective use in patients with limited mouth opening. They also suggested that the Combitube be used on a more regular basis in the operating room so that it is a familiar device when needed emergently.[34,94]

The ease of learning the use of the Combitube has been recently published. Enlund et al.[23] reported a case where conventional endotracheal intubation failed. The patient was ventilated by a face mask in the sitting position, while the Combitube was brought to the operating room. Although the authors were inexperienced in Combitube use, they read the manufacturer's instructions in the OR and successfully inserted the Combitube. The device worked well throughout the entire surgical procedure.

Since tracheal suctioning is impossible with the Combitube placed in the esophageal position, the Combitube was redesigned.[55] The two anterior, proximal perforations of regular Combitubes were replaced by a larger, ellipsoid-shaped hole. Twenty patients with normal airways (Mallampati I or II) were studied. During general anesthesia, patients were esophageally intubated with the Combitube. A flexible bronchoscope was inserted and guided via the modified hole and glottic opening down the trachea. For the replacement procedure, a J tip guide wire was introduced through the bronchoscope. The bronchoscope and the Combitube were removed and a standard ET was advanced over a guide catheter. Bronchoscopic evaluation of the trachea and guided replacement of the Combitube by an ET was successful in all 20 patients. The average time needed to perform airway exchange was 90 +/− 20 seconds (mean +/− SD). Arterial oxygen saturation and $EtCO_2$ levels remained normal in all patients. No case of laryngeal trauma was observed during intubation or the airway exchange procedure. The redesigned Combitube enables fiberoptic bronchoscopy, fine-tuning of its position in the esophagus, and guided airway exchange in patients with normal airways. Further studies are warranted to demonstrate the value of this redesigned Combitube in patients with abnormal airways. This version has not been manufactured for sale.

2. Gynecologic Laparoscopy

Airway management during gynecologic laparoscopy is complicated by intraperitoneal CO_2 inflation, Trendelenburg tilt, increasing airway pressures and pulmonary aspiration risk. Hartmann et al.[43] investigated whether the SA Combitube is a suitable airway during laparoscopy. One hundred patients were randomly allocated to receive either the SA Combitube ($n = 49$) or ET ($n = 51$). Esophageal placement of the Combitube was successful at the first attempt [16 ± 3 sec]. Peak airway pressures were 25 ± 5 cm H_2O. An airtight seal was obtained using air volumes of 55 ± 13 mL (oropharyngeal balloon) and 10 ± 1 mL (esophageal cuff). Significant correlations were observed between patient's height and weight and the balloon volumes necessary to produce a seal. Similar findings were recorded for the control group, with tracheal intubation being difficult in three patients. The SA Combitube provided a patent airway during laparoscopy. Non-traumatic insertion was possible and an airtight seal was provided at airway pressures of up to 30 cm H_2O.

Exposure to sevoflurane (SEVO) and nitrous oxide (N_2O) during ventilation using an SA Combitube was compared with waste gas exposure using conventional ET.[45]

Trace concentrations of SEVO and N_2O were assessed using a direct reading spectrometer during 40 gynecologic laparoscopic procedures under general anesthesia. Measurements were made at the patients' mouth and in the anesthesiologists' breathing zone. Mean (SD) concentrations of SEVO and N_2O measured at the patients' mouth were comparable in the SA Combitube (SEVO 0.6 ± 0.2 p.p.m.; N_2O 9.7 (8.5) p.p.m.) and ET group (SEVO 1.2 ± 0.8 p.p.m.; N_2O 17.2 ± 10.6 p.p.m.). These values caused comparable contamination of the anesthesiologists' breathing zone (SEVO 0.6 ± 0.2 p.p.m. and N_2O 4.3 ± 3.7 p.p.m. for the SA Combitube group, compared with SEVO 0.5 ± 0.2 p.p.m. and N_2O

4.1 (1.8) p.p.m. for the ET group). It is concluded that the use of the SA Combitube during positive pressure ventilation is not necessarily associated with increased waste gas exposure, especially when air conditioning and scavenging devices are available. Finally, the Combitube worked well in another study in which it was used in 22 patients scheduled for elective laparotomy.[67,81]

3. Obstetric Anesthesia

Airway-related problems represent the most frequent cause of death among women who die from a complication of general anesthesia for cesarean section (GACS).[96] The authors reported two cases of emergency cesarean section under general anesthesia in which an SA Combitube was used for airway management as primary device. In a 17-year-old, obese pregnant woman an acute severe fetal bradycardia did not allow time for spinal blockade. Therefore, general anesthesia was induced, maternal airway management was performed using a facemask airway and applying the Sellick maneuver. After childbirth, an SA Combitube was blindly inserted into the esophagus while maintaining cricoid pressure. Ventilation and oxygenation were adequate. In a 27-year-old deaf-mute pregnant woman, fetal heart rate suddenly became pathologic suggesting acute fetal distress. She was taken to the OR for cesarean section and a spinal blockade was performed. Soon after beginning of surgery, the patient demonstrated clear signs of pain. Therefore, general anesthesia was induced and ventilation was performed via the SA Combitube inserted in the esophagus under laryngoscopic guidance. No postoperative pharyngeal symptoms and no respiratory complications were detected in both cases. The main communication of this report is that Combitube allowed adequate ventilation and airway protection for emergency GACS in this group of patients. In addition, the Combitube was quickly inserted both blindly and with laryngoscopic guidance.

Wissler has used the Combitube in obstetric anesthesia.[101] He states that the Combitube is most easily and atraumatically inserted into the esophagus under direct vision using a laryngoscope. In his practice of obstetric anesthesia, the Combitube is his first choice for the anesthetized parturient who cannot be intubated or mask ventilated with cricoid pressure. His reasoning is that it provides a better barrier against regurgitation and aspiration than the LMA.[101]

In a pilot study performed by Hagberg and colleagues, the Combitube was determined to be comparable to the LMA regarding the incidence of gastroesophageal reflux (GER) and tracheal acid aspiration, as detected by pH monitoring.[41] Fifty-seven patients were randomly assigned to receive either an LMA or a Combitube for their elective surgical procedure. All patients were paralyzed and received positive pressure ventilation. Two monocrystalline antimony catheters were used for pH monitoring of the trachea, oropharynx and esophagus. One episode of GER occurred with the Combitube in place upon extubation, yet there were no pH changes reflected in the oropharyngeal or tracheal regions. There were three patients in the LMA group who met the pH criterion for aspiration (pH below 4.0 that lasted at least 15 sec), as compared to only one patient in the Combitube group, yet no patient developed any clinical signs of aspiration. Thus, by providing reliable airway protection, the Combitube provides another alternative in managing a difficult airway.

Additionally, ideal insertion conditions for the LMA include lubrication and a special method of cuff deflation, whereas the Combitube is ready to use in its package. In an obstetric patient with increased oxygen consumption, decreased functional residual capacity, and airway obstruction, these differences in preparation time may be clinically important.

4. Comparison of the Combitube with Other Alternative Airway Techniques (Table 25-1)[101]

The design of the Combitube has several advantages over other devices, including an open distal tip that allows decompression and suctioning of the esophagus and stomach in the esophageal position and ventilation in the tracheal position. As opposed to other devices, the double-lumen design of the Combitube prevents lumen occlusion if the patient bites the tube, avoiding ventilation emergencies during the awakening period.

When compared to the LMA, Laryngeal Tube (LT, VBM, Sulz, Germany) and other similar devices, the Combitube provides a decompression barrier (the tracheoesophageal lumen) to minimize regurgitation of gastric contents[20] and allows controlled mechanical ventilation with ventilation pressures higher than 20 cm H_2O.[33,69]

Since the Combitube has been shown to be safe against aspiration and avoids gastric insufflation during positive pressure ventilation, the use of the LMA is recommended in elective cases only without danger of aspiration. The LT is a new device simulating the design of the Combitube. While the LT bears no lumen for active decompression, the new laryngeal tube (LTS, VBM) does allow for decompression of gastric contents. However, the device, as currently manufactured, is very bulky and therefore may be difficult to place in patients with a small interincisor distance. Another disadvantage is that analogous to the LMA, several sizes need to be available to meet the needs for different sized patients.

V. GUIDELINES AND REFERENCES REGARDING THE COMBITUBE

The Combitube has gained worldwide interest[14,15,65] and is now considered to be an adjunct to standard airway equipment in many anesthesiology departments and ambulance services. The Combitube has been recommended in the difficult airway algorithm of the "Practice Guidelines for Management of the Difficult Airway" of the American Society of Anesthesiologists[5,71] for use when an anesthetized patient can be neither intubated nor mask ventilated. Since 1992, it is also included in the "Guidelines for Cardiopulmonary Resuscitation and Emergency Cardiac Care" of the American Heart Association as the first alternate airway, replacing the esophageal-obturator as alternative to ET.[3,4] In the section "Adult Advanced Cardiac Life Support," the

Table 25-1 **Comparisons of Emergency Airway Equipment**

Description	Esophageal-Tracheal Combitube	Laryngeal Mask Airway	Esophageal Obturator Airway	Esophageal Gastric Tube Airway	Pharyngotracheal Lumen Airway
Provides barrier to minimize regurgitation of gastric contents	Yes	Yes	Yes	Yes	Yes
Allows buildup in esophagus of pressure and gastric contents during use	No	Yes	Yes	No	No
Functions when blindly passed into esophagus	Yes	NA	Yes	Yes	Yes
Functions when blindly passed into trachea	Yes	NA	No	No	Yes
Requires effective mask fit on face	No	No	Yes	Yes	No
Available in pediatric sizes	No	Yes	No	No	No

NA, not applicable.
From Wissler RN: The esophageal-tracheal Combitube. Anesthesiol Rev 20:147, 1993.

Combitube is described as a valuable tool for emergency intubation.[4] In 2000, the Combitube has been upgraded as a class IIa device.[3] Furthermore, the Combitube has been included in the Guidelines of the European Resuscitation Council[8] as well as in many National Guidelines.[56]

The Combitube is cited in many review articles[1,2,35,74,75,97] as an alternative method for artificial ventilation and is recommended for patients with massive regurgitation or airway hemorrhage when visualization of the vocal cords may be impossible.[15] Gaitini et al.[36] described the Combitube as an easily inserted, double-lumen/double-balloon supraglottic airway device. The major indication of the Combitube is as a back-up device for airway management. It is recommended as an excellent option for rescue ventilation in both in- and out-of-hospital environments and in situations of difficult ventilation and intubation, useful especially in patients with massive airway bleeding or limited access to the airway and in patients in whom neck movement is contraindicated.

Continued airway management with a Combitube that has been placed is a reasonable option in many cases. Having thus secured the airway, it may not be necessary to abort the anesthetic or to continue with further airway management efforts. Additionally, the Combitube is the perfect solution in places where a fiberoptic device is not available or when fiberoptic intubation fails.

Similarly, Agrò and colleagues[2] emphasized that the Combitube is an easily inserted and highly efficacious device to be used as an alternative airway whenever conventional ventilation fails. The Combitube allows ventilation and oxygenation whether the device locates in the esophagus (very common) or the trachea (rare). In this report the reviewed studies suggest the Combitube is a valuable and effective airway in the emergency and prehospital settings, in cardiopulmonary resuscitation, in elective surgery, and in critically ill patients in the intensive care unit. Also reviewed are studies that demonstrate the superiority of the Combitube over other supraglottic ventilatory devices in resuscitation with respect to success rates with insertion and ventilation. Contrary to the LMA, the Combitube may help in patients with limited mouth opening. The Combitube may be of special benefit in patients with massive bleeding or regurgitation, and it minimizes the risk of aspiration.

Finally, as the Combitube is one of the three alternatives approved by the ASA for managing the "cannot intubate-cannot ventilate" situation, its continued use would be highly advisable especially for trainees in order to become familiar and to allow its successful use during an emergency.

VI. EASYTUBE

The Easytube (Teleflex Medical Ruesch, Bannockburn, IL) is a new airway device similar to the Combitube.[86] It has a pharyngeal lumen providing a supraglottic ventilation outlet ending just below the oropharyngeal balloon, thereby allowing passage of a bronchoscope for inspection of the trachea, suctioning of tracheal secretions, or replacement if necessary (Fig. 25-10). Because of this design, the longer tracheo-esophageal lumen has a smaller outer tube together with a larger inner diameter and ends like an ET, thereby decreasing the chance of injury to the pharyngeal and tracheal mucosa. The distal end of the Easytube is designed like a standard tracheal tube, with a tip diameter of 7.5 mm (41 Fr) and 5.5 mm (28 Fr). Furthermore, the device has kink-resistant outer tubes. It is a latex-free, sterile, single-use double-lumen tube and is available in two sizes: a larger adult 41 Fr for patients with a height taller than 130 cm, and a 28 Fr pediatric size for patients measuring 90 to 130 cm. It provides sufficient ventilation whether placed in the esophagus or the trachea. The Easytube may be positioned with the help of a laryngoscope or blindly. Laryngoscopic insertion is similar to that used for a standard tracheal tube. After placing the patient's head in a sniffing position and performing direct laryngoscopy, the trachea is intubated with the Easytube. A black mark at the distal end of the tube indicates correct depth of insertion. Ventilation is performed via the transparent No. 2 lumen. In a cannot-ventilate, cannot-intubate situation, the Easytube can be inserted into the esophagus using a laryngoscope. Ventilation is then performed using the colored No. 1 lumen. The Easytube may also be inserted blindly as health care providers especially in the prehospital setting usually perform it. While the patient's head is kept in a neutral position, the tube is inserted in a straightforward movement, parallel to the frontal axis of the patient, until the proximal black ring mark is positioned at the level of the upper incisor teeth. In the esophageal position, the transparent No. 2 lumen may serve to drain gastric contents or to insert a gastric tube. The pharyngeal and the distal cuff are inflated with 80 and 10 mL of air, respectively, using the two prefilled

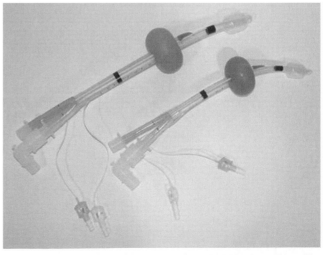

Figure 25-10 Two sizes of the Easytube (41 Fr large, 28 Fr small).

syringes in the package. The oropharyngeal cuff of the Easytube prevents aspiration of blood or secretions from the oral or nasal cavity, while the distal cuff seals the esophagus.

A preliminary study by Thierbach and coworkers[87] was undertaken to report early experiences with the Easytube in prehospital and in-hospital emergency airway management procedures. All airway management procedures with the Easytube were recorded for a period of 18 months. The Easytube was successfully used in 15 patients with unanticipated airway difficulties during anesthesia induction or prehospital airway management. In all patients, the Easytube was positioned successfully at the first attempt, with a median time of 31 seconds until start of ventilation. Effective supraglottic ventilation and oxygenation were achieved within 25 to 40 seconds. In three patients, the Easytube needed one additional repositioning maneuver. On removal of the Easytube, no blood was observed on the surface of the device, and no injuries were observed in the patients' mouth, pharynx, or esophagus. The authors concluded that the device successfully established sufficient ventilation and oxygenation.

In another study by Thierbach and colleagues[88] 30 adult patients (ASA class I-II, Mallampati class I and II, between 50 and 80 kg) undergoing minor surgery were randomly allocated to the esophageal Easytube insertion group using the blind or laryngoscopy-guided technique. Data were collected for number of attempts, time taken to provide an effective airway, blood staining, and postoperative airway morbidity. The time to obtain an effective airway was noted from the removal of the face mask to confirmation of normal ventilation, evaluated by bilateral chest movement and normal capnography curve. There were no failures on inserting the device with either technique. First attempt/second attempt insertion rates were 86%/14% for the blind insertion technique and 93%/7% for the laryngoscopy-guided technique. Time to achieve an effective airway was 31 ± 4 seconds for the blind technique and 33 ± 6 seconds for the laryngoscopy-guided technique. After removal of the device, blood stains were observed in eight patients, four patients in each group. Sore throat in the postanesthesia care unit was 20% for both groups, and no patient required treatment. Data suggest that insertion of the Easytube has the same success rate with or without using a laryngoscope. A recent study determined that pressures exerted on the oropharyngeal mucosa were lower than with laryngeal masks.[89]

VII. FUTURE ASPECTS

The studies demonstrate that the Combitube is an effective alternative to traditional intubation techniques. It has been shown to be as effective as an endotracheal tube in emergency situations. Further studies, especially with respect to management of difficult airways, are needed to elucidate this device fully. The wide range of applications and ease of insertion make it a valuable piece of equipment in the wards, in operating theaters, and in prehospital conditions. Being a rescue device, it is highly advisable that operators involved in airway management should be familiar with the techniques described in order to successfully manage an emergency and to avoid using it for the first time during a crisis. The device may be reused.[59] Recent data[73] suggest that the Combitube can be inserted successfully during microgravity. Since the Combitube requires less training than endotracheal intubation and is easier to insert than an endotracheal airway, it is recommended for further study as an alternative airway to what is currently on the shuttle. The results of this study might aid in developing future protocols for managing airway emergencies while on space missions. Studies demonstrate that the Combitube is superior to other supraglottic devices in the emergency situation.[78,85]

REFERENCES

1. Agro F, Frass M, Benumof J, et al: The esophageal tracheal Combitube as a non-invasive alternative to endotracheal intubation. A review. Minerva Anestesiol 2001;67:863-874.
2. Agro F, Frass M, Benumof JL, Krafft P: Current status of the Combitube: A review of the literature. J Clin Anesth 2002;14:307-314.
3. American Heart Association (AHA) Emergency Cardiac Care (ECC) Guidelines, Part 6: Advanced Cardiovascular Life Support, Section 3: Adjuncts for Oxygenation, Ventilation, and Airway Control. Airway Adjuncts. Circulation 2000;102:I-95-I-104.
4. American Heart Association: Combination esophageal-tracheal tube. In Guidelines for cardiopulmonary resuscitation and emergency cardiac care: recommendations of the 1992 National Conference of the American Heart Association, JAMA 268:2203, 1992.
5. American Society of Anesthesiologists' Task Force on Management of the Difficult Airway: Practice guidelines for management of the difficult airway. Anesthesiology 78:597, 1993.
6. Atherton GL, Johnson JC: Ability of paramedics to use the Combitube in prehospital cardiac arrest. Ann Emerg Med 22:1263, 1993.
7. Banyai M, Falger S, Roggla M, et al: Emergency intubation with the Combitube in a grossly obese patient with bull neck. Resuscitation 26:271, 1993.
8. Baskett PJF, Bossaert L, Carli P, et al: Guidelines for the advanced management of the airway and ventilation during resuscitation. A statement by the Airway and Ventilation Management Working Group of the European Resuscitation Council. Resuscitation 31:201-230, 1996.
9. Benumof JL: Management of the difficult adult airway. Anesthesiology 75:1087, 1991.
10. Bigenzahn W, Pesau B, Frass M: Emergency ventilation using the Combitube in cases of difficult intubation. Eur Arch Otorhinolaryngol 248:129, 1991.
11. Blostein PA, Koestner AJ, Hoak S: Failed rapid sequence intubation in trauma patients: Esophageal tracheal Combitube is a useful adjunct. J Trauma 44:534-537, 1998.

12. Blouin D, Topping C, Moore S, Stiell I, Afilalo M: Out-of-hospital defibrillation with automated external defibrillators: postshock analysis should be delayed. Ann Emerg Med 38:256-261, 2001.

13. Bryson TK, Benumof JL, Ward CF: The esophageal obturator airway: A clinical comparison of ventilation with a mask and oropharyngeal airway. Chest 74:537-539, 1978.

14. Clinton JE, Ruiz E: Emergency airway management procedures. In Roberts JR, Hedges JR (eds): Clinical Procedures in Emergency Medicine, 2nd ed. Philadelphia, WB Saunders, 1991, pp 7-8.

15. Cozine K, Stone G: The take-back patient in ear, nose, and throat surgery. In Benumof JL (ed): Anesthesiology Clinics of North America, vol 11, no 3. Philadelphia, WB Saunders, 1993.

16. Crippen D, Olvey S, Graffis R: Gastric rupture: An esophageal obturator airway complication. Ann Emerg Med 10:370, 1981.

17. Davis DP, Valentine C, Ochs M, Vilke GM, Hoyt DB: The Combitube as a salvage airway device for paramedic rapid sequence intubation. Ann Emerg Med 42:697-704, 2003.

18. Della Puppa A, Pittoni G, Frass M: Tracheal esophageal combitube: A useful airway for morbidly obese patients who cannot intubate or ventilate. Acta Anaesthesiol Scand 46:911-913, 2002.

19. Deroy R, Ghoris M: The Combitube™ elective anesthetic airway management in a patient with cervical spine fracture. Anesth Analg 87:1441-1442, 1998.

20. Don Michael TA, Lambert EH, Mehran A: Mouth-to-lung airway for cardiac resuscitation. Lancet 2:1329, 1968.

21. Dunham CM, Barraco RD, Clark DE, et al: EAST Practice Management Guidelines Work Group. Guidelines for emergency tracheal intubation immediately after traumatic injury. J Trauma 55:162-179, 2003.

22. Eichinger S, Schreiber W, Heinz T, et al: Airway management in a case of neck impalement: use of the oesophageal tracheal Combitube airway. Br J Anaesth 68:534, 1992.

23. Enlund M, Miregard M, Wennmalm K: The Combitube for failed intubation—instructions for use. Acta Anaesthesiol Scand 45:127-8, 2001.

24. Frass M, Frenzer R, Zahler J, et al: First experimental studies with a new device for emergency intubation (esophageal tracheal Combitube). Intensivmed Notfallmed 24:390-392, 1987.

25. Frass M, Frenzer R, Rauscha F, et al: Evaluation of esophageal tracheal Combitube in cardiopulmonary resuscitation. Crit Care Med 15:609, 1987.

26. Frass M, Frenzer R, Rauscha F, et al: Ventilation with the esophageal tracheal Combitube in cardiopulmonary resuscitation: Promptness and effectiveness. Chest 93:781, 1988.

27. Frass M, Frenzer R, Ilias W, et al: The esophageal tracheal Combitube (ETC): Animal experiment results with a new emergency tube. [German] Anasthesiol Intensivther Notfallmed Schmerzther 22:142-144, 1987.

28. Frass M, Frenzer R, Mayer G, et al: Mechanical ventilation with the esophageal tracheal Combitube (ETC) in the intensive care unit. Arch Emerg Med 4:219-225, 1987.

29. Frass M, Frenzer R, Zahler J: Respiratory tube or airway. U.S. Patent no. 4,688,568, 1987.

30. Frass M, Frenzer R, Zdrahal F, et al: The esophageal tracheal Combitube: Preliminary results with a new airway for CPR. Ann Emerg Med 16:768, 1987.

31. Frass M, Johnson JC, Atherton GL, et al: Esophageal tracheal Combitube (ETC) for emergency intubation: anatomical evaluation of ETC placement by radiography. Resuscitation 18:95, 1989.

32. Frass M, Lackner FX, Frenzer R, Hofbauer R: Analysis of 500 uses of the Combitube: Safety, efficacy, and maximum ventilatory pressures during routine surgery. Difficult Airway 2:84-90, 2001.

33. Frass M, Rodler S, Frenzer R, et al: Esophageal tracheal Combitube, endotracheal airway and mask: comparison of ventilatory pressure curves. J Trauma 29:1476, 1989.

34. Frass M: Development, patent procedure, and 15 years experience: combitube-from bench to bedside. Curr Opin Clin Exp Res 2:31-38, 2000.

35. Gaitini LA, Vaida SJ, Agro F.:The Esophageal-Tracheal Combitube. Anesthesiol Clin North America. 20:893-906, 2002.

36. Gaitini LA, Vaida SJ, Mostafa S, et al: The Combitube in Elective Surgery: A Report of 200 Cases. Anesthesiology 94:79-82, 2001.

37. Gaitini LA, Vaida SJ, Somri M, Fradis M, Ben-David B: Fiberoptic-guided airway exchange of the Esophageal-Tracheal Combitube in spontaneously breathing vs. mechanically ventilated patients. Anesth and Analg 88:193-196, 1999.

38. Gertler JP, Cameron DE, Shea K, Baker CC: The esophageal obturator airway: obturator or obtundator? J Trauma 25:424, 1985.

39. Green K, Beger T: Proper use of the Combitube. Anesthesiology 81:513, 1994.

40. Hagberg C, Johnson S, Pillai D: Effective use of the esophageal tracheal Combitube following severe burn injury. J Clin Anesth 15:463-466, 2003.

41. Hagberg C, Vartazarian TN, Chelkly JE, Ovassapian A: The incidence of gastroesophageal reflux and tracheal aspiration detected with pH electrodes is similar with the Laryngeal Mask Airway® and Esophageal Tracheal Combitube® - a pilot study. Can J Anaesth 51:243-249, 2004.

42. Hammargren Y, Clinton JE, Ruiz E: A standard comparison of esophageal obturator airway and endotracheal tube ventilation in cardiac arrest. Ann Emerg Med 14:953, 1985.

43. Hartmann T, Krenn CG, Zoeggeler A, et al: The oesophageal-tracheal Combitube Small Adult.© An alternative support during gynaecological laparoscopy. Anaesthesia 55:670-675, 2000.

44. Haynes BE, Pritting J: A rural emergency medical technician with selected advanced skills. Prehospital Emergency Care 3:343-346, 1999.

45. Hoerauf KH, Hartmann T, Acimovic S, et al: Waste gas exposure to sevoflurane and nitrous oxide during anaesthesia using the oesophageal-tracheal Combitube small adult.™ Br J Anaesth 86:124-126, 2001.

46. Hofbauer R, Röggla M, Staudinger T, et al: Emergency intubation with the Combitube in a patient with persistent vomiting. Anästhesiolog - Intensivmed - Notfallmed - Schmerzther 29:306-308, 1994.

47. Johnson JC, Atherton GL: The esophageal tracheal Combitube: An alternate route to airway management. J Emerg Med Services 5:23-34, 1991.

48. Johnson JC: Personal communication, 1995.

49. Johnson KR, Genovesi MG, Lassar KH: Esophageal obturator airway: use and complications, JACEP 5:36, 1976.

50. Keller C, Brimacombe J, Boehler M, Loeckinger A, Puehringer F: The influence of cuff volume and anatomic location on pharyngeal, esophageal, and tracheal mucosal pressures with the esophageal tracheal combitube. Anesthesiology 96:1074-1077, 2002.

51. Klein H, Williamson M, Sue-Ling HM, Vucevic M, Quinn AC: Esophageal rupture associated with the use of the Combitube. Anesth Analg 85:937-939, 1997.

52. Klein U, Rich JM, Seifert A, Tesinsky P: Use of the Combitube as a rescue airway during a case of "can't ventilate—can't intubate (CVCI)" in the operating room when a laryngeal mask failed. Difficult Airway 3:4-7, 2002.

53. Knacke P: Personal communication, 2003.

54. Krafft P, Frass M: Der schwierige Atemweg (The difficult airway). Wien Klin Woch 112:260-270, 2000.

55. Krafft P, Röggla M, Fridrich P, Locker GJ, Frass M, Benumof JL: Bronchoscopy via a re-designed Combitube™ in the esophageal position. A clinical evaluation. Anesthesiology 86:1041-1045, 1997.

56. L'intubazione difficile e la difficoltá di controllo delle vie aeree nell'adulto. Linea Guida SIIARTI, Il Coordinatore Prof. Giulio Frova. Minerva Anestesiol 64:361-371, 1998.

57. Lefrancois DP, Dufour DG: Use of the esophageal tracheal combitube by basic emergency medical technicians. Resuscitation 52:77-83, 2002.

58. Liao D, Shalit M: Successful intubation with the Combitube in acute asthmatic respiratory distress by a parkmedic. J Emerg Med 14:561-563, 1996.

59. Lipp M, Jaehnichen G, Golecki N, Fecht G, Reichl R, Heeg P: Microbiological, microstructure, and material science examinations of reprocessed Combitubes after multiple reuse. Anesth Analg 91:693-697, 2000.

60. Lipp M, Thierbach A, Daubländer M, Dick W: Clinical evaluation of the Combitube. 18th Annual Meeting of the European Academy of Anaesthesiology, August 29 to September 1, 1996, Copenhagen, Denmark, p 43.

61. Lorenz V, Frass M: Securing the airway with the help of the Combitube in a patient trapped in a car. Difficult Airway 2:64-67, 2001.

62. Mercer M, Gabbott D: The influence of neck position on ventilation using the Combitube airway. Anaesthesia 53:146-150, 1998.

63. Mercer MH, Gabbott DA: Insertion of the Combitube airway with the cervical spine immobilised in a rigid cervical collar. Anaesthesia 53:971-974, 1998.

64. Morimoto F, Yoshioka T, Ikeuchi H, Inoue Y, Higashi T, Abe Y: Use of Esophageal Tracheal Combitube to control severe oronasal bleeding associated with craniofacial injury: Case report. J Trauma 51:168-169, 2001.

65. Niemann JT: Cardiopulmonary resuscitation: current concepts. N Engl J Med 327:1075, 1992.

66. Ochs M, Vilke GM, Chan TC, Moats T, Buchanan J: Successful prehospital airway management by EMT-Ds using the combitube. Prehosp Emerg Care 4:333-337, 2000.

67. Oczenski W, Krenn H, Dahaba AA, et al: Hemodynamic and catecholamine stress responses to insertion of the Combitube, laryngeal mask airway or tracheal intubation. Anesth Analg 88:1389-1394, 1999.

68. Ovassapian A, Liu S, Krejcie T: Fiberoptic tracheal intubation with Combitube in place. Abstract für 67th Congress of International Anesthesia Research Society to be held at the San Diego Marriott Hotel and Marina, March 19-23, 1993. Anesth Analg 76:S315, 1993.

69. Paning, Personal communication, 1998.

70. Piotrowski D, Gaszynski W, Wacowska-Szewczyk M, Kaszynski Z: Intubation with the oesophageal tracheal combitube for elective laparatomy. Anaesthesiol Intens Ther 27:25-30, 1995.

71. Practice Guidelines for Management of the Difficult Airway. An Updated Report by the American Society of Anesthesiologists Task Force on Management of the Difficult Airway. Anesthesiology 98:1269-1277, 2003.

72. Rabitsch W, Krafft P, Lackner FX, et al: Evaluation of the oesophageal-tracheal double-lumen tube (Combitube) during general anaesthesia. Wien Klin Wochenschr 116:90-93, 2004.

73. Rabitsch W, Moser D, Inzunza MR, et al: Airway management with endotracheal tube versus Combitube during parabolic flights. Anesthesiology, in press.

74. Rich JM, Mason AM, Bey TA, Krafft P, Frass M: The critical airway, rescue ventilation, and the combitube: Part I. AANA J 72:17-27, 2004.

75. Rich JM, Mason AM, Bey TA, Krafft P, Frass M: The critical airway, rescue ventilation, and the combitube: Part II. AANA J 72:115-124, 2004.

76. Rich JM, Mason AM, Ramsay MA: AANA journal course: update for nurse anesthetists. The SLAM Emergency Airway Flowchart: A new guide for advanced airway practitioners. AANA J 72:431-439, 2004.

77. Rich M, Thierbach A, Frass M: The Combitube, Self-Inflating Bulb, and Colorimetric Carbon Dioxide Detector to Advance Airway Management. In the first Echelon of the Battlefield. Mil Med 171:389-395, 2006.

78. Rumball CJ, MacDonald D: The PTL, Combitube, laryngeal mask, and oral airway: A randomized prehospital comparative study of ventilatory device effectiveness and cost-effectiveness in 470 cases of cardiorespiratory arrest. Prehospital Emergency Care 1:1-10, 1997.

79. Schofferman J, Oill P, Lewis AJ: The esophageal obturator airway: a clinical evaluation. Chest 69:67, 1976.

80. Scholl DG, Tsai SH: Esophageal perforation following the use of the esophageal obturator airway. Radiology 122:315, 1977.

81. Schreier H, Papousek A, Aram L, et al: Use of the esophageal-tracheal Combitube in children. Proceedings of the Vienna International Anesthesiology & Intensive Care Congress, Vienna, Oct 2-5, 1996. Acta Anaesthesiol Scand 40:246, 1996.

82. Shea SR, MacDonald JR, Gruzinski G: Prehospital endotracheal tube airway or esophageal gastric tube airway: a critical comparison. Ann Emerg Med 14:102, 1985.

83. Staudinger T, Brugger S, Watschinger B, et al: Emergency intubation with the Combitube: comparison with the endotracheal airway. Ann Emerg Med 22:1573, 1993.

84. Tamblay J: Insertion of the Esophageal-Tracheal Combitube® using inhalational anesthetic induction with sevoflurane. Difficult Airway 3:51-57, 2002.

85. Tanigawa K, Shigematsu A: Choice of airway devices for 12,020 cases of nontraumatic cardiac arrest in Japan. Prehospital Emergency Care 2:96-100, 1998.

86. Thierbach AR, Piepho T, Maybauer MO: A new device for emergency airway management: the EasyTube.™ Resuscitation 60:347, 2004.

87. Thierbach AR, Piepho T, Maybauer M: The EasyTube™ for airway management in emergencies. Prehosp Emerg Care 9:445-448, 2005.

88. Thierbach AR, Werner C: Infraglottic airway devices and techniques. Best Pract Res Clin Anaethesiol 19:595-609, 2005.

89. Ulrich-Pur H, Hrska F, Krafft P, et al: Comparison of mucosal pressures induced by cuffs of different airway devices. Anesthesiology 104:933-938, 2006.

90. Urtubia R, Aguila C: Combitube: A new proposal for a confusing nomenclature. Anesth Analg 89:803, 1999.

91. Urtubia R, Lorca E, De la Fuente D: Rescate exitoso de emergencia extrahospitalaria de la vía aérea mediante el uso del Combitubo por un operador no entrenado. Rev Méd Chile 129:119-120, 2001.

92. Urtubia R, Medina J, Marshall J, et al: Insertion of Esophageal Tracheal Combitube® using inhalational anesthetic induction with sevoflurane. Difficult Airway 3:51-57, 2002.

93. Urtubia RM, Aguila CM, Cumsille MA: Combitube: A study for proper use. Anesth Analg 90:958-962, 2000.

94. Urtubia RM, Aguila M: New thoughts on the difficult airway. Curr Opin Clin Exp Res 2:61-67, 2000.

95. Urtubia RM, Frass M, Agro F: New insertion technique of the Esophageal-Tracheal Combitube®. Acta Anaesthesiol Scand 46:341, 2002.

96. Urtubia RM, Medina JN, Alzamora R, et al: Combitube for emergency cesarean section under general anesthesia. Case reports. Difficult Airway 2:78-83, 2001.

97. Urtubia RM: Combitubo para el manejo electivo de la vía aérea. Revista Chilena Anestesia 31:221-232, 2002.

98. Vezina D, Lessard MR, Bussieres J, Topping C, Trepanier CA: Complications associated with the use of the Esophageal-Tracheal Combitube. Can J Anaesth. 45:76-80, 1998.

99. Walz R, Davis S, Panning B: The Combitube™: A useful emergency airway device for anesthesiologists? Anesth Analg 88:233, 1999.

100. Wiltschke C, Kment G, Swoboda H, et al: Ventilation with the Combitube during tracheotomy. Laryngoscope 104:763-765, 1994.

101. Wissler RN: The esophageal-tracheal Combitube. Anesth Review 20:147, 1993.

26

TRANSTRACHEAL JET VENTILATION VIA PERCUTANEOUS CATHETER AND HIGH-PRESSURE SOURCE

William H. Rosenblatt
Jonathan L. Benumof

I. INTRODUCTION

The published incidence of the cannot-ventilate, cannot-intubate (CNV/CNI) situation has ranged from 0.01 to 2.0 per 10,000 anesthetics.[7,14,25,29,63] Although the cause of this dire apneic or obstructive state may be fully or partially related to patients' disease, it often has an iatrogenic component, being recognized at the time of anesthetic induction. The clinician caring for the patient in this acutely life-threatening state must be prepared to act swiftly in order to sustain or recover oxyhemoglobin saturation and ensure ventilation.

A completely obstructed state does not have to exist for the patient to be at jeopardy. Any time the clinician cannot provide adequate, life-sustaining upper airway gas exchange, further actions, noninvasive or invasive, are mandatory.

There is widespread agreement in the literature that percutaneous transtracheal jet ventilation (TTJV), using a large-bore catheter placed through the cricothyroid membrane (CTM), is a simple, relatively safe, and extremely effective treatment for the desperate cannot-ventilate-by-mask, cannot-intubate situation.[47] Compared with surgical cricothyrotomy and tracheostomy, the establishment of

TTJV (with a high-pressure oxygen source and noncompliant tubing) is ordinarily quicker, simpler, and therefore more efficacious for most anesthesiologists, who may not be practiced in more formal surgical techniques.[47]

The literature is replete with the descriptions of the TTJV technique as well a number of devices, both commercial and "operating room rigged."[15,38,40,53,61] As discussed here, many of these TTJV "setups" have not undergone objective testing and, although easy to construct, may not be life sustaining.

The goal of this chapter is to present a clinically applicable discussion of the technique of TTJV. This is presented in a manner that will give the clinician the tools to perform TTJV rapidly. It is important that the clinician give some advanced consideration to the technique (e.g., appropriate cannulas, availability of connectors and tubing, as well as an accessible high-pressure oxygen source). These materials, as well as the knowledge to use them, must be immediately available.

The difficult airway algorithm of the American Society of Anesthesiologists (ASA) includes TTJV in the emergency pathway.[1,10] The significance of its placement in the algorithm is the ASA's encouragement of a minimally invasive procedure where surgical cricothyrotomy or tracheostomy has been the standard, accepted procedure. It is generally accepted that TTJV, although incapable of providing the same pulmonary toilet and in some cases as adequate ventilation as a cricothyrotomy, is rapid and requires comparatively little training.

II. TRANSTRACHEAL JET VENTILATION AND THE DIFFICULT AIRWAY ALGORITHM OF THE AMERICAN SOCIETY OF ANESTHESIOLOGISTS

The ASA's algorithm lists three techniques that should be employed when circumstances are encountered in which one cannot mask ventilate, cannot intubate by direct laryngoscopy, and cannot effectively use the laryngeal mask airway (LMA): insertion of an esophageal-tracheal Combitube (ETC), TTJV, and emergency surgical airway. Both supraglottic airways, the LMA and ETC, should be considered first during supraglottic obstruction, unfavorable natural anatomy, and other CNV/CNI situations because one or both are familiar to the vast majority of anesthesiologists. Both have been demonstrated to be highly effective in this situation.[1,46] In addition, both are noninvasive, occupying natural airway spaces, and are associated with little trauma.[5] As such, one or both of these devices should be readily available wherever a CNV/CNI situation may arise.[5] If insertion of the LMA or ETC or another supraglottic device does not affect gas exchange quickly, the ASA difficult airway algorithm recommends that the clinician move to an more invasive maneuver without delay. Of the maneuvers suggested, TTJV may be the most familiar to the anesthesiologist. Although surgical cricothyrotomy and tracheostomy are historical standards

of care in emergency medicine, they may be technically challenging. Along with the ease of performance, an advantage of TTJV is that it may be practiced in nonemergency clinical care; the anesthesiologist practicing elective, awake intubation may choose to make percutaneous transtracheal injection of lidocaine a routine technique, thereby practicing laryngeal catheter placement.

III. MECHANISM OF ACTION

The insufflation of oxygen at high pressure and through a large-bore cannula within the lumen of the trachea can provide alveolar oxygenation by two mechanisms: bulk flow of oxygen through the catheter and the Venturi effect.

A. INSPIRATORY PHASE

Although the therapeutic effect of TTJV is ideally both alveolar oxygenation and carbon dioxide removal (ventilation), the latter effect is dependent on the ability to supply adequate tidal volumes as well as provide both a pathway and adequate time for passive gas egress. Contrary to this, the former effect, oxygenation, is dependent on adequate gas flow alone and is, therefore, more reliably achieved. The earliest reports of TTJV in both animals and humans focused on short-term oxygenation, appreciating that a definitive airway was required to achieve adequate ventilation.[24] There is general agreement that when a size 14G catheter or smaller is employed, oxygen flow must be driven by pressures of 50 psi (equivalent to 3420 cm H_2O) or oxygen flows of 15 L/min in order to achieve adequate gas flow.[24,42] Neff and colleagues insufflated gas through multiple catheters.[42] The smallest diameter catheter that this group employed had a 1.4 mm inner diameter (ID) (15G). This catheter provided marginal oxygenation with 15 L/min constant gas flow as well as 50 psi "pulsed flow." Gas flow is further affected by factors such as airway resistance and pulmonary compliance. Although flow through various cannulas has been measured during simulated TTJV, actual flow varies in the clinical situation. Table 26-1 lists experimental data on flow rates through catheters of various sizes with a 50 psi gas supply.

Studies using low-pressure systems (e.g., self-inflating ventilating bags) have shown inadequate oxygenation unless very large (3 to 4 mm) cannulas are used.[42] Likewise, spontaneous breathing through a small cannula is likely to be inadequate. Ooi and coworkers considered the work of breathing through relatively small catheters (compared with 5 to 6 mm ID "tracheostomy" cannulas).[45] Using a mechanical lung model, this group found the inspiratory workload excessively high compared with cannulas of 4.0 mm ID or greater. This has been noted by others, although the oxygenation achieved is typically noted as "marginal" even through these large lumens.[42] This is not surprising in that spontaneous inspiratory forces produce only 7 to 35 cm H_2O (0.1 to 0.5 psi) of negative pressure.[13]

Table 26-1   **Flow Rates through Cannulas in Various Models**

Cannula Gauge	Internal Diameter (mm)	Flow (mL/sec)	Model	Reference
18*	1.4	50	Sheep (46-54 kg)	40
15*	2	150	Sheep (46-54 kg)	40
13*	2.5	250	Sheep (46-54 kg)	40
12*	3	340	Sheep (46-54 kg)	40
9*	4	800	Sheep (46-54 kg)	40
20	0.89*	400	Lung model	23
16	1.65*	500	Animal	58
14	2.1*	1600	Lung model	23

*Approximate conversion.

In an attempt to overcome the limitation of small catheters, authors have successfully inserted more than one cannula in order to improve gas exchange during spontaneous ventilation and upper airway obstruction.[13]

In the 1700s, Bernoulli described the drop in pressure that occurs as a flow of gas in a tube exits a narrow orifice.[41] This phenomenon is responsible for the Venturi effect, in which a second gas may be entrained into a system because of the drop in surrounding pressure. Rapidly flowing gas injected into the trachea during TTJV can cause a subatmospheric pressure in the upper airway, leading to room air entrainment from the mouth or nose, or both. This has been observed in ex vivo, experimental models.[23,24] In the presence of a completely patent glottis, gas entrainment by the Venturi effect could, in theory, significantly contribute to total tracheal gas flow, adding as much as 40% to 50% more gas to that delivered from the TTJV cannula alone.[23,24,60] In the clinical situation, this gas entrainment may either be insignificant compared with that delivered by the transtracheal catheter or not occur at all secondary to airway collapse above the point of insufflation (also because of the pressure decrease described by Bernoulli).[31,60,64,68] This has been substantiated by the finding that the arterial blood gas data in animals, as well as healthy patients managed with TTJV, demonstrate arterial oxygen tension (PaO_2) values consistent with the insufflation of 100% oxygen (no entrainment of room air).[31,64,68]

B. EXPIRATORY PHASE

The expiratory phase of TTJV is often passive, relying on the elasticity of the chest wall and intra-abdominal pressure as the driving force. Thus, no significant egress of gas is expected from the transtracheal catheters unless large-bore (e.g., >3 mm ID) devices are used.[42] Expiration is, therefore, by the upper airway route, which must be patent, although some investigators have had moderate success using a second transtracheal catheter to facilitate expiration.[13,50] Detection of air movement from the mouth and nose, detection of exhaled CO_2, rise and fall of

the chest, and maintenance of cardiovascular stability are, apart from stable or improving oxyhemoglobin saturation, qualitative signs of ventilation.

The use of high-pressure insufflation during TTJV facilitates ventilation through expansion of the pulmonary circuit and the resultant elastic recoil. In the original studies on TTJV, using 15 L/min oxygen flow through 13G catheters, Jacoby and colleagues were unable to maintain dogs for greater than 30 minutes because of CO_2 retention.[28] It was the introduction of high-pressure (30 to 50 psi) TTJV by Spoerel and others in 1971 that finally overcame this problem.[60] In the nonobstructed ventilation during high pressure, TTJV appears to be similar in the spontaneous ventilation or muscle-relaxed state.[65]

C. TRANSTRACHEAL JET VENTILATION IN COMPLETE AIRWAY OBSTRUCTION

Experimental models have demonstrated that partial upper airway obstruction may facilitate ventilation during high-pressure TTJV by virtue of increased tracheal pressure and resultant augmentation of the tidal volume.[11] Complete or near-complete airway obstruction results in more serious consequences during TTJV.[11] In a controlled trial of graded airway obstruction in dogs with 45 psi inflation pressures through a 13G catheter, tracheal pressures of 24 cm H_2O were associated with decreasing blood pressure and increased central venous pressure even in the absence of pneumothorax.[11] In complete upper airway obstruction (laryngeal web, upper airway edema, foreign body), barotrauma has been reported during the use of TTJV.[11,42] Complete airway obstruction, therefore, demands a different technique of resuscitation. Although controversial and based on animal models, insufflation of oxygen into the pulmonary circuit, without active or passive ventilation, has been proposed as a mechanism of maintaining *oxygenation*, not ventilation, in the obstructed patient.[11,20,21]

Frame and associates, using a canine model (20 to 29 kg), found that with complete airway obstruction, oxygen flows of 5 to 7 L/min through large catheters (10 and 12G) could maintain oxygenation with 1 second/ 4 second inspiration/expiration phases and provide reasonable ventilation ($PaCO_2 < 75$).[20] When flow rates of 3 L/min were used, CO_2 tension increased rapidly after 5 to 20 minutes. Although this study demonstrated the successful use of low-pressure oxygen flow in complete airway obstruction (in an effort to avoid barotrauma), it must be cautioned that small animals and large insufflation catheters were employed.

D. TRANSTRACHEAL JET VENTILATION AND THE PATIENT WITH A FULL STOMACH

Emergency surgery is associated with a higher incidence of the CNV/CNI situation.[1,10] Likewise, the incidence of emergency tracheostomy is higher in the emergency department compared with the operating room (OR).[51] This is not surprising when one considers the relative lack of time for decision making and alternatives for the critical patient. In addition, the relative inexperience with airway evaluation and intubation of many emergency medicine physicians helps to explain this difference. A complicating aspect of the emergency patient is the likelihood of a nonfasted state. When laryngoscopy and intubation fail, regurgitation and aspiration may ensue. Difficult mask ventilation with gastric insufflation, as well as the time incurred during attempts to control the airway, can increase this likelihood. Interestingly, one study in dogs, using methylene blue instilled into the oral cavity, demonstrated reduced aspiration of oral contents in dogs undergoing TTJV compared with control dogs.[8,30] The authors concluded that this was due to the continuous retrograde egress of air from the larynx. A similar phenomenon has been noted in humans during oxygen insufflation through an endotracheal tube (ET) exchange catheter.[35]

Another important aspect of the upper airway changes that may be induced by the introduction of oxygen by transtracheal catheter is the potential for partial relief of upper airway obstruction. In a controlled study, Okazaki and colleagues demonstrated that induced airway obstruction (by simple neck flexion) was partially relieved by the insufflation of 10 L/min O_2, although not as well as by the chin lift–jaw thrust maneuver.[43] This finding may imply a use of transtracheal insufflation in the patient at high risk for airway obstruction during postanesthetic recovery.[3,43]

IV. INDICATIONS

There are both emergency (inadequate gas exchange) and elective (gas exchange may become inadequate) indications for the use of TTJV. In both situations, TTJV is an alternative only if the clinician has prepared for its use. In this regard, the clinician should assess his or her anesthetizing or resuscitation location and facilities for TTJV should it become necessary.

A. EMERGENCY INDICATIONS

Inability to provide adequate oxygenation by routine or other noninvasive means is the primary indication for the use of TTJV. (Although it is not within the scope of this chapter or within the practice of most anesthesiologists, transtracheal oxygenation has been used on a chronic basis in patients with hypoxemia related to chronic lung disease.)[26]

1. Cannot-Ventilate, Cannot-Intubate Situations

Acute indications for TTJV include the inability to (adequately) face mask or LMA oxygenate or to perform endotracheal intubation with or without a trial with ETC ventilation.[1] Even when some gas exchange is evidenced (e.g., detection of end-tidal CO_2, chest movement, auscultation of breath sounds), oxygen delivery at the level of the alveolus and subsequent diffusion into the pulmonary capillary blood may not meet the metabolic demands of the patient. In these cases, TTJV is also a viable method of oxygenation.

2. Lack of Equipment or Trained Personnel for Conventional Airway Management

When trained personnel are unavailable to secure an airway rapidly in an agitated, gasping patient or if the proper armamentarium to perform endotracheal intubation, tracheostomy, or bronchoscopy is not immediately at hand, institution of percutaneous transtracheal ventilation may be lifesaving.

B. ELECTIVE INDICATIONS
1. To Facilitate Operations Involving the Upper Airway

There are several reports and recommendations for the use of TTJV in planned surgical situations either to avoid tracheostomy or to facilitate safe endotracheal intubation. Singh and coworkers[56] reported 1500 cases of TTJV for diagnostic and surgical procedures of the upper airways. There were 1257 cases for bronchoscopy and esophagoscopy and 135 cases for endolaryngeal surgery. Postoperative ventilatory support was carried out with this technique in 108 cases, with the patients ventilated for periods of 24 to 48 hours.

Spoerel and Greenway,[59] describing ventilation techniques during endolaryngeal surgery, similarly found adequate pulmonary ventilation with excellent conditions for microscopic surgery. Smith and colleagues[57] reported elective transtracheal ventilation in children undergoing surgical procedures involving the head and neck. They described the use of this technique in two children, one undergoing an operation for laryngeal stenosis and one who became obstructed and cyanotic in the recovery room. $PaCO_2$ determinations at the end of the procedures indicated that the patients were moderately hyperventilated.

Similarly, because percutaneous TTJV leaves the entire airway from the vocal cords to the face accessible for surgical manipulation, it is not surprising that it has been used for virtually every conceivable type of operation on these structures in adults.[32] In addition, Wagner and coauthors[66] described a case in which high-frequency ventilation was used with success (thus avoiding tracheostomy) in a patient with a partial upper airway obstruction caused by a hypopharyngeal foreign body with four sharp appendages.

Dhara and colleagues reported two cases in which a triple-lumen central venous catheter was placed through the CTM prior to induction of anesthesia. This allowed the clinicians to measure tracheal CO_2 and intra-airway pressure as well as provide jet oxygenation.[17] In both cases, an upper airway egress for insufflated oxygen was maximized: by use of a nasopharyngeal airway in one and tongue retraction in the other.

Depierraz and associates[16] investigated the elective use of TTJV in pediatric patients (younger than 1 to 12 years) with significant upper airway obstruction. They expounded on the major advantages of this technique: improved surgical exposure of the upper airway obstructive lesion, reduced manipulation of the lesion, reduced operative field movement during laser surgery, reduced danger of airway fire, and reduced risk of blowing particles into the distal airway.[16]

2. To Permit Safe Intubation of the Trachea with a Standard Endotracheal Tube by Another Route (Prevent the CNV/CNI Situation)

In situations in which an increased risk of a CNV/CNI situation can be identified, elective institution of TTJV may prevent the development of a life-threatening gas exchange problem while a more secure, permanent airway is being established. Elective placement of an intravenous catheter through the CTM and use of TTJV are entirely compatible with a subsequent conventional orotracheal or nasotracheal intubation, fiberoptic-aided intubation, and retrograde intubation technique as well as with formal tracheostomy. Indeed, one report described prophylactic TTJV to provide adequate oxygenation in a patient who was known to be difficult to intubate. The TTJV enabled the patient to be anesthetized, muscle relaxed, and intubated in a safe, nonemergent manner.[36] In another report of a 13-year-old girl with ankylosis of the temporomandibular joint secondary to a fractured mandible, TTJV was electively instituted before the induction of anesthesia. The trachea was subsequently intubated with the aid of a fiberoptic bronchoscope (FOB).[4] In a third report, a TTJV catheter allowed enough spontaneous ventilation (in addition to the natural airway) in a patient with a massive upper airway tumor so that the airway could be secured in a safe and nonemergent manner.[13] Thus, it appears that TTJV can prevent the development of life-threatening gas exchange inadequacies in patients who

are difficult to ventilate and intubate and who require general anesthesia. The technique permits uninterrupted ventilation and oxygenation while allowing the operator unhurried access to the patient's upper airway.

3. To Facilitate Training

A not-to-be-ignored benefit of the elective use of transtracheal techniques is training of students and residents of anesthesiology as well as affording critical practice to attending physicians themselves. The ASA difficult airway algorithm suggests four alternatives in the CNV/CNI situation: LMA, ETC, TTJV, and surgical airway.[1] The first two techniques can be practiced electively (the cost of the single-use ETC may be decreased by reprocessing).[33] Although a surgical airway can be electively practiced in appropriate patients (e.g., upper airway pathology when a tracheostomy is surgically planned and an otolaryngologist is available as a supervising physician), transtracheal catheter placement has definite clinical indications that can be employed for training purposes (e.g., awake intubation procedures and retrograde intubation). Many authors agree with this approach, especially because total airway obstruction may not be relieved by the supralaryngeal devices.[48,52,67]

V. EQUIPMENT

The literature is replete with manufactured and OR-rigged devices for delivering oxygen to a translaryngeal catheter. The great advantage of using a preassembled, commercially made TTJV system is the quality assurance built into a commercial product and freedom from having to assemble the system yourself. In addition, because low-pressure systems (e.g., utilizing the anesthesia breathing circuit, a self-inflating resuscitation bag) are typically ineffective and manufacturers are limiting the utility of the anesthesia machine common gas outlet (CGO) for TTJV, commercial systems offer specifically designed components and joints for use with high pressure.[42] Many of the OR-rigged devices remain untested, and although they may resemble working systems, performance in a true clinical emergency is unknown. In addition, a working system should be assembled or made before the need for it arises. In the CNV/CNI situation, small increments of time can contribute to devastating effects. Not only can it take many seconds to minutes to assemble a device, not all anesthetizing or resuscitating locations contain uniform equipment. Basic characteristics of a TTJV system are listed in Table 26-2.

Table 26-3 lists some of the assemblies described in the literature. There are many possible configurations, and, as already mentioned, not all have been thoroughly researched. Not all parts may be available at a particular institution.[15] Table 26-3 is meant not to be a definitive list but only to give examples of the ingenuity of

Table 26-2 Characteristics of an Ideal Transtracheal Jet Ventilation Device

Has undergone clinical or laboratory validation studies
Minimum of 14G cannula size
Low-compliance tubing, fixed component joints
Can connect to a high-pressure (50 psi) oxygen source
Can connect to anesthesia circuit/self-inflating bag (if ≥ 3 mm inner diameter)
Kink resistant
Intratracheal pressure measurable
End-tidal CO_2 measurable
Flow controllable
Pressure regulation
Available preassembled
Available sterile

some clinicians. All of the assemblies described in Table 26-3 utilize the anesthesia machine CGO.[54] As discussed later, the CGO of a particular anesthesia machine may not be adequate for TTJV. Not shown in Table 26-3 are systems that use very low pressure delivery systems (self-inflating resuscitation bags and the anesthesia circuit).[37,40]

One study has examined the efficacy of OR-rigged devices, including one in which the drip chamber of an intravenous infusion device is cut to fit on the hose of an anesthesia machine CGO and the bag spike fit into a transtracheal catheter.[40] The gas volume delivered by each system was dependent on the pressure delivered to it. This was limited in the anesthesia circuit or resuscitation bag types of systems. The cut intravenous infusion set provided the best performance by virtue of high gas pressures that were applied. In conclusion, this study recognized that, regardless of the conveying devices, the ability to provide high pressure within the device dictated its efficacy. A similar study testing four different OR-rigged devices arrived at a similar conclusion: only devices employing high pressure were capable of delivering adequate transcannula flows and maintaining oxygenation, although there was inadequate ventilation.[53] A study applying the technique of using an intravenous bag spike as a large-bore cannula on a full-body physiologic simulator showed that it provides adequate high pressure as well as anesthesia circuit bag ventilation.[54]

Given the proliferation of OR-rigged devices, it is interesting to note the variety in practice among clinicians. In two studies, investigators surveyed their colleagues to determine what devices might be preferred by each.[40,53] In Morley and Thorpe's[40] survey, three different configurations were described, and the survey by Ryder and colleagues[53] described seven different configurations. In these studies, 5% and 10%, respectively, of practitioners could not assemble any device, and only 5% and 40%, respectively, of devices were considered adequate for TTJV.[40,53] When clinicians were asked to assemble a device of their own choosing, 20 to 365 seconds (mean 90 seconds) were required to produce a functional device.[53] Thus, anesthesiologists need to become educated in the use of the equipment in their clinical practice in order to perform TTJV properly.

A. OXYGEN SOURCE

The most critical element in the setup used for TTJV may be the availability of pressurized gas. There are three acceptable systems that can be used: central supply ("wall"), oxygen flowmeters, and an anesthesia machine fresh gas outlet that is capable of providing high pressure.

Central wall oxygen, supplied at 50 psi, is ubiquitous in ORs, intensive care units, and other areas of the hospital. Some anesthesia machines provide an outlet that is tied into their high-pressure gas supply (Fig. 26-1). High-pressure gas is best further regulated (20 to 50 psi, on-off switching) by the delivery device (Fig. 26-2).

Table 26-3 Examples of Operating Room–Rigged Transtracheal Jet Ventilation Gas Delivery Systems in the Case Report Literature

Connection to O_2 Source A	Tubing from Source B	Luer-Lok Connector to Transtracheal Catheter C	Flow Regulation	Advantage	Disadvantage	Reference
4.0-mm endotracheal tube adapter	Nasal O_2 tubing (cut)	Cut 1-mL syringe	Anesthesia machine Flush valve	Simple, available	Need to have specific pieces	36
Endotracheal tube adapter	O_2 tubing	Luer to nipple piece	Anesthesia machine Flush valve	Simple	Several pieces Need egress for gas	59

*CGO, anesthesia machine common gas outlet.

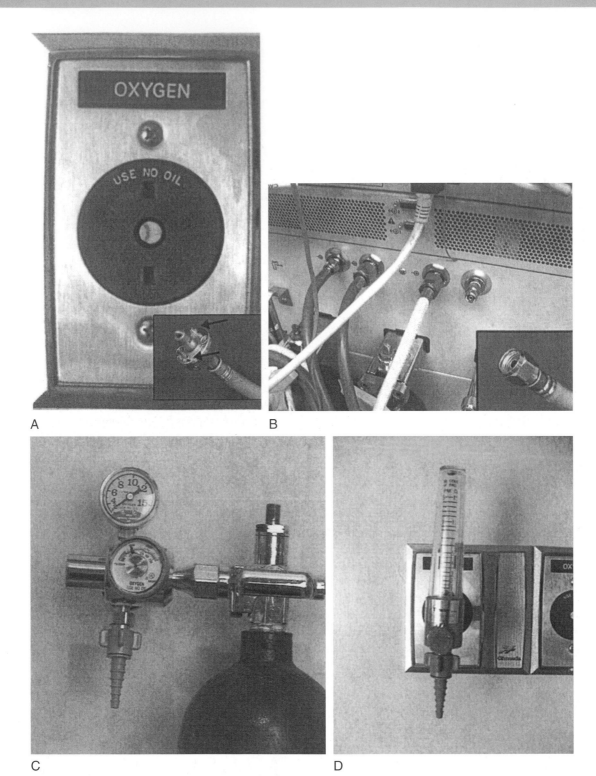

Figure 26-1 **A,** Pin-indexed 50 psi central oxygen supply. Pins on the male connector *(arrows, inset)* are uniquely placed so that this connector cannot interface with the female wall plate for other gases or vacuum. **B,** DSS-type indexed 50 psi central supply oxygen. The male supply pictured is provided on the back of the Aestiva/5 anesthesia machine (Datex-Ohmeda, Finland) for use with transtracheal jet ventilation. **C,** Oxygen tank flowmeter. **D,** Central oxygen supply flowmeter.

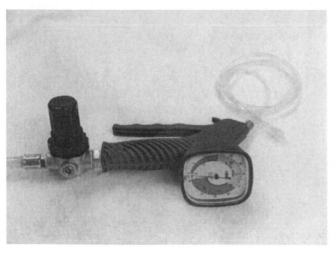

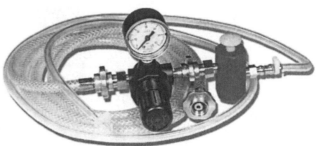

A

B

Figure 26-2 Three jet ventilators with regulators. **A,** Manujet III (Acutronic Medical Systems, Hirzel, Switzerland). **B,** Manual jet ventilator (Instrumentation Industries, Bethel Park, PA). **C,** Jet ventilator (Anesthesia Associated, San Marco, CA). (**B,** Courtesy of Instrumentation Industries.)

C

The advantage of regulated wall pressure (0 to 50 psi) is the ability to minimize barotrauma, especially in pediatrics. Only medical-grade delivery devices should be used. Similar high-pressure devices are manufactured for industrial use and may contain oil lubricants. Ventilators that deliver oxygen through injector catheters can be used during bronchoscopy. These devices automate the respiratory cycle of jet ventilation. TTJV could be performed using the Muallem jet ventilator (Dr. Muallem, Lebanon) (Fig. 26-3).[41]

The second TTJV system consists of a jet injector powered by an oxygen-tank regulator (see Fig. 26-1C). Tank regulators can be classified as high flow or low flow with respect to the steady-state pressure (pounds per square inch) and corresponding flow rates that each can generate. High-flow tank regulators can achieve maximum steady-state pressures of 100 psi and flow rates of 320 L/min and, therefore, present no problem with respect to providing adequate TTJV, although they must have an adjustable flow regulator. A low-flow regulator (such as those that are commonly available on small [E-cylinder] oxygen transport tanks, some anesthesia machines, and attached to central

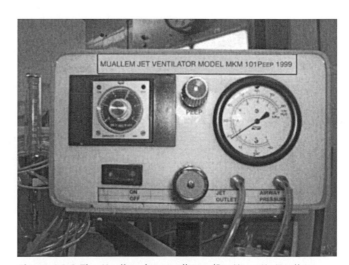

Figure 26-3 The Muallem jet ventilator (Dr. Musa K. Muallem, American University of Beirut, Beirut, Lebanon) uses a 50 psi oxygen source. Automated jet ventilator device devised for bronchoscopy. Inspiratory and expiratory times, respiratory rate (0 to 300/min), inspiratory pressure, and positive end-expiratory pressure can all be controlled.

supply oxygen; see Fig. 26-1D) can achieve a maximum pressure of 50 psi when the flowmeter is set at the maximum of 15 L/min but no flow is allowed to occur. When flow is allowed to commence (i.e., the button on the jet injector is pressed), very high flows occur for a moment and then decay exponentially as the pressure in the regulator decreases exponentially to steady-state values of 0 to 5 psi that permit the flow that was preset on the flowmeter (0 to 15 L/min). Satisfactory tidal volumes with the 16 and 14G TTJV catheters may be achieved within the first 0.5 second.[24]

The advantage of a low-flow regulator is that it is mobile and can be used in locations that do not have a central (wall) source of high-pressure oxygen (e.g., in patients' rooms, hallways, and out-of-hospital situations). In other situations, central supply (50 psi) oxygen may be available, but a delivery apparatus fitting the pin-indexed or Diameter Indexed Safety System (DISS) connectors does not allow connection. If a low-flow regulator must be used, the flow should be set at the maximum of 15 L/min and an inspiration/expiration ratio of 1:1 used to ensure adequacy of tidal volume. But the inspiratory time should be limited to 1 second or less to allow the pressure in the regulator to restore itself so that the initial high-burst flow rate may once again be achieved with the next breath.[24]

A study by Preussler and colleagues compared the two aforementioned source systems that are ubiquitous in the hospital environment.[49] This group compared hospital-supplied oxygen at 50 psi applied using a hand-triggered

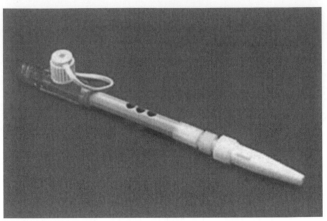

Figure 26-4 Enk oxygen flow modulator (Cook Critical Care, Bloomington, IN). "Thumb holes" are covered to direct the flow of oxygen to the patient. Pharmaceuticals may be delivered through Luer-Lok port during the inspiratory phase.

emergency jet injector (Manujet III, VBM Medizintechnik, Sulz, Germany) (see Fig. 26-2A) with 15 L/min flowmeter oxygen supplied through an Enk oxygen flow modulator (Cook, Bloomington, IN) (Fig. 26-4).[19] Both setups were tested in anesthetized pigs using a specialized 15G transtracheal catheter (Fig. 26-5A). The upper airway of the pigs was kept patent with an ET and a 20 cm H_2O positive end-expiratory pressure valve in order to simulate a clinical "partially obstructed airway." These investigators found that both device setups performed equally well,

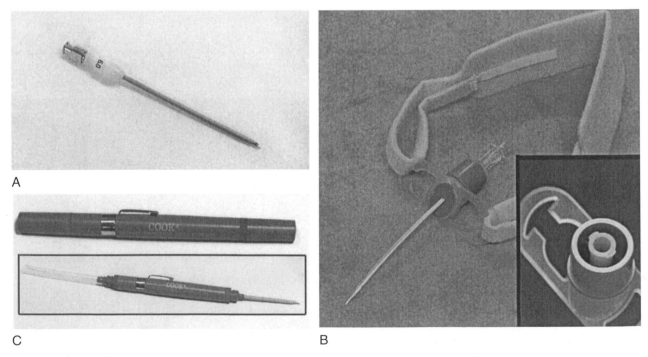

A

C

B

Figure 26-5 A, Cook transtracheal jet ventilation catheter (Cook Critical Care, Bloomington, IN) is a 15G, 5- or 7.5-cm wire-reinforced, kink-resistant cannula. The proximal end has a female Luer-Lok type of adapter. **B,** The Acutronic transtracheal jet cannula (Acutronic Medical Systems, Switzerland) is 13 or 14G and has rings for securing the cannula to the patient, both Luer-Lok and 15-mm proximal adapters (inset), and a preformed curve. **C,** The Wadhwa (Cook Critical Care) is a transtracheal cannula device designed to be carried by the physician in a shirt pocket.

maintaining end-tidal CO_2, PcO_2, and PaO_2 in acceptable ranges. Interestingly, the Enk flow modulator includes a Luer-Lok syringe port for administration of drugs into the trachea without interruption of ventilation or oxygenation. The Manujet III has a variable pressure regulator and pressure gauge (see Fig. 26-2A).

The third type of TTJV pressure supply system often cited in the literature uses the anesthesia-machine flush valve as the jet injector. The anesthesia-machine flush valve can be powered by either a central supply or a tank high-pressure oxygen source.[23] The fresh-gas outlet of the anesthesia machine (now an industry-wide standard 15-mm male outlet) is connected to noncompliant oxygen-supply tubing by a standard 15-mm tracheal tube adapter that fits a 4-mm ID ET (see Fig. 23-12). The noncompliant oxygen-supply tubing allows bypass of the compliant reservoir bag and corrugated tubing of the anesthesia circle system. This third TTJV system is completed by connecting the oxygen-supply tubing to the TTJV catheter, although this may be accomplished in many ways (see Table 26-2).

Caution must be exercised in using the CGO of the anesthesia machine as a TTJV oxygen source. The CGO–flush valve mechanisms of the anesthesia machine were not intended for this use.[41] Manufacturers have incorporated pressure relief valves into the circuitry of newer machines. The primary intent of these valves is protection of the vaporizers from the pumping effect whereby back pressure can cause an increase in the delivered concentration of the volatile agent. Some manufacturers, such as Dräger Medical (Telford, PA), have eliminated the CGO altogether. The Aestiva series of machines from Datex-Ohmeda supply an accessory CGO, located within a panel under the breathing circle inspiratory and expiratory limb connectors, which is limited to a pressure of 20 psi (Fig. 26-6). The Aestiva does include an accessory gas outlet on the rear of the machine, which supplies oxygen at a constant 50 psi (see Fig. 26-1B). An oxygen line Y connector is available from Dräger Medical to allow access to 50 psi central supply oxygen when using newer anesthesia machines from this manufacturer.

B. CONVEYANCE TUBING

Tubing used to convey the jetted oxygen from the pressure source to the transtracheal cannula should be of low compliance. A chief reason that the anesthetic breathing circle or a self-inflating resuscitation bag is incapable of generating high pressures is the compliance of the components. In addition, incorporation of devices with small-bore lumens (e.g., intravenous line valves) can critically restrict flow.[54]

C. CONVEYANCE TO CANNULA CONNECTION

A crucial aspect of the TTJV device setup is the connection to the transtracheal cannula. Most authors suggest

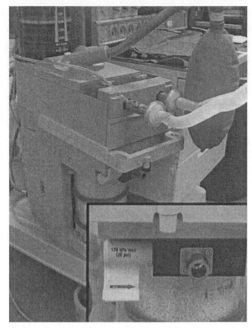

Figure 26-6 The accessory common gas outlet of the Aestiva/5 anesthesia machine (Datex-Ohmeda) is limited to 20 psi.

a tight-fitting male Luer-Lok connector that interfaces with the cannula (generally female). A variety of alternative approaches have been described, including the spike of intravenous drip chamber and the male end of a non–Luer-Lok, 1-mL syringe. Many alternative systems have been plagued by critical air leaks that impede their effectiveness.[40]

D. CANNULA

As discussed earlier, flow, pressure and on-off regulators can be incorporated along the course of the conveyance tubing. All connections should be secure with either Luer-Loks or cable ties (Fig. 26-7).

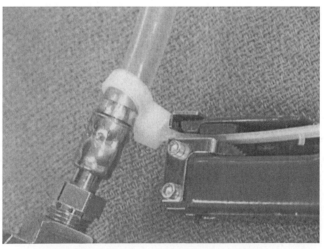

Figure 26-7 A joint is secured with a cable tie.

The last critical device in the TTJV setup is the transtracheal cannula itself. Historically, a variety of intravenous catheter-over-needle devices have been employed.[13,15,37,38,52,60] Others, in attempts to measure expired CO_2 and intratracheal pressure, have used alternative devices such as triple-lumen central venous catheters.[17] Garry and colleagues used a needle-in-needle catheter assembly (14G or 16G internal, 3 mm ID, externally).[22] Oxygen was insufflated in the central needle, and suction and CO_2 monitoring were applied to the annular space. Newer catheters have been constructed from kink-resistant materials (see Fig. 26-5A), which have a preformed tip angulation, Luer-Lok connectors, 15-mm circuit adapters, or securing rings (see Fig. 26-5B).

VI. TECHNIQUE OF TRANSTRACHEAL JET VENTILATION

A. INSERTION OF TRANSTRACHEAL CATHETER

The CTM is palpated with the neck of the patient extended (Fig. 26-8A). A 12 to 16G cannula with the needle pointed 30 degrees caudad off the perpendicular is used to puncture the CTM (see Fig. 26-8B). If it is not already pre-shaped by the manufacturer (see Fig. 26-5B), a small-angle bend (15 degrees) is placed 2.5 cm from the distal end (Fig. 26-9; see Fig. 26-8B).[55] This angulation helps in preventing intratracheal cannula kinking or cephalad travel. The cannula should be connected to either an empty or a partly clear fluid-filled 20-mL syringe.[55] As the needle-cannula is advanced through the CTM, constant withdrawal of the syringe-plunger creates a negative pressure that aids in identifying the trachea when air fills the syringe. Syringes smaller than 20 mL may not be as revealing; the smaller cross-sectional space in the plunger easily allows the operator to pull back the plunger before entering the trachea. The CTM is a relatively avascular structure, although blood is occasionally drawn into the syringe (this should not deter the operator from completing this lifesaving procedure). The vascular structures adjacent to the membrane can be avoided by performing the puncture in the midline of the neck in the lower third of the membrane just above the cricoid cartilage.[27,34] Resistance to needle advancement may be due to contact with the cricoid or thyroid cartilage, and the landmarks of the airway should be rapidly reassessed.

Once entry into the trachea has been performed, the catheter can be threaded over the needle stylet into the trachea (see Fig. 26-8C, method 3). A 14G intravenous cannula has enough structural strength to be pushed into the trachea itself, and therefore the needle stylet of a 14G catheter may be completely withdrawn prior to feeding the cannula into the trachea (see Fig. 26-8C, method 1). The needle stylet *should not* be withdrawn a short distance back into the lumen of the cannula and advanced together with the cannula—this causes the catheter to hit the posterior membrane of the trachea, increasing the risk of the needle stylet perforating the cannula or the posterior membrane of the trachea, or both (see Fig. 26-8C, method 2). When the hub of the cannula reaches the skin line (see Fig. 26-8D), air should once again be aspirated to reconfirm the intratracheal location of the cannula (see Fig. 26-8E). From the moment the cannula is inserted into the trachea, a human hand should be dedicated to holding the transtracheal cannula exactly in place until a definitive airway is established (see Fig. 26-8D).

B. MAINTENANCE OF THE NATURAL AIRWAY

The only driving pressure for exhalation is the elastic recoil of the lung (10 to 20 cm H_2O). Thus, the inspiratory gas is driven through a relatively small catheter under high pressure, but the expiratory gas must escape through as large a channel as possible (i.e., the natural airway) under a relatively low driving pressure. Therefore, during TTJV the natural airway must be maintained as well as possible to avoid trapping of air and hyperexpansion of the lungs. Oropharyngeal and nasopharyngeal airways as well as a maximal jaw thrust maneuver should be employed when not contraindicated.

VII. COMPLICATIONS

The incidence of serious complications resulting from elective use of TTJV is relatively low and appears to be primarily limited to tissue emphysema.[39] High-pressure oxygen insufflation can be hazardous, especially when no clear egress for gas exists.[9,22,42] Peak inspiratory intra-airway pressures during TTJV depend upon the cross-sectional area of the trachea; driving pressure; diameter, length, and cross-sectional area of the orifice of the cannula; degree of outflow obstruction; compliance of the lungs and chest wall; and inspiratory time.

In a series of elective TTJV cases, there was an overall minor complication rate of 3%.[52] These complications (minor bleeding, subcutaneous emphysema) were typically seen when multiple attempts had to be made during cannula placement. The authors recommend no more than two attempts.

In studies in animals (normal dogs) in which distal airway pressure was measured during TTJV through a 16G needle, it was demonstrated that low-frequency ventilatory rates (<30 breaths/min) produced peak airway pressures of 20 to 50 cm H_2O.[60] These peak airway pressures varied linearly with driving pressure when inspiratory time was held constant. Tidal volume also varied linearly with driving pressure. In addition, the tidal volumes and peak inspiratory pressures observed during TTJV were similar to those observed with conventional positive-pressure ventilation through an ET.

When complete airway obstruction was simulated in dogs, intratracheal airway pressure rose precipitously as

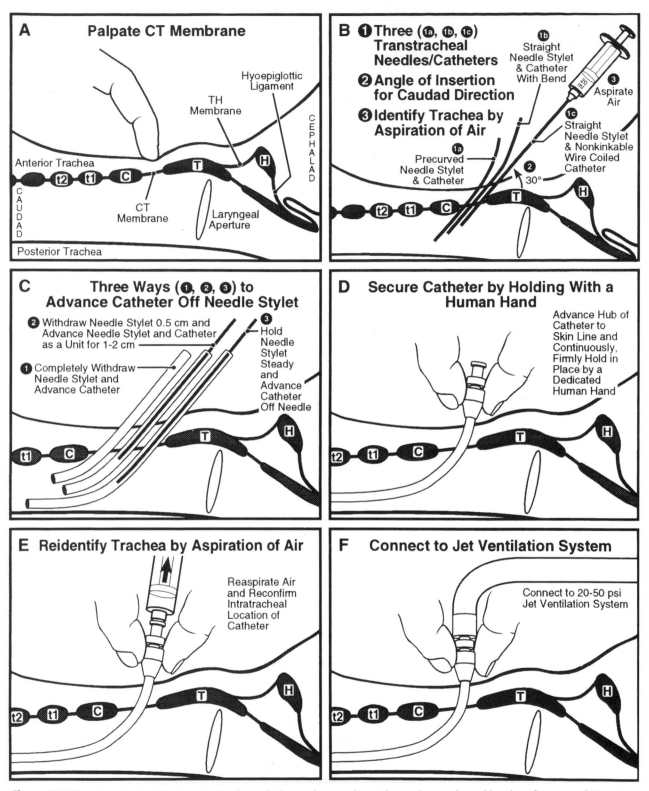

Figure 26-8 The steps involved in transtracheal ventilation and some alternative options and considerations for some of the steps (**B** and **C**). **A,** Cricothyroid (CT) membrane is palpated. **B,** 1. Transtracheal needle is inserted through CT membrane. Transtracheal needle/cannula can be 1a, precurved (see Fig. 26-5B); 1b, straight with a distal small-angle bend; or 1c, straight with a wire coiled nonkinkable catheter (see Fig. 26-5A). 2. Angle between distal end of needle/catheter and skin (i.e., angle of insertion for caudad direction) should be 30 degrees. 3. Entry into trachea should be confirmed by aspirating air. **C,** The three ways to advance catheter off needle (1, 2, and 3) are explained by labeling. **D,** Once catheter has been advanced so that hub is at skin line, it must be held in place continuously by a human hand (do not try to tape or suture hub of catheter in place). **E,** Intratracheal location should be reconfirmed by reaspirating air. **F,** Transtracheal jet-ventilation catheter is connected to jet ventilator. C, cricoid cartilage; H, hyoid bone; T, thyroid cartilage; TH, thyrohyoid membrane; t1, first tracheal cartilage; t2, second tracheal cartilage.

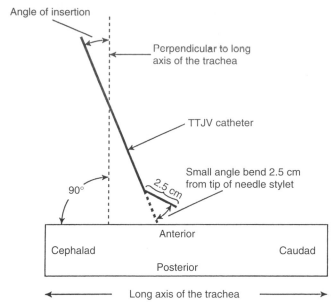

Figure 26-9 Definition of angle of insertion and small-angle bend 2.5 cm from the distal end of needle stylet. TTJV, transtracheal jet ventilation.

soon as the total lung capacity was exceeded. This was accompanied by a fall in systolic blood pressure. Rupture of the pulmonary system occurred when an intratracheal pressure of 250 cm H_2O (4 psi) was achieved (pneumothoraces, pneumomediastinum, subcutaneous emphysema, cardiac fibrillation).[42]

Ideally, intratracheal pressures should be monitored during high-pressure insufflation. Although this is not possible with standard angiocatheters or dedicated transtracheal cannulas, some authors have developed dual-lumen transtracheal catheters that serve this purpose.[22] A cannula employed by Garry and colleagues consisted of a 14 to 16G insufflation catheter within the lumen of a 3 mm ID needle.[22] Suction could be applied to the resulting annular space to facilitate gas removal. In vitro studies, employing dual-lumen catheters and an artificial lung model, have demonstrated the efficacy of these arrangements in providing adequate (and safe) airway pressures and tidal volumes in a variety of lung compliance and airway resistance settings. In addition, continuous measurement of airway pressures and measurement of end-tidal CO_2 should be possible.[22]

Smith and coworkers[58] also reported a 29% incidence of complications in 28 patients managed with TTJV to provide an emergency airway. These complications included subcutaneous emphysema (7.1%), mediastinal emphysema (3.6%), exhalation difficulty (14.3%), and arterial perforation (3.6%). None of these complications were fatal. Subcutaneous emphysema may be caused not only by aberrant placement of the distal tip of the cannula but also by cannula shaft lacerations.[2]

Barotrauma with resultant pneumothorax has been reported with both TTJV and translaryngeal jet ventilation.[12,18,44,58,62,68] Therefore, it is clearly necessary to document breath sounds as well as chest inflation and deflation following institution of TTJV and to assume that any change in cardiovascular parameters, such as hypotension, tachycardia, or bradycardia, may be secondary to pneumothorax. Clearly, the risk of pneumothorax is much increased in cases of total airway obstruction because gas cannot escape from the lungs in a normal manner. Other complications, such as esophageal puncture, bleeding, hematoma, and hemoptysis, have been reported following TTJV.[6] In addition, it appears that damage to tracheal mucosa may occur following TTJV, especially if the gas is not humidified. In pigs managed with TTJV for approximately 2 hours with single-orifice transtracheal catheters, using three different methods of nonhumidified gas delivery to the cannula, the posterior wall of the trachea clearly demonstrated macroscopic evidence of irritation and microscopic evidence of mucosal erosion.[64] However, Klain and Smith[31] did not find any tracheal damage in dogs whose lungs were subjected to 50 hours of nonhumidified high-frequency TTJV in which 14G multi-orifice catheters were used. Nonetheless, the possibility of causing tracheal mucosal ulceration should certainly be considered, particularly if TTJV is attempted through single-orifice catheters without humidification for prolonged periods of time.

VIII. CONCLUSION

The incidence of the CNV/CVI situation is 1 per 10,000 patients presenting to the OR and higher in the emergency room. The degree to which the supralaryngeal airway devices have reduced the occurrence of this critical situation has yet to be defined. Percutaneous TTJV is a simple, easily mastered procedure that offers a remedy for this dire situation. The lungs of healthy and critically ill patients have been successfully oxygenated and ventilated by this method, and it has a place in every anesthetizing position. The systems of choice, in descending order of preference, are a jet injector powered by regulated wall or tank oxygen pressure, a jet injector powered by unregulated wall or tank oxygen pressure, and an anesthesia machine flush valve using noncompliant tubing from the fresh-gas outlet, if allowed by the available machine. Much less efficacious transtracheal ventilation systems utilize the anesthesia circle system (with reservoir bag) and self-inflating resuscitation bags. These systems are helpful only if very large (>3 mm) cannulas are used. Additional applications of TTJV are to facilitate upper airway surgery; intubation by conventional laryngoscopy, antegrade FOB, or in conjunction with a retrograde intubation technique; cricothyrotomy; and tracheostomy. Nevertheless, there are a number of serious TTJV complications; thus, this lifesaving procedure should be undertaken only in desperate emergencies or in carefully thought-out elective situations. However, because desperate CNV/CNI emergencies continue to occur in association with the practice of anesthesia, we recommend that every anesthetizing location have the immediate availability of TTJV and that anesthesiologists become familiar with the technique.

REFERENCES

1. American Society of Anesthesiologists Task Force on Management of the Difficult Airway: Practice guidelines for the management of the difficult airway. Anesthesiology 98:1269, 2003.
2. Ames W, Venn P: Complication of the transtracheal catheter. Br J Anaesth 81:825, 1998.
3. Asai T, Koga K, Vaughan RS: Respiratory complications associated with tracheal intubation and extubation. Br J Anaesth 80:767, 1998.
4. Baraka A: Transtracheal jet ventilation during fiberoptic intubation under general anesthesia. Anesth Analg 65:1091, 1986.
5. Benumof JL: Laryngeal mask airway and the ASA difficult airway algorithm. Anesthesiology 84:686, 1996.
6. Benumof JL, Scheller MS: The importance of transtracheal jet ventilation in the management of the difficult airway. Anesthesiology 71:769, 1989.
7. Bolander FMF: Deaths associated with anesthesia. Br J Anaesth 47:36, 1975.
8. Bruno J, Cheung HK, Chong ZK, et al: Aspiration and tracheal jet ventilation with different pressures and depths and chest compressions. Crit Care Med 27:142, 1999.
9. Campbell CT, Harris RC, Cook MH, et al: A new device for emergency percutaneous transtracheal ventilation in partial and complete airway obstruction. Ann Emerg Med 17:927, 1988.
10. Caplan R, Benumof JL, Berry FA, et al: Practice guidelines for management of the difficult airway: A report by the ASA Task Force on Management of the Difficult Airway. Anesthesiology 78:597, 1993.
11. Carl ML, Rhee KJ, Schelegle ES, et al: Effects of graded upper-airway obstruction on pulmonary mechanics during transtracheal jet ventilation in dogs. Ann Emerg Med 24:1137, 1994.
12. Cote CJ, Eavey RD, Todres D, et al: Cricothyroid membrane puncture: Oxygenation and ventilation in a dog model using an intravenous catheter. Crit Care Med 16:615, 1988.
13. Dallen LT, Wine R, Benumof JL: Spontaneous ventilation via transtracheal large-bore intravenous catheters is possible. Anesthesiology 75:531, 1991.
14. Davis DA: An analysis of anesthetic mishaps from medical liability claims. Int Anesthesiol Clin 22:31, 1984.
15. DeLisser EA, Muravchick S: Emergency transtracheal ventilation. Anesthesiology 55:606, 1981.
16. Depierraz B, Ravussin P, Brossard E, et al: Percutaneous transtracheal jet ventilation for paediatric endoscopic laser treatment of laryngeal and subglottic lesions. Can J Anaesth 41:1200, 1994.
17. Dhara SS, Liu EH, Tan KH: Monitored transtracheal jet ventilation using a triple lumen central venous catheter. Anaesthesia 57:578, 2002.
18. Egol A, Culpepper JA, Snyder JV: Barotrauma and hypotension resulting from jet ventilation in critically ill patients. Chest 88:98, 1985.
19. Enk D, Busse H, Meissner A, et al: A new device for oxygenation and drug administration by transtracheal jet ventilation. Anesth Analg 86:s203,1998.
20. Frame SB, Simon JM, Kerstine MD, et al: Percutaneous transtracheal catheter ventilation in complete airway obstruction—An animal model. J Trauma 29:774, 1989.
21. Frame SB, Timberlake GA, Kerstine MD, et al: Transtracheal needle catheter ventilation incomplete airway obstruction—An animal model. Ann Emerg Med 18:127, 1989.
22. Garry B, Woo P, Perrault DF Jr, et al: Jet ventilation in upper airway obstruction: Description and model lung testing of a new jetting device. Anesth Analg 87:915,1998.
23. Gaughan SD, Benumof JL, Ozaki GT: Can an anesthesia machine flush valve provide for effective jet ventilation? Anesth Analg 76:800, 1993.
24. Gaughan SD, Ozaki GT, Benumof JL: Comparison in a lung model of low- and high-flow regulators for transtracheal jet ventilation. Anesthesiology 77:189, 1992.
25. Harrison GG: Death attributable to anesthesia. Br J Anaesth 50:1041, 1978.
26. Heimlich HJ, Carr GC: Transtracheal catheter technique for pulmonary rehabilitation. Ann Otol Rhinol Laryngol 94:502, 1985.
27. Holst M, Hertegard S, Persson A: Vocal dysfunction following cricothyrotomy: A prospective study. Laryngoscope 100:179, 1990.
28. Jacoby JJ, Reed JP, Hamelberg W, et al: A simple method of artificial respiration. Am J Physiol 167: 789, 1951.
29. Keenan RL, Boyan CP: Cardiac arrest due to anesthesia. JAMA 253:2373, 1985.
30. Klain M, Keszler H, Stool S: Transtracheal high frequency jet ventilation prevents aspiration. Crit Care Med 11:170, 1983.
31. Klain M, Smith RB: High frequency percutaneous transtracheal jet ventilation. Crit Care Med 5:280, 1977.
32. Layman PR: Transtracheal ventilation in oral surgery. Ann R Coll Surg Engl 65:318, 1983.
33. Lipp MD, Jaehnichen G, Golecki N, et al: Microbiological, microstructure, and material science examinations of reprocessed Combitubes after multiple reuse. Anesth Analg 91:693, 2000.
34. Little C, Parker M, Tarnopolsky R: The incidence of vasculature at risk during cricothyroidostomy. Ann Emerg Med 15:805, 1986.
35. Loudermilk EP, Hartmannsgruber M, Stoltzfus DP, et al: A prospective study of the safety of tracheal extubation using a pediatric airway exchange catheter for patients with a known difficult airway. Chest 111:1660, 1997.

36. McLellan I, Gordon P, Khawaja S, et al: Percutaneous transtracheal high frequency jet ventilation as an aid to difficult intubation. Can J Anaesth 35:404, 1988.

37. Metz S, Parmet JL, Levitt JD: Failed emergency transtracheal ventilation through a 14-gauge intravenous catheter. J Clin Anesth 8:58, 1996.

38. Meyer PD: Emergency transtracheal jet ventilation system. Anesthesiology 73:787, 1990.

39. Monnier PH, Ravussin P, Savary M, et al: Percutaneous transtracheal ventilation for laser endoscopic treatment of laryngeal and subglottic lesions. Clin Otolaryngol 13:209, 1988.

40. Morley D, Thorpe CM: Apparatus for emergency transtracheal ventilation. Anaesth Intensive Care 25:675, 1997.

41. Muallem MK: Muallem jet ventilator. Middle East J Anesthesiol 15:575, 2000.

42. Neff CC, Pfister RC, Van Sonnenberg E: Percutaneous transtracheal ventilation: Experimental and practical aspects. J Trauma 23:84, 1983.

43. Okazaki J, Isono S, Atsuko T, et al: Usefulness of continuous oxygen insufflation into trachea for management of upper airway obstruction during anesthesia. Anesthesiology 93:62, 2000.

44. Oliverio R, Ruder CB, Fermon C, et al: Report on pneumothorax secondary to ball-valve obstruction during jet ventilation. Anesthesiology 51:255, 1979.

45. Ooi R, Fawcett J, Soni N, et al: Extra inspiratory work of breathing imposed by cricothyrotomy devices. Br J Anaesth 70:17, 1993.

46. Parmet JL, Colonna-Romano P, Horrow JC, et al: The laryngeal mask airway reliably provides rescue ventilation in cases of unanticipated difficult tracheal intubation along with difficult mask ventilation. Anesth Analg 87:661, 1998.

47. Patel RG: Percutaneous transtracheal jet ventilation: A safe, quick, and temporary way to provide oxygenation and ventilation when conventional methods are unsuccessful. Chest 116:1689, 1999.

48. Patel SK, Whitten CW, Ivy R, et al: Failure of the laryngeal mask airway: An undiagnosed laryngeal carcinoma. Anesth Analg 86:438, 1998.

49. Preussler NP, Schreiber T, Huter L, et al: Percutaneous transtracheal ventilation: Effects of a new oxygen flow modulator on oxygenation and ventilation in pigs compared with a hand triggered emergency jet injector. Resuscitation 56:329, 2003.

50. Rone CA, Pavlin EG, Cummings CW, et al: Studies in transtracheal ventilation catheters. Laryngoscope 92:1259, 1982.

51. Rosenblatt WH, Murphy M: The intubating laryngeal mask: Use of a new ventilating intubating device in the emergency department. Ann Emerg Med 33:234, 1999.

52. Russell WC, Maguire AM, Jones GW: Cricothyroidotomy and transtracheal high frequency jet ventilation for elective laryngeal surgery: An audit of 90 cases. Anaesth Intensive Care 28:62, 2000.

53. Ryder IG, Paoloni CC, Harle CC: Emergency transtracheal ventilation: Assessment of breathing systems chosen by anaesthetists. Anaesthesia 51:764, 1996.

54. Sanders J, Haas RE, Geisler M, et al: Using the human patient simulator to test the efficacy of an experimental emergency percutaneous transtracheal airway. Mil Med 163:544, 1998.

55. Sdrales L, Benumof JL: Prevention of kinking of percutaneous transtracheal intravenous catheter. Anesthesiology 82:288, 1995.

56. Singh NP, Agrawal AR, Dhawan R: Resuscitation centre for management of respiratory insufficiency cases. Indian J Chest Dis 13:99, 1971.

57. Smith RB, Myers EN, Sherman H: Transtracheal ventilation in pediatric patients. Br J Anaesth 46:313, 1974.

58. Smith RB, Schaer WB, Pfaeffle H: Percutaneous transtracheal ventilation for anesthesia: A review and report of complications. Can J Anaesth 22:607, 1975.

59. Spoerel WE, Greenway RE: Technique of ventilation during endolaryngeal surgery under general anesthesia. Can J Anaesth 20:369, 1973.

60. Spoerel WE, Narayanan PS, Singh NP: Transtracheal ventilation. Br J Anaesth 43:932, 1971.

61. Sprague D: Transtracheal jet oxygenator from capnographic monitoring components. Anesthesiology 73:788, 1990.

62. Sullivan TJ, Healy GB: Complications of Venturi jet ventilation during microlaryngeal surgery. Arch Otolaryngol Head Neck Surg 111:127, 1985.

63. Taylor G, Larson CP, Prestwich R: Unexpected cardiac arrest during anesthesia and surgery: An environmental study. JAMA 236:2758, 1976.

64. Thomas T, Zornow M, Scheller MS, et al: The efficacy of three different modes of transtracheal ventilation in hypoxic hypercarbic swine. Can J Anaesth 35(Suppl): 61, 1988.

65. Tran TP, Rhee KJ, Schultz HD, et al: Gas exchange and lung mechanics during percutaneous transtracheal ventilation in an unparalyzed canine model. Acad Emerg Med 5:320, 1998.

66. Wagner DJ, Coombs DW, Doyle SC: Percutaneous transtracheal ventilation for emergency dental appliance removal. Anesthesiology 62:664, 1985.

67. Warmington A, Hughes T, Walker J, et al: Cricothyroidotomy and transtracheal high frequency jet ventilation for elective laryngeal surgery: An audit of 90 cases. Anaesth Intensive Care 28:711, 2000.

68. Weymuller EA, Paugh D, Pavlin EG, et al: Management of the difficult airway problems with percutaneous transtracheal ventilation. Ann Otol Rhinol Laryngol 96:34, 1987.

27

PERFORMANCE OF RIGID BRONCHOSCOPY

Kevin D. Pereira
Amy C. Hessel

I. HISTORICAL BACKGROUND

Rigid bronchoscopy is a surgical technique that allows visualization of the upper aerodigestive tract from the larynx to the proximal pulmonary branches. Through the use of today's bronchoscopes, it is possible to visualize and manipulate within the airway during spontaneous ventilation. This technique was perfected throughout the 1900s. Because of limitations with lighting, it was difficult to visualize the body's cavities through optical scopes. It was not until 1879 that incandescent light was developed and endoscopy could become more advanced.[16] In addition, the advent of local anesthesia in 1880 made it possible to consider visualizing the aerodigestive tract. In 1881, Mukulicz developed a rigid esophagoscope, and in 1897, Gustave Killian used that esophagoscope and cocaine local anesthesia to remove a foreign body from the bronchus.[10,16] He later developed a rigid bronchoscope that used a reflected light source. Further adjustments have since been made, including the incorporation of a light carrier within the bronchoscope and a separate lumen for administration of inhalational agents.[3] The most significant development was that of telescopic lenses by Hopkins in 1954, which opened the door for fiberoptic bronchoscopy.[9]

II. INDICATIONS FOR BRONCHOSCOPY

Direct examination of the tracheobronchial tree in adults can be preformed with either a rigid or a flexible bronchoscope. Although the flexible bronchoscope has had an increasing role in diagnostic procedures in the adult lower airway, there remain distinct advantages to using the rigid instrument. With its open lumen and rigid construction, this instrument is ideal for operative procedures and stabilization of the airway. The rigid bronchoscope allows relatively rapid access to the airway and can be positioned in any location along the trachea; thus, it can be utilized for patients who are having difficulty with ventilation. Because the bronchoscope can be connected directly to the anesthesia ventilator, it is a valuable tool for maintaining an airway while performing airway procedures. It is this major advantage of the rigid scope over the flexible one, being able to control ventilation safely in a moribund patient, that has led to rigid bronchoscopy being included in the practice guidelines for the management of a difficult airway.[4]

Other indications for adult rigid bronchoscopy include foreign body removal; large diagnostic biopsies; removal of secretions, debris, or obstructing neoplasms; use of an endobronchial laser; control of hemorrhage; control of airway from stenoses or trauma; and placement of airway stents.[16] The indications for endoscopic examination of the pediatric airway are summarized in Table 27-1. An *absolute* contraindication to rigid bronchoscopy is unstable cervical spine injury or disease, or both. Because of the rigid nature of the scopes, it is necessary to hyperextend and turn the neck in order to reach the distal airway. If the patient's neck is too stiff to extend or if there is concern about neurologic injury with spine manipulation, flexible bronchoscopy is the better option for visualizing the trachea and bronchi. However, in both adults and children, the rigid scopes offer a better conduit for surgical procedures involving the airway and foreign body retrieval.

III. INSTRUMENTATION

It is of vital importance that the endoscopist has a full selection of rigid and flexible laryngoscopes and bronchoscopes, including biopsy and extraction forceps, telescopes, a backup light source, and a tracheostomy set readily available in the endoscopy suite. A rigid bronchoscope is a nonflexible metal tube that is tapered and beveled at one end for introduction into the airway. It has ventilating ports at the leading end that facilitate delivery of oxygen and anesthesia. The proximal end has three well-defined openings and a metallic channel that bifurcates the angle between the leading and superior ports. The main opening is the working channel for introduction of telescopes, laser fibers, forceps, and rigid suction cannulas. The inferior port receives the light source and optical prism, and the superior one is usually connected to the anesthetic circuit. Flexible suction catheters and thin wire instruments may be introduced through the metal channel, which is generally kept closed to prevent air leaks and egress of anesthetic gases.

There are different methods of visualizing the airway through a bronchoscope. The older endoscopes have a channel through which a light carrier rod can be placed that illuminates the distal end of the instrument. This is usually attached to a fiberoptic cable connected to an incandescent light source. The more recent ones have a port that allows a prismatic light deflector to be inserted, providing proximal and distal illumination. The amount of illumination produced is directly dependent on the quality and integrity of the fiberoptic cable and the cold light source. Telescopes of various diameters and lengths are introduced into the airway through the bronchoscope for wide-angled and detailed examination of the airway. Their lengths are usually matched with those of the bronchoscopes, and they do not extend beyond the tip of the rigid scope. These can also be used directly through a laryngoscope for a preliminary examination of the airway or instead of the rigid bronchoscope. Most diagnostic bronchoscopies in the pediatric population can be performed without the rigid scope. Bronchoscopes are sized according to their inner diameter and range from 2.5 to 10 mm. The standard adult sizes are 7, 8, and 9 mm in diameter and 40 cm long. The smaller 6- and 6.5-mm scopes are shorter in length, usually 30 to 35 cm. Guidelines for selection of pediatric laryngoscopes and bronchoscopes are given in Table 27-2. A range of suction equipment including rigid metallic cannulas and flexible suction catheters, mucus traps, and filters should be readily available during bronchoscopy. A selection of biopsy and extraction forceps including those with an optical carrier should also be readily available for the procedure.

IV. PREOPERATIVE CONSIDERATIONS

As with many of the otolaryngology procedures, rigid bronchoscopy carries special challenges. Because of the small spaces involved and the need to share the airway, there must be good communication and cooperation between the surgeon and the anesthesiologist. The preoperative evaluation needs to consider not only the status of the airway but also the patient's comorbid conditions. Many adults requiring this type of procedure have underlying pulmonary and cardiac risk factors. It is

Table 27-1 **Indications for Endoscopic Examination of the Airway**

Acute upper airway obstruction
    Inflammatory causes
    Vocal cord dysfunction
    Benign tumors of the larynx (papillomas, hemangiomas)
    Trauma to the laryngotracheal complex

Removal of foreign bodies
Management of tracheal strictures, webs, granulomas
To facilitate laser surgery of the airway
Placement of stents
Evaluation of bronchial obstruction and bronchial biopsy
Bronchoalveolar lavage
Bronchopulmonary toilet

Table 27-2 **Guidelines for Airway Endoscopic Equipment in Children**

Patient's Age	Bronchoscope Size (Karl Storz)	Laryngoscope Size (Parsons)
Premature infant	2.5	8
Full term-6 mo	3-3.5	9
6-18 mo	3.5-3.7	9
2-6 yr	4-5	11
> 6 yr	5-6	13

important to acknowledge the effects of long-term smoking on the lungs and to assess patients appropriately. Routine pulmonary function tests are not always necessary, and much information can be obtained by assessing the patient's tolerance for daily routines such as climbing stairs and walking. Pulmonary reserve should be optimized before the procedure by treating preoperative bronchospasm or infection. Patients who do require formal pulmonary function tests and have forced expiratory volumes less than 50% may be at risk for carbon dioxide retention and hypoxia.

Cardiac function is best screened by assessing the patient's response to daily activities. Patients with daily angina or hypertension with baseline electrocardiographic findings of left ventricular hypertrophy may be at higher risk for cardiac complications. If possible, these issues should be evaluated and optimized before the procedure. Bronchoscopy is occasionally performed as an urgent procedure, and knowledge of risk factors may help both intraoperative and postoperative management. The goal of the preoperative airway evaluation should be to identify the patient with any abnormality that may interfere with mask ventilation or intubation, or both.

Langeron and colleagues[11] outlined several risk factors that may predict difficult bag-mask ventilation (DMV). In a prospective study, they assessed patients for potential risk factors for DMV and then assessed the patients' ability to be mask ventilated and intubated. These risk factors included presence of a beard, body mass index (BMI), age, sex, Mallampati class, mouth opening, thyromental distance, macroglossia, receding mandible, and history of snoring. The only criteria found to be statistically significant for increased difficulty with mask ventilation were age older than 55 years, BMI greater than 26 km/m^2, lack of teeth, presence of a beard, and a history of snoring. The presence of two or more risk factors indicated a high likelihood of DMV (sensitivity 0.72, specificity 0.73). In addition, it was shown in this study, as well as others, that there is a significantly higher incidence of difficult intubation in patients with DMV (30%).[11]

Therefore, special attention should be paid to the patient's neck mobility, mouth opening, and dentition status and the presence of obesity. The Mallampati classification used routinely by anesthesiologists cannot be used alone to predict difficult intubations. Ideally, patients should be kept without anything by mouth for at least 6 hours prior to the procedure in order to reduce the risk of aspiration. However, in the case of emergency, precautions such as cricoid pressure, evacuation of gastric contents, and rapid sequence induction may be necessary.[16]

V. ANESTHESIA FOR BRONCHOSCOPY

Safe bronchoscopy requires excellent communication between the anesthesiologist and the surgeon. The procedure should be discussed in advance and agreed upon by both parties to ensure safe airway management. If required,

a preliminary flexible laryngoscopy can be performed to establish patency of the upper airway and confirm vocal cord mobility. Preoperative sedation, especially with a narcotic agent, is avoided in a patient with signs of airway obstruction or foreign body. An inhalational induction is often performed while vascular access is established. Anesthesia can then be maintained by spontaneous respiration or neuromuscular paralysis followed by positive-pressure ventilation, jet ventilation, or apneic anesthesia with intermittent intubation. Spontaneous assisted ventilation can also be used, and patients have been managed with negative-pressure ventilation techniques.[12]

The goals of anesthesia during bronchoscopy are to keep the patient asleep and reduce reactivity of the airway to permit instrumentation while maintaining adequate oxygen saturation and preventing carbon dioxide retention and acidosis. These goals can be difficult to achieve because of the constant stimulation of the airway by the endoscope, the periodic loss of ventilatory capacity related to the position of the scope in the main stem bronchi, and the inevitable leaks that occur with opening the ports to allow instrumentation and suction. Typically, the induction of anesthesia for a patient undergoing rigid bronchoscopy is similar to a routine intravenous induction and intubation with the exception of using topical lidocaine in the airway before introducing the endoscope. Once the scope is placed, the patient is connected to the ventilator circuit. If positive-pressure ventilation is used, the patient is paralyzed and apneic and the airway maintained entirely through the anesthetic circuit.

Disadvantages of this approach include difficulty with maintaining adequate oxygen saturation because of leaks around the endoscope either from the distal end or whenever instruments are placed through the proximal ports. To avoid this, a widely used alternative is spontaneous assisted ventilation, in which the patient is allowed to breathe spontaneously but is supported with ventilation when the oxygen saturation declines.[12] Another alternative is high-frequency jet ventilation, which allows optimal visibility and easy access for surgical instruments into the airway.[2] A disadvantage of this technique is carbon dioxide retention and acidosis. In addition, the high airway pressures generated can worsen distal airway obstruction by tumors or foreign bodies and increase the risk of air embolism, pneumothorax, and particle dissemination into the lungs.[12] For successful jet ventilation, it is important to predict the patients who may be at risk for hypercapnia (male, overweight, abnormal preoperative lung function) and to monitor both CO_2 levels and airway pressures throughout the procedure.[2]

Children differ from adults in their anesthetic requirements. Premedication is usually not administered to any child younger than 6 months or with impending airway obstruction. For routine diagnostic bronchoscopy, midazolam may be used, depending on the child's response to parental separation. If vascular access has been established, induction may proceed with fentanyl, propofol, oxygen, and sevoflurane (or any other inhalant anesthetic).

Sevoflurane is a fast and safe inhalational agent that is well accepted by children. Additional propofol is used if the anesthesia is not deep enough as assessed clinically by the eye position according to the Guedel classification. Lidocaine spray on the vocal cords helps decrease the overall anesthetic requirements as it reduces airway reactivity. Anticholinergic agents help decrease secretions and reduce operative time. Relaxants are usually administered after cord motion has been confirmed or patency of the upper airway ascertained. Because inhaled anesthetics can be administered only during the periods of ventilation, supplemental propofol has to be administered if the apneic technique is used. During the periods of ventilation, higher concentrations of longer acting inhalational anesthetics such as isoflurane or halothane are administered in order to increase the depth of anesthesia and prolong its effect to cover the apneic periods. Full relaxation is helpful in limiting the amount of inhaled and intravenous anesthetic administered. If the rigid bronchoscope is used, ventilation is carried out through the side port of the bronchoscope and an inhalational technique is used to maintain the depth of anesthesia. In situations where air leaks prevent achieving the proper depth of anesthesia, intermittent boluses of intravenous propofol may be used. For emergence, all inhaled anesthetics are switched off, muscle relaxants are reversed, and the patient is converted to spontaneous ventilation. Lidocaine may be administered to control coughing and laryngospasm. Dexamethasone is used to decrease postoperative edema resulting from instrumentation of the airway and also to help prevent postoperative nausea and vomiting.

VI. SURGICAL TECHNIQUE

Rigid bronchoscopy involves sharing the airway between the surgeon and the anesthesiologist. The patient must be positioned at the head of the bed with a shoulder roll under the shoulders. The neck is flexed on the body and the head extended on the neck. A foam donut is used to stabilize the head in the midline. The occiput is higher than the plane of the table in older children, but an infant or a child can be positioned without a roll under the shoulders and with its head flat on the table in a small donut.[8] Hyperextension of the head tends to displace the larynx anteriorly and misaligns the straight laryngotracheal axis. The patient's eyes should be protected with lubricant and tape, and the upper dentition should be covered with a dental guard. All instruments required for the procedure are placed within reach of the surgeon. In addition to the telescopes, laryngoscopes, and bronchoscope, two endotracheal tubes (ETs) are placed on the Mayo stand or tray (Fig. 27-1). In children, one of these is age and weight appropriate and the other is one or two sizes smaller, depending on the nature of the case.

When the anesthesiologist is comfortable with all medical aspects of the case, anesthesia is induced with

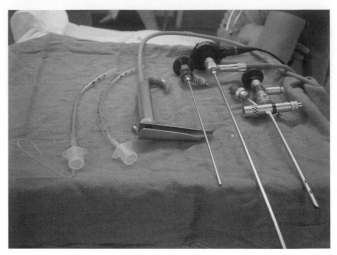

Figure 27-1 Instruments for the initial examination of the lower airway.

mask ventilation (Fig. 27-2). The airway is then turned over to the surgeon, who generally commences the procedure with a preliminary examination using a laryngoscope. The oral and oropharyngeal airway is examined in detail before exposing the supraglottic larynx. After the vocal cords have been seen and patency of the airway confirmed, topical lidocaine may be sprayed on the vocal cords and below to reduce laryngeal reactivity, especially if spontaneous ventilation is to maintained. In children, a slotted laryngoscope may be used to expose the larynx and then 0 degrees and angled telescopes are usually used to perform a detailed examination of the larynx and tracheobronchial airway (Fig. 27-3). This is especially helpful when the airway is compromised and the introduction of a rigid bronchoscope could precipitate complete obstruction. Oxygen may be insufflated through a nasopharyngeal airway or flexible large-bore catheter with its tip through the laryngeal inlet. This gives the surgeon additional working time in the airway.

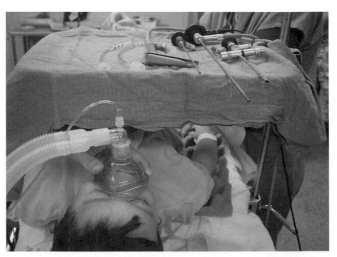

Figure 27-2 Induction of anesthesia with mask ventilation.

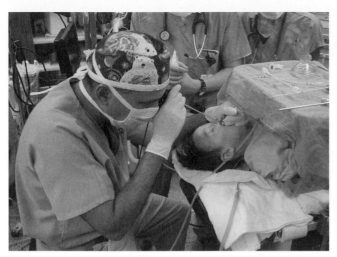

Figure 27-3 Preliminary examination with a laryngoscope and 0-degree telescope.

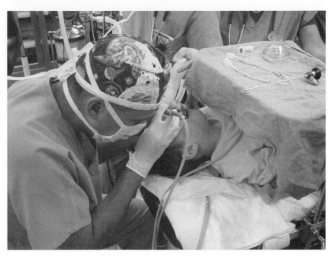

Figure 27-4 Examination with a rigid ventilating bronchoscope connected to the anesthetic circuit.

In an adult, the airway can be accessed by a slotted laryngoscope or by the bronchoscope directly. Often, the size of the adult bronchoscopes precludes the ability to use both instruments in the upper airway at the same time. The light source and suction are once again checked prior to placing the rigid bronchoscope through the right corner of the mouth and deflecting the tongue to the left. The left thumb should be positioned over the maxillary dentition or gingiva in order to prevent the instrument from injuring the maxillary structures as well as guide the scope into the airway. Starting with the scope perpendicular to the plane of the patient, the uvula and posterior pharynx are visualized. As the posterior tongue is picked up by the bronchoscope, it is then rotated to be parallel with the patient's neck and airway. The scope is then guided past the base of the tongue and under the epiglottis. Gently lifting up, the arytenoids and posterior larynx are visualized. The tip of the bronchoscope is then gently passed under the laryngeal surface of the epiglottis and into the posterior larynx. Care is taken not to rock the instrument on the patient's dentition but to protect the dentition with the left thumb and forefinger. This allows the bronchoscope to be guided through the oral cavity and into the upper airway.

The bronchoscope is then directed through the vocal cords and into the immediate subglottis. When the scope is positioned directly above or immediately below the vocal cords, the ventilator can be connected to the appropriate side port on the scope (Fig. 27-4). For ventilation, it is necessary to apply the lens cap to the proximal port in order to prevent anesthetic gas from escaping from the end of the scope. Secretions are usually suctioned with rigid cannulas with vents passed directly through the lumen of the bronchoscope. This can be accomplished only by removing the lens or telescope, or both, and sealing the open end of the scope, resulting in loss of the closed ventilating system. Flexible suction catheters may be introduced through the superior metallic side port without loss of the closed circuit. Although frequent suctioning keeps the airway free of secretions and improves visualization, it can cause mucosal edema and inflammation. In addition, it can result in earlier oxygen desaturation. The lumen of the trachea and bronchi should always be in the center of the operating field in order to avoid inadvertent trauma to the airway. When the carina has been identified, the main stem bronchi can be examined either directly or with telescopes by turning the patient's head in the direction *opposite* to the bronchus being examined. Telescopes can be placed within the bronchoscope at any time after passing through the vocal cords in order to visualize the trachea, carina, or bronchi. The lobar bronchi and segmental airways are better examined with telescopes with straight and angled optical systems.

When the anesthesiologist is comfortable with the patient's gas exchange and ventilation, instrumentation of the airway can begin. For procedures, the bronchoscope can be rested on the protected maxillary gingiva in the edentulous patient or carefully brought to the lateral gingival-labial sulcus in order to protect the dentition. When using larger forceps and suction through the proximal end, ventilation should be stopped to avoid exposing operating room personnel to the inhaled anesthetic gas. The bronchoscope has to be withdrawn periodically to a level above the carina and the instrument sealed to enable maintenance of anesthesia and oxygenation. It is a good rule to reserve all biopsies and other procedures within the lumen of the airway until after a complete examination has been carried out. Bleeding is controlled with neurosurgical cotton pledgets soaked in an oxymetazoline solution. A thorough suction of the tracheobronchial tree should be performed after *any* procedure on the airway to prevent postoperative atelectasis. At the end of the procedure, the bronchoscope is withdrawn under direct vision after notifying the anesthesiologist in advance and the patient ventilated by a mask or ET until emergence from anesthesia.

VII. COMPLICATIONS

The complications of rigid bronchoscopy can occur either intraoperatively or after the procedure. They are usually directly related to the condition of the patient, the anesthetic technique used, the duration and type of procedure, and the expertise of the involved physicians. The complication rate for rigid pediatric bronchoscopy ranges from 2% to 4%.[6] Intraoperative complications include loss of airway, iatrogenic injury to the upper aerodigestive tract, tracheobronchial hemorrhage, and cardiac dysrhythmias including asystole. The loss of the airway is a serious problem that is usually caused by lack of communication between anesthesiologist and surgeon. In a patient with a difficult airway, it is imperative that any repositioning or removal of the bronchoscope be discussed with the anesthesiologist so that he or she is prepared for the transfer of airway responsibility. The patient should be preoxygenated and positioned appropriately to change to mask ventilation.

Iatrogenic injury during bronchoscopy can occur at any level in the upper aerodigestive tract along the course of bronchoscope insertion. The dentition can be damaged, loosened, or lost if not adequately protected with a guard. The bronchoscope can also cause injury to the larynx if improperly inserted. This can include vocal cord edema, hemorrhage, laceration, and even arytenoid dislocation. Hemorrhage usually occurs during biopsies or with inadvertent injury to major vascular structures that may be in an abnormal position or exposed by disease. Poor outcomes are usually due not to blood loss but to aspiration.[6] Immediate changeover to a cuffed ET to seal off tracheal bleeding or protect the uninjured lung may rescue the situation. Dysrhythmias are more often seen in patients with preexisting cardiac disease, and a careful preoperative evaluation should identify those at risk. This is also true for children with congenital heart disease.

Later complications include airway edema, pneumothorax, and pulmonary atelectasis.[16] Edema of the larynx is more likely to be problematic in younger patients in whom the airway is smaller. However, this may be managed without intubation by using humidified oxygen, racemic epinephrine, and systemic steroids. Pneumothorax is rare but may occur with patients requiring high-pressure ventilation or if significant trauma or surgery is taking place within the tracheal lumen. Atelectasis is more likely in the patient with an obstructed distal airway. Both of these complications can be quickly diagnosed with a routine postoperative chest radiograph.

VIII. SPECIAL CONSIDERATIONS

A. FOREIGN BODY REMOVAL

Foreign body removal is probably the most common indication for use of rigid bronchoscopy in the surgical population. Aspiration of a foreign body is common and accounts for approximately 300 to 2000 deaths per year.[8] Most of the aspiration complications occur in children; but regardless of the age, it can lead to serious respiratory problems. The most specific and frequent presenting symptom for foreign body aspiration is a witnessed sudden onset of choking and cough with or without vomiting (penetration syndrome).[15] Other suggestive symptoms include persistent cough, fever, breathlessness, and wheezing. Plain radiographs of the neck and chest are basic preliminary investigations that can be performed, but when they are normal, foreign body ingestion cannot be definitively ruled out. In a multi-institutional review of 1269 foreign body events, 85% were correctly diagnosed in a single physician encounter. However, chest radiographs were reported as normal in 30% of true aspirations. They also found that hyperinflation was more common than atelectasis or pneumonia in patients with a foreign body in the lower airway. In addition, they noted radiopaque objects in 63% of esophageal foreign bodies as opposed to 15% of those in the airway.[1] It is imperative that chest films are taken during both inspiration (Fig. 27-5) and expiration (Fig. 27-6). Obstructive emphysema is noted on the side of the obstruction as the bronchus dilates during inspiration, allowing air to enter around the foreign body but preventing its exit during expiration, producing a ball-valve effect. When in doubt, a fluoroscopic examination of the chest may help locate the area of obstruction. Late radiologic signs include pneumonia, bronchiectasis, and lung abscess.

The diagnosis of a foreign body in the airway requires reasonably prompt removal without compromising safety.

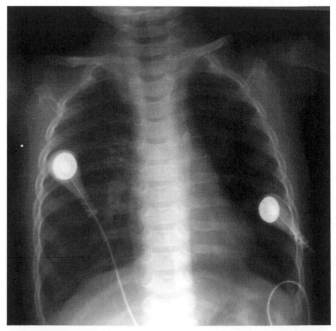

Figure 27-5 Inspiratory chest radiograph of a 5-year-old with a bean lodged in the left main stem bronchus.

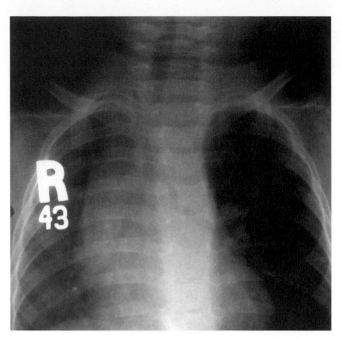

Figure 27-6 Expiratory film of the same patient showing hyperinflation of the left lung with mediastinal shift to the right.

Most patients who are examined in the emergency room with a suspected foreign body have passed the stage of acute airway obstruction and are in relatively stable condition. Frequently, foreign bodies in the airway are considered emergencies, leading to inadequate investigation and preparation of the patient as well as improper attempts at removal.[13] If the patient is not in immediate danger, the procedure can be scheduled for the earliest time when trained operating room personnel, experienced surgeons, and anesthesiologists are available. However, undue delay can result in poor outcomes because of the nature of the foreign body or its movement from the initial site of impaction. This is especially true in the case of organic or vegetative foreign bodies, which may swell as they absorb water and can cause a significant mucosal reaction and obstruction within the lumen of the airway. Aspiration of a disc battery can be considered an absolute emergency as catastrophic complications can occur in as few as 6 to 8 hours. The most common foreign bodies in children are peanuts, carrots, seeds, and plastic toys. In adults, food is most common followed by dental pieces (teeth, dentures) and other objects that may be placed between the lips (e.g., pins, pen caps).[15]

Rigid bronchoscopy under general anesthesia is still the mainstay therapeutic option for removal of airway foreign bodies. This technique is superior to flexible bronchoscopy in that it allows ventilation throughout the procedure as well as allowing various types of instruments into the airway in order to remove the object. It is important to know the characteristics of the foreign body (e.g., sharp, round, plastic, vegetable matter) before the procedure in order to be prepared with the appropriate instruments.

Smaller foreign bodies can be removed through the lumen of the bronchoscope, but larger objects may need to be pulled out as the scope is withdrawn. This may create an unstable airway situation if the foreign body becomes lodged at the level of the larynx. Excellent communication between the surgeon and anesthesiologist is necessary in this situation. If the airway becomes obstructed during the attempt to remove a foreign body, the object may need to be pushed distally in order to reestablish the patency of the airway. If repeated attempts to remove a foreign body fail, a tracheostomy can be made in the proximal trachea in order to remove an object too large to fit through the glottis. Vegetable matter may become edematous and obstruct the airway. In addition, this type of foreign body can cause a granulation tissue reaction, resulting in bleeding and local mucosal trauma. If necessary, staged bronchoscopies can be can be done to accommodate complete removal.

B. HEMORRHAGE

Rigid bronchoscopy is often the technique of choice in the presence of massive hemoptysis. Because the lumen is larger and there is direct access to the lumen of the airway, rigid bronchoscopy is superior to flexible bronchoscopy. It is possible to clear secretions and blood rapidly from the airway and to reestablish ventilation during the procedure. Therapeutic as well as diagnostic procedures can be done, including hemostasis with epinephrine pledgets, balloon tamponade, laser cauterization, and relief of tumor obstruction.[16] In addition, rigid bronchoscopy can assist in endotracheal intubation by directly visualizing the placement of a catheter into the tracheal lumen that can serve as a guidewire for ET placement.

C. AIRWAY STENOSES

The airway below the larynx is divided into the immediate subglottis (starting 5 mm below the vocal cords and extending to the base of the cricoid) and the trachea. Stenoses in these areas can result from a primary disease or a secondary complication related to a mechanical injury. Subglottic stenosis is a finding in diseases such as Wegener's granulomatosis, respiratory papillomatosis, amyloidosis, hemangioma, and various infectious processes such as tuberculosis, syphilis, and diphtheria. The stenoses caused by mechanical trauma may be from endotracheal intubation injury or surgical injury (such as previous laser or tracheotomy).

The mechanism for endotracheal intubation injury is thought to be a pressure erosion of the posterior laryngeal and subglottic mucosa. This can lead to an ischemic process or a mucosal tear, or both. Although most heal spontaneously without incident, ulceration and inflammation sometimes occur. This results in perichondritis, chondritis, and possibly necrosis. Healing from this can lead to scar formation and subsequently narrowing of the airway.

There are many treatment options for subglottic and tracheal stenoses. The most conservative therapy is steroids. These are given systemically or injected locally in an attempt to decrease scar formation. Local injection is done through a direct laryngoscope or rigid bronchoscope. Dilation is another treatment option for stenoses. Dilation is done by performing rigid bronchoscopy and using dilators of increasing diameter or progressively larger ventilating bronchoscopes. Because there is some risk of further iatrogenic injury, this technique is used in very selected cases. Stenting is another option for airway stenoses. The stents are placed by rigid or flexible bronchoscopy. Laser-assisted endoscopic resection of stenoses can also be performed. When stenoses are in the immediate subglottic area, the CO_2 laser can be used with a direct laryngoscope. However, farther into the airway, the neodymium-yttrium-aluminum-garnet (Nd:YAG) laser through an optical fiber is used through a rigid bronchoscope. Despite all of these options for stenoses, this disease process is difficult to treat and often recurs. The only proven successful technique is airway expansion using cartilage grafts or resection of the stenotic segment and direct thyrotracheal anastomosis.

D. STENT PLACEMENT

Stenting the airway has been successful in relieving airway distress with both tumor and benign stenoses as well as tracheal cartilage collapse.[14] The stents used today are usually made of silicon or self-expanding wire mesh. Both types of stents can be placed by bronchoscopy and are utilized to maintain airway patency. Because there are complications with the long-term use of intraluminal stents, they are usually reserved for patients who are not candidates for a surgical procedure or have stenoses not amenable to surgical treatment.

Complications from stents are mostly related to malposition, migration, or obstruction of the stent. Migration tends to occur more frequently with the silicon stents, and various fixation techniques have been tried to prevent the stent from moving. With wire stents, there is less of a problem with migration but a higher risk of obstruction. These lumens can become obstructed by the ingrowth of tumor or granulation tissue. The newer mesh stents have been designed with a thin layer of silicon overlying the wire in order to decrease granulation tissue formation.

All in all, this technique, with or without laser resection, has been successful in relieving ventilatory distress and restoring airway patency.[14] However, because of the possible long-term complications with an indwelling airway stent, it is often used only to improve quality of life and prevent suffocation in otherwise life-threatening conditions.

E. LASER

Lasers are routinely used to relieve airway masses and obstructions. They can be used to cut, coagulate, and vaporize with precise accuracy. As the technology and instrumentation have evolved, it has become possible to use the laser in all parts of the airway and for a variety of different lesions. The CO_2 laser is most commonly used because its wavelength of 10,600 nm can vaporize soft tissues without creating collateral tissue injury. However, it is not possible to send the CO_2 laser wavelength through a fiberoptic cable. In order to access the subglottic and immediate trachea with the CO_2 laser, a bronchoscope coupler must be used.[5]

In order to gain better access to the distal airway, the Nd:YAG laser, with a wavelength of 1060 nm, has become popular for the distal trachea and bronchi. This laser can be passed through a fiberoptic cable, which can pass through a port on a rigid bronchoscope. In addition, it has excellent coagulation properties. However, with this laser there is a risk of deeper penetration and injury to the wall of the airway causing perforation or further scarring. In summary, lasers have become invaluable for relieving airway obstruction caused by stenoses or mass lesions. They can successfully vaporize and cauterize to regain airway patency.

IX. CONCLUSIONS

Rigid bronchoscopy is a surgical technique that has a variety of applications. Despite the advances with flexible bronchoscopy, rigid bronchoscopy is still used for visualization and direct manipulation of the airway. Because of the wide lumen of the rigid bronchoscope, it is possible to perform biopsies, remove foreign bodies, and use lasers to relieve obstructions. In addition, it is possible to ventilate through the bronchoscope, allowing the patient to be under general anesthesia with adequate airway protection during the procedure. It is an excellent tool for emergent airway situations such as acute hemorrhage or impending airway compromise. Despite the advantages, performing rigid bronchoscopy requires training in anatomy and instrumentation as well as a well-trained anesthesia team familiar with the problems of sharing the airway with the operating surgeon. Communication between the surgeon and the anesthesiologist is as important as the performance of the procedure itself. When appropriate, rigid bronchoscopy is a valuable tool for airway management.

REFERENCES

1. Baharloo F, Veyckemans F, Francis C, et al: Tracheobronchial foreign bodies: Presentation and management in children and adults. Chest 115:1357-1362, 1999.
2. Biro P, Layer M, Wiedemann K, et al: Carbon dioxide elimination during high-frequency jet ventilation for rigid bronchoscopy. Br J Anaesth 84:635-637, 2000.
3. Boyd AD: Chevalier Jackson: The father of American bronchoesophagology. Ann Thorac Surg 57:502-505, 1994.
4. Caplan RA, Benumof JL, Berry FA, et al: Practice guidelines for management of the difficult airway. Anesthesiology 98:1269-1277, 2003.
5. Colt HG, Harrell JH: Therapeutic rigid bronchoscopy allows level of care changes in patients with acute respiratory failure from central airway obstruction. Chest 112:202-206, 1997.
6. Hoeve LJ, Rombout J, Meursing AEE: Complications of rigid laryngobronchoscopy in children. Int J Pediatr Otorhinolaryngol 26:47-56, 1993.
7. Holinger LD: Diagnostic endoscopy of the pediatric airway. Laryngoscope 99:346-348, 1989.
8. Holinger LD : Foreign bodies of the airway and esophagus. In Holinger LD, Lusk RP, Green CG (eds): Pediatric Laryngology and Bronchoesophagology. Philadelphia, Lippincott-Raven, 1997, pp 233-251.
9. Ikeda S, Yanai N, Ishikawa S: Flexible bronchofiberscope. Keio J Med 17:1-16, 1968.
10. Killian G: Ein vier Jahre lang in der rechten lunge steckendes Knochenstuck auf natulichem Wege enfernt. Dtsch Med Wochenschr 25:161-163, 1900.
11. Langeron O, Masso E, Huraux C, et al: Prediction of mask ventilation. Anesthesiology 92:1229-1236, 2000.
12. Natalini G, Cavaliere S, Vitacca M, et al: Negative pressure ventilation vs. spontaneous assisted ventilation during rigid bronchoscopy. Acta Anaesthesiol Scand 42:1063-1069, 1998.
13. Reilly J, Thompson J, MacArthur C, et al: Pediatric aerodigestive foreign body injuries are complications related to timeliness of diagnosis. Laryngoscope 107:17-20, 1997.
14. Shapshay SM, Valdez TA: Bronchoscopic management of benign stenosis. Chest Surg Clin North Am 11:749-768, 2001.
15. Swanson KL, Edell ES: Tracheobronchial foreign bodies. Chest Surg Clin North Am 11:861-871, 2001.
16. Wain JC: Rigid bronchoscopy: The value of a venerable procedure. Chest Surg Clin North Am 11:691-699, 2001.

PERCUTANEOUS DILATIONAL CRICOTHYROTOMY AND TRACHEOSTOMY

Richard J. Melker
Karen M. Kost

I. CONTROL OF THE AIRWAY

In the vast majority of instances, anesthesiologists control and maintain the airway by endotracheal intubation. However, despite extensive training and skill, every anesthesiologist occasionally encounters an airway that cannot be managed by endotracheal intubation or in which it is contraindicated. In the operating room (OR), three general scenarios have been repeatedly observed and reported during attempts to control the airway: (1) the airway can be easily controlled by mask ventilation and endotracheal intubation; (2) the airway can be mask ventilated but cannot be intubated; and (3) rarely, the airway cannot be mask ventilated or intubated. It is every anesthesiologist's nightmare to encounter a difficult airway (DA) that he or she is unable to establish and maintain.

A. ADVERSE OUTCOMES

Adverse outcomes related to respiratory events accounted for the largest class of injury in the American Society of Anesthesiologists (ASA) closed claims study, with brain damage or death occurring in 85% of cases.[22] Three mechanisms of injury were responsible for three fourths of the adverse respiratory events: inadequate ventilation (38%), esophageal intubation (18%), and difficult endotracheal intubation (17%). Inadequate ventilation and esophageal intubation are largely preventable with better monitoring; failed endotracheal intubation is not.

There are several clinical situations (i.e., orofacial or neck injury, patients who are assessed preoperatively to have DAs, and those who have an unexpected DA after induction of general anesthesia) that may require alternative means of airway management. Five to 35 of 10,000 patients (0.05% to 0.35%) reportedly cannot be endotracheally intubated.[29,41,68,95] Approximately 0.01 to 2.0 of 10,000 patients are difficult to mask ventilate and intubate.[9,108] Failure to provide adequate ventilation and oxygenation is the primary cause of cardiac arrest during general anesthesia.[49,61,104]

B. AMERICAN SOCIETY OF ANESTHESIOLOGISTS PRACTICE GUIDELINES

Because some degree of airway difficulty is often encountered during attempted intubation and serious adverse outcomes occur, the ASA Task Force on Management of the Difficult Airway published "Practice guidelines for management of the difficult airway" in 1993.[103] Since publication of the first edition of this textbook, these guidelines have been updated to reflect the availability of new airway adjuncts and additional knowledge gained since 1993.[3] The ASA guidelines contain a DA algorithm and provide strategies for evaluating, preparing for, and intubating the DA. They also consider the relative merits and feasibility of alternative management choices, such as nonsurgical versus surgical techniques for the initial approach to ventilation, awake intubation versus intubation after induction of general anesthesia, and preservation versus ablation of spontaneous ventilation. Development of primary and alternative strategies for awake intubation and intubation after the induction of general anesthesia is emphasized. The algorithm describes both emergency and nonemergency pathways of managing the airway if intubation fails. Both ASA guidelines also suggest that equipment suitable for "emergency surgical airway access" be among the contents of a portable storage unit readily available in the OR. Among the suggested emergency airway procedures is cricothyrotomy, a technique for gaining and securing airway access through the cricothyroid space. Although the ASA guidelines offer a stepwise approach to the patient with a DA, they primarily focus on difficulties encountered in the OR, with strategies to anticipate and treat in this environment.

C. HOSPITAL-WIDE ROLE OF THE ANESTHESIOLOGIST

As the recognized airway expert, the anesthesiologist is often called upon to manage the airways of critically ill patients in other hospital environments, such as the emergency department (ED), wards, diagnostic areas (i.e., radiology), or intensive care units (ICUs). The anesthesiologist may be called either immediately or after other physicians have attempted unsuccessfully to secure the airway or failed to recognize the futility of standard intubation techniques. In rare instances, the availability of a physician skilled in the technique of cricothyrotomy may be lifesaving. It is altogether appropriate that this individual be the anesthesiologist. Appropriate equipment for cricothyrotomy should be available throughout the hospital or as part of an emergency airway kit. No data exist regarding how frequently anesthesiologists are called to secure an airway outside the OR, but in many hospitals this responsibility seems to be handled more frequently by emergency medicine physicians. No studies have attempted to compare the skills and success rates among anesthesiologists and critical care medicine, emergency, and ear, nose, and throat physicians in handling the DA, nor are they likely to be performed. Suffice it to say, each institution should have a clear plan for alerting qualified individuals when emergency airway support is required in different areas of the hospital.

D. ROLE OF THE OTOLARYNGOLOGIST

The otolaryngologist plays a critical role in airway management by contributing a skill set that is different from yet complementary to that of the anesthesiologist. Circumstances may range from well-controlled elective situations to near-panic "last-ditch" attempts to establish an airway when all else has failed. The otolaryngologist possesses an unparalleled knowledge of the three-dimensional anatomy of the upper aerodigestive tract and the variations encountered in pathologic circumstances. This, as well as expert endoscopy skills, may assist the anesthesiologist in establishing a DA.

E. RENEWED INTEREST IN CRICOTHYROTOMY

Chevalier Jackson was largely responsible for discouraging the use of cricothyrotomy for almost five decades.[56] Only in the 1970s, when surgeons sought a safe, effective alternative to surgical tracheostomy, did cricothyrotomy begin to gain generalized acceptance.[18,19]

Interest in cricothyrotomy as an alternative to endotracheal intubation is largely the result of the development of emergency medicine as a distinct specialty and the frequent treatment of patients with DAs in the prehospital and ED environments. Emergency physicians and prehospital providers often encounter patients with life-threatening injuries who cannot be intubated by conventional routes and who need immediate and definitive treatment. The majority of literature dealing with the use of cricothyrotomy in emergent situations appears in the emergency medicine literature. The first edition of this textbook focused on a lengthy and sometimes contentious debate concerning which *surgical* technique is preferable in the prehospital and ED settings.* Sadly, only two publications, both cadaver studies, compared surgical with percutaneous dilational cricothyrotomy, one of which used a device that is no longer commercially available.[23,32]

For anesthesiologists, interest in percutaneous dilational tracheostomy and cricothyrotomy increased as part of a trend toward less invasive surgical procedures, often performed over guidewires. Although anesthesiologists are familiar with the Seldinger technique for the insertion of vascular catheters, many may still be unaware that airway devices using the same technology have been developed. Surveys performed in both the United States and the United Kingdom indicate that many anesthesiologists lack formal training in cricothyrotomy, although more do in the United Kingdom.[34,86]

Cricothyrotomy can be performed surgically, percutaneously with or without a guidewire, or by placement of a transtracheal catheter. There remain many questions about which of these techniques is best suited for a particular clinical situation. Cricothyrotomy is an alternative to a "surgical" airway (tracheostomy) in the emergency and nonemergency limbs of the ASA DA algorithm. In the nonemergency sequence, it may be elected when intubation is unsuccessful but the patient can be adequately mask ventilated. If other alternatives of airway management such as fiberoptic bronchoscopy (FOB) or blind intubation fail, either nonsurgical or surgical cricothyrotomy can be employed to secure the airway. Likewise, cricothyrotomy can be used in the emergency situation when the airway cannot be ventilated or intubated.

No guidelines similar to the ASA guidelines exist for treatment of the DA outside the OR. The algorithm could be modified and adapted for non-OR settings (i.e., in the ED or ICU). This chapter reviews the various approaches to cricothyrotomy (used interchangeably in the medical literature with coniotomy, cricothyroidotomy, cricothyrostomy, intercricothyrotomy, and minitracheostomy) with an emphasis on percutaneous dilational techniques and also percutaneous dilational tracheostomy. Use in truly emergent situations is stressed. Areas of continuing controversy regarding the timing and appropriateness of cricothyrotomy by anesthesiologists are discussed.

F. INTEREST IN PERCUTANEOUS TRACHEOSTOMY

In 1909, Chevalier Jackson described the technical details of tracheostomy and in so doing standardized

---

*References 5, 7, 17, 20, 22, 30, 31, 36, 45, 50, 65.

the procedure. The subsequent dramatic decrease in morbidity and mortality was such that tracheostomy became solidly integrated into the surgical armamentarium. This original description has stood the test of time and persists as the "gold standard" against which other techniques are compared to this day.

Interest in percutaneous techniques emerged 20 years ago for a variety of reasons. These ranged from rapid airway access in emergency situations to converting from intubation to tracheostomy in the ICU setting. The rationale for developing such a procedure stemmed, at least in part, from changes in the delivery, accessibility, and cost of health care. Over half of modern-day tracheotomies are performed on intubated ICU patients.[78] Traditionally, these patients are taken to the OR. Transporting these critically ill individuals is not without risk.[34,56] Furthermore, such an approach uses precious OR resources and time, all at a substantial cost. Performing the procedure percutaneously at the bedside in the ICU obviates the necessity for the OR, possibly reduces the cost, and eliminates transport risks. Several different techniques of percutaneous tracheostomy were developed, described, and published, with mixed results. Early reports of serious complications dampened enthusiasm, particularly among surgeons. Only when the differences between techniques were elucidated, the indications for the procedure clarified, and technical refinements introduced did percutaneous tracheostomy regain credibility as a worthy procedure. Percutaneous dilatational tracheostomy with endoscopic guidance has emerged as the technique of choice and is a simple and safe bedside procedure.

II. DEFINITION AND CLASSIFICATION OF CRICOTHYROTOMY

A. CRICOTHYROTOMY

Cricothyrotomy is a technique for providing an opening in the space between the anterior inferior border of the thyroid cartilage and the anterior superior border of the cricoid cartilage for the purpose of gaining access to the airway.[21] This area is considered to be the most accessible part of the respiratory tree below the glottis.

There are many classification schemes for cricothyrotomy. The procedure has been classified, based on the urgency of the clinical situation, as either emergent or elective. Emergent cricothyrotomy may be done in the prehospital setting, in the ED, ICU, or OR. Elective cricothyrotomy is usually done prior to surgery in the OR. It may also be performed in critically ill patients in the ICU at the bedside. Depending on the technique used, the procedure may also be classified as nonsurgical or surgical. The nonsurgical approach can be achieved either by needle puncture or percutaneously over a guidewire after a small skin incision, with or without cricothyroid membrane (CTM) incision.

We choose to classify cricothyrotomy into three broad technical categories, considering emergent techniques only. The first and least invasive are techniques utilizing a needle or over-the-needle catheter placed directly into the cricothyroid space without a skin incision. We prefer to call these techniques transtracheal catheter ventilation, without reference to the frequency of ventilation or the pressures required to ventilate by these techniques. Although transcricoid ventilation is a more descriptive term, we bow to the convention of using the term *transtracheal ventilation*. The techniques have in common insertion without prior skin incision and use devices with a caliber insufficient to deliver tidal volumes and flow rates at peak inspiratory pressures usually provided by conventional ventilators. Therefore, special high-pressure systems are often required to provide adequate ventilation with the use of this technique.

The second category includes techniques requiring an initial skin incision (and often an incision of the CTM), followed by introduction of a guidewire inserted through a needle or catheter placed through the incision into the cricothyroid space. An airway catheter is then introduced over a dilator threaded over the guidewire. (We use the term *airway catheter* to describe "cricothyrotomy" tubes or tracheostomy tubes inserted through the cricothyroid space.) These techniques allow the ultimate insertion of an airway considerably larger than the initial needle or catheter, often of sufficient internal diameter (ID) to allow ventilation with conventional ventilation devices, suctioning, and spontaneous ventilation. We refer to this as percutaneous dilational cricothyrotomy. Some authors substitute the term *dilatational* for dilational; we use them interchangeably.

The last category of cricothyrotomy techniques is surgical cricothyrotomy. This involves the use of a scalpel and other surgical instruments to create an opening between the skin and the cricothyroid space. A tracheostomy or endotracheal tube (ET) is then inserted. When properly performed, this technique allows insertion of a tube of an ID sufficient to allow conventional ventilation, suctioning, and spontaneous ventilation.

B. TRACHEOSTOMY

1. Surgical or "Open" Tracheostomy

Surgical tracheostomy, as described by Chevalier Jackson, is a means of providing an airway through the cervical trachea, and it remains the standard against which all other procedures must be compared. Classically, the procedure is performed in the OR under general or local anesthesia, as dictated by the clinical situation. Open tracheostomy may also be performed at the bedside in the ICU or in the ED in urgent situations. Following an initial skin incision, sharp dissection is carried out to the thyroid isthmus, which is divided. The cervical trachea is then incised and a tracheostomy tube inserted.

2. Percutaneous Tracheostomy

Percutaneous tracheostomy also provides an airway through the cervical trachea but differs technically. Although there are many different described methods of performing percutaneous tracheostomy, they all begin with an initial puncture through the skin into the trachea, which is then "enlarged," by either dilatation or some sort of spreading forceps, to a size that allows placement of an appropriate tracheostomy tube. These techniques are used only in patients with an established airway (ET or laryngeal mask airway) and are therefore most suitable for intubated ICU patients. Use in emergency situations is contraindicated and indeed is an invitation to disaster.

The Fantoni technique is based on retrograde dilatation of an initial tracheal puncture. During the procedure dilatation is carried out alongside the ET, which must be changed once, with potential loss of the airway. The tracheostomy tube is brought out in a retrograde fashion through the cervical trachea and skin. This technique is used primarily in Italy, its site of origin, but has found little applicability in North America because it is lengthy to perform and involves potential loss of the airway.

The Griggs guidewire dilating forceps technique involves placing a guidewire through an initial puncture site. The area is forcibly enlarged with the use of a speculum-like instrument inserted over the guidewire and into the trachea. The procedure as originally described is blind and subject to complications such as false passage and subcutaneous emphysema. Concurrent endoscopic visualization reduces these risks, although bleeding[65] may be a problem because of "tearing" of adjacent structures when inserting and opening the forceps. This technique, although used in Europe, is used infrequently, if at all, in North America.

The Ciaglia technique, also known as percutaneous dilatational tracheostomy, involves making a very small skin incision, introducing a needle into the trachea, and subsequently bluntly dilating the aperture to allow insertion of the preselected tracheostomy tube. As originally described, this procedure is blind, but it is increasingly performed under continuous endoscopic guidance, with step-by-step visualization from beginning to end. Of the percutaneous approaches described, the Ciaglia technique with continuous endoscopic visualization is probably the safest and is the most widely used in North America.

III. HISTORICAL PERSPECTIVE

A. EARLY HISTORY OF SURGICAL AIRWAY CONTROL

Surgical manipulation of the trachea for emergent airway control is one of the oldest invasive procedures documented.[78] It was performed in ancient Egypt and India over 3000 years ago. Tracheostomy was mentioned in the writings and illustrations of the great Greek physician Galen (AD 130 to 200). He provided anatomic drawings of the airway and favored a vertical rather than horizontal incision in emergencies. He based his anatomic knowledge on dissections of animals and assumed that the structures were identical in the human body.[77] Galen also stated that Asclepiades (124 to 56 BC), who practiced in Rome, recommended opening the trachea in its upper part to prevent suffocation.[96] Antyllus (approximately AD 150) detailed both the indications and technique of tracheostomy, advocating a transverse incision between two rings.[96]

Galenic teaching persisted for over 1300 years until Andreas Wesele Vesalius (AD 1515 to 1564) published *de Humani Corporis Fabrica*, detailing the first correct description of human anatomy.[77] Vesalius secretly conducted extensive dissection of human cadavers and, at age 28, published his landmark work in seven volumes. Included was a detailed description of tracheostomy—control of the airway with the use of a cane or reed and assisted ventilation of the lung. Interestingly, he allegedly performed a tracheostomy and experimentally inflated the lungs of a dead Spanish nobleman. The nobleman's heart was reported to beat again. His action brought outrage in the medical and clerical community. He was condemned by the Spanish Inquisition to a pilgrimage to the Holy Land, and he died along the way in a shipwreck on an island near Greece. During the next 300 years, very few reports were published regarding the surgical control of the airway and were primarily limited to experimental control of breathing in laboratory animals. In *Respiratory Changes of Intrathoracic Pressure*, published in 1892, Samuel Meltzer described the insertion of breathing tubes through tracheostomy and successfully controlling ventilation in curarized animals.[77] In France, Armand Trousseau recognized the importance of emergency tracheostomy in airways compromised by upper airway obstruction, diphtheria, and massive infection in the oropharynx and neck.

B. CONDEMNATION OF "HIGH" TRACHEOSTOMY

In 1909, Chevalier Jackson, Sr,[57] published his first critical assessment of the airway management techniques of that time. He advocated formal tracheostomy as the preferred method of surgical airway management and emphasized that surgical incision, rather than a tracheal stab, should be performed in cases of an obstructed larynx. Jackson observed many of his tracheotomized patients for over 30 years. In 1921, he published the results of 200 cases of chronic laryngeal and subglottic stenosis.[56] Thirty cases of laryngeal stenosis were attributed to laryngeal inflammation and cartilage necrosis associated with the primary disease process necessitating the tracheostomy. The remaining 170 patients had subglottic stenosis judged to be due to the surgical procedure, of whom 158 had a previous "high" tracheostomy. In 32 cases, the opening was made through the CTM and thyroid cartilage. He condemned this type of procedure and advocated that emergency tracheostomy be performed lower over the cervical trachea. Unfortunately, the high tracheostomy that Jackson referred to involved division of the cricoid (or thyroid) cartilage. Modern techniques of cricothyrotomy utilize only division or dilatation of the CTM, or both.[115] In addition, the underlying pathology for which cricothyrotomy was indicated in 1920 differs greatly from modern indications. Most of Jackson's patients had inflammatory lesions involving the upper airway (acute laryngeal edema from diphtheria, epiglottitis, streptococcal laryngitis, syphilis, tuberculosis of the larynx, Ludwig's angina, angioneurotic edema, and other oropharyngeal infection), predisposing them to subsequent airway stenosis. Furthermore, there were no antibiotics or biocompatible ETs available at that time.

C. RENEWED INTEREST IN CRICOTHYROTOMY

For over half a century, the use of cricothyrotomy was almost universally condemned, largely because of fear of chronic subglottic stenosis. In 1969, Toye and Weinstein[105] first described a technique for percutaneous tracheostomy. It was based on the premise that a functional tracheal airway could be more rapidly and safely achieved percutaneously than with Jackson's method of surgical dissection. The technique involves inserting a needle into the trachea and dilating the resultant needle tract to allow placement of a breathing catheter.

Cricothyrotomy made a popular comeback when, in 1976, two Denver cardiothoracic surgeons, Brantigan and Grow,[18] published the results of 655 consecutive cricothyrotomies in which there were minimal complications and no reported incidence of subglottic stenosis. Subsequently, other clinical and experimental series have been reported, and cricothyrotomy has become generally accepted. The procedure was found to be faster, simpler, less invasive, and less likely to cause bleeding than tracheostomy. It also involves less morbidity and mortality than emergency tracheostomy, making it desirable as an emergency technique for gaining immediate airway control. Various modifications of the original technique have been developed. The use of the Seldinger technique for insertion, as described by Corke and Cranswick in 1988,[28] enhances the safety of the procedure. The use of a guidewire and the passing of a dilator to create a channel reduce the chance of incorrect placement and damage to surrounding blood vessels. Detailed insertion instructions for a variety of cricothyrotomy and tracheostomy devices are given later in this chapter.

IV. ANATOMY AND PHYSIOLOGY

Safe and rapid performance of cricothyrotomy requires a thorough knowledge of cricothyroid space anatomy and its relationship to other structures in the neck. The CTM (ligament) measures 10 mm in height and 22 mm in width and is composed mostly of yellow elastic tissue.[21]

It covers the cricothyroid space and is located in the anterior neck between the thyroid cartilage superiorly and the cricoid cartilage inferiorly. The cricothyroid space can be readily identified by palpating a slight dip or indentation in the skin immediately below the laryngeal prominence.

The CTM consists of a central anterior triangular portion (conus elasticus) and two lateral parts. The thicker and stronger conus elasticus narrows above and broadens out below, connecting the thyroid to the cricoid cartilage. It lies subcutaneously in the midline and is often crossed horizontally in its upper third by the superior cricothyroid vessels. To minimize the possibility of bleeding, the CTM should be incised at its inferior third. The two lateral parts are thinner, lie close to the laryngeal mucosa, and extend from the superior border of the cricoid cartilage to the inferior margin of the true vocal cords. On either side, the CTM is bordered by the cricothyroid muscle. Also lateral to the membrane are venous tributaries from the inferior thyroid and anterior jugular veins. Because the vocal cords usually lie a centimeter above the cricothyroid space, they are not commonly injured, even during emergency cricothyrotomy. The anterior jugular veins run vertically in the lateral aspect of the neck and are usually spared injury; however, tributaries may occasionally course over the cricothyroid space and be damaged during the procedure. Characteristically, the CTM does not calcify with age and lies immediately underneath the skin.

Variations in the anatomy and dimensions of the CTM are common. A comprehensive study of the anatomy of the cricothyroid space was reported by Caparosa and Zavatsky,[21] describing the detailed structure of 51 human larynges. They showed that the anterior cricothyroid space is trapezoidal in shape and has a cross-sectional area of approximately 2.9 cm. The mean distance between the anterior borders of the inferior thyroid cartilage and the superior cricoid cartilage is 9 mm (range 5 to 12 mm), whereas the width of the anterior cricothyroid space ranges from 27 to 32 mm. Kirchner[62] demonstrated that the cricothyroid space is not much larger than 7 mm in its vertical dimension and that the space may be narrowed further by contraction of the cricothyroid muscle. The vertical distance between the undersurface of the true vocal cords and the lower anterior edge of the thyroid cartilage has been reported to be 5 to 11 mm.[64] Bennett and colleagues[10] studied 13 fresh adult cadavers and found the vertical height of the CTM from the superior border of the cricoid cartilage to the inferior border of the thyroid cartilage in the midline to vary from 8 to 19 mm with a mean of 13.69 mm, a somewhat greater distance that can probably be explained by the fresh rather than fixed state of the specimens.

There is also considerable variation in both the arterial and venous vessel pattern in the neck area surrounding the CTM. Although the arteries always lie deep to the pretracheal fascia and are easily avoided during a skin incision, veins may be found in the pretracheal fascia and between the pretracheal and superficial cervical fascia.[66]

Little and coworkers[66] showed that the classical pattern of small bilateral cricothyroid arteries was seen only in a minority of the 27 cadavers dissected. Sixty-two percent of the cadavers had one or more vascular structures vertically crossing anterior to the CTM, predisposing them to damage during cricothyrotomy.

Bennett and colleagues[10] also confirmed the frequent presence of a small cricothyroid artery, which is a branch of the superior thyroid artery crossing the upper portion of the CTM and anastomosing with the artery on the other side. To locate the CTM, external visible and palpable anatomic landmarks are utilized (Fig. 28-1).[48] The laryngeal prominence (thyroid cartilage, Adam's apple) and the hyoid bone above it are readily palpable. The CTM usually lies one to one-and-a-half fingerbreadths below the laryngeal prominence. The cricoid cartilage is also easily felt below the CTM. It should take less than 5 seconds to identify these landmarks. Their importance must be emphasized because it is disastrous to place the cricothyroid tube into the thyrohyoid space instead of the cricothyroid space. Conscious effort to identify these landmarks reduces the possibility of committing this preventable error. There are instances in which the normal anatomy may be distorted and identification of these landmarks is difficult. In such cases, the suprasternal notch may be used as an alternative marker. The small finger of the right hand should be placed in the patient's suprasternal notch, followed by placement of the ring, long, and index fingers adjacent to each other in a stepwise fashion up the neck, with each finger touching the one below it.[113] When the head is in the neutral position, the index finger is usually on or near the CTM.

V. INDICATIONS AND CONTRAINDICATIONS

A. CRICOTHYROTOMY

Cricothyrotomy is considered by many to be the standard approach to airway management when orotracheal or nasotracheal intubation and FOB have failed.[68,90,113] In the ED, cricothyrotomy is indicated for immediate airway control in patients with maxillofacial, cervical spine, head, neck, and multiple trauma and in other patients in whom endotracheal intubation is impossible to perform or contraindicated. It is also used for the immediate relief of upper airway obstruction. In the OR and in the ICU, the technique is indicated when conventional methods of intubation fail, such as in patients with traumatic facial injuries, in whom other techniques of airway access are difficult or impossible to perform. Cricothyrotomy can also be used as an alternative to tracheostomy in patients with recent sternotomy who need airway access because the incision does not communicate with the mediastinal tissue planes.

Emergency cricothyrotomy has largely replaced emergency tracheostomy in an ED setting because of its simplicity, rapidity, and minimal morbidity. Use of emergency tracheostomy is limited and indicated only in instances

Figure 28-1 Anatomic landmarks of the neck. (From Heffner JE, Sahn SA: The technique of tracheostomy and cricothyroidotomy. J Crit Illness 2:79, 1987. Illustration by William B. Westwood, MS, AMI, copyright 1987.)

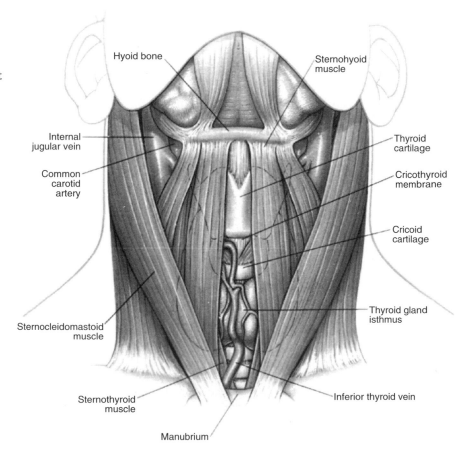

of direct laryngeal fractures and emergent airway management in infants and small children.[84] Laryngeal trauma may be accompanied by local edema, hemorrhage, subcutaneous emphysema, and damage to either thyroid or cricothyroid cartilage, precluding the performance of cricothyrotomy. Cricothyrotomy is difficult to perform in pediatric patients because the larynx is smaller and funnel shaped with the narrowest portion at the cricoid cartilage. Their airways contain less fibrous supporting tissue and have only loose mucous membrane attachments in the airway inlet.[69]

Absolute and relative contraindications to cricothyrotomy are rare. Patients who have been intubated translaryngeally for more than 3 days (many authors state 7 days) should not undergo cricothyrotomy because of the propensity to develop subglottic stenosis. Also, those with preexisting laryngeal diseases, such as cancer, acute or chronic inflammation, or epiglottitis, have a higher morbidity when cricothyrotomy is performed. Distortion of the normal neck anatomy by disease or injury may render the technique impossible. Normal anatomic landmarks may be distorted, making identification of the CTM difficult. Lastly, bleeding diathesis and history of coagulopathy predispose the patient to hemorrhage, making the procedure extremely dangerous.

As previously stated, infants and children in whom anatomic landmarks are difficult to identify are largely precluded. Cricothyrotomy is technically problematic to perform in the pediatric population and should be performed with extreme caution in children younger than 10 years. It should not be performed at all in children younger than 6 years unless a wire can be placed in the cricothyroid space and placement within the trachea can be verified. Emergency tracheostomy under controlled OR conditions is the preferred choice.[72,98]

Physicians who are unfamiliar or inexperienced with the technique are discouraged from performing the procedure without adequate supervision from a more senior or knowledgeable member of the medical team. Inexperience has been implicated as the most important contributory factor in cricothyroid complications.[35,48]

B. PERCUTANEOUS DILATIONAL TRACHEOSTOMY

Percutaneous dilatational tracheostomy (PCT) is indicated only in adult intubated patients (Table 28-1). Significantly, this population of patients accounts for close to two thirds of all tracheostomies performed today.[78] The more common reasons for converting from endotracheal or nasotracheal intubation to tracheostomy include:

- Removing the ET
- Aid in weaning from mechanical respiration
- Facilitating pulmonary toilet
- Upper airway obstruction

Anatomic suitability for this procedure must be determined preoperatively with the patient's neck extended.

Table 28-1 **Indications and Contraindications for Percutaneous Tracheostomy**

Indications
Adult intubated intensive care unit patients
Contraindications
Inability to palpate cricoid
Midline neck mass
High innominate artery
Uncorrected coagulopathy
Unprotected airway
Children
Positive end-expiratory pressure ≥ 20 cm H_2O

Maximum neck extension increases the length of the cervical trachea and defines critical anatomic landmarks such as the cricoid cartilage and sternal notch. A contraindication to the procedure is the inability to palpate the cricoid cartilage above the sternal notch. Similarly, the patient with a midline neck mass, high innominate artery, or large thyroid gland should undergo open surgical tracheostomy in the OR. Coagulopathies are common in this population of patients and should be corrected preoperatively. Platelets should be 50,000 or greater (and functional) and the International Normalized Ratio (INR) corrected to 1.5 or less. Patients requiring a positive end-expiratory pressure (PEEP) of 20 cm H_2O or greater are at high risk for complications such as subcutaneous emphysema and pneumothorax and should undergo surgical tracheostomy in the OR.

PCT is absolutely contraindicated in nonintubated patients with acute airway compromise. The procedure is too lengthy (2 to 10 minutes) and requires bronchoscopic visualization through an ET. PCT is completely unsuitable in the pediatric population. Reasons include the different airway anatomy and dimensions in children and the technical difficulties of maintaining adequate ventilation with a bronchoscope within a small ET (see Table 28-1).

VI. CRICOTHYROTOMY TECHNIQUES AND DEVICES

The focus of this chapter is percutaneous dilational techniques. Surgical cricothyrotomy and transtracheal catheter ventilation are discussed in detail elsewhere in this text. However, these techniques are described briefly in the context of relative ease of use and comparative complication rates. To some extent, these procedures overlap. Similarities and differences are emphasized. Direct needle puncture cricothyrotomy, a technique that has largely fallen into disfavor, is also briefly discussed.

A. DIRECT NEEDLE PUNCTURE CRICOTHYROTOMY

Numerous large-bore, straight and curved metal needles have been developed and described for direct puncture cricothyrotomy (Fig. 28-2). With some sets, an incision is recommended before insertion; with others, it is not. The tip may have a sharp cutting edge for use without a skin incision or may be blunted, in which case an incision is needed. A sharp-tipped trocar coaxially loaded inside the cannula is another variation. The cannulas described by Safar and Penninckx[93] and Pridmore[85] and the Abelson device discussed subsequently are typical.

Abbrecht and coauthors[1] evaluated the insertion forces and risk of complications caused by a number of cricothyrotomy devices, including the Abelson (Gilbert Surgical Instruments, Bellmawr, NJ) direct puncture device. The Abelson required higher initial penetration forces, was the only device that required torquing, and had the highest complication rate of the devices tested. (It is unclear whether this device is still commercially available.) Ravlo and associates[87] compared another direct puncture device (essentially a large, straight hypodermic needle) with the Nu-Trake (Smiths Medical, Keene, NH) device. Both previously trained and untrained users had significantly lower success rates with the direct puncture devices. Fortunately, these have largely fallen out of favor but may still be found on "crash carts" or in other emergency equipment sets.

Rusch (Duluth, GA) presently markets the QuickTrach, which features a stainless steel needle loaded inside a plastic breathing tube and attached to a syringe. The device is used by puncturing the skin and CTM with the needle, aspirating air to verify placement in the airway, and leaving the plastic breathing tube (similar to a tracheostomy tube) in place as the needle is withdrawn. A single reference (in German) from 1990 evaluated this

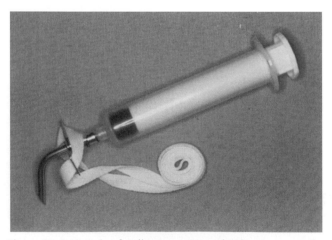

Figure 28-2 Example of a direct puncture cricothyrotomy needle.

device,[37] but no references compare it with other devices used for cricothyrotomy.

B. SURGICAL CRICOTHYROTOMY

Most authors state that surgical cricothyrotomy is more time consuming than percutaneous methods and requires an experienced surgeon to perform or assist the anesthesiologist. However, compared with emergency tracheostomy, it is safer, faster, and easier to perform.[15,33,40,81] The technique is performed as follows: after aseptically preparing the neck, the anatomic landmarks are identified, and the larynx is held in place by holding the upper pole of the thyroid cartilage firmly with the thumb and middle finger of the dominant hand. The cricothyroid space is palpated with the index finger, and, if time allows, local anesthetic is injected. A 2.0- to 3.0-cm skin incision is made in the midline of the cricothyroid space. Some authors recommend spreading the incision with Mayo scissors and making a 1.5- to 2.0-cm transverse incision at the inferior third of the CTM. Others recommend a single midline incision through both layers. In either case, the thyroid cartilage is identified, and the tracheal hook is inserted, applying gentle traction on the inferior margin of the thyroid cartilage. A Trousseau dilator is then inserted through the incision into the airway and spread vertically to enlarge the diameter of the cricothyroid space. If needed, the Mayo scissors can be used to enlarge the space in the transverse direction. Once the dilator is in place, the tracheal hook is removed, and an appropriately sized tracheostomy tube and stylet are inserted into the airway. After the tube is inserted, the stylet is removed, and the inner cannula (if supplied) is inserted. The cuff is inflated, and the tube is attached to a breathing circuit for positive-pressure ventilation. Clinical signs and radiographic verification are observed for proper tube placement. A suction catheter may be passed through the ET. If the catheter passes easily, the tube is in the airway.

Since publication of the first edition of this textbook, a new surgical cricothyrotomy technique, the rapid four-step technique (RFST), has been introduced. It consists of (1) identification of the CTM, (2) stab incision through the skin and membrane, (3) caudal traction on the cricoid membrane with a tracheal hook, and (4) intubation of the trachea.[45] In cadaver studies, this technique has been shown to take less time than traditional surgical cricothyrotomy (43 versus 134 seconds) but to have equal success rates.[50] The technique has been further refined by the development of the "Bair claw," a modified hemostat with "dual hooks dispersing the traction force (on the cricoid cartilage) across a wider surface area," thus reducing cricoid injury.[6,31]

The inventor (Aaron Bair) and colleagues have published the 5-year experience with cricothyrotomy at their institution.[7] Cricothyrotomy was indicated in 1.1% of ED patients requiring airway management and 10.9% of patients encountered by the institution's aeromedical transport service. Of these, 77% had cricothyrotomy performed with RFST and the remainder by other surgical techniques. The authors report no complications when RFST was used in the ED and a 25% complication rate when other surgical techniques were employed. Overall complication rates were 14% in the ED and 54.5% in the aeromedical setting. Attempts to determine whether this device is available commercially have been unsuccessful.

C. TRANSTRACHEAL CATHETER VENTILATION

Transtracheal catheter ventilation is a relatively safe and easy method to oxygenate temporarily patients who cannot be mask ventilated or intubated.[12] We consider it to be a bridge technique that "buys time" until the patient is awakened or a definitive airway can be secured. The CTM is punctured percutaneously with a needle or, preferably, an over-the-needle catheter. In the latter case, the needle is removed, and the catheter is attached to either a high-pressure oxygen source or a high-frequency jet ventilator. The mechanism by which this technique works is thought to be air entrainment and mass movement of gas. It is preferable during initial resuscitation to emergency surgical cricothyrotomy and tracheostomy because it is a much quicker procedure, the patient may not be well positioned, correct instruments for the surgical procedure may not be readily available, or the patient's anatomy may not be normal.[11,12,43,106]

As early as 1956, Jacoby and colleagues[59] showed that patients with complete respiratory obstruction undergoing general anesthesia could be adequately oxygenated using an oxygen flow of 4 L/min through an 18G cricothyrotomy catheter. However, the technique was limited by unacceptable carbon dioxide (CO_2) retention and respiratory acidosis. Alternatively, high-frequency jet ventilation has been used successfully in patients without airway obstruction in the OR and in the ICU, providing more stable hemodynamic conditions than positive-pressure ventilation.[38,99,109] Spoerel and coworkers[101] combined the concept of a percutaneously placed tracheal catheter and intermittent jet oxygen delivery into the respiratory tree of adults undergoing general anesthesia. They used a 16G catheter connected to a 50 pounds per square inch gauge (PSIG) oxygen source to deliver gas at an insufflation rate of 12 L/min and an inspiratory duration of 1 to 1.5 seconds. Tidal volume was estimated to be between 400 and 750 mL. Ventilation was adequate, and no significant damage to the tracheal mucosa or excessive buildup of airway pressure was noted. Other investigators, such as Ravussin and Freeman[88] and Nakatsuka and MacLeod,[79] have demonstrated that percutaneous cricothyrotomy combined with high-frequency jet ventilation provided adequate oxygenation and ventilation during general surgery on patients known to be difficult to intubate or with known distorted upper airway anatomy.

Benumof and Scheller[12] and Benumof[11] proposed that percutaneous transtracheal jet ventilation using a larger bore intravenous catheter inserted through the CTM be used as the treatment of choice in situations in which the patient cannot be ventilated or intubated. Until recently, kits containing the required high-pressure circuits and equipment were not readily available. The equipment is now readily available and consists of a 16G or larger intravenous cannula and an acceptable high-pressure (50 PSIG) oxygen source from either a jet injector powered by regulated wall or oxygen tank pressure (preferred) (Mercury Medical), a jet injector powered by unregulated wall or oxygen tank pressure, or the anesthesia machine flush valve using noncompliant oxygen tubing from the fresh gas outlet.

The technique is simple and can be performed rapidly. The patient should be continuously oxygenated with 100% oxygen by mask. After stabilizing the trachea and locating the cricothyroid cartilage by finger palpation, the CTM is punctured with the intravenous catheter. To confirm proper intratracheal position, air should be aspirated. The needle stylet is then withdrawn, discarded, and the catheter advanced to the hub. Intratracheal position should be rechecked again by air aspiration.

Although oxygenation may be adequate with transtracheal catheter ventilation, with near-total to total upper airway obstruction, passive exhalation may be insufficient to sustain ventilation, and air trapping and excessive hypercarbia may result. Provisions should be made to secure the airway in a more permanent fashion. Other problems associated with prolonged use of nonhumidified transtracheal jet ventilation include subcutaneous or mediastinal emphysema, pneumothorax, esophageal puncture, sore throat, infection, bleeding, hematoma formation, and mucosal ulceration. The needle or catheter may break or bend if the patient coughs or moves, resulting in respiratory obstruction. Of these complications, catheter kinking and subcutaneous air injection (sometimes massive) with loss of anatomic landmarks and pneumothorax appear to be the most serious and widely encountered. In our opinion, use of this technique with a needle or standard intravenous catheter for more than short intervals for bridging to another technique is inappropriate because it is extremely difficult to secure and maintain them in the proper position, and displacement with subcutaneous air or kinking can both be lethal.

D. PERCUTANEOUS TRACHEOSTOMY

For completeness, the currently used techniques of percutaneous tracheostomy are briefly described, although emphasis is placed on the percutaneous dilatational method.

The Ciaglia technique, also known as PCT, involves making a very small skin incision, introducing a needle into the trachea, and subsequently bluntly dilating the aperture to allow insertion of the preselected tracheostomy tube. The entire procedure is performed under continuous endoscopic guidance, with step-by-step visualization from beginning to end. As originally described, dilatation was accomplished by using a series of graduated dilators until the tracheal opening allowed insertion of the desired tracheostomy tube. In 1999, a modification was introduced whereby the series of dilators was replaced with a single, sharply tapered dilator, permitting complete dilatation in one step. Although the multiple dilators are still commercially available, they have been largely supplanted by the single dilator. Of the percutaneous approaches described, the Ciaglia technique, endoscopically guided, is probably the safest and is the most widely used in North America.

The Fantoni technique is based on retrograde dilatation of an initial tracheal puncture. Upon completion of the dilatation, the tracheostomy tube is also brought out in a retrograde fashion through the cervical trachea and skin. During the procedure the ET must be changed once, with potential loss of the airway. This technique is used primarily in Italy, its site of origin, but has found little applicability in North America because it is technically more involved, lengthy to perform, and involves potential loss of the airway.

The Griggs guidewire dilating forceps technique involves placing a guidewire through an initial puncture site. The area is forcibly enlarged with the use of a speculum-like instrument inserted over the guidewire and into the trachea. The procedure as originally described is blind and subject to complications such as false passage and subcutaneous emphysema. Concurrent endoscopic visualization reduces these risks, although bleeding[65] may be a problem because of tearing of adjacent structures when inserting and opening the forceps. Furthermore, the forceps may be difficult to use in patients with a short, thick neck, where the distance through the subcutaneous tissue to the trachea may be increased relative to the fixed length of the forceps. This technique, although used in Europe, is used infrequently, if at all, in North America.

VII. PERCUTANEOUS DILATIONAL CRICOTHYROTOMY

A. GENERAL PRINCIPLES

Percutaneous dilational cricothyrotomy is fast and usually easy to perform, even on patients with short necks or with spinal injury. Rehm and colleagues[89] recommend cricothyrotomy for elective airway management in trauma patients with "technically challenging neck anatomy" in lieu of tracheostomy. It does not require a surgeon's skill to gain airway access and has fewer operative and postoperative complications. A number of commercially available devices use this technology. These devices have in common the insertion of an airway catheter over a dilator, which is usually introduced over a guidewire. The guidewire is inserted through a needle or over-the-needle catheter (the Seldinger technique) after an initial skin incision. This technique, often used for the insertion of

catheter introducer sheaths and central lines, is familiar to anesthesiologists. We prefer insertion of an airway over a dilator and guidewire because of the inherent safety of this technique and the ability to insert an airway of far greater diameter than the initial catheter. One device (the Nu-Trake device) introduces a "housing" similar to a dilator but made in two parts, with the needle loaded coaxially within it. After the needle is withdrawn, metal airways with obturators are serially introduced inside the housing until the desired diameter tube is reached.

Several devices have been introduced that allow insertion of the dilator directly over a needle or directly into the skin incision. Although they lack the step of introducing a guidewire, they are included here because they require both a skin incision and a dilator for insertion of the airway. Percutaneous dilational cricothyrotomy is gaining popularity in the ED, ICU, and OR. It is very similar to another popular ICU technique, percutaneous dilational tracheostomy, an elective procedure.[26,46,47,106] Airways can be introduced rapidly by the Seldinger over-the-wire technique, which allows positive-pressure ventilation without modification of standard ventilation devices.[73,115] Although the technique requires more time to perform than needle cricothyrotomy, it may be more effective in providing adequate ventilation and oxygenation.

A number of cricothyrotomy sets are available that are inserted by the percutaneous dilational cricothyrotomy technique (e.g., Melker Emergency Cricothyrotomy Catheter Set, Cook Critical Care, Bloomington, IN; Portex Mini-Trach II, Smiths Medical, Keene, NH; and Pertrach, Tri-anim, Sylmar, CA). The Melker device uses a skin incision, followed by insertion of a guidewire and insertion of a dilator and airway catheter (cricothyrotomy tube). The Melker set is available in 3.5, 4.0, and 6.0 mm ID *uncuffed* airway catheter sizes with lengths of 3.8, 4.2, and 7.5 cm, respectively. The Melker set also comes in a "military version" that is modified for direct insertion through an incision without use of a guidewire. The 4.0 mm ID airway catheter is 7.5 cm long. This allows the use of a smaller diameter tube of sufficient length for an adult neck. The military version is available with both cuffed and uncuffed airway catheters. In addition, a cuffed 5.0 mm ID airway catheter 9 cm in length was introduced to the market. These sets are available with adapters so that both jet ventilators and conventional ventilators can be attached to the airway device. Pertrachs are available with 5.5 and 7.1 mm ID.

Chan and coauthors[23] compared wire-guided cricothyrotomy with the 6.0 mm ID Melker uncuffed catheter set with surgical cricothyrotomy using cadavers. Emergency medicine attending physicians and residents received a 15-minute training session on the use of the Melker set and then practiced both techniques on a fresh cadaver. They were then randomly assigned to which technique they would perform first. Thirteen of 15 airways were placed successfully with a standard surgical technique and 14 of 15 with the wire-guided technique. Complication rates were equal, as were times to insertion. A significantly smaller skin incision (0.53 versus 2.53 cm) was made using the wire-guided technique, and 14 of 15 physicians preferred the wire-guided technique.

Eisenburger and colleagues[32] compared conventional surgical cricothyrotomy with wire-guided cricothyrotomy with a group of intensive care physicians using cadavers. The wire-guided set (which is no longer available) required puncturing the CTM with an 18G needle with a water-filled syringe attached to a side arm. A guidewire was then inserted through the needle into the trachea, the needle removed, a skin incision made at the site of the guidewire, and an uncuffed tube loaded on a dilator placed over the wire and advanced into the airway. This device is far more cumbersome than the Melker device. The study demonstrated poor results, with only 66% successful placement with both techniques. However, failures with surgical cricothyrotomy were due to tube misplacement and with the wire-guided technique due to kinks in the guidewire and difficulty manipulating the components. The authors do not state why they chose to use this technically difficult set rather than the Melker device, which is favored by a majority of users.

Of particular interest is the survey conducted by Ratnayake and Langford[86] in the United Kingdom. Although the purpose of the survey was to evaluate anesthesiologist training in various DA techniques, they provide data from practicing anesthesiologists of an extremely high complication rate (73.3%) with the Protex Mini-Trach, with over 50% of the complications considered serious. These complications included failure to gain airway access, multiple attempts at cannulation, pneumothorax,

and severe bleeding. The high complication rate was attributed to the device being too flexible, which increased the likelihood that it would deviate from the midline during placement.

The Portex device was most frequently used in the United Kingdom (58.6%); the William-Cook device, which is similar to the Melker set, was used in only 8.5% of cases but had a reported major complication rate of 27.3%. A similar complication rate of 22.2% was found using 14G intravenous cannulas.

Wain and associates[112] reported successful use of the Portex device in 60 patients. Only one insertion was for acute airway obstruction; the others were for suctioning of secretions. Intratracheal placement was possible in every case. Two major episodes of intratracheal bleeding occurred, which necessitated endotracheal intubation. There were few minor complications.

B. INSERTION INSTRUCTIONS

1. Melker, Percutaneous Dilational Cricothyrotomy Device

The Melker set contains a scalpel blade, a syringe with an 18G over-the-needle catheter or a thin-wall introducer needle or both, a guidewire, a dilator of appropriate length and diameter, and a polyvinyl airway catheter with or without a cuff (Fig. 28-3).[35] Detailed insertion instructions for this type of device are as follows (Fig. 28-4):

1. Position the patient supine and, if there is no contraindication, slightly extend the neck, using a roll

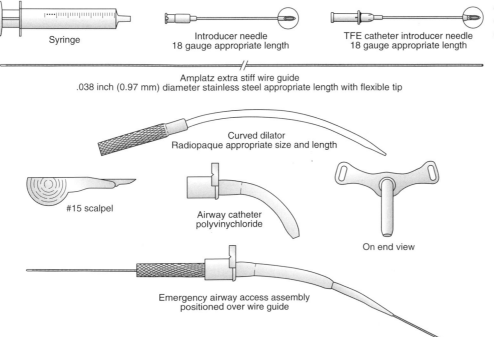

Syringe

Introducer needle
18 gauge appropriate length

TFE catheter introducer needle
18 gauge appropriate length

Figure 28-3 Melker percutaneous dilational cricothyrotomy set (Cook Critical Care, Bloomington, IN).

Amplatz extra stiff wire guide
.038 inch (0.97 mm) diameter stainless steel appropriate length with flexible tip

Curved dilator
Radiopaque appropriate size and length

#15 scalpel

Airway catheter
polyvinylchloride

On end view

Emergency airway access assembly
positioned over wire guide

SET CONSISTS OF ITEMS SHOWN ABOVE AND CLOTH TRACHEOSTOMY
TAPE STRIP FOR FIXATION OF AIRWAY CATHETER

under the neck or shoulders. If cervical spine injury is suspected, properly immobilize the head and neck and maintain a neutral position.

2. Open the prepackaged cricothyrotomy set and assemble the components. Whenever possible and appropriate, use aseptic technique and local anesthetic.

3. Identify the CTM between the cricoid and thyroid cartilages (see Fig. 28-4A).

4. Carefully palpate the CTM, and, while stabilizing the cartilage, make a vertical skin incision (about 1.0 to 1.5 cm) in the midline using the scalpel blade. Next make a vertical stab incision through the lower third

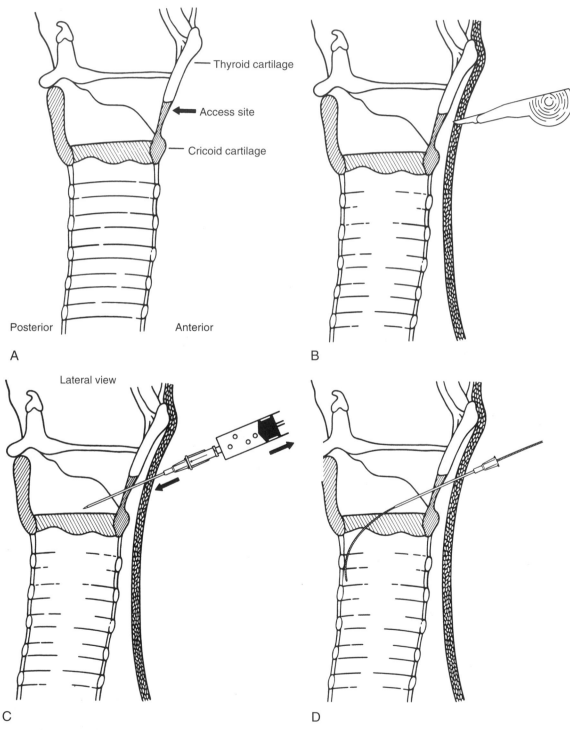

Figure 28-4 A to H, Detailed instructions (see text) for insertion of the Melker, percutaneous dilational cricothyrotomy sets. (From Melker emergency cricothyrotomy sets: Suggested instructions for placement, instruction pamphlet. Cook Critical Care, Bloomington, IN, 1988.)

Continued

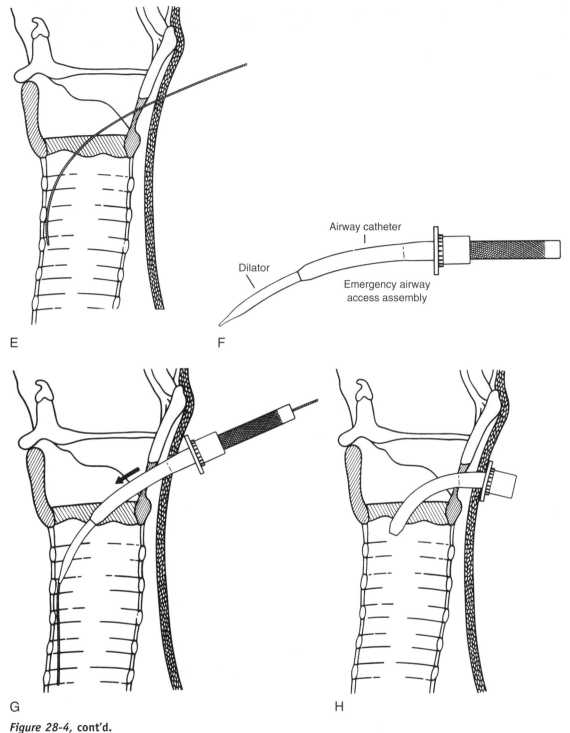

E

F

Airway catheter

Dilator

Emergency airway access assembly

G

H

Figure 28-4, cont'd.

of the CTM. An adequate incision eases introduction of the dilator and airway (see Fig. 28-4B). See comments a and b following.

5. With the supplied syringe attached to the 18G plastic (over-the-needle) catheter introducer needle (or alternatively, to the introducer needle), advance it through the incision into the airway at a 45-degree angle to the frontal plane in the midline in a caudad direction. When advancing the needle forward, entrance into the

airway can be confirmed by aspiration on the syringe resulting in free air return (see Fig. 28-4C). (Some users fill the syringe with fluid so that bubbles can be observed when the needle enters the airway. We find this unnecessary and time consuming.)

6. Remove the syringe and needle, leaving the plastic catheter or introducer needle in place. Do not attempt to advance the plastic catheter completely into the airway, which may result in kinking of the catheter and

inability to pass the guidewire. Advance the soft, flexible end of the guidewire through the catheter or needle and into the airway several centimeters (see Fig. 28-4D). See comment c following.

7. Remove the plastic catheter or needle, leaving the guidewire in place (see Fig. 28-4E).

8. Advance the handled dilator, tapered end first, into the connector end of the airway catheter until the handle stops against the connector. With other sets, insert the dilator to the recommended depth (see Fig. 28-4F).

Note: This step may be performed before beginning the procedure. Use of lubrication on the surface of the dilator may enhance fit and placement of the emergency airway catheter.

9. Advance the emergency airway access assembly over the guidewire until the proximal stiff end of the guidewire is completely through and visible at the handle end of the dilator. It is important always to visualize the proximal end of the guidewire during the airway insertion procedure to prevent its inadvertent loss into the trachea. Maintaining the guidewire position, advance the emergency airway access assembly over the guidewire with an in-and-out motion. (Note: in the first edition it was recommended that the dilator be advanced with a reciprocating as well as in-and-out motion. It has been determined that simply using an in-and-out motion, especially so that the junction of the dilator and airway catheter advances through the incision, is all that is needed for airway placement.) Initially, advance and retract only the dilator completely into the incision several times, then advance the dilator–airway catheter combination through the incision with an in-and-out motion. Once the tract has been dilated, continue to advance the dilator and airway catheter into the airway. Care should be taken not to advance the tip of the dilator beyond the tip of the guidewire within the trachea (see Fig. 28-4G).

10. As the airway catheter is fully advanced into the trachea, remove the guidewire and dilator simultaneously.

11. If a cuffed tube is inserted, inflate with 10 mL of air with the syringe provided.

12. Fix the emergency airway catheter in place with the cloth tracheostomy tape strip in a standard fashion (see Fig. 28-4H).

13. Connect the emergency airway catheter, using its standard 15-22 adapter, to an appropriate ventilatory device.

a. Recommendation for Skin Incision prior to Needle Insertion

We recommend an incision before introducing the catheter for two reasons. First, the catheter is more likely to kink when the needle is removed if there is no skin incision, making it difficult to pass the guidewire, and second, we have had cases reported of inability to advance the dilator because the skin incision was not next to the guidewire. Extending the incision to the guidewire solved the problem. Although anesthesiologists and critical care physicians usually make a skin incision after wire introduction, we strongly recommend skin and membrane incision as the first step. We have had no cases of catheter kinking or inability to pass the dilator when the incision is made first. The set includes an additional introducer needle of sufficient ID to allow the guidewire to be advanced directly through a needle without the need for placing the catheter. This eliminates any chance of kinking but increases the risk of shearing the guidewire.

b. Vertical versus Horizontal Incision

It is unclear whether a horizontal or vertical skin incision is superior. The literature is evenly divided on this matter but usually refers to surgical cricothyrotomy. However, it can be argued that a vertical incision is better during emergency cricothyrotomy because it can be extended superiorly or inferiorly if the relationship of the skin and CTM changes (as frequently happens). We recommend a vertical stab through the CTM in the inferior third to ease placement of the dilator and avoid the cricothyroid arteries, which often anastomose in the midline superiorly.

c. Use of Over-the-Needle Catheter versus Introducer Needle

We studied the success rate of 32 anesthesiology residents at guidewire introduction with or without skin incision and with an over-the-needle catheter or an introducer needle in 16 cadavers. Residents were asked to judge the ease of delineating the pretracheal anatomy and then attempted to pass a guidewire through the 18G over-the-needle catheter supplied with the set, a stiff 16G over-the-needle catheter, or a thin-walled introducer needle prior to skin incision. After skin incision, the 18G catheter was again introduced, and guidewire insertion was again attempted. The results are shown in Table 28-2.

This study shows insertion of the guidewire through a needle to be superior when a skin incision is not used but similar in success rate to an over-the-needle catheter if an incision is used initially. Also, it appears that catheters kinked only when attempts were made to pass the total length of the catheter into the airway.

In a second study, we evaluated the rate of successfully advancing a guidewire into the airway through an over-the-needle catheter with or without a skin incision. The catheters were either advanced into the airway just to the point where air could be aspirated or totally into the airway, as with insertion of a transtracheal catheter for jet ventilation. In seven cadavers, the guidewire was successfully inserted on all attempts, with or without a skin incision, when the catheter was advanced only to the point where it entered the airway. When attempts were made

Table 28-2   **Success Rate of Guidewire Introduction with or without Skin Incision and with an Over-the-Needle Catheter or an Introducer Needle in 16 Cadavers**

	Easy	Difficult	Impossible
18G over-the-needle catheter	8	6	2
16G over-the-needle catheter	8	6	2
18G needle	11	3	0
18G over-the-needle catheter after incision	12	4	0

G, gauge.

to advance the catheter completely into the airway, it was unsuccessful three of seven times without a skin incision and two of seven times with a skin incision. The catheter was successfully advanced in cases in which the catheter-needle assembly could be placed at a 45-degree angle and the needle was maintained inside the airway when the catheter was advanced.

2. Pertrach Percutaneous Dilational Cricothyrotomy Device

The Pertrach (Fig. 28-5) is similar to the previously described devices except that the guidewire and dilator are a single unit, and, therefore, the introducer needle must be split after the distal end of the guidewire is advanced so that the dilator can be introduced (a catheter cannot be used). This is cumbersome, especially in emergency situations, and requires that the guidewire and dilator be

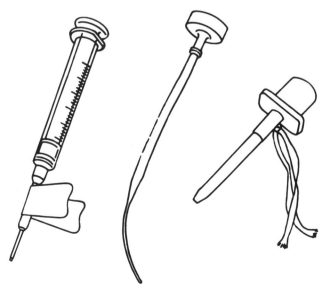

Figure 28-5 Pertrach percutaneous dilational cricothyrotomy set (Pertrach, Long Beach, CA).

advanced far down the airway. A study in cadavers showed equal success for percutaneous dilational cricothyrotomy with the Pertrach and surgical cricothyrotomy. Surgical cricothyrotomy was faster, but it was impossible to predict whether bleeding complications would have been higher with the surgical cricothyrotomies.[60] Both the manufacturer and users have reported difficulty with the needle, which is occasionally difficult or impossible to split.

Detailed insertion instructions for the Pertrach percutaneous dilational cricothyrotomy device are as follows (Fig. 28-6):

1. Test cuffed tube on dilator, lubricate cuff, deflate.
2. Make a 1- to 2-cm incision in skin over CTM.
3. Insert needle into incision, with syringe attached, perpendicular to the cricoid, and advance until tip is in airway (see Fig. 28-6A). Aspirate for air to establish position in the airway. Note: Before use, test the needle for air leaks by placing one finger over the end and aspirating with the attached syringe. If there is an air leak, the preceding technique for insuring correct needle placement cannot be relied upon. Instead, one must adjust the needle placement by:
   a. Seeing that the needle moves freely back and forth in the tracheal lumen.
   b. Seeing that the dilator tubing can be threaded easily through the needle into the trachea.
   c. A useful sign that the needle is correctly placed is the patient coughing when the tubing is threaded in.
4. Advance needle at 45-degree angle into airway, toward the carina (see Fig. 28-6B).
5. Remove syringe and insert Teflon guide of dilator in needle, guiding the tubing through it (see Fig. 28-6C). Squeeze wings to split needle. The needle may not completely separate at this point but will enable the dilator to be advanced into the slot created by squeezing the wings. As the tubing passes down the slot, it will complete the splitting of the needle. When the tip of the dilator reaches skin level, pull out the needle and discard.
6. Exert pressure and force dilator into the airway until the tube is in position, with face plate against the skin (see Fig. 28-6D).
7. Remove dilator and secure tube to patient. Inflate cuff, and attach respirator if needed (see Fig. 28-6E).

3. Nu-Trake Percutaneous Dilational Cricothyrotomy Device

The Nu-Trake device (Fig. 28-7) is more complicated to use, has a rigid airway, and is difficult to secure. In a study comparing it with the Pertrach, the Nu-Trake was found to require far greater insertion forces, often resulting in the introducer-stylet embedding in the posterior wall of the trachea.[1] Another study reported numerous complications with this device; however, these are

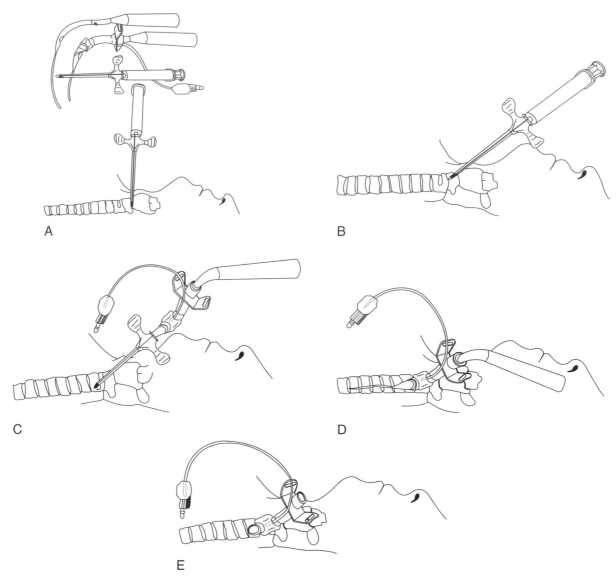

Figure 28-6 **A** to **E,** Detailed instructions (see text) for insertion of the Pertrach percutaneous dilational cricothyrotomy set. (From Cricothyroidotomy, instruction sheet. Pertrach, Long Beach, CA.)

not documented or referenced.[114] Unfortunately, the authors experienced difficulty with percutaneous dilational tracheostomy because of poor selection of patients and condemn all percutaneous techniques. Bjoraker and colleagues[13] had anesthesiologists and residents attempt cricothyrotomy in 11 dogs with the Nu-Trake device. There was difficulty inserting the stylet and blunt needle, resulting in slippage and two subcricoid insertions. There were also frequent air leaks, and the lumen had a tendency to occlude on the posterior wall of the trachea. Subcutaneous emphysema, cricoid cartilage injury, cricotracheal ligament perforation, posterior wall perforation, and incidental submucosal airway hemorrhage were found in 8 of 11 dogs. Hulsey[53] concluded that the Nu-Trake device "needs further development or solid clinical evidence of safety and efficacy before it can be recommended for use in emergency medicine practice."

No additional references to the Nu-Trake have been found since the first edition of this textbook. Direct comparisons of all devices presently available have not been performed. Detailed insertion instructions for the Nu-Trake percutaneous dilational cricothyrotomy device are as follows (Fig. 28-8):

1. Patient's head is hyperextended, if possible, and the CTM identified; palpate (see Fig. 28-8A).
2. Pinch 1 cm of skin, and insert sharp tip of knife blade through skin. Cut in an outward motion (see Fig. 28-8B).
3. The needle should puncture the membrane just beyond the entry at approximately the same angles as the lower edge of the housing. Aspirate; easily moving spring obturator denotes tracheal entrance (see Fig. 28-8C).

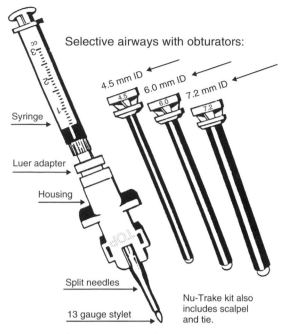

Selective airways with obturators:

4.5 mm ID   6.0 mm ID   7.2 mm ID

Syringe

Luer adapter

Housing

Split needles

13 gauge stylet

Nu-Trake kit also includes scalpel and tie.

Figure 28-7 Nu-Trake percutaneous dilational cricothyrotomy set (International Medical Devices, Northridge, CA).

4. The stylet and syringe are removed as a unit by twisting the Luer adapter counterclockwise and lifting out (see Fig. 28-8D).
5. The blunt needle is gently moved further into the trachea until the housing rests on the overlying skin. A freely rocking motion confirms proper depth of insertion (see Fig. 28-8E).
6. In all cases, begin with the smallest airway (4.5 mm), and insert airway and obturator together, *pushing with the thenar eminence* resting against the cap of the obturator. Airway and obturator are *pushed* (not squeezed) downward into the needle, which is divided lengthwise and spreads apart to accommodate them (see Fig. 28-8F).
7. Obturator is removed, leaving a clear passage for air to reach the lungs. If airway size requires change, this can be easily performed by leaving the housing and needle guide in place while removal and insertion of airways are performed. Ties are threaded through the brackets on the sides of the housing (see Fig. 28-8G).
8. System in operation: bag valve or universal (15-mm) adapter may be fitted to the top of the housing. Expansion of lungs can also be started by mouth-to-mouth respiration, with fingers closing off the vents in the housing (see Fig. 28-8H).

4. Portex and Melker Military Percutaneous Dilational Cricothyrotomy Devices

The Portex Mini-Trach and the military variation of the Melker set are sold without the guidewire. In this design, only a scalpel, dilator, and airway catheter are supplied. The devices are inserted by passing the dilator and airway catheter directly through the incision. They may lend

themselves to use by prehospital providers who are unfamiliar with the Seldinger technique and often work under difficult environmental conditions. The Portex set is designed primarily for "management of sputum retention." The dilator ("introducer") is rigid and malleable, and the breathing tube is not tapered. The instructions recommend insertion of the dilator, followed by loading and passage of the breathing tube. Detailed insertion instructions for the Portex percutaneous dilational cricothyrotomy device are as follows:

1. Attach needle introducer assembly to the cricothyrotomy catheter. Lubricate the catheter (Fig. 28-9A).
2. Prepare anterior neck of patient.
3. Identify CTM between the cricoid and thyroid cartilages, and stabilize trachea with thumb and index finger (see Fig. 28-9B).
4. Make a skin incision with the no. 15 scalpel large enough to admit the catheter, over the CTM, close to the cricoid cartilage.
5. Cannulate the trachea with the catheter tip facing caudad. A loss of resistance is felt when the trachea is entered (see Fig. 28-9C).
6. Aspirate air into a water-filled 5-mL syringe to confirm catheter position within the tracheal lumen (see Fig. 28-9D).
7. Remove the needle, and advance the catheter and dilator caudad. Aspirate again to confirm position.
8. Remove the dilator, and aspirate once again to ensure correct placement within the trachea (see Fig. 28-9E).
9. Connect the catheter to oxygen source, and secure catheter with the tape provided.

The preceding instructions are designed for OR insertion under controlled circumstances. Instructions for the military design intended for emergent field use are as follows:

1. Identify the cricothyroid space by palpating between the thyroid and the cricoid cartilage.
2. Under strict aseptic technique, infiltrate the cricothyroid space with anesthetic, if clinically indicated.
3. While stabilizing the cricoid cartilage, make an incision with the no. 15 scalpel blade through all layers of the cricothyroid space down to the airway.
4. Insert the 18 French (Fr) curved dilator with the cricothyrotomy tube loaded over it into the incision in a caudad direction.
5. Advance and withdraw the dilator a few times to dilate the tract for insertion of the cricothyrotomy tube.
6. Applying steady pressure, advance the tube into the airway.
7. Maintaining the tube in the airway, withdraw the dilator.
8. If a cuffed airway catheter is supplied, inflate the cuff with 10 mL of air with the syringe provided.
9. Secure tube in place with tape provided.

Most presently available sets (excluding the Pertrach and the cuffed airway catheter available with the Melker set) have uncuffed airway catheters. In situations in which a cuffed tube is desirable, the airway catheter can be changed to a soft plastic tracheostomy tube of the same ID. For instance, a Shiley 6SCT can be used in place of the 6.0 mm ID uncuffed airway catheter supplied with the Melker set.

VIII. PERCUTANEOUS DILATIONAL TRACHEOSTOMY

A. PREOPERATIVE PLANNING

As with any procedure, proper planning begins with a history and physical examination. Palpation of critical landmarks such as the cricoid cartilage and sternal notch is mandatory. The neck must also be inspected for the occasional high innominate artery or midline neck mass. It is at this stage that suitability for the procedure is determined, not once an incision has been made. Preoperative testing is minimal and includes a recent chest radiograph and serum determination of hemoglobin, prothrombin time (PT), partial thromboplastin time, and platelets. Currently, the INR, which is calculated to reflect the PT, best reflects coagulation status. Although 1 is a normal value, an INR corrected to less than 1.5 is acceptable. Because bleeding is usually minimal, crossmatching is not necessary, even in the presence of a low hemoglobin. A fully equipped intubation cart should be available nearby in the event of accidental extubation during the procedure. In patients with short thick necks, consideration should be given to placement of an extra long tracheostomy tube to prevent accidental decannulation or displacement into the pretracheal soft tissues.

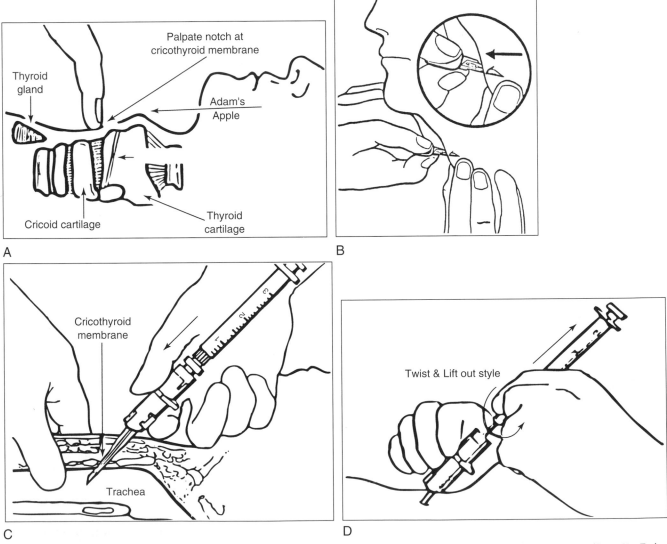

Figure 28-8 A to H, Detailed instructions (see text) for insertion of Nu-Trake percutaneous dilational cricothyrotomy set. (From Nu-Trake cricothyrotomy device, instruction pamphlet. International Medical Devices, Northridge, CA.)

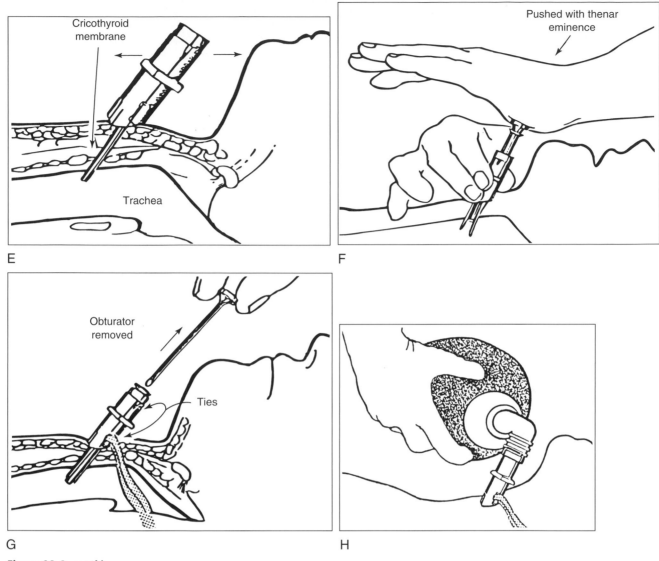

Figure 28-8, cont'd.

B. PERSONNEL

Generally, four people are required, including the operating physician, a resident or critical care colleague to perform the bronchoscopy, a respiratory technician to assist in adjusting ventilator settings and to hold the ET firmly in position, and a nurse to administer medication, monitor vital signs, and assist in obtaining necessary materials and instruments. The surgeon and necessary instruments are positioned to the patient's right, the respiratory technician to the left, and the bronchoscopist at the head of the bed.

C. INSTRUMENTS

At present, two kits are commercially available for this procedure: the original Cook kit based on the use of graduated tapered dilators and the more recent Cook single-dilator kit.

The Cook kit in its original form includes seven curved dilators sized from 12 to 36 Fr. A 38 Fr dilator is available separately and is highly recommended for routine use. The 24 Fr dilator can be used to insert a no. 6 Shiley or no. 9 Portex tracheostomy tube, and a 28 Fr dilator can be used to insert a no. 8 Shiley or no. 11 Portex tracheostomy tube. The size of the tube can be determined at the time of the procedure.

The Cook single-dilator kit contains a single, sharply tapered curved dilator designed to achieve dilatation sufficient to accommodate a no. 8 Shiley tracheostomy tube in one step. The tip is soft, to prevent soft tissue injury, and its surface has a hydrophilic coating to facilitate dilatation. The kit also contains three loading dilators, size 24, 26, and 28 Fr, to allow placement of a no. 6 or no. 8 ID Shiley tracheostomy tube, respectively. Also included is a scalpel, a 10-mL syringe, a 1.32-mm guidewire, a 17G introducer needle with sheath, a 14 Fr introducer dilator,

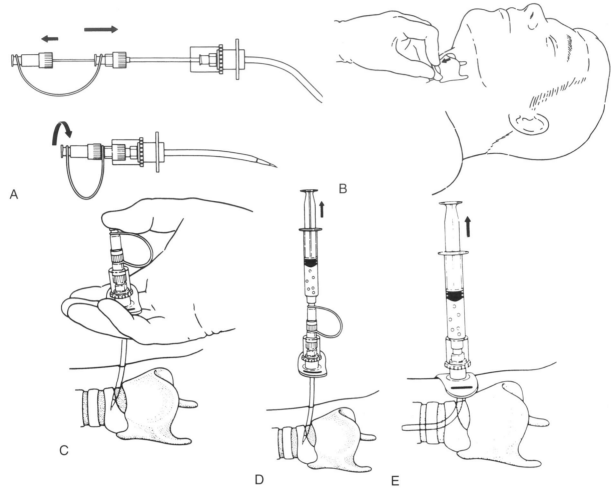

Figure 28-9 A to **E** Detailed instructions (see text) for insertion of Patil, Portex, and Melker military percutaneous dilational cricothyrotomy sets. (From Patil emergency cricothyrotomy catheter set: Suggested instructions for use. Cook Critical Care, Bloomington, IN, 1993.) Patil device shown is no longer commercially available.

and a 12 Fr guiding catheter. Other required instruments include a curved hemostat, straight scissors, needle driver, nonresorbable sutures, water-based lubricant, two 10-mL syringes, and an appropriately sized tracheostomy tube.

The instruments should be placed on a stand over the patient's bed in the order in which they are to be used. An appropriately sized bronchoscope with a suction port must be chosen to fit within the ET or nasotracheal tube while still allowing adequate ventilation. A pediatric broncho-scope must be used when the ET is less than 7 mm. A video monitor, if available, may be connected to the bronchoscope, allowing full visualization of the intra-tracheal portion of the procedure by the operating surgeon and staff.

D. ANESTHESIA

Any procedure involving manipulation of the trachea is highly stimulating to the patient and requires adequate local anesthesia supplemented by intravenous sedation. Local anesthesia, consisting of 1% or 2% lidocaine with 1:100,000 epinephrine, is used for generous infiltration

of the incision site down to the level of the trachea. Topical anesthesia in the form of 2% to 4% lidocaine may be injected through the bronchoscope and is useful in decreasing the cough reflex during intratracheal instru-mentation. Intravenous sedation is also required, with the particular drug combination dependent on the individ-ual patient and the institution. Frequently used medica-tions include morphine, midazolam, fentanyl (Sublimaze), and propofol. Pancuronium bromide may be used as an adjunct when agitation is a problem. The presence of an anesthesiologist is optional and may depend on hospital policy. Care should be exercised in administering these medications, particularly in elderly patients, because large fluctuations in blood pressure and heart rate may occur even with small doses.

E. TECHNIQUE

The patient is positioned as for conventional tracheostomy with the head extended on the neck, and a standard preparation and drape are applied. The skin and subcu-taneous tissues are infiltrated with 2% lidocaine and

1:100,00 epinephrine one or two fingerbreadths below the previously palpated cricoid cartilage. A 1.5-cm horizontal skin incision is made and the subcutaneous tissues are bluntly separated with a curved hemostat. No attempt is made to manipulate the strap muscles or thyroid gland. At this point, the bronchoscope is advanced until its tip is flush with the ET. Any ties securing the ET are loosened and the bronchoscope and ET are withdrawn slowly in unison until the incision is maximally transilluminated. The bronchoscope, which may be connected to a monitor when available, is maintained in this position throughout the procedure, allowing direct visualization of every step. The 16 or 17G introducer needle is then inserted between the first and second or second and third tracheal rings. A midline intercartilaginous placement is verified bronchoscopically. The needle is withdrawn, leaving the overlying catheter sheath through which the guidewire can then be inserted. This sheath is removed and replaced by a 14 Fr introducer dilator, which is advanced over the guidewire; this maneuver enlarges the tracheal aperture sufficiently to allow easy placement of the 12 Fr guiding catheter. The guiding catheter and guidewire are left in place and form the backbone over which the single dilator is used. The single dilator (with the hydrophilic coating moistened) is advanced over this unit, several times if necessary, until resistance is minimal. The dilator is then replaced by the preloaded tracheostomy tube, which is advanced into the trachea. Some resistance may be encountered at the interface between the dilator and tracheostomy tube. The guidewire, guiding catheter, and dilator are removed and replaced by the inner cannula. The ventilatory apparatus is connected to the tracheostomy, which is secured with four corner sutures. When ventilation is adequate, the ET is removed while examining the vocal folds. A postoperative chest radiograph is obtained to rule out the presence of a pneumothorax. In a patient with a short, thick neck, a longer tracheostomy tube should be used to prevent accidental displacement of the tube into the pretracheal soft tissue. In the event of accidental decannulation within 5 days of the procedure, the ICU staff is advised to reintubate the patient orally rather than attempt to reinsert the tracheostomy tube.

IX. POSTOPERATIVE CONSIDERATIONS

A. CRICOTHYROTOMY

Cricothyrotomy is usually performed emergently to secure a DA. It is rarely performed electively, although Brantigan and Grow[18] and others have reported lower complication rates with elective cricothyrotomy than with elective tracheostomy.

Because cricothyrotomy is usually performed under less than ideal circumstances, it should be considered a temporizing measure, and when the patient is stabilized either endotracheal intubation with or without a fiberoptic

bronchoscope or a tracheostomy should be performed. FOB affords an opportunity to evaluate the airway, especially at the site of the cricothyrotomy.

The cricothyrotomy site should be examined frequently for signs of infection, and all patients should have a careful neurologic and airway evaluation prior to discharge from the hospital to ensure that there has been no damage to the vocal cords or other proximate structures. There is no consensus of opinion on what work-up is necessary after emergency cricothyrotomy, but clearly any complaints by the patient of difficulty swallowing or phonating should be carefully evaluated. As discussed later in this chapter, complication rates from properly performed emergent cricothyrotomy are acceptably low.

B. PERCUTANEOUS TRACHEOSTOMY

With the termination of the intense stimulation produced by the procedure, the effects of the sedation may become more pronounced, and particular care must be taken in monitoring for changes in vital signs such as hypotension, tachycardia, or O_2 desaturation. In some cases, pharmacologic intervention may be required. Excess secretions or blood may compromise ventilation and result in an O_2 saturation drop, requiring suctioning. A postoperative chest radiograph is required to ensure the absence of pneumothorax and pneumomediastinum.

Many of these patients have copious secretions from the tracheostomy site from their associated pulmonary condition. A tracheostomy tube with an inner cannula facilitates care and hygiene and ensures added safety by easy removal should obstruction from secretions occur. The PCT technique is primarily dilational with minimal tissue dissection resulting in a tighter tract and a very snug fit of the tracheostomy tube. The technique does not allow placement of traction sutures at the level of the trachea. Because of these factors, the patient should be reintubated orally in the event of accidental decannulation within the first 5 days of the procedure while the tract is still relatively immature. Attempts at replacing the tracheostomy tube in an emergent situation could result in bleeding, the creation of a false passage, pneumomediastinum, hypoxia, and even death.

X. COMPLICATIONS AND OUTCOME DATA

A. CRICOTHYROTOMY

The reported complication rate associated with elective cricothyrotomy is between 6% and 8% and for emergent procedures between 10% and 40%.[63,98] The morbidity and mortality of elective cricothyrotomy are similar to those with elective tracheostomy. Boyd and colleagues[15] found 10 complications (6.8%) in 147 cricothyrotomies, but no differentiation was made between elective and emergency procedures. Brantigan and Grow[18] reported a

6.1% complication rate in 655 cases, most of which were correctable and self-limited, and this compared favorably with the complication rate associated with tracheostomy. The same authors also implicated the presence of acute laryngeal pathology (especially prolonged intubation prior to cricothyrotomy) as the predisposing factor in the subsequent development of subglottic obstruction.[19]

Adverse effects of cricothyrotomy can be categorized into two groups: those that occur early and those that occur late in the postoperative period (Box 28-1). Early complications include asphyxia related to failure to establish the airway, hemorrhage, improper or unsuccessful tube placement, subcutaneous and mediastinal emphysema, prolonged procedure time, pneumothorax, and airway obstruction. Esophageal or mediastinal perforation, vocal cord injury, aspiration, and laryngeal disruption may also occur. Long-term complications include tracheal and subglottic stenosis (especially in the presence of preexisting laryngeal trauma or infection), aspiration, swallowing dysfunction, tube obstruction, tracheoesophageal fistula, and voice changes. Voice change is the most common complication, occurring in up to 50% of cases.[27] Voice problems include hoarseness, weak voice, or decreased pitch. This dysfunction in voice may be due to injury to the external branch of the superior laryngeal nerve, decreased cricothyroid muscle contractility, or mechanical obstruction related to narrowing of the anterior parts of the thyroid and cricoid cartilages.[52] Infection, late bleeding, persistent stoma, and tracheomalacia have also been reported.

Box 28-1   Complications of Cricothyrotomy

Early
Asphyxia
Hemorrhage
Improper or unsuccessful tube placement
Subcutaneous and mediastinal emphysema
Pneumothorax
Airway obstruction
Esophageal or mediastinal perforation
Vocal cord injury
Aspiration
Laryngeal disruption
Prolonged procedure time
Late
Tracheal and subglottic stenosis
Aspiration
Swallowing dysfunction
Tube obstruction
Tracheoesophageal fistula
Voice change
Infection
Late bleeding
Persistent stoma
Tracheomalacia

Although subglottic stenosis is the most frequently reported major complication after cricothyrotomy, it is rare after tracheostomy. Pneumothorax and major blood vessel erosion are also associated with tracheostomy. Other complications associated with tracheostomy include mediastinal emphysema, accidental extubation, cardiac arrest, and death.

The complication rate for cricothyrotomy is higher in the pediatric population. Pneumothorax is the most common complication in children (5% to 7%) and is rarely seen in adults. One percent to 2% of adults develop subglottic stenosis following tracheostomy compared with 2% to 8% of children. The mortality rate in children is up to 8.7%.

Numerous reports describing various complications associated with cricothyrotomy have appeared since the landmark paper of Brantigan and Grow.[18] Habel[44] claimed to have no major complications in his series of 30 patients who had elective cricothyrotomy. Similarly, Morain[76] found no significant complications attributable to cricothyrotomy performed in his series of 16 patients. Greisz and colleagues[42] had 61 elective cricothyrotomy cases, of which 30 eventually died (of unrelated causes) and 20 underwent postmortem laryngeal evaluation. They demonstrated histologic abnormalities, including overt inflammation and granular tissue formation in the majority of cases. Of the 21 extubated survivors, none had subglottic stenosis, although 14% had permanent voice change. On the other hand, Holst and associates[51] reported a 52% incidence of hoarseness, weakness, and fatigue in a series of 103 elective cricothyroidotomies. Ten percent of their patients also complained of dysphagia. Van Hasselt and coauthors[110] reported a similar incidence of dysphonia in their 61 elective cricothyrotomy cases.

Sise and coworkers[98] reported a prospective analysis of morbidity and mortality in 76 critically ill and injured patients: 46 patients (61%) died, and postmortem examination was performed on 85% of them. Twenty-eight percent had airway pathologies such as ulceration, hemorrhage, and abscess at the stoma or cuff site, subglottic erosion, and mucosal separation. Seven percent had major complications, including one death, two with subglottic stenosis, and two with reversible subglottic granulation—one with partial obstruction and one with tracheomalacia. Minor complications were noted in 30% of the survivors. These included transient hoarseness, aspiration pneumonia, chronic aspiration, pain at the stoma scar, bleeding, stoma site abscess, and subglottic ulceration.

Prehospital cricothyrotomy performed by emergency medical services (EMS) personnel carries a higher risk of morbidity than the in-hospital procedure. Spaite and Joseph[100] reported an overall acute complication rate of 31% in 20 emergency patients. Failure to secure the airway accounted for the major complication (12%). Minor complications included right main stem intubation, infrahyoid placement, and thyroid cartilage fracture. On the other hand, 60 surgical cricothyrotomies performed by trained aeromedical system personnel had a complication rate of 8.7%.[16] These complications included significant hemorrhage or soft tissue hematoma and incorrect placement.

Problems and complications associated with percutaneous cricothyrotomy include difficulties with insertion, esophageal or mediastinal misplacement, and bleeding.[92] The overall reported complication rate is 5%. CTM calcification and blockage by secretion may make insertion difficult. Pedersen and colleagues[83] reported a case in which a repeated minitracheostomy could not be performed 2 months after the initial procedure. Postmortem examination of the larynx showed calcification of the CTM. This abnormal change was believed to be due to dystrophic ossification and heterotrophic bone formation. Displacement of the tube into the mediastinum may occur and can cause emphysema, respiratory distress, and pneumothorax.[97,102,107] Bleeding occurs in 2% of cases, and significant hemorrhage requiring surgical intervention has been reported.[4,111] The Seldinger technique appears to lessen the incidence of bleeding and promote a more precise technique of insertion.[58]

B. PERCUTANEOUS TRACHEOSTOMY

Potential complications of tracheostomy, whether performed openly or percutaneously, are the same and are listed in Table 28-3. In practice, however, complications

Table 28-3 **Complications of Tracheostomy**

Intraoperative
Hemorrhage
Tracheoesophageal fistula
Pneumothorax
Pneumomediastinum
Recurrent laryngeal nerve injury
Cricoid cartilage injury
Cardiopulmonary arrest
Postoperative
Hemorrhage
Wound infection
Subcutaneous emphysema
Swallowing problems
Tube obstruction
Displaced tracheostomy tube
Granuloma
Tracheocutaneous fistula
Laryngotracheal stenosis

such as tracheoesophageal fistula, recurrent laryngeal nerve injury, cricoid cartilage injury, tracheoinnominate fistula, and cardiopulmonary arrest are extremely rare with either technique. The use of endoscopy in PCT has largely eliminated the risk of subcutaneous emphysema, pneumothorax, and pneumomediastinum.

Any discussion of PCT raises first and foremost the issue of safety. Addressing this concern requires an understanding of the population of patients involved. Almost two thirds of modern tracheotomies are performed in intubated ICU patients.[78] ICU patients are critically ill with frequent multisystem disease and as such are at an increased risk for complications. In a retrospective review of 281 tracheostomies, Zeitouni and Kost[78] noted a 30% complication rate in tracheostomies performed in ICU patients compared with a 17% complication rate in non-ICU patients. This finding has been substantiated in other studies as well.[23,41] Although an early study by Wang reported unacceptably high complication rates for PCT, a closer look shows that selection of patients was poor, and the procedure was performed without the benefit of endoscopic guidance. This author's prospective data on 191 endoscopically guided tracheotomies using the multiple dilator technique shows a complication rate of 12%, with most of these complications being minor. A more recent prospective evaluation of endoscopically guided PCT using the single-dilator technique in 150 patients showed a low complication rate of 7%.[45]

Comparing individual complications between surgical tracheostomy and PCT shows a substantially reduced incidence of bleeding and stomal infection in the percutaneous technique compared with the standard operative technique.[45] The decreased incidence of bleeding may be related to the lack of sharp dissection and the tamponading effect of the dilator. The much smaller wound created with the PCT technique reduces the surface area available for bacterial colonization and may explain the relative rarity of wound infection.

A number of studies [17,30,32,95] have consistently shown that PCT performed under continuous bronchoscopic control is at least as safe as conventional open tracheostomy. Specifically, the incidence of serious complications, such as pneumothorax, false passage, and subcutaneous emphysema, appears to be significantly reduced with endoscopic visualization.[6,19,95] Late outcome studies evaluating serious long-term complications associated with PCT indicate that the incidence of clinically significant tracheomalacia or stenosis requiring corrective intervention is low. Fischler and colleagues evaluated 16 patients after decannulation by means of physical examination, standardized interviews, and fiberoptic laryngotracheoscopy. The subjective rating was good in all patients. Laryngotracheoscopy showed incidental tracheal changes in two patients consisting of soft tissue swelling and a membranous scar, respectively. Neither of these findings required treatment. Stoeckli and coworkers conducted histologic studies on 21 laryngotracheal specimens from patients who had undergone PCT or standard open tracheostomy. In the percutaneous group, cartilage fractures associated with a strong inflammatory response were noted in one third of cases, compared with a more limited inflammatory response in the standard group. There was no clinical evidence of laryngotracheal stenosis in either group.

XI. PRACTICAL APPLICATIONS OF CRICOTHYROTOMY

A. OPERATING ROOM AND INTENSIVE CARE UNIT SETTINGS

Brantigan and Grow[18] reported the largest single series of elective long-term cricothyrotomy, involving 655 patients. The procedure was initially used to decrease the incidence of sternotomy-related wound infection and subsequently expanded for long-term mechanical ventilation. Cricothyrotomy was performed either in the OR or under local anesthesia in the patient's room. They did not observe any subglottic stenosis, and there was only a 2.6% incidence of tracheal stenosis and an overall complication rate of 6.1%. Only one patient died after a tracheostomy tube change. The authors attributed their success to the elective use of the procedure, proper usage of antibiotics, lack of laryngeal inflammation, anatomic dissection, and better, less irritating tracheostomy tubes. They concluded that cricothyrotomy is a benign, safe, well-tolerated procedure that is not significantly associated with subglottic stenosis and offers advantages over standard tracheostomy: technical simplicity, faster performance, low complication rate, ability to be done at the bedside, and better isolation from the median sternotomy. They recommended cricothyrotomy as the method of choice for all elective or emergency tracheal airway access. However, the authors were subsequently faulted for their lack of detailed follow-up of patients.[75] Therefore, Brantigan and Grow published a follow-up paper[19] in which they reviewed 17 patients with subglottic stenosis after cricothyrotomy. They recommended that all patients have endoscopic airway assessment prior to elective placement. They also suggested tracheostomy for patients with significant laryngotracheal injury.

Other authors reported higher complication rates. Boyd and associates[15] reported a series of 147 cricothyrotomies. Fifteen cases were emergent, and the remaining 132 were done electively on postoperative median sternotomy patients. Severe glottic and subglottic stenosis was noted in 2 of the 105 survivors. Subglottic stenosis was not observed in those intubated less than 7 days prior to cricothyrotomy but was seen in 9.1% of survivors intubated for more than 7 days before the procedure. Esses and Jafek[33] found an overall complication rate of 28%. Kuriloff and colleagues[64] performed elective surgical cricothyrotomies in 48 patients undergoing

cardiothoracic surgery. They showed a 52% incidence of airway complications, and six of their patients died while still cannulated. Morbidity was highest among diabetics, elderly patients, and patients in whom cricothyroid cannulation lasted more than 1 month.

PCT (and cricothyrotomy) was first described by Toye and Weinstein in 1969.[105] Subsequently, they reported their results with tracheostomy and cricothyrotomy in 100 patients.[106] Ninety-four of these were tracheotomies, and only six were cricothyrotomies. Airway access was obtained in 30 seconds to 2 minutes. Compared with standard surgical tracheostomy, there was less bleeding and a smaller resulting scar. Stoma formation was observed to develop within 24 hours and, with time, increasingly larger ETs could be inserted through the stoma. The complication rate was 14%, and there was one death directly attributed to the use of the device. No long-term complications were reported on subsequent follow-ups.

A literature search for additional references to the use of cricothyrotomy in the OR or ICU settings published since the first edition of this textbook found no additional publications.

B. EMERGENCY DEPARTMENT SETTING

There is significantly less information available on the use of cricothyrotomy in the ED. McGill and coauthors[71] reviewed their experience with emergent surgical cricothyrotomies performed in the ED on 38 patients. The majority of the procedures (82%) were done after other forms of airway management failed. The remaining five patients (18%) had surgical cricothyrotomy performed as the first airway control maneuver because of severe facial or neck injury or airway hemorrhage, or both. Almost a third of their patients developed immediate complications, the most common of which was incorrect placement of the tracheostomy tube. Other complications observed included prolonged insertion, unsuccessful tracheostomy tube insertion, and significant bleeding. Thirty-two percent survived and were discharged from the hospital. Only one long-term complication was reported. The patient had a longitudinal fracture of the thyroid cartilage during placement of an oversized tube through the cricoid membrane, requiring operative repair and leaving the patient with permanent dysphonia.

In the first edition of this textbook, we had reports of 15 airway control attempts using a cricothyrotomy set (Melker) in an emergency setting (Table 28-4). Thirteen were successful, and all salvageable patients did well without complications attributable to the procedure. Three attempts failed initially because of inability to pass the guidewire through the catheter. No skin incision was used in these cases. In two, kinking was recognized, and the guidewire was introduced through larger, stiffer catheters without further difficulty. In the third, the patient was intubated from above in the interim. The other failure was related to passing the dilator into the incision

Table 28-4 **Clinical Experience with Cricothyrotomy Set (Melker Emergency Cricothyrotomy Catheter Set, Cook Critical Care, Bloomington, IN) in 15 Attempted Placements in Adult Patients**

	Number of Patients
Diagnosis	
Multitrauma with severe facial injuries	4
Respiratory failure	3
Cardiac arrest	3
Head and neck tumor	1
Massive subcutaneous and intraoral	1
Emphysema	1
Gunshot to chest	1
Inability to intubate	2
Setting	
Prehospital	6
Emergency department	3
Intensive care unit	3
Operating room	3
Technique	
Over-the-wire	13
Direct insertion	2
Long-term complications	0
Complications during insertion	
Kinked intravenous catheter	3
Initial incision not at wire site	1

without placing the guidewire first. This was attempted during helicopter transport of a patient in extremis. The airway catheter was placed in the subcutaneous tissue. This was immediately recognized, and the airway catheter was removed. This technique had been used successfully on a previous patient and was felt to be as safe as the wire-guided technique. In another case, the physician attempted to pass the dilator over the wire without making a skin incision with the scalpel. He was unaware that a scalpel was provided or that an incision was necessary. We do not consider this to be a failure of the technique. We continue to receive numerous reports of successful insertion of the Melker device, but the postcard enclosed with the set does not provide enough detailed information to report success or problems encountered.

Isaacs[54] reviewed the long-term outcome of 27 survivors who had surgical cricothyrotomy performed emergently in the ED (65 patients initially). The average length of follow-up was 37 months. In 13 patients, no airway problems were found. In the remaining 14, only minor problems related to the procedure were noted, including hoarse voice and mild untreated stenosis. He concluded that emergency cricothyrotomy is effective in obtaining an airway with a low incidence of later airway problems.

Sakles and colleagues[94] evaluated 610 attempted intubations during a single year in one ED. Rapid sequence induction (RSI) was used in 515 (84%). Six hundred and three patients (98.9%) were successfully intubated; seven patients could not be intubated and underwent cricothyrotomy. In 33 patients, inadvertent esophageal intubation occurred but was immediately recognized and corrected. However, eight esophageal intubations resulted in an immediate complication. All cricothyrotomies were successful, and the rate was comparable to that reported in other studies.

Bair and coworkers[14] in a multicenter trial, evaluated 7712 attempted emergency intubations. Two hundred and seven (2.7%) were unsuccessful and required a rescue procedure. In 102 cases (49% of total failed intubations) RSI was used successfully, and in 43 (21%) cricothyrotomy was required. Complication rates for cricothyrotomy were not reported. The remaining patients were "rescued" with other airway adjuncts including the laryngeal mask airway, Trachlight, and other devices.

Chang and others[24] expressed concern that implementation of emergency medicine residencies has reduced the need for cricothyrotomy in trauma patients and that ED physicians are becoming less proficient in the technique. They looked at three time periods, 1985 to 1989, 1990 to 1992, and 1993 to 1994. The rate of cricothyrotomy declined from 1.8% of emergency airway procedures during the first time period to 1.1% during the second and 0.2% during the third. They recommended alternative means to train ED physicians in cricothyrotomy. It is important to point out that these results were from a level 1 trauma center and that other EDs do not report similar declines in the use of cricothyrotomy.

Gerling and associates[40] evaluated the effect of surgical cricothyrotomy on the unstable cervical spine using a cadaver model. A complete C5-6 transection was performed on 13 fresh-frozen cadavers and surgical cricothyrotomy performed. From 1 to 2 mm anteroposterior displacement and less than 1 mm axial compression was noted, with no angular displacement. These findings were considered to be clinically insignificant. No similar studies have been performed using percutaneous dilational cricothyrotomy.

C. AEROMEDICAL ENVIRONMENT

We have chosen to discuss cricothyrotomy performed by hospital-based aeromedical system personnel separately from cricothyrotomy performed by EMS personnel because of the differences in training and skill levels between the groups. In general, hospital-based aeromedical providers have significantly greater training and are more familiar and comfortable with cricothyrotomy, in no small part because of active involvement of medical directors. Statistics of success and complication rates support this contention.

Boyle and colleagues[16] reported a 98.5% success rate in 69 patients transported by a regional helicopter program. All procedures were performed by flight nurses, and the complication rate was 8.7%. A number of other studies involving flight nurses or flight nurse–physician teams reported similar results.[74,80,116]

Gerich and coauthors[39] prospectively analyzed 383 acutely injured patients who required emergent airway control. Three hundred seventy-three (97%) were successfully orally intubated, but two (0.5%) were found to be intubated in the esophagus on arrival in the ED. Eight patients (2.4%) underwent cricothyrotomy in the field, six without previous attempts at intubation. All attempts were successful.

No studies have yet addressed the use of percutaneous dilational cricothyrotomy, although we are aware from postcards provided with the Melker cricothyrotomy catheter set that many have been performed by aeromedical transport services.

D. PREHOSPITAL SETTING

Efficacy of cricothyrotomy is difficult to evaluate in the prehospital setting. However, it is not uncommon for paramedics to encounter clinical situations in which the airway cannot be secured by conventional means (i.e., endotracheal intubation). Training in cricothyrotomy is mandatory in most paramedic training programs, although its use is usually at the discretion of the medical director. The complication and mortality rates are higher for patients treated with surgical cricothyrotomy, owing largely to late application of the technique and the severity of injuries.[80,100] The long-term complication rates resulting from prehospital surgical cricothyrotomy have not yet been established. Johnson and coworkers[60] studied the proficiency of paramedic students in performing percutaneous dilational cricothyrotomy versus surgical cricothyrotomy in human cadavers. Forty-four paramedic students performed the two techniques on cadavers, but analysis of data was limited to procedures performed on subjects with intact cricoid membranes. There was no significant difference in the success rate on the first attempt between the two approaches, but the surgical procedure was significantly faster than percutaneous cricothyrotomy. Surgical cricothyrotomy was also judged to be easier to perform. However, one must be cautious in interpreting the data because the study did not consider the presence of bleeding, which may prolong the performance of surgical cricothyrotomy. In addition, there is a marked difference between the tone of the cricoid musculature and surrounding structures in an alive subject and in a cadaver—cadaver models may favor surgical cricothyrotomy. Also, the procedures were performed under optimal lighting conditions, all equipment was ready for use, and there was no anatomic distortion of the neck structures.

Spaite and Joseph[100] reported 20 cases of emergency prehospital surgical cricothyrotomies performed by EMS personnel. They had an 88% success rate, comparable to the success rate for cricothyrotomy performed by physicians (92%). All patients had major injuries, and the majority had massive facial trauma or failed oral intubation with no other alternative means of airway control. They had a low incidence of serious complications (12%), primarily related to inability to secure the airway.

Two studies address the use of cricothyrotomy by EMS personnel. Fortune and coworkers[36] reported that of 376 patients requiring intubation in the prehospital setting, 56 had surgical cricothyrotomies performed. In most (79%) endotracheal intubation was attempted first. Cricothyrotomy was successful in 89% of attempts, and 62% of patients receiving cricothyrotomy were discharged from the ED. The authors concluded that cricothyrotomy can be performed effectively with few complications with adequate training of EMS personnel.

Marcolini and associates[70] reported the results of 68 cricothyrotomies performed over an 8-year period by prehospital providers using a standing-order protocol. Hospital records of 61 patients were reviewed. Fifty-six patients received surgical cricothyrotomy, six were ventilated by jet ventilation, and one received both methods. Sixty-one percent of procedures were performed on trauma victims, with the remainder of patients with medical problems. Of 13 trauma patients who arrived alive in the ED, 8 survived to discharge, but only 2 had minimal or no neurologic impairment. Most patients were dead on arrival at the ED.

A committee of emergency medicine, anesthesiology, and neurologic surgery physicians at our institution developed a protocol for prehospital emergency airway control in trauma patients (Fig. 28-10). Many patients can be assisted or ventilated with a bag-valve-mask. The major indications for intubation include inability to ventilate the apneic patient who has absent airway reflexes, major facial trauma precluding airway control, and severe head injury requiring hyperventilation. Orotracheal intubation is the preferred route for definitive airway control. When contraindicated, cricothyrotomy or blind nasotracheal intubation should be considered. Blind nasotracheal intubation should be performed only if the patient is breathing spontaneously. It should not be performed at all in patients with significant facial trauma above or including the maxilla, in those with nasal trauma, or in those with suspected basilar skull fractures. Placement of an intravenous catheter in the cricothyroid space is a stopgap measure. Appropriately trained rescuers should always have proper equipment available.

XII. TRAINING MODELS

Because percutaneous dilational cricothyrotomy is so rarely performed, there is a need for quality teaching and

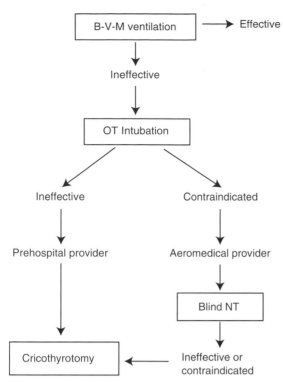

Figure 28-10 Emergency airway protocol for prehospital care. B-V-M, bag-valve-mask; NT, nasotracheal; OT, orotracheal.

training aids. Although the technique closely mimics over-the-wire vascular insertion methods, it is sufficiently different that, ideally, anesthesiologists should practice on a regular basis.

Of the available animal models, dogs appear to be most similar to humans. Ruhe and associates[91] found the canine CTM, muscles, and cricothyroid area in toto to be similar to those in humans. The tracheal dimensions of the 25-kg dog are comparable to those of the adult human.[2]

We have performed cricothyrotomy on other animals, including pigs, sheep, and goats. Sheep and goats are acceptable, but even in adult animals, the larynx is significantly smaller, and 3.5 or 4.0 mm ID sets must be used for teaching. Our experience with pigs has been poor. When we attempted to pass a needle or over-the-needle catheter into the cricothyroid space, we invariably hit cartilage. The space could be entered only by directing the needle cephalad, not caudad. Dissection of the larynx revealed a projection on the inferior surface of the thyroid cartilage articulating with the cricoid cartilage. This cornu had been previously described and had to be removed in order to perform cricothyrotomy studies.[52]

Our experience with cadavers has been excellent. We use both fresh and embalmed specimens. The former are superior but much harder to find. The laryngeal structures of embalmed specimens are somewhat constricted because of muscle contraction, and it is more difficult to discern the cricothyroid space. Despite this, we have found them to be an excellent training aid.

Mannequins are a less acceptable model, although several new products are more realistic. The original Laerdal Intubation Head (Laerdal Medical, Armonk, NY) has palpable cricoid and thyroid cartilages and a separate larynx and tracheal model. These are good for teaching anatomy but cannot be used for practicing cricothyrotomy. Medical Plastics Laboratory (MPL) is now owned by Laerdal and several new products allow practice in transtracheal jet ventilation and cricothyrotomy, including AirMan, which is specifically designed for DA training and procedures. The Deluxe Difficult Airway head is an intubation mannequin with a large hole at the level of the cricothyroid space. It is covered with a replaceable soft latex covering. Although this device is not very good for discerning anatomy, it allows easy passage of even large cricothyrotomy devices. The MPL cricothyrotomy model has rigid cricoid and thyroid cartilages and a narrow cricothyroid space. It works well for teaching anatomy but is not lifelike for cricothyrotomy, and the rigid plastic limits insertion of needles and small airway catheters.

Nasco (Fort Atkinson, WI) manufactures a simulator that can be used for teaching cricothyrotomy. It has a replaceable latex larynx with the cricoid and thyroid cartilages molded in. The system works well for needle cricothyrotomy, but it is difficult to insert large dilators and airway catheters; the latex tends to split and needs replacement frequently when used for percutaneous dilational cricothyrotomy. It is, however, one of the best models available.

XIII. MISCELLANEOUS

A. CUFF PRESSURES

Tracheostomy tube cuffs have two functions: (1) to create a seal against the tracheal mucosa, thereby minimizing aspiration, and (2) to facilitate positive-pressure ventilation by preventing leakage of air.

Tracheal stenosis from low-volume, high-pressure, low-compliance cuffs was a major complication of tracheostomy during the 1960s. These cuffs may exert pressures as high as 180 to 250 mm Hg on the tracheal mucosa, far in excess of the normal capillary perfusion pressures of 20 to 30 mm Hg. The result is a time-related progressive ischemic injury ranging from inflammatory changes all the way to chondronecrosis and tracheal stenosis or tracheomalacia.[103] With the accumulated evidence attesting to the injurious effects of low-volume, high-pressure cuffs, there has been a gradual shift in the past three decades toward the use of high-volume, low-pressure cuffs with the correct assumption that the latter are safer and to a great extent problem free.

The transition in the 1970s to high-volume, low-pressure cuffs decreased the incidence of cuff-related tracheal stenosis by 10-fold[103] because of the ability of the cuff to seal the airway at pressures below mucosal capillary perfusion pressure. These cuffs inflate symmetrically, adapt to tracheal contour, and allow pressure distribution over a wide area. It must be understood that overinflating these high-volume, low-pressure cuffs alters their characteristics to those of low-pressure, high-volume cuffs.

The risk of overinflation with resultant high intracuff pressures may be minimized by:

- Having a pressure-controlled cuff with a pressure pop-off valve, which prevents inflation beyond 20 mm Hg.
- Regular measurement of intracuff pressure with a manometer attached to a three- or four-way stopcock; the latter gives more accurate results.
- Cuff deflation for as long as safely possible in patients who do not require mechanical ventilation.

B. INFECTIONS

1. Risk Factors

a. Disruption of Host Defenses

Performing a tracheostomy requires a skin incision, thereby breaching this highly effective natural barrier to infection. The resultant open surgical wound provides a wide surface area for colonization, which may occur from surrounding skin, preexisting infected pulmonary secretions, aspiration of oropharyngeal secretions, or instrumentation or handling of the tracheostomy tube.

The nose, paranasal sinuses, and pharynx, where filtration and humidification as well as local leukocyte antibacterial activity occur under normal circumstances, are all bypassed in the patient with a tracheostomy. Impaired vocal fold adduction in patients with tracheostomies and the presence of the tube prevent the generation of an effective cough. Oropharyngeal secretions, often colonized with potentially pathogenic gram-negative organisms, are ineffectively cleared or swallowed, allowing some degree of aspiration and contamination of the tracheobronchial tree.

b. Tracheostomy Tubes

The majority of tracheostomy tubes, ETs, and cuffs are made of polyvinyl chloride, a plastic to which bacteria readily adhere. Clumps of rod-shaped and coccoid bacteria have been identified projecting from the surface of the ET and, by extension, from tracheostomy tubes.[5] Cultures of this material have grown a variety of gram-negative and gram-positive bacteria, including *Pseudomonas aeruginosa*, *Proteus mirabilis*, *Staphylococcus aureus*, and *Staphylococcus epidermidis*. These bacterial clumps may reach the tracheobronchial tree and lungs through detachment and aspiration or be dislodged during suction or bronchoscopy. Tracheostomy tubes that are made of polyvinyl chloride may therefore serve as reservoirs for persistent contamination of the tracheobronchial tree.

2. INFECTION SITES

a. Stomal infection

Colonization of the surgical wound after tracheostomy occurs within 24 to 48 hours with primarily gram-negative organisms including *Klebsiella*, *P. aeruginosa*, *Escherichia coli*, and occasionally, *S. aureus*.[18,50] Wound edges may demonstrate mild erythema and yellow or green secretions from the area may be copious, particularly in the first 7 to 10 days. These findings are much more marked after standard open tracheostomy than PCT, probably because of the very small incision and tight tract in the latter procedure. Frequent meticulous wound care, with mechanical débridement if necessary, is the best way to deal with this situation. Progressive cellulitis, despite aggressive local care, indicates infection, usually polymicrobial, and warrants systemic antibiotics. Rarely, necrotizing stomal infections may occur, with substantial loss of soft tissue down to and including the tracheal wall. This may create difficulties in maintaining adequate mechanical ventilation. Progression of the process may result in carotid artery exposure, with its attendant risks. Management involves replacing the tracheostomy tube with an ET and aggressive wound débridement and cleaning with antiseptic dressings.[5] Rarely, local flaps may be necessary to provide soft tissue coverage to vital structures.

b. Tracheitis

Colonization of the wound, along with mechanical irritation from the tube, cuff, and tube tip, means that there is always some degree of localized reversible tracheitis that is often manifest by increased secretions. Progression of this situation may lead to loss of tracheal support, resulting in tracheal stenosis or tracheomalacia. Full-thickness loss may result in life-threatening complications such as tracheoesophageal or tracheoinnominate fistula. Selecting appropriate tube size, material, and cuff can minimize mechanical irritation. The cuff should be inflated only when necessary.

The known bacterial colonization of polyvinyl chloride devices makes a strong argument in favor of more frequent tube changes, perhaps weekly, in ventilator-dependent, critically ill patients.

c. Nosocomial Pneumonia

The most important risk factors in the development of nosocomial pneumonia include the presence of a tracheostomy tube, a colonized trachea, and mechanical ventilation.[67] Nosocomial pneumonia occurs in 9% to 21% of patients in this subset and proves fatal in 30% of these.[50] Up to 40% of infections are polymicrobial with organisms resembling those found in the colonized trachea (*P. aeruginosa*, *S. aureus*, *Klebsiella pneumoniae*, *E. coli*, and *Enterobacter* species).[31,104]

Distinguishing between colonization and development of pneumonia may be difficult because fever, leukocytosis, purulent secretions, and pulmonary infiltrates are all common nonspecific findings in the ICU population. Quantitative cultures of the lower airways obtained bronchoscopically and bronchoalveolar lavage techniques may increase diagnostic accuracy.

C. CLEANING AND SUCTIONING

Under normal circumstances the nose efficiently warms, humidifies, and filters inspired air; in the patient with a tracheostomy, these functions must be restored artificially. Dehydration of the respiratory tract results in impaired mucociliary function, causing inspissated secretions and atelectasis. Providing adequate humidification, whether or not the patient requires mechanical ventilation, is therefore essential.

Suctioning of secretions to maintain pulmonary toilet and patency of the tracheostomy tube constitutes an integral component of the care of the tracheostomy patient receiving mechanical ventilation and should be carried out according to the patient's needs. In the early days after tracheostomy, this may be necessary as frequently as every hour or two. Some patients are able and should be encouraged to expectorate and clear their airways independently. Indications for suctioning are given in Table 28-5.[3,108]

Hypoxia, cardiac dysrhythmia, injury to the tracheobronchial tree, atelectasis, hypoxemia, and infection have all been reported in association with suctioning.[29] These events can be minimized by strict attention to technical detail. Factors that may contribute to hypoxia include the suctioning of oxygen-rich air for too long and the use of inappropriately large catheters. This can be prevented by applying suction for 12 seconds or less with a catheter less than half the size of the tracheostomy tube and ventilating the patient with 100% O_2 for at least five breaths before and after suctioning. A strictly aseptic technique using disposable catheters is mandatory to reduce the risk of cross-contamination.

Meticulous care of the tracheostomy tube and peristomal area is important in maintaining a patent airway and preventing infection and breakdown of the skin. Placement of a tracheostomy tube with an inner cannula

Table 28-5 **Indications for Suctioning**

Visible secretions in the tracheostomy tube
Audible gurgling
Coarse or diminished breath sounds
Dyspnea
Increased airway pressure
Unexplained decrease in O_2 saturation levels

is mandatory. This cannula should be removed several times daily in the early postoperative period for cleaning. Complete occlusion of the lumen with blood, crusts, and secretions may occur, resulting in oxygen desaturation, hypoxia, and even death; in this circumstance, rapid removal of the inner cannula is potentially lifesaving.

Bacterial colonization of the peristomal area is known to occur and cannot be prevented with antibiotics. The wound should be cleaned of accumulated secretions and crusts with hydrogen peroxide to prevent breakdown of the skin and the progression from wound colonization to infection. The skin under the tracheostomy neck plate should be kept dry with a thin nonadherent dressing such as Telfa. Petroleum-based products are best avoided on open wounds as they may stimulate granulation tissue and result in myospherulosis.

D. COMMUNICATION AND SWALLOWING

In patients requiring mechanical ventilation with tracheostomies in place, the incidence of swallowing dysfunction approaches 80%.[86] The etiology in most cases is multifactorial and may include the following:

- Glottic injury from previous orotracheal or nasotracheal intubation, or both
- Limitation of normal laryngeal excursion by the tethering effect of the tracheostomy tube
- Compression of the esophagus, particularly in the presence of an inflated cuff
- Desensitization of the larynx and loss of protective reflexes related to chronic diversion of air through the tube
- Impaired vocal fold adduction
- The use of anxiolytics or neuromuscular blocking agents, or both
- Altered mental status or underlying neuromuscular illness

For patients on ventilators with minimal swallowing abnormalities and negligible aspiration, oral feedings may be possible, particularly with the help of the speech-language pathologist (SLP). Selection of appropriate food consistencies and emphasis on specific head positions may minimize or prevent aspiration. In the presence of mild or moderate aspiration, eligible patients on or off the ventilator may benefit from the use of a Passy-Muir valve. This device may reduce aspiration and improve deglutition by restoring subglottic air pressure.

Unfortunately, for the majority of ventilator-dependent patients with a tracheostomy, the degree of swallowing dysfunction is such that oral intake is not an option. In these cases enteral feeding is preferred when the gastrointestinal tract can be used safely because it is convenient, there are fewer metabolic and infectious complications, and the cost is lower than that of parenteral nutrition.[36]

Placement of a cuffed, nonfenestrated tracheostomy tube necessarily results in aphonia. Every effort should be made to reestablish effective communication. To this end, involving the SLP and adequately assessing the patient's cognitive and linguistic skills is essential. Before establishing the best form of communication, the SLP may seek the assistance of an otolaryngologist in confirming that the upper airway is patent and physiologically intact. Where clinically possible, cuffed tracheostomy tubes may be exchanged for cuffless or fenestrated tubes, allowing speech either by manual occlusion of the tube on expiration or by placement of a device such as a Passy-Muir valve. The latter device may also assist the patient in coughing and swallowing. Successful implementation of communication strategies or devices depends on detailed instruction as well as encouragement and support by the SLP toward the nursing staff, patient, and family.

XIV. UNANSWERED QUESTIONS AND CONTROVERSY

A. CRICOTHYROTOMY

Considerable controversy exists regarding the role of cricothyrotomy in the emergency setting. This is largely due to the lack of controlled clinical trials to evaluate differences in efficacy and morbidity among various emergency airway techniques.

Clearly, the situations in which an anesthesiologist would consider using cricothyrotomy techniques are quite different from those encountered by an emergency medicine physician, trauma surgeon, or a prehospital or aeromedical provider. We believe percutaneous dilational cricothyrotomy to be the procedure of choice for anesthesiologists. It is performed in a manner very similar to the Seldinger technique for vascular access. We believe it to be safer than both transtracheal catheter ventilation and surgical cricothyrotomy. If an anesthesiologist can pass a catheter into the airway, it is relatively simple to pass a guidewire, dilator, and airway catheter. We feel it is also safer to establish an airway with a device that can be secured in place and used with conventional ventilation devices. The addition of a cuffed airway catheter eliminates the objection that the airway is unprotected and that it is difficult to ventilate some patients with poor compliance or increased airway resistance.

The cadaver studies performed in our laboratory suggest a relatively high failure rate related to kinking during insertion when conventional over-the-needle catheters are used. We have experienced and received reports of massive subcutaneous emphysema after attempted transtracheal ventilation with over-the-needle catheters.

A key issue is the determination of what size airway catheter to use. In situations in which the patient can awaken quickly or a definitive airway is likely before the patient attempts to breathe spontaneously, a small, 3.0 mm ID, kink-resistant airway catheter is a reasonable choice. With an airway catheter of this size, ventilation can be performed with conventional equipment, and passive exhalations are likely to be complete if adequate time is permitted.

In emergency settings in which endotracheal intubation is impossible or contraindicated, particularly maxillofacial trauma, we suggest using a larger airway catheter, which allows unimpeded air exchange and spontaneous ventilation without increased imposed work of breathing. We and others have shown that a 6.0 mm ID, 7.0-cm-long cricothyrotomy tube imposes the same work as a 7.0 mm ID ET.[8,73,82] We make a clear distinction between the truly emergent airway requiring cricothyrotomy and the DA that can be treated with a number of airway adjuncts, each attempted in a controlled, orderly manner. The addition of the cuffed 5.0 mm ID airway catheter set makes it the clear choice in the majority of instances.

There are clearly other methods for emergency airway control. It is probably more important for an anesthesiologist to become familiar and facile with one, and to practice it periodically, than to know a myriad of techniques.

B. PERCUTANEOUS TRACHEOSTOMY

1. Use of Bronchoscopy

The issue of bronchoscopy has been hotly debated in the literature over the past decade. Those in favor argue that it is easy to perform and adds to the safety of the procedure by significantly decreasing or eliminating the risk of false passage, pneumomediastinum, pneumothorax, and subcutaneous emphysema. Furthermore, bronchoscopy allows early detection and suctioning of intratracheal blood and secretions.

Opponents argue that bronchoscopy increases the length and cost of the procedure and does not add to safety in experienced hands. Moreover, the presence of the bronchoscope within the ET may result in CO_2 retention and difficulty ventilating the patient.

The accumulated weight of evidence in the literature points irrefutably to the advantages of bronchoscopy for safety reasons.[6,19,45,95] The risk of serious, life-threatening complications, although perhaps not completely eliminated, is indeed dramatically reduced when the procedure is endoscopically visualized from beginning to end. In terms of additional advantages, the bronchoscope allows proper midline needle placement between the second and third tracheal rings and prevents injury to the posterior tracheal wall. This author has performed PCT using multiple dilators in 191 patients and PCT using the single dilator in 150 cases. Bronchoscopy was used in all 341 patients (unpublished data) with no instances of false passage, pneumothorax, or pneumomediastinum. The era of minimally invasive surgery champions working in small operative fields without sacrificing visualization or safety. In PCT, bronchoscopy is a key element in providing visualization and safety, and its use should be mandatory in all cases.

2. Patient's Habitus

Controversy exists regarding the suitability of percutaneous tracheostomy in obese patients. It is believed by some that obesity may preclude adequate palpation of critical landmarks and increase the risk of false passage or accidental decannulation into the soft tissues of the neck. Optimal positioning of the neck almost always permits localization of the cricoid cartilage and sternal notch. Vigorous spreading of the subcutaneous tissues during the procedure facilitates palpation of the tracheal rings for precise needle placement. The risk of false passage may be addressed by always using a bronchoscope and ensuring step-by-step visualization. Accidental decannulation in these patients is more likely to occur because of the excessive length of the tube in the soft tissues. Using proximally extended tracheostomy tubes dramatically reduces the risk of this complication. In a series of 150 patients undergoing PCT, we noted that almost 25% of patients were obese or morbidly obese using body mass index criteria. There was no increased incidence of false passage, accidental decannulation, or other complications.

XV. PERCUTANEOUS DILATIONAL TRACHEOSTOMY

Toye and Weinstein[105] are credited with conceiving of percutaneous dilational tracheostomy. They published their initial results and a description of the Pertrach device in 1969. Their subsequent paper, published in 1988,[106] reported 94 cases of tracheostomy and 6 cases of cricothyrotomy. Only six cases were emergent, the remainder elective. Despite their results, interest in percutaneous dilational tracheostomy was sporadic, at best, until Ciaglia and colleagues refined the technique and published their initial findings.[26] Today, percutaneous dilational tracheostomy is an accepted alternative to formal surgical tracheostomy and is gaining in popularity, particularly for patients in the ICU who have been intubated for extended periods of time.

Percutaneous dilational tracheostomy is an elective procedure. It is included in this chapter because many anesthesiologists provide airway consultation in the ICU. Ivatury and coworkers[55] reported on the use of an emergency tracheostomy device (RapiTrac, Premier Medical Products, Norristown, PA) in 61 patients. Although the device uses the Seldinger technique and a dilator, we feel cricothyrotomy to be the preferred route for emergent airway access.

The Ciaglia percutaneous tracheostomy introducer (Cook Critical Care, Bloomington, IN) set (Fig. 28-11) is typical of devices used for this procedure. Unlike the Pertrach, which may be used for cricothyrotomy or tracheostomy, the Ciaglia and other sets are intended for subcricoid tracheostomy only. The technique is intended for use in controlled settings with the assistance of a respiratory therapist and nursing personnel.

This device is contraindicated for emergency placement, in patients with enlarged thyroids or nonpalpable cricoid cartilage, and in pediatric patients.

Detailed insertion instructions for the Ciaglia percutaneous dilational tracheostomy are as follows (Fig. 28-12):

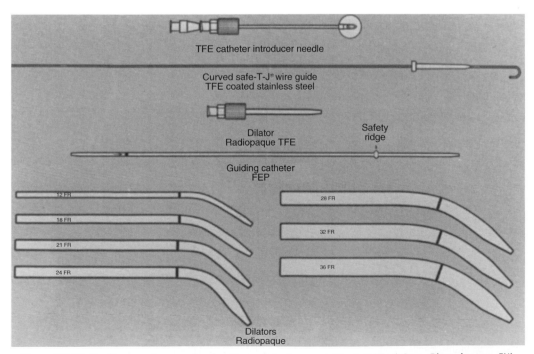

TFE catheter introducer needle

Curved safe-T-J® wire guide
TFE coated stainless steel

Dilator
Radiopaque TFE

Safety
ridge

Guiding catheter
FEP

12 FR

18 FR

21 FR

24 FR

28 FR

32 FR

36 FR

Dilators
Radiopaque

Figure 28-11 Ciaglia percutaneous tracheostomy introducer set (Cook Critical Care, Bloomington, IN).

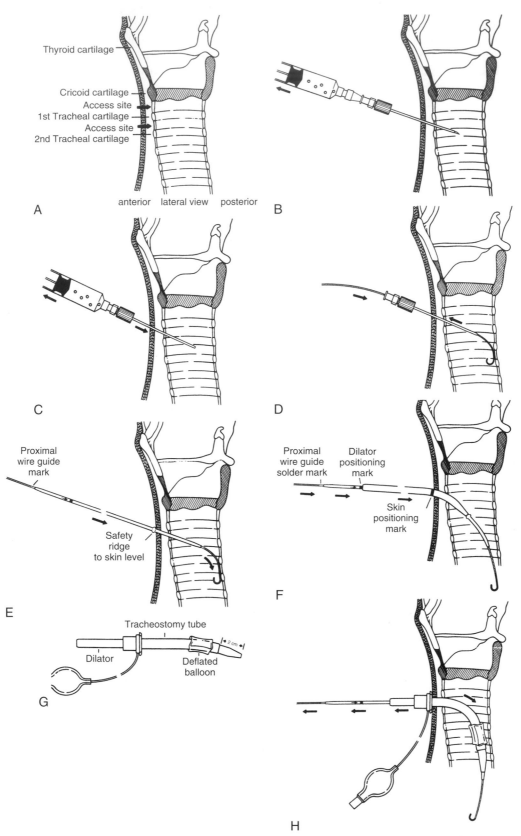

Figure 28-12 **A** to **H,** Detailed instructions (see text) for insertion of the Ciaglia percutaneous tracheostomy introducer set. (From Ciaglia P: Suggested instructions for percutaneous tracheostomy introducer set. Cook Critical Care, Bloomington, IN, 1988.)

A. PREPARATION OF THE PATIENT

1. Place the patient in the tracheostomy position. Position a pillow under the shoulders to permit full extension of head and neck. Elevate the head of the patient's bed 30 to 40 degrees.
2. Use ventilator changes and sedation to control patient's respiration. A PEEP level of 5 to 10 cm H_2O is recommended.
3. Instruct the respiratory therapist to loosen the fixation tapes of the in-place ET and deflate the cuff, making necessary changes in tidal volume, frequency, and so forth to evaluate compensation needed for air lead. Continuous oximetry monitoring should be employed.
4. Prepare and drape the anterior neck area.

B. PROCEDURE

1. Palpate landmark structures (thyroid notch, cricoid cartilage) to ascertain proper location for intended tracheostomy tube placement. Access and ultimate tube placement are made at the level between the cricoid and the first tracheal cartilage or between the first and second tracheal cartilages whenever feasible (see Fig. 28-12A).
2. After introduction of local anesthesia (1% lidocaine with epinephrine), make a vertical incision from the lower edge of the cricoid cartilage downward, in the midline, for a distance of 1 to 1.5 cm.
3. If desired, use a curved mosquito clamp to dissect gently vertically and transversely down to the anterior tracheal wall. With the tip of the finger, dissect the front of the trachea, in the midline, free of any tissues, and identify the cricoid cartilage. Displace the isthmus of the thyroid downward, if present.
4. Inject additional local anesthesia to the area, and seek the tracheal air column by directing the needle, in the midline, posterior and caudad. Again, this should be done after the respiratory therapist has deflated the ET cuff and withdrawn the ET 1 cm. When advancing the needle forward, entrance into the tracheal lumen can be confirmed by aspiration on the syringe resulting in air bubble return.
5. With the needle tip positioned in the trachea, inject 1.0 mL of lidocaine into the trachea, and remove the needle.
6. Attach a syringe half filled with lidocaine to the 17G sheathed introducer needle hub, and, using the technique described in step 4, seek the tracheal air column (see Fig. 28-12B). It is important not to impale the ET with the needle. This can be checked by having the respiratory therapist gently move the ET in and out 1 cm. If impaled, the needle is also seen and felt to move. It will be necessary to withdraw the needle and have the respiratory therapist pull back the ET 1 cm and then reinsert the needle.
7. When free flow of air is obtained with no impalement of the ET, remove the inner needle of the introducer needle assembly and advance the outer Teflon sheath several millimeters. Attach a syringe and confirm position within the tracheal lumen by visualizing free flow of air into the syringe when aspirated (see Fig. 28-12C).
8. Remove the syringe, and introduce the 0.052 inch (1.32 mm) diameter J guidewire several centimeters into the trachea. Remove the Teflon sheath while maintaining the guidewire position within the tracheal lumen (see Fig. 28-12D).
9. Maintaining the guidewire position at the skin level mark on the guidewire, advance the short, 11 Fr introducing dilator over the guidewire to dilate the initial access site into the trachea using a slight twisting motion. Remove the dilator while maintaining the guidewire in position with the skin level mark on the guidewire at its proper level.
10. Following the direction of the arrow on the guiding catheter, advance the 8.0 Fr Teflon guiding catheter over the guidewire to the skin level mark on the guidewire. Insert the guiding catheter and guidewire as a unit into the trachea until the safety ridge on the guiding catheter is at the skin level. The end of the guiding catheter with the safety ridge should be introduced toward the patient. Align the proximal end of the Teflon guiding catheter at the mark on the proximal portion of the guidewire. This ensures that the distal end of the guiding catheter is properly positioned back on the guidewire, preventing possible trauma to the posterior tracheal wall during subsequent manipulations. Position the guiding catheter and guidewire as a unit so that the safety ridge on the guiding catheter is at the skin level (see Fig. 28-12E).
11. Begin to dilate serially the access site into the trachea. This is accomplished by first advancing the 12 Fr blue dilator over the guidewire–guiding catheter assembly. To align the dilator properly on the guidewire–guiding catheter assembly, position the proximal end of the dilator at the single positioning mark on the guiding catheter. This ensures that the distal tip of the dilator is properly positioned at the safety ridge on the guiding catheter to prevent possible trauma to the posterior tracheal wall during introduction. While maintaining the visual reference points and positioning relationships of the guidewire, guiding catheter, and dilator, advance them as a unit, with a twisting motion, to the skin level mark on the blue dilator. Advance and pull back the dilating assembly several times, while twisting, to perform effective dilatation of the tracheal entrance site. Remove the blue dilator, leaving the guidewire–guiding catheter assembly in position (see Fig. 28-12F).
12. Continue the dilatation procedure by advancing, in sizing sequence (small to large), the supplied dilators.

Positioning of the dilators on the guidewire–guiding catheter assembly and dilatation of the tracheal entrance site should be done as described in step 11.

13. Slightly overdilate the tracheal entrance site to a size appropriate for passage of the tracheostomy tube of choice to allow easy passage of the balloon portion of the tracheostomy tube into the trachea.

Tracheostomy Tube Inner Diameter (mm)	Appropriate Dilator for Initial Overdilation (Fr)
6	24
7	28
8	32
9	36

14. Preload the flexible tracheostomy tube to be inserted on the appropriate size blue dilator by first generously lubricating the surface of the dilator. Position the tracheostomy tube onto the dilator so that its tip is approximately 2 cm back from the distal tip of the dilator. Make sure the balloon is totally deflated. Thoroughly lubricate tracheostomy tube assembly prior to insertion (see Fig. 28-12G). The sizing chart should be used as a guide to ensure correct fit.

Tracheostomy Tube Inner Diameter (mm)	Appropriate Dilator for Initial Overdilation (Fr)
6	18
7	21
8	24
9	28

Note: Dual-cannula tracheostomy tubes may also be placed using this technique. The inner cannula must be removed for introduction. Always check fit of dilator to tracheostomy tube prior to insertion. Follow tracheostomy tube manufacturer's instructions for testing of balloon cuff and inflation system prior to insertion.

15. Advance the preloaded, lubricated tracheostomy tube over the guiding catheter assembly to the safety ridge, and then advance as a unit into the trachea. As soon as the deflated balloon enters the trachea, withdraw the blue dilator, guiding catheter, and guidewire (see Fig. 28-12H).

16. Advance the tracheostomy tube to its flange. Note: If using a dual-cannula tracheostomy tube, insert the inner cannula at this point.

17. Connect the tracheostomy tube to the ventilator, inflate the balloon cuff, and remove the ET. Note: Prior to complete removal of the ET, test ventilation through tracheostomy tube.

18. Perform suction to determine whether any significant bleeding or possible obstruction exists that has not been noted to this point.

19. If necessary, one suture may be taken at the bottom of the initial incision.

C. POSTPLACEMENT INSTRUCTIONS

Apply antibiotic ointment and dressing to the stoma site three times a day for 3 days. Elevate the head of the patient's bed 30 to 40 degrees for 1 hour.

D. PRECAUTIONS

1. Always confirm access into trachea by air bubble aspiration.
2. Maintain safety positioning marks of guidewire, guiding catheters, and dilators during dilating procedure to prevent trauma to posterior wall of the trachea.
3. Tracheostomy tubes should fit snugly to dilator for insertion. Generous lubrication of the surface of the dilator enhances fit and placement of the tracheostomy tube.

To date, most studies report excellent success and low complication rates with percutaneous dilational tracheostomy. A follow-up study by Ciaglia and Graniero[25] and a study of 55 patients by Hazard and colleagues[47] demonstrate the utility of this procedure. A subsequent study by Hazard and colleagues[46] compared percutaneous tracheostomy with conventional tracheostomy in 46 patients. Complication rates were higher for conventional tracheostomy than for the percutaneous method (58% versus 25%); pre-decannulation problems were higher for conventional tracheostomy (46% versus 13%), as were late sequelae (88% versus 27%) in survivors.

Only Wang and associates[114] reported a high incidence of complications with percutaneous tracheostomy. However, they used a different device, which is no longer on the market, and a review of their selection of patients demonstrates that they used patients who would probably not meet inclusion criteria in most protocols.

XVI. CONCLUSION

In the 1970s, after a 50-year hiatus, cricothyrotomy became recognized as an important procedure for emergency airway management. Despite considerable evidence that cricothyrotomy can be lifesaving and has an acceptable low complication rate, controlled trials comparing various techniques have not been and are unlikely to be performed. This is largely the result of the infrequency with which physicians and other health care providers encounter patients requiring emergency cricothyrotomy.

The lack of opportunity to perform cricothyrotomy or other emergency airway procedures is a particular problem for anesthesiologists, who are the recognized airway experts. Although the opportunity to perform a cricothyrotomy is rare, it must be performed expeditiously and correctly when required. We believe that percutaneous dilational cricothyrotomy should be easy for anesthesiologists to learn because it is so similar to the Seldinger technique for insertion of catheters and sheaths, a technique used on a daily basis. The anesthesiologist should be well trained in emergency airway techniques and have appropriate equipment available at all times.

Although anesthesiologists practice primarily in the OR, there is a significant likelihood that they will be called upon to perform emergency airway procedures in other settings. In addition, they are often asked by colleagues to lecture on the subjects of the DA and the emergency airway. The purpose of this chapter is to familiarize anesthesiologists with the cricothyrotomy options available.

PCT is a safe and technically simple alternative to open surgical tracheostomy. It may be performed independently of OR schedules and eliminates the need to move critically ill patients from one location to another. The simplicity of the procedure, however, does not alter the need for proper preoperative planning, meticulous preparation and execution of the procedure, and appropriate postoperative care. PCT is the technique of choice in adult, intubated ICU patients.

REFERENCES

1. Abbrecht PH, Kyle RR, Reams WH, Brunette J: Insertion forces and risk of complications during cricothyroid cannulation. J Emerg Med 10:417, 1992.
2. Altman PL, Dittmer DS (eds): Respiration and Circulation. Bethesda, Md, Federation of American Societies for Experimental Biology, 1972.
3. An Updated Report by the American Society of Anesthesiologists Task Force on Management of the Difficult Airway: Practice guidelines for management of the difficult airway. Anesthesiology 98:1269, 2003.
4. Au J, Walker WS, Inglis D, Cameron EW: Percutaneous cricothyroidostomy (minitracheostomy) for bronchial toilet: Results of therapeutic and prophylactic use. Ann Thorac Surg 48:850, 1989.
5. Bair AE: Safety and efficacy of the rapid four-step technique for cricothyrotomy using a Bair claw [letter]. J Emerg Med 20:301, 2001.
6. Bair AE, Sakles JC: A comparison of a novel cricothyrotomy device with a standard surgical cricothyrotomy technique. Acad Emerg Med 6:1172, 1999.
7. Bair AE, Panacek EA, Wisner DH, et al: Cricothyrotomy: A 5-year experience at one institution. J Emerg Med 24:151, 2003.
8. Banner MJ, Blanch PB, Blackshear RH, et al: Excessive work imposed during spontaneous breathing through transtracheal catheters [abstract]. Anesthesiology 77:A1231, 1992.
9. Bellhouse CP, Dore C: Criteria for estimating likelihood of difficulty of endotracheal intubation with Macintosh laryngoscope. Anaesth Intensive Care 16:329, 1988.
10. Bennett JDC, Guha SC, Sankar AB: Cricothyrotomy: The anatomical basis. J R Coll Surg Edinb 41:57, 1996.
11. Benumof JL: Management of the difficult airway: with special emphasis on the awake tracheal intubation. Anesthesiology 75:1087, 1991.
12. Benumof JL, Scheller MS: The importance of transtracheal jet ventilation in the management of the difficult airway. Anesthesiology 71:769, 1989.
13. Bjoraker DJ, Kumar NB, Brown ACD: Evaluation of the Nu-Trake emergency cricothyrotomy device. Anesthesiology 59:A517, 1983.
14. Bair AE, Filbin MR, Kulkarni RG, Walls RM: The failed intubation attempt in the emergency department: Analysis of prevalence, rescue techniques, and personnel. J Emerg Med 23:131, 2002.
15. Boyd AD, Romita MC, Conlan AA, et al: A clinical evaluation of cricothyroidotomy. Surg Gynecol Obstet 149:365, 1979.
16. Boyle MF, Hatton D, Sheets C: Surgical cricothyrotomy performed by air ambulance flight nurses: A 5-year experience. J Emerg Med 11:41, 1993.
17. Bramwell KJ, Davis DP, Cardall TV, et al: Use of the Trousseau dilator in cricothyrotomy. J Emerg Med 17:433, 1999.
18. Brantigan CO, Grow JB: Cricothyroidotomy: Elective use in respiratory problems requiring tracheostomy. J Thorac Cardiovasc Surg 71:72, 1976.
19. Brantigan CO, Grow JB: Cricothyroidotomy revisited again. Ear Nose Throat J 59:289, 1980.
20. Brofeldt T, Panacek EA, Richards JR: An easy cricothyrotomy approach: The rapid four-step technique. Acad Emerg Med 3:1060, 1996.
21. Caparosa RJ, Zavatsky AR: Practical aspects of the cricothyroid space. Laryngoscope 67:577, 1957.
22. Caplan RA, Posner KL, Ward RJ, Cheney FW: Adverse respiratory events in anesthesia: A closed claims analysis. Anesthesiology 72:828, 1990.
23. Chan TC, Vilke GM, Bramwell KJ, et al: Comparison of wire-guided cricothyrotomy versus standard surgical cricothyrotomy technique. J Emerg Med 17:957, 1999.
24. Chang RS, Hamilton RJ, Carter WA: Declining rate of cricothyrotomy in trauma patients with an emergency medicine residency: Implications for skills training. Acad Emerg Med 5:247, 1998.
25. Ciaglia P, Graniero KD: Percutaneous dilatational tracheostomy—Results and long-term follow-up. Chest 101:464, 1992.

26. Ciaglia P, Firsching R, Syniec C: Elective percutaneous dilatational tracheostomy: A new simple bedside procedure-preliminary report. Chest 87:715, 1985.

27. Cole RR, Aguilar EA: Cricothyroidotomy versus tracheostomy: An otolaryngologist's perspective. Laryngoscope 98:131, 1988.

28. Corke C, Cranswick P: A Seldinger technique for minitracheostomy insertion. Anaesth Intensive Care 16:206, 1988.

29. Cormack RS, Lehane J: Difficult tracheal intubation in obstetrics. Anaesthesia 39:1105, 1984.

30. Davis DP, Bramwell KJ, Hamilton RS, et al: Safety and efficacy of the rapid four-step technique for cricothyrotomy using a Bair claw. J Emerg Med 19:125, 1999.

31. Davis DP, Bramwell KJ, Vilke GM, et al: Cricothyrotomy technique: Standard versus the rapid four-step technique. J Emerg Med 17:17, 1999.

32. Eisenburger P, Laczika K, List M, et al: Comparison of conventional surgical versus Seldinger technique emergency cricothyrotomy performed by inexperienced clinicians. Anesthesiology 92:687, 2000.

33. Esses BA, Jafek BW: Cricothyroidotomy: A decade of experience in Denver. Ann Otol Rhinol Laryngol 96:519, 1987.

34. Ezri T, Szmuk P, Warters RD, et al: Difficult airway management practice patterns among anesthesiologists practicing in the United States: Have we made any progress? J Clin Anesth 15:418, 2003.

35. Florete OG Jr: Airway management. In Civetta JM, Taylor RW, Kirby RR (eds): Critical Care. Philadelphia, JB Lippincott, 1992, pp 1419-1436.

36. Fortune JB, Judkins DG, Scanzaroli D, et al: Efficacy of prehospital surgical cricothyrotomy in trauma patients. J Trauma 42:832, 1997.

37. Frei FJ, Meier PY, Lang FJ, Fasel JH: [Cricothyreotomy using the Quicktrach coniotomy instrument set]. Anasth Intensivther Notfallmed 25(Suppl 1):44, 1990.

38. Fusciardi J, Rouby JJ, Barakat T, et al: Hemodynamic effects of high frequency jet ventilation in patients with and without circulatory shock. Anesthesiology 65:485, 1986.

39. Gerich TG, Schmidt U, Hubrich V, et al: Prehospital airway management in the acutely injured patient: The role of surgical cricothyrotomy revisited. J Trauma Injury Infect Crit Care 45:312, 1998.

40. Gerling MC, Davis DP, Hamilton RS, et al: Effect of surgical cricothyrotomy on the unstable cervical spine in a cadaver model of intubation. J Emerg Med 20:1, 2001.

41. Glassenburg R, Vaisrub N, Albright G: The incidence of failed intubation in obstetrics: Is there an irreducible minimum abstracted? Anesthesiology 73:A1061, 1990.

42. Greisz H, Qvarnstorm O, Willen R: Cricothyroidotomy: A clinical and histopathological study. Crit Care Med 10:387, 1982.

43. Griggs WM, Worthley LI, Gilligan JE, et al: A simple percutaneous tracheostomy technique. Surg Gynecol Obstet 170:543, 1990.

44. Habel DW: Cricothyroidotomy as a site for elective tracheostomy. Trans Pac Coast Otoophthalmol Soc Annu Meet 58:181, 1977.

45. Hawkins ML, Shapiro MB: Emergency cricothyrotomy: A reassessment. Am Surg 61:52, 1995.

46. Hazard PB, Garrett HE Jr, Adams JW, et al: Bedside percutaneous tracheostomy: Experience with 55 elective procedures. Ann Thorac Surg 46:63, 1988.

47. Hazard P, Jones C, Benitone J: Comparative clinical trial of standard operative tracheostomy with percutaneous tracheostomy. Crit Care Med 19:1018, 1991.

48. Heffner JE, Sahn SA: The technique of tracheostomy and cricothyroidotomy. J Crit Illness 2:79, 1987.

49. Holland R: Anesthesia related mortality in Australia. Int Anesthesiol Clin 22:61, 1984.

50. Holmes JF, Panacek EA, Sakles JC, Brofeldt BT: Comparison of 2 cricothyrotomy techniques: Standard method versus rapid 4-step technique. Ann Emerg Med 32:442, 1998.

51. Holst M, Hedenstiema G, Kumlein JA, et al: Five years' experience with elective coniotomy. Intensive Care Med 11:202, 1985.

52. Holst M, Halbig I, Persson A, Schiratzki H: The cricothyroid muscle after cricothyroidotomy. Acta Otolaryngol (Stockh) 107:136, 1989.

53. Hulsey S: Cricotomes. In Dailey RH, Simon B, Young GP (eds): The Airway: Emergency Management. St Louis, Mosby, 1992.

54. Isaacs JH Jr: Emergency cricothyrotomy: Long-term results. Am Surg 67:346, 2001.

55. Ivatury R, Siegel JH, Stahl WM, et al: Percutaneous tracheostomy after trauma and critical illness. J Trauma 32(2):133, 1992.

56. Jackson C: High tracheostomy and other errors: The chief causes of chronic laryngeal stenosis. Surg Gynecol Obstet 32:392, 1921.

57. Jackson C: Tracheostomy. Laryngoscope 18:285, 1909.

58. Jackson IJB, Choudhry AK, Ryan DW, et al: Minitracheostomy: Seldinger—Assessment of a new technique. Anaesthesia 46:475, 1991.

59. Jacoby JJ, Flory FA, Jones JR: Transtracheal resuscitation. JAMA 162:625, 1956.

60. Johnson DR, Dunlap A, McFeeley P, et al: Cricothyrotomy performed by prehospital personnel: A comparison of two techniques in a human cadaver model. Am J Emerg Med 11:3:207, 1993.

61. Keenan RL, Boyan CP: Cardiac arrest due to anesthesia. JAMA 253:2373, 1985.

62. Kirchner JA: Cricothyroidotomy and subglottic stenosis. Plast Reconstr Surg 68:828, 1981.

63. Kress TD, Balasbramanian S: Cricothyroidotomy. Ann Emerg Med 11:197, 1982.

64. Kuriloff DB, Setzen M, Portnoy W, Gadaleta D: Laryngotracheal injury following cricothyroidotomy. Laryngoscope 99:125, 1989.

65. Linsdey D: Emergency cricothyrotomy [letter]. Am J Emerg Med 12:124:1994.

66. Little CM, Parker MG, Tarnopolsky R: The incidence of vasculature at risk during cricothyroidostomy. Ann Emerg Med 15:805, 1986.

67. Lyons G: Failed intubation. Anaesthesia 40:759, 1985.

68. Mace SE: Cricothyrotomy. J Emerg Med 6:309, 1988.

69. Malhotra V: Pyloric stenosis. In Yao FSF, Artusio JF Jr (eds): Anesthesiology: Problem-Oriented Patient Management. Philadelphia, JB Lippincott, 1993.

70. Marcolini EG, Burton JH, Bradshaw JR, Baumann MR: A standing-order protocol for cricothyrotomy in prehospital emergency patients. Prehosp Emerg Care 8:23, 2004.

71. McGill J, Clinton JE, Ruiz E: Cricothyrotomy in the emergency department. Ann Emerg Med 11:361, 1982.

72. McLaughlin J, Iserson KV: Emergency pediatric tracheostomy: A usable technique and model for instruction. Ann Emerg Med 15:463, 1986.

73. Melker RJ, Banner MJ: Work imposed by breathing through cricothyrotomy tube. Presented at the Sixth World Congress on Emergency and Disaster Medicine, Hong Kong, Sept 6-18, 1989.

74. Miklus RM, Elliott C, Snow N: Surgical cricothyrotomy in the field: Experience of a helicopter transport team. J Trauma 29:506, 1989.

75. Mitchell SA: Cricothyroidotomy revisited. Ear Nose Throat J 58:54, 1979.

76. Morain WD: Cricothyroidotomy in head and neck surgery. Plast Reconstr Surg 65:424, 1980.

77. Morch ET: History of mechanical ventilation. In Kirby RR, Banner MJ, Downs JB (eds): Clinical Applications of Ventilatory Support. New York, Churchill Livingstone, 1990, pp 1-62.

78. Mulder DS, Marelli D: The 1991 Fraser Gurd lecture: Evolution of airway control in the management of injured patients. J Trauma 33:856, 1992.

79. Nakatsuka M, MacLeod AD: Hemodynamic and respiratory effects of transtracheal high frequency jet ventilation during difficult intubation. J Clin Anesth 4:321, 1992.

80. Nugent WL, Rhee KJ, Wisner DH: Can nurses perform surgical cricothyrotomy with acceptable success and complication rates? Ann Emerg Med 20:367, 1991.

81. O'Connor JV, Reddy K, Ergin MA, et al: Cricothyroidotomy for prolonged ventilatory support after cardiac operations. Ann Thorac Surg 39:353, 1988.

82. Ooi R, Fawcett WJ, Soni N, Riley B: Extra inspiratory work of breathing imposed by cricothyrotomy devices. Br J Anaesth 70:17, 1993.

83. Pedersen J, Lou H, Schurizek BA, et al: Ossification of the cricothyroid membrane following minitracheostomy. Intensive Care Med 15:272, 1989.

84. Piotrowski JJ, Moore EE: Emergency department tracheostomy. Emerg Med Clin North Am 6:737, 1988.

85. Pridmore SA: A new cricothyrotomy cannula. Med J Aust 1:532, 1979.

86. Ratnayake B, Langford RM: A survey of emergency airway management in the United States. Anaesthesia 51:908, 1996.

87. Ravlo O, Bach V, Lybecker H, et al: A comparison between two emergency cricothyroidotomy instruments. Acta Anaesthesiol Scand 31:317, 1987.

88. Ravussin P, Freeman J: A new transtracheal catheter for ventilation and resuscitation. Can Anaesth Soc J 32:60, 1985.

89. Rehm CG, Wanek SM, Gagon EB, et al: Cricothyroidotomy for elective airway management in critically ill trauma patients with technically challenging neck anatomy. Crit Care 6:531, 2002.

90. Roven AN, Clapham MC: Cricothyroidotomy. Ear Nose Throat J 62:68, 1983.

91. Ruhe DS, Williams GV, Proud GO: Emergency airway by cricothyroid puncture or tracheostomy. Trans Am Acad Ophthalmol Otolaryngol 64:182, 1960.

92. Ryan DW: Minitracheostomy. Intensive Care World 8:128, 1991.

93. Safar P, Penninckx JJ: Cricothyroid membrane puncture with special cannula. Anesthesiology 28:943, 1967.

94. Sakles JC, Laurin EG, Rantapaa AA, Panacek EA: Airway management in the emergency department: A one-year study of 610 tracheal intubations. Ann Emerg Med 31:325, 1998.

95. Samsoon GLT, Young JRB: Difficult tracheal intubation: A retrospective study. Anaesthesia 42:487, 1987.

96. Shapiro SL: Emergency airway for acute laryngeal obstruction. Eye Ear Nose Throat Mon 49:35, 1970.

97. Silk JM, Marsh AM: Pneumothorax caused by minitracheostomy. Anaesthesia 44:663, 1989.

98. Sise MJ, Shackford SR, Cruickshank JC, et al: Cricothyroidotomy for long-term tracheal access: A prospective analysis of morbidity and mortality in 76 patients. Ann Surg 200:13, 1984.

99. Sladen A, Guntupalli K, Marquez J, Klain M: High frequency jet ventilation in the postoperative period: A review of 100 patients. Crit Care Med 12:782, 1984.

100. Spaite D, Joseph M: Prehospital cricothyrotomy: An investigation of indications, technique, complications and patient outcome. Ann Emerg Med 19:279, 1990.

101. Spoerel WE, Narayanan PS, Singh NP: Transtracheal ventilation. Br J Anaesth 43:932, 1971.

102. Stokes DN: Re-insertion of a minitracheostomy tube. Anaesthesia 42:782, 1987.

103. Task Force on Guidelines for Management of the Difficult Airway: Practice guidelines for management of the difficult airway. Anesthesiology 78:597, 1993.

104. Tiret L, Desmonts JM, Hatton F, Vourc'h G: Complications associated with anesthesia: A prospective survey in France. Can Anaesth Soc J 33:336, 1986.

105. Toye FJ, Weinstein JD: A percutaneous tracheostomy device. Surgery 65:384, 1969.

106. Toye FJ, Weinstein JD: Clinical experience with percutaneous tracheostomy and cricothyroidotomy in 100 patients. J Trauma 26:1034, 1988.

107. Tran Y, Hedley R: Misplacement of a minitracheostomy tube. Anaesthesia 42:783, 1987.

108. Tunstall ME: Failed intubation in the parturient [editorial]. Can J Anaesth 36:611, 1989.

109. Turnbull AD, Carlon G, Howland WS, Beattie EJ Jr: High frequency jet ventilation in major airway or pulmonary disruption. Ann Thorac Surg 32:468, 1981.

110. Van Hasselt EJ, Bruining HA, Hoeve LJ: Elective cricothyroidotomy. Intensive Care Med 11:207, 1985.

111. Wagstaff A, Spraling R, Ryan DW: Minitracheostomy. Anaesthesia 42:216, 1987.

112. Wain JC, Wilson DJ, Mathisen DJ: Clinical experience with minitracheostomy. Ann Thorac Surg 49:881, 1990.

113. Walls RM: Cricothyroidotomy. Emerg Med Clin North Am 6:725, 1988.

114. Wang MB, Berke GS, Ward PH, et al: Early experience with percutaneous tracheostomy. Laryngoscope 102:157, 1992.

115. Ward Booth RP, Brown J, Jones K: Cricothyroidotomy, a useful alternative to tracheostomy in maxillofacial surgery. Int J Oral Maxillofac Surg 18:24, 1989.

116. Xeropotamos NS, Coats TJ, Wilson AW: Prehospital surgical airway management: One year's experience from the helicopter emergency medical service. Injury 24:222, 1993.

29

SURGICAL AIRWAY

Michael A. Gibbs
Ron M. Walls

I. INTRODUCTION

A. GENERAL PRINCIPLES

Emergency surgical airway management comprises four distinct but related techniques that gain access to the infraglottic airway. These are needle cricothyrotomy, percutaneous cricothyrotomy, surgical cricothyrotomy, and surgical tracheostomy. In emergency situations, cricothyrotomy is greatly preferred over tracheostomy because of its relative simplicity, speed, and lower complication rate. The airway is very superficial at the level of the cricothyroid membrane (CTM), separated from the skin only by the subcutaneous fat and anterior cervical fascia. The trachea moves progressively deeper in the neck as it travels caudally, making anterior access more difficult and introducing additional anatomic barriers (e.g., thyroid isthmus.) Needle cricothyrotomy with percutaneous transtracheal ventilation may provide temporary oxygenation in some patients, but the technique does not provide a secure (protected) airway and cannot support ventilation. Needle cricothyrotomy is reviewed elsewhere in this textbook (see Chapter 28). The emphasis in this chapter is on surgical and percutaneous cricothyrotomy; as the former, and in some cases the latter, places a cuffed endotracheal tube (ET) in the trachea.

Any discussion of surgical airway management techniques must account for three important concepts:

1. *Most clinicians with responsibility for airway management have either limited, or no, experience with these procedures.* Whether in the prehospital setting, the emergency department, the operating room, the inpatient unit, or the intensive care unit, surgical airway management is simply not required very often, largely because of high proficiency with direct laryngoscopy, increasing capability of identifying difficult airways (DAs) in advance, and the multitude of sophisticated alternative intubation devices that can be used when direct laryngoscopy is not possible or successful. The progressive diminution in use of emergency surgical airway procedures over the past two decades has, therefore, multifactorial causes but is primarily the result of two evolutionary changes: the shift in emphasis in trauma airway management from avoidance of oral laryngoscopy to widespread acceptance of gentle, controlled, oral laryngoscopy with in-line cervical spine immobilization and the growing proficiency of clinicians from multiple specialties with rapid sequence intubation (RSI). Contemporary emergency department studies using RSI demonstrate high success rates (97% to 99%) and an infrequent need for surgical airway rescue (0.5% to 2.0%) even though the unselected nature of the patients and the large percentage with trauma result in a high proportion of DAs compared with those seen in elective surgery.[5,23,54,56] Despite increasing familiarity with alternative airway rescue devices (e.g., flexible and semirigid fiberoptic bronchoscopy, video laryngoscopy, retroglottic airways, supraglottic airways, retrograde intubation, lighted stylet) that further reduce the need for cricothyrotomy, the surgical airway remains the final pathway on *all* failed airway algorithms.[60] Therein lies the dilemma. As clinicians embrace new technologies and devices that make the need for surgical airway management increasingly rare, acquisition and maintenance of the skills necessary to perform surgical airway management, which in some cases is the only method capable of sustaining the patient's life, become increasingly elusive.

2. *Surgical airway management is infrequently, if ever, performed in the stable patient and is most often needed in a "can't-intubate, can't-ventilate" situation, when failure to perform the technique properly and in a timely fashion may prove disastrous.* The patient in need of emergency cricothyrotomy is typically one with significantly distorted airway anatomy or who has been subjected to multiple failed intubation attempts, or both. Thus, the operator is required to establish an airway in the presence of potentially overwhelming difficulty and very little time.

3. *If a surgical approach fails, few, if any, options remain and there may not be sufficient time for an alternative attempt.* Most would consider surgical cricothyrotomy to be the ultimate consideration among a series of airway management options. In addition, a failed surgical cricothyrotomy may result in bleeding, loss of airway integrity, or further airway distortion, making the success of subsequent rescue attempts highly unlikely.

Thus, emergency cricothyrotomy is a rarely performed procedure; done under duress by clinicians who may have limited experience, in patients in whom it is difficult to perform and who are likely to die if it fails. These challenges speak powerfully to those involved in airway management, counseling them to invest the time required to master this crucial technique. Fortunately, although it has been unfairly cloaked in mystique and represented as dramatic and difficult, cricothyrotomy is a relatively straightforward procedure that can be accomplished with a high success rate and low rate of complications by providers with adequate, but not extensive, training. This training can be achieved using various animal models (not whole animals) and by medical simulation.

1. Historical Perspective

The surgical airway as a lifesaving procedure has been appreciated for thousands of years. The first depictions of surgical tracheostomy have been found on Egyptian tablets dating from 3600 BC.[40] In the second century AD, Galen suggested tracheostomy, utilizing a vertical incision, as an emergency treatment for airway obstruction.[11,40] Vesalius later published the first detailed descriptions of tracheostomy in the 16th century, using a reed to ventilate the lungs. Ironically, his alleged resuscitation of a Spanish nobleman through tracheostomy and ventilation led to condemnation by the Spanish Inquisition and his ultimate death.[43] The first record of a successful tracheostomy performed in the United States was in 1852. Unfortunately, the patient later died of airway stenosis, a common complication at that time. A paper from 1886 described a mortality rate of 50% for tracheostomy and a high incidence of stenosis, which accounted for many of the deaths.[17]

Chevalier Jackson published a landmark paper on tracheostomy in 1909, which described principles still relevant today.[32] He described a surgical mortality rate of 3%, which he attributed to several factors: optimal airway control prior to surgery, the use of local anesthesia rather than sedation, using a well-designed tube, and meticulous surgical and postoperative care. Jackson achieved international recognition; however, so did his condemnation of "high tracheostomy" as the cause of subglottic stenosis. The high tracheostomy he referred to was cricothyrotomy, but at that time it involved division of the cricoid or thyroid cartilage. Modern cricothyrotomy involves incision of the CTM only. In 1921, Jackson published a study of 200 patients referred to him for postcricothyrotomy stenosis. Aside from the obvious referral bias, the indication for a surgical airway at that time was primarily inflammatory lesions of the upper airway, which probably accounted for the high incidence of subglottic stenosis.[31]

Although, in retrospect, it was the technique and the underlying condition that were largely responsible for the high rate of stenosis, fear of this complication condemned the technique of cricothyrotomy for over half a century. In the interest of developing a technique that was safer and quicker than Jackson's open dissection, Toye and Weinstein described the first percutaneous tracheostomy in 1969.[58] However, cricothyrotomy was not widely reconsidered as a surgical airway option until 1976, when Brantigan and Grow published the results of cricothyrotomy for long-term airway management in 655 patients.[13] In this series, the rate of stenosis was 0.01%, no major complications were described, and the procedure was found to be faster, simpler, and less likely to cause bleeding than tracheostomy. Subsequent studies have supported their conclusions that cricothyrotomy is a safe and effective surgical airway procedure and, in fact, the preferred technique when emergent surgical airway control is needed.[9,26,42] Contemporary case series have shown that cricothyrotomy can be performed with a high success rate and reasonably low complication rate by hospital-based physicians and other clinicians (i.e., nurses, paramedics) providing prehospital care.[10,25,32,37,45,55,62]

2. Definitions of the Surgical Airway

The definition of surgical airway can be so broad as to comprise all forms of airway management that require the creation of a new opening into the airway. Cricothyrotomy is the establishment of a surgical opening in the airway through the CTM and placement of a cuffed tracheostomy tube or endotracheal tube (ET). Cricothyrotomy has also been referred to as cricothyroidotomy, cricothyroidostomy, cricothyrostomy, laryngostomy, or laryngotomy; however, cricothyrotomy is presently the preferred term. Tracheostomy differs from cricothyrotomy in the anatomic location of entry into the airway. Tracheostomy is the establishment of a surgical opening in the airway at any level including or caudal to the first tracheal ring.

Surgical airways may be further subclassified by the technique used:

1. Surgical (sometimes referred to as "open" or "full open" or "full surgical")

2. Percutaneous (more precisely described by the actual technique, e.g., Seldinger)
3. Dilational (a distinct percutaneous approach)
4. Transtracheal catheter

Surgical cricothyrotomy and surgical tracheostomy refer to the use of a scalpel and other surgical instruments to create an opening in the airway.[41,61] This technique allows the creation of a definitive, protected airway by the insertion of a cuffed tracheostomy tube with an internal diameter sufficient for ventilation, oxygenation, and suctioning.

The percutaneous dilational technique utilizes a kit or device that is intended to establish a surgical airway without requiring a formal surgical cricothyrotomy. Following a small skin incision, the airway is accessed by a small needle through which a flexible guidewire is passed using the Seldinger technique. The airway device is then introduced over a dilator and passed over the guidewire and into the airway in a manner analogous to that of central line placement. An alternative percutaneous technique has been used that relies on placement of an airway device using a direct puncture into the airway (e.g., Nu-Trake, Smith Medical, Keene, NH). A large-bore metal needle or a sharp trocar within the catheter is used to puncture the airway directly, without the use of a guidewire. Direct puncture devices are more hazardous and have fallen out of favor because of the higher incidence of complications and lower success rates compared with other percutaneous techniques.[1,49]

Transtracheal catheter ventilation, considered the least invasive surgical technique, involves the direct placement of a moderate-bore catheter through the CTM.[8] The small caliber of these devices does not allow adequate oxygenation without attachment to a high-pressure oxygen source or jet ventilator, except in small children, and does not support adequate ventilatory gas exchange. A 6.0 Fr reinforced fluorinated ethylene propylene, kink-resistant, emergency transtracheal airway catheter (Cook Critical Care, Bloomington, IN) has been designed as a kink-resistant catheter for this purpose.

3. Role of the Surgical Airway

The relative merit of percutaneous dilatational tracheostomy versus open surgical tracheostomy continues to be a subject of debate. Although formal open tracheostomies are primarily performed by surgeons, the percutaneous dilatational tracheostomy is frequently performed by anesthesiologists and other nonsurgical intensivists, particularly in the intensive care unit setting. This technique was originally described by Toye and Weinstein in 1969, but it did not gain popularity until the results with a modified device were reported by Ciaglia and colleagues in 1985.[17,58]

There have been no clinical studies to date demonstrating the superiority of any one approach over another or of any of these devices over formal surgical cricothyrotomy.

II. ANATOMY

An understanding of the anatomy of the upper airway and the neck is required for the successful and rapid performance of a surgical airway. Most emergent surgical techniques involve surgical fields that become rapidly obscured by blood and are, therefore, essentially "blind" procedures. The identification of anatomic landmarks is critical.

A. BONES AND CARTILAGES

The horseshoe-shaped hyoid bone is the most cephalad rigid structure in the anterior neck, palpable approximately a fingerbreadth cephalad to the laryngeal prominence. It suspends the larynx during phonation and respiration by the thyrohyoid membrane and muscle.

The thyroid cartilage is the largest structure of the larynx and consists of two laminae fused in the midline to form the laryngeal prominence. The angle of this fusion is more acute in males, creating the more distinct prominence known as the Adam's apple. The separation of the laminae superiorly forms the palpable superior thyroid notch. The laryngeal prominence of the thyroid cartilage represents the most readily and consistently identified landmark in the neck when performing a surgical airway. The superior and inferior cornua of the thyroid cartilage are the posterior extensions of the upper and lower edges of the lamina. The thyrohyoid ligament attaches to the superior cornu and the posterior cricoid cartilage articulates with the inferior cornu.

The cricoid cartilage is the only complete cartilaginous ring in the upper airway and defines the inferior aspect of the larynx (Fig. 29-1). It is shaped like a signet ring with the wider lamina posterior. Superiorly, the lamina has synovial articulations with the arytenoids and thyroid cartilage. Anteriorly, the cricoid ring is attached to the inferior thyroid cartilage by the CTM.

B. CRICOTHYROID MEMBRANE

The CTM is a fibroelastic tissue that covers the cricothyroid space, between the thyroid cartilage and the cricoid ring. It is trapezoidal in shape and in the average adult is 1 cm high and 2 to 3 cm wide. It is located in the midline, approximately 2 to 3 cm below the laryngeal prominence. The vocal cords are located 1 cm above the CTM and are, therefore, rarely injured during a cricothyrotomy.

Several anatomic characteristics make this membrane an ideal choice for emergency airway access. It is a subcutaneous structure located just beneath the skin, a small amount of subcutaneous fat, and the anterior cervical fascia in most patients. Accordingly, it is easily palpated as a depression inferior to the thyroid cartilage, bounded on its inferior aspect by a hard ridge, the cricoid cartilage. The ligament does not calcify with age. It has no overlying muscles, major vessels, or nerves. It is supported by the anterior cervical fascia, which is not robust at this level.

C. VASCULAR STRUCTURES

The major arteries of the neck always lie deep to the pretracheal fascia and should not present a concern when incising the skin over the CTM. The paired superior thyroid arteries arise from the external carotid arteries, superior and lateral to the cricoid cartilage. The anterior branches of these arteries run along the upper thyroid isthmus to anastomose in the midline. The unpaired inferior thyroid artery also anastomoses with the superior thyroid artery at the isthmus. In 10% of the population, the potentially large thyroid ima artery ascends anterior

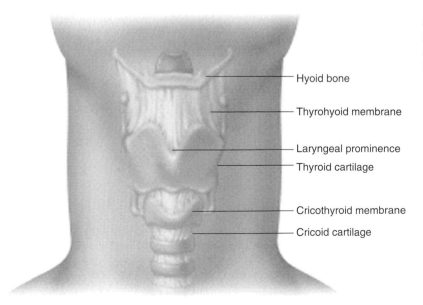

Figure 29-1 Surface anatomy of the larynx. (From Walls RM, et al: Manual of Emergency Airway Management, 2nd ed. Philadelphia, Lippincott Williams & Wilkins, 2004.)

Hyoid bone

Thyrohyoid membrane

Laryngeal prominence
Thyroid cartilage

Cricothyroid membrane
Cricoid cartilage

to the trachea to join the anastomoses. A large venous plexus is found over the thyroid isthmus.

The right and left cricothyroid arteries are branches of the right and left superior thyroid arteries, respectively, and in the majority of patients cross the superior aspect of the CTM to anastomose in the midline.[38] Although at risk for injury during a cricothyrotomy, they do not appear to be clinically significant. Bleeding is often self-limited and easily controlled with gauze packing. There is no venous plexus over the CTM.

D. THYROID GLAND

The isthmus of the thyroid gland lies anterior to the trachea, generally between the second and third tracheal rings, although it may extend to the first and fourth rings. Its size and location can be variable; however, its average height and thickness are 1.25 cm. A pyramidal lobe of the thyroid gland is present in one third of the population and extends superiorly from the isthmus, over the cricoid membrane and larynx to the left of the midline.

E. ANATOMIC VARIATIONS

In infants, the hyoid bone and cricoid cartilage are the most prominent structures in the neck. The laryngeal prominence does not develop until adolescence. The larynx also starts higher in the neck of the child and descends from the level of the second cervical vertebra at birth to the level of the fifth or sixth in the adult.[19] The laryngeal prominence is more acute and therefore more prominent in males. This also results in longer vocal cords and accounts for the deeper voices of males.

The CTM can vary in size among adults and be as small as 5 mm in height. This space may narrow further with contraction of the cricothyroid muscle.[33] The CTM in the child is disproportionately smaller in area than that in the adult (Fig. 29-2). In an infant, the width of the membrane constitutes only one fourth of the anterior tracheal diameter, as opposed to three fourths in the adult. Because of this smaller area and the difficulty in identifying landmarks in children, emergency surgical cricothyrotomy is difficult and hazardous in small children and is not recommended in children younger than 10 years. In this age group, placement of a needle catheter with percutaneous transtracheal ventilation is the preferred method.

Identification of landmarks in the obese, edematous, or traumatized neck may be difficult. The CTM usually lies 1½ of the patient's fingerbreadths below the laryngeal prominence. Alternatively, its location may be estimated to be three to four of the patient's fingerbreadths above the suprasternal notch with the neck in a neutral position.

There can be significant variation in the arterial and venous pattern in the anterior vessels of the neck, which

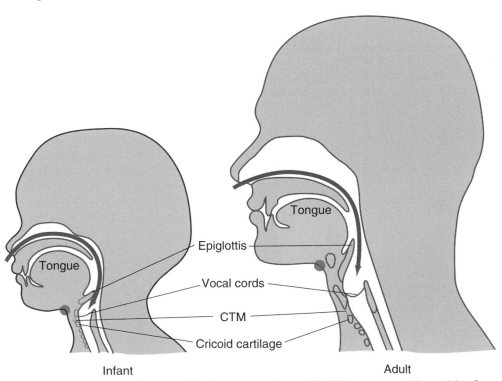

Figure 29-2 The anatomic differences in the pediatric airway: (1) Higher, more anterior position for the glottic opening. (2) Relatively larger tongue in the infant, which lies between the mouth and glottic opening. (3) Relatively larger and more floppy epiglottis in the child. (4) The cricoid ring is the narrowest portion of the pediatric airway versus the vocal cords in the adult. (5) Position and size of the cricothyroid membrane in the infant. (6) Sharper, more difficult angle for nasotracheal intubation. (7) Larger relative size of the occiput in the infant. See text for details. (From Walls RM, et al: Manual of Emergency Airway Management, 2nd ed. Philadelphia, Lippincott Williams & Wilkins, 2004.)

can result in a major artery crossing the midline. This is rarely a problem for cricothyrotomy, as most anomalous vessels are present lower in the neck.

III. SURGICAL CRICOTHYROTOMY

A. INDICATIONS AND CONTRAINDICATIONS

The primary indication for an emergent surgical airway (Table 29-1) is the failure of endotracheal intubation or alternative noninvasive airway techniques in a patient requiring immediate airway control. The American Society of Anesthesiologists (ASA) DA algorithm advocates a surgical airway as the final endpoint for the unsuccessful arm of the emergency pathway.[3,48] There are a number of other DA algorithms in the literature, as well as numerous modifications of the ASA guidelines; however, all comprehensive pathways include the surgical airway as the technique of choice when others have failed.[7,44,48] Despite the introduction of numerous alternative rescue devices, the most common error in the management of the DA is persistent attempts at laryngoscopy in a failed airway situation.[51-53] This behavior has been associated with increased morbidity and mortality.[51] Identification of the can't-intubate, can't-ventilate scenario should result in immediate consideration of surgical airway access. If alternative methods are tried when there is inability to oxygenate and ventilate the patient by bag and mask, precious time may be lost in what are ultimately futile attempts, and by the time cricothyrotomy is undertaken

Table 29-1   Indications for Cricothyrotomy

Indications
Inability to Secure the Airway Using a Less Invasive Technique
1. Massive upper airway hemorrhage
2. Massive regurgitation
3. Maxillofacial trauma
4. Structural abnormalities of the airway (congenital or acquired)
Airway Obstruction
1. Traumatic
a. Airway edema (includes thermal/inhalation injury)
b. Foreign body
c. Airway stenosis or disruption
2. Nontraumatic
a. Airway edema
b. Mass effect (e.g., tumor, hematoma, abscess)
c. Upper airway infection (supraglottitis)

and accomplished, delays in achieving airway control and oxygenation will have led to hypoxic brain injury.

In most circumstances, cricothyrotomy is regarded as an emergency rescue technique for the failed, airway when other noninvasive rescue techniques, such as the laryngeal mask airway, have either failed, are predicted to fail, or are unavailable.[5] There are occasions, however, when a cricothyrotomy is the primary airway of choice. An example would be the patient with such severe facial trauma that nasal or oral approaches to the airway are deemed impossible. There also has been a renewed interest in the role of elective cricothyrotomy in the operative setting. Some cardiothoracic surgeons prefer this to a tracheostomy in their patients with a median sternotomy, suggesting that the higher location of the airway wound reduces the potential for contamination of the sternal wound.[46] A study described the use of elective cricothyrotomy instead of tracheostomy in the intensive care unit for trauma patients who had technically challenging neck anatomy. The procedure was described as simpler with no difference in short- or long-term complications.[50]

Cricothyrotomy is considered safe in trauma patients with unstable cervical spine injuries provided that cervical spine immobilization is maintained.[2,24] Although coagulopathy has been described as a relative contraindication, there are reports of successful cricothyrotomy after systemic fibrinolytic therapy for acute myocardial infarction.[59]

The primary indication for cricothyrotomy is failure of intubation by oral or nasal means in the presence of an immediate need for definitive airway management. A second indication is as a method of primary airway management in patients for whom nasotracheal or orotracheal intubation is contraindicated or thought to be impossible. Thus, cricothyrotomy should be thought of as a rescue technique in most circumstances and is only infrequently used as the primary method of airway management.

Often, the main hurdle to performing cricothyrotomy is simply making the initial decision to forgo further attempts at laryngoscopy or with other rescue devices and to proceed with a surgical airway. Noninvasive airway management methods are used so successfully that cricothyrotomy is often viewed as a procedure that will never be required. However, the single-minded pursuit of multiple noninvasive airways with the resultant delay in the initiation of a surgical airway can result in hypoxic disaster, particularly if the patient is not able to be oxygenated and ventilated adequately with a bag and mask between attempts.

The decision to proceed to a surgical airway must also consider some other important variables. The airway provider must appreciate whether the surgical airway will bypass the airway problem anatomically. For example, if the obstructing lesion is infraglottic, performing a cricothyrotomy may be a critical waste of time. The patient's anatomy or pathology must be considered when weighing the difficulty of performing a cricothyrotomy. Placement of the initial skin incision is based on palpating the pertinent anatomy. Adiposity, burns, trauma, or infection may make this difficult; they do not represent absolute contraindications, but the strategy may need to be adjusted. The operator must also consider the type of invasive technique (i.e., open surgical or percutaneous). This consideration takes into account provider preference based on experience, the patient's presentation, and equipment availability.

Contraindications for surgical airway management are few and, with one exception, are relative. That one exception is young age. Children have a small, pliable, mobile larynx and cricoid cartilage, making cricothyrotomy extremely difficult. For children younger than 10 years, unless the larynx and cricoid cartilage are teenage or adult sized, percutaneous transtracheal ventilation should be used as the surgical airway management technique of choice. Two other situations have been proposed as absolute contraindications: tracheal transection and laryngeal fracture.[39] In either situation, tracheostomy is recommended as the preferred method. Although anatomically and philosophically appealing, this assertion is clinically impractical. First, these injuries may not be readily apparent at the bedside. Second, there may be no other means of securing the airway in a dying patient. Third, expert surgical backup may not be readily available and tracheostomy is a much more complicated procedure than cricothyrotomy. Therefore, these, too, should be considered relative contraindications, and cricothyrotomy should be recognized as carrying significant risk in these situations and used when there is thought to be no other method to secure the airway. Relative contraindications include preexisting laryngeal or tracheal pathology such as tumor, infections, or abscess in the area in which the procedure will be performed; hematoma or other anatomic destruction of the landmarks that would render the procedure difficult or impossible; coagulopathy; and lack of operator expertise.

The presence of an anatomic barrier in particular should prompt consideration of alternative techniques that might result in a successful airway. However, in cases in which no alternative method of airway management is likely to be successful or timely enough, cricothyrotomy should be performed without hesitation. The same principles apply for both the cricothyrotomy and percutaneous transtracheal ventilation. Percutaneous transtracheal ventilation is the surgical airway method of choice for children younger than 10 years. The cricothyrotomes have not been demonstrated to improve success rates or time or to decrease complication rates when compared with surgical cricothyrotomy. As with formal cricothyrotomy, experience, skill, knowledge of anatomy, and adherence to proper technique are essential for success when a cricothyrotome is used. The large size and cutting characteristics of the insertion part of the cricothyrotome may be likely to cause more damage in the neck than either an open cricothyrotomy or Seldinger-based technique.

B. PROCEDURE

1. Equipment

Tracheostomy tubes are made in a variety of designs and materials.[58] They may have a single lumen, but many have an inner cannula that can easily be removed to allow routine cleaning and prevention of mucous obstruction. Most tubes also come with a blunt-tipped obturator that is used to facilitate insertion and reduce trauma. The tubes may also be rigid or flexible and kink resistant and of variable curves, angles, and sizes, depending upon the anatomic needs of the patient. Tracheostomy tubes are secured with twill or a padded fastener that goes around the neck and attaches to the neck plate of the tube. Tubes may be cuffed or uncuffed. Cuffs should be kept at inflation pressures of 20 to 25 mm Hg, but over the short term, inflation can be judged by palpation of the reservoir balloon.[27] Underinflation can increase aspiration, whereas high cuff pressures can cause mucosal ischemia and subsequent tracheal stenosis or tissue necrosis.

It is critical that whatever surgical technique is chosen, the instrument and its location are familiar to the airway providers. The kit needs to be easily accessible, compact, and ideally located in a DA cart positioned in the room or readily accessible (Fig. 29-3). The operating room tracheostomy surgical trays are not appropriate for this purpose because of their size and complexity. It is recommended that a custom cricothyrotomy kit be assembled with the components in Box 29-1 or a commercial kit designed for this purpose be utilized. A commercial kit has become available that offers both the Seldinger technique and the necessary instruments for a surgical cricothyrotomy with a cuffed tracheostomy tube all in one system (Fig. 29-4).

2. Landmarks

The CTM is the anatomic site of access in the emergent surgical airway, regardless of the technique used. The CTM is identified by first locating the laryngeal prominence of the thyroid cartilage. This may be easier to appreciate in males because of their more prominent

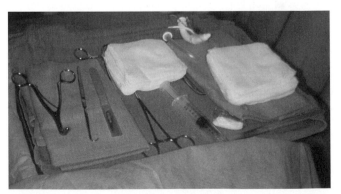

Figure 29-3 Simply organized cricothyrotomy tray with tracheal hook, Trousseau dilator, scalpel, and tracheostomy tube. (Photo courtesy of R.M. Walls, MD.)

thyroid notch. Approximately 1 to 1½ of the patient's fingerbreadth below the laryngeal prominence, the membrane may be palpated in the midline of the anterior neck, as a soft depression between the inferior aspect of the thyroid cartilage above and the rigid cricoid ring below. The thyrohyoid space, which lies superior to the laryngeal prominence and inferior to the hyoid bone, should also be identified. This space should be distinguished from the CTM to avoid misplacement of the tracheostomy tube above the vocal cords. In children, the CTM is disproportionately smaller because of a greater overlap of the thyroid cartilage over the cricoid cartilage. Because of this, cricothyrotomy is not recommended in children younger than 10 years.

Unfortunately, the same anatomic or physiologic abnormalities (i.e., trauma, morbid obesity, congenital anomalies) that precipitated the surgical airway may also hinder easy palpation of landmarks. The location of the CTM can be estimated by placing four fingers on the neck, vertically, with the small finger in the sternal notch. The membrane is approximately located under the index finger and can serve as a point at which the initial

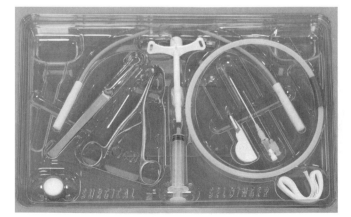

Figure 29-4 A new cricothyrotomy set (Melker Universal Cricothyrotomy Set, Cook Critical Care) combines capability for a percutaneous, Seldinger-based cricothyrotomy *(right)* with a simple instrument set for a full surgical cricothyrotomy *(left)*. The same cuffed tracheostomy tube is used for either technique, but a blunt introducing cannula is substituted when surgical insertion is desired. (Photograph© Cook Critical Care, Bloomington, IN, 2004.)

incision is made. A vertical skin incision is preferred in the emergent situation because of the location of major blood vessels as well as ease in locating the membrane. Palpation through the vertical incision can then confirm the location. Identification may be assisted by using a locator needle attached to a syringe containing saline or lidocaine. Aspiration of air bubbles suggests entry into the airway, but this does not distinguish between the CTM and an intertracheal space.

Although palpation of the CTM is easily performed on most patients, the particular condition creating the airway difficulty may obscure traditional landmarks. The urgency and anxiety associated with a failed airway may further compound this difficulty. Because of this, it is the practice of some anesthesiologists to mark the skin overlying the approximate location of the CTM prior to the procedure if a possible DA is anticipated. Routinely palpating the CTM on patients is also recommended to become familiar with the landmarks.

C. SURGICAL CRICOTHYROTOMY TECHNIQUES

1. Traditional Surgical Cricothyrotomy: The "No-Drop" Technique

a. Preparation of the Neck

Appropriate antiseptic solution should be applied and sterile technique observed as much as possible. The procedure should not be delayed if time does not allow ideal preparation. Suction, a bag-valve-mask, and oxygen should be immediately available. The tracheostomy tube should be opened and prepared for insertion at this time. There may be circumstances, such as the conscious patient, in which it is desirable to infiltrate the skin and subcutaneous tissues with 1% lidocaine. The operator may wish to localize the membrane at this time using a 20G needle. Upon aspiration of air into syringe, lidocaine can be injected into the airway. The injection precipitates a cough in the patient with intact airway reflexes; however, this serves to disperse the lidocaine and diminish further stimulation in the conscious patient. Caution is advised in patients with potentially unstable cervical spine injuries.

b. Landmark Identification

An emergent cricothyrotomy is best thought of as a procedure that is done by touch rather than by visualization. The identification of the external landmarks before initiating the incision and the use of a method to maintain knowledge of the anatomic relationships (see later) are keys to success. The operator should be positioned on the same side of the patient as the operator's dominant hand (the hand that will be used to make the incisions; i.e., a right-handed operator stands to the patient's right). After identification of the laryngeal prominence, the superior horns of the thyroid cartilage are firmly grasped between the thumb and long finger of the nondominant hand. This leaves the index finger ideally positioned to localize the CTM and re-identify its location at any time during the

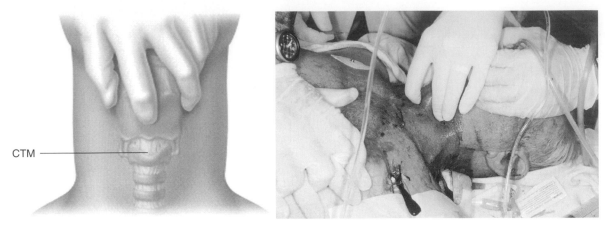

Figure 29-5 With the superior cornua of the larynx firmly immobilized by the thumb and long finger of the nondominant hand the index finger is free to palpate and locate the cricothyroid membrane. (From Walls RM, et al: Manual of Emergency Airway Management, 2nd ed. Philadelphia, Lippincott Williams & Wilkins, 2004.)

procedure by capitalizing on the constancy of the relationship as long as the thyroid cartilage is not released. Thus, it is critical that control of the larynx with this hand be maintained until the placement of the tracheal hook (Fig. 29-5).

c. Vertical Skin Incision
Using the operator's dominant hand, a generous vertical incision is made in the midline, with its center over the CTM. The incision should be at least 2 cm in length and may need to be extended in patients with significant obesity or where identification is difficult. The incision should go through subcutaneous tissues down to, but not into, the thyroid and cricoid cartilages (Fig. 29-6).

d. Confirmation of Membrane Location
With the thumb and long finger maintaining control of the thyroid cartilage, the index finger may now be inserted into the incision. Without interposed skin and tissues, it is much easier to appreciate the structures of the anterior neck and confirm the location of the CTM. The index finger can be left in the wound, resting on the inferior aspect of the anterior larynx, indicating the superior limit of the CTM (Fig. 29-7).

e. Horizontal Incision of the Cricothyroid Membrane
The index finger may be withdrawn just prior to the incision or left in the wound to serve as a guide. The CTM should be incised horizontally 1 to 2 cm in length (Fig. 29-8). It is recommended to attempt to incise the lower half of the membrane to avoid the superiorly placed cricothyroid artery and vein. This may be difficult to achieve, and inadvertent injury to these vessels is rarely clinically significant. Despite the exposure obtained with the skin incision, bleeding from the skin and various vascular structures eliminates a clear view of the field in most cases. Time does not permit the operator to attempt to deal with bleeding in order to achieve a bloodless field. Maintenance of the anatomic relationships outlined previously allows the procedure to be completed expeditiously without the need for direct visualization of the structures of interest. If significant

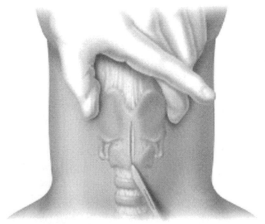

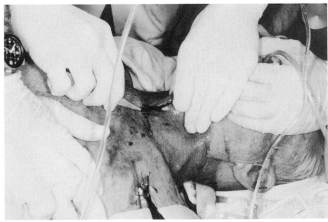

Figure 29-6 A vertical skin incision is made down to, but not through, the airway. (From Walls RM, et al: Manual of Emergency Airway Management, 2nd ed. Philadelphia, Lippincott Williams & Wilkins, 2004.)

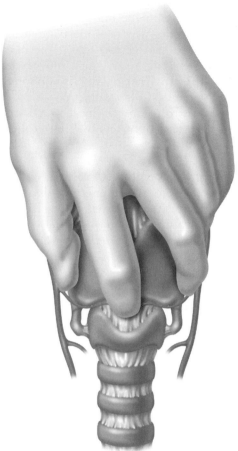

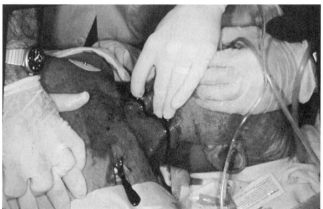

Figure 29-7 The index finger can now directly palpate and relocate the cricothyroid membrane. (From Walls RM, et al: Manual of Emergency Airway Management, 2nd ed. Philadelphia, Lippincott Williams & Wilkins, 2004.)

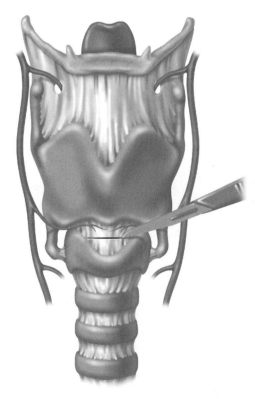

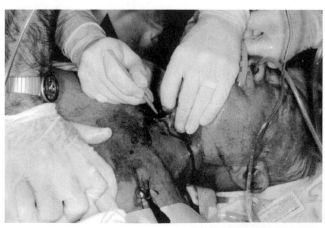

Figure 29-8 A transverse incision is made in the cricothyroid membrane staying low to attempt to avoid the cricothyroid artery and vein.

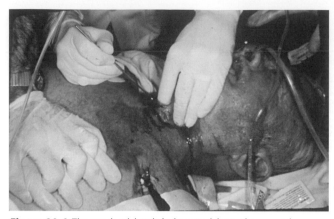

Figure 29-9 The tracheal hook is inserted into the wound, oriented transversely, and then rotated to pick up the inferior edge of the thyroid cartilage.

bleeding occurs, it can be dealt with (usually by simple wound packing) after the airway is secured.

Attempts at ventilation (which have to be discontinued at this point) may result in the presence of air bubbles appearing in the wound and tissues of the neck in synchrony with respirations. The index finger may also be reinserted into the opening to confirm the proper location of the incision in the membrane.

f. Insertion of the Tracheal Hook

Laryngeal control should be maintained with the thumb and long finger of the nondominant hand. The hook is held in the dominant hand and turned so that it is oriented transversely and then inserted into the trachea through the surgical opening (Fig. 29-9). The index finger of the nondominant hand can serve as a guide to help place the hook into the incision. Once through the CTM, the hook is rotated so that the hook is oriented in the cephalad direction. The hook is firmly applied to the inferior

border of the thyroid cartilage, and gentle upward and anterior traction with the hook handle at a 45-degree angle to the anterior neck skin can be used to bring the airway up to the skin (Fig. 29-10). The hook may be passed to an assistant to maintain immobilization and control of the larynx. The operator's nondominant hand may now be released for completion of the procedure with the proviso that the tracheal hook is maintaining control and should not be removed until confirmation of tube placement.

g. Dilation of the Opening with Dilator

The Trousseau dilator is then inserted using the dominant hand. It is our preference to insert the dilator so that the prongs are oriented to dilate the opening in the rostral-caudal direction rather than transversely (Fig. 29-11). Although the dilator appears to be designed to insert directly into the airway and dilate transversely, in fact it is the rostral-caudal dimension of the CTM that provides the most resistance to cannulation and thus it is desirable to dilate in this plane. The Trousseau dilator is inserted only a couple of millimeters into the airway and then opened to dilate the airway. With the airway thus opened, the dilator, in situ, is transferred from the operator's dominant hand to the nondominant hand, where it can be held from underneath (see Fig. 29-11). This frees the dominant hand to insert the tracheostomy tube.

h. Insertion of the Tracheostomy Tube

The tracheostomy tube is then inserted with the obturator in place (Fig. 29-12). To avoid unnecessary delays at this juncture, the tube should have been removed from its packaging prior to initiation of the procedure and the blunt-tipped obturator already inserted. The tube is oriented along the handle of the dilator (i.e., at a 90-degree angle to the patient) and inserted between the dilator blades following their natural curve. As the tracheostomy

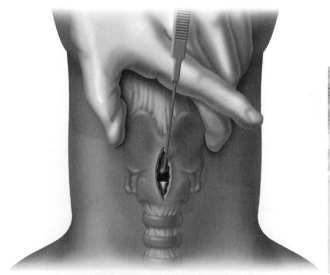

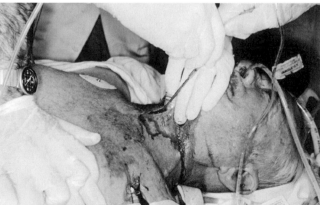

Figure 29-10 The tracheal hook exerts light traction on the inferior aspect of the thyroid cartilage.

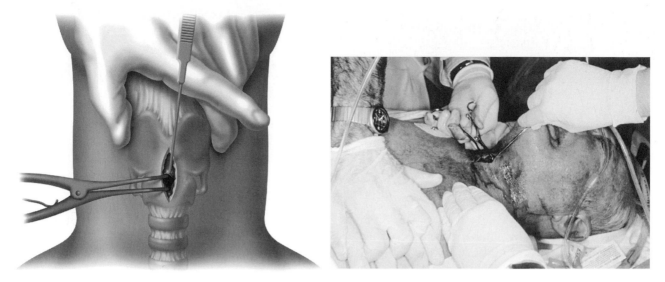

Figure 29-11 The Trousseau dilator is used to enlarge the vertical dimension of the membrane, the aspect providing the most resistance to insertion of the tube.

tube gains the airway and is passing between the prongs of the Trousseau dilator, it is helpful to rotate the dilator handle counterclockwise 90 degrees (see Fig. 29-12) so that the dilation is now occurring in the transverse rather than the rostral-caudal dimension. The reason is that when the tracheostomy tube has gained access into the airway, the prongs of the Trousseau dilator may themselves inhibit successful passage of the tip of the tracheostomy tube down the trachea. By rotating the Trousseau dilator, the prongs are moved out of the way to either side of the tube but dilation is continued to assist in placing the tracheostomy tube until it is firmly seated against the anterior neck. The dilator is gently

removed as the tube is being advanced, just before it is seated in its final position (Fig. 29-13).

i. Cuff Inflation and Securing the Tracheostomy Tube

The cuff should be inflated. The obturator is then removed, and if there is an inner cannula, this must be inserted now to allow the attachment of the ventilation bag. Care must be taken during the initial assembly of the tracheostomy tube not to lose track of the inner cannula, as this is necessary for the attachment of ventilation devices. The tracheostomy tube can be secured with twill or a padded fastener that goes around the neck and attaches to the neck plate of the tube.

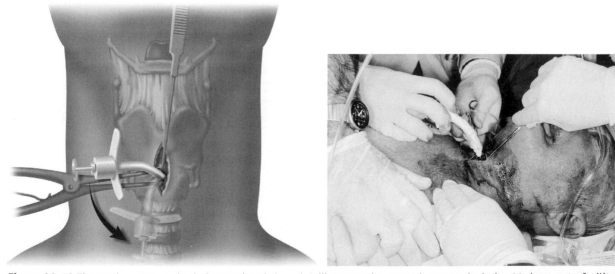

Figure 29-12 The tracheostomy tube is inserted and then the dilator can be rotated counterclockwise 90 degrees to facilitate passage of the tube.

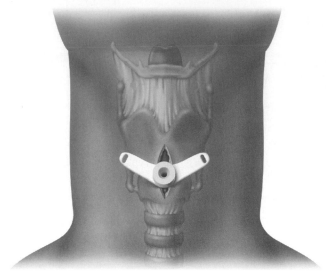
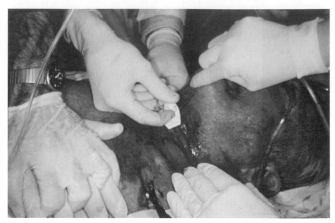

Figure 29-13 The tube is firmly seated and the dilator can be removed. It is best to leave the hook in place until placement is confirmed and the cuff inflated.

j. Confirmation of Tube Position

The tracheostomy tube position can be confirmed using the same methods as those for ET position. Carbon dioxide detection can be used to confirm correct placement in the airway. If there is concern that the tube is placed outside the trachea, a nasogastric tube may be gently inserted. In the airway the tube advances easily, but resistance is met if the tube is in a false passage. Auscultation of both lungs and the epigastric area is also recommended, although esophageal placement of the tube is highly unlikely. A chest radiograph can be helpful in the identification of barotrauma. Only when the position of the tube is certain should the tracheal hook be removed. This should be done with great care in order to avoid hooking a part of the tracheostomy tube and inadvertently extubating the patient. If the tube was inadvertently placed in a false passage, the correction of this is greatly facilitated with the hook still in place.

2. Rapid Four-Step Technique

The rapid four-step technique (RFST) is an attempt to simplify the procedure by using a horizontal stab incision through the skin and membrane simultaneously, followed by tracheal hook traction applied caudad at the cricoid ring.[13] Cadaveric studies have shown RFST to be simple to learn and faster in obtaining a surgical airway than the open technique just described.[18,28] Other advantages are that (1) less equipment is necessary (it is performed with a scalpel, hook, and tracheostomy tube), (2) it may be performed independently, and (3) the operator is positioned at the head of the bed, similar to the performance of orotracheal intubation.

Acute complications from RFST may be more common, however. The stab technique may increase the incidence of trauma to the posterior trachea and anterior aspect of the esophagus. In cadaveric models an increase in damage to the cricoid ring has been found because of direct traction on the ring with the tracheal hook.[5,18,28] This may be remedied through the use of a double-hook device that disperses the forces across the cricoid ring.[5,18] RFST may not be as desirable in patients in whom landmark identification is difficult. In this circumstance, the authors recommend beginning with a vertical incision, similar to the traditional technique described previously.[13] There are no clinical studies that report the success rates and associated acute and delayed complications of RFST compared with traditional methods in live patients. The choice between the RFST and the traditional technique, often called the "no-drop" technique, is an individual one, as there is no clear evidence that either method is superior or more likely to bring success than the other.

As with other techniques, attempts should be made to oxygenate and ventilate the patient maximally prior to and during the procedure. The anterior neck should be prepared as described earlier for the "no-drop" technique. From a position at the head of the bed, RFST is performed in the following manner:

a. Landmark Identification

As in traditional cricothyrotomy, the airway is accessed through the CTM. Therefore, the identification of landmarks is exactly the same as described previously (see Figs. 29-5 and 29-14). Because of the horizontal stab incision, however, it is even more critical to be confident of the location of membrane. If there is uncertainty, it is

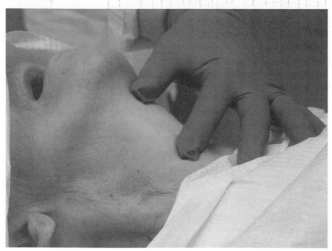

Figure 29-14 The landmarks are palpated as for the "no-drop" technique, but the horizontal skin incision leaves little room for error, so extra care is needed. (From Walls RM, et al: Manual of Emergency Airway Management, 2nd ed. Philadelphia, Lippincott Williams & Wilkins, 2004.)

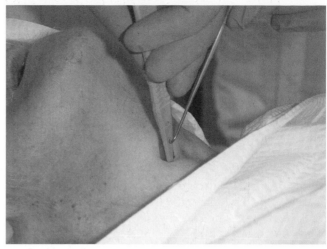

Figure 29-16 The hook is oriented transversely and inserted alongside the scalpel before the scalpel is removed. (From Walls RM, et al: Manual of Emergency Airway Management, 2nd ed. Philadelphia, Lippincott Williams & Wilkins, 2004.)

recommended to begin with a vertical incision first, as described earlier.

b. Horizontal Stab Incision

A single horizontal stab incision using a no. 20 scalpel is made directly through the skin, subcutaneous tissues, and CTM. The incision should be approximately 1.5 cm wide, and because of the size of the no. 20 blade, widening of the opening is rarely required (Fig. 29-15). If the anatomy is not readily palpable through the skin, an initial vertical incision should be created to allow subsequent palpation of the anatomy and identification of the CTM. Once the CTM is incised, the no. 20 blade is maintained in the airway until the tracheal hook is secured.

c. Stabilization of the Larynx with the Tracheal Hook

A tracheal hook is placed parallel to the scalpel on the caudal side of the blade (Fig. 29-16). The hook is then rotated to secure and control the cricoid ring. The scalpel is then removed from the airway. The tracheal hook is now used to apply gentle traction on the cricoid ring to lift the airway up toward the surface of the skin and to provide modest stoma dilation (Fig. 29-17). The direction of force on the hook is reminiscent of the "up and away" direction employed with laryngoscopy. The amount of traction force required for easy intubation (18 newtons) is significantly lower than the force that is associated with breakage of the cricoid ring (54 newtons); however, the

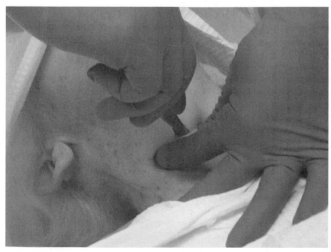

Figure 29-15 A single, horizontal, stab incision is made through skin and membrane. (From Walls RM, et al: Manual of Emergency Airway Management, 2nd ed. Philadelphia, Lippincott, Williams & Wilkins, 2004.)

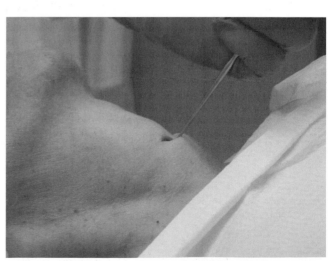

Figure 29-17 The hook exerts traction on the superior aspect of the cricoid cartilage and skin, pulling the airway up into the field. (From Walls RM, et al: Manual of Emergency Airway Management, 2nd ed. Philadelphia, Lippincott Williams & Wilkins, 2004.)

chance of trauma may be further reduced by using a double-tined hook.[5] Utilization of the hook in this direction generally provides sufficient widening of the incision to obviate the need for further dilation (i.e., Trousseau dilator). Placement of the hook on the cricoid ring may also reduce the possibility of intubating the pretracheal potential space, which is essentially eliminated by the apposition of the airway and the subcutaneous fat by the traction on the hook.

d. Insertion of the Tracheostomy Tube

With adequate control of the airway using the hook placed on the cricoid ring, a tracheostomy tube is gently inserted through the cricothyroid space into the trachea (Fig. 29-18). The cuff is then inflated, the tube secured, and its location confirmed by the same methods described earlier.

3. Percutaneous Cricothyrotomy Techniques

Numerous commercial cricothyrotomy devices are available, many of which utilize a modified Seldinger technique to assist in the placement of a tracheal airway (see Fig. 29-4). There are aspects of this technique that may make it appealing to the anesthesiologist. This method is similar to the one commonly utilized in the placement of central venous catheters and offers some familiarity to the operator uncomfortable or inexperienced with the surgical cricothyrotomy technique described earlier. This technique can be learned quickly. By the fifth practice attempt on a mannequin model, 96% of anesthesiologists achieved success within 40 seconds.[60] However, the technique still requires knowledge of the anatomy and the ability to localize the membrane and has several steps, so it approaches the open technique in complexity. When compared with the standard open technique in cadavers and dog models,

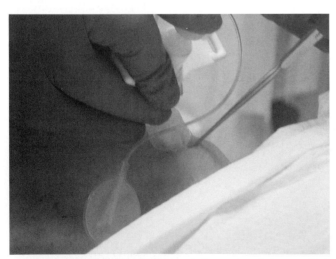

Figure 29-18 The tracheostomy tube is inserted and then verified and secured in the usual fashion. (From Walls RM, et al: Manual of Emergency Airway Management, 2nd ed. Philadelphia, Lippincott Williams & Wilkins, 2004.)

there were no differences in performance times or complications.[4,14,20] It is estimated that the procedure may be accomplished in 40 to 100 seconds.[4,14,20,60] Also, the percutaneous cricothyrotomy kits are preassembled and commercially available, whereas at present the surgical tools used in the traditional approach are not (except in the combination kit shown in Fig. 29-4). It seems intuitive that the technique should result in less bleeding, but no studies have been performed to assess the significance of this. One of the limitations is the relatively smaller lumen, which is of no real concern in an emergency, and in some models the absence of a cuff, which could be an issue if airway protection from emesis or hemorrhage is needed. When selecting a device, it is suggested to choose one with a cuff, as many of these procedures are performed on patients who have not been fasted or are actively hemorrhaging and require further airway protection. The Melker Cuffed Emergency Cricothyrotomy Catheter Set and the Melker Universal Cricothyrotomy Set both are available with a cuffed airway catheter (Cook Critical Care).

As with other techniques, attempts should be made to preoxygenate and ventilate the patient maximally prior to and during the procedure. The anterior neck should be prepared as described earlier. Although the kits may vary, most of the percutaneous cricothyrotomy kits use the Seldinger technique and share the following steps:

a. Landmark Identification

The CTM is identified using the same methods described previously. The nondominant hand is then used to control the larynx and maintain identification of the landmarks.

b. Insertion of Locator Needle

The introducer needle is then inserted through the skin and the CTM in a slightly caudal direction. The needle is attached to a syringe and advanced with the dominant hand, while negative pressure is maintained on the syringe. The sudden aspiration of air indicates placement of the needle into the tracheal lumen (Fig. 29-19).

c. Insertion of the Guidewire

The syringe is then removed from the needle and a soft-tipped guidewire is inserted through the needle into the trachea in a caudal direction. The needle is then removed, leaving the wire in place. As with most Seldinger techniques, control of the wire must be maintained at all times (Fig. 29-20).

d. Skin Incision

A small skin incision is then made adjacent to the wire. This facilitates passage of the airway device through the skin. Alternatively, the skin incision may be made vertically over the membrane before insertion of the needle and guidewire.

e. Insertion of the Airway

The airway catheter provided in the kit (3 to 6 mm internal diameter), with an introducing dilator in place, is then

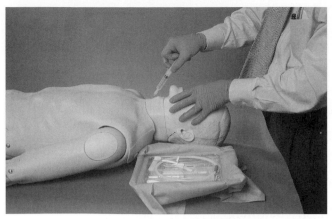

Figure 29-19 The finder needle is inserted through the cricothyroid membrane. A small, vertical skin incision may be made prior to insertion of the needle or later, just before insertion of the airway and dilator. (Photo from STRATUS Center for Medical Simulation, Brigham & Women's Hospital, with permission.)

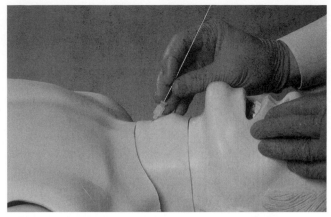

Figure 29-20 The wire is fed through in a caudad direction; then the needle is removed. (Photo from STRATUS Center for Medical Simulation, Brigham & Women's Hospital, with permission.)

inserted over the wire into the trachea. If resistance is met, the skin incision should be deepened and a gentle twisting motion applied to the airway device (Fig. 29-21). When the airway device is firmly seated against the skin, the wire and obturator are removed together, leaving the tracheostomy tube in place. Tube location should then be confirmed as described previously and secured properly. The devices are radiopaque on radiographs.

IV. TRAINING ISSUES

A survey published in 1995 found that although 80% of anesthesiology programs taught cricothyrotomy as part of their curriculum, most of them did so through lectures only, with no practical experience.[37] A survey published in 2003 demonstrated only 21% of anesthesiologists claimed skills to perform cricothyrotomy.[22] Most anesthesiology graduates have never performed a cricothyrotomy during their training.[60]

The merits of a procedure are irrelevant if hesitancy on the part of the provider leads to a significant delay in establishing a definitive airway. Discomfort with a procedure is usually overcome with technical proficiency obtained through stepwise practice; however, this procedure is performed so rarely that proficiency must be obtained through scheduled, simulated learning. Invasive airway methods, like any other invasive procedures, must be learned and practiced at regular intervals to maintain proficiency.

The advent of emergency medicine as a specialty with its own airway expertise has resulted in a significant decrease in exposure to emergency airways for anesthesiology trainees. The success of RSI in the emergency setting, as well as advances in airway management techniques in anesthesiology, have prompted editorials concerned with the

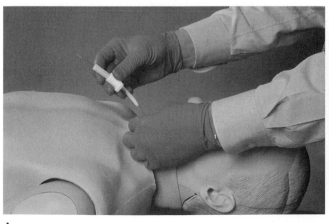

A

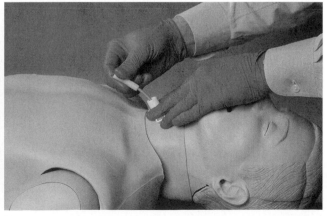

B

Figure 29-21 A, The airway is inserted over the guidewire with the dilator in place. **B,** The dilator and wire are then removed together. (Photo from STRATUS Center for Medical Simulation, Brigham & Women's Hospital, with permission.)

current problem of gaining and maintaining competence in invasive airway management.[16,35,36] Studies suggest a current cricothyrotomy rate of approximately 1% of all emergency airways and a dramatically lower rate in the operating suite. Regardless of the setting, this incidence is too low to ensure adequate training, but it highlights the probability that most airway managers will be called upon to perform an invasive airway at some point in their career.

The practice required to obtain familiarity with the equipment and technique must take place outside the clinical setting. Of anesthesiology programs that instruct their residents on cricothyrotomy, 60% use lectures only, which is a poor teaching technique for developing proficiency in manual skills.[37] One study using a mannequin model determined that five cricothyrotomies are necessary to reach a steady performance state in which the procedure can be completed in 40 seconds.[62] There are no studies that have identified the optimal interval between training episodes for retention, although one small report suggested increased retention when repeated monthly versus every 3 months.[48] Studies in cadavers performed primarily to compare different surgical airway techniques incidentally identified a similar rapid learning curve.[15,21]

There are no studies examining the clinical correlation of these training techniques, but the high success rate of emergency cricothyrotomy suggests that retention and competence have occurred. On the basis of the limited available literature, some recommendations regarding the learning and retention of invasive airway techniques can be made: Identify a preferred method of invasive airway management that is immediately available; become trained in the procedure by performing a sufficient number of repetitions under the supervision of a qualified instructor, using an animal or simulator model, or both; and practice the technique in one to two "refresher sessions" per year on animal or simulator models, with five repetitions per session.

Animal tracheas may be obtained from a slaughterhouse at relatively low cost, and the technique may be attempted multiple times on each specimen (pigs and sheep are most commonly used). Simulators represent a significant capital investment, but newer simulators are much less expensive and much simpler to operate than older models. Models specifically for cricothyrotomy training are also available. Formal training under expert guidance is available through some difficult airway continuing medical education (CME) courses.

V. COMPLICATIONS

The rate of complications associated with emergency cricothyrotomy is difficult to quantify with precision. A critical review of the literature reveals that many of these "complications" are the result of the patient's underlying illness or occur as a consequence of the unsuccessful attempts at airway management *preceding* cricothyrotomy. In addition, the definition of complications, variations in technique, and skill of the operators vary widely from study to study.

With these limitations in mind, the complication rate following surgical cricothyrotomy is highly variable, ranging from 14% to 50%, depending on the technique, clinical setting, definition of complications, and experience of the operator.[7,23,26,30,63]

A. HEMORRHAGE

When performing surgical cricothyrotomy, venous hemorrhage is the rule rather than the exception. This seldom interferes with successful completion of the procedure, and bleeding can usually be controlled with direct pressure or postprocedure suture closure of the incision. Major arterial hemorrhage can result from inadvertent laceration of the thyroid ima artery located near the isthmus of the thyroid, but this would require considerable misplacement of the skin incision from that described here. If the dissection strays far from the midline, the carotid artery or jugular vein can be injured. Arterial bleeding is distinctly unusual if the procedure is performed as described previously. Although it may seem intuitive that bleeding would be less likely following percutaneous cricothyrotomy, this has never been assessed in randomized human trials.

B. TUBE MISPLACEMENT

Tracheostomy tube misplacement is the most important potential complication of both surgical and percutaneous cricothyrotomy. Whether it is considered a complication or a failure of the procedure, inadvertent placement of the tube in either the pretracheal or paratracheal soft tissue can be a lethal error. If ventilation is attempted before misplacement is recognized, massive subcutaneous emphysema and distortion of the neck can ensue, making subsequent efforts to gain the airway extremely difficult. This is perhaps the strongest argument for using surgical (rather than percutaneous) cricothyrotomy, where the entry into the airway is confirmed by palpation and by direct insertion of the hook, dilator, and tracheostomy tube through an open incision.

C. ACCIDENTAL EXTUBATION

Replacing a decannulated tube into a recently performed tracheostomy can be extremely difficult, and all care must be taken to ensure that decannulation does not occur. Tracheostomy ties should be applied immediately after tracheal entry is confirmed by capnography and under the direct supervision of the operator. Additional care should be taken to prevent excessive neck movement or entanglement by monitor lines or intravenous tubing if the patient is being transported. Violent coughing or exaggerated neck movement may also cause the tube to dislodge, and the patient should be appropriately sedated. Finally, self-extubation can occur if the patient is not unconscious or sedated.

D. OTHER COMPLICATIONS

Injury to the posterior laryngeal wall or esophagus can occur if an excessively deep incision is made when entering the airway. This is easily avoidable, provided careful technique is used. Insertion of a cricothyrotome adjacent to or through the airway can result in significant local tissue damage, including vascular injury and esophageal injury.

REFERENCES

1. Abbrecht PH, Kyle RR, Reams WH, Brunette J: Insertion forces and risk of complications during cricothyroid cannulation. J Emerg Med 10:417-426, 1992.
2. American College of Surgeons Committee on Trauma: Advanced Trauma Life Support Providers' Manual. ACS, Chicago, IL 2003.
3. ASA Task Force on the Management of the Difficult Airway: Practice guidelines for the management of the difficult airway. Anesthesiology 98:1269-1277, 2003.
4. Bainton CR: Cricothyrotomy. Int Anesthesiol Clin 32:95-108, 1994.
5. Bair AE, Filbin MR, Kulkarni RG, et al: The failed intubation attempt in the emergency department: Analysis of prevalence, rescue techniques, and personnel. J Emerg Med 23:131-140, 2002.
6. Bair AE, Laurin EG, Karchin A, et al: Cricoid ring integrity: Implications for cricothyrotomy. Ann Emerg Med 41:331-337, 2003.
7. Bair AE, Panacek EA, Wisner DH, et al: Cricothyrotomy: A 5-year experience at one institution. J Emerg Med 24:151-156, 2003.
8. Benumof JL: Management of the difficult adult airway with special emphasis on awake tracheal intubation. Anesthesiology 75:1087-1110, 1991.
9. Benumof JL: Transtracheal jet ventilation via percutaneous catheter and high-pressure source. In Benumof JL (ed): Airway Management: Principles and Practice. St Louis, Mosby, 1996, pp 455-474.
10. Boyd AD, Romita MC, Conlan AA: A clinical evaluation of cricothyrotomy. Surg Gynecol Obstet 149:365-368, 1979.
11. Boyle MF, Hatton D, Sheets C: Surgical cricothyrotomy performed by air ambulance flight nurses: A 5-year experience. J Emerg Med 11:41-45, 1993.
12. Bradby M: History of tracheostomy. Nurs Times 62:1548-1550, 1966.
13. Brantigan CO, Grow JB: Cricothyrotomy: Elective use in respiratory problems requiring tracheostomy. J Thorac Cardiovasc Surg 71:72-81, 1976.
14. Brofeldt BT, Panacek EA, Richards JR: An easy cricothyrotomy approach: The rapid four-step technique. Acad Emerg Med 3:1060-1063, 1996.
15. Chan TC, Vilke GM, Bramwell KJ, et al: Comparison of wire-guided cricothyrotomy versus standard surgical cricothyrotomy technique. J Emerg Med 17:957-962, 1999.
16. Chang RS, Hamilton RJ, Carter WA: Declining rate of cricothyrotomy in trauma patients with an emergency medicine residency: Implications for skills training. Acad Emerg Med 5:247-251, 1998.
17. Ciaglia P, Firsching R, Syneic C: Elective percutaneous dilatational tracheostomy: A new simple bedside procedure—Preliminary report. Chest 87:715-719, 1985.
18. Colles CJ: On stenosis of the trachea after tracheostomy for croup, diphtheria. Ann Surg 3:499, 1886.
19. Davis DP, Bramwell KJ, Hamilton RS, et al: Safety and efficacy of the rapid four-step technique for cricothyrotomy using a Bair Claw. J Emerg Med 19:125-129, 2000.
20. Dickinson AE: The normal and abnormal pediatric upper airway: Recognition and management of obstruction. Clin Chest Med 8:583-596, 1987.
21. Eisenberger P, Laczika K, List M, et al: Comparison of conventional surgical versus Seldinger technique emergency cricothyrotomy performed by inexperienced clinicians. Anesthesiology 92:687-690, 2000.
22. Ezri T, Szmuk P, Warters RD, et al: Difficult airway management practice patterns among anesthesiologists practicing in the United States: Have we made any progress? J Clin Anesth 15:418-422, 2003.
23. Francois B, Clavel M, Desachy A, et al: Complications of tracheostomy performed in the ICU: Subthyroid tracheostomy versus surgical cricothyroidotomy. Chest 123:151-158, 2003.
24. Gerich TG, Schmidt U, Hubrich V, et al: Prehospital airway management in the acutely injured patient: The role of surgical cricothyrotomy revisited. J Trauma 45:312-314, 1988.
25. Gerling MC, Davis DP, Hamilton RS, et al: Effect of surgical cricothyrotomy on the unstable cervical spine in a cadaver model of intubation. J Emerg Med 20:1-5, 2001.
26. Gillespie MB, Eisele DW: Outcomes of emergency surgical airway procedures in a hospital-wide setting. Laryngoscope 109:1766-1769, 1999.
27. Greisz H, Qvarnstorm O, Willen R: Elective cricothyrotomy: A clinical and histopathological study. Crit Care Med 10:387-389, 1982.
28. Heffner JE, Hess D: Tracheostomy management in the chronically ventilated patient. Clin Chest Med 22:55-69, 2001.
29. Holmes JF, Panacek EA, Sackles JC, Brofeldt BT: Comparison of 2 cricothyrotomy techniques: Standard method versus rapid 4-step technique. Ann Emerg Med 32:442-447, 1998.

30. Isaacs JH Jr: Emergency cricothyrotomy: Long-term results. Am Surg 67:349-350, 2001.

31. Jackson C: High tracheostomy and other errors: The chief causes of chronic laryngeal stenosis. Surg Gynecol Obstet 32:392, 1921.

32. Jackson C: Tracheotomy. Laryngoscope 18:285, 1909.

33. Jacobson LE, Gomez GA, Sobieray RJ, et al: Surgical cricothyrotomy in trauma patients: Analysis of its use by paramedics in the field. J Trauma 41:15-20, 1996.

34. Kirchner JA: Cricothyroidotomy and subglottic stenosis. Plast Reconstr Surg 68:828-829, 1981.

35. Knopp RK: Practicing cricothyrotomy on the newly dead. Ann Emerg Med 25:694-695, 1995.

36. Knopp RK, Waeckerle JF, Callaham ML: Rapid sequence intubation revisited. Ann Emerg Med 31:398-400, 1998.

37. Koppel J, Reed A: Formal instruction in difficult airway management. Anesthesiology 83:1343-1346, 1995.

38. Leibovici D, Fredman B, Gofrit ON, et al: Prehospital cricothyrotomy by physicians. Am J Emerg Med 15:91-93, 1997.

39. Little CM, Parker MG, Tarnopolsky R: The incidence of vasculature at risk during cricothyroidostomy. Ann Emerg Med 15:805-807, 1986.

40. Mace SE: Blunt laryngotracheal trauma: The recognition and management of acute laryngeal fracture. Ann Emerg Med 15:836-839, 1986.

41. Mace SE: Cricothyrotomy and translaryngeal jet ventilation In: Roberts JR, Hedges JR (eds): Clinical Procedures in Emergency Medicine, 3rd ed. Philadelphia, WB Saunders, 1998, pp 57-74.

42. Mace SE: Cricothyrotomy. J Emerg Med 6:309-319, 1988.

43. Morain WD: Cricothyroidostomy in head and neck surgery. Plast Reconstr Surg 65:424-428, 1980.

44. Morch ET: History of mechanical ventilation. In Kirby RR, Banner MJ, Downs JB (eds): Clinical Applications of Ventilatory Support. New York, Churchill Livingstone, 1990, pp 1-61.

45. Murphy MF, Walls RM: The difficult and failed airway. In Walls RM (ed): Manual of Emergency Airway Management. Philadelphia, Lippincott Williams & Wilkins, 2000, pp 31-39.

46. Nugent WL, Rhee KJ, Wisner DH, et al: Can nurses perform surgical cricothyrotomy with acceptable success and complication rates? Ann Emerg Med 20:367-370, 1991.

47. Pierce WS, Tyers GFO, Walhausen JA: Effective isolation of a tracheostomy from a sternal wound. J Thorac Cardiovasc Surg 96:178-193, 1973.

48. Prabhu AJ, Correa R, Wong DT, et al: What is the optimal training interval for a cricothyrotomy? Can J Anaesth 48:A59, 2001.

49. Practice guidelines for the management of the difficult airway: A report by the American Society for Anesthesiologists Task Force on the Management of the Difficult Airway. Anesthesiology 78:597-602, 1993.

50. Ravlo O, Bach V, Lybecker H, et al: A comparison between two emergency cricothyroidotomy instruments. Acta Anaesthesiol Scand 31:317-319, 1987.

51. Rehm CG, Wanek SM, Gagnon EB, et al: Cricothyroidotomy for elective airway management in critically ill trauma patients with technically challenging neck anatomy. Crit Care 6:531-535, 2002.

52. Rose DK, Cohen MM: Has the practice of airway management changed? Can J Anaesth 44:A51B, 1997.

53. Rose DK, Cohen MM: The airway: Problems and predictions in 18,500 patients. Can J Anaesth 41:372-383, 1994.

54. Rosenblatt WH, Wagner PJ, Ovassapian A, et al: Practice patterns in managing the difficult airway by anesthesiologists in the United States. Anesth Analg 87:153-157, 1998.

55. Sakles JC, Laurin EG, Ranatapaa AA, et al: Airway management in the emergency department: A one year study of 610 tracheal intubations. Ann Emerg Med 31:398-400, 1998.

56. Salvino CK, Dries D, Gamelli R, et al: Emergency cricothyrotomy in trauma victims. J Trauma 34:503-505, 1993.

57. Tayal VS, Riggs RW, Marx JA, et al: Rapid-sequence intubation at an emergency medicine residency: Success rates and adverse events during a two-year period. Acad Emerg Med 6:31-37, 1999.

58. Toye FJ, Weinstein JD: A percutaneous tracheostomy device. Surgery 65:384-389, 1969.

59. Vissers RJ: Tracheostomy issues. In Meldon S (ed): Geriatric Emergency Medicine. New York, McGraw-Hill, 2004, pp 485-489.

60. Walls RM, Gibbs MA: Surgical Airway. In: Katz RL, Patel RV (eds): Seminars in Anesthesia, Perioperative Medicine and Pain: The Difficult Airway. Philadelphia, Saunders, 2000.

61. Walls RM, Pollack CV: Successful cricothyrotomy after thrombolytic therapy for acute myocardial infarction: A report of two cases. Ann Emerg Med 35:188-191, 2000.

62. Wong DT, Prabhu AJ, Coloma M, et al: What is the minimum training required for successful cricothyrotomy? Anesthesiology 98:349-353, 2003.

63. Xeropotamos NS, Coats TJ, Wilson AW: Prehospital surgical airway management: 1 year's experience from the Helicopter Emergency Medical Service. Injury 24:222-224, 1993.

30

CONFIRMATION OF TRACHEAL INTUBATION

M. Ramez Salem

Anis Baraka

I. OVERVIEW

A. ASA CLOSED CLAIMS STUDIES

In the past two decades, the Committee on Professional Liability of the American Society of Anesthesiologists (ASA) has studied adverse anesthetic outcome based on closed claims files of nationwide insurance carriers.[21] Since the inception, it became evident that adverse outcomes involving the respiratory system constitute the single largest class of injury, representing one third of the overall claims. Generally involving healthy adults undergoing nonemergency surgery with general anesthesia, three mechanisms of injury accounted for approximately three fourths of the adverse respiratory events in the 1970s and early 1980s: inadequate ventilation (38%), esophageal intubation (18%), and difficult tracheal intubation (17%).[21] The remaining adverse respiratory events were produced by a variety of low-frequency (≤2%) mechanisms, including airway obstruction, bronchospasm, aspiration, premature and unintentional extubation, inadequate inspired oxygen delivery, and endobronchial intubation.[21]

Care was judged substandard in more than 80% of inadequate ventilation and esophageal intubation cases.[21] Almost all (>90%) claims for inadequate ventilation and esophageal intubation were considered preventable with better monitoring opposed to only 36% of claims for difficult tracheal intubation.[21] Death and permanent brain damage were more frequent in claims for inadequate ventilation and esophageal intubation (>90%) than in claims for difficult tracheal intubation (56%). Median payment was $240,000 for inadequate ventilation, $217,000 for esophageal intubation, and $76,000 for difficult tracheal intubation.[21]

In 23% of the claims for esophageal intubation, there was documentation of difficult intubation; in 73%, there was sufficient information to reconstruct the time to detection of esophageal intubation.[21] Within this subset, 3% of esophageal intubations were detected before 5 minutes, 61% in 5 to 10 minutes, and 36% after 10 minutes.[21] Auscultation of breath sounds (presumed) was documented in 63% of the claims for esophageal intubation. In 48% of cases, auscultation led to the erroneous conclusion that the tube was in the trachea.[21] This diagnostic error was eventually recognized in a variety of ways including reexamination with direct laryngoscopy, absence of the tube in the trachea at the time of an emergency tracheostomy, resolution of cyanosis after reintubation, and discovery of esophageal intubation at autopsy. Cyanosis was documented in 52% of the claims and preceded the recognition of esophageal intubation in only 34% of the cases.

Because pulse oximetry and capnography have been used since the mid-1980s, data from the closed claims project were analyzed to determine whether these monitoring modalities correlate with improvement in patients' safety.[23] Respiratory events have decreased primarily in claims for injuries caused by inadequate ventilation and, to a lesser extent, esophageal intubation (Fig. 30-1).[23]

Figure 30-1 The incidence of respiratory, cardiovascular, and equipment-related damaging events as a percentage of total claims for death and brain damage in each time period (P≤0.5, Z test) (compared with 1970-1979). (Modified from Cheney FW: The American Society of Anesthesiologists Closed Claims Project: What have we learned, how has it affected practice, and how will it affect practice in the future? Anesthesiology 91:552, 1999.)

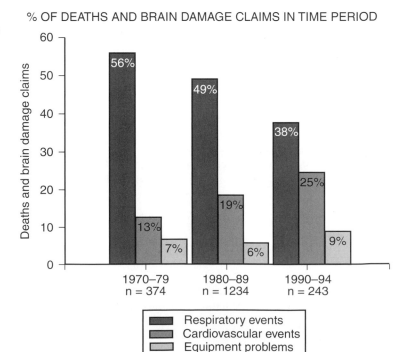

% OF DEATHS AND BRAIN DAMAGE CLAIMS IN TIME PERIOD

Table 30-1 **Comparison of Pediatric and Adult Damaging Events with Special Reference to the Respiratory System**

Damaging Event	Pediatric (n = 238) (%)	P	Adult (n = 1953) (%)
Respiratory system	43	≤.01	30
Inadequate ventilation	20	≤.01	9
Esophageal intubation	5	NS	6
Airway obstruction	5	NS	2
Difficult intubation	4	NS	6
Inadvertent extubation	3	NS	1
Premature extubation	3	NS	1
Aspiration	2	NS	2
Endobronchial intubation	1	NS	1
Bronchospasm	0	NS	2
Inadequate FIO_2	0	NS	<0.5

FIO_2, fraction of inspired oxygen; NS, not significant.
Data from Morray JP, Geiduschek JM, Caplan RA, et al: A comparison of pediatric and adult anesthesia closed malpractice claims. Anesthesiology 78:461, 1993.

1. Pediatric versus Adult Anesthesia Closed Malpractice Claims

Outcome studies in pediatric patients revealed that adverse respiratory events constitute a leading cause of morbidity and mortality.[62,79,104] The ASA closed claims study provided a database to compare pediatric and adult cases in which an adverse outcome occurred.[79] The pediatric claims presented a different distribution of damaging events compared with adults (Tables 30-1 and 30-2). Respiratory events and mortality rate were greater in pediatric claims.[79] Anesthetic care was more often judged "less than appropriate," and the complications more frequently were considered preventable with better monitoring. The median payment to the plaintiff was greater for pediatric claims than for adult claims. Cyanosis (49%), bradycardia (64%), or both often preceded cardiac arrest in pediatric claims, resulting in death (50%) or brain damage (30%) in previously healthy children.[79]

B. THE MAGNITUDE OF THE PROBLEM OF TRACHEAL TUBE MISPLACEMENT

Outcome studies during the past three decades have repeatedly identified adverse respiratory events including unrecognized esophageal intubation as a leading and recurring cause of injury in anesthetic practice.[40,47,54,78,135,136] The report on confidential enquiries into maternal deaths in England and Wales in 1979 to 1981 revealed that

Table 30-2 **Comparison of Pediatric and Adult Demographic, Injury, and Payment Data**

	Pediatric (n = 238) (%)	P	Adult (n = 1953) (%)
Age			
0-14	28	—	—
Sex			
Male	65	≤.01	38
Female	32	≤.01	62
Unknown	3	≤.05	<0.5
ASA physical status			
1	35	≤.01	22
2	14	≤.01	22
3	6	≤.01	13
4	4	NS	3
5	<0.5	NS	1
Unknown	40	NS	40
Poor medical condition and/or obesity	6	≤.01	41
Death	50	≤.01	35
Brain damage	30	≤.01	11
Less than appropriate anesthetic care	54	≤.01	44
Preventable with better monitoring	45	≤.01	30
Median payment	$111,234	≤.05	$90,000

ASA, American Society of Anesthesiologists; NS, not significant.
Data from Morray JP, Geiduschek JM, Caplan RA, et al: A comparison of pediatric and adult anesthesia closed malpractice claims. Anesthesiology 78:461, 1993.

8 of 22 deaths attributable to anesthesia were related to difficulty in tracheal intubation.[78] In four patients, the tube proved to be misplaced in the esophagus.[78] An investigation of anesthesia mortality in Australia revealed that 69% of the deaths were related to airway management, with esophageal intubation once again identified as an important contributing factor.[54]

Virtually all anesthesiologists have experienced esophageal intubation sometime in their career, especially during their training and when they encountered difficulty in visualizing the larynx. Fortunately, most unintentional esophageal intubations are immediately and easily recognized. What has been intriguing is the rare situation in which misplacement of the tube in the esophagus was not recognized, resulting in grave consequences. Failure to recognize esophageal intubation is not limited to junior residents or inexperienced personnel. It has occurred with experienced and skilled anesthesiologists. A case was reported in which three "consultant anaesthetists" failed to recognize that the tracheal tube was in the esophagus.[40] There are also many case reports in the literature describing anesthetic catastrophes and near disasters in patients whose esophagus had been unintentionally intubated and in whom some or many of the commonly used signs indicative of proper tube placement were misleading.[12,52,54,56,90,96,97,121]

Unintentional esophageal intubation may occur more frequently in emergency airway management, in critically ill patients, and in patients who suffer cardiac arrest during out-of-hospital paramedic intubation.[112,114,120] Esophageal intubation occurred in 8% of intubation attempts in critically ill patients.[112] In a study of paramedics trained in direct laryngoscopic tracheal intubation, there were 14 esophageal intubations in 779 patients, an incidence of 1.8%.[120] Esophageal tube placement was recognized and corrected in 11 patients. Three of the 14 esophageal intubations (0.4% of the total) were not recognized and remained uncorrected. Contributing factors to this relatively high incidence of esophageal intubation include intubation under less than optimal conditions, unavailability of appropriate monitoring equipment, violation of the standard technique of auscultation of lung fields and epigastrium, and nonexpert personnel attempting intubations.

It is obvious that intubation of the trachea can produce grave consequences if the tube is misplaced in the esophagus or a main stem bronchus or if inadvertent extubation occurs. Thus, whenever tracheal intubation is performed clinicians should verify (1) that the tube is placed in the airway (not in the esophagus) and (2) that the tube is positioned at an appropriate depth inside the trachea.

II. CONFIRMATION OF TRACHEAL TUBE PLACEMENT

A. IS THERE AN IDEAL TEST FOR CONFIRMATION OF TRACHEAL TUBE PLACEMENT?

Over the years, the search continued for an ideal test for confirmation of tracheal tube placement. Such a test would be simple, quick, reliable, safe, inexpensive, and repeatable and would require minimal training. It would function reliably in patients of different age groups, in various locations, and during difficult intubation. It should not yield false results and should function in the patient with cardiac arrest.

Unfortunately, such a perfect test does not yet exist. Over the years, many clinical signs and technical aids have been described to confirm tracheal intubation. Many of the studies used to assess these tests involve the placement of two tubes, one in the trachea and the other in the esophagus.[22,144] This scenario makes the observer's decision as to which tube was in the trachea or esophagus much easier and helps the recognition of esophageal intubation. The clinician does not have the luxury of choice between two tubes in the clinical situation.[144] In the assessment of any of these tests, the reader must understand what is meant by false-negative and false-positive results. Although not all articles are in agreement, most use the term false-negative as the tube is in the trachea but the test fails and false-positive as the tube is in the esophagus but the result mimics that of tracheal intubation. In case of capnography, false-negative refers to the tube in the trachea but absent waveform; false-positive implies the tube in the esophagus but present waveform. To avoid confusion and to maintain conformity with previously used terms, these definitions are retained throughout the discussion.

B. METHODS OF VERIFICATION OF TRACHEAL TUBE PLACEMENT

Methods of verification of tracheal tube placement (or detection of esophageal intubation) can be classified into non-failsafe, almost failsafe, and failsafe, depending on their reported reliability and specificity.

1. Non-Failsafe Methods

a. Observation and Palpation of Chest Movements
Commonly used maneuvers to confirm tracheal intubation are observation of symmetric bilateral chest movements and palpation of upper chest excursions during compression of the reservoir bag. These signs can easily distinguish tracheal from esophageal intubation in most patients. However, in obese patients, women with large breasts, and patients with a rigid chest wall, barrel chest, or less compliant lungs, observation and palpation of chest excursions can be misinterpreted to indicate that the tube is in the esophagus.[17] More important, upper chest wall movements simulating ventilation of the lungs can be seen and felt with an esophageally placed tube. This phenomenon has been described in many instances of what ultimately proved to be esophageal intubation[12,56,90,96,97,121] and has been reported in patients with intrathoracic hiatal hernia and after gastric pull-up operations.[52]

Chest movements during esophageal ventilation were studied in a male cadaver after a cuffed tube was placed into the esophagus and attached to an inflating bag.[97] It was noted that "the chest and epigastric movements observed when the bag was compressed were indistinguishable from those normally seen in ventilation of the lungs even in the upper chest area." When the body was dissected starting with the epigastrium, it was noted that "the stomach was being inflated and was spontaneously deflating via the esophagus, the feel of the inflating bag being indistinguishable from normal pulmonary ventilation." Even when the lower end of the esophagus was occluded, "chest movements still appeared identical to those seen when the lungs are inflated." After the chest was entered, it was observed that "chest movements were caused by the flat esophagus distending into a firm tube that lifted the heart and upper mediastinal structures forward, thus elevating the sternum and ribs." The lifting of the chest wall by the distended esophagus is the most plausible explanation for the "chest movements" occurring during "esophageal ventilation."[97] A second possible mechanism is that gastric insufflation causes upward displacement of the diaphragm and outward movement of the lower chest. With release of bag compression, gas escapes from the stomach up the esophagus, allowing the diaphragm to move downward and the lower chest to move inward.[56,97]

b. Auscultation of Breath Sounds

Auscultation of bilateral breath sounds is the most common method used to ensure proper tracheal tube placement. It can be done repeatedly anywhere tracheal intubation is performed and whenever changes in the position of the tube are suspected. In almost all cases, breath sounds heard near the midaxillary lines leave very little doubt regarding the position of the tube. However, in numerous anecdotal reports, "deceptive" breath sounds were heard in cases that proved to be esophageal intubation.

There are several reasons why sounds heard with esophageal intubation may mimic breath sounds from the lungs. The combination of esophageal wall oscillations with gas movement and acoustic filtering can produce inspiratory or expiratory wheezes indistinguishable from sounds arising from gas movement in the airway.[5,37,56] The high flow rate, distribution, and volume of gas delivered through the esophagus may lead to auscultation of predominantly bronchial breath sounds.[56] In infants and children, esophageal sounds can be easily transmitted to wide areas of the chest wall.[134] The quality of breath sounds may also differ depending on whether the chest is auscultated near the middle line or laterally near the axilla and may vary with the presence of pulmonary disease and from patient to patient. It should be noted that sounds retrieved by an esophageal stethoscope are different from those heard with a precordial stethoscope, and thus an esophageal stethoscope should not be used to differentiate tracheal from esophageal intuation.[97] In patients with a thoracic stomach or hiatal hernia, many of the clinical signs of esophageal intubations may be obscured. Because of the intrathoracic location of a large distensible viscera, bilateral breath sounds may be heard during manual ventilation.[52] For these reasons, it is recommended that whenever abnormal breath sounds are heard, they should not be relied on to confirm tracheal intubations.

c. Endobronchial Intubation

Intentional endobronchial intubation has been used to discriminate between tracheal and esophageal intubation when doubt exists.[142] The tube is advanced until breath sounds are lost on one side and unilateral breath sounds are heard on the other side. That should not happen if the tube is in the esophagus. The tube is then gradually withdrawn to 1 to 2 cm beyond the point at which bilateral breath sounds are heard. This technique has been used in infants and children, particularly in infants with tracheoesophageal fistulas.[108] However, it is not recommended for routine use because it can precipitate carinal irritation and bronchospasm.[133]

d. Epigastric Auscultation and Observation for Abdominal Distention

Auscultation of the epigastric area to elicit air movement in the stomach has been recommended as a routine maneuver after tracheal intubation even before auscultating the chest.[90,96] However, normal vesicular breath sounds from the lungs can be transmitted to the epigastric area in tracheally intubated thin and small patients.[17] On rare occasions, esophageal intubation may not be easily distinguishable from tracheal intubation if epigastric auscultation alone is used. Furthermore, there are circumstances, such as obstetric emergencies, in which the abdomen is prepared before induction of anesthesia that may preclude epigastric auscultation after intubation.

Abdominal distention caused by gastric insufflation after compression of the breathing bag in cases of esophageal intubation can be readily observed in most patients. Occasionally, this sign may not be a reliable indicator of esophageal intubation for the following reasons[17,66,97]: (1) gastric insufflation and abdominal distention might have occurred during prior mask ventilation, (2) gastric distention may not be apparent in obese patients, (3) a previously placed nasogastric tube can cause intermittent decompression of the stomach, and (4) gradual gastric filling can be difficult to distinguish from normal abdominal movements because of the esophageal reflux of gases. Conversely, gastric distention can occur in patients with congenital or acquired tracheoesophageal fistula despite the placement of a tube in the trachea.[108]

e. Combined Auscultation of Epigastrium and Both Axillae

In a study of 40 adult patients who had both their trachea and esophagus intubated, "blinded" observers auscultating both axillae failed to diagnose esophageal intubation in 15% of cases.[1] When movement of the abdominal wall alone was used to assess tube position, false results were obtained in 90% of cases. In contrast, the combination of auscultation of the epigastrium and both axillae was found to be totally reliable in diagnosing esophageal intubation.[1] These findings emphasize the importance of combining tests to achieve a high degree of reliability in assessing tracheal tube placement.

Detection of misplaced tubes by auscultation of the chest and epigastrium is probably more difficult in infants than in adults. Uejima[134] reported two cases, a 7-month-old and a 5-year-old, in whom esophageal intubation occurred. In both cases, bilateral chest movements and "breath sounds" were heard over four areas of the chest and over the epigastrium. However, these "breath sounds" were not vesicular in nature. The ease of transmission of sounds from the esophagus to the chest and epigastrium may thus mimic breath sounds, especially in infants, emphasizing again that whenever any but normal vesicular breath sounds are heard, they should not be relied on to confirm tracheal intubation.

f. Reservoir Bag Compliance and Refilling

Manual compression of the reservoir bag after tracheal intubation and cuff inflation yields a characteristic feel of the compliance of the lungs and chest wall, whereas passive exhalation on release of bag compression is accompanied by rapid bag refilling. In almost all esophageal intubations, compressing the reservoir bag does not inflate the chest and is not followed by appreciable refilling. However, exceptions to this rule do occur, as has been shown in reports of accidental esophageal intubations. In these cases, repeated filling and emptying of the stomach resulted in concomitant emptying and refilling of the reservoir bag, leading to the erroneous conclusion that the tube was in the trachea.[56,66,90,97,121] It is possible that high, fresh gas flow might have contributed to reservoir bag refilling in these cases. To enhance the reliability of this test, it has been suggested that the fresh gas flow should be shut off temporarily.[9] If this is done, chest inflation and rapid bag refilling can be repeatedly done (three to five times) in tracheally intubated patients but not in esophageally intubated patients. Because changes in lung or chest wall compliance can be misinterpreted by the clinician compressing the reservoir bag and high airway resistance can lead to slow refilling, this test used alone should not be relied upon in distinguishing esophageal from tracheal intubation.[17]

g. Reservoir Bag Movements with Spontaneous Breathing

Movement of the reservoir bag during spontaneous breathing has been considered one of the signs indicative of tracheal intubation. However, it has been demonstrated that this sign can be unreliable. In a group of anesthetized patients, the trachea and esophagus were intubated and the patients were allowed to breathe spontaneously.[100] With the tracheal tube intentionally occluded, the high negative intrapleural pressures generated with spontaneous breathing efforts were transmitted to the esophagus, resulting in reservoir bag movements and measurable tidal volumes up to 180 mL. Therefore, slight reservoir bag movements or measurements of small tidal volumes during spontaneous breathing are not reliable indicators of tracheal intubation.[100]

h. Cuff Maneuvers and Neck Palpation

The higher pitched sound produced by leakage around a tube placed in the trachea with the cuff deflated during compression of the reservoir bag compared with the "flatus-like" sound of leakage around a tube placed in the esophagus has been used as a distinguishing test.[17] As has been shown in many case reports, when the cuff of an esophageally placed tube is inflated close to the cricoid cartilage, the characteristic guttural sound may be absent or may become higher pitched, resembling leakage around a tracheally placed tube.[97]

Palpation of the cuff on each side of the trachea between the cricoid cartilage and suprasternal notch while moving the tube has been proposed to confirm tracheal intubation.[33] After intubation and cuff inflation, two or three fingers are placed above the suprasternal notch. Several rapid inflations of the cuff are performed (up to 10 mL of air). An outward force is felt by the palpating fingers if the tracheal tube is in correct position. Intermittent squeezing of the pilot balloon of a slightly overinflated cuff with the thumb and index finger while sensing the transmitted pulsations in the neck has been suggested as a sign for confirming tracheal tube placement.[80] A maneuver using the pilot balloon as a sensor has also been proposed.[133] A low-pressure, large-volume prestretched cuff may not be palpable despite correct placement.[133] Conversely, an inflated cuff can be palpated in the neck in cases of esophageal intubations.[121] Therefore, these maneuvers should not be relied upon in verifying tracheal intubation.

If an assistant gently palpates the trachea in the suprasternal notch or applies cricoid compression during tracheal intubation, "an old washboard-like" vibration is appreciated as the tube rubs against the tracheal rings.[102] It has been suggested that there should be no false-positive results of this sign if the tube is misplaced in the esophagus because the esophagus is soft and lies posterior to the trachea. Thus far, there have been no controlled studies to confirm the validity of this sign.

i. Sound of Expelled Gases during Sternal Compression

Pressing sharply on the sternum while listening over the proximal end of the tube to detect a characteristic feel and sound of expelled gases from the airway is occasionally used to distinguish esophageal from tracheal intubation.[97] This test is mistrusted by many because of the (1) inability to distinguish gases expelled passing through the tracheal tube from gases passing through or around a tube misplaced in the esophagus, (2) inability to distinguish gases being expelled through the nose, and (3) inability to distinguish esophageal and stomach gases present from prior mask ventilation.[97]

j. Tube Condensation of Water Vapor

The principle of this sign is that water vapor seen in clear plastic tubes is more likely to be present in gases exhaled through a tracheally placed tube than gases emanating from the stomach through a tube in the esophagus (Fig. 30-2). Two studies have demonstrated the observation of water condensation in all cases in which tubes were placed in the trachea.[1] Unfortunately, water condensation can and does occur when tubes are placed in the esophagus. The fact that condensation was noticed in

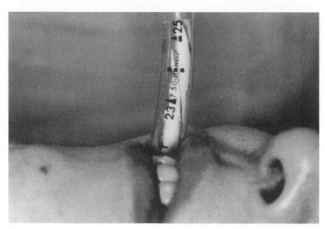

Figure 30-2 Condensation of water vapor seen in a clear plastic tube after tracheal intubation during exhalation.

85% in one study[1] and 28% in another study[44] of all cases of esophageal intubations should strongly discourage its presence from being interpreted as a reliable indicator of a successful intubation.

k. Nasogastric Tubes, Gastric Aspirates, Introducers, and Other Devices

A test devised to distinguish between placement of a tube in the trachea and a tube in the esophagus involves threading a lubricated nasogastric tube (NGT) through the tube in question, applying continuous suction, and attempting to withdraw the NGT.[60] This test exploits the distinguishing features that the esophagus will collapse around the NGT when suction is applied, whereas free suction continues if applied in the trachea. In a study of 20 patients in whom both the trachea and esophagus were intubated, the ability to maintain suction and the ease of withdrawal while continuous suction is applied clearly distinguished between the two positions.[60] When the NGT was in the trachea, suction applied to it could be maintained easily because the trachea remained patent and air was entrained through the open end of the tube. This allowed the NGT to be withdrawn easily despite suctioning. In contrast, when suction was applied to the NGT in the esophagus, the esophageal wall collapsed around it, thereby obstructing suction, and interfered with easy withdrawal of the NGT.[60]

Although the length of the NGT that could be easily inserted in conjunction with feeling an impediment or resistance (5 to 15 cm distal to the tip of the tube) identified correct tracheal placement, it was found less useful in identifying esophageal intubation.[60] Similarly, the nature of the aspirate (mucus versus bile or gastric juice) was found to be of limited value in most patients.[60] Because the total time spent to make these observations was 20 to 30 seconds, the authors concluded that the test is reliable.[60] Despite their enthusiasm, this test is rarely used because of the availability of other better methods but may have a place when other tests are unavailable.

The Eschmann introducer is a 60-cm-long device composed of two layers: a core of tube woven from Dacron polyester threads and an outer resin layer to provide stiffness, flexibility, and a slippery, water impervious surface. Frequently, the device is referred to as a "gum elastic bougie"—despite the fact that it is not gum, elastic, or a bougie. The introducer has a 35-degree kink 2.5 cm from its distal end. Because its external diameter is 5 mm, it can be used with tracheal tubes with an inner diameter of 6 mm or greater. The device has been used for many years to facilitate intubation and has been introduced to differentiate tracheal from esophageal intubation in emergencies when there is doubt about the location of the tube.[17] When inserted through the lumen of the tube, the curved tip of the lubricated introducer may be felt rubbing over the tracheal rings, and resistance is encountered as the tip of the introducer meets the carina or a main stem bronchus at approximately 28 to 32 cm in the adult.[17] If the tube is in the esophagus, the introducer passes without resistance to the distal end of the esophagus or stomach.[17] As yet, there are no studies verifying the reliability and safety of this technique in a large number of patients. Forceful insertion of an excessive length of the introducer could conceivably result in bronchial rupture or other injuries. This led the manufacturer to discourage its use as a tracheal tube changer because other devices specifically designed for this purpose are now available.

l. Transtracheal Illumination

The success of transillumination of the soft tissues of the neck anterior to the trachea in accomplishing guided oral or nasal intubation has culminated in the development of improved lighted stylets and introducers[34,39,149] (see Chapter 20). It also prompted investigators to use transtracheal illumination to differentiate esophageal from tracheal tube placement and to position the tube accurately inside the trachea. Transmission of light through tissues depends on thickness, compactness, color, density, and light absorption characteristics of the tissue; wavelength, quality, and intensity of light; proximity of the tissue to the light source; and the ambient lighting condition in the room.[76] Typically, tracheal intubation with the lighted stylet or introducer inside the tube or placement of the stylet in the lumen of the tube after intubation gives off an intense circumscribed midline glow in the region of the laryngeal prominence and sternal notch (Fig. 30-3). The illumination is mostly seen opposite the thyrohyoid, cricothyroid, and cricotracheal membranes. In the event of esophageal intubation, the light is either absent or perceived as dull and diffuse.

To enhance transillumination, darkening the room, dimming the overhead lights, and cricoid pressure (to approximate the tracheal wall to the light source and stretch the soft tissues anterior to the light source) have been recommended.[34,39,76,149] Newer lighted stylets or introducers, battery operated or incorporating a

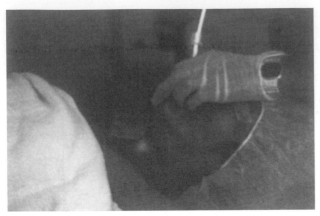

Figure 30-3 When the lighted stylet (or introducer) enters the larynx, an intense circumscribed midline glow seen in the region of the laryngeal prominence is suggestive of tracheal intubation.

fiberoptic light source, have brighter lights than earlier prototypes. Consequently, dimming the overhead lights or cricoid pressure may not be necessary. The reliability of transtracheal illumination in distinguishing esophageal from tracheal intubation in adults has been demonstrated.[76,119] In one study conducted on five cadavers, only 1 of 56 intratracheal placements was misidentified as esophageal, whereas of 112 extratracheal placements (esophageal or pyriform fossa), 1 was misidentified as intratracheal.[119] In another study of 420 adult patients, tracheal transillumination was graded as excellent in 81% of patients and as good in the remaining 19%.[76] In contrast, transesophageal illumination could not be demonstrated in any patient. Despite these reports, we have noticed occasional false-negative results (tube in trachea but no transillumination) with the use of the newer lighted stylets and introducers in patients with neck swelling or dark skin and in obese patients. Similarly, occasional false-positive results have been noted in thin patients. Nonetheless, the use of transillumination could reduce, if not eliminate, unrecognized esophageal intubation, especially outside the operating room where other technical aids are not available.[76,119]

Reports delineated several complications with these transillumination devices.[27,122,127] Loss of the bulb into the lung necessitating bronchoscopic removal has been reported.[122] A change in design involving encasing the bulb in a plastic retaining cover has virtually eliminated the possibility of this complication recurring.[34] Other reports described arytenoid subluxation.[27,127] However, no evidence exists that there is an increased incidence of this complication with the use of lighted stylets because it can also occur after conventional intubation.

m. Pulse Oximetry and Detection of Cyanosis

Although unrecognized esophageal intubation ultimately leads to severe decreases in oxygen saturation (and detectable cyanosis), minutes may elapse before this happens. A disturbing finding that emerged from the

ASA closed claims study is that detection of esophageal intubation required 5 minutes or more in 97% of cases.[21] Furthermore, detectable cyanosis preceded the recognition of esophageal intubation in only one third of cases. Several factors contribute to the delay in diagnosing esophageal intubation by pulse oximetry or the detection of cyanosis, or both.

Reliance on the appearance of cyanosis as a clue to esophageal intubation can contribute to such a delay. Recognition of cyanosis usually necessitates the presence of greater than 5 g/dL of reduced hemoglobin, which corresponds to 75% to 85% oxygen saturation.[85] However, the detection may also depend on the concentration and type of hemoglobin and the observer's own interpretations. With severe anemia, cyanosis may not be apparent until the oxygen saturation falls to 60%. Conversely, cyanosis is usually detectable at 80% to 85% oxygen saturation when the hemoglobin concentration is normal or elevated. The infant with a high proportion of fetal hemoglobin may still look "pink" at an arterial partial pressure of oxygen (PaO_2) near 40 mm Hg because of the increased blood affinity of oxygen and leftward shifting of the fetal oxyhemoglobin dissociation curve, and thus a serious reduction in PaO_2 may develop before cyanosis is apparent. Recognition of cyanosis is influenced by the limited exposure of the patient's body and the insensitivity of the human eye to changes in skin color or even the color of the blood that occurs during arterial desaturation. It could also be affected by variations in room lighting and the color of the surgical drapes.

Noninvasive monitoring of oxygen saturation (SaO_2) by pulse oximetry has proved to be a reliable indicator of arterial hemoglobin saturation.[20,150] It is undoubtedly quicker to detect accurate changes in SaO_2 by pulse oximetry than to rely on clinical detection of cyanosis. The main limitation of pulse oximetry is that it does not measure PaO_2, which may fall long before SaO_2 is affected in case of interruption of oxygen delivery.

Preoxygenation of the patient's lungs before anesthetic induction extends the period of time before a significant decrease in SaO_2 occurs in case of esophageal intubation.[10,74] In general, oxygen deprivation or apnea after air breathing results in a substantial fall in PaO_2 in 90 seconds, whereas PaO_2, after oxygen breathing, remains above 100 mm Hg for at least 3 minutes of apnea and thus SaO_2 does not change during this period.[85] Consequently, pulse oximetry after preoxygenation does not immediately indicate that the esophagus has been intubated.[74] Because of this prolonged interval with normal SaO_2 being recorded initially after the intubation attempt, misplacement of the tube may not be suspected later when SaO_2 begins to decrease.[21,74] Furthermore, the risk of misinterpretation of clinical findings suggestive of esophageal intubation may be greater when other clues such as decrease in SaO_2 or cyanosis are not yet manifest.[21] This "hazard" of preoxygenation has led a few clinicians to abandon such a practice before intubation so that the recognition of esophageal intubation would be more readily appreciated.[55] One does not need to go to such extremes as to abandon a practice that has definite merits. However, it must be borne in mind that normal pulse oximetry readings after intubation should not be taken as evidence of successful tracheal intubation and that after preoxygenation, oxyhemoglobin desaturation as indicated by pulse oximetry is a relatively late manifestation of esophageal intubation.[21,48,55,74,116,143]

Both oxygen consumption and cardiac output can influence the SaO_2 through their effect on mixed venous oxygen tension ($P\bar{v}O_2$) and mixed venous oxygen content ($C\bar{v}O_2$).[85] A decrease in oxygen consumption associated with anesthetic induction, an increase in cardiac output, or both leads to an increase in $P\bar{v}O_2$ and $C\bar{v}O_2$. The high $P\bar{v}O_2$ retards the decrease in PaO_2 in the event of oxygen deprivation resulting from esophageal intubation and consequently may delay its recognition. Conversely, in patients with low SaO_2 and in patients whose oxygen consumption is high (children, women in labor, and the morbidly obese) or functional residual capacity (FRC) is decreased, oxyhemoglobin desaturation may occur faster.

With the vocal cords open, manual ventilation into the esophagus can result in alveolar gas exchange. In 18 of the 20 patients studied after intentional intubation of both the esophagus and trachea, ventilation into the esophagus caused cyclic compression of the lungs by the distending stomach and esophagus, leading to some gas exchange evidenced by CO_2 recording at the proximal end of the tracheal tube.[66] Although in this situation esophageal ventilation causes ventilation of the lungs with room air, it considerably delays the onset of cyanosis and oxyhemoglobin desaturation.[66] Similarly, respiratory efforts by the spontaneously breathing patient through the unintubated trachea may delay the recognition of esophageal intubation. Esophageal ventilation may also be effective in yielding apneic oxygenation if the cords are open and there is a leak around the cuff of the misplaced esophageal tube.

n. The Beck Airway-Air Flow Monitor

The Beck Airway-Air Flow Monitor (BAAM) consists of a cylindrical plastic whistle with a 2-mm aperture diameter (Fig. 30-4). When it is connected to the proximal end of a tracheal tube in a spontaneously breathing patient, the airflow is forced through the small lumen, producing a loud whistle.[25] The pitch during inspiration and exhalation differs because of varying airflow velocities. The BAAM has been used to assist blind intubation techniques to guide the tube into the trachea.[25] The loudness of the whistle indicates proximity to the tracheal air column, whereas cessation of the sound implies esophageal intubation, obstruction of the tracheal tube, or excessive leak around the tube. In patients who are not breathing spontaneously, a gentle squeeze of the chest produces whistling in tracheally intubated patients. It should be noted that

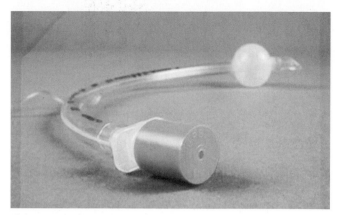

Figure 30-4 The Beck Airway-Air Flow Monitor (BAAM) attaches to a standard 15-mm endotracheal tube connector and magnifies airway-airflow sounds. (Courtesy of Life-Assist, Inc., Rancho Cordova, CA.)

because the whistle is produced by the airflow, a tube in the pharynx can produce a whistle. Reports on this device have been limited to case reports and a study in neonates.[25] More studies are needed to determine its validity.

o. Chest Radiography

A chest radiograph can diagnose esophageal intubation if the tube is located in the lower esophagus distal to the carina (Fig. 30-5).[70] Because a tube in the esophagus is often projected over the tracheal air column on anteroposterior chest radiographs, the radiologic features of esophageal intubation are usually difficult to assess.[116] However, it should be suspected (1) if any part of the tube's borders is seen outside or lateral to the air column of the tracheobronchial tree (in the absence of a pneumomomediastinum); (2) in the presence of esophageal air and gastric distention, particularly in the presence of an NGT; and (3) if there is noticeable deviation of the trachea caused by an overinflated cuff.[70,116]

Although a lateral view of the chest could precisely reveal esophageal intubation, such views are often difficult to obtain. However, the tube location could be identified correctly in 92% of the films taken with the patients in a 25-degree right posterior oblique position with the head turned to the right side.[116] Because the esophagus is located slightly to the left as well as behind the trachea, this projection presents the relationship en face with respect to the radiologic beam, resulting in avoidance of superimposition of the trachea over the esophagus (Fig. 30-6). Because radiography is time consuming, cumbersome, and not failsafe, it should never be relied upon for diagnosing esophageal intubation, even in the critical care setting.

2. Almost Failsafe Methods

a. Identification of Carbon Dioxide in Exhaled Gas

The availability of capnometry (measurement of CO_2 in expired gas) and capnography (instantaneous display of

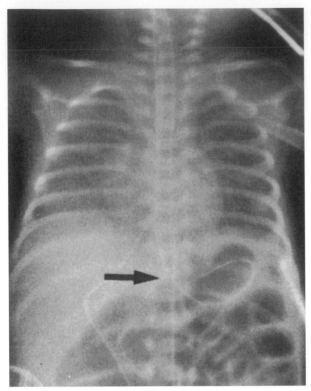

Figure 30-5 Tracheal tube malposition. Tube at the gastroeso-phageal junction *(arrow)*. Moderate intestinal dilation is seen. (From Mandel GA: Neonatal intensive care radiology. In Goodman LR, Putman CE [eds]: Intensive Care Radiology: Imaging of the Critically Ill. Philadelphia, WB Saunders, 1983, p 290.)

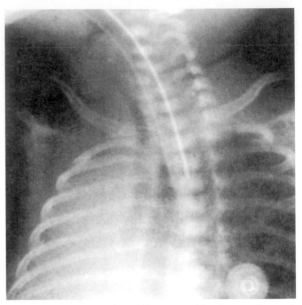

Figure 30-6 Right posterior oblique portable chest radiograph with patient's head turned to right shows air-filled trachea projecting to right of endotracheal tube. Tube aligns with air-filled distal esophagus. This is the best position for diagnosis of esophageal intubation. (From Smith GM, Reed JC, Choplin RH: Radiographic detection of esophageal malpositioning of endotracheal tubes. AJR Am J Roentgenol 154:23, 1990.)

the CO_2 waveform during the respiratory cycle) for intraoperative monitoring has prompted clinicians to extend their use to facilitate detection of esophageal intubation.[11,31,66,82,95,116] The principle of use stems from the fact that exhaled CO_2 can be reliably detected during controlled or spontaneous ventilation in patients with adequate pulmonary flow whose trachea is properly intubated, whereas no CO_2 would be detected in gases emanating from a tube in the esophagus. Studies revealed that the combined use of capnography and pulse oximetry could avert more than 80% of mishaps considered preventable.[129] In an amendment to its original basic intraoperative monitoring standards, the ASA stated,* "When an endotracheal tube is inserted, its correct positioning in the trachea must be verified by clinical assessment and by identification of carbon dioxide in the expired gas. End-tidal CO_2 analysis, in use from the time of endotracheal tube placement, is strongly encouraged." Identification of CO_2 in the exhaled gas has emerged as the standard for verification of proper tracheal tube placement. Furthermore, interruption of CO_2 sampling in the exhaled gas because of disconnection, obstruction, accidental tracheal extubation, or total loss of ventilation is immediately detected. Two main methods are currently used: capnography and colorimetric detection of CO_2.

i. Capnography

Currently available CO_2 analyzers use various principles to measure CO_2 in the inspired and exhaled gases on a breath-to-breath basis and display the CO_2 waveform: (1) mass spectrometry, (2) infrared absorption spectrometry, and (3) Raman scattering. A normal capnographic waveform in relation to the respiratory cycle is shown in Figure 30-7.[73] A mass spectrometric tracing showing a

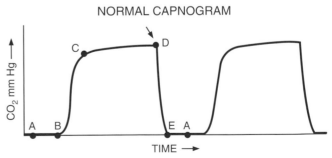

Figure 30-7 The CO_2 waveform. A, Expiratory pause begins. A → B, Clearance of anatomic dead space. B → C, Dead space air mixed with alveolar air. C → D, Alveolar plateau. D, Level of end-tidal CO_2 *(arrow* indicates end-tidal CO_2 registered by capnogram) and beginning of inspiratory phase. D → E, Clearance of dead space air. E → A, Inspiratory gas devoid of CO_2. (Modified from May WS, Heavner JE, McWorther D, Racz G: Capnography in the Operating Room. An Introductory Directory. New York, Raven Press, 1985, p 1.)

---

*Standards for Basic Anesthetic Monitoring. 2003 Directory of Members. American Society of Anesthesiologists, Park Ridge, Ill, p 493.

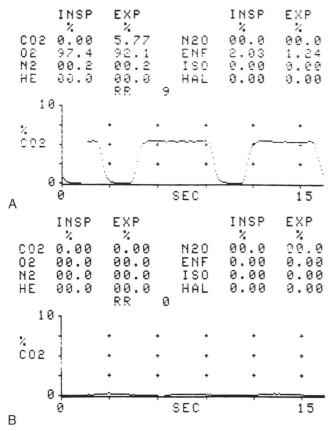

Figure 30-8 **A,** Normal capnograph, tube in trachea. **B,** Absent capnograph, tube in esophagus.

CO_2 waveform after esophageal intubation and after correct placement of the tube in the trachea is shown in Figure 30-8. Although capnography typically distinguishes tracheal from esophageal intubation, false-negative results (tube in trachea, absent waveform) and false-positive results (tube in esophagus or pharynx, present waveform) have been reported.

Since the advent of capnography in confirming tracheal tube placement, there have been reports of markedly different problems yielding unexpected false-negative results. Disconnection of the tracheal tube from the breathing apparatus, apnea, and equipment failure may be misinterpreted as absent waveform caused by esophageal intubation.[32] A kinked or obstructed tracheal tube interferes with sampling of exhaled gas and may lead to an absent or distorted waveform. Lack of a CO_2 waveform because of severe bronchospasm has also been reported.[32] Unintentional application of positive end-expiratory pressure (PEEP) to a loosely fitted or uncuffed tracheal tube may cause exhaled gases to escape around the distal lumen of the tube and result in a sampling error and absent waveform.[72] Dilution of exhaled gases by high fresh gas flow in a Mapleson D system when proximal sidestream sampling is used in infants smaller than 10 kg leads to erroneous sampling.[3,4] This problem could be corrected by distal sampling from the tracheal tube, up to the 12-cm mark; use of a mainstream sampling device;

or use of special ventilators.[4] Dilution of exhaled gases with fresh gas flow has also been demonstrated during use of the Dryden disposable absorber in adult patients.[15] This dilution can be similarly corrected by distal sampling or by alteration of absorber design.[15] Lower sampling flow rates[46] and gas sampling line leaks[153] can result in artifactually low exhaled CO_2 values and an abnormal waveform.

Marked diminution of pulmonary blood flow increases the alveolar component of the dead space.[64,85] Low cardiac output, hypotension, pulmonary embolism, pulmonary stenosis, tetralogy of Fallot, and kinking or clamping of the pulmonary artery during pulmonary surgery all cause a decrease in end-tidal carbon dioxide partial pressure ($P_{ET}CO_2$), reflecting an increase in alveolar dead space.[85,103] Other factors contributing to the increased alveolar dead space during anesthesia include patient's age, tidal volume, use of negative phase during exhalation, short inspiratory phase, and the presence of pulmonary disease.[85,103] As a result of the widespread destruction of alveolar capillaries in patients with chronic obstructive lung disease, an increased alveolar dead space ensues. An increase in alveolar dead space is manifested as a decrease in $P_{ET}CO_2$ and an increase in $PaCO_2$ to $P_{ET}CO_2$ difference (normally 0 to 5 mm Hg).[85,103] If one depends on capnography alone in confirming tracheal tube placement in patients who have a very large alveolar dead space, the low $P_{ET}CO_2$ values might mislead the clinician into thinking that the tube was not placed in the trachea.

An abrupt reduction in cardiac output reduces $P_{ET}CO_2$ by two mechanisms: (1) a reduction in venous return causes a decrease in CO_2 delivered to the lungs and (2) the increase in alveolar dead space dilutes the CO_2 from normally perfused alveoli, thus decreasing $P_{ET}CO_2$.[57,59,115] When cardiac arrest ensues, CO_2 is no longer delivered to or eliminated through the lungs, even if ventilation is adequate, and consequentially $P_{ET}CO_2$ values exponentially decrease to remarkably low values (<0.5%). Ninety seconds after experimentally induced ventricular fibrillation, $P_{ET}CO_2$ is usually decreased by 90%.[131] Thus, a decision regarding the location of the tracheal tube based on capnographic findings alone during cardiac arrest may lead to a misdiagnosis.

Experimental cardiac arrest studies demonstrated a remarkably high correlation between $P_{ET}CO_2$, cardiac output, and coronary perfusion pressure during closed-chest precordial compression, open-chest cardiac massage, and after resuscitation.[35,109] Similar observations were reported during episodes of cardiac arrest in critically ill patients.[35,41] The restoration of spontaneous circulation was heralded by a rapid increase in $P_{ET}CO_2$ within 30 seconds. This overshoot in $P_{ET}CO_2$, which is characteristic of successful resuscitation, may exceed the prearrest value and reflects washout of CO_2 that accumulated in venous blood and in tissues during circulatory arrest.[35,41] In patients in whom resuscitative efforts failed to restore spontaneous circulation, $P_{ET}CO_2$ remained low or even declined, whereas in those who eventually regained

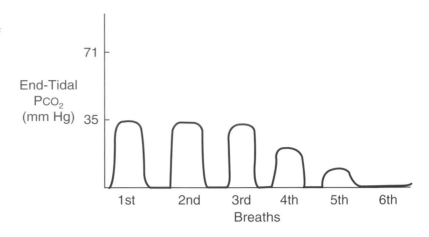

Figure 30-9 CO_2 waveforms obtained in a 10-year-old boy with an esophageal intubation. The waveform of the first three breaths looks virtually normal before becoming flat very quickly. (From Sum Ping ST: Esophageal intubation. Anesth Analg 66:481, 1987.)

spontaneous circulation, P_{ETCO_2} was 19 mm Hg or greater. These observations suggest that capnography can be used for monitoring the adequacy of blood flow generated by precordial compression during cardiopulmonary resuscitation and can serve as a prognostic indicator of successful resuscitation.[35,41]

False-positive results can occur when the tube is misplaced in the esophagus after exhaled gases are forced into the stomach during bag-and-mask ventilation preceding intubation attempts.[66,124] If enough alveolar gas reaches the stomach, CO_2 concentration higher than 2% may be initially detected, and the CO_2 waveform may be indistinguishable from that of tracheal intubation.[66,124,125] In fact, CO_2 waveforms have been observed in one third of esophageal intubations,[125] but repeated ventilation results in rapidly diminishing CO_2 levels while the waveform becomes rather flat and irregular (Fig. 30-9).[66,124] As a result of the dilution with successive ventilation, it is very unlikely that any CO_2 would be detected after the sixth breath or after 1 minute in case of esophageal intubation, making it easy to distinguish esophageal from tracheal intubation.[66] It has also been observed that compression of the chest caused clear, peaked CO_2 elevation in 18 of 20 tracheally intubated patients but no changes in esophageal intubation.[66] This simple, quick maneuver together with other signs can confirm proper tracheal tube placement.

False-positive results can potentially occur in the case of esophageal intubation after ingestion of carbonated beverages or antacids.[101,126,152] High CO_2 levels (20%) are present in all carbonated beverages.[126] Sodium bicarbonate, an ingredient found in most antacids (except sodium citrate), reacts with hydrochloric acid in the stomach, releasing CO_2 levels comparable to that found in alveolar gas. With carbonated beverages, CO_2 levels as high as 5.3% can be measured initially, with esophageal ventilation rendering correct assessment of tracheal tube placement rather difficult.[126] However, rapid decline in CO_2 levels occurs with successive ventilations (Fig. 30-10). The abnormal CO_2 waveform may give an important

clue in the early detection of esophageal intubation.[126] Because the observation of a normal-looking CO_2 waveform during the first few ventilations is no guarantee of correct tube placement, the waveform must be watched closely for at least 1 minute after placement of the tube.

It should be emphasized that a normal waveform is not synonymous with "the tube in the trachea."[124] A normal waveform may be observed without a tube being in the trachea during spontaneous or controlled ventilation in the following situations: face mask anesthesia, the use of a laryngeal mask airway, and the use of the esophageal-tracheal Combitube because ventilation is carried out through the pharyngeal perforations.[139] A normal waveform may also be present and sustained if the distal end of the tracheal tube is in the pharynx but not necessarily in the trachea.[28] This should be suspected by the unusual volume of cuff air required to stop the leak and an increased peak inspiratory pressure.

Although capnography has been widely used in operating rooms, its use in emergency rooms, intensive care units, and hospital floors has been rather limited for the following reasons: (1) need for warm-up and careful calibration time; (2) requirement for an external power source, which further decreases the ability to be used in emergency situations; and (3) not easily transferable to the patient's side. Portable apnea monitors that use infrared spectrometry for sensing CO_2 have been used for confirmation of tracheal tube placement.[93] Although they do not accurately quantify CO_2 concentration, a moving-bar indicator with seven light-emitting diodes does provide an estimate of 1.5 percentage points per illuminated diode. Gas is aspirated through plastic tubing attached to the elbow connector proximal to the tracheal tube (Fig. 30-11), allowing it to sense CO_2 in the first exhalation after intubation. The device is cheap, portable, operates for 90 minutes on batteries, and requires neither warm-up time nor calibration. This electronic instrument can also function as a breathing circuit disconnection alarm.[93]

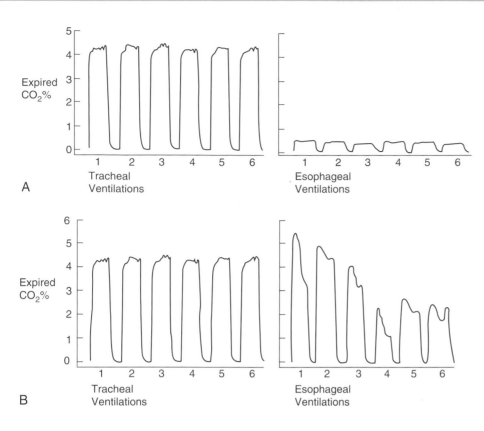

A

B

Figure 30-10 Expired CO_2 waveform during tracheal and esophageal ventilations before **(A)** and after **(B)** addition of a carbonated beverage in the stomach. (From Sum Ping ST, Mehta MP, Symreng T: Reliability of capnography in identifying esophageal intubation with carbonated beverage or antacid in the stomach. Anesth Analg 73:333, 1991.)

ii. Colorimetric End-Tidal Carbon Dioxide Detection

Early studies attempted to use techniques to quantitate the amount of CO_2 in exhaled gas and relied on the reaction of CO_2 with another substance such as barium hydroxide to produce a color change.[118] Thereafter, chemical indicators that change colors in the presence of increased hydrogen ion concentrations were used. The Einstein CO_2 detector was constructed by attaching a 15-mm adapter to one end of a De Lee mucus trap containing a mixture of 3 mL of phenolphthalein and 3 mL of cresol. When the exhaled gas is bubbled through the chamber, carbonic acid formation causes a dramatic color change from red to yellow within seconds. Failure of the solution to change from red to yellow should suggest esophageal intubation.[16]

A disposable CO_2 detector device (Easy Cap Endtidal CO_2 Detector)* that can be connected between a tracheal tube and a breathing circuit or a bag-and-mask assembly is now available (Fig. 30-12).[29,45,58,68,88,89,123] The detector contains filter paper impregnated with a colorless liquid base and pH-sensitive indicator (metacresol purple) that reversibly changes from purple to yellow as a result of pH change when exposed to CO_2 and reverts to purple when CO_2 is no longer present. The color changes are made visible through a transparent

---

*Nellcor, Inc., New York, NY.

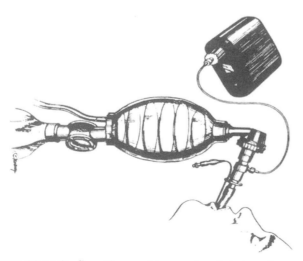

Figure 30-11 Configuration used to sample exhaled gas from an endotracheal tube. (From Owen RL, Cheney FW: Use of an apnea monitor to verify endotracheal intubation. Respir Care 30:974, 1985.)

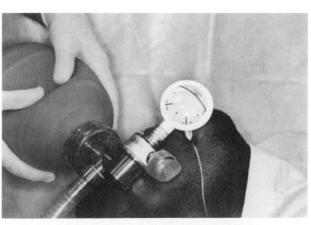

Figure 30-12 The colorimetric carbon dioxide detector.

dome in the plastic housing unit of the device. In general, a purple color (A range) indicates a CO_2 level less than or equal to 0.5%. The B range is a dusty tan color, reflecting 0.5% to 2% CO_2 levels. When the detector is exposed to CO_2 levels higher than 2%, the color brightens to a yellow-tan color, the C range.

Studies have shown that colorimetric $PETCO_2$ monitoring is reliable in verifying proper tracheal tube placement in nonarrested patients.[29,45,58,68,88,89,123] In one study,[58] the mean minimum CO_2 concentration required for detection of the perceivable color change was 0.54% (4.1 mm Hg) and ranged from 0.25% to 0.60% (1.9 to 4.6 mm Hg). When a tracheal tube is correctly placed in a patient with adequate pulmonary blood flow, the detector should register C. The color change occurs immediately with the first breath in almost all patients. In the nonarrested patient when the device registers low or absent CO_2 (A reading), esophageal intubation should be strongly suspected. If a C is obtained in an arrested patient, proper tube placement is confirmed. In contrast, an A reading (absence of color change) during manual ventilation in a patient with cardiac arrest is consistent with either an esophageal or a tracheal intubation in patients with profound low-flow state resulting from prolonged arrest or inadequate resuscitation. In another study, for 28 of 106 tracheal intubations in "pulseless" patients, the detector did not show any color change, indicating a $PaCO_2$ less than 4 mm Hg.[68] A multicenter trial of a colorimetric CO_2 detection device found that all cardiac arrest patients who survived to admission had a value of C registered on the monitor.[92] No patient in whom the detector failed to register color change survived. Thus, the device may be useful as a prognostic indicator of successful resuscitation.[68]

Although the availability of such a device is considered a great leap forward, it has its own pitfalls and thus is not a substitute for assessment skills. The manufacturer suggests an algorithm in case of color ranges, A, B, and C. Following such an algorithm certainly detracts from the simplicity of the detector. Because the device has a dead space of 38 mL, the manufacturer does not recommend its use in children weighing less than 15 kg, although its efficacy in verifying tracheal intubation has been confirmed in infants older than 6 months.[63] The color change may be difficult to discern under low-light conditions and may be misinterpreted by color-blind individuals. The color chart in the detector dome is color matched to fluorescent lighting. The manufacturer provides a separate color chart for use in lighting other than fluorescent, such as incandescent lighting.

Although the detector is not sensitive to temperature, it is eventually affected by humidity. Water vapor interferes with the chemical reaction and inactivates the device. It can be rendered ineffective within 15 minutes if the patient is receiving humidified gases. It has been suggested that trapping the humidity with a passive moisture exchanger may extend the useful life of the device.[63]

The manufacturer cautions against the use of the device in conjunction with a heated humidifier or nebulizer and emphasizes that it is not intended to be used for longer than 10 minutes after intubation. Because the indicator permanently changes colors if exposed for prolonged period to low CO_2 or other acids in the air, the device is packaged in a gas-impermeable metallic foil and is marketed as a one-time-one-use item. The packaged detector has a shelf life of 15 months if left unopened but may not function properly if the package is accidentally opened and the device is exposed to room air for several hours. For this reason, it is essential to verify that the indicator color is purple before use.

Widespread use of colorimetric CO_2 detectors has been hampered by limitations in their performance characteristics. However, new colorimetric CO_2 indicators seem to have overcome some of these limitations.[42] With this improved technology,[42] it is expected that newer colorimetric CO_2 detectors will be more durable during prolonged exposure to heat, humidity, and CO_2. Furthermore, they will be cheaper and will have a longer shelf life. Even in the nonarrested patient, there are potential sources of rare errors with the use of colorimetric CO_2 monitoring. After manual ventilation with bag and mask before intubation, CO_2 from the exhaled air may be blown into the stomach and may result in detectable CO_2 levels, yielding a false-positive yellow color if the tracheal tube is misplaced in the esophagus. Ventilating the patient with six breaths results in a washout of CO_2 to near zero if the tube is misplaced in the esophagus. Close observation of the color of the detector is essential during and after the delivery of six quick breaths so that false-positive results are avoided.

Concerns over inadvertent detection of gastric CO_2 from ingested beverages after esophageal intubation and potentially vitiating colorimetric CO_2 detection have been raised.[89] In a study of carbonated beverage ingestion and esophageal intubation in the cardiac arrest porcine model, the amount of CO_2 released did not result in spurious color change of the detector in the four animals studied and did not cause difficulty in interpretation of the readings.[53] Therefore, concern that false-positive results might be caused by esophageal placement in a patient who had recently ingested carbonated beverages appears to be unwarranted.[53,68]

Colorimetric CO_2 is a simple, safe, highly sensitive, reliable, and quick method for confirming tracheal tube placement in the nonarrested patient. Unlike capnography, it is portable (pocket sized) and does not require calibration or a power source. It is useful in places where capnography is unavailable, such as hospital floors, emergency departments, and prehospital settings. As with capnography, false-negative results (tube in trachea, no color change) may occur. Although very rare, false-positive results (tube in esophagus, with color change) can occur with the first few breaths. In the arrested patient, interpretation of no color change requires caution because it may indicate circulatory arrest, inadequate resuscitation, or esophageal intubation.

b. Esophageal Detector Device/Self-Inflating Bulb

The principle of use of the esophageal detector device (EDD) is based on anatomic differences between the trachea and the esophagus.[145] The trachea in the adult is about 10 to 12 cm long and its diameter can vary from 13 to 22 mm. The trachea remains constantly patent because of C-shaped rigid cartilaginous rings joined vertically by fibroelastic tissue and closed posteriorly by unstriped trachealis muscle. The esophagus is a fibromuscular tube, 25 cm long in adults, that extends from the cricopharyngeal sphincter to the gastroesophageal junction, and there is no intrinsic structure to maintain its patency. Wee[145] and O'Leary and colleagues[91] introduced a new method using a simple device to distinguish esophageal from tracheal intubation. The principle underlying the use of the device is that the esophagus collapses when a negative pressure is applied to its lumen, whereas the trachea does not. The device consists of a 60-mL syringe fitted by an adapter that can be attached to a tracheal tube connector.[91,145]

When the syringe is attached to a tube placed in the trachea, withdrawal of the plunger of the syringe aspirates gas freely from the patient's lungs without any resistance apart from that inherent in the device (Fig. 30-13).[91,145] If the tube is in the esophagus, withdrawal of the plunger causes apposition of the walls of the esophagus, occluding its lumen around the tube, and a negative pressure or resistance is felt when the plunger is pulled back. Wee[145] conducted a study in 100 patients in whom placement of tracheal and esophageal tubes was assessed using the EDD. There were 99 first-time correct identifications of tube placement, and the mean time taken by the observer to diagnose tube placement was 6.9 seconds. The application of constant but slow aspiration has been recommended to avoid the suction effect and prevent mucosal damage. Tracheal intubation is confirmed if 30 to 40 cm³ of gas is aspirated without resistance in adults[91,145] and 5 to 10 cm³ in children older than 2 years.[146]

Nunn[86] simplified the EDD by replacing the syringe with an Ellik evacuator, which is a self-inflating bulb (SIB) with a capacity of 75 to 90 mL. After intubation, the device is connected to the tube, and the bulb is compressed. Compression is silent and refill is instantaneous if the tube is in the trachea. In contrast, if the tube is in the esophagus, compression of the SIB is accompanied by a characteristic flatus-like noise, and the SIB remains collapsed on release. It has been shown that the test can be accomplished easily within 3 seconds, and the outcome is unmistakable.[148] This technique has been further modified by compressing the SIB before, rather than after, connection to the tracheal tube connector.[7] Investigations that used the latter technique confirmed earlier studies and demonstrated that the sensitivity,

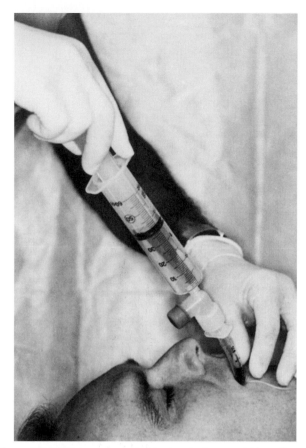

Figure 30-13 The esophageal detector device consisting of a 60-mL syringe fitted by an adapter to a tracheal tube connector.

specificity, and predictive value of the SIB are 100%[87,105,106,151] (Figs. 30-14 and 30-15).

Despite the efficacy of both the EDD and the SIB in differentiating esophageal from tracheal intubation, false-negative results (tube in the trachea, but gas cannot be aspirated by the EDD or the SIB does not reinflate)

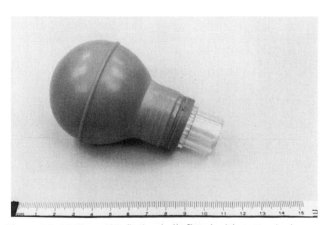

Figure 30-14 The self-inflating bulb fitted with a standard 15-mm adapter. (From Salem MR, Wafai Y, Joseph NJ, et al: Efficacy of the self-inflating bulb in detecting esophageal intubation. Does the presence of a nasogastric tube or cuff deflation make a difference? Anesthesiology 80:42, 1994.)

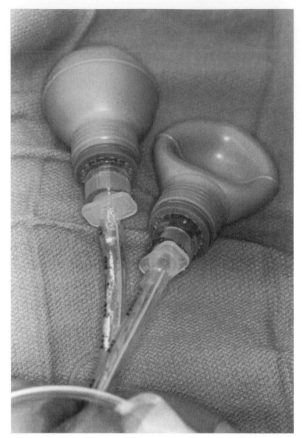

Figure 30-15 In a demonstration, collapsed self-inflating bulbs were connected simultaneously to tracheally and esophageally placed tubes in the presence of a nasogastric tube. The bulb connected to the tube in the trachea instantaneously reinflated, whereas that connected to the tube in the esophagus remained collapsed. (From Salem MR, Wafai Y, Joseph NJ, et al: Efficacy of the self-inflating bulb in detecting esophageal intubation. Does the presence of a nasogastric tube or cuff deflation make a difference? Anesthesiology 80:42, 1994.)

Table 30-3   Demographics of False-Negative Results

Technique	T1	T2
Morbid obesity	45	20
Severe bronchospasm	2	2
Elderly with chronic obstructive pulmonary disease	2	2
Main stem intubation	1	0
Pulmonary secretions	1	0
Pulmonary edema	0	1
Totals	51	25

T1, The self-inflating bulb (SIB) is compressed before it is connected to the tracheal tube.
T2, The SIB is first connected to the tube and is then compressed. See text for details.
From Wafai Y, Salem MR, Joseph NJ, et al: The self-inflating bulb for confirmation of tracheal intubation: Incidence and demography of false negatives. Anesthesiology 81:A1303, 1994.

have been reported. The EDD or the SIB may fail to confirm tracheal tube placement in infants in whom the tracheal wall is not held open by rigid cartilaginous rings, if the tube is obstructed by kinking or the presence of material in the tube, and in patients with severe bronchospasm.[6,50,117] Slow or no reinflation of the SIB may be encountered if the tube bevel is at the carina or in the right main stem bronchus.[144] Slight retraction or rotation of the tube usually corrects the position of the tube and orientation of the bevel, resulting in instantaneous reinflation of the SIB.[141,144] The SIB may also fail to reinflate or may reinflate slowly when connected to a properly placed tracheal tube in morbidly obese patients[65,141] and in other patients who have a marked reduction in expiratory reserve volume, such as those with pulmonary edema or adult respiratory distress syndrome or parturients undergoing cesarean section.[8,65]

In a study involving 2140 consecutive anesthetized adult patients,[141] the overall incidence of false-negative results with the SIB (no reinflation or delayed reinflation

> 4 seconds) was 3.6%. It was apparent that the technique used can contribute to false-negative results. When the SIB was fully compressed before connection to the tracheal tube, the incidence was 4.6%, whereas it was reduced to 2.4% when the SIB was compressed after connection to the tube.[141] Most of the patients (85.5%) in whom false-negative results were obtained were morbidly obese (body mass index > 35 kg/m^2) (Table 30-3). We surmise that this phenomenon seen in morbidly obese patients and pregnant women is related to marked reduction in FRC after anesthetic induction and muscular paralysis in the supine position leading to reduced caliber of intrathoracic airways and collapsibility of the trachea on the application of subatmospheric pressure by the SIB.[8,65,141] It is also possible that the negative pressure generated (>−50 cm H$_2$O) may cause collapse and invagination of the posterior tracheal wall. Further compression can occur as a result of mediastinal compression.[8,65] The chain of events that may lead to failure of the SIB to confirm tracheal intubation is presented in Figure 30-16. If the SIB is compressed after connection to the tracheal tube rather than before, a volume of gas is first introduced in the airway before subatmospheric pressure is generated by the SIB and thus would limit the collapse of the SIB seen when it is compressed before connection to the tracheal tube.[8,65,141]

Advantages of the SIB include low cost, unlimited shelf life, no power source, usability with one hand, and usability in areas of low light. It is quicker to use (<10 seconds) and is unaffected by ingested carbonated beverages, antacids, or exhaled CO$_2$, in the event of esophageal intubation. It can confirm tracheal intubation before initiating manual ventilation. The performance of the SIB should not be affected by a cardiac arrest, an NGT, or cuff deflation.[106] Studies found the EDD/SIB to be

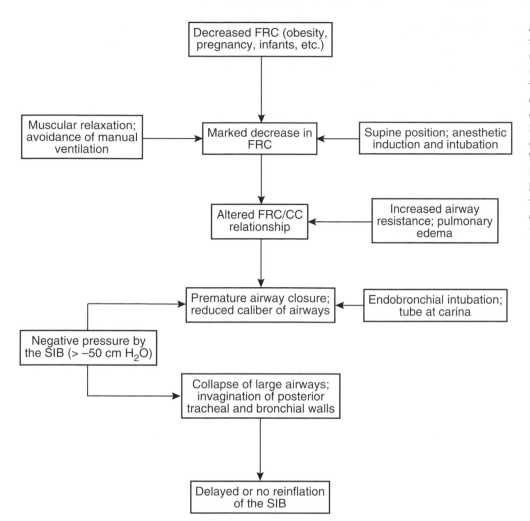

Figure 30-16 Chain of events in false-negative results when using the self-inflating bulb (SIB) to confirm tracheal intubation in patients with decreased functional residual capacity. CC, closing capacity; FRC, functional residual capacity. (From Lang DJ, Wafai Y, Salem MR, et al: Efficacy of the self-inflating bulb in confirming tracheal intubation in the morbidly obese. Anesthesiology 85:246, 1996.)

more accurate in verifying proper tube placement in out-of-hospital cardiac arrest patients and during emergency intubations than CO_2 detection methods.[19,30,106,110] Indeed, it has been the method preferred by emergency medical personnel.[30,106,110] Verification of tracheal tube placement using the SIB would enable physicians and emergency personnel to proceed with other resuscitation duties. Other studies found the SIB to be complementary to CO_2 detection.[61,128]

Concern has been raised that false-positive results (tube in esophagus, but SIB reinflates) may occur as a result of gastric insufflation after bag-and-mask ventilation before intubation. In 72 patients, it has been demonstrated that even after the intentional delivery of three small breaths (300 to 350 mL each), the SIB was effective in detecting esophageal intubation in all 72 patients.[105] In another study, despite the use of mask ventilation before intubation, the authors did not observe a single instance of instantaneous reinflation of the SIB from the esophagus.[148] In a study of one pig, Foutch and colleagues[38] used a syringe similar to that of Wee[145] and found that the device is effective in detecting esophageal intubation even after 1 minute of bag-and-mask ventilation. Although these studies lead us to believe that the SIB is

effective in detecting esophageal intubation after mask ventilation (and modest gastric insufflation), it may fail occasionally in cases of massive gastric insufflation[2] and if the lower esophageal tone is decreased.[8] It is recommended that when the SIB is used to confirm tracheal intubation the test should be undertaken before ventilation is initiated through the tube.

It is essential that the SIB be of an appropriate size.[105,107,140] Although a smaller SIB (capacity 20 mL) generates a higher negative pressure (because of its smaller radius) (Fig. 30-17), it is unreliable in detecting esophageal intubation if the SIB is compressed after

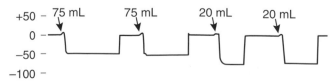

Figure 30-17 Representative tracing of negative pressure generated by large (75 mL) and small (20 mL) SIBs when the SIB is compressed before it is connected to the tubes placed in the esophagus. The small SIB generates greater negative pressure than the large SIB. See text for details.

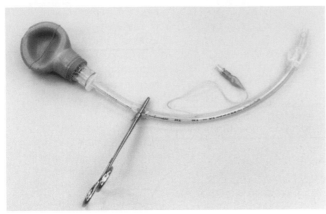

Figure 30-18 Testing the self-inflating bulb for leakage. The compressed bulb is connected to a clamped tracheal tube. The absence of reinflation is indicative of airtightness. This test reveals leakage from the bulb and the connector (cracked connector or loose fitting).

connection to the tube.[140] The larger SIB (capacity 75 mL) is recommended because it does not yield false-positive results when either technique is used.[107] Although SIBs can be constructed by fitting bulbs with a standard 15-mm adapter, they are commercially available for single use. The devices are checked before use by connecting the compressed SIB to a clamped tracheal tube; the absence of reinflation is an indication of airtightness (Fig. 30-18). We have found that proper function of the device is not affected when a bacterial or viral filter is placed between the device and the tracheal tube connector.

The use of the SIB has been extended to identify the location of the esophageal-tracheal Combitube (ETC) and facilitate its proper positioning using a simple algorithm (Figs. 30-19 and 30-20).[139] This may be of importance if the ETC is used in patients whose lungs cannot be ventilated by mask and whose trachea cannot be intubated.[139] After blind placement, the compressed SIB is connected to the distal lumen. Instantaneous reinflation implies that the ETC is in the trachea and ventilation is carried out through the distal lumen, whereas the absence of reinflation is indicative of esophageal placement (very common). In this position, the pharyngeal balloon and the distal cuff are inflated and the compressed SIB is connected to the proximal lumen; instantaneous reinflation is expected to occur because the compressed SIB aspirates gas from the lungs through the pharyngeal perforations. If slow or no reinflation of the SIB occurs, repositioning the ETC (1 to 2 cm pullback) may be indicated, and rechecking with the SIB confirms proper placement. Controlled ventilation is then carried out through the proximal lumen. Proper positioning and adequacy of ventilation can be further confirmed by the presence of breath sounds, absence of gastric insufflation, capnography or colorimetric CO_2 detection, and pulse oximetry.[139]

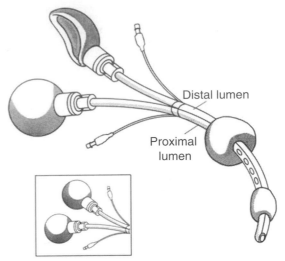

Figure 30-19 Schematic diagram depicting outcome when the compressed self-inflating bulb is connected to the distal and proximal lumen of an esophageal-tracheal Combitube in the esophageal position. Note that the bulb connected to the distal lumen remains collapsed, whereas that connected to the proximal lumen instantaneously reinflates. The insert depicts outcome when the esophageal-tracheal Combitube is in the trachea. Both bulbs instantaneously reinflate. (From Wafai Y, Salem MR, Baraka A, et al: Effectiveness of the self-inflating bulb for verification of proper placement of the esophageal tracheal Combitube. Anesth Analg 80:122, 1995.)

c. Acoustic Devices/Reflectometry

Devices utilizing sonic techniques as the basis for distinguishing tracheal from esophageal intubation have been developed. The mechanism of action of the sonomatic confirmation of tracheal intubation (SCOTI) device is

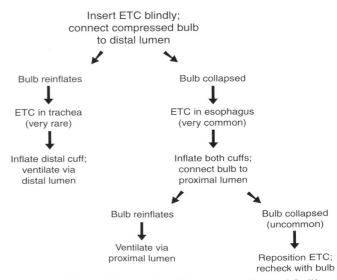

Figure 30-20 Algorithm for identifying the position and facilitating proper placement of the esophageal-tracheal Combitube (ETC) after blind placement. (From Wafai Y, Salem MR, Baraka A, et al: Effectiveness of the self-inflating bulb for verification of proper placement of the esophageal tracheal Combitube. Anesth Analg 80:122, 1995.)

based on the recognition of the resonating frequencies, which vary according to whether the tube is in an open structure (trachea) or a closed structure (esophagus).[49,67,81,83,132] Although the concept is intriguing, the inability to configure the device correctly with all types and lengths of tracheal tubes limited the usefulness of the device as an indicator of tracheal intubation.[49,67,83,132] The disappointing sales led to the withdrawal of the device from the market in 1996.[69]

The principle of acoustic reflectometry was applied by using a series of sonic impulses into the airway with a miniature microphone placed in the tracheal tube wall to monitor sound pressure.[71] The presence of deflection at the tracheal tube tip allowed discrimination between esophageal and tracheal intubation.[71] Acoustic reflectometry allowed the construction of a one-dimensional image of a cavity, such as the airway or the esophagus.[98] The reflectometric area-distance profile consists of a constant cross-sectional area segment (length of the tube), followed either by a rapid increase in the area beyond the tube in case of tracheal intubation or by an immediate decrease in the area in case of esophageal intubation.[98] In a study of 200 tracheal intubations confirmed by capnography, acoustic reflectometry correctly identified 198 (Figs. 30-21, 30-22, and 30-23).[99] In two patients, tracheal intubations were interpreted as an esophageal intubation. In contrast, all 14 esophageal intubations were correctly identified.[99] Because it is noninvasive and rapid (<3 seconds), acoustic imaging may become popular in the near future in the determination of the location of tube placement in patients with cardiac arrest, particularly when visualization of the glottis may not be visible. With technical improvement of the computer-based system, acoustic reflectometry may have use as an imaging adjunct device that can be used in the diagnosis and treatment of airway emergencies.[99]

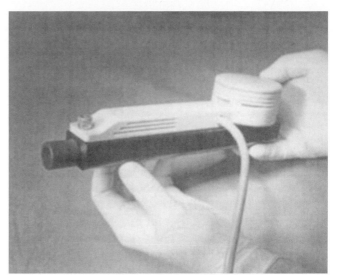

Figure 30-21 A Hood Labs (Pembroke, MA) two-microphone acoustic reflectometer.

3. Failsafe Methods

a. Direct Visualization of the Tracheal Tube between the Cords

Sighting the tube passage through the larynx during intubation or confirmation of the presence of the tube between the cords after intubation is one of the most reliable methods to ensure correct tube placement. Two maneuvers can be helpful to assist direct visual confirmation of tracheal intubation, one during and the other after intubation.

If the tube is introduced directly posterior to the laryngoscope blade as shown in Figure 30-24A, the laryngoscopist's view of the cords may be obscured and the tube may inadvertently enter the esophagus. This can be avoided by directing the tube from the right corner of

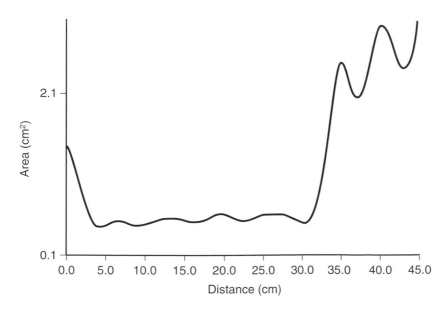

Figure 30-22 An acoustic reflectometry area-distance profile consists of a plot of the total cross-sectional area of the cavity versus axial length down into the cavity. For an endotracheal tube (ET) in the trachea, the reflectometric profile consists of a constant cross-sectional area segment (length of ET), followed by a rapid increase in the area beyond the carina. (From Raphael DT, Benbassat M, Arnaudov D, et al: Validation study of two-microphone acoustic reflectometry for determination of breathing tube placement in 200 adult patients. Anesthesiology 97:1371, 2002.)

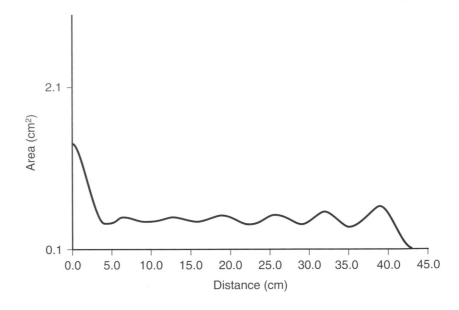

Figure 30-23 For a breathing tube in the esophagus, the reflectometric profile consists of a constant cross-sectional area segment (length of endotracheal tube), followed by an immediate decrease in the area distal to the tube. (From Raphael DT, Benbassat M, Arnaudov D, et al: Validation study of two-microphone acoustic reflectometry for determination of breathing tube placement in 200 adult patients. Anesthesiology 97:1371, 2002.)

the mouth toward the larynx. As seen in Figure 30-24B, this maneuver can allow visualization of the tube entering the larynx, thus confirming tracheal intubation. The other maneuver that can be performed after intubation but before removing the laryngoscope from the mouth involves gentle posterior displacement of the tube toward the palate (Fig. 30-25).[36] The backward push on the tube against the forward traction of the laryngoscope blade exposes the cords by altering the direction of the tube as it enters the larynx.[36] This maneuver can be helpful

in cases in which the cords are obscured by the tube as it enters the larynx.

Viewing the tube entering the larynx cannot be performed in all cases of direct laryngoscopy, especially if intubation is difficult and during blind nasal intubation. Even after visualization of the tube entering the larynx, the tube may slip out of the larynx while the laryngoscope is being removed, during taping of the tube, while positioning the patient, or during transportation. This tends to occur more frequently if the distal end

Figure 30-24 **A,** When the tube is introduced directly posterior to the blade, the view of the cords may be obscured and the tube may enter the esophagus instead of the trachea.
B, Directing the tube from the right corner of the mouth toward the larynx can allow better visualization of the tube entering the larynx.

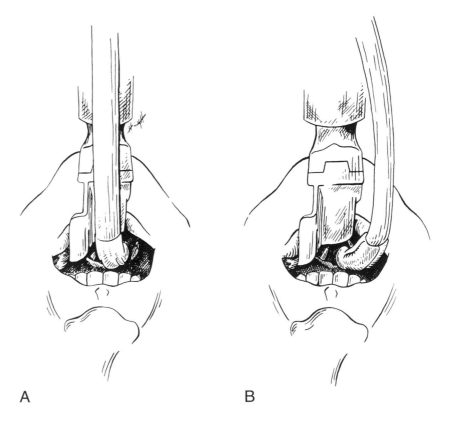

A   B

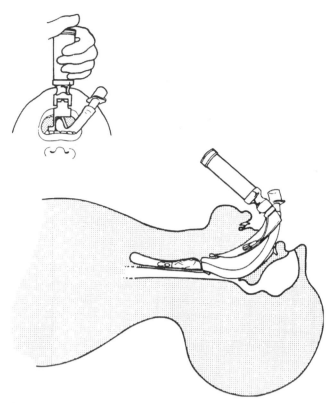

Figure 30-25 Posterior displacement of tracheal tube restores view of larynx. (From Ford RW: Confirming tracheal intubation: A simple manoeuvre. Can Anaesth Soc J 30:191, 1983.)

of the tube lies just below the cords or high in the trachea.

b. Flexible Fiberoptic Bronchoscopy

A sure method for confirmation of tracheal intubation is visualization of the tracheal rings and carina with a fiberoptic scope after intubation.[14,147] This is convenient only when a fiberoptic scope is readily available or when the instrument is used to aid intubation (see Chapter 18). It should be emphasized that visualization of the vocal cords and tracheal rings through the fiberoptic scope before threading the tube over it does not guarantee tracheal intubation. There are three reasons why the tube may not follow the path of the scope into the trachea.[14,77,84,113] First, a stiff, large tube may carry a relatively thin scope into the esophagus even though the tip of the scope was originally placed in the larynx and trachea.[14,77] Second, the tip of the tube and its Murphy eye are at 90 degrees to the right when the concavity of the tube is facing anteriorly.[14,113] Consequently, the tip of the tube may be blocked from entering the larynx by the right arytenoid cartilage, vocal cord, or both. If excessive force is used, the tube may slip into the esophagus. This problem can be corrected by a 90-degree counterclockwise rotation.[14,113] Third, if the scope is inserted through a tube placed nasally, the scope may exit the tube through the Murphy eye and may actually enter the trachea, but it will be impossible to thread the

tube over the scope.[14,84] To ensure that tracheal intubation has been accomplished, the scope should be withdrawn after placement of the tube and then reintroduced to visualize the tracheal rings and carina and to determine the distance from the distal end of the tube to the carina.[14]

III. VERIFICATION OF TRACHEAL TUBE INSERTION DEPTH

According to the ASA closed claims analysis, the combination of inadvertent extubation and main stem intubation accounts for 2% of all the adverse respiratory events in adults and 4% in pediatric patients.[21,79] The incidence of main stem intubation in anesthetic practice is unknown, but it is probably more frequent than the literature indicates. The incidence of main stem intubation in the critical care setting, not detected by clinical examination but discovered on the chest radiograph after intubation, is 4%.[111] Applying a strict definition of "acceptable tracheal tube placement" as greater than 2 cm and less than or equal to 6 cm above the carina (with the head in a neutral position) in adult patients after emergent intubation, Schwartz and coworkers[111] found an incidence of 15.5% of inappropriately placed tubes according to radiologic assessment, with a higher incidence in women than in men.

Fortunately, endobronchial intubation is not a common cause of death, but, if unrecognized, it can lead to hypoxemia secondary to collapse of the contralateral lung and hyperinflation of the intubated lung with resultant tension pneumothorax. The ensuing hypoxemia depends on the degree of venous admixture ($\dot{V}/\dot{Q} > 0$), the magnitude of intrapulmonary shunting where ($\dot{V}/\dot{Q} = 0$), fraction of inspired oxygen, degree of inhibition of hypoxic pulmonary vasoconstriction, and the level of $S\bar{v}O_2$. An atelectatic lung can also be the site of infection.

Unintentional main stem intubation can result in one of several scenarios depending on the location of the distal end of the tube (Fig. 30-26). Placement of the tube high in the right main bronchus (or even at the carina) may result in preferential ventilation of the right lung. Retrograde gas flow may lead to partial ventilation of the left lung if the tracheal tube cuff does not provide a tight seal (see Fig. 30-26A).[75] A biphasic CO_2 waveform may be noticed (the two lungs have different time constants). Ventilation with high flow rates through a tube whose tip is placed just proximal to the orifice of the right upper lobe bronchus promotes negative pressure (Bernoulli effect) and atelectasis of the right upper lobe (see Fig. 30-26B). Placement of the tube further down the right main bronchus prevents ventilation of the left lung and occludes the right upper lobe bronchus (see Fig. 30-26C). A tube placed in the lower portion of the trachea may obstruct a congenital tracheal bronchus,

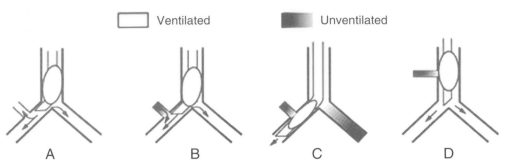

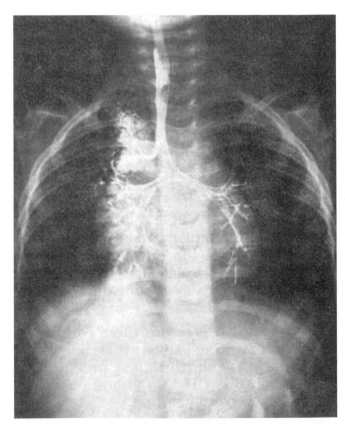

Figure 30-26 Unintentional main stem intubation can result in one of several scenarios, depending on the location of the distal end of the tube. **A,** Placement of the tube high in the right main bronchus may result in preferential ventilation of the right lung. Retrograde gas flow may lead to partial ventilation of the left lung if the tracheal tube cuff does not provide a tight seal. **B,** Ventilation with high flow rates through a tube whose tip is placed just proximal to the orifice of the right upper lobe bronchus promotes negative pressure and atelectasis of the right upper lobe. **C,** Placement of the tube further down the right main bronchus prevents ventilation of the left lung and occludes the right upper lobe bronchus. **D,** A tube placed in the lower portion of the trachea may obstruct a congenital tracheal bronchus causing upper right lobe atelectasis. (Modified from Mecca RS: Management of the difficult airway. In Kinby RR, Gravenstein N [eds]: Clinical Anesthesia Practice, 2nd ed. Philadelphia, Saunders, 2002, pp 921-954.)

causing upper right lobe atelectasis (Fig. 30-27; see Fig. 30-26D).[137,138] In this rare anomaly, the bronchus to the right apical lung segment or the bronchus to the right upper lobe arises directly from the trachea—usually less than 2 cm from the carina.

A. METHODS OF VERIFICATION OF TRACHEAL TUBE INSERTION DEPTH

To decrease the likelihood of main stem intubation and unintentional extubation, clinicians should aim at positioning the distal end of the tube in the middle third of the trachea. Various methods can be used before, during, or after intubation in order to locate the tube at an appropriate depth in the trachea.

1. Referencing the Marks on the Tube before and after Intubation

In one method, the tube is placed alongside the patient's face and neck with the tip of the tube lying at the suprasternal notch and the tube aligned to conform externally to the position of the nasal or oral tube. The centimeter markings at which the tube intersects with the teeth or gums for oral intubation, or the nare for nasal intubation, are noted so that the tube is secured in that position after intubation. Another method is securing orally placed tracheal tubes at the upper incisor teeth (or gums) at the 23-cm mark in men and the 21-cm mark in women of average adult size.[94] This method has been found to be reliable in anesthetized patients[94] but not in critically ill patients.[94,112] We have observed that in tall men and in patients in whom excessive head extension is needed, the tube may need to be secured at the 24- or

Figure 30-27 Bronchographic study revealing the presence of an apical displaced, right tracheal bronchus. The left tracheal shadow at the level of the first rib is suggestive of a vascular ring, although this is not verified by cardiac catheterization or esophagograms. The potential for inadvertent intubation or occlusion of this lower airway anomaly is apparent. (From Venkateswarlu T, Turner CJ, Carter JD, Morrow DH: The tracheal bronchus: An unusual airway problem. Anesth Analg 55:746, 1976.)

25-cm mark; in some shorter women it may need to be secured at the 19-cm mark for optimal placement of the distal end of the tube in the middle of the trachea. Formulas regarding the appropriate length of tracheal tubes are available for infants and children. The reader is referred to pediatric anesthesia texts for this information.

2. Direct Visualization of the Tube and Its Cuff

Positioning the distal end of the tube in the middle of the trachea is a relatively easy maneuver when the tube can be seen entering the larynx during direct laryngoscopy. Because the length of the trachea is 10 to 13 cm in an average adult, placing the upper end of the cuff of a tube (size 7 or 8 inside diameter) 2 cm below the vocal cords positions the distal end of the tube approximately 4 cm from the carina. In a simple study based on measurements,[26] it has been found that except in cases of short tracheas, placing the upper end of the cuff 2 cm below the cords predictably positions the distal end of the tube in the middle of the trachea.[26] This maneuver should be used whenever orotracheal intubation is performed under direct laryngoscopy.

3. Prevention of Tracheal Tube Displacement after Intubation

Despite initial proper positioning, the tube can still slip out of the larynx (or move closer to the carina) while the laryngoscope blade is being removed, during taping of the tube, after changing the position of the head, while positioning the patient, or during transportation. Several precautions should be undertaken to prevent tube displacement (Table 30-4).

4. Influence of Positioning on Tracheal Tube Insertion Depth

Excessive movement of the tube can occur during extension and flexion of the head. In a radiologic study

Table 30-4 Precautions to Prevent Tracheal Tube Displacement

The laryngoscope blade should be gently removed after intubation while securing the tube in position.
The tube should be taped or anchored carefully in place.
An oropharyngeal airway (or a bite block) placed adjacent to the tube can minimize the movement of the tube inside the mouth and prevent its dislodgement, especially during coughing.
The head should be kept in neutral position unless head extension or flexion is needed for the surgical procedure.

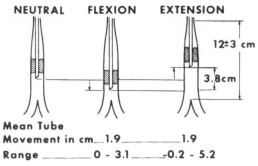

Figure 30-28 Mean endotracheal tube movement with flexion and extension of the neck from neutral position. The mean tube movement between flexion and extension is about one third to one fourth the length of an adult trachea (12 ± 3 cm). (From Conrardy PA, Goodman LR, Lainge F, Singer MM: Alteration of endotracheal tube position: Flexion and extension of the neck. Crit Care Med 4:7, 1976.)

in adults, Conrardy and associates[24] demonstrated an average 3.8 cm movement of the tube toward the carina when the head was moved from full extension to full flexion (Fig. 30-28). In some patients this movement reached as much as 6.4 cm. With lateral head rotation, the tube moved an average of 0.7 cm away from the carina. Because the average movement of the tube when the head is moved from the neutral position to full extension or full flexion is 1.9 cm in the adult, it is unlikely that extubation or main stem intubation would occur during this movement if the distal end of the tube was in the middle of the trachea, but it could occur if it was too high or too low in the trachea.

Malpositioning of the tube can occur with changes in patient's positioning,[51] displacement of the diaphragm, and during surgical manipulations of the trachea or esophagus, especially if the tube is not initially placed in the middle of the trachea. A high incidence of main stem intubation has been reported after the institution of a 30-degree Trendelenburg position. This is due to cephalad shift of the carina causing a taped tube to relocate into a main stem bronchus. The opposite can happen when the reverse Trendelenburg position is used. Because the trachea and the esophagus are invested in the same cervical fascia, pulling on either structure during surgery can misplace a previously correctly placed tracheal tube. This can occur during repair of esophageal atresia in infants and during esophagoscopy. Excessive movement of the head and neck of intubated patients must be avoided; however, if such movements are necessary, they should be done carefully. The position of the tube should be rechecked when the patient's position is altered; when the head is moved; after surgical manipulation of the trachea or esophagus; whenever displacement of the diaphragm is suspected (e.g., changes in FRC); and when an unexplained decrease in SaO_2,

Figure 30-29 Radiographs illustrate the effect of head position on endotracheal tube placement in newborn infants. The upper arrow indicates the tip of the endotracheal tube; the lower arrow indicates the tip of the carina. Note the marked excursion of the tip of the tube with head flexion (right). (From Todres ID, deBros F, Kramer SS: Endotracheal tube displacement in the newborn infant. J Pediatr 89:126, 1976.)

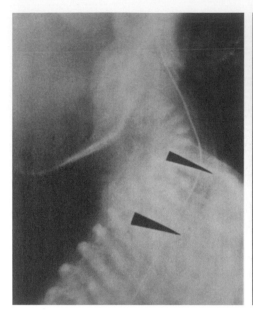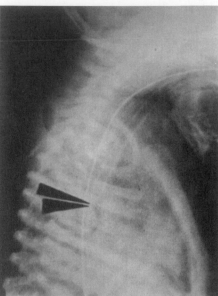

increased airway pressure, cuff leak, or biphasic CO_2 waveform is noticed.

The ease with which main stem intubation can occur with head flexion and unintentional extubation with head extension is of particular concern in the infant, especially in the neonate, whose trachea is only 4.7 to 5.7 cm in length (Fig. 30-29).[18,130] When tracheal intubation is performed in infants, precautions should be taken to ensure that the tube is placed far enough in the trachea but not in a main stem bronchus. One precaution is to use tubes that have circumferential marks at 2.2 cm from the distal end and introduce the marker on the tube as far as the cords in term infants, to slightly above the cords in preterm infants, and to slightly below the cords in older infants. Another alternative that has been recommended is to use tubes with marks 2.2, 2.4, and 2.6 cm from the distal end in tubes with diameters of 2.5, 3.0, and 3.5 mm, respectively. The reader is referred to pediatric anesthesia texts for more details.

5. Observation and Palpation of Chest Movements and Auscultation of Breath Sounds

Observation or palpation of an asymmetric chest movement and detection of unequal bilateral breath sounds should alert the clinician to the possibility of a main stem intubation (usually right side). In addition, absences of right apical movement or breath sounds, or both, imply that the tube and its cuff are obstructing the right upper lobe bronchus. Gradual withdrawal of the tube should correct the problem. Unless auscultation of bilateral breath sounds is repeated, main stem intubation may go unrecognized for hours.

6. Cuff Maneuvers and Neck Palpation

Various maneuvers of palpation of the tracheal tube cuff on each side of the trachea above the suprasternal notch (rapid cuff inflations, intermittent squeezing of the pilot balloon of a slightly overinflated cuff, and using the pilot balloon as a sensor while palpating the cuff in the neck) have been proposed to ensure that the tube is not in a main bronchus.[13] Suprasternal palpation of the cuff provides a high degree of confidence that the distal tip of the tube is greater than 2 cm from the carina, whereas if the cuff is not palpable, the tip is probably close to the carina.

7. Use of Fiberoptic Bronchoscopes

During fiberoptic-aided intubation, the distance from the distal end of the tube to the carina can be determined and the position of the tube easily corrected, if necessary.[14,147] The distal end of the tube is usually positioned at approximately 4 cm from the carina. The use of fiberoptic scopes to evaluate the position of the tube has been extended to the critical care setting to obviate the necessity of frequent chest radiographs.

8. Transtracheal Illumination

Transillumination techniques can help position the tracheal tube tip at a reliable distance above the carina. Two methods have been suggested. In one, the flexible lighted stylet is placed inside the tube so that the stylet bulb is positioned at the tube's distal opening prior to intubation.[76,120] By observing maximal illumination at the sternal notch (a consistent anatomic landmark) during intubation, the tip of the tube can be placed consistently 5.0 ± 1.0 cm from the carina.[120] In the other, the tip of the lighted stylet is placed inside the tube, just proximal to the cuff, before intubation. Visualization of transillumination distal to the cricoid cartilage is indicative of proper cuff positioning. In this position, the distance between the tip of the tube and the carina varies between 3.7 and 4 cm in adults.[76,150] Use of either method can reduce the need for radiographic confirmation of tracheal tube positioning.

9. Capnography

In cases of main stem intubation, the capnographic waveform usually shows a normal pattern. Main stem intubation or a tube impinging on the carina, however, should be suspected whenever a biphasic waveform is noticed.[43] Under these circumstances, other causes of biphasic waveforms should be excluded, such as lateral decubitus position, kyphoscoliosis causing compression of the lung, pulmonary disease, spontaneous breathing efforts, hiccups, and sampling line leak.

10. Use of the Esophageal Detector Device/Self-Inflating Bulb

The use of the EDD/SIB is of no value in diagnosing main stem intubation. However, it should be suspected in cases of slow reinflation of the SIB.[107] Rotation or

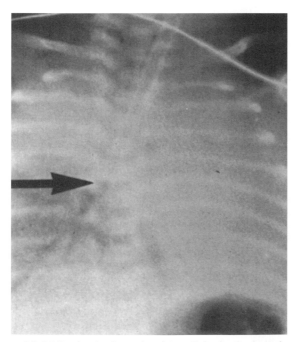

Figure 30-30 Tracheal tube malposition. Tube in the bronchus intermedius *(arrow)*. Note the airless left lung and right upper lobe. (From Mandel GA: Neonatal intensive care radiology. In Goodman LR, Putman CE [eds]: Intensive Care Radiology: Imaging of the Critically Ill. Philadelphia, WB Saunders, 1983, p 290.)

gradual pull-back of the tube, or both, may lead to instantaneous reinflation of the SIB.

11. Chest Radiography

In critically ill patients, a portable chest radiograph can easily detect main stem intubation and can determine the location of the distal end of the tube in relation to the carina (Fig. 30-30).[111,112,116] Because malpositioned tracheal tubes may not be detected by routine clinical assessment, some investigators are recommending that chest radiographs should remain the standard practice in the critical care setting.[111]

IV. CONCLUSIONS

The goals of tracheal intubation are to place the tube in the trachea and to position the tube at an appropriate depth inside the trachea. Unfortunately, unrecognized esophageal intubation and tracheal tube malposition have been a leading cause of injury involving the respiratory system in anesthetic practice and in the prehospital setting. Although they are rare events, the outcome is so devastating that awareness of their occurrence is essential whenever tracheal intubation is performed. A vast array of methods has been described to verify tracheal tube placement. In the majority of patients, these methods (alone or in combination) can successfully and quickly differentiate esophageal from tracheal intubation. Nevertheless, almost all these methods have been documented to fail under certain circumstances. It is crucial that the clinicians involved in tracheal intubation have the necessary airway management skills, perform these tests accurately, and interpret their results correctly. Obviously, not all these tests can be applied in every situation, but the clinician should be familiar with and use as many tests as possible. Prioritization of these tests depends on many factors, including experience, availability of devices, condition of the patient, and the location where tracheal intubation is performed. Viewing the tube passing between the cords during direct laryngoscopy and visualization of the tracheal rings and carina with a fiberoptic scope after intubation are the only foolproof methods of confirming tracheal intubation. In the nonarrested patient, CO_2 monitoring can quickly differentiate tracheal from esophageal intubation. In the arrested patient, however, CO_2 monitoring can be unreliable, although it can be useful as a prognostic indicator of the efficacy of resuscitation. Devices such as the SIB/EDD may be more useful in patients with cardiac arrest, but they can also yield false results.

Placing the distal tip of the tube in the middle of the trachea can be accomplished by positioning the upper end of the cuffed tube 2 cm below the cords during direct laryngoscopy or by placing the distal tip of the tube 4 cm

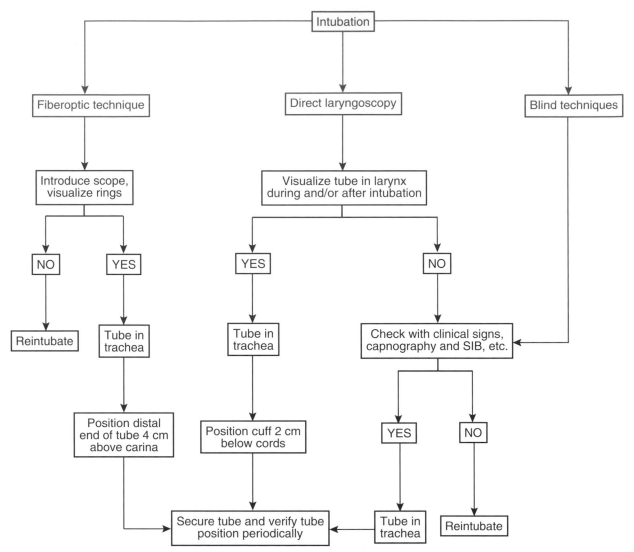

Figure 30-31 Proposed algorithm for verification of tracheal tube position and insertion depth during elective tracheal intubation. Intubation—using a tube of appropriate size and length. Blind techniques include blind nasal or oral intubation and intubation with introducers or with intubating stylets. Verify tube position periodically, especially in the following situations: changes in tube position, changes in head or body position, suspected decrease in functional residual capacity or displacement of the diaphragm, traction on trachea or esophagus, unexpected fall in Sao_2, biphasic CO_2 waveform, and unexpected cuff leak. Cuff leak after adequate cuff inflation can be due to leak around the cuff or loss of air from the cuff: cuff protruding above cords, tube too small, extremely compliant airway, tracheomalacia, tracheoesophageal fistula (very rare), defective cuff or damage to cuff during intubation, defective pilot-balloon system, and kinking of connecting tubing. SIB, self-inflating bulb. (From Salem MR: Verification of endotracheal tube position. Anesthesiol Clin North Am 19:813, 2001.)

above the carina with the aid of a fiberoptic scope in adults. The position of the tube should always be verified by clinical assessment (auscultation of both axillae and epigastrium). If direct visualization cannot be done, referencing the marks on the tube, transillumination techniques, or cuff maneuvers can be helpful. In the emergency and critical care settings, a chest radiograph can easily detect malpositioned tracheal tubes that may not be detected by routine clinical assessment. Other techniques (use of fiberoptic scopes, cuff maneuvers,

transillumination) can obviate the necessity of frequent chest radiographs.

On the basis of available information, two algorithms are proposed: one for verification of tracheal tube position in elective intubation (Fig. 30-31) and the other for emergency intubation (Fig. 30-32). These algorithms are designed to assist the clinician and should not be a substitute for clinical judgment. Under no circumstances should clinical signs be ignored in the presence of conflicting information from monitors and technical aids.

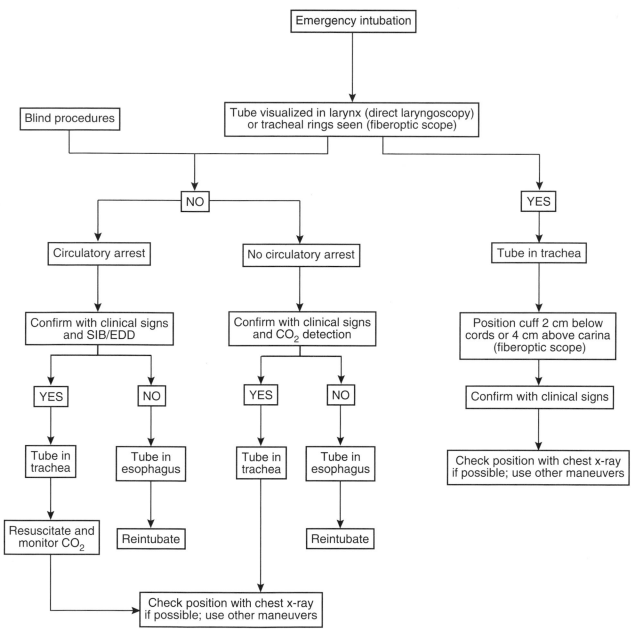

Figure 30-32 Proposed algorithm for verification of tracheal tube position and insertion depth during emergency intubation. In the emergency and critical care settings, a chest radiograph (frequently obtained) can easily detect malpositioning of tracheally placed tubes. Other techniques (fiberscopes, cuff maneuvers, transillumination) can decrease the need for frequent chest radiographs. In patients with circulatory arrest, CO_2 monitoring can be unreliable despite tracheal tube placement. In these patients, devices such as the self-inflating bulb/esophageal detector device (SIB/EDD) are more helpful. During cardiopulmonary resuscitation, monitoring CO_2 can serve as a prognostic indicator of the efficacy of resuscitation. (From Salem MR: Verification of endotracheal tube position. Anesthesiol Clin North Am 19:813, 2001.)

REFERENCES

1. Andersen KH, Hald A: Assessing the position of the tracheal tube: The reliability of different methods. Anaesthesia 44:984, 1989.
2. Andres AH, Langenstein H: The esophageal detector device is unreliable when the stomach has been ventilated. Anesthesiology 91:566, 1999.
3. Badgwell JM, Heavner JE, May WS, et al: End-tidal PCO_2 monitoring in infants and children ventilated with either a partial rebreathing or a nonrebreathing circuit. Anesthesiology 66:405, 1987.
4. Badgwell JM, McLoed ME, Lerman J, et al: End-tidal PCO_2 measurements sampled at the distal and proximal ends of the endotracheal tube in infants and children. Anesth Analg 66:959, 1987.
5. Banaszak EF, Kory RC, Snider GL: Phonopneumography. Am Rev Respir Dis 107:449, 1973.

6. Baraka A: The oesophageal detector device [letter]. Anaesthesia 45:697, 1991.

7. Baraka A, Muallem M: Confirmation of correct tracheal intubation by a self-inflating bulb. Middle East J Anesthesiol 11:193, 1991.

8. Baraka A, Khoury PJ, Siddik SS, et al: Efficacy of the self-inflating bulb in differentiating esophageal from tracheal intubation in the parturient undergoing cesarean section. Anesth Analg 84:533, 1997.

9. Baraka A, Tabakian H, Idriss A, et al: Breathing bag refilling [letter]. Anaesthesia 44:81, 1989.

10. Baraka AS, Salem MR: Preoxygenation. In Hagberg C: Benumof's Airway Management: Principles and Practice. 2nd ed. New York, Elsevier Science, 2004.

11. Bashein G, Cheney FW: Carbon dioxide detection to verify intratracheal placement of a breathing tube. Anesthesiology 61:782, 1984.

12. Batra AK, Cohn MA: Uneventful prolonged misdiagnosis of esophageal intubation. Crit Care Med 11:763, 1983.

13. Bednarek FJ, Kuhns LR: Endotracheal tube placement in infants determined by suprasternal palpation: A new technique. Pediatrics 56:224, 1975.

14. Benumof JL: Management of the difficult adult airway: With special emphasis on awake tracheal intubation. Anesthesiology 75:1087, 1991.

15. Benyamin RM, Salem MR, Joseph NJ: Sampling errors during use of the Dryden disposable absorber circuit. Can they be corrected? [abstract] Anesthesiology 80:A585, 1994.

16. Berman JA, Burgiuele JJ, Marx GF: The Einstein carbon dioxide detector [letter]. Anesthesiology 60:613, 1984.

17. Birmingham PK, Cheney FW, Ward RJ: Esophageal intubation: A review of detection techniques. Anesth Analg 65:886, 1986.

18. Bosman YK, Foster PA: Endotracheal intubation and head posture in infants. S Afr Med J 52:71, 1977.

19. Bozeman WP, Hexter D, Liang HK, et al: Esophageal detector device versus detection of end-tidal carbon dioxide level in emergency intubation. Ann Emerg Med 27:595, 1996.

20. Brodsky JB, Shulman MS, Swan M, et al: Pulse oximetry during one-lung ventilation. Anesthesiology 63:212, 1985.

21. Caplan RA, Posner KL, Ward RJ, et al: Adverse respiratory events in anesthesia: A closed claims analysis. Anesthesiology 72:828, 1990.

22. Charters P, Wilkinson K: Confirmation of tracheal tube placement [reply]. Anaesthesia 43:72, 1988.

23. Cheney FW: The American Society of Anesthesiologists Closed Claims Project: What have we learned, how has it affected practice, and how will it affect practice in the future? Anesthesiology 91:552, 1999.

24. Conrardy PA, Goodman LR, Lainge F, et al: Alteration of endotracheal tube position: Flexion and extension of the neck. Crit Care Med 4:7, 1976.

25. Cook RT, Maglia BA: The Beck air flow monitor as an aid for evaluation of endotracheal tube placement in neonatal patients. J Pediatr 128:568, 1996.

26. Cristoloveanu C, Salem MR, Joseph NJ: Does positioning the upper end of the tracheal tube cuff 2 cm below the vocal cords assure proper tracheal tube positioning? [abstract] Anesthesiology 99:A1239, 2003.

27. Debo RF, Colonna D, Dewerd G, et al: Cricoarytenoid subluxation: Complication of blind intubation with a lighted stylet. Ear Nose Throat J 68:517, 1989.

28. Deluty S, Turndorf H: The failure of capnography to properly assess endotracheal tube location. Anesthesiology 78:783, 1993.

29. Denman WT, Hayes M, Higgins D, et al: The Fenem CO_2 detector device: An apparatus to prevent unnoticed oesophageal intubation. Anaesthesia 45:465, 1990.

30. Donahue PL: The oesophageal detector device. An assessment of accuracy and ease of use by paramedics. Anaesthesia 49:863, 1994.

31. Duberman SM, Bendixen HH: Concepts of fail-safe in anesthesia practice. Int Anesthesiol Clin 22:149, 1984.

32. Dunn SM, Mushlin PS, Lind LJ, et al: Tracheal intubation is not invariably confirmed by capnography. Anesthesiology 73:1285, 1990.

33. Ehrenwerth J, Nagle S, Nirsch N, et al: Is cuff palpation a useful tool for determining endotracheal tube position? [abstract] Anesthesiology 65:A137, 1986.

34. Ellis DG, Jakymec A, Kaplan RM, et al: Guided orotracheal intubation in the operating room using a lighted stylet: A comparison with direct laryngoscopic technique. Anesthesiology 64:823, 1986.

35. Falk JL, Rackow EC, Weil MH: End-tidal carbon dioxide concentration during cardiopulmonary resuscitation. N Engl J Med 318:607, 1988.

36. Ford RWJ: Confirming tracheal intubation: A simple manoeuvre. Can Anaesth Soc J 30:191, 1983.

37. Forgacs P: The functional basis of pulmonary sounds. Chest 73:399, 1978.

38. Foutch RG, Magelssen MD, MacMillan JG: The esophageal detector device: A rapid and accurate method for assessing tracheal versus esophageal intubation in a porcine model. Ann Emerg Med 21:43, 1992.

39. Fox DJ, Castro T Jr, Rastrelli AJ: Comparison of intubation techniques in the awake patient: The Flexi-lum surgical light (lightwand) versus blind nasal approach. Anesthesiology 66:69, 1987.

40. Gannon K: Mortality associated with anaesthesia: A case review study. Anaesthesia 46:962, 1991.

41. Garnett AR, Ornato JP, Gonzalez ER, et al: End-tidal carbon dioxide monitoring during cardiopulmonary resuscitation. JAMA 257:512, 1987.

42. Gedeon A, Krill P, Mebius C: A new colorimetric breath indicator (Colobri): A comparison of the performance of two carbon dioxide indicators. Anaesthesia 49:798, 1994.

43. Gilbert D, Benumof JL: Biphasic carbon dioxide elimination waveform with right mainstem bronchial intubation. Anesth Analg 69:829, 1989.

44. Gillespie JH, Knight RG, Middaugh RE, et al: Efficacy of endotracheal tube cuff palpation and humidity in distinguishing endotracheal from esophageal intubation [abstract]. Anesthesiology 69:A265, 1988.

45. Goldberg JS, Rawle PP, Zehnder IL, et al: Colorimetric end-tidal carbon dioxide monitoring for tracheal intubation. Anesth Analg 70:191, 1990.

46. Gravenstein N: Capnometry in infants should not be done at lower sampling flow rates [letter]. J Clin Monit 5:63, 1989.

47. Green RA, Taylor TH: An analysis of anesthesia medical liability claims in the United Kingdom, 1977-1982. Int Anesthesiol Clin 22:73, 1984.

48. Guggenberger H, Lenz G, Federle R: Early detection of inadvertent oesophageal intubation: Pulse oximetry vs. capnography. Acta Anaesthesiol Scand 33:112, 1989.

49. Haridas RP, Chesshire NJ, Rocke DA: An evaluation of the SCOTI device. Anaesthesia 52:453, 1997.

50. Haynes SR, Morten NS: Use of the oesophageal detector device in children under one year of age. Anaesthesia 45:1067, 1991.

51. Heinonen J, Takki S, Tammisto T: Effect of the Trendelenburg tilt and other procedures on the position of endotracheal tubes. Lancet 26:850, 1969.

52. Heiselman D, Polacek DJ, Snyder JV, et al: Detection of esophageal intubation in patients with intrathoracic stomach. Crit Care Med 13:1069, 1985.

53. Heller MB, Yealy DM, Seaberg DC, et al: End-tidal CO_2 detection. Ann Emerg Med 18:12, 1989.

54. Holland R, Webb RK, Runciman WB: Oesophageal intubation: An analysis of 2000 incident reports. Anaesth Intensive Care 21:608, 1993.

55. Howells TH: A hazard of pre-oxygenation [letter]. Anaesthesia 40:86, 1985.

56. Howells TH, Riethmuller RJ: Signs of endotracheal intubation. Anaesthesia 35:984, 1980.

57. Isserles SA, Breen PH: Can changes in end-tidal P_{CO_2} measure changes in cardiac output? Anesth Analg 73:808, 1991.

58. Jones BR, Dorsey MJ: Sensitivity of a disposable end-tidal carbon dioxide detector. J Clin Monit 7:268, 1991.

59. Kalenda Z: The capnogram as a guide to the efficacy of cardiac massage. Resuscitation 6:259, 1978.

60. Kalpokas M, Russell WJ: A simple technique for diagnosing oesophageal intubation. Anesth Intensive Care 17:39, 1989.

61. Kasper CL, Deem S: The self-inflating bulb to detect esophageal intubation during emergency airway management. Anesthesiology 88:898, 1998.

62. Keenan RL, Boyan CP: Cardiac arrest due to anesthesia: A study of incidence and causes. JAMA 253:2373, 1985.

63. Kelly JS, Wilhoit RD, Brown RE, et al: Efficacy of the FEF colorimetric end-tidal carbon dioxide detector in children. Anesth Analg 75:45, 1992.

64. Kern KB, Sanders AB, Voorhees WD, et al: Changes in expired end-tidal carbon dioxide during cardiopulmonary resuscitation in dogs: A prognostic guide for resuscitation. J Am Coll Cardiol 13:1184, 1989.

65. Lang DJ, Wafai Y, Salem MR, et al: Efficacy of the self-inflating bulb in confirming tracheal intubation in the morbidly obese. Anesthesiology 85:246, 1996.

66. Linko K, Paloheimo M, Tammisto T: Capnography for detection of accidental oesophageal intubation. Acta Anaesthesiol Scand 27:199, 1983.

67. Lockey DJ, Woodward W: SCOTI vs. Wee. An assessment of two oesophageal intubation detection devices. Anaesthesia 52:242, 1997.

68. MacLeod GJ, Heller MB, Gerard J, et al: Verification of endotracheal tube placement with colorimetric end-tidal CO_2 detection. Ann Emerg Med 20:267, 1991.

69. Maleck WH: Distinguishing endotracheal and esophageal intubation. Anesthesiology 94:539, 2001.

70. Mandel GA: Neonatal intensive care radiology. In Goodman L, Putman CE (eds): Intensive Care Radiology: Imaging of the Critically Ill. Philadelphia, WB Saunders, 1983, p 290.

71. Mansfield JP, Lyle RP, Voorhees WD, Wodicka GR: An acoustical guidance and position monitoring system for endotracheal tubes. IEEE Trans Biomed Eng 40:1330, 1993.

72. Markovitz BP, Silverberg M, Godinez RI: Unusual cause of an absent capnogram. Anesthesiology 71:992, 1989.

73. May WS, Heavner JE, McWhorter D, et al: Capnography in the Operating Room: An Introductory Directory. New York, Raven Press, 1985.

74. McShane AJ, Martin JL: Preoxygenation and pulse oximetry may delay detection of esophageal intubation. J Natl Med Assoc 79:987, 1987.

75. Mecca RS: Management of the difficult airway. In Kirby RR, Gravenstein N (eds): Clinical Anesthesia Practice. 2nd ed. Philadelphia, WB Saunders, 2002, p 921.

76. Mehta S: Transtracheal illumination for optimal tracheal tube placement: A clinical study. Anaesthesia 44:970, 1989.

77. Moorthy SS, Dierdorf SF: An unusual difficulty in fiberoptic intubation [letter]. Anesthesiology 63:229, 1985.

78. Morgan M: The confidential enquiry into maternal deaths in England and Wales [editorial]. Anaesthesia 41:698, 1986.

79. Morray JP, Geiduschek JM, Caplan RA, et al: A comparison of pediatric and adult anesthesia closed malpractice claims. Anesthesiology 78:461, 1993.

80. Munro TN: Oesophageal misplacement of a tracheal tube [letter]. Anaesthesia 40:919, 1985.

81. Murray D, Ward ME, Sear JW: SCOTI—A new device for identification of tracheal intubation. Anaesthesia 50:1062, 1995.

82. Murray IP, Modell JH: Early detection of endotracheal tube accidents by monitoring carbon dioxide concentration in respiratory gas. Anesthesiology 59:344, 1983.

83. Nandwani N, Caranza R, Lin ES, Raphael JH: Configuration of the SCOTI device with different tracheal tubes. Anaesthesia 51:932, 1996.

84. Nichols KP, Zornow MH: A potential complication of fiberoptic intubation. Anesthesiology 70:562, 1989.

85. Nunn JF: Applied Respiratory Physiology. 4th ed. Oxford, Butterworth-Heinemann, 1994.

86. Nunn JF: The oesophageal detector device [letter]. Anaesthesia 43:804, 1988.

87. Oberly D, Stein S, Hess D, et al: An evaluation of the esophageal detector device using a cadaver model. Am J Emerg Med 10:317, 1992.

88. O'Callaghan JP, Williams RT: Confirmation of tracheal tube intubation using a chemical device [abstract]. Can J Anaesth 33:S59, 1988.

89. O'Flaherty D, Adams AP: The end-tidal carbon dioxide detector: Assessment of a new method to distinguish oesophageal from tracheal intubation. Anaesthesia 45:653, 1990.

90. Ogden PN: Endotracheal tube misplacement [letter]. Anaesth Intensive Care 11:273, 1983.

91. O'Leary JJ, Pollard BJ, Ryan MJ: A method of detecting oesophageal intubation or confirming tracheal intubation. Anaesth Intensive Care 16:299, 1988.

92. Ornato JP, Shipley JB, Racht EM, et al: Multicenter study of a portable, hand-size, colorimetric end-tidal carbon dioxide detection device. Ann Emerg Med 21:518-523, 1992.

93. Owen RL, Cheney FW: Use of an apnea monitor to verify endotracheal intubation. Respir Care 30:974, 1985.

94. Owen RL, Cheney F: Endobronchial intubation: A preventable complication. Anesthesiology 67:255, 1987.

95. Peters RM: Monitoring of ventilation in the anesthetized patient. In Gravenstein JS, Newbower RS, Ream AK, et al (eds): Monitoring Surgical Patients in the Operating Room. Springfield, Ill, Charles C Thomas, 1989.

96. Peterson AW, Jacker LM: Death following inadvertent esophageal intubation: A case report. Anesth Analg 52:398, 1973.

97. Pollard BJ, Junius F: Accidental intubation of the oesophagus. Anaesth Intensive Care 8:183, 1980.

98. Raphael DT: Acoustic reflectometry profiles of endotracheal and esophageal intubation. Anesthesiology 92:1293, 2000.

99. Raphael DT, Benbassat M, Arnaudov D, et al: Validation study of two-microphone acoustic reflectometry for determination of breathing tube placement in 200 adult patients. Anesthesiology 97:1371, 2002.

100. Robinson JS: Respiratory recording from the esophagus. Br Med J 26:225, 1974.

101. Rosenblatt WH, Kharatian A: Capnography: Never forget the false positives! [letter] Anesth Analg 73:509, 1991.

102. Roy RC: Esophageal intubation [letter]. Anesth Analg 66:482, 1987.

103. Salem MR: Hypercapnia, hypocapnia, and hypoxemia. Semin Anesthesiol 6:202, 1987.

104. Salem MR, Bennet EJ, Schweiss JF, et al: Cardiac arrest related to anesthesia: Contributing factors in infants and children. JAMA 233:238, 1975.

105. Salem MR, Wafai Y, Baraka A, et al: Use of the self-inflating bulb for detecting esophageal intubation after "esophageal ventilation." Anesth Analg 77:1227, 1993.

106. Salem MR, Wafai Y, Joseph NJ, et al: Efficacy of the self-inflating bulb in detecting esophageal intubation. Does the presence of a nasogastric tube or cuff deflation make a difference? Anesthesiology 80:42, 1994.

107. Salem MR, Wafai Y, Joseph NJ, et al: The esophageal detector device: Ellick's evacuator versus syringe [reply]. Anesthesiology 82:314-316, 1995.

108. Salem MR, Wong AY, Lin YH, et al: Prevention of gastric distension during anesthesia for newborns with tracheoesophageal fistula. Anesthesiology 38:82, 1973.

109. Sanders AB, Atlas M, Ewy GA, et al: Expired P_{CO_2} as an index of coronary perfusion pressure. Am J Emerg Med 3:147, 1985.

110. Schaller RJ, Huff JS, Zahn A: Comparison of a colorimetric end-tidal CO_2 detector and an esophageal aspiration device for verifying endotracheal tube placement in the prehospital setting: A six-month experience. Prehospital Disaster Med 12:57, 1997.

111. Schwartz DE, Lieberman JA, Cohen NJ: Women are at greater risk than men for malpositioning of the endotracheal tube after emergent intubation. Crit Care Med 22:1127, 1994.

112. Schwartz DE, Matthay MA, Cohen NH: Death and other complications of emergency airway management in critically ill adults. Anesthesiology 82:367, 1995.

113. Schwartz KD, Johnson C, Roberts J: A maneuver to facilitate flexible fiberoptic intubation. Anesthesiology 71:470, 1989.

114. Shea SR, MacDonald JR, Gruzinski G: Prehospital endotracheal tube airway or esophageal gastric tube airway: A critical comparison. Ann Emerg Med 14:102, 1985.

115. Shibutani K, Whelan G, Zung N, Ferlazzo P: End-tidal CO_2: A clinical noninvasive cardiac output monitor. Anesth Analg 72:S2251, 1991.

116. Smith GM, Reed JC, Choplin RH: Radiographic detection of esophageal malpositioning of endotracheal tubes. AJR Am J Roentgenol 154:23, 1990.

117. Smith I: Confirmation of correct endotracheal tube placement [letter]. Anesth Analg 72:263, 1991.

118. Smith RH, Volpitto PP: Simple method of determining CO_2 content in alveolar air [letter]. Anesthesiology 20:702, 1959.

119. Stewart RD, LaRosee A, Stoy WA, et al: Use of a lighted stylet to confirm correct endotracheal tube placement. Chest 92:900, 1987.

120. Stewart RD, Paris PM, Winter PM, et al: Field endotracheal intubation by paramedical personnel: Success rates and complications. Chest 85:341, 1984.

121. Stirt JA: Endotracheal tube misplacement. Anaesth Intensive Care 10:274, 1982.

122. Stone DJ, Stirt JA, Kaplan MJ, et al: A complication of lightwand-guided nasotracheal intubation. Anesthesiology 61:780, 1984.

123. Strunin L, Williams T: The FEF end-tidal carbon dioxide detector [letter]. Anesthesiology 71:621, 1989.

124. Sum Ping ST: Esophageal intubation [letter]. Anesth Analg 66:481, 1987.

125. Sum Ping ST, Mehta MP, Anderton JM: A comparative study of methods of detection of esophageal intubation. Anesth Analg 69:627, 1989.

126. Sum Ping ST, Mehta MP, Symreng T: Reliability of capnography in identifying esophageal intubation with carbonated beverage or antacid in the stomach. Anesth Analg 73:333, 1991.

127. Szigeti CL, Baeuerle JJ, Mongan PD: Arytenoid dislocation with lighted stylet intubation: Case report and retrospective review. Anesth Analg 78:185, 1994.

128. Tanigawa K, Takeda T, Goto E, et al: Accuracy and reliability of the self-inflating bulb to verify tracheal intubation in out-of-hospital cardiac arrest. Anesthesiology 93:1432, 2000.

129. Tinker JH, Dull DL, Caplan RA, et al: Role of monitoring devices in prevention of anesthetic mishaps: A closed claims analysis. Anesthesiology 71:541, 1989.

130. Todres ID, deBros F, Dramer SS, et al: Endotracheal tube displacement in the newborn infant. J Pediatr 89:126, 1976.

131. Trevino RP, Bisera J, Weil MH, et al: End-tidal CO_2 as a guide to successful cardiopulmonary resuscitation: A preliminary report. Crit Care Med 13:910, 1985.

132. Trikha A, Singh C, Rewari V, Arora MK: Evaluation of the SCOTI device for confirming blind nasal intubation. Anaesthesia 54:347, 1999.

133. Triner L: A simple maneuver to verify proper positioning of an endotracheal tube [letter]. Anesthesiology 57:548, 1982.

134. Uejima T: Esophageal intubation [letter]. Anesth Analg 66:481, 1987.

135. Utting JE: Pitfalls in anaesthetic practice. Br J Anaesth 59:877, 1987.

136. Utting JE, Gray TC, Shelley FC: Human misadventure in anesthesia. Can Anaesth Soc J 26:472, 1979.

137. Venkateswarlu T, Turner CJ, Carter JD, Morrow DH: The tracheal bronchus: An unusual airway problem. Anesth Analg 55:746:1976.

138. Vredevoe LA, Brechner T, Moy P: Obstruction of anomalous tracheal bronchus with endotracheal intubation. Anesthesiology 55:581, 1981.

139. Wafai Y, Salem MR, Baraka A, et al: Effectiveness of the self-inflating bulb for verification of proper placement of the esophageal tracheal Combitube. Anesth Analg 80:122, 1995.

140. Wafai Y, Salem MR, Czinn EA, et al: The self-inflating bulb in detecting esophageal intubation: Effect of bulb size and technique used [abstract]. Anesthesiology 79:A496, 1993.

141. Wafai Y, Salem MR, Joseph NJ, et al: The self-inflating bulb for confirmation of tracheal intubation: Incidence and demography of false negatives [abstract]. Anesthesiology 81:A1303, 1994.

142. Wallace CT, Cooke JE: A new method of positioning endotracheal tubes [letter]. Anesthesiology 44:272, 1976.

143. Warden JC: Accidental intubation of the oesophagus and preoxygenation [letter]. Anaesth Intensive Care 8:377, 1980.

144. Wee MY: Comments on the oesophageal detector device [letter]. Anaesthesia 44:930, 1989.

145. Wee MYK: The oesophageal detector device: Assessment of a method to distinguish oesophageal from tracheal intubation. Anaesthesia 43:27, 1988.

146. Wee MYK, Walker KY: The oesophageal detector device: An assessment with uncuffed tubes in children. Anaesthesia 46:869, 1991.

147. Whitehouse AC, Klock LE: Evaluation of endotracheal tube position with the fiberoptic intubation laryngoscope [letter]. Chest 68:848, 1975.

148. Williams KN, Nunn JF: The oesophageal detector device: A prospective trial in 100 patients. Anaesthesia 44:984, 1989.

149. Williams RT, Stewart RD: Transillumination of the trachea with a lighted stylette. Anesth Analg 65:542, 1986.

150. Yelderman M, New W: Evaluation of pulse oximetry. Anesthesiology 59:349, 1983.

151. Zaleski L, Abello D, Gold MI: The esophageal detector device. Does it work? Anesthesiology 79:244, 1993.

152. Zbinden S, Schupfer G: Detection of esophageal intubation: The cola complication [letter]. Anaesthesia 44:81, 1989.

153. Zupan J, Martin M, Benumof JL: End-tidal CO_2 excretion waveform and error with gas sampling line leak. Anesth Analg 67:579, 1988.

SECTION V

DIFFICULT AIRWAY SITUATIONS

DIFFICULT AIRWAY ALGORITHM

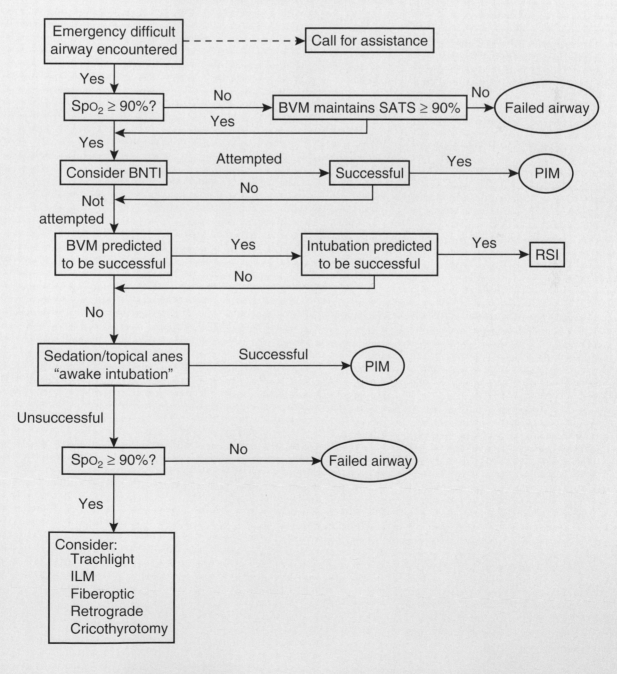

31

PREHOSPITAL AIRWAY MANAGEMENT

Andreas R. Thierbach
Michael F. Murphy

I. INTRODUCTION

Complications related to airway management in the prehospital setting are frequent and, because of the importance and vulnerability of the ventilatory system, can be life threatening within a very short time.[51,73] Therefore, airway management is perhaps the most vital component in the early treatment of any patient in critical condition.[200]

This chapter is intended to give an overview of prehospital airway management in Europe and North America, particularly advanced prehospital airway management (APAM) procedures. For the most part, prehospital advanced airway care is undertaken by physicians in central Europe and nonphysician paramedical personnel in North America, although overlap exists. In much of Europe, particularly Germany, these physicians are often trained as anesthesiologists.[198]

Although the training and credentials of those performing airway evaluation, management, and rescue may vary widely around the world, the *issues* related to prehospital emergency airway management demonstrate consistent themes, such as:

- Should patients be intubated in the field?
- Endotracheal intubation versus alternative (e.g., supraglottic) devices
- The use of neuromuscular blocking drugs in APAM
- What is the standard of care with respect to the verification of intratracheal placement of the endotracheal tube (ET) in prehospital care?

Airway management in an emergency situation is stressful and anxiety provoking. Crucial decisions must be made rapidly and often without the benefit of a detailed history or physical examination. The environment of care is therefore "error prone." Strategies designed to minimize error must do so reproducibly in a time-sensitive fashion. Clear definitions and simple evaluation and management memory tools, including algorithms, taken together represent such strategies. This imperative has led to the development of specialized programs dealing with airway management education, particularly the cognitive and technical aspects of the recognition and management of the "difficult airway" (DA) and the "failed airway," and they have seen rapid growth in emergency medicine and anesthesia. The same is likely to occur in prehospital care.

Identifying the DA, managing the failed airway, and performing a cricothyrotomy are no different in the prehospital arena than they are in hospital. Thus, the thinking and doing in the prehospital environment are identical to those that occur in an emergency department or operating room. However, the *environment of care* is much different in the prehospital arena and often presents unique features. Alternative and innovative methods must at times be employed in these unique situations.

II. THE PREHOSPITAL SITUATION

A. UNIQUE PREHOSPITAL PROBLEMS

In comparison with the in-hospital setting of the emergency department or the operating room, the prehospital setting presents specific problems that may directly influence the outcome of airway management procedures. Table 31-1 shows the unique factors that may directly or indirectly challenge emergency medical service (EMS) personnel in successfully managing the airway on each and every mission.

B. TASKS OF PREHOSPITAL AIRWAY MANAGEMENT

The fundamental priorities of APAM are no different from those in the hospital: the optimization of oxygenation and ventilation and airway protection. Endotracheal intubation still remains the "gold standard" intervention when one fails to meet these imperatives. However, there has been considerable rethinking of endotracheal intubation as the gold standard, particularly in the hands of individuals tasked with first response and resuscitation who infrequently perform this technical task. Nonetheless, it remains the current standard for many prehospital care professionals.

The term advanced prehospital airway management, rather than simply endotracheal intubation, is intended to encompass all levels of personnel, the equipment they might use, and the techniques they might employ in accomplishing advanced airway management in the field.

C. AVAILABILITY OF PERSONNEL AND EQUIPMENT

In an ideal situation, the prehospital airway management team comprises three individuals:

- The airway manager
- An assistant to stabilize the head and neck in trauma patients

Table 31-1 **Unique Problems Related to the Prehospital Environment**

Availability of information (e.g., knowledge of cause and extent of acute medical problem, patient's history, prescriptions)
Availability of personnel
Availability of equipment (limited resources in multiple-patient incidents)
Accessibility of the patient (e.g., entrapped victim)
Specific medical problems (e.g., cervical spine trauma)
Awkward surrounding conditions (e.g., weather, temperature, lighting)

- An assistant to apply cricoid pressure, assist with suctioning, administer medications as needed, assist with selected equipment, and perform the backward, upward, rightward pressure (BURP) maneuver[201]

Equipment for APAM should be stored in mobile packs such as backpacks or shoulder-carried trauma packs, offering a maximum of flexibility to fit the unique needs of patients and be adaptable to changing surroundings and conditions. Essential items of equipment must have paired redundancy.

The specific equipment that ought to be available for APAM depends on a variety of factors, such as:

- The proficiency and level of training of the medical care provider (e.g., emergency medical technician [EMT], paramedic, emergency physician, anesthesiologist)
- The system infrastructure: response configuration (e.g., basic followed by advanced), duration of transport, trip destination policies, trauma system design
- The specific medical or traumatic problem presented by the individual patient

In addition to the tools required to provide preliminary oxygenation of the apneic patient (bag-valve-mask ventilation) and perform endotracheal intubation, at least one supraglottic device (e.g., EasyTube, esophageal-tracheal Combitube [ETC], laryngeal mask airway [LMA]) must be available as an alternative to a surgical airway.

III. THE PREHOSPITAL PATIENT

A. URGENCY OF PREHOSPITAL AIRWAY MANAGEMENT

In contrast to most operating room situations, most airway management procedures in emergency medicine and the prehospital setting have to be performed under substantial time pressure. Table 31-2 categorizes the degree of urgency

Table 31-2 **Time Priorities for Prehospital Airway Management**

1. *Immediate* intervention in apneic patients
2. *Emergency* intervention, for example, in patients having respiratory distress
3. *Urgent* intervention, for example, in patients currently stable but with increased risk for aspiration because of bleeding after maxillofacial trauma or airway swelling related to smoke inhalation and airway burns
4. *Delayed* intervention in all other patients, for example, with a high risk for developing pulmonary problems such as adult respiratory distress syndrome

in performing APAM.[201] These categories reflect the available time to chose the appropriate algorithm, prepare equipment and drugs, and perform the selected APAM technique. Patients in need of immediate intervention ("crash airway") require the least time-consuming technique offering the highest success rate, recognizing that proper preoxygenation of the patient, risk evaluation, and preparation of equipment may not be possible.

B. INDICATIONS FOR PREHOSPITAL AIRWAY MANAGEMENT

The indications for APAM (preferably endotracheal intubation) in an emergency remain[215]:

- Failure to maintain adequate oxygenation
- Failure to maintain adequate ventilation (CO_2 removal)
- Failure to protect the airway (e.g., from aspiration)
- The need for neuromuscular blockade
- The anticipated clinical course

Adequate oxygenation is generally considered to be the maintenance of oxygen saturation in excess of 90% in adults and 92% in children. This may be altered if the baseline saturation of a patient is ordinarily lower. The adequacy of ventilation is usually based on an evaluation of chest excursion and palpable airflow at the nose and mouth, although quantitative carbon dioxide devices and techniques are rapidly invading the prehospital environment. The observed ability to coordinate a swallow is replacing the gag reflex as evidence that the patient can protect the airway. Finally, the need to administer neuromuscular blocking agents to facilitate airway management, establish control of the patient, or institute hyperventilation (among others) is a recognized indication for endotracheal intubation in an emergency.

That the anticipated clinical course may represent an indication for endotracheal intubation is somewhat specific to those who care for emergency airways. Even though there may not be a compelling reason to intubate the trachea *immediately*, one must evaluate the risk of an insidiously progressive condition advancing to the point that intubation becomes more hazardous or physically impossible.[215] The best example in prehospital care often relates to the transport environment, where access to the airway may be severely limited. For example, some rotary aircraft used for air medical transport position the patient so that access to the head and neck, and thus the airway, is compromised.

Once the decision to intubate has been made, and ordinarily this decision is made rapidly by prehospital care providers, one must decide how to proceed. First responders and basic rescuers are typically limited to simple upper airway adjuncts and bag-valve-mask ventilation. Intermediate rescuers may employ supraglottic devices such as the ETC, LMA (American Heart Association, the

International Guidelines 2000 class IIa recommendation[20]) or, more recently, the EasyTube or laryngeal tube to facilitate bag ventilation and provide some element of airway protection. Their decision is typically a simple one: will the victim tolerate insertion of the device or not?

C. RISK EVALUATION

Perhaps most important of all, the emergency personnel must be able to recognize patients in whom airway management may be difficult and be able to formulate and implement alternative plans adapted to various patients and prehospital situations.[200]

Patients who have suffered major trauma or have life-threatening conditions can present the most complex airway management problems, especially in the prehospital setting. Because the treatment is time critical, the evaluation of the airway for difficulty is at risk of being incomplete at the time airway management is undertaken.

Decisions regarding emergency airway management must be made rapidly and the course of action selected be designed to minimize error. The decision matrix is even more complex if neuromuscular blockade is permitted and utilized, as the specter of "taking something away from the patient that the caregiver cannot replace" presents itself.

1. How to Proceed

Figure 31-1[216] represents graphically how this decision-making process ought to proceed.

- Is this a "crash situation" in which the patient is unconscious and near death or at the very least predicted to be unresponsive to direct laryngoscopy? If so, the patient has a crash airway and the crash airway algorithm ought to be used.
- If not, is difficulty anticipated? If so, the patient is *anticipated* to have a DA and the difficult airway algorithm ought to be used.
- If neither of the preceding exists, neuromuscular blocking agents should be employed by qualified personnel in a rapid sequence intubation framework.
- Should any of these fail, that failure must be rapidly identified and managed appropriately and the failed airway algorithm followed.

Thus, each airway situation is associated with a different management approach, or algorithm.

2. Difficult Airway Management (Box 31-1)

Recognizing the crash airway is not difficult, nor is defining the failed airway. Failure is simply defined[138]:

1. Failure to intubate on three attempts *and*
2. Any failure to intubate, no matter the number of attempts, in the presence of oxygen saturations less than 90%.

The same cannot be said of the DA. The definition of "difficulty" has proved elusive. Most authorities have chosen to use surrogates for difficulty, almost always retrospectively applied, such as failure to intubate on three attempts by a skilled operator, more than 10 minutes having elapsed during the attempts, or difficulty experienced in visualizing the glottis during laryngoscopy (Cormack-Lehane grade 3 or 4 view).[46] No clear definition has emerged.

Experts agree that a comprehensive physical examination of the patient's dentition and airway should be performed in every patient before *nonemergency* endotracheal intubation (see Table 31-2, time priorities 3 and 4). Although other authors in this text provide a detailed discussion of the features and conditions that may predict a DA, summary lists useful in APAM are shown in Tables 31-3 and 31-4. Approximately 2% to 3% of patients have anatomic features that cause difficulties during APAM.

Likewise, it is agreed that the use of paralytics and a rapid sequence technique mandates an evaluation of the airway for difficulty. In an emergency, one must possess techniques to assess the patient rapidly for airway management difficulty.

An essential step in the evaluation of a patient for intubation is determining whether the patient has attributes

Figure 31-1 Decision-making process prior to airway management procedures. (From Afilalo M, Guttman A, Stern E, et al: Fiberoptic intubation in the emergency department: A case series. J Emerg Med 11:387-391, 1993.)

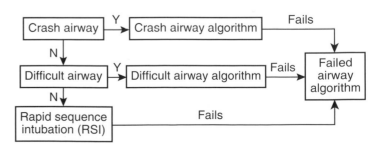

Table 31-3   Findings That Suggest a Difficult Intubation Using Standard Direct Laryngoscopy

Small mouth, inability to open mouth, temporomandibular joint abnormalities
Narrow receding mandible
Protuberant maxilla (overbite)
Large tongue or one whose mobility is limited
Less than 6 cm distance between the tip of the mentum and the thyroid prominence
Inability to place the head in the "sniff position"; for example, cervical spine trauma
Short, full, or bull neck or the presence of a neck mass

Table 31-4   Direct and Indirect Trauma to the Airways

Direct Airway Trauma
Mandibular fractures
Maxillary fractures
Penetrating wounds (e.g., gunshot, stab injury) of the neck or face
Indirect Airway Trauma
Cervical spine trauma
Bleeding into the airway
Subcutaneous emphysema and edema of the soft tissues of the neck or face
Pneumothorax
Burns of neck and upper chest

that would make oral intubation, bag and mask ventilation (BMV), or airway rescue maneuvers difficult to achieve. This evaluation usually includes some assessment of how effective preoxygenation will be in preserving oxygen saturation during the intubation attempt. The effects of various physical and physiologic attributes on time to desaturation to 90% were described by Benumof and colleagues and are depicted in Figure 31-2.[23]

Airway management difficulty has *four dimensions*[139]:

- Difficult bag and mask ventilation
- Difficult laryngoscopy
- Difficult intubation
- Difficult surgical airway management (ordinarily, cricothyrotomy)

These four dimensions can be further reduced to *three operations*:

- Bag and mask ventilation
- Laryngoscopy and intubation
- Cricothyrotomy

Although numerous physical features, measurements, and scores have been identified, none have proved to be failsafe in predicting intubation failure and none have undergone rigorous scientific evaluation in the setting of emergency airway management. Time pressures and the reality of the emergency setting require any airway evaluation for difficulty to be simple and easily remembered; thus, three strategies are required:

- Will bag and mask ventilation be difficult?
- Will laryngoscopy and orotracheal intubation be difficult?
- Will a surgical airway be difficult to create?

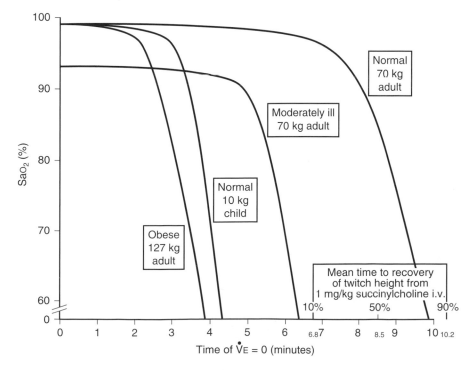

Figure 31-2 Time to hemoglobin desaturation with initial alveolar oxygen fraction (F_{AO_2}) = 0.87 for various circumstances of patients. Note the bars indicating recovery from succinylcholine paralysis on the bottom right. (From Akhtar TM, Street MK: Risk of aspiration with the laryngeal mask. Br J Anaesth 72:447-450, 1994.)

3. Bag and Mask Ventilation

Langeron and colleagues have published their findings with respect to predicting difficulty with bag and mask oxygenation and ventilation[114]:

- The bearded
- The obese (body mass index > 26 kg/m²)
- The edentulous
- The elderly (age older than 55)
- The snorers

Over the years, most experienced airway managers have identified these characteristics of patients as predictive of difficult BMV; however, it is useful to have scientific validation. A useful memory aid for evaluating difficulty of BMV is the mnemonic BONES (Box 31-2), standing for *b*eard, *o*bese, *n*o teeth, *e*lderly, and *s*nores.[139] Another mnemonic, MOANS, can be used (see Chapter 38, Box 38-7).

4. Laryngoscopy and Endotracheal Intubation

It is often possible to identify the patients with whom difficulty performing oral laryngoscopy and intubation will be encountered. Direct laryngoscopy is a key step in the identification process. It is clear that repeated attempts at laryngoscopy may lead to upper airway edema and bleeding, compounding the degree of difficulty. In the words of Benumof, "it is imperative that an optimal *best attempt* at laryngoscopy be made as early as possible, and if that fails *Plan B* should immediately be activated." Table 31-5 lists the features that Benumof would say characterize an optimal intubation attempt.[22] Anesthesiologists from Canada, the United Kingdom, and much of the rest of the world would probably include failure of Eschmann

Table 31-5 **Definition of Optimal Intubation Attempt**

Reasonably experienced endoscopist
No significant muscle tone
Optimal sniff position
Optimal external laryngeal pressure (OELM or BURP)
Change of length of blade once
Change of type of blade once
Intubating stylet (e.g., gum elastic bougie [Eschmann] or Frova) failed

BURP, backward, upward, rightward pressure; OELM, optimal external laryngeal manipulation.

stylet (gum elastic bougie) or Frova-guided intubation in this list, so it has been added to Benumof's six criteria as a seventh. The authors believe that in an emergency the *first* attempt should take all of these factors into account and be the *best* attempt.

Through many iterations, the developers of the Airway Course, an educational initiative focused on emergency airway management (Airway Management Education Center, Wellesley, MA), have developed the LEMON law for identification of the DA (Box 31-3)[138]: *l*ook externally for features of difficulty; *e*valuate the geometry of the airway; perform a *M*allampati examination; look for upper airway *o*bstruction; and assess *n*eck mobility for positioning purposes. Although yet to be scientifically validated, it is a commonsense approach well suited to the prehospital and emergency setting.

a. Look Externally

Most of the time, difficult laryngoscopy and intubation can be identified simply by looking: if it looks difficult, it probably is.

b. Evaluate Geometry of the Airway

Evaluate 3-3-2: Three of the patient's own fingers of mouth opening, three fingers distance from the hyoid bone to the tip of the chin, and two fingers from the hyoid to the thyroid notch. The first 3 assesses access to the airway. The second 3 and the 2 evaluate the geometry of the upper airway, in particular, the adequacy of the mandibular space (where the tongue goes during conventional laryngoscopy) and the location of the larynx in relation to the base of the tongue. Patil described the concept of the thyromental distance in 1983, associating a distance of less than 6 cm with difficult intubation.[150] In the normal adult, the distance from the tip of the chin to the thyroid notch is 6.5 cm and forms the hypotenuse of a triangle. Analyzing the axis (3) and the abscissa (2) of this triangle focuses the intubator on evaluating these important geometric relationships so as not to miss risk factors heralding a difficult laryngoscopy and intubation.

c. Mallampati

Although prospective analyses have failed to validate more than a moderate correlation of Mallampati score with laryngeal view, the examination remains easily and quickly done in an emergency and a good indicator of adequate mouth opening (access).[131] A slightly modified score by Samsoon and Young uses four instead of Mallampati's three grades to define the mouth opening.[167]

The Mallampati score assesses access and the degree to which the oropharynx can be visualized. Another aspect of mandibular mobility, the degree to which the mandible can be jutted ("translated") forward, has been identified as an indicator of potential intubation difficulty (Box 31-4).[107] The upper lip bite test (ULBT) is a rapid and valid assessment of this ability, competing favorably against the modified Mallampati score in predicting difficult endotracheal intubation.

d. Upper Airway Obstruction

Upper airway obstruction demands that only direct vision techniques of airway management be employed lest a blind intrusion into the airway trigger total obstruction. Even indirect verification of tracheal placement techniques such as digital and light-guided intubations is ill advised in the setting of upper airway obstruction. Evaluation of upper airway obstruction should be focused on three questions:

- Where is the obstruction? Lesions above the level of the larynx may be amenable to rescue devices that are positioned supralaryngeally such as the EasyTube, the ETC, the LT, and the LMA. Laryngeal lesions that cannot be bypassed under direct vision from above (e.g., carcinomas, laryngeal edema) require a surgical airway.
- Is the obstruction fixed or pliable? Fixed lesions such as malignancies, foreign bodies, and hematomas usually prevent BMV in the event that total airway obstruction supervenes. On the other hand, inflammatory disorders such as croup, epiglottitis, and angioedema are often amenable to BMV.
- What is the pace of change of the obstruction? The timing of airway intervention in the presence of upper airway obstruction is crucial. Lesions that are static or changing slowly, as is often the case with malignancies and other laryngeal lesions, may not require immediate management. However, the upper airway lesion leading or potentially leading to sudden total airway obstruction, such as an expanding neck hematoma, must be managed immediately. The venue for managing this type of airway may be the field or the emergency department, mandating a complete armamentarium of surgical and nonsurgical airway management rescue devices in the field and the emergency department. Movement of such patients to the operating room or intensive care unit prior to airway management to cater to the comfort of the airway manager is unacceptable.

e. Neck Mobility

The cervical spine is often immobilized in the prehospital environment, precluding optimal airway positioning (see Table 31-5, item 3) and introducing an element of difficulty with respect to laryngoscopy and intubation. This needs to be considered in the total evaluation for difficulty scheme.

5. Creating a Surgical Airway

Surgical airway management is defined as the creation of an airway by surgical techniques. Although this may include a formal or dilatational tracheostomy under local anesthesia, it also includes the urgent creation of an opening to the trachea by formal surgical cricothyrotomy, the use of a cricothyrotome (e.g., Melker, Cook Critical Care, Bloomington, IN), and percutaneous transtracheal ventilation. The latter two techniques are ordinarily considered "rescue" airway techniques and are the predominant surgical techniques utilized in prehospital care.

An examination of the patient for features indicating that a surgical airway may be difficult or impossible is essential as it may eliminate a rescue technique that one has counted on should some other technique fail (e.g., the patient has been paralyzed and now cannot be intubated or ventilated by bag and mask).

Surgical airway management may be considered difficult or even contraindicated in the following circumstances, summarized by the acronym SHORT (Box 31-5):

- Neck *s*urgery in the past on the neck or a disrupted airway
- The presence of a *h*ematoma or neck abscess over the anterior neck; consider whether thrombolytic therapy has been instituted
- A patient who is *o*bese or other situations or conditions in which access to the anterior neck is compromised (e.g., patient in the prone position, fixed flexion deformity of the cervical spine)
- Prior *r*adiation therapy
- *T*umors or preexisting laryngeal or tracheal pathology (e.g., neoplasia in the area of the intended procedure)

D. INTUBATING PATIENTS IN THE FIELD

Inadequate airway management has been identified as a primary contributor to preventable mortality, both in hospital and out of hospital. It would seem intuitive that endotracheal intubation ought to mitigate these deaths, and because of this thinking endotracheal intubation has become the gold standard in APAM.

However, there has been considerable controversy about whether patients demonstrating indications for endotracheal intubation should be intubated in the field or have intubation deferred until hospital arrival. There are several dimensions to this controversy:

Trauma victims: There continues to be skepticism concerning whether intubation of trauma victims improves survival. Through the 1980s it was generally thought that invasive airway management was ineffective in improving survival in urban environments but that it might be effective in longer transport environments.[153] Although many conflicting studies populate the literature through the 1990s,[5,59,65,102,160,164,170] a meta-analysis by Liberman and coworkers published in 2000 (although not specifically investigating the effects of airway management) found that the aggregated data failed to demonstrate a benefit of on-site advanced life support (ALS) procedures in general and supported a "scoop and run" or "load and go" approach.[125] In a multicenter comparison of ALS with basic life support rendered by EMTs, Liberman described similar results but admitted the dependence of the findings on the regional medical infrastructure.[124]

It might be anticipated that endotracheal intubation would clearly benefit patients with acute, severe head injury, but the literature provides no clear direction.[29,74,75,140,144,227]

Solving the controversies, evidenced-based guidelines for emergency endotracheal intubation immediately after traumatic injury[58] state in a *level I recommendation* that endotracheal intubation is needed in trauma patients with the following traits:

- Airway obstruction
- Hypoventilation
- Severe hypoxemia (despite supplemental oxygen)
- Severe cognitive impairment (Glasgow Coma Scale score 8)
- Cardiac arrest
- Severe hemorrhagic shock
- Smoke inhalation with specific conditions (traits mentioned previously, 40% burns, prolonged transport time, and impending airway obstruction).

In nontrauma patients, the issue of efficacy has also been discussed extensively.[4,27,60,135,155,156]

Children: The intubation of children in emergency situations is usually even more anxiety provoking than that of adults. Early studies suggested that the intubation of children by paramedics was associated with higher failure and complication rates than in adults.[11] Some subsequent studies have challenged these early findings,[39,212] although most have tended to support them.[30,77,190] Most studies and authorities maintain that the results of the latter studies may reflect a lack of sufficient training in pediatric intubation. Furthermore, the literature does not resolve whether the prehospital intubation of head-injured children improves their outcome.[45,191]

Undoubtedly, the question whether or not to perform APAM including intubating the patient's trachea in the field depends on several factors, such as:

- The proficiency and experience of the medical care provider (e.g., EMT, paramedic, emergency physician, anesthesiologist)
- The immediate availability of required personnel and airway equipment
- The medical infrastructure (e.g., access to qualified hospitals, means and duration of patient's transport, availability of emergency departments)
- The patient's specific injury or medical problem
- Other factors (e.g., threats to the EMS team on scene, mass casualty incidents without sufficient resources)

Comparative, prospective studies are needed to resolve the controversy.

IV. PREHOSPITAL AIRWAY TECHNIQUES

Airway management involves more than just proficiency with endotracheal intubation techniques. With an ever increasing number of devices and techniques available, the method chosen is that which best matches the needs of the patient, depending on the availability of equipment, the level of training and expertise, and the patient's specific injury or disease (see Table 31-1).

Standard monitoring of emergency patients presenting with airway problems includes pulse oximetry, noninvasive automated blood pressure monitoring, electrocardiography, and, in ventilated patients, capnography.

Generally, BMV is employed to ensure immediate oxygenation, although supraglottic devices may be used in specific situations. Although standard laryngoscope blades are the norm, modifications of such blades (e.g., Henderson, McCoy), and flexible or rigid fiberoptic intubation techniques (e.g., Bonfils) may offer alternatives to the expert, even in the prehospital environment. Needle or surgical cricothyrotomy is rarely required, but they remain crucial techniques in the event that other techniques fail.[200]

A. MONITORING THE PREHOSPITAL PATIENT

In addition to the comprehensive clinical evaluation of the patient, standard monitoring should be employed including pulse oximetry, noninvasive automated blood pressure monitoring, and electrocardiography.

Ordinarily, a decrease in oxygen saturation, especially in preoxygenated patients, becomes manifest within 3 to 5 minutes. It may take even longer in patients who are vasoconstricted or hypovolemic (i.e., many trauma patients) or may occur more rapidly in seriously ill patients. Pulse oximetry is not a reliable method of verifying the proper or improper placement of ETs[209] or supraglottic devices, although it does provide a valuable method of identifying trends of oxygen saturation.

Carbon dioxide detection devices should be applied as soon as airway management procedures (e.g., endotracheal intubation, use of supraglottic airways) have been accomplished to prove the presence of exhaled carbon dioxide. Carbon dioxide detection is regarded as the most reliable method to confirm ET placement in emergency conditions in the prehospital setting.[83] Quantitative capnometry and capnography may also be of use in spontaneously breathing patients in the prehospital setting to help quantify severe hypoventilation or hyperventilation.[213]

1. Bag-Mask Ventilation

BMV is used worldwide to administer oxygen and to ventilate apneic patients or patients in severe respiratory distress.[56] Its efficacy is most often related to the operator's skill. Inadequate ventilation related to mask leakage, airway obstruction, and gastric distention is common.[48,145] High pharyngeal pressures are likely to result from ventilation using excessive tidal volumes or rapid inspiratory flow rates, especially in the presence of airway obstruction. Gastric inflation occurs during positive-pressure exhaled air or bag-valve-mask ventilation when inspiratory airway pressure exceeds esophageal opening pressure (approximately 15 to 18 cm H_2O). Furthermore, Bowman and associates demonstrated a rapid and severe decrease in lower esophageal sphincter (LES) tone to less than 5 cm H_2O during prolonged cardiac arrest in an animal model.[31] The decreasing LES pressure and the relatively high pharyngeal pressures both contribute to the high risk of gastric regurgitation and subsequent pulmonary aspiration. Patients ventilated during cardiopulmonary resuscitation (CPR) with BMV alone have a significantly higher incidence of regurgitation (12.4%) compared with patients ventilated with an LMA (3.5%).[189]

Several other disadvantages of BMV during CPR dictate early APAM:

- Thoracic compressions are less efficient because they need to be synchronized with BMV.[189]
- BMV offers no access to the patient's trachea (e.g., endotracheal suctioning and intratracheal administration of drugs cannot be performed).
- Respiratory system compliance decreases significantly during CPR. This may have a significant impact on peak airway pressure and distribution of gas during ventilation of unintubated patients with cardiac arrest.[225]

Distention of the stomach may be minimized during BMV in emergency patients by[84]:

- Application of bimanual cricoid pressure (Sellick's maneuver) by an assistant

- Using slow inspiratory flow rates (each breath given over a 1.0- to 1.5-second inspiratory time)
- Avoiding unnecessary continuous positive airway pressure or positive end-expiratory pressure
- Limiting tidal volume to that producing observable chest expansion
- Relieving airway obstruction.

After endotracheal intubation is accomplished, the stomach should be decompressed by orogastric or nasogastric tube insertion.

B. SUPRAGLOTTIC DEVICES

1. EasyTube

A new airway device, the EasyTube (EzT), was introduced in 2003. The EzT is a sterile, single-use, double-lumen tube with an oropharyngeal proximal cuff and a distal cuff. The device is latex free and available in an adult size (to be used in patients taller than 130 cm [4 feet 3 inches]) and a pediatric size (to be used in patients from 90 [3 feet] to 130 cm [4 feet 3 inches] in height). The device has a locking valve with Luer adapter and color-coded pilot balloon for sealing each of the two cuffs. One of the device's lumens opens at the distal (lower) end; the other lumen opens between the balloons into the pharynx. A 15-mm standard connector is fitted to each lumen for connection to ventilatory equipment.

The distal end of the EzT is designed like a standard ET, including a Murphy eye. The device provides sufficient ventilation whether it is placed into the esophagus or into the trachea. Because of the design of the pharyngeal aperture (Fig. 31-3), the EzT allows the passage of a flexible fiberoptic bronchoscope (FOB), bougies, or suction catheters into the trachea.

The EzT is intended to be used for emergency airway management, difficult intubation, and intubation for general anesthesia. It may be placed using a laryngoscope

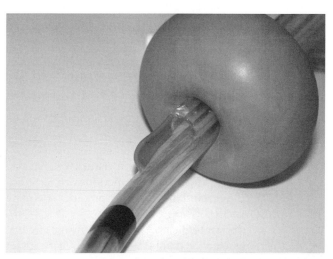

Figure 31-3 EasyTube: design of pharyngeal opening, providing access to the trachea, when tip of tube has been positioned in the esophagus.

or blindly. Using a laryngoscope may ease positioning of the device as well as confirm the position of its tip.

Emergency indications may include conditions such as emergency surgery, CPR, and facial trauma. Difficult intubation indications include "cannot intubate, cannot ventilate" situations, patient with obstructed or DA access, poor visibility during laryngoscopy, and bleeding into the upper airways.

The EzT is contraindicated in patients suffering from complete upper airway obstruction as well as responsive patients with intact gag reflexes. In patients suffering from esophageal diseases or ingestion of caustic substances, the EzT should be inserted only under direct visual control (e.g., by use of a laryngoscope).

2. Esophageal-Tracheal Combitube

The ETC is a single-use, double-lumen tube that may be introduced blindly or with the aid of a laryngoscope into the mouth. It combines the functions of an esophageal obturator airway and a conventional endotracheal airway.[68] It is manufactured in two sizes: Combitube 37 Fr SA (small adult) and Combitube 41 Fr.[70]

The device is designed to ventilate the lungs whether the distal end enters the esophagus or the trachea. The longer channel has an open distal end; the other channel has a blind end with eight small openings corresponding to the supraglottic level when the device is correctly positioned. There are a small-volume distal cuff (esophageal or tracheal) and a large-volume proximal cuff designed to create a seal in the hypopharynx.

The ETC has been used successfully as an artificial airway during cardiorespiratory arrest.[55,66,68,69,79,109,158,173] The device has also been evaluated for use by intensive care unit nurses and paramedics in the prehospital setting.[18,41,53,67,119,123,173,193,228] The ETC is an effective substitute for tracheal intubation in cases in which there is a lack of expertise or familiarity with endotracheal intubation, there is an inability to intubate caused by difficult anatomy, or patients are entrapped in unusual positions. [25,49,93,99,120,181,185,218]

A disadvantage of the ETC, especially for APAM, is that suctioning of the trachea is impossible with the device in its intended esophageal position because of the design of the air outlets, eight small openings above the glottic opening.[113] Endotracheal intubation through this device is not possible.

Complications of the device include lacerations of the pharyngeal and hypopharyngeal soft tissues, esophageal or tracheal perforation (not in conjunction with laryngoscopic positioning), and inability to provide adequate ventilation.[82,98,110-112,208,210]

The ETC is contraindicated in the following circumstances: patients smaller than 4 feet, patients with intact gag reflexes irrespective of their level of consciousness, patients with known esophageal pathology, patients who have ingested caustic substances, and patients with obstruction of the upper airways (e.g., foreign bodies and tumors).

3. Laryngeal Mask Airways

The classical LMA offers a method of establishing an airway in the unconscious patient before personnel trained in APAM techniques have arrived. The LMA is not intended to replace endotracheal intubation by skilled providers or to provide a long-term airway for APAM in emergency patients. It may be used to provide rapid oxygenation and ventilation in patients in whom intubation has failed but BMV is possible. The device does not provide airway protection and may be ineffective in ventilating patients with abnormal resistance or compliance. Originally, the device was designed to serve as a substitute for mask ventilation during anesthesia.

Favorable experience with the LMA has been reported in adults and children. In addition to hundreds of reports of its use in patients having elective surgery, the device has been employed in emergency situations when endotracheal intubation was impossible or not yet available.[53,56,99,132,142,148,161,189,205]

The use of the LMA is not without problems in the emergency setting; difficulties in placement and aspiration have been reported.[12,16,36,127,143] The LMA may, however, be used for a brief period as a bridge to reestablish airway patency and buy time to permit intubation aided by a flexible fiberscope or perform a surgical airway. Its major disadvantage of special importance in emergencies is the fact that it seals the airway only up to ventilation pressures of approximately 20 mbar.[17,37,116]

The intubating LMA (Fastrach or ILMA) device is a modification of the LMA. The tube is bent and fixed at a 90-degree angle by a metal shaft. It may be used like a conventional LMA and inserted with the patient in almost any position or used as a guide path to the glottic opening through which a specially designed silicon-tipped ET may be passed blindly. For APAM, it has been recommended as a rescue device in a variety of situations, such as entrapped patients and difficult direct laryngoscopy.[34,71,100,132,157] Although it has been recommended in patients suffering from cervical spine trauma,[137,149,217] a rigid collar restricting mouth opening prevents endotracheal intubation through the ILMA.[214]

The new ProSeal LMA was designed as a double-lumen LMA that has a modified cuff designed to enhance the seal and a second tube that acts as a drain opening into the upper esophageal sphincter. It offers a higher airway seal pressure, compared with the standard LMA, of well above 30 mbar and may therefore provide better protection against aspiration.[38,62,105]

The ProSeal insertion technique is unique, and its size (as in the LMA Classic and ILMA) needs to be chosen carefully.[108,188] Special techniques and "tricks of the trade" are recommended to evaluate the correct position of the ProSeal in addition to the usual techniques.[9,95,146]

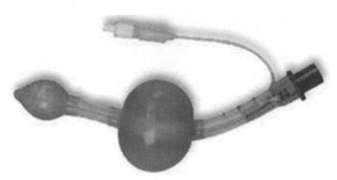

Figure 31-4 Laryngeal tube: multiuse, supralaryngeal device.

Table 31-6 Benefits of Endotracheal Intubation

Best protection against aspiration
Providing a route to administer drugs without intravenous access (e.g., epinephrine, lidocaine, atropine, naloxone)
Facilitated ventilation (assisted or controlled mechanical ventilation, application of positive end-expiratory pressure)
Allows endotracheal suctioning and bronchial toilet

4. Laryngeal Tube and Laryngeal Tube-S

The laryngeal tube (LT) is a relatively new, multiuse, supralaryngeal device for airway management (Fig. 31-4). Its oropharyngeal and esophageal soft silicon cuffs are connected and can be inflated using a single pilot tube. An outlet in front of the vocal cords between these cuffs enables ventilation of the patient. The LT is available in five sizes to fit patients from newborns to large adults.

The LT has been recommended as an emergency device to be used in cases of difficult intubation and cannot intubate, cannot ventilate situations[10,57] while one is preparing to perform a surgical airway.

A potential disadvantage of the LT is the blind ending, which may provoke esophageal rupture in the case of vomiting.[54] Accordingly, the LT was fitted with a second lumen to provide a channel for gastric drainage and suctioning. The laryngeal tube-S (LTS) is a multiple-use, double-lumen modification of the LT. It is available in three sizes to fit patients from small to large adults. A relatively high airway sealing pressure of up to 40 cm H_2O has been reported.[54]

C. TRACHEAL DEVICES AND TECHNIQUES

1. Direct Laryngoscopy

Endotracheal intubation is the most common technique for securing the airway in an emergency situation by suitable trained and experienced individuals. A cuffed ET in the trachea is the most effective conduit to facilitate oxygenation and ventilation in patients with abnormal resistance and compliance and provides the most secure protection against aspiration of foreign material.[21] Securing the airway with an ET and inflated cuff offers several advantages in the management of critically ill patients, such as those listed in Table 31-6. It is indicated in a variety of acute medical conditions as well as trauma. Contraindications to orotracheal intubation are relative (e.g., the intubation attempt may provoke total airway obstruction, orotracheal intubation is judged to be impossible) and precautions are few (e.g., patients with facial, laryngeal, or tracheal injuries).

Nonfixed dental prostheses may facilitate BMV but should always be removed before direct laryngoscopy.

Barring any concerns about cervical spine trauma, in the adult, a pillow or pad is usually placed under the occiput to elevate the patient's head approximately 10 cm and thereby align the oral, pharyngeal, and laryngeal structures (so-called sniffing position). The sniffing position may improve the laryngeal view in cases of difficult direct laryngoscopy. The standard sniffing position has been questioned in an anatomic[2] and a clinical[1] study; therefore, a modified position of the patient with an increased head and neck elevation to improve the laryngeal view is recommended.[171]

Because children have relatively large heads, it is not necessary to use a pillow.

When performing orotracheal intubation in patients with potential injury of the cervical spine, manipulations of the cervical spine must be minimized and an assistant should always apply manual axial in-line stabilization, being careful to maintain the neck in a neutral position. Other adjuncts for immobilization of the cervical spine (e.g., rigid collar or head rolls and tape) must be removed if they limit the mouth opening and therefore threaten to impede direct laryngoscopy. If the patient's cervical spine is stabilized by a rigid two-part collar, the ventral portion should be removed after stabilizing the neck with one hand underneath the dorsal part of the collar. Alternative techniques designed to minimize movement of the cervical spine include supralaryngeal devices such as the ILMA[217] or rigid intubation fiberscopes such as the Bonfils,[52] although their utility in prehospital airway management needs further evaluation.

The duration of attempts to intubate the patient's trachea without interposed BMV should not exceed 30 to 40 seconds.[197]

Many laryngoscope blade modifications have been introduced into clinical practice. Few experts advocate straying from conventional Macintosh and Miller blades and conventional techniques for APAM. Of note, some have advocated a technique called inverse intubation, or the "ice pick" technique, whereby entrapped patients are intubated from the front holding the laryngoscope in the right hand and inserting the tube with the left hand.[85] Blades of alternative design such as the Henderson straight blade[90] and the CLM laryngoscope[133] have been demonstrated to be of benefit in selected patients presenting with a difficult intubation. A modification of the

Macintosh blade, the Dörges blade,[80] combines the advantages of the Macintosh with the straight blade, enabling one to use the same blade in both children and adults. It is narrower and has a lower profile than Macintosh blade size 3 and 4 blades, requiring 30% less mouth opening and facilitating maneuvering of the blade in the mouth.

2. Endotracheal Intubation versus Alternative Devices

The accepted gold standard for definitive airway control, correct tracheal placement of a cuffed ET, is proving to be a double-edged sword when wielded by prehospital care providers of limited skill.[13] Moreover, there is evidence that endotracheal intubation is not a benign intervention in the hands of inexperienced personnel who apply the technique infrequently.[49,142] The trade-offs—ease of placement, airway protection, and effective ventilation and oxygenation—seem to be tilting in favor of abandoning endotracheal intubation in the field, particularly in this latter, inexpert group.

Over the past 20 years and particularly over the past 7 years, airway management during emergency resuscitation has undergone a dramatic transformation, with widespread use of neuromuscular blocking agents, refinement and dissemination of the technique of rapid sequence intubation (RSI), and an increasing focus on predicting and managing the difficult and failed airway, including rescue skills and techniques. Although new, simple airway devices have been introduced and validated,[28,41,50,53,55,78,166,193] studies of traditional endotracheal intubation have raised doubts about the benefit of prehospital intubation, the ability of prehospital providers to intubate the trachea successfully, and the retention of infrequently exercised skills.

Newer devices and techniques that are easy to teach and learn have been shown to provide effective airway management, even when wielded by providers inexperienced in endotracheal intubation. Furthermore, some of the same devices and techniques are effective in managing the difficult and failed airway.[28,41,50] To ascertain the values, advantages, and disadvantages of the new supraglottic devices for APAM (EasyTube, LT-S, ProSeal) and compare them with the established ones[20] (ETC, LMA), further comparative studies are needed.

D. SURGICAL TECHNIQUES

1. Cricothyrotomy

Rarely, surgical cricothyrotomy may be necessary.[203] In the event that endotracheal intubation or the use of a supraglottic device is not possible or contraindicated, the most rapid way to secure an airway is by emergency cricothyrotomy.[64] Common indications for this procedure are foreign body obstruction, facial or laryngotracheal trauma, inhalation thermal or caustic injury of the upper airway, angioedema, upper airway hemorrhage,

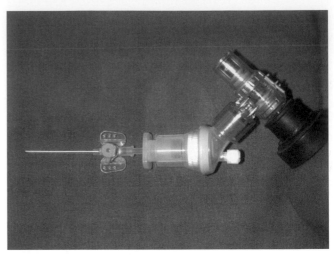

Figure 31-5 Transtracheal ventilation: large-bore venous catheter, fixed to the adapter of an endotracheal tube 3.5.

and epiglottitis. Although cricothyrotomy is an excellent method of securing an airway rapidly, it risks significant blood loss and damage to the cricoid cartilage, thyroid cartilage, and vocal cords.[182]

2. Transtracheal Ventilation

Although fraught with serious complications and less fervently advocated by today's experts, transtracheal ventilation may be a lifesaving measure when neither ventilation by mask nor endotracheal intubation nor cricothyrotomy is possible. This technique is especially valuable for children up to 10 years of age, in whom a sufficient ventilatory volume may be accomplished through small catheters.[180] Necessary equipment comprises a large-bore venous catheter and the adapter of an ET 3.5 (Fig. 31-5). To puncture the trachea, a syringe filled with saline or water is helpful.

It must be remembered that the only way insufflated gases can be expired is through the upper airway. In the case of total upper airway obstruction, percutaneous transtracheal ventilation must be converted to a surgical cricothyrotomy or tracheostomy so that conventional intermittent positive-pressure ventilation can be initiated. The major complications of transtracheal (jet) ventilation are subcutaneous emphysema and barotrauma with resultant pneumothorax.

E. ADVANCED TECHNIQUES

1. Rigid and Semirigid Intubation Fiberscopes

Rigid intubation fiberscopes such as the Bonfils[165] (Fig. 31-6), the Bullard,[44,88,221] the Upsher scope, or the Wu-scope and semirigid devices such as the Shikani Optical Stylet not only improve the view of the larynx, especially in patients with difficult anatomy, but also permit endotracheal intubation with less head and cervical spine movement than is often generated by

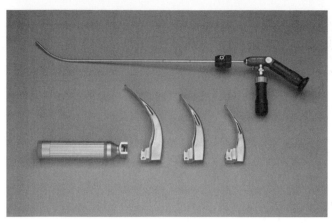

Figure 31-6 Bonfils rigid intubation fiberscope with battery-driven light source.

direct laryngoscopy. However, success in the timely fashion demanded by APAM with these devices requires experience and proficiency. Furthermore, the fragility and expense of the instruments mitigate against more than their occasional use in the prehospital setting.

2. Flexible Fiberoptic Intubation

Although the experienced endoscopist makes the procedure appear simple, flexible fiberoptic intubation (FFI) requires skill and practice, especially in the emergency patient.[8,86,136] A remarkable improvement in terms of versatility for emergency use of FFI techniques is achieved by fiberscopes with a battery-driven light source in the handle.

Flexible FOBs are expensive, fragile instruments, and therefore this technique has been used only occasionally for APAM.[202] Although this technique is one of the cornerstones for the in-hospital management of the DA, its success may be limited in the prehospital setting because of the lack of proper preparation of the patient, presence of secretions and blood that blur the field, and the practical realities of having the necessary equipment immediately available to handle the emergency patient.

Caution must be exercised when administering sedation sufficiently heavy to permit FFI to patients with full stomachs (virtually all emergency patients). Furthermore, producing topical anesthesia sufficiently profound to permit FFI, although perhaps preferable to deep sedation, is virtually impossible in patients with wet upper airways. Thus, the utility of this technique in APAM is severely limited.

F. RAPID SEQUENCE INTUBATION IN PREHOSPITAL CARE

1. Rapid Sequence Intubation

Because emergencies are unplanned, these patients may have eaten or drunk immediately before the event. A delay or even arrest of gastric emptying is caused by the trauma itself, anxiety, and pain as well as alcohol and drug consumption.[127] All patients requiring APAM must be considered to have a full stomach and to be at high risk for vomiting, regurgitation, and aspiration.

Several methodologies are utilized to minimize and prevent an acid aspiration syndrome[128,196] (aspiration pneumonitis or Mendelson's syndrome) in hospitalized patients at risk for acid aspiration: patients are fasted; the intravenous administration of H_2-receptor blockers (cimetidine [400 mg] or ranitidine [100 mg]) 30 to 60 minutes prior to induction reduces the rate of accumulation and increases the pH of gastric secretions; antacids such as sodium citrate (15 to 30 mL orally) shortly before induction increase the pH of existing gastric fluid without producing an excessive increase in volume; and, finally, the endotracheal intubation can be done awake or with an RSI, using induction agents and muscle paralysis.[3,184]

The classical rapid sequence or so-called crash induction technique with muscle paralysis and oral endotracheal intubation is preferred by the authors in emergency situations in which a difficult mask ventilation and intubation is not anticipated (see BONES, LEMON, and SHORT earlier) and adequate preoxygenation or ongoing oxygenation of the patient is feasible. Mask ventilation is avoided if possible because of a theoretical risk of air being forced into the stomach and inducing regurgitation.

Placing the patient in a 40-degree head-up position may be preferable because gravity minimizes the risk of passive regurgitation of gastric contents. Optimally, the patient should breathe 100% oxygen for 3 to 5 minutes, at normal tidal volumes, to denitrogenate the functional residual capacity of the lungs. If time is limited, almost the same degree of preoxygenation can be accomplished with eight vital capacity breaths of 100% oxygen. An induction dose of intravenous anesthetic drugs is then given rapidly, followed immediately by an appropriate dose of a rapid-acting muscle relaxant (succinylcholine or rocuronium).[14,183] After the patient loses consciousness, cricoid pressure (the Sellick maneuver) is applied and maintained until the trachea is intubated and the cuff inflated.

More recently, the so-called modified rapid sequence technique has been increasingly used.[169] The modified RSI technique may be performed in uncooperative patients, patients in shock or with pulmonary contusion and ventilation-perfusion mismatch, and any patient in whom preoxygenation and denitrogenation are difficult or impossible. In this special setting, induction agents and neuromuscular blocking drugs can be given intravenously, followed by unconsciousness and then the application of cricoid pressure. After the onset of apnea from the anesthetic drugs, these patients should be ventilated gently with 100% oxygen until muscle relaxation is adequate. Inflation pressures below 18 cm H_2O and maintenance of cricoid pressure while mask ventilating are essential to minimize the risk of passive regurgitation and consecutive aspiration of gastric contents.

This is a reasonable modification of the rapid sequence induction technique for special groups of patients because

- The use of pulse oximetry and capnography has revealed that a significant percentage of trauma patients treated with the classical RSI approach have unacceptably low oxygen saturation during the induction procedure and
- Properly applied cricoid pressure is very effective in preventing both gastric distention and passive regurgitation during mask ventilation.

2. Cricoid Pressure

Cricoid pressure (Sellick's maneuver) should always be applied after the patient loses consciousness in RSI.[117] By placing the thumb and index finger on the cricoid cartilage and exerting 44 newtons of pressure in an antero-posterior direction, the esophagus is occluded, although this much pressure may also obstruct the airway.[87,92,174,179] Proponents of the bimanual technique have the assistant place one hand behind the patient's neck, flexing it into the sniffing position, while applying conventional cricoid pressure with the other hand. Bimanual cricoid pressure should be the initial technique of choice during rapid sequence induction provided the cervical spine has been cleared. In a minority of cases, switching to a single-handed technique may improve the laryngoscopic view.[229]

Cricoid pressure to prevent regurgitation and aspiration is maintained until proper placement of the ET is confirmed (by visualizing the tube passing through the glottis, noting that the ET cuff has been inflated, auscultating breath sounds, and detecting carbon dioxide). Prematurely releasing the cricoid pressure prior to confirming the correct placement of the tracheal tube is a common error and places the patient at risk for aspiration, particularly if an inadvertent esophageal intubation has occurred. Cricoid pressure must be released immediately should active vomiting occur; otherwise, there is danger of esophageal rupture.[172]

In addition to cricoid pressure, the importance of using a properly functioning suction apparatus for prehospital RSI cannot be overemphasized.

In trauma patients with the potential for cervical spine trauma[47] (e.g., falls, motor vehicle or bicycle accidents), manual axial in-line stabilization should always be combined with bimanual[72] cricoid pressure.

3. Use of Neuromuscular Blocking Drugs

Acting as physician extenders, nonphysician paramedical personnel (e.g., paramedics, nurses, respiratory therapists) have been using advanced airway management skills, including endotracheal intubation, in North America since the early to middle 1970s and in Europe since the late 1980s.[61,76,97,121,152,187,226] The ability of such physician extenders to use the skill reliably and successfully has

been repeatedly supported in the literature, provided they are trained and retrained appropriately.[26,51,81,115,178,204,207,220]

Neuromuscular blockade greatly facilitates orotracheal intubation. On balance, the literature supports the use of neuromuscular blockade by nonanesthesiologist physicians and physician extenders to facilitate endotracheal intubation, provided patients with DAs are recognized and managed appropriately, extensive training in the technique has been provided and the intubator is skilled in a variety of rescue techniques should intubation failure occur.[19,40,42,129,134,162,163,176,177,211,222,223]

Sedative-hypnotic agents used alone as adjuncts to facilitate intubation have also been studied in the prehospital care setting,[159,219] although their limitation when used without neuromuscular blockade has been identified, consistent with findings in the anesthesia literature.[6]

V. CONFIRMATION OF ENDOTRACHEAL INTUBATION

A. NONDEFINITIVE METHODS

1. Physical Examination and Auscultation

Physical examination as well as chest and abdomen auscultation techniques to verify placement of an ET in the trachea, although neither sensitive nor specific, remain important adjuncts to more elaborate techniques, particularly in the patient with cardiopulmonary arrest.

Auscultation of the chest for breath sounds and of the epigastrium for absence of air entry into the stomach and observation of chest motion during ventilation are common but notoriously inaccurate methods of ascertaining proper ET placement.[83,104,192] These tests have very limited value, particularly in obese patients and those with lung disease. The periodic presence of condensed water vapor (coinciding with exhalation) in the ET lumen is not reliable.

B. SEMIDEFINITIVE METHODS

The American Heart Association 2000 guidelines require secondary confirmation of proper tube placement in all patients by exhaled CO_2 or an esophageal detector device immediately after intubation and during transport.[84] CO_2 detection and esophageal detector devices have become the standard of care in APAM to verify correct placement of the ET in the trachea, although both techniques have shortcomings.[24,32,43,63,83,89,91,103,104,106,122,130,147,151,168,192,194,195,206,230]

1. Capnometry and Capnography

Detection of expired carbon dioxide provides reliable evidence of tracheal rather than esophageal intubation.

A single-use device, the colorimetric end-tidal carbon dioxide detector, can be used in the emergency room as well as in the prehospital setting where endotracheal intubations are performed.[168] It is interposed between the ET and the bag to indicate the presence of carbon dioxide in the exhaled gases by a colorimetric change.[15]

As might be expected, carbon dioxide detection techniques tend to be less accurate in identifying correct placement of the ET in patients with circulatory arrest, with reported false-negative rates (carbon dioxide not detected, tube in the trachea) as high as 30% to 35%.[130] In nonarrested patients, carbon dioxide detection is highly reliable, indicating correct placement 99% to 100% of the time.[83,122,147,192]

Soft drinks in the stomach containing carbon dioxide may mimic the exhaled carbon dioxide from the lungs for a couple of breaths, the so-called cola complication,[15] although this confounding result ought not to persist beyond six breaths.

Finally, the migration of an ET from the trachea to the esophagus during the tosses and turns of transport is an ever present hazard. It has been demonstrated that continuous monitoring of exhaled carbon dioxide during the prehospital phase of care minimizes the risk of such displacement going unrecognized.[231]

2. Esophageal Detector Devices

The correct endotracheal placement of the tube can be evaluated by the esophageal detector device or Wee device, which consists of a self-inflating suction bulb or syringe and an attached adapter to fit it to a standard ET connector. The collapsed bulb or syringe rapidly fills with air if the ET is in the trachea; it does not inflate if the tube is in the collapsed esophagus[32,101] with a specificity of about 99%.[228]

Unlike carbon dioxide detection techniques, the esophageal detector device is not dependent on the presence of pulmonary blood flow. Although some prehospital care systems use this device instead of carbon dioxide detection, the rate of failure to detect esophageal intubation as high as 20% suggests that it not be the only verification method used.[91]

C. DEFINITIVE METHODS

1. Direct Laryngoscopy

Visualization of the ET entering the larynx provides a reliable method of verifying correct position of the tube. Furthermore, this technique helps to distinguish between unilateral endobronchial and correct endotracheal intubation by having the black ring mark printed on some ETs used for APAM between the vocal cords.

2. Fiberoptic Bronchoscopy

Although rarely available in the prehospital setting, FOB remains the gold standard of verifying correct ET placement in adults[141] and pediatric patients[118] by permitting the direct visualization of tracheal rings. This technique

can also be applied to verify the position of the ET in the trachea following emergency airway management.[96]

In summary, although carbon dioxide detection remains the most reliable method of verifying tracheal placement of the ET in prehospital care, multiple methods of confirmation are superior to any single method.

VI. PUTTING IT ALL TOGETHER: THE ALGORITHMS

The optimal method of managing the patient in whom laryngoscopy and endotracheal intubation cannot be easily accomplished depends on the cause of the difficulty, whether it is anticipated, the nature and urgency of securing the airway, the patient's condition, and the personnel and equipment available. Having an organized approach to alternative methods of securing the airway provides a basis for determining the type of equipment required and minimizes time lost in emergency situations.

It is fair to say that after years of formal medical education, most of us harbor an aversion to algorithms. Memorized by rote and seldom used, most of the algorithms we have memorized have disappeared from recall. However, there is no question that having a logical and simple approach in a clinical *crisis* is an economical strategy leading rapidly to a series of actions most likely to lead to a positive outcome.[216]

The most important and influential airway management algorithm is the American Society of Anesthesiologists (ASA) difficult airway algorithm, updated in 2003.[154] The ASA, in an attempt to prevent the occurrence of airway management disasters, has produced several iterations of the ASA difficult airway algorithm since 1993. The algorithm guides the preoperative evaluation of the airway, management strategies when difficulty is predicted, and rescue tactics in the event of failure. It emphasizes the importance of airway managers possessing expertise in more than one airway management technique (plan B and plan C). The take-home messages from the ASA difficult airway algorithm are as follows:

- If suspicious of trouble—secure the airway awake
- If you get into trouble—awaken the patient
- Think ahead—have plans B and C immediately available or in place
- Intubation choices—do what you do best

An additional take-home message from the ASA closed claims project and the medical-legal experience accumulating in anesthesia is that if the technique you do best has not and is not working after several attempts (e.g., three), use some other technique.

The ASA algorithm has served to highlight the importance of predicting the DA and managing the failed airway and has probably led to a reduction in adverse events related to airway management disasters in the operating room setting. However, the nonbinary nature of the decision matrices and the multiplicity of pathways have limited the clinical usefulness of the algorithm in guiding day-to-day practice, particularly when faced with an airway management failure (i.e., plans B and C). Most authorities on DA management agree that simplified clinical pathways with binary decision points are required, particularly for guiding decision making during emergency management of the DA and management of the failed airway. Finally, the option of canceling the case or awakening the patient does not exist in prehospital and emergency situations, although it is present in most anesthesia airway management algorithms!

Because the ASA difficult airway algorithm has been developed to suit the necessities of the intrahospital anesthesia patient, it may serve only as a general guideline to develop algorithms designed to meet the requirements of the prehospital patient.

The algorithms presented in this chapter, although consistent with the thinking embedded in the ASA algorithm, are tailored for urgent and emergent clinical situations and adhere to the principles we believe to be fundamental to managing the airway in such clinical scenarios. They are not meant to be memorized and followed slavishly as a recipe. Rather, they represent ways of thinking rapidly through urgent clinical situations, guiding crucial decisions and actions.

Fundamental to a successfully designed algorithm to be used in crisis situations are the following design elements:

- Entry and exit points must be easily recognized.
- It must be based on the best available evidence.
- It must simplify branch points to binary directions.
- Options for actions at each step must be limited.
- It must be easy to remember and represent graphically.

The algorithms for managing the crash situation, the DA, and the failed airway are drawn directly from the Airway Course, mentioned earlier in this chapter. The reader may wish to refer to the figures (Figs. 31-7, 31-8, and 31-9) while reading the text descriptions. The algorithms do not attempt to define the need for intubation and do not deal with the decision to intubate. Therefore, the entry point to the algorithms is immediately after the decision to intubate has been made.

A. THE CRASH AIRWAY ALGORITHM

Entry at this point in the crash airway algorithm (see Fig. 31-7) connotes an unconscious patient unresponsive to direct laryngoscopy with immediate need for endotracheal intubation.

- Attempt oral intubation.

The first step in the crash algorithm is to attempt oral intubation immediately by direct laryngoscopy without pharmacologic assistance.

- Is the oral intubation successful?

CRASH AIRWAY ALGORITHM

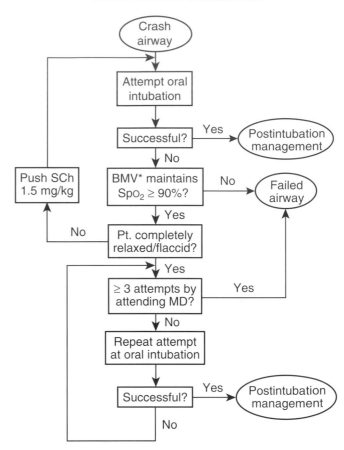

* BMV = bag mask ventilation

Figure 31-7 The crash airway algorithm: unconscious patient, unresponsive to direct laryngoscopy; immediate need for endotracheal intubation. BMV, bag-mask ventilation; SCh, succinylcholine.

If yes, one proceeds to postintubation management. If not, why not? Consider the seven features of an optimal intubation attempt described in Table 31-5.

- Is bag and mask ventilation successful?

In other words, "Do I have time?" If bag ventilation is successful, one has time and further attempts at oral intubation are possible. If bag ventilation is unsuccessful in the context of a failed oral intubation with a crash airway, a *failed airway* is present. One further attempt at intubation may be indicated provided preparations are under way to perform a surgical airway, but no more than one, because intubation has failed and the failure of bag ventilation places the patient in serious and immediate jeopardy. This is a cannot intubate, cannot oxygenate scenario, and in such circumstances, the failed airway algorithm (see Fig. 31-8) mandates surgical airway management. If surgical airway management is not *immediately* possible, temporizing methods such as placement of an LMA, ETC, or LT may be attempted, but such attempts should not delay creation of a surgical airway.

- Failed airway (see Fig. 31-8)

FAILED AIRWAY ALGORITHM

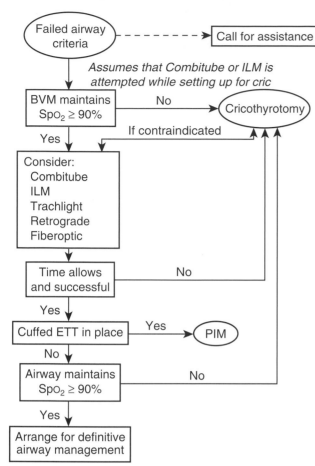

Figure 31-8 The failed airway algorithm. BVM, bag-mask ventilation; ETT, endotracheal tube; SpO_2, oxygen saturation from pulse oximetry; ILM, intubating laryngeal mask; PIM, postintubation management.

This circle leads directly to the failed airway algorithm.

- Is the patient completely relaxed and flaccid?

During the first attempt at orotracheal intubation in the unconscious, unresponsive patient, the patient is assessed for degree of relaxation to permit intubation. If the impression is one of absolute, complete skeletal muscle relaxation, further intubation attempts are indicated. If the patient is felt to be exhibiting any resistance to intubation, a single dose of succinylcholine, 1.5 mg/kg, should be given and oral intubation attempted again.

- Succinylcholine 1.5 mg/kg

Succinylcholine is given to ensure complete relaxation of the patient for intubation. Usually only one dose is indicated. No induction agent is required.

- Have there been three or more attempts at intubation by an experienced clinician?

If the answer to this question is yes, consistent with the preceding definition, the situation represents a failed airway (see Fig. 31-8). If fewer than three attempts have been made by an experienced intubator, repeated attempts at oral intubation are justified. Between intubation attempts, defined by a single laryngoscopy, the patient should receive ventilation and oxygenation by bag and mask as one contemplates why the attempt has failed (see Table 31-5).

- Repeat attempt at oral intubation.

It is appropriate to repeat attempts at oral intubation until three attempts have failed. The failure of three attempts indicates a very low likelihood of ultimate success with oral intubation.

- Successful?

If intubation is achieved, one proceeds to postintubation management; if not, one cycles back to make another attempt or proceed to the failed airway algorithm, depending on the number of attempts that have already been made.

- Postintubation management

This is undertaken in the event of a successful intubation.

B. THE DIFFICULT AIRWAY ALGORITHM

This algorithm (Fig. 31-9), although appearing fairly busy with some 16 boxes and circles, in reality poses a series of simple, straightforward considerations:

- Is the airway difficult?

The clinician must be confident in the wake of a BONES, LEMON, and SHORT analysis that BMV, laryngoscopy, and intubation or cricothyrotomy, or both, are possible following neuromuscular blockade.

- Do I have time?

Are the oxygen saturations reasonable, or can I make them reasonable? If not, it is a failed airway situation, and the failed airway algorithm should be used.

- Is blind nasal intubation reasonable?

This is probably the only place that this once preeminent APAM technique might be considered indicated in this day and age.

- Reconsider the use of neuromuscular blocking agents?

The decision to proceed with a rapid sequence technique utilizing neuromuscular blockade in the patient with a predicted DA must be attended by a high degree of certainty that it will be successful in securing the airway. Alternatively, the clinician must be confident that adequate BMV can be achieved or cricothyrotomy performed rapidly.

- Topical anesthesia, sedation, and awake laryngoscopy?

A variety of techniques are available to obtund the airway, the patient, or both without burning any bridges.

Figure 31-9 The difficult airway algorithm poses a series of simple, straightforward considerations. BNTI, blind nasal intubation; BVM, bag-mask ventilation; ILM, intubating laryngeal mask; PIM, postintubation management; RSI, rapid sequence intubation; SATS, oxygen saturations; SpO₂, oxygen saturation from pulse oximetry.

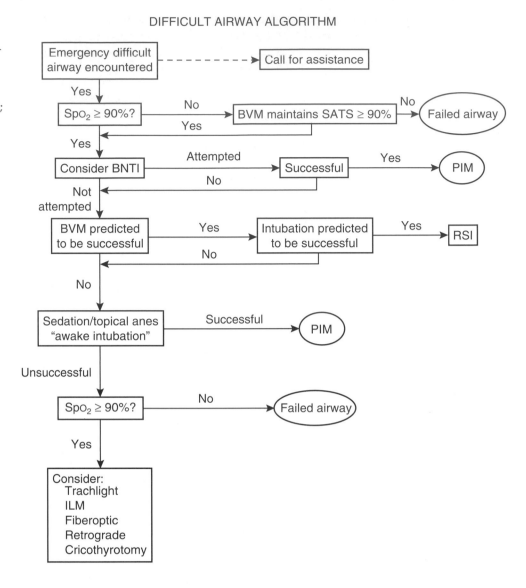

DIFFICULT AIRWAY ALGORITHM

The condition of the patient and the clinical situation dictate the aggressiveness of this maneuver (how much does one need to see?). It may be that the airway manager simply needs to verify that the epiglottis is in the midline to make the decision to back off and move to a rapid sequence technique. At other times, it may progress to an awake intubation.

In the event that none of the preceding techniques are possible and failed criteria have not been met, the box at the bottom of the algorithm suggests a variety of techniques that might be attempted. It should be noted that all of the devices and techniques listed in this box result in the placement of a tube *in* the trachea.

C. THE FAILED AIRWAY ALGORITHM

Failure to intubate is rarely accompanied by failure to ventilate and oxygenate. This situation has variously been termed cannot intubate, cannot ventilate or cannot intubate, cannot oxygenate, the latter being the more precise term. It is a clinical emergency of such magnitude that, if not rectified, it rapidly leads to neurologic compromise and death. Decisive action in selecting a technique most likely to lead to a secure airway (i.e., an emergency surgical airway) is a sine qua non for success in such a situation.

More often, the failure to intubate is associated with some degree of BMV or oxygenation being possible, giving the clinician time to consider alternative techniques. This cannot intubate, can ventilate/oxygenate situation is amenable to nonsurgical rescue techniques such as the ETC, LMA, LT, and light wand, depending on the presumed etiology of the failure. It should be noted that some of the devices recommended in the failed airway situation do not result in the placement of a tube *in* the trachea.

The take-home message from the failed airway algorithm is that the decision to move to a surgical airway must be made early when the failure to maintain oxygenation is recognized. Wasting valuable time attempting a variety of devices or techniques is to be avoided at all costs unless it is while one is *concurrently preparing to perform a surgical airway*.

- Failed airway criteria have been met.

This is the entry point of the failed airway algorithm. The criteria are either three failed attempts at intubation by oral laryngoscopy by an experienced clinician or a single failed attempt at oral intubation with inability to maintain oxygen saturation from pulse oximetry (SpO_2) greater than 90% using a bag and mask. A mandated intubation in a patient with a DA or crash airway in whom BMV fails also represents a failed airway. As with the DA, it is advisable to call for assistance when a failed airway has occurred. This is especially true if BMV has also failed and if there is qualified help *immediately* available, which is usually not the case in the prehospital environment.

- Is BMV possible and adequate?

In the circumstance of a failed airway, if BMV is not adequate, immediate cricothyrotomy is mandatory. Further attempts at intubation or use of alternative devices merely prolongs the patient's hypoxemic state. The only exception to this recommendation is the use of a temporizing technique, such as the LMA, ETC, or LT, when cricothyrotomy is not immediately possible. If surgical airway management is itself contraindicated, alternative methods may be tried first. For example, if the patient has known laryngeal pathology, such as a tumor or hematoma, alternative techniques may be preferred. However, if these methods are not successful, cricothyrotomy should be performed immediately, even in the presence of relative contraindications.

- Consider EasyTube, ETC, LT, LMA.
- If qualified using the specific technique and it is immediately available, consider rigid or flexible fiberoptic method, lighted stylet, or transtracheal jet ventilation.

If ventilation and oxygenation by bag and mask can maintain SpO_2 greater than 90%, a number of different devices and procedures may be attempted to rescue the failed airway. At all times, the patient must be monitored for adequate oxygenation. If oxygenation becomes inadequate at any time and cannot be restored by BMV, cricothyrotomy is mandatory. Likewise, failure to rescue the airway with the alternative devices indicates that cricothyrotomy should be undertaken. Fiberoptic methods may include flexible FOB with intubation, the Bonfils, Bullard, or Wu laryngoscope, or others, although most are seldom available in the prehospital environment.

- Time allows and successful?

If there is sufficient time to achieve oxygenation and ventilation using one of these devices or techniques, one proceeds down the main path of the algorithm. If not, cricothyrotomy is mandated.

- Was an ET placed?

If the technique that was successful resulted in the placement of an ET in the trachea, a definitive airway has been placed and postintubation management may be undertaken. If supralaryngeal devices or percutaneous transtracheal ventilation has been used, the airway should be considered to be temporary, at best.

- Airway as placed adequate to ventilate?

If adequate ventilation and oxygenation are achieved by the airway that has been placed, arrangements must be initiated for definitive airway management. If the airway as placed is inadequate and there is a failure of oxygenation, immediate cricothyrotomy is indicated.

REFERENCES

1. Adnet F, Baillard C, Borron SW, et al: Randomized study comparing the "sniffing position" with simple head extension for laryngoscopic view in elective surgery patients. Anesthesiology 95:836-841, 2001.
2. Adnet F, Borron SW, Dumas JL, et al: Study of the "sniffing position" by magnetic resonance imaging. Anesthesiology 94:83-86, 2001.
3. Adnet F, Borron SW, Lapostolle F: The safety of rapid sequence induction. Anesthesiology 96:517, 2002.
4. Adnet F, Jouriles NJ, Le Toumelin P, et al: Survey of out-of-hospital emergency intubations in the French prehospital medical system: A multicenter study. Ann Emerg Med 32:454-460, 1998.
5. Adnet F, Lapostolle F, Ricard-Hibon A, et al: Intubating trauma patients before reaching hospital—Revisited. Crit Care 5:290-291, 2001.
6. Adnet F, Minadeo JP, Finot MA, et al: A survey of sedation protocols used for emergency endotracheal intubation in poisoned patients in the French prehospital medical system. Eur J Emerg Med 5:415-419, 1998.
7. Adult Basic Life Support: Guidelines 2000 for Cardiopulmonary Resuscitation and Emergency Cardiovascular Care—International Consensus on Science. Circulation (Suppl): I22-I59, 2000.
8. Afilalo M, Guttman A, Stern E, et al: Fiberoptic intubation in the emergency department: A case series. J Emerg Med 11:387-391, 1993.
9. Agro F, Antonelli S, Cataldo R, et al: The ProSeal laryngeal mask airway: Fiberoptic visualization of the glottic opening is associated with ease of insertion of the gastric tube. Can J Anaesth 49:867-870, 2002.
10. Agro F, Cataldo R, Alfano A, et al: A new prototype for airway management in an emergency: The laryngeal tube. Resuscitation 41:284-286, 1999.
11. Aijian P, Tsai A, Knopp R, et al: Endotracheal intubation of pediatric patients by paramedics. Ann Emerg Med 18:489-494, 1989.

12. Akhtar TM, Street MK: Risk of aspiration with the laryngeal mask. Br J Anaesth 72:447-450, 1994.

13. American Heart Association: ACLS Provider Manual. 2002.

14. Andrews JI, Kumar N, van den Brom RH, et al: A large simple randomized trial of rocuronium versus succinylcholine in rapid-sequence induction of anaesthesia along with propofol. Acta Anaesthesiol Scand 43:4-8, 1999.

15. Anton WR, Gordon RW, Jordan TM, et al: A disposable end-tidal CO_2 detector to verify endotracheal intubation. Ann Emerg Med 20:271-275, 1991.

16. Asai T, Barclay K, Power I, et al: Cricoid pressure impedes placement of the laryngeal mask airway and subsequent endotracheal intubation through the mask. Br J Anaesth 72:47-51, 1994.

17. Asai T, Howell TK, Koga K, et al: Appropriate size and inflation of the laryngeal mask airway. Br J Anaesth 80:470-474, 1998.

18. Atherton GL, Johnson JC: Ability of paramedics to use the Combitube in prehospital cardiac arrest. Ann Emerg Med 22:1263-1268, 1993.

19. Austin PN: A literature review of the prehospital use of neuromuscular blocking agents by air medical personnel to facilitate endotracheal intubation. Air Med J 19:90-97, 2000.

20. Barnes TA, MacDonald D, Nolan J, et al: Cardiopulmonary resuscitation and emergency cardiovascular care. Airway devices. Ann Emerg Med 37:145-151, 2001.

21. Baskett PJF, Bossaert L, Carli P, et al: Guidelines for the advanced management of the airway and ventilation during resuscitation. Resuscitation 31:201-230, 1996.

22. Benumof JL: The ASA difficult airway algorithm: New thoughts and considerations. American Society of Anesthesiologists 51st annual refresher course lecture, 2000.

23. Benumof JL, Dagg R, Benumof R: Critical hemoglobin desaturation will occur before return to an unparalyzed state following 1 mg/kg intravenous succinylcholine. Anesthesiology 87:979-982, 1997.

24. Bhende MS, LaCovey DC: End-tidal carbon dioxide monitoring in the prehospital setting. Prehosp Emerg Care 5:208-213, 2001.

25. Bigenzahn W, Pesau B, Frass M: Emergency ventilation using the Combitube in cases of difficult intubation. Eur Arch Otorhinolaryngol 248:129-131, 1991.

26. Bishop MJ, Michalowski P, Hussey JD, et al: Recertification of respiratory therapists' intubation skills one year after initial training: An analysis of skill retention and retraining. Respir Care 46:234-237, 2001.

27. Bissell RA, Eslinger DG, Zimmerman L: The efficacy of advanced life support: A review of the literature. Prehospital Disaster Med 13:77-87, 1998.

28. Blostein PA, Koestner AJ, Hoak S: Failed rapid sequence intubation in trauma patients: Esophageal tracheal Combitube is a useful adjunct. J Trauma 44:534-537, 1988.

29. Bochicchio GV, Ilahi O, Joshi M, et al: Endotracheal intubation in the field does not improve outcome in trauma patients who present without an acutely lethal traumatic brain injury. J Trauma 54:307-311, 2003.

30. Boswell WC, McElveen N, Sharp M, et al: Analysis of prehospital pediatric and adult intubation. Air Med J 14:125-127, 1995.

31. Bowman FP, Menegazzi JJ, Check BD, et al: Lower esophageal sphincter pressure during prolonged cardiac arrest and resuscitation. Ann Emerg Med 26:216-219, 1995.

32. Bozeman WP, Hexter D, Liang HK, et al: Esophageal detector device versus detection of end-tidal carbon dioxide level in emergency intubation. Ann Emerg Med 27:595-599, 1996.

33. Brain A: A new concept: The Proseal LMA. 2001.

34. Brain AI, Verghese C, Addy EV, et al: The intubating laryngeal mask. II: A preliminary clinical report of a new means of intubating the trachea. Br J Anaesth 79:704-709, 1997.

35. Brain AI, Verghese C, Strube PJ: The LMA 'ProSeal'—A laryngeal mask with an oesophageal vent. Br J Anaesth 84:650-654, 2000.

36. Brimacombe JR, Berry A: The incidence of aspiration associated with the laryngeal mask airway: A meta-analysis of published literature. J Clin Anesth 7:297-305, 1995.

37. Brimacombe J, Keller C: The cuffed oropharyngeal airway vs. the laryngeal mask airway: A randomised cross-over study of oropharyngeal leak pressure and fibreoptic view in paralysed patients. Anaesthesia 54:683-685, 1999.

38. Brimacombe J, Keller C, Brimacombe L: A comparison of the laryngeal mask airway ProSeal and the laryngeal tube airway in paralyzed anesthetized adult patients undergoing pressure-controlled ventilation. Anesth Analg 95:770-776, 2002.

39. Brownstein D, Shugerman R, Cummings P, et al: Prehospital endotracheal intubation of children by paramedics. Ann Emerg Med 28:34-39, 1996.

40. Bulger EM, Copass MK, Maier RV, et al: An analysis of advanced prehospital airway management. J Emerg Med 23:183-189, 2002.

41. Calkins MD, Robinson TD: Combat trauma airway management: Endotracheal intubation versus laryngeal mask airway versus combitube use by Navy SEAL and Reconnaissance combat corpsmen. J Trauma 46:927-932, 1999.

42. Cantineau JP, Tazarourte K, Merckx P, et al: [Tracheal intubation in prehospital resuscitation: Importance of rapid-sequence induction anesthesia]. Ann Fr Anesth Reanim 16:878-884, 1997.

43. Cardoso MM, Banner MJ, Melker RJ, et al: Portable devices used to detect endotracheal intubation during emergency situations: A review. Crit Care Med 26:957-964, 1998.

44. Cohn AI, Hart RT, McGraw SR, et al: The Bullard laryngoscope for emergency airway management in a morbidly obese parturient. Anesth Analg 81:872-873, 1995.

45. Cooper A, DiScala C, Foltin G, et al: Prehospital endotracheal intubation for severe head injury in children: A reappraisal. Semin Pediatr Surg 10:3-6, 2001.

46. Cormack RS, Lehane J: Difficult endotracheal intubation in obstetrics. Anaesthesia 39:1105-1111, 1984.

47. Criswell JC, Parr MJ, Nolan JP: Emergency airway management in patients with cervical spine injuries. Anaesthesia 49:900-903, 1994.

48. Cummins RO, Austin D, Graves JR, et al: Ventilation skills of emergency medical technicians: A teaching challenge for emergency medicine. Ann Emerg Med 15:1187-1192, 1986.

49. Deakin CD: Prehospital management of the traumatized airway. Eur J Emerg Med 3:233-243, 1996.

50. Della PA, Pittoni G, Frass M: Tracheal esophageal combitube: A useful airway for morbidly obese patients who cannot intubate or ventilate. Acta Anaesthesiol Scand 46:911-913, 2002.

51. Doran JV, Tortella BJ, Drivet WJ, et al: Factors influencing successful intubation in the prehospital setting. Prehosp Disaster Med 10:259-264, 1995.

52. Dörges V, Gerlach K: Endotracheal intubation using the Bonfils fibrescope and the intubating laryngeal mask airway—A comparison in a model of cervical spine injury. Eur J Anaesthesiol 20:170, 2003.

53. Dörges V, Ocker H, Wenzel V, et al: Emergency airway management by non-anaesthesia house officers—A comparison of three strategies. Emerg Med J 18:90-94, 2001.

54. Dörges V, Ocker H, Wenzel V, et al: The Laryngeal Tube S: A modified simple airway device. Anesth Analg 96:618-621, table, 2003.

55. Dörges V, Sauer C, Ocker H, et al: Airway management during cardiopulmonary resuscitation—A comparative study of bag-valve-mask, laryngeal mask airway and combitube in a bench model. Resuscitation 41:63-69, 1999.

56. Dörges V, Wenzel V, Knacke P, et al: Comparison of different airway management strategies to ventilate apneic, nonpreoxygenated patients. Crit Care Med 31:800-804, 2003.

57. Dörges V, Wenzel V, Neubert E, et al: Emergency airway management by intensive care unit nurses with the intubating laryngeal mask airway and the laryngeal tube. Crit Care 4:369-376, 2000.

58. Dunham CM, Barraco RD, Clark DE, et al: Guidelines for emergency endotracheal intubation immediately after traumatic injury. J Trauma 55:162-179, 2003.

59. Eckstein M, Chan L, Schneir A, et al: Effect of prehospital advanced life support on outcomes of major trauma patients. J Trauma 48:643-648, 2000.

60. Eisen JS, Dubinsky I: Advanced life support vs basic life support field care: An outcome study. Acad Emerg Med 5:592-598, 1998.

61. Eisenberg MS, Bergner L, Hallstrom A: Out-of-hospital cardiac arrest: Improved survival with paramedic services. Lancet 1:812-815, 1980.

62. Evans NR, Gardner SV, James MF: ProSeal laryngeal mask protects against aspiration of fluid in the pharynx. Br J Anaesth 88:584-587, 2002.

63. Falk JL, Sayre MR: Confirmation of airway placement. Prehosp Emerg Care 3:273-278, 1999.

64. Fortune JB, Judkins DG, Scanzaroli D, et al: Efficacy of prehospital surgical cricothyrotomy in trauma patients. J Trauma 42:832-836, 1997.

65. Frankel H, Rozycki G, Champion H, et al: The use of TRISS methodology to validate prehospital intubation by urban EMS providers. Am J Emerg Med 15:630-632, 1997.

66. Frass M: Use of the Combitube in resuscitation and trauma. Trauma Care 9:24-26, 1999.

67. Frass M, Frenzer R, Mayer G, et al: Mechanical ventilation with the esophageal tracheal Combitube (ETC) in the intensive care unit. Arch Emerg Med 4:219-225, 1987.

68. Frass M, Frenzer R, Rauscha F, et al: Evaluation of the esophageal tracheal combitube in cardiopulmonary resuscitation. Crit Care Med 15:609-611, 1986.

69. Frass M, Frenzer R, Rauscha F, et al: Ventilation with the esophageal tracheal Combitube in cardiopulmonary resuscitation. Chest 93:781-784, 1988.

70. Frass M, Frenzer R, Zdrahal F, et al: The esophageal tracheal combitube: Preliminary results with a new airway for CPR. Ann Emerg Med 16:768-772, 1987.

71. Fukutome T, Amaha K, Nakazawa K, et al: Tracheal intubation through the intubating laryngeal mask airway (LMA-Fastrach) in patients with difficult airways. Anaesth Intensive Care 26:387-391, 1998.

72. Gabbott DA: The effect of single-handed cricoid pressure on neck movement after applying manual in-line stabilisation. Anaesthesia 52:586-588, 1997.

73. Gabram SG, Jacobs LM, Schwartz RJ, et al: Airway intubation in injured patients at the scene of an accident. Conn Med 53:633-637, 1989.

74. Garner A, Crooks J, Lee A, et al: Efficacy of prehospital critical care teams for severe blunt head injury in the Australian setting. Injury 32:455-460, 2001.

75. Garner A, Rashford S, Lee A, et al: Addition of physicians to paramedic helicopter services decreases blunt trauma mortality. Aust N Z J Surg 69:697-701, 1999.

76. Gatrell CB: The prehospital airway. J Emerg Med 2:301-302, 1985.

77. Gausche M, Lewis RJ, Stratton SJ, et al: Effect of out-of-hospital pediatric endotracheal intubation on survival and neurological outcome: A controlled clinical trial. JAMA 283:783-790, 2000.

78. Genzwuerker HV, Dhonau S, Ellinger K: Use of the laryngeal tube for out-of-hospital resuscitation. Resuscitation 52:221-224, 2002.

79. Genzwuerker HV, Finteis T, Krieter H, et al: Supraglottic airway devices with oesophageal access: Comparison of Combitube, LMA-Proseal and LTS in a resuscitation model. Eur J Anaesthesiol 20:171, 2003.

80. Gerlach K, Wenzel V, von Knobelsdorff G, et al: A new universal laryngoscope blade: A preliminary comparison with Macintosh laryngoscope blades. Resuscitation 57:63-67, 2003.

81. Gray AJ, Cartlidge D, Gavalas MC: Can ambulance personnel intubate? Arch Emerg Med 9:347-351, 1992.

82. Green KS, Beger TH: Proper use of the Combitube. Anesthesiology 81:513, 1994.

83. Grmec S: Comparison of three different methods to confirm tracheal tube placement in emergency intubation. Intensive Care Med 28:701-704, 2002.

84. Guidelines 2000 for cardiopulmonary resuscitation and emergency cardiovascular care: Adjuncts for oxygenation, ventilation and airway control. Circulation 102:I-95-I-104, 2000.

85. Gürtner I, Kanz KG, Lackner C, et al: [Inverse intubation in multiple traumatized patients: Indication, technique, experiences]. Intensivmed 30:426-427, 1993.

86. Hamilton PH, Kang JJ: Emergency airway management. Mt Sinai J Med 64:292-301, 1997.

87. Hartsilver EL, Vanner RG: Airway obstruction with cricoid pressure. Anaesthesia 55:208-211, 2000.

88. Hastings RH, Vigil AC, Hanna R, et al: Cervical spine movement during laryngoscopy with the Bullard, Macintosh, and Miller laryngoscopes. Anesthesiology 82:859-869, 1995.

89. Hayden SR, Sciammarella J, Viccellio P, et al: Colorimetric end-tidal CO_2 detector for verification of ET placement in out-of-hospital cardiac arrest. Acad Emerg Med 2:499-502, 1995.

90. Henderson JJ: The use of paraglossal straight blade laryngoscopy in difficult tracheal intubation. Anaesthesia 52:552-560, 1997.

91. Hendey GW, Shubert GS, Shalit M, et al: The esophageal detector bulb in the aeromedical setting. J Emerg Med 23:51-55, 2002.

92. Ho AM, Wong W, Ling E, et al: Airway difficulties caused by improperly applied cricoid pressure. J Emerg Med 20:29-31, 2001.

93. Hofbauer R, Roggla M, Staudinger T, et al: [Emergency intubation with the Combitube in a patient with persistent vomiting]. Anasthesiol Intensivmed Notfallmed Schmerzther 29:306-308, 1994.

94. Benumof JL: Definition and incidence of the difficult airway. In Benumof JL (ed): Airway Management—Principles and Practice. St. Louis, Mosby-Year Book, 1996, pp 121-125.

95. Howath A, Brimacombe J, Keller C: Gum-elastic bougie-guided insertion of the ProSeal laryngeal mask airway: A new technique. Anaesth Intensive Care 30:624-627, 2002.

96. Hutton KC, Verdile VP, Yealy DM, et al: Prehospital and emergency department verification of endotracheal tube position using a portable, non-directable, fiber-optic bronchoscope. Prehospital Disaster Med 5:131-136, 1990.

97. Jacobs LM, Berrizbeitia LD, Bennett B, et al: Endotracheal intubation in the prehospital phase of emergency medical care. JAMA 250:2175-2177, 1983.

98. Jaehnichen G, Golecki N, Lipp MD: A case report of difficult ventilation with the Combitube—Valve-like upper airway obstruction confirmed by fibreoptic visualisation. Resuscitation 44:71-74, 2000.

99. Janssens M, Hartstein G: Management of difficult intubation. Eur J Anaesthesiol 18:3-12, 2001.

100. Joo H, Rose K: Fastrach—A new intubating laryngeal mask airway: Successful use in patients with difficult airways. Can J Anaesth 45:253-256, 1998.

101. Kapsner CE, Seaberg DC, Stengel C, et al: The esophageal detector device: Accuracy and reliability in difficult airway settings. Prehosp Disaster Med 11:60-62, 1996.

102. Karch SB, Lewis T, Young S, et al: Field intubation of trauma patients: Complications, indications, and outcomes. Am J Emerg Med 14:617-619, 1996.

103. Kasper CL, Deem S: The self-inflating bulb to detect esophageal intubation during emergency airway management. Anesthesiology 88:898-902, 1998.

104. Katz SH, Falk JL: Misplaced endotracheal tubes by paramedics in an urban emergency medical services system. Ann Emerg Med 37:32-37, 2001.

105. Keller C, Brimacombe J, Kleinsasser A, et al: Does the ProSeal laryngeal mask airway prevent aspiration of regurgitated fluid? Anesth Analg 91:1017-1020, 2000.

106. Kelly JJ, Eynon CA, Kaplan JL, et al: Use of tube condensation as an indicator of endotracheal tube placement. Ann Emerg Med 31:575-578, 1998.

107. Khan ZH, Kashfi A, Ebrahimkhani E: A comparison of the upper lip bite test (a simple new technique) with modified Mallampati classification in predicting difficulty in endotracheal intubation: A prospective blinded study. Anesth Analg 96:595-599, table, 2003.

108. Kihara S, Brimacombe J: Sex-based ProSeal laryngeal mask airway size selection: A randomized crossover study of anesthetized, paralyzed male and female adult patients. Anesth Analg 97:280-284, table, 2003.

109. Kofler J, Sterz F, Hofbauer R, et al: Epinephrine application via an endotracheal airway and via the Combitube in esophageal position. Crit Care Med 28:1445-1449, 2000.

110. Krafft P, Frass M: A complication of percutaneous tracheostomy while using the Combitube for airway control. Eur J Anaesthesiol 15:616, 1998.

111. Krafft P, Frass M, Reed AP: Complications with the Combitube. Can J Anaesth 45:823-824, 1998.

112. Krafft P, Nikolic A, Frass M: Esophageal rupture associated with the use of the Combitube. Anesth Analg 87:1457, 1998.

113. Krafft P, Roggla M, Fridrich P, et al: Bronchoscopy via a redesigned Combitube in the esophageal position. A clinical evaluation. Anesthesiology 86:1041-1045, 1997.

114. Langeron O, Masso E, Huraux C, et al: Prediction of difficult mask ventilation. Anesthesiology 92:1229-1236, 2000.

115. Larmon B, Schriger DL, Snelling R, et al: Results of a 4-hour endotracheal intubation class for EMT-basics. Ann Emerg Med 31:224-227, 1998.

116. Latorre F, Eberle B, Weiler N, et al: Laryngeal mask airway position and the risk of gastric insufflation. Anesth Analg 86:867-871, 1998.

117. Lawes EG, Campbell I, Mercer D: Inflation pressure, gastric insufflation and rapid sequence induction. Br J Anaesth 59:315-318, 1987.

118. Lee YS, Soong WJ, Jeng MJ, et al: Endotracheal tube position in pediatrics and neonates: Comparison between flexible fiberoptic bronchoscopy and chest radiograph. Zhonghua Yi Xue Za Zhi (Taipei) 65:341-344, 2002.

119. Lefrancois DP, Dufour DG: Use of the esophageal tracheal combitube by basic emergency medical technicians. Resuscitation 52:77-83, 2002.

120. Levitan RM: Myths and realities: The "difficult airway" and alternative airway devices in the emergency setting. Acad Emerg Med 8:829-832, 2001.

121. Lewis RP, Stang JM, Warren JV: The role of paramedics in resuscitation of patients with prehospital cardiac arrest from coronary artery disease. Am J Emerg Med 2:200-203, 1984.

122. Li J: Capnography alone is imperfect for endotracheal tube placement confirmation during emergency intubation. J Emerg Med 20:223-229, 2001.

123. Liao D, Shalit M: Successful intubation with the Combitube in acute asthmatic respiratory distress by a paramedic. J Emerg Med 14:561-563, 1996.

124. Liberman M, Mulder D, Lavoie A, et al: Multicenter Canadian study of prehospital trauma care. Ann Surg 237:153-160, 2003.

125. Liberman M, Mulder D, Sampalis J: Advanced or basic life support for trauma: Meta-analysis and critical review of the literature. J Trauma 49:584-599, 2000.

126. Lipp MDW, Thierbach AR: Prehospital airway management in the trauma patient. TraumaCare 9:11-13, 1999.

127. Lockey DJ, Coats T, Parr MJ: Aspiration in severe trauma: A prospective study. Anaesthesia 54: 1097-1098, 1999.

128. Lomotan JR, George SS, Brandstetter RD: Aspiration pneumonia. Strategies for early recognition and prevention. Postgrad Med 102:225-226, 1997.

129. Ma OJ, Atchley RB, Hatley T, et al: Intubation success rates improve for an aeromedical program with use of neuromuscular blocking agents. 1996.

130. MacLeod BA, Heller MB, Gerard J, et al: Verification of endotracheal tube placement with colorimetric end-tidal CO_2 detection. Ann Emerg Med 20:267-270, 1991.

131. Mallampati RS, Gatt SP, Gugino LD: A clinical sign to predict difficult tracheal intubation: A prospective study. Can Anaesth Soc J 32:429-431, 1985.

132. Martel M, Reardon RF, Cochrane J: Initial experience of emergency physicians using the intubating laryngeal mask airway: A case series. Acad Emerg Med 8:815-822, 2001.

133. McCoy EP, Mirakhur RK: The levering laryngoscope. Anaesthesia 48:516-519, 1993.

134. McDonald CC, Bailey B: Out-of-hospital use of neuromuscular-blocking agents in the United States. Prehosp Emerg Care 2:29-32, 1998.

135. Mitchell RG, Guly UM, Rainer TH, et al: Can the full range of paramedic skills improve survival from out of hospital cardiac arrests? J Accid Emerg Med 14:274-277, 1997.

136. Mlinek EJJ, Clinton JE, Plummer D, et al: Fiberoptic intubation in the emergency department. Ann Emerg Med 19:359-362, 1990.

137. Moller F, Andres AH, Langenstein H: Intubating laryngeal mask airway (ILMA) seems to be an ideal device for blind intubation in case of immobile spine. Br J Anaesth 85:493-495, 2000.

138. Murphy MF, Walls RM: The difficult and failed airway. In Walls RM (ed): Manual of Emergency Airway Management. Philadelphia, Lippincott Williams & Wilkins, 2000, pp 42-58.

139. Murphy MF, Walls RM: The difficult and failed airway. In Murphy MF (ed): Syllabus for the Difficult Airway Course: Anesthesia. Boston, Airway Management Education Center, 2001, pp 96-105.

140. Murray JA, Demetriades D, Berne TV, et al: Prehospital intubation in patients with severe head injury. J Trauma 49:1065-1070, 2000.

141. Nielsen LH, Kristensen J, Knudsen F, et al: Fibre-optic bronchoscopic evaluation of tracheal tube position. Eur J Anaesthesiol 8:277-279, 1991.

142. Nolan JD: Prehospital and resuscitative airway care: Should the gold standard be reassessed? Curr Opin Crit Care 7:413-421, 2001.

143. Norton A, Germonpre J, Semple T: Pulmonary aspiration of blood following traumatic laryngeal mask airway insertion. Anaesth Intensive Care 26:213-215, 1998.

144. Ochs M, Davis D, Hoyt D, et al: Paramedic-performed rapid sequence intubation of patients with severe head injuries. Ann Emerg Med 40:159-167, 2002.

145. Ocker H, Wenzel V, Schmucker P, et al: Effectiveness of various airway management techniques in a bench model simulating a cardiac arrest patient. J Emerg Med 20:7-12, 2001.

146. O'Connor CJ Jr, Stix MS: Bubble solution diagnoses ProSeal insertion into the glottis. Anesth Analg 94:1671-1672, 2002.

147. Ornato JP, Shipley JB, Racht EM, et al: Multicenter study of a portable, hand-size, colorimetric end-tidal carbon dioxide detection device. Ann Emerg Med 21:518-523, 1992.

148. Parmet JL, Colonna-Romano P, Horrow JC, et al: The laryngeal mask airway reliably provides rescue ventilation in cases of unanticipated difficult tracheal intubation along with difficult mask ventilation. Anesth Analg 87:661-665, 1998.

149. Parr MJ, Gregory M, Baskett PJ: The intubating laryngeal mask. Use in failed and difficult intubation. Anaesthesia 53:343-348, 1998.

150. Patil VU: Predicting the difficulty of intubation utilizing an intubation guide. Anesthesiol Rev 10:32, 1983.

151. Pelucio M, Halligan L, Dhindsa H: Out-of-hospital experience with the syringe esophageal detector device. Acad Emerg Med 4:563-568, 1997.

152. Pepe PE, Copass MK, Joyce TH: Prehospital endotracheal intubation: Rationale for training emergency medical personnel. Ann Emerg Med 14:1085-1092, 1985.

153. Pepe PE, Stewart RD, Copass MK: Prehospital management of trauma: A tale of three cities. Ann Emerg Med 15:1484-1490, 1986.

154. Practice guidelines for management of the difficult airway: An updated report by the American Society of Anesthesiologists Task Force on Management of the Difficult Airway. Anesthesiology 98:1269-1277, 2003.

155. Rainer TH, Houlihan KP, Robertson CE, et al: An evaluation of paramedic activities in prehospital trauma care. Injury 28:623-627, 1997.

156. Rainer TH, Marshall R, Cusack S: Paramedics, technicians, and survival from out of hospital cardiac arrest. J Accid Emerg Med 14:278-282, 1997.

157. Reardon RF, Martel M: The intubating laryngeal mask airway: Suggestions for use in the emergency department. Acad Emerg Med 8:833-838, 2001.

158. Reed AP: Current concepts in airway management for cardiopulmonary resuscitation. Mayo Clin Proc 70:1172-1184, 1995.

159. Reed DB, Snyder G, Hogue TD: Regional EMS experience with etomidate for facilitated intubation. Prehosp Emerg Care 6:50-53, 2002.

160. Regel G, Stalp M, Lehmann U, et al: Prehospital care, importance of early intervention on outcome. Acta Anaesthesiol Scand Suppl 110:71-76, 1997.

161. Reinhart DJ, Simmons G: Comparison of placement of the laryngeal mask airway with endotracheal tube by paramedics and respiratory therapists. Ann Emerg Med 24:260-263, 1994.

162. Ricard-Hibon A, Chollet C, Leroy C, et al: Succinylcholine improves the time of performance of a tracheal intubation in prehospital critical care medicine. Eur J Anaesthesiol 19:361-367, 2002.

163. Rose WD, Anderson LD, Edmond SA: Analysis of intubations. Before and after establishment of a rapid sequence intubation protocol for air medical use. Air Med J 13:475-478, 1994.

164. Ruchholtz S, Waydhas C, Ose C, et al: Prehospital intubation in severe thoracic trauma without respiratory insufficiency: A matched-pair analysis based on the Trauma Registry of the German Trauma Society. J Trauma 52:879-886, 2002.

165. Rudolph C, Schlender M: [Clinical experiences with fiber optic intubation with the Bonfils]. Anaesthesiol Reanim 21:127-130, 1996.

166. Rumball CJ, MacDonald D: The PTL, Combitube, laryngeal mask, and oral airway: A randomized prehospital comparative study of ventilatory device effectiveness and cost-effectiveness in 470 cases of cardiorespiratory arrest. Prehosp Emerg Care 1:1-10, 1997.

167. Samsoon GLT, Young JRB: Difficult tracheal intubation: A retrospective study. Anaesthesia 14:17-27, 1987.

168. Schaller RJ, Huff JS, Zahn A: Comparison of a colorimetric end-tidal CO_2 detector and an esophageal aspiration device for verifying endotracheal tube placement in the prehospital setting: A six-month experience. Prehospital Disaster Med 12:57-63, 1997.

169. Schlesinger S, Blanchfield D: Modified rapid-sequence induction of anesthesia: A survey of current clinical practice. AANA J 69:291-298, 2001.

170. Schmidt U, Frame SB, Nerlich ML, et al: On-scene helicopter transport of patients with multiple injuries—Comparison of a German and an American system. J Trauma 33:548-553, 1992.

171. Schmitt HJ, Mang H: Head and neck elevation beyond the sniffing position improves laryngeal view in cases of difficult direct laryngoscopy. J Clin Anesth 14:335-338, 2002.

172. Sellick BA: Rupture of the oesophagus following cricoid pressure? Anaesthesia 37:213-214, 1982.

173. Shirk T, Fuller F, Taillac PP, et al: Comparison of the esophageal-tracheal Combitube in the out-of-hospital management of cardiac arrest. Prehospital Disaster Med 10:S52, 1995.

174. Shorten GD, Alfille PH, Gliklich RE: Airway obstruction following application of cricoid pressure. J Clin Anesth 3:403-405, 1991.

175. Silvestri S, Ralls G, Rothrock S, et al: Improvement in misplaced endotracheal tube recognition within a regional EMS system. Conference Proceedings: Society for Academic Emergency Med, 2003.

176. Sing RF, Reilly PM, Rotondo MF, et al: Out-of-hospital rapid-sequence induction for intubation of the pediatric patient. Acad Emerg Med 3:41-45, 1996.

177. Sloane C, Vilke GM, Chan TC, et al: Rapid sequence intubation in the field versus hospital in trauma patients. J Emerg Med 19:259-264, 2000.

178. Smale JR, Kutty K, Ohlert J, et al: Endotracheal intubation by paramedics during in-hospital CPR. Chest 107:1655-1661, 1995.

179. Smith KJ, Dobranowski J, Yip G, et al: Cricoid pressure displaces the esophagus: An observational study using magnetic resonance imaging. Anesthesiology 99:60-64, 2003.

180. Smith RB, Schaer WB, Pfaeffle H: Percutaneous transtracheal ventilation for anaesthesia and resuscitation: A review and report of complications. Can Anaesth Soc J 22:607-612, 1975.

181. Sofferman RA, Johnson DL, Spencer RF: Lost airway during anesthesia induction: Alternatives for management. Laryngoscope 107:1476-1482, 1997.

182. Spaite DW, Joseph M: Prehospital cricothyrotomy: An investigation of indications, technique, complications, and patient outcome. Ann Emerg Med 19:279-285, 1990.

183. Sparr HJ: Choice of the muscle relaxant for rapid-sequence induction. Eur J Anaesthesiol Suppl 23:71-76, 2001.

184. Speirs M, Webster RE: Pre-hospital emergency rapid sequence induction of anaesthesia. J Accid Emerg Med 15:286, 1998.

185. Staudinger T, Tesinsky P, Klappacher G, et al: Emergency intubation with the Combitube in two cases of difficult airway management. Eur J Anaesthesiol 12:189-193, 1995.

186. Stewart RD, LaRosee A, Stoy WA, et al: Use of a lighted stylet to confirm correct endotracheal tube placement. Chest 92:900-903, 1987.

187. Stewart RD, Paris PM, Pelton GH, et al: Effect of varied training techniques on field endotracheal intubation success rates. Ann Emerg Med 13:1032-1036, 1984.

188. Stix MS, O'Connor CJ Jr: Depth of insertion of the ProSeal laryngeal mask airway. Br J Anaesth 90:235-237, 2003.

189. Stone BJ, Chantler PJ, Baskett PJ: The incidence of regurgitation during cardiopulmonary resuscitation: A comparison between the bag valve mask and laryngeal mask airway. Resuscitation 38:3-6, 1998.

190. Su E, Mann NC, McCall M, et al: Use of resuscitation skills by paramedics caring for critically injured children in Oregon. Prehosp Emerg Care 1:123-127, 1997.

191. Suominen P, Baillie C, Kivioja A, et al: Intubation and survival in severe paediatric blunt head injury. Eur J Emerg Med 7:3-7, 2000.

192. Takeda T, Tanigawa K, Tanaka H, et al: The assessment of three methods to verify tracheal tube placement in the emergency setting. Resuscitation 56:153-157, 2003.

193. Tanigawa K, Shigematsu A: Choice of airway devices for 12,020 cases of nontraumatic cardiac arrest in Japan. Prehosp Emerg Care 2:96-100, 1998.

194. Tanigawa K, Takeda T, Goto E, et al: Accuracy and reliability of the self-inflating bulb to verify tracheal intubation in out-of-hospital cardiac arrest patients. Anesthesiology 93:1432-1436, 2000.

195. Tanigawa K, Takeda T, Goto E, et al: The efficacy of esophageal detector devices in verifying tracheal tube placement: A randomized cross-over study of out-of-hospital cardiac arrest patients. Anesth Analg 92:375-378, 2001.

196. Tasch MD, Stoelting RK: Aspiration prevention, prophylaxis and treatment. In Benumof JL (ed): Airway Management—Principles and Practice. St. Louis, Mosby-Year Book, 1996, pp 183-201.

197. Thierbach A: [Maintaining a patent airway in cardiopulmonary resuscitation]. Notfall Rettungsmed 6:14-18, 2003.

198. Thierbach A, Brachlow J, Lipp M: [Emergency Medical Center of the Clinic of Anesthesiology, Johannes Gutenberg University, Mainz]. Notfall Rettungsmed 3:180-184, 2000.

200. Thierbach AR: Advanced prehospital airway management techniques. Eur J Emerg Med 9:298-302, 2002.

201. Thierbach AR, Lipp MDW: Airway management in trauma patients. In Grande CM, Smith CE (eds): Trauma. Philadelphia, WB Saunders, 1999, pp 63-81.

202. Thierbach A, Lipp M: [Fiberoptic intubation in prehospital emergency medicine]. Notfall Rettungsmed 2:105-110, 1999.

203. Thierbach A, Lipp M, Dick W: [Airway management in emergency patients]. Notfallmedizin 23:352-361, 1997.

204. Thomas SH, Harrison T, Wedel SK: Flight crew airway management in four settings: A six-year review. Prehosp Emerg Care 3:310-315, 1999.

205. Tobias JD: The laryngeal mask airway: A review for the emergency physician. Pediatr Emerg Care 12:370-373, 1996.

206. Tong YL, Sun M, Tang WH, et al: The tracheal detecting-bulb: A new device to distinguish tracheal from esophageal intubation. Acta Anaesthesiol Sin 40:159-163, 2002.

207. Ummenhofer W, Scheidegger D: Role of the physician in prehospital management of trauma: European perspective. Curr Opin Crit Care 8:559-565, 2002.

208. Urtubia RM, Gazmuri RR: Is the combitube traumatic? Anesthesiology 98:1021-1022, 2003.

209. Vaghadia H, Jenkins LC, Ford RW: Comparison of end-tidal carbon dioxide, oxygen saturation and clinical signs for the detection of oesophageal intubation. Can J Anaesth 36:560-564, 1989.

210. Vezina D, Lessard MR, Bussières J, et al: Complications associated with the use of the esophageal-tracheal Combitube. Can J Anaesth 45:76-80, 1998.

211. Vilke GM, Hoyt DB, Epperson M, et al: Intubation techniques in the helicopter. J Emerg Med 12:217-224, 1994.

212. Vilke GM, Steen PJ, Smith AM, et al: Out-of-hospital pediatric intubation by paramedics: The San Diego experience. J Emerg Med 22:71-74, 2002.

213. Wahlen BM, Wolcke BB, Thierbach A: Measurement of end-tidal carbon dioxide in spontaneously breathing patients in the pre-hospital setting: A prospective evaluation of 350 patients. Resuscitation 55:61, 2002.

214. Wakeling HG, Nightingale J: The intubating laryngeal mask airway does not facilitate tracheal intubation in the presence of a neck collar in simulated trauma. Br J Anaesth 84:254-256, 2000.

215. Walls RM: The decision to intubate. In Walls RM (ed): Manual of Emergency Airway Management. Philadelphia, Lippincott Williams & Wilkins, 2000, pp 11-19.

216. Walls RM: The emergency airway algorithms. In Walls RM (ed): Manual of Emergency Airway Management. Philadelphia, Lippincott Williams & Wilkins, 2000, pp 30-41.

217. Waltl B, Melischek M, Schuschnig C, et al: Tracheal intubation and cervical spine excursion: Direct laryngoscopy vs. intubating laryngeal mask. Anaesthesia 56:221-226, 2001.

218. Walz R, Davis S, Panning B: Is the Combitube a useful emergency airway device for anesthesiologists? Anesth Analg 88:227, 1998.

219. Wang HE, O'Connor RE, Megargel RE, et al: The utilization of midazolam as a pharmacologic adjunct to endotracheal intubation by paramedics. Prehosp Emerg Care 4:14-18, 2000.

220. Wang HE, Sweeney TA, O'Connor RE, et al: Failed prehospital intubations: An analysis of emergency department courses and outcomes. Prehosp Emerg Care 5:134-141, 2001.

221. Watts AD, Gelb AW, Bach DB, et al: Comparison of the Bullard and Macintosh laryngoscopes for endotracheal intubation of patients with a potential spine injury. Anesthesiology 87:1335-1342, 1997.

222. Wayne MA, Friedland E: Prehospital use of succinylcholine: A 20-year review. Prehosp Emerg Care 3:107-109, 1999.

223. Wayne MA, Slovis CM, Pirrallo RG: Management of difficult airways in the field. Prehosp Emerg Care 3:290-296, 1999.

224. Wee MY: The oesophageal detector device. Assessment of a new method to distinguish oesophageal from tracheal intubation. Anaesthesia 43:27-29, 1988.

225. Wenzel V, Idris AH, Banner MJ, et al: Respiratory system compliance decreases after cardiopulmonary resuscitation and stomach inflation: Impact of large and small tidal volumes on calculated peak airway pressure. Resuscitation 38:113-118, 1998.

226. White RD: Controversies in out-of-hospital emergency airway control: Esophageal obstruction or endotracheal intubation? Ann Emerg Med 13:778-781, 1984.

227. Winchell RJ, Hoyt DB: Endotracheal intubation in the field improves survival in patients with severe head injury. Trauma Research and Education Foundation of San Diego. Arch Surg 132:592-597, 1997.

228. Yardy N, Hancox D, Strang T: A comparison of two airway aids for emergency use by unskilled personnel. Anaesthesia 54:172-197, 1999.

229. Yentis SM: The effects of single-handed and bimanual cricoid pressure on the view at laryngoscopy. Anaesthesia 52:332-335, 1997.

230. Zaleski L, Abello D, Gold MI: The esophageal detector device. Does it work? Anesthesiology 79:244-247, 1993.

231. Zbinden S, Schüpfer G: Detection of oesophageal intubation: The cola complication. Anaesthesia 44:81, 1989.

32

THE PATIENT WITH A FULL STOMACH

Maya S. Suresh
Uma Munnur
Ashutosh Wali

I. INTRODUCTION

Anesthetic intervention in patients considered to have a full stomach presents the anesthesia provider with three challenges: (1) prevention of gastric regurgitation, (2) prevention of pulmonary aspiration, and (3) appropriate airway management. The accepted safe anesthetic management plan for reducing pulmonary aspiration in patients with a full stomach involves (1) identifying patients at risk for gastric regurgitation and pulmonary aspiration, (2) utilizing practice guidelines for preoperative fasting, (3) implementing prophylactic pharmacologic therapies, and (4) applying appropriate airway management techniques that may reduce pulmonary aspiration risk. A review of the relevant literature suggests that the incidence of perioperative pulmonary aspiration is declining; further, the mortality from this dreaded complication has dramatically decreased.[182]

II. DEFINITION OF PULMONARY ASPIRATION

Perioperative pulmonary aspiration is defined as the presence of bilious secretions or particulate matter in the tracheobronchial tree. Perioperative pulmonary aspiration can occur at any time preoperatively until 2 hours after discontinuing anesthesia. Diagnosis is made by either direct examination of the airway, bronchoscopic assessment of the tracheobronchial tree, or postoperative radiograph demonstrating the presence of lung infiltrates not previously identified on the preoperative radiograph.[272]

The incidence, morbidity, and mortality from aspiration are considered in detail in Chapter 11.

III. TIMING OF PULMONARY ASPIRATION

Patients with a full stomach are considered to be at higher risk for pulmonary aspiration, which may occur either before or during induction or at extubation. In adults, the majority of cases involving pulmonary aspiration occur either during induction of anesthesia, that is, prior to laryngoscopy and endotracheal intubation (50%), or during laryngoscopy (29%). Only a minority of cases occur at the onset of the surgical procedure.[182,273] Conversely, in the pediatric population, the majority of cases of pulmonary aspiration occur during induction with an inhalation anesthetic or endotracheal intubation without muscle relaxant, and more than 30% take place during extubation.[272]

Although most instances of pulmonary aspiration coincide with anesthetic induction, laryngoscopy, or surgery, they can also occur postoperatively.[130] Patients who are at risk before surgery are also at risk during the postoperative period because residual effects of anesthetic agents, muscle relaxants, and narcotic analgesics act to decrease protective airway reflexes.

IV. PHYSIOLOGIC RISK FACTORS IN THE PERIOPERATIVE PATIENT

Physiologic risk factors predisposing to aspiration pneumonitis (Table 32-1) include:

1. Increased gastric fluid volume (GFV) with either acidic pH, increased bacterial count, or solid material
2. Delayed gastric emptying
3. Impaired protective physiologic mechanisms, which include reduction in lower esophageal sphincter (LES) and upper esophageal sphincter (UES) pressure
4. Loss of protective airway (laryngeal-pharyngeal) reflexes

A. GASTRIC VOLUME AND pH

The widely cited criteria for aspiration pneumonitis (GFV 0.4 mL/kg and pH < 2.5), generated from a study done on a single Rhesus monkey and extrapolated to humans, have been refuted.[199] Current evidence supports a dose-response relationship for both gastric volume instilled directly into the lung and gastric acidity. The lethal dose for acid pulmonary aspiration has been studied in numerous animal models.[130,180,190] James and colleagues[111] demonstrated that hydrochloric (HCl) acid instilled directly into rat trachea resulted in high mortality. Late mortality rates were 90% with a volume of 0.3 mL/kg at a pH of 1 and 14% with a volume of 1 to 2 mL/kg at a pH less than 1.8. An investigation involving primates demonstrated that aspiration of large volumes (0.8 to 1.0 mL/kg) of acid at a pH of 1 was associated with severe pneumonitis. Instillation of smaller volumes (0.4 to 0.6 mL/kg) produced mild radiologic and clinical changes but no mortality. The median lethal dose for acid aspiration into the lungs was 1.0 mL/kg. Extrapolation of these data to humans provides a critical volume for severe pulmonary aspiration in adult humans of approximately 50 mL.[194] The effect of aspiration of milky products into the lungs has also been studied in animals.[33]

Acidification of human milk to a pH of 1.8 with HCl acid increased the severity of aspiration pneumonitis, compared with 5% dextrose acidified to a pH of 1.8 with HCl acid. Acidification of human breast milk with gastric juice instead of HCl acid did not increase the severity of lung injury. Instillation of soy-based formula or other dairy milk formula into the lungs caused a less severe form of acute injury.[48] They determined that human milk is particularly noxious when aspirated compared with other types of milk.

In normal, healthy children, the range of residual gastric volume at the time of anesthetic induction is quite wide. Cote and coauthors[54] reported values of 0.11 to 4.72 mL/kg compared with the values reported by Splinter and associates[231] (0.01 to 4.08 mL/kg). Children in clinical studies typically have average gastric volumes greater than 0.4 mL/kg, with acidic pH

Table 32-1   **Physiologic Risk Factors for Regurgitation and Aspiration of Gastric Contents**

Increased gastric volume, pressure, acidity	<6 hours NPO (recent meal, drink, alcohol) Gastric insufflation (mask ventilation)
	Acid hypersecretion (hypoglycemia, alcohol, ↑gastrin secretion)
Delayed gastric emptying	Intestinal obstruction (opioids, anticholinergics)
	Drugs
	Pregnancy
	Obesity
	Diabetes, peptic ulcer disease, trauma
	Sympathetic stimulation (acute pain, anxiety, and stress)
Impaired protective physiologic mechanism	Autonomic neuropathy (diabetic gastroparesis)
Decreased LES tone	Pregnancy, gastroesophageal reflux, hiatus hernia, laryngoscopy, cricoid pressure
Decreased UES tone	General anesthesia and sedation
Loss of protective airway (laryngeal-pharyngeal) reflexes	Altered mental state or head injury
	CNS-depressant drugs
	Cerebral hemorrhage or infarct
	Neurologic diseases (multiple sclerosis, Guillain-Barré, cerebral palsy, Parkinson's disease)
	Neuromuscular diseases (muscular dystrophies, myasthenia gravis)

CNS, central nervous system; LES, lower esophageal sphincter; UES, upper esophageal sphincter.

levels,[57,109,133,140,154,214,219,230,231] and yet have a rare occurrence (1 in 10,000) of aspiration pneumonia in association with anesthesia.[218]

Therefore, instead of focusing on GFV at induction, the emphasis to prevent pulmonary aspiration should be on characteristics of the aspirate, patients' comorbidities, anesthetic practice, and patients' risk.

B. DELAYED GASTRIC EMPTYING

Patients who have delayed gastric emptying are considered as having a full stomach and are considered to be at risk for pulmonary aspiration. Patients' conditions that delay gastric emptying include obesity, pregnancy, diabetes, peptic ulcer disease, trauma, stress, and acute pain.

C. IMPAIRED PROTECTIVE PHYSIOLOGIC MECHANISMS

1. Lower Esophageal Sphincter Tone

The LES forms a border between the stomach and the esophagus with the lower esophagus creating a sling around the abdominal esophagus.[225] Barrier pressure is the difference between LES pressure and gastric pressure. Gastric pressure is normally less than 7 mm Hg. Normal resting LES pressure in conscious individuals is 15 to 25 mm Hg higher than intragastric pressure. The presence of an incompetent LES reduces barrier pressure and increases the risk of regurgitation of gastric contents.

LES tone reduction is the major problem in patients with gastroesophageal reflux during anesthesia and disease states. In patients presenting with hiatal hernia, the maximum pressure at the gastroesophageal junction was lower (17.1 mm Hg) than pressures in healthy volunteers (28 mm Hg).[115] Intragastric pressure increases to 35 mm Hg when the stomach is distended.[34] Gastric distention with increased intragastric pressure and reflex relaxation of LES causes spontaneous gastroesophageal reflux. When esophageal pressure equals gastric pressure, the development of a common cavity leads to spontaneous gastroesophageal reflux.[61]

Patients with coexisting gastroesophageal pathology presenting for anesthesia are susceptible to gastroesophageal reflux. The mechanism for reflux is transient relaxation of the LES.[61,217] Anesthetic agents and techniques also relax the LES, reduce barrier pressure, and predispose the patient to gastroesophageal reflux.[55] Cricoid pressure and laryngoscopy during anesthesia also lower LES tone.[245] Drugs that lower LES tone include anticholinergics, benzodiazepines, dopamine, sodium nitroprusside, ganglion blockers, thiopental, tricyclic antidepressants, β-adrenergic stimulants, halothane, enflurane, opioids, and propofol.[55]

Inhalation agents can also reduce the LES pressure below intragastric pressure, depending on the degree of relaxation.[46,55] Propofol has no effect on barrier pressure except for a transient decrease in LES tone and gastric pressure at 1 minute, which return to basal values later.[86]

Drugs that increase LES pressure include antiemetics, cholinergic drugs, succinylcholine, pancuronium, metoclopramide, domperidone, edrophonium, neostigmine, metoprolol, α–adrenergic stimulants, and antacids.[55,86]

2. Upper Esophageal Sphincter Tone

The cricopharyngeus muscle acts as the functional UES. It is one of the two inferior constrictor muscles of the pharynx. It extends around the pharynx from one end of the cricoid arch to the other and is continuous with the circular, muscular coat of the esophagus.[225] In the conscious, healthy patient, the UES helps prevent pulmonary aspiration by sealing off the upper esophagus from the hypopharynyx.[114]

Various anesthetic techniques and agents (except ketamine) reduce the UES tone and predispose the patient to the risk of regurgitation of material from the esophagus into the hypopharynx. Residual neuromuscular blockade (even with train of four of 0.7) also puts the patient at risk for pulmonary aspiration because of a reduction in UES tone and impaired swallowing.[17,153,237,240,262]

D. LOSS OF PROTECTIVE AIRWAY (LARYNGEAL-PHARYNGEAL) REFLEXES

There are four well-defined reflexes in the upper airway that protect the lungs from aspiration. These reflexes include apnea with laryngospasm, coughing, expiration, and spasmodic panting that involves the glottic area and the true or false vocal cords.[170]

Impaired laryngeal-pharyngeal function generally occurs secondary to an altered consciousness level. Patients with central nervous system disorders, cerebrovascular injuries, head trauma, alcohol intoxication, and neuromuscular disorders (particularly myotonia dystrophica and scleroderma) have an increased pulmonary aspiration risk secondary to diminished pharyngeal sensation as well as diminished protective airway reflexes.[70]

Anesthetic agents that result in the loss of UES tone impair protective reflexes.[40] The prevention of protective laryngeal closure permits entry of this foreign matter into the tracheobronchial passages, resulting in regurgitation of gastroesophageal contents into the pharynx.

V. PATIENTS AT RISK FOR PULMONARY ASPIRATION

Thus, recognizing patients who have any of the aforementioned risk factors for pulmonary aspiration is the first step toward minimizing the incidence of perioperative

pulmonary aspiration. These patients can be broken down into two groups:

1. Patients with a full stomach—history of recent ingestion of a meal with less than 6 hours fasting time[1]
2. Patients designated as having a "full stomach" despite prolonged preoperative fast

The groups of patients who are at higher than normal risk for pulmonary aspiration include patients with the following characteristics:

- Extremes of age
- Altered consciousness
- Failure to follow nothing by mouth (NPO) orders
- Pregnant (particularly those in labor)
- Sustained trauma. Trauma, even if nonabdominal in nature, delays gastric emptying.[23,186] Trauma patients (especially those in acute pain scheduled for emergency surgery) have decreased gastrointestinal motility and increased gastrointestinal secretion despite fasting preoperatively.[113] The incidence of pulmonary aspiration increases markedly after trauma because of factors such as recent ingestion of food, depression of consciousness, diminished or absent airway reflexes, and gastric stasis induced by raised sympathoadrenal influx of catecholamines. In 53 adults with Glasgow Coma Scale score less than 8 intubated by the London Helicopter Emergency Medical Service, the incidence of gross pulmonary aspiration was 38%.[135,165]
- Taking medications that delay gastric emptying affects protective physiologic mechanisms. Patients receiving narcotics are expected to have delayed gastric emptying[173,174]; however, it has also been demonstrated that administration of opioids in a single dose to healthy patients did not delay gastric emptying or acidity.[143,145,211]
- Presenting with long-standing diabetes and gastroparesis. Diabetic gastroparesis impairs gastric emptying and may also compromise LES function.[116,156,182,254]
- Morbidly obese. These patients potentially have delayed gastric emptying, increased abdominal pressure, and a difficult airway (DA), all of which are potential risks for pulmonary aspiration. The gastric volumes in 71% of these patients are in the at-risk range compared with normal levels.[265]
- Presenting with stress and acute pain
- Presenting with raised intracranial pressure
- Presenting with neuromuscular disorders
- Undergoing certain types of surgery. The incidence of silent gastric regurgitation is higher in esophageal,[182,273] upper abdominal,[2] and emergency laparoscopic surgeries.[19,41]
- Presenting with comorbidities (American Society of Anesthesiologists [ASA] IV and V)
- Undergoing emergency surgery, especially at night
- Presenting with a DA, followed by failed endotracheal intubation, leading to hypoxia associated with gastric

regurgitation and pulmonary aspiration. General anesthesia administration in patients with a full stomach necessitates tracheal intubation in order to protect the airway from pulmonary aspiration. This procedure of tracheal intubation (which is undertaken to isolate the airway and avoid pulmonary aspiration), if proved to be difficult, can itself become a problem leading to pulmonary aspiration. A difficult intubation (DI) can be predicted in only two thirds of cases; therefore, problems with anesthetic induction, compounded with difficult tracheal intubation, difficult mask ventilation, or inadequate anesthesia with coughing or straining, constitute prime conditions for gastric regurgitation and pulmonary aspiration and have been reported in up to 77% of these cases.[18,122]

- Undergoing regional anesthesia (RA), followed by complications. RA is usually considered safe in patients at risk for pulmonary aspiration because they are awake and have intact protective airway reflexes.[155] After administration of spinal anesthesia, some patients develop extensive sympathetic block followed by hypotension, vomiting, difficulty swallowing, or impaired cough reflex.[182] The pulmonary aspiration risk is further exacerbated by difficulty in swallowing secondary to a high level of sympathetic block. Further, concomitant administration of narcotics or sedatives compounds the effects of obtunding the protective airway reflexes, thus leading to gastric regurgitation and pulmonary aspiration.[166,170,249] Vomiting associated with sympathetic blockade–induced hypotension requires turning the patient's head to the lateral position to avoid the risk of pulmonary aspiration.

VI. PERIOPERATIVE ANESTHETIC CONSIDERATIONS IN FULL-STOMACH PATIENTS

Anesthetic management in patients with a full stomach involves preemptive methods to minimize pulmonary aspiration and its morbidity. Goals are to minimize the volume of gastric contents, reduce gastroesophageal reflux, and prevent perioperative pulmonary aspiration. Preemptive measures targeted to accomplish these goals include preoperative starvation, pharmacologic therapies (to decrease gastric acidity), facilitation of gastric emptying or drainage, and competent LES tone maintenance. Full-stomach "precautions" dictate the anesthetic induction technique. Appropriate airway management techniques involve cricoid pressure (CP) application, endotracheal intubation, or the use of other airway devices.

A. PREOPERATIVE FASTING

Historically, adult patients have fasted 8 to 12 hours before surgery to reduce the volume of gastric contents and the aspiration pneumonitis risk. The National Confidential

Enquiry into Perioperative Deaths[235] highlighted the issue of preoperative starvation. Thus, NPO (Latin, *nulla per os* or "nothing by mouth") after midnight is an accepted preoperative order. Long fasting, prior to an elective operation, is uncomfortable and creates detrimental effects by causing thirst, hunger, irritability, noncompliance, and resentment in adult patients.[2] Prolonged fasting is especially deleterious in children because it also produces dehydration or hypoglycemia.[179,219] During the last 10 years, several papers have challenged the traditional practice of preoperative fasting for more than 8 hours. Further, new understanding of gastric emptying physiology has generated revised preoperative fasting policies.[71,75,92,108,134,142,143,144,158,187,219,272]

Despite knowledge that the stomach handles emptying solids and liquids differently, physicians traditionally lumped consideration for both together in the standard preoperative order: NPO after midnight the day before surgery. After an extensive review, the ASA task force has now revised policies and has published specific practice guidelines for preoperative fasting.[1]

1. Liquids

Residual gastric volume is directly related to regurgitation and pulmonary aspiration. However, the ASA task force, despite an extensive scrutiny of the existing data, has been unable to establish a link between residual gastric volume and pulmonary aspiration.[191]

a. Clear Liquids

Clear liquids in healthy patients empty exponentially. The emptying half-life ($t_{1/2}$) of clear liquids is 12 minutes, which is considerably faster than for solids. Theoretically, this means that, for a patient who consumes 500 mL of clear liquid, almost 97% of the liquid is eliminated from the stomach after five half-lives (60 minutes).[12,104,106] The rate of gastric emptying after a liquid meal has been well studied in adults.[142,158,191] The studies demonstrated that after drinking 750 mL of pulp-free orange drink, mean gastric emptying $t_{1/2}$ ranged from 10 ± 7 to 20 ± 11 minutes. The fastest $t_{1/2}$ for an individual subject was 2.9 minutes and the slowest $t_{1/2}$ was 41.6 minutes, indicating that almost complete gastric emptying could be accomplished in 2 hours (approximately five half-lives) after a clear liquid drink was given. Thus, even in individuals with the slowest emptying rates, only 10% or less of the original liquid would be retained in the stomach after 2 hours.[108,144,152,216,223]

The ASA task force now supports a fasting period of 2 hours following the ingestion of clear liquids for all patients. Clear liquids include, but are not limited to, water and fruit juices without pulp, carbonated beverages, clear tea, and black coffee. The clear liquid category does not include alcohol. The volume of liquid ingested is less important than the type of liquid.

b. Milk

In term and preterm infants, breast milk leaves the stomach more rapidly than formula milk. The emptying $t_{1/2}$ for breast milk is approximately 25 minutes; for formula milk, it is twice as long.[42,43] Consultants and the ASA task force now recommend fasting 4 hours after breast milk and 6 hours after infant formula.

2. Solids and Nonhuman Milk

Gastric emptying for solids occurs in a linear pattern with time, and 10% to 30% of ingested solids may still remain in a patient's stomach after 6 hours.[102] Gastric emptying is inhibited when (1) the duodenum is distended; (2) the chyme contains a high concentration of acid, proteins, or fats; or (3) the osmolarity is not iso-osmolar. Gastric emptying after solid ingestion is also dependent on body posture after intake, exercise, meal weight, size of food particles, and the amount of food.[161,164] Lack of readily available, appropriate methodology makes the assessment of stomach contents in the perioperative period difficult.

Miller and coworkers[157] investigated patients who ate a light breakfast of a slice of buttered toast and a cup of tea or coffee with milk 2 to 4 hours before surgery. Gastric contents were measured by inserting a gastric tube after anesthetic induction. There was no significant difference in gastric volume or pH between the control group (fasting) and the study group. Soreide and associates[229] investigated a group of healthy, female volunteers who ingested a standard hospital breakfast of one slice of white bread with butter or jam, one cup (150 mL) of coffee without milk or sugar, and one glass (150 mL) of pulp-free orange juice. These gastric contents were measured by repeated ultrasonography and paracetamol absorption techniques. No solid food was detected in any volunteer 240 minutes after breakfast. The latter test determined that at least 4 hours between eating and surgery are needed for solid foods to empty from the stomach.

3. Patients with Diabetes

It has been shown, using radioisotopic techniques and electrical impedance tomography, that type 1 diabetic patients have delayed gastric emptying.[254] After ingestion of a semisolid meal, the mean $t_{1/2}$ of gastric emptying was 54.8 ± 26.6 minutes in diabetic patients compared with 40.4 ± 8.6 minutes in nondiabetic control subjects. Thus, the diabetic patient requires a longer fasting period (8 hours) than nondiabetic patients.

4. Ambulatory Patients and Anxiety

Anxiety delays gastric emptying and increases acid secretion.[93,224] Ambulatory surgery increases anxiety; a background study showed that the mean gastric volume was 69 mL in outpatients versus 33 mL in inpatients with the average pH less than 2.5 in both groups.[183]

To test the hypothesis that preoperative stress would affect residual GFV and pH in children, children aged 3 to 17 years were randomly assigned to three groups: outpatients, inpatients, and patients who had multiple surgeries.[54] There were no differences in the residual GFV between the three groups and no differences in gastric contents between inpatients and outpatients.

Further, the relationship between oral premedication, preoperative anxiety, and gastric contents showed that premedication reduces anxiety. However, there was no correlation between the type of premedication, level of anxiety, gastric volume, and gastric pH.[9]

B. FASTING GUIDELINES SUMMARY

Almost 80% of elective surgeries today are in ambulatory patients or those with same-day admittance. The ASA task force practice guidelines for preoperative fasting time[191] recommend avoiding anesthetizing a patient with a full stomach to reduce the risk of pulmonary aspiration. A recap of the aforementioned guidelines about minimum fasting period for ingested material is as follows: clear liquids, 2 hours; breast milk, 4 hours; infant formula, nonhuman milk, and light meal, 6 hours (ASA practice guidelines). A fast should precede elective procedures requiring general anesthesia, RA, or sedation or analgesia (i.e., monitored anesthesia care). The guidelines also recommend a fasting period for a meal that includes fried foods, fatty foods, or meat of 8 hours or more before elective procedures. Diabetic patients need 8 hours or more for gastric emptying after ingesting semisolid material.

Most anesthesiologists practicing outpatient anesthesia in the United States have conformed to the recommendation of the ASA task force practice guidelines for preoperative fasting time.[187] Similar opinions from associations linked to the World Federation of Societies of Anesthesiologists and from current literature have led to changes in preoperative fasting guidelines worldwide.[68,71,75,92,189]

C. PHARMACOTHERAPY

The ASA task force does not recommend the routine preoperative use of gastrointestinal stimulants, medications that block gastric acid secretion, antacids, prokinetics, antiemetics, or anticholinergics to reduce the risk of pulmonary aspiration.[191]

Surveys on pulmonary aspiration prophylaxis in the full-stomach, nonobstetric population are rare. The accepted pharmacologic regimens include an attempt to manipulate the gastric pH and volume as well as barrier pressure.[72,123,146,162,175,176,181,246,269] Other existing surveys on antacid prophylaxis are limited to obstetric anesthesia.[50,73,90,228,236,285] Most studies *suggest* improved safety from reduced gastric volume or increase in gastric pH, or both.* However, there are no data to show evidence of improved outcome after the use of antacids, H_2-receptor blockers, proton pump inhibitors, or prokinetics. Because of the paucity of data and a lack of evidence to prove the value of pharmacologic therapies for preventing pulmonary aspiration, it is not possible to analyze a cost-benefit ratio.[191]

D. PREOPERATIVE GASTRIC EMPTYING

Preoperative stomach emptying through a gastric tube is beneficial for patients at risk for pulmonary aspiration (e.g., small bowel obstruction). Any contents emptied from the stomach make anesthesia induction safer for the patient.

Preoperative gastric emptying concerns include the: (1) effect of routine gastric tube insertion prior to emergency surgery for at-risk patients, (2) effect of in situ gastric tube on efficacy of CP application during induction of anesthesia, and (3) effect of the gastric tube on gastroeophageal reflux and pulmonary aspiration in mechanically ventilated patients.

1. Preoperative Gastric Tube Insertion in Patients Scheduled for Emergency Surgery

The first concern is that preoperative gastric emptying is not without hazards. Preoperative insertion of a gastric tube and subsequent gastric emptying in an awake, unsedated patient elicit a profound sympathetic response and oxygen desaturation.[126] This response, which is similar to the cardiovascular response after endotracheal intubation without analgesia,[78,117] puts the patient with cardiac problems at risk for cardiac ischemia. Routine preoperative nasogastric tube placement is *not* recommended except in selected patients with small bowel or gastric outlet obstruction. Although the gastric tube helps reduce intragastric volume and pressure, it does not guarantee that the stomach is completely empty. Therefore, preoperative nasogastric tube insertion and stomach decompression are recommended only in patients with a distended stomach (e.g., bowel obstruction).

2. In Situ Presence of a Gastric Tube during Induction

What one does with a gastric tube that is already in place during induction is a debatable issue. Once the stomach is decompressed, the gastric tube can be removed or left in situ during a rapid sequence induction. Although the presence of the gastric tube may impair the function of both the UES and LES,[222] studies with cadavers have shown that the efficacy of CP application during induction of anesthesia is not impaired.[208,260] Thus, if the patient

---

has a nasogastric tube, it need not be withdrawn before induction of anesthesia as it acts as an overflow valve and prevents pressure buildup in the stomach; it also allows drainage during anesthesia induction.[98]

3. Possible Detrimental Effects of Gastric Tube Placement in Mechanically Ventilated Patients

The third concern was tested in mechanically ventilated, intensive care unit (ICU) patients to determine the effect of the nasogastric tube size on the incidence of gastroesophageal reflux.[76] The concern with gastroesophageal reflux is that it can result in pulmonary aspiration and bacterial pneumonias. Investigators found no significant difference in gastroesophageal reflux and pulmonary aspiration with the use of small- and large-gauge nasogastric tubes.

4. Sealing the Esophagus by Inflatable Cuffs

The concept design to prevent reflux regurgitation by inflating a cuff at the gastroesophageal junction, as previously described, is now considered unsafe. A newly designed, but similar, nasogastric device with an inflatable cuff to occlude the gastric cardia (Aspisafe, Braun, Melsungen, Germany) was studied in pigs (Fig. 32-1).[201] After gastric filling with large volumes, despite maneuvers and drugs used to promote regurgitation, the new nasogastric device did not produce gastroesophageal reflux.[201] The same experiment was duplicated in healthy volunteers and surgical patients considered at risk for pulmonary aspiration, with similar findings.[201] Use of this device is considered safe because there was no test evidence of gastroesophageal reflux following rapid sequence induction.[170]

The device was subsequently studied in conjunction with the use of a laryngeal mask airway (LMA). A dye indicator injected into the stomach revealed that the balloon tube prevented gastroesophageal reflux.[221] Future clinical studies should decidedly prove balloon tube safety and usefulness in preventing regurgitation during induction and extubation.

VII. GENERAL ANESTHESIA MANAGEMENT

The goals of general anesthesia in full-stomach patients include skillful airway management and prevention of pulmonary aspiration of gastric contents.

Airway management techniques used to isolate the trachea from the gastrointestinal tract with a cuffed endotracheal tube (ET) include (1) intubation of the trachea in an awake patient using a rigid or fiberoptic bronchoscope (FOB) and (2) rapid sequence induction and endotracheal intubation technique following preoxygenation and CP application.

---

*References 32, 51, 64, 110, 160, 171, 178, 182, 184, 234, 279, 284.

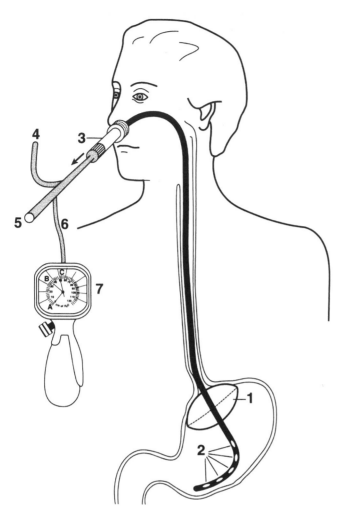

Figure 32-1 Schematic representation of a nasogastric balloon tube in a patient; 1, inflatable balloon; 2, lateral openings to aspirate stomach contents and equilibrate pressure between the stomach and the outside air; 3, pliable nose stopper with foam ring and locking device (overdimensional drawing for purpose of illustration); 4, separate lumen ("slurp lumen"); 5, main lumen with aspiration connection; 6, branch tube with the subsidiary lumen leading into the inside of the balloon; and 7, pressure monitoring device (A = pressure level in the deflated state of the balloon, B = pressure level in the inflated state of the balloon, and C = pressure level when the aspiration tube is pulled tight resulting in close appositional contact of the balloon with the cardia). (From Roewer N: Can pulmonary aspiration of gastric contents be prevented by balloon occlusion of the cardia? A study with a new nasogastric tube. Anesth Analg 80:378-383, 1995.)

A. AWAKE INTUBATION IN PATIENTS AT HIGH RISK FOR ASPIRATION

The distinct advantages of securing the airway with the patient awake versus rapid sequence induction and intubation in patients with a full stomach and a DA are the avoidance of (1) loss of protective reflexes, (2) the failure of CP to prevent pulmonary aspiration, (3) failed endotracheal intubation leading to hypoxia and brain death, and (4) cardiovascular collapse.

A full-stomach patient with a DA warrants an awake intubation (AI). The potential for a DA (i.e., either a DI or a difficult mask ventilation) may be self-evident because of preexisting or acquired condition. However, normal individual anatomic variation may also contribute to difficulty with either endotracheal intubation or mask ventilation. Various physical characteristics are associated with DA, including small mouth, limited mouth opening, short interincisor distance, prominent upper incisors with overriding maxilla, short neck, limited neck mobility, receding mandible or mandibular hypoplasia, high arched and narrow palate, temporomandibular joint dysfunction, rigid cervical spine, obesity, and congenital anomalies found in infancy. Morbidly obese patients and infants, particularly, are at risk for both DA and pulmonary aspiration. No single feature on physical examination accurately predicts a DI, but a variety of simple diagnostic tests have been suggested to identify patients with DAs.*

A major priority in managing patients with a DA and a full stomach is securing the airway with an ET while the patient is awake. There are several advantages for this, including (1) maintenance of protective airway reflexes, (2) uncompromised airway exchange and oxygenation, and (3) maintenance of normal muscle tone, which helps in the identification of anatomic landmarks.

Intubation of the trachea while the patient is awake is a very useful technique with a high degree of acceptance by patients and is considered a failsafe method of choice when gastric regurgitation and pulmonary aspiration are likely.[20] The AI method is useful not only in situations of anticipated difficulties in intubation but also in patients with intestinal obstruction, gastrointestinal hemorrhage, or upper airway obstruction; in seriously ill or moribund patients; and in those with respiratory failure.[66]

In patients with intestinal obstruction, paralytic ileus with abdominal distention, or upper gastrointestinal hemorrhage, the timing of regurgitation of gastric contents into the pharynx, particularly between the loss of consciousness and endotracheal intubation, is greatly increased. Therefore, intubation of the trachea while the patient is awake is a sound practice affording protection against inhalation of gastric contents, loss of the airway, hypoxia, and cardiovascular collapse.

Successful accomplishment of AI in patients at risk for pulmonary aspiration is dependent on several factors, including adequate psychological preparation, topicalization of the airway, skills and experience of the endoscopist, and the nature and urgency of the surgery.

Prior to topicalization of the airway, the administration of anticholinergic drugs minimizes secretions, thereby allowing adequate penetration of local anesthetic through the mucosa and thus enhancing the local anesthetic effects and enabling better visualization through the scope. The drawback of using anticholinergic drugs in patients

*References 16, 37, 67, 82, 141, 172, 177, 200, 202, 213, 215, 247, 278.

with a full stomach is that it can reduce LES tone and barrier pressure, creating a potential risk for pulmonary aspiration.

Efficacy and safety of AI in full-stomach patients can be accomplished with the use of minimal sedation, administration of oxygen by nasal cannula during intubation, and application of local anesthetic to the pharynx, larynx, and trachea. The premise of conscious sedation is to balance the comfort of the patient and tolerance of the procedure and yet have a patient responsive to commands. Judicious sedation with small amounts of short-acting benzodiazepines and narcotics helps allay anxiety and helps the patient who is awake tolerate any discomfort that occurs during endotracheal intubation. Ovassapian and colleagues[185] presented the concept of awake fiberoptic intubation using judicious sedation and topicalization of upper and lower airways in patients at high risk for pulmonary aspiration. An accompanying editorial stated that this study of 121 patients was too small to accept the safety of the technique of AI, sedation, and topicalization of the airway.

Topicalization of the lower airway (i.e., below the vocal cords) in an awake patient, at risk for pulmonary aspiration, is controversial. However, topicalization of the airway adds to the patient's comfort and enhances the chances of successful AI. There are a number of ways to anesthetize the upper and lower airway, including administering local anesthetic spray to the mucosa, administering lidocaine jelly to the base of the tongue, bilateral blockade of the internal branch of the superior laryngeal nerve (sensory to the base of the tongue, vallecula, epiglottis, and larynx up to the level of the cords), bilateral glossopharyngeal nerve blocks (eliminates gag reflex), and transtracheal injection of local anesthetic through the cricothyroid membrane (anesthetizes the airway below the vocal cords).

After judicious sedation and topicalization of the airway, a number of techniques can be used to accomplish AI, including blind nasal intubation, FOB intubation, use of rigid scopes, intubating laryngeal mask airways (ILMAs), light wand–guided intubation, and retrograde intubation. There are advantages and drawbacks with each of these techniques.

B. RAPID SEQUENCE INDUCTION

Rapid sequence induction (RSI) of anesthesia to protect the airway from pulmonary aspiration of gastric contents has evolved since the introduction of succinylcholine in 1951 and the first description of CP by Sellick in 1961.[222]

The primary objective of RSI is to minimize the time interval between loss of consciousness and endotracheal intubation. The essential features of RSI include preoxygenation with 100% oxygen, administration of a predetermined induction dose, application of CP, and avoidance of positive-pressure ventilation until the airway is secured[53] with a cuffed ET.[242] Many emergency physicians use RSI of anesthesia as their technique of choice to facilitate orotracheal intubation in patients presenting to the emergency room.[89,124,139,149,168,207] Having specialized

equipment for management of failed intubation is also an integral part of RSI.[1,4,163,257]

RSI plays a major role in emergency anesthesia and is used almost universally for obstetric general anesthesia in both the United Kingdom[53] and United States; however, it is practiced less widely in mainland Europe.[13] A survey of French anesthetists showed that only 23% used a full complement of measures to prevent pulmonary aspiration, and CP was rarely used,[14,182] yet the incidence of fatal aspiration in France is lower than in other countries (1.4 per 10,000 anesthetics versus 4.7 per 10,000 anesthetics).[14,182]

Currently, there are no prospective studies that identify either the efficacy of RSI in preventing morbidity or its safety. In the past decade, changes in available induction agents, muscle relaxants, and airway aids and increased research in airway management have led to opportunities for RSI in general anesthesia practice to evolve further.

Preoxygenation is a standard component of RSI.[242] Preoxygenation with fresh gas flows of 100% oxygen through a mask with a good fit for 3 to 5 minutes is recommended. Alternatively, a series of four vital capacity breaths of 100% may be used in an emergency.[242] Thiopental remains the most popular induction agent for RSI,[242] although propofol is now used extensively. Other intravenous induction agents include ketamine[8] and etomidate.[83]

Succinylcholine remains the muscle relaxant of choice for use in RSI.[242] Certain conditions may preclude the use of succinylcholine (e.g., burns and spinal cord injuries, because the administration of succinylcholine can result in adverse effects such as hyperkalemia and dysrhythmias). Several studies have demonstrated that rocuronium in adequate doses (0.8 to 1.2 mg/kg) rapidly produces intubation conditions comparable to those with succinylcholine 1 mg/kg.[69,283] However, this large dose leads to prolonged duration of action of up to 1 hour.[21] In a patient with a DA, this drug may allow less margin for error than succinylcholine.[38] Fifty percent of cases of DI occur without preoperative predictive signs and can increase the risks of gastric regurgitation and pulmonary aspiration in full-stomach patients.[277]

1. Modified Rapid Sequence Induction

RSI is a well-established technique in anesthesia practice. During standard RSI, patients are made apneic and unconscious without establishing the ability to ventilate the lungs. Positive pressure is generally avoided to prevent pulmonary aspiration and gaseous distention of the stomach in RSI. This, theoretically, avoids distention of the stomach and subsequent pulmonary aspiration. However, avoidance of ventilation of lungs during RSI precludes the ability to "test the airway" and verify that a patient's lungs can be ventilated by mask before the administration of a muscle relaxant. Therefore, the technique of RSI involves inherent risks to the patient. These risks include potential inability to secure an airway or to ventilate and oxygenate the lungs in a patient who is unconscious and apneic. Further, during RSI, failure to secure the airway can lead to multiple attempts at endotracheal intubation and trauma to the airway, and failure to ventilate the lungs can lead to hypoxia, hypercarbia, and alteration in heart rate and blood pressure resulting in significant morbidity. These risks may not be warranted or appropriate, particularly in patients who are at risk for gastric regurgitation and pulmonary aspiration. For these patients, a modification of the standard RSI technique consisting of preoxygenation, induction of anesthesia, CP, and the added step of gentle positive-pressure ventilation of lungs before endotracheal intubation may be appropriate.

The technique of a modified RSI technique allows the anesthesia provider to affirm that the patient's lungs can be ventilated and oxygenated by mask before insertion of a cuffed ET. Positive pressure is provided by a face mask before and after the administration of the muscle relaxant. However, the risks and benefits of modified RSI have to be considered in a patient with a full stomach and a potential DA. The risks of being unable to intubate the trachea and ventilate the lungs have to be weighed against the risk of pulmonary aspiration; the results of both complications could be disastrous if they are not managed appropriately.

2. Cricoid Pressure

CP is an integral part and key component of RSI and is accepted as a standard of care during anesthesia[30,203,242] and to a lesser extent during resuscitation[232] in patients with a full stomach. As early as the 1770s, CP was recognized as an important method to occlude the esophagus and prevent gastric distention during lung ventilation of drowned victims.[209] However, it was almost 200 years later that Sellick first introduced CP into clinical anesthesia practice.[222] Although studies cite increasing concerns regarding the safety and efficacy of CP, it is still widely practiced.[127,220,244]

The cricoid cartilage (CC) is signet ring shaped and is a complete ring. It is attached superiorly to the thyroid cartilage by the cricothyroid ligament and inferiorly to the first tracheal ring. The esophagus begins at the lower border of the CC, and the cricopharyngeus muscle guards the esophageal opening. The CC differs in size and location in adults and children.

The CP, a force measured in newtons (N), must be of sufficient amount applied during induction to prevent regurgitation from the esophagus and stomach. Regurgitation of stomach contents is dependent on esophageal pressure, gastrointestinal pathology, intragastric pressure, UES and LES pressures, and the effectiveness of occluding the esophageal lumen. On the basis of several studies,[74,129,208,210,261,282] a cricoid force (CP) of 44 N (9.8 N = 1 kg = 2.2 lb) was accepted as the "gold standard" for the prevention of gastric regurgitation in adults, in the standard or tonsillectomy position.[282] CP greater than 44 N was shown to prevent gastric regurgitation. When appropriate force is applied, the upper end of the esophagus is occluded and compressed against the C6 vertebra. In paralyzed intubated patients, lowering the CP to 40 N increased

esophageal pressure to more than 38 mm Hg.[263] In a study using the double-lumen Salem sump tube in 20 females undergoing emergency cesarean delivery under general anesthesia,[100] the mean gastric pressure was 11 mm Hg (range, 4 to 19 mm Hg). It was predicted that 99% of women undergoing emergency cesarean delivery having a gastric pressure of 25 mm Hg are unlikely to have regurgitation of fluid. Evidence from a cadaver study showed that a CP of 30 N prevents regurgitation of esophageal fluid even with gastric pressure at 42 mm Hg. Anatomic studies suggest that CP of 30 N is adequate and should reduce the risk of esophageal rupture.[260,263]

The CP necessary to provide an adequate occlusive effect in children of different age groups is debatable. There are no data available to clarify this issue. An observational study, using the bench model, indicated that the mean cricoid force applied clinically to a 5-year-old should be 22.4 to 25.1 N.[79]

a. Head and Neck Position

Sellick made the original recommendation to use the tonsillectomy position, without a pillow, with CP applied at C5 vertebra.[222] The rationale for the tonsillar position is that it increases the concavity of the cervical spine, stretches the esophagus, and prevents lateral displacement of the esophagus. Unfortunately, this mode of CP application often worsens the view at laryngoscopy.[15] The head position must be ideal for intubating with head extension, neck flexion, and a pillow beneath the occiput.[11]

b. Timing of Cricoid Pressure Application

The timing and amount of force of CP applied during induction are also important. The original recommendation was synchronous CP application; moderate pressure in an awake, conscious individual; and a gradual increase to a full force of 44 N immediately on loss of consciousness. Applying a full force of 44 N prior to induction in a conscious individual is detrimental; it produces significant discomfort, complete airway obstruction,[258] retching, and vomiting.[30] Vomiting with continued CP application can cause death from pulmonary aspiration[276] or a ruptured esophagus.[195]

A cricoid yoke has also been used to apply pressure in awake volunteers without considerable pain or coughing.[129] The current accepted practice is to apply a lower CP (20 N) prior to induction of anesthesia and increase it to 30 N as the patient loses consciousness.[259]

Reluctance to use CP stems from faulty technique of CP application and its effect on airway management, reported cases of pulmonary aspiration, and esophageal rupture. Application of CP causes anatomic distortion of the upper airway, making airway management more difficult. The majority of the data were collected with a CP of 40 N. Studies[259] show that a CP of 30 N in an upward and backward manner improves the laryngoscopy view during intubation. Similarly, Randell and colleagues[196] have shown that CP, modified to backward, upward, rightward pressure (BURP), improved the view in 57 of 68 cases.

c. Single-Handed Cricoid Pressure

For single-handed CP, the thumb and middle finger are placed on either side of the CC, and the index finger is placed above to prevent lateral movement of the cricoid.[222] The laryngoscopic view is better with the head in the Magill position and with single-handed CP as compared with double-handed CP.[52]

Another single-handed method is to place the palm of the hand on the sternum, applying pressure with only the index and middle fingers.[56] This technique improves the laryngoscopic view of the glottis. In infants and children, the single-handed technique compressing the CC is performed with the little or middle finger while the same hand holds the face mask.[212]

It is recommended that the application of CP should be performed with the left hand from the left side of the patient, thus preventing interference with laryngoscopy, specifically when the laryngoscope blade is inserted from the right corner of the mouth.

d. Double-Handed Cricoid Pressure

The bimanual or two-handed CP technique uses the single-handed technique, as previously described, in addition to using the assistant's right hand to provide counterpressure beneath the cervical vertebra for neck support. The purpose of this maneuver is to provide support to the hyperextended arch of the vertebral column to maintain the efficacy of CP and optimize the laryngoscopic view. Variations of this technique include placing the left hand behind the head and holding the extended head to maintain the Magill intubating position.[58]

e. Cricoid Pressure in Clinical Practice

In clinical practice, the application of a predetermined CP can be sustained for only a short period of time. The application of CP with a flexed arm could be sustained only for a mean time of 3.7 minutes at 40 N, with considerable onset of pain at 2.3 minutes. In view of the fact that sustained CP cannot be maintained for more than a few minutes, it has important clinical implications in the situation of failed endotracheal intubation in the presence of a full stomach. Further, an important clinical limitation to the application of CP in clinical practice is that it may interfere with airway management (endotracheal intubation, face mask ventilation, and LMA placement), and failure to manage the airway appropriately is a more frequent cause of morbidity and mortality compared with the risk of pulmonary aspiration.[39]

VIII. MANAGEMENT OF A DIFFICULT AIRWAY IN THE PATIENT WITH A FULL STOMACH

The management of difficulty with intubation at RSI is little studied. Airway catastrophes occur predominantly when airway difficulty is not recognized before anesthesia is administered.[35,121] Although airway difficulty should be anticipated in 90% of cases, a prospective study showed that only approximately 51% of DIs were recognized and expected.[128] Also, difficult and failed intubations occur more frequently during emergency than during elective surgery.[9,101,239] Unanticipated DI in full-stomach patients undergoing emergency surgery poses additional problems. There is no option for anesthesiologists to postpone surgery, and the risk of pulmonary aspiration of gastric contents is much greater.

In full-stomach patients, not only do repeated attempts to intubate the trachea increase the risk of airway trauma, bleeding, and laryngeal edema but also failure to secure the airway can increase the incidence of pulmonary aspiration. Hypoxia and death can result from failure to oxygenate and ventilate the patient's lungs or from unrecognized intubation of the esophagus, neither of which is caused solely by failed endotracheal intubation.[16]

Significant advances in airway management have been made in the past two decades. New airway devices and adjuncts to assist in the intubation of DAs are now available. In majority of cases of DI, a partial view of the glottis is possible (grade III laryngoscopic view).[9,101,163] In the United Kingdom and Canada, of the many airway devices available to physicians, the gum elastic bougie is most frequently used to facilitate endotracheal intubation in more than 95% of grade III laryngoscopic views.[88] Another commonly utilized device is the McCoy laryngoscope (CLM, Mercury Medical, Clearwater, FL), which has been shown to improve visualization of the larynx in up to 50% of difficult laryngoscopic views.[49,248]

Additional levering laryngoscopes include the Flipper (Rusch, Duluth, GA) and the Heine Flex Tip (Heine Optotechnik, Herrsching, Germany). These laryngoscopes were designed to provide greater flexibility and improved visualization of the larynx in instances in which a DA is present, mouth opening is decreased, or head and neck movement is restricted.[95]

A. DIFFICULT AIRWAY MANAGEMENT USING THE LARYNGEAL MASK AIRWAY

Before 1990, the choice of airway devices essentially was limited to the face mask or the ET. The LMA (LMA North America, San Diego, CA) is one of the most significant and important airway devices introduced for airway management. Since then, a number of supraglottic airway devices, such as the pharyngeal airway express (PAxpress, or PAX, Vital Signs, Totowa, NJ) have been developed. Other devices now available for airway management include the esophageal-tracheal Combitube (ETC, Tyco Healthcare, Mansfield, MA) and the laryngeal tube (LT, King Systems, Noblesville, IN).

Dr. Archie Brain, the inventor of the LMA, continues to develop variations of the original device. These modifications include eight sizes of the original LMA-Classic (cLMA), a single-use LMA (LMA-Unique), a reinforced/flexible LMA (LMA-Flexible), an LMA specifically designed for blind endotracheal intubation (Intubating LMA-Fastrach), and an LMA fitted with an integral gastric access/venting port (LMA-ProSeal).

The LMA is now a recognized part of the ASA difficult airway algorithm. As a ventilatory device or intubating conduit, or both, the LMA fits into the DA algorithm in several places.

1. LMA-Classic Device

The use of the cLMA is contraindicated in full-stomach patients and patients at high risk for pulmonary aspiration (i.e., patients presenting with gastrointestinal pathology, obesity, gastroesophageal reflux, emergency surgery).

The main disadvantage of using the cLMA device in patients with a full stomach or obstetric patients is an increased risk for gastric regurgitation and pulmonary aspiration. The design of the cLMA is such that even when correctly placed, the cLMA tip lies against the UES and the cLMA does not isolate the respiratory tract from the gastrointestinal tract. Because the esophagus is included in the rim of the cLMA, it does not protect the lungs from regurgitated gastric contents. Thus, full-stomach and pregnant patients are vulnerable to gastric regurgitation and pulmonary aspiration with the use of this device.[169]

Studies of gastric regurgitation and pulmonary aspiration rates associated with using these new supraglottic devices have mainly focused on the cLMA. A meta-analysis of 547 publications suggested that the overall incidence of pulmonary aspiration with the cLMA is probably in the region of 2 per 10,000,[31] a figure corroborated by a large number of studies. This rate is comparable to that of outpatient anesthesia administered with a face mask and ET,[116] as seen in Table 32-2. Studies have also demonstrated that the use of cLMA is associated with a reduction in barrier pressure at the LES.[193] In comparing the cuffed ET with the cLMA during general anesthesia with positive-pressure ventilation, Valentine and colleagues[256] (using a pH electrode placed in the midesophageal zone) determined that there were significantly more episodes

of reflux in the cLMA group of patients. In contrast, Agro and associates[3] found no episodes of reflux with the use of cLMA in patients undergoing elective orthopedic surgery. The association between gastroesophageal reflux and the cLMA is not clear. However, there is insufficient evidence to support the hypothesis that the reduction in lower esophageal pH is influenced directly by either the pressure or the volume in the cuff of the cLMA.[206] The application of CP causes a reduction in LES pressure[245]; a similar reflux may also occur because of the increased pharyngeal pressure exerted by the cLMA. There is controversy about the effect of the cLMA on LES tone, with some studies reporting a reduction in tone[193] and others reporting no change[36]; however, it has been generally accepted that UES function is relatively unimpaired by the cLMA. Therefore, some anesthesiologists believe that the cLMA is contraindicated in patients with a full stomach and in obstetric patients.

Despite the pulmonary aspiration risks with a cLMA (with or without CP) being the same as those encountered with a face mask,[31,267] particularly in patients with a full stomach, there are a number of case reports documenting the use of cLMA after failed intubation attempts during emergency cesarean section. These case reports have shown that after failed endotracheal intubation during emergency cesarean section, the use of the cLMA device not only provided a clear airway but also was useful in rapidly providing oxygenation and relieving hypoxia. There were no reports of pulmonary aspiration.[45,31,87,150,151,192] In addition, in 1346 elective cesarean sections, the cLMA was used in obstetric patients as an alternative to ET intubation to ventilate lungs. The ET was blindly inserted with minimal cardiovascular responses, and there was no incidence of pulmonary aspiration in 98% of cases.[148] In another study, the cLMA was used in 1067 patients undergoing elective cesarean sections.[88] After RSI with CP, the cLMA was inserted and an effective airway was obtained in 1060 patients (99%). There were no episodes of pulmonary aspiration, hypoxia, laryngospasm, or gastric insufflation.[97]

The major benefit of using the cLMA device after failed intubation attempts in a patient with a full stomach is that it serves as a rescue device and provides oxygenation.[60] However, because of the potential for gastric regurgitation and the risk for pulmonary aspiration, a choice must be made about whether to use the cLMA as a definitive airway or as a conduit for endotracheal intubation. The technical problems associated with the cLMA include the less than ideal position of the LMA in relation to the glottic opening and the downfolding of epiglottis in the LMA aperture bars. The blind passage of an ET through the cLMA has an unacceptably low degree of success. Difficulties include catching the ET tip on the aperture bars or the anterior commissure because of the natural bend in a standard polyvinyl chloride ET and the natural bend where the tube exits the LMA. Heath and Allagain[103] could intubate the trachea blindly through the cLMA

Table 32-2 **Incidence of Aspiration with the Laryngeal Mask Airway**

Authors	Ratio
Haden (1994)	1:3500
Wainwright (1995)	0:1877
Verghese (1996)	1:11910
Brimacombe (1996)	0:1500
Lopez-Gil (1996)	0:2000

Data from Haden,[94] Wainwright,[270] Verghese,[267] Brimacombe,[24] and Lopez-Gil.[136]

when CP was not applied in 72% of patients at first attempt and in a majority of patients when time was not limited. However, the blind technique of intubation through the cLMA often requires significant manipulation of the head and neck to accomplish the intubation. A gum elastic bougie can be used to aid endotracheal intubation. A high success rate was obtained with patients in whom DI was not anticipated by inserting the bougie with its angulated end pointing anteriorly until it passed through the grille of the cLMA and then rotating the bougie 180 degrees.[5] Failures, however, have been reported with this visually unassisted guided technique of endotracheal intubation through the cLMA.[275] Because of these potential problems, in an urgent situation, blind intubation through the cLMA may not be advisable. Fiberoptic-guided intubation through the cLMA has been shown to be the most reliable technique, which has a much higher success rate (Fig. 32-2).[103,239]

If the cLMA is used as a definitive airway without the passage of an ET, the timing of the removal of the device in a patient with a full stomach becomes crucial. A previous randomized, controlled trial demonstrated that the pH in the lower esophagus was significantly higher in patients in whom the cLMA remained in situ until the end of the case (at which point the patient was able to follow commands). It is suggested, therefore, that the cLMA should be removed only when the patient has fully regained consciousness at the end of the anesthetic.[47]

2. Intubating Laryngeal Mask Airway-Fastrach

After attempts to intubate the trachea of patients with a full stomach have failed, an alternative to using the cLMA is to use the LMA-Fastrach or ILMA. The ILMA is designed specifically to overcome the problems associated with (blind) endotracheal intubation using the cLMA. The ILMA-Fastrach consists of a rigid, anatomically curved airway tube made of stainless steel with a standard 15-mm connector. The tube is wide enough to accommodate an 8.0 ET and short enough to ensure passage of the ET beyond the vocal cords.

The highest degree of success in intubating the trachea blindly through the ILMA can be achieved by using the special endotracheal tube supplied with the ILMA (Euromedical ILM endotracheal tube, Euromedical, Malaysia). This silicon tube is soft tipped, straight, wire reinforced, and cuffed. Ferson and coauthors[77] reported their clinical experience with the ILMA in 254 patients with DA, including patients with Cormack-Lehane grade 4 views; patients with immobilized cervical spines; those with airways distorted by tumors, surgery, or radiation therapy; and those wearing stereotactic frames. The device was particularly useful in the emergency and elective surgery of patients in whom intubation with a rigid laryngoscope had failed.[7,137,274] There are similar multicenter trials and reports involving the use of an ILMA in patients with DAs and failed endotracheal intubation (including emergency cases at risk for aspiration).[10,112,131,188,226,227,271] The ILMA has also been used as a rescue device by emergency

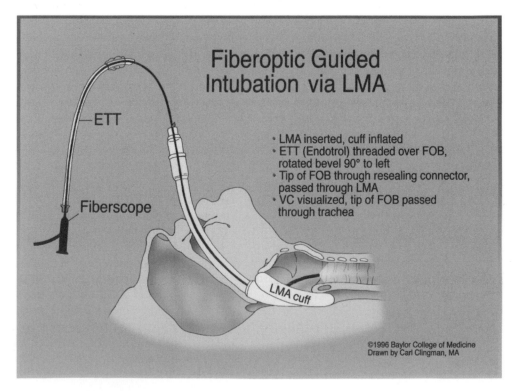

Figure 32-2 Fiberoptic-guided intubation. The fiberscope is inserted through the laryngeal mask airway (LMA), vocal cords (VC), and into trachea. The endotracheal tube (ETT) is mounted on the fiberscope. The endotracheal tube is threaded over the fiberscope into the LMA shaft with the bevel pointed to the left; as it enters through the maximum aperture bars, it is rotated anteriorly. Once it is located in the trachea, the placement is confirmed with presence of end-tidal CO_2. FOB, fiberoptic bronchoscope. (From Publications and Creative Services–Baylor College of Medicine.)

Fiberoptic Guided Intubation via LMA

—ETT

Fiberscope

- LMA inserted, cuff inflated
- ETT (Endotrol) threaded over FOB, rotated bevel 90° to left
- Tip of FOB through resealing connector, passed through LMA
- VC visualized, tip of FOB passed through trachea

LMA cuff

©1996 Baylor College of Medicine
Drawn by Carl Clingman, MA

room physicians after failed RSI.[204] We have described a case report in which the ILMA proved to be a lifesaving rescue device following failed endotracheal intubation during emergency cesarean section.[238]

3. ProSeal LMA

The ProSeal LMA (PLMA) recently introduced into clinical practice is a complex and potentially useful device for patients particularly at risk for gastric regurgitation and pulmonary aspiration. Some anesthesiologists refuse to use the classic LMA because of their concerns regarding gastric distention with positive-pressure ventilation and the potential risk of pulmonary aspiration. To address these issues, the primary goal of designing the PLMA was to construct a device with improved ventilatory characteristics that also offered protection against gastric insufflation and regurgitation. The principal feature of the PLMA is a double mask forming two end-to-end junctions: one with the respiratory tract and the other with the gastrointestinal tract. In contrast, the original cLMA forms a single end-to-end junction with the respiratory tract. The PLMA has a modified posterior cuff that provides a high seal at low pressures. The PLMA also offers a better airway seal at a given pressure than the cLMA.[138] When properly positioned, the distal orifice of the PLMA lies against the UES and separates the esophagus and stomach from the glottic area. It has an integral gastric access–venting port that allows passage of a 14 Fr gastric tube, allowing suctioning of gastric contents.

In awake volunteers, neither the PLMA nor the cLMA appeared to interfere with UES or LES tone.[120] There have been no manometric studies performed to assess LES function in anesthetized patients, but FOB inspection of the PLMA drainage tube showed that the UES is completely open in 3% to 7% of paralyzed patients[26] and in 9% of nonparalyzed patients.[29] This effect, which may have implications for the frequency of regurgitation into the drainage tube, may be mechanical, a local reflex, or result from direct exposure to atmosphere through the drainage tube.

The PLMA is easy to insert and is a more effective ventilatory device when using positive-pressure ventilation. A meta-analysis using Fisher's method[205] has shown that the PLMA forms a more effective seal with the respiratory tract than the cLMA. The efficacy of the seal with the gastrointestinal tract has been determined by measuring the airway pressure at which air leaks into the drainage tube in anesthetized adults. Depending on cuff volume,[28] the efficacy of the seal for air is at least 27 to 29 cm H_2O[27,138]; for fluid, the efficacy is 19 to 73 cm H_2O, with the seal mechanism being similar for the respiratory tract.

The drainage tube provides a conduit to the gastrointestinal tract. It is also possible to insert a gastric balloon tube to reduce further the risk of pulmonary aspiration.[221] The success rate for gastric tube insertion is 88% to 100%.[27,29] The advantages of inserting a gastric tube are that (1) the tube allows removal of gas or fluid from the stomach, (2) the process of insertion provides information about the position or patency of the drainage tube, and (3) the tube can function as a guide for PLMA reinsertion if accidental displacement occurs.[65]

The incidence of gastric insufflation seems to be low, even at high airway pressures.[118,138] In fact, gastric insufflation has been detected in only 1 of 572 patients (data collected from seven studies).[22,26,27,29,105,118,138] Gastric insufflation is less common with the PLMA than with the cLMA[138] when high airway positive-pressure ventilation is used.

There are reports of this device being used in the DA scenario. Keller and colleagues,[118] in a prospective study of morbidly obese patients (i.e., patients at risk for gastric regurgitation and pulmonary aspiration), found that the PLMA was successful in 11 of 11 patients who were either difficult or impossible to intubate with a laryngoscope. However, there are two case reports of pulmonary aspiration of gastric contents using the PLMA. In the first patient, brownish fluid was seen ejecting from the drainage tube of PLMA after administration of reversal agents at the end of surgery. There were clinical signs of pulmonary aspiration without any radiologic changes.[125] In the second patient, foldover malposition of the distal cuff against the posterior oropharyngeal wall (confirmed later by FOB) during insertion was cited as the reason for pulmonary aspiration.[25]

There are two reports of the successful use of the PLMA in obstetric patients following failed endotracheal intubation.[119] Keller and colleagues showed that the PLMA not only was a rescue device following failed endotracheal intubation in an obstetric patient with the hemolysis, elevated liver enzymes, and low platelets (HELLP) syndrome but also proved to be useful for postoperative respiratory support for 8 hours until the platelet count had increased and the patient was hemodynamically stable.[119]

Emergence characteristics for the PLMA seem to be similar to those for the cLMA.[26] The main practical considerations are to suction and remove the gastric tube and to reverse any residual neuromuscular blockade before beginning of emergence. As with the cLMA, the patient should not be disturbed and the PLMA should be removed only when the patient is conscious and obeys commands.

B. USE OF THE ESOPHAGEAL-TRACHEAL COMBITUBE (ETC) IN THE FULL-STOMACH PATIENT

The ETC, developed by Frass and colleagues, is a disposable, polyvinyl chloride, double-lumen airway device that combines the features of an esophageal obturator airway and an ET.[84] It functions well in both the esophageal and tracheal positions.[81] Using the Lipp maneuver,[132] the ETC is inserted blindly. Insertion usually results in esophageal placement (Fig. 32-3) and ventilation is initiated through the gastric lumen.[250] With both cuffs inflated, ventilation through the proximal lumen allows airflow through eight oval fenestrations from the hypopharynx into the trachea.

Figure 32-3 Esophageal-tracheal Combitube (ETC) in esophagus. The tube is advanced until the black rings are at the level of the teeth. The distal cuff is inflated with 15 mL of air to seal the esophagus, and the proximal cuff is inflated with 80 to 100 mL of air; this serves to secure the tube in position and occlude the nasal and oral passages. Ventilation is attempted through lumen No. 1. (From Publications and Creative Services–Baylor College of Medicine.)

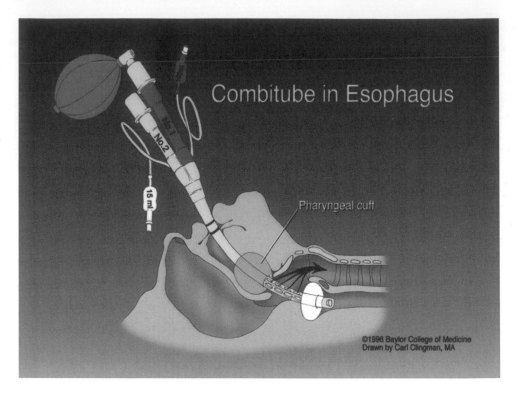

The effective seal of the oropharyngeal balloon prevents the escape of air from the mouth and nose. Instead, air is forced into the trachea and lungs. If the ETC is placed in the esophagus, gastric fluids can be aspirated through the gastric lumen. If breath sounds are not heard, the ETC has more than likely been placed in the trachea (Fig. 32-4). Without removing the ETC, ventilation is switched to the tracheoesophageal lumen and confirmed with auscultation and capnography.

Unsatisfactory ventilation through either lumen indicates that the ETC is too far advanced into the esophagus to produce airway obstruction by the oropharyngeal balloon (Fig. 32-5A). In this situation, both the distal cuff and the oropharyngeal balloon are deflated and the

Figure 32-4 Esophageal-tracheal Combitube (ETC) placement in trachea. The ETC is placed in trachea; the ventilation is shifted to lumen No. 2. (From Publications and Creative Services–Baylor College of Medicine.)

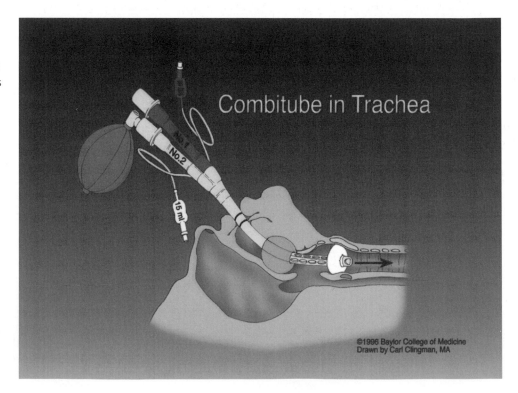

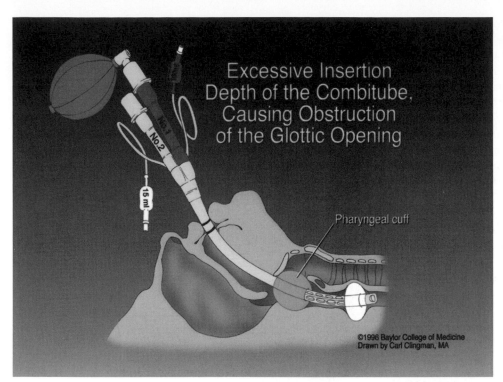

A

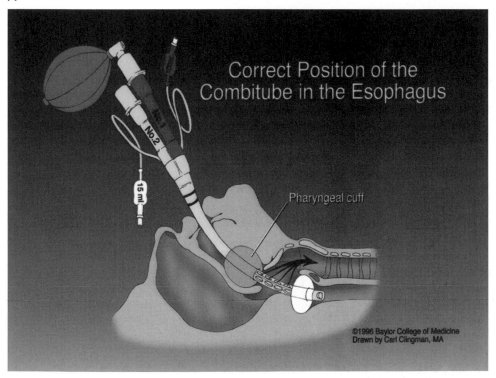

B

Figure 32-5 Improper placement of esophageal-tracheal Combitube (ETC). **A,** Excessive insertion depth of the ETC, causing obstruction of the glottic opening. Ventilation is not possible. **B,** Readjustment of ETC, which is pulled back 2 to 3 cm (indicated by the two black rings), and ventilation through lumen No. 1 allow the passage of gas from the side orifices into the trachea. (From Publications and Creative Services–Baylor College of Medicine.)

ETC is withdrawn approximately 2 to 3 cm (Fig. 32-5B). The distal cuff and the oropharyngeal balloon are then reinflated and pulmonary ventilation is resumed.[236]

The ETC serves as a rescue device for establishing an airway in "cannot intubate" and "cannot intubate, cannot ventilate" situations, and it is particularly useful in the full-stomach patient. It is inserted blindly or under direct laryngoscopy,[80] is shown to secure the airway easily and rapidly, and requires minimal preparation (i.e., the device can be properly used even with relatively little formal training).[18] ETC placement by inexperienced personnel (e.g., ICU nurses) under medical supervision was found to be as safe and efficacious in providing effective oxygenation and ventilation of lungs as endotracheal intubation performed by ICU physicians during cardiopulmonary resuscitation.[233] As a rescue device, it is helpful in securing the airway if vocal cord visualization is compromised or if oropharyngeal bleeding has occurred.

The ETC prevents pulmonary aspiration during cardiopulmonary resuscitation,[81] especially when protective airway reflexes are absent, and therefore it protects the airway from pulmonary aspiration of gastric contents.[251] Frass and coworkers[81] noted that the tracheoesophageal lumen served as a conduit for decompression of gastric contents and allowed gastric suctioning. Urtubia and associates[251] administered methylene blue orally to 25 patients before induction of anesthesia and found no evidence of methylene blue in the hypopharynx during laryngoscopy prior to ETC placement or after its removal. In addition, Hagberg and colleagues[96] determined that the ETC and the cLMA are comparable with regard to the incidence of pulmonary aspiration.

C. USE OF THE ESOPHAGEAL-TRACHEAL COMBITUBE AND PREVENTION OF PULMONARY ASPIRATION

Multiple case reports attest to the safety of use of the ETC and the use of the tracheoesophageal lumen as an effective decompression channel for regurgitated gastric contents that prevents pulmonary aspiration during cardiopulmonary resuscitation[241] or during anesthesia.[63,96] The 10 Fr orogastric tube, available in the prepackaged ETC kit, can be readily used for esophageal and gastric suctioning. The ETC has been used successfully as a primary airway device in seven patients (R. M. Urtubia, personal communication), two of whom were reported.[252] They did not

have a history of difficult endotracheal intubation in the past but underwent general anesthesia for emergency cesarean section. The ETC was used as the initial airway device and allowed adequate oxygenation-ventilation and protection from pulmonary aspiration of gastric contents.[252] Wissler[280] reported the use of the ETC under direct laryngoscopy during obstetric anesthesia and stated that the ETC is the primary device of his choice in an anesthetized parturient whose trachea cannot be intubated or whose lungs cannot be mask ventilated while applying CP.

If endotracheal intubation becomes necessary, it can be achieved using the FOB with the ETC in place. The fiberscope is passed alongside the ETC, the oropharyngeal balloon is partially deflated, and endotracheal intubation is achieved visually and is followed by removal of the ETC without interruption of airway control, oxygenation, or ventilation (Fig. 32-6). This technique has been used for both spontaneously breathing[85] and mechanically ventilated patients.[186] We report a case of a morbidly obese, 550-lb female patient with obstructive sleep apnea, who had been in the ICU with an ETC in situ. Endotracheal intubation was needed to help with weaning the patient from the ventilator. Using the hybrid technique of direct laryngoscopy and fiberoptic bronchoscopy, we safely performed endotracheal intubation followed by ETC removal.

Video film recordings of 25 patients undergoing laparoscopic cholecystectomy under general anesthesia and mechanical ventilation using the ETC revealed no gastric insufflation at the beginning or end of surgery.[253] A large retrospective survey of 12,020 cases of nontraumatic cardiac arrest in Japan revealed 1594 instances of ETC use without any evidence of pulmonary aspiration of gastric contents.[241]

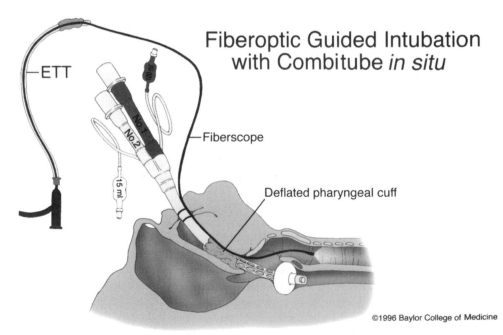

Figure 32-6 Replacement of esophageal-tracheal Combitube with fiberoptic scope guides endotracheal intubation. ETT, endotracheal tube. (From Publications and Creative Services–Baylor College of Medicine.)

ETT

Fiberoptic Guided Intubation with Combitube in situ

Fiberscope

Deflated pharyngeal cuff

©1996 Baylor College of Medicine

Advantages of using the ETC compared with the LMA include the following:

1. Preparation time is minimal.
2. The device is ideal for full-stomach patients and pregnant patients, especially after failed endotracheal intubation. In these patients, oxygenation, avoidance of arterial desaturation, and pulmonary aspiration are key factors.
3. Lubrication is not required.
4. No special method is required for cuff inflation/deflation.

There are, however, a few case reports of complications related to the use of the ETC. These reports primarily involve the previous version of the device and are attributed to the stiffer, rather large (41 Fr), and potentially traumatic[99] design of the device. These complications have included esophageal rupture, subcutaneous emphysema, piriform sinus rupture, pneumomediastinum, and pneumoperitoneum.[198,268] Common factors in all of these complications included difficult ambient conditions in the field or prehospital environment, multiple attempts to insert the device, resistance with insertion, and the use of excessive force.

The following recommendations help both minimize the complications and enhance the rate of successful placement of the ETC: (1) use the smaller Combitube SA (small adult) universally for patients between 4 and 6 ft tall; (2) dip the device in warm saline, briefly, prior to use; (3) use the Lipp maneuver (holding the two ends of the ETC together to bend it into a semicircle for a few seconds prior to insertion) during placement of the device; (4) place the device under direct laryngoscopy[80]; (5) use a gentle technique to reduce the hemodynamic response from stimulation of the proprioceptors at the base of the tongue[99]; (6) inflate the oropharyngeal balloon slowly and to the minimum volume necessary for an airtight seal to reduce soft tissue injury[99]; and (7) and employ a reliable technique, using direct laryngoscopy as an aid to ETC placement, if necessary.[80] Even though there are no large, randomized studies available that indicate the relative safety of the ETC in preventing pulmonary aspiration of gastric contents, the preceding recommendations are useful and appealing to health care personnel managing patients who have a full stomach, with or without a DA.

IX. EXTUBATION

When an AI or RSI is indicated to prevent pulmonary aspiration, an awake tracheal extubation is also indicated.[91] The patient should be awake, conscious, and appropriately responding to commands prior to extubation. Daley and colleagues[59] performed a survey of tracheal extubation of adult surgical patients who were still deeply anesthetized. The majority of the respondents in the survey, who otherwise used the technique for extubation, considered risk of pulmonary aspiration a contraindication to deep tracheal extubation.

X. MANAGEMENT OF PULMONARY ASPIRATION

When a fully conscious person aspirates substances into the tracheobronchial tree, a brief but effective bout of coughing can clear the aspirate. Patients with an observed pulmonary aspiration under sedation should have their mouth and pharynx suctioned immediately so that patency of upper airway is restored. Suctioning solid or liquid material allows recovery of the aspirated material so that it is not absorbed by the lungs and also stimulates coughing to expel the aspirate further. Once asphyxiation has been averted, bronchoscopy can be performed to clear the obstructing material from the lower airways. Bronchoscopy should not be routinely performed but rather reserved for patients who have aspirated sufficient solid material to cause significant airway obstruction.[91] Damage to the mucosa of the tracheobronchial tree occurs within seconds, but the bronchial secretions neutralize the aspirated acid within minutes.[286] Attempts to neutralize the acid aspirate with saline or bicarbonate lavage have proved to be futile and have been hypothesized to increase any damage.[107]

The treatment of pulmonary aspiration of gastric contents is aimed at restoring pulmonary function to normal as soon as possible. If the patient is awake and able to maintain a reasonable arterial oxygen tension (PaO_2), a conservative approach would be to provide supplemental oxygen through a face mask. The inspired oxygen concentration (FIO_2) can be increased to maintain PaO_2 at approximately 60 mm Hg. This may suffice in a patient with a mild condition, but more aggressive therapy is indicated if aspiration is more severe. Severe bronchospasm may be treated by aminophylline infusion or the inhalation of a β-adrenergic bronchodilator.[107,264]

When severe pulmonary aspiration is suspected, early ventilatory support is the mainstay of treatment. Early continuous positive airway pressure (CPAP) is indicated in awake and alert patients who do not respond to a face mask. CPAP can be administered through a tight-fitting mask up to 12 to 14 mm Hg. If higher levels are required, mechanical ventilation should be considered. The level of CPAP can be reduced as the patient improves, but it should not be completely withdrawn before the alveoli can maintain stability. A high FIO_2 can be utilized initially but should be decreased as soon as possible.[167]

If the patient is obtunded, an ET should be placed and mechanical ventilation initiated. Positive end-expiratory pressure (PEEP) should be applied, and, again, FIO_2 should be decreased as soon as possible while adequate oxygenation is maintained. PEEP is commonly used to elevate functional residual capacity and prevent atelectasis resulting from poor ventilatory efforts.[264] It also improves the ventilation/perfusion ($\dot{V}/\dot{Q}$) ratio and allows the use of less toxic levels of oxygen to be administered, thus giving the lungs a chance to recover.[286] Caution should be exercised when using PEEP as high levels can worsen pulmonary damage by causing increased transudation of fluid through injured capillary beds.[243] Cereda and coworkers investigated the effect of PEEP in patients with acute lung injury and found that a PEEP of at least 15 cm H_2O was needed to prevent a decay in the respiratory system compliance.[44]

Despite these measures, if hypoxemia persists along with bilateral lung infiltrates and poor lung compliance, management should be similar to that for the acute respiratory distress syndrome (ARDS). A large, National Institutes of Health–sponsored, multicenter, randomized trial was performed comparing ventilation with lower versus traditional tidal volumes in patients with ARDS.[266] Smaller tidal volumes (6 mL/kg predicted body weight) and hypoventilation with permissive hypercapnia were associated with a 10% reduction in mortality, along with a shorter period of time using mechanical ventilation. The lower tidal volume ventilation approach protected the lungs from excessive stretch, resulting in improvement in several important clinical indicators of outcome in patients with ARDS.[266] An alveolar recruitment maneuver using a CPAP of 40 cm H_2O for 40 seconds has been shown to improve oxygenation in patients with early ARDS who do not have impairment of the chest wall.[255] A recruitment maneuver with a smaller tidal volume was associated with a survival rate of 62%, compared with a rate of 29% when using conventional ventilation without the recruitment maneuver.[6]

Use of prophylactic antibiotics is not recommended.[147] Antibiotics alter the normal flora of the respiratory tract, which predisposes the susceptible patient to secondary infection with resistant organisms. Mitsushima and colleagues[159] demonstrated that acid aspiration induced epithelial injury leading to subsequent bacterial infection in mice. Approximately 20% to 30% of patients who manifest initial gastric content aspiration eventually develop a secondary infection.[196] Antibiotics should be reserved for patients who show signs of clinical infection and for patients who have aspirated grossly contaminated material into their lungs.

Wolfe and coauthors[281] found that pneumonia resulting from gram-negative bacteria was more frequent after pulmonary aspiration among patients treated with corticosteroids than those who were not treated. Corticosteroids interfered with the healing of granulomatous lesions in experimental rabbits.[287] The current consensus appears to be that corticosteroids play no role in the treatment of aspiration pneumonitis.[62]

XI. CONCLUSION

Anesthetic intervention in patients with a full stomach presents the anesthesiologist with three challenges: prevention of gastric regurgitation, prevention of pulmonary aspiration, and appropriate airway management. Large surveys of pulmonary aspiration in general surgical patients found a low incidence of pulmonary aspiration of gastric contents with only a slightly greater risk in obstetric and pediatric patients. The resulting morbidity is also low, and mortality is rare. Changes in anesthetic practice and training have probably contributed to the decline in this dreaded complication. Preoperative fasting was introduced to reduce the risk and severity of aspiration pneumonitis. Adequate time (6 hours) must still be allowed before surgery for solid foods to be emptied; however, there is overwhelming weight of support to reduce the preoperative fluid fast for pediatric patients and to allow free clear fluids until 2 hours before any scheduled surgery. The routine preoperative use of multiple pharmacologic agents in patients who have no apparent risk for pulmonary aspiration is not recommended. Meticulous attention to airway management of patients at risk for pulmonary aspiration is crucial. RSI and CP, although accepted in routine practice, have never had scientific validation. In addition, a large number of patients at risk for pulmonary aspiration (e.g., pregnant, obese, extremes of age, and patients with comorbidities) are likely to desaturate more rapidly during prolonged periods of apnea associated with difficult endotracheal intubation during RSI. Awake endotracheal intubation and preparedness to deal with difficult or failed intubation in patients with a full stomach are crucial to successful management of these patients.

REFERENCES

1. Adams AP: General principles of emergency anaesthesia. In Adams AP, Hewitt PB, Rogers MC (eds): Emergency Anaesthesia. London, Edward Arnold, 1986, pp 1-13.
2. Agarwal A, Chari P, Singh H: Fluid deprivation before operation. The effect of a small drink. Anaesthesia 44: 632-634, 1989.
3. Agro F, Brimacombe J, Verghese C, et al: Laryngeal mask airway and incidence of gastro-oesophageal reflux in paralysed patients undergoing ventilation for elective orthopaedic surgery. Br J Anaesth 81:537-539, 1998.
4. Aitkenhead AR, Smith G: Textbook of Anaesthesia. Edinburgh, Churchill Livingstone, 1996, pp 523-525.
5. Allison A, McCrory J: Tracheal placement of a gum elastic bougie using the laryngeal mask airways. Anaesthesia 45: 419-420, 1990.
6. Amato MB, Barbas CS, Medeiros DM, et al: Effect of a protective-ventilation strategy on mortality in the acute respiratory distress syndrome. N Engl J Med 338:347-354, 1998.
7. Asai T, Hirose T, Shingu K: Failed tracheal intubation using a laryngoscope and intubating laryngeal mask. Can J Anaesth 47:325-328, 2000.
8. Baraka AS, Sayyid SS, Assaf BA: Thiopental-rocuronium versus ketamine-rocuronium for rapid-sequence intubation

in parturients undergoing cesarean section. Anesth Analg 84:1104-1107, 1997.

9. Barnard P, Jenkins J: Failed tracheal intubation in obstetrics: A 6-year review in a UK hospital. Anaesthesia 55:685-694, 2000.

10. Baskett PJ, Parr MJ, Nolan JP: The intubating laryngeal mask. Results of a multicentre trial with experience of 500 cases. Anaesthesia 53:1174-1179, 1998.

11. Baxter AD: Cricoid pressure in the sniffing position. Anaesthesia 46:327, 1991.

12. Beaumont W: Experiments and Observation on the Gastric Juice and Physiology of Digestion. Boston, Lily, Wait, 1834, pp 159-160.

13. Benhamou D: French obstetric anaesthetists and acid aspiration prophylaxis. Eur J Anaesthesiol 10:27-32, 1993.

14. Benhamou D: Controversies in obstetric anaesthesia. Cricoid pressure is unnecessary in obstetric general anaesthesia. Int J Obstet Anaesth 4:30-33, 1995.

15. Benumof JL: Difficult laryngoscopy: Obtaining the best view. Can J Anaesth 41:361-365, 1994.

16. Benumof JL: Management of the difficult adult airway. With special emphasis on awake tracheal intubation. Anesthesiology 75:1087-1110, 1991.

17. Berg H: Is residual neuromuscular block following pancuronium a risk factor for postoperative pulmonary complications? Acta Anaesthesiol Scand Suppl 110: 156-158, 1997.

18. Bishop MJ, Kharasch ED: Is the Combitube a useful emergency airway device for anesthesiologists? Anesth Analg 86:1141-1142, 1998.

19. Blitt CD, Gutman HL, Cohen DD, et al: "Silent" regurgitation and aspiration during general anesthesia. Anesth Analg 49:707-713, 1970.

20. Bonica JJ: Transtracheal anaesthesia for endotracheal intubation. Anesthesiology 10:736-738, 1949.

21. Booth MG, Marsh B, Bryden FM, et al: A comparison of the pharmacodynamics of rocuronium and vecuronium during halothane anaesthesia. Anaesthesia 47:832-834, 1992.

22. Brain AI, Verghese C, Strube PJ: The LMA 'ProSeal TM'—A laryngeal mask with an oesophageal vent. Br J Anaesth 84:650-654, 2000.

23. Bricker SR, McLuckie A, Nightingale DA: Gastric aspirates after trauma in children. Anaesthesia 44: 721-724, 1989.

24. Brimacombe J: Analysis of 1500 laryngeal mask uses by one anaesthetist in adults undergoing routine anaesthesia. Anaesthesia 51:76-80, 1996.

25. Brimacombe J, Keller C: Aspiration of gastric contents during use of a ProSeal™ laryngeal mask airway secondary to unidentified foldover malposition. Anesth Analg 97:1192-1194, table, 2003.

26. Brimacombe J, Keller C: Stability of the LMA-ProSeal and standard laryngeal mask airway in different head and neck positions: A randomised crossover study. Eur J Anaesthesiol 20:65-69, 2003.

27. Brimacombe J, Keller C: The ProSeal™ laryngeal mask airway: A randomized, crossover study with the standard laryngeal mask airway in paralyzed, anesthetized patients. Anesthesiology 93:104-109, 2000.

28. Brimacombe J, Keller C: The ProSeal™ laryngeal mask airway. Anesthesiol Clin North Am 20:871-891, 2002.

29. Brimacombe J, Keller C, Fullekrug B, et al: A multicenter study comparing the ProSeal and Classic laryngeal mask airway in anesthetized, nonparalyzed patients. Anesthesiology 96:289-295, 2002.

30. Brimacombe JR, Berry AM: Cricoid pressure. Can J Anaesth 44:414-425, 1997.

31. Brimacombe JR, Berry A: The incidence of aspiration associated with the laryngeal mask airway: A meta-analysis of published literature. J Clin Anesth 7:297-305, 1995.

32. Brock-Utne JG, Downing JW, O'Keefe SJ, Gjessing J: Protection against acid pulmonary aspiration with cimetidine. Anaesth Intensive Care 11:138-140, 1983.

33. Brodsky JB, Brock-Utne AJ, Levi DC, et al: Pulmonary aspiration of a milk/cream mixture. Anesthesiology 91:1533-1534, 1999.

34. Broussard CN, Richter JE: Treating gastro-oesophageal reflux disease during pregnancy and lactation: What are the safest therapy options? Drug Saf 19:325-337, 1998.

35. Lunn JN, Devlin HB: Lessons from the confidential enquiry into perioperative deaths in three NHS regions. Lancet 2:1384-1386, 1987.

36. Bunchungmongkol N, Chumpathong S, Catto-Smith AG, et al: Effects of the laryngeal mask airway on the lower oesophageal barrier pressure in children. Anaesth Intensive Care 28:543-546, 2000.

37. Butler PJ, Dhara SS: Prediction of difficult laryngoscopy: An assessment of the thyromental distance and Mallampati predictive tests. Anaesth Intensive Care 20:139-142, 1992.

38. Cadamy AJ, Booth MG, Cademy AJ: Rapid sequence induction. Anaesthesia 54:817, 1999.

39. Caplan RA, Posner KL, Ward RJ, Cheney FW: Adverse respiratory events in anesthesia: A closed claims analysis. Anesthesiology 72:828-833, 1990.

40. Caranza R, Nandwani N, Tring JP, et al: Upper airway reflex sensitivity following general anaesthesia for day-case surgery. Anaesthesia 55:367-370, 2000.

41. Carlsson C, Islander G: Silent gastropharyngeal regurgitation during anesthesia. Anesth Analg 60:655-657, 1981.

42. Cavell B: Gastric emptying in preterm infants. Acta Paediatr Scand 68:527-531, 1979.

43. Cavell B: Gastric emptying in infants fed human milk or infant formula. Acta Paediatr Scand 70:639-641, 1981.

44. Cereda M, Foti G, Musch G, et al: Positive end-expiratory pressure prevents the loss of respiratory compliance during low tidal volume ventilation in acute lung injury patients. Chest 109:480-485, 1996.

45. Chadwick IS, Vohra A: Anaesthesia for emergency caesarean section using the Brain laryngeal airway. Anaesthesia 44:261-262, 1989.

46. Chassard D, Tournadre JP, Berrada KR, et al: Effect of halothane, isoflurane and desflurane on lower oesophageal sphincter tone. Br J Anaesth 77:781-783, 1996.

47. Cheong YP, Park SK, Son Y, et al: Comparison of incidence of gastroesophageal reflux and regurgitation associated with timing of removal of the laryngeal mask airway: On appearance of signs of rejection versus after recovery of consciousness. J Clin Anesth 11:657-662, 1999.

48. Chin C, Lerman J, Endo J: Acute lung injury after tracheal instillation of acidified soya-based or Enfalac formula or human breast milk in rabbits. Can J Anaesth 46:282-286, 1999.

49. Chisholm DG, Calder I: Experience with the McCoy laryngoscope in difficult laryngoscopy. Anaesthesia 52: 906-908, 1997.

50. Cohen SE, Jasson J, Talafre ML, et al: Does metoclopramide decrease the volume of gastric contents in patients undergoing cesarean section? Anesthesiology 61:604-607, 1984.

51. Colman RD, Frank M, Loughnan BA, et al: Use of i.m. ranitidine for the prophylaxis of aspiration pneumonitis in obstetrics. Br J Anaesth 61:720-729, 1988.

52. Cook TM: Cricoid pressure: Are two hands better than one? Anaesthesia 51:365-368, 1996.

53. Cook TM, McCrirrick A: A survey of airway management during induction of general anaesthesia in obstetrics. Int J Obstet Anesth 3:143-145, 1994.

54. Cote CJ, Goudsouzian NG, Liu LM, et al: Assessment of risk factors related to the acid aspiration syndrome in pediatric patients—Gastric pH and residual volume. Anesthesiology 56:70-72, 1982.

55. Cotton BR, Smith G: The lower oesophageal sphincter and anaesthesia. Br J Anaesth 56:37-46, 1984.

56. Cowling J: Cricoid pressure—A more comfortable technique. Anaesth Intensive Care 10:93-94, 1982.

57. Crawford M: Fasting in children prior to surgery. Anesth Analg 71:402-403, 1990.

58. Crowley DS, Giesecke AH: Bimanual cricoid pressure. Anaesthesia 45:588-589, 1990.

59. Daley MD, Norman PH, Coveler LA: Tracheal extubation of adult surgical patients while deeply anesthetized: A survey of United States anesthesiologists. J Clin Anesth 11:445-452, 1999.

60. DeMello WF, Kocan M: The laryngeal mask in failed intubation [letter]. Anaesthesia 45:689-690, 1990.

61. Dent J, Dodds WJ, Friedman RH, et al: Mechanism of gastroesophageal reflux in recumbent asymptomatic human subjects. J Clin Invest 65:256-267, 1980.

62. DePaso WJ: Aspiration pneumonia. Clin Chest Med 12:269-284, 1991.

63. Deroy R, Ghoris M: The Combitube elective anesthetic airway management in a patient with cervical spine fracture. Anesth Analg 87:1441-1442, 1998.

64. Dive A, Miesse C, Galanti L, et al: Effect of erythromycin on gastric motility in mechanically ventilated critically ill patients: A double-blind, randomized, placebo-controlled study. Crit Care Med 23:1356-1362, 1995.

65. Drolet P, Girard M: An aid to correct positioning of the ProSeal™ laryngeal mask. Can J Anaesth 48:718-719, 2001.

66. Duncan JA: Intubation of the trachea in the conscious patient. Br J Anaesth 49:619-623, 1977.

67. el Ganzouri AR, McCarthy RJ, Tuman KJ, et al: Preoperative airway assessment: Predictive value of a multivariate risk index. Anesth Analg 82:1197-1204, 1996.

68. Emerson BM, Wrigley SR, Newton M: Pre-operative fasting for paediatric anaesthesia. A survey of current practice. Anaesthesia 53:326-330, 1998.

69. Engbaek J, Viby-Mogensen J: Can rocuronium replace succinylcholine in a rapid induction of anaesthesia? Acta Anaesthesiol Scand 43:1-3, 1993.

70. Engelhardt T, Webster NR: Pulmonary aspiration of gastric contents in anaesthesia. Br J Anaesth 83: 453-460, 1999.

71. Eriksson LI, Sandin R: Fasting guidelines in different countries. Acta Anaesthesiol Scand 40:971-974, 1996.

72. Escolano F, Castano J, Lopez R, et al: Effects of omeprazole, ranitidine, famotidine and placebo on gastric secretion in patients undergoing elective surgery. Br J Anaesth 69:404-406, 1992.

73. Ewart MC, Yau G, Gin T, et al: A comparison of the effects of omeprazole and ranitidine on gastric secretion in women undergoing elective caesarean section. Anaesthesia 45:527-530, 1990.

74. Fanning GL: The efficacy of cricoid pressure in preventing regurgitation of gastric contents. Anesthesiology 32: 553-555, 1970.

75. Fasting S, Soreide E, Raeder JC: Changing preoperative fasting policies. Impact of a national consensus. Acta Anaesthesiol Scand 42:1188-1191, 1998.

76. Ferrer M, Bauer TT, Torres A, et al: Effect of nasogastric tube size on gastroesophageal reflux and microaspiration in intubated patients. Ann Intern Med 130:991-994, 1999.

77. Ferson DZ, Rosenblatt WH, Johansen MJ, et al: Use of the intubating LMA-Fastrach in 254 patients with difficult-to-manage airways. Anesthesiology 95: 1175-1181, 2001.

78. Fox EJ, Sklar GS, Hill CH, et al: Complications related to the pressor response to endotracheal intubation. Anesthesiology 47:524-525, 1977.

79. Francis S, Enani S, Shah J, et al: Simulated cricoid force in paediatric anaesthesia. Br J Anaesth 85:164, 2000.

80. Frass M: The Combitube: esophageal/tracheal double lumen airway. In Benumof JL (ed): Airway Management—Principles and Practice. St. Louis, Mosby, 1996, pp 444-455.

81. Frass M, Frenzer R, Rauscha F, et al: Evaluation of esophageal tracheal Combitube in cardiopulmonary resuscitation. Crit Care Med 15:609-611, 1987.

82. Frerk CM: Predicting difficult intubation. Anaesthesia 46:1005-1008, 1991.

83. Fuchs-Buder T, Sparr HJ, Ziegenfuss T: Thiopental or etomidate for rapid sequence induction with rocuronium. Br J Anaesth 80:504-506, 1998.

84. Gaitini LA, Vaida SJ, Agro F: The Esophageal-Tracheal Combitube. Anesthesiol Clin North Am 20:893-906, 2002.

85. Gaitini LA, Vaida SJ, Somri M, et al: Fiberoptic-guided airway exchange of the esophageal-tracheal Combitube in spontaneously breathing versus mechanically ventilated patients. Anesth Analg 88:193-196, 1999.

86. Gardaz JP, Theumann N, Guyot J, et al: Effects of propofol on lower oesophageal sphincter pressure and barrier pressure. Eur J Anaesthesiol 13:203, 1996.

87. Gataure PS, Hughes JA: The laryngeal mask airway in obstetrical anaesthesia. Can J Anaesth 42:130-133, 1995.

88. Gataure PS, Vaughan RS, Latto IP: Simulated difficult intubation. Comparison of the gum elastic bougie and the stylet. Anaesthesia 51:935-938, 1996.

89. Gerardi MJ, Sacchetti AD, Cantor RM, et al: Rapid-sequence intubation of the pediatric patient. Pediatric Emergency Medicine Committee of the American College of Emergency Physicians. Ann Emerg Med 28:55-74, 1996.

90. Gibbs CP, Banner TC: Effectiveness of Bicitra as a preoperative antacid. Anesthesiology 61:97-99, 1984.

91. Gibbs CP, Modell JH: Pulmonary aspiration of gastric contents: Pathophysiology, prevention, and management. In Miller RD (ed): Anesthesia. New York, Churchill Livingstone, 1994, pp 1437-1464.

92. Green CR, Pandit SK, Schork MA: Preoperative fasting time: Is the traditional policy changing? Results of a national survey. Anesth Analg 83:123-128, 1996.

93. Haavik PE, Soreide E, Hofstad B, Steen PA: Does preoperative anxiety influence gastric fluid volume and acidity? Anesth Analg 75:91-94, 1992.

94. Haden RM, Pinnock CA, Scott PV: Incidence of aspiration with the laryngeal mask airway [letter]. Br J Anaesth 72:496, 1994.

95. Hagberg CA: Special devices and techniques. Anesthesiol Clin North Am 20:907-932, 2002.

96. Hagberg CA, Vartazarian TN, Chelly JE, Ovassapian A: The incidence of gastroesophageal reflux and tracheal aspiration detected with pH electrodes is similar with the Laryngeal Mask Airway and Esophageal Tracheal Combitube—A pilot study. Can J Anaesth 51:243-249, 2004.

97. Han TH, Brimacombe J, Lee EJ, Yang HS: The laryngeal mask airway is effective (and probably safe) in selected healthy parturients for elective cesarean section: A prospective study of 1067 cases. Can J Anaesth 48:1117-1121, 2001.

98. Hardy JF, Lepage Y, Bonneville-Chouinard N: Occurrence of gastroesophageal reflux on induction of anaesthesia does not correlate with the volume of gastric contents. Can J Anaesth 37:502-508, 1990.

99. Hartmann T, Krenn CG, Zoeggeler A, et al: The oesophageal-tracheal Combitube Small Adult. Anaesthesia 55:670-675, 2000.

100. Hartsilver EL, Vanner RG, Bewley J, Clayton T: Gastric pressure during emergency caesarean section under general anaesthesia. Br J Anaesth 82:752-754, 1999.

101. Hawthorne L, Wilson R, Lyons G, Dresner M: Failed intubation revisited: 17-yr experience in a teaching maternity unit. Br J Anaesth 76:680-684, 1996.

102. Heading RC: Gastric motility and emptying. In Sireus W, Smith AN (eds): Scientific Foundations of Gastroenterology. London, Heinemann, 2003, pp 287-296.

103. Heath ML, Allagain J: Intubation through the laryngeal mask. A technique for unexpected difficult intubation. Anaesthesia 46:545-548, 1991.

104. Horowitz M, Pounder DJ: Is the stomach a useful forensic clock? Aust NZ J Med 15:73-76, 1985.

105. Howath A, Brimacombe J, Keller C: Gum-elastic bougie–guided insertion of the ProSeal laryngeal mask airway: A new technique. Anaesth Intensive Care 30:818, 2002.

106. Hunt JN: Some properties of an alimentary osmoreceptor mechanism. J Physiol 132:267-288, 1956.

107. Hupp JR, Peterson LJ: Aspiration pneumonitis: Etiology, therapy, and prevention. J Oral Surg 39:430-435, 1981.

108. Hutchinson A, Maltby JR, Reid CR: Gastric fluid volume and pH in elective inpatients. Part I: Coffee or orange juice versus overnight fast. Can J Anaesth 35:12-15, 1988.

109. Ingebo KR, Rayhorn NJ, Hecht RM, et al: Sedation in children: Adequacy of two-hour fasting. J Pediatr 131:155-158, 1997.

110. Jahr JS, Burckart G, Smith SS, et al: Effects of famotidine on gastric pH and residual volume in pediatric surgery. Acta Anaesthesiol Scand 35:457-460, 1991.

111. James CF, Modell JH, Gibbs CP, et al: Pulmonary aspiration—Effects of volume and pH in the rat. Anesth Analg 63:665-668, 1984.

112. Joo H, Rose K: Fastrach—A new intubating laryngeal mask airway: Successful use in patients with difficult airways. Can J Anaesth 45:253-256, 1998.

113. Jorgensen NH, Byer DE, Gould AB Jr: Aspiration pneumonitis. Prevention and treatment. Minn Med 72:517-519, 530, 1989.

114. Kahrilas PJ, Dodds WJ, Dent J, et al: Effect of sleep, spontaneous gastroesophageal reflux, and a meal on upper esophageal sphincter pressure in normal human volunteers. Gastroenterology 92:466-471, 1987.

115. Kahrilas PJ, Lin S, Chen J, Manka M: The effect of hiatus hernia on gastro-oesophageal junction pressure. Gut 44:476-482, 1999.

116. Kallar SK, Everett LL: Potential risks and preventive measures for pulmonary aspiration: New concepts in preoperative fasting guidelines. Anesth Analg 77:171-182, 1993.

117. Katz RL, Bigger JT Jr: Cardiac arrhythmias during anesthesia and operation. Anesthesiology 33:193-213, 1970.

118. Keller C, Brimacombe J, Kleinsasser A, Brimacombe L: The laryngeal mask airway ProSeal as a temporary ventilatory device in grossly and morbidly obese patients before laryngoscope-guided tracheal intubation. Anesth Analg 94:737-740, 2002.

119. Keller C, Brimacombe J, Lirk P, Puhringer F: Failed obstetric tracheal intubation and postoperative respiratory support with the ProSeal laryngeal mask airway. Anesth Analg 98:1467-1470, 2004.

120. Keller C, Brimacombe J: Resting esophageal sphincter pressures and deglutition frequency in awake subjects after oropharyngeal topical anesthesia and laryngeal mask device insertion. Anesth Analg 93:226-229, 2001.

121. King TA, Adams AP: Failed tracheal intubation. Br J Anaesth 65:400-414, 1990.

122. Kluger MT, Short TG: Aspiration during anaesthesia: A review of 133 cases from the Australian Anaesthetic Incident Monitoring Study (AIMS). Anaesthesia 54:19-26, 1999.

123. Kluger MT, Willemsen G: Anti-aspiration prophylaxis in New Zealand: A national survey. Anaesth Intensive Care 26:70-77, 1998.

124. Knopp RK: Rapid sequence intubation revisited. Ann Emerg Med 31:398-400, 1998.

125. Koay CK: A case of aspiration using the ProSeal™ LMA. Anaesth Intensive Care 31:123, 2003.

126. Kristensen MS, Gellett S, Bach AB, Jensen TK: Hemodynamics and arterial oxygen saturation during preoperative emptying of the stomach. Acta Anaesthesiol Scand 35:342-344, 1991.

127. Kron SS: Questionable effectiveness of cricoid pressure in preventing aspiration. Anesthesiology 83:431-432, 1995.

128. Latto I: Management of difficult intubation. In Latto I, Rosen M (eds): Difficulties in Tracheal Intubation. London, Baillière Tindall, 1987, pp 99-141.

129. Lawes EG, Duncan PW, Bland B, et al: The cricoid yoke—A device for providing consistent and reproducible cricoid pressure. Br J Anaesth 58: 925-931, 1986.

130. Leigh JM, Tytler JA: Admissions to the intensive care unit after complications of anaesthetic techniques over 10 years. 2. The second 5 years. Anaesthesia 45: 814-820, 1990.

131. Lim CL, Hawthorne L, Ip-Yam PC: The intubating laryngeal mask airway (ILMA) in failed and difficult intubation. Anaesthesia 53:929-930, 1998.

132. Lipp M, Thierbach A, Daublander M, Dick W: Clinical evaluation of the Combitube [abstract]. 18th Annual Meeting of the European Academy of Anaesthesiology, Copenhagen, Denmark, 43, 1996.

133. Litman RS, Wu CL, Quinlivan JK: Gastric volume and pH in infants fed clear liquids and breast milk prior to surgery. Anesth Analg 79:482-485, 1994.

134. Ljungqvist O, Soreide E: Preoperative fasting. Br J Surg 90:400-406, 2003.

135. Lockey DJ, Coats T, Parr MJ: Aspiration in severe trauma: A prospective study. Anaesthesia 54: 1097-1098, 1999.

136. Lopez-Gil M, Brimacombe J, Alvarez M: Safety and efficacy of the laryngeal mask airway. A prospective survey of 1400 children. Anaesthesia 51:969-972, 1996.

137. Lu PP, Brimacombe J, Ho AC, et al: The intubating laryngeal mask airway in severe ankylosing spondylitis. Can J Anaesth 48:1015-1019, 2001.

138. Lu P, Brimacombe J, Yang C, et al: The ProSeal™ versus the Classic laryngeal mask airway for positive pressure ventilation during laparoscopic cholecystectomy. Br J Anaesth 88:824-827, 2002.

139. Ma OJ, Bentley B, Debehnke DJ: Airway management practices in emergency medicine residencies. Am J Emerg Med 13:501-504, 1995.

140. Maekawa N, Mikawa K, Yaku H, et al: Effects of 2-, 4- and 12-hour fasting intervals on preoperative gastric fluid pH and volume, and plasma glucose and lipid homeostasis in children. Acta Anaesthesiol Scand 37:783-787, 1993.

141. Mallampati SR, Gatt SP, Gugino LD, et al: A clinical sign to predict difficult tracheal intubation: A prospective study. Can Anaesth Soc J 32:429-434, 1985.

142. Maltby JR, Lewis P, Martin A, Sutherland LR: Gastric fluid volume and pH in elective patients following unrestricted oral fluid until three hours before surgery. Can J Anaesth 38:425-429, 1991.

143. Maltby JR, Reid CR, Hutchinson A: Gastric fluid volume and pH in elective inpatients. Part II: Coffee or orange juice with ranitidine. Can J Anaesth 35: 16-19, 1988.

144. Maltby JR, Sutherland AD, Sale JP, Shaffer EA: Preoperative oral fluids: Is a five-hour fast justified prior to elective surgery? Anesth Analg 65:1112-1116, 1986.

145. Manchikanti L, Canella MG, Hohlbein LJ, Colliver JA: Assessment of effect of various modes of premedication on acid aspiration risk factors in outpatient surgery. Anesth Analg 66:81-84, 1987.

146. Manchikanti L, Colliver JA, Marrero TC, Roush JR: Assessment of age-related acid aspiration risk factors in pediatric, adult, and geriatric patients. Anesth Analg 64:11-17, 1985.

147. Marik PE: Aspiration pneumonitis and aspiration pneumonia. N Engl J Med 344:665-671, 2001.

148. Martinez EJ: Use of laryngeal mask in obstetrics and gynecology [abstract]. Argentinian Congress of Anaesthesiology, 247[I, II], 1997.

149. McAllister JD, Gnauck KA: Rapid-sequence intubation of the pediatric patient. Fundamentals of practice. Pediatr Clin North Am 46:1-32, 1999.

150. McClure S, Regan M, Moore J: Laryngeal mask airway for caesarean section. Anaesthesia 45:227-228, 1990.

151. McFarlane C: Failed intubation in an obese obstetric patient and the laryngeal mask airway. Int J Obstet Anaesth 2:183-185, 1992.

152. McGrady EM, Macdonald AG: Effect of the preoperative administration of water on gastric volume and pH. Br J Anaesth 60:803-805, 1988.

153. McGrath JP, McCaul C, Byrne PJ, et al: Upper oesophageal sphincter function during general anaesthesia. Br J Surg 83:1276-1278, 1996.

154. Meakin G, Dingwall AE, Addison GM: Effects of fasting and oral premedication on the pH and volume of gastric aspirate in children. Br J Anaesth 59:678-682, 1987.

155. Mellin-Olsen J, Fasting S, Gisvold SE: Routine preoperative gastric emptying is seldom indicated. A study of 85,594 anaesthetics with special focus on aspiration pneumonia. Acta Anaesthesiol Scand 40:1184-1188, 1996.

156. Merio R, Festa A, Bergmann H, et al: Slow gastric emptying in type I diabetes: Relation to autonomic and peripheral neuropathy, blood glucose, and glycemic control. Diabetes Care 20:419-423, 1997.

157. Miller M, Wishart HY, Nimmo WS: Gastric contents at induction of anaesthesia. Is a 4-hour fast necessary? Br J Anaesth 55:1185-1188, 1983.

158. Minami H, McCallum RW: The physiology and pathophysiology of gastric emptying in humans. Gastroenterology 86:1592-1610, 1984.

159. Mitsushima H, Oishi K, Nagao T, et al: Acid aspiration induces bacterial pneumonia by enhanced bacterial adherence in mice. Microb Pathog 33:203-210, 2002.

160. Momose K, Shima T, Haga S, et al: [The effect of preoperative oral administration of ranitidine on pH and volume of gastric juice]. Masui 41:1482-1485, 1992.

161. Moore JG, Christian PE, Coleman RE: Gastric emptying of varying meal weight and composition in man. Evaluation by dual liquid- and solid-phase isotopic method. Dig Dis Sci 26:16-22, 1981.

162. Morison DH, Dunn GL, Fargas-Babjak AM, et al: A double-blind comparison of cimetidine and ranitidine as prophylaxis against gastric aspiration syndrome. Anesth Analg 61:988-992, 1982.

163. Morris J, Cook TM: Rapid sequence induction: A national survey of practice. Anaesthesia 56: 1090-1097, 2001.

164. Moukarzel AA, Sabri MT: Gastric physiology and function: Effects of fruit juices. J Am Coll Nutr 15(5 Suppl):18S-25S, 1996.

165. Moulton C, Pennycook AG: Relation between Glasgow coma score and cough reflex. Lancet 343:1261-1262, 1994.

166. Murphy PJ, Langton JA, Barker P, Smith G: Effect of oral diazepam on the sensitivity of upper airway reflexes. Br J Anaesth 70:131-134, 1993.

167. Nader-Djalal N, Knight PR, Davidson BA, Johnson K: Hyperoxia exacerbates microvascular lung injury following acid aspiration. Chest 112:1607-1614, 1997.

168. Nakayama DK, Waggoner T, Venkataraman ST, et al: The use of drugs in emergency airway management in pediatric trauma. Ann Surg 216:205-211, 1992.

169. Nanji GM, Maltby JR: Vomiting and aspiration pneumonitis with the laryngeal mask airway. Can J Anaesth 39:69-70, 1992.

170. Ng A, Smith G: Gastroesophageal reflux and aspiration of gastric contents in anesthetic practice. Anesth Analg 93:494-513, 2001.

171. Ng WL, Glomaud D, Hardy F, Phil S: Omeprazole for prophylaxis of acid aspiration in elective surgery. Anaesthesia 45:436-438, 1990.

172. Nichol HC, Zuck D: Difficult laryngoscopy—The "anterior" larynx and the atlanto-occipital gap. Br J Anaesth 55:141-144, 1983.

173. Nimmo WS: Aspiration of gastric contents. Br J Hosp Med 34:176-179, 1985.

174. Nimmo WS, Heading RC, Wilson J, et al: Inhibition of gastric emptying and drug absorption by narcotic analgesics. Br J Clin Pharmacol 2:509-513, 1975.

175. Nishina K, Mikawa K, Maekawa N, et al: A comparison of lansoprazole, omeprazole, and ranitidine for reducing preoperative gastric secretion in adult patients undergoing elective surgery. Anesth Analg 82:832-836, 1996.

176. Nishina K, Mikawa K, Takao Y, et al: A comparison of rabeprazole, lansoprazole, and ranitidine for improving preoperative gastric fluid property in adults undergoing elective surgery. Anesth Analg 90:717-721, 2000.

177. Oates JD, Macleod AD, Oates PD, et al: Comparison of two methods for predicting difficult intubation. Br J Anaesth 66:305-309, 1991.

178. O'Connor TA, Basak J, Parker S: The effect of three different ranitidine dosage regimens on reducing gastric acidity and volume in ambulatory surgical patients. Pharmacotherapy 15:170-175, 1995.

179. O'Flynn PE, Milford CA: Fasting in children for day case surgery. Ann R Coll Surg Engl 71:218-219, 1989.

180. O'Hare B, Lerman J, Endo J: Acute lung injury after instillation of human breast milk or infant formula into rabbit's lungs. Anesthesiology 90:1112-1118, 1996.

181. Olsson GL, Hallen B: Pharmacological evacuation of the stomach with metoclopramide. Acta Anaesthesiol Scand 26:417-420, 1982.

182. Olsson GL, Hallen B, Hambraeus-Jonzon K: Aspiration during anaesthesia: A computer-aided study of 185,358 anaesthetics. Acta Anaesthesiol Scand 30:84-92, 1986.

183. Ong BY, Palahniuk RJ, Cumming M: Gastric volume and pH in out-patients. Can Anaesth Soc J 25:36-39, 1978.

184. Ormezzano X, Ganansia MF, Arnould JF, et al: [Prevention of aspiration pneumonia in obstetrical anesthesia with the effervescent combination of cimetidine and sodium citrate]. Ann Fr Anesth Reanim 9:285-288, 1990.

185. Ovassapian A, Krejcie TC, Yelich SJ, et al: Awake fiberoptic intubation in the patient at high risk of aspiration. Br J Anaesth 62:13-16, 1989.

186. Ovassapian A, Liu S, Krejcie T: Fiberoptic tracheal intubation with Combitube in place. Anesth Analg 76:S315, 1993.

187. Pandit SK, Loberg KW, Pandit UA: Toast and tea before elective surgery? A national survey on current practice. Anesth Analg 90:1348-1351, 2000.

188. Parr MJ, Gregory M, Baskett PJ: The intubating laryngeal mask. Use in failed and difficult intubation. Anaesthesia 53:343-348, 1998.

189. Phillips S, Daborn AK, Hatch DJ: Preoperative fasting for paediatric anaesthesia. Br J Anaesth 73:529-536, 1994.

190. Plourde G, Hardy JF: Aspiration pneumonia: Assessing the risk of regurgitation in the cat. Can Anaesth Soc J 33:345-348, 1986.

191. Practice guidelines for preoperative fasting and the use of pharmacologic agents to reduce the risk of pulmonary aspiration: Application to healthy patients undergoing elective procedures: A report by the American Society of Anesthesiologist Task Force on Preoperative Fasting. Anesthesiology 90:896-905, 1999.

192. Priscu V, Priscu L, Soroker D: Laryngeal mask for failed intubation in emergency caesarean section. Can J Anaesth 39:893, 1992.

193. Rabey PG, Murphy PJ, Langton JA, et al: Effect of the laryngeal mask airway on lower oesophageal sphincter pressure in patients during general anaesthesia. Br J Anaesth 69:346-348, 1992.

194. Raidoo DM, Rocke DA, Brock-Utne JG, et al: Critical volume for pulmonary acid aspiration: Reappraisal in a primate model. Br J Anaesth 65:248-250, 1990.

195. Ralph SJ, Wareham CA: Rupture of the oesophagus during cricoid pressure. Anaesthesia 46:40-41, 1991.

196. Randell T, Maattanen M, Kytta J: The best view at laryngoscopy using the McCoy laryngoscope with and without cricoid pressure. Anaesthesia 53:536-539, 1998.

197. Rebuck JA, Rasmussen JR, Olsen KM: Clinical aspiration-related practice patterns in the intensive care unit: A physician survey. Crit Care Med 29:2239-2244, 2001.

198. Richards CF: Piriform sinus perforation during Esophageal-Tracheal Combitube placement. J Emerg Med 16:37-39, 1998.

199. Roberts RB, Shirley MA: Reducing the risk of acid aspiration during cesarean section. Anesth Analg 53:859-868, 1974.

200. Rocke DA, Murray WB, Rout CC, Gouws E: Relative risk analysis of factors associated with difficult intubation in obstetric anesthesia. Anesthesiology 77:67-73, 1992.

201. Roewer N: Can pulmonary aspiration of gastric contents be prevented by balloon occlusion of the cardia? A study with a new nasogastric tube. Anesth Analg 80:378-383, 1995.

202. Rose DK, Cohen MM: The airway: Problems and predictions in 18,500 patients. Can J Anaesth 41:372-383, 1994.

203. Rosen M: Anesthesia for obstetrics [editorial]. Anaesthesia 36:145-146, 1981.

204. Rosenblatt WH, Murphy M: The intubating laryngeal mask: Use of a new ventilating-intubating device in the emergency department. Ann Emerg Med 33:234-238, 1999.

205. Rosenthal R: Combining results from independent studies. Psychol Bull 85:185-193, 1978.

206. Roux M, Drolet P, Girard M, et al: Effect of the laryngeal mask airway on oesophageal pH: Influence of the volume and pressure inside the cuff. Br J Anaesth 82:566-569, 1999.

207. Sakles JC, Laurin EG, Rantapaa AA, Panacek EA: Airway management in the emergency department: A one-year study of 610 tracheal intubations. Ann Emerg Med 31:325-332, 1998.

208. Salem MR, Joseph NJ, Heyman HJ, et al: Cricoid compression is effective in obliterating the esophageal lumen in the presence of a nasogastric tube. Anesthesiology 63:443-446, 1985.

209. Salem MR, Sellick BA, Elam JO: The historical background of cricoid pressure in anesthesia and resuscitation. Anesth Analg 53:230-232, 1974.

210. Salem MR, Wong AY, Fizzotti GF: Efficacy of cricoid pressure in preventing aspiration of gastric contents in paediatric patients. Br J Anaesth 44:401-404, 1972.

211. Salem MR, Wong AY, Mani M, et al: Premedicant drugs and gastric juice pH and volume in pediatric patients. Anesthesiology 44:216-219, 1976.

212. Salem MR, Wong AY, Mani M, Sellick BA: Efficacy of cricoid pressure in preventing gastric inflation during bag-mask ventilation in pediatric patients. Anesthesiology 40:96-98, 1974.

213. Samsoon GL, Young JR: Difficult tracheal intubation: A retrospective study. Anaesthesia 42:487-490, 1987.

214. Sandhar BK, Goresky GD, Maltby JR, et al: Effects of oral liquids and ranitidine on gastric fluid volume and pH in children undergoing outpatient surgery. Anesthesiology 71:402-403, 1989.

215. Savva D: Prediction of difficult tracheal intubation. Br J Anaesth 73:149-153, 1994.

216. Scarr M, Maltby JR, Jani K, Sutherland LR: Volume and acidity of residual gastric fluid after oral fluid ingestion before elective ambulatory surgery. CMAJ 141:1151-1154, 1989.

217. Schoeman MN, Tippett MD, Akkermans LM, et al: Mechanisms of gastroesophageal reflux in ambulant healthy human subjects. Gastroenterology 108: 289-291, 1995.

218. Schreiner M: The preop fast: Not quite so fast. Contemp Pediatr 6:45-52, 1992.

219. Schreiner MS, Triebwasser A, Keon TP: Ingestion of liquids compared with preoperative fasting in pediatric outpatients. Anesthesiology 72:593-597, 1990.

220. Schwartz DE, Cohen NH: Questionable effectiveness of cricoid pressure in preventing aspiration [letter]. Anesthesiology 83:432, 1995.

221. Schwarzmann G, Wurmb T, Greim C, Roewer N: Difficult airway management: combination of the laryngeal mask airway with a new gastric balloon tube [abstract]. Anesthesiology 89:A1237, 1998.

222. Sellick BA: Cricoid pressure to prevent regurgitation of stomach contents during induction of anaesthesia. Lancet 2:404-406, 1961.

223. Shevde K, Trivedi N: Effects of clear liquids on gastric volume and pH in healthy volunteers. Anesth Analg 72:528-531, 1991.

224. Simpson KH, Stakes AF: Effect of anxiety on gastric emptying in preoperative patients. Br J Anaesth 59: 540-544, 1987.

225. Sinnatamby CS: Abdomen. Last's Anatomy Regional and Applied. Edinburgh, Churchill Livingstone, 1999, pp 215-320.

226. Skinner HJ, Ho BY, Mahajan RP: Gastro-oesophageal reflux with the laryngeal mask during day-case gynaecological laparoscopy. Br J Anaesth 80:675-676, 1998.

227. Smart NG, Varveris DA, Jacobs P: Use of the intubating laryngeal mask in failed intubation associated with amyloid macroglossia. Br J Anaesth 89:186-187, 2002.

228. Solanki DR, Suresh M, Ethridge HC: The effects of intravenous cimetidine and metoclopramide on gastric volume and pH. Anesth Analg 63:599-602, 1984.

229. Soreide E, Hausken T, Soreide JA, Steen PA: Gastric emptying of a light hospital breakfast. A study using real time ultrasonography. Acta Anaesthesiol Scand 40:549-553, 1996.

230. Splinter WM, Schaefer JD: Ingestion of clear fluids is safe for adolescents up to 3 h before anaesthesia. Br J Anaesth 66:48-52, 1991.

231. Splinter WM, Stewart JA, Muir JG: Large volumes of apple juice preoperatively do not affect gastric pH and volume in children. Can J Anaesth 37:36-39, 1990.

232. Standards and guidelines for cardiopulmonary resuscitation [CPR] and emergency cardiac care. JAMA 255:2905-2985, 1985.

233. Staudinger T, Brugger S, Watschinger B, et al: Emergency intubation with the Combitube: Comparison with the endotracheal airway. Ann Emerg Med 22:1573-1575, 1993.

234. Strain JD, Moore EE, Markovchick VJ, Duzer-Moore S: Cimetidine for the prophylaxis of potential gastric acid aspiration pneumonitis in trauma patients. J Trauma 21:49-51, 1981.

235. Strunin L: In the Report of the National Confidential Enquiry into Perioperative Deaths. London, NCEPOD, 1995, pp 76-78.

236. Stuart JC, Kan AF, Rowbottom SJ, et al: Acid aspiration prophylaxis for emergency caesarean section. Anaesthesia 51:415-421, 1996.

237. Sundman E, Witt H, Olsson R, et al: The incidence and mechanisms of pharyngeal and upper esophageal dysfunction in partially paralyzed humans: Pharyngeal videoradiography and simultaneous manometry after atracurium. Anesthesiology 92:977-984, 2000.

238. Suresh M, Gardner M, Key E: Intubating Laryngeal Mask Airway (ILMA): A life saving rescue device following failed tracheal intubation during cesarean section (CS) [abstract]. Presented at the 36th Annual Meeting of the Society for Obstetric Anesthesia and Perinatology (SOAP), Fort Myers, Fla, May 12-16, 2004.

239. Suresh M, Wali A: Failed intubation in obstetrics—Airway management strategies. Anesthesiol Clin North Am 16:477-498, 1998.

240. Tagaito Y, Isono S, Nishino T: Upper airway reflexes during a combination of propofol and fentanyl anesthesia. Anesthesiology 88:1459-1466, 1998.

241. Tanigawa K, Shigematsu A: Choice of airway devices for 12,020 cases of nontraumatic cardiac arrest in Japan. Prehosp Emerg Care 2:96-100, 1998.

242. Thwaites AJ, Rice CP, Smith I: Rapid sequence induction: A questionnaire survey of its routine conduct and continued management during a failed intubation. Anaesthesia 54:376-381, 1999.

243. Toung T, Saharia P, Permutt S, et al: Aspiration pneumonia: Beneficial and harmful effects of positive end-expiratory pressure. Surgery 82:279-283, 1977.

244. Tournadre JP, Chassard D, Berrada K, et al: Lower oesophageal sphincter pressure during application of cricoid pressure in conscious volunteers. Br J Anaesth 76:A50, 1996.

245. Tournadre JP, Chassard D, Berrada KR, Bouletreau P: Cricoid cartilage pressure decreases lower esophageal sphincter tone. Anesthesiology 86:7-9, 1997.

246. Tryba M, Yildiz F, Zenz M, Schwerdt M: [Prevention of aspiration pneumonia with cimetidine]. Anaesthesist 31:584-587, 1982.

247. Tse JC, Rimm EB, Hussain A: Predicting difficult endotracheal intubation in surgical patients scheduled for general anesthesia: A prospective blind study. Anesth Analg 81:254-258, 1995.

248. Tuckey JP, Cook TM, Render CA: Forum. An evaluation of the levering laryngoscope. Anaesthesia 51:71-73, 1996.

249. Tweedle D, Nightingale P: Anesthesia and gastrointestinal surgery. Acta Chir Scand Suppl 550:131-139, 1989.

250. Urtubia R, Aguila C: Combitube: A new proposal for a confusing nomenclature. Anesth Analg 89:803, 1999.

251. Urtubia RM, Aguila CM, Cumsille MA: Combitube: A study for proper use. Anesth Analg 90:958-962, 2000.

252. Urtubia R, Medina J, Alzamora R: Combitube for emergency cesarean section under general anesthesia. Case reports. Difficult Airway 4:78-83, 2001.

253. Vaida S: The effectiveness of the Esophageal Tracheal Combitube in mechanically ventilated patients undergoing laparoscopic cholecystectomy. Anaesthesiol Intensivmed 34:S121, 1999.

254. Vaisman N, Weintrob N, Blumental A, et al: Gastric emptying in patients with type I diabetes mellitus. Ann NY Acad Sci 873:506-511, 1999.

255. Valente Barbas CS: Lung recruitment maneuvers in acute respiratory distress syndrome and facilitating resolution. Crit Care Med 31(4 Suppl):S265-S271, 2003.

256. Valentine J, Stakes AF, Bellamy MC: Reflux during positive pressure ventilation through the laryngeal mask. Br J Anaesth 73:543-544, 1994.

257. Van Maren GA: Emergency anaesthesia in the unprepared patient. In Prys-Roberts C, Brown BR (eds): International Practice of Anaesthesia. Oxford, Butterworth-Heinemann, 1996, pp 1291-1297.

258. Vanner RG: Tolerance of cricoid pressure by conscious volunteers. Int J Obstet Anaesth 1:195-198, 1992.

259. Vanner RG: Mechanisms of regurgitation and its prevention with cricoid pressure. Int J Obstet Anaesth 2:207-215, 1993.

260. Vanner RG, Pryle BJ: Regurgitation and oesophageal rupture with cricoid pressure: A cadaver study. Anaesthesia 47:732-735, 1992.

261. Vanner RG, Pryle BJ: Nasogastric tubes and cricoid pressure. Anaesthesia 48:1112-1113, 1993.

262. Vanner RG, Pryle BJ, O'Dwyer JP, Reynolds F: Upper oesophageal sphincter pressure and the intravenous induction of anaesthesia. Anaesthesia 47:371-375, 1992.

263. Vanner RG, Pryle BJ, O'Dwyer JP, Reynolds F: Upper oesophageal sphincter pressure during inhalational anaesthesia. Anaesthesia 47:950-954, 1992.

264. Vaughan GG, Grycko RJ, Montgomery MT: The prevention and treatment of aspiration of vomitus during pharmacosedation and general anesthesia. J Oral Maxillofac Surg 50:874-879, 1992.

265. Vaughan RW, Bauer S, Wise L: Volume and pH of gastric juice in obese patients. Anesthesiology 43:686-689, 1975.

266. Ventilation with lower tidal volumes as compared with traditional tidal volumes for acute lung injury and the acute respiratory distress syndrome. The Acute Respiratory Distress Syndrome Network. N Engl J Med 342:1301-1308, 2000.

267. Verghese C, Brimacombe JR: Survey of laryngeal mask airway usage in 11,910 patients: Safety and efficacy for conventional and nonconventional usage. Anesth Analg 82:129-133, 1996.

268. Vezina D, Lessard MR, Bussieres J, et al: Complications associated with the use of the Esophageal-Tracheal Combitube. Can J Anaesth 45:76-80, 1998.

269. Viegas OJ, Ravindran RS, Shumacker CA: Gastric fluid pH in patients receiving sodium citrate. Anesth Analg 60:521-523, 1981.

270. Wainwright AC: Positive pressure ventilation and the laryngeal mask airway in ophthalmic anaesthesia [letter]. Br J Anaesth 75:249-250, 1995.

271. Wakeling HG, Bagwell A: The intubating laryngeal mask (ILMA) in an emergency failed intubation. Anaesthesia 54:305-306, 1999.

272. Warner MA, Warner ME, Warner DO, et al: Perioperative pulmonary aspiration in infants and children. Anesthesiology 90:66-71, 1999.

273. Warner MA, Warner ME, Weber JG: Clinical significance of pulmonary aspiration during the perioperative period. Anesthesiology 78:56-62, 1993.

274. Watson NC, Hokanson M, Maltby JR, Todesco JM: The intubating laryngeal mask airway in failed fibreoptic intubation. Can J Anaesth 46:376-378, 1999.

275. White A, Sinclair M, Pillai R: Laryngeal mask airway for coronary artery bypass grafting. Anaesthesia 46:234, 1991.

276. Whittington RM, Robinson JS, Thompson JM: Fatal aspiration (Mendelson's) syndrome despite antacids and cricoid pressure. Lancet 2:228-230, 1979.

277. Wilson ME: Predicting difficult intubation. Br J Anaesth 71:333-334, 1993.

278. Wilson ME, Spiegelhalter D, Robertson JA, Lesser P: Predicting difficult intubation. Br J Anaesth 61:211-216, 1988.

279. Wilson SL, Mantena NR, Halverson JD: Effects of atropine, glycopyrrolate, and cimetidine on gastric

secretions in morbidly obese patients. Anesth Analg 60:37-40, 1981.

280. Wissler RN: The esophageal-tracheal Combitube. Anesthesiol Rev 20:147-152, 1993.

281. Wolfe JE, Bone RC, Ruth WE: Effects of corticosteroids in the treatment of patients with gastric aspiration. Am J Med 63:719-722, 1977.

282. Wraight WJ, Chamney AR, Howells TH: The determination of an effective cricoid pressure. Anaesthesia 38:461-466, 1983.

283. Wright PM, Caldwell JE, Miller RD: Onset and duration of rocuronium and succinylcholine at the adductor pollicis and laryngeal adductor muscles in anesthetized humans. Anesthesiology 81:1110-1115, 1994.

284. Wrobel J, Koh TC, Saunders JM: Sodium citrate: An alternative antacid for prophylaxis against aspiration pneumonitis. Anaesth Intensive Care 10:116-119, 1982.

285. Wyner J, Cohen SE: Gastric volume in early pregnancy: Effect of metoclopramide. Anesthesiology 57:209-212, 1982.

286. Wynne JW, Modell JH: Respiratory aspiration of stomach contents. Ann Intern Med 87:466-474, 1977.

287. Wynne JW, Reynolds JC, Hood I, et al: Steroid therapy for pneumonitis induced in rabbits by aspiration of foodstuff. Anesthesiology 51:11-19, 1979.

33

THE DIFFICULT PEDIATRIC AIRWAY

Mary F. Rabb

Peter Szmuk

I. INTRODUCTION

One of the most challenging aspects facing anesthesiologists is maintaining the technical skills that are necessary for the management of the difficult airway (DA). A DA is defined in the American Society of Anesthesiologists (ASA) guidelines as the clinical situation in which a conventionally trained anesthesiologist experiences difficulty with face mask ventilation of the upper airway, difficulty with endotracheal intubation, or both.[297] Recent reports demonstrate how important skilled airway management is to the practice of pediatric anesthesia. Data from the ASA Pediatric Closed Claims Data Base demonstrate a greater frequency of adverse respiratory events in the pediatric population.[257] In the pediatric closed claims analysis, respiratory events accounted for 43% of all adverse events. These were most frequently related to inadequate ventilation (20%). Esophageal intubation, airway obstruction, and difficult intubation (DI) combined accounted for 14% of the remaining adverse respiratory events. In the Pediatric Perioperative Cardiac Arrest (POCA) registry, 20% of all cardiac arrests were attributed to the respiratory system.[258] Airway obstruction and DI were responsible for 27% and 13% of these events, respectively. Most of the patients who experienced arrests from airway obstruction or DI had underlying diseases or syndromes.

In addition, infants and small children display anatomic differences when compared with adults. Knowledge of the anatomic differences, congenital syndromes, as well as different disease states is required for management of the DA.

II. ANATOMY OF THE PEDIATRIC AIRWAY

The pediatric airway, particularly in infants, is different from the adult airway. Understanding the differences between the two is important when managing the pediatric airway. Following is a brief review of the anatomy of the normal pediatric airway.[82,85,106,399]

A. LARYNX

The larynx is situated more cephalad at C3-4 in the infant and migrates to the adult level of C5 by 6 years.[106] Because the infant's larynx is more rostral (higher), the tongue is located closer to the palate and more easily apposes the palate. As a result, airway obstruction may occur during induction of or emergence from anesthesia. A common misnomer is that the infant's larynx is more "anterior" when it is really more "rostral" or "superior" in the neck (compared with the adult larynx). In syndromes associated with mandibular hypoplasia, such as Pierre Robin, the larynx is actually positioned more *posteriorly* than normal. This results in a greater acute angulation between the laryngeal inlet and the base of the tongue. In this circumstance, direct visualization of the glottis may be difficult or impossible. Because of the cephalad position of the larynx and the large occiput, the "sniffing" position does not assist in visualization of the larynx.[82,399] Elevating the head only moves the larynx into a more anterior position. Infants should be positioned with the head and shoulders on a flat surface with the head in a neutral position and the neck neither flexed nor extended.[85]

B. EPIGLOTTIS

The infant epiglottis is longer, stiff, and often described as omega or U shaped.[106] It projects posteriorly above the glottis at a 45-degree angle. Because the epiglottis is more obliquely angled, visualization of the vocal cords may be difficult during direct laryngoscopy. It may be necessary to lift the tip of the epiglottis with a laryngoscope blade in order to visualize the vocal cords. Straight laryngoscope blades are often preferred for this reason.

C. SUBGLOTTIS

The cricoid cartilage is the narrowest portion of the infant's airway (about 5 mm in diameter) versus the vocal cords of the adult airway.[106] The infant's larynx is funnel shaped with a narrow cricoid cartilage, whereas the adult airway is cylindrical. Tight-fitting endotracheal tubes (ETs) that compress the mucosa at this level may cause edema and increase resistance to flow. Resistance to flow is inversely proportional to the radius of the lumen to the fourth power. One millimeter of edema can reduce the cross-sectional area of the infant trachea by 75% versus 44% in the adult trachea.

III. EVALUATION OF THE PEDIATRIC AIRWAY

The evaluation of the pediatric airway should begin with a history and physical examination of the head and neck. Clues to a potentially DA include snoring, noisy breathing, difficulty breathing with feeding or an upper respiratory tract infection, and recurrent croup. Review of previous anesthesia records should be performed if they are available. In the event a DA is encountered, documentation of events and the ability to mask ventilate is helpful for future caregivers. A prior uneventful anesthesia does not guarantee success the next time.[82,399]

Knowledge of syndromes that may adversely affect the airway is crucial to the management of the difficult pediatric airway. The presence of one anomaly mandates a search for others. A common feature in many of these syndromes is micrognathia. Micrognathia creates more difficulty with displacement of the tongue during direct laryngoscopy, thus increasing the chance that the glottis will be difficult to visualize.[82,399] The ability to intubate often changes as the child grows. Intubation often becomes easier with time in patients with syndromes associated with micrognathia such as Pierre Robin syndrome.[85] In patients with mucopolysaccharide disorders or abnormalities involving the cervical spine (e.g., Klippel-Feil syndrome), intubation may become more difficult as the child grows older.[85]

Abnormalities of the ear or the presence of ear tags has been suggested as an indicator of DI.[85] In one study, bilateral microtia was associated with an increased incidence of DI (42% versus 2% in unilateral microtia). Mandibular hypoplasia was associated with bilateral microtia more than with unilateral microtia (50% versus 5%), thus enabling bilateral microtia to be used as an indirect predictor of DI.[376]

Physical examination must focus on the head, neck, and cervical spine. Many of the evaluations used for predicting a DA in adults have not been extrapolated to the pediatric population. Cooperation of the patient is necessary for precise evaluation to take place. In the young or uncooperative child, appropriate evaluation is limited. Preliminary data indicate that the Mallampati classification may be an insensitive predictor of DI in the pediatric population.[202] Pediatric anesthesiologists are at a disadvantage because they are anesthetizing patients with less objective airway information available. This underscores the need for a skilled approach to the difficult pediatric airway.

Evaluations should focus on the size and shape of the mandible, size of the mouth and tongue, absence or prominence of teeth, presence of loose teeth, and the neck length and range of motion. Berry has suggested that the appropriate thyromental distance in infants is one fingerbreadth (1.5 cm).[34] Lateral examinations of the head and neck may provide clues to the presence of micrognathia. Mandibular enlargement has also been identified as a risk factor for DI. Cherubism is a disease of early childhood, consisting of painless mandibular enlargement with or without maxillary involvement, that progresses rapidly in early childhood and then regresses during puberty.[240] In cherubism, the potential displacement space is encroached upon by mandibular enlargement.[240] Palpation of the soft tissue of the potential displacement area may reveal the problem.

A. DIAGNOSTIC EVALUATION

Magnetic resonance imaging (MRI) and computed tomography (CT) may be extremely helpful in the evaluation of airway pathology. Flexible fiberoptic endoscopy may be of benefit prior to intubation when visualization of vocal cords is thought to be difficult or when airway pathology is suspected. In patients with unilateral hemifacial microsomia, radiographic classification of the mandibular anatomy has been shown to help predict ease of intubation.[269]

Radiographic evaluation of patients with airway obstruction may be obtained in patients who present to the emergency room *only if they are not in respiratory distress.* Radiographs should be obtained in the upright position because obstruction may become worse in the supine position.[388] In this situation, it is mandatory that a person skilled in airway management and capable of managing a difficult pediatric airway accompany the patient along with the appropriate equipment.

Radiographs have high sensitivity (greater than 86%) for the diagnosis of airway foreign body, exudative tracheitis, and innominate artery compression. For laryngomalacia and tracheomalacia, they have a much lower sensitivity (5% and 62%, respectively).[388]

Radiologic evaluation should not take precedence over airway control in patients with a compromised airway.

IV. CLASSIFICATION OF THE DIFFICULT PEDIATRIC AIRWAY

Difficulty with ventilation, intubation, or both is the definition of a DA according to the ASA DA management guidelines.[297] Recognition of the DA along with the circumstances that predispose to airway problems is crucial to the safe management of the pediatric airway. Classification of the difficult pediatric airway may be made according to the anatomic location affected. Major anomalies of the head, face, mouth and tongue, nasopharynx, larynx, trachea, and neck are listed.

V. PEDIATRIC AIRWAY EQUIPMENT

In order to manage a DA successfully, the appropriate equipment should be immediately available. We recommend the creation of a *difficult pediatric airway cart* stocked with equipment for patients ranging from premature infants to small adults. In addition, the American Academy of Pediatrics, Section on Anesthesiology recommends the creation of a DA cart for all locations anesthetizing children.[6] This cart should be dedicated only for use in a DA or "cannot intubate, cannot ventilate" scenario (Table 33-1).

A. FACE MASK

When managing the DA, the ability to ventilate with a mask is more important than endotracheal intubation. When dealing with the pediatric airway, and especially the difficult pediatric airway, it is important to have a selection

Table 33-1 **Pediatric Difficult Airway Cart**

Assortment of laryngoscope handles or blades
Oxyscope
Endotracheal tubes 2.0 to 7.0 mm
Oral/nasopharyngeal airways
Masks
Stylets
Endotracheal tube exchangers
Laryngeal mask airways—all sizes
Fiberoptic intubation equipment
Bronchoscopic swivel connector
Retrograde intubation kit
McGill forceps
Percutaneous cricothyrotomy kit
Advanced equipment: Bullard laryngoscope, light wand, Shikani scope, angulated video-intubation laryngoscope

of masks readily available. Disposable clear plastic masks with an inflatable rim are commonly used. These masks should extend from the chin to the bridge of the nose. A leak-free seal should be obtained with minimal pressure applied to the face or mandible. Transparent masks allow visualization of secretions or vomitus during induction. These masks can be purchased in different flavors or scented prior to induction so that they are less intimidating.

Face masks have been modified for fiberoptic intubation in a variety of ways.[108,117,118,198] Frei and colleagues described modifying a commercially available mask (Vital Signs) by drilling a hole into the lateral aspect of the mask and attaching a corrugated silicon tube. The center of the mask is fitted with a plastic ring covered by a silicon membrane. A hole, 1 to 2 mm smaller than the outer diameter (OD) of the bronchoscope, is punched into the membrane.[117,118] This airway endoscopy mask has been used to facilitate fiberoptic bronchoscopy (FOB) in patients ranging in age from 3 days to 12 months with spontaneous ventilation and propofol sedation.[108] A commercially available face mask with a ventilation side port (MERA, Senko Ika Kogyo, Tokyo, Japan) was modified and used successfully to intubate fiberoptically nine patients ranging in age from 3 months to 11 years under inhalational anesthesia with continuous manual ventilation.[198]

B. OROPHARYNGEAL AIRWAY

Upper airway obstruction may occur during induction of anesthesia because the infant's tongue is large in relation to the oropharynx. Appropriately sized oropharyngeal airways are necessary for air exchange. Guedel and Berman airways are the most common airways available. By holding the airway next to the child's face, the correct size can be estimated.[82] If the airway is too short, obstruction may be worsened. If the airway is too long, the epiglottis or uvula may be damaged. Use of a tongue depressor to insert the oropharyngeal airway is recommended to avoid impaired lymphatic drainage of the tongue.[82]

A modified Guedel airway, the cuffed oropharyngeal airway or COPA, is a supraglottic anesthesia device developed by Greenberg in 1990. It has a distal inflatable end cuff and a proximal end connector that may be attached to the anesthesia circuit.[136] The COPA is disposable and available in four sizes, 8, 9, 10, and 11. The size corresponds to the distance in centimeters between the flange and distal tip.[59] The use of the COPA in pediatric patients was examined; successful insertion on the first attempt was 90%. The most frequent airway manipulations were head tilt in 27.5% and chin lift in 5%. In that same study, COPA sizing based on weight recommendations was made[59] (Table 33-2).

In another study, comparing the COPA with the laryngeal mask airway (LMA) in children, more positional maneuvers such as repositioning of the airway and airway manipulations (chin lift, jaw thrust) were required with the COPA (28.6%) versus the LMA (2.9%). There was no difference in the incidence of laryngospasm or bronchospasm in the two groups.[230]

C. NASOPHARYNGEAL AIRWAY

Nasopharyngeal airways are available in sizes from 12 to 36 Fr. They are to be used with caution in pediatric patients with hypertrophied adenoids.

D. ENDOTRACHEAL TUBE

ETs in a variety of sizes (2.5 to 7.0 mm) should be available for the pediatric patient. Laser-resistant, nasal/oral Ring-Adair-Elwyn (RAE), and wire-reinforced ETs are available for use depending on the surgical requirement. Determination of correct ET size is based on the patient's age and weight. ETs one half size larger and smaller than the calculated size should be available. Traditional teaching

advocates the use of uncuffed ETs in patients younger than 8 years. Pediatric ETs with low-pressure, high-volume cuffs are available for use in patients with low lung compliance or those who are at risk for aspiration. For cuffed ETs, one half size smaller tube should be used as the OD of the tube is larger because of the cuff.[382] Maintenance of a leak with or without a cuff is recommended in order to minimize the occurrence of postintubation croup. The incidence of postintubation croup has been cited as 1% by Koka and coauthors.[201] This has been challenged by Litman and Keon. In a prospective study of over 5000 children, 7 patients developed croup, defined as inspiratory stridor of at least 30 minutes duration, for an incidence of 0.1%. In that study, ETs with air leaks greater than 40 cm H_2O were replaced with the next smaller size.[216] The presence or absence of a leak depends on the level of anesthesia and the use of muscle relaxants. Many clinicians use the degree of difficulty in passing the ET below the vocal cords as the indicator of proper fit.

In general, there are many formulas to calculate the appropriate size of ET. Formulas for selecting an uncuffed ET in children older than 2 years include (age + 16)/4 or (age/4) + 4. The use of cuffed ETs in newborns and children younger than 8 years has been studied. In a group of 488 patients, patients were randomly allocated to receive a cuffed or an uncuffed ET.[194] The formula for the cuffed tube was (age/4) + 3. This formula was appropriate for 99% of patients. In that study, three patients in each group were treated for croup symptoms. Formulas for length of insertion of an oral ET include length (cm) = 3 × internal diameter (mm) or length (cm) = age(years)/2 + 12.[382] In the premature or newborn infant, the rule is tip-to-lip distance in cm = 6 + weight (kg).[46] Whatever method is chosen, correct ET position should be confirmed by auscultation of bilateral breath sounds (Tables 33-3 and 33-4).

Double-lumen tubes are not available for use in pediatric patients younger than 6 to 8 years. The Arndt Endobronchial Blocker (Cook Critical Care, Bloomington, IN) has been used to provide one-lung

Table 33-2 **Cuffed Oropharyngeal Airway (COPA) Sizing Based on Weight**

COPA Size	Weight (kg)
8	12-20
9	20-40
10	40-60
11	>60

Table 33-3 **Suggested Endotracheal Tube Size for Infants**

Age	Size (mm ID)
Preterm < 1000 g	2.5
Preterm 1000 to 2500 g	3.0
Newborn to 6 months	3.0-3.5
6 months to 1 year	3.5-4.0
1 to 2 years	4.0-4.5
>2 years	(age + 16)/4

ID, internal diameter.

Table 33-4   **Formula for Endotracheal Tube Size and Depth of Insertion**

Uncuffed Endotracheal Tube > 2 Years	(Age + 16)/4 or Age/4 + 4
Cuffed endotracheal tube	Age/4 + 3
Length of insertion (oral)	Age (years)/2 + 12 or 3 × ID (mm)
Length of insertion (nasal)	3 × ID (mm) + 2

ventilation in infants.[148] The 5.0 Fr blocker is available; the recommended ET size is 4.5 mm. The Univent tube (Fuji Systems Corporation, Tokyo, Japan) is a single-lumen tube with an incorporated movable bronchial blocker inside.[146] Pediatric sizes of the Univent tube are available: 3.5 mm internal diameter (ID) and 4.5 mm ID. The 3.5-mm Univent tube does not have a lumen for suctioning or administration of oxygen to the blocked lung. FOB is needed for placement. Further detail regarding one-lung ventilation is provided in Chapter 24.

E. ENDOTRACHEAL TUBE EXCHANGERS

ET exchangers have multiple uses; they can be used to exchange damaged ETs and provide a conduit for reintubation, if necessary. Many different types of exchangers are available for use in adult patients. These tube exchangers are long, semirigid, catheters that fit inside ETs. The Frova Intubating Introducer (Cook Critical Care) is available in a pediatric size (8 Fr) that allows placement of a 3.0-mm ET.[144] It is 33 cm in length with a hollow lumen and a blunt curved tip that is shaped like the gum elastic bougie. The blunt curved tip can be passed "blindly" into the trachea in cases in which visualization of the glottis is inadequate. The Frova catheter has a hollow lumen and two side ports; it is packaged with removable Rapi-Fit adaptors that allow ventilation and a stiffening cannula[144] (Fig. 33-1).

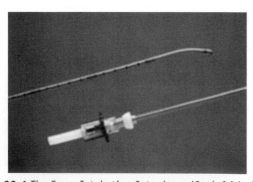

Figure 33-1 The Frova Intubating Introducer (Cook Critical Care, Bloomington, IN) catheter is available in a pediatric size (8 Fr) that allows placement of a 3.0-mm endotracheal tube. It is hollow with two side ports, is blunt tipped, and has a Rapi-Fit adaptor.

Cook also manufactures airway exchange catheters in four sizes. These catheters are blunt tipped, hollow with distal side ports, and have a Rapi-Fit adaptor as well. The 8 Fr size is 45 cm in length and can be used in 3.0-mm ETs.[144]

F. LARYNGOSCOPE BLADES

Laryngoscope blades in different sizes and shapes should be available prior to induction of anesthesia. Laryngoscope blades fall into two categories: straight and curved. Because the epiglottis is angled posteriorly, visualization of the glottis may be difficult. Straight laryngoscope blades are often recommended for use in neonates and infants in order to lift the epiglottis. The most common straight blades include the Miller, Wisconsin, Wis-Hipple, and Wis-Foregger blades. Curved blades are also available for use; they are more suitable for older children.

G. OXYSCOPE

The Oxyscope is a fiberoptic Miller 1 blade with a port for insufflation of oxygen during intubation. Oxygen insufflation during laryngoscopy in spontaneously breathing, anesthetized infants has been shown to minimize the decrease in transcutaneous oxygen tension, thus making airway instrumentation safer.[208]

H. ANTERIOR COMMISSURE LARYNGOSCOPE

The anterior commissure laryngoscope is commonly used by otolaryngologists for visualization of the glottis. It is a rigid tubular straight-blade laryngoscope with a distally located recessed light source. This design permits enhanced visualization by preventing the tongue from obscuring the field of view.[95]

I. BULLARD LARYNGOSCOPE

The Bullard laryngoscope (Circon ACMI, Stanford, CT), developed by Dr. Roger Bullard at the Medical College of Georgia, is an indirect laryngoscope that utilizes fiberoptic and mirror technology to visualize the larynx.[48] Use of fiberoptics and a curved blade enable visualization of the larynx "around the corner" of the blade, thus eliminating the need to align the oral, pharyngeal, and tracheal axes. A standard laryngoscope handle or a flexible fiberoptic cable connected to a light source powers the fiberoptic light source. This laryngoscope is manufactured in three sizes: adult, pediatric, and pediatric long.[57] The adult size, with a blade that is 2.5 cm wide, is suitable for children older than 10 years. The pediatric version (newborn to age 2) has a blade that is 1.3 cm wide that extends 0.6 cm beyond the fiberoptics. This blade is recommended for use in neonates, infants, and smaller children. The pediatric long version is available for use in infants and small children up to age 10; it has a longer blade (1.4 cm) and a wider flange (1.6 cm). In the pediatric long version, a multifunctional stylet is attached to the fiberoptic bundle between the eyepiece and handle and aligns the tip of the ETT beneath the flange of the blade. The smallest ET that passes over the stylet in the pediatric long version is 4.5 mm.[57] The Bullard laryngoscope requires minimal mouth opening for its insertion (0.64 cm in the cephalad-caudad axis). It has been used to intubate patients with unstable cervical spines, Pierre Robin syndrome, Treacher Collins, Noonan's syndrome, and Klippel-Feil syndrome, to name a few.[48] The adult Bullard laryngoscope has been used successfully to intubate patients older than 12 months with normal airways.[348] Contact with the right aryepiglottic fold and, in children, contact with the anterior vocal cord occurred.[347,348] When compared with the Wis-Hipple 1½, the adult Bullard laryngoscope provided a similar view and required a slightly longer time for intubation in children 1 to 5 years of age.[347]

J. ANGULATED VIDEO-INTUBATION LARYNGOSCOPE

The angulated video-intubation laryngoscope (AVIL), invented by Dr. Marcus Weiss of Zurich, Switzerland, is a new endoscopic intubation device. The AVIL consists of a cast plastic Macintosh 4 laryngoscope, with the blade angulated distally, and an integrated fiberoptic endoscope (1.8 m long, OD 2.8 mm, VOLPI AG, Schlieren, Switzerland). The distal blade tip is angulated about 25 degrees to provide increased viewing for the fiberoptic lens. With the angulated tip, the AVIL resembles an activated McCoy blade. Flattening of the blade's vertical flange enables the device to be used in children. The fiberoptic endoscope runs from the handle to the tip of the blade. The AVIL uses conventional laryngoscopy techniques coupled with video monitoring from the blade tip. Styletted ETs, in a "hockey stick" configuration, are passed along the vertical flange of the blade under video control.[104] The AVIL has been used in patients ranging in age from 3 months to 17 years old with manual in-line neck stabilization. In infants and small children, care should be taken with insertion of the blade; initial insertion of the blade was too deep in these patients.[396] Several reports document the use of this device in pediatric patients with a DA. The video laryngoscope has been used successfully to intubate children with Morquio's syndrome as well as a 3-day-old neonate with Pierre Robin syndrome.[104,333]

K. STYLETS

Stylets should be available for the DA. The stylet is inserted into the ET until the distal end of the stylet is at the tip of the ET. The ET and stylet are bent into the desired shape—usually a hockey stick configuration. Complications associated with use of stylets include tracheal trauma, ET obstruction, and shearing of the stylet. When difficulty with removal of a stylet is encountered, the tip should be examined.[304]

L. VIDEO-OPTICAL INTUBATION STYLET

The video-optical intubating stylet (Acutronic Medical Systems, AG, Hirzel, Switzerland), consisting of a flexible fiberoptic endoscope, was developed by Dr. Marcus Weiss of Zurich, Switzerland. A sliding connector locks the video stylet onto the ET adaptor. One report documents successful use of the video-optical intubating stylet in patients age 6 to 16 years with a simulated grade III laryngoscopic view. Forty-six of 50 patients were intubated on the first attempt; four attempts were considered failures because of a prolonged intubation time (more than 60 seconds).[395]

M. LIGHTED STYLETS

Many different types of lighted stylets or light wands are currently commercially available. Pediatric versions are available for use with ETs as small as 2.0 to 4.0 mm (Trachlight, Laerdal Medical, Armonk, NY).[114] The use of the lighted stylet to guide blind endotracheal intubation relies on the principle of transillumination.[114] The presence of a well-defined glow in the neck indicates tracheal placement. Esophageal placement is indicated by the absence of a glow in the neck. Several different reports describe successful intubation of pediatric patients with the light wand.[166,205] Several important facts for a successful technique have been reported[114]: (1) A small shoulder roll should be used to keep the head in a neutral to slightly extended position. This is extremely important in a small infant, whose neck naturally flexes when lying on a flat surface because of the large occiput. (2) The light wand should be advanced in the midline; if the light deviates to one side, the light wand should be withdrawn and repositioned. (3) The epiglottis is elevated by lifting the jaw with the nondominant hand. (4) Transillumination should be assessed before advancing the light wand too far. (5) Blind nasal intubation in children is often easier with the rigid stylet left in place. The wand is bent less sharply than for an oral intubation.[114] As with any new technique, experience in patients with normal anatomy should be obtained prior to attempts in patients with a DA.

N. OPTICAL STYLET

The first optical stylet, described in 1979, was a Hopkins telescope with a fiberoptic external light source (Karl Storz, Tuttlingen, Germany).[190] The Seeing Optical Stylet (SOS) system (Clarus Medical, Minneapolis, MN) is a new, reusable, high-resolution fiberoptic endoscope with a malleable stainless steel stylet.[1] It combines the features of an FOB and a light wand. The Shikani Seeing

Stylet is portable, lightweight, and available in pediatric and adult versions. The pediatric version is compatible with ETs in the 3.0 to 5.0 mm size range. The SOS can be inserted directly into an ET, allowing intubation to be performed under direct vision. Illumination is provided by a standard green line fiberoptic laryngoscope handle or the included SITElite halogen handle. An adjustable tube stop with an oxygen port, which goes over the shaft of the stylet, allows supplemental oxygen to be delivered. Many factors such as cervical spine injury, small mouth, large tongue, and reduced jaw mobility do not affect the SOS.[1] Pfitzner and colleagues described the use of the Shikani SOS on eight occasions in seven patients with DA.[289] There were seven successful intubations; one patient, who had previous surgery and radiotherapy for a retropharyngeal rhabdomyosarcoma, could not be intubated by any method. Two patients with limited mouth opening and one patient with a C1-C2 subluxation were intubated on the first attempt. A patient with Hunter's syndrome was intubated on the second attempt. A potential difficulty mentioned with the SOS is loss of the visual field, which occurs when the lens is next to a mucosal surface.[343] Maneuvers to increase the operating space available are use of a laryngoscope to retract the base of the tongue, lifting the mandible, and pulling the tongue forward.[343]

The Shikani stylet is inserted into the ET after lubrication with silicon spray. The fiberoptic cable can be connected to a video monitor. The mandible is lifted with the left hand and displaced anteriorly until the lower teeth are anterior to the upper teeth.[343] The stylet with the loaded ET is advanced into the trachea under direct vision. Laryngoscopy may be useful in cases of DI (Fig. 33-2).

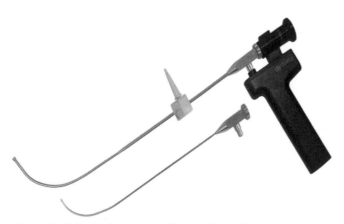

Figure 33-2 The Shikani Seeing Optical Stylet (Clarus Medical, Minneapolis, MN) is a reusable, high-resolution fiberoptic endoscope. The pediatric version is compatible with endotracheal tubes in the range 3.0 to 5.0 mm. Supplemental oxygen can be delivered through the oxygen port. It can be used with the SITElite halogen handle (as shown) or a standard green line fiberoptic laryngoscope handle.

O. LARYNGEAL MASK AIRWAY

The LMA[53] (LMA North America., San Diego CA), introduced in 1983 and approved for use in 1991 by the Food and Drug Administration, is a standard part of the ASA DA algorithm.[297] Pediatric versions of the LMA Classic, as well as the disposable LMA, are available for use and are part of the pediatric DA algorithm, as described by Steward and coauthors.[353] This device requires minimum training and has been shown to be useful in neonatal resuscitation.[288] The LMA Flexible is available in a size 2 and 2.5 and the LMA ProSeal is available in a size 2. The size of the LMA in children is determined by the patient's weight. A new method to determine the size of the LMA in children has been suggested. With the hand extended and palm side facing up, the thumb and little finger are extended. The second, third, and fourth fingers are placed together. The fully inflated LMA is placed against the palmar side of the patient's fingers, keeping the widest part of the LMA in line with the widest part of the three fingers. In a study of 163 children aged birth to 14 years old, this method was correct 78% of the time. In the remaining patients, a difference of only one size was observed.[122]

The LMA has been described as a conduit for blind intubation as well as a conduit for fiberoptic intubation.[107, 283, 291,305,335] Awake placement of the LMA has been described in an infant with Pierre Robin syndrome.[236] Anterograde intubation through the LMA with a guidewire has also been described. In that case, an infant with micrognathia could not be intubated with conventional methods. A soft-tipped guidewire was advanced through the LMA and the position confirmed by fluoroscopy. An ET was inserted over the guidewire, followed by removal of the LMA.[325] A review of the literature demonstrates different insertion techniques.

The standard technique described with the cuff deflated for adults has also been advocated for children. In addition, a rotational or reverse technique has been described. The LMA is inserted with the cuff facing the hard palate and then rotated and advanced simultaneously. An alternative technique involves inserting the LMA with the cuff partially inflated. There are conflicting reports concerning placement of the LMA with the different techniques. In children, one study compared two insertion techniques. The partially inflated cuff insertion technique does not increase the incidence of downfolding of the epiglottis and is an acceptable alternative to the standard technique.[374] In another study, insertion of the partially inflated LMA required less time and was associated with a higher success rate on first attempts compared with the standard (deflated) technique.[275] Results from a study detailing the fiberoptic positioning of the LMA in children with a DA show that 29.5% of patients had a grade I (full) view of the glottis, 29.5% of patients had a grade II (partial) view, and 41% of patients had a grade III (epiglottis only) view. Children with a mucopolysaccharide disorder had a grade III view 54% of the time and a grade I view 14% of the time.[387]

The ProSeal LMA is now available in pediatric sizes. This LMA has a second mask to isolate the upper esophagus with a second dorsal cuff to increase the seal against the glottis.[224] Lopez-Gill and coworkers[224] found that it was easily inserted and the oropharyngeal leak pressure was greater than 40 cm H_2O (Table 33-5).

P. RIGID VENTILATING BRONCHOSCOPE

The rigid ventilating bronchoscope is extremely useful for ventilating patients with a DA and is included in the most recent version of the ASA DA algorithm as an alternative device in the cannot ventilate, cannot intubate situation. In any situation of potential airway collapse, the otolaryngologist and the rigid ventilating bronchoscope should be immediately available.

VI. INDUCTION TECHNIQUE

The principles outlined in the ASA guidelines for DA management apply to the pediatric patient. Evaluation, recognition, and preparation are key elements.[297] Preoxygenation of pediatric patients, although difficult, should be attempted if possible prior to any DA intervention. Studies have demonstrated that the optimal time for preoxygenation in pediatric patients is different from that in adults. Values ranging from 80 to 100 seconds have been reported for adequate preoxygenation in healthy children.[61,260] Summoning help early, awake intubation (AI) and preservation of spontaneous ventilation during intubation attempts are also important when managing the DA. The awake or awake sedated approach would be the preferred method in most circumstances when managing the DA. However, in pediatric patients, the patient's cooperation may limit the usefulness of AIs. One technique that is well tolerated is placement of a lubricated LMA in awake infants, which provides an airway for inhalational induction.[236]

The traditional approach to the difficult pediatric airway has been maintenance of spontaneous ventilation under inhalational anesthesia. Premedication with oral or intravenous atropine (0.01 to 0.02 mg/kg) is indicated for vagolytic and antimuscarinic effects. Inhalation induction may be performed with either halothane or sevoflurane in 100% oxygen. Sevoflurane has been used in the management of the DA with success.[188,389] The low blood-gas solubility of sevoflurane and consequent rapid induction and emergence are advantageous when managing the DA. Steward and associates recommended converting from sevoflurane to halothane when induction is complete.[353] When the ability to ventilate the patient by mask is demonstrated, a small dose of muscle relaxant or propofol may be given to facilitate intubation.

For patients who can tolerate an awake sedated technique, a variety of drugs can be used. One must always keep in mind the risk-benefit ratio when sedating a patient with a DA. Sedatives may further compromise an airway. Sedatives should not be given to any patient in acute distress or with the potential for acute obstruction. The use of sedative agents should be based on a careful physical examination, the anesthesiologist's experience with the agents involved, and the overall condition of the patient. If there are no other options available, slow titration of pharmacologic agents to effect without loss of spontaneous ventilation should be performed. Use of pharmacologic agents that are easily antagonized is recommended. For older children and adolescents, a combination of midazolam and fentanyl may be used. Remifentanil has been used successfully to perform an awake fiberoptic intubation in a morbidly obese patient with facial, cervical, and upper thoracic edema.[300] In extreme circumstances,

Table 33-5 **Laryngeal Mask Airway Classic Mask Size with Corresponding Cuff Volumes, Endotracheal Tube, and Fiberoptic Scope Size**

Mask Size	Weight	Maximum Cuff Volume (mL)	Maximum ET Size	Maximum FOB (mm)
1	Infants up to 5 kg	Up to 4	3.5 uncuffed	2.7
1.5	5 to 10 kg	Up to 7	4.0 uncuffed	3.0
2	10 to 20 kg	Up to 10	4.5 uncuffed	3.5
2.5	20 to 30 kg	Up to 14	5.0 uncuffed	4.0
3	30 to 50 kg	Up to 20	6.0 cuffed	5.0
4	50 to 70 kg	Up to 30	6.0 cuffed	5.0
5	70 to 100 kg	Up to 40	7.0 cuffed	5.0
6	Over 100 kg	Up to 50	7.0 cuffed	5.0

ET, endotracheal tube; FOB, fiberoptic bronchoscope.

parental presence at induction may be allowed. Careful preparation of the parent must be performed prior to induction. As soon as the patient separates or begins to lose consciousness, a designated member of the operating room staff should immediately escort the parent out of the operating room.

Another important aspect for successful airway management is topicalization of the airway with local anesthesia. In pediatric patients, this may be obtained by nebulizing, spraying, or swabbing local anesthetic solution or by applying viscous gel to a gloved finger. FOB with suction ports can be used to spray local anesthesia on the vocal cords under direct vision. The maximum dose of local anesthetic allowed should be calculated before topicalization. The drug of choice is lidocaine because it has the best safety profile. Maximum doses of lidocaine are 5 mg/kg. Agents containing benzocaine, such as Cetacaine spray, Americaine ointment, and Hurricaine ointment, gel, or spray, should be avoided in infants and young children because of the risk of methemoglobinemia.[399]

VII. AIRWAY MANAGEMENT TECHNIQUES

A. TECHNIQUES FOR VENTILATION

Obstruction of the upper airway is a common occurrence in pediatric patients undergoing an inhalation induction. Techniques for overcoming this type of obstruction include insertion of an oropharyngeal airway or a nasopharyngeal airway, or both. Choosing the correct size is important, as previously described, or the obstruction may worsen. Another common mistake is occlusion of the submandibular space with incorrect placement of the anesthesiologist's hand. Care should be taken to position the hand on the tip of the mandible and not on the submandibular space. Chin lift or jaw thrust combined with continuous positive airway pressure (CPAP) at 10 cm H_2O has been shown to improve upper airway patency.[309]

Additional techniques are available for mask ventilation. The two-person technique involves either one person holding the mask with both hands while an assistant compresses the reservoir bag or a second person assisting in jaw lift while the first person continues to compress the reservoir bag. Another option is using the anesthesia ventilator to provide ventilation so that one person can hold the face mask with both hands.[33]

B. TECHNIQUES FOR INTUBATION

1. Direct Laryngoscopy

Tips for successful visualization of the larynx include proper use of external laryngeal pressure and positioning. Direct laryngoscopy involves alignment of the oral, pharyngeal, and laryngeal axes in order to visualize the glottis.

Because the larynx is situated in a more cephalad position and the occiput is large, the sniffing position in infants does not assist in visualization of the larynx.[82,399] The infant should be positioned with the head in a neutral position with the neck neither flexed or extended.[58] A small shoulder or neck roll may be beneficial. Optimum external laryngeal manipulation (OELM) should also be used with a poor laryngoscopic view in order to improve visualization. OELM may improve the laryngoscopic view by at least one whole grade in adults. This is not cricoid pressure but rather pressing posteriorly and cephalad over the thyroid, hyoid, and cricoid cartilages.[32] Benumof and Cooper suggested that OELM should be an instinctive and reflex response to a poor laryngoscopic view.[32] This maneuver has also proved effective in pediatric patients.[292] The main mechanism seems to be shortening of the incisor-to-glottis distance.

The two-anesthesiologist technique involves manipulating the larynx under direct vision by the laryngoscopist and intubation by a second anesthesiologist. This technique has been used successfully to intubate a 6-month-old infant with Pierre Robin syndrome and concomitant tongue tie.[184]

The retromolar or paraglossal technique has been advocated as useful in cases of DI related to a small mandible.[159] A straight laryngoscope blade is introduced into the extreme right corner of the mouth overlying the molars, thus reducing the distance to the vocal cords. It is advanced in the space between the tongue and lateral pharyngeal wall until the epiglottis or glottis is visualized. The head is rotated to the left to improve visualization while applying external laryngeal pressure displacing the larynx to the right. Advancement of the ET is facilitated by retracting the corner of the mouth to allow placement of the ET. The styletted ET should be shaped into the classical hockey stick configuration. An alternative approach involves placement of the ET from the left side of the mouth.[99] Lateral placement of the laryngoscope blade reduces the soft tissue compression because the tongue is essentially bypassed. The maxillary structures are also bypassed by the lateral blade placement, thus improving the view.[82] As there is a reduced space for displacement of the tongue in syndromes with micrognathia, this approach may be useful. The retromolar technique has been described as an alternative method for intubation of patients with Pierre Robin syndrome.[47] A pediatric version of the Bonfils Retromolar Intubation Fiberscope (Karl Storz) should be available soon. It is an optical stylet that allows a retromolar approach to the DA.[144]

In adults, the left molar approach with a Macintosh blade and OELM has been reported to improve the glottic view in cases of difficult laryngoscopy.[410]

Suspension laryngoscopy is often employed by otolaryngologists as an alternative technique for visualization of the difficult larynx. Intubation of an infant with Goldenhar's syndrome was accomplished by suspension laryngoscopy.[68] This method is similar to standard laryngoscopy by the retromolar technique.

Finally, with any direct laryngoscopy technique, limitation of attempts is recommended. Edema can rapidly occur and create a cannot ventilate, cannot intubate scenario.

2. Blind Intubation Technique

a. *Blind Nasotracheal Intubation*

Blind nasotracheal intubation requires preservation of spontaneous ventilation either under general anesthesia or with adequate vasoconstriction and topicalization of the nasal mucosa. The tip of the ET is directed toward the larynx by listening to the intensity of the breath sounds or by the capnograph tracing. This technique requires extensive practice prior to use. Tips for this technique include external pressure on the neck, which may direct the glottis toward the ET; placement of a stylet through the ET after passage through the nasopharynx to direct the tip to the glottis; inflating the ET cuff with air to center it at the glottis and then deflating it for actual passage; and repositioning of the head (flexion/extension) if the initial intubation attempt fails.[353] Pediatric patients with enlarged adenoids may be at risk for bleeding and trauma with this technique. Blind nasotracheal intubation of a neonate with Pierre Robin syndrome has been described.[294]

b. *Digital Endotracheal Intubation*

Digital intubation is a blind technique that is relatively easy to learn. Intubation of an 8-day-old, 3.3-kg neonate with Pierre Robin syndrome has been reported.[364] The left index finger is passed midline along the surface of the tongue until it passes the epiglottis. The left thumb may apply cricoid pressure to steady the larynx. The ET, using the left index finger as a guide, is advanced into the trachea. This technique has been used as the primary method of intubating neonates in some neonatal centers.[149] As with any new technique, practice is required.

c. *Light Wand*

Intubation with a light wand is a blind technique that has found success in management of the difficult pediatric airway.[114,166,205] The success rate increases with experience; thus, practice is required. As with any new technique, experience with patients who have normal anatomy should be gained first. Contraindications to the use of the light wand include tumors, infections, trauma, and foreign bodies of the upper airway.[2] Causes of failed intubation include entrapment in the vallecula or the aryepiglottic folds.[114] A shoulder roll helps to extend the head and neck and increase the exposure of the anterior neck. Following preparation of the light wand, the jaw is lifted with the nondominant hand or a laryngoscope blade. The light wand is inserted in the midline into the patient's mouth. It is rotated around the patient's tongue and then gently rocked backward and forward. If the ET-wand is in the trachea, a well-defined bright light (size of a quarter) is visible at the level of the subglottis on the anterior surface of the neck.

3. Fiberoptic Laryngoscopy

Aids for fiberoptic intubation include face masks, oropharyngeal airways, guidewires, and the LMA.[403] The Frei mask previously described or variations of commercially available masks have been used with success.[117,108,136,189] The Patil-Syracuse mask is available in a size 2, but it is difficult to achieve a good seal with this mask. An endoscopy mask can be made by attaching a swivel FOB adaptor to a pediatric face mask in one of two ways.[403] First, a commercially available swivel adaptor (Instrumentation Industries, Bethel Park, PA) can be attached directly to the mask. Next, an adaptor designed for attachment to the ET, such as the Portex bronchoscope adaptor, can be connected to the face mask with a 15- to 22-mm adaptor.

Oropharyngeal airways may also be modified for use in pediatric fiberoptic intubations. A strip may be cut from the convex surface of a Guedel-style airway in order to produce an aid for oral fiberoptic laryngoscopy, creating a channel. The fiberscope is placed in the channel, which helps maintain a midline position. The use of a smaller airway than predicted is suggested so that one may visualize the base of the tongue and epiglottis. Modified oropharyngeal airways are not effective as bite blocks, and one must be careful.[403] Finally, a nipple from a baby bottle has been modified to act as a conduit for fiberoptic intubation in an infant with an unstable cervical spine. In this case, a hole was cut obliquely into the end of the nipple. After topicalization of the airway with 2% lidocaine, fiberoptic intubation was performed with a 4.0-mm uncuffed ET.[131]

Flexible fiberoptic laryngoscopy is one of the cornerstones of DA management. Preparation for fiberoptic laryngoscopy should include preparation of the patient (antisialogue) and checking of the fiberscope, light source, and suction as well as standard airway equipment. An assistant is necessary for monitoring of the patient and providing a jaw lift. A jaw lift is useful because it elevates the tongue from the posterior pharynx.[399] For older children and adolescents who will be sedated for the procedure, explanation and reassurance in a calm manner are helpful. A method of delivering oxygen is necessary as well. This can be accomplished in a variety of ways: either blowby from the anesthesia circuit or by nasal cannula. For patients who are anesthetized, an LMA or an endoscopy mask may be used to ventilate the patient while the intubation is being performed. Tips for successful oral intubation include midline placement of the fiberscope, advancement of the fiberscope only when recognizable structures are visualized, and retraction of the tongue with gauze or clamps if needed.[399]

If the view from the fiberscope is pink mucosa, the fiberscope is slowly pulled back until a recognizable structure is seen. If the nasal route is chosen, a topical vasoconstrictor may be used to reduce the chance of bleeding. In a series of 46 patients with DA, fiberoptic nasal intubation was successful on the first attempt in 37 patients (80.4%) and on the second or third attempt in 7 patients (15.2%). Two failures occurred: one related to bleeding and the other to inability to introduce the scope nasally.[43]

Flexible fiberoptic laryngoscopy may be performed in a variety of ways. The standard technique involves passage of the ET over the fiberscope. The ultrathin fiberoptic laryngoscope with a directable tip allows fiberoptic intubation to be performed with ETs as small as 2.5 mm. Intubation of a 3-month-old infant with the Pierre Robin syndrome has been successfully performed with an ultrathin fiberscope.[199] A new 2.5-mm ultrathin flexible FOB with a 1.2-mm suction channel has been used to intubate a newborn with a DA.[38] This bronchoscope has a 2.5 mm OD, a 1.2 mm working suction channel, an angle of deflection of 160 degrees up and 130 degrees down, and a working length of 450 mm.

In scenarios where the available bronchoscope is too large for the required ET, a staged technique may be employed.[356] A fiberscope with a working channel, a cardiac catheter, and a guidewire are required. The guidewire is passed into the working channel of the fiberscope prior to the intubation. The fiberscope-guidewire assembly is then introduced into the mouth and positioned above the larynx. The guidewire is advanced into the trachea under direct visualization, followed by removal of the fiberscope. A cardiac catheter (used to stiffen the wire) is threaded over the guidewire. Finally, an ET is advanced into the trachea over the guidewire-catheter assembly, which is then removed. A modification of this technique involves passage of the ET over the guidewire without the reinforcing cardiac catheter. This has been used to intubate nasotracheally a 3-day-old infant with Pierre Robin syndrome.[168]

The fiberscope may also be used as an aid for nasal intubation either under direct vision or with the use of a guide. In these cases, the FOB is introduced into one of the nares while the ET is advanced into the trachea through the other naris.[3] Alternatively, if the ET cannot be manipulated into the glottis, a guide may be placed in the opposite naris and directed into the trachea. The ET is then removed and threaded over the guide. A urethral catheter has been used in this manner to assist in the intubation of a 2-week-old neonate with Klippel-Feil syndrome, occipital meningocele, and microretrognathia.[132] Another variation of the staged technique involves placement of a larger ET into the larynx under fiberoptic visualization followed by removal of the fiberscope, leaving the larger ET in the larynx. A bougie is placed through the larger ET into the trachea, and then the ET is removed. An ET of the appropriate size is then advanced over the bougie into the trachea.[35]

Flexible FOB intubation through the LMA has been reported with success.[271, 283,291] Staged intubation techniques involving the LMA, fiberscope, guidewires, and catheters (dilators) have been reported. An example of this is the use of LMA-assisted wire-guided fiberoptic endotracheal intubation.[157] In a series of 15 cases, Heard and colleagues[157] demonstrated that this technique was safe, successful, and easy to learn. After the bronchoscope is placed through the LMA and the vocal cords are visualized, the guidewire is passed through the suction port of the bronchoscope and into the trachea. The LMA and bronchoscope are carefully removed and the ET is advanced over the wire. A variation of this theme involves fiberoptic visualization of the glottis through the LMA followed by passage of a guidewire through the suction port of a bronchoscope into the trachea as before. The fiberscope is then removed and an airway catheter or a ureteral dilator is passed over the wire into the trachea through the LMA. The LMA is then removed and an ET is advanced over the catheter into the trachea.[386] This technique has been used successfully to manage the airway in children with mucopolysaccharidoses. The use of an LMA, an airway exchange catheter, and a 2.2 mm OD FOB has also been described.[367] After placement of the LMA and visualization of the vocal cords, the fiberscope is removed. The fiberscope is placed into the lumen of a size 11 airway exchange catheter, which had been cut to 25 cm. This combination was advanced through the LMA into the trachea by a connector. The LMA and fiberscope are removed and an ET is advanced over the Cook airway exchange catheter.

Przybylo and coauthors[299] reported the performance of a retrograde fiberoptic intubation through a tracheocutaneous fistula in a child with Nager's syndrome. The ultrathin fiberscope was passed through the tracheocutaneous fistula in a cephalad direction past the vocal cords and exiting the nares. The ET was then advanced over the bronchoscope into the trachea.

4. Bullard Laryngoscope

The pediatric Bullard laryngoscope is placed into the oropharynx in the horizontal plane. After passing the tongue, the handle is rotated to a vertical position. One must be careful to stay in the midline as the blade slides around the tongue. Then the handle is lifted in order to visualize the glottis.[48] Once the glottis is visualized, a styletted ET is advanced under direct vision into the trachea.

5. Dental Mirror–Assisted Laryngoscopy

The dental mirror can be used as an adjunct to direct laryngoscopy in order to view an anterior larynx. After direct laryngoscopy is performed, the dental mirror is inserted on the right side of the mouth and angled so that the vocal cords are seen. The handle of the mirror is moved to the left and held by the left hand. Then an appropriately shaped styletted ET is advanced into the trachea while looking at the dental mirror. Practice is required to develop the necessary coordination. A Stortz No. 3 dental mirror and a Macintosh No. 1 laryngoscope have been used to intubate a 2.5-month, 3.9-kg infant.[284]

6. Retrograde Intubation

The classical retrograde technique involves percutaneous placement of an intravenous catheter through the cricothyroid membrane into the trachea followed by placement of a guidewire. The guidewire exits the mouth or nose and the ET is then exchanged over the guidewire. If resistance to ET passage occurs, counterclockwise rotation of the ET may facilitate placement. This technique has been used for intubation of an infant with Goldenhar's syndrome.[81] A 14 Fr retrograde intubation set is commercially available from Cook for use with ETs with an ID of 5.0 mm or larger.

A combined technique utilizing the FOB and retrograde intubation has been used successfully in management of the difficult pediatric airway as well, as previously mentioned.[100]

A bronchoscope with a working channel is necessary for the combined technique. The guidewire is threaded into the suction port of an intubating bronchoscope that has a preloaded softened ET on it. The bronchoscope is passed along the guidewire until it is past the vocal cords. When the scope is past the vocal cords, the wire is withdrawn and the ET is correctly positioned. This technique allows passage without obstruction from the arytenoid cartilage or epiglottis. Oxygen insufflation can be performed through the suction port as well, even with the wire in place. Care must be taken to limit flow to avoid tracheobronchial injury from excessive gas velocity. Audenaert and coworkers[17] reported this technique in 20 patients with DAs ranging in age from 1 day to 17 years old.[17] In that series, no major complications were reported. Retrograde wire-guided direct laryngoscopy has also been reported for airway management in a 1 month old.[332] In that case, attempts to pass a 2.5-mm ET over the wire itself were unsuccessful, yet endotracheal intubation was achieved over the wire with the aid of direct laryngoscopy.

7. Emergency Access

Emergency access is divided into the emergency surgical and the nonsurgical airway.[297] Emergency surgical airway access is often very difficult and requires the presence of a skilled anesthesiologist. It is the last resort in the cannot ventilate, cannot intubate arm of the ASA DA algorithm.[406] Three procedures are referred to in this category—emergency tracheostomy, emergency cricothyroidotomy, and percutaneous needle cricothyroidotomy. In children younger than 6 years, emergency tracheostomy is usually the procedure of choice because the cricothyroid membrane is too small for cannulation.[17] In older children, percutaneous needle cricothyroidotomy is often preferred over a surgical approach because most anesthesiologists can rapidly perform this technique. Also, there is less chance of injury to surrounding structures.[82] Emergency cricothroidotomy kits are available from Cook with 3.5, 4, and 6 mm ID airway catheters.

The emergency nonsurgical pathway includes use of the LMA, esophageal-tracheal Combitube, and transtracheal jet ventilation (TTJV).[297] The Combitube is available in a small adult size and is contraindicated in patients less than 4 feet tall.[399] The LMA is a device that is very useful in the management of the difficult pediatric airway. As stated previously, it can be used as an SVD or as a conduit for intubation. However, in the presence of glottic or subglottic obstruction, the LMA is ineffective. TTJV is considered to be the technique of choice in this situation. This has been reported in two cases for laser endoscopic surgery.[308] Caution with this technique is urged as serious complications may result from the use of jet ventilation.[354] Jet ventilation below a glottic or subglottic obstruction may result in barotrauma because the pathway for egress of air and oxygen is limited. Tension pneumothorax has been reported with jet ventilation through an airway exchange catheter in an adult.[25]

VIII. COMPLICATIONS OF AIRWAY MANAGEMENT

Complications that result from intubation in adults can occur in the pediatric population as well. Airway injury accounted for 6% of claims in the ASA closed claims database.[102] Four percent of the airway injury claims involved pediatric patients younger than 16 years. The most frequent sites of injury reported were the larynx (33%), pharynx (19%), and esophagus (18%). Injuries to the esophagus and trachea were more frequently associated with DI. Laryngeal injuries included vocal cord paralysis, granuloma, arytenoid dislocation, and hematoma. Pharyngeal injuries included lacerations, perforation, infection, sore throat, and miscellaneous injuries (foreign body, burn, hematoma, and diminished taste). An oropharyngeal burn related to the laryngoscope lamp occurred in a term baby weighing 3.6 kg who was easily intubated at birth.[200] The laryngoscope was switched on prior to intubation. Light bulb laryngoscopes, in contrast to fiberoptic laryngoscopes, can reach temperatures that would result in burns to the oropharynx. As the filaments age, they may overlap, and it is common for two or more coils to touch.[200] The resistance of the lamp decreases and current increases, thus increasing the temperature. These authors recommend that all light bulb laryngoscopes be switched on for less than 1 minute; if they are left on, the temperature of the bulb should be manually checked prior to intubation.

DI accounted for 62% of all esophageal injuries. Most of the esophageal injuries involved esophageal perforation (90%). Esophageal perforation following DI has been reported in a neonate.[334]

Laryngotracheal stenosis may be classified as glottic, subglottic, or tracheal. Prolonged intubation seems to be the major etiology. The mechanism responsible seems to be ischemic necrosis caused by pressure from the ET against the glottic and subglottic mucosa. This results in an inflammatory reaction with a secondary bacterial infection and scar formation. Risk factors include too large an ET, prolonged intubation, repeated intubation, laryngeal trauma, sepsis, and chronic inflammatory disease.[222]

The incidence of postintubation croup varies from 0.1% to 1%.[201,216] Risk factors include age younger than 4, tight-fitting ET, repeated intubation attempts, duration of surgery greater than 1 hour, patient's position other than supine, and previous history of croup. Reports are conflicting concerning the risk from a concurrent upper respiratory tract infection. Classical treatment consists of humidified air, nebulized racemic epinephrine, and dexamethasone. In pediatric trauma patients, absence of an air leak at the time of extubation was the strongest predictor of postextubation stridor requiring treatment.[193]

IX. AIRWAY DISEASES AND IMPLICATIONS

A. HEAD ANOMALIES

Airway management can be adversely affected by conditions that involve enlargement of the head. Mass lesions and macrocephaly can interfere with mask ventilation or direct laryngoscopy, or both.

1. Airway Implications

Airway management in children with macrocephaly requires proper head and neck positioning and care of the associated airway anomalies that are a frequent finding in patients with mucopolysaccharidosis. If preoperative evaluation suggests presence of a DA, awake methods of endotracheal intubation should be initially attempted.

In children, AI may require careful use of sedatives in addition to topical anesthesia to the oropharynx, larynx, and nasopharynx (for nasotracheal intubation). A limited number of attempts at direct laryngoscopy may be made. If these are not successful, one of the various techniques of nonvisual or indirect laryngoscopy as detailed earlier may be used to secure the airway. If the patient does not comply with awake endotracheal intubation without the use of an amount of sedative that risks respiratory compromise, general anesthesia may be induced as long as mask ventilation is possible. The patient may breathe a potent vapor anesthetic until a level of anesthesia is achieved that allows endotracheal intubation. Other options include

fiberoptic laryngoscopy in a patient breathing spontaneously through a mask or an LMA, use of a lighted stylet, use of a Bullard laryngoscope, and the retrograde technique. In children in whom mask ventilation is known to be easy, muscle relaxants may be used if their use notably improves the chance of endotracheal intubation.

The pathologic conditions that involve enlargement of the head and affect the airway are encephalocele, hydrocephalus, and mucopolysaccharidosis together with other less frequent conditions such as phakomatoses, cranioskeletal dysplasias, or conjoint twins with face-to-face encroachment of the heads or close proximity of the chests (thoracopagus).

2. Specific Anomalies

a. Encephalocele

Patients with encephaloceles may have other diseases that complicate airway management. The only two syndromes associated with encephalocele in which survival past infancy is likely are Roberts-SC phocomelia syndrome (includes pseudothalidomide syndrome, hypomelia-hypertrichosis-facial hemangioma syndrome) and facioauriculovertebral spectrum (includes first and second brachial arch syndrome, oculoauricular vertebral dysplasia, hemifacial microsomia, Goldenhar's syndrome).

Encephaloceles, or neural tube defects of the head, usually occur in the occipital area, although they may involve the frontal and nasal regions. When large, they affect airway management by interfering with mask fit or laryngoscopy.[237]

b. Hydrocephalus

Hydrocephalus is associated with over 30 malformation syndromes. Some of the craniosynostosis syndromes are associated with hydrocephalus and result from bone compression that prevents free flow of the cerebrospinal fluid. Examples of these include achondroplasia, Apert's syndrome, and Pfeiffer's syndrome.

Some of these diseases may affect the airway by more than one mechanism (e.g., children with hydrocephalus who also have Arnold-Chiari malformation). Difficulties with airway management are usually associated with the underling pathology and interference with face mask ventilation.

c. Mucopolysaccharidosis (Storage Diseases)

The mucopolysaccharidoses (MPSs) are a group of seven inherited lysosomal storage disorders caused by the deficiency of specific lysosomal enzymes required for the degradation of glycosaminoglycans (GAGs), which are complex macromolecules. The inability to degrade GAGs leads to their lysosomal accumulation and the subsequent clinical features of the disorders, which can include facial coarsening, corneal clouding, valvular heart disease, hepatosplenomegaly, and dysostosis multiplex accompanied by short stature.

MPS type I, which results from the deficiency of L-iduronidase activity, can manifest as one of three different clinical phenotypes: Hurler's syndrome (i.e., MPS type IH), Scheie's syndrome (i.e., MPS type IS), and Hurler-Scheie syndrome (i.e., MPS type I H/S). Of these, Scheie's syndrome is the mildest form of the metabolic defect. The other MPSs are Hunter's syndrome (type II), Sanfilippo's syndrome (type III), Morquio's syndrome (type IV), Maroteaux-Lamy syndrome (type VI), and Sly's syndrome (type VII).

The anesthetic morbidity of the MPSs is 20% to 30%.[26] Morbidity is almost always related to respiratory difficulties. Intubation and maintenance of the airway might be difficult because of a variety of upper airway abnormalities, including micrognathia, macroglossia, patulous lips, restricted motion of the temporomandibular joints, friable tissues, and the presence of copious viscous secretions. Semenza and Pyeritz,[336] in a retrospective study on 21 patients with the diagnosis of MPS, found that the anatomic factors affecting respiratory status included (1) upper airway narrowing by hypertrophied tongue, tonsils, adenoids, and mucous membranes; (2) lower airway narrowing by GAG deposition within the tracheobronchial mucosa; (3) decreased thoracic dimensions related to scoliosis and thoracic hyperkyphosis; and (4) decreased abdominal dimensions because of lumbar hyperlordosis, gibbus formation, and hepatosplenomegaly. In addition, a short neck and an anterior and narrowed larynx may lead to an increased incidence of difficult or failed intubations.[385]

A particularity of the patients with Hunter, Hurler, and Maroteaux-Lamy syndromes is that they have significantly more airway difficulties as they grow older compared with patients in this group with other syndromes.[254]

The incidence of DI is high. In one review[385] of 34 patients who underwent 89 anesthesias, the overall incidence of DI was 25% and failed intubation 8%. In children with Hurler's syndrome, the DI incidence was 54% and failed intubation incidence 23%. In another study,[163] 38 anesthetics were administered to nine patients with MPSs, specifically the Hunter, Hurler, Sanfilippo, and Morquio's syndromes. The authors found an overall incidence of airway-related problems of 26%. In patients with the Hurler's or Hunter's syndrome the incidence of airway-related problems was 53%.

Belani and associates[30] reported their experience with 141 anesthetics in 30 patients with MPSs. It is worthwhile to note that it was easier to see the vocal cords during laryngoscopy in children with Hurler's syndrome when they were younger (23 versus 41 months, $P \leq .01$) and smaller (12 versus 15 kg, $P \leq .05$). Also, children with preoperative obstructive breathing had a significantly higher incidence of postextubation obstruction. A total of 28 children underwent bone marrow transplantation; this reversed upper airway obstruction and also reversed intracranial hypertension.

Failure to insert an LMA[207,386] or nasopharyngeal airway[207] as well as fatal outcomes[121] have been reported. Consequently, nasotracheal intubation is not recommended, owing to difficulties with the anatomy of nasal passages and potential hemorrhage from soft tissue trauma. Accumulation of mucopolysaccharides in the trachea may require a much smaller ET than usual.[207] Tracheostomy can also be difficult technically in these patients and in one case was impossible even postmortem.[167]

Cervical instability, potential spinal cord damage, and severe thoracic and lumbar skeletal abnormalities make positioning and intubation difficult. In their series, in children with Hurler's syndrome, Belani and associates[30] found an incidence of odontoid dysplasia of 94%, whereas 38% demonstrated anterior C1-C2 subluxation. To avoid cervical cord damage in patients with cervical instability, Walker and colleagues[385] described manual in-line stabilization during intubation and concluded that a pediatric FOB should be available for all known DIs. Tzanova and coworkers[375] reported successful anesthesia in a 23-month-old girl with Morquio's syndrome and unstable neck. The authors suggested the use of fiberoptic nasal intubation with spontaneous ventilation as the method of choice.

Apart from the aforementioned problems, a number of other skeletal deformities should be considered in these patients. Chest cage dysfunction related to kyphoscoliosis leads to reduction in vital capacity and a restrictive pulmonary disorder.[58]

Cardiac diseases are common in patients with MPSs. Both clinical and histologic studies of the cardiovascular system show progressive involvement of the coronary arteries, heart valves, and myocardium. The lumen of the coronary arteries is narrowed owing to deposition of collagen and mucopolysaccharides in the intima. Coronary artery involvement[110,254] and valvular involvement[170] in patients with Hurler's syndrome have been reported.

Belani and coauthors[30] reported their complications with 141 anesthetics in 30 patients with MPSs. One child suffered an intraoperative stroke; another, pulmonary edema. Severe and extensive coronary obstruction was responsible for two intraoperative deaths. Coronary angiography underestimated coronary artery disease.

Considering the high rate of DI in these patients, regional anesthesia would seem to be a good alternative. Failed epidural anesthesia[207] was reported in one patient. The deposition of mucopolysaccharides in either the general epidural space or the sheath of the nerve fibers preventing direct access of the local anesthetic to the nerve was suspected.

B. FACIAL ANOMALIES: MAXILLARY AND MANDIBULAR DISEASE

The pediatric airway may be complicated by a large number of syndromes involving the head, neck, and cervical spine. The airway and associated structures are deviated from the branchial arches. The first arch develops into the maxilla, mandible, incus, malleus, zygoma, and a portion of the temporal bone. The second arch develops into stapes, the styloid process of the temporal bone, and a portion of the hyoid. The third arch develops into the reminder of the hyoid. The fourth and six arches fuse to form the laryngeal structures including the thyroid, cricoid, and arytenoid cartilages. The pharyngeal muscle develops from the fourth arch, whereas the sixth arch gives rise to the laryngeal musculature. Failure of any of these to develop properly may lead to characteristic anomalies.

1. Tumors

a. Cystic Hygroma

Cystic hygromas are multiloculated cystic structures that are benign in nature. They form as the result of budding lymphatics and, thus, may occur anywhere in the body, although they are most frequently encountered in the neck (75%) and axilla (20%). As the tumor grows, it may cause symptoms from pressure on the trachea, pharynx, blood vessels, tongue, and nerves and eventually may severely compromise the airway. The tongue often protrudes outside the mouth and prevents its closure, making maintenance of the airway difficult if not impossible. Airway obstruction is the most critical complication of the cystic hygroma in the neck. The safest approach in these children seems to be nasal intubation,[397] either blind or with fiberoptic assistance with the patient awake. In extreme cases, tracheostomy may be necessary.

b. Neck Teratoma

Teratomas of the head and neck are interesting because of their obscure origin, bizarre microscopic appearance, unpredictable behavior, and often dramatic clinical presentation. The reported incidence of cervical teratomas ranges from 2.3% to 9.3% of all teratomas. A teratoma is a true neoplasm, which includes four groups: dermoid cysts, teratoid cysts, true teratomas, and epignathi (pharyngeal teratomas).

Teratomas of the head and neck frequently arise with respiratory distress or even asphyxia at delivery, and a well-established plan for early airway management should be prepared. If they are untreated, the mortality of patients with these masses is 80% to 100%.[331] Fetal ultrasonography has been used since the 1970s to aid in the prenatal diagnosis. Antenatal diagnosis is important for two reasons. First, elective cesarean section should be planned to avoid dystocia and fetal trauma. Second, because immediate establishment of a patent airway is essential for survival, a team of pediatric airway experts must be available.

The ex utero intrapartum technique (EXIT) allows the continuance of fetoplacental circulation during cesarean section. Initially, only the infant's head and shoulders (but not the placenta) are delivered, thus maintaining uteroplacental blood flow. After the infant's airway is secured, the umbilical cord is clamped and delivery of the infant is completed. The EXIT has proved useful in cases of anticipated DA instrumentation of the neonate (e.g., large fetal neck masses causing airway obstruction).[342] Once the head of the neonate is delivered, a multitude of choices are available for airway management: direct laryngoscopy, fiberoptic intubation, pediatric Bullard laryngoscopy,[331] or tracheostomy. The EXIT procedure has proved to be safe and efficacious, allowing establishment of an airway in a controlled manner as the placenta allows continued gas exchange during airway manipulation.[266,412] Early identification of these masses allows controlled delivery of the neonate in a setting where pediatric anesthesiologists, surgeons, and neonatologists can develop strategies to minimize the risk of a postnatal respiratory death.

c. Cherubism

Cherubism is a familial disease of childhood in which patients acquire mandibular and sometimes maxillary enlargement. The mandibular rami hypertrophy, limiting the submandibular space for displacement of the tongue and making visualization of the glottis during direct laryngoscopy difficult.[240]

2. Congenital Hypoplasia

a. Acrocephalosyndactyly

Maxillary hypoplasia results from premature synostosis of facial and cranial sutures and usually manifests as one of multiple abnormal features in a group of rare but complex syndromes called acrocephalosyndactylies. Acrocephalosyndactyly encompasses a number of dysostoses, not all of which can be distinguished clearly. The midface retrusion gives the appearance of prognathia, although in reality the mandible is smaller than normal. In addition, there may be associated anomalies of the central nervous system (CNS) (increased intracranial pressure and absent corpus callosum), the extremities, and, in a small percentage of patients, the heart.[238] Both the upper and lower airways may be compromised in these patients.[78]

Multiple pathologic conditions may be associated: maxillary regression may be associated with choanal stenosis or atresia, reduction in nasopharyngeal space,[243] and palate deformity (narrow, high arched, or cleft). These features may cause respiratory compromise or obstructive apnea[77,178, 252,287] early in life, although as the child grows obstruction can become worse because of continued restriction in growth of the maxillary region. In one series, upper airway obstruction arose more frequently in Crouzon's and Pfeiffer's syndrome than in Apert's syndrome.

The incidence of airway obstruction has been addressed.[221] Of a total of 40 patients with severe "syndromic" craniosynostosis (13 had Apert's syndrome and 27 had Crouzon's disease), 40% presented with airway obstruction (12.5% severe and 27.5% mild obstruction). There was no significant difference in the distribution of airway status between patients with Apert's syndrome and Crouzon's disease. Causes for the five patients with severe obstruction were midface hypoplasia, lower airway obstruction, tonsillar and adenoid hypertrophy, and choanal atresia.

Lower airway disease in the acrocephalosyndactylies occurs in the form of tracheomalacia, bronchomalacia, solid cartilaginous trachea lacking tracheal rings, and tracheal stenosis. Patients with tubular cartilaginous tracheas have displayed a propensity for easy tracheal injury, edema, and stenosis and a potential for lower airway infection (tracheitis and bronchitis) and mucous plugging because tracheal ciliary activity may be deficient. Sleep apnea was described in association with tracheal cartilaginous sleeve in a patient with Pfeiffer's syndrome.[272]

Airway problems can be divided into those arising from the nasal passages, nasopharynx, palate, or trachea. Nasal septal deviation is a common feature of craniosynostosis patients and is considered a principal finding in Saethre-Chotzen syndrome. Narrowing of the nasal passages arises from maxillary hypoplasia. Although choanal atresia can occur, the usual picture is one of generalized narrowing. The nasopharynx is very shallow because of hypoplasia of the maxilla and the altered angulation of the skull base. Finally, palatal abnormalities further impinge on the nasopharynx. These deformities may consist of arched or ridged palates or increased thickness of the soft tissue. The degree of airway obstruction is variable in these patients, being among the worst in Apert's syndrome. Complications including cor pulmonale and even death from airway obstruction have been reported. Lower airway obstruction may result from a number of abnormalities, including subglottic stenosis and vertically fused tracheal cartilage. Subglottic stenosis is especially common in Crouzon's patients. Vertically fused tracheal cartilage has been reported in cases of Apert's, Crouzon's, and Pfeiffer's. With this abnormality, the entire trachea is encased in a tube of nonsegmented cartilage. These children can be quite difficult to manage and usually present with episodes of recurrent lower respiratory tract infections, reactive airway disease, and chronically retained secretions.

Acrocephalosyndactyly disorders include:

- Apert's syndrome (type I)
- Apert-Crouzon disease

Acrocephalosyndactyly also occurs with other diseases:

- Chotzen's syndrome
- Pfeiffer-type acrocephalosyndactyly

Apert Syndrome. Apert's syndrome is characterized by agenesis or premature closure of the cranial sutures, midface hypoplasia, and syndactyly of the hands and feet that is symmetrical and involves at least the second, third, and fourth digits. Prevalence is estimated as 1 in 65,000 (approximately 15.5 in 1,000,000) live births. Apert's syndrome accounts for 4.5% of all cases of craniostenosis.

Concerning CNS abnormalities, intelligence varies from normal to mental deficiency, although a significant number of patients are mentally retarded. Malformations of the CNS may be responsible for most cases. Papilledema and optic atrophy with loss of vision may be present in cases of subtle increased intracranial pressure.

Other abnormalities include cervical spine fusion, which is common and almost always involves C5-C6; osseous fusions may also be evident in other joints of the extremities and in the spine, tracheal cartilage anomalies, and diaphragmatic hernia.[405]

Airway anomalies result from facial abnormalities, which include small nasopharynx and hypoplastic and retropositioned maxilla. DI in Apert's syndrome has been reported. One of the suggested mechanisms is trismus related to temporalis muscle fibrosis.[259] Both upper and lower airway can be compromised by complete or partial cartilage sleeve abnormalities of the trachea and obstructive sleep apnea.[78]

Crouzon's Syndrome. Crouzon's syndrome is closely related to Apert's syndrome. In 1912, Crouzon[89] described the triad of skull deformities, facial anomalies, and exophthalmos. Crouzon's syndrome is an autosomal dominant disorder with complete penetrance and variable expressivity.[290,383] Approximately 50% of cases represent sporadic mutations, and 40% are familial. In the United States, the prevalence is 1 case per 60,000 (approximately 16.5 cases per million population) live births. Crouzon's syndrome makes up approximately 4.8% of all cases of craniosynostosis at birth.[76]

Crouzon's syndrome is associated with acanthosis nigricans (5%) and CNS defects as chronic tonsillar herniation (73%), progressive hydrocephalus[103] (30%), and syringomyelia.

Multiple sutural synostoses frequently involve premature fusion of the skull base sutures, causing midfacial hypoplasia, shallow orbits, a foreshortened nasal dorsum, maxillary hypoplasia, and occasional upper airway obstruction.[28]

Airway anomalies. Crouzon's syndrome is characterized by premature closure of calvarial and cranial base sutures as well as those of the orbit and maxillary complex (craniosynostosis). Other features include beaked nose; short upper lip; mandibular prognathism; overcrowding of upper teeth; malocclusions; V-shaped maxillary dental arch; narrow, high, or cleft palate and bifid uvula; hypoplastic maxilla; and relative mandibular prognathism. Cervical fusions of C2-C3 and C5-C6 are present in 18% of cases.

Saethre-Chotzen Syndrome. Saethre-Chotzen syndrome is an autosomal dominant acrocephalosyndactyly syndrome that affects between 1 and 2 of every 50,000 people. Craniosynostosis, facial asymmetry, low frontal hairline, ptosis, brachydactyly, and cutaneous syndactyly of the fingers and of the second and third toes are characteristic features.[72]

b. Acrocephalopolysyndactyly

Acrocephalopolysyndactyly includes four types of syndromes:

I—Noack's syndrome: similar to acrocephalosyndactyly type V (Pfeiffer type)
II—Carpenter's syndrome: mental retardation, bradydactyly
III—Sakati-Nyhan syndrome: hypoplastic tibias; deformed, displaced fibulas
IV—Goodman's syndrome: congenital heart defect, clinodactyly, camptodactyly, ulnar deviation, intact intelligence

Pfeiffer's Syndrome (Type I). Pfeiffer's syndrome (type I) is also a close relative of Apert's syndrome, although it is less severe. Pfeiffer's syndrome has three clinical subtypes and is manifested by craniosynostosis, broad thumbs and toes, variable maxillary retrusion, and partial soft tissue syndactyly. Type I is classical Pfeiffer's syndrome; affected patients have normal intelligence and a good prognosis. Type II disease is associated with cloverleaf skull, severe proptosis, and ankylosis of the elbows (Fig. 33-3). Type III is manifested by the absence of cloverleaf skull but the presence of elbow ankylosis and high morbidity in infancy. Other abnormalities are severe exorbitism that puts patients at risk for corneal exposure and damage, high-arched palate, crowded teeth, hydrocephalus, and seizures.[251]

Airway implications. As with Apert's syndrome, Pfeiffer's syndrome can arise with upper and lower airway obstruction. Congenital tracheal stenosis,[358] tracheal obstruction related to congenital tracheomalacia,[326] and

obstructive sleep apnea[249] have been reported. A high incidence of vertebral fusion (73%) has been reported[8] together with other radiologic abnormalities, which included hypoplasia of the neural arches, hemivertebrae, and a "butterfly" vertebra. C2-C3 was the level most commonly involved, although fusion was noted at all levels of the cervical spine.

Carpenter's Syndrome (Type II). Carpenter's syndrome (type II) is typically evident at or shortly after birth. Because of craniosynostosis, the top of the head may appear unusually conical (acrocephaly) or the head may seem short and broad (brachycephaly). In addition, the cranial sutures often fuse unevenly, causing the head and face to appear dissimilar from one side to the other (craniofacial asymmetry). Additional malformations of the skull and facial (craniofacial) region may include downslanting eyelid folds (palpebral fissures); a flat nasal bridge; malformed (dysplastic), low-set ears; small dental malformations[44]; and underdeveloped (hypoplastic) upper or lower jaw (maxilla or mandible), or both.

Additional abnormalities such as short stature, structural heart malformations (congenital heart defects), mild to moderate obesity, protrusion of portions of the intestine through an abnormal opening in the abdominal wall near the navel (umbilical hernia), or failure of the testes to descend into the scrotum (cryptorchidism) in affected males can be present. Both normal intellect[313] and mild mental retardation[75] have been reported in these patients.

Airway implications. DI might be expected in case of hypoplastic upper or lower jaw, oral malformations, and obesity.

c. Mandibular Hypoplasia

Mandibular hypoplasia is one of the main anomalies of the mandible with a profound effect on airway management.

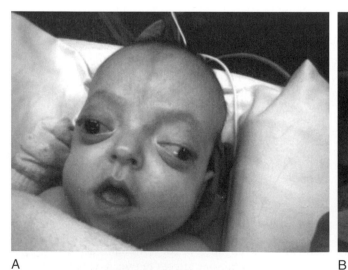

A

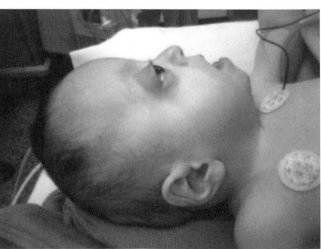

B

Figure 33-3 Pfeiffer's syndrome. Craniosynostosis, marked proptosis, and maxillary retrusion are present in Pfeiffer's syndrome. Upper and lower airway obstruction may be present as well.

Micrognathia results in posterior regression of the tongue and a small hyomental space. The mandible develops from the first branchial arch and is a feature in many rare syndromes,[183] including Pierre Robin, Treacher Collins, Goldenhar's, and Nager's syndrome. Although micrognathia is a feature commonly shared by these syndromes, they often present additional specific features with adverse effects on the airway.

The finding of periauricular skin tags or abnormally developed external ears, which also develop from the first branchial arch, may be used as a marker for a potentially DA.

Micrognathia may affect the airway in several ways: first, the tongue may not be easily moved during laryngoscopy; second, if the tongue is not pulled forward in the normal developmental fashion, the laryngeal inlet appears more anterior and difficult to visualize; and third, the oral aperture is not opened as easily or as widely.[379] Glossoptosis may further complicate the airway in micrognathic children. Glossoptosis makes displacement of the tongue to the left difficult, so that the airway is difficult to visualize.

Pierre Robin Syndrome. Pierre Robin sequence, which affects 1 in 8500 newborns,[355] was described in 1923 by Pierre Robin as airway obstruction associated with glossoptosis and hypoplasia of the mandible. At present, this syndrome is characterized by retrognathia or micrognathia, glossoptosis, and airway obstruction. An incomplete cleft of the palate is associated with the syndrome in approximately 50% of these patients (Fig. 33-4).

Pierre Robin sequence results from failure of mandibular growth during the first several weeks of embryogenesis. This causes posterior displacement of the tongue, which prevents normal growth and closure of the palate.

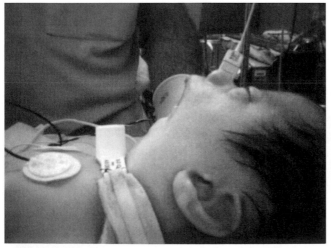

Figure 33-4 Pierre Robin syndrome. Marked micrognathia, glossoptosis, and cleft palate are evident in Pierre Robin syndrome. The micrognathia causes posterior displacement of the tongue, preventing normal development of the palate. Because of the upper airway obstruction present, an elective tracheostomy was performed.

The Pierre Robin sequence represents a spectrum of anatomic anomalies whose common features include mandibular hypoplasia, glossoptosis, and cleft palate. Four types of airway obstruction have been described in patients with Pierre Robin sequence; in only 50% is the obstruction totally related to posterior positioning of the tongue.[346] Therefore, glossopexy fails to relieve airway obstruction in approximately half of all symptomatic patients with the Pierre Robin sequence. This may explain why the use of an oral or nasopharyngeal airway alone may not improve an already difficult mask airway. Patients who fail to improve after glossopexy or nasopharyngeal airway placement, or both, usually require tracheostomy.[236]

Airway implications. There is a large body of literature concerning airway management of patients with Pierre Robin sequence. Preoperative or postoperative airway obstruction and mask ventilation difficulties have been a frequent problem in these patients.

In a 10-year retrospective study of 26 infants with Pierre Robin syndrome, Benjamin and Walker found that AI without general anesthesia proved to be safer and less difficult when a special-purpose slotted laryngoscope was used.[31] Li and colleagues[212] reviewed the airway management in 110 children with Robin sequence. Prone posturing was effective in the treatment of mild airway obstruction in 82 patients (90.2%) who had noisy breathing sounds. Only 30% of the patients required endotracheal intubation and 6.6% required tracheostomy (all were eventually decannulated).

A large array of alternative intubation techniques have been used successfully in patients with Pierre Robin: LMA,[67,150,236,398] FOB intubation,[168,329,363] fiberoptic intubation through an LMA,[283] rigid nasoendoscope with video camera[307] or video intubation laryngoscope,[333] Trachlight[171] with a homemade lighted stylet,[80] and retrograde intubation.[295] Digitally assisted endotracheal intubation[364] and elective endotracheal intubation in prone position[294] have also been reported.

Treacher Collins Syndrome. Treacher Collins syndrome (also called mandibulofacial dysostosis or Franceschetti syndrome) results from a deficient vascular supply to the first visceral arch during the initial 3 to 4 weeks of gestation and is believed to be caused by a change in the gene on chromosome 5 that affects facial development and leads to hypoplasia of the facial bones, especially the zygoma and the mandible. There is a 50% chance that the child will pass the trait on to future generations. It is often associated with DI and airway obstruction, mainly related to micrognathia.

Facial clefting causes a hypoplastic facial appearance, with deformities of the ear, orbital, midface, and lower jaw regions. The clinical appearance is a result of the zygoma (malar bone) failing to fuse with the maxilla, frontal, and temporal bones. Highly variant degrees of involvement (complete, incomplete, and abortive forms) can be seen, but common facial features may include hypoplastic cheeks, zygomatic arches, and mandible; microtia with possible hearing loss; high-arched or cleft palate; antimongoloid slant to the eyes; colobomas; increased anterior facial height; malocclusion (anterior open bite); small oral cavity and airway with a normal-sized tongue; and pointed nasal prominence.

Most children with Treacher Collins syndrome have normal development and intelligence; however additional physical findings can be present: a 40% hearing loss, dry eyes, cleft palate, and breathing problems. Both acute[337] and obstructive sleep apneas[181] have been described.

An extensive array of complications can affect management. Because of the small jaw and airway, combined with the normal size of the tongue, breathing problems can occur at birth and during sleep when the base of the tongue obstructs the small hypopharynx. This can also cause serious problems during the induction of general anesthesia. Consequently, a tracheostomy may be required to control the airway adequately.

Airway implications. The airway of children with Treacher Collins syndrome was successfully managed with an LMA,[21,105,357] the Bullard intubating laryngoscope,[57] the Augustine stylet,[203] and FOB. Rasch and coauthors[306] recommended that children with obstructive symptoms have laryngoscopy prior to anesthetic induction. If the glottic opening is visualized, inhalational induction can proceed. If the glottic structures cannot be visualized, the anesthetist must choose between awake oral or nasal intubation, elective tracheostomy, or fiberoptic intubation.

Goldenhar's Syndrome/Hemifacial Microsomia. Synonyms of Goldenhar's syndrome/hemifacial microsomia are first and second branchial arch syndrome, facioauricular vertebral spectrum, oculoauricular vertebral dysplasia, and oculoauriculovertebral spectrum disorder.

The main feature of this condition is unilateral underdevelopment of one ear (which may not even be present) associated with underdevelopment of the jaw and cheek on the same side of the face. When this is the only problem, it is normally referred to as hemifacial microsomia, but when associated with other abnormalities, particularly of the vertebrae (hemivertebrae or underdeveloped vertebrae, usually in the neck), it is referred to as Goldenhar's syndrome. It is likely, however, that these are two ends of the spectrum of the same condition.

The muscles of the affected side of the face are underdeveloped and there are often skin tags or pits in front of the ear or in a line between the ear and the corner of the mouth.

Children with the Goldenhar end of the spectrum may have congenital heart diseases in 5% to 58% of cases (ventricular septal defect, patent ductus arteriosus, tetralogy of Fallot, coarctation of the aorta). A variety of kidney abnormalities (ectopic kidneys, renal agenesis, hydronephrosis) may also be present.

Airway implications. Difficulties in airway management result from mandibular hypoplasia, cleft or high-arched palate, cervical vertebral anomalies, and scoliosis.[191] Various airway management approaches have been suggested, such as using a lighted stylet,[280] suspension laryngoscopy,[68] or LMA[20] under anesthesia or using awake fiberoptic intubation through a laryngeal mask.[180]

Nager's Syndrome. Nager's syndrome, otherwise known as mandibulofacial dysostosis, is a rare craniofacial disorder with fewer than 100 cases reported in the medical literature. The morphologic features of Nager's syndrome include down-slanted palpebral fissures, malar hypoplasia, a high nasal bridge, atretic external auditory canals, and micrognathia (severe underdevelopment of the lower jaw). Proximal limb malformations include absent or hypoplastic thumbs, hypoplasia of the radius, and shortened humeral bones.[139] Many of the characteristic facial features may be similar to those of Treacher Collins syndrome. However, patients with Treacher Collins syndrome have more severe maxillary and zygomatic hypoplasia, downward-slanting palpebral fissures, and lower lid coloboma.

Among the additional problems of children with Nager's syndrome are stomach and kidney reflux and hearing loss. Cardiac and spine defects have been also reported.[93] Four patients in the report of Danziger and coworkers[93] had a cardiac defect (type unspecified), and tetralogy of Fallot has been reported in another patient.[183]

Airway implications. Difficulties with airway management and postoperative airway obstruction may occur secondary to mandibular hypoplasia with micrognathia, restricted jaw mobility, and microstomia. Associated cleft lip or cleft palate, or both, and maxillary hypoplasia with midface deformities may further complicate airway management and appropriate mask fit during mask ventilation. The airway was successfully managed with LMA,[267] retrograde intubation,[299] and fiberoptic intubation.[384]

d. Smith-Lemli-Opitz Syndrome

Smith-Lemli-Opitz syndrome (SLOS) is an autosomal recessive syndrome characterized by congenital anomalies affecting the airway; cardiorespiratory, gastrointestinal, and genitourinary systems; and CNS. SLOS has an incidence between 1 in 26,500 pregnancies in Canada and 1 in 50,000 pregnancies in the United States.[192,274] The syndrome results from an inborn error of cholesterol biosynthesis involving a deficiency of 3β-hydroxysterol Δ^7-reductase, the enzyme that catalyzes the reduction of 7-dehydrocholesterol to cholesterol.[370] Patients with SLOS can have severe growth failure, congenital anomalies affecting most organ systems, early death, developmental delay, and self-injurious and ritualistic behavior.[9,213,281]

Airway implications. Patients with SLOS can be a challenge for airway management because of the presence of typical dysmorphic facial features, including micrognathia, prominent incisors, cleft palate, and a small and abnormally hard tongue. There are several reports of DI and abnormal laryngoscopic views in patients with SLOS.[60,70,145] An LMA was used successfully in managing the airway in a newborn infant with SLOS.[278]

In one publication,[302] experience from a series of 20 anesthesias in 14 SLOS patients was presented. The authors prospectively decided to use fiberoptic laryngoscopy as the initial technique of intubation in spite of the possible gastroesophageal reflux,[192] muscle rigidity,[145] and behavioral abnormalities[281] in these patients. In all cases, adequate spontaneous ventilation was maintained throughout the airway management. There was one case of laryngospasm during induction, and one patient was intubated by an otolaryngologist.

e. Cornelia de Lange (Cryptophthalmos) Syndrome

Cornelia de Lange syndrome (CDLS) is a syndrome of multiple congenital anomalies transmitted in an autosomal dominant pattern, characterized by a distinctive facial appearance, prenatal and postnatal growth deficiency, feeding difficulties, psychomotor delay, behavioral problems, and associated malformations mainly involving the upper extremities. The incidence is 1 per 30,000 to 50,000 live births.[276] A most important feature is a striking delay in the maturation of structure and function of most organ systems, including the CNS.[327] CDLS patients are short in stature (the syndrome is also called Amsterdam dwarfism[112]), have microcephaly (98%), and the facial features are perhaps the most diagnostic of all the physical signs. It has been reported that cardiac defects occur in 15% of these patients.[261]

Airway implications. Intubation may be difficult because of a short (86%), often webbed neck; a high-arched (66%), sometimes cleft palate; and a small mouth with micrognathia (84%). There is also a high incidence of gastroesophageal reflux (58%) and hiatal hernia. There are a number of case reports of DI in CDLS. In one of these reports the airway was successfully managed by blind nasal intubation.[411] Respiratory arrest was reported in a 3-year-old child after caudal injection of bupivacaine.[225] The authors hypothesized that changes in intracranial pressure secondary to caudal injection might be the cause of the cardiac arrest.

f. Hallermann-Streiff Syndrome

Hallermann-Streiff syndrome (oculomandibulodyscephaly syndrome) is rare, with approximately 150 cases reported.[317] Cardinal features are dyscephaly with bird facies; frontal or parietal bossing; dehiscence of sutures with open fontanelles; hypotrichosis of scalp, eyebrows, and eyelashes; cutaneous atrophy of scalp and nose; mandibular hypoplasia; forward displacement of temporomandibular joints; high-arched palate; small mouth; multiple dental anomalies; and proportionate small stature.[94,227] Children with Hallermann-Streiff syndrome can have a multitude of cardiorespiratory problems. The incidence of cardiac anomalies is 4.8% and includes septal defects, patent ductus arteriosus, and tetralogy of Fallot.

Upper airway obstruction may result from small nares and glossoptosis secondary to micrognathia, which may lead to cor pulmonale.[317]

Airway implications. The patients have natal teeth, which are brittle and may be easily broken or avulsed during laryngoscopy. The temporomandibular joint may be easily dislocated. At times, the temporomandibular joint is absent, making placement of the ET by the oral route impossible. Small nostrils, deviated nasal septum, high-arched palate, and anterior larynx preclude blind nasotracheal intubation. The ascending ramus of the mandible is either underdeveloped or absent, resulting in a small mouth cavity.

Intubation was achieved with difficulty in two cases with the patient under inhaled anesthesia. In both cases, mask ventilation was impossible.[195,227] Most of the patients may require elective tracheostomy because of respiratory difficulty.[94]

g. Turner's Syndrome

Turner's syndrome (gonadal dysgenesis) is due to the absence of a second X chromosome. Manifestations of the syndrome include primary amenorrhea, genital immaturity, and short stature; intelligence is usually normal. Additional associated features that may influence the management of anesthesia include hypertension, short neck, high palate, micrognathia, the occasional presence of aortic stenosis or coarctation of aorta, and an absent kidney.

Airway implications. In spite of the micrognathia and the short neck, only one case of DI has been published.[101] Because of the small stature, unexpected unilateral endobronchial intubation was reported.[219]

3. Inflammatory

a. Juvenile Rheumatoid Arthritis (Still's Disease)

Juvenile rheumatoid arthritis (JRA) is a systemic disease of mesenchymal tissues, which may affect collagen and connective tissue of any organ and in which arthritis is but one manifestation. Although it is beyond the scope of this review to describe this complex disease, the possible involvement of the heart (36% pericarditis confirmed by echocardiography) should be mentioned.

Abnormalities predisposing to DA management include temporomandibular ankylosis, mandibular hypoplasia, and cricoarytenoid arthritis. Atlantoaxial or low cervical subluxation may occur. The vertebrae may fail to grow, and ankylosis of the apophyseal joints may result.

Difficulty in maintaining the airway patency and inability to intubate the trachea are the most serious anesthetic problems in these children. Severe respiratory distress requiring endotracheal intubation in children with JRA has been reported.[128,176,228,381] Vetter[381] reported a case with an acute exacerbation of JRA, manifesting as acute arytenoiditis and resulting in marked upper airway obstruction. Symmetrical swelling of the arytenoids and moderate swelling of the epiglottis were noted at laryngoscopy. In another case, direct laryngoscopy demonstrated immobile vocal cords, which were approximated to each other in the midline secondary to arthritis of the cricoarytenoid joints.[228] In both cases intubation was achieved with some difficulty during direct laryngoscopy and both patients recovered after large doses of steroids. Nevertheless, an FOB should always be available in case of failure.

C. MOUTH AND TONGUE ANOMALIES

1. Microstomia

Microstomia (a small mouth opening) is uncommon and may be congenital or acquired. Pediatric microstomia may be congenital (in Freeman-Sheldon [whistling face], Hallermann-Streiff, and otopalatodigital syndrome) but is more often acquired after accidental thermal injuries such as biting an electrical extension cord or ingesting household lye.[100]

a. Congenital Microstomia

Freeman-Sheldon Syndrome. Freeman-Sheldon syndrome (also known as whistling face syndrome, windmill-vane-hand syndrome, craniocarpotarsal dysplasia, and distal arthrogryposis type 2) is a rare congenital disorder defined by facial and skeletal abnormalities. The three basic abnormalities are microstomia with pouting lips, camptodactyly with ulnar deviation of the fingers, and talipes equinovarus.

Airway implications. There are several anesthetic challenges including DA management, intravenous cannulation, and regional technique. Patients may be at increased risk for malignant hyperthermia and postoperative pulmonary complications. Oral fiberoptic intubation is considered the preferred airway management technique (the nasal route cannot be used because of small nostrils[378]). An LMA was used successfully[91] in one case after direct laryngoscopy proved to be impossible.[265]

Hallermann-Streiff Syndrome. Hallermann-Streiff syndrome, also known as oculomandibulodyscephaly with hypotrichosis, is a rare congenital disorder characterized by dyscephaly with bird facies, frontal or parietal bossing, dehiscence of sutures with open fontanelles, mandibular hypoplasia, forward displacement of temporomandibular joints, high-arched palate, small mouth, multiple dental anomalies, and proportionate small stature.[227] The presence of mandibular hypoplasia and microstomia makes intubation difficult.

Airway implications. These patients have brittle natal teeth that may be easily broken or avulsed during laryngoscopy. The temporomandibular joint may be easily dislocated.[50] At times, the temporomandibular joint is absent, making oral intubation impossible. The small nostrils, deviated nasal septum, high-arched palate, and anterior larynx preclude blind nasotracheal intubation. The ascending ramus of the mandible may

either be underdeveloped or absent, resulting in a small mouth cavity.

The options available to circumvent these problems are AI, intubation over a fiberoptic bronchoscope, retrograde intubation,[50] and intubation under inhalational anesthesia. Even tracheostomy proved to be difficult in these cases; thus, an experienced pediatric otolaryngologist should be available.[49]

b. Acquired Microstomia

Epidermolysis Bullosa Hereditaria Dystrophica. See "Pharyngeal Bullae or Scarring" under "Nasal and Palatal Anomalies" in Section IX.D.7 in this chapter.

Burns. *Airway implications.* Postburn contractures of the neck may hamper cervical hyperextension and lifting of the mandible. Direct laryngoscopy may also be difficult because of the presence of rigid scar tissue, which obscures the mandibular and laryngeal anatomy, or the presence of microstomia following retraction of scar tissue in facial burns.[204]

Fiberoptic intubation is the method of choice for securing the airway,[62] but LMA can also be used successfully. Kreulen and colleagues[204] described a quick surgical neck release of contractures to facilitate endotracheal intubation in postburn patients. Bilateral commissurotomy to allow insertion of the laryngoscope into the mouth was also reported.[100]

Burns from Lye Ingestion. Microstomia from lye ingestion may be associated not only with limited mouth opening but also with such severe intraoral scarring that common landmarks guiding either rigid or flexible fiberoptic laryngoscopy are obscured, rendering oral and nasal intubation difficult or impossible.[100,255]

2. Disease of the Tongue

Increase in tongue size is known as macroglossia. Macroglossia is defined as a resting tongue that extends beyond the teeth or alveolar ridge.[394]

a. Congenital

Hemangioma and Lymphangioma. Hemangiomas are the most common tumor seen during infancy and affect between 10% and 12% of white children.[264] Most hemangiomas (70%) are seen during the first weeks of life as an erythematous macula or a telangiectasia. All hemangiomas proliferate during the first year of life. Complications include ulceration, high-output cardiac failure, airway obstruction, and the Kasabach-Merritt syndrome, which results from platelet sequestration and destruction within the hemangioma as well as consumptive coagulopathy. It is fatal in 60% of children.

Lymphangioma is a rare congenital disease of unknown etiology.[79] Cystic hygroma of the head and neck, with large lymphatic endothelium-lined cysts, is amenable to surgical excision. Cavernous or microcystic lymphangioma, however, is composed of small lymphatic spaces and poses a therapeutic dilemma by its propensity to cause airway and feeding difficulties and by its tendency to recur despite extensive surgery. All lymphangiomas are present at birth even though they may not become apparent until the first or second year of life. Although the lymphatic malformation affects preferentially the submandibular space and the neck, it may extend cephalad and invade the tongue and surrounding structures.[79]

Airway implications. Lymphangiomatous involvement of the tongue is generally diffuse and may result in dramatic macroglossia, extending the tongue outside the mouth beyond the lip margins. It is associated with airway obstruction as well as dysphagia and speech, orthodontic, and aesthetic problems. Acute enlargement of the tongue has been reported following trauma or upper respiratory tract infections. Of the multiple therapeutic methods advocated, surgical laser resection is the mainstay. Laser resection may have to be repeated because there is tendency for recurrence. Spontaneous resolution is uncommon. In many patients, if it is left untreated for extended periods, pulmonary hypertension and cor pulmonale may develop.

In one series,[152] 9 (50%) of 18 patients reviewed required tracheostomy because of the size of the lymphoma and the tendency for recurrence. Nasal fiberoptic intubation was used successfully in these cases.[187]

Down Syndrome. See "Neck and Spine Anomalies" Section IX.G.

b. Traumatic

Burn. *Airway implications.* With burns of the face and mouth, the tongue and pharynx can be affected. Aspiration of hot liquid can occur in conjunction with upper body scald burns, leading to acute compromise of the airway "thermal epiglottitis" with clinical features similar to those of acute infectious epiglottitis. Clinical and radiologic findings are similar to those in acute infectious epiglottitis.[206] This can be a very difficult problem if subtle signs of impending airway compromise are not appreciated. The treatment should be approached with the same caution and preparedness for emergency airway management as in acute infectious epiglottitis. Immediate endotracheal intubation should be performed in those with acute respiratory distress, and prompt investigation by direct laryngoscopy in the operating room is appropriate in those who have not yet developed overt respiratory distress.[341] Surprisingly only 9.2% of 1092 burn patients admitted to the Shriners Burns Institute in Galveston over a 5-year period needed endotracheal intubation or tracheostomy for more than 24 hours.[63] A similar incidence of endotracheal intubation (10%) was found after accidental inhalation of caustic substances.[263]

Lymphatic or Venous Obstruction. Tongue swelling may occur as a result of prolonged surgical traction and local mechanical pressure. This may be caused by transesophageal echocardiography probe[409] or by dentures in adults.[365] Angioneurotic edema[245] or other reactions to drugs[71,185] can cause marked swelling of the tongue leading to life-threatening airway emergencies.

c. Metabolic Disorders

Beckwith-Wiedemann Syndrome. The Beckwith-Wiedemann syndrome (BWS) comprises a constellation of clinical features including the presence of omphalocele, macroglossia, hypoglycemia (related to hyperinsulinism), inguinal hernia with gigantism, organomegaly, renal medullary dysplasia, cardiac defects, and embryonic tumors occurring less frequently.[130]

Airway implications. The anesthetic management of children with BWS may be complicated by a potentially DA related to macroglossia.[361,366,372] Because of the high rate of omphalocele in this syndrome, anesthetic care is frequently required during the neonatal period.

The LMA was used successfully in children with BWS.[130] Even though endotracheal intubation was possible in most of the published case reports,[196,361,372] airway obstruction presented a major concern, especially after extubation. Swelling, secretions, and blood may precipitate complete airway obstruction. Because of the size of the tongue, additional pathology (tongue hematoma and bleeding[366]) can increase the difficulty of airway management and cause postoperative obstruction.

Mucopolysaccharidosis. See "Head Anomalies" in Section IX.A earlier in this chapter.

Glycogen Storage Diseases. Glycogen storage diseases (GSDs) are a heterogeneous group of inherited disorders involving one of the several steps of glycogen synthesis or degradation. They occur in approximately 1 in 20,000 live births. Isolated deficiencies of virtually all of the enzymes involved in glycogen processing have been described. The glycogen present in patients with GSD is abnormal in structure, amount, or both.

Of the 10 Cori-type GSDs, only Cori's type II (Pompe's disease, also known as generalized glycogenosis or [lysosomal] acid maltase deficiency) is associated with glycogen infiltration of the skeletal muscle of the tongue, which can lead to macroglossia and potential airway issues.[248]

Airway implications. Severe macroglossia may lead to airway obstruction during anesthetic induction, emergence from anesthesia, or the postoperative period. Associated cardiomyopathy, myopathy, nervous system involvement (especially the motor neurons in the brain stem and spinal cord), and alterations in the regulation of serum glucose concentrations are part of the clinical presentation. There are only a few reports regarding airway problems related to macroglossia in GSD.[84,250]

Lipid Storage Diseases. Lipid storage diseases are characterized by abnormal sphingolecithin metabolism, which results in an abnormal amount of lipid products being stored in the cells of the reticuloendothelial system. The lipids include cholesterol (xanthomatosis), cerebroside (Gaucher's disease), and sphingomyelin (Niemann-Pick disease).

In Gaucher's disease, accumulation of the substrate leads to multiorgan dysfunction involving the brain, spleen, liver, lymph node, and bone marrow. Airway difficulties may arise because of trismus, limited neck extension, and upper airway infiltration with glucocerebroside. Kita and coauthors[197] reported a case in which it was impossible to insert an LMA in a 9-year-old child with Gaucher's disease because of trismus and a narrowed oral cavity. Subsequently, fiberoptic intubation was performed successfully.

Neurofibromatosis. Neurofibromatoses are a group of hereditary diseases transmitted in an autosomal dominant fashion and are characterized by a tendency to formation of tumors of ectodermal and mesodermal tissues. Two distinct forms have been recognized on clinical and genetic grounds. These are designated neurofibromatosis type 1 (NF1) and neurofibromatosis type 2 (NF2).[164] Von Recklinghausen's neurofibromatosis (NF1) is one of the most common genetic disorders related to an autosomal dominant mutation and occurs at a frequency of 1 in 3000 to 1 in 4000 live births.[127]

The clinical features of NF1 include café-au-lait spots; neurofibromas involving the skin, deeper peripheral nerves, nerve roots, and blood vessels; intracranial and spinal cord tumors; kyphoscoliosis; short stature; and learning disability. One feature common to all patients is progression of the disease with time. There is also a higher incidence of malignant disease in association with NF1 compared with NF2.

Airway implications. Possible problems in airway management of the patient with NF1 include the presence of intraoral lesions, tumors compromising the airway, and the presence of thoracic deformities or neurologic lesions. Although the presence of neurofibromas in the upper airway is rare, they may pose a serious problem in the management of the airway. It is estimated that 5% of NF1 patients have intraoral manifestations of the disease.[90] Discrete neurofibromas may involve the tongue[339] or the larynx.[113] This may cause obstruction, and symptoms of dyspnea, stridor, loss or change of voice, or dysphagia and should warn the anesthetist of potential airway problems.[310] Airway obstruction after induction of anesthesia has been reported in patients with a tongue neurofibroma[90] and a neurofibroma involving the laryngeal inlet.[310] Both patients required emergency tracheostomy. Even if intraoral pathology is recognized preoperatively, elective awake fiberoptic endotracheal intubation may fail because of a grossly distorted anatomy.[164] In addition, the presence of macroglossia, macrocephaly, mandibular abnormalities, and cervical spine involvement may contribute to difficulties of airway management.[164]

d. Tongue Tumors

Lingual Tonsils. The lingual tonsil, a normal component of Waldeyer's ring, consists of lymphoid tissue located at the base of the tongue. Acute inflammation and hypertrophy can occur and has been reported to be one of the unusual causes of unexpected difficulties with both mask ventilation and endotracheal intubation.[12,141]

Hypertrophy of the lingual tonsil (LTH) has occasionally been reported in children[142] but more often occurs in adults, particularly in atopic individuals.[129] The etiology is unclear. However, it is speculated to be a compensatory mechanism following removal of the palatine tonsils[179] or secondary to a chronic, low-grade infection of the tonsils.[129]

Airway implications. Clinically, LTH is not detectable on routine preoperative physical examination.[182] Although many patients are asymptomatic, others may complain of a globus sensation, alteration of voice, chronic cough, choking, or dyspnea.[373]

Jones and Cohle[182] were the first to report a death secondary to failed airway management in a patient with unrecognized LTH. Asai and colleagues[12] reported a case of suboptimal ventilation and failed endotracheal intubation using various intubation strategies including the intubating LMA and FOB.

Enlarged lingual tonsils can impinge against the epiglottis, displacing it posteriorly. This can make mobilization of the epiglottis difficult during direct laryngoscopy. Similarly, fiberoptic intubation is often equally difficult because the posterior displacement of the epiglottis causes interference with the insertion of the tip of the endoscope under it. These difficulties may be compounded by the presence of redundant pharyngeal tissue interfering with fiberoptic exposure and the use of muscle relaxants.[182] With the onset of neuromuscular blockade the pharyngeal musculature relaxes, causing further posterior movement of the tongue and epiglottis.[88]

In a retrospective study of unexpected DI in 33 patients, Ovassapian and coworkers[282] reported that the only finding common to all patients was LTH observed on fiberoptic pharyngoscopy. Most of the patients had normal airway measurements (Mallampati class of I or II) and 36% of patients were difficult to ventilate.

The LMA has been used in cannot intubate, cannot ventilate situations caused by LTH with both success[40, 87,96] and partial success.[120] The case report by Asai and colleagues[12] highlights the fact that the LMA cannot always solve a truly glottic or subglottic problem; rather, the ventilatory mechanism must get below the lesion. If an airway cannot be established with an LMA, transtracheal jet ventilation and cricothyrotomy are other options. Crosby and Skene[87] recommended the Bullard laryngoscope (which can be fitted with a camera) as the airway device of choice for these cases because its robust construction permits gentle manipulation of airway tissues, allowing it to create the necessary endoscopic airspace.

Cystic Hygroma. See "Facial Anomalies" Section IX.B.

Other Tongue Masses. Other masses situated at the base of the tongue may displace the epiglottis and may distort the airway anatomy. Such masses include thyroglossal duct cysts and thyroid tumors.

D. NASAL AND PALATAL ANOMALIES

Nasal obstruction in pediatrics may result from a number of causes, including choanal atresia or stenosis, nasal masses, foreign body, trauma, adenoidal hypertrophy, and a combination of choanal stenosis with nasal mucosal edema.[74,98] These lesions may become evident at the time of birth or later in childhood. They can result in airway obstruction and feeding difficulty and complicate airway management.

1. Choanal Atresia

Choanal atresia is a congenital anomaly of the nasal choana that results in lack of continuity between the nasal cavity and the pharynx. This entity is rare and develops as a result of failure of resorption of the nasobuccal membrane at the sixth to seventh week of gestation. Congenital choanal atresia is most commonly bony and unilateral, as opposed to membranous and bilateral. Complete nasal obstruction in a newborn may cause death from asphyxia. During attempted inspiration, the tongue is pulled to the palate, and obstruction of the oral airway results. Vigorous respiratory efforts produce marked chest retraction. Death may occur if appropriate treatments are not available; however, if the infant cries and takes a breath through the mouth, the airway obstruction is momentarily relieved. Then the crying stops, the mouth closes, and the cycle of obstruction is repeated.

Many patients have associated narrowed nasopharynx, widened vomer, medialized lateral nasal wall, or arched hard palate. Associated malformations occur in 47% of infants without chromosome anomalies. Such malformations include cleft palate, cleft lip, and Treacher Collins syndrome. The upper airway abnormalities have been found to be present in 56% of these patients.[143] Nonrandom association of malformations can be demonstrated using the CHARGE association, which appears to be overused in clinical practice. The components of the CHARGE association are as follows: coloboma, 80%; heart disease, 58%; atresia choanae, 100%; retarded growth, 87%; development, or CNS anomalies, 97%; genital hypoplasia, 75%; and ear anomalies or deafness, 88%. Other airway abnormalities, as part of the CHARGE association, may be present.[352]

A high level of suspicion is required to diagnose bilateral choanal atresia. Symptoms of severe airway obstruction and cyclical cyanosis are the classical signs of neonatal bilateral atresia. If bilateral, choanal atresia is a medical emergency that becomes evident after birth with severe respiratory distress and cyanosis. These signs resolve with cry and recur when crying stops or the infant attempts to feed. In unilateral disease, the signs and symptoms are less evident and thus may result in delayed diagnosis. These patients come to medical attention with unilateral nasal discharge and mouth breathing. Respiratory distress occurs when the second nostril becomes obstructed, as during an upper respiratory tract infection. Older children display nasal discharge, inability to blow the nose on the affected side, nasal speech, and mouth breathing.

The diagnosis is based on history and physical examination, inability to pass a nasal catheter into the nasopharynx, flexible fiberoptic examination, and radiologic studies. CT scan is useful in demonstrating the atretic area. Endotracheal intubation is usually not needed unless there are associated congenital anomalies, and tracheostomy is not necessary.

Airway implications. Treatment of the choanal atresia is directed at providing the patient with a patent airway. Infants may benefit from the placement of an oral airway. Feeding may take place in the form of gavage. Endotracheal intubation is usually not needed unless there are associated congenital anomalies, and tracheostomy is not necessary. Surgical correction is not an emergency and is carried out by an endonasal or a transpalatal approach. It is aimed at removing the bony or membranous obstruction and part of the vomer and stenting the newly created path. In infants, the transpalatal approach is less common because of the risk of injury to the palatal growth center.

Roger and associates[318] evaluated the need for a tracheostomy and its timing in 45 patients during the evolution of CHARGE association. They found a high percentage of associated airway abnormalities: pharyngolaryngeal anomalies leading to dyspnea (58%) (discoordinate pharyngolaryngomalacia, glossoptosis, retrognathia, laryngeal paralysis, and DI) and tracheobronchial anomalies (40%) (tracheoesophageal fistula, esophageal atresia, and tracheomalacia). Tracheostomy was necessary in 13 patients (29%) in spite of the fact that the posterior nasal choanae were patent in 10 patients. They concluded that often a tracheostomy could not be avoided in these patients, regardless of choanal patency, and that tracheostomy needs to be performed early to avoid hypoxic events. Asher and coworkers[14] studied the association between catastrophic airway events and developmental delay in patients with CHARGE association. They found that children with CHARGE association have a propensity for airway instability and that cerebral hypoxia contributed to the developmental delay in some of the patients, and they recommended early tracheostomy rather than early choanal atresia repair in these patients to protect the CNS.

If micrognathia or subglottic stenosis is present, a difficult endotracheal intubation should be anticipated. Awake endotracheal intubation, direct laryngoscopy, indirect visual techniques, or nonvisual intubation techniques may be tried. Should tracheal stenosis exist, a smaller than usual ET must be available.

2. Nasal Masses

Nasal mass lesions are rare disorders in the pediatric population, with an incidence from 1 in 20,000 to 1 in

40,000 live births.[151,169] Nasal mass lesions are a diverse group of lesions that include anomalies of embryogenesis, such as encephaloceles, dermal and nasolacrimal duct cysts, tumors, and inflammatory processes.[151] Encephaloceles represent herniation of CNS tissue at the level of the cranium. Although most encephaloceles are located in the occipital area, some occur anteriorly and may contain various quantities of brain tissue. Encephaloceles may be associated with midline defects. Dermal cysts become evident as hard intranasal masses that result from herniation of dura and subsequent contact with the skin. These midline defects may manifest as a nasal obstruction without a facial mass. There is a risk of local abscess formation and intracranial infection.

Tumors located in the nasal area in children are rare occurrences. They include hemangiomas, neurofibromas, angiofibromas, hamartomas, lipomas, and rhabdomyosarcomas. Radiologic studies such as CT, MRI, and angiography can elucidate the size and position of the mass and display coexistence of any cranial bone defect. The mainstay of treatment is surgery.

A foreign body in the nostril is a finding in small children. These may be various toy objects or food particles. It is typically manifest as nasal discharge, which may be purulent, foul smelling, or bloody, and obstruction of the affected side. Diagnosis is made by history, examination of the nares, and, occasionally, radiologic evaluation.

Airway implications. Nasal masses can affect the management of the airway by interfering with mask ventilation or with direct laryngoscopy and endotracheal intubation. Nasotracheal intubation in these cases should be avoided. Extension of a cephalocele through a palatal defect interfered with endotracheal intubation in one case.[64] All of the airway implications discussed under choanal atresia with unilateral (or even bilateral) obstruction are valid in patients with nasal airway obstruction.

3. Palatal Anomalies

Cleft lip and cleft palate are the most common of the craniofacial anomalies, with an incidence of approximately 1 in 800 live births. Twenty-five percent of cases of cleft lip are bilateral, and 85% of these are associated with cleft palate. There has been a move toward earlier surgical repair of both cleft lip and palate, with cleft lip repair being performed in the neonatal period in some centers.

Anomalies of the palate include cleft and high-arched deformities and hypertrophy of the alveolar ridge area. In children undergoing palate repair, the incidence of difficult laryngoscopy (Cormack and Lehane grade III and IV) was found to be 6.5% in one study[315] and 7.4% in a more recent report.[143] Of the 59 patients with difficult laryngoscopy in Gunawardana's study,[143] 2.95% had unilateral cleft lip, 45.76% had bilateral cleft lip, and 34.61% had retrognathia. Interestingly, endotracheal intubation was successful in 99% of patients in whom laryngoscopy was difficult (failed intubation was 1%). There was a significant association between age and laryngoscopic view: 66.1% of patients with difficult laryngoscopies were younger than 6 months, 20.3% were 6 to 12 months, and 13.6% were 1 to 5 years old.

The presence of other associated congenital anomalies, including cardiac and renal anomalies, should always be remembered, particularly in children with isolated cleft palate. Over 150 syndromes have been described in association with cleft lip or palate, but fortunately all are rare. Some, however, have considerable anesthetic implications, and many involve potential airway problems. The most well known of these are the Pierre Robin, Treacher Collins, and Goldenhar syndromes. Other, such as the Klippel-Feil syndrome, may include abnormalities of the cervical spine.[155]

Henriksson and Skoog[160] reviewed the records of 154 patients who underwent closure of the palate. They found that 84% of patients had isolated cleft palate, 12% had Pierre Robin syndrome, and the rest had other identified syndromes. The risk of anesthetic complications was four times greater when the operation was done to children younger than 1 year and there was a sixfold increase when a more elaborate velopharyngoplasty technique was used.

The postoperative airway complications ranged between 5.6%[10] and 8%[286] in two surveys. As a rule, patients with cleft palate with the Pierre Robin sequence or other additional congenital anomalies had an increased risk for airway problems following palatoplasty.

Palatal edema or hematoma may also develop. Swelling limited to the soft palate or uvula can cause posture-dependent airway obstruction in children.[16] Edema may result from a variety of insults, such as instrumentation of the airway, burn injury, allergy, and infectious agents.

Many methods of management of DA in patients with cleft palate have been described. The use of firm pressure over the larynx (cricoid pressure) to aid laryngoscopy with a bougie as a guide to endotracheal intubation is relatively simple to perform by any competent anesthetist and is successful in most cases.[143] Other techniques (e.g., LMA, FOB) have been described,[155] especially when cleft palate is associated with different syndromes.

4. Adenotonsillar Disease

Together, the lingual tonsils anteriorly, the palatine tonsils laterally, and the pharyngeal tonsils (adenoids) posterosuperiorly form a ring of lymphoid or adenoid tissue at the upper end of the pharynx known as Waldeyer's tonsillar ring. All the structures of Waldeyer's ring have similar histology and function, and from the airway management point of view, they produce similar symptoms and require treatment. In response to recurrent infections, adenoids and tonsils can hypertrophy and lead to airway obstruction.[401]

Adenoidal hypertrophy peaks at 4 to 6 years of age and disappears by adolescence. Although it is a disease of the older child, it can occur in the infant. One of the major complications of adenoidal hyperplasia is obstructive sleep apnea.[329] Signs and symptoms of airway obstruction include snoring and restless sleep, somnolence during the day, noisy breathing, mouth breathing, hyponasal speech, persistent nasal secretions, apnea, choking during feeding, respiratory distress, and behavioral disturbances.[329] If the condition is left untreated, failure to thrive; a characteristic long adenoid facies with open mouth, palate, and dental malformations; and cardiovascular changes (cor pulmonale) reflective of chronic hypoxemia and hypercapnia may develop.[56,329]

Airway obstruction resulting from adenoid tissue is determined not by the absolute size of the adenoids but rather by their size relative to the volume of the pharynx.[141] Patients with preexisting diseases that reduce nasopharyngeal size or alter its integrity may have airway obstruction with only mild degrees of adenoidal hyperplasia. Examples are children with craniofacial anomalies (in whom the nasopharynx may be reduced in size) and those with nasal polyps, septal or turbinate malformations, MPSs, or deficient pharyngeal support (Down syndrome).

Tonsillar hyperplasia is a physiologic phenomenon of childhood that peaks at about 7 years of age. It can cause obstructive sleep apnea with restless sleep and an irregular breathing pattern, snoring, and intermittent periods of apnea as well as daytime somnolence, irritability, and poor school performance.[351] Long-standing partial obstruction of the airway can be associated with repeated hypoxic episodes and may result in pulmonary hypertension, cor pulmonale, and right-sided heart failure. Acute exacerbation of adenotonsillar hypertrophy may necessitate an emergency securing of the airway.[220,340]

The treatment of adenoidal and tonsillar hyperplasia is adenoidectomy and tonsillectomy. These are among the most common surgical procedures in children. There are multiple indications for excision of tonsils and adenoids.[401] Upper airway obstruction is of most concern for the anesthesiologist because these patients may have airway obstruction both during induction of anesthesia and in the postoperative period.

Airway implications. Upper airway obstruction may occur after premedication, during induction of anesthesia, or following tracheal extubation. Visualization of the glottis during direct laryngoscopy may be difficult with tonsillar hypertrophy. Resection of tonsils and adenoids may not result in immediate relief of airway obstruction. Bleeding and edema can make the child susceptible to postoperative airway obstruction. Although it usually causes chronic upper airway obstruction, adenotonsillar hypertrophy can result in acute airway obstruction.[45,220,340] Airway assessment and management of patients with obstructive sleep apnea caused by adenotonsillar hypertrophy are detailed in the obstructive sleep apnea section.

Peritonsillar abscess in children manifests as a purulent mass surrounded by the tonsillar capsule. It occurs more frequently in untreated children with chronic tonsillitis or those who have been inadequately treated.[401] Signs and symptoms include fever, sore throat, tonsillar mass, dysphagia, drooling (caused by odynophagia and dysphagia), muffled voice, trismus (caused by irritation of the pterygoid muscle by the pus and inflammation), and variable degrees of toxic state. Peritonsillar abscess requires intravenous antibiotic therapy. If symptoms of airway obstruction develop or the patient fails to respond to medical therapy, needle aspiration, incision, and drainage with tonsillectomy are recommended.[401] In a prospective study of 50 adult patients with peritonsillar abscess, the Mallampati score did not correlate with the Cormack and Lehane glottic view during laryngoscopy because of palatopharyngeal arch distortion. There were no DIs in this study group.[111]

Peritonsillar abscess affects the airway in a manner similar to tonsillar hypertrophy, except that the patients may have trismus. There may be associated edema of the supraglottic area, uvula, and soft palate that exacerbates airway obstruction. Patients are susceptible to airway obstruction during either spontaneous breathing or manual mask ventilation. During direct laryngoscopy, care should be taken not to rupture the abscess. When the abscess is large, it may interfere with visualization of the vocal cords.

5. Obstructive Sleep Apnea

a. Definition
Obstructive sleep apnea syndrome (OSAS) in children is a disorder of breathing during sleep characterized by prolonged partial upper airway obstruction or intermittent complete obstruction (obstructive apnea) that disrupts normal ventilation during sleep and normal sleep patterns.[247]

b. Prevalence of Snoring and Obstructive Sleep Apnea
The prevalence of primary snoring ranges from 3.2%[124] to 12.1%,[4] whereas the prevalence of OSAS ranges from 0.7%[4] to 10.3%.[311]

The ability to maintain upper airway patency during the normal respiratory circle is the result of a delicate equilibrium between various forces that promote airway closure and dilatation. This "balance of pressure" concept was first proposed independently by Remmers and colleagues[312] in 1978 and Brouillette and Thach[55] in 1979 and represents the current line of thought regarding the pathophysiologic mechanisms of OSAS.

The four major predisposing factors for upper airway obstruction are as follows:

Anatomic Narrowing. The upper airway behaves as predicted by the Sterling resistor model; that is, the maximal inspiratory flow is determined by the pressure changes upstream (nasal) to a collapsible site of the upper airway and flow is independent of downstream (tracheal) pressure generated by the diaphragm.

Children with OSAS were found to close their airways at the level of enlarged adenoids and tonsils at low positive pressures, whereas healthy children required subatmospheric pressures to induce upper airway closure.[173]

Abnormal Mechanical Linkage between Airway Dilating Muscles and Airway Walls. Control of the upper airway size and stiffness depends on the relative and rhythmic contraction of a host of paired muscles, which include palatal, pterygoid, tensor palatini, genioglossus, geniohyoid, and sternohyoid. With contraction, these muscles promote motion of the soft palate, mandible, tongue, and hyoid bone. The activity of these muscles is dependent in particular on the brain stem respiratory network. Wakefulness conveys a supervisory function that ensures airway patency, and sedative agents that compromise genioglossal muscle activity may result in significant upper airway compromise. Roberts and coauthors demonstrated that mechanoreceptor- and chemoreceptor-mediated genioglossal activity is critical for maintenance of upper airway patency in both normal and micrognathic infants.[316]

Muscle Weakness. There is little evidence to suggest that intrinsic muscle weakness is a major contributor to upper airway dysfunction. Nevertheless, in patients with neuromuscular disorders, airway obstruction is frequently observed during sleep.[66]

Abnormal Neural Regulation. Subtle alterations in central chemoreceptor activity were found by different researchers. Gozal and others[133] reported that arousal to hypercapnia was blunted, whereas Onal and coworkers[279] found that upper airway musculature is more stimulated than the diaphragm.

c. Pathophysiology and Clinical Picture

The etiology and pathophysiology of obstructive sleep apnea in children are multifactorial, with anatomic and neuromuscular abnormalities playing a major role in the disorder.[24,231,233,234,344] Others, however, downplay the role of neuromuscular factors because the vast majority of children with OSAS can be cured by correcting anatomic obstructions. The narrowing of the airway lumen by hypertrophied lymphoid tissue, compliance, elasticity of the pharyngeal soft tissue, facial morphology, and the physiologic changes that occur in the pharyngeal dilators during sleep determine the severity of airway collapse.

Patients with dysmorphic constricted craniofacial development, such as those with Pierre Robin sequence; Treacher Collins, Apert's, and Crouzon's syndromes; and those with neuromuscular abnormalities as in cerebral palsy and anoxic encephalopathy, have a much higher incidence of severe OSAS.

Adenotonsillar hypertrophy plays a major role in the pathogenesis of OSAS in children. The volume of lymphoid tissue in the upper airway increases from about 6 months of age up to puberty, with the maximum

proliferation occurring in the preschool years, which coincides with the peak incidence of OSAS in children. Despite this narrowing of the upper airway by lymphoid tissue, most children do not develop OSAS. A normal child's airway is less likely to collapse in sleep than the adult airway.

One of the hallmarks of sleep-disordered breathing is fragmentation and disruption of normal sleep architecture. By definition, deeper levels of sleep, especially rapid eye movement (REM) sleep, are less susceptible to arousal from various stimuli, including adverse ventilatory events.[125] Oxyhemoglobin desaturations therefore tend to be more frequent and more severe during REM sleep. The hypercapnia and hypoxemia and the resulting arousals that are associated with OSAS, at least in part, often result in a reduction in REM sleep.[125,134]

Although OSAS and hypertension are commonly associated in adults, children with OSAS also tend to have higher diastolic blood pressures. The cardiovascular changes appear to be the result of an increase in sympathetic tone that results from the sleep arousals, which in turn are related to the obstructive respiratory events.[232] The clinical presentation of OSAS in children has many similarities and important differences when compared with the disorder in adults[109,134,339] (Table 33-6).

Unlike findings in adults, obesity is not a common factor in pediatric OSAS, although its role increases with the age of the child.[229] Abnormal sleep positions with preference for an upright position and hyperextension of the neck have been noted in children with sleep-related breathing disorders.[215]

Table 33-6   Differences between Adult and Childhood Obstructive Sleep Apnea Syndrome

Features	Adult	Child
Snoring	Intermittent	Continuous
Mouth breathing	Uncommon	Common
Obesity	Common	Uncommon
Failure to thrive		Common
Daytime hypersomnolence	Common	Uncommon
Gender predilection	Male	None
Most common obstructive event	Apnea	Hypopnea
Arousal	Common	Uncommon
Treatment		
Nonsurgical	CPAP in majority	CPAP in minority
Surgery	Selected cases	T & A in the majority

CPAP, continuous positive airway pressure; T & A, tonsillectomy and adenoidectomy.

Prolonged exposure to hypoxia and hypercarbia results in compensatory changes in the pulmonary vasculature. Pulmonary vascular resistance increases, causing increased right ventricular strain.[345] Severe cases may progress to pulmonary hypertension, dysrhythmias, and cor pulmonale.[211]

d. Laboratory Evaluations

Polysomnography (PSG) remains the "gold standard" for the diagnosis of OSAS in adults and children. In 1995, the American Thoracic Society adopted guidelines for performing PSG in children.[7] It was recommended in order to differentiate primary snoring, which does not require any form of treatment, from OSAS, which, if left untreated, can lead to cardiopulmonary dysfunction and functional impairment.[175] In general, studies have shown that history alone does not have sufficiently high diagnostic sensitivity or specificity to be the basis for recommending therapy.[65]

Normal PSG values for the various respiratory events have been reported by Marcus and colleagues in a study of 50 healthy children.[235] The apnea indices (number of apneas per hours of total sleep time) were 0.1 ± 0.5, with the minimum oxygen saturation being 96%, maximal drop in saturation 4%, and CO_2 over 55 mm Hg no more than 0.5% of the total sleep time. An abnormal study includes an apnea index greater than 1, oxygen desaturation greater than 4% more than three times an hour or associated with a greater than 25% change in heart rate, oxygen desaturation less than 92%, and elevation of end-tidal CO_2 to more than 52 mm Hg for more than 8% of total sleep time or 45 mm Hg for more than 60% of sleep time (Table 33-7).

e. Airway Implications

Medical therapy of pediatric obstructive sleep apnea is not considered to be consistently effective. Systemic or topical steroids may shrink lymphoid tissue, but the long-term effectiveness is not known, and a short course of systemic corticosteroids appears to be ineffective. Topical intranasal steroids appear to reduce the severity of OSAS.[54] Adenotonsillectomy remains the mainstay of treatment for pediatric obstructive sleep apnea.[296] The optimal age for adenotonsillectomy is between 4 and 7 years; yet young age, even younger than 1 year, is not a contraindication for surgery for airway obstruction or sleep apnea. Children with Down syndrome deserve further comment because they frequently have severe obstructive sleep apnea.[209] Although there are conflicting data on the usefulness of adenotonsillectomy in this group, it appears worthwhile if the tonsils or adenoids are obstructing the airway. If an adenotonsillectomy fails or is not considered appropriate therapy, uvulopalatopharyngoplasty may be effective.[4]

Several studies demonstrated the relative safety of this procedure performed on an outpatient basis with a suitable period of postoperative observation and hydration.

Table 33-7 Normal Sleep Study Measurements in Children

Measurement	Normal Values
Sleep latency (min)	>10
TST (hours)	>5.5
% REM sleep	>15% TST
% stage 3-4 non-REM sleep	>25% TST
Respiratory arousal index (No./hour TST)	<5
Periodic leg movements (No./hour TST)	<1
Apnea index (No./hour TST)	<1
Hypopnea index (nasal/esophageal pressure catheter; No./hour TST)	<3
Respiratory disturbance index (RDI) (Apnea/hypopnea index)	<1
Nadir oxygen saturation (%)	>92
Mean oxygen saturation (%)	>95
Desaturation index (>4% for 5 sec; No./hour TST)	<5
Highest CO_2 (mm Hg)	52
CO_2 > 45 mm Hg	<20% TST

REM, rapid eye movement; TST, total sleep time.

It appears that if children meet standard discharge criteria (normal respiratory parameters, no bleeding, adequate oral intake and pain control, and normal mental status) at 4 to 6 hours after surgery, they can be safely discharged home regardless of age or preoperative diagnoses.

There is little specific evidence for or against the use of opiates and sedatives in the perioperative period in children with OSAS. To date, there are only anecdotal reports of respiratory depression in children in response to sedatives such as chloral hydrate[37] and respiratory depression in the postoperative period,[390] including hypoxia.[158,241,298] Children with OSAS appear to have increased sensitivity to opioids.

Waters and associates[391] found that children with OSAS develop more pronounced respiratory depression than with aged-matched control subjects when breathing spontaneously under anesthetic with the upper airway secured. Addition of a small dose of opioids additionally increased the respiratory depression in children with OSAS. The low dose of fentanyl used ($0.5 \mu g/kg$) precipitated central apnea in 46% of the OSAS group. In this study, the best predictor of opioid-induced central apnea was an increase in end-tidal CO_2 to levels greater than 50 mm Hg during spontaneous breathing after anesthetic induction.

In contrast to the previous studies[36,241,320,391] Wilson and coauthors[402] found no correlation between the preoperative cardiorespiratory sleep study (PSG and home sleep studies) parameters and opioid administration and postoperative outcome.

Few studies provide data pertaining to complications of surgery in children undergoing adenotonsillectomy for upper airway obstruction. All specifically address the risk of postoperative respiratory obstruction.[36,123,158,241,244,298,320,321,402] These papers are listed in Table 33-8. The authors define respiratory compromise in various ways but generally consider the need for supplemental oxygen as a minimum criterion. The papers report a wide range for the incidence of postoperative respiratory complications (0% to 27%), primarily because their populations include different proportions of children with neuromuscular, chromosomal, and craniofacial disorders.

Young age (younger than 3 years) and associated medical problems were found in most studies to define the highest risk groups. A high preoperative respiratory disturbance index (apnea/hypopnea index) also seems to be a risk factor for postoperative complications.[241,298] Time to onset of respiratory compromise after adenotonsillectomy appears to be brief, although McColley and others[241] reported that for one patient it took 14 hours to manifest respiratory symptoms. Postobstructive pulmonary edema may develop in some children undergoing adenotonsillectomy for relief of upper airway obstruction. The incidence of this complication is unknown, and it is often manifested immediately after endotracheal intubation.

The patient's position, especially after extubation, seems to be important for the development of airway obstruction.

Table 33-8 **Respiratory Compromise after Adenotonsillectomy in Children with Obstructive Sleep Apnea Syndrome**

Author	Year	Methodology and Rating	Inclusion Criteria	N	Rate of Respiratory Compromise	Comments
McGowan [244]	1992	Case series, level IV	Clinical upper airway obstruction	53	25%	Risk factors for complications were prematurity, adenoidal facies, preoperative respiratory distress.
McColley [241]	1992	Case series, level IV	Abnormal PSG	69	23%	Onset up to 14 hours postop. Main risk factors were age and preop RDI.
Price [298]	1993	Case series, level IV	Clinical upper airway obstruction, nap PSG	160	19%	Associations with risk factors (age, preop PSG) asserted but not quantitated
Rosen [320]	1994	Case series, level IV	Abnormal PSG	37	27%	Postop obstruction occurred within hours of surgery. All patients with complications were complex and had a higher mean RDI preop.
Helfaer [158]	1996	Case series, level IV	Mild OSAS by PSG (no severe cases)	15	0%	No postop desaturation or obstruction in children with mild OSAS
Gerber [123]	1996	Case series, level IV	Questionnaire	292	15% (38% if younger than 3 years)	Included complex patients. Respiratory compromise developed only in patients who snored preoperatively.
Rothschild [321]	1994	Case series, level IV	Clinical diagnosis	69	7%	Specific diagnostic criteria for OSAS not specified.
Biavati [36]	1997	Case series, level IV	Clinical diagnosis	3552 3 with PSG	25% (36% with abnormal PSG)	Included complex patients. No patient with normal PSG had postop respiratory complications.
Wilson [402]	2002	Case series, retrospective	Abnormal PSG	163	21%	96% were managed in a recovery room or ward setting.

OSAS, obstructive sleep apnea syndrome; postop, postoperative; preop, preoperative; PSG, polysomnography; RDI, respiratory disturbance index.

Ishikawa and colleagues found that prone position increases upper airway collapsibility in anesthetized infants.[172] Isono and associates, in a study of adult patients, reported that lateral position structurally improves maintenance of the passive pharyngeal airway in patients with obstructive sleep apnea.[174] These findings are in concordance with the current practice of extubating and transporting children in the lateral position.

In a retrospective study of 163 OSAS children, Wilson and coworkers[402] found a 21% incidence of respiratory compromise requiring medical interventions after adenotonsillectomy. Ninety-six percent of the children with OSAS were managed in a recovery room or ward setting. Six children required postoperative admission to the intensive care unit.

Most of the polysomnographic studies done weeks after adenotonsillectomy in children with OSAS reported a cure rate between 85%[362] and 100%.[414] A major concern in the immediate postoperative period is the effect of residual anesthesia, pain, sedative and analgesic medication, and edema of the pharyngeal tissues on the complication rate in this category of patients. Helfaer and coauthors[158] tried to respond to this question by comparing preoperative and first night postoperative polysomnograms in children with mild OSAS. Surprisingly, most of the children had improvements in their sleep studies on the night of surgery. These findings were not affected by the choice of intraoperative anesthetic. Specifically, intraoperative administration of narcotics was not associated with postoperative respiratory impairment. Even though this study was performed on a relatively small number of patients with mild disease, it was concluded that children with mild OSAS can be safely discharged home on the day of surgery (see Table 33-8).

In our institution, the criteria for postoperative admission are severe OSAS; age younger than 3 years; associated craniofacial anomalies (including Down syndrome); associated neuromotor, cardiac, or pulmonary diseases; upper airway burn; hypotonia; morbid obesity; or children with recent upper respiratory tract infection.

In conclusion, the anesthetic management of OSAS should be directed toward assessing and managing the coexisting cardiac or pulmonary diseases; managing the airway, especially in syndromic children; minimizing the amount of opiates used intraoperatively; and preventing and managing the possible postoperative complications. Preoperative sleep studies are necessary for a positive diagnostic and for decisions regarding postoperative monitoring. In consequence, anesthesiologists need to be familiar with reading a sleep study and interpreting the results of PSG.

6. Retropharyngeal and Parapharyngeal Abscesses

The various cavities and virtual spaces in the pharynx and neck are in anatomic continuity with one another. The retropharyngeal, parapharyngeal, peritonsillar, and submandibular spaces intercommunicate, and infection in one can extend to the others. The superior limit of the retropharyngeal space is the base of the skull; inferiorly, it extends into the mediastinum to the level of the tracheal bifurcation. Retropharyngeal abscess is a rare but potentially fatal infection of the pharyngeal wall. It occurs primarily in pediatric patients; in one study[83] more than half of the patients were younger than 12 months. In children it commonly results from suppurative involvement of lymph nodes located in the retropharyngeal space. These nodes drain lymph from the pharynx, nasopharynx, paranasal sinuses, and middle ear. The most common pathogens are *Staphylococcus aureus* (25%), *Klebsiella* species (13%), group A streptococcus (8%), and a mixture of gram-negative and anaerobic organisms (38%).[73,83] Other causes of retropharyngeal abscess include spread of infection from pharyngitis or peritonsillar abscess, penetrating trauma, and foreign body ingestion.

Clinical presentation varies with the patient's age. Most children have fever, some degree of toxic appearance, a hyperextended or stiff neck, dysphagia, drooling, trismus, muffled voice, and respiratory distress. Infants and young children may have stridor. Older children with mediastinal involvement may, in addition, complain of chest pain. Physical examination may reveal cervical lymphadenopathy and pharyngeal swelling. A lateral radiograph of the neck typically shows widening of the retropharyngeal prevertebral soft tissue. CT is helpful in the diagnosis of retropharyngeal abscess but has difficulties in differentiating cellulites and abscess. Lateral neck radiography was found to be very specific when the air sign was present.[51] Ultrasound imaging can also distinguish between suppurative and presuppurative stage.[303] Chest radiographs may show mediastinal involvement and tracheal deviation.[153]

Complications of retropharyngeal abscess include airway obstruction, abscess rupture, pneumonia, sepsis, and extension of the disease into the mediastinum and the carotid sheath, causing mediastinitis, jugular vein thrombosis, or penetration into the carotid artery. Treatment consists of airway support, antibiotic therapy, and early incision and drainage.

Airway implications. The danger of retropharyngeal abscess is related to the potential for rapid progression to airway obstruction. In one report, 5 of 65 patients required tracheostomy.[368] There is also an ever-present risk of abscess rupture and aspiration of pus into the airway. The clinical presentation of children with retropharyngeal abscess can mimic that of children with epiglottitis and croup. The mortality rate is high. The exact incidence is not known. In a retrospective study, Ameh[5] reported two deaths among 10 children surveyed: one child died before the abscess was drained and the other died in the postoperative period because of laryngospasm. Coulthard and Isaacs[83] reported two deaths in 31 children with retropharyngeal abscess.

All patients with the diagnosis of retropharyngeal abscess must be considered to have a DA. The management depends on the severity of airway distress and degree of patient's cooperation. In most children, general anesthesia is required for airway management because few patients, if any, accept an awake technique. General anesthesia may be induced by inhalation of sevoflurane (or halothane) and oxygen with emergency plans for securing the airway in case airway obstruction develops. If not in place, an intravenous line should be secured and atropine administered. It is advantageous to maintain spontaneous ventilation because neuromuscular blockade may relax the pharyngeal musculature and potentiate airway obstruction with an already reduced pharyngeal space. After adequate anesthetic depth is achieved, gentle direct laryngoscopy should be attempted, taking care not to rupture the abscess. If endotracheal intubation is not possible following limited attempts at direct laryngoscopy, a surgical airway should be considered for those with large lesions. In children with minimal respiratory distress and adequate mask air exchange, other intubation techniques (indirect visual or nonvisual) may be tried first. It is important to take special precautions not to traumatize the abscess during endotracheal intubation. Blind attempts at intubation, insertion of an LMA or oral airway, or overzealous direct laryngoscopy may result in rupture of the abscess.

7. Pharyngeal Bullae or Scarring

Epidermolysis bullosa (EB) describes a group of genetically determined mechanobullous disorders that vary in course and severity, ranging from relatively minor disability to death in early infancy.[15,408] They are characterized by an excessive susceptibility of the skin and mucosa to separate from the underlying tissues and form bullae following minimal mechanical trauma. The affected areas can be considerable in size as the bullae enlarge by expanding and tracking along the natural tissue planes. Like all blisters, they can be extremely painful. There are over 20 types of EB described,[262] with three major subtypes: dystrophic EB (DEB), EB simplex (EBS), and junctional EB (JEB), with each broad category of EB containing several subtypes.

a. Dystrophic Epidermolysis Bullosa

DEB, which was first described by Fox in 1879, is probably the most frequent type of EB to have surgical treatment.[161,162] The prevalence of DEB is approximately 2 in 100,000.[19] The majority of DEB sufferers have wounds that are present at birth or very shortly after, with a variety of blister sizes seen, some even exceeding 10 cm in diameter. The blisters of DEB are usually flaccid and filled with either a clear or blood-stained fluid. New blisters tend to develop less frequently as the child ages. Scarring is unusual after a single episode of blistering, but blistering is much more easily provoked in previously blistered areas and it is this recurrence that causes atrophic scars to form. As a result of repeated skin infection,

injury, and healing, patients with the dystrophic form develop contractures. Contractures may involve the skin of the neck and mouth. Oral, pharyngeal, and esophageal blistering is common in DEB. The recurrent blistering leads to progressive contraction of the mouth (causing limited opening) and fixation of the tongue. The associated pain and resulting dysphagia lead to a reduction of nutritional intake as eating is a painful, slow, and exhausting experience. Gastroesophageal reflux is common in patients with DEB. Esophageal scarring leads to dysmotility and the formation of strictures or webs, which contributes to the dysphagia by exacerbating oral, pharyngeal, and esophageal ulceration and also by increasing dental decay.

b. Epidermolysis Bullosa Simplex

Almost all cases of EBS are inherited in an autosomal dominant manner.[161] Although the exact prevalence of EBS is not known, it is thought to be approximately 1 or 2 in 100,000.[15] There are three major subtypes: Dowling-Meara, Weber-Cockayne, and Koebner.

Only the Dowling-Meara type (EBS herpetiformis) has airway implications. The onset of this type of EBS is usually in early infancy. There is a great range in the severity of Dowling-Meara, from relatively mild to exceptionally severe with death during the neonatal period. Oral involvement is usually not prominent, but a number of severely affected neonates exhibit extreme oropharyngeal involvement, which interferes with feeding. They may also have a tendency for gastroesophageal reflux and also aspiration. Laryngeal involvement, causing a hoarse cry, is also regularly seen in Dowling-Meara EBS.

c. Junctional Epidermolysis Bullosa

There are three major subtypes of JEB: Herlitz, non-Herlitz, and JEB with pyloric atresia. Junctional epidermolysis bullosa Herlitz type is the commonest form of JEB. Formerly known as lethal JEB, it affects the larynx, producing a characteristic hoarse cry in infancy. This hoarseness is usually followed by recurrent bouts of stridor (caused by granulation tissue and not usually fresh blisters), each with the potential risk of fatal asphyxiation. The mouth and pharynx are often severely affected, causing substantial pain and feeding difficulties, which in turn leads to a profound failure to thrive. Death in the first 2 years of life is usual in Herlitz JEB, either from acute respiratory obstruction or from overwhelming sepsis related to a poor nutritional state.

Airway implications. Children with EB, especially DEB, are more likely to have airway management problems, with the risk of DI secondary to contracture formation. In addition to oral, pharyngeal, and laryngeal problems, head and neck skin involvement and contractures may make positioning for laryngoscopy difficult.[330] A DI should always be suspected and contingency plans made prior to embarking upon anesthesia. To avoid prolonged facial manipulation during the procedure, airway maintenance by intubation is often preferred.[407] To reduce the risk of new laryngeal bullae formation, an ET a half to one size smaller than predicted may be necessary. If a cuffed tube is required, the cuff should be slightly inflated. The risk of bullae formation following intubation is low because the larynx and trachea are lined with ciliated columnar epithelium rather than the squamous epithelium that lines the oropharynx and esophagus.[177]

Although securing the ET by wiring it to a tooth has been advocated,[350] a more conservative approach would be to tie the tube in place with either ribbon gauze or Vaseline gauze and a collar of adhesive tape around the ET to prevent the ties from slipping. Nasal intubation can be performed, preferably with a fiberoptic scope, but blind nasal intubation should be avoided. Blind techniques (e.g., blind oral intubation or lighted stylet) have been used successfully[138] but may result in trauma to the laryngeal structures if multiple unsuccessful attempts are required and probably should be avoided.

The lips are lined with lubricated gauze at the place they touch the ET and also underneath the tie to prevent chafing. An intravenous cannula should be secured with a nonadhesive dressing. Central venous and arterial cannulas, if required, should be sutured in place.

In caring for patients with EB, it is important to take general precautions to protect the integrity of the skin from trauma, friction injury, and adhesive products. Areas susceptible to pressure (e.g., below the face mask) should be generously lubricated. Patients receiving systemic corticosteroid therapy may need perioperative supplementation.

E. LARYNGEAL ANOMALIES

1. Laryngomalacia

Laryngomalacia is the most common congenital abnormality of the larynx and is characterized by a long narrow epiglottis and floppy aryepiglottic folds.[19] It is the most common cause of noninfective stridor in children.[19] Stridor, usually present at birth, may appear after weeks or months. It may appear only with crying or in the presence of an acute upper respiratory infection. The stridor is inspiratory, high pitched and more obvious in the supine position.[112] In the mild form, stridor peaks at 9 months and then levels off, declines, and disappears by 2 years of age.[27] Severe laryngomalacia may cause upper airway obstruction, cyanosis, failure to thrive, and cor pulmonale. Gastroesophageal reflux has been reported as well, and antireflux therapy is recommended.[39]

Diagnosis is by endoscopy, particularly laryngoscopy. Indirect laryngoscopy is not practical for infants and children. Flexible endoscopy or rigid endoscopy may be necessary. General anesthesia is necessary.

Airway implications. These patients are at risk for airway obstruction, and preparations for management of the difficult pediatric airway must be made. A gradual inhalation induction with 100% oxygen is performed, maintaining spontaneous ventilation. CPAP with 10 cm H_2O may be necessary to overcome obstruction, along with an oral airway and jaw lift. The time required for an adequate depth of anesthesia may be delayed in cases of airway obstruction. When deep levels of anesthesia are achieved, direct laryngoscopy may be performed. Topicalization of the vocal cords prior to laryngoscopy decreases the incidence of coughing. As stated previously, one should calculate the maximum dose prior to topicalization so that toxic doses are avoided. Surgical treatment consists of either aryepiglottoplasty or laser excision of redundant supraglottic tissue.[165] Endoscopic division of the aryepiglottic folds has been suggested as the first-line therapy for severe laryngomalacia.[223]

2. Epiglottitis

Epiglottitis, more appropriately called supraglottitis, is a serious life-threatening infection of the epiglottis, aryepiglottic folds, and arytenoids. It is a true airway emergency because supraglottitis may progress rapidly to complete airway obstruction. Supraglottitis is classically described as occurring between 2 and 8 years of age, although it can occur in infants, older children, and adults.[322] *Haemophilus influenzae* type B (Hib) is the most common causative agent although other organisms have been reported. *Pseudomonas*, group A beta hemolytic *Streptococcus*, and *Candida* have been reported in the literature as etiologies of epiglottitis as well.[42,242,322] The introduction of the *H. influenzae* conjugate vaccine has dramatically reduced the incidence of supraglottitis, but vaccine failure does occur.[242] A high index of suspicion for the diagnosis of supraglottitis should be maintained as the disease has not been completely eliminated.

Children with epiglottitis often present with the four Ds of supraglottitis: drooling, dyspnea, dysphagia, and dysphonia. These children are described as "toxic appearing" and anxious, preferring to rest in the tripod position (upright sitting position, leaning forward with the mouth open).[42] High fevers and signs of respiratory distress evolve over a few hours. Stridor, if present, is usually inspiratory.[380]

Diagnosis is usually based on clinical findings. Radiographs are indicated only if the child has no respiratory distress and a physician capable of controlling the DA is in attendance. A lateral neck radiograph obtained with hyperextension during inspiration is the single best exposure. Classical findings include round thick epiglottis (thumb sign), loss of the vallecular air space, and thickening of the aryepiglottic folds.[322] Definitive diagnosis is made at laryngoscopy in the operating room. No one should attempt to visualize the posterior pharynx in the emergency room. Dynamic airway collapse may occur and complete obstruction ensues.

Airway implications. The mainstay of therapy for supraglottitis is to obtain an airway, usually with a multidisciplinary approach in an organized and controlled manner. An otolaryngologist, capable of performing an emergency tracheostomy, is present at the time of induction. The difficult pediatric airway cart, a rigid bronchoscope, and the tracheostomy set must be in the operating room. When dealing with the child with epiglottitis, it is vital that the child remain calm. If separation from the parents is too stressful, parental presence at induction, after proper preparation, should be considered. Sedation is not advised in this situation. After placement of a precordial stethoscope and pulse oximeter, a gradual inhalation induction with 100% oxygen is performed with the child in the sitting position. Maintenance of spontaneous ventilation is crucial; CPAP 10 cm H_2O may be beneficial in maintaining a patent airway. Once anesthesia is induced, an intravenous line is placed and a volume bolus of 10 to 30 mL/kg of lactated Ringer's solution is given. The rest of the monitors are applied, and atropine or glycopyrrolate is given intravenously prior to laryngoscopy for its antimuscarinic effect. After an adequate depth of anesthesia is obtained, direct laryngoscopy is performed and an oral ET is placed. Identification of a cherry-red edematous epiglottis is diagnostic. A tip for successful intubation is that gentle pressure applied to the chest may reveal expiratory gas bubbles. A styletted ET, one or two sizes smaller than predicted, is placed into the trachea.[380] If the patient cannot be intubated, the DA algorithm is followed. Rigid FOB may be attempted if the condition permits or a surgical airway is obtained.

After the appropriate cultures are obtained, antibiotic therapy is initiated. Some advocate changing the oral ET to a nasotracheal tube because of the greater stability of the nasotracheal tube. The mean duration of intubation ranges from 30 to 72 hours.[322] Extubation is performed when the patient demonstrates clinical improvement and there is evidence of an air leak around the ET. Some clinicians advocate the use of dexamethasone before extubation to reduce the incidence of postextubation stridor.[322]

3. Congenital Glottic Lesions

Congenital laryngeal anomalies include laryngomalacia, vocal cord paralysis, laryngeal web, and atresia. Vocal cord paralysis is the second most common cause of congenital laryngeal malformations.[400] Bilateral vocal cord paralysis is often associated with CNS abnormalities such as Arnold-Chiari malformation. Birth trauma may also induce vocal cord paralysis. The presentation of bilateral vocal cord paralysis is high-pitched inspiratory stridor and a normal or mildly hoarse cry. Severe airway obstruction may develop that requires emergency intubation or tracheostomy.[400] Occasionally, vocal cord paralysis resolves spontaneously or after a ventriculoperitoneal shunt is placed.[349] In unilateral paralysis, the left side is more commonly affected. Cardiovascular and mediastinal problems are often associated with unilateral paralysis.[400] Unilateral paralysis arises with a weak cry.[401] It seldom requires surgery.[349]

Laryngeal webs occur when there is failure of recanalization of the larynx during embryologic development.[400] In general, webs occur at the level of the glottis, causing respiratory distress at birth. They may be very thin and limited to the glottis with minimal airway obstruction. Significant airway obstruction is usually the result of more extensive webs. These webs are thick, extending into the subglottis.[400] Surgical treatment is endoscopic division of the web for smaller webs. Laryngotracheal reconstruction may be needed for extensive webs. Laryngeal atresia is a rare and often fatal anomaly. Survival depends on the presence of an associated tracheoesophageal fistula or immediate tracheostomy at birth.[400]

Airway implications. The degree of obstruction determines the method used for airway management. Severe forms require a surgical airway; milder cases may be managed with intubation. Intubation may be performed either awake or after inhalation induction, depending on the patient and the situation. Preparations for a failed intubation should be made.

4. Recurrent Respiratory Papillomatosis

Laryngeal papillomatosis or recurrent respiratory papillomatosis is the most frequent benign tumor of the larynx, with an incidence in the United States of 4.3 per 100,000 children.[97] It is caused by the human papilloma virus types 6 and 11. It is also the second most common cause of hoarseness in children.[97] Laryngeal papillomas are located primarily in the larynx on the vocal cord margins and epiglottis; however, any part of the respiratory tract may be affected.[135] Recurrent respiratory papillomatosis (RRP) may affect children and adults. The juvenile form is often more aggressive than the adult form of the disease. Pediatric patients with RRP often wheeze and the diagnosis may be delayed. The primary symptom of RRP is hoarseness or a weak cry. Stridor is often the second symptom to develop, usually starting as inspiratory and progressing to biphasic with advancing disease.[97] Other symptoms may include chronic cough, paroxysms of choking, failure to thrive, and respiratory fatigue.[135] Diagnosis is made with a flexible fiberoptic nasopharyngoscope. If patient's cooperation limits the examination, general anesthesia may be needed. Treatment consists of CO_2 laser microlaryngoscopy, which vaporizes the lesions and causes minimal bleeding. Frequent surgical procedures may be required to control the disease. Medical management includes the use of acyclovir, alpha interferon, cidofovir, and indole 3-carbinol.[135]

Airway implications. Airway obstruction has been reported with induction of anesthesia in patients with recurrent respiratory papillomatosis.[92] Anesthetic evaluation should include careful preoperative assessment of the airway and the emotional status of the child.[314] Sedation is necessary because these patients require frequent surgeries, but it should be avoided in patients with respiratory compromise. In appropriate instances, parental presence in the operating room may be beneficial. Anesthesia should be induced with an inhalational induction in 100% oxygen while maintaining spontaneous respirations. Patients may be apprehensive about the mask, and an alternative technique such as cupping the hands around the circuit to increase the concentration of the inhalational agent may be useful.[314] This is a recognized DA, and appropriate equipment and personnel should be in the operating room prior to induction.

5. Laryngeal Granulomas

Laryngeal granulomas are frequently the result of prolonged endotracheal intubation.[222] However, granuloma formation has been reported after short-term intubation as well.[189] Other factors contributing to granuloma formation include female gender, size of the ET, position of the ET, traumatic intubation, and excessive cuff pressure.[189] The incidence in adults has been described as 1 in 800 to 1 in 20,000.[392] Typically, granulomas form in the posterior glottis on the medial aspect of the arytenoids.[200] Hoarseness is a common feature. Treatment consists of inhaled steroids, antireflux measures, antibiotics, and surgical removal under direct visualization.[189]

Airway implications. If the granulomas are large or pedunculated, airway obstruction may be seen. AI may be indicated in the adult population or, rarely, inhalation induction with intubation in the pediatric population. ETs smaller than predicted should be immediately available.

6. Congenital and Acquired Subglottic Disease

a. Subglottic Stenosis

Subglottic stenosis may be classified as congenital or acquired. It is defined as the presence of an abnormally small subglottic lumen (less than 3.5 mm in diameter in a newborn infant).[400] Congenital subglottic stenosis is the third most common congenital anomaly.[349] Patients may present with mild or severe airway obstruction. Another common presentation is recurrent croup.[400] Patients who develop recurrent croup with upper respiratory tract infections during the first years of life should be evaluated for congenital subglottic stenosis. Acquired subglottic stenosis is usually the result of endotracheal intubation. Definitive diagnosis is made with rigid endoscopy. Treatment consists of anterior or multiple cricoid splitting with cartilage graft interpositioning. The success rate for these procedures has been shown to be approximately 90%.[349]

b. Croup

Croup or laryngotracheobronchitis is the most common cause of infectious airway obstruction in children. The incidence of croup in the United States is 18 per 1000 children annually. The peak incidence is 60 per 1000 among children 1 to 2 years of age.[322] Croup affects children between the ages of 6 months and 4 years, with peak incidence in early fall and winter. Parainfluenza type I is the most common etiologic agent responsible for croup. This is a viral infection that affects the subglottic region of the larynx, causing edema. The disease has a gradual onset, usually arising after an upper respiratory tract infection. Symptoms include inspiratory stridor; suprasternal, intercostal, and subcostal retractions; and a croupy or barking cough. Anteroposterior films of the neck show the classical church steeple sign (symmetrical narrowing of the subglottic air).[322]

For mild cases, treatment consists of breathing humidified air or oxygen.[322] In severe cases, treatment with nebulized racemic epinephrine (0.25 to 0.5 mL in 2 mL of saline) is indicated. Repeated treatments, every 1 to 2 hours, may be necessary. Because the duration of action is brief (less than 2 hours), rebound respiratory distress may develop after treatment, and observation is necessary. Studies suggest that patients may be discharged from the emergency room after a 3-hour observation period provided that the parents are reliable and easy access to the emergency room is available.[360] Racemic epinephrine should be used with caution in patients with tachycardia or underlying cardiac abnormalities, such as tetralogy of Fallot or idiopathic hypertrophic subaortic stenosis.[360]

After years of debate, the use of steroids in the treatment of mild to moderate viral croup has gained acceptance.[226,319,324] Treatment with steroids has been associated with a reduction in admissions and length of stay.[324] Dexamethasone 0.6 mg/kg (maximum dose, 10 mg) intravenously is the standard dose.[226] Dexamethasone (0.6 mg/kg) given orally was associated with more rapid resolution of symptoms than nebulized dexamethasone.[226] Heliox, a mixture of helium and oxygen, has also been used in the treatment of viral croup.[29] Helium is an inert, nontoxic gas that has low specific gravity, low viscosity, and low density. Because of these properties, helium reduces airway resistance by decreasing turbulent flow in the airway.[29] If the preceding measures fail, intubation is necessary.

Airway implications. As with all cases of upper airway obstruction, preparations for management of a difficult pediatric airway must be made. The appropriate equipment and personnel must be in the operating room at the time of induction. A gradual inhalation induction is performed with 100% oxygen maintaining spontaneous respirations. Intubation is performed with an ET that is one or two sizes smaller than predicted in order to decrease the risk of subglottic stenosis. Extubation is performed after an adequate air leak around the ET is demonstrated.

F. TRACHEOBRONCHIAL ANOMALIES

1. Tracheomalacia

Tracheomalacia is characterized by weakness of the tracheal wall related to softness of the cartilaginous support.

This allows the affected portion to collapse under conditions where the extraluminal pressure exceeds the intraluminal pressure.[18] Tracheomalacia may be classified into either congenital (primary) or acquired (secondary). Congenital tracheomalacia may be further subdivided into idiopathic or syndromic conditions. Tracheoesophageal fistula, CHARGE syndrome, and DiGeorge's syndrome are associated with congenital tracheomalacia. Acquired tracheomalacia is typically due to extrinsic compression of great vessels or secondary to bronchopulmonary dysplasia. Symptoms include episodic respiratory distress, persistent dry cough, wheezing, dysphagia, and recurrent respiratory infections. Failure to wean from the ventilator or failure of extubation may also be indicative of tracheomalacia.[18]

Airway implications. Airway obstruction has been reported in patients with tracheomalacia during general anesthesia, even in asymptomatic patients.[13,277] Collapse of the affected segment occurs during expiration and particularly forceful expiration or coughing. CPAP with or without intermittent positive-pressure ventilation can alleviate the obstruction.[404] Noninvasive positive-pressure ventilation through a face mask has been used successfully to prevent reintubation in an infant with tracheomalacia postoperatively.[52]

2. Croup

See "Laryngeal Anomalies" Section IX.E.6b.

3. Bacterial Tracheitis

Bacterial tracheitis, formerly called pseudomembranous tracheitis or membranous laryngotracheobronchitis, is a potentially life-threatening disease.[86] It is an infection of the subglottic region and progression to full airway obstruction is possible. Bacterial tracheitis is believed to be due to a bacterial superinfection preceded by a viral upper respiratory tract infection.[86] The peak incidence is in the fall and winter, affecting children from age 6 months to 8 years.[322] *S. aureus, H. influenzae,* alpha-hemolytic *Streptococcus,* and group A *Streptococcus* are the usual causative agents.[322] Patients usually present with a several day history of viral upper respiratory symptoms followed by rapid deterioration. The patient develops high fever, respiratory distress, and a toxic appearance. In contrast to those with supraglottitis, these patients have a substantial cough, appear comfortable when supine, and tend not to drool.[322] In contrast to those with laryngotracheobronchitis, patients with bacterial tracheitis do not respond to racemic epinephrine or corticosteroids. Radiographs of the airway often show irregular tracheal densities and subglottic narrowing.[86] Patients with severe respiratory distress should be taken to the operating room for rigid endoscopy and intubation.

Airway implications. Patients with bacterial tracheitis have the potential for airway obstruction. Preparations for management of the difficult pediatric airway must be made, including a rigid bronchoscope. Inhalation induction with maintenance of spontaneous respirations is preferred. Endoscopy is performed with removal of the sloughed mucosa. Intubation is performed and specimens for culture and Gram stain are taken. Broad-spectrum antibiotics are started and continued for 10 to 14 days. Intubation is usually required for 3 to 7 days.[322]

4. Mediastinal Masses

Anesthesia for patients with mediastinal masses, usually anterior mediastinal masses, is associated with a high risk of airway obstruction, hemodynamic instability, or even death from extrinsic compression of three structures: the heart, great vessels (primarily superior vena cava), and the trachea and bronchi.[268] Induction of anesthesia and positive-pressure ventilation may exacerbate the airway compression in a variety of ways. Loss of intrinsic muscle tone, reduced lung volumes, and a reduced transpleural pressure gradient combine to increase the effects of extrinsic compression. Cardiac arrest, superior vena cava syndrome, and airway occlusion are problems that can occur during induction of anesthesia.[210,270,273] Airway compression during induction of anesthesia can occur even in asymptomatic patients.[270] These complications may be unresponsive to position changes or open cardiac massage. Mediastinal masses may be divided into anterosuperior, visceral, and posterior. The anatomic location of the mediastinal mass varies with age. In children, mediastinal masses are predominately found in the posterior mediastinum. Neurogenic tumors, especially neuroblastomas, are the most common mediastinal tumor in young children. Germ cell tumors are the second most common anterior mediastinal mass in children.[268] In adolescents, lymphomas are the most common anterior mediastinal mass.[268]

Symptoms such as orthopnea, stridor, and wheezing are ominous signs of airway obstruction.[126] Positional dyspnea, tachyarrhythmia, and syncope are suggestive of right heart and pulmonary vascular compression. Syncope during a Valsalva maneuver is suggestive of significant vascular encroachment.[268] Children usually display symptoms earlier than adults. Small decreases in airway diameter result in an increase in resistance. Preoperative evaluation should focus on symptoms of respiratory compromise in the supine and standing position. Intolerance of the supine position indicates compression by the mass on the trachea, heart, pulmonary artery, or superior vena cava. Shamberger stated that the minimum criteria for safe administration of general anesthesia are a tracheal cross-sectional area at least 50% of predicted and a peak expiratory flow rate at least 50% of predicted.[338]

Airway implications. In regard to the DA, patients with a mediastinal mass are considered difficult to ventilate. Avoidance of general anesthesia, muscle relaxants, and positive-pressure ventilation are the mainstay of anesthetic management for patients presenting for biopsy prior to irradiation or chemotherapy. Biopsies should be performed if at all possible under local anesthesia.[137] Ketamine, local anesthesia, and 50:50 mixture of O_2 and N_2O while maintaining spontaneous ventilation have been used successfully for a diagnostic biopsy in a 13-year-old.[369] Positioning the patient in the reverse Trendelenburg position may help.

In the case of pediatric patients, general anesthesia may be needed for biopsy. Recommendations for a rigid pediatric bronchoscopy and femoral-to-femoral bypass standby have been made.[270,413] If possible, irradiation of the mass prior to general anesthesia may reduce the risk associated with anesthesia. Peripheral shielding of the mediastinum may allow subsequent tissue biopsy.[371] For older children, an awake fiberoptic intubation or FOB should be performed to assess the degree of obstruction following topicalization of the airway. In small infants and children, an AI is not practical. In these cases, an inhalation induction with maintenance of spontaneous ventilation is recommended. Intravenous access must be obtained in a lower extremity prior to induction.[413] Induction of anesthesia in the lateral semi-Fowler position has been recommended.[273] Maintenance of spontaneous ventilation is vital; however, this is not foolproof. Heliox (80% helium and 20% oxygen) has been used for induction with halothane and an LMA for successful airway management in a 3-year-old with severe respiratory distress related to a massive mediastinal mass.[293]

If airway obstruction or hemodynamic collapse occurs with induction, the following steps are suggested. First, one attempts to pass the ET down the least obstructed bronchus. If passage of the ET is not possible, rigid bronchoscopy to bypass the obstruction is attempted. Position changes to the lateral or prone position may alleviate the obstruction by changing the weight distribution of the tumor. Finally, cardiopulmonary bypass has been recommended.[270] Airway obstruction may occur during emergence as well. Extubation should be performed with the patient awake. These patients should be monitored postoperatively in the intensive care unit.

5. Vascular Malformations

Vascular malformations result from an abnormal development of the arterial component of the branchial arch system resulting in complete or incomplete encirclement of the trachea, esophagus, or both.[23] In 1945, Gross introduced the term vascular ring to describe this anomaly.[140] Patients with vascular rings may present with symptoms of respiratory distress or dysphagia because of tracheoesophageal compression. Patients may present with respiratory distress after birth or be asymptomatic for life. Most children with vascular rings present with nonspecific symptoms such as stridor, dyspnea, cough, or recurrent respiratory tract infection.[377] Dysphagia is often the primary symptom in adults with vascular ring.[23]

In a retrospective review of vascular rings, 74% of the malformations were symptomatic, with inspiratory stridor and wheezing as the main complaints.[377]

Various types of vascular rings have been described. Double aortic arch and right aortic arch with aberrant left subclavian artery are a few of the vascular rings described. The double aortic arch usually arises earlier than other varieties requiring surgical correction.[23] Associated cardiac anomalies are often present with the vascular ring.

Diagnosis is confirmed by radiologic studies. A chest radiograph may indicate the site of the ascending and descending aorta. A barium esophagogram may disclose extrinsic compression of the esophagus. Angiography has been considered the gold standard for identifying vascular rings.[377] CT and MRI scans are able to assist in the diagnosis of vascular ring and determine the anatomy. There may be a delay in the diagnosis of vascular ring because of the nonspecific symptoms.[377] Patients who are symptomatic should undergo surgery. Surgical correction is by a left thoracotomy, a right thoracotomy, or a median sternotomy.[23]

Airway implications. Patients with a vascular ring are at risk of airway obstruction from compression of the trachea. Tracheomalacia may be present as well. Maintenance of spontaneous ventilation until the trachea is intubated with a reinforced ET may be beneficial. A rigid bronchoscope should be available to serve as an airway stent in the event of airway collapse.

6. Foreign Body Aspiration

Foreign body aspiration is a cause of significant morbidity and mortality in the pediatric population. Young children are at increased risk for foreign body aspiration, with children younger than 2 years being the most commonly affected.[186] There is a second peak of aspiration that occurs between ages 10 and 11.[119] Most of the deaths occur in children younger than 1 year. The objects most frequently aspirated are food products. There is only a slight propensity for the object to lodge on the right side because of symmetrical bronchial angles in children younger than 15 years.[323] The left main stem bronchus is displaced by the aortic knob by the age of 15, creating a more obtuse angle at the carina.[323]

Witnessed events are easier to diagnose. A history of choking, gagging, or coughing is usually given. Patients may be asymptomatic at the time or develop symptoms of acute distress. A persistent cough, wheezing, or recurrent pneumonia may be the initial sign if the aspiration occurred in the past. The American Academy of Pediatrics has developed guidelines for the management of choking episodes. For children younger than 1 year, back blows and abdominal thrusts with the child in a head-down position are recommended. The Heimlich maneuver is reserved for older children and adults.[359]

Classically, peanuts should be removed promptly because of the inflammatory reaction to the peanut oil.

Emergency removal is indicated if the patient is in distress or if the foreign body is in a precarious location. If the patient is stable, radiographs may be taken to assist in localizing and identifying the foreign body. If the foreign body is radiopaque, it is easily identified. Radiolucent foreign bodies may demonstrate soft tissue density in or narrowing of the airway.[388] Indirect signs of air trapping, mediastinal shift, or atelectasis may be present. Lateral decubitus films are helpful in infants and younger children because they cannot cooperate with expiratory films.[323] The down-side lung should be deflated unless it is obstructed with a foreign body.[119]

Airway implications. In general, inhalation induction without cricoid pressure is the favored technique for removal of foreign bodies in the airway regardless of the type of object according to a postal survey of members of the Society for Pediatric Anesthesia.[186] For foreign bodies in the upper esophagus, a rapid sequence induction without cricoid pressure was the preferred technique; whereas for objects in the lower esophagus and stomach, a rapid sequence induction with cricoid pressure was chosen.[186] Cricoid pressure may cause harm if the foreign body is sharp or positioned in the larynx. If the case is not an emergency, one can wait until the appropriate nothing-by-mouth time has passed. In a retrospective review of anesthetic management for tracheobronchial foreign body removal, neither spontaneous nor controlled ventilation was associated with an increased incidence of adverse events.[217]

With an inhalation induction, a prolonged induction may occur because of airway obstruction. CPAP 5 to 10 cm H_2O and assisted ventilation may be needed at times in order to maintain a patent airway. After an adequate level of anesthesia is obtained, topicalization of the airway may decrease the incidence of coughing or laryngospasm. Use of a ventilating rigid bronchoscope allows ventilation during the procedure. High oxygen flow rates may be needed to overcome the presence of an air leak around the bronchoscope. Communication between the anesthesiologist and the endoscopist is crucial because this is a shared airway. The patient may require intermittent ventilation if desaturation occurs during the FOB. When the foreign body is grasped, the glottis should be relaxed for removal. Short-acting muscle relaxants, propofol, or deeper inhalational anesthesia may be used. The forceps and the bronchoscope are removed from the trachea as a single unit.[380] Dislodgement of foreign bodies at the glottic or subglottic area has been reported.[285] If a foreign body is dislodged and obstructs the trachea, the bronchoscope must be used to push the foreign body into a main stem bronchus to enable ventilation of one lung.[115] FOB with tracheotomy removal of a bronchial foreign body has been used successfully to remove a foreign body that was too large to pass through the subglottis.[115]

When the foreign body is removed, the patient is usually intubated with an appropriate size of ET. Depending on the amount of edema from the procedure, the patient should be able to be extubated. Postoperatively, racemic epinephrine (0.5 mL of 2.25% solution in 3 mL of saline) may be used for stridor. Dexamethasone is often given for edema.

7. Other Tracheal Disease

Tracheal stenosis is either a congenital or acquired disease. Congenital stenosis may be associated with congenital airway malformations such as tracheoesophageal fistula, hypoplastic lungs, and tracheomalacia. Congenital complete tracheal rings are also a cause of tracheal stenosis. In this condition, the rings are fused posteriorly and there is no posterior membranous wall.[401] Acquired stenosis is usually attributed to prolonged intubation, inhalational injuries, trauma, or tumors. Symptoms include stridor, wheezing, croup, tachypnea, and cough. For mild lesions, conservative therapy is warranted.[401] Surgical treatment involves tracheal resection with primary reanastomosis for short segment lesions. Anterotracheal split procedures may be used for longer segmental lesions. Laser excision of granulation tissue at the repair site may be needed.[401]

Airway implications. These cases may cause difficulty with ventilation or advancement of the ET. Minimal trauma to the airway can lead to acute airway obstruction.[401] The use of an LMA has been described in two cases of subglottic stenosis in which the stenotic areas were 2 mm or less.[11,22] Passage of the rigid bronchoscope should be performed only at the time of definitive repair.

G. NECK AND SPINE ANOMALIES

1. Neck

2. Limited Cervical Spine Mobility

Limited cervical spine mobility may be due to congenital or acquired disorders. The two congenital disorders that limit the mobility of the cervical spine are Klippel-Feil and Goldenhar's syndrome (see "Mandibular Hypoplasia" Section IX.B.2c).

a. Klippel-Feil Syndrome

Klippel-Feil syndrome is characterized by fusion of two or more cervical vertebrae. Other features of the Klippel-Feil syndrome include short neck, a low posterior hairline, scoliosis, and congenital heart disease.[214] Difficulty with airway management usually arises in the latter half of the first decade. The degree of difficulty with airway management depends on the severity of neck fixation.

b. Goldenhar's Syndrome

See "Mandibular Hypoplasia" on page 800.

c. Juvenile Rheumatoid Arthritis

JRA is a chronic arthritis with variable manifestations. Several different subgroups of disease have been identified—systemic onset (Still's disease), polyarticular, and oligoarticular (see "Facial Anomalies: Maxillary and Mandibular Disease: Juvenile Rheumatoid Arthritis").

Airway implications. Careful preoperative evaluation of these patients must be done before anesthetic induction. Previous anesthetic records, if available, should be reviewed for any relevant information. Because a DA is presumed to exist, preparation for management of the difficult pediatric airway must be made. In cases of limited cervical mobility, the ability to align the oral, pharyngeal, and laryngeal axes for visualization of the glottis is hampered. The presence of temporomandibular joint involvement may limit mouth opening as well. Awake endotracheal intubation is recommended in this scenario. There are many techniques available for use: FOB, Bullard laryngoscope, retrograde wire technique, and light wand. This may not be suitable in younger patients. For patients who will not cooperate with an awake technique, a mask induction with 100% oxygen and spontaneous ventilation is indicated. Retrograde intubation, the use of suspension laryngoscopy, and fiberoptic intubation through the LMA have all been reported in pediatric patients with Goldenhar's syndrome.[68,81,156] The light wand was used to intubate an 18-day-old infant with right hemifacial microsomia.[205]

3. Congenital Cervical Spine Instability

Cervical spine instability, if unrecognized, is a potential cause of serious morbidity and even mortality during airway management. Cervical spine instability or subluxation most often involves the atlanto-occipital joint. Congenital syndromes such as trisomy 21, Hurler's syndrome, Hunter's syndrome, and Morquio's syndrome are associated with cervical spine instability.[116] Of these, trisomy 21 is the syndrome most commonly encountered by anesthesiologists.

a. Down Syndrome

Down syndrome occurs in approximately 1 of every 660 live births. Mental retardation, congenital heart disease, obstructive sleep apnea, and congenital subglottic stenosis may be present. Approximately 20% of patients have ligamentous laxity of the atlantoaxial joint, which may allow atlantoaxial instability. This may predispose them to cervical spinal cord compression. Children are at risk for injury during hyperextension, hyperflexion, or increased rotation of the neck.[16,253] Signs of cervical spinal cord compression include loss of ambulatory function, spasticity, hyperreflexia of the lower extremities, extensor plantar reflexes, and loss of bowel and bladder control. Other signs may include increased fatigue with walking and torticollis.[253] Preoperative evaluation of the patient with Down syndrome must attempt to discover any preexisting signs or symptoms of spinal cord compression. The issue of screening for atlantoaxial instability in patients with Down syndrome is controversial. The American Academy of Pediatrics Committee on Sports Medicine and Fitness decided that uncertainty exists concerning the value of cervical spine radiographs in screening for possible catastrophic neck injury in athletes with Down syndrome.[253] However, Pueschel argued that patients should be screened for atlantoaxial instability.[301] In a survey of members of the Society of Pediatric Anesthesia, respondents obtain preoperative radiographs (18%) or subspecialty consultation (8%), or both, for asymptomatic patients. For symptomatic patients, radiographs and preoperative consultations are obtained 64% and 74% of the time, respectively. The majority of respondents attempt to maintain the head in a neutral position for both symptomatic and asymptomatic patients.[218]

Airway implications. Airway management for patients with Down syndrome should take into consideration the possibility of cervical spine instability with cord compression. In addition, the large tongue and potential for obstructive sleep apnea can lead to upper airway obstruction. Patients who have symptoms of cord compression should have radiographic evaluation prior to any elective surgical procedure. Lateral extension and flexion radiographs of the upper cervical spine can reveal atlantoaxial subluxation. An odontoid process (axis) to anterior arch (atlas) distance greater than 4.5 mm indicates abnormal instability.[253]

For emergency surgery, cervical spine precautions should be used in patients who are symptomatic. In-line stabilization of the cervical spine for direct laryngoscopy should be used. Techniques for airway management that require minimal neck movement such as the Bullard laryngoscope, light wand, the angulated video laryngoscope, or the SOS may be useful.

4. Acquired Cervical Spine Instability

Acquired cervical spine instability in pediatric patients can result from multiple trauma or head and neck trauma. Any pediatric patient with a severe head injury should be treated as though a cervical spine injury is present.[41] It has been estimated that 1% to 2% of pediatric patients with multiple trauma have a cervical spine injury.[359] Pediatric patients with underlying medical conditions such as Down syndrome may be more susceptible to cervical cord injury.[359] Pediatric patients younger than 8 years are at increased risk for injury to the upper cervical spine and craniovertebral junction. Only 30% of cervical spine injuries occur below C3 in children younger than 8 years. They also have a higher incidence of spinal cord injury without radiographic abnormality (SCIWORA).[239] Immobilization of a patient with suspected cervical spine injury is crucial so that further damage to the cord is prevented. A hard collar, spine board, and soft spacing devices between the head and securing straps are needed. The occiput is large, and a blanket under the torso allows the neck to rest in a neutral position.

Airway implications. The choice of airway management depends on the degree of urgency associated with the intubation. Techniques that minimize head extension and cervical flexion are mandatory. Trauma patients are considered at risk for aspiration, and appropriate measures need to be taken.

For an urgent airway in a patient with a DA or facial fractures, a surgical airway may be the best option. If time allows, a limited number of attempts at direct laryngoscopy may be performed. The Bullard laryngoscope may be useful in this situation. In an emergency, the LMA may be used to ventilate or oxygenate the patient until a formal airway is established. This does not provide protection against aspiration.

For a nonurgent intubation, further evaluation of the cervical spine is warranted. When the cervical spine has been "cleared" by the neurosurgeon or trauma surgeon, a rapid sequence induction with cricoid pressure may be performed after adequate preoxygenation if the airway appears reasonable. If the cervical spine is unstable, a rapid sequence induction with cricoid pressure may be performed with in-line stabilization. Fluoroscopy was used to assist the intubation of an 11-year-old with an unstable subluxation of C1-C2 after a motor vehicle accident.[256] Awake techniques such as flexible fiberoptic laryngoscopy, the Bullard laryngoscope, light wand, SOS, or retrograde intubation may be indicated if the patient has an unstable cervical spine and a DA.

X. PEDIATRIC TRAUMA

All pediatric trauma patients are considered to have a cervical spine injury until proved otherwise. In addition, these patients are at risk for aspiration. Oxygen should be administered and ventilation assisted if needed as soon as possible. Trauma patients should be immobilized on a spine board with a rigid collar as previously described. After an evaluation of the airway, one should decide on the method of intubation. If the airway is judged to be adequate, a rapid sequence induction with cricoid pressure and manual in-line stabilization should be employed. The front of the collar and strapping should be removed prior to laryngoscopy. If the airway cannot be secured, the ASA DA algorithm should be followed. In a DA scenario, one of the previously described awake techniques may be used. In certain cases, awake tracheostomy or surgical cricothyrotomy may be indicated. A multidisciplinary approach to the management of the difficult pediatric trauma airway is necessary.

XI. EXTUBATION OF THE DIFFICULT AIRWAY

The management of the difficult pediatric airway does not end until the plan for extubation has been established. Choices include extubation over an airway catheter or guidewire or extubation when an air leak develops as in the case of epiglottitis. Preparations for the difficult pediatric airway must be made because an extubation may lead to a reintubation. If airway edema is suspected at the end of the surgery, because of either the intubation process or the surgery, dexamethasone may be of benefit. Postoperative ventilation may be indicated as well until the edema resolves. Extubation has been successfully performed over an airway exchange catheter in an adolescent with a DA.[69] Alternatively, a 0.018' guidewire has been used to maintain airway access in a 2-year-old with severe micrognathia and tetralogy of Fallot.[147]

REFERENCES

1. Agro F, Cataldo R, Carassiti M, et al: The Seeing Stylet: A new device for tracheal intubation. Resuscitation 44: 177-180, 2000.

2. Agro F, Hung OR, Catalda R, et al: Lightwand intubation using the Trachlight: A brief review of current knowledge. Can J Anaesth 48:592-599, 2001.

3. Alfrey DD, Ward CF, Harwood IR, et al: Airway management for a neonate with congenital fusion of the jaws. Anesthesiology 51:340-342, 1979.

4. Ali NJ, Pitson DJ, Stradling JR: Snoring, sleep disturbance, and behavior in 4-5 year olds. Arch Dis Child 68:360-366, 1993.

5. Ameh EA: Acute retropharyngeal abscess in children. Ann Trop Paediatr 19:109-112, 1999.

6. American Academy of Pediatrics, Section on Anesthesiology: Guidelines for the pediatric perioperative anesthesia environment. Pediatrics 103:512-515, 1999.

7. American Thoracic Society: Standards and indications for cardiopulmonary sleep studies in children. Am J Respir Crit Care Med 153:866-878, 1996.

8. Anderson PJ, Hall CM, Evans RD, et al: Cervical spine in Pfeiffer's syndrome. J Craniofac Surg 7:275-279, 1996.

9. Andersson HC, Frentz J, Martinez JE, et al: Adrenal insufficiency in Smith-Lemli-Opitz syndrome. Am J Med Genet 82:382-384, 1999.

10. Antony AK, Sloan GM: Airway obstruction following palatoplasty: Analysis of 247 consecutive operations. Cleft Palate Craniofac J 39:145-148, 2002.

11. Asai T, Fujise K, Uchida M: Use of the laryngeal mask in a child with tracheal stenosis. Anesthesiology 75: 903-904, 1991.

12. Asai T, Hirose T, Shingu K: Failed tracheal intubation using a laryngoscope and intubating laryngeal mask. Can J Anaesth 47:325-328, 2000.

13. Asai T, Shingu K: Airway obstruction in a child with asymptomatic tracheobronchomalacia. Can J Anaesth 48:684-687, 2001.

14. Asher BF, McGill TJ, Kaplan L, et al: Airway complications in CHARGE association. Arch Otolaryngol Head Neck Surg 116:594-595, 1990.

15. Atherton DJ, Denyer J: Epidermolysis Bullosa: An Outline for Professionals. London, DEBRA, 1997.

16. Atlantoaxial instability in Down syndrome: Subject review. American Academy of Pediatrics Committee on Sports Medicine and Fitness. Pediatrics 96:151-154, 1995.

17. Audenaert SM, Montgomery CL, Stone B, et al: Retrograde-assisted fiberoptic intubation in children with difficult airways. Anesth Analg 73:660-664, 1991.

18. Austin J, Ali T: Tracheomalacia and bronchomalacia in children: Pathophysiology, assessment, treatment and anesthesia management. Paediatr Anaesth 13:3-11, 2003.

19. Badgwell JM, McLeod ME, Friedberg J: Airway obstruction in infants and children. Can J Anaesth 34:90-98, 1987.

20. Bahk JH, Han SM, Kim SD: Management of difficult airways with a laryngeal mask airway under propofol anaesthesia. Paediatr Anaesth 9:163-166, 1999.

21. Bahk JH, Kim JK, Kim CS: Use of the laryngeal mask airway to preoxygenate in a paediatric patient with Treacher-Collins syndrome. Paediatr Anaesth 8:274-275, 1998.

22. Bahk JH, Rhee KY: Assisted ventilation through a laryngeal mask airway for severe subglottic stenosis. Paediatr Anaesth 8:523, 1998.

23. Bakker DAH, Berger RMF, Witsenburg M, et al: Vascular rings: A rare cause of common respiratory symptoms. Acta Paediatr 88:947-952, 1999.

24. Bar A, Tarasiuk A, Segev Y, et al: The effect of adenotonsillectomy on serum insulin-like growth factor-I and growth in children with obstructive sleep apnea syndrome. J Pediatr 135:76-80, 1999.

25. Baraka AS: Tension pneumothorax complicating jet ventilation via a Cook airway exchange catheter. Anesthesiology 91:557-558, 1999.

26. Bartz HJ, Wiesner L, Wappler F: Anaesthetic management of patients with mucopolysaccharidosis IV presenting for major orthopaedic surgery. Acta Anaesthesiol Scand 43:679-683, 1999.

27. Baxter MRN: Congenital laryngomalacia. Can J Anaesth 41:332-339, 1994.

28. Beck R, Sertie AL, Brik R, Shinawi M: Crouzon syndrome: association with absent pulmonary valve syndrome and severe tracheobronchomalacia. Pediatr Pulmonol 34:478-481, 2002.

29. Beckman KR, Brueggemann WM: Heliox treatment of severe croup. Am J Emerg Med 18:735-736, 2000.

30. Belani KG, Krivit W, Carpenter BL, et al: Children with mucopolysaccharidosis: Perioperative care, morbidity, mortality, and new findings. J Pediatr Surg 28:403-408, 1993.

31. Benjamin B, Walker P: Management of airway obstruction in the Pierre Robin sequence. Int J Pediatr Otorhinolaryngol 22:29-37, 1991.

32. Benumof JL, Cooper SD: Quantitative improvement in laryngoscopic view by optimal external laryngeal manipulation. J Clin Anesth 8:136-140, 1996.

33. Benyamin RM, Wafai Y, Salem MR, et al: Two-handed mask ventilation of the difficult airway by a single individual. Anesthesiology 88:1134, 1998.

34. Berry FA: Anesthesia for the child with a difficult airway. In Berry FA (ed): Anesthetic Management of Difficult and Routine Pediatric Patients, 2nd ed. New York, Churchill Livingstone, 1990.

35. Berthelsen P, Prytz S, Jacobsen E: Two-stage fiberoptic nasotracheal intubation in infants: A new approach to difficult pediatric intubation. Anesthesiology 63:457-458, 1985.

36. Biavati MJ, Manning SC, Phillips DL: Predictive factors for respiratory complications after tonsillectomy and adenoidectomy in children. Arch Otolaryngol Head Neck Surg 123:517-521, 1997.

37. Biban P, Baraldi E, Pettennazzo A, et al: Adverse effect of chloral hydrate in two young children with obstructive sleep apnea. Pediatrics 92:461-463, 1993.

38. Biban P, Rugolotto S, Zoppi G: Fiberoptic endotracheal intubation through an ultra thin bronchoscope with suction channel in a newborn with difficult airway. Anesth Analg 90:1007, 2000.

39. Bibi H, Khvolis E, Shoseyov D, et al: The prevalence of gastroesophageal reflux in children with tracheomalacia and laryngomalacia. Chest 119:409-413, 2001.

40. Biro P, Shahinian H: Management of difficult intubation caused by lingual tonsillar hyperplasia. Anesth Analg 79:389, 1994.

41. Bissonette B, Sadeghi P: Anesthesia for neurosurgical procedures. In Gregory G (ed): Pediatric Anesthesia, 4th ed. New York, Churchill Livingstone, 2002.

42. Blackstock D, Adderley RJ, Steward DJ: Epiglottitis in young infants. Anesthesiology 67:97-100, 1987.

43. Blanco G, Melman E, Cuairan V, et al: Fibreoptic nasal intubation in children with anticipated and unanticipated difficult intubation. Paediatr Anaesth 11:49-53, 2001.

44. Blankenstein R, Brook AH, Smith RN, et al: Oral findings in Carpenter syndrome. Int J Paediatr Dent 11:352-360, 2001.

45. Bleovsky LT, Prinsley PR: Acute tonsillar airway obstruction after adenoidectomy. Anaesth Intensive Care 17:516, 1989.

46. Bloom RS, Cropley C: Textbook of Neonatal Resuscitation. Dallas, AHA, 1994.

47. Bonfils P: Schwierge Intubation bei Pierre-Robin-Kindern, eine neue Methode: Der retromolare Weg. Anaesthesist 32:363-367,1983.

48. Borland L, Casselbrandt M: The Bullard laryngoscope: A new indirect oral laryngoscope (pediatric version). Anesth Analg 70:105-108, 1990.

49. Borland LM, Swan DM, Leff S: Airway management in Hallermann-Streiff syndrome. Am J Otolaryngol 5:64-67, 1984.

50. Borland LM, Swan DM, Leff S: Difficult paediatric endotracheal intubation: A new approach to the retrograde technique. Anaesthesiology 55:577-578, 1981.

51. Boucher C, Dorion D, Fisch C: Retropharyngeal abscesses: A clinical and radiologic correlation. J Otolaryngol 28:134-137, 1999.

52. Bouchut JC, Stamm D, Floret D: Postoperative ventilatory management with noninvasive positive pressure ventilation in a child with severe tracheomalacia. Anesthesiology 93:1562-1563, 2000.

53. Brain AIJ: The laryngeal mask airway—A new concept in airway management. Br J Anaesth 55:801-805, 1983.

54. Brouillette RT, Manoukian JJ, Ducharme FM, et al: Efficacy of fluticasone nasal spray for pediatric obstructive sleep apnea. J Pediatr 138:838-844, 2001.

55. Brouillette RT, Thach BT: A neuromuscular mechanism maintaining extrathoracic airway patency. J Appl Physiol 46:772-779, 1979.

56. Brown OE, Manning SC, Ridenour B: Cor pulmonale secondary to tonsillar and adenoidal hypertrophy: Management considerations. Int J Pediatr Otorhinolaryngol 16:131, 1988.

57. Brown RE Jr, Vollers JM, Rader GR, Schmitz ML: Nasotracheal intubation in a child with Treacher Collins syndrome using the Bullard intubating laryngoscope. J Clin Anesth 5:492-493, 1993.

58. Buhain WJ, Rammohan G, Berger HW: Pulmonary function in Morquio's disease: A study of two siblings. Chest 68:41-45, 1975.

59. Bussolin L, Busoni P: The use of the cuffed oropharyngeal airway in paediatric patients. Paediatr Anaesth 12:43-47, 2002.

60. Butler MG, Hayes BG, Hathaway MM, Begleiter ML: Specific genetic diseases at risk for sedation/anesthesia complications. Anesth Analg 91:837-855, 2000.

61. Butler PJ, Munro HM, Kenny MB: Preoxygenation in children using expired oxygraphy. Br J Anaesth 77:333-334, 1996.

62. Buttner J, Klose R: Peculiarities of anesthesia in severely burned patients. Langenbecks Arch Chir 364:213-217, 1984.

63. Calhoun KH, Deskin RW, Garza C, et al: Long-term airway sequelae in a pediatric burn population. Laryngoscope 98:721-725, 1988.

64. Carlan SJ, Angel JL, Leo J, et al: Cephalocele involving the oral cavity. Obstet Gynecol 75:494, 1990.

65. Carroll, JL, McColley SA, Marcus CL, et al: Inability of clinical history to distinguish primary snoring from obstructive sleep apnea syndrome in children. Chest 108:610-618, 1995.

66. Cerveri I, Fanfulla F, Zoia MC, et al: Sleep disorders in neuromuscular diseases. Monaldi Arch Chest Dis 48:318-321, 1993.

67. Chadd GD, Crane DL, Phillips RM, Tunell WP: Extubation and reintubation guided by the laryngeal mask airway in a child with the Pierre-Robin syndrome. Anesthesiology 76:640-641, 1992.

68. Chen PP, Cheng CK, Abdullah V, Chu CP: Tracheal intubation using suspension laryngoscopy in an infant with Goldenhar's syndrome. Anaesth Intensive Care 29:548-551, 2001.

69. Chipley PS, Castresana M, Bridges MT, et al: Prolonged use of an endotracheal tube changer in a pediatric patient with a potentially compromised airway. Chest 105:961-962, 1994.

70. Choi PT, Nowaczyk MJ: Anesthetic considerations in Smith-Lemli-Opitz syndrome. Can J Anaesth 47:556-561, 2000.

71. Clark RJ: Tongue-swelling with droperidol. Anaesth Intensive Care 21:898, 1993.

72. Clauser L, Galie M, Hassanipour A, Calabrese O: Saethre-Chotzen syndrome: Review of the literature and report of a case. J Craniofac Surg 11:480-486, 2000.

73. Cmejrek RC, Coticchia JM, Arnold JE: Presentation, diagnosis, and management of deep-neck abscesses in infants. Arch Otolaryngol Head Neck Surg 128:1361-1364, 2002.

74. Coates H: Nasal obstruction in the neonate and infant. Clin Pediatr (Phila) 31:25-29, 1992.

75. Cohen DM, Green JG, Miller J, et al: Acrocephalopolysyndactyly type II—Carpenter syndrome: Clinical spectrum and an attempt at unification with Goodman and Summit syndromes. Am J Med Genet 28:311-324, 1987.

76. Cohen MM, Kreiborg S: Birth prevalence studies of the Crouzon syndrome: Comparison of direct and indirect methods. Clin Genet 41:12-15, 1992.

77. Cohen MM Jr: Jackson-Weiss syndrome. Am J Med Genet 100:325-329, 2001.

78. Cohen MM Jr, Kreiborg S: Upper and lower airway compromise in the Apert syndrome. Am J Med Genet 44:90-93, 1992.

79. Cohen SR, Thompson JW: Lymphangiomas of the larynx in infants and children: A survey of pediatric lymphangioma. Ann Otol Rhinol Laryngol Suppl 127:1-20, 1986.

80. Cook-Sather SD, Schreiner MS: A simple homemade lighted stylet for neonates and infants: A description and case report of its use in an infant with the Pierre Robin anomalad. Paediatr Anaesth 7:233-235, 1997.

81. Cooper CM, Murray-Wilson A: Retrograde intubation. Management of a 4.8-kg, 5-month infant. Anaesthesia 42:1197-1200, 1987.

82. Coté CJ, Todres ID: The pediatric airway. In Coté CJ, Todres ID, Goudsouzian NG, Ryan JF (eds): A Practice of Anesthesia for Infants and Children, 3rd ed. Philadelphia, WB Saunders, 2001.

83. Coulthard M, Isaacs D: Retropharyngeal abscess. Arch Dis Child 66:1227-1230, 1991.

84. Cox J: Anesthesia and glycogen-storage disease. Anesthesiology 29:1221-1223, 1964.

85. Creighton RE: The infant airway. Can J Anaesth 41:174-176, 1994.

86. Cressman WR, Myer CM: Diagnosis and management of croup and epiglottitis. Pediatr Clin North Am 41:265-275, 1994.

87. Crosby E, Skene D: More on lingual tonsillar hypertrophy. Can J Anaesth 49:758, 2002.

88. Crosby ET, Cooper RM, Douglas MJ, et al: The unanticipated difficult airway with recommendations for management. Can J Anaesth 45:757-776, 1998.

89. Crouzon O: Dysostose cranio-faciale héréditaire. Bull Mem Soc Med Hop Paris 33:545-555, 1912.

90. Crozier WC: Upper airway obstruction in neurofibromatosis. Anaesthesia 42:1209-1211, 1987.

91. Cruickshanks GF, Brown S, Chitayat D: Anesthesia for Freeman-Sheldon syndrome using a laryngeal mask airway. Can J Anaesth 46:783-787, 1999.

92. Dalmeida RE, Mayhew JF, Driscoll B, et al: Total airway obstruction by papillomas during induction of general anesthesia. Anesth Analg 83:1332-1334, 1996.

93. Danziger I, Brodsky L, Perry R, et al: Nager's acrofacial dysostosis: Case report and review of the literature. Int J Pediatr Otorhinolaryngol 20:225-240, 1990.

94. David LR, Finlon M, Genecov D, Argenta LC: Hallermann-Streiff syndrome: Experience with 15 patients and review of the literature. J Craniofac Surg 10:160-168, 1999.

95. Davies R, Balachandran S: Anterior commissure laryngoscope. Anaesthesia 58:721-722, 2003.

96. Davies S, Ananthanarayan C, Castro C: Asymptomatic lingual tonsillar hypertrophy and difficult airway management: A report of three cases. Can J Anaesth 48:1020-1024, 2001.

97. Derkay CS, Darrow DH: Recurrent respiratory papillomatosis of the larynx. Otolaryngol Clin North Am 33:1127-1142, 2000.

98. Derkay CS, Grundfast KM: Airway compromise from nasal obstruction in neonates and infants. Int J Pediatr Otorhinolaryngol 19:241, 1990.

99. Dhakshinomoorthi P: Straight blade laryngoscopy. Anaesthesia 54:202-203, 1999.

100. Diaz JH, Guarisco JL, LeJeune FE: Perioperative management of pediatric microstomia. Can J Anaesth 38:217, 1991.

101. Divekar VM, Kothari MD, Kamdar BM: Anaesthesia in Turner's syndrome. Can Anaesth Soc J 30:417-418, 1983.

102. Domino KB, Posner KL, Caplan RA, et al: Airway injury during anesthesia. Anesthesiology 91:1703-1711, 1999.

103. Dubey AK, Gupta RK: Crouzon's syndrome with hydrocephalus. Indian Pediatr 38:200, 2001.

104. Dullenkopf A, Holzman D, Feurer R, et al: Tracheal intubation in children with Morquio syndrome using the angulated video-intubation laryngoscope. Can J Anaesth 49:198-202, 2002.

105. Ebata T, Nishiki S, Masuda A, Amaha K: Anaesthesia for Treacher Collins syndrome using a laryngeal mask airway. Can J Anaesth 38:1043-1045, 1991.

106. Eckenhoff JE: Some anatomic considerations of the infant larynx influencing endotracheal anesthesia. Anesthesiology 12:401, 1951.

107. Ellis DS, Potluri PK, O'Flaherty JE et al: Difficult airway management in the neonate: A simple method of intubating through a laryngeal mask airway. Paediatr Anaesth 9:460-462, 1999.

108. Erb T, Hammer J, Rutishauer M, et al: Fibreoptic bronchoscopy in sedated infants facilitated by an airway endoscopy mask. Paediatr Anesth 9:47-52, 1999.

109. Everett AD, Koch WC, Saulsbury FT: Failure to thrive due to obstructive sleep apnea. Clin Pediatr 26:90-92, 1987.

110. Factor SM, Biempica L, Goldfischer S: Coronary intimal sclerosis in Morquio's syndrome. Virchows Arch A Pathol Anat Histol 379:1-10, 1978.

111. Fagan JJ, James MF: A prospective study of anaesthesia for quinsy tonsillectomy. Anaesthesia 50:783-785, 1995.

112. Filippi G: The de Lange syndrome: Report of 15 cases. Clin Genet 35:343-363, 1989.

113. Fisher MM: Anaesthetic difficulties in neurofibromatosis. Anaesthesia 30:648-650, 1975.

114. Fisher QA, Tunkel DE: Lightwand intubation of infants and children. J Clin Anesth 9:275-279, 1997.

115. Fraga JC, Neto AM, Seitz E, et al: Bronchoscopy and tracheotomy removal of bronchial foreign body. J Pediatr Surg 37:1239-1240, 2002.

116. Frankville DD: Uncommon malformation syndromes of infants and pediatric patients. In Benumof JL (ed): Anesthesia and Uncommon Diseases, 4th ed. Philadelphia, WB Saunders, 1998.

117. Frei FJ, aWengen D, Rutishauser GE, et al: The airway endoscopy mask: Useful device for fiberoptic evaluation and intubation of the paediatric airway. Paediatr Anaesth 5:319-324, 1995.

118. Frei FJ, Ummenhofer W: A special mask for teaching fiber-optic intubation in pediatric patients. Anesth Analg 76:458-459, 1993.

119. Friedman EM: Tracheobronchial foreign bodies. Otolaryngol Clin North Am 33:179-185, 2000.

120. Fundingsland BW, Benumof JL: Difficulty using a laryngeal mask airway in a patient with lingual tonsil hyperplasia [letter]. Anesthesiology 84:1265-1266, 1996.

121. Gaitini L, Fradis M, Vaida S, et al: Failure to control the airway in a patient with Hunter's syndrome. J Laryngol Otol 112:380-382, 1998.

122. Gallart L, Mases A, Martinez J: Simple method to determine the size of the laryngeal mask airway in children. Eur J Anaesthesiol 20:570-574, 2003.

123. Gerber ME, O'Connor DM, Adler E, Myer CM III: Selected risk factors in pediatric adenotonsillectomy. Arch Otolaryngol Head Neck Surg 122:811-814, 1996.

124. Gislason T, Benediktsdottir B: Snoring, apneic episodes, and nocturnal hypoxemia among children 6 months to 6 years old. An epidemiological study of lower limit of prevalence. Chest 107:963-966, 1995.

125. Goh DYT, Marcus CL: Changes in obstructive sleep apnea characteristics in children through the night. Am J Respir Crit Care Med 157:A533, 1998.

126. Goh MH, Liu XY, Goh YS: Anterior mediastinal masses: An anesthetic challenge. Anaesthesia 54:670-682, 1999.

127. Goldberg Y, Dibbern K, Klein J, et al: Neurofibromatosis type 1—An update and review for the primary pediatrician. Clin Pediatr 35:545-561, 1996.

128. Goldhagen JL: Cricoarytenoiditis as a cause of acute airway obstruction in children. Ann Emerg Med 17:532-533, 1988.

129. Golding-Wood DG, Whittet HB: The lingual tonsil. A neglected symptomatic structure? J Laryngol Otol 103:922-925, 1989.

130. Goldman LJ, Nodal C, Jimenez E: Successful airway control with the laryngeal mask in an infant with Beckwith-Wiedemann syndrome and hepatoblastoma for central line catheterization. Paediatr Anaesth 10:445-448, 2000.

131. Goskowicz R, Colt HG, Voulelis LD: Fiberoptic tracheal intubation using a nipple guide. Anesthesiology 85:1210-1211, 1996.

132. Gouverneur JM: Using an ureteral catheter as a guide in difficult neonatal fiberoptic intubation. Anesthesiology 66:436-437, 1987.

133. Gozal D, Arens R, Omlin KJ, et al: Ventilatory response to consecutive short hypercapnic challenges in children with obstructive sleep apnea. J Appl Physiol 79:1608-1614, 1995.

134. Gozal D: Sleep-disordered breathing and school performance in children. Pediatrics 102:616-620, 1998.

135. Green GE, Bauman NM, Smith RJ: Pathogenesis and treatment of juvenile onset recurrent respiratory papillomatosis. Otolaryngol Clin North Am 33:187-207, 2000.

136. Greenberg RS, Mullin AM, Summer AB: COPA Instruction Manual. St. Louis, Mallinckrodt, 1997.

137. Greengrass R: Anaesthesia and mediastinal masses. Can J Anaesth 37:596, 1990.

138. Griffin RP, Mayou BG: The anaesthetic management of patients with dystrophic epidermolysis bullosa: A review of forty-four patients over a 10-year period. Anaesthesia 48:810, 1993.

139. Groeper K, Johnson JO, Braddock SR, Tobias JD: Anaesthetic implications of Nager syndrome. Paediatr Anaesth 12:365-368, 2002.

140. Gross RF: Surgical relief for tracheal obstruction from a vascular ring. N Engl J Med 233:586-590, 1945.

141. Guarisco JL: Congenital head and neck masses in infants and children. Ear Nose Throat J 70:40, 1990.

142. Guarisco JL, Littlewood SC, Butcher RB III: Severe upper airway obstruction in children secondary to lingual tonsil hypertrophy. Ann Otol Rhinol Laryngol 99:621-624, 1990.

143. Gunawardana RH: Difficult laryngoscopy in cleft lip and palate surgery. Br J Anaesth 76:757-759, 1996.

144. Hagberg CA: Special devices and techniques. Anesthesiol Clin North Am 20:907-932, 2002.

145. Haji-Michael PG, Hatch DL: Smith-Lemli-Opitz syndrome and malignant hyperthermia. Anesth Analg 83:200, 1996.

146. Hammer GB, Brodsky JB, Redpath JH, et al: The Univent tube for single-lung ventilation in paediatric patients. Paediatr Anaesth 8:55-57, 1998.

147. Hammer GB, Funck N, Rosenthal DN, et al: A technique for maintenance of airway access in infants with a difficult airway following tracheal extubation. Paediatr Anaesth 11:622-625, 2001.

148. Hammer GB, Harrison TK, Vricella LA, et al: Single lung ventilation in children using a new paediatric bronchial blocker. Paediatr Anaesth 12:69-72, 2002.

149. Hancock PJ, Peterson G: Finger intubation of the trachea in newborns. Pediatrics 89:325-326, 1992.

150. Hansen TG, Joensen H, Henneberg SW, Hole P: Laryngeal mask airway guided tracheal intubation in a neonate with the Pierre Robin syndrome. Acta Anaesthesiol Scand 39:129-131, 1995.

151. Harley EH: Pediatric congenital nasal masses. Ear Nose Throat J 70:28, 1991.

152. Hartl DM, Roger G, Denoyelle F, et al: Extensive lymphangioma presenting with upper airway obstruction. Arch Otolaryngol Head Neck Surg 126:1378-1382, 2000.

153. Hartmann RW: Recognition of retropharyngeal abscess in children. Am Fam Physician 46:193, 1992.

154. Haselby KA, McNiece WL: Respiratory obstruction from uvular edema in a pediatric patient. Anesth Analg 62:1127, 1983.

155. Hatch DJ: Airway management in cleft lip and palate surgery. Br J Anaesth 76:755-756, 1996.

156. Haxby E, Liban J: Fiberoptic intubation via a laryngeal mask in an infant with Goldenhar syndrome. Anesth Intensive Care 23:753, 1995.

157. Heard CMB, Caldicott LD, Fletcher JE, et al: Fiberoptic-guided endotracheal intubation via the laryngeal mask airway in pediatric patients: A report of a series of cases. Anesth Analg 82:1287-1289, 1996.

158. Helfaer MA, McColley SA, Pyzik PL, et al: Polysomnography after adenotonsillectomy in mild pediatric obstructive sleep apnea. Crit Care Med 24:1323-1327, 1996.

159. Henderson JJ: The use of paraglossal straight blade laryngoscopy in difficult tracheal intubation. Anaesthesia 52:552-560, 1997.

160. Henriksson TG, Skoog VT: Identification of children at high anaesthetic risk at the time of primary palatoplasty. Scand J Plast Reconstr Surg Hand Surg 35:177-182, 2001.

161. Herod J, Denyer J, Goldman A, Howard R: Epidermolysis bullosa in children: Pathophysiology, anaesthesia and pain management. Paediatr Anaesth 12:388-397, 2002.

162. Herod J, Denyer J, Howard R: Reply to Ames and Levine. Paediatr Anaesth 13:4, 371-371, 2003.

163. Herrick IA, Rhine EJ: The mucopolysaccharidoses and anaesthesia: A report of clinical experience. Can J Anaesth 35:67-73, 1988.

164. Hirsch NP, Murphy A, Radcliffe JJ: Neurofibromatosis: Clinical presentations and anaesthetic implications. Br J Anaesth 86:555-564, 2001.

165. Holinger LD, Konier RJ: Surgical management of severe laryngomalacia. Laryngoscope 99:136-142, 1989.

166. Holzman RS, Nargozian CD, Florence FB: Lightwand intubation in children with abnormal upper airways. Anesthesiology 69:784-787,1988.

167. Hopkins R, Watson JA, Jones JH, Walker M: Two cases of Hunter's syndrome—The anaesthetic and operative difficulties in oral surgery. Br J Oral Surg 10:286-299, 1973.

168. Howardy-Hansen P, Berthelsen P: Fibreoptic bronchoscopic nasotracheal intubation of a neonate with Pierre Robin syndrome. Anaesthesia 43:121-122, 1988.

169. Hughes GB, Shapiro G, Hunt W, et al: Management of the congenital midline mass. Head Neck Surg 2:222, 1980.

170. Ireland MA, Rowlands DB: Mucopolysaccharidosis type IV as a cause of mitral stenosis in an adult. Br Heart J 46:113-115, 1981.

171. Iseki K, Watanabe K, Iwama H: Use of the Trachlight for intubation in the Pierre-Robin syndrome. Anaesthesia 52:801-802, 1997.

172. Ishikawa T, Isono S, Aiba J, et al: Prone position increases collapsibility of the passive pharynx in infants and small children. Am J Respir Crit Care Med 166:760-764, 2002.

173. Isono S, Shimada A, Utsugi M, et al: Comparison of static mechanical properties of the passive pharynx between normal children and children with sleep-disordered breathing. Am J Respir Crit Care Med 157:1204-1212, 1998.

174. Isono S, Tanaka A, Nishino T: Lateral position decreases collapsibility of the passive pharynx in patients with obstructive sleep apnea. Anesthesiology 97:780-785, 2002.

175. Jacob SV, Morielli A, Mograss MA, et al:. Home testing for pediatric obstructive sleep apnea syndrome secondary to adenotonsillar hypertrophy. Pediatr Pulmonol 20:241-252, 1995.

176. Jacobs JC, Hui RM: Cricoarytenoid arthritis and airway obstruction in juvenile rheumatoid arthritis. Pediatrics 59:292-294, 1977.

177. James I, Wark H: Airway management during anesthesia in patients with epidermolysis bullosa dystrophica. Anesthesiology 56:323-326, 1982.

178. Jarund M, Lauritzen C: Craniofacial dysostosis: Airway obstruction and craniofacial surgery. Scand J Plast Reconstr Surg Hand Surg 30:275-279, 1996.

179. Jesberg N: Chronic, hypertrophic, lingual tonsillitis. Arch Otolarygol 64:3-13, 1956.

180. Johnson CM, Sims C: Awake fibreoptic intubation via a laryngeal mask in an infant with Goldenhar's syndrome. Anaesth Intensive Care 22:194-197, 1994.

181. Johnston C, Taussig LM, Koopmann C, et al: Obstructive sleep apnea in Treacher-Collins syndrome. Cleft Palate J 18:39-44, 1981.

182. Jones DH, Cohle SD: Unanticipated difficult airway secondary to lingual tonsillar hyperplasia. Anesth Analg 77:1285-1288, 1993.

183. Jones KL: Smith's Recognizable Patterns of Human Malformation. Philadelphia, WB Saunders, 1997, pp 258-259.

184. Jones SEF, Derricin GM: Difficult intubation in an infant with Pierre-Robin syndrome and concomitant tongue tie. Paediatr Anaesth 8:510-511, 1998.

185. Jungling AS, Shangraw RE: Massive airway edema after azathioprine. Anesthesiology 92:888-890, 2000.

186. Kain ZN, O'Conner TZ, Berde CB: Management of tracheobronchial and esophageal foreign bodies in children: A survey study. J Clin Anesth 6:28-32, 1994.

187. Kanai M, Horimoto Y, Yoshioka H, et al: Perioperative management for partial resection of a lymphangioma of the tongue. Masui 45:869-872, 1996.

188. Kandasamy R, Sivalingam P: Use of sevoflurane in difficult airways. Acta Anaesthesiol Scand 44:627-629, 2000.

189. Kaneda N, Goto R, Ishijima S, et al: Laryngeal granuloma caused by short term endotracheal intubation. Anesthesiology 90:1482-1483, 1999.

190. Katz RL, Berci G: The optical stylet—A new intubation technique for adults and children with specific reference to teaching. Anesthesiology 51: 251-254, 1979.

191. Kaymak C, Gulhan Y, Ozcan AO, et al: Anaesthetic approach in a case of Goldenhar's syndrome. Eur J Anaesthesiol 19: 836-838, 2002.

192. Kelley RI: A new face for an old syndrome. Am J Med Genet 68:251-256, 1997.

193. Kemper KJ, Benson MS, Bishop MJ: Predictors of postextubation stridor in pediatric trauma patients. Crit Care Med 19:352-355, 1991.

194. Khine HH, Corddry DH, Kettrick RG, et al: Comparison of cuffed and uncuffed endotracheal tubes in young children during general anesthesia. Anesthesiology 86:627-631, 1997.

195. Kim S, Nishizawa M, Kasama S, et al: [Management of difficult airway during induction of anesthesia in a patient with Hallermann-Streiff syndrome]. Masui 47:865-867, 1998.

196. Kim Y, Shibutani T, Hirota Y, et al: Anesthetic considerations of two sisters with Beckwith-Wiedemann syndrome. Anesth Prog 43:24-28, 1996.

197. Kita T, Kitamura S, Takeda K, et al: Anesthetic management involving difficult intubation in a child with Gaucher disease. Masui 47:69-73, 1998.

198. Kitamura S, Fukumitsu K, Kinouchi K, et al: A new modification of anaesthesia mask for fiberoptic intubation in children. Paediatr Anaesth 9:119-122, 1999.

199. Kleeman PP, Jantzen J-PAH, Bonfils P: The ultra-thin bronchoscope in management of the difficult paediatric airway. Can J Anaesth 34:606-608, 1987.

200. Koh THHG, Coleman R: Oropharyngeal burn in a newborn baby: New complication of light-bulb laryngoscopes. Anesthesiology 92:277-279, 2000.

201. Koka BV, Jeon IS, Andre JM, et al: Postintubation croup in children. Anesth Analg 56:501-505, 1977.

202. Kopp VJ, Bailey A, Valley RD, et al: Utility of the Mallampati classification for predicting difficult intubation in pediatric patients. Anesthesiology 83:A1147, 1995.

203. Kovac AL: Use of the Augustine stylet anticipating difficult tracheal intubation in Treacher-Collins syndrome. J Clin Anesth 4:409-412, 1992.

204. Kreulen M, Mackie DP, Kreis RW, Groenevelt F: Surgical release for intubation purposes in postburn contractures of the neck. Burns 22:310-312, 1996.

205. Krucylak CP, Schreiner MS: Orotracheal intubation of an infant with hemifacial microsomia using a modified lighted stylet. Anesthesiology 77:826-827, 1992.

206. Kulick RM, Selbst SM, Baker MD, Woodward GA: Thermal epiglottitis after swallowing hot beverages. Pediatrics 81:441-444, 1988.

207. Lakshmi Vas, Naregal F: Failed epidural anaesthesia in a patient with Hurler's disease. Paediatr Anaesth 10:95-98, 2000.

208. Ledbetter JL, Rasch DK, Pollard TG, et al: Reducing the risks of laryngoscopy in anaesthetized infants. Anaesthesia 43:151-153, 1988.

209. Levanon A, Tarasiuk A, Tal A: Sleep characteristics in children with Down's syndrome. J Pediatr 134:755-760, 1999.

210. Levin H, Bursztein S, Heifetz M: Cardiac arrest in a child with an anterior mediastinal mass. Anesth Analg 64:1129-1130, 1985.

211. Levy AM, Tabakian BS, Hanson JS, et al: Hypertrophied adenoids causing pulmonary hypertension and severe congestive heart failure. N Engl J Med 277:506, 1967.

212. Li HY, Lo LJ, Chen KS, et al: Robin sequence: Review of treatment modalities for airway obstruction in 110 cases. Int J Pediatr Otorhinolaryngol 65:45-51, 2002.

213. Lin AE, Ardinger HH, Ardinger RH Jr, et al: Cardiovascular malformations in Smith-Lemli-Opitz syndrome. Am J Med Genet 68:270-278, 1997.

214. Lin YC: Cervical spine disease and Down syndrome in pediatric anesthesia. Anesthesiol Clin North Am 16:911-923, 1998.

215. Lind MG, Lundell BP: Tonsillar hyperplasia in children. A cause of obstructive sleep apneas, CO_2 retention and retarded growth. Arch Otolaryngol 108:650-654, 1982.

216. Litman RS, Keon TF: Postintubation croup in children. Anesthesiology 75:1122-1123, 1991.

217. Litman RS, Ponnuri J, Trogan I: Anesthesia for tracheal or bronchial foreign body removal in children: An analysis of ninety-four cases. Anesth Analg 91:1389-1391, 2000.

218. Litman RS, Zerngast BA, Perkins FM: Preoperative evaluation of the cervical spine in children with trisomy-21: Results of a questionnaire study. Paediatr Anaesth 5:355-361, 1995.

219. Liu WC, Hwang CB, Cheng RK, et al: Unexpected left endobronchial intubation in a case of Turner's syndrome. Acta Anaesthesiol Sin 35:253-256, 1997.

220. Livesey JR, Solomons NB, Gillies EAD: Emergency adenotonsillectomy for acute postoperative upper airway obstruction. Anaesthesia 46:36, 1991.

221. Lo LJ, Chen YR: Airway obstruction in severe syndromic craniosynostosis. Ann Plast Surg 43:258-264, 1999.

222. Loh KS, Irish JC: Traumatic complications of intubation and other airway management procedures. Anesthesiol Clin North Am 20:953-969, 2002.

223. Loke D, Ghosh S, Panarese A, et al: Endoscopic division of the ary-epiglottic folds in severe laryngomalacia. Int J Pediatr Otorhinolaryngol 60:59-63, 2001.

224. Lopez-Gill M, Brimacombe J, Brain AIJ: Preliminary evaluation of a new prototype laryngeal mask in children. Br J Anaesth 82:132-134, 1999.

225. Lumb AB, Carli F: Respiratory arrest after a caudal injection of bupivacaine. Anaesthesia 44:324-325, 1989.

226. Luria JW, Gonzalez-del-Rey JA, DiGiulio GA, et al: Effectiveness of oral or nebulized dexamethasone for children with mild croup. Arch Pediatr Adolesc Med 155:1340-1345, 2001.

227. Malde AD, Jagtap SR, Pantvaidya SH: Hallermann-Streiff syndrome: Airway problems during anaesthesia. J Postgrad Med 40:216-218, 1994.

228. Malleson P, Riding K, Petty R: Stridor due to cricoarytenoid arthritis in pauciarticular onset juvenile rheumatoid arthritis. J Rheumatol 13:952-953, 1986.

229. Mallory GB, Fiser DH, Jackson R: Sleep associated breathing disorders in morbidly obese children and adolescents. J Pediatr 115:892-897, 1989.

230. Mamaya B: Airway management in spontaneously breathing anaesthetized children: Comparison of the laryngeal mask airway with the cuffed oropharyngeal airway. Paediatr Anaesth 12:411-415, 2002.

231. Marcus CL: Pathophysiology of childhood obstructive sleep apnea: Current concepts. Respir Physiol 119:143-154, 2000.

232. Marcus CL, Greene MG, Carroll JL: Blood pressure in children with obstructive sleep apnea. Am J Respir Crit Care Med 157:1098-1103, 1998.

233. Marcus CL, McColley SA, Carroll JL, et al: Upper airway collapsibility in children with obstructive sleep apnea syndrome. J Appl Physiol 77:918-924, 1994.

234. Marcus CL, Moreira GA, Bamford O, Lutz J: Response to inspiratory resistive loading during sleep in normal children and children with obstructive apnea. J Appl Physiol 87:1448-1454, 1999.

235. Marcus CL, Omlin KJ, Basinki DJ, et al: Normal polysomnographic values for children and adolescents. Am Rev Respir Dis 146:1235-1239, 1992.

236. Markakis DA, Sayson SC, Schreiner MS: Insertion of the laryngeal mask airway in awake infants with the Robin sequence. Anesth Analg 75:822-824, 1992.

237. Marquez X, Roxas R: Induction of anesthesia in infants with frontonasal dysplasia and meningoencephalocele: A case report. Anesth Analg 56:736, 1977.

238. Marsh JL, Galic M, Vannier MW: The craniofacial anatomy of Apert syndrome. Clin Plast Surg 18:237, 1991.

239. Martz DG, Schreibman DL, Matjasko MJ: Neurologic diseases. In Benumof JL (ed): Anesthesia and Uncommon Diseases, 4th ed. Philadelphia, WB Saunders, 1998.

240. Maydew RP, Berry FA: Cherubism with difficult laryngoscopy and tracheal intubation. Anesthesiology 62:810, 1985.

241. McColley SA, April MM, Carroll JL, et al: Respiratory compromise after adenotonsillectomy in children with obstructive sleep apnea. Arch Otolaryngol Head Neck Surg 118:940-943, 1992.

242. McEwan J, Giridharan W, Clarke RW, et al: Paediatric acute epiglottitis: Not a disappearing entity. Int J Pediatr Otorhinolaryngol 67:317-321, 2003.

243. McGill T: Otolaryngologic aspects of Apert syndrome. Clin Plast Surg 18:309, 1991.

244. McGowan FX, Kenna MA, Fleming JA, O'Connor T: Adenotonsillectomy for upper airway obstruction carries increased risk in children with a history of prematurity. Pediatr Pulmonol 13:222-226, 1992.

245. Mchaourab A, Sarantopoulos C, Stowe DF: Airway obstruction due to late-onset angioneurotic edema from angiotensin-converting enzyme inhibition. Can J Anaesth 46:975-978, 1999.

246. Meier S, Geiduschek, Paganoni R, et al: The effect of chin lift, jaw thrust, and continuous positive airway pressure on the size of the glottic opening and on stridor score in anesthetized, spontaneously breathing children. Anesth Analg 94:494-499, 2002.

247. Messner AH, Pelayo R: Pediatric sleep related breathing disorders. Am J Otolaryngol 21:98-107, 2000.

248. Miller JD, Rosenbaum H: Muscle diseases. In Benumof JL (ed): Anesthesia and Uncommon Diseases, 4th ed. Philadelphia, WB Saunders, 1998, pp 338-344.

249. Mixter RC, David DJ, Perloff WH, et al: Obstructive sleep apnea in Apert's and Pfeiffer's syndromes: More than a craniofacial abnormality. Plast Reconstr Surg 86:457-463, 1990.

250. Mohart D, Russo P, Tobias JD: Perioperative management of a child with glycogen storage disease type III undergoing cardiopulmonary bypass and repair of an atrial septal defect. Paediatr Anaesth 12:649-654, 2002.

251. Moore MH, Cantrell SB, Trott JA, David DJ: Pfeiffer syndrome: A clinical review. Cleft Palate Craniofac J 32:62-70, 1995.

252. Moore MH: Upper airway obstruction in the syndromal craniosynostoses. Br J Plast Surg 46:355-362, 1993.

253. Moore RA, McNicholas KW, Warran SP: Atlantoaxial subluxation with symptomatic spinal cord compression in a child with Down's syndrome. Anesth Analg 66:89-90, 1987.

254. Moores C, Rogers JG, McKenzie IM, Brown TC: Anaesthesia for children with mucopolysaccharidosis. Anaesth Intensive Care 24:459-463, 1996.

255. Mordjikian E: Severe microstomia due to burn by caustic soda. Burns 28:802-805, 2002.

256. Morell RC, Colonna DM, Mathes DD, et al: Fluoroscopy-assisted intubation of a child with an unstable subluxation of C1/C2. J Neurosurg Anesthesiol 9:25-28, 1997.

257. Morray JP, Geiduschek JM, Caplan RA, et al: A comparison of adult and pediatric anesthesia closed malpractice claims. Anesthesiology 78:461-467, 1993.

258. Morray JP, Geiduschel JM, Ramamoorthy C, et al: Anesthesia-related cardiac arrest in children. Anesthesiology 93:6-14, 2000.

259. Morris GP, Cooper MG: Difficult tracheal intubation following midface distraction surgery. Paediatr Anaesth 10:99-102, 2000.

260. Morrison JE, Collier E, Friesen RH, et al: Preoxygenation before laryngoscopy in children: How long is enough? Paediatr Anaesth 8:293-298, 1998.

261. Moschini V, Ambrosini MT, Sofi G: [Anesthesiologic considerations in Cornelia de Lange syndrome]. Minerva Anestesiol 66:799-806, 2000.

262. Moss C: Hereditary bullous disorders. Curr Paediatr 5:252-257, 1995.

263. Moulin D, Bertrand JM, Buts JP, et al: Upper airway lesions in children after accidental ingestion of caustic substances. J Pediatr 106:408-410, 1985.

264. Mulliken JB, Glowacki J: Hemangiomas and vascular malformations in infants and children: A classification based on endothelial characteristics. Plast Reconstr Surg 69:412-422, 1982.

265. Munro HM, Butler PJ, Washington EJ: Freeman-Sheldon (whistling face) syndrome. Anaesthetic and airway management. Paediatr Anaesth 7:345-348, 1997.

266. Mychaliska GB, Bealer JF, Graf JL, et al: Operating on placental support: The ex utero intrapartum treatment procedure. J Pediatr Surg 32:227-231, 1997.

267. Nagahama H, Suzuki Y, Tateda T, et al: [The use of a laryngeal mask in a newborn infant with Nager acrofacial dysostosis]. Masui 44:1555-1558, 1995.

268. Narang S, Harte BH, Body SC: Anesthesia for patients with a mediastinal mass. Anesthesiol Clin North Am 19:559-579, 2001.

269. Nargozian C, Ririe DG, Bennun RD, et al: Hemifacial microsomia: Anatomical predictors of difficult intubation. Paediatr Anaesth 9:393-398, 1999.

270. Neuman GG, Weingarten AE, Abramowitz RM, et al: The anesthetic management of the patient with an anterior mediastinal mass. Anesthesiology 60:144-147, 1984.

271. Nguyen NH, Morvant EM, Mayhew JF: Anesthetic management for patients with arthrogryposis multiplex congenita and severe micrognathia: Case reports. J Clin Anesth 12:227-230, 2000.

272. Noorily MR, Farmer DL, Belenky WM, Philippart AI: Congenital tracheal anomalies in the craniosynostosis syndromes. J Pediatr Surg 34:1036-1039, 1999.

273. Northrup DR, Bohman BK, Tsueda K: Total airway occlusion and superior vena cava syndrome in a child with an anterior mediastinal mass. Anesth Analg 65:1079-1082, 1986.

274. Nowaczyk MJ, McCaughey D, Whelan DT, Porter FD: Incidence of Smith-Lemli-Opitz syndrome in Ontario, Canada. Am J Med Genet 102:18-20, 2001.

275. O'Neil B, Templeton JJ, Caramico L, et al: The laryngeal mask airway in pediatric patients: Factors affecting ease of use during insertion and emergence. Anesth Analg 78:659-662, 1994.

276. O'Donnell D, Davis PJ, King NM: Management problems associated with Cornelia de Lange syndrome. Spec Care Dentist 5:160-163, 1985.

277. Okuda Y, Sato H, Kitajima T, et al: Airway obstruction during general anesthesia in a child with congenital tracheomalacia. Eur J Anaesth 17:642-644, 2000.

278. Oliva P, Fernandez-Liesa JI, Sanchez Tirado JA, et al: [Use of the laryngeal mask in a newborn infant with Smith-Lemli-Opitz syndrome and a difficult airway]. Rev Esp Anestesiol Reanim 49:339-340, 2002.

279. Onal E, Lopata M, O'Connor TD: Diaphragmatic and genioglossal electromyogram responses to CO_2 rebreathing in humans. J Appl Physiol 50:1052-1055, 1981.

280. Ono S, Takeda K, Nishiyama T, Hanaoka K: [Endotracheal intubation with a lighted stylet in a patient with difficult airway from the first and second brancheal arch syndrome]. Masui 50:1239-1241, 2001.

281. Opitz JM: RSH (so-called Smith-Lemli-Opitz) syndrome. Curr Opin Pediatr 11:353-362, 1999.

282. Ovassapian A, Glassenberg R, Randel GI, et al: The unexpected difficult airway and lingual tonsil hyperplasia: A case series and a review of the literature. Anesthesiology 97:124-132, 2002.

283. Patel A, Venn PJH, Barham J: Fiberoptic intubation through a laryngeal mask airway in an infant with Robin sequence. Eur J Anaesthesiol 15:237-239, 1998.

284. Patil VU, Sopchak AM, Thomas PS: Use of a dental mirror as an aid to tracheal intubation in an infant. Anesthesiology 78:619-620, 1993.

285. Pawar DK: Dislodgement of bronchial foreign body during retrieval in children. Paediatr Anaesth 10:333-335, 2000.

286. Pena M, Choi S, Boyajian M, Zalzal G: Perioperative airway complications following pharyngeal flap palatoplasty. Ann Otol Rhinol Laryngol 109:808-811, 2000.

287. Perkins JA, Sie KC, Milczuk H, Richardson MA: Airway management in children with craniofacial anomalies. Cleft Palate Craniofac J 34:135-140, 1997.

288. Peterson S, Byrne P, Molesky M, et al: Neonatal resuscitation using the laryngeal mask airway. Anesthesiology 80:1248-1253, 1994.

289. Pfitzner L, Cooper MG, Ho D: The Shikani Seeing Stylet for difficult intubation in children: Initial experience. Anaesth Intensive Care 30:462-466, 2002.

290. Pinkerton OD, Pinkerton FJ: Hereditary craniofacial dysplasia. Am J Ophthalmol 35:500-506, 1952.

291. Pivalizza EG, McGraw-Wall BL, Khalil SN: Alternative approach to airway management in Nager's syndrome. Can J Anaesth 44:228, 1997.

292. Podraza AG, Ansari-Winn D, Salem MR, et al: Tracheolaryngeal cephalad displacement facilitates tracheal intubation in pediatric patients. Anesth Analg 80:S377, 1995.

293. Polaner DM: The use of heliox and the laryngeal mask airway in a child with an anterior mediastinal mass. Anesth Analg 82:208-210, 1996.

294. Populaire C, Lundi JN, Pinaud M, et al: Elective tracheal intubation in the prone position for a neonate with Pierre-Robin syndrome. Anesthesiology 62:214, 1985.

295. Poradowska-Jeszke M, Falkiewicz H: [Retrograde intubation in an infant with Pierre Robin syndrome]. Cah Anesthesiol 37:605-607, 1989.

296. Potsic WP, Shah UK: Non surgical and surgical management of infants and children with obstructive sleep apnea syndrome. Otolaryngol Clin North Am 31:969-997, 1997.

297. Practice guidelines for management of the difficult airway: An updated report by the American Society of Anesthesiologists Task Force on Management of the Difficult Airway. Anesthesiology 98:1269-1277, 2003.

298. Price SD, Hawkins DB, Kahlstrom EJ: Tonsil and adenoid surgery for airway obstruction: Perioperative respiratory morbidity. Ear Nose Throat J 72:526-531, 1993.

299. Przybylo HJ, Stevenson GW, Vicari FA, et al: Retrograde fiberoptic intubation in a child with Nager's syndrome. Can J Anaesth 43:697-699, 1996.

300. Puchner W, Obwegeser J, Puhringer FK: Use of remifentanil for awake fiberoptic intubation in a morbidly obese patient with severe inflammation of the neck. Acta Anaesthesiol Scand 46:473-476, 2002.

301. Pueschel SM: Should children with Down syndrome be screened for atlantoaxial instability? Arch Pediatr Adolesc Med 152:123-125, 1998.

302. Quezado ZM, Veihmeyer J, Schwartz L, et al: Anesthesia and airway management of pediatric patients with Smith-Lemli-Opitz syndrome. Anesthesiology 97:1015-1019, 2002.

303. Quraishi MS, O'Halpin DR, Blayney AW: Ultrasonography in the evaluation of neck abscesses in children. Clin Otolaryngol 22:30-33, 1997.

304. Rabb MF, Larson SM, Greger JR: An unusual cause of partial ETT obstruction. Anesthesiology 88:548, 1998.

305. Rabb MF, Minkowitz HS, Hagberg CA: Blind intubation through the laryngeal mask airway for management of the difficult airway in infants. Anesthesiology 84:1510-1511, 1996.

306. Rasch DK, Browder F, Barr M, Greer D: Anaesthesia for Treacher Collins and Pierre Robin syndromes: A report of three cases. Can Anaesth Soc J 33:364-370, 1986.

307. Ravishankar M, Kundra P, Agrawal K, et al: Rigid nasendoscope with video camera system for intubation in infants with Pierre-Robin sequence. Br J Anaesth 88:728-731, 2002.

308. Ravussin P, Bayer-Berger M, Monnier P, et al: Percutaneous transtracheal ventilation for laser endoscopic procedures in infants and small children with laryngeal obstruction: Report of two cases. Can J Anaesth 34: 83-86, 1987.

309. Reber A, Paganoni R, Frei FJ: Effect of common airway manoeuvres on upper airway dimensions and clinical signs in anaesthetized, spontaneously breathing children. Br J Anaesth 86:217-222, 2001.

310. Reddy ARR: Unusual case of respiratory obstruction during induction of anaesthesia. Can Anaesth Soc J 19:192-197, 1972.

311. Redline S, Tishler PV, Schluchter M, et al: Risk factors for sleep-disordered breathing in children. Associations with obesity, race, and respiratory problems. Am J Respir Crit Care Med 159:1527-1532, 1999.

312. Remmers JE, deGroot WJ, Sauerland EK, Anch AM: Pathogenesis of upper airway occlusion during sleep. J Appl Physiol 44:931-938, 1978.

313. Richieri-Costa A, Pirolo Junior L, Cohen MM Jr: Carpenter syndrome with normal intelligence: Brazilian girl born to consanguineous parents. Am J Med Genet 47:281-283, 1993.

314. Rietz CS, Tobias JD: Anesthetic management of children with recurrent, viral laryngeal papillomatosis: A case report. J Am Assoc Nurs Anesth 64:362-368, 1996.

315. Rinaldi PA, Dogra S, Sellman GL: Difficult intubation in paediatric palatoplasty. Anaesthesia 48:358, 1993.

316. Roberts JL, Reed WR, Mathew OP, et al: Assessment of pharyngeal airway stability in normal and micrognathic infants. J Appl Physiol 58:290-299, 1985.

317. Robinow M: Respiratory obstruction and cor pulmonale in the Hallermann-Streiff syndrome. Am J Med Genet 41:515-516, 1991.

318. Roger G, Morisseau-Durand MP, Van Den Abbeele T, et al: The CHARGE association: The role of tracheotomy. Arch Otolaryngol Head Neck Surg 125:33-38, 1999.

319. Rosekrans JA: Viral croup: Current diagnosis and treatment. Mayo Clin Proc 73:1102-1107, 1998.

320. Rosen GM, Muckle RP, Mahowald MW, et al: Postoperative respiratory compromise in children with obstructive sleep apnea syndrome: Can it be anticipated? Pediatrics 93:784-788, 1994.

321. Rothschild MA, Catalano P, Biller HF: Ambulatory pediatric tonsillectomy and the identification of high-risk subgroups. Otolaryngol Head Neck Surg 110:203-210, 1994.

322. Rotta AT, Wiryawan B: Respiratory emergencies in children. Respir Care 48:248-260, 2003.

323. Rovin JD, Rodgers BM: Pediatric foreign body aspiration. Pediatr Rev 21:86-90, 2000.

324. Rowe BH: Corticosteroid treatment for acute croup. Ann Emerg Med 40:353-355, 2002.

325. Sahin A, Cekirge S, Aypar U: Anterograde endotracheal intubation with a laryngeal mask airway and guidewire in an infant with micrognathia. Turk J Pediatr 45: 78-79, 2003.

326. Santoli E, Di Biasi P, Vanelli P, Santoli C: Tracheal obstruction due to congenital tracheomalacia in a child. Case report. Scand J Thorac Cardiovasc Surg 25:227-220, 1991.

327. Sargent WW: Anesthetic management of a patient with Cornelia de Lange syndrome. Anesthesiology 74:1162-1163, 1991.

328. Schechter MS; Section on Pediatric Pulmonology, Subcommittee on Obstructive Sleep Apnea Syndrome: Technical report: Diagnosis and management of childhood obstructive sleep apnea syndrome. Pediatrics 109:e69, 2002.

329. Scheller JG, Schulman SR: Fiber-optic bronchoscopic guidance for intubating a neonate with Pierre-Robin syndrome. J Clin Anesth 3:45-47, 1991.

330. Scherhag A, Dick W: Special aspects of anesthesia in patients with epidermolysis bullosa based on a case example. Anaesthesiol Reanim 23:129-133, 1998.

331. Schulman SR, Jones BR, Slotnick N, Schwartz MZ: Fetal tracheal intubation with intact uteroplacental circulation. Anesth Analg 76:197-199, 1993.

332. Schwartz D, Singh J: Retrograde wire-guided direct laryngoscopy in a 1-month old infant. Anesthesiology 77:607-608, 1992.

333. Schwrz U, Weiss M: Endotracheal intubation of patients with Pierre-Robin sequence. Successful use of video intubation laryngoscope. Anaesthesist 50:118-121, 2001.

334. Seefelder C, Elango S, Rosbe KW, et al: Oesophageal perforation presenting as oesophageal atresia in a premature neonate following difficult intubation. Paediatr Anaesth 11:112-118, 2001.

335. Selim M, Mowafi H, Al-Ghamdi A, et al: Intubation via LMA in pediatric patients with difficult airways. Can J Anaesth 46:891-893, 1999.

336. Semenza GL, Pyeritz RE: Respiratory complications of mucopolysaccharide storage disorders. Medicine (Baltimore) 67:209-219, 1988.

337. Shah FA, Ramakrishna S, Ingle V, et al: Treacher Collins syndrome with acute airway obstruction. Int J Pediatr Otorhinolaryngol 54:41-43, 2000.

338. Shamberger RC: Preanesthetic evaluation of children with anterior mediastinal masses. Semin Pediatr Surg 8:61-68, 1999.

339. Sharma SC, Srinivasan S: Isolated plexiform neurofibroma of tongue and oropharynx: A rare manifestation of von Recklinghausen's disease. J Otolaryngol 27: 81-84, 1998.

340. Shechtman FG, Lin PT, Pincus RL: Urgent adenotonsillectomy for upper airway obstruction. Int J Pediatr Otorhinolaryngol 24:83, 1992.

341. Sheridan RL: Recognition and management of hot liquid aspiration in children. Ann Emerg Med 27: 89-91, 1996.

342. Shih GH, Boyd GL, Vincent RD Jr, et al: The EXIT procedure facilitates delivery of an infant with a pretracheal teratoma. Anesthesiology 89:1573-1575, 1998.

343. Shikani AH: New "seeing" stylet-scope and method for the management of the difficult airway. Otolaryngol Head Neck Surg 120:113-116, 1999.

344. Shintani T, Asakura K, Katuaura A: Adenotonsillar hypertrophy and skeletal morphology of children with obstructive sleep apnea syndrome. Acta Otolaryngol Suppl 523:222-224, 1996.

345. Shiomi T, Guilleminault C, Stoohs R, Schnittger I: Obstructed breathing in children during sleep monitored by echocardiography. Acta Paediatr 82:863-871, 1993.

346. Shprintzen RJ: Pierre Robin, micrognathia, and airway obstruction: The dependency of treatment on accurate diagnosis. Int Anesthesiol Clin 26:64-71, 1988.

347. Shulman B, Connelly NR: The adult Bullard laryngoscope as an alternative to the Wis-Hipple 1½ in paediatric patients. Paediatr Anaesth 10: 41-45, 2000.

348. Shulman GB, Connelly NR, Gibson C: The adult Bullard laryngoscope in paediatric patients. Can J Anaesth 44:969-972, 1997.

349. Sichel JY, Dungoor E, Eliashar R, et al: Management of congenital laryngeal malformations. Am J Otolaryngol 21:22-30, 2000.

350. Smith GB, Shibman AJ: Anaesthesia and severe skin disease. Anaesthesia 39:443-455, 1984.

351. Spector S, Bautista AG: Respiratory obstruction caused by acute tonsillitis and acute adenoiditis. NY State J Med 56:2118, 1956.

352. Stack CG, Wyse RKH: Incidence and management of airway problems in the CHARGE association. Anaesthesia 46:582, 1990.

353. Steward DJ, Lerman J: Techniques and procedures of pediatric anesthesia. In Steward DJ, Lerman J (eds): Manual of Pediatric Anesthesia, 5th ed. New York, Churchill Livingstone, 2001.

354. Steward DJ: Percutaneous transtracheal ventilation for laser endoscopic procedures in infants and small children. Can J Anaesth 34:429-430, 1987.

355. St-Hilaire H, Buchbinder D: Maxillofacial pathology and management of Pierre Robin sequence. Otolaryngol Clin North Am 33:1241-1256, 2000.

356. Stiles CM: A flexible fiberoptic bronchoscope for endotracheal intubation of infants. Anesth Analg 53:1017-1019, 1974.

357. Stocks RM, Egerman R, Thompson JW, Peery M: Airway management of the severely retrognathic child: Use of the laryngeal mask airway. Ear Nose Throat J 81:223-226, 2002.

358. Stone P, Trevenen CL, Mitchell I, Rudd N: Congenital tracheal stenosis in Pfeiffer syndrome. Clin Genet 38:145-148, 1990.

359. Strange GR: Respiratory distress. In Strange GR (ed): APLS the Pediatric Emergency Medicine Course, 3rd ed. 2000.

360. Stroud RH, Friedman NR: An update on inflammatory disorders of the pediatric airway: Epiglottitis, croup, and tracheitis. Am J Otolaryngol 22:268-275, 2001.

361. Suan C, Ojeda R, Garcia Perla JR, et al: Anaesthesia and the Beckwith-Wiedemann syndrome. Paediatr Anaesth 6:231-233, 1996.

362. Suen JS, Arnold JE, Brooks LJ: Adenotonsillectomy for treatment of obstructive sleep apnea in children. Arch Otolaryngol Head Neck Surg 121:525-530, 1995.

363. Suriani RJ, Kayne RD: Fiberoptic bronchoscopic guidance for intubating a child with Pierre-Robin syndrome. J Clin Anesth 4:258-259, 1992.

364. Sutera PT, Gordon GJ: Digitally assisted tracheal intubation in a neonate with Pierre-Robin syndrome. Anesthesiology 78:983-985, 1993.

365. Tan WK, Liu EH, Thean HP: A clinical report about an unusual occurrence of post-anesthetic tongue swelling. J Prosthodont 10:105-107, 2001.

366. Thomas ML, McEwan A: The anaesthetic management of a case of Kawasaki's disease (mucocutaneous lymph node syndrome) and Beckwith-Weidemann syndrome presenting with a bleeding tongue. Paediatr Anaesth 8:500-502, 1998.

367. Thomas PB, Parry MC: The difficult paediatric airway: A new method of intubation using the laryngeal mask airway, Cook airway exchange catheter and tracheal intubation fiberscope. Paediatr Anaesth 11:618-621, 2001.

368. Thompson JW, Ahmed AR, Dudley JP: Epidermolysis bullosa dystrophica of the larynx and trachea. Ann Otol Rhinol Laryngol 89:428, 1980.

369. Tinker TD, Crane DL: Safety of anesthesia for patients with anterior mediastinal masses: I. Anesthesiology 73:1060, 1990.

370. Tint GS, Irons M, Elias ER, et al: Defective cholesterol biosynthesis associated with the Smith-Lemli-Opitz syndrome. N Engl J Med 330:107-113, 1994.

371. Tobias JD: Anesthesia for thoracic surgery in children. Chest Surg Clin North Am 3:357-374, 1993.

372. Tobias JD, Lowe S, Holcomb GW 3rd: Anesthetic considerations of an infant with Beckwith-Wiedemann syndrome. J Clin Anesth 4:484-486, 1992.

373. Tokumine J, Sugahara K, Ura M, et al: Lingual tonsil hypertrophy with difficult airway and uncontrollable bleeding. Anaesthesia 58:390-391, 2003.

374. Tsujimura Y: Downfolding of the epiglottis induced by the laryngeal mask airway in children: A comparison between two insertion techniques. Paediatr Anaesth 11:651-655, 2001.

375. Tzanova I, Schwarz M, Jantzen JP: Securing the airway in children with the Morquio-Brailsford syndrome. Anaesthesist 42:477-481, 1993:

376. Uezono S, Holzman RS, Goto T, et al: Prediction of difficult airway in school-aged patients with microtia. Paediatr Anaesth 11:409-413, 2001.

377. van Son JAM, Julsrud PR, Hagler DJ, et al: Surgical treatment of vascular rings: The Mayo Clinic experience. Mayo Clin Proc 68:1056-1063, 1993.

378. Vas L, Naregal P: Anaesthetic management of a patient with Freeman Sheldon syndrome. Paediatr Anaesth 8:175-177, 1998.

379. Vener DF, Lerman J: The pediatric airway and associated syndromes. Anesth Clin North Am 13:585-614, 1995.

380. Verghese ST, Hannallah RS: Pediatric otolaryngologic emergencies. Anesthesiol Clin North Am 19:237-255, 2001.

381. Vetter TR: Acute airway obstruction due to arytenoiditis in a child with juvenile rheumatoid arthritis. Anesth Analg 79:1198-1200, 1994.

382. Veycekemans F: Equipment, monitoring and environmental conditions. In Bissonnette B, Dalens B (eds): Pediatric Anesthesia: Principles and Practice. New York, McGraw-Hill, 2002.

383. Vulliamy DG, Normandale PA: Cranio-facial dysostosis in a Dorset family. Arch Dis Child 41:375-382, 1966.

384. Walker JS, Dorian RS, Marsh NJ: Anesthetic management of a child with Nager's syndrome. Anesth Analg 79:1025-1026, 1994.

385. Walker RW, Darowski M, Morris P, Wraith JE: Anaesthesia and mucopolysaccharidoses. A review of airway problems in children. Anaesthesia 49:1078-1084, 1994.

386. Walker RWM, Allen DI, Rothera MR: A fiberoptic intubation technique for children with mucopolysaccharidoses using the laryngeal mask airway. Paediatr Anaesth 7:421-426, 1997.

387. Walker RWM: The laryngeal mask airway in the difficult paediatric airway: An assessment of positioning and use in fiberoptic intubation. Paediatr Anaesth 10:53-58, 2000.

388. Walner D, Ouanounou S, Donnelly LF, et al: Utility of radiographs in the evaluation of pediatric upper airway obstruction. Ann Otol Rhinol Laryngol 108:378-383, 1999.

389. Wang CY, Chiu CL, Dellkan AE: Sevoflurane for difficult intubation in children. Br J Anaesth 80:408, 1998.

390. Waters KA, Everett FM, Bruderer JW, Sullivan CE: Obstructive sleep apnea: The use of nasal CPAP in 80 children. Am J Respir Crit Care Med 152:780-785, 1995.

391. Waters KA, McBrien F, Stewart P, et al: Effects of OSA, inhalational anesthesia, and fentanyl on the airway and

ventilation of children. J Appl Physiol 92:1987-1994, 2002.

392. Weber S: Traumatic complications of airway management. Anesthesiol Clin North Am 20:503-512, 2002.

393. Weider DJ, Sateia MJ, West RP: Nocturnal enuresis in children with upper airway obstruction. Otolaryngol Head Neck Surg 105:427-432, 1991.

394. Weiss LS, White JAJ: Macroglossia: A review. La State Med Soc 142:13-16, 1990.

395. Weiss M, Hartmann K, Fisher J, et al: Video-intuboscopic assistance is a useful aid to tracheal intubation in pediatric patients. Can J Anaesth 48:691-696, 2001.

396. Weiss M, Hartmann K, Fisher JE, et al: Use of angulated video-intubation laryngoscope in children undergoing manual in-line neck stabilization. Br J Anaesth 87:453-458, 2001.

397. Weller RM: Anaesthesia for cystic hygroma in a neonate. Anaesthesia 29:588-594, 1974.

398. Wheatley RS, Stainthorp SF: Intubation of a one-day-old baby with the Pierre-Robin syndrome via a laryngeal mask. Anaesthesia 49:733, 1994.

399. Wheeler M: The difficult pediatric airway. In Hagberg CA (ed): Handbook of Difficult Airway Management, 1st ed. Philadelphia, Churchill Livingstone, 2000.

400. Wiatrak BJ: Congenital anomalies of the larynx and trachea. Otolarygol Clin North Am 33:91-108, 2000.

401. Wiatrak BJ, Woolley AL: Pharyngitis and adenotonsillar disease. In Cummings CW, Frederickson JM, Harker LA, et al (eds): Otolaryngology Head and Neck Surgery, 3rd ed. St Louis, Mosby–Year Book, 1998, pp 188-215.

402. Wilson K, Lakheeram I, Morielli A, et al: Can assessment for obstructive sleep apnea help predict postadenotonsillectomy respiratory complications? Anesthesiology 96:313-322, 2002.

403. Wilton NCT: Aids for fiberoptically guided intubation in children. Anesthesiology 75:549-550, 1991.

404. Wiseman NE, Duncan PG, Cameron CB: Management of tracheomalacia with continuous positive airway pressure. J Pediatr Surg 20:489-493, 1985.

405. Witters I, Devriendt K, Moerman P, et al: Diaphragmatic hernia as the first echographic sign in Apert syndrome. Prenat Diagn 20:404-406, 2000.

406. Wong MEK, Bradrick JP: Surgical approaches to airway management for anesthesia practitioners. In Hagberg CA (ed): Handbook of Difficult Airway Management, 1st ed. Philadelphia, Churchill Livingstone, 2000.

407. Wright JT: Comprehensive dental care and general anesthetic management of hereditary epidermolysis bullosa. A review of fourteen cases. Oral Surg Oral Med Oral Pathol 70:573-578, 1990.

408. Wright JT, Fine JD: Hereditary epidermolysis bullosa. Semin Dermatol 13:102-107, 1994.

409. Yamamoto H, Fujimura N, Namiki A: Swelling of the tongue after intraoperative monitoring by transesophageal echocardiography. Masui 50:1250-1252, 2001.

410. Yamamoto K, Tsubokawa T, Ohmura S, et al: Left-molar approach improves the laryngeal view in patients with difficult laryngoscopy. Anesthesiology 92:70-74, 2000.

411. Yokoyama T, Tomoda M, Nishiyama T, et al: [General anesthesia for a patient with Cornelia de Lange syndrome]. Masui 49:785-787, 2000.

412. Zerella JT, Finberg FJ: Obstruction of the neonatal airway from teratomas. Surg Gynecol Obstet 170: 126-131, 1990.

413. Zornow MH, Benumof JL: Safety of anesthesia for patients with anterior mediastinal masses: II. Anesthesiology 73:1061, 1990.

414. Zucconi M, Strambi LF, Pestalozza G, et al: Habitual snoring and obstructive sleep apnea syndrome in children: Effects of early tonsil surgery. Int J Pediatr Otorhinolaryngol 26:235-243, 1993.

34

THE DIFFICULT AIRWAY IN OBSTETRIC ANESTHESIA

Edward T. Crosby

Airway management and difficulties related to it continue to represent the single largest risk factor for anesthetic-related maternal mortality. General anesthesia for cesarean section, in particular emergency cesarean section, represents the highest risk anesthetic intervention in obstetric anesthesia and accounts for the bulk of the poor maternal outcomes reported. A difficult or failed intubation increases the risk of both pulmonary aspiration and cardiorespiratory arrest with subsequent maternal morbidity or mortality. Physician recognition of the factors associated with or predisposing to maternal airway disasters and appropriate preparation for dealing with difficulties are essential to reduce anesthesia-attributable maternal injury. The following discussion offers insights into the occurrence of anesthesia-related maternal mortality as well as assessment and management guidelines related to airway care in obstetric anesthesia.

I. THE OBSTETRIC AIRWAY IN PERSPECTIVE

A. MATERNAL MORBIDITY AND MORTALITY

The Confidential Enquiries into Maternal Deaths (in England and Wales and the United Kingdom) represent the most accurate and in-depth analyses of maternal mortality. They have charted the causes and incidence of maternal mortality since 1952. Maternal mortality in the United Kingdom decreased between 1970 and 1993 but increased from 1994 to 1996.[146-149,196] This was not necessarily related to a detrimental change in care but was probably due to increased case ascertainment.[196] Maternal mortality attributable to anesthetic care decreased from 12.8 deaths to 0.5 deaths per million estimated pregnancies from 1970 to 1996 (Fig. 34-1).

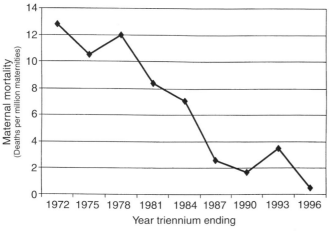

Figure 34-1 Anesthesia-attributable maternal mortality, 1970 to 1996, England and Wales. (Data from [1] Report on Confidential Enquiries into Maternal Deaths in the United Kingdom 1985-87. London, Her Majesty's Stationery Office, 1991 and [2] Why Mothers Die. Report on Confidential Enquiries into Maternal Deaths in the United Kingdom 1994-96. London, Stationery Office, 1999.)

The majority of anesthetic-attributable deaths in recent reports have been associated with induction of general anesthesia and result from two main causes, inhalation of gastric contents and failure to intubate the trachea with resultant cardiac arrest.[146-149] Deaths from aspiration pneumonitis became less common in latter reports, but when they occurred, they often followed difficult or failed intubation. Hypoxemic cardiac arrest following failed endotracheal intubation was a more common cause of anesthetic maternal mortality than aspiration. Two factors appear to predominate in these deaths, failure to acknowledge that the patient cannot be intubated and must be oxygenated and a reluctance to accept that the tracheal tube is in the esophagus. Surprisingly, even the advent of capnography has not eliminated the occurrence of esophageal intubation. The operative procedure most commonly involved with episodes of mortality across the last decade was emergency cesarean section, accounting for up to three quarters of all deaths. The majority of anesthesia-attributable maternal mortalities are deemed to be avoidable, and anesthesia care provided in these cases has been consistently, although not uniformly, rated as substandard. Finally, it has also been a consistent conclusion in these reports that many of the problems associated with avoidable maternal mortality involved a failure of communication between the obstetrician and the anesthesiologist.

An accurate assessment of maternal mortality is more difficult to derive from North American sources as there are no data comparable in scope or detail to the Confidential Enquiries. Reports have tended to reflect experience on a state or regional basis, although more recent initiatives have broadened the reporting base. The Maternal Mortality Collaborative, a special interest group of the American College of Obstetricians and Gynecologists, established voluntary surveillance of maternal mortality in 1985.[150] The first detailed report was published in 1988. Maternal mortality was estimated by the collaborative at 14.1 deaths per 100,000 live births, and anesthesia complications were recorded as the sixth leading cause of maternal mortality. Unfortunately, the specific details of the anesthetic-attributable mortality are not available from the published reports of the Collaborative. The Centers for Disease Control and Prevention (CDC) also reviewed pregnancy-related mortality in the United States for the years 1987 to 1990.[100] The CDC again identified anesthesia complications as the sixth leading cause of maternal mortality, accounting for 2.5% of maternal deaths. The ranking of anesthesia as the sixth leading cause of maternal mortality was also consistent with that reported a decade earlier by Kaunitz and colleagues, reviewing countrywide (U.S.) data.[97] Kaunitz and colleagues noted that anesthesia care contributed to 4% of maternal mortalities and the rates were highest in both the smallest (<300 deliveries per year) and largest (>3001 deliveries per year) centers. These findings were attributed to the presumed decreased capabilities (both physician and institutional) in the smaller centers and a higher incidence of referred cases and high-risk parturients seen in the larger centers. The CDC reported a contrary finding, noting that the women who delivered in smaller hospitals had better outcomes overall but had worse outcomes after pulmonary embolism than women in larger hospitals.[100] It was suggested that the smaller hospitals were increasingly selecting low-risk populations but perhaps lacked the resources to salvage patients in the event of serious complications.

Reviews of state-maintained databases have reported that anesthesia was responsible for or contributed to 4.2% of all maternal deaths in the state of Massachusetts from 1954 to 1985 and 5.2% of maternal deaths in Maryland from 1984 to 1997.[136,160] The primary causes of anesthesia-attributable deaths were aspiration and cardiorespiratory arrest. Aspiration deaths during mask anesthesia occurred exclusively in the early part of the experience and were largely supplanted by deaths related to failed intubation or aspiration associated with difficult endotracheal intubation.

After analysis of data reported to the CDC, Hawkins and coauthors determined that anesthesia-related complications remained the sixth leading cause of pregnancy-related death in the United States from 1979 to 1990.[79] Consistent with other reports, most maternal deaths related to complications of anesthesia occurred during general anesthesia for cesarean sections. The anesthesia-related maternal mortality rate decreased from 4.3 per million live births in the first triennium (1979 to 1981) to 1.7 per million in the last (1988 to 1990). The number of deaths involving general anesthesia remained stable, but the number of regional anesthesia-related deaths decreased since 1984. The case-fatality risk ratio for general anesthesia was 2.3 times that for regional anesthesia before 1985, increasing to 16.7 times that after 1985.

Finally, malpractice claims filed against anesthesiologists for care involving obstetric anesthesia taken from the American Society of Anesthesiologists Closed Claim Database provide an alternative, albeit biased, assessment of maternal anesthetic risk in the United States.[28] Among the claims, difficult endotracheal intubation, inadequate ventilation, aspiration, and esophageal intubation were the most common events cited. Half of the cases of pulmonary aspiration were associated with difficult endotracheal intubation, esophageal intubation, or inadequate ventilation. In over half the cases in which the anesthesiologist was considered to be responsible for the outcome and liable for damages, the delivered care was deemed by the assessors to be substandard.

Maternal deaths related to anesthesia have been significantly reduced over the past decades. There is evidence that further reductions are possible, as avoidable deaths predominantly involving management of the airway account for most maternal deaths attributed to anesthetic care in North America and the United Kingdom.[28,146]

In addition, care rated as substandard continues to be a consistent finding in enquiries into maternal deaths in the reports reviewed and others.[15,28,127,146-149,196]

B. DIFFICULT INTUBATION IN OBSTETRIC ANESTHESIA

The incidences of the difficult airway, difficult laryngoscopy, and difficult intubation in obstetric anesthesia have not been well defined. In the largest review published to date, Rocke and coworkers reported that some difficulty was experienced during intubation in 7.9% (119 of 1500) of parturients undergoing general anesthesia for cesarean section.[151] Two percent of the patients (30 of 1500) were deemed to be very difficult to intubate. In a nonobstetric surgical population, Rose and Cohen noted that 2.5% of patients required two laryngoscopies to achieve endotracheal intubation and that 1.8% required more than three.[155] These data suggest that some degree of difficulty with intubation is experienced more frequently during obstetric anesthesia than general surgical anesthesia (7.9% versus 2.5%) but that very difficult intubations are seen with a similar frequency in the two populations (2% versus 1.8%). The incidence of difficult mask ventilation is again not well defined but appears to be much less than that of difficult intubation.

There are a number of factors that may conspire to yield the perceived higher incidence of intubation difficulties and failure in the obstetric population. The adoption of a failed intubation drill probably occurs earlier in obstetric anesthesia than in the general surgical population. Pregnant patients are more likely to have full and intact dentition, reducing the interdental distance in which the laryngoscopist maneuvers. Obesity is common in parturients, and morbid obesity is not rare. Obesity results in relative neck extension when the patient is supine, leading to more anterior placement of the larynx.[30,47] The neck is somewhat foreshortened and redundant pharyngeal and palatal folds are evident in the airways of obese patients. The breasts of the parturient are enlarged and engorged and may interfere with placement of the laryngoscope in the mouth.[98] Further, the hand of the assistant providing cricoid pressure is by necessity situated higher in the field (placed above the breasts) and may also interfere with laryngoscopy. Proper application of cricoid pressure, as described by Sellick, requires some degree of neck extension, resulting in anterior displacement of the larynx.[167] The supine wedged position may result in a change in orientation of the trachea relative to the underlying cervical spine, and cricoid pressure may be more likely to result in tracheal displacement and intubation difficulties.

Pregnancy is an edematous state and the tongue and supraglottic soft tissues may be engorged.[30] Although not usually a problem, severe airway edema has been associated with excessive weight gain in pregnancy, preeclampsia, iatrogenic fluid overload, excess airway manipulations, and maternal expulsive efforts.* Severe airway edema may develop over a short period of time, especially when associated with maternal efforts.[56] As tissues of the supraglottic airway expand because of edema, the airway lumen is compromised and mask ventilation, laryngoscopy, and endotracheal intubation are more difficult. Edema of the face and neck may alert the physician to the potential for significant but asymptomatic airway edema, but these features are not consistently present.[16] Because of mucosal congestion and the increased friability of the airway tissues, repeated attempts at intubation may result in airway bleeding and edema and a rapidly worsening situation.

Physician anxiety has also been cited as a factor in failed obstetric intubations. In commentary on the Confidential Enquiries, it has been suggested that, in the haste to achieve rapid intubation, laryngoscopy is attempted too early, by inexperienced physicians assisted by untrained aides.[121] This opinion is supported by the finding that less experienced physicians are more likely to attempt laryngoscopy well before adequate muscle relaxation has been achieved in obstetric patients than in general surgical patients.[26] During these premature intubation attempts, the mouth is more difficult to open, interdental distance is reduced, laryngoscopy is compromised, and there is increased potential for patients' retching, gastric regurgitation, and aspiration. As the frequency of general anesthesia for cesarean section continues to decrease, this may become an increasingly relevant issue.

1. Assessment of the Airway—Prediction of Difficult Intubation

Multiple strategies have been proposed to assess the airway. These range from using simple anatomic descriptors, ranking and summating anatomic factor scores, using logistic regression to create predictive scales, and the derivation of performance indices. The different strategies share some common characteristics; they have high sensitivity but low specificity. The low specificity of the tests, when combined with the low incidence of difficult airway, leads to the poor positive predictive value. In addition, many of the tests have only moderate interobserver reliability.[95] This may further explain why the assessment strategies often fail to predict difficult endotracheal intubation. Despite careful preoperative evaluation, difficulties are not predicted in many instances and strategies to manage the unanticipated difficult airway should be preformulated and practiced.

Parturients whose tracheas were difficult to intubate were often reported not to present with the features of a difficult airway; intubation difficulties were thus unanticipated.[55] The question of whether an adequate assessment was made in these patients is a pertinent one as follow-up evaluation of parturients who presented as unanticipated difficult intubations demonstrated features of the patient suggesting that difficulties should have been anticipated on the basis of the patient's examination.[55,163]

Involving the obstetric team to identify parturients at high risk for difficult intubation was a novel strategy evaluated by Gaiser and associates.[65] The airways of 160 parturients were assessed by four physicians, one attending and one resident obstetrician and one attending and one resident anesthesiologist. Obstetricians tended to underpredict difficult airway compared with the attending anesthesiologist. Although the attending obstetricians were not more likely to ask for antepartum consultation for identified high-risk patients, they were more likely to request early epidural analgesia. Obstetricians clearly may play a role in identifying at-risk patients and relaying this information to their colleagues in anesthesia.

C. ACID ASPIRATION SYNDROME IN OBSTETRIC ANESTHESIA

1. The Effects of Pregnancy on Gastroesophageal Physiology

The physiologic changes of pregnancy include a number of hormonal alterations that influence gastroesophageal physiology. Maternal gastrin levels are elevated in pregnancy.[8] Gastrin induces copious secretions of water, electrolytes, and enzymes from the stomach, pancreas, and small intestine. Decreased plasma motilin levels have also been reported in pregnant patients.[34] Motilin is a hormonal peptide that has gastrointestinal smooth muscle stimulating effects. It accelerates gastric emptying, stimulates the lower esophageal sphincter (LES), and reduces intestinal transit time. Finally, the increased serum progesterone levels seen in pregnancy are associated with a reduction of the LES pressure and an increase in gastrointestinal transit time.[24,58,193]

Published works have demonstrated no consistent delays in gastric emptying across populations of term parturients.[87,135,164] However, Sandhar and coworkers recorded a doubling of gastric emptying time at term in two of the patients studied when compared with control values measured 6 weeks postpartum.[164] Hirschheimer and coauthors also reported that gastric emptying slowed in some mothers during early labor.[87] Established labor may cause unpredictable delays in gastric emptying that are further potentiated by the use of narcotic analgesics. Once labor is initiated, solid foodstuffs may remain in the stomach for prolonged periods.[27] There is ultrasound documentation of solid food in the stomachs of 66% of laboring parturients, irrespective of the time of last oral intake.[194] Gastric emptying has returned to normal by 24 hours postpartum.[194] However, the pattern of emptying during the first postpartum day has not been elucidated and the same precautions against aspiration should be

---

*References 16, 21, 48, 51, 56, 94, 110, 143, 153, 162, 166, 175, 196.

taken with newly delivered mothers as with laboring patients. Mothers undergoing tubal ligation within 9 hours of delivery had gastric aspirates of pH less than 2.5, and 60% had gastric volumes greater than 25 mL.[93] The high incidence of reflux as measured by lower esophageal pH studies returns to normal by the second postpartum day.[186]

Symptoms suggestive of gastroesophageal reflux occur in almost 80% of pregnant women at term.[85] The symptom of heartburn correlates with reflux, and moderate to severe reflux occurs in 80% of parturients with heartburn and in 30% of those without symptoms.[9] Pregnant women suffering from heartburn have the longest delay in gastric emptying.[34] The LES pressure is also lower in parturients with heartburn than in those without the symptom.[187] The presence of heartburn indicates an increased risk of regurgitation, particularly when the supine position is assumed.[31] Gastroesophageal reflux occurs when the LES pressure is inadequate to prevent retrograde flow of gastric contents across the sphincter into the esophagus. During pregnancy, the growth of the uterus from the pelvis into the abdomen may increase average intragastric pressures from 7 to 17 cm H_2O.[108] The supine position and especially the lithotomy and Trendelenburg positions may further increase intragastric pressures. The presence of multiple gestations, polyhydramnios, or gross obesity may be associated with intragastric pressures in excess of 40 cm H_2O.[108] However, the LES tone increases to average values of 44 cm H_2O during pregnancy, providing some protection from the increased intragastric pressure. Medications commonly used in anesthesia that reduce the LES tone and barrier pressures include narcotics, benzodiazepines, and anticholinergic agents.[22,23,70,84] Intravenous anticholinergic administration may cause sufficiently large decrements in LES pressure to allow free reflux into the esophagus.[50]

2. Airway Pressure and Gastric Distention

The average intragastric pressure in spontaneously breathing, nonpregnant subjects is 11 cm H_2O (range 9 to 16 cm H_2O).[154] In paralyzed, anesthetized patients, the average intragastric pressure required to cause reflux is 23 to 35 cm H_2O, consistent with pressures known to exist in normal pregnant patients.[36,39,108,174] There is a relationship between the airway pressures required to ventilate the lungs and those that force air into the stomach. In subjects ventilated by bag and mask without cricoid pressure, airway pressures below 15 cm H_2O rarely cause stomach inflation, pressures between 15 and 25 cm H_2O result in gastric insufflation in some patients, and pressures greater than 25 cm H_2O do so in most patients.[105,158] Application of cricoid pressure during mask-bag ventilation increases the maximum pressure reached during mask ventilation without air entering the stomach, to about 45 cm H_2O.[105] Gastric distention, as may occur with forceful mask ventilation, may increase

intragastric pressures by 10 mm Hg.[171] A requirement for high-pressure mask and bag ventilation in the difficult to ventilate pregnant patient results in increased intragastric pressure and an augmented risk of regurgitation.

3. Aspiration Pneumonitis in Obstetrics

In 1946, Mendelson published his classical treatise on acid aspiration pneumonitis in parturients and calculated an incidence of 0.15%; the syndrome occurred in 66 of the 44,016 parturients reviewed.[118] All aspirations occurred in patients receiving face mask anesthesia for labor and delivery. More than half of the patients who aspirated required longer administration and greater depth of anesthesia for the operative intervention than was the norm for his institution. Sixty-eight percent of the aspirations were recognized at the time that they occurred; the remainder were not known to have occurred (silent aspiration) until the patients subsequently became symptomatic. Patients who had liquid aspiration developed a syndrome characterized by bronchospasm, hypoxemia, and atelectasis. They were acutely ill, but their condition gradually stabilized over 24 to 36 hours, and then they recovered. Two patients who died aspirated solid material, obstructing their airways. Three others who aspirated solid material either had partial obstruction or their obstruction was relieved and they survived. The incidence of fatal pulmonary aspiration syndrome reported by Mendelson was 0.005% (1 in 22,008 parturients). Mendelson concluded his report by encouraging the oral administration of warm alkaline solutions during labor to balance gastric acidity, discouraging the involvement of new and inexperienced anesthesia personnel as the primary care providers in obstetric anesthesia, and advocating the wider use of local anesthesia in obstetric anesthesia practice.

Krantz and Edwards retrospectively reviewed their experience with general anesthesia for vaginal delivery and cesarean section from 1962 to 1972.[101] Of 37,282 patients who delivered vaginally during this time, approximately 85% (31,600) received nurse-administered general anesthesia without endotracheal intubation. Oral intake during labor was not restricted, nor was anesthesia withheld if patients had recently ingested food or fluid by mouth. Five patients (0.017%, 1 in 6000) developed aspiration pneumonitis; all cases were mild and responded to limited medical therapy. More than 90% of cesarean sections were performed with the patients having anesthesiologist-delivered general anesthesia. Aspiration during cesarean section occurred seven times (0.2%, 1 in 430) and one patient died. Although not advocating the use of general anesthesia without airway protection, Krantz and Edwards did note that the incidence of clinically significant pulmonary aspiration was low. Four decades after Mendelson, Olsson and colleagues, after reviewing 2643 operations, reported that the incidence of aspiration associated with cesarean section was also 0.15%, no different from that noted by either Mendelson or Krantz.[101,132]

Ezri and associates estimated the incidence of pulmonary aspiration during general anesthesia for obstetric procedures (excluding cesarean section) performed in the peripartum period.[54] In their study, 1870 parturients received general anesthesia without endotracheal intubation and a single case (0.05%) of mild aspiration was detected. All the patients underwent emergency procedures during labor or within 30 minutes of delivery. Most patients had received meperidine (Demerol) for analgesia during labor. Anesthesia was induced with either ketamine and a benzodiazepine or methohexital and fentanyl and maintained with additional boluses of the induction agents. Ezri and associates noted that this incidence was similar to that reported following mask anesthesia in nonobstetric populations.

4. Cricoid Pressure

Sellick proposed the application of cricoid pressure as a simple maneuver, employed during induction of anesthesia, to control regurgitation of gastric or esophageal contents and also to prevent inflation of the stomach, a potent cause of regurgitation.[167] To perform the maneuver, the neck was extended, increasing the anterior convexity of the cervical spine and stretching the esophagus. This prevented lateral displacement of the esophagus when cricoid pressure was applied. Before induction of anesthesia, the cricoid was palpated and lightly held between the thumb and second finger. As induction commenced, pressure was exerted on the cricoid cartilage, mainly by the index finger. As the patient lost consciousness, Sellick recommended firm pressure, sufficient to seal the esophagus without obstructing the airway. Sellick suggested that during the application of cricoid pressure, the lungs may be ventilated without the risk of gastric distention.

Cricoid pressure was initially thought to be contraindicated by Sellick in the setting of active vomiting, in the belief that the esophagus may be damaged by vomit under high pressure. He later modified this stand, stating that he felt the risk of rupture to be almost nonexistent.[168] This particular item has continued to represent a focus of controversy in anesthesia. There are reports in which fatal aspiration has occurred because cricoid pressure was released when the patient began vomiting during induction of anesthesia.[195] There is also a single case report in the literature attributing rupture of the esophagus to cricoid pressure.[145] It involved an elderly woman subjected to laparotomy after repeated episodes of hematemesis. The patient vomited on induction; the patient was positioned laterally, cricoid pressure was released, and the trachea was intubated after pharyngeal aspiration. At surgery, a longitudinal split was found in the lower esophagus. It was concluded by the reporting authors that the esophageal rupture represented an esophageal injury attributable to the cricoid pressure. However, the diagnosis of spontaneous rupture of the esophagus as a result of the repeated episodes of hematemesis is more likely as the stomach adjacent to the area of esophageal injury was noted to be bruised and swollen during the surgery, suggesting a temporally more remote injury. Other authors are in agreement with Sellick's revised views on releasing cricoid pressure during induction should the patient vomit.[59,131,187] That is, although there is ample evidence that fatal aspiration may result if cricoid pressure is released should vomiting occur at induction, there is no evidence that esophageal rupture is a significant risk should the pressure be maintained.

Following publication of Sellick's report, the use of cricoid pressure became perceived by many as the most important mechanism to prevent pulmonary aspiration in parturients undergoing general anesthesia. Rapid sequence induction with cricoid pressure has become the accepted standard of care for the parturient undergoing general anesthesia in many parts of the world. However, the effectiveness of cricoid pressure in preventing aspiration has been challenged by Whittington and others, who reported two cases of aspiration in parturients despite cricoid pressure having been employed at induction.[195] In both instances, muscle relaxation was maintained during anesthesia maintenance for cesarean section by large doses of pancuronium. The first patient vomited and aspirated after extubation, and the second demonstrated signs of inadequate relaxant reversal, then respiratory failure, and subsequently manifested signs of pulmonary aspiration. In neither case was there any intraoperative evidence of the massive, fatal aspirations that were clearly evident after extubation.

a. How Much Cricoid Pressure Is Needed to Prevent Gastroesophageal Reflux?

Values of 40 to 44 newtons (N; about 4 kg applied pressure) were recommended as the cricoid force that would prevent regurgitation with a theoretical maximum gastric pressure of 59 mm Hg.[188,197] Hartsilver and colleagues measured gastric pressure and volume in 20 pregnant women during emergency cesarean section under general anesthesia with neuromuscular block.[75] Mean gastric pressure was 11 mm Hg (range 4 to 19 mm Hg), and they predicted that 99% of women undergoing emergency cesarean section with neuromuscular block are likely to have gastric pressures less than 25 mm Hg (mean + 3 SD). If it is accepted that gastric and therefore esophageal pressures are unlikely to be above 25 mm Hg, what cricoid force would be adequate? Wraight and associates reported that 34 N occluded a manometry catheter behind the cricoid cartilage at a pressure greater than 30 mm Hg in all patients.[197] In another study of anesthetized patients, a cricoid force of 30 N occluded a manometry catheter with a pressure greater than 25 mm Hg in all patients.[189] A study of 10 cadavers showed that 20 N of cricoid force prevented the regurgitation of esophageal fluid at a pressure of 25 mm Hg in all cases and 30 N prevented regurgitation at a pressure of 40 mm Hg in all cases.[189] Therefore, 20 N of cricoid pressure is probably enough and 30 N is more than enough to prevent regurgitation into the pharynx in the majority of patients; pressures greater than 30 N are unlikely to be necessary.

b. How Well Is the Application of Cricoid Pressure Performed?

There are probably two elements to this question. First, how well is the maneuver performed, and second, how long can it effectively be maintained once applied? Meek and coworkers investigated the cricoid pressure technique of anesthetic assistants.[115] A large variation in the force applied (from <10 N to >90 N) was observed. Performance was improved markedly by providing simple instruction and further improved by practical training in the application of target force on a simulator.

Meek and coworkers also studied six operating department assistants performing simulated cricoid pressure (on a model of the larynx) to determine how long and under what conditions cricoid pressure could be sustained.[116] Subjects were asked to maintain forces of 20, 30, and 40 N for a target time of 20 minutes, with the arm either extended or flexed; most could not do so. Mean times to release of cricoid pressure varied from 3.7 (flexed) to 7.6 minutes (extended) at 40 N, 6.4 to 10.2 minutes at 30 N, and 13.2 to 14.6 minutes at 20 N. These findings are relevant to the management of cricoid pressure during failed intubation and suggest that the ability to generate forces sufficient to provide esophageal occlusion and airway protection for prolonged periods is limited.

c. Does Cricoid Pressure Complicate Airway Interventions?

A concern about cricoid pressure in general and the higher applied pressures in particular has been the potential for compromise of either the quality of the airway or the effectiveness of airway interventions. Ventilation of the lungs is imperative following failure to intubate the trachea, and cricoid pressure may interfere with or prevent ventilation.[3,123,190] In a report of 23 failed intubations over a 17-year period in one maternity unit, cricoid pressure was maintained during the failed intubation drill.[80] In 14 patients (60%), ventilation by a face mask was not difficult, indicating that cricoid pressure was at least not harmful in these patients. In the remaining nine patients, ventilation was difficult in seven patients (30%) and impossible in two (9%). It is possible that cricoid pressure contributed to the difficult ventilation in these patients.

Vanner and coauthors reported that difficulty breathing occurred in about half of awake patients with 40 N forces applied, and Lawes and colleagues reported that airway obstruction occurred in about 10%.[106,190] Hartsilver and Vanner investigated whether airway obstruction is related strictly to the force applied or whether the technique of application was also relevant.[74]

Airway obstruction occurred in only 2% of patients with cricoid pressure applied in the usual fashion at 30 N but in 56% when the pressure was applied in an upward and backward direction. MacG Palmer and Ball studied the effect of cricoid pressure (20, 30, and 44 N) on airway anatomy in 30 anesthetized patients examined fiberoptically through a laryngeal mask airway (LMA).[109] At 20 N, 23% had cricoid deformation, 43% did so at 30 N, and at 44 N it occurred in 90% of patients. Associated difficulty in ventilation was present in 50% of patients, and 60% had vocal cord closure with associated difficult ventilation at higher applied forces.

Generally speaking, cricoid pressure has a limited impact on the ability to ventilate the lungs, the quality of the airway, or the effectiveness of airway interventions. However, there is an effect, and as application technique worsens or applied pressures are increased, the potential for airway compromise is increased.

d. Is Bimanual Cricoid Pressure Better than a One-Handed Technique?

Flexion of the head on the neck may occur as a result of cricoid pressure, and this may impede laryngoscopy. Bimanual (two-handed) cricoid pressure with the free hand of the assistant placed behind and supporting the neck or, alternatively, with the use of a small support placed behind the patient's neck has been recommended to overcome the tendency to head flexion (Fig. 34-2).[44] Cook studied 121 patients to compare the view of the larynx at laryngoscopy with one- or two-handed cricoid pressure applied.[42] In 81 cases the laryngeal view was the same with either type of cricoid pressure, in 28 cases the laryngeal view was better with one-handed cricoid pressure, and in 11 cases the laryngeal view was better with two-handed cricoid pressure. Two-handed cricoid pressure was not demonstrated by Cook to provide an advantage

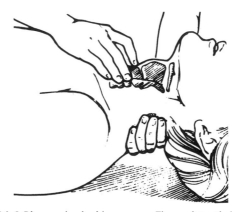

Figure 34-2 Bimanual cricoid pressure. The assistant's left hand is placed behind the neck lifting up and the right hand is used to apply cricoid pressure. The lifting action (countercricoid pressure) places the head in an improved sniffing position for laryngoscopy. (From Crowley DS, Giesecke AH. Bimanual cricoid pressure. Anaesthesia 45:588-589, 1990, and Benumof JL [ed]: Airway Management: Principles and Practice, 1st ed. St. Louis, Mosby, 1996.)

routinely over the one-hand technique. Yentis also studied the effects of two different methods of cricoid pressure on laryngoscopic view in 94 healthy patients and reached conclusions contrary to those of Cook.[198] In 21 cases, a better laryngoscopic view was obtained with the bimanual technique; in 8 cases it was better with the single-handed technique; and in 65 cases, the method of cricoid pressure made no difference.

The technique of cricoid pressure that produces the best laryngoscopic view in an individual patient cannot be predicted. The alternative technique should be considered if it is suspected that the technique of cricoid pressure application is having a deleterious effect on direct laryngoscopy. Switching to the alternative technique may improve the laryngoscopic view.

II. ISSUES IN MANAGEMENT OF PATIENTS

A. AIRWAY ASSESSMENT

All parturients being considered for an anesthetic, whether regional or general, or presenting with a condition that predisposes them to higher risk for cesarean section should undergo airway evaluation and have a Mallampati-Samsoon classification assigned. Davies and colleagues encouraged evaluation of the airway in the supine position, although Tham and associates reported that there is little difference in the class assigned with supine versus upright position.[46,178] In fact, on the basis of Tham's data, routine assessment in the supine position would result in decreased specificity of the Mallampati assessment. Further airway evaluation should include determination of the patient's body habitus, mouth opening (interdental distance), prominence of upper incisors, ability to protrude the lower jaw beyond the upper incisors, mandibular length, thyromental distance, and neck extension. After airway assessment, a summary conclusion should be generated about the anticipated difficulty in both ventilating the patient and performing laryngoscopy; the patient can be advised of both the conclusion and its implications. A body mass index greater than 26 kg/m^2, absence of teeth, and a history of snoring are relevant findings predictive of difficult mask ventilation.[102] Rocke and colleagues constructed a figure predicting the probability of difficult intubation in parturients based on the findings of preoperative evaluation (Fig. 34-3).[151]

B. ACID ASPIRATION—STRATEGIES FOR RISK REDUCTION IN THE PARTURIENT

There are four major risk factors for acid aspiration: (1) a full stomach with acid gastric contents, (2) an increased intra-abdominal or intragastric pressure, (3) a decreased LES barrier pressure, and (4) a delay or inability to protect the airway should the upper esophageal sphincter fail. Strategies to reduce the risk of acid aspiration

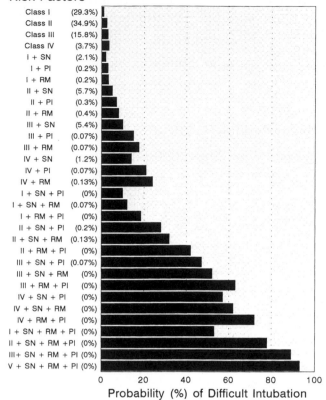

Risk Factors

Figure 34-3 The probability of experiencing a difficult intubation (grades 3 and 4 combined) for the varying combinations of risk factors and the observed incidence of these combinations. PI, protruding maxillary incisors; RM, receding mandible; SN, short neck. (From Rocke DA, Murray WB, Rout CC: Relative risk analysis of factors associated with difficult intubation in obstetric anesthesia. Anesthesiology 77:67-73, 1992, and Benumof JL [ed]: Airway Management: Principles and Practice, 1st ed. St. Louis, Mosby, 1996.)

focus on (1) reducing the potential for significant gastric volume and acidity in parturients, (2) reducing the use of general anesthesia in obstetrics, (3) appropriate assessment of the maternal airway (even when urgent interventions are otherwise required), and (4) evolving management schemes to deal with failures to ventilate and/or intubate.

The concept of critical or threshold volumes and pH of gastric contents is debated.[31] However, that the incidence and intensity or severity of aspiration pneumonitis increase as pH decreases and gastric volume increases is widely accepted. Reduction of the acidity of the gastric contents may reduce morbidity should aspiration occur, although there is no direct evidence to support this supposition. There are two mechanisms to reduce gastric acidity, direct neutralization of gastric acids already present in the stomach and reduction of the volume of acid produced. Antacids effectively neutralize acid contents of the stomach. Nonparticulate antacids are favored as there is evidence that particulate antacids are themselves capable of causing lung injury should aspiration occur.[181] Sodium citrate is the most widely used and recommended antacid in obstetric anesthesia practice.[31] Thirty milliliters of 0.3 M sodium citrate given 15 to 20 minutes before induction of general anesthesia is effective in raising the pH of stomach contents, beginning about 5 minutes after administration and lasting for 40 to 60 minutes.[67,191] The effect may be relatively prolonged in anesthetized patients with beneficial effects persisting several hours after administration.[192]

The histamine (H$_2$) blocking agents cimetidine and ranitidine have also been consistently shown to reduce gastric volume and acidity in parturients.[31] The use of ranitidine is favored because of its longer duration of action, fewer side effects, and lesser inhibition of the mixed function oxidase system when compared with cimetidine. An orally administered dose of ranitidine 150 mg given 90 minutes before surgery reliably increases pH in the majority of parturients. A small number of patients continue to have gastric pH below 2.5 despite ranitidine administration. The incidence of at-risk patients increases in the setting of urgent cesarean section compared with elective surgeries, despite ranitidine administration.[40] The coadministration of sodium citrate with intravenous ranitidine provides more effective prophylaxis than antacid alone, although 30 minutes is required from the time of injection to see this enhanced effect.[157] The use of effervescent cimetidine–sodium citrate is also more effective than sodium citrate alone in increasing and maintaining maternal gastric pH above 2.5.[133]

Omeprazole, which selectively blocks the proton pump in the gastric parietal cell (the terminal step in the production of gastric acid), is more effective than ranitidine in decreasing pH in parturients presenting for elective cesarean section when given orally both the evening before and the morning of surgery.[53] Intravenous omeprazole reduces both the gastric pH and volume in parturients presenting for emergency cesarean section but, once again, about 30 minutes is required for this effect.[152] Maternal and fetal side effects have not been a significant issue with respect to the use of the acid-suppressing agents. The use of anticholinergics to reduce gastric acid secretion has been widely and wisely abandoned.[181] Their effect on gastric secretion is variable, and there is little evidence that they reduce gastric acid secretion. Further, anticholinergics adversely affect the esophageal sphincter pressure, thus reducing the barrier to esophageal reflux.

Finally, metoclopramide is a prokinetic agent that, when administered to parturients undergoing cesarean section, results in an increased barrier pressure at the LES and may promote gastric emptying.[37] Whether metoclopramide consistently promotes gastric emptying in all parturients has not been fully resolved. Metoclopramide (10 mg administered intramuscularly) decreased gastric emptying time in primigravid women, including some who had received meperidine during labor.[89] Cohen and colleagues were unable to demonstrate this effect in individual parturients, although overall there was a decrease in the number of patients with gastric volumes greater than 25 mL and pH less than 2.5.[37] Despite the narcotic antagonism to the gastric emptying effects of metoclopramide, there is still evidence for enhanced gastric emptying after administration of metoclopramide in laboring patients who have received narcotics.[125] The usual dose of metoclopramide is 10 mg given either orally, intravenously, or intramuscularly, 60 to 90 minutes before surgery. In an emergency, 10 mg injected slowly intravenously begins to have an effect in 1 to 3 minutes.

C. MANAGEMENT OF GENERAL ANESTHESIA IN OBSTETRIC CARE

As a general rule, regional anesthesia is to be advocated over general anesthesia in elective situations. In particular, patients in whom difficulty with intubation is anticipated should undergo operative delivery under regional anesthesia. However, there are some circumstances that either encourage or demand the use of general anesthesia. If general anesthesia is deemed to be specifically indicated in a high-risk patient, consideration should be given to the induction of general anesthesia after awake endotracheal intubation.

1. Aspiration Prophylaxis (Table 34-1)

Patients presenting for elective cesarean section under general anesthesia should receive oral ranitidine (150 mg) the evening before surgery and 90 minutes before surgery. Oral sodium citrate or its equivalent administered 10 to 20 minutes before surgery is a commonly used supplement. Metoclopramide 10 mg may be administered in the same manner as ranitidine to parturients who experience symptomatic reflux.

2. Equipment

Clinicians engaged in anesthetic practice should be experienced with a device that could serve as an alternative airway in the event that ventilation with a face mask fails, as well as adjuncts and alternatives to the direct laryngoscope should it fail to facilitate endotracheal intubation. Obviously, it is recommended that clinicians familiarize themselves with these items in elective scenarios before they are required in emergent situations. There are a number of items of equipment that should be immediately available for all cases and brought into the room for anticipated difficulties or once difficulties are experienced. Equipment specifically modified for use in obstetric anesthesia has also been described and may be of particular use in some situations.[45] A list of essential items to be included in a difficult intubation kit is provided in Table 34-2.

3. Positioning

The table should be at a height that is most convenient for the anesthesiologist performing laryngoscopy. The height

Table 34-1 **Pharmacologic Prophylaxis—Aspiration Pneumonitis**

Labor
All women in active labor are under restricted oral intake—primarily clear fluids and ice chips.
Patients in normal or augmented labor do not receive routine prophylaxis.
Ranitidine or metoclopramide or both are administered to parturients who have significant reflux symptoms or excess nausea and vomiting while in labor.
Elective Cesarean Section
For patients who have significant symptoms of reflux, ranitidine 150 mg with or without metoclopramide 10 mg is given orally at hour of sleep the night before surgery and 90 minutes before surgery.
Sodium citrate (30 mL of 0.3 M solution) may be given by mouth 10 to 20 minutes preoperatively irrespective of the type of anesthesia planned.
Nonelective Cesarean Section
Parenteral ranitidine or metoclopramide or both may be given to parturients for whom nonelective surgery is planned irrespective of the type of anesthesia planned.
Sodium citrate (30 mL of 0.3 M solution) may be given by mouth before moving the patient to the operating room, irrespective of the type of anesthesia planned.
Emergency Cesarean Section
Sodium citrate (30 mL of 0.3 M solution) may be given by mouth in the labor suite before transporting the patient to the operating room.
Ranitidine and metoclopramide are not routinely given before induction but may be administered intraoperatively or on specific indication.

Table 34-2 **The Difficult Intubation Kit for Obstetric Anesthesia—Essential Elements**

Adjuncts to the face mask for assisted ventilation   Airways, oral and pharyngeal

Alternatives to the face mask for assisted ventilation (at least one of)
    Laryngeal mask airways size 3 and 4
    Combitube

Adjunct to the direct laryngoscope
    Straight and levering blade
    Short (polio-type) handles
    Bougie
    Stylets

Alternative to the direct laryngoscope (at least one of)
    Lighted stylet
    Rigid fiberoptic (Bullard type) laryngoscope
    Fiberoptic laryngoscope or bronchoscope

Surgical airway kit (one of)
    Retrograde catheter kit
    Cricothyrotomy kit (preassembled oxygen insufflation kit)

of the table can be adjusted to suit the obstetrician when the airway has been secured. The patient is placed in the wedged-supine position. The head should be positioned in the sniffing position with a small pillow under the occiput. Although the benefit of the sniffing position compared with simple extension was challenged by Adnet and colleagues, it did provide an advantage in patients who were obese or in whom there was at least one factor predictive of difficult intubation present.[1] Thus, the use of the sniffing position in obstetrics is still advocated at this time. Folded sheets or flannels may be used to accomplish this positioning and are particularly useful in the very obese parturient (Fig. 34-4). The obstetric patient is typically prepared and draped for surgery before the induction of general anesthesia to minimize the induction-delivery interval. The drapes on the ether screen (or its equivalent) should be arranged such that they do not overlie the neck and head region so as not to interfere with laryngoscopy. Delaying the fixing of the drapes until after the airway has been secured is a common practice and one to be encouraged.

4. Preoxygenation

Denitrogenation occurs more quickly in parturients because of the decreased functional residual capacity (FRC) and higher minute ventilation that occur in pregnancy.[25,130,159] Oxygen consumption is also higher in parturients and lung stores of oxygen are reduced because of the decreased FRC.[35,114] The parturient sustains a threefold more rapid reduction in arterial oxygen content during apneic periods, as would occur following induction of anesthesia, before endotracheal intubation is achieved.[6] The usual method for preoxygenating patients before anesthetic induction involves having the patient breathe 100% oxygen through a snug-fitting face mask for 3 to 5 minutes. Norris and Dewan reported that four maximal capacity breaths are as effective in preoxygenating parturients, although an additional study by Norris and colleagues disputed this finding.[129,130] Further, nonpregnant patients preoxygenated with four vital capacity breaths desaturate more quickly than patients preoxygenated for 3 minutes.[66] For these reasons and whenever possible, it is recommended that the tidal breathing technique be employed and that the four-breath technique be reserved for situations that require haste. Two to 3 minutes of tidal breathing provides adequate denitrogenation in parturients.[25]

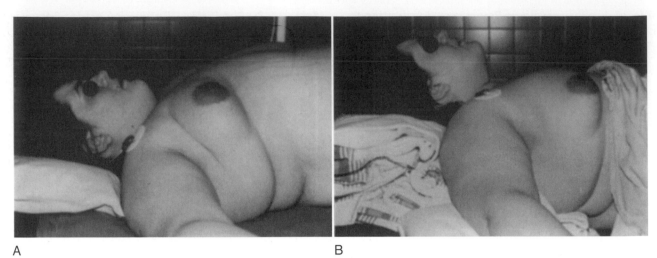

Figure 34-4 Enhanced positioning of the obese parturient for laryngoscopy. **A,** Standard positioning on the operating table. **B,** Improved positioning achieved with elevation of the torso and head. (From Davies JM, Weeks SA, Crone LA, et al: Difficult intubation in the parturient. Can J Anaesth 36:668-674, 1989, and Benumof JL [ed]: Airway Management: Principles and Practice, 1st ed. St. Louis, Mosby, 1996.)

5. Cricoid Pressure

The cricoid cartilage should be identified by the assistant during preoxygenation, before induction of anesthesia, and the accuracy of the landmark should be confirmed by the anesthesiologist. Cricoid pressure may be gently applied at the start of the induction sequence and the pressure increased to that required concurrent with induction of anesthesia. The pressure should not be released until the intratracheal position of the tube has been confirmed. Should the patient make retching motions after administration of anesthetic induction agents, this author asks that the assistant maintain cricoid pressure. The risk of esophageal rupture, albeit real, appears extremely small. The risk of aspiration should cricoid pressure be released, although also undefined, seems of greater magnitude.

6. Induction of Anesthesia

Rapid sequence induction implies rapid administration of both the induction agent and muscle relaxant. Succinylcholine remains for most practitioners the muscle relaxant of choice in rapid sequence induction in obstetric anesthesia.[179] Adequate time should be allowed for muscle relaxation before attempting laryngoscopy. If sufficient time is not allowed, masseter muscle tone may be increased, making mouth opening more difficult and compromising laryngoscopy.[26,161]

There has been increasing enthusiasm to employ nondepolarizing neuromuscular blockers in the place of succinylcholine during rapid sequence induction, both in general surgical anesthesia and in obstetric anesthesia. The use of vecuronium for rapid sequence induction in patients undergoing cesarean section has been reported.[78]

Patients were given 10 μg/kg as a priming dose followed 4 to 6 minutes later by 100 or 200 μg/kg as a single bolus. Onset time to 100% twitch suppression was 177 and 175 seconds, respectively. Duration of effect, measured to 25% twitch height recovery, was 73 and 115 minutes, respectively.

Rocuronium has been the most extensively studied of the nondepolarizing drugs for use during rapid sequence induction because it has a more rapid onset than the other nondepolarizing relaxants. Intubating conditions were compared after rocuronium (0.6 mg/kg) and succinylcholine (1 mg/kg) following rapid sequence induction of anesthesia in patients scheduled for elective, nonobstetric surgery.[173] Intubation time did not differ, and conditions were clinically acceptable in all patients given succinylcholine and in 96% of the patients given rocuronium. Baraka and associates investigated the neuromuscular effects and conditions of endotracheal intubation after administration of rocuronium (0.6 mg/kg) in parturients undergoing elective cesarean section.[10] Anesthesia was induced by either thiopental or ketamine and rocuronium was then administered. The time to 50% neuromuscular block (45 ± 10 seconds for thiopental and 42 ± 14 seconds for ketamine) and the time to maximum block (105 ± 35 seconds and 101 ± 5 seconds, respectively) were not different between the two groups. Endotracheal intubation at 50% neuromuscular block was easily performed in all patients in the ketamine-rocuronium group but was difficult in 75% of the thiopental-rocuronium group.

The pharmacologic profile for rocuronium is such that a similar time to onset of relaxation during rapid sequence induction can be expected compared with succinylcholine, although recovery is longer with rocuronium. Its effect is enhanced when larger doses are employed, when ketamine is used as the induction agent, and if narcotics are employed as supplements.

a. Should the Lungs Be Ventilated during Rapid Sequence Induction Using Cricoid Pressure?

The conventional pattern of practice in obstetric anesthesia has been to manage rapid sequence induction by aggressively preoxygenating the patient's lungs and then, with cricoid pressure applied, inducing general anesthesia and administering a muscle relaxant. Before performing laryngoscopy, while awaiting the onset of the muscle block, the patient is left apneic. Despite the fact that this practice is not supported by any evidence base, there seems to be little enthusiasm to challenge or change the practice.[122,179] However, there is evidence not only that there is a benefit to ventilating the patient's lungs during the period of apnea but also that it can be done safely. The average time to return to 50% of twitch height following an intubating dose of succinylcholine is 8 to 9 minutes; for return to 90% twitch height, 10 to 11 minutes is required. This is considerably longer than it takes most nonpregnant patients to desaturate, even under ideal circumstances.[57] Thus, it is likely that, at some point, mask bag ventilation will be required if difficulties are encountered during laryngoscopy. However, the time at which it would be necessary to intervene to prevent desaturation would be predictably longer if the patient's lungs had been ventilated during the induction-laryngoscopy interval.

There is a relationship between the airway pressures required to ventilate the lungs and those that force air into the stomach.[105] In subjects ventilated by bag and mask without cricoid pressure, airway pressures below 15 cm H_2O rarely cause stomach inflation, pressures between 15 and 25 cm H_2O result in gastric insufflation in some patients, and pressures greater than 25 cm H_2O do so in most patients.[158] Application of cricoid pressure during mask-bag ventilation increases the maximum pressure reached during mask ventilation without air entering the stomach, to about 45 cm H_2O.

Petito and Russell measured the ability of cricoid pressure to prevent gastric inflation during mask and bag ventilation of the lungs.[140] Fifty patients were randomly assigned to either have or not have cricoid pressure applied during a 3-minute period of standardized mask ventilation. Patients who had cricoid pressure applied had less gas in the stomach after mask ventilation. However, more patients who had cricoid pressure applied (36% versus 12%) were considered difficult to ventilate, and these patients tended to have larger volumes of air in the stomach than the patients considered easy to ventilate with applied cricoid pressure. The application of cricoid pressure reduces the volume of air entering the stomach at low to moderate ventilation pressures. It allows continued ventilation of the lungs even in situations in which past

convention would have discouraged it, such as in rapid sequence inductions. Ventilating the lungs after induction of anesthesia, while awaiting the onset of muscle block, is a useful maneuver to prevent maternal oxygen desaturation.

III. THE FAILED INTUBATION—MANAGEMENT OPTIONS

A. THE FAILED INTUBATION DRILL IN OBSTETRIC ANESTHESIA—A HISTORICAL PERSPECTIVE

A number of authors have advanced protocols for the management of failed intubation in obstetric anesthesia.[83,107,156,169,182-184] Two conclusions have been consistent through most protocols. First, an early acceptance of failure to intubate must occur, and a maximum of two to three intubation attempts have been recommended. Second, it is desirable to evolve and implement a standard protocol for managing failed intubation that recognizes the paramount importance of ensuring oxygenation. If the fetus is in good condition, the mother should be allowed to awaken after failed intubation and an alternative method of anesthesia should be employed. In the absence of a threat to maternal health, it has even been argued that there are no compelling reasons to carry on with a general anesthetic despite fetal concerns.[72]

B. GENERAL CONSIDERATIONS

A simple approach is proposed to aid in the management of the unanticipated difficult airway. It is based on a strategy that encourages the immediate diagnosis of the specific airway problem encountered and a directed response determined by the clinical scenario. The diagnostic choices for unanticipated difficult airway are limited to three: (1) difficult or failed mask ventilation, (2) difficult laryngoscopy, and (3) difficult or failed intubation. The clinical problems arising are that (1) the lungs cannot be ventilated, (2) the laryngoscope cannot be passed into the mouth, (3) the larynx cannot be seen, or (4) the tracheal tube cannot be passed. The response is determined by both the underlying diagnosis and the physician's chosen alternative for managing the condition. The chosen alternative is directed specifically at the underlying problem and is likely to be effective. The following discussion outlines the nature of the response.

Techniques and technologies directed toward the management of the difficult airway continue to proliferate. Although in many cases their specific roles and efficacy have not been rigorously defined to date, some conclusions may be drawn from the experience thus accumulated: success with all devices relies more on the operator's experience and skill than on the tools themselves, and the success of any technique depends on proper selection of patients, meticulous preparation, good technique, and regular practice, regardless of the device employed.

1. Problems and Solutions

In some patients, mask ventilation is difficult, yet endotracheal intubation is achieved readily. If mask ventilation seems difficult, before endotracheal intubation is attempted, consideration should be given to reducing the magnitude of the cricoid force and inserting an oral airway. If ventilation remains very difficult and sufficient time has elapsed to allow muscle relaxation, an attempt at endotracheal intubation is a prudent next intervention. Given that the compelling clinical imperative in this setting is to establish a patent airway and not to effect intubation, attempts at intubation must not be persistent in this setting. All physicians responsible for airway management should be practiced in at least one alternative to mask-bag ventilation. New technology intuitively useful in this setting includes the LMA and the Combitube. Transtracheal techniques should be considered early if alternative transoral techniques are not available or do not achieve ventilation.

If the laryngoscopic view is inadequate to permit visual intubation (grade 3 or 4), efforts can be made to improve the view and consideration given to utilizing either an adjunct or an alternative to the direct laryngoscope. The best laryngoscopic view is dependent on optimal positioning of the patient, an experienced practitioner with capable assistance, and a technique designed to ensure that the best view is obtained. For direct laryngoscopy, the patient should be in a sniff position (slight flexion of the neck and extension of the head on the neck) to best align the oral, pharyngeal, and laryngeal axes. If the best laryngoscopic view is grade 2 to 4, optimal external laryngeal manipulation (OELM) or backward, upward, rightward laryngeal displacement (BURP maneuver) should be used.[13,177] OELM is described as pressing posteriorly and cephalad over the thyroid, hyoid, and cricoid cartilages in an attempt to improve the laryngeal view.[13] The BURP maneuver requires the manual displacement of the larynx posteriorly against the cervical vertebrae, superiorly as far as possible and to the right.[177] These maneuvers can improve a poor laryngoscopic view, are readily and rapidly performed, and should be the initial response to a poor view.

2. Adjuncts to Direct Laryngoscopy

Adjuncts to the direct laryngoscope should be introduced early during management of the unanticipated difficult intubation; they are probably most useful when applied in the setting of a grade 3 or better view. Repeated attempts at endotracheal intubation using adjuncts to the direct laryngoscope are not warranted. One adjunct to direct laryngoscopy for the unanticipated difficult intubation meriting attention is the gum elastic bougie.[49,99,128]

Kidd and associates reported the use of the bougie in 98 patients with simulated and 2 with genuine grade 3 laryngoscopy.[99] The bougie entered the trachea in 78 patients and the esophagus in 22. Tracheal clicks were noted in 90% of the tracheal placements and no clicks were noted with the esophageal placements. Hold-up of the bougie at 24 to 40 cm occurred in all tracheal placements as the tip made contact with the smaller airways, and this was not seen in any of the esophageal placements. Both signs were advanced as useful indicators of tracheal placement.

A vast number of laryngoscope blades are available; many are subtle variations on earlier designs. Few have undergone a controlled assessment to determine whether they provide improved glottic visualization in patients with difficult laryngoscopy. A new blade introduced into anesthetic practice, the McCoy articulating blade, has undergone such assessments, albeit not in obstetric patients. In 50 patients, in whom difficult laryngoscopic conditions were simulated by neck immobilization in the neutral position, the laryngoscopic view obtained with the McCoy blade was better by at least one grade in most of the patients with a grade 2 (70% improved) or 3 (83% improved) compared with the view obtained with the Macintosh blade.[185] However, in the patients with a grade 4 view, there was no improvement in view. Similar findings of improvements on grade 2 and 3 views were reported by others.[64,104] Laurent and coworkers[104] also determined that cricoid pressure does not interfere with use of the McCoy blade and that similar improvements in view can still be expected, an important finding relevant to obstetric anesthesia practice.[64]

3. Alternatives to the Direct Laryngoscope

If no view of laryngeal structures (grade 4) is obtainable with the direct laryngoscope, it is the author's opinion that an alternative to the direct laryngoscope rather than an adjunct is the optimum second intervention. Both the literature and clinical experiences support the conclusion that adjuncts have the highest utility (improving intubating conditions and efficiency) when a poor grade 2 or grade 3 view is obtained as they typically improve these views by one grade. They are less successful at improving conditions when the best view is a nonconvertible grade 4.

The alternatives to the direct scope useful in these circumstances are indirect techniques. They, in effect, "turn the corner" in the airway and it is not necessary to establish a line of view. They may provide a view (fiberoptic endoscopes) or facilitate a blind intubation by providing a cue (tracheal illumination). There are increasing data that they present a significant advantage to the experienced practitioner in situations in which the direct scope is found lacking. Alternatives to the direct laryngoscope include the light stylet and the rigid and flexible fiberoptic endoscopes.

C. MANAGEMENT GUIDELINES—SCENARIO-SPECIFIC CONSIDERATIONS

1. Failed Intubation—Elective Cesarean Section

No approach to the failed intubation in obstetric anesthesia may be formulated that does not have some limitations. The following comments represent guidelines for the management of the parturient, presenting for elective or nonemergent cesarean section, whose trachea is ascertained to be very difficult or impossible to intubate. If laryngoscopy is difficult, cricoid pressure may be transiently reduced or released. It can be determined whether or not this maneuver will facilitate laryngoscopy and intubation. If not, cricoid pressure probably should be reapplied and maintained. The surgical team is alerted to the situation and experienced help is summoned immediately, if possible. The position of the patient is not changed initially, and the face mask is reapplied and positive-pressure ventilation with 100% oxygen commenced. Maternal oxygenation and airway protection are the paramount goals from this point forward. Many intubation difficulties may be overcome if positioning is optimized and two-handed cricoid pressure may be employed to offset the flexion of the head caused by application of cricoid pressure. The efficacy of these maneuvers can be ascertained.

Positioning of the patient, cricoid pressure, the intubating instrument, and the personnel (second practitioner) may all be modified during subsequent attempts at intubation. Early consideration should be given to the use of alternative devices if the physician is practiced in their use. If three properly controlled attempts at intubation have failed, a decision must be taken on further management. In the absence of fetal compromise, the procedure is abandoned and the mother is allowed to awaken. If ventilation is easy with mask and bag, it can be artificially maintained until spontaneous ventilation returns. Cricoid pressure is sustained during this period. Positioning the mother in the left lateral, head-down position can be considered when spontaneous ventilation has resumed and is encouraged. If ventilation is initially or becomes impossible, insertion of a either a laryngeal mask or a Combitube should be considered. It may be necessary to release cricoid pressure transiently to insert these devices. Transtracheal oxygenation through a cricothyroid puncture should be reserved for the unlikely event that neither an LMA nor a Combitube is available or effective.

2. Failed Intubation—Nonelective Cesarean Section

The decision to abandon the anesthetic or surgery and awaken the mother is influenced by both the ability to oxygenate the mother and the degree of urgency of the cesarean section. It is difficult to justify putting the mother at continued risk by persisting with an anesthetic after failed intubation has occurred when there is no threat to fetus or mother. However, in situations where the mother, the fetus, or both are at risk because of obstetric circumstances, continuation of the anesthetic and delivery may be lifesaving to one or both. If a decision is made to continue with the procedure, the best possible airway is sought. A tenuous airway is not acceptable, and it is prudent to proceed to the next step to ensure a secure airway.

Once a decision has been taken to carry on following failed intubation, mask and bag ventilation is attempted, facilitated by an airway if necessary, with cricoid pressure maintained. If ventilation is successful, spontaneous ventilation is allowed to return and the cesarean section may be carried out with the patient under face mask general anesthesia. Minimal fundal pressure to effect delivery of the fetus is encouraged to reduce intragastric pressures, and the use of a vacuum to facilitate fetal extraction may permit lower fundal pressures. If ventilation is difficult (a tenuous airway) or impossible, either an LMA or a Combitube should be employed without delay. A transtracheal or translaryngeal (retrograde) intubation is generally reserved for situations in which an acceptable airway cannot otherwise be obtained nonsurgically. However, rather than tolerate an undue delay in achieving a nonsurgical airway, earlier invasive airway intervention is readily defensible.

Emergency induction of general anesthesia for urgent cesarean section, the "crash section," is a particularly high-risk intervention in obstetric anesthesia, with much of the measured maternal mortality resulting from this intervention.[79,146-149,196] Because of the inherent risk involved, it should be reserved for situations where such haste and risk are warranted. A strategy for identifying patients likely to deliver by cesarean section early in labor and initiating epidural anesthesia reduces the requirement for urgent induction of general anesthesia (Table 34-3).[119] The need for nonelective or emergency cesarean section could be anticipated in 87% of parturients reviewed by

Table 34-3 **Factors Increasing the Likelihood of Nonelective Cesarean Section**

Obstructed labor—failed augmentation
Abnormal fetal heart rate trace
Abnormal fetal blood sampling
Breech presentation
Persistent malpresentation other than breech
Nonengaged fetal head
Multiple gestation pregnancy
Suspected intrauterine growth retardation
Fetal macrosomia
Vaginal birth after cesarean section
Suspected cephalopelvic disproportion
Obesity

Morgan and colleagues, and epidural anesthesia was provided in 70% of patients.[119] However, not all epidural blocks established for labor analgesia could be rapidly or successfully converted to provide surgical anesthesia for cesarean delivery. In 194 patients an epidural catheter was placed and activated after they were deemed likely to deliver by cesarean section, and a catheter was placed in a further 57 patients when the decision to deliver them by cesarean section was actually made. Twenty-seven (12%) of these patients were given general anesthesia for delivery, 15 because the epidural block was inadequate for surgery, the rest for reasons not explicitly stated. Ostheimer reported that epidural blockade provided inadequate anesthesia for cesarean delivery in 18.2% of patients.[134] Preston and colleagues reported that 5% of functioning labor epidural blocks could not be extended to provide adequate anesthesia for cesarean delivery.[141] Many of the blocks performed in the latter two series were performed by residents and fellows, and these failure rates may have been influenced by the experience of the anesthesiologist. Subarachnoid block is typically associated with significantly lower failure rates than epidural anesthesia.

3. Emergency Cesarean Section for Fetal Distress

The normal fetal heart rate (FHR) pattern has a baseline rate of 120 to 160 beats per minute. FHR variability is represented by the variation in the FHR, and it is a marker of fetal well-being. The presence of normal FHR variability is almost invariably associated with fetal vigor at birth.[139] If the FHR demonstrates normal variability, the fetus is at low risk for immediate morbidity from asphyxia even in the presence of decelerations and bradycardia. A decrease or loss of variability in the presence of these patterns is a sign that the physiologic compensations available to the fetus are being overwhelmed as a result of the severity of asphyxia.

Heart rates below 120 bpm are arbitrarily deemed to be bradycardia and those above 160, tachycardia. The severity and duration of bradycardia are proportional to the duration and severity of the asphyxial insult to the fetus. Bradycardia between 100 and 120 bpm with normal variability is generally well tolerated. Rates of 80 to 100 bpm, again with preserved variability, can be managed conservatively. Rates below 80 and especially below 60 bpm represent obstetric emergencies that necessitate immediate delivery if they are persistent and cannot be resolved by other measures. Tachycardia is caused by a large number of fetal and maternal conditions, the most common of which is maternal fever, and it is nonspecific with respect to the fetal condition.[90,96] If variability is preserved and tachycardia is the isolated finding, it is thought by many authors to be well tolerated by the fetus.[4,138]

Fetal distress as applied to interpretation of FHR traces is a widely used but poorly defined term. A normal FHR recording correctly predicts a healthy newborn in 95% of cases, yet the predictive value of tracings defined as pathologic lacks diagnostic specificity, and in 50% of cases *fetal distress* is diagnosed in a completely healthy fetus.[96] This fact should be balanced against the maternal risks inherent in emergency surgical interventions carried out for fetal distress. This poor predictive value has also encouraged the abandonment of the term fetal distress and its replacement with nondiagnostic terms such as "nonreassuring fetal heart trace."

Should operative delivery be deemed necessary based on the finding of a nonreassuring fetal heart trace, the presence of FHR variability and a heart rate persistent above 80 bpm implies that sufficient time exists for both maternal assessment and regional anesthesia. Absent variability and severe decelerations (either late or variable type) imply poor fetal condition and a more rapid delivery is mandated. However, there is still time for assessment of the maternal airway, and if difficulty is anticipated, regional anesthesia or awake intubation can still be recommended. Subarachnoid anesthesia is an appropriate option if maternal assessment suggests that maternal airway difficulties are probable in the setting of a nonreassuring fetal heart trace.[111,139] Rapid induction of general anesthesia is an option if maternal assessment is consistent with no anticipated airway difficulties.

The severity of the FHR abnormality should be considered when the urgency of the delivery and the type of anesthesia to be administered are determined. As noted, cesarean deliveries that are performed for a nonreassuring fetal heart pattern do not necessarily preclude the use of regional anesthesia, a conclusion endorsed by the American College of Obstetricians and Gynecologists.[41] Emergency induction of general anesthesia for nonreassuring fetal heart pattern should be reserved for situations in which it is likely that the fetus is at risk for imminent asphyxial morbidity or mortality. These situations could include bradycardia with heart rates persisting below 80 bpm or severe, deep, and prolonged decelerations, either late or variable, with absent FHR variability. However, regional anesthesia is not contraindicated and subarachnoid anesthesia in particular is recommended if it is recognized that the airway is likely to be difficult. If the trachea cannot be intubated when general anesthesia has been induced, alternative methods of airway management should be employed to effect prompt delivery of the infant. If the airway cannot be controlled or maintained despite multiple attempts, consideration should be given to waking the mother up and proceeding with regional anesthesia, despite the perception of fetal compromise.

4. Maternal Hemorrhagic Emergencies

Obstetric hemorrhage as a cause of maternal death remains prominent in mortality reports.[79,146-149,196] The most common causes of maternal hemorrhage include placenta previa, abruptio placentae, placenta accreta, and uterine rupture. Placenta previa is defined as a placenta implanted in the lower uterine segment with varying degrees of encroachment on the internal cervical os. The primary presenting complaint is painless vaginal bleeding with the initial bleeding usually being self-limited and rarely fatal. However, 10% to 25% of parturients with placenta previa develop hypovolemic shock, and shock is more common in patients with total previa.[86,120] Abruptio placentae is defined as the separation of all or part of the normally implanted placenta after the 20th week of gestation and before the birth of the fetus. The presentation and clinical manifestations of abruptio placentae depend primarily on the degree of placental separation and the amount of hemorrhage. Uterine rupture may occur spontaneously in a uterus with no scars but is more commonly manifest as scar separation through a previous cesarean scar. The rupture may be initially silent, particularly in the case of a scar dehiscence, but abdominal pain, maternal shock, and fetal distress or demise can result.

Emergent cesarean section may be required to achieve fetal or maternal salvage in these hemorrhagic syndromes. Regional anesthesia may be employed for delivery in parturients with abruptio placentae or placenta previa when there is limited hemorrhage without evidence of significant ongoing loss and no maternal hemodynamic instability. In these instances, the fetus is often not compromised. However, general anesthesia is often indicated as maternal hemodynamic instability, hypovolemic shock, clotting abnormalities, and severe fetal compromise may all contraindicate regional anesthesia. Provided that an airway may be obtained after failed intubation, general anesthesia can be continued, the fetus delivered, and the hemorrhagic condition surgically ablated. A second, experienced anesthesiologist should be summoned to assist with care of the patient as the primary physician is likely to be well occupied with the airway.

Retained or adherent placenta is a common early postpartum complication. The intravenous administration of nitroglycerin may allow spontaneous or assisted removal of a placenta trapped by a closed cervix but is often ineffective for adherent placenta.[29] If bleeding is limited and the mother is stable hemodynamically, spinal saddle block provides good conditions for assisted removal. Conscious sedation and analgesia using nitrous oxide supplemented with intravenous narcotics (fentanyl 1 to 2 µg/kg) and low-dose ketamine (0.25 mg/kg) incrementally also provide good conditions for manual removal and uterine curettage. A patient and gentle obstetrician and an encouraging anesthesiologist do much to complement this technique. In the event that hemorrhage has been considerable and is persistent, ketamine induction of general anesthesia may be lifesaving. Again, provided that an airway can be maintained after failed intubation, general anesthesia should be continued and the uterus evacuated. A second anesthesiologist is again invaluable in this setting and should be summoned immediately when failed intubation is recognized.

5. Emergent Vaginal Delivery

There are a number of obstetric scenarios for which there is an immediate requirement for vaginal delivery. The most commonly encountered situation is that of severe fetal decompensation as manifest by FHR abnormalities. These are often a result of head compression as the fetus negotiates the terminal portion of the passageway. In many instances a saddle block or a pudendal block with perineal infiltration allows forceps extraction. If there are any concerns about the maternal airway, this management scheme is encouraged. Incremental low-dose ketamine or fentanyl supplementation may also be used. Less commonly, immediate induction of general anesthesia is required to effect vaginal delivery. An assessment of the maternal airway must precede induction. If there is concern about difficult intubation, general anesthesia should be avoided. In the event that intubation is difficult or impossible when general anesthesia has been established, the patient should be managed as would be the patient presenting for emergent cesarean section. That is, the airway should be controlled and protected and the delivery effected.

Shoulder dystocia and a trapped after-coming head during breech delivery are two less commonly encountered situations requiring immediate vaginal delivery. Incremental intravenous boluses of nitroglycerin (50 to 400 µg) may provide sufficient uterine relaxation to release the trapped breech head. Because of the nature of the occurrence and the urgency of the situation, general anesthesia is often required to facilitate delivery. Failure of a second twin to deliver after the uneventful delivery of the first or acute deterioration in the condition of the second twin may also prompt a request for immediate induction of anesthesia to allow delivery, either vaginal or abdominal. Ideally, this scenario is anticipated and an epidural catheter is placed, tested, and activated. However, it may happen that the mother presents to hospital already having delivered the first infant or delivers precipitously soon after admission, with no time available to establish epidural anesthesia. Electronic FHR monitoring should be initiated and may provide reassurance about the condition of the second fetus. Concurrent with the initiation of the FHR monitoring, an evaluation of the maternal airway must be made. In many instances and particularly if the maternal airway is suspect, subarachnoid anesthesia remains the technique of choice to allow prompt operative delivery. If there are no concerns about the maternal airway, general anesthesia remains a prudent alternative choice. If general anesthesia is induced and endotracheal intubation cannot be achieved, the ability to manage the airway and the condition of the fetus determine the next step.

6. The Morbidly Obese Parturient

Morbidly obese parturients experience more antenatal medical complications and are more likely to be delivered by cesarean section than nonobese parturients.[91,146] Intrapartum complications occur more frequently in obese patients; thus, the likelihood of an urgent or emergent cesarean section is also greater.[47] Morbid obesity is implicated as a risk factor for maternal mortality, and it is likely that both antepartum and intrapartum factors figure in the deaths.[47,79,146-149,196] Expiratory reserve volume, FRC, and residual volume are all decreased in obesity and further decreased in pregnancy.[47] The resultant decreased alveolar size reduces lung compliance and shunts ventilation to the nondependent, more compliant portions of the lung. Obese patients tend to breathe at smaller tidal volumes and faster respiratory rates. The smaller tidal volumes tend to exaggerate this shift in ventilation away from the more dependent, well-perfused portions of the lungs.[47] Ventilation-perfusion mismatch results and maternal partial pressure of oxygen in arterial blood (PaO_2) is reduced in the obese parturient compared with nonobese mothers.[47] There is a greater tendency to hypoxemia in the obese parturient, and the supine portion exaggerates the hypoxemia.

Morbidly obese parturients are more likely to become hypoxemic during induction of general anesthesia, and if intubation is delayed, severe hypoxemia results. Although there is a correlation between increasing body mass index and difficult intubation, obesity alone is not a strong predictor of difficult intubation.[151] Airway assessment of all laboring morbidly obese parturients is recommended early in the labor. The use of regional anesthesia is encouraged for the provision of both labor analgesia and anesthesia for operative delivery. If general anesthesia is to be employed in the morbidly obese parturient, consideration can be given to awake intubation, especially if other characteristics of the maternal airway enhance the possibility of difficult intubation. (The author does not consider morbid obesity alone to be an indication for routine awake intubation.) Positioning is all important to optimize the conditions for laryngoscopy and intubation in the morbidly obese patient, and considerable effort (and laundry!) may be required to achieve optimum positioning (see Fig. 34-4). Three to 5 minutes of preoxygenation is recommended. It is often difficult to achieve adequate response to peripheral nerve stimulation in the morbidly obese parturient, and this author performs laryngoscopy at 45 seconds elapsed time after administration of the succinylcholine. Failed intubation should prompt immediate consideration of awakening the patient.

IV. APPLICATION OF TECHNOLOGY IN THE FAILED MATERNAL AIRWAY: WHICH DEVICE, WHEN?

A. ALTERNATIVES TO THE FACE MASK AND BAG IN ESTABLISHING AN AIRWAY

1. The Role of the Laryngeal Mask Airway

The most outstanding feature of the LMA is its ability to provide a clear airway rapidly. The bulk of the literature regarding the use of the LMA in obstetric anesthesia relates to the original LMA, the LMA Classic. Two newer modified versions of the LMA are now marketed, and although they have some advantages compared with the Classic model and may prove to have greater utility with time, there is currently only a modest literature base regarding these devices. They are discussed subsequently.

There are now numerous reports of the LMA relieving hypoxia after failed intubation and ventilation in obstetric anesthesia.[18,33,76,112,113,175] It has also been utilized in parturients who could not be intubated but whose airways could be managed with face mask anesthesia.[29,142] The latter application has generated controversy for two reasons. First, there is evidence that the LMA is more likely to promote gastric regurgitation than face mask anesthesia.[11,144] The LMA results in a decrease in the LES barrier pressure in anesthetized, spontaneously breathing patients. Although El Mikatti and colleagues did not find an increased incidence of regurgitation in patients managed with an LMA compared with face mask anesthesia, it was commented that two LMA patients not included in the study analysis had signs of regurgitation after vigorous coughing during light anesthesia.[52] There were no similar events in the patients managed with a face mask. Second, it has been suggested that the inflated cuff of the LMA may prevent escape of regurgitated material into the pharynx and deflect it instead into the airway.[126] This effect would diminish or negate the protective effect of the left lateral position during a failed intubation drill.

Finally, Han and coauthors reported the use of LMA elective airway management during cesarean section in 1067 consecutive parturients presenting for elective cesarean section.[71] Patients were excluded if they had pharyngeal reflux, a body mass index greater than 30, and known or anticipated difficult airway. They had been fasted for at least 6 hours and all were treated with ranitidine and sodium citrate. Rapid sequence induction was performed with pentothal and succinylcholine, and cricoid pressure was maintained until delivery. An effective airway was obtained in 1060 patients, 1051 on the first attempt and 9 on the second or third attempt. Six patients required intubation for airway control. There were no recognized episodes of hypoxia, aspiration, regurgitation, bronchospasm, or gastric insufflation. Han and coauthors concluded that the LMA provided an effective and safe airway for elective cesarean section in healthy, selected patients.

When the patients' lungs can be ventilated adequately with a face mask after failed intubation, the LMA Classic probably confers little advantage and may promote gastric regurgitation. The liberal use of an LMA in this scenario has been discouraged, but it is probably a low-risk intervention.[63] The airway can be maintained with a face mask and cricoid pressure and spontaneous ventilation allowed to resume. Once spontaneous ventilation has returned through an open airway, there again would be little advantage to be gained by passing an LMA. However, when adequate ventilation cannot be maintained after failed intubation, placement of an LMA should be immediately considered. An attempt to pass it should be made early in the course of management after it has been determined that intubation is impossible and ventilation is difficult or impossible with the face mask. The laryngeal reflexes are likely still to be blunted by the residual effects of the anesthetic induction and the patient is less likely to respond unfavorably to airway placement if it is attempted early.[81] The stimulation related to passage of a laryngeal mask is approximately the same as that for an oropharyngeal airway.[172] Because there should be less gastric distention if there have not been persistent and forceful attempts to ventilate a patient with an obstructed airway, the risk of regurgitation may be reduced.

Whether or not cricoid pressure should be released during insertion of the LMA is controversial, but it is reasonable and prudent to do so and, in fact, it may be necessary to facilitate placement. The presence of the LMA does not appear to compromise effective application of cricoid pressure, although cricoid pressure may make the insertion of the LMA more difficult.[5,7,81] It is also more difficult to pass an endotracheal tube through the LMA and into the trachea, both blindly and assisted by a fiberoptic scope, with cricoid pressure applied.[7,19] Cricoid pressure causes an anterior tilt to the larynx, and this is probably the cause of the difficulty intubating the trachea.[19] The anterior angulation of the larynx may also result in closure of the vocal cords and airway obstruction and, although this has been reported, it is presumably rare.[17]

If ventilation is reestablished with the LMA, the mother should be allowed to awaken. The option to wake the patient should be excluded only by urgency to proceed for fetal or maternal welfare. In this circumstance, general anesthesia may be provided by the LMA, with cricoid pressure maintained and the mother breathing spontaneously. Other factors, such as the mother's preoperative reluctance to undergo elective cesarean delivery with regional anesthesia, should in no way compel the anesthesiologist to carry on with general anesthesia with a controlled but relatively unprotected airway. Once the airway has been opened with the LMA and the decision made to proceed with general anesthesia for cesarean delivery because of compelling maternal or fetal factors, it is controversial whether further steps should be taken to protect the airway. Intubation through the LMA with a small-gauge (6.0-mm) endotracheal tube, blind or assisted with a bougie, tube changer, or fiberoptic scope, has been described.[2,7,76,82] Such interventions are compromised by the maintenance of cricoid pressure, and it is difficult to justify release of the pressure if an adequate airway has already been achieved with the LMA and the airway is protected by cricoid pressure. Clearly, if not readily successful, attempts to pass an endotracheal tube should not be persistent, given that an adequate airway has already been established with the LMA.

As noted previously, two modified laryngeal masks are now available commercially in addition to the original model (LMA Classic). An intubating laryngeal mask (ILMA) designed to facilitate endotracheal intubation is available. There is also a mask with both a modified cuff to improve the seal and a port to provide a channel for gastric drainage (ProSeal LMA). There is evidence that the ILMA is easier to insert than the standard mask and more readily achieves an airway, even when used by practitioners inexperienced in its use.[12,32] Again, cricoid pressure would probably have to be released transiently to allow mask placement and facilitate passage of the tracheal tube.[73] The ILMA could then be used to facilitate endotracheal intubation, and there is published evidence attesting to its efficacy in this regard.[103] There is some evidence that the ProSeal LMA is more difficult to insert than the conventional mask unless an insertion device is used but also that it effectively isolates the glottis from the upper esophagus when properly positioned.[20] Although there are theoretical advantages to the use of the modified LMAs in securing a maternal airway, as compared with the LMA Classic, there is no published experience that would support a strong recommendation for any particular type or style of LMA as a salvage airway.

2. The Role of the Combitube

The Combitube is a double-lumen tube combining the function of an esophageal obturator airway and a conventional endotracheal airway.[60-62] Although anesthetic experience with the Combitube is limited to date and its use in obstetric anesthesia has yet to be reported, it is clearly an alternative to the LMA in the parturient in whom intubation has failed and ventilation is difficult. It can be placed quickly and allows protection of the airway, thus preventing aspiration. The stomach can be evacuated, usually through the tracheal lumen. Cricoid pressure would have to be released transiently to allow placement of the Combitube and the airway would be at risk from aspiration during the brief period before cuff inflation. It probably offers a greater degree of airway protection than the LMA Classic but may be similar to the ProSeal in this regard, although formal comparisons are lacking.

B. ALTERNATIVES TO THE DIRECT LARYNGOSCOPE IN ACHIEVING ENDOTRACHEAL INTUBATION

1. The Role of the Light Stylet

The light stylet (LS) or light wand uses the principle of transillumination of the soft tissues of the anterior neck to guide the tip of the endotracheal tube into the trachea.[92] The largest published series related to the use of the LS in patients with difficult intubation is that of Hung and colleagues, using the Trachlight LS, describing their experience with 265 patients.[91] There were 206 patients with a history of difficult airway (105) or anticipated difficult airway (101) and 59 were anaesthetized patients, with an unanticipated difficult but failed laryngoscopic intubation. In the first group, endotracheal intubation was achieved in all but two, with a mean time to intubation of 25.7 ± 20.1 seconds (range 4 to 120 seconds). In the second group (failed direct laryngoscopic intubation), endotracheal intubation was successful in all patients with a mean time to intubation of 19.7 ± 13.5 seconds (range 5 to 75 seconds). Apart from mucosal bleeding in patients who had multiple unsuccessful direct laryngoscopic attempts, no complications were noted.

The particular advantage of the LS is in its application to patients with anatomic characteristics that interfere with aligning the axes to obtain a line of view during direct laryngoscopy. These characteristics include limited mouth opening from any cause, a hypoplastic mandible, prominent upper incisors, restricted cervical spine movement or spinal immobilization, glossoptosis or glossomegaly, or restricted access to the airway (halo traction, stereotaxic frames). The LS may be less effective in patients in whom transillumination of the anterior neck may not be adequate, such as those who are morbidly obese or patients with limited neck extension. The use of the LS may also be compromised by the application of cricoid pressure. Hodgson and associates reported that successful first-attempt intubation with an LS took longer and intubation required more attempts when cricoid pressure was being applied than when there was none.[88] Intubation was successful in 97% of patients and all failures occurred in the first patients studied, suggesting that practice improved performance. In the author's experience, a split-fingered technique of cricoid pressure allows easier visualization of the transilluminated light and may facilitate the use of the LS when cricoid pressure is being used.

2. The Role of the Rigid Fiberoptic Laryngoscopes

The Bullard laryngoscope (BL) is representative of the indirect, rigid fiberoptic laryngoscopes and its use has been most widely reviewed.[14,38,39,43,68,77,112,165] Minimal mouth opening is required for insertion of the blade of the BL, and there is no need to align the oral, pharyngeal, and laryngeal axes in order to view the larynx. Its use has been reported in a variety of circumstances, including patients with both normal and abnormal airways, cervical spine instability, rapid sequence intubations, and awake patients. The time to successful intubation is not affected by the laryngoscopic grade.[43]

The BL is a viable alternative in the difficult maternal airway setting. There are a number of conditions in which an indirect, rigid laryngoscope may be advantageous. These include limitation of mouth opening from any cause as well as congenital or acquired conditions that lead to distortion of the upper airway and inability to align the airway axes. The rigid structure of the BL allows it to achieve an "endoscopic airspace" to allow anatomic visualization, a property not characteristic of flexible endoscopes. This may facilitate the manipulation of excess pathologic (tumor) or nonpathologic tissue (obesity, lingual

tonsil, edematous tissues) in the airway. The BL is more resistant to the effects of cricoid pressure than is a flexible fiberoptic endoscope.[170]

3. The Role of the Flexible Fiberoptic Endoscopes

Tracheal intubation with a flexible fiberoptic endoscope (FFE) is a technique particularly well suited for endotracheal intubation in the awake patient, although intubation can be done in the unconscious or anesthetized patient. In Rose and Cohen's review of 18,500 patients, the FFE was the most commonly utilized alternative to the direct laryngoscope, electively or in the event of unanticipated difficult intubation.[155] Unfortunately, use of the FFE may be rendered more difficult by induction of general anesthesia. Loss of consciousness is associated with a loss of tone in the muscles that support the tongue and indirectly support the epiglottis. Posterior movement of the tongue and epiglottis can then obstruct the airway at the level of the pharynx and larynx, respectively. The degree of obstruction is influenced by variations in airway anatomy, body habitus, and depth of coma. In addition, in the unconscious individual, reduction of the caliber of the pharyngeal lumen makes fiberoptic visualization more difficult. Contact of the lens with the mucosa results in complete loss of the visual field, and thus one's ability to maneuver past an epiglottis in contact with the posterior pharyngeal wall is limited. Although the FFE is a useful device in the hands of experienced operators for the management of the difficult airway, its effectiveness may be somewhat compromised in the unconscious or anesthetized patient and when cricoid pressure is being applied.[137]

V. SUMMARY

Muir posed the question, "Is general anesthesia for obstetric patients obsolete?"[124] In response to her own query, she noted that, although uncommonly used in academic centers, general anesthesia remains a widely employed technique for operative delivery, including elective cesarean section. General anesthesia may be induced rapidly, provides reliably good operative conditions, maintains hemodynamic stability, and usually renders the patient unaware. Further, there remain situations in obstetric anesthesia for which general anesthesia represents the anesthetic technique of choice and many more for which it is an ideal, although not exclusively so, choice. General anesthesia continues to be a useful, occasionally lifesaving (fetal and maternal) technique that will occupy the anesthetic landscape for the foreseeable future.

The major limitation to the use of general anesthesia is the requirement to maintain the airway and protect it from the threat of acid aspiration. Rapid sequence induction, cricoid pressure, and endotracheal intubation are the mechanisms usually employed to achieve these goals.

However, it must be recognized that the appropriate endpoints are maintaining and protecting the airway and ensuring maternal oxygenation and not necessarily achieving endotracheal intubation. These goals can be achieved through a variety of techniques and modalities, some recently introduced to anesthesia. The safety of general anesthesia will be enhanced with assessment of at-risk patients by obstetricians and appropriate referral for anesthetic consultation, routine preoperative (elective and emergent situations) maternal airway assessments, strict avoidance of general anesthesia when the airway is deemed to be difficult, automatic implementation of a practiced failed intubation drill when intubation difficulties become manifest, and ensuring physician familiarity with new and novel equipment designed to aid in the management of the difficult airway. Such cooperative management schemes are effective in identifying at-risk patients and will be instrumental in reducing maternal morbidity and mortality in the future.

REFERENCES

1. Adnet F, Baillard C, Borron SW, et al: Randomized study comparing the "sniffing position" with simple head extension for laryngoscopic view in elective surgery patients. Anesthesiology 95:836-841, 2001.
2. Allison A, McCrory J: Tracheal placement of a gum elastic bougie using the laryngeal mask airway. Anaesthesia 45:419-420, 1990.
3. Allman KG: The effect of cricoid pressure on airway patency. J Clin Anesth 7:197-199, 1995.
4. American College of Obstetricians and Gynecologists: Intrapartum Fetal Heart Rate Monitoring. Technical Bulletin 132, 1989.
5. Ansermino JM, Blogg CE: Cricoid pressure may prevent insertion of the laryngeal mask airway. Br J Anaesth 69:465-467, 1992.
6. Archer GW Jr, Marx GF: Arterial oxygen tension during apnoea in parturient women. Br J Anaesth 46:358-360, 1974.
7. Asai T, Barclay K, Power I, et al: Cricoid pressure impedes placement of the laryngeal mask airway and subsequent tracheal intubation through the mask. Br J Anaesth 72:47-51, 1994.
8. Attia RR, Ebeid AM, Fischer JE, et al: Maternal, fetal and placental gastrin concentrations. Anaesthesia 37:18-21, 1982.
9. Bainbridge ET, Temple JG, Nicholas SP, et al: Symptomatic gastro-oesphageal reflux in pregnancy: A comparative study of white Europeans and Asians in Birmingham. Br J Clin Pract 37:53-57, 1983.
10. Baraka AS, Sayyid SS, Assaf BA: Thiopental-rocuronium versus ketamine-rocuronium for rapid-sequence intubation in parturients undergoing cesarean section. Anesth Analg 84:1104-1107, 1997.
11. Barker P, Langton JA, Murphy PJ, et al: Regurgitation of gastric contents during general anaesthesia using the laryngeal mask airway. Br J Anaesth 69:314-315, 1992.
12. Baskett PJ, Parr MJ, Nolan JP: The intubating laryngeal mask. Results of a multicentre trial with an experience of 500 cases. Anaesthesia 53:1174-1179, 1998.
13. Benumof JL, Cooper SD: Quantitative improvement in laryngoscopic view by optimal external laryngeal manipulation. J Clin Anesth 8:136-140, 1996.
14. Bjoraker DG: The Bullard intubating laryngoscopes. Anesth Rev 17:64-70, 1990.
15. Bouvier-Colle MH, Varnoux N, Breart G: Maternal deaths and substandard care: The results of a confidential survey in France. Medical Experts Committee. Eur J Obstet Gynecol Reprod Biol 58:3-7, 1995.
16. Brimacombe J: Acute pharyngolaryngeal oedema and pre-eclamptic toxaemia. Anaesth Intensive Care 20:97-98, 1992.
17. Brimacombe J: Cricoid pressure and the laryngeal mask airway. Anaesthesia 46:986-987, 1991.
18. Brimacombe J, Berry A: Mechanical airway obstruction after cricoid pressure with the laryngeal mask airway. Anesth Analg 78:604-605, 1994.
19. Brimacombe J, Berry A: The laryngeal mask airway— The first ten years. Anaesth Intensive Care 21:225-226, 1993.
20. Brimacombe J, Keller C: The ProSeal laryngeal mask airway: A randomized, crossover with the standard laryngeal mask airway in paralyzed, anesthetized patients. Anesthesiology 93:104-109, 2000.
21. Brock-Utne JG, Downing JW, Seedat F: Laryngeal oedema associated with pre-eclamptic toxaemia. Anaesthesia 32:556-558, 1977.
22. Brock-Utne JG, Rubin J, Welman S, et al: The action of commonly used anti-emetics on the lower oesophageal sphincter. Br J Anaesth 50:295-298, 1978.
23. Brock-Utne JG, Rubin J, Welman S, et al: The effect of glycopyrrolate (Robinul) on the lower oesophageal sphincter. Can Anaesth Soc J 25:144-146, 1978.
24. Bruce LA, Behsudi FM: Progesterone effects on three regional gastrointestinal tissues. Life Sci 25:729-734, 1979.
25. Byrne F, Odeno-Dominah A, Kipling R: The effect of pregnancy on pulmonary nitrogen washout: A study of pre-oxygenation. Anaesthesia 42:148-150, 1987.
26. Carnie JC, Street MK, Kumar B: Emergency intubation of the trachea facilitated by suxamethonium. Observations in obstetric and general surgical patients. Br J Anaesth 58:498-501, 1986.
27. Carp H, Jayaram A, Stoll M: Ultrasound examinations of the stomach contents of parturients. Anesth Analg 74:683-687, 1992.
28. Chadwick HS: An analysis of obstetric anesthesia cases from the American Society of Anesthesiologists closed claims project database. Int J Obstet Anesth 5:258-263, 1996.
29. Chadwick IS, Vohra A: Anaesthesia for emergency caesarean section using the Brain laryngeal airway. Anaesthesia 44:261-262, 1989.
30. Cheek TG, Gutsche BB: Maternal physiologic alterations during pregnancy. In Shnider SM, Levinson G (eds): Anesthesia for Obstetrics, 3rd ed. Baltimore, Williams & Wilkins, 1993, pp 3-19.

31. Cheek TG, Gutsche BB: Pulmonary aspiration of gastric contents. In Shnider SM, Levinson G (eds): Anesthesia for Obstetrics, 3rd ed. Baltimore, Williams & Wilkins, pp 407-432.

32. Choyce A, Avidan MS, Patel C, et al: Comparison of laryngeal mask and intubating laryngeal mask insertion by the naive intubator. Br J Anaesth 84:103-105, 2000.

33. Christian AS: Failed obstetric intubation. Anaesthesia 45:995, 1990.

34. Christofides ND, Ghatei MA, Bloom SR, et al: Decreased plasma motilin concentrations in pregnancy. Br Med J 285:1453-1454, 1982.

35. Clapp JF III: Oxygen consumption during treadmill exercise before, during and after pregnancy. Am J Obstet Gynecol 161:1458-1464, 1989.

36. Clark CG, Riddoch ME: Observations on the human cardia at operation. Br J Anaesth 34:875-883, 1962.

37. Cohen SE, Jasson J, Talafre ML, et al: Does metoclopramide decrease the volume of gastric contents in patients undergoing cesarean section? Anesthesiology 61:604-607, 1984.

38. Cohn AI, Hart RT, McGraw SR, Blass NH: The Bullard laryngoscope for emergency airway management in a morbidly obese parturient. Anesth Analg 81:872-873, 1995.

39. Cohn AI, McGraw SR, King WH: Awake intubation of the adult trachea using the Bullard laryngoscope. Can J Anaesth 42:246-248, 1995.

40. Colman RD, Frank M, Loughnan BA, et al: Use of IM ranitidine for the prophylaxis of aspiration pneumonitis in obstetrics. Br J Anaesth 61:720-729, 1988.

41. Committee on Obstetrics. Maternal and Fetal Medicine: Anesthesia for emergency deliveries. American College of Obstetricians and Gynecologists, Committee Opinion 104, 1992.

42. Cook TM: Cricoid pressure: Are two hands better than one? Anaesthesia 51:365-368, 1996.

43. Cooper SD, Benumof JL, Ozaki GT: Evaluation of the Bullard laryngoscope using the new intubating stylet: Comparison with conventional laryngoscopy. Anesth Analg 79:965-970, 1994.

44. Crowley DS, Giesecke AH: Bimanual cricoid pressure. Anaesthesia 45:588-589, 1990.

45. Datta S, Briwa J: Modified laryngoscope for endotracheal intubation of obese patients. Anesth Analg 60:120-121, 1981.

46. Davies JM, Weeks S, Crone LA, et al: Difficult intubation in the parturient. Can J Anaesth 36:668-674, 1989.

47. Dewan DM: Anesthesia for the morbidly obese parturient. Prob Anesth 3:56-68, 1989.

48. Dobb G: Laryngeal oedema complicating obstetric anaesthesia. Anaesthesia 33:839-840, 1978.

49. Dogra S, Falconer R, Latto IP: Successful difficult intubation: Tracheal tube placement over a gum-elastic bougie. Anaesthesia 45:774-776, 1990.

50. Dow TGB, Brock-Utne JG, Rubin J, et al: The effect of atropine on the lower oesophageal sphincter in late pregnancy. Obstet Gynecol 51:426-430, 1978.

51. Ebert RJ: Post partum airway obstruction after vaginal delivery. Anaesth Intensive Care 20:365-367, 1992.

52. El Mikatti N, Luthra D, Healy TEJ, Mortimer AJ: Gastric regurgitation during general anaesthesia in the supine position with the laryngeal and face mask airways. Br J Anaesth 69:529P-530P, 1992.

53. Ewart MC, Yau G, Gin T, et al: A comparison of the effects of omeprazole and ranitidine on gastric secretion in women undergoing elective Caesarean section. Anaesthesia 45:527-530, 1990.

54. Ezri T, Szmuk P, Stein A, et al: Peripartum general anesthesia without tracheal intubation; incidence of aspiration pneumonia. Anaesthesia 55:421-426, 2000.

55. Fahy L, Horton WA, Sprigge JS, et al: X-ray laryngoscopy in patients with a history of difficult laryngoscopy during pregnancy. Br J Anaesth 62:234P, 1989.

56. Farcon EL, Kim MH, Marx GF: Changing Mallampati score during labour. Can J Anaesth 41:50-5, 1994.

57. Farmery AD, Roe PG: A model to describe the rate of oxyhemoglobin desaturation during apnoea. Br J Anaesth 76:284-291, 1996.

58. Fisher RS, Roberts GS, Grabowski CJ, et al: Inhibition of lower esophageal sphincter circular muscle by female sex hormones. Am J Physiol 23:E243-E247, 1978.

59. Forrester PC: Active vomiting during cricoid pressure. Anaesthesia 40:388, 1985.

60. Frass M, Frenzer R, Mayer G, et al: Mechanical ventilation with the esophageal tracheal Combitube (ETC) in the intensive care unit. Arch Emerg Med 94:219-225, 1987.

61. Frass M, Frenzer R, Rauscha F, et al: Evaluation of esophageal tracheal Combitube in cardiopulmonary resuscitation. Crit Care Med 15:609-611, 1986.

62. Frass M, Frenzer R, Zahler J: Ventilation via the esophageal tracheal combitube in a case of difficult intubation. J Cardiothor Anesth 1:565-568, 1987.

63. Freeman R, Baxendale B: Laryngeal mask airway for Caesarean section. Anaesthesia 45:1094-1095, 1990.

64. Gabbott DA: Laryngoscopy using the McCoy laryngoscope after application of a cervical collar. Anaesthesia 51:812-814, 1996.

65. Gaiser RR, McGonigal ET, Litts P, et al: Obstetricians' ability to assess the airway. Obstet Gynecol 93:648-652, 1999.

66. Gamber AM, Hertzka RE, Fisher DM: Preoxygenation techniques: Comparison of three minutes and four breaths. Anesth Analg 66:468-470, 1987.

67. Gibbs CP, Banner TC: Effectiveness of Bicitra as a preoperative antacid. Anesthesiology 61:97-99, 1984.

68. Gorback MS: Management of the challenging airway with the Bullard laryngoscope. J Clin Anesth 3:473-477, 1991.

69. Greenan J: The cardio-oesophageal junction. Br J Anaesth 33:432-439, 1961.

70. Hall AW, Moossa AR, Clark J, et al: The effects of premedication drugs on the lower oesophageal high pressure zone and reflux status of rhesus monkeys and man. Gut 16:347-352, 1975.

71. Han TH, Brimacombe J, Lee EJ, Yang HS: The laryngeal mask is effective (and probably safe) in selected healthy parturients for elective Cesarean section: A prospective study of 1067 cases. Can J Anaesth 48:1117-1121, 2001.

72. Harmer M, Rubin AP: Only maternal, not fetal, survival should persuade the anaesthetist to proceed with general anaesthesia for caesarean section after failed intubation. Int J Obstet Anesth 2:100-102, 1993.

73. Harry RM, Nolan JP: The use of cricoid pressure with the intubating laryngeal mask. Anaesthesia 54:656-659, 1999.

74. Hartsilver EL, Vanner RG: Airway obstruction with cricoid pressure. Anaesthesia 55:208-211, 2000.

75. Hartsilver EL, Vanner RG, Bewley J, Clayton T: Gastric pressure during emergency caesarean section under general anaesthesia. Br J Anaesth 82:752-754, 1999.

76. Hashman FM, Andrews PJD, Juneja MM, et al: The laryngeal mask airway facilitates intubation at cesarean section. A case report of difficult intubation. Int J Obstet Anesth 2:181-183, 1993.

77. Hastings RH, Vigil AC, Hanna R, et al: Cervical spine movement during laryngoscopy with the Bullard, Macintosh and Miller laryngoscopes. Anesthesiology 82:859-869, 1995.

78. Hawkins JL, Johnson TD, Kubicek MA, et al: Vecuronium for rapid-sequence intubation for cesarean section. Anesth Analg 71:185-190, 1990.

79. Hawkins JL, Koonin LM, Palmer SK, Gibbs CP: Anesthesia-related deaths during obstetric delivery in the United States, 1979-1990. Anesthesiology 86: 277-284, 1997.

80. Hawthorne L, Wilson R, Lyons G, Dresener M: Failed intubation revisited: 17-yr experience in a teaching maternity unit. Br J Anaesth 76:680-684, 1996.

81. Heath ML: Endotracheal intubation through the laryngeal mask airway: Helpful when laryngoscopy is difficult or dangerous. Eur J Anaesth Suppl 4:41-42, 1991.

82. Heath ML, Allagain J: Intubation through the laryngeal mask. A technique for unexpected difficult intubation. Anaesthesia 46:545-548, 1991.

83. Hewett E, Livingstone P: Management of failed endotracheal intubation at caesarean section. Anaesth Intensive Care 18:330-335, 1990.

84. Hey VMF, Cowley DJ, Ganguli PC, et al: Gastro-esophageal reflux in late pregnancy. Anaesthesia 32: 372-377, 1977.

85. Hey VMF, Ostick DG, Mazumder JK, et al: Pethidine, metoclopramide and the gastro-oesophageal sphincter: A study in healthy volunteers. Anaesthesia 36:173-176, 1981.

86. Hibbard LT: Placenta previa. Am J Obstet Gynecol 104:172-184, 1969.

87. Hirschheimer A, January D, Daversa JJ: An X-ray study of gastric function in labor. Am J Obstet Gynecol 36:671-673, 1938.

88. Hodgson RE, Gopalan PD, Burrows RC, Zuma K: Effect of cricoid pressure on the success of endotracheal intubation with a lightwand. Anesthesiology 94:259-262, 2001.

89. Howard FA, Sharp DS: Effect of metoclopramide on gastric emptying during labour. Br Med J 1:446-448, 1973.

90. Huddleston JF: Electronic fetal monitoring. In Eden RD, Boehm FH, Haire M (eds): Assessment and Care of the Fetus. Physiological, Clinical and Medicolegal Principles. Norwalk, Conn, Appleton & Lange, 1990, pp 449-457.

91. Hung OR, Pytka S, Morris I, et al: Lightwand intubation: II. Clinical trial of a new lightwand for tracheal intubation in patients with difficult airways. Can J Anaesth 42:826-830, 1995.

92. Hung OR, Stewart RD: Lightwand intubation: I—A new lightwand device. Can J Anaesth 42:820-825, 1995.

93. James CF, Gibbs CP, Banner T: Postpartum perioperative risk of aspiration pneumonia. Anesthesiology 61:756-759, 1984.

94. Jouppila R, Jouppila P, Hollmén A: Laryngeal oedema as an obstetric anaesthesia complication. Acta Anaesthesiol Scand 24:97-98, 1980.

95. Karkouti K, Rose DK, Ferris LE, et al: Inter-observer reliability of ten tests used for predicting difficult tracheal intubation. Can J Anaesth 43:554-559, 1996.

96. Katz M, Meizner I, Insler V: Fetal Well-Being. Physiological Basis and Methods of Clinical Assessment. Boca Raton, Fla, CRC Press, 1990, pp 129-159.

97. Kaunitz AM, Hughes JM, Grimes DA, et al: Causes of maternal mortality in the United States. Am J Obstet Gynecol 65:605-612, 1985.

98. Kay NH: Mammomegaly and intubation. Anaesthesia 37:221, 1982.

99. Kidd JF, Dyson A, Latto IP: Successful difficult intubation. Use of the gum elastic bougie. Anaesthesia 43:437-438, 1988.

100. Koonin LM, Mackay AP, Berg CJ, et al: Pregnancy-related mortality surveillance—United States, 1987-90. MMWR CDC Surveill Summ 46(4):17-36, 1997.

101. Krantz ML, Edwards WL: The incidence of nonfatal aspiration in obstetric patients. Anesthesiology 39:359, 1973.

102. Langeron O, Masso E, Huraux C, et al: Prediction of difficult mask ventilation. Anesthesiology 92:1229-1236, 2000.

103. Langeron O, Semjen F, Bourgain JL, et al: Comparison of the intubating laryngeal mask with the fiberoptic intubation in anticipated difficult airway management. Anesthesiology 94:968-972, 2001.

104. Laurent SC, de Melo AE, Alexander-Williams JM: The use of the McCoy laryngoscope in patients with simulated cervical spine injuries. Anaesthesia 51:74-75, 1996.

105. Lawes EG, Campbell I, Mercer D: Inflation pressure, gastric insufflation and rapid sequence induction. Br J Anaesth 59:315-318, 1987.

106. Lawes EG, Duncan PW, Bland B, et al: The cricoid yoke—A device for providing consistent and reproducible cricoid pressure. Br J Anaesth 58:925-931, 1986.

107. Lawlor M, Johnson C, Weiner M: Airway management in obstetric anesthesia. Int J Obstet Anaesth 3:225-230, 1993.

108. Lind JF, Smith A, McIver DR, et al: Heartburn in pregnancy: A manometric study. Can Med Assoc J 98:571-574, 1968.

109. MacG Palmer JH, Ball DR: The effect of cricoid pressure on the cricoid cartilage and vocal cords: An endoscopic study in anaesthetised patients. Anaesthesia 55:263-268, 2000.

110. MacKenzie AI: Laryngeal oedema complicating obstetric anaesthesia. Anaesthesia 33:271-272, 1978.

111. Marx GF, Luykx WM, Cohen S: Fetal-neonatal status following caesarean section for fetal distress. Br J Anaesth 56:1009-1013. 1984.

112. McClune S, Regan M, Moore J: Laryngeal mask airway for Caesarean section. Anaesthesia 45:227-228, 1990.

113. McFarlane C: Failed intubation in the obese obstetric patient and the laryngeal mask. Int J Obstet Anaesth 2:183-185, 1993.

114. McMurray RG, Katz VL, Berry MJ, et al: The effect of pregnancy on metabolic responses during rest, immersion and aerobic exercise in the water. Am J Obstet Gynecol 158:481-486, 1988.

115. Meek T, Gittins N, Duggan JE: Cricoid pressure: Knowledge and performance amongst anaesthetic assistants. Anaesthesia 54:59-62, 1999.

116. Meek T, Vincent A, Duggan JE: Cricoid pressure: Can protective force be sustained? Br J Anaesth 80:672-674, 1998.

117. Mendel P, Bristow A: Anaesthesia for procedures on the larynx and pharynx. The use of the Bullard laryngoscope in conjunction with high frequency jet ventilation. Anaesthesia 48:263-265, 1993.

118. Mendelson CL: The aspiration of stomach contents into the lungs during obstetric anesthesia. Am J Obstet Gynecol 52:191-205, 1946.

119. Morgan BM, Magni V, Goroszenuik T: Anaesthesia for emergency caesarean section. Br J Obstet Gynecol 97:420-424, 1990.

120. Morgan J: Placenta previa, report on a series of 538 cases. J Obstet Gynecol Br Commonw 72:700, 1965.

121. Morgan M: Anaesthetic contribution to maternal mortality. Br J Anaesth 59:842-855, 1987.

122. Morris J, Cook TM: Rapid sequence induction: A national survey of practice. Anaesthesia 56:1090-1115, 2001.

123. Moynihan RJ, Brock-Utne JG, Archer JH, et al: The effect of cricoid pressure on preventing gastric insufflation in infants and children. Anesthesiology 78:652-656, 1993.

124. Muir HA: General anaesthesia for obstetrics, is it obsolete? Can J Anaesth 41:R20-R25, 1994.

125. Murphy DF, Nally B, Gardiner J, et al: Effect of metoclopramide on gastric emptying before elective and emergency Caesarean section. Br J Anaesth 56:1113-1116, 1984.

126. Nanji GM, Maltby JR: Vomiting and aspiration pneumonitis with the laryngeal mask airway. Can J Anaesth 39:69-70, 1992.

127. National Committee on Confidential Enquiries into Maternal Deaths: A review of maternal deaths in South Africa during 1998. S Afr Med J 90:367-373, 2000.

128. Nolan JP, Wilson ME: Orotracheal intubation in patients with potential cervical spine injuries. An indication for the gum elastic bougie. Anaesthesia 48:630-633, 1993.

129. Norris MC, Dewan DM: Preoxygenation for cesarean section: A comparison of two techniques. Anesthesiology 62:827-829, 1985.

130. Norris MC, Kirkland MR, Torjman MC, et al: Denitrogenation in pregnancy. Can J Anaesth 36:523-525, 1989.

131. Notcutt WG: Rupture of the oesphagus following cricoid pressure? Anaesthesia 36:911, 1981

132. Olsson GL, Hallen B, Hambraeus-Jonzon K: Aspiration during anaesthesia: A computer-aided study of 185,358 anaesthetists. Acta Anaesthesiol Scand 30:84-92, 1986.

133. Ormezzano X, Francois TP, Viaud JY, et al: Aspiration pneumonitis prophylaxis in obstetric anesthesia: Comparison of effervescent-sodium citrate mixture and sodium citrate. Br J Anaesth 64:503-506, 1990.

134. Ostheimer GW: The labor and delivery suite. In Ostheimer GW (ed): Manual of Obstetric Anesthesia. New York, Churchill Livingstone, 1984, pp. 399-412.

135. O'Sullivan G: Gastric emptying during pregnancy and the puerperium. Int J Obstet Anaesth 2:216-224, 1993.

136. Panchal S, Arria AM, Labhsetwar SA: Maternal mortality during hospital admission for delivery: A retrospective analysis using a state-maintained database. Anesth Analg 93:134-141, 2001.

137. Pandit JJ, Dravid RM, Iyer R, Popat MT: Orotracheal fiberoptic intubation for rapid sequence induction of anaesthesia. Anaesthesia 57:123-127, 2002.

138. Parer JT: Diagnosis and management of fetal asphyxia. In Shnider SM, Levinson G (eds): Anesthesia for Obstetrics, 3rd ed. Baltimore, Williams & Wilkins, 1993, pp 657-670.

139. Parer JT, Livingstone EG: What is fetal distress? Am J Obstet Gynecol 162:1421-1427, 1990.

140. Petito SP, Russell WJ: The prevention of gastric insufflation—A neglected benefit of cricoid pressure. Anaesth Intensive Care 16:139-143, 1988.

141. Preston R, Halpern SH, Petras A: Quality assurance in obstetrical anaesthesia. Can J Anaesth 41:A28, 1994.

142. Priscu V, Priscu L, Soroker D: Laryngeal mask for failed intubation in emergency cesarean section. Can J Anaesth 39:893, 1992.

143. Procter AJM, White JB: Laryngeal oedema in pregnancy. Anaesthesia 38:167, 1983.

144. Rabey PG, Murphy PJ, Langton JA, et al: Effect of the laryngeal mask airway on lower oesophageal sphincter pressure in patients during general anaesthesia. Br J Anaesth 69:346-348, 1992.

145. Ralph SJ, Wareham CA: Rupture of the oesophagus during cricoid pressure. Anaesthesia 46:40-41, 1991.

146. Report on Confidential Enquiries into Maternal Deaths in England and Wales 1982-84. London, Her Majesty's Stationery Office, 1989.

147. Report on Confidential Enquiries into Maternal Deaths in the United Kingdom 1985-87. London, Her Majesty's Stationery Office, 1991.

148. Report on Confidential Enquiries into Maternal Deaths in the United Kingdom 1988-90. London, Her Majesty's Stationery Office, 1994.

149. Report on Confidential Enquiries into Maternal Deaths in the United Kingdom 1991-93. London, Her Majesty's Stationery Office, 1996.

150. Rochat RW, Koonin LM, Atrash HK, et al: Maternal mortality in the United States: Report from the maternal mortality collaborative. Obstet Gynecol 72:91-97, 1989.

151. Rocke DA, Murray WB, Rout CC, et al: Relative risk analysis of factors associated with difficult intubation in obstetric anesthesia. Anesthesiology 77:67-73, 1992.

152. Rocke DA, Rout CC, Gouws E: Intravenous administration of the proton pump inhibitor omeprazole reduces the risk of acid aspiration at emergency cesarean section. Anesth Analg 78:1093-1098, 1994.

153. Rocke DA, Scoones GP: Rapidly progressive laryngeal oedema associated with pregnancy aggravated hypertension. Anaesthesia 47:141-143, 1992.

154. Roe RB: The effect of suxamethonium on intragastric pressure. Anaesthesia 17:179-185, 1962.

155. Rose DK, Cohen MM: The airway: Problems and predictions in 18,500 patients. Can J Anaesth 41: 372-383, 1994.

156. Rosen M: Difficult and failed intubation in obstetrics. In Latto IP, Rosen M (eds): Difficulties in Tracheal Intubation. London, Bailliére Tindall, 1985.

157. Rout CC, Rocke DA, Gouws E: Intravenous ranitidine reduces the risk of acid aspiration of gastric contents at emergency cesarean section. Anesth Analg 73:156-161, 1993.

158. Ruben H, Krudsen EJ, Carngati G: Gastric inflation in relation to airway pressure. Acta Anaesthesiol Scand 5:107-112, 1961.

159. Russell GN, Smith CL, Snowden SL, et al: Preoxygenation and the parturient patient. Anaesthesia 42:346-351, 1987.

160. Sachs BP, Oriol NE, Ostheimer GW, et al: Anesthetic-related maternal mortality, 1954 to 1985. J Clin Anesth 1:333-338, 1989.

161. Saddler JM, Bevan JC, Plumley MH, et al: Jaw tension after succinylcholine in children undergoing strabismus surgery. Can J Anaesth 37:21-22, 1990.

162. Salt PJ, Nutbourne PA, Park GR, et al: Laryngeal oedema after Caesarean section. Anaesthesia 38: 693-694, 1983.

163. Samsoon GLT, Young JRB: Difficult tracheal intubation: A retrospective study. Anaesthesia 42: 487-490, 1987.

164. Sandhar BK, Elliott RH, Windram I, et al: Peripartum changes in gastric emptying. Anaesthesia 47:196-198, 1992.

165. Saunders PR, Geisecke AH: Clinical assessment of the adult Bullard laryngoscope. Can J Anaesth 36:S118-S119, 1989.

166. Seager SJ, MacDonald R: Laryngeal oedema and pre-eclampsia. Anaesthesia 35:360-362, 1980.

167. Sellick BA: Cricoid pressure to control regurgitation of stomach contents during induction of anaesthesia. Lancet 2:404-406, 1961.

168. Sellick BA: Rupture of the oesophagus following cricoid pressure? Anaesthesia 37:213-214, 1982.

169. Shnider SM, Levinson G: Anesthesia for cesarean section. In Shnider SM, Levinson G (eds): Anesthesia for Obstetrics, 3rd ed. Baltimore, Williams & Wilkins, 1993, pp 211-246.

170. Shulman GB, Connelly NR: A comparison of the Bullard laryngoscope versus the flexible fiberoptic bronchoscope during intubation in patients afforded inline stabilization. J Clin Anesth 13:182-185, 2001.

171. Smith G, Dalling R, Williams TIR: Gastroesophageal pressure gradients produced by induction of anaesthesia and suxamethonium. Br J Anaesth 50:1137-1143, 1978.

172. Smith I, White PF: Use of the laryngeal mask airway as an alternative to a face mask during outpatient arthroscopy. Anesthesiology 77:850-855, 1992.

173. Sparr HJ, Luger TJ, Heidegger T, Putensen-Himmer G: Comparison of intubating conditions after rocuronium and succinylcholine following "rapid-sequence induction" with thiopentone in elective cases. Acta Anaesthesiol Scand 40:425-430, 1996.

174. Spence AA, Moir DD, Finlay WEI: Observations on intragastric pressure. Anaesthesia 22:249-253, 1967.

175. Spotoft H, Christensen P: Laryngeal oedema accompanying weight gain in pregnancy. Anaesthesia 36:71, 1981.

176. Storey J: The laryngeal mask for failed intubation at caesarean section. Anaesth Intensive Care 20:118-119, 1992.

177. Takahata O, Kubota M, Mamiya K, et al: The efficacy of the "BURP" maneuver during a difficult laryngoscopy. Anesth Analg 84:419-421, 1997.

178. Tham EJ, Gildersleve CD, Sanders LD, et al: Effects of posture, phonation and observer on Mallampati classification. Br J Anaesth 68:32-38, 1992.

179. Thwaites AJ, Rice CP, Smith I: Rapid sequence induction; a questionnaire survey of its routine conduct and continued management during a failed intubation. Anaesthesia 54:376-381, 1999.

180. Tillmann Hein HA: Cardiorespiratory arrest with laryngeal oedema in pregnancy-induced hypertension. Can Anaesth Soc J 31:210-212, 1984.

181. Tordoff SG, Sweeney BP: Acid aspiration prophylaxis in 288 obstetric anaesthetic departments in the United Kingdom. Anaesthesia 45:776-780, 1990.

182. Tunstall ME: Failed intubation drill. Anaesthesia 31:850, 1976.

183. Tunstall ME, Geddes C: Failed intubation in obstetric anaesthesia. An indication for use of the "esophageal gastric tube airway." Br J Anaesth 56: 659-661, 1984.

184. Tunstall ME, Sheikh A: Failed intubation protocol: Oxygenation without aspiration. Clin Anaesth 4: 171-187, 1986.

185. Uchida T, Hikawa Y, Saito Y, Yasuda K: The McCoy levering laryngoscope in patients with limited neck extension. Can J Anaesth 44:674-676, 1997.

186. Vanner RG: Mini-symposium on the gastrointestinal tract and pulmonary aspiration: Mechanisms of regurgitation and its prevention with cricoid pressure. Int J Obstet Anaesth 2:207-215, 1993.

187. Vanner RG: Tolerance of cricoid pressure by conscious volunteers. Int J Obstet Anesth 1; 195-198, 1992.

188. Vanner RG, Goodman NW: Gastro-oesophageal reflux in pregnancy at term and after delivery. Anaesthesia 44:808-811, 1989.

189. Vanner RG, O'Dwyer JP, Pryle BJ: Upper oesophageal sphincter pressure and the effect of cricoid pressure. Anaesthesia 47:95-100, 1992.

190. Vanner RG, Pryle BJ: Regurgitation and oesophageal rupture with cricoid pressure: A cadaver study. Anaesthesia 47:732-735, 1992.

191. Viegas OJ, Ravindran RS, Schumacker CA: Gastric fluid pH in patients receiving sodium citrate. Anesth Analg 60:521-523, 1981.

192. Viegas OJ, Ravindram RS, Stoops CA: Duration of action of sodium citrate as an antacid. Anesth Analg 61:624, 1982.

193. Wald A, Van Thiel DH, Hoechspetter L, et al: Gastrointestinal transit: The effect of the menstrual cycle. Gastroenterology 80:1497-1500, 1981.

194. Whitehead EM, Smith M, Dean Y, et al: An evaluation of gastric emptying times in pregnancy and the puerperium. Anaesthesia 48:53-57, 1993.

195. Whittington RM, Robinson JS, Thompson JM: Fatal aspiration (Mendelson's) syndrome despite antacids and cricoid pressure. Lancet 2:228-230, 1979.

196. Why Mothers Die. Report on Confidential Enquiries into Maternal Deaths in the United Kingdom 1994-96. London, Stationery Office, 1999.

197. Wraight WJ, Chamney AR, Howells TH: The determination of an effective cricoid pressure. Anaesthesia 38:461-466, 1983.

198. Yentis SM: The effects of single-handed and bimanual cricoid pressure on the view at laryngoscopy. Anaesthesia 52:332-335, 1997.

35

ANESTHESIA AND AIRWAY MANAGEMENT OF LARYNGOSCOPY AND BRONCHOSCOPY

Ian R. Morris

I. INTRODUCTION

Anesthetic and airway management for laryngoscopy and bronchoscopy has inherent risks and requires an organized approach. As time and circumstances permit, airway pathology should be defined prior to any airway intervention and a primary plan of airway management developed, as well as alternative plans should the primary technique fail.

Anesthetic requirements include airway control, adequate ventilation, attenuation of unwanted reflexes, appropriate monitoring, prevention of aspiration, and, in most circumstances, prompt emergence.[14,42,78,89,109] Surgical or endoscopic requirements include adequate visualization of and access to the airway, immobility of the larynx for microsurgery, mobility to permit assessment of laryngeal function, adequate time for diagnostic evaluation and therapeutic intervention, and safety during laser deployment.[14,42,89]

As the anesthesiologist and endoscopist must share the airway during laryngoscopic and bronchoscopic procedures, a high level of communication and cooperation is required if the patient's safety is to be optimized. The anesthesiologist must understand the surgical requirements, equipment, and technique; and conversely, the endoscopist must understand the principles of anesthetic and airway management.[14] No single anesthetic or airway management technique is suitable for all circumstances, and each has inherent advantages and disadvantages.[14,26,42,69,89] The technique chosen should be individualized to the age of the patient, the site and extent of the pathology, the clinical setting, and the expertise of the operator.[14,17,42,105] Familiarity with a variety of techniques is desirable.

II. PATIENT EVALUATION

Patients presenting for laryngoscopic and bronchoscopic procedures require the same meticulous systematic preoperative airway evaluation, as do any other patients presenting for anesthetic and airway management. Anatomic variation and limitation of joint movement, which may be associated with difficult intubation or difficult mask ventilation, should be identified on physical examination. Any history of previous airway management should be reviewed, including prior anesthetic records, and the operator should proceed with caution should there be a history of past intubation difficulties.[145]

In addition to the presence of anatomic variants and limitation of joint movement, the patient presenting for airway endoscopy may have airway pathology that can make intubation and mask ventilation more difficult. Upper airway pathology includes *supraglottic* lesions such as benign and malignant tumors, infection, and laryngomalacia; *glottic* abnormalities such as vocal cord palsy, papillomatosis, neoplasm, or edema; and *subglottic* disease such as tumor, stenosis, or tracheomalacia. On preoperative evaluation, the location, size, and mobility of the airway disease should be assessed as precisely as possible.[42] The extent of airway obstruction and the site of the obstruction (supraglottic, glottic, or subglottic) should be determined, as should the rapidity of its progression.[14,42]

Stridor is produced by partial airway obstruction at the level of the larynx or trachea[37,43,97] and occurs at rest when the diameter of the airway has been reduced to 4 mm.[43,97] Stridor on exertion occurs when the diameter of the airway has been reduced to 4 to 6 mm.[43,97] Stridor may also be positional if the causative lesion is mobile.[42] Inspiratory stridor is usually associated with supraglottic or glottic lesions, whereas expiratory stridor is more commonly associated with subglottic obstruction.[42,70,97] *Hoarseness* implies dysfunction, or pathology at the level of the vocal cords, whereas a weak voice can be produced by decreased airflow insufficient to produce normal phonation.[42] *Aphonia* occurs in the presence of complete airway obstruction.[57,97] *Snoring* sounds are associated with

obstruction at the level of the pharynx, and *expiratory wheezing* implies bronchial obstruction.[97,119] *Cough* can be voluntary or due to mechanical, thermal, or chemical stimulation of cough receptors.[77,97] A cough with a barking or croupy quality is typically associated with subglottic pathology, whereas a "brassy" cough implies tracheobronchial disease.[77,97] *Drooling* in the context of respiratory distress is classically associated with acute epiglottitis but also occurs in association with esophageal obstruction and organophosphate poisoning.[97]

The presence of surgical scars should be noted, as should evidence of induration and fibrosis associated with previous radiotherapy.[42] Edema secondary to irradiation of the larynx may require 6 to 12 months to resolve.[51] In the setting of airway trauma, the presence or absence of external bruising, hematoma, and subcutaneous emphysema should also be noted and cervical spine integrity evaluated as required. Clinical evaluation of the *degree* of airway obstruction and respiratory distress includes assessment of the level of consciousness, agitation, cyanosis, respiratory rate and chest wall excursion, heart rate and blood pressure, voice quality, and upper airway noise.

In the elective setting, additional information with regard to the location, size, and mobility of the airway disease may be obtainable by means of special radiographic studies, such as computed tomographic (CT) scans and magnetic resonance imaging.[42] Indirect, telescopic, or fiberoptic laryngoscopy performed in the awake patient under local anesthesia can also be used to define the airway pathology further.[14,42]

Following evaluation of the patient, an assessment of the likelihood of increased airway obstruction following sedation or the induction of general anesthesia (GA), as a result of a decrease in muscle tone or a change in position of a mobile lesion, should be performed.[42,89] The likelihood of difficult mask ventilation, difficult laryngoscopy, and difficult intubation should also be assessed.[42,89]

Comorbidities must also be evaluated. In particular, ischemic heart disease, hypertension, and chronic obstructive lung disease are frequently found in adult patients presenting for airway endoscopy.[42]

III. MONITORING

During GA for laryngoscopy and bronchoscopy, the continuous presence of a vigilant, appropriately trained, and experienced anesthesiologist is indispensable.[14,58] Monitoring should include heart rate, blood pressure, electrocardiogram, pulse oximetry, and, where possible, end-tidal CO_2 waveforms.[14,42,58] During supraglottic jet ventilation, measurement of end-tidal CO_2 is problematic. End-tidal CO_2 can be measured during subglottic jet ventilation utilizing a modified Benjamin jet tube that incorporates a carbon dioxide and pressure monitoring port.[26,69] Chest excursions must be observed during manual jet ventilation, and an assessment of intrathoracic pressure is necessary during high-frequency ventilation (HFV). A precordial, esophageal, or paratracheal stethoscope should be exclusively available, as should equipment to measure temperature.[58] When technically possible, measurement of tidal volume can be useful and a spirometer should be immediately available.[58]

When neuromuscular blocking agents are administered, a peripheral nerve stimulator should be utilized. The response of the orbicularis oculi to muscle relaxants correlates more closely with the response of the laryngeal muscles than does the adductor pollicis.[40,42,121] Monitoring the response of the orbicularis oculi may therefore be more appropriate during endoscopy.[40,42,121] However, monitoring neuromuscular blockade at the orbicularis oculi may underestimate the level of blockade at the muscles of respiration.[42] Additional clinical evidence of adequate reversal of muscle relaxants should exist before extubation. Gastric distention can occur during supraglottic jet ventilation.[69] Abdominal distention during the procedure should be noted and the stomach decompressed as necessary.[143] Adequate lighting to visualize an exposed portion of the patient must be available, and, where feasible, the use of agent-specific anesthesia gas monitors is encouraged.[58] Mechanical and electronic devices are, however, at best aids to monitoring and constant vigilance by the anesthesiologist is essential.[14,58]

IV. PREPARATION OF THE PATIENT

Comorbidities should be optimized preoperatively. Because airway secretions impair visualization and reduce the effectiveness of topically applied local anesthetics,[42] administration of antisialagogues can be of great benefit. Although these agents can be given intravenously (IV) immediately before operation, they are optimally given intramuscularly (IM) or subcutaneously (SC) 30 minutes prior to airway manipulation to permit drying of the mucosa to occur.[98,99] Either atropine or glycopyrrolate is effective, although glycopyrrolate is the more potent drying agent.[94,99] The appropriate dosage of glycopyrrolate in the adult is 0.2 to 0.4 mg IM (children, 0.01 mg/kg)[94] and of atropine 0.4 to 0.6 mg IM (children 0.01 to 0.03 mg/kg, maximum 0.6 mg).[82] Glycopyrrolate can also be administered subcutaneously.[88] It is not recommended for use in newborns when packaged in multidose vials.[116]

Local anesthesia of the airway can be used to perform brief direct laryngoscopy, the "awake look," to evaluate a potentially difficult airway.[42] Local anesthesia can also be administered preoperatively as a supplement to GA. When used prior to GA, local anesthetics can be administered by various aerosol or injection techniques.[14,42,98,99]

Preoperative sedation must be used with extreme caution in the presence of airway compromise and, if used at all, titrated carefully to effect. Either narcotics or benzodiazepines can produce useful sedation and are reversible but may precipitate increased airway obstruction.

V. LARYNGOSCOPY

A. INTRODUCTION

Since its introduction into clinical practice in the late 1800s, direct laryngoscopy has evolved into a sophisticated technique for the diagnosis and treatment of laryngeal pathology.[143,153] In its modern form, direct laryngoscopy usually includes three distinct stages.[17] Initially, a handheld direct laryngoscopy is performed for preliminary examination of the laryngopharynx with the naked eye or a telescope. The laryngoscope is then fixed in position utilizing a suspension or fulcrum device to permit a more detailed examination and diagnostic and therapeutic procedures as indicated.[17,153] Telescopes with a selection of viewing angles permit visualization of the laryngeal ventricles, posterior surface of the epiglottis, the anterior commissure, the posterior glottic space, and the subglottic region.[17,117] Finally, the operating microscope can be positioned to allow more precise microlaryngoscopy and microlaryngeal surgery.[17] Indications for operative laryngoscopy include (1) direct examination of the larynx in a patient with signs or symptoms of laryngeal disease; (2) evaluation of malignant laryngeal lesions as part of a complete endoscopic survey in the presence of a known primary carcinoma of the aerodigestive tract or metastatic neck cancer from an occult primary; (3) removal of benign, premalignant, and limited malignant laryngeal lesions; (4) evaluation of laryngeal trauma; (5) insertion or removal of laryngeal stents; (6) treatment of vocal cord paralysis; and (7) removal of foreign bodies.[14,74]

B. EQUIPMENT

The rigid laryngoscopes used by otolaryngologists consist of a tapered stainless steel tube or spatula fixed to a rigid steel handle, which forms an L- or C-shaped configuration with the barrel of the scope (Fig. 35-1). The laryngoscope is typically fitted with distal or proximal illumination and a working channel, which can be used for insufflation, suction, or jet ventilation (Fig. 35-2).[17,153] Operative laryngoscopes can be classified into general-purpose and special-purpose instruments, such as the anterior commissure scope and the subglottiscope,[14,106,153] and a selection of appropriately sized scopes is available for infants and children. If the caliber of the proximal lumen is adequate, binocular vision can be obtained.[17,106,153] In an effort to overcome the design shortcomings of preexisting operative laryngoscopes, the universal modular laryngoscope has been introduced.[153] This modification has a detachable handle, a triangular barrel, and proximal lateral slots to facilitate instrumentation of the larynx (Fig. 35-3).[153]

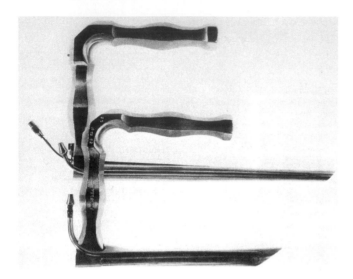

Figure 35-1 Side view of an Ossoff-Karlan modified Dedo laryngoscope (foreground) and the subglottiscope (background), demonstrating the elongated tube of the subglottiscope. (From Ossoff RH, Duncavage JA, Dere H: Microsubglottoscopy. An expansion of operative microlaryngoscopy. Otol Hand Neck Surg 104:842, 1991, Fig. 2.)

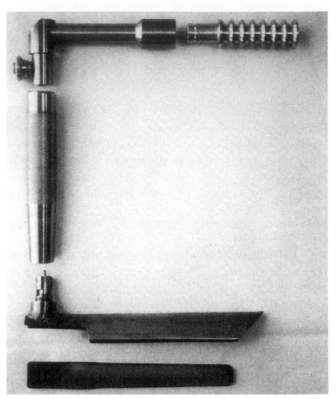

Figure 35-3 Modularity of universal modular glottiscope is well seen in this prototype. (From Zeitels SM: Universal modular glottoscope system: The evolution of a century of design and technique for direct laryngoscopy. Ann Otol Rhinol Laryngol Suppl 179:2, 1999, Fig. 41.)

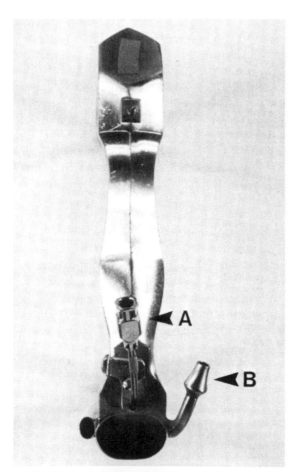

Figure 35-2 Proximal view of the subglottiscope shows (A) jet ventilation and (B) smoke evacuation ports. (From Ossoff RH, Duncavage JA, Dere H: Microsubglottoscopy. An expansion of operative microlaryngoscopy. Otol Hand Neck Surg 104:842, 1991, Fig. 3.)

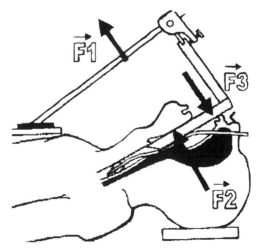

Figure 35-4 Vectorial forces applied to the patient by the standard laryngoscope holder. FI, force applied to the long lever arm; F2, force within the larynx and tongue; F3, force directed into the upper alveolus or teeth. (From Morgado PF, Abrahao M: Angled telescopic surgery, an approach for laryngeal diagnosis and surgery without suspension. Sao Paolo Med J 17:224, 1999, Fig. 1.)

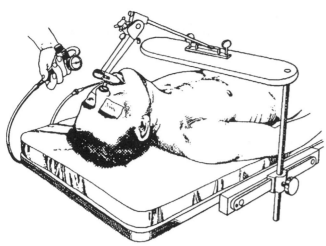

Figure 35-5 A self-retaining laryngoscope holder is securely in position, supported free of the patient's chest by a Mustard table. (From Benjamin B: Endolaryngeal Surgery. London, Martin Dunitz, 1998, Fig. 6.13.)

Once manually positioned in the larynx, the laryngoscope can be suspended to maintain or achieve optimal visualization,[17] using a fulcrum or true suspension device.[153] A fulcrum device such as the Lewy laryngoscope stabilizer is more commonly used[39,66,153] and exerts traction on the supraglottic structures by applying force to the maxilla (Fig. 35-4). The base of the device is placed on an overtable fixed to the operating room table or a free-standing support such as a Mayo stand (Fig. 35-5).[17,66,74,112] Placing the base of the device on the patient's chest can limit respiratory excursion.[17,66,112] True suspension devices that do not use the maxilla as a fulcrum such as the Boston University gallows exist and can provide better surgical exposure but are not widely used (Fig. 35-6).[153]

The ideal position of the patient for microlaryngoscopy is generally considered to be the Boyce-Jackson or sniffing position, although glottic exposure is not difficult in most patients despite suboptimal positioning.[66] Visualization of the anterior glottic commissure during direct laryngoscopy has been shown to be improved with the head and neck in flexion, but this position is not feasible for microlaryngoscopic procedures.[66] Pure flexion may, however, be the position of choice for difficult endotracheal intubation by direct laryngoscopy.[153]

C. ANESTHESIA FOR DIRECT LARYNGOSCOPY

No method of anesthesia and airway management is universally applicable to all direct laryngoscopic procedures.[14] Options include local anesthesia with or without sedation and GA utilizing endotracheal intubation, apneic oxygenation, insufflation, jet ventilation, or some combination of techniques.

1. Local Anesthesia

Direct laryngoscopy was performed almost exclusively under regional, usually topical, anesthesia until the late 1950s, when GA for direct laryngoscopy became popular.[13,27,112] Indications for direct laryngoscopy under local anesthesia include brief diagnostic examination of the airway, a requirement for phonation or a dynamic airway, minimal instrumentation, and no expected bleeding.[42]

Indirect endolaryngeal surgery under local anesthesia has been suggested as a safe, convenient, effective, and economical alternative to direct laryngoscopy in selected clinical situations.[13] In 1996, Bastian and Delsupehe reported a series of 192 indirect endolaryngopharyngeal surgeries performed in an outpatient videoendoscopy laboratory under topical anesthesia with a success rate of 96% and no complications.[13] Intravenous sedation (midazolam) was used in 39% of the patients.[13] The use of topical anesthesia for transnasal endoscopic examination of the supraglottic larynx, subglottis, and trachea with

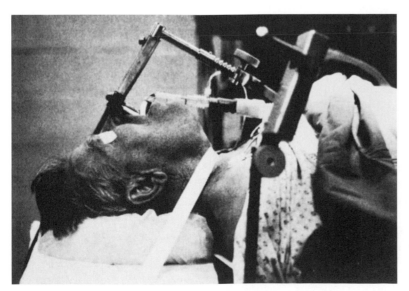

Figure 35-6 Patient in Boyce-Jackson position being maintained by Boston University gallows to achieve elevated-vector suspension. External counterpressure is applied with silk tape. (From Zeitels SM: Universal modular glottoscope system: The evolution of a century of design and technique for direct laryngoscopy. Ann Otol Rhinol Laryngol Suppl 179:2, 1999, Fig. 32.)

visualization to the level of the carina has also been reported.[67]

Clinical judgment must be used when indirect staging or biopsy procedures are performed under local anesthesia in the presence of some degree of airway obstruction.[13] In the circumstance of rapidly progressive or near-total airway obstruction, the equipment and personnel necessary to secure the airway must be immediately available, and diagnostic procedures under local anesthesia may have limited application. However, evaluation of difficult or compromised airways under local anesthesia by direct or indirect means can be critically important in making airway management decisions, especially when the administration of GA or muscle relaxants is considered.[42]

Various aerosol techniques have been used to administer topical anesthesia, and lidocaine ointment can be used on the posterior third of the tongue.[42] The glossopharyngeal nerve can be blocked by a transmucosal injection,[19,27,42,98,99,145,149] and the superior laryngeal nerve can be blocked using either an external or internal approach.[19,42,98,99,145] Pressure on the root of the tongue can elicit a gag reflex mediated by submucosal pressure receptors not susceptible to topical anesthesia, and transmucosal glossopharyngeal nerve block may be required to obliterate this response.[146] Topical anesthetics can also be administered by cricothyroid puncture and through the suction channel of the fiberoptic bronchoscope. Lidocaine, 2% to 10%,[19,23] and tetracaine 0.5% to 2%,[19,23] are both commonly used for topical anesthesia of the airway. Nebulized tetracaine appears to be more potent, and 0.5% tetracaine may provide a more complete block than 4% lidocaine.[19] However, tetracaine has a narrower margin of safety[89] and has a higher incidence of allergic reactions.[19,89] A chemical laryngitis has been reported with the use of benzocaine-tetracaine-butamben (Cetacaine) in the larynx.[13]

Cocaine has been traditionally used for nasal anesthesia.[97-99] Benzocaine is also an effective topical anesthetic, but methemoglobinemia has been associated with its use.[23] Local anesthetics applied to the mucous membranes of the airway are rapidly absorbed into the circulation, producing peak blood levels 15 to 20 minutes after application.[31,97] The maximum safe dosage of topical lidocaine has been stated by various authors to be 3 to 4 mg/kg or 6 mg/kg.[9,41,45,98,128] However, the use of topical lidocaine doses of 11 mg/kg[132] and up to 19 mg/kg[4] has also been reported. Absorption of lidocaine from the trachea and more distal airways is more efficient than absorption from the larynx, and higher blood levels are achieved more rapidly.[36,42,151] It has been recommended that the amount of lidocaine administered to the trachea be limited to 1 to 1.5 mg/kg.[42] The maximum dosage of topical tetracaine when applied to the adult airway has been reported to be 50 mg,[128] 80 mg,[45] and 100 mg,[130,145] although the maximum safe dosage of topical tetracaine has never been clearly defined.[101] Other recommended maximum dosages include 50 mg in the healthy 70-kg adult[23] and 100 mg in the adult over 15 minutes.[19] A dose of 1 mg/kg of topical tetracaine has also been used.[69] Fatalities have been reported following the topical application of 100 mg of tetracaine to mucous membranes.[145]

Adequate sedation for direct laryngoscopy under local anesthesia in the adult can be achieved with midazolam given in aliquots of 0.5 to 1 mg IV and titrated to effect.[13] The use of narcotics in addition to midazolam for conscious sedation during direct laryngoscopy can provide additional analgesia, but the risk of respiratory depression is increased. If a narcotic is used for conscious sedation, fentanyl given in aliquots of 25 to 50 μg may be a reasonable choice.

2. General Anesthesia

The current consensus is that GA is superior to local anesthesia for microlaryngoscopy,[89] and the vast majority of direct laryngoscopic procedures are performed under GA using endotracheal intubation, apneic techniques, insufflation, or jet ventilation. When the site of the lesion and the degree of airway obstruction are not well defined, inhalation induction with maintenance of spontaneous ventilation is generally thought to be a safer technique than intravenous induction.[14,105] Should airway obstruction occur during induction, a prompt response is required including mask ventilation with 100% oxygen and the establishment of a patent airway by endotracheal intubation, rigid bronchoscopy, an alternative rescue technique, or a surgical airway as required.

a. Microlaryngoscopy Tube

The overwhelming majority of direct laryngoscopic procedures under GA can be adequately and safely performed without compromising the surgeon's view using a small (4 to 6 mm internal diameter) endotracheal tube (ET) that is 30 cm in length, a so-called microlaryngoscopy tube (MLT) (Mallinckrodt, St. Louis, MO).[14,42] The MLT is manufactured from polyvinyl chloride and is fitted with a high-volume, low-pressure cuff.[14,78] In situ, the tube lies between the arytenoid cartilages, leaving at least the anterior two thirds of the glottis unobscured, and can be lifted forward out of the posterior commissure using the beak of the laryngoscope to view this area.[78,142] Endotracheal intubation provides a secure airway protected against aspiration, permits positive-pressure ventilation that can be monitored by spirometry and capnography,[38,42,78,89] and is the easiest and safest way to secure the airway.[35] It may be the technique of choice in the presence of preexisting upper airway obstruction[35] or if loss of airway patency is a possibility; when bleeding, edema, or excess secretions are expected; when there is a risk of regurgitation and aspiration (gastroesophageal reflux, full stomach, or vocal cord paralysis); when the duration of the procedure is uncertain or likely to be prolonged; or when assisted or positive-pressure ventilation may be required to ensure adequate gas exchange in high-risk patients with obesity or respiratory or cardiovascular disease.[2,6]

GA can be induced by inhalation or intravenous agents, individualized to the clinical setting and operator preference. Equipment and personnel necessary to secure the airway by an alternative technique if laryngoscopy is difficult should be immediately available.[1] As a general rule, spontaneous ventilation should not be abolished unless it is certain that an airway can be established, and if there is serious doubt about effective airway control, the airway should be secured under local anesthesia.[14] Appropriate attention should be directed to the attenuation of the tachycardic and hypertensive response to direct laryngoscopy. Following induction, topical anesthesia applied to the larynx under direct vision may attenuate the risk of laryngospasm and coughing at emergence. Anesthesia can be maintained using a volatile or intravenous technique or some combination, and muscle relaxants can be used as necessary. A smooth emergence with a rapid return of protected airway reflexes is desirable,[4,6] and drugs such as remifentanil and propofol and the newer volatile agents may be particularly useful in this setting. Vocal cord mobility may be observed prior to emergence if required.[5] Awake extubation of a spontaneously breathing patient provides a wide margin of safety. Airway obstruction at emergence can occur, and rarely reintubation is necessary to maintain airway patency.[55] When airway obstruction following extubation can be predicted, intubation continued into the postoperative period may be necessary or tracheostomy required.

The posterior commissure is not involved in about 95% of patients with airway disease presenting for microlaryngoscopy.[6] However, the use of an MLT may not be appropriate when surgical access to the posterior glottis or subglottic area is necessary[2,6] or in the presence of subglottic or posterior glottic stenosis.[2] The MLT also prevents visualization of the full range of laryngeal mobility, distorts the laryngeal structures, and is associated with the risk of fire if laser treatment is performed.[2,6,54] Alternative anesthetic and airway management techniques are therefore required.

b. Apneic Techniques

Apneic techniques can be used in conjunction with an MLT during direct laryngoscopy.[7,53,56] During suspension laryngoscopy and muscle relaxation, the patient is hyperventilated with 100% oxygen and the MLT removed under direct vision to obtain visualization of, and surgical access to, the larynx and subglottic area.[53,56] The duration of apnea is limited by hypoxia and hypercarbia and requires continuous pulse oximetry monitoring. End-tidal carbon dioxide levels can be measured following reintubation. The carbon dioxide pressure (P_{CO_2}) can be expected to rise 6 to 7 mm Hg in the first minute of apnea and 3 to 4 mm Hg per minute thereafter.[53] In a series reported by Weisberger and Miner, the apneic technique was used for laser resection of laryngeal papillomatosis.[142]

The median number of apneic episodes required was two and the mean length of an apneic episode was 2.6 minutes.[53] The technique is not appropriate in the presence of a marginal airway[56] or limited cardiorespiratory reserve and is relatively contraindicated in the presence of severe anemia and increased oxygen utilization.[53]

c. Insufflation

An anesthetic technique employing spontaneous ventilation with insufflation of anesthetic agents has been described by several authors.[2,6,7,51,57,58] Insufflation techniques are best suited to brief diagnostic examinations, especially in the pediatric population when minimal instrumentation is required, minimal bleeding is expected, and the airway is relatively unobstructed with a fixed lesion.[6] The technique is useful when there is a need to evaluate the dynamics of the airway during spontaneous ventilation, when a full view of the glottis is required,[6] and eliminates the risk of airway fire during laser surgery.[35,51] The insufflation technique is not useful in the presence of large or mobile supraglottic lesions that may cause increased airway obstruction with the induction of GA.[6] Insufflation has been used for excision of a laryngeal polyp and stripping of a vocal cord lesion under microlaryngoscopy, biopsy, and vocal cord Teflon injection.[57]

GA can be induced intravenously or by inhalation of a potent volatile agent administered by mask, as appropriate.[2,6,7,57,58] When an adequate depth of GA has been achieved, topical anesthesia can be administered to the larynx and trachea during direct laryngoscopy.[2,6,7,57,58] An appropriately sized nasopharyngeal airway attached to a standard ET connector[2,57] or a shortened ET[7] can then be positioned in the nasopharynx and used for insufflation of anesthetic gases. Alternatively, gases can be administered through a suction catheter positioned in the trachea,[58] through the suction channel of an Andrews anterior commissure retractor positioned at the level of the cords,[51] or through the working channel or side port of the suspension laryngoscope.[2,7] An adequate depth of anesthesia may be more easily maintained in children up to 10 to 12 years of age,[2] although the technique has been used in adults.[57] Inadequate anesthesia can result in laryngospasm, whereas apnea and hypoventilation can occur if the depth of GA is excessive.[7,57] Assessment of tidal volume is difficult.[57] Inhalational anesthesia can be supplemented with an intravenous infusion of propofol,[7,35] and total intravenous anesthesia using infusions of propofol and remifentanil have also been used.[7] Following the endoscopic procedure under insufflation, intubation may be desirable to secure the airway during emergence, or conversely emergence can proceed without intubation.

Disadvantages associated with insufflation include pollution of the operating room with anesthetic gases,[35] no protection of the airway against aspiration, and gastric distention if the tip of the insufflation tube directs its flow into the esophagus.[6,35,51,57,58] Intermittent apnea can also be combined with insufflation techniques.[6]

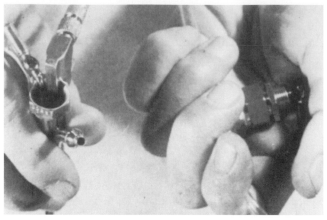

Figure 35-7 Vapor entrainment adapter applied to 3.5 × 30 bronchoscope. Control valve for intermittent application of oxygen pressure. (From Sanders RD: Two ventilating attachments for bronchoscopes. Del Med J 39:170, 1967, Fig. III.)

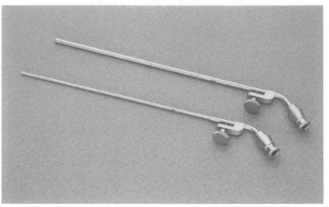

Figure 35-8 Proximal jet cannulas. The cannulas have a working length of 13.5 cm. There is a choice of tubes with an outside diameter of 2 or 3 cm. The cannula is slightly malleable to permit adjustment of the direction of the jet to be aimed at the glottic opening. (From Benjamin B: Endolaryngeal Surgery. London, Martin Dunitz, 1998, Fig. 5.17.)

d. Jet Ventilation

Jet ventilation was introduced by Sanders in 1967, when he reported the use of a jet injector attached to a rigid bronchoscope[120] (Fig. 35-7). The jet stream entrains ambient air, a phenomenon commonly attributed to the Venturi principle, although Newton's law of motion may more accurately describe the physics involved.[8] When the moving jet of gas encounters the ambient stationery gas, viscous shearing occurs between the moving and static fluid layers, an exchange of velocity occurs, and ambient gas is dragged into the moving stream or entrained.[8] The amount of gas entrained is proportional to the jet velocity and flow volume.[8] The use of jet ventilation for suspension laryngoscopy was described by Oulton and Donald in 1971,[107] and it has subsequently become a well-established technique.[18]

Jet ventilation for direct laryngoscopy can be subdivided into supraglottic and subglottic techniques. Ventilation can be delivered manually or by means of a mechanical ventilator.[19,61-64] Low- or high-frequency ventilation, or a combination of the two, can be used.

i. Supraglottic Jet Ventilation Supraglottic (or proximal) jet ventilation can be achieved using a jet cannula that is securely attached within the lumen of the laryngoscope proximally by means of a screw clamp.[2,63] Use of a slightly malleable cannula allows adjustment of the direction of the jet and alignment with the glottis[2] (Fig. 35-8). Alternatively, the jet injector can be inserted into the light source or side channel within the laryngoscope[63-65] (Fig. 35-9). Typically, oxygen at 50 psi is attached by means of high-pressure tubing to a reducing valve and toggle switch, which is then connected by additional tubing to the injector nozzle. Manually depressing the toggle switch then permits gas at a reduced pressure to flow to the jet injector. Flow through the injector increases with the driving pressure.[64] At a given driving pressure using a supraglottic jet, tidal volume has been

shown to increase with the size of the injector.[64,66] Various sizes of injectors have been used: 13G, 14G (adults), 16G (infants and children),[63] 2 to 3 mm outside diameter (OD)[14], and 3 mm inside diameter (ID).[64] Jet ventilation can be initiated using a jet pressure of 5 to 10 psi in children and 20 psi in adults.[63] The pressure is then increased until adequate chest excursions are noted.[63] Infants can be ventilated at driving pressures of 6 to 12 psi, most children at 10 to 16 psi, and most adults at 12 to 18 psi.[64]

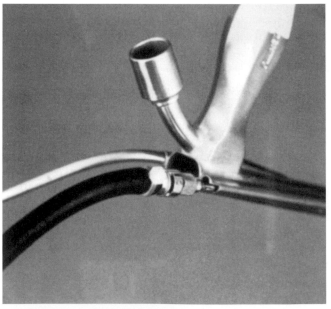

Figure 35-9 Jet injector inserted into the right laryngoscope light channel. (From Crockett DM, Scamman FL, McCabe BF, et al: Venturi jet ventilation for microlaryngoscopy: Technique, complications, pitfalls. Laryngoscope 97:1326, 1987, Fig. 2.)

The tracheal pressure generated depends on the driving pressure, the diameter of the jet, and the cross-sectional area of the trachea.[50] In a laboratory model of jet ventilation using an adult ventilating laryngoscope and driving pressures of 10 to 45 psi, a rate of 20 breaths per minute (bpm), and an inspiratory time of 1 second, distal tracheal pressures were measured and found to be never greater than the known highest pressures generated by a conventional anesthesia circuit.[64] In a canine model of supraglottic jet ventilation, at an insufflation pressure of 45 psi, distal tracheal pressure was found to be between 30 and 35 cm H_2O.[66] In a series of 500 patients ventilated using a *combination* of high- and low-frequency supraglottic ventilation, the inspiratory pressures measured at the tip of the jet laryngoscope were 5.8 ± 2.2 cm H_2O.[62] Entrained ambient air dilutes the oxygen delivered by the jet nozzle[6] and when 100% oxygen is used the effective FIO_2 is 80% to 90%.[6] Sanders used a rate of 8 bpm at 50 psi driving pressure through a 14 to 16G jet and demonstrated adequate oxygenation and ventilation.[120] Adequate oxygenation and PCO_2 levels during jet ventilation have subsequently been demonstrated by multiple investigators.[60,64,65,67,68] Furthermore, a 100% correlation has been demonstrated between the clinician's assessment of chest wall movement and the adequacy of ventilation.[64] Oxygen or oxygen–nitrous oxide mixtures can be utilized.[64] Koufman and colleagues recommended a 1- to 1.5-second inspiratory time and a ventilation rate of about 20 bpm.[79] An inspiratory/expiratory (I:E) ratio of 1:3 has also been recommended.[1] A driving pressure of 30 to 50 psi[1,6] and a frequency of 8 to 10 jets/min can also be used.[6]

Advantages associated with jet ventilation include an unobstructed view of, and access to, the larynx and trachea as well as the absence of a potentially flammable ET during laser surgery.[2] The use of supraglottic jet ventilation in the presence of upper airway obstruction may be associated with an increased risk of barotrauma[1,6,7,63]; however, it has been used successfully in this setting.[64] Jet ventilation can be extremely difficult in the presence of obesity or poor pulmonary compliance[63] and may be contraindicated in this setting.[69] Supraglottic jet ventilation may also be inappropriate when proper placement of the laryngoscope, and therefore alignment of the supraglottic jet with the glottis, is difficult.[63] Precise alignment of the jet is critical.[8]

GA for direct laryngoscopy and supraglottic jet ventilation can be induced intravenously or by inhalation. Once an appropriate depth of anesthesia has been achieved and adequate mask ventilation demonstrated, a muscle relaxant can be administered and direct laryngoscopy performed.[63,64] If the glottic airway is judged to be adequate for jet ventilation, the jet nozzle is attached to the laryngoscope and jet ventilation initiated. If, however, the airway is not judged to be adequate, an MLT tube can be placed and positive-pressure ventilation begun. Partial surgical resection of a glottic or supraglottic lesion such as a papilloma may be required before jet ventilation

is appropriate.[63] Manual jet ventilation is initiated with gentle depression of the toggle valve while observing for appropriate chest wall motion.[63] The inspiratory phase is terminated about 0.1 second before maximum chest rise is noted, and the chest is then observed to fall appropriately.[63] No further jetting is done until adequate expiration has occurred.[63] Vigilance and hand-eye coordination are necessary.[63] Anesthesia is maintained intravenously, and adequate muscle relaxation is essential.[5] The use of a video monitor permits both the anesthesiologist and the laryngoscopist to visualize the glottis and monitor the airway.[64] On completion of the surgical procedure, the laryngoscope can be removed and ventilation maintained by mask, or alternatively an ET can be placed for emergence.[63]

Disadvantages associated with supraglottic jet ventilation techniques include vocal cord vibration produced by the jet; drying of the laryngeal mucosa; distal spread of particulate material with potential tracheobronchial viral or tumor seeding; barotrauma (subcutaneous emphysema, pneumothorax) especially in the presence of expiratory obstruction or malalignment of the scope[8]; gastric distention related to scope malalignment, or excess pressure; inability to monitor end-tidal CO_2 ($EtCO_2$); and possible hyper- or hypoventilation.[6,8,63,64]

ii. Subglottic Jet Ventilation Jet ventilation for endolaryngeal surgery can also be performed using a subglottic technique. Advantages associated with subglottic jetting include minimal movement of the vocal cords, expulsion of blood or tissue debris from the trachea during expiration,[2,8,51] and excellent surgical access to the larynx and subglottis.[2] Obstruction to expiratory outflow can, however, rapidly produce severe barotrauma during subglottic jetting[51] and the technique is considered to be contraindicated in the presence of significant laryngeal obstruction,[6,8] although it has been used successfully in the presence of a 4- to 5-mm diameter laryngeal stenosis.[2] Other contraindications include obesity and poor chest compliance.[8] Benjamin has described the use of the subglottic jet technique for more than 15 years without complication.[14]

Subglottic jet ventilation was initially performed using a 3.5 mm OD or a metal supraglottic cannula inserted below the level of the glottis.[8,61] A plastic tube tends to whip around in the trachea during jetting and a rigid cannula, if malaligned, can cause submucosal injection.[8] In 1979, Benjamin and Gronow developed 2.8 and 4.0 mm OD flexible polyvinyl chloride tubes fitted with four distal petals that centered the tube in the midtrachea and stabilized it following transglottic insertion.[15]

Hunsaker subsequently modified the Ben-Jet tube by attaching a 1 mm ID monitoring channel that opened 3 mm proximal to the distal end of the tube.[69] The petals of the Ben-Jet tube were also modified to form a flange or basket configuration, and the device was constructed of highly flame-resistant fluoroplastic[69] (Fig. 35-10).

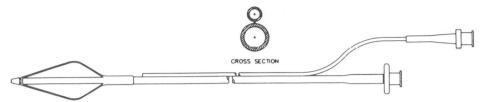

CROSS SECTION

Figure 35-10 Xomed-Treace Mon-Jet tube. Distal flanges for centering tube in trachea and monitor side port for monitoring tracheal pressures and end-tidal carbon dioxide. Constructed entirely of highly flame-resistant fluoroplastic. (From Hunsaker DH: Anesthesia for microlaryngeal surgery: The case for subglottic jet ventilation. Laryngoscope 104[8 pt 2 Suppl 65]:1, 1994.)

This 3.5-mm self-centering jet tube was then evaluated in patients undergoing suspension microlaryngoscopy.[69,70] The jet tube was inserted 5 to 8 cm below the glottis and connected to an automatic ventilator set to shut down if tracheal pressure exceeded 35 cm H_2O.[69] Tracheal pressure was monitored continuously and $EtCO_2$ intermittently using a three-way valve connected to the monitor channel. The jet ventilator was set to deliver 100% O_2 at a jet pressure of 24 to 30 cm H_2O, inspiratory time at 30% of the respiratory cycle, and the respiratory rate was adjusted between 10 and 15 bpm to maintain O_2 saturation above 95%.[69] This subglottic group was compared with a supraglottic group who underwent jet ventilation by means of a rigid cannula attached to the laryngoscope and positioned 1 cm above the glottis.[69] On one occasion during subglottic ventilation, proximal obstruction occurred and triggered ventilator shutdown. Oxygenation and ventilation were found to be adequate. The monitoring channel satisfactorily measured $EtCO_2$ with a correlation of 0.82 with $PaCO_2$.[68] Subglottic ventilation was found to be more efficient than supraglottic jet ventilation.[69]

Brooker and colleagues subsequently reported 36 adult patients who underwent suspension microlaryngeal surgery using the Hunsaker Mon-Jet tube (Xomed-Treace, Jacksonville, FL) to perform subglottic jet ventilation using an automatic jet ventilator set to deliver 100% oxygen with an inspiratory time of 20% to 50% of the respiratory cycle, a driving pressure of 15 psi, an end-expiratory pressure limit of 10 cm H_2O, and a peak pressure limit of 35 to 40 cm H_2O. A respiratory rate of 10 to 20 bpm was used.[26] $EtCO_2$ varied between 31 and 42 mm Hg.[26] Mean case length was 48 minutes, and oxygen saturation greater than 95% was maintained.[26] Proximal obstruction triggered ventilator shutdown on one occasion. No barotrauma occurred. Anesthesia was induced intravenously, and following muscle relaxation, intubation was achieved primarily with a styletted Hunsaker Mon-Jet tube or a standard ET, which was replaced with the Mon-Jet following suspension. Anesthesia was maintained by intravenous infusion. A standard ET or mask ventilation was used for emergence.[26]

Barotrauma occurs more commonly during subglottic than supraglottic jet ventilation and a single jet has produced massive emphysema.[8] It may be possible to minimize the risk of barotrauma by avoiding the use of rigid tubes, using an automatic ventilator with an adjustable automatic shutoff valve, initiating jet ventilation with low jetting pressures that are then slowly increased observing chest excursions, using muscle relaxation, using I:E ratios less than or equal to 1:2, and using HFV.[8]

iii. Transtracheal Jet Ventilation Endolaryngeal surgery can also be performed using transtracheal jet ventilation, and this mode of ventilation may be useful in certain emergency or other special airway problems such as subglottic stenosis.[8,54] In the circumstance of failed intubation and failed mask ventilation, transtracheal jet ventilation can also be lifesaving.[71] However, the incidence of barotrauma is greater than that associated with supra- and subglottic techniques.[8] Advantages include unobstructed surgical visibility, reduced ignition hazard during laser surgery, and diminished risk of distal movement of blood and tissue debris.[54] Safety may be enhanced by insertion of the transtracheal catheter under endoscopic control.[54] Constant clinical surveillance of chest movement and exhalation is necessary if barotrauma is to be minimized.[54]

iv. High-Frequency Ventilation HFV can be subdivided into high-frequency positive-pressure ventilation (HFPPV), high-frequency jet ventilation (HFJV), and high-frequency oscillation,[8] although only HFJV is discussed here.

HFJV employs a narrow cannula or injector to deliver jets of gas under high pressure (25 to 400 kPa) into an open system.[8,72,73] Tidal volumes are typically 2 to 3 cm^3/kg and respiratory rates 60 to 180 bpm.[73] The important clinical variables are driving pressure, frequency, and the inspiratory time.[72] Mechanisms proposed for gas exchange include direct alveolar ventilation, asymmetric velocity profiles, Taylor dispersion, pendelluft, cardiogenic mixing, and accelerated diffusion.[72] Problems associated with HFV include barotrauma, inadequate humidification, tracheobronchitis, and bronchospasm.[1] Measurement of proximal airway pressure is a poor indicator of intrathoracic pressure during HFV, and measurement of esophageal pressure may be more useful.[72]

In 1980, Babinski and colleagues reported a series of 87 patients who underwent HFJV through a subglottic catheter during operative laryngoscopy.[10] Driving pressures of 6 to 50 psi, respiratory rates of 60 to 100 bpm, and an FIO_2 of 30% to 100% were used. Oxygenation was adequate, although hypercarbia occurred in seven patients. Intratracheal pressures were less than or equal to 7 mm Hg.[74] Further experience with subglottic HFJV was reported in 1994 by Evans and coauthors, who noted the positive end-expiratory pressure (PEEP) associated with the technique and the risk of barotrauma in the presence of expiratory obstruction.[48]

HFJV has also been used concomitantly with jet ventilation at conventional respiratory rates.[62,76,77] In 2000, Lanzenberger-Schragl and associates reported a series of 500 patients who underwent laryngoscopic procedures and who were ventilated using a supraglottic superimposed high-frequency jet ventilation (SHFJV) technique.[81] An operative laryngoscope was fitted with two jet nozzles and a pressure-monitoring cannula that opened into the lumen of the scope[62] (Fig. 35-11). The distal nozzle was used for jet ventilation at 8 to 20 bpm and the proximal nozzle for HFJV at 400 to 800 bpm. A ventilator capable of simultaneously providing two jet streams at different frequencies was utilized and set to shut off the gas supply and sound an alarm if a preset inspiratory peak pressure was exceeded. GA was induced and maintained intravenously. Mask ventilation was performed prior to insertion of the laryngoscope and at emergence. In 497 patients, adequate oxygenation of hemoglobin and ventilation was achieved. Three high-risk patients required intubation because of oxygen saturation less than or equal to 90%. The measured inspiratory pressures were 5.7 ± 2.2 millibar and PEEPs were 2.1 ± 0.8 millibar. No barotrauma occurred, and no adverse hemodynamic effects were observed. Benefits of SHFJV include diminished vocal cord movements

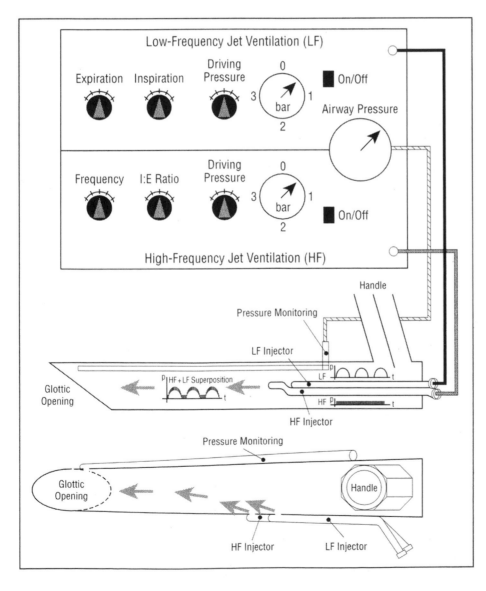

Figure 35-11 Technical diagram of the jet laryngoscope, with arrow indicating the flow of the jet stream. I:E, inspiration-expiration; P, pressure. (From Lanzenberger-Schragl E, Donnor A, Grasl MC, et al: Superimposed high frequency jet ventilation for laryngeal and tracheal surgery. Arch Otolaryngol Head Neck Surg 126:43, 2000, Fig. 1.)

caused by the low-frequency jet stream,[62,76] maintenance of excellent surgical exposure, reduced risk of barotrauma in the presence of laryngeal stenosis, and superiority over single-frequency techniques in the obese and in patients with respiratory disease.[62] Supraglottic combined frequency jet ventilation has also been found to be superior to subglottic combined frequency jet ventilation, which is itself more effective than subglottic low-frequency jet ventilation.[78] Contraindications to SHFJV include inability to hyperextend the neck and bleeding in the larynx or tracheobronchial system.[62,76]

Percutaneous transtracheal high-frequency jet ventilation (TTHFJV) has also been used during anesthesia for laryngeal microsurgery.[54,79,80] It can provide excellent operative conditions, adequate gas exchange, and a low ignition hazard during laser surgery.[54] When glottic visualization through the jet laryngoscope is not possible, TTHFJV has been said to be the technique of choice.[62] However, barotrauma can occur and constant clinical surveillance of chest movement and exhalation, as well as adequate monitoring of end-expiratory pressure, is critically important if this risk is to be minimized.[54] TTHFJV delivered by a ventilator with an automatic pressure sensitive cutoff device is a reliable ventilation technique when performed by experienced practitioners.[54,80] However, the risk of pneumothorax is present despite automatic control of airway pressure.

It is unclear whether HFV techniques possess any clear advantage over traditional ventilation modalities.[1] However, HFV continues to evolve and the precise role of these techniques in laryngoscopy has yet to be defined.[1]

D. HEMODYNAMIC RESPONSE TO DIRECT LARYNGOSCOPY

Suspension laryngoscopy stretches the laryngeal structures, maximally stimulates sensory receptors in the larynx, and can produce marked increases in blood pressure and heart rate.[81] This reflex response appears to vary with the depth of anesthesia, the duration of the procedure, and the maximal force applied to expose the larynx adequately.[81] The transient tachycardia and hypertension produced are generally without sequelae but can be deleterious in the presence of cardiovascular and intracranial comorbidity.[81-83] Numerous studies have investigated attenuation of the hemodynamic response to direct laryngoscopy and endotracheal intubation.[82] Lidocaine, chloroprocaine, narcotics, β-blockers, intravenous induction drugs, inhalational agents, α-agonists, vasodilators, adenosine phosphate, magnesium sulfate, and calcium channel blockers have all been used to obtund this hemodynamic reflex with varying degrees of success.[82,84] Fewer studies have been carried out on attenuation of the hemodynamic response during microlaryngeal surgery; however, labetalol and esmolol have been found to be effective in limiting increases in heart rate and blood pressure in this setting.[81] Remifentanil 2 μg/kg was reported to block the hemodynamic response

to direct laryngoscopy and endotracheal intubation,[85] whereas 1 μg/kg[85,86] and a bolus dose of 1 μg/kg followed by an infusion of 0.5 μg/kg/min[87] attenuated but did not completely block the response. The ultrafast onset and offset of remifentanil may make this drug particularly useful for the purpose of obtunding a brief but noxious stimulus such as suspension laryngoscopy[85]; however, hypotension and bradycardia can occur.[87]

Ultimately, the method or drug chosen to attenuate the hypertension and tachycardia associated with suspension laryngoscopy should be individualized to the clinical setting and operator preference.[82]

E. COMPLICATIONS

Although usually brief in duration, suspension laryngoscopy is not a trivial procedure and has been associated with cardiovascular, ventilatory, and airway complications.

In 1974, Strong and colleagues reported a 1.47% overall incidence of myocardial ischemia associated with endolaryngeal surgery and, in the presence of a preoperative history of heart disease, an incidence of 4%.[131] In 1986, Wenig and coworkers reported a prospective study of 100 consecutive suspension laryngoscopy patients.[140] Twenty-six patients experienced an elevation in systolic blood pressure greater than 20% and four intraoperative arrhythmias occurred. Postoperative electrocardiographic (ECG) changes occurred in three patients; however, cardiac enzymes were normal.[83] In 1994, Hendrix and coauthors reported major complications in 24% of 200 adult patients who underwent direct laryngoscopy and associated endoscopic procedures.[63] Major complications included respiratory difficulty, pneumothorax, chest pain, arrhythmias, ECG changes, pulmonary edema, and hypertension, among others.[90]

Recovery room reintubation rates of 1.2% in patients who had undergone direct laryngoscopy alone and 3% in those who had also undergone other endoscopic procedures have also been reported.[91] Twelve of 13 endoscopy patients who required reintubation had undergone laryngeal biopsy and 10 had cancer of the larynx or piriform sinus. Nine required reintubation within 1 hour of extubation.[91] In a series of 589 direct laryngoscopies, five airway emergencies occurred within 30 minutes of extubation.[55] Three of the five patients required reintubation, whereas respiratory distress resolved with racemic epinephrine in the remaining two.[55] An emergency tracheostomy rate of 0.4% has also been reported after multiple endoscopy.[92]

In a 1991 survey, data for 15,701 patients who underwent laser endolaryngeal procedures using jet ventilation or an ET were analyzed for associated complications.[93] In 4151 patients who received jet ventilation, 49 (1.2%) complications occurred, of which 18 (0.43%) were serious or life threatening and 24 (0.43%) were ventilation related. In 11,550 patients in the ET group, 42 (0.36%) complications occurred, of which 17 (0.15%) were serious or life threatening and 17 (0.15%) were ventilation related. Overall complications, ventilation-related complications, serious or life threatening ventilation-related complications, and barotrauma were more prevalent in the jet ventilation group.[93] The overall complication rate associated with jet ventilation was found to be three times that of ventilation by an ET,[93] and the occurrence of complications associated with jet ventilation was higher at institutions that used the technique less frequently.[93] Thirty-six percent of the complications associated with jet ventilation were potentially life threatening and included pneumothorax, mediastinal air, and transient hypoxemia.[93] Other studies have reported complication rates of 0% to 7% associated with jet ventilation.[93]

Specific pathology or surgical procedures may favor a particular ventilatory mode or anesthetic technique. Teamwork and a methodical approach with careful attention to detail are necessary if complications are to be minimized.

F. PEDIATRIC DIRECT LARYNGOSCOPY

The general principles of adult laryngoscopy can be applied to infants and children, although anatomic, physiologic, and pathologic differences exist. The infant larynx is about one third the size of the adult larynx, is located high in the neck at the level of the fourth cervical vertebra, is easily irritated, and is susceptible to laryngospasm.[94] The infant epiglottis falls posteriorly, is omega shaped, and extends into the oropharynx with its tip behind the soft palate.[94] The infant airway is narrowest in the subglottis at the level of the cricoid cartilage and is susceptible to obstruction secondary to edema at this location.[94] The high metabolic rate, high cardiac output, and small functional residual capacity of children predispose them to the rapid development of hypoxia in the presence of airway obstruction or apnea.[6,94] Vagal stimulation with airway manipulation can also produce profound bradycardia in the pediatric age group, and atropine 10 to 20 µg/kg or glycopyrrolate 5 to 10 µg/kg can be used prophylactically to block or attenuate this vagally mediated reflex.[3,6,94] Preterm infants are also predisposed to apneic spells both during and after GA.[94] Causes of airway obstruction in infants include bilateral choanal atresia, laryngomalacia, pharyngeal or laryngeal cysts or masses, bilateral vocal cord paralysis, cystic hygroma, subglottic hemangioma, and subglottic stenosis.[94,95] In older children, causes of airway obstruction include croup, acute epiglottitis, glottic or supraglottic papillomas, foreign bodies, and trauma.[94]

Options for anesthesia and airway management for pediatric endoscopy include awake techniques and GA with spontaneous or controlled ventilation. Ventilation techniques include insufflation, endotracheal intubation, jet ventilation, and intermittent apnea.[2,3,6,7,54,94] The anesthetic technique chosen is dependent on the age and health status of the patient, the site of the lesion, the degree of obstruction, the requirements of the endoscopic procedure, as well as the preference and experience of the anesthesiologist and endoscopic surgeon.[3,7,94]

Awake transnasal fiberoptic laryngoscopy can be performed in the neonate without anesthesia.[96] Topical lidocaine (0.5% to 2%) up to 5 mg/kg or tetracaine (0.2% to 0.5%) up to 1 mg/kg has also been used to facilitate endoscopy in children.[3] Intravenous sedation with drugs such as fentanyl 0.5 µg/kg or midazolam 0.03 mg/kg can also be used in an appropriately monitored setting and titrated to effect.[6] However, in the presence of potential or actual airway obstruction or respiratory failure, the administration of any sedation can exacerbate airway compromise.

Most pediatric endoscopy procedures and virtually all direct endoscopic examinations are performed with the patient under GA.[6,94] A spontaneous ventilation inhalation induction is commonly employed in smaller children.[94] If airway compromise is not anticipated, premedication with midazolam 0.5 mg/kg given orally or rectally can be used.[7] Halothane has been the traditional inhalation induction agent, although sevoflurane may be better tolerated and is associated with very rapid induction and emergence times.[94] When an adequate depth of anesthesia has been established, lidocaine up to 5 mg/kg can be applied to the mucosa of the larynx and upper trachea under direct laryngoscopy to attenuate laryngospasm, cough, and breath holding.[94] Inhalation anesthesia can be maintained by insufflation using a metal cannula in the suspension laryngoscope, a nasopharyngeal airway or a shortened ET positioned in the pharynx, or a small-diameter ET positioned in the trachea.[7,94] Supplemental intravenous anesthesia or total IV anesthesia using propofol-remifentanil can also be used.[7] Alternatively, endotracheal intubation, muscle relaxants, and intermittent positive-pressure ventilation can be used. Intermittent apnea can be induced using muscle relaxants or intravenous anesthetics.[7] Jet ventilation has also been used in small children,[54,62-64,76] although its use in this age group is controversial because of the incidence of associated barotrauma.[94] Anesthetic and airway management techniques in older children are similar to those described for adults.

On occasion, awake intubation of a sick, unstable neonate or an infant with a difficult airway problem, without the use of adjunctive medication, may be the safest technique.[2] Awake intubation of children with upper airway obstruction using local anesthesia and sedation is also theoretically attractive but difficult to achieve in practice.[94] Because most pediatric patients do not tolerate awake intubation, an inhalation induction of GA with preservation of spontaneous ventilation is usually performed in this setting.[7] Intravenous access is secured as early as possible. Preliminary awake fiberoptic examination may assist in diagnosis but may not be adequate to determine the full extent of airway encroachment.[7] The equipment and personnel necessary to establish an airway by means of a variety of techniques, including the use of a rigid bronchoscope or a surgical approach, should be immediately available.

During inhalation induction, application of 5 to 10 cm H_2O constant positive airway pressure may help to maintain an open airway.[94] Direct laryngoscopy at an appropriate depth of GA can then be performed to determine the nature and extent of pathology and further airway management choices.[94] Options include endotracheal intubation either directly or indirectly using flexible or rigid fiberscopes, a laryngeal mask airway (LMA), retrograde or blind techniques, jet ventilation (if exhalation can be ensured), intubation with a rigid bronchoscope, intermittent mask ventilation, or tracheostomy.[7,94] Aspiration of an obstructing cyst or removal of a mass or foreign body may also be indicated.[94] Should complete airway obstruction occur and intubation not be possible, a surgical airway is immediately required. In the presence of tracheal pathology that precludes tracheostomy, the use of femoral cardiopulmonary bypass may be a possibility.[7] Following inhalation induction, if manual mask ventilation can be achieved, muscle relaxants may facilitate further airway management; however, spontaneous ventilation should not be abolished until it is certain that an airway can be established.[94]

Anesthesia and airway management for pediatric endoscopy require an understanding of the causes of airway pathology in this age group and the ability to individualize the appropriate technique to the clinical setting. In most circumstances, a spontaneous ventilation induction of GA maintains airway control and provides a wide margin of safety.

VI. BRONCHOSCOPY

Bronchoscopy has become the most common invasive procedure used in the diagnosis and treatment of respiratory disease.[1,40] Rigid bronchoscopes were used exclusively until the introduction of flexible fiberoptic bronchoscopes in the 1960s, following which the utilization of rigid scopes declined.[97] Since the mid-1980s, however, there has been renewed interest in rigid bronchoscopy associated with the development of a number of endobronchial treatment modalities for carcinoma of the lung.[97] Rigid bronchoscopy and flexible bronchoscopy are complementary, and each has inherent advantages and disadvantages.[98,99]

A. RIGID BRONCHOSCOPY

1. History

The first rigid bronchoscopy was performed by Gustav Killian in 1897, when he used a Mikulicz-type esophagoscope to remove a pork bone from a farmer's bronchus under topical cocaine anesthesia.[99,100] He subsequently designed the first rigid bronchoscope using a reflected incandescent light source.[99] Chevalier Jackson later incorporated an auxiliary tube within the lumen of the scope to serve as a light carrier.[41,99] Other modifications have included the addition of a ventilating side arm to permit administration of oxygen or anesthetic gases.[99] In 1954, Hopkins developed a telescopic rod-lens system to improve visualization,[99] and in 1967 Sanders described manual jet ventilation using the rigid bronchoscope.[120] In the last five decades, the rigid bronchoscope has undergone only minor structural changes,[40] and modern scopes closely resemble those used in the early years of the 20th century.[97]

2. Equipment

The rigid bronchoscope consists of a round, straight stainless steel tube with a beveled and sometimes flared distal tip[97,99] (Fig. 35-12). The proximal aspect of the bronchoscope consists of a central opening and a side port to permit assisted or controlled ventilation.[97,98]

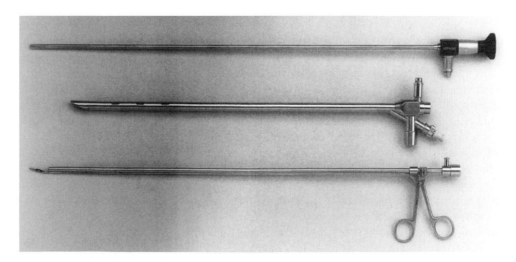

Figure 35-12 A typical rigid bronchoscope (middle) with Hopkins rod rigid telescope (top) and optical biopsy forceps. (From Ayers ML, Beamis JF: Rigid bronchoscopy in the twenty-first century. Clin Chest Med 22:355, 2001, Fig. 1A.)

A detachable eyepiece or telescope gasket can be placed over the open central proximal end of the scope to produce a closed system for positive-pressure ventilation.[98] Rigid telescopes and accessory instruments can be passed through the central proximal opening.[97] Additional proximal ports may also be used to insert suction catheters, laser fibers, and biopsy forceps.[97] Illumination is typically conducted to the distal tip of the bronchoscope by means of a thin glass rod contained in an eccentrically placed cannula, attached to the inner aspect of the shaft of the scope. The light carrier is then connected to a light source by means of a fiberoptic cable attached to a proximal side port.[97,99] Slitlike openings in the distal aspect of the shaft of the bronchoscope function as auxiliary ventilation ports.[97,99] Rigid telescopes with 0- to 90-degree lenses passed through the rigid bronchoscope improve visualization in the more distal and upper lobe bronchi.[97,98] Charge-coupled device (CCD) chip video cameras can also be attached to these telescopes.[97] The standard adult rigid bronchoscope is 40 cm in length and has an internal diameter of 8 mm.[98] The nominal diameter of a rigid bronchoscope is determined by the internal diameter of the barrel and is typically 2 to 3 mm less than the corresponding external diameter.[99] A standard set of adult rigid bronchoscopes includes 7-, 8-, and 9-mm scopes.[99]

3. Technique

The rigid bronchoscope can be inserted with the patient's head and neck in the sniffing position as in routine endotracheal intubation.[99,100] The operator grasps the bronchoscope at its proximal end using the right thumb and index and middle fingers in a pencil-like grip.[99] The left hand is positioned at the patient's maxilla with the thumb extended parallel to and just above the patient's upper gingiva or dental arch.[99] The left thumb then serves as a rest or fulcrum for the bronchoscope, and the fingers of the left hand are used to guide the scope through the upper airway.[99] The lubricated scope with the leading edge of the bevel oriented anteriorly is then introduced into the oral cavity over the operator's left thumb either in the midline or along the right side of the tongue.[99,100] In the supine patient, the scope is held almost vertically as it enters the oral cavity and is then rotated into an increasingly horizontal position as the pharynx is entered.[100] With the tip of the scope midline, the epiglottis is then visualized.[99,100] The distal leading edge of the scope is then passed into the hypopharynx posterior to the epiglottis and lifted using the left thumb at the maxilla to elevate the epiglottis anteriorly and expose the larynx.[99,100]

As the vocal cords are approached, the bronchoscope is rotated 90 degrees to align the leading edge of the bevel with the vocal cords and advanced through the glottis into the proximal trachea.[89,99] Once the trachea is entered, the scope is rotated 90 degrees back into its original position with the leading edge anteriorly.[97]

Intubation of the right or left main stem bronchus is facilitated by rotating the patient's head to the contralateral side and moving the bronchoscope to the contralateral side of the mouth.[100] The head may need to be raised or lowered as well to facilitate visualization of the bronchial tree.[100] With the aid of angled telescopes, visualization to the level of the segmental bronchial orifices can be achieved.[99] A flexible bronchoscope can be passed through the rigid instrument to visualize the more distal airway.[97,99] The rigid bronchoscope can also be inserted using a direct laryngoscope to expose the larynx, as in routine endotracheal intubation.[97,100] On occasion, rigid bronchoscopy is required in a patient who is already intubated.[97,100] In this setting, the rigid bronchoscope can be inserted to the level of the vocal cords using the ET as a guide.[97,100] The vocal cords can then be visualized through the rigid scope, the ET removed, and the scope advanced through the glottis into the trachea.[97,100]

4. Anesthesia for Rigid Bronchoscopy

Rigid bronchoscopy can be performed under local anesthesia. However, insertion of the rigid bronchoscope typically requires extremes of head and neck positioning and produces considerable pressure and mucosal stimulation.[1,6] Sudden movement of the patient as a result of a noxious stimulus during rigid bronchoscopy can produce significant airway damage.[1,6] GA is therefore usually preferred.[1,6,40,99,100] If a local technique must be used, regional anesthesia of the airway can be achieved using nerve blocks or topical anesthesia. Local anesthesia of the airway can also be used to supplement GA.[100]

The GA technique used for rigid bronchoscopy should be individualized to the expertise of the anesthesiologist and surgeon, the surgical requirements, and the patient's medical status.[1,40] Rigid bronchoscopy should be performed in an appropriately equipped operating room or endoscopy suite with full capabilities for cardiopulmonary resuscitation, adequate monitoring, suction, an oxygen source, and an anesthetic machine capable of delivering 30 L/min of gas flow.[99]

In the presence of upper airway obstruction, induction of GA using an inhalation agent such as sevoflurane and maintaining spontaneous ventilation are preferred.[98,99] Alternatively, an intravenous induction can be utilized if uneventful passage of the rigid bronchoscope is anticipated. In the absence of significant airway stenosis, the rigid bronchoscope is commonly inserted following IV induction and the administration of muscle relaxants.[99] Should insertion of the rigid bronchoscope fail following intravenous induction and mask ventilation not be satisfactory, an alternative technique to establish an airway is immediately required. GA can be maintained using inhalational or intravenous techniques. Manual ventilation can be performed by attaching the anesthesia circuit to the proximal side arm of the bronchoscope[40] (Fig. 35-13). With this technique, a variable leak usually occurs around

Figure 35-13 Schematic diagram showing a rigid ventilating bronchoscope system, which consists of the anesthesia circle system attached to a flexible connector that is attached to the side arm of the bronchoscope. With the proximal eyepiece in place, most of the inspired gas goes into the patient. However, because the bronchoscope cannot fully fill the area of the trachea, there is a variable leak out the distal end of the bronchoscope. Exhaled gases are through the anesthesia circle system. When the eyepiece is removed, there is a very large leak out the proximal end of the bronchoscope. (From Benumof JL: Anesthesia for Thoracic Surgery, 2nd ed. Philadelphia, WB Saunders, 1995, Fig. 14-10.)

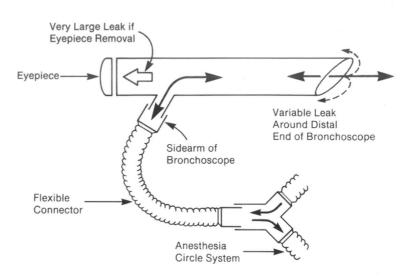

Rigid Ventilating Bronchoscope

the bronchoscope at the level of the larynx, and interruption of ventilation occurs when the proximal eyepiece is removed to permit suction and manipulation of surgical instruments.[6,40] If inhalational anesthetic agents are used, some operating room pollution inevitably occurs. The leak at the level of the larynx can be compensated for by using high gas flow rates and attenuated by using laryngeal packing.[40] Brief intermittent apnea may be required to permit diagnostic and therapeutic surgical maneuvers.[40] In the presence of a reduced bronchoscopic lumen related to surgical instruments and telescopes, the resistance to airflow is increased and the potential for air trapping and barotrauma exists.[6]

Muscle relaxants must be titrated to effect and the duration of the procedure; however, providing adequate relaxation of short duration can be problematic. One option is the use of a succinylcholine infusion.[99] A spontaneous ventilation technique using the ventilating bronchoscope can also be used. However, a satisfactory depth of anesthesia, such that hypoventilation with deep anesthesia and patient movement with light anesthesia are avoided, can be difficult to achieve.[1,40] Alternatively, ventilation during rigid bronchoscopy can be provided using a manual jet technique (Fig. 35-14). With this mode of ventilation, the endoscopist has continuous access to the open proximal end of the bronchoscope for surgical instrumentation.[6,40,98,99,102] In the original description of this technique, Sanders attached a 0.035-inch diameter jet injector to the proximal open end of the rigid bronchoscope.[120] The jet injector was attached to a high-pressure oxygen source (50 psi) by means of tubing with an in-line pressure regulator and a levered on-off valve to permit flow. Jet ventilation was provided at about 20 times/min and the adequacy of ventilation assessed by chest wall excursion.

Figure 35-14 Schematic diagram of a rigid Venturi bronchoscope showing that the jet of gas exiting from a Venturi needle placed within the lumen and parallel to the long axis of the bronchoscope entrains gas from the environment. The jetted gas comes from a high-pressure source and an intermittent (12 L/min) injector. The flow of gas from the tube into the patient is equal to the volume of gas through the jet plus the air entrained. (From Benumof JL: Anesthesia for Thoracic Surgery, 2nd ed. Philadelphia, WB Saunders, 1995, Fig. 14-11.)

Rigid Venturi Bronchoscope

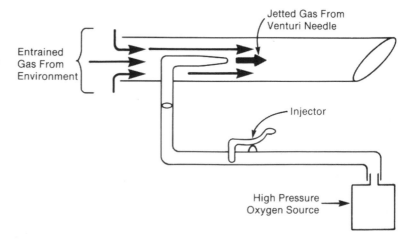

No specific problems with oxygenation or ventilation were reported. The pressure measured at the distal tip of the bronchoscope varied from 21 cm H_2O using an 8×40 bronchoscope to 36 cm H_2O using a 3.5×30 scope.[59] Subsequent modifications of the technique included use of the proximal side arm to inject oxygen.[1,6,40] Nitrous oxide–oxygen jet mixtures have also been used, although environmental pollution occurs, and the nitrous oxide can produce optical distortion because of an alteration of the refractive index of the gas mixture.[1]

Using a 50-psi source, oxygen jets usually entrain two to three times their own volume of ambient air.[40] The tidal volume and tracheal pressure produced are a function of the jet diving pressure, the size of the injector, and the diameter, length, and type of bronchoscope.[40] Tidal volumes produced with jet ventilation also vary with thoracic compliance,[6] and chest wall excursions must be observed to assess the adequacy of ventilation.[6] Ventilatory rates of 10 to 20 bpm are generally satisfactory. The reducing value pressure can be adjusted in accordance with chest wall movement and measured tracheal pressures.[40] A tracheal pressure of 30 cm H_2O usually results in normocarbia.[40] Adequate time and sufficient lumen patency for egress of injected gases are necessary if the risk of barotrauma is to be minimized.[6] The inspired oxygen concentration is uncertain because of the variable amount of air entrained.[1,97] Anesthesia during manual jet ventilation can be maintained using intravenous agents such as remifentanil 0.1 to 0.15 µg/kg/min combined with propofol 80 to 100 µg/kg/min.[99] Paralysis can be useful to improve chest wall compliance and ensure adequate ventilation.[40] Attenuation of the hemodynamic response to rigid bronchoscopy is analogous to that described for direct laryngoscopy.

HFJV and HFPPV have also been used during rigid bronchoscopy.[1,6,40,103] Adequate oxygenation, lower inspiratory pressures, and a quiet surgical field can be achieved.[1] Carbon dioxide retention can, however, occur with HFJV at frequencies above 300 to 360/min.[1,103] At frequencies of 150 to 300 bpm, HFJV produced adequate but not superior gas exchange when compared with manual jet ventilation at 20 bpm.[103]

At the completion of rigid bronchoscopy, the airway can be maintained during emergence by means of an ET, LMA, or mask ventilation, as appropriate for the particular clinical setting.

5. Indications for Rigid Bronchoscopy

The intrinsic advantages of the rigid bronchoscope include its ability to serve as an instrument for ventilation, the size of its operative lumen, and its inherent rigidity.[99] Indications for rigid bronchoscopy include (1) control and management of massive hemoptysis, (2) foreign body removal, (3) securing an airway in the presence of stenosis or obstruction, (4) endoscopic removal of neoplastic and benign tracheobronchial obstruction, (5) placement of endobronchial stents, and (6) laser bronchoscopy.[1,97-99] Rigid bronchoscopy can also be used to obtain larger biopsy specimens when specimens obtained using the fiberoptic scope are inadequate,[98,99] to dilate tracheal structures, and to remove large amounts of secretions or endobronchial debris.[97,99] The rigid bronchoscope can be used for diagnosis of airway lesions to the level of the segmental bronchi[99] and for therapeutic interventions such as electrocautery, cryotherapy, argon beam coagulation, balloon dilatation, and brachytherapy.[97,98]

6. Contraindications

The characteristics that make the rigid bronchoscope useful (contour, stiffness, and size) also limit its usefulness.[99] Cervical spine pathology may preclude the positioning required for rigid bronchoscopy, and upper airway disease or variant anatomy can make visualization of the larynx using the rigid bronchoscope impossible. Bleeding disorders are a relative contraindication.[98,99] Comorbid disease can also increase the risk associated with rigid bronchoscopy and in some settings may contraindicate the procedure.[97] A flexible bronchoscope is required for diagnostic and therapeutic procedures beyond the segmental bronchi.[99]

7. Complications

Complications associated with rigid bronchoscopy include dental and gingival injury,[40,98] vasovagal reactions associated with positioning,[40,98,99] arrhythmias, mucosal perforation with subcutaneous emphysema, pneumomediastinum[40] and pneumothorax,[98,99] hypoxemia and hypercarbia,[40] bronchospasm,[98] laryngospasm,[98] bleeding,[40,98] and subglottic edema in pediatrics and patients with subglottic stenosis.[99] Blood and tumor particles can also be blown into the distal airway during jet ventilation.[40] However, when it is performed in a controlled setting by experienced operators, complications associated with rigid bronchoscopy are rare.[97]

B. FLEXIBLE BRONCHOSCOPY

The flexible fiberoptic bronchoscope (FOB) was initially conceptualized as an extended telescope for use with the rigid bronchoscope to permit more distal inspection of the bronchial tree.[99] However, since its introduction, it has revolutionized the practice of pulmonary medicine[104] and has become the instrument of choice for most diagnostic and therapeutic bronchoscopic procedures in adults.[104] Visualization can be achieved as far as fifth-generation subsegmental bronchi.[1,41]

1. Equipment

The standard adult bronchoscope has a distal diameter of 5.9 to 6.0 mm, a working channel of 2.2 to 2.8 mm diameter, and a shaft length of 58 cm.[41] A lever located at the handle of the scope controls flexion of the tip of the shaft in a single plane. The working channel can be used for suctioning, instilling solutions, and passing various biopsy instruments.[41] Illumination is provided by a xenon or halogen light source.[41] Video bronchoscopes contain high-resolution CCD chips that provide superior images compared with fiberoptic scopes.[41]

2. Indications

Flexible fiberoptic bronchoscopy has essentially replaced rigid bronchoscopy in the diagnosis of chest disease.[41] Diagnostic indications include the identification, tissue diagnosis, and determination of the endobronchial extent of lung cancer; hemoptysis; pleural effusion; pulmonary infiltrates; ventilator-associated pneumonia; airway trauma; uncertain tracheal patency; smoke inhalation injury; and confirmation of ET position and patency.[41] Therapeutic indications include acute lobar collapse, mucous plug removal, selected foreign body removal, difficult intubation, hemoptysis, brachytherapy, laser ablation, electrocautery, balloon dilation, and selected stent placement.[41] Newer applications include bronchoscopic ultrasonography.[104]

3. Anesthesia for Flexible Bronchoscopy

Fiberoptic bronchoscopy can be performed under either local anesthesia or GA. Although infrequently required, GA may be indicated if the procedure is prolonged or if the patient is uncooperative.[6]

Regional anesthesia for flexible bronchoscopy can be achieved utilizing various aerosol or atomizer techniques. Topical lidocaine or tetracaine administered using an atomizer such as the DeVilbiss (DeVilbiss Manufacturing Company, Toledo, OH) works particularly well. Glossopharyngeal and superior laryngeal nerve blocks can also be used,[24,25,40] and local anesthetic can be injected by cricothyroid puncture or through the suction channel of the bronchoscope.[40] Hypoxemia occurs frequently during and for several hours after fiberoptic bronchoscopy and appears to be due to a ventilation-perfusion mismatch related to suctioning, airway obstruction, bronchospasm, and alveolar filling with lavage or anesthetic solutions.[41] The average decrease in Po_2 is 20 mm Hg, which persists for 1 to 4 hours following the procedure.[40] Supplemental oxygen is highly desirable[40] and can be administered by nasal prongs or a modified face mask.[1] Flexible bronchoscopy can also be performed with the awake patient in the sitting or semisitting position, and ventilatory mechanics may thereby be improved compared with the supine position.[1]

Sedation is not necessary during fiberoptic bronchoscopy under local anesthesia but can be used to minimize the patient's discomfort, provide anxiolysis, and attenuate recall. A 1991 survey performed by the American College of Chest Physicians revealed that intravenous sedation was used routinely by 50.7%, sometimes by 23.2%, and rarely by 23.8% of bronchoscopists.[105] The sedative agent chosen is largely dependent on the preference and expertise of the operator and should be individualized to the clinical setting and carefully titrated to effect. A benzodiazepine, such as midazolam 0.02 to 0.04 mg/kg, and a narcotic, such as fentanyl 1 to 2 µg/kg, can both be given in IV increments.[6]

Adverse reactions to local anesthetics and respiratory depression from excessive sedation can occur; thus, bronchoscopy should be performed in areas that are adequately equipped for airway management and cardiopulmonary resuscitation.[41] Monitoring should include level of consciousness, respirations, pulse oximetry, electrocardiogram, and blood pressure.[6] Standard guidelines with regard to preoperative fasting should be followed.

Fiberoptic bronchoscopy under GA is almost always performed following endotracheal intubation. Flexible FOBs with ODs of 5.0, 5.7, and 6.0 mm occupy only 6%, 10%, and 11%, respectively, of the cross-sectional area of the average adult trachea.[40] However, a 5.7 mm OD bronchoscope reduces the cross-sectional area of an 8.0 mm ID ET by 51%[106] (Fig. 35-15). The remaining cross-sectional area is equivalent to that of a 5.5-mm ET.[103] As a result of this increased airway resistance, inadequate ventilation can occur and ventilation should be controlled or vigorously assisted.[1,40] However, if the bronchoscope occupies too much of the cross-sectional area of the ET, the elastic recoil of the lungs may not be sufficient to force tidal gas out of the lungs, resulting in high PEEP and potential barotrauma.[1,40] No PEEP values above 20 cm H_2O were observed when a 5.7-mm bronchoscope was used with an 8.0- to 8.5-mm ET.[1] Therefore, depending on the size of the bronchoscope, an ET no smaller than 8.0 to 8.5 should be used during fiberoptic bronchoscopy in the average adult.[1] If a smaller tube must be used, the use of helium-oxygen mixtures should be considered.[40] In addition, sufficient time must be allowed for expiration to occur.[6,40] Intermittent removal of the bronchoscope and hyperventilation with oxygen may also be required to maintain adequate ventilation.[1] Fiberoptic bronchoscopy can also be performed through an LMA in anesthetized children and under general or topical anesthesia in adults.[40,107] Size 3 and 4 LMAs have both been used for fiberoptic bronchoscopy in adults under topical anesthesia and sedation.[107] The shaft of a size 4 LMA has an ID of 9 to 10 mm.[40] Subglottic HFJV has also been used during interventional fiberoptic bronchoscopy.[108]

GA for flexible bronchoscopy can be administered using an intravenous, inhalational, or combined technique. Local anesthesia of the airway can be used to supplement GA and is most effective when administered by nebulizer prior to induction.[90] When used alone, high concentrations of potent volatile anesthetics (1.7 minimum alveolar

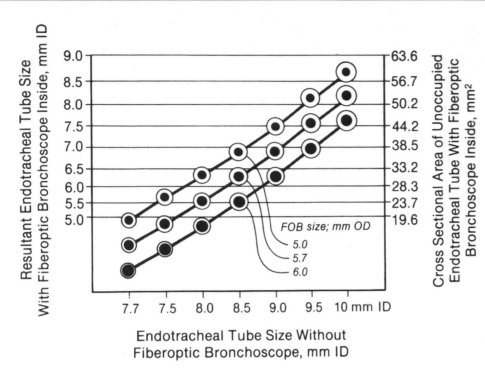

Figure 35-15 Diagram relating the size of an endotracheal tube without an indwelling fiberoptic bronchoscope (x-axis) to the resultant functional size that the endotracheal tube would have with an indwelling fiberoptic bronchoscope (left-hand y-axis) (three fiberoptic bronchoscope sizes are shown: 5.0, 5.7, and 6.0 mm outside diameter). The cross-sectional area of unoccupied endotracheal tube in mm² that is responsible for the resultant functional size is shown on the right-hand y-axis. ID, inside diameter. (Modification of Fig. 7 from Lindholm CE, Ollman B, Snyder JV, et al: Cardiorespiratory effect of flexible fiberoptic bronchoscopy in critically ill patients. Chest 74;362,1978, and Benumof JL: Anesthesia for Thoracic Surgery, 2nd ed. Philadelphia, WB Saunders, 1995, Fig. 14-1.)

concentration [MAC]) may be required to suppress airway reflexes.[6] Nitrous oxide concentrations should be limited to ensure adequate oxygenation.[6] Short-acting muscle relaxants and intravenous agents such as propofol, alfentanil, and remifentanil can be used. Achieving an adequate depth of anesthesia to suppress airway reflexes and appropriate relaxation, without prolonging recovery, can be a challenge.

4. Contraindications

The risk of bronchoscopy is increased in the presence of unstable cardiopulmonary disease, coagulopathy, uremia, pulmonary hypertension, and severe anemia.[41] Absolute contraindications include absence of consent, inadequate facilities and personnel, and inability to oxygenate the patient during the procedure.[41]

5. Complications

Complications associated with fiberoptic bronchoscopy include hypoxemia, excessive sedation, local anesthetic toxicity, hypoventilation, bronchospasm, laryngospasm, barotrauma, bleeding, fever, hypertension, tachycardia, and arrhythmias.[1,6,40,41] In a review of 156,064 anesthetics, bronchospasm associated with bronchoscopy occurred in up to 16.4 per 1000 patients, whereas the overall incidence of bronchospasm during anesthesia was found to be 1.6 per 1000 anesthetics.[109] The incidence of bronchospasm associated with bronchoscopy has also been reported to be 6 per 24,521 (0.2 per 1000).[110] Laryngospasm occurred in 3 of these 24,521 bronchoscopies (1.3 per 1000).[110]

High airway pressures occurring during bronchoscopy are an indication for a postoperative chest radiograph to rule out pneumothorax and mediastinal emphysema. Studies from the 1970s reported a mortality associated with flexible bronchoscopy of 0.01% to 0.5% and a major complication rate of 0.08% to 5.0%.[41] A 1995 retrospective review of 4273 flexible bronchoscopies reported no associated mortality, a major complication rate of 0.5%, and a minor complication rate of 0.8%.[111]

C. PEDIATRIC BRONCHOSCOPY

Bronchoscopy in the pediatric age group is performed using both rigid and flexible instruments. Historically, pediatric bronchoscopy was performed exclusively with the rigid bronchoscope prior to the introduction of fiberoptic scopes small enough for use in infants and children. Since the initial English literature report of its clinical utility in the pediatric age group in 1978, the use of fiberoptic airway endoscopy has expanded dramatically in the evaluation and management of airway and pulmonary disorders in children.[112] However, rigid bronchoscopy and flexible bronchoscopy continue to be complementary techniques, and each has advantages and disadvantages when applied to the pediatric population.[113]

1. Indications

Indications for bronchoscopy in children include evaluation of stridor, chronic cough, foreign body aspiration, laryngomalacia, subglottic and tracheal stenosis, gastroesophageal reflux, persistent wheezing, atelectasis, pneumonia, hemoptysis, and tracheostomy care.[113,114] Rigid bronchoscopy is particularly useful for the documentation of glottic and subglottic pathology, such as cleft palates and high fistulas, evaluation of hemoptysis, biopsy, and interventions such as foreign body extraction, laser surgery, stent placement,[113,115] and dilation of strictures.[113] The flexible bronchoscope is indispensable if functional assessment of dynamic airway movement is required and is particularly useful in the removal of secretions, evaluation of airway trauma, bronchoalveolar lavage, tracheostomy care, difficult intubations,[113,115] and visualization of the anterior glottis.[117] The rigid bronchoscope may be required for removal of tenacious central mucous plugs, whereas the flexible scope is required when the distal airways must be evaluated.[114]

2. Equipment

Pediatric rigid bronchoscopes are similar to adult rigid bronchoscopes except that the sheaths are shorter and have a smaller diameter. Pediatric bronchoscopes are classified by the length of the sheath into infant and child sizes; for Storz (Karl Storz, Culver City, CA) instruments, 20- and 30-cm sheaths, respectively.[51] A range of diameters is available for both sheath lengths. The "nominal size" of the instrument is related to diameter but does not correspond exactly to the internal diameter.[51] The *infant* sheaths are designated 2.5, 3.0, and 3.5; the *child* sheaths 3.5, 4.0, 5.0 and 6.0. The external diameters of the Storz sheaths are slightly larger than the corresponding size of ET.[51] The 2.5 rigid bronchoscope has an internal diameter of 3.2 mm and an external diameter of 4.0 mm.[51] During bronchoscopy, gas exchange occurs through the lumen of the bronchoscope and, when a telescope is in place, through the circumferential space between the telescope and the sheath.[51]

The standard telescope for infant sheaths has a diameter of 2.8 mm and when inserted into the 2.5 sheath, the 0.2-mm circumferential space is inadequate for gas exchange.[51] When using this instrumentation, the telescope must be removed frequently, and only occasional positive pressure breaths administered with low-flow oxygen (1 L/min) and a pressure relief valve that must be kept open.[51] The 3.0 infant sheath-telescope system has a resistance to flow comparable to that of a 3.0-mm ET, and should be adequate for most infants.[51] Resistance to gas flow through a tube is related to the length of the tube and the fourth power of the radius, and under conditions of turbulent flow it increases with flow rates.[51] The telescopes used in child sheaths have diameters of 2.8 to 4.0 mm.[51] In paralyzed patients, exhalation is passive and the recoil of the infant lungs and chest wall may not be sufficient to avoid air trapping and barotrauma, and hemodynamic compromise can occur.[51] The risk of barotrauma can be minimized by permitting spontaneous ventilation under anesthesia such that exhalation

is active, allowing adequate expiratory times, and intermittent removal of the telescope.[51] Interference with gas exchange is usually of major consequence only when using the 2.5-mm sheath with the telescope in place.

The size of the bronchoscopic sheath must also be considered when jet ventilation is used during rigid bronchoscopy. As the lumen of the bronchoscope decreases, it approximates an extension of the jet injector,[51] as there is less gas contained within the lumen for entrainment.[51] The smaller bronchoscopic lumen produces high inflation pressures, and instruments occupying the lumen of the bronchoscope have the same effect.[51] Jet ventilation techniques also require unimpeded egress of gas from the lung through the bronchoscopic lumen, and if the lumen is significantly narrowed, exhalation is inhibited.[51] The use of jet techniques in pediatric patients has been associated with barotrauma and requires a high level of expertise, an extensive knowledge of the particular system utilized, and a high degree of vigilance.[51]

Flexible FOBs are now available in pediatric sizes ranging from 2.2 to 4.9 mm OD.[114] The 2.2-mm scope can be passed through a number 2.5 to 3.0 ET and can be used in premature and term infants.[114] Scopes with an external diameter of 3.2 to 3.5 can be used in term infants and children up to 7 years of age (and can be passed through 4.0 to 5.5 ETs).[114] Scopes with an external diameter of 4.5 to 4.9 mm are suitable for children 7 years of age and older and can be passed through 5.5 to 6.5 ETs.[114] Flexible bronchoscopes with a diameter of 3.2 mm or more have working channels, whereas bronchoscopes that are 2.2 mm or less in diameter do not.[114] A 1.8-mm flexible scope has been manufactured that does not have a movable tip or a suction channel.[51]

In contrast to the rigid bronchoscope, which provides a lumen through which ventilation can occur, the flexible FOB introduces a solid foreign body into the pediatric airway that increases resistance to gas flow and disturbs ventilation-perfusion relationships.[118,119] An appropriately sized scope should be used and the duration of airway obstruction limited such that adequate ventilation can occur.

3. Anesthesia for Pediatric Bronchoscopy

Although it can be performed in awake, stridorous newborns,[6] rigid bronchoscopy in the pediatric age group is typically performed under GA.[113,115,120] Anesthetic management should be individualized to the site and extent of pathology, comorbid disease, and physical status of the patient. Inhalation or intravenous induction and maintenance can be utilized as appropriate in the clinical setting. Anticholinergic medication can be used to decrease airway secretions and attenuate vagally mediated reflexes.[51] Ventilation can be spontaneous, manually assisted, or controlled. Attention must be directed to adequate exhalation when small bronchoscopes and telescopes are used, and interruption of ventilation, when the proximal end of the bronchoscope is open, must be limited to permit adequate ventilation. Following removal of the bronchoscope, the airway can be maintained by means of mask ventilation, ET, or LMA until airway reflexes have returned and the child is awake.

Postoperative stridor related to airway edema can occur following bronchoscopy, is usually related to the extent of airway manipulation, and is usually apparent within 30 minutes.[51] Treatment includes racemic epinephrine, steroids, and airway management including reintubation as required.[51] Local anesthesia can be used as a supplement to GA for rigid bronchoscopy. Lidocaine up to 3 to 5 mg/kg can be applied to the mucous membranes of the airway above the vocal cords.[51] When used below the vocal cords, doses of 1.5[6] to 2[51] mg/kg have been recommended. The use of topical lidocaine in doses up to 8 mg/kg has also been reported.[114] A reduction in lidocaine dosage by 25% to 50% in newborns, particularly premature infants, has been recommended.[51] Standard monitors for pediatric patients undergoing bronchoscopy include a pulse oximeter, electrocardiogram monitor, noninvasive blood pressure, a precordial stethoscope, a capnograph, and gas monitors.[51] Doppler ultrasound devices are also used in some settings.[51]

Flexible fiberoptic bronchoscopy in children is commonly performed under GA in many centers.[113,115,118,121] Inhalation induction with halothane or sevoflurane or intravenous induction with agents such as propofol can be used.[114] Supplemental local anesthesia can be applied to the larynx and trachea and, at an adequate depth of anesthesia, an LMA or ET can be inserted. The bronchoscope can be passed through a self-sealing swivel connector attached to a face mask, LMA, or ET.[114] The bronchoscope can be passed through the nostril in patients who have not been intubated.[114] Standard monitors are employed and ventilation can be spontaneous, assisted, or controlled. Again, attention must be directed to the presence of a foreign body in the airway producing increased resistance to gas flow and adequate exhalation. Bronchoscopic suctioning can also adversely affect oxygenation.

Flexible bronchoscopy in children is also commonly performed under local anesthesia and sedation.[112,115,116,117,119] Preoperative antisialagogues have been advocated, but the efficacy of these agents in adult fiberoptic endoscopy has been disputed and their role in pediatric fiberoptic endoscopy has not been clearly established.[112] Local anesthetics can be administered by a variety of techniques; however, inhalation of topical anesthetics through a face mask can be difficult in children because of the bad taste of lidocaine.[115] A handheld nebulizer or atomizer can be used, and lidocaine jelly can be applied to the nasal cavity.[119] Additional aliquots of lidocaine can be administered through the suction channel of the bronchoscope.[119] A maximum total dose of 4 mg/kg has been recommended.[115]

Sedation can be achieved with a variety of agents; benzodiazepines and narcotics are commonly used. Sedatives should be administered in aliquots or by intravenous infusion and carefully titrated to effect. Appropriate choices include IV fentanyl 0.5 µg/kg[6] or 1 to 3 µg/kg/hr,[114] morphine 0.07 mg/kg,[6] midazolam 0.1 mg/kg[114,115] to a maximum of 0.2 to 0.3 mg/kg[115] or 0.03 mg/kg,[6] alfentanil 0.5 µg/kg/min,[115] or remifentanil 0.05 to 0.1 µg/kg/min.[115] If necessary, excessive narcotic and benzodiazepine effects can be reversed by naloxone (Narcan) and flumazenil, respectively.[6] Propofol has also been used for sedation for flexible bronchoscopy,[115] as has ketamine, although a 20% incidence of complications has been reported with the use of ketamine.[122] Monitoring during conscious sedation should be consistent with current guidelines and include pulse oximetry and ECG monitoring. Oxygen can be administered by nasal prongs or modified face mask. Oxygen can also be insufflated through the suction channel of the bronchoscope, but a risk of pulmonary barotrauma and gastric distention exists with this technique.[115,123,124] Oversedation can be associated with respiratory depression, whereas inadequate sedation can be associated with inadequate operating conditions. Inadequate local anesthesia can result in bradycardia and laryngospasm.[114]

Continuous observation of the patient by someone other than the bronchoscopist is essential,[117] and a health care professional skilled in the monitoring of the patient's cardiopulmonary status and capable of handling airway emergencies should be present when sedation is administered.[122] Appropriate selection of patients for bronchoscopy under conscious sedation is necessary if complications are to be minimized. When potential clinical difficulty is suggested by the patient's physical status, underlying disease, or comorbidity, GA with airway support by an LMA or ET may be required.[115,119]

4. Complications

Complications of bronchoscopy in the pediatric age group include arrhythmias, pneumothorax, laryngospasm, bleeding, dental injury, pneumomediastinum, bronchial perforation, bronchospasm, and fever.[113,114] A 2001 survey of rigid and flexible pediatric bronchoscopy reported a complication rate of 0.4%.[113]

VII. SPECIAL CIRCUMSTANCES

A. AIRWAY FOREIGN BODIES

Foreign body aspiration is a common problem worldwide and in the United States accounts for 300 to 2000 deaths annually, with more than half of these deaths occurring in children 6 months to 4 years of age.[125,126] Aspiration of a foreign body occurs most frequently in the toddler age group (1 to 3 years), and about 75% to

85% of all foreign body aspiration occurs in children younger than 15 years of age.[126,127] In the adult age group, foreign body aspiration occurs most commonly in the sixth or seventh decade of life, and is associated with a failure of airway protective mechanisms that can occur in primary neurologic disorders or with a decreased level of consciousness.[125,126] In children, the most common foreign bodies aspirated are food products, especially peanuts.[125,128] In adults, aspirated foreign bodies include dental and medical appliances as well as organic material.[125-127] Foreign bodies may lodge in the laryngeal inlet, but most pass through the larynx and trachea to reach the more distal airways[129]; 7.4% to 20% become impacted in the larynx or trachea, 30% to 40% in the left bronchial tree, and 40% to 70% in the right bronchial tree.[126,129]

The clinical presentation can be acute or chronic and depends on the location as well as the degree of obstruction and inflammatory response caused by the foreign body. Complete airway obstruction is more likely to be caused by foreign bodies lodged in the larynx than those located below the glottis.[6] Bronchial foreign bodies may be dislodged by cough or a change in body position to produce subglottic or contralateral main stem bronchus obstruction[50] (Fig. 35-16). Complete airway obstruction can be recognized as the onset of sudden respiratory distress associated with an inability to speak or cough.[129] Adults and older children may use the universal distress

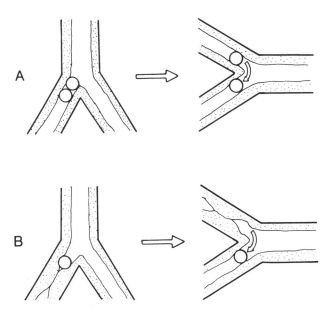

Figure 35-16 Mechanisms of bilateral bronchial obstruction following foreign body aspiration. **A,** Two objects are in the right main bronchus and when the patient assumes the left lateral decubitus position, one of them enters the opposite bronchus (**B**). There is swelling distal to a foreign body. When the object is dislodged and enters the opposite bronchus, total obstruction results. (From Woods AM: Pediatric endoscopy. In Berry FA [ed]: Anesthetic Management of Difficult and Routine Pediatric Patients, 2nd ed. New York, Churchill Livingstone, 1990, p 199.)

signal of choking (the hand clasped to the throat) or gesticulate wildly. With a laryngeal foreign body, severe coughing, choking, hoarseness, and gagging are frequently seen.[126] A subglottic or tracheal foreign body causing incomplete obstruction produces inspiratory stridor and cough.[126] Bronchial foreign bodies may produce minimal symptoms other than localized or unilateral wheezing.[126] Retained foreign bodies can produce obstructive pneumonia, emphysema, and bronchiectasis.[125,127] The classical triad of choking, cough, and wheezing is present in only a small percentage of patients[126]; however, a choking crisis is one of the most accurate indications of foreign body aspiration with a sensitivity of 96% and a specificity of 76%.[125] Physical findings include stridor, chest retractions, fever, and decreased breath sounds.[125] Radiographic imaging can be helpful if the aspirated foreign body is radiopaque or if hyperexpansion is seen on expiration.[125] Atelectasis, recurrent pneumonia, and bronchiectasis can also be seen.[125] Negative radiographs do not rule out aspirated foreign bodies.[125]

The emergency management of foreign body obstruction is directed by the degree of airway compromise and should follow the current guidelines for cardiopulmonary resuscitation and emergency cardiovascular care.[16]

A foreign body in the airway may or may not be a true medical emergency, as determined by the location, chronicity, and reactivity of the object; however, prompt endoscopic removal is the treatment of choice.[51,125,128] The timing of bronchoscopy requires clinical judgment, weighing the risks of increased airway obstruction against the risk of aspiration of gastric contents, should a full stomach exist. In the pediatric age group, the rigid bronchoscope has traditionally been the primary tool for removal of tracheobronchial foreign bodies,[125,128] and extraction of a foreign body by means of a rigid bronchoscope under GA is said to be the standard of care.[130] Although the flexible bronchoscope has been used successfully to remove aspirated foreign bodies in children under GA, the equipment and personnel necessary to convert to rigid bronchoscopy were immediately available.[125,126,131] Flexible bronchoscopy can also be useful for diagnostic purposes in patients with suspected foreign bodies.[125] GA can be induced using halothane or sevoflurane and oxygen during spontaneous ventilation.[6,129] Spontaneous ventilation is preferred to positive-pressure ventilation to avoid the potential risk of forcing the foreign body deeper into the airway, or into the glottis or trachea, and producing total airway obstruction.[6,130] When an adequate depth of anesthesia has been achieved, direct laryngoscopy can be performed. If the foreign body is visualized, it may be possible to extract it using appropriate forceps, or the introduction of the operating laryngoscope may be required.[6] If no foreign body is seen in the larynx, topical lidocaine spray can be applied to attenuate further unwanted airway reflexes.[6,127,129] The appropriately sized rigid bronchoscope is then introduced by the surgeon in the usual manner. Should complete airway obstruction occur during induction, direct laryngoscopy may permit extraction of a laryngeal foreign body or intubation around it. It may also be possible to push a tracheal foreign body distally into a bronchus and achieve ventilation or intubate around it.[51] In the cannot-intubate, cannot-ventilate situation, a surgical airway is immediately indicated.

GA can be maintained using inhalational or intravenous agents. Spontaneous ventilation can be used throughout the procedure, although a risk of patient movement exists.[6,129] Controlled or jet ventilation and muscle relaxants can be also be used,[6,128,132] although the foreign body can be forced more distally into the airway with this technique.[6] Placement of the bronchoscope deep into a bronchus can also be associated with inadequate ventilation, and it may be necessary to pull the scope back intermittently into the trachea.[6]

When the foreign body is too large to withdraw through the lumen of the bronchoscope (or as a standard technique), the bronchoscope, forceps, and the foreign body can be removed as a single unit.[127,128] Communication and coordination between the surgeon and anesthesiologist are critical throughout the procedure.[127] Should the foreign body become lost in the subglottic area, causing life-threatening obstruction, and immediate extraction not be possible, the object can be pushed distally into a main stem bronchus to permit ventilation before a second attempt at removal.[128] Following extraction of the foreign body and inspection of the airways, endotracheal intubation and positive-pressure ventilation can be performed to reexpand atelectatic lung segments, as appropriate to the clinical setting. Postinstrumentation airway edema can occur, and treatment with inhaled racemic epinephrine and intravenous steroids may be required.[6,127,128] Significant airway edema may require the presence of an ET into the postoperative period.[6]

In the adult, although the rigid bronchoscope has been the traditional instrument used for removal of tracheobronchial foreign bodies,[125] the flexible bronchoscope has gained acceptance as the preferred initial instrument for diagnosis as well as extraction of foreign bodies in the airway.[126] Fiberoptic bronchoscopy can be performed under local anesthesia and conscious sedation.[126] Various techniques for foreign body removal including the use of grasping forceps, balloon catheters, and baskets have been described.[126] During foreign body extraction by flexible bronchoscopy, the airway is not secure. Should the foreign body become lost in the subglottic area, airway obstruction is possible and thoracic surgery and anesthesia services may be emergently required.[126] A success rate of 80% in more than 400 fiberoptic extractions by flexible bronchoscopy has been reported.[126]

Endoscopic removal of aspirated foreign bodies has been reported to be successful in 98% to 99% of cases with an associated complication rate of 0.2% and a mortality rate less than 0.1%.[133] Foreign bodies that cannot be removed by bronchoscopy require tracheostomy or open thoracotomy and bronchotomy or lung resection.[130,134] Thoracotomy has been reported to be necessary in less than 1% to 2.5% of cases.[134,135]

B. AIRWAY TRAUMA

Laryngotracheal trauma is rare. Blunt and penetrating laryngeal injury has been reported to occur in less than 0.04% to 0.3% of trauma victims.[136,137] Review of a 54 million trauma admission database revealed an incidence of blunt laryngeal trauma of 1 in 137,000.[138] Tracheobronchial injuries are also rare. In emergency department admissions with blunt trauma, tracheobronchial injury occurred in less than 1%.[139] The anatomic location of the larynx between the mandible and the sternum, its cartilaginous resilience, and its mobility confer some protection against injury.[140] In the pediatric population, the higher cervical position of the larynx behind the mandibular arch, the relatively short neck, and the increased pliability of the cartilaginous structures provide further protection against blunt trauma.[141-145] However, the relatively small size of the laryngotracheal airway and the loose perichondrial attachment of submucosal tissue in children may predispose to airway obstruction.[141,143,144] The mobility, elasticity, and cartilaginous support of the trachea also make it a difficult structure to injure.[135] Injuries to the larynx and cervical trachea are usually caused by direct blows to the neck.[142,146] Common mechanisms include motor vehicle accidents, falls onto handlebars, "clothesline" injuries, sports injuries, and assaults.[142,146] Penetrating injury occurs secondary to gunshot or stab wounds, animal bites, or falls onto sharp objects and is less common in children.[142]

Laryngeal injury may be limited to minor endolaryngeal hematoma or laceration or include massive trauma to laryngeal mucosa, fractures, and laryngotracheal separation.[42,140,143] Laryngotracheal separation is frequently associated with recurrent laryngeal nerve injury and bilateral vocal cord paralysis.[20,143] Tracheobronchial injury can be produced by a crush injury to the chest that produces a rapid increase in intratracheal pressure against a closed glottis, compression of the tracheobronchial tree between the sternum and vertebral column, or rapid deceleration-acceleration that results in a shearing force at points of tracheal fixation (cricoid cartilage and carina).[139,142] Eighty percent of tracheobronchial tears occur within 2.5 cm of the carina.[139,142] Tracheobronchial injuries occur almost exclusively in association with major trauma, such as high-speed motor vehicle accidents or falls from heights.[142] Injuries associated with blunt laryngeal trauma include head injury 13%[138] to 29%,[137] esophageal or pharyngeal injury 3%[138] to 14%,[137] open neck injury 9%,[138] and spine or spinal cord injury 8%[138] to 14%.[137] Cervical spine injury has been reported in 9% of patients with blunt trauma to the cervical trachea.[145,147] Injuries associated with tracheobronchial injury include vascular, esophageal, head, chest, spinal cord, and facial injury.[139] The most commonly associated organ to be injured is the esophagus.[139]

The presenting symptoms of acute laryngeal trauma include voice change, dysphagia, odynophagia, cough, hemoptysis, and dyspnea.[140,142,143,145] Findings on examination include respiratory distress, stridor, crepitance, subcutaneous emphysema, palpable cartilage fracture, loss of thyroid prominence, open neck wound, and anterior neck pain on palpation.[140,142,143,145] External signs of injury, however, may not correlate with the site or extent of injury.[145] Tracheobronchial injury should be suspected in trauma victims with increasing subcutaneous emphysema or failure to reexpand a pneumothorax or large air leak following chest tube placement.[142] Crepitus indicates an air leak from the larynx, trachea, pharynx, or esophagus.[145]

The airway should be considered to be potentially unstable in the presence of laryngotracheal trauma, and urgent evaluation and management are required.[141,144] The order and pace of evaluation and intervention are dictated by the level of respiratory distress.[145] Cervical spine injury must be assumed until it can be ruled out by examination or radiologically.[146] If cervical spine injury is identified or cannot be ruled out, in-line stabilization of the cervical spine is required. Emergent or urgent airway management can be difficult, and the optimal technique is controversial. In the presence of laryngotracheal injury, endotracheal intubation can convert a partial tear into a complete transection, cannulate a false passage,[140,141,145,146] and otherwise exacerbate an existing injury.[141] Coughing or gagging during intubation can dislodge clots and produce massive bleeding[146] and can worsen subcutaneous emphysema with further airway deterioration.[143] However, when conditions permit, oral intubation can be attempted[140] and in the presence of respiratory distress can be lifesaving.[146] Awake intubation over an FOB under local anesthesia is a valuable option. Intubation should be undertaken only with the ability to perform emergency tracheostomy.[142]

Tracheostomy has been advocated as the airway of choice in patients with laryngotracheal injury[140,142,144] and is ideally performed awake during spontaneous ventilation under local anesthesia.[142] Cricothyrotomy has been performed when time did not permit a controlled tracheostomy[140]; however, instrumentation at this level may increase the severity of injury.[142] Also, cricothyrotomy is not recommended in children younger than 6 to 12 years of age.[142,149] As a last resort in the emergent setting, needle cricothyrotomy may provide airway control until a more permanent airway can be established.[142] Awake tracheostomy or intubation may not be practical in children.[142] Therefore, when possible, the traumatized pediatric airway should be secured in the operating room under GA induced with an inhalational agent during spontaneous ventilation.[141-143] Cricoid pressure may completely disrupt a partially injured cricothyroid junction and should be avoided.[142] Following induction, the airway can be evaluated by endoscopy and intubation or tracheostomy performed as required.[141,142] In the presence of a disruption in the upper airway, administration of nitrous oxide and positive-pressure ventilation can exacerbate subcutaneous emphysema,[143] and positive-pressure ventilation should be avoided until distal airway control can be achieved.

If on initial assessment there is no immediate need for airway control, further evaluation by flexible laryngoscopy and radiologic examination can be performed. Free air in the deep spaces of the neck on radiographs implies injury to the upper airway or esophagus.[142] Injuries to the tracheobronchial tree are associated with pneumomediastinum and pneumothorax.[142] CT is the imaging modality of choice for laryngeal injury[142]; however, the benefits of CT scanning must be weighed against the potential risk of worsening respiratory status.[145] During radiologic evaluation, the patient must be accompanied by individuals capable of managing the airway.[145] Endoscopic evaluation is mandatory for suspected laryngeal, tracheal, or bronchial injury.[142,145] Both rigid and flexible bronchoscopes can be utilized.[145] Esophageal injury can also be evaluated or ruled out using rigid or flexible scopes.[142] When GA is required for trauma endoscopy, the same principles including the use of spontaneous ventilation apply, as described in the emergent setting. The information obtained on flexible endoscopy can be used to determine whether panendoscopy is required.[141] In a review of 392 patients with laryngeal trauma, 63% required surgical intervention including endoscopy, tracheostomy, or surgical repair.[138] Direct laryngoscopy or bronchoscopy was performed in 45% of the patients.[138] Patients with tracheobronchial injuries can be safely intubated, but the use of positive-pressure ventilation can increase the air leak and ventilation can be inadequate.[142] Selective bronchial intubation and emergent surgical repair may be required.[142]

Although laryngotracheal trauma is rare, it is potentially lethal. Airway management is controversial and options are limited. Tracheostomy under local anesthesia is considered to be the method of choice for securing the airway.[140] However, endotracheal intubation may be effective[145] and acceptable in certain circumstances.[140] When GA is required to permit emergent airway control or airway evaluation in trauma, spontaneous ventilation and inhalational induction should be employed.[139,141-143]

C. MASSIVE HEMOPTYSIS

Massive hemoptysis has been variously defined as the expectoration of more than 100 to more than 1000 mL of blood in 24 hours or more than 600 mL in 48 hours.[40,148,150,151] A commonly used criterion is more than 600 mL in 24 hours.[99,150,151] The clinical effects of the hemoptysis (airway obstruction, hypotension, blood loss) can also be used to define its magnitude.[148,150] Massive hemoptysis is uncommon, accounting for 1.5%[147] to 4.8% to 14%[148] of all cases of hemoptysis. The source of bleeding in 90% of cases is the bronchial arteries, which are branches of the aorta and have systemic pressures.[150]

The most common cause of massive hemoptysis is infection, which accounts for 45% to 90% of cases,[40] the three most common infections being bronchitis, tuberculosis, and bronchiectasis.[40] Neoplasm accounts for 7% to 19% of cases.[40] Other causes include cardiovascular diseases such as mitral stenosis, collagen vascular diseases, foreign bodies, and pulmonary artery catheterization.[40,148,150] In 2% to 15% of cases, the cause is indeterminate.[148,150]

The degree of respiratory distress associated with massive hemoptysis is variable. Acute airway hemorrhage can be immediately life threatening, and death from massive hemoptysis is usually from asphyxiation.[40,150] Immediate resuscitative measures include the administration of oxygen, ensuring intravenous access, and volume administration.[148,150] Monitoring the patient in a sitting or semisitting position may attenuate the level of respiratory distress. If airway compromise exists, endotracheal intubation is indicated and may be more easily performed in the semiupright position, as cough and blood in the upper airway are minimized.[40] An ET greater than or equal to 8.0 mm ID should be used to permit bronchoscopy.[150,151] If the side of bleeding can be lateralized by history and physical examination, positioning the patient with the bleeding side down will theoretically protect the uninvolved lung.[148,150,151] When time permits, plain chest radiography can identify the side of bleeding in 60% of cases.[150]

Bronchoscopy, in the setting of active hemoptysis, is the single most important technique for determining the cause and location of bleeding.[40] The timing of bronchoscopy is, however, controversial.[148,151] The consensus opinion is that urgent bronchoscopy should be performed in patients who manifest rapid clinical deterioration, whereas the performance of bronchoscopy within 24 to 48 hours is preferred in stable patients.[151] When performed within 48 hours, rigid bronchoscopy has been shown to identify the source of bleeding in up to 86% of cases.[150] Success rates with early flexible bronchoscopy range from 34% to 93%.[150] Whether rigid or flexible bronchoscopy should be used in the setting of massive hemoptysis is also controversial.[148,152] Rigid bronchoscopy has been traditionally recommended as the technique of choice[150] because of its greater suctioning capability and its ability to secure an airway and provide ventilation.[150] Flexible bronchoscopy has, however, become more accepted as an initial procedure, particularly in patients who are already intubated.[150] The FOB permits better access to the distal airways[148] and upper lobe bronchi,[40,152] but limitations include less effective suction and difficult visualization in the presence of active bleeding.[150,152] Excessive use of suction can steal tidal volume and adversely affect ventilation.[150] In the presence of ongoing severe bleeding or hemodynamic instability, when possible, the patient should be transferred to the operating room, where rigid and flexible bronchoscopy can be performed.[150] The technique selected ultimately depends on operator preference.[148] Although rigid bronchoscopy can be performed under local anesthesia, it is most commonly performed under GA.[151]

If the patient has not already been intubated during resuscitation, endotracheal intubation can be achieved in the operating room awake or after appropriately dosed rapid sequence induction, with ongoing hemodynamic resuscitation as required. During rigid bronchoscopy or jet ventilation, if the proximal end of the bronchoscope is occluded, positive-pressure controlled ventilation can be utilized. GA can be maintained intravenously or in a closed system using inhalation agents. The primary goal during rigid bronchoscopy is to clear the airways of gross blood and then lateralize and locate the bleeding site.[150] Control of bleeding may be obtained by use of iced saline lavage or topical epinephrine (1:20,000) administered through the flexible bronchoscope[40,148] passed through the rigid instrument. Topical thrombin and thrombin-fibrinogen can also be used.[150] Other techniques used to control endobronchial bleeding include use of balloon catheter tamponade,[151] direct pressure with swabs,[99] neodymium:yttrium-aluminum-garnet (Nd:YAG) laser phototherapy,[148,150] electrocautery, endobronchial tumor resection through the rigid scope, and cryotherapy.[150]

If bleeding cannot be controlled, the bleeding side or site should be isolated with endobronchial techniques utilizing a bronchial blocker positioned under fiberoptic control or a double-lumen tube.[150] A single-lumen tube may also be advanced into the nonbleeding side.[150] However, if a single-lumen tube is advanced into the right main stem bronchus, occlusion of the right upper lobe bronchus often occurs.[150] Endobronchial tamponade can be utilized for up to 24 hours and may control bleeding without further therapy.[150] However, these selective intubation techniques can also be considered palliative and used with the anticipation of further therapeutic intervention.[150,151] Complications of tamponade include local ischemia and obstructive pneumonitis.[150] Double-lumen tubes can also be used during initial resuscitation to achieve lung isolation and prevent asphyxiation prior to emergent bronchoscopy.[40] Systemic therapy during resuscitation can include intravenous vasopressin (0.2 to 0.4 U/min) and tranexamic acid.[150]

If bleeding is not localized by bronchoscopy or is localized but not adequately controlled, angiography and angioembolization can be used to identify the source of bleeding and achieve hemostasis.[151] Surgical resection may be required when (1) embolization is unavailable, fails, or is technically impossible; (2) the extent of hemoptysis precludes angiography; or (3) the cause of the bleeding is unlikely to be controlled by embolization.[148] Radiation therapy is occasionally used in the treatment of massive hemoptysis.[148]

Mortality rates associated with the usual definition of massive hemoptysis range from 12% to 50% with medical management.[150] Overall mortality with surgical resection is as much as 50%.[150] Overall mortality is influenced by the presence of malignancy and the bleeding rate.[151] A rate of bleeding greater than 1000 mL in 24 hours in the presence of malignancy is associated with a mortality rate of 80%.[151]

D. TRACHEOBRONCHIAL STENTS

The increasing number of patients presenting with central airway obstruction from carcinoma of the lung over the past two decades has stimulated the development of endobronchial treatment modalities including tracheobronchial stents.[97] Although stents may be used to treat benign airway obstruction, they are most commonly used as palliative therapy in major airway obstruction related to unresectable malignancy.[153] Stents may also be used in the palliative treatment of malignant tracheoesophageal or bronchoesophageal fistulas.[153,154] Expandable metal stents can be placed using the rigid or flexible bronchoscope; however, silicone stents can be placed only using the rigid bronchoscope.[97,99] Under GA, a ventilating laryngotracheoscope can be inserted under telescopic guidance with the tip placed proximal to the lesion.[153] This suspendable rigid scope provides airway control and a conduit for ventilation and passage of telescopes and other instruments as well as the stent.[153] Alternatively, the rigid bronchoscope can be used. If, on initial presentation, airway compromise exists and emergent intervention is required, patients should be immediately transferred to the operating room for airway control using the rigid bronchoscope following induction of general anesthesia. Rigid bronchoscopic ventilation techniques, as previously described, are employed. GA can be maintained intravenously or by using inhalational agents if the proximal end of the scope is occluded. The flexible bronchoscope can be inserted through the rigid instrument to inspect the lesion further, and laser therapy, balloon dilation, and mechanical debulking with optical forceps may be performed prior to stent placement.[153] Potential complications include bleeding and pneumothorax.[153] Following removal of the bronchoscope or laryngotracheoscope, mask or LMA ventilation can be used during emergence from GA.

Relief of airway obstruction with endoluminal tracheobronchial stents can provide a meaningful addition to life expectancy.[153] Expertise in airway management and anesthesia administration for these complex bronchoscopic procedures is integral to their success.

VII. CONCLUSION

The administration of anesthesia and airway management for laryngoscopy and bronchoscopy can be demanding because of the inherent airway pathology and the necessity of sharing the airway with the operator. Familiarity with the underlying pathophysiology and communication and cooperation between the anesthesiologist and the surgeon or pulmonologist are essential. Various airway management and ventilatory techniques exist and should be individualized to the clinical setting and the expertise of the operator. As the endoscopic treatment of airway lesions continues to evolve, both anesthetic and airway management considerations will continue to present new challenges.

REFERENCES

1. Ahmad M, Dweik RA: Flexible bronchoscopy in the 21st century. Future of flexible bronchoscopy. Clin Chest Med 20:1, 1999.
2. Albert SN, Shibuya J, Albert CA: Ventilation with an oxygen injector for suspension laryngoscopy. Anesth Analg 51:866, 1972.
3. Aloy A, Schachner M, Cancura W: Tubeless translaryngeal superimposed jet ventilation. Eur Arch Otorhinolaryngol 248:475, 1991.
4. Ameer B, Burlingame MB, Harman EM: Systemic absorption of topical lidocaine in elderly and young adults undergoing bronchoscopy. Pharmacotherapy 9:74, 1989.
5. Armstrong M, Mark LJ, Snyder DS, et al: Safety of direct laryngoscopy as an outpatient procedure. Laryngoscope 107:1060, 1997.
6. Atkins JP, Keane WM, Young KA, et al: Value of panendoscopy in determination of second primary cancer. Arch Otolaryngol 110:533, 1984.
7. Atkinson RS, Rushman GB, Lee JA: A Synopsis of Anaesthesia, 8th ed. Bristol, John Write and Sons, 1977.
8. Ayers ML, Beamis JF: Rigid bronchoscopy in the twenty-first century. Clin Chest Med 22:355, 2001.
9. Ayuso A, Luis M, Sala X, et al: Effects of anesthetic technique on the hemodynamic response to microlaryngeal surgery. Am Otol Laryngol 106:863, 1997.
10. Babinski M, Smith RB, Klain M: High frequency jet ventilation for laryngoscopy. Anesthesiology 52:178, 1980.
11. Bacher A, Lang T, Webber J, et al: Respiratory efficacy of subglottic low frequency, subglottic combined frequency, and supraglottic combined frequency, jet ventilation during microlaryngeal surgery. Anesth Analg 91:1506, 2000.
12. Barclay K. Kluger MT: Effect of bolus dose of remifentanil on hemodynamic response to tracheal intubation. Anesth Intensive Care 28:403, 2000.
13. Bastian RW, Delsupehe KG: Indirect larynx and pharynx surgery: A replacement for direct laryngoscopy. Laryngoscope 106:1280, 1996.
14. Benjamin B: Anaesthesia techniques. In Benjamin B: Endolaryngeal Surgery. London, Martin Dunitz, 1998, pp 45-68.

15. Benjamin B, Gronow D: A new tube for microlaryngeal surgery. Anesth Intensive Care 7(3):258-263, 1979.

16. Benjamin B: Anesthesia for pediatric airway endoscopy. Otolaryngol Clin North Am 33:29, 2000.

17. Benjamin B: Direct laryngoscopy. In Benjamin B: Endolaryngeal Surgery. London, Martin Dunitz, 1998, pp 69-81.

18. Bent JP, Silver JR, Porubsky ES: Acute laryngeal trauma: A review of 77 patients. Otolaryngol Head Neck Surg 109:441, 1993.

19. Benumof JL: Anesthesia for Thoracic Surgery, 2nd ed. Philadelphia, WB Saunders, 1995.

20. Benumof JL: Management of the Difficult Airway. Ann Acad Med Singapore 23:589, 1994.

21. Berkowitz RG: Neonatal upper airway assessment by awake flexible laryngoscopy. Ann Otol Rhinol Laryngol 107:75, 1998.

22. Black RE, Johnson DG, Matlak ME: Bronchoscopic removal of aspirated foreign bodies in children. J Pediatr Surg 29:682, 1994.

23. Borchers SD, Beamis JF: Flexible bronchoscopy. Chest Clin North Am 6:169, 1996.

24. Bourgain JL, Desruennes E, Fischler M, et al: Transtracheal high frequency jet ventilation for endoscopic airway surgery: A multicentre study. Br J Anaesth 87:870, 2001.

25. Brimacombe J, Tucker P, Simons S: The laryngeal mask airway for awake diagnostic bronchoscopy. A retrospective study of 200 consecutive patients. Eur J Anesth 12:357, 1995.

26. Brooker CR, Hunsaker DH, Zimmerman AA: A new anesthetic system for microlaryngeal surgery. Otolaryngol Head Neck Surg 118:55, 1998.

27. Calcaterra TC, House J: Local anesthesia for suspension microlaryngoscopy. Trans Pac Coast Otoophthalmol Soc Annu Meet 55:29, 1974.

28. Castro M, Midthun DE, Edell ES, et al: Flexible bronchoscopic removal of foreign bodies from pediatric airways. J Bronchol 1:92, 1994.

29. Catterall W, Mackie K: Local anesthetics. In: Hardman JC, Linbird LE, Molinoff PS, Ruddon RW (eds): Goodman and Gilman's the Pharmacological Basis of Therapeutics, 9th ed. New York, McGraw-Hill, 1996, pp 331-347.

30. Chhajed PN, Cooper P: Pediatric flexible bronchoscopy. Indian Pediatr 38:1382, 2001.

31. Chu SS, Rah KH, Brannan MD, Cohen JL: Plasma concentrations of lidocaine after endotracheal spray. Anesth Analg 54:438, 1975.

32. Cohen S, Pine H, Drake A: Use of rigid and flexible bronchoscopy among pediatric otolaryngologists. Arch Otolaryngol Head Neck Surg 5:505, 127.

33. Cohen SR, Herbert WI, Thompson JW: Anesthesia management of microlaryngeal laser surgery in children: Apneic technique anesthesia. Laryngoscope 98:347, 1988.

34. Cozine K, Stone JG, Shulman S, et al: Ventilatory complications of carbon dioxide laser laryngeal surgery. J Clin Anesth 3:20, 1991.

35. Crockett DM, Scamman FL, McCabe BF, et al: Venturi jet ventilation for microlaryngoscopy: technique, complications, pitfalls. Laryngoscope 97:1326, 1987.

36. Curran J, Hamilton C, Taylor T: Topical anesthesia before tracheal intubation. Anaesthesia 30:765, 1975.

37. DeGowan EL, DeGowan RL: Bedside Diagnostic Examination, 2nd ed. New York, Macmillan, 1969.

38. Depierraz B, Brossard E: Percutaneous transtracheal jet ventilation for paediatric endoscopic laser treatment of laryngeal and subglottic lesions. Can J Anaesth 41:1200, 1994.

39. Deslodge RB, Zeitels SM: Endolaryngeal microsurgery at the anterior glottal commissure: Controversies and observations. Ann Otol Rhinol Laryngol 109:385, 2000.

40. Donati F, Meitelman C, Benoit P: Vecuronium neuromuscular blockade at the adductor muscles of the larynx and adductor pollicis. Anesthesiology 74:833, 1991.

41. Donlon JV Jr: Anesthesia for eye, ear, nose and throat surgery. In Miller RD (ed): Anesthesia, 2nd ed. New York, Churchill Livingstone, 1986, pp 1837-1894.

42. Donlon JV Jr: Anesthetic and airway management of laryngoscopy and bronchoscopy. In Benumof JL (ed): Airway Management: Principles and Practice. St. Louis, Mosby, 1996, pp 666-685.

43. Donlon JV Jr: Anesthetic management of patients with compromised airways. Anesth Rev 7:22, 1980.

44. Doyle PJ, Blokmanis A, Oulton JL: Anesthesia for microlaryngoscopy. Trans Pac Coast Otoophthalmol Soc Annu Meet 57:199, 1976.

45. Dripps RD, Eckenhoff JE, Vandam LD: Introduction to Anesthesia: The Principles of Safe Practice, 6th ed. Philadelphia, WB Saunders, 1982.

46. Durrani M, Barwise JA, Johnson RE, et al: Intravenous chloroprocaine attenuates hemodynamic changes associated with direct laryngoscopy and tracheal intubation. Anesth Analg 90:1208, 2000.

47. Dweik RA, Stoller JK: Role of bronchoscopy in massive hemoptysis. Clin Chest Med 20:89, 1999.

48. Evans KL, Keene MH, Bristow ASE: High-frequency jet ventilation—A review of its role in laryngology. J Laryngol Otol 108:23, 1994.

49. Fitzpatrick PC, Guarisco JL: Pediatric airway foreign bodies. J La State Med Soc 4:138, 1998.

50. Friedman EM: Tracheobronchial foreign bodies. Otolaryngol Clin North Am 1:179, 2000.

51. Gaitini LA, Fradis M, Vaida SJ, et al: Pneumomediastinum due to venturi jet ventilation used during microlaryngeal surgery in a previously neck-irradiated patient. Ann Otol Rhinol Laryngol 109:519, 2000.

52. Goddon DJ, Willey RF, Fergusson RJ: Rigid bronchoscopy under intravenous GA with oxygen venturi ventilation,. Thorax 37:532, 1982.

53. Gold SM, Gerber ME, Shott SR et al: Blunt laryngotracheal trauma in children. Arch Otolaryngol Head Neck Surg 123:83, 1997.

54. Granholm T, Farmer DL: The surgical airway. Respir Care Clin North Am 1:13, 2001.

55. Grasl MC, Donner A, Schragl E, et al: Tubeless laryngeal surgery in infants and children via jet ventilation laryngoscope. Laryngoscope 107:277, 1997.

56. Gredle WF, Smidely JE, Elliott RC: Complications of fiberoptic bronchoscopy. Am Rev Respir Dis 109:67, 1972.

57. Guidelines 2000 for cardiopulmonary resuscitation and emergency cardiovascular care. International Consensus on Sciences. Circulation 102:8, 2000.

58. Guidelines to the practice of anesthesia—2002. Can J Anaesth 49:9, 2002.

59. Gussack GS, Jurkovich GT, Luterman A: Laryngotracheal trauma: A protocol approach to a rare injury. Laryngoscope 96:660, 1986.

60. Hadaway EG, Page J, Shortridge RT: Anaesthesia for microsurgery of the larynx. Ann R Coll Surg Engl 4:279, 1982.

61. Hautmann H: High frequency jet ventilation in international fiberoptic bronchoscopy. Anesth Analg 90:1436, 2000.

62. Helmers RA, Sanderson DR: Rigid bronchoscopy: The forgotten art. Clin Chest Med 16:393, 1995.

63. Hendrix RA, Ferouz A, Bacon CK: Admission planning and complications of direct laryngoscopy. Otolaryngol Head Neck Surg 110:510, 1994.

64. Hershey MD, Hannenberg AA: Gastric distention and rupture from oxygen insufflation during fiberoptic intubation. Anesthesiology 85:1479, 1996.

65. Hill RS, Koltai PJ, Parnes SM: Airway complications from laryngoscopy and panendoscopy. Ann Otol Rhinol Laryngol 96:691, 1987.

66. Hochman H, Zeitels SM, Heaton JT: Analysis of the forces and position required for direct laryngoscopic exposure of the anterior vocal cords. Ann Otol Rhinol Laryngol 108:715, 1999.

67. Hogikyan ND: Transnasal endoscopic examination of the subglottis and trachea using topical anesthesia in the otolaryngology clinic. Laryngoscope 109:1170, 1999.

68. Huang J, Needs RE, Miller HAB, et al: Unsuspected tracheal rupture in blunt thoracic trauma. Can J Anaesth 41:1208, 1994.

69. Hunsaker DH: Anesthesia for microlaryngeal surgery: The case for subglottic jet ventilation. Laryngoscope 104(8 pt 2 Suppl 65):1, 1994.

70. Jacobson S: Upper airway obstruction. Emerg Med Clin North Am 7:205, 1989.

71. Jean-Baptiste E: Clinical assessment and management of massive hemoptysis. Crit Care Med 28:1642, 2000.

72. Jewett BS, Shockley WW, Rutledge R: External laryngeal trauma analysis of 392 patients. Arch Otolaryngol Head Neck Surg 125:877, 1999.

73. Johnson JT, Cheng J-L, Myers EN: Jet ventilation for operative laryngoscopy. Laryngoscope 92:1194, 1982.

74. Johnson JT, Myers EN: Recent advances in operative laryngoscopy. Otolaryngol Clin North Am 17:35, 1984.

75. Jones LM, Mair EA, Fitzpatrick TM, et al: Multidisciplinary airway stent team: A comprehensive approach and protocol for tracheobronchial stent treatment. Ann Otol Rhinol Laryngol 109:889, 2000.

76. Karmy-Jones R, Cushieri J, Vallieres E: Role of bronchoscopy in massive hemoptysis. Chest Surg Clin North Am 11:873, 2001.

77. Kastendieck J: Airway management. In Rosen P (ed): Emergency Medicine: Concepts and Clinical Practice, 2nd ed. St. Louis, Mosby, 1988, pp 26-53.

78. Keen RI, Kotak PK, Ramsden RT: Anesthesia for microsurgery of the larynx. Ann R Coll Surg Engl 64:111, 1982.

79. Koufman JA, Little FB, Weeks DB: Proximal large-bore jet ventilation for laryngeal laser surgery. Arch Otolaryngol Head Neck Surg 113:314, 1987.

80. Kovac AL: Controlling the hemodynamic responses to laryngoscopy and endotracheal intubation. J Clin Anesth 8:63, 1996.

81. Lanzenberger-Schragl E, Donnor A, Grasl MC, et al: Superimposed high-frequency jet ventilation for laryngeal and tracheal surgery. Arch Otolaryngol Head Neck Surg 126;40, 2000.

82. Levin RM: Pediatric Anesthesia Handbook, 2nd ed. Garden City, NY, Medical Examination Publishing, 1980.

83. Lieber JM, Markin CJ: Fiberoptic bronchoscopy for diagnosis and treatment. Crit Care Clin 16:83, 2000.

84. Lindholm CE, Bengt O, Snyder JV, et al: Cardiorespiratory effects of flexible fiberoptic bronchoscopy in critically ill patients. Chest 74:362, 1978.

85. Marks SC, Marsh BR, Dudgeon DL: Indications for open surgical removal of airway foreign bodies. Ann Otol Rhinol Laryngol 102:690, 1993.

86. Mechenbier JA: Jet ventilation in microlaryngoscopy reduces anesthesia risks. Clin Laser Mon 10:23, 1992.

87. McAtamney D, O'Hare R, Hughes D, et al: Evaluation of remifentanil for control of hemodynamic response to tracheal intubation. Anaesthesia 53:1209, 1998.

88. McEvoy GK: Glycopyrrolate. In AHFS Drug Information. Bethesda, American Society of Health System Pharmacists Inc., 2005, pp 1243-1244.

89. McGoldrick KE, Ho MD: Endoscopy procedures and laser surgery of the airway. In McGoldrick K (ed): Anesthesia for Ophthalmic and Otolaryngologic Surgery. Philadelphia, WB Saunders, 1992, pp 37-63.

90. Mehta AC, Desgupta A: Flexible bronchoscopy in the 21st century. Airway stents. Clin Chest Med 20:139, 1999.

91. Merritt RM, Bent JP, Porubsky ES: Acute laryngeal trauma in the pediatric patient. Ann Otol Rhinol Laryngol 107:104, 1998.

92. Miller JI: Rigid bronchoscopy. Chest Surg Clin North Am 6:161, 1996.

93. Minard G, Kudsk KA, Croce MA, et al: Laryngotracheal trauma. Am Surg 58:181, 1992.

94. Mirakhur RK, Dundee JW: Glycopyrrolate: Pharmacology and clinical use. Anaesthesia 38:1195, 1983.

95. Monnier PH, Ravussin P, Savory M, Freeman J: Percutaneous transtracheal ventilation for laser endoscopic treatment of laryngeal and subglottic lesions. Clin Otolaryngol Allied Sci 13:209, 1988.

96. Morgado PF, Abrahao M: Angled telescopic surgery, an approach for laryngeal diagnosis and surgery without suspension. Sao Paulo Med J 117:224, 1999.

97. Morris IR: Airway management. In Rosen P (ed): Emergency Medicine: Concepts and Clinical Practice, 3rd ed. St. Louis, Mosby–Year Book, 1992, pp 79-105.

98. Morris IR: Fiberoptic intubation. Can J Anaesth 41:996, 1994.

99. Morris IR: Pharmacologic aids to intubation and the rapid sequence induction. Emerg Med Clin North Amer 6:753, 1988.

100. Nicolai T: Pediatric bronchoscopy. Pediatr Pulmonol 31:150, 2001.

101. Noorily AD, Noorily SH, Oho RA: Cocaine, lidocaine, tetracaine: Which is best for topical nasal anesthesia? Anesth Analg 81:724-727, 1995.

102. Nussbaum E, Zagnoev M: Pediatric fiberoptic bronchoscopy with a laryngeal mask airway. Chest 120:2, 2001.

103. Olney DR, Greinwald JH, Smith RJH: Laryngomalacia and its treatment. Laryngoscope 109:1770, 1999.

104. Olsson GL: Bronchospasm during anesthesia: A computer aided incidence study of 136,529 patients. Acta Anaesthesiol Scand 31:244, 1987.

105. Orr RJ, Elwood T: Special challenging problems in the difficult pediatric airway. Lymphoma, laryngeal papillomatosis, and subglottic hemangioma. Anesthesiol Clin North Am 16:869, 1998.

106. Ossoff RH, Duncavage JA, Dere H: Microsubglottiscopy. An expansion of operative microlaryngoscopy. Otol Head Neck Surg 104:842, 1991.

107. Oulton J, Donald DM: A ventilating laryngoscope. Anesthesiology 35:540, 1971.

108. Ovassapian A, Mesnick PS, Hannberg AA, et al: Oxygen insufflation through the fiberscope to assist intubation is not recommended. Anesthesiology 87:183, 1997.

109. Parsons DS, Lockett JS, Martin TW: Pediatric endoscopy: Anesthesia and surgical techniques. Am J Otolaryngol 13:271, 1992.

110. Prakash UB, Offord KP, Stubbs SE: Bronchoscopy in North America: The ACCP survey. Chest 100:1668, 1991.

111. Pue CA, Pacht ER: Complications of fiberoptic bronchoscopy at a university hospital. Chest 107:430, 1995.

112. Quintal MC, Cunningham MJ, Ferrari LR: Tubeless spontaneous ventilation technique for pediatric microlaryngeal surgery. Arch Otol Laryngol Head Neck Surg 123:209, 1997.

113. Rafanan AL, Mehta AC: Adult airway foreign body removal. Clin Chest Med 22:2, 2001.

114. Rajagopalan R, Smith F, Ramachandran PR: Anaesthesia for microlaryngoscopy and definitive surgery. Can Anaesth Soc J 19:83, 1972.

115. Reece GP, Shatney CH: Blunt injuries of the cervical trachea. Review of 51 patients,. South Med J 91:1542, 1988.

116. Repchinsky C, Welborks L, Bisson R, et al (eds): Compendium of Pharmaceuticals and Specialties. The Canadian Drug Reference for Health Professionals. Ottawa, Canadian Pharmacists Association 2004, pp 201-204.

117. Richtsmeier WJ, Scher RL: Telescopic laryngeal and pharyngeal surgery. Ann Otol Rhinol Laryngol 106:995, 1997.

118. Rovin JD, Rodgers BM: Pediatric foreign body aspiration. Pediatr Rev 21:86, 2000.

119. Safar P: Sequential steps of emergency airway control. In Safer P (ed): Advances in Cardiopulmonary Resuscitation. New York, Springer Verlag, 1977.

120. Sanders RD: Two ventilating attachments for bronchoscopes. Del Med J 39:170, 1967.

121. Sayson SC, Mongan PD: Onset of action of mivacurium chloride. Anesthesiology 81:34, 1994.

122. Schellhouse DE: Pediatric flexible airway endoscopy. Curr Opin Pediatr 14:327, 2002.

123. Schoem SR, Choi SS, Zalzal GH: Pneumomediastinum and pneumothorax from blunt cervical trauma in children. Laryngoscope 107:351, 1997.

124. Slonim AD, Ognibene FP: Amnestic agents in pediatric bronchoscopy. Chest 16:1802, 1999.

125. Slonim AD, Ognibene FP: Enhancing patient safety for pediatric bronchoscopy. Alternatives to conscious sedation. Chest 120:2, 2001.

126. Smith BE: Developments in the safe use of high frequency jet ventilation. Br J Anaesth 65:735, 1990.

127. Smith BE: High frequency ventilation: Past, present, and future? Br J Anaesth 65:130, 1990.

128. Snow JC: Manual of Anesthesia. Boston, Little, Brown, 1977.

129. Stacey S, Hurley E, Bush A: Sedation for pediatric bronchoscopy. Chest 119:1, 2001.

130. Stoelting RK: Pharmacology and Physiology in Anesthetic Practice, 2nd ed. Philadelphia, JB Lippincott, 1991.

131. Strong MS, Vaughn CW, Mahler DL, et al: Cardiac complications of microsurgery of the larynx. Laryngoscope 84:908, 1974.

132. Sutherland AD, Williams RT: Cardiovascular responses and lidocaine absorption in fiberoptic assisted awake intubation. Anesth Analg 65:389, 1986.

133. Swanson KL, Edell ES: Tracheobronchial foreign bodies. Chest Surg Clin North Am 11:861, 2001.

134. Swor RA: Penetrating and blunt neck trauma. In Tintinolli JE (ed): Emergency Medicine. A Comprehensive Study Guide, 4th ed. New York, McGraw-Hill, 1996, pp 1153-1156.

135. Tan HKK, Brown K, McGill T, et al: Airway foreign bodies (FB): A 1-year review. Int J Pediatr Otorhinolaryngol 1:91, 2000.

136. Thompson JP, Hall AP, Russell J, et al: Effect of remifentanil on the hemodynamic response to orotracheal intubation. Br J Anaesth 80:467, 1998.

137. Thuang MK: Tubeless anesthesia for microlaryngoscopy. Anaesth Intensive Care 17:111, 1989.

138. Verghese ST, Hannallah RS: Pediatric otolaryngologic emergencies. Anesthesiology Clin North Am 1912, 2001.

139. Vourc'h G, Fischler M, Michon F, et al: High frequency jet ventilation v. manual jet ventilation during bronchoscopy in patients with tracheo-bronchial stenosis. Br J Anaesth 55:969, 1983.

140. Wain JC: Rigid bronchoscopy: The value of a venerable procedure. Chest Surg Clin North Am 11:691, 2001.

141. Wei-chung H, Tsung-shiann S, Chia-der L, et al: Clinical experiences of removing foreign bodies in the airway and esophagus with a rigid endoscope: A series of 3217 cases from 1970 to 1996. Otolaryngol Head Neck Surg 122:450, 2000.

142. Weisberger EC, Miner JD: Apneic anesthesia for improved endoscopic removal of laryngeal papillomata. Laryngoscope 98:693, 1988.

143. Welty P: Anesthetic concerns and complications during suspension microlaryngoscopy procedures. CRNA 3:113, 1992.

144. Wenig BL, Raphael N, Stern JR, et al: Cardiac complications of suspension laryngoscope. Arch Otolaryngol Head Neck Surg 112:860, 1986.

145. Wheeler M, Ovassapian A: Prediction and evaluation of the difficult airway. In Hagberg CA (ed): Handbook of Difficult Airway Management. Philadelphia, Churchill Livingstone, 2000, pp 15-30.

146. Wiseman NE, Sanchez I, Powell RE: Rigid bronchoscopy in the pediatric age group: Diagnostic effectiveness. J Pediatr Surg 27:1294, 1992.

147. Wong MEK, Bradrick JP: Surgical approaches to airway management for anesthesia practitioners. In Hagberg CA (ed): Handbook of Difficult Airway Management. Philadelphia, Churchill Livingstone, 2000, pp 185-218.

148. Woo P, Eurenius S: Dynamics of venturi jet ventilation through the operating laryngoscope. Ann Otol Rhinol Laryngol 91:615, 1982.

149. Wood RE: Pitfalls in the use of the flexible bronchoscope in pediatric patients. Chest 97:199, 1990.

150. Woods AM, Lander CJ: Abolition of gagging and the hemodynamic response to awake laryngoscopy. Anesthesiology 67:A220, 1987.

151. Woods AM: Pediatric endoscopy. In Berry FA (ed): Anesthetic Management of Difficult and Routine Pediatric Patients, 2nd ed. New York, Churchill Livingstone, 1990, pp 199-242.

152. Zatoun GM, Rauadi PW, Baki DHA: Endoscopic management of foreign in the tracheobronchial tree: Predictive factors for complications. Otolaryngol Head neck Surg 123:311, 2000.

153. Zeitels SM: Universal modular glottiscope system: The evolution of a century of design and technique for direct laryngoscopy. Ann Otol Rhinol Laryngol 108(Suppl 179):2, 1999.

154. Zimmerman AA: Supraglottic vs subglottic jet ventilation. Anesth Analg 78:S1, 1994.

36

THE DIFFICULT AIRWAY IN CONVENTIONAL HEAD AND NECK SURGERY

Nasir I. Bhatti
David Goldenberg

I. INTRODUCTION

Airway management in head and neck surgery is unique as the operative field is the upper airway itself or the adjacent structures, and therefore the anesthesiologist has to share the access during all phases of the procedure. The head and neck surgeon is uniquely qualified to help diagnose and manage the compromised airway, and a collegial relationship and ongoing communication with the surgeon are of paramount value to the anesthesia team.

Acute airway situations in head and neck surgery should be approached in a systematic manner. The simplest adequate form of control should be selected and the lowest level of airway obstruction should be ascertained;

control should be established by securing an airway below that level. In addition, it is important to recognize that acute airway problems often evolve in association with other medical problems.

The spectrum of head and neck surgery is vast and includes so-called simple procedures such as tonsillectomy and major head and neck ablative and reconstructive procedures. The potential for a compromised airway is nowhere as great as it is in head and neck surgery. Mask ventilation and endotracheal intubation may be potentially or obviously difficult because of the nature of the patient's underlying condition.

Current principles and techniques for securing and safely managing the airways of patients undergoing conventional head and neck surgery are discussed in this chapter, with an emphasis on the prevention of airway problems associated with these kinds of operations. The severity or completeness of airway obstruction is categorized as follows:

Complete obstruction: No detectable airflow in or out of lungs.

Partial obstruction: The patient has stridor or respiratory difficulty because of narrowing of the major airway.

Potential or impending airway obstruction: The potential or fear that a patient will develop airway compromise because of a known anatomic or physical condition if the respiratory physiology or the consciousness level is altered.

II. AERODIGESTIVE ONCOLOGIC SURGERY

A. PREOPERATIVE AIRWAY ASSESSMENT

The preoperative airway assessment must include a comprehensive general medical history, focused history related to upper airway symptoms, general and head and neck physical examination, a thorough assessment of previous anesthetic records, details of surgical steps and alternative plans, and laboratory and imaging studies.

1. History

Heavy smoking and alcohol abuse are responsible for most cases of head and neck cancer and predispose these patients to chronic obstructive pulmonary disease, pneumonia, hypertension, coronary artery disease, and alcohol withdrawal. Information about previous surgical and anesthetic procedures with an emphasis on history of anesthetic or intubation difficulties, or both, must be obtained and communicated. Patients with a history of obstructive sleep apnea, especially those without an obvious anatomic abnormality, need careful assessment as a vallecular mass may hinder mask ventilation and ability to intubate.

The most common symptoms of acute airway obstruction are voice change, dyspnea, and cough. Physical findings may include stridor; hoarseness; restlessness; and intercostal, suprasternal, and supraclavicular retraction. Voice changes provide an early suggestion of the anatomic level and severity and progression of the lesion. A muffled voice indicates a supraglottic disease, whereas glottic lesions result in a coarse, scratchy voice.

Anesthetizing a patient with an anterior mediastinal, pharyngeal, or neck mass in the supine position without first securing the airway may lead to severe airway obstruction and therefore deserves special preoperative evaluation.

2. Physical Examination

A systematic and comprehensive evaluation of the patient's upper airway is mandatory. The condition of dentition, size and mobility of the tongue, and presence and character of stridor should be addressed (Table 36-1). Postradiation changes, neck masses, and previous neck surgery may result in reduced neck mobility, causing difficulty with mask ventilation and intubation. A thyrocervical distance less than 6 cm in a fully extended adult neck is a good indicator of difficulty with direct laryngoscopy and inability to visualize the vocal cords. Lower cranial nerve dysfunction from tumor or previous surgery may also result in airway difficulty related to aspiration or obstruction.

Obvious and potential difficulties with ventilation and intubation should be discussed with the head and neck surgeon, and thoughtful discussion about sequential steps of anesthesia and surgery and all available alternatives

Table 36-1 Evaluation of Stridor

Definition	Harsh High-Pitched Sound from Partial Obstruction of Upper Airway
Typical characteristics	Inspiratory Monophonic High pitched
Airway obstruction Inspiratory versus expiratory	Inspiratory stridor suggests that the lesion is extrathoracic Expiratory stridor suggests that the lesion is intrathoracic
Awake versus asleep	Obstruction worse awake or with exertion suggests a laryngeal, tracheal, or bronchial origin Obstruction worse asleep suggests a pharyngeal origin

should take place before anesthetic induction and especially before attempting intubation.

3. Laboratory and Imaging Studies

Assessments of arterial blood gas and pulmonary function are important in patients with chronic pulmonary diseases. Flexible laryngoscopy or indirect laryngoscopy done by an otolaryngologist head and neck surgeon may help with anticipation and planning for a difficult airway. Computed tomography and magnetic resonance imaging may help in determining the size, location, and nature of the obstruction.

B. OPTIONS FOR SECURING THE AIRWAY

One third of all severe complications encountered in analyses of anesthesia-related cardiorespiratory arrests are due to inability to establish an optimal airway following the induction of general anesthesia.[8,21]

1. Option 1: Tracheal Intubation after Induction of General Anesthesia

In patients with no obvious or expected airway compromise, the endotracheal tube (ET) can be placed during direct laryngoscopy after induction with a short-acting paralyzing agent such as succinylcholine.

2. Option 2: Examination of the Airway in the Awake Patient

a. Preparation of the Patient

In case of a potentially difficult airway, the anesthesiologist may elect to evaluate the airway in an awake patient with the help of judicious intravenous sedation and topical anesthesia. This assessment helps determine the best possible approach to securing the airway without compromising the patient's spontaneous breathing. The successful execution of this technique requires constant meaningful contact with the patient and adequate use of topical agents such as 4% lidocaine spray with the ultimate goal of not compromising the ability of the patient to breathe spontaneously as well as protect the airway. Percutaneous blocks of the superior laryngeal nerves or translaryngeal instillation of lidocaine is best avoided in patients with a head and neck tumor.

b. Choice of Tracheal Intubation Technique

Once the patient is adequately prepared, a careful but timely direct laryngoscopy is performed to assess whether to proceed with the intubation in an awake patient or to induce general anesthesia for subsequent intubation. It should always be remembered that a reasonable airway in an awake patient may change to a compromised airway immediately after induction of general anesthesia with anterior displacement of the larynx.[35]

3. Option 3: Tracheal Intubation in the Awake Patient

In case of an anticipated difficult airway or intubation from the preoperative work-up or after the awake assessment of the airway has mandated an awake intubation, one of the techniques of tracheal intubation of an awake patient is performed.

a. Fiberoptic-Guided Nasotracheal or Orotracheal Intubations

The choice of route is directed by the surgical requirement as well as the physical condition of the patient. Constant administration of supplemental oxygen during the entire process is mandatory. The nasotracheal route is useful in cases of small mouth opening, severe trismus, large tongue, receding lower jaw, or tracheal dilatation.

Orotracheal intubation is facilitated with an airway intubator such as a Williams or Ovassapian oral airway. The lubricated ET with its connector removed is loaded onto the proximal end of the fiberoptic scope. The tip of the scope is then introduced through the oral airway and passed behind the epiglottis into the glottic opening leading into the trachea. The tube is then eased into the trachea over the scope and the placement is confirmed with a combination of bilateral chest auscultation and end-tidal CO_2. After confirmation of the placement, general anesthesia is induced.

For nasal intubation, the nose is prepared with a nasal decongestant spray such as pseudoephedrine (Afrin) and topical 4% cocaine. Cocaine is advantageous over lidocaine as it is a vasoconstrictor in addition to being a very effective surface anesthetic. The potential for abuse by the personnel is occasionally a deterrent for its routine use. In placing the tube through the nose, it is necessary to remember that the nasal floor is slanted inferiorly as one proceeds posteriorly and the angle is approximately 30 degrees from the front to the back of the nose. The ET is advanced to approximately the 15-cm mark and the connector is removed. The fiberoptic scope is then used to visualize the glottic opening and to introduce the tube into the trachea.

b. Alternative Techniques

The rigid bronchoscope, basically a hollow stainless steel tube through which a rigid telescope is placed, provides excellent access to the airways. The distal end of the rigid bronchoscope is usually beveled to facilitate intubation and lifting of the epiglottis. The updated American Society of Anesthesiologists (ASA) protocol states that in the presence of inadequate face mask ventilation after induction in a situation in which the patient cannot be intubated, "A rigid bronchoscope for difficult airway management reduces airway-related adverse outcomes." In addition, this modality is recommended as a technique for cases of difficult ventilation. Other indications for rigid bronchoscopy include massive airway hemoptysis, foreign body retrieval, laser or photodynamic therapy, and placement of airway stents.

Other awake intubation techniques including retrograde intubation can be used in case of bleeding in the airway or when reasonable (three or four) attempts have failed. This technique can also be used in case of trismus, temporomandibular joint ankylosis, or upper airway masses that are not large and friable.

A combination of conventional, fiberoptic, and retrograde techniques can be used to intubate successfully.[5] A fiberoptic laryngoscope with a suction port can be used as an anterograde guide over a retrograde wire. A direct laryngoscopic view can facilitate placement of the tip of a fiberoptic scope into or near the glottic aperture.

4. Option 4: Tracheostomy with Local Anesthesia

If the patient is in acute respiratory distress because of upper airway obstruction, the best choice is to perform a planned but urgent awake tracheostomy. This is done under local anesthesia with minimal intravenous sedation to avoid loss of spontaneous breathing. Tracheostomy under local anesthesia in an awake patient is also an excellent way to secure the airway in the following situations: (1) patient with an upper airway abscess that may be in the way of or distorting the pathway for endotracheal intubation and (2) patient with a bulky friable supraglottic or glottic mass. In these situations, attempts at direct laryngoscopy and intubation may result in abscess rupture or aspiration of purulent material, blood, or material from a friable tumor.

5. Difficult or Failed Intubation

An unanticipated difficult or failed intubation is not an uncommon occurrence in head and neck surgery. When this situation is encountered after induction of general anesthesia, a very systematic and thought-out plan should be followed. Maintenance of oxygenation is paramount, and mask ventilation should be continued between the attempts at intubation. Repeated attempts at intubation carry the risk of traumatizing the larynx and therefore should be minimized. Three to four attempts with different neck positions and different laryngoscope blades should be the limit.

The time and ability to think clearly are limited under these circumstances, and therefore each anesthesia team should have a algorithm to follow routinely. The subsequent course of action depends upon the team's ability to achieve satisfactory mask ventilation.

a. Options When Mask Ventilation Is Adequate

If mask ventilation is adequate, a potent inhalational agent is used to continue general anesthesia and a Holinger anterior commissure laryngoscope should be used to visualize the vocal cords. This laryngoscope has a flared superior flange that is able to lift the epiglottis to visualize anteriorly placed vocal cords. An Eschmann stylet is passed through the glottic opening, and an ET is then passed over it after withdrawing the laryngoscope. The anesthesiology team should practice visualizing the larynx with this laryngoscope, which is available on the otolaryngology head and neck surgeon's laryngoscopy cart.

As an alternative, in a patient who is adequately mask ventilated, the ET may be passed with oral fiberoptic-guided laryngoscopy. An airway intubator bite block[32] is placed in the patient's mouth and the regular mask is replaced with an endoscopy port (Patil-Syracuse endoscopy mask).[34] The lubricated flexible fiberoptic laryngoscope is passed through the mask's diaphragm into the airway intubator and into the trachea through the glottis. The tube is then threaded over the laryngoscope into the patient's trachea.

A fiberoptic flexible scope can also be used to pass an ET through the nose. The nose is decongested with topical Afrin and topical 4% cocaine is used to anesthetize the nose. The appropriately sized well-lubricated ET is then placed along the floor of the nose and a fiberoptic scope is passed through the tube. An assistant occludes the other nostril and the mouth, and a triple connector is used so that the scope and oxygen delivery can be simultaneously introduced.

It is critical to remember that despite multiple attempts and use of the preceding techniques, the intubation attempts may continue to be unsuccessful. If mask ventilation is still possible, anesthesia should be discontinued and the patient allowed to awaken. One should then proceed with an awake intubation as discussed in option 3.

b. Options in Case of Failed Mask Ventilation

In situations of inadequate mask ventilation of an anesthetized patient, the ASA algorithm should be followed.[34] The laryngeal mask airway (LMA) was integrated into the ASA difficult airway algorithm in different locations in 1996,[4] either as a ventilatory device or as an intubation conduit. If LMA ventilation is not adequate or feasible, the emergency pathway should be followed and a call made for help. See Chapter 9 for further detail.

Use of LMAs is increasing in many situations of inadequate ventilation,[7,15] but they should be used with extreme caution in conventional head and neck surgery even by those with adequate experience with these devices.

6. Cricothyrotomy (Coniotomy)

Cricothyrotomy is a procedure for establishing an emergency airway when other methods are unsuitable or impossible. Emergency cricothyrotomy is performed in approximately 1% of all emergency airway cases in the emergency room.[1,2] The access site is the cricothyroid membrane. This procedure is especially suited for gaining control of the airway in cases of severe hemorrhage or massive facial trauma, foreign bodies, or emeses not permitting visualized intubation. Other cases arise when teeth are clenched, there is repeated failed intubation, and there is a possibility of cervical spine injury. In these

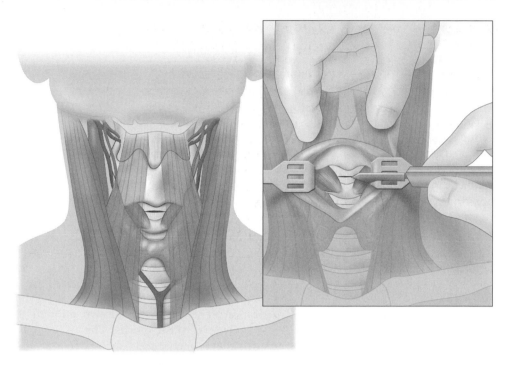

Figure 36-1 Cricothyrotomy: the cricothyroid membrane is palpated through the skin using the thyroid notch and cricoid cartilage as reference points.

cases, cricothyrotomy becomes the safest and quickest way to obtain an airway.[11] If a patient has sustained a respiratory insult associated with burns or smoke inhalation, it may be indicated to perform an elective prophylactic cricothyrotomy early to prevent fatal respiratory obstruction occurring during transport.[26]

a. Cricothyrotomy Surgical Technique

The cricothyroid membrane is identified by palpating a slight indentation in the skin inferior to the laryngeal prominence. The membrane is immediately subcutaneous in location with no overlying large veins, muscles, or fascial layers, allowing easy access. A vertical skin incision and a horizontal entrance into the cricothyroid membrane are advised. For incision into the cricothyroid membrane itself, a low horizontal stab is made to avoid laterally placed vessels.[24] Either a small tracheotomy tube or a small standard ET can be used in cricothyrotomy. Tube size is important in ensuring successful cannulation without excessive trauma. Once the patient is stabilized, the cricothyrotomy should be converted to a formal tracheotomy for adequate ventilation (Fig. 36-1). This technique is contraindicated in patients with an increased risk for subglottic stenosis, preexisting laryngeal disease, malignancy, inflammatory processes in near proximity, epiglottitis, severe distortion of normal anatomy, or a bleeding diathesis and in infants and children.

b. Needle Cricothyrotomy

Needle cricothyrotomy is performed in dire emergencies when either the appropriate equipment or knowledge to perform a formal emergency cricothyrotomy or intubation is unavailable. A large-gauge needle and cannula with a syringe attached are introduced through the cricothyroid

membrane until air can be aspirated. The cannula is then advanced off the needle down the airway (Fig. 36-2). The cannula is connected to an oxygen supply. The patient can then be oxygenated, but ventilation to remove CO_2 is not achieved and respiratory acidosis may ensue rapidly.

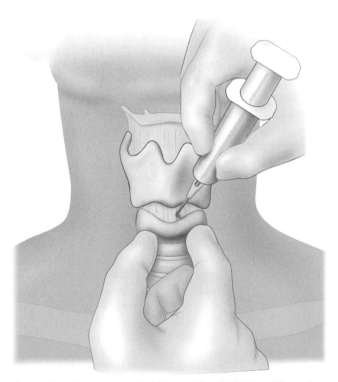

Figure 36-2 Needle cricothyrotomy: a large-gauge needle and cannula with a syringe attached is introduced through the cricothyroid membrane until air can be aspirated.

A needle cricothyrotomy ensures a supply of oxygen for a short time only, and it must be converted to a surgical cricothyrotomy or tracheotomy in a timely fashion to allow adequate ventilation.[19]

i. Transtracheal Needle Ventilation The transtracheal needle ventilation technique can be used to great advantage in the emergency setting. This technique requires access to 100% oxygen at 50 psi and a Luer-Lok connector. Adequate ventilation through the catheter is not possible with a conventional ventilator or handheld anesthesia bag.[6] The airway is controlled by puncturing the trachea or cricothyroid membrane with a 16-gauge plastic-sheathed needle. The needle is withdrawn, leaving the sheath in the trachea; the sheath is then attached to the high-pressure line through a pressure regulator control, and ventilation is accomplished using a manual interrupter switch.

The patient can be fully ventilated with this technique for only 45 minutes. In addition, the only way the oxygen inspired through transtracheal jet ventilation (TTJV) can escape is through the patient's own airway, and attempts at securing the airway must continue. The equipment to perform adequate TTJV should be available in the operating room, and the anesthesia team should familiarize themselves with its assembly.

7. Percutaneous Dilatational Tracheostomy

Percutaneous dilatational tracheostomy (PDT) is a procedure for placement of a tracheotomy tube without direct surgical visualization of the trachea. The general consensus is that PDT should be performed only on intubated patients. It is considered to be a minimally invasive, bedside procedure that is easily performed in the intensive care unit or ward, with continuous monitoring of the patient's vital signs.[18] The criteria for PDT are more stringent than those for open surgical tracheotomy.[12] PDT should be performed on patients whose cervical anatomy can be clearly defined by palpation through the skin. The two critically important preoperative criteria are the ability to hyperextend the neck and ensuring that the patient can be reintubated in case of accidental extubation. Obese patients, children, and those with severe coagulopathies should not be considered candidates for this procedure (Table 36-2).[12]

A number of different systems and approaches to performing a "percutaneous tracheotomy" have been described and marketed since the inception of the idea. Many comprehensive accounts of the evolution of this approach are available in the literature. Controversy surrounding this approach still lingers, but there have been many large series with acceptable rates of complications as long as selection of patients and adherence to a procedural protocol are assured.[9]

Ciaglia and colleagues[10] described a technique in which there is no sharp dissection beyond the skin incision. The patient is positioned and prepared in the same way as for standard operative tracheotomy. The procedure is done with the patient under general anesthesia, and all steps are done under bronchoscopic vision. A skin incision is made and the pretracheal tissue is cleared with the help of blunt dissection. The ET is withdrawn enough to place the cuff at the level of the glottis. The endoscopist places the tip of the bronchoscope such that the light from the tip shines through the surgical wound. The operator then enters the tracheal lumen below the second tracheal ring with an introducer needle. The track between the skin and the tracheal lumen is then serially dilated over a guidewire and stylet. A tracheotomy tube is then placed under direct bronchoscopic vision over a dilator. The placement of the tube is confirmed again by visualizing the tracheobronchial tree through the tube. The tube is then secured to the skin with sutures and the tracheostomy tape.

In the second technique, known as the Schachner (Rapitrac) method, following a small skin incision a dilator tracheotome is passed over a guidewire into the trachea to dilate the tract fully in one step.[36] The tracheotome has a beveled metal core with a hole through its center that accommodates a guidewire. Once inside the trachea, the tracheotome is dilated. A conventional tracheotomy cannula, fitted with a special obturator, is passed through the tracheal opening. The dilator and obturator are then removed. A novel method is called translaryngeal tracheostomy (Fantoni's technique). For Fantoni's tracheostomy, in contrast to the other techniques, the initial puncture of the trachea is carried out with the needle directed cranially and the tracheal cannula inserted with a pull-through technique along the orotracheal route in a retrograde fashion. The cannula is then rotated downward using a plastic obturator. The main advantage of Fantoni's tracheostomy is that hardly any skin incision is required, and therefore practically no bleeding is observed.[17,30] The procedure can be carried out only under endoscopic guidance, and rotating the tracheal cannula downward may pose a problem, demanding more experience.

The routine use of bronchoscopy during PDT, apart from Fantoni's tracheostomy, is still controversial. There are reports of lower rates of acute complications

Table 36-2   Contraindications to Percutaneous Dilatational Tracheostomy

Absolute	Relative
Emergent airway access	Anatomic abnormalities
Infants	(e.g., deviated trachea,
Infection at insertion site	enlarged superficial veins)
High positive end-expiratory pressure or oxygenation requirements	Enlarged thyroid or other neck mass
	Coagulopathy
	Previous neck surgery
	Obesity

under endoscopic guidance. In addition, the resultant hypercarbia should be considered when choosing endoscopically guided PDT for critically ill patients or those with head injuries. However, endoscopic guidance plays a critical role in the training of physicians, during percutaneous tracheostomy in patients with difficult anatomy, and to remove aspirated blood.

Another consideration that supports the use of bronchoscopy is the ability to better define the exact location of tracheal puncture. A number of cadaver studies in autopsies of patients who had undergone PDT found that the puncture site of the trachea varied greatly. It seems logical that bronchoscopic guidance during PDT can confirm the initial airway puncture site, although a controlled study is necessary to settle this issue.[29]

The technique of PDT is relatively easy to learn, but it has been repeatedly reported that a learning curve exists, which may be overcome by performing a number of supervised procedures. The time required for performing bedside PDT is considerably shorter than that required for performing an open tracheotomy.[23] In critical care patients, one of the major advantages of PDT is the elimination of scheduling difficulty associated with the operating room and anesthesiology teams. Bedside PDT also precludes the necessity to schedule the surgery and to transport critically ill patients who require intensive monitoring to and from the operating room. Therefore, PDT actually expedites the performance of the procedure in most cases. Lastly, the cost of performing PDT is roughly half that of open surgical tracheotomy. The major components of the savings in these series were operating room charges and anesthesia fees.

C. INTRAOPERATIVE AIRWAY MANAGEMENT

1. Positioning of the Endotracheal Tube

Otolaryngology head and neck surgical procedures have a need for very specific positioning of the ET, as the operative field is shared between the anesthesia and surgical teams. In addition, procedures such as oropharyngeal tumor resection and reconstruction mandate the nasal placement of the ET. The ala of the nose has to be well protected from the risk of necrosis by pressure from the ET. For operations with direct access to the trachea, the ET has to be converted to a reinforced tube (anode tube) so that kinking of the tube can be avoided.

2. Surgical Field Requirements

Head and neck surgery often requires that the operative team be on both sides of the table, and the operating table has to be positioned to accommodate this need. In addition, bulky anesthetic equipment has to be kept clear of the surgical field. The ET and the connectors have to be nonkinking, of low profile, and secured to the head so that head movement does not compromise the anesthetic circuit.

The exact positioning of the ET should be planned with the head and neck surgeon. The tube should be taped to the oral commissure or around the nose so as not to exert downward pressure leading to the risk of accidental extubation or pressure necrosis of the nasal ala or the tip. The position of entry of the tube into the airway has to be switched during certain head and neck procedures such as tracheostomy. It is imperative to ensure correct positioning of the second tube before removing the first tube.

3. Tracheostomy

Administration of 100% oxygen is advised prior to the actual tracheal opening so that in case of loss of airway at the time of placement of a tracheostomy tube, there is sufficient reserve in the lungs to prevent hypoxemia.

Most head and neck procedures on the neck and around the upper airway involve routine use of Bovie cautery. As the dissection approaches the trachea, it is advisable to avoid the use of Bovie cautery directly over the airway to avoid an airway fire. If Bovie cautery is necessary, it is mandatory to reduce the fraction of inspired oxygen to the lowest possible level compatible with optimal oxygen saturation.

Once the trachea is entered and the surgeon is able to visualize the ET, the anesthesiologist should loosen the tape and should be able to withdraw the ET so that the distal tip is just above the opening into the trachea. An adapter and a short flexible tube (Jolly tube) are placed onto the cuffed tracheostomy tube to avoid pull on the trachea. This maneuver requires excellent communication and planning on the part of anesthesia and surgical teams to avoid mishaps.

Correct placement of the tracheostomy tube is confirmed by the appearance of an end-tidal CO_2 waveform and by the presence of bilateral breath sounds on auscultation. In order to prevent contamination of the tracheobronchial tree with blood and secretions above the tracheostomy site, this area should be meticulously suctioned at the time of changing to a more permanent tracheostomy tube.

In situations where the tracheostomy is performed as part of a head and neck resection and reconstructive procedure and when a reinforced tube is placed, it is mandatory to secure it to the chest wall with sutures. This prevents accidental slipping of the tube into a main stem bronchus, which can result in oxygenation problems or bronchospasm if the anesthesia is light at that point.

III. EXTUBATION IN HEAD AND NECK SURGERY

Accidental extubation is a real risk in head and neck surgery, as the surgical team is mostly working around the oral and nasal cavities. The anesthesiologist should be extremely aware of this possibility and remain in constant communication with the surgical team to avoid inadvertent extubation. In addition, the preparations and plans to reintubate should be in place if the situation arises.

In head and neck procedures in which the patient does not have a tracheostomy, there is a definite risk of supraglottic and glottic edema because of the presence of an ET and intraoperative manipulation. Intraoperative measures such as administration of short-acting intravenous steroids (i.e., dexamethasone [Decadron]), minimizing the movement of the ET, and keeping the head of the patient slightly elevated can reduce this risk. Avoiding overzealous intravenous fluid administration is another important consideration.

Patients undergoing lengthy ablative and reconstructive procedures should be kept lightly sedated and should remain intubated overnight in the intensive care unit. The extubation can then be planned for the next day in the presence of experienced anesthesia and surgical personnel with equipment for securing the airway available. This may include instruments to be able to perform a bedside cricothyrotomy or tracheostomy.

Extubation is straightforward in most situations. In others, it may be more challenging than the original intubation. It may not be possible to mask ventilate because of the postsurgical edema and changes related to the reconstruction. The use of oral and nasal airway devices may not be feasible because of the fear of disrupting delicate surgical repair in the oropharynx or nasopharynx.

In order to ensure a safe extubation, the anesthesia team should take into consideration the following questions. First, is there an air leak around the tube after deflating the cuff? Second, if the patient develops acute airway obstruction on extubation, are the equipment and personnel at hand to secure an airway to prevent hypoxia? This may include options for emergency cricothyrotomy, TTJV, or tracheostomy. If the answer is an affirmative, one should proceed with extubation.

If the preceding criteria cannot be met, one should wait another 24 hours or consider extubating over a tube exchanger or a jet stylet,[22] which can be left in place up to 72 hours, while maintaining nothing by mouth status. A hollow tube exchanger with a small internal diameter is inserted through the ET into the patient's trachea. The ET is then withdrawn over the stylet; the catheter can be used as a means of jet ventilation, a reintubation guide, or both.[5] This approach is especially useful in situations in which an ET needs to be exchanged or replaced.

A. MANAGING ACCIDENTAL DECANNULATION OF FRESH TRACHEOSTOMY

Accidental decannulation of a fresh tracheostomy, especially during the first 48 hours after the initial surgery, can be a challenging situation. This is an even bigger problem in obese patients or those with a short thick neck, small retrognathic jaw, intermaxillary fixation, or a deep

and posterior airway. It should be managed as a potentially life-threatening emergency. The patient should be immediately mask ventilated and a call for help initiated.

The patient should be placed supine with the neck extended and a shoulder roll in place. A tracheal dilator or cricoid hook, or both, and good light can enable replacement of a one size smaller tracheostomy tube or an ET. No more than one or two attempts should be made, especially if the mask ventilation is optimal. An experienced anesthesiologist should place an orotracheal tube with direct laryngoscopy. A Holinger anterior commissure laryngoscope and Eschmann stylet can be a lifesaving combination in this situation in experienced hands. When the airway is secured from above, the patient can be taken back to the operating room for replacement of the tracheostomy tube in a relatively elective manner.

IV. UPPER AERODIGESTIVE SURGERY

A. PREOPERATIVE CONSIDERATIONS

Patients with an upper aerodigestive tract malignancy, such as esophageal carcinoma, may have limited cardiopulmonary reserve because of the disease process, dysphagia, and toxic effects of the chemotherapeutic agents. The risk of regurgitation and aspiration should be considered at the time of induction of general anesthesia.

B. MANAGEMENT OF THE AIRWAY

As it is difficult or impossible to empty out the stomach with a nasogastric tube in case of a large pharyngeal or esophageal tumor, the patient is assumed to have a full stomach.[3] The options for securing the airway are rapid sequence induction or awake fiberoptic-guided intubation after topical analgesia.

Risk of aspiration is reduced by preinduction administration of ranitidine, metoclopramide, and oral sodium citrate–citric acid buffer (Bicitra, Willen Drug Company, Baltimore, MD).

In order to ensure placement of the ET beyond the fistula site in case of tracheoesophageal fistula, an awake fiberoptic-guided intubation is an excellent choice. A similar technique may be used to place a reinforced tube beyond the narrowing in case of external compression on the trachea by an enlarged mediastinal lymph node or mass.

V. TONSILLECTOMY AND INTRAORAL PROCEDURES

A. PREOPERATIVE CONSIDERATIONS

Tonsillectomy is one of the commonest procedures performed by the otolaryngologist head and neck surgeon. Most of these operations are performed on otherwise healthy adults and children. The current indications include history of recurrent tonsillitis, tonsillar hypertrophy, snoring, obstructive sleep apnea, asymmetric tonsils, recurrent peritonsillar abscess, and tonsillar malignancy.[14] The performance of these procedures in patients with coagulation disorders is uncommon but can be challenging if diagnostic work-up fails to alert the surgical and anesthesia team about the presence, nature, and extent of the problem.

B. OBSTRUCTIVE SLEEP APNEA

Obstructive sleep apnea (OSA) can lead to serious and potentially life-threatening conditions if left untreated. These include hypertension, pulmonary hypertension, coronary artery disease, cor pulmonale, and congestive heart failure.[20] There are various nonsurgical options for patients with mild to moderate sleep apnea, but most patients with severe sleep apnea, tonsillar hypertrophy, and soft palate redundancy benefit from tonsillectomy, uvulectomy, and uvulopalatopharyngectomy.

Adults with this disorder must have a preoperative assessment of the severity of the problem with an overnight polysomnogram. The severity of OSA and the extent of desaturation and number and duration of apneic episodes have significant implications, especially for postoperative monitoring of these patients.

Induction of general anesthesia relaxes the pharyngeal muscles in a manner similar to the effect of rapid-eye-movement sleep.[22] This makes mask ventilation difficult to maintain, and the oral and nasal airways do not seem to improve the situation significantly.

Excessive pharyngeal tissue exacerbates the obstruction caused by the redundant soft palate and base of the tongue, hindering a good view of the cords at laryngoscopy. Patients with OSA are more sensitive to sedative and narcotic analgesics. This necessitates extreme caution and need for slow titration in using these agents. A fiberoptic-guided awake intubation should be attempted prior to induction of general anesthesia.

C. PERITONSILLAR AND PARAPHARYNGEAL ABSCESS

Anesthetic management of patients with peritonsillar abscess is a challenging task in anesthesia for head and neck surgery. These patients have severe odynophagia, upper airway edema, and distortion of the normal anatomy. In addition, the limited mouth opening resulting from local pain and inflammation makes securing the airway an even more daunting task.

The anesthesiologist should expect a difficult airway on induction of general anesthesia and therefore make alternative plans to be able to achieve a secure airway. A spontaneous or traumatic rupture of the abscess is a real risk, and the consequential aspiration of pus into an unprotected airway remains a possibility. One option is for the head and neck surgeon to attempt needle aspiration for decompression of the abscess under local anesthetic.[16]

Awake intubation on direct laryngoscopy is a safe option only if the abscess is relatively small and does not distort the route of intubation. A possible alternative is fiberoptic tracheal intubation using topical anesthesia. Topical anesthesia can be accomplished using the spray-as-you-go technique or translaryngeal injection of 3 to 4 mL of 4% lidocaine.[32] In case of a sizable abscess or airway distortion, a tracheostomy done under local anesthesia with minimal, if any, sedation is the safest approach.

D. MANAGEMENT OF THE AIRWAY DURING ROUTINE TONSILLECTOMY AND ORAL PROCEDURES

The surgeon places a mouth gag (Crowe-Davis) into the mouth to increase exposure of the oropharynx. The ET is held in a groove under the blade of this gag. There is a small but real danger of extubation during placement, adjustment, and removal of this blade. The ET should, therefore, always be secured with a tape to the lower lip. In order to monitor for any kinking or obstruction of the ET, the anesthesiologist must pay extremely close attention to end-tidal CO_2, bilateral chest auscultation, and peak airway pressures.

The oral cavity and oropharynx should be gently but meticulously suctioned at the end of the procedure to prevent aspiration of blood causing laryngospasm. The patient's head should be to the side at the end of the procedure to avoid blood trickling onto the vocal cords.[36]

E. POSTOPERATIVE AIRWAY PROBLEMS AFTER TONSILLECTOMY

Monitoring of patients for OSA after tonsillectomy has been a controversial issue. Children with severe and mixed (obstructive and central) sleep apnea should be monitored overnight in a postanesthesia care unit (PACU). Relief of airway obstruction does not ensure cessation of apneic episodes as the central component may be unmasked and result in oxygen desaturation as well as loss of respiratory drive.[25] The postoperative care of adults with OSA after tonsillectomy and similar procedures should be individualized. This should be based on the severity of sleep apnea preoperatively and performance in the PACU in the immediate postoperative period.

F. MANAGEMENT OF POST-TONSILLECTOMY BLEEDING

Post-tonsillectomy bleeding may take place in the immediate postoperative period (reactionary) or between 7 and 10 days after the surgery (secondary, infection). Preventive measures such as meticulous hemostasis (reactionary) and hydration and administration of oral antibiotics (secondary) are routinely recommended by surgeons. Obstruction of the airway by a combination of bleeding and postoperative airway edema is the commonest cause of post-tonsillectomy morbidity.[13]

Post-tonsillectomy bleeding is usually a slow ooze, and a large volume of blood may be swallowed by the patient. Postoperative nausea, vomiting, and loss of blood may result in severe hypovolemia before a fall in hemoglobin level is detected. Reduced hemoglobin level and aspiration of blood may result in hypoxemia in the patient, especially in a young child. Careful serial monitoring of hemoglobin levels and judicious use of packed cell transfusions are important considerations, particularly in children.

If surgical treatment is required for post-tonsillectomy hemorrhage, the patient should be assumed to have a full stomach with blood in the airway.[22] Awake intubation under direct laryngoscopy in adults or rapid sequence induction of anesthesia with etomidate or ketamine is the preferred choice in this situation. A work-up for coagulation disorders should take place in case of recurrent hemorrhage. An angiogram or a computed tomography scan to rule out a pseudoaneurysm of the carotid may occasionally be needed in rare cases of recurrent and severe post-tonsillectomy hemorrhage.

VI. SURGERY ON THE ANTERIOR SKULL BASE

The scope of head and neck surgery has expanded to include craniofacial, maxillofacial, and anterior skull base surgery. The indications may include trauma, syndromic skeletal abnormalities, sleep apnea, orthognathic deformities, and tumor removal. It is critical for the anesthetic team to discuss and understand the approach, nature, and extent of the proposed surgical procedure to be able to anticipate airway problems.[27]

Most patients undergoing these procedures are previously healthy adults or children, but a few have anatomic abnormalities that predispose them to challenging airway problems. These include limited mouth opening, retrognathia, protruded maxilla, and presence of orthodontic appliances.[28]

A. AIRWAY MANAGEMENT

Anesthesiologists should be prepared for fiberoptic-guided intubation if a difficult airway is anticipated during the preoperative work-up. The nasal route is preferred as the access for most of these procedures involves intraoral incisions. The possibility of maxillo-mandibular fixation at the end of the case is another reason for considering nasotracheal intubation.

Nasotracheal intubation is achieved using the technique previously mentioned. The regular adapter of the ET is replaced with a curved adapter with a flexible extension, which is connected to the ventilator. The extension is then padded and taped over the patient's forehead so as to come off the top of the head.

B. EXTUBATION IN SKULL BASE SURGERY

In case of maxillomandibular fixation, an attempt at extubation should be considered only if the patient is fully awake, following commands, with intact airway reflexes. Appropriate wire-cutting instruments should always be at hand for patients with such an impediment to access to the airway.

REFERENCES

1. Bair AE, Laurin EG, Karchin A, et al: Cricoid ring integrity: Implications for cricothyrotomy. Ann Emerg Med 41: 331-337, 2003.
2. Bair AE, Panacek EA, Wisner DH, et al: Cricothyrotomy: A 5-year experience at one institution. J Emerg Med 24:151-156, 2003.
3. Banoub MN, Nugent M: Thoracic anesthesia. In Rogers MC, Tinker JH, Covino BG, et al (eds): Principles and Practice of Anesthesia, vol 2. St Louis, Mosby, 1993, pp 1719-1930.
4. Benumof JL: Laryngeal mask airway and the ASA difficult airway algorithm. Anesthesiology 84:686-699, 1996.
5. Benumof JL: Management of the difficult adult airway. With special emphasis on awake tracheal intubation. Anesthesiology 75:1087-1110, 1991.
6. Benumof JL, Scheller MS: The importance of transtracheal jet ventilation in the management of the difficult airway. Anesthesiology 71:769-778, 1989.
7. Calder I, Ordman AJ, Jackowski A, Crockard HA: The Brain laryngeal mask airway. An alternative to emergency tracheal intubation. Anaesthesia 45:137-139, 1990.
8. Caplan RA, Posner KL, Ward RJ, Cheney FW: Adverse respiratory events in anesthesia: A closed claims analysis. Anesthesiology 72:828-833, 1990.
9. Ciaglia P: Differences in percutaneous dilational tracheostomy kits. Chest 117:1823, 2000.
10. Ciaglia P, Firschling R, Syniec C: Elective percutaneous dilatational tracheostomy. A new, simple bedside procedure: Preliminary report. Chest 87(6):715-719, 1985.
11. Collicott P, A AC, Carrico CJ: Upper airway management. In Advanced Trauma Life Support. Chicago, American College of Surgeons, 1984, pp 155-161.
12. Couch ME, Bhatti N: The current status of percutaneous tracheotomy. Adv Surg 36:275-296, 2002.
13. Crysdale WS, Russel D: Complications of tonsillectomy and adenoidectomy in 9409 children observed overnight. CMAJ 135:1139-1142, 1986.
14. Davidson TM, Calloway CA: Tonsillectomy and adenoidectomy—Its indications and its problems. West J Med 133:451-454, 1980.

15. de Mello WF, Ward P: The use of the laryngeal mask airway in primary anaesthesia. Anaesthesia 45:793-794, 1990.
16. Donlon JV Jr: Anesthesia for ear, nose, and throat surgery. In Miller RD (ed): Anesthesia, vol 2. New York, Churchill Livingstone, 1990, pp 2001-2023.
17. Fantoni A, Ripamonti D: A non-derivative, non-surgical tracheostomy: The translaryngeal method. Intensive Care Med 23:386-392, 1997.
18. Goldenberg D, Golz A, Huri A, et al: Percutaneous dilation tracheotomy versus surgical tracheotomy: Our experience. Otolaryngol Head Neck Surg 128:358-363, 2003.
19. Goldenberg D. Bhatti N: Management of the impaired airway in the adult. In Cummings CW (ed): Otolaryngology—Head and Neck Surgery. Philadelphia, Elsevier, 2005, pp 2441-2453.
20. Hall JB: The cardiopulmonary failure of sleep-disordered breathing. JAMA 255:930-933, 1986.
21. Keenan RL, Boyan CP: Cardiac arrest due to anesthesia. A study of incidence and causes. JAMA 253:2373-2377, 1985.
22. Kirk GA: Anesthesia for ear, nose, and throat surgery. In Rodgers MC, Tinker JH, Covino BG, et al (eds): Principles and Practice of Anesthesia, vol 2. St Louis, Mosby, 1993, pp 2257-2274.
23. Massick DD, Powell DM, Price PD, et al: Quantification of the learning curve for percutaneous dilatational tracheotomy. Laryngoscope 110:222-228, 2000.
24. Matthews HR, Hopkinson RB: Treatment of sputum retention by minitracheotomy. Br J Surg 71:147-150, 1984.
25. McColley SA, April MM, Carroll JL, et al: Respiratory compromise after adenotonsillectomy in children with obstructive sleep apnea. Arch Otolaryngol Head Neck Surg 118:940-943, 1992.
26. Milner SM, Bennett JD: Emergency cricothyrotomy. J Laryngol Otol 105:883-885, 1991.
27. Munro IR: Craniofacial surgery: Airway problems and management. Int Anesthesiol Clin 26:72-78, 1988.
28. Murphy A, Donoff B: Anesthesia for orthognathic surgery. Int Anesthesiol Clin 27:98-101, 1989.
29. Oberwalder M, Weis H, Nehoda H, et al: Videobronchoscopic guidance makes percutaneous dilational tracheostomy safer. Surg Endosc 18:839-842, 2004.
30. Oeken J, Adam H, Bootz F: [Fantoni translaryngeal tracheotomy (TLT) with rigid endoscopic control]. HNO 50:638-643, 2002.
31. Ovassapian A: Topical anesthesia of the airway. In Ovassapian A (ed): Fiberoptic Airway Endoscopy in Anesthesia and Critical Care. New York, Raven Press, 1990, pp 45-56.
32. Ovassapian A, Tuncbilek M, Weitzel EK, Joshi CK: Airway management in adult patients with deep neck infections: A case series and review of the literature. Anesth Analg 100:585-589, 2005.
33. Patil VU: Concerning the complications of the Patil-Syracuse mask. Anesth Analg 76:1165-1166, 1993.
34. Practice guidelines for management of the difficult airway: An updated report by the American Society of Anesthesiologists Task Force on Management of the Difficult Airway. Anesthesiology 98:1269-1277, 2003.
35. Sivarajan M, Fink BR: The position and the state of the larynx during general anesthesia and muscle paralysis. Anesthesiology 72:439-442, 1990.
36. Schachner A, Ovil Y, Sidi J, et al: Percutaneous tracheostomy: A new method. Crit Care Med 17(10): 1052-1056, 1989.

ANESTHESIA FOR LASER AIRWAY SURGERY

Lorraine J. Foley
Roy D. Cane

I. INTRODUCTION

Laser, an acronym for light application by stimulated emission of radiation, is used both in medicine and surgery. Maiman developed the first ruby laser in 1960.[76] This first working laser is the prototype for other lasers today. Clinical applications of laser technology are used in ophthalmology, dermatology, plastic surgery, cardiovascular disease, general surgery, gynecology, gastrointestinal surgery, urology, and otolaryngology, with continuation of research for further applications. Lasers serve as a source of radiant power or energy that is focused onto tissue. This energy is absorbed by tissue, causing a localized increase in temperature, and used to cut, coagulate, or vaporize tissue. Advantages of laser surgery are a dry field and good homeostasis, rapid healing and minimal scarring, surgical accuracy and preservation of normal tissue, a high degree of sterility, and decreased postoperative edema and pain with shorter surgery time and recovery. The high energy of the laser and its potential for combustion pose special problems when the surgical field is in proximity to the airway (Fig 37-1).

> "Fire in breathing tube kills surgery patient in Rome, Italy." An Italian man died after an operation in which surgeons accidentally set fire to a breathing tube in his throat with a laser they were using to remove a tumor (Reuters)" Circa 1999, *Boston Globe*, Boston, Massachusetts.

It is thought that operating room fires are underreported and that there are probably between 100 and 200 operating room fires in the United States per year. Of the reported fires, 20% result in serious injury to the patient. The one or two deaths per year are usually secondary to airway fire.[6] To provide care to patients undergoing laser surgery, the anesthesiologist who works with lasers should be familiar with the elements of laser operation, the types of lasers available, and special anesthesia considerations for

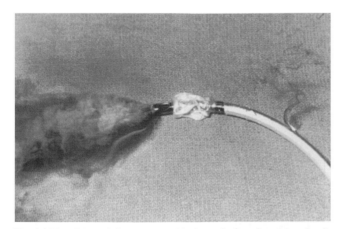

Figure 37-1 Potentially catastrophic laser-induced endotracheal tube (ET) fire. Polyvinyl chloride ET that had been wrapped with Radio Shack no. 44-1155 tape is pictured. The site of the laser's impingement on the wrapped ET can be seen at the right. This ET had 100% O_2 flowing through it. A CO_2 laser with a power output of 70 W in the continuous mode was used. (From Sosis M: Adv Anesth 6:175, 1989.)

safe laser surgery. This chapter reviews both laser technology and the special anesthesia considerations essential for safe care of patients.

II. PRINCIPLES OF LASER TECHNOLOGY

Einstein in 1917 developed the quantum theory.[46] This theory states that when an atom or molecule is in an excited state and spontaneously returns to a stable state, it emits a of light with a specific wavelength. Should that photon collide with another similarly excited atom, the atom will return to its stable state, emitting a photon that will travel in exactly the same direction with the same wavelength and be in phase with the first photon. This is the process of stimulated emission (Fig 37-2).[52]

In the laser instrument, there are several components: (1) a power source (flash lamp or chemical reactions) and (2) an active medium, a source of laser radiation that may be gaseous, liquid, or solid between two parallel mirrors. When the power source is activated, the electrons of the atoms of the laser medium absorb energy. They are elevated to energy levels above their ground state. The electrons then decay to lower energy levels and emit photons that are not in phase with one another and are traveling in all directions. However, a photon striking one of the laser's mirrors is reflected back through the laser medium, where it stimulates the emission of more photons of the same energy, phase, and direction. The parallel mirrors reflect these in turn. The result is a large number of photons of the same energy that are in phase and traveling in the same direction. In practice, one of the mirrors allows a small portion of light to pass through it, thus a laser radiation beam (Fig. 37-3).

Laser radiation has the following properties that normal light does not (see Fig. 37-3):

1. It is monochromatic (one color); all the photons have the same energy, frequency, and wavelength.
2. It is coherent; the peaks and troughs of the waves are in phase, travel in the same direction.
3. It is collimated; the beam does not usually diverge (unlike the radiation from an incandescent light source).
4. It has a high energy density.

The wavelength of emission (nanometers) of the laser and spectral absorption characteristics of the tissue determine the effectiveness of laser on tissue. In addition, the power density

$$\text{Power density (W cm}^{-2}) = \text{power output of laser/area of laser strike (cm}^2)$$

affects the amount of tissue vaporization or coagulation. Surgical lasers are operated in various modes[52,86]:

1. Continuous mode: a steadily emitting laser beam
2. Pulsed mode: a single brief emission of laser radiation (fraction of a second)

Figure 37-2 The processes of absorption, spontaneous emission, and stimulated emission necessary for a laser to operate. A photon or light packet with energy *(hν)* or other power source can provide the energy necessary to raise the energy level of electrons from the ground state to an excited state *(absorption)*. In the excited state the electron is unstable and reemits this energy *(spontaneous emission)*. A photon of the appropriate energy impinging on an electron in the excited state causes the release of a second photon of the same energy *(stimulated emission)*. The latter photon travels in the same direction and is in phase with the first photon. (From Saunders ML, Young HF, Becker DP, et al: The use of the laser in neurological surgery. Surg Neurol 14:1, 1980.)

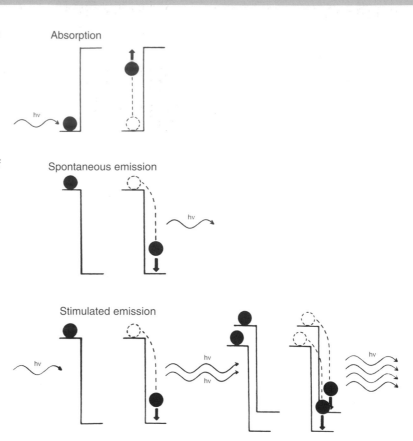

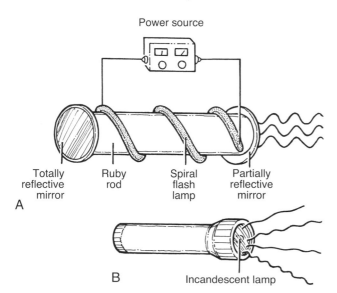

Figure 37-3 In the laser **(A)** a power source (power supply and flash lamp) stimulates the lasing medium, in this case a ruby rod. The spontaneous emission of photons from electrons in the excited state stimulates the emission of more photons. The parallel mirrors reflect the photons traveling along the axis of the laser, amplifying the intensity of the radiation. This results in a coherent monochromatic laser beam emerging from the partially reflective mirror that can produce high power densities. In contrast, an incandescent lamp **(B)** produces radiation of many wavelengths and directions, which is difficult to focus. (From Sosis M: Anesthesia for laser surgery. Int Anesthesiol Clin 28:119, 1990.)

3. Q-switching: release of laser radiation in a short burst of high peak power, thus reducing the interval of the pulse and increasing high peak power

The selection of an operating mode is dependent on the type of laser (medium) and the clinical application.

A. TYPES OF LASERS

There are six types of lasers used in the operating room for airway surgery ranging from turbinate surgery to tracheobronchial tumors. The differences between these laser types depend on the laser emitted wavelength, output power, mode of operation (pulsed or continuous mode), and whether it is a contact or noncontact application.

1. Carbon Dioxide Laser

The carbon dioxide (CO_2) laser has been used for a wide variety of otolaryngology and head and neck surgical procedures and in gynecologic surgery for the treatment of intraepithelial neoplasms, condylomata acuminata, and other lesions. The CO_2 laser uses carbon dioxide mixed with nitrogen and helium as its laser medium. The nitrogen is used to aid in energy transfer to the upper excitation level of the carbon dioxide molecule. The CO_2 laser emits invisible infrared light at a wavelength of 10,600 nm. Carbon dioxide lasers usually incorporate a visible helium-neon (He-Ne) laser for aiming purposes because the CO_2

laser is invisible. The low-intensity (0.8 mW) He-Ne laser has a red color (wavelength, 0.6328 μm). Its mode of delivery is either continuous or pulsed. CO_2 radiation is highly absorbed by water, thus by all tissues. It is readily absorbed by the first 200 μm depth in all biologic materials independent of tissue pigmentation (Table 37-1). The CO_2 laser's radiation cannot be transmitted through ordinary fiberoptic bundles. Also, injuries to the eyes from the CO_2 laser are confined to the cornea.[68] There is no risk to the retina.

The CO_2 laser has advantages that make it a very effective surgical tool. Its use with an operating microscope allows the surgeon to destroy precisely targets approximately 2 mm in diameter under binocular vision (Fig. 37-4). This degree of precision may be impossible to achieve with conventional cautery.[145] Also, during CO_2 laser surgery, the surgical field is usually bloodless because of the laser's considerable hemostatic action. Vessels up to 0.5 mm in diameter can usually be sectioned without bleeding.[145] The CO_2 laser has been used successfully to excise vascular lesions, even in patients with a bleeding diathesis.[86] The use of more traditional surgical tools such as cautery usually results in considerable postoperative edema. Edema does not usually occur after using the CO_2 laser because of the sharp line of tissue destruction with virtually no injury to surrounding tissue. Ninety percent of the laser's energy is absorbed within 0.03 mm.[3] In addition, there is no manipulation of tissues because laser treatment is usually a noncontact technique. Microscopic examination of tissue after CO_2 laser surgery revealed a discrete line of destruction, with preservation of capillaries and normal features of adjacent tissues. The preservation of adjacent tissues is thought to account for the rapid healing, minimal scarring, and lack of pain often observed after CO_2 laser surgery.[145]

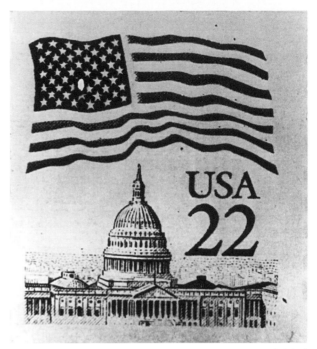

Figure 37-4 The hole made by a CO_2 laser in the starry field of the flag in this stamp illustrates the precision afforded by laser surgery. (From Sosis M: Adv Anesth 6:175, 1989.)

The carbon dioxide laser is preferred for laryngeal lesions. Carbon dioxide lasers allow precise cutting and shallow penetration of tissues. These qualities are imperative for removal of lesions situated in the supraglottic or immediate subglottic regions. The CO_2 laser is a safe and extremely useful surgical modality in the airways and the digestive tract.[58] It is best suited for widening benign tracheal stenoses and for removal of granulation tissues.[13]

2. Argon Laser

The applications of the argon laser include ophthalmologic surgery, especially for retinal and anterior chamber procedures. Its applications in dermatologic and plastic surgery include the removal of port wine stains, hemangiomas, and tattoos because of the laser's absorption by hemoglobin and other pigments. The argon laser uses an argon gas medium. It emits visible blue-green radiation at wavelengths of 488 and 514 nm (see Table 37-1). Fiberoptic bundles readily transmit the radiation in a continuous mode. It is absorbed selectively by hemoglobin and melanin or other pigments. It can be transmitted through clear substances. Because the tissue penetration is 0.5 to 2 mm, it is useful for superficial coagulation and capillary vessels. Port wine stains are lightened without scarring after treatment with the argon laser.[86]

3. Ruby Laser

The ruby laser uses a solid medium of a crystal aluminum oxide (sapphire) containing chromium ions. It emits visible red radiation at a wavelength of 0.695 μm (see Table 37-1).

Table 37-1 **Characteristics of Commonly Used Medical Lasers**

Type of Laser	Laser Wavelength (μm)	Color	Fiberoptic Transmission
Gas			
Helium-neon	0.633	Red	Yes
Argon	0.5	Blue-green	Yes
Carbon dioxide	10.6	Invisible	No
Solid			
Ruby	0.695	Red	Yes
Nd:YAG	1.06	Invisible	Yes
KTP	0.532	Green	Yes

KTP, potassium titanyl phosphate; Nd:YAG, neodymium:yttrium-aluminum-garnet.
From Sosis M: Probl Anesth 7:160, 1993.

The ruby laser is used only in the pulse mode. The radiation is not readily absorbed by water but is significantly absorbed by pigments such as melanin and hemoglobin. The ruby laser can easily penetrate the anterior structures of the eye. It is used to photocoagulate vascular and pigmented retinal lesions. Ruby laser use has decreased with the newer lasers available.

4. Neodymium:Yttrium-Aluminum-Garnet Laser

The neodymium:yttrium-aluminum-garnet (Nd:YAG) or "YAG" laser has been used for photocoagulation and deep thermal necrosis for the treatment of gastrointestinal bleeding and obstructing bronchial lesions. The Nd:YAG laser uses a clear solid crystalline medium that emits radiation in the infrared region of the electromagnetic spectrum; the radiation has a wavelength of 1.06 μm and thus is invisible (see Table 37-1). Conventional fiberoptic bundles readily transmit Nd:YAG laser radiation at high power. It is applied in either a continuous or pulsed mode. The radiation is more readily absorbed by dark tissue. However, blue and black pigmentation enhances Nd:YAG absorption, whereas pale colors enhance its penetration.[52,68,118,145] Nd:YAG radiation penetrates tissues to a depth of 2 to 6 mm and provides good homeostasis for blood vessels up to 0.5 cm in diameter. However, the depth of penetration is less predictable than that of the CO_2 laser. The power density below the tissue surface depends on the color of that surface, which makes laser penetration more difficult than that noted with the CO_2 laser.

The Nd:YAG laser is recommended for lesions distal to the larynx and bulky vascular endobronchial neoplasms. The advantage of the Nd:YAG laser is that the radiation can be transmitted through fiberoptic bundles. Excision of lesions that are located distal to the larynx is complicated because it is difficult to reach the tumor with the laser beam. In these situations the Nd:YAG laser is preferred because it can be used with either the rigid or fiberoptic bronchoscope (FOB).[117] Nd:YAG lasers are less precise in cutting, penetrate the tissue deeper, and have improved photocoagulation and superior hemostasis.

Dumon and coauthors,[42] reporting on a large series of cases, recommended the use of rigid rather than flexible bronchoscopy for treating obstructive pulmonary lesions by means of endoscopic Nd:YAG laser surgery (Fig. 37-5). Brutinel and associates[23] have reported difficulty ventilating and oxygenating patients' lungs through an endotracheal tube (ET) during Nd:YAG surgery with an indwelling FOB in place. Casey and colleagues[27] reported a complication during which there was combustion of the FOB and ET in a patient undergoing Nd:YAG laser airway surgery. The use of a rigid bronchoscope for the treatment of obstructing pulmonary lesions facilitates the removal of tissue and the treatment of complications.[24] Power levels less than 50 watts (W) in short pulsations decrease the chances of impingement on vital underlying structures.[24]

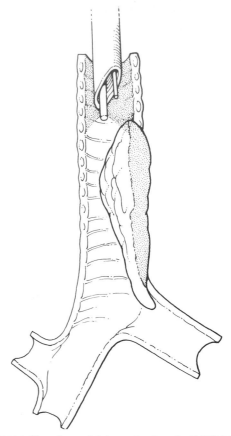

Figure 37-5 A fiber (*top, right*) conducting the Nd:YAG laser radiation through a rigid bronchoscope for the resection of a tracheal lesion. A light source is depicted to its left. (From Sosis M: Adv Anesth 6:175, 1989.)

McDougall and Cortese[77] reported two patients who died during Nd:YAG laser endoscopic treatment of airway obstructions using very high power. At high power, the penetration of tissues by the Nd:YAG laser cannot be readily controlled, and the perforation of a large blood vessel is possible.

5. KTP Laser

The potassium titanyl phosphate (KTP) laser is used in otolaryngology, vascular diseases, and hemorrhages.[63] Passing the light of a rapidly pulsed Nd:YAG laser through a potassium titanyl phosphate crystal creates the KTP laser. This doubles the frequency and thus halves the wavelength to 532 nm in the bright green visible spectrum. The radiation is able to pass through a flexible fiberoptic bundle and is used in a pulsed mode. KPT laser radiation is strongly absorbed by hemoglobin and melanin. It is also transmitted through clear substances. The tissue penetration is 0.5 to 2 mm.[63]

6. Diode Laser

The diode laser is the most recent addition to a growing array of tools of laser surgery. This laser is effective for treatment of hyperplastic inferior nasal turbinates and provides good hemostasis and a sufficient reduction of tumors in otolaryngology.[63] It is a continuous-wave semi-conductor diode laser emitting radiation at wavelengths of 810 and 940 nm in the near infrared. The radiation is delivered by a flexible fiber coupled with an aiming beam. The diode laser depth of penetration of tissue is 1 to 3 mm.

III. OPERATING ROOM HAZARDS

Many hazards that must be taken into consideration during the surgical procedure can occur in the operating room when using laser surgery. Use of lasers can place patients, surgeons, anesthesiologists, and other operating room and ancillary personnel at risk when inadvertently exposed to the hazards of laser radiation. The risks to personnel and patients may be damage to the retina, cornea, and skin depending upon the type of laser. Other hazards associated with laser surgery are electric shock and explosions of volatile gases in the operating room. The environmental hazard from the plume or fumes of the vaporized tissue also places personnel at risk.[118] It is necessary to be aware of these hazards, and strict safety precautions must be followed to prevent them from occurring.

Eye protection is very important for all personnel and the patient. The laser easily damages eyes. The damage to the eye from exposure to radiation emitted by the CO_2 laser is limited to the cornea. Its radiation is largely absorbed by water, and the cornea is more than 75% water.[108] With the Nd:YAG laser, unprotected eyes may absorb and focus laser light at the ocular fundus, resulting in irreparable damage. The endoscopist is at greatest risk because of the Nd:YAG laser's potential for backscatter.[118] Radiation from the KTP and other lasers such as Nd:YAG can penetrate the cornea and lens of the eye, resulting in severe retinal damage.[118]

Except for the carbon dioxide laser, conventional eyeglasses are inadequate protection from laser radiation. Contact lenses are inadequate even for carbon dioxide lasers. The use of eyeglasses with side guards is recommended, if not mandatory, to protect the eyes from stray rays. All protective eyewear should be labeled clearly with the optical density value, the wavelengths against which protection is afforded, and maximum radiant exposure or irradiance to which eyewear is exposed (Fig 37-6).[26] The patient's eyes should be closed during surgery and covered with moist eye patches. Protective goggles or glasses may also be placed on the patient. The Nd:YAG and argon lasers can penetrate glass; therefore, any windows in the operating room should have an opaque covering to prevent penetration by laser radiation. A warning sign should be placed on the operating room door so that anyone entering is informed that the laser is in use (Fig. 37-7). Extra goggles should be available for personnel entering the operating room.

Burns to the skin can occur. The patient's face should be protected with wet towels and drapes. Preparation solution should not contain alcohol. Oxygen saturation monitors are a standard of care and should be used because detection of cyanosis is difficult with the patient's face covered.

The plume of smoke produced by vaporization of tissues in either electrocautery or laser surgery may be hazardous. The smoke contains fine particles (mean size 0.31 µm, range of sizes 0.1 to 0.8 µm) that can be efficiently transported and deposited in the alveoli.[84] In rat lungs, the deposition of laser plume particles appeared capable of producing interstitial pneumonia, bronchiolitis, a reduction in mucociliary clearance, inflammation, and emphysema.[12,50] The laser's smoke plume acting as a vector for viruses is controversial. Viral DNA has been detected in plumes from condyloma and skin warts but not from laryngeal papilloma.[2,47,48,115] Carbon dioxide lasers seem to produce the most smoke related to vaporization of tissue. A precaution to protect the operating room personnel is to use an efficient smoke evacuator at the surgical site.[126,127] Ordinary operating room masks are efficient to filter particles only down to about 3.0 µm. Laser masks that are more highly efficient should be used to protect the operating room personnel from plume particles.

Disposable surgical drapes are a potential fire hazard. They are treated with flame-retardant chemicals and are water resistant. Even so, all types of surgical drapes can be potentially flammable. Multiple cases of drapes catching on fire have been reported. When the drapes catch on fire, it is difficult to extinguish because the drapes are water resistant and the water rolls off them. Therefore, a CO_2 fire extinguisher should be available. Drapes, once ignited, go up in flames immediately, causing the operating

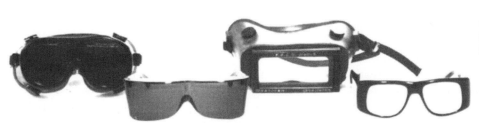

Figure 37-6 A variety of glasses and goggles designed for laser use. (From Sosis M: Adv Anesth 6:175, 1989.)

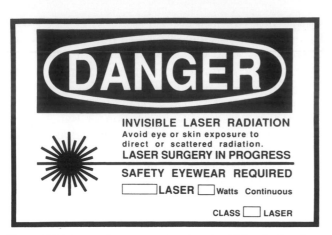

Figure 37-7 A conspicuous warning sign should be displayed on the operating room door whenever the laser is used. (Courtesy of Sharplan Lasers.)

room to be inundated with smoke and making it difficult for everyone to see and breathe.[72,82,96] The following case report illustrates the severity of a laser-induced drape fire: "During a craniotomy for the removal of a brain tumor, the patient's drapes were set on fire when a carbon dioxide laser accidentally discharged. The patient had approximately 10% second-degree and third-degree burns to her chest, neck, and arm. The patient survived, but after the operation, had to be treated for the burns and underwent skin grafts to the arms and upper chest. Also, as a result of the fire, three nurses and two physicians had to be treated for smoke inhalation."[71] As a result, the government and various standard-setting organizations (Association of Operating Room Nurses, Consumer Product Safety Commission, and National Fire Protection Agency) have flammability standards for all fabric and paper material in the operating room. It has been recommended that a minimum amount of surgical draping be used during laser surgery. Also, towels moistened with water can be used to decrease combustion. It is important to keep the towels moist or they can become flammable.

ET fires are another serious hazard, mainly to the patient. Airway fires with laser surgery have been underreported. Special anesthetic considerations, types of ETs, and management are discussed further in this chapter.

Overall, the intensity of the laser and its potential for tissue damage and combustion necessitate that strict safety precautions are followed whenever it is used. Lasers should always be set to the "standby" mode, except when they are ready to fire, so that inadvertent actuation is impossible. They should be used in the pulsed (shuttered) mode rather than the continuous mode whenever possible to limit the energy delivered by the laser and to allow the area being lased to cool between firings. The laser radiation should never be allowed to strike highly polished or mirror-like surfaces. For this reason, most instrumentation for use with lasers has a dull or matte finish, and blackened instruments are widely used. This is important because reflection of the coherent laser beam may not disperse it. Thus, injury

to the patient or operating room personnel is possible, even from a reflected laser beam. Any instruments that become hot as a result of laser radiation may cause burns.[26,71] Tracheal laceration, tooth damage, injury to soft tissue, and cutaneous burns to operating room personnel have been described during laser surgery.[95]

IV. MANAGEMENT OF ANESTHESIA

Laser airway surgery requires an airway shared between the surgeon and the anesthesiologist. The most important thing is communication and cooperation between the surgeon and the anesthesiologist on the surgical and anesthetic management of the patient. The surgeon needs maximal free access to the airway and an unobstructed surgical field with little or no interference from an ET. Meanwhile, the anesthesiologist must provide adequate ventilation and oxygenation to the patient, giving the surgeon optimal conditions for surgery in a patient who preoperatively has an airway that is compromised and most likely has significant comorbidities. During the course of surgery, the surgeon and anesthesiologist should continue to communicate throughout the procedure. Rontal and colleagues used a video monitor during all laser endoscopic procedures so that the entire operating room team could observe the procedure.[112] This allows the operating room nurses to anticipate the surgeons' needs. More important, it allows the anesthesiologist to communicate better and adjust the anesthetic accordingly as well act quickly if there is an airway fire.

A. PREOPERATIVE EVALUATION

A thorough medical evaluation is essential for all patients coming to surgery. Patients requiring laser surgery of the airway usually have increased risk for medical problems. They probably have history of tobacco use and are likely to have cardiovascular and respiratory dysfunction. A detailed history and physical examination should be obtained as well as any relevant tests. Also, the patient's old anesthetic records should be available for history of prior intubations.

The major concerns of preoperative assessment by review of systems for such patients are as follows.

1. Head and neck: The anesthesiologist should know the underlying pathology of the lesion, anatomic characteristics, and severity of obstruction. An extensive evaluation of the degree of airway obstruction should be undertaken. A history should be obtained of signs of airway obstruction possibly related to edema or tumor, such as obstructive sleep apnea, difficulty breathing, difficulty swallowing, shortness of breath, snoring, stridor, wheezing, or difficulty clearing secretions. An airway examination should be done including the Mallampati classification, mouth

opening, prognathia, size of tongue, neck range of motion, prominent teeth, and tracheal deviation from external compression. The precise location and extent of the tumor should be defined by chest radiography, computed tomography, and magnetic resonance imaging (MRI).[99] However, the patient's general condition may preclude obtaining all of the excellent images that can be provided by modern radiologic techniques. The test results should be reviewed looking at the luminal size of the trachea and assessing tracheobronchial obstruction. Such studies should include chest radiography (anteroposterior and lateral for possible pulmonary collapse and consolidation, presence of air-filled lung bullae, or pneumothorax), computed tomography or MRI, flow-volume loops, and barium swallow.

2. Respiratory: The concerns are upper airway obstruction and coexisting pulmonary problems such as a history of chronic obstructive pulmonary disease, emphysema, or even newly diagnosed asthma; wheezing; and exercise tolerance. Whether the patient requires home O_2 should be determined. Physical examination includes auscultation of the lungs for wheezing or decreased breath sounds and looking for clubbing or cyanosis. One should review the chest radiograph, percent O_2 saturation, baseline arterial blood gas, flow-volume loop, and pulmonary function tests to determine the amount of pulmonary reserve and involvement of the extrabronchial structures.

3. Cardiovascular: The concerns are related to potential cardioarterial disease. History of chest pain, shortness of breath with exertion, exercise tolerance, and previous myocardial infarction or congestive heart failure are of interest. Examination includes auscultation of the heart for rate, rhythm, and heart murmurs and the lungs for rales. One should look for jugular venous distention not only for congestive heart failure but also for possible subclavian venous occlusion secondary to the tumor. Tests that may be needed are a 12-lead electrocardiogram, cardiac echocardiogram, dipyridamole (Persantine) thallium, and exercise stress test.

4. Other systems include the gastrointestinal system for aspiration potential such as hiatal hernia, acid reflux, nighttime cough, and obesity. Routine blood work should be done unless otherwise indicated.

The patient's physical status should be optimized before surgery. Patients receiving methylxanthine bronchodilators should have their serum levels checked and their dosages changed as required. It should be remembered that many airway procedures may cause sustained hypertension and tachycardia, both of which stress the cardiovascular system. Patients should receive nothing by mouth according to the American Society of Anesthesiologists (ASA) recommendation or hospital policy.

B. PREMEDICATION

Patients are in a precarious medical state. They are at risk for respiratory obstruction. Any premedications given to patients should be given in the holding area of the operating room, where they can be monitored. During the preoperative visit, the anesthesiologist should attempt to allay the patient's fears. An antisialagogue to minimize oral and tracheobronchial secretions may be given, glycopyrrolate, 0.2 mg intravenously or 0.4 mg intramuscularly, or atropine, 0.4 to 0.5 mg subcutaneously or intramuscularly. Caution should be taken if the patient has difficulty mobilizing secretions because the antisialagogue thickens pulmonary secretions. If the patient has a severe history of coronary artery disease, there is a possible increase in heart rate.

For patients with moderate obstruction, decreasing anxiety may be beneficial as quieter breathing results in a fall in airway resistance.[53] For patients with severely narrowed airways, respiratory depression must be avoided. Thus, careful deliberation is needed before giving any anxiolytic or opioids or combination thereof, which can act synergistically toward respiratory depression. Midazolam 0.5 to 1 mg intravenously with repeated doses may be given for anxiolysis.

Patients should be monitored with a three- or five-lead electrocardiogram depending on the cardiac history, pulse oximetry, capnography, oxygen analyzer, precordial stethoscope, peripheral nerve stimulator, and noninvasive blood pressure (BP) cuff. An invasive arterial BP line, preferably in the left arm, should be considered for patients with cardiovascular instability to monitor closely hemodynamic changes and arterial blood gases intraoperatively.[104] Compression or rarely division of an innominate artery results in inaccurate BP readings if the line is placed in the right arm.

A difficult airway cart should be in the room that contains a complement of airway equipment and local anesthetics for topicalization. Airway equipment that should be available includes different laryngoscopes, oral and nasal airway, laryngeal mask airway (LMA), intubating LMA, fiberoptic scope, retrograde and cricothyrotomy kits, and jet ventilation. A rigid bronchoscopy and tracheostomy tray should also be in the room.

Correct eyeglass protection for patient and personnel should also be in the room. Sterile water or saline should be immediately available. A CO_2 fire extinguisher should be nearby.

C. INDUCTION AND MAINTENANCE OF ANESTHESIA

1. General Anesthesia

Choice of anesthesia depends upon the condition of the patient, the location of the tumor, and the nature of the planned procedure. Any technique that maintains spontaneous ventilation is safest in the presence of airway obstruction.[114] Spontaneous breathing is critical with intrathoracic obstructive lesions of the large airways.

In spontaneous breathing, large airways are stented open during inspiration by the negative intrathoracic pressure that is generated. This permits some inspired tidal volume to get past the obstruction. In addition, when the chest wall expands during inspiration, the negative pressure generated is beneficial in preventing collapse of the tumor mass onto the large airways and vessels. These two safeguards are removed when spontaneous ventilation ceases. Caution is needed if muscle relaxants are to be used. The airway can collapse with loss of muscle tone and this may not be overcome by positive-pressure ventilation, resulting in total loss of the airway. Before abolishing the ability to breath spontaneously by administering a muscle relaxant or inducing a deep plane of anesthesia, it is prudent to establish that patient can be ventilated with positive pressure by face mask.

In pediatric patients, general anesthesia is used. In small children with airway obstruction, attempting bronchoscopic procedures with sedation alone is not recommended. General anesthesia using inhalation agents allows better airway control and permits the operator to concentrate on the procedure.[143] In a retrospective review of pediatric patients undergoing diagnostic bronchoscopic procedures in the intensive care unit with sedation, ketamine was associated with 20% of adverse reactions. Complications were mostly in children younger than 3 years with severe underlying disease.[125]

A tubeless spontaneous respiration technique has been used for pediatric microlaryngeal surgery. It allows an unrestricted view and surgical access to the larynx. This can be accomplished by delivering inhalation agents proximal to the larynx or by using propofol. Halothane 0% to 5% at 4 to 10 L/min is delivered by the suction channel of the microlaryngoscope. Propofol 2 mg/kg as a bolus is followed by an infusion of 100 µg/kg/min. In pediatric microsurgery, satisfactory results were obtained in two groups of children using either halothane or propofol.[107]

General anesthesia is preferred in most adults to the same extent. Airway control that is possible with general anesthesia is fundamental in situations of airway obstruction and severe respiratory distress. There is better control of the airway and easier clearance of blood and mucus with use of a rigid bronchoscope.[54] For the insertion of a rigid bronchoscope, general anesthesia is necessary.

Rigid bronchoscopy can be performed in a spontaneously breathing patient using an inhalation technique. This is a safe technique in the presence of significant airway obstruction. However, a deep plane of anesthesia is needed to prevent coughing. Laryngospasm or bronchospasm can complicate induction if the instrumentation is attempted too hastily. This can disastrously worsen the situation, causing total airway obstruction resulting in hypoxemia and hypotension. Because the uptake of any inhalation agent is delayed by airway obstruction, induction times are always longer than usual. Sufficient time must be spent making sure that the patient is "deep enough"

for intubation. Judging the appropriate depth of anesthesia is often difficult. Excess anesthesia may result in hypoventilation in a spontaneously breathing patient.[81] Heightened caution should be exercised in monitoring the patient when using inhalation agents at such critical periods. The concentration required for an adequate depth of anesthesia to permit instrumentation of the trachea may not be tolerated by the cardiovascular system, causing hypotension and hemodynamic instability. Consequently, the margin of safety for inhalation agents may be very narrow. This is especially true in infants and in elderly patients. In children, sevoflurane seems to cause less complications such as dysrhythmias and laryngospasm than halothane.

Patients with significant tracheal obstruction benefit from sitting up and receiving supplementary humidified oxygen. A coughing spell may critically exacerbate the obstruction and should be avoided. Glycopyrrolate (0.2 to 0.3 mg) is helpful in controlling secretions, and midazolam (2 to 4 mg intravenously) is given for sedation. If an inhalation induction is chosen, the patient is preoxygenated with 100% oxygen, gradually induced with sevoflurane, and allowed to breath spontaneously. For total intravenous anesthesia, the patient is induced with a sleep bolus of 2 mg/kg propofol followed by a propofol infusion of 100 to 150 µg/kg/min. Before administering a muscle relaxant, it is prudent to establish the ability to ventilate the patient by positive pressure through a face mask. Positive-pressure ventilation may become impossible in the presence of certain large lesions in the airway. Urgent measures are necessary when the situation deteriorates to acute central airway obstruction. An ET may be inserted to bypass the obstruction. Positive-pressure ventilation and suctioning may not be enough in certain situations. Rigid bronchoscopy may be required urgently to force the tube and establish an airway under direct vision.[34]

Muscle relaxation is often necessary to hold a quiescent surgical field for laser excisions. Medium- or short-acting muscle relaxants are preferred. Mivacurium (0.2 to 0.25 mg/kg intubating dose, 3 to 15 µg/kg/min infusion), rocuronium (0.6 mg/kg), and cisatracurium (0.15 to 0.25 mg/kg) have been used. Anesthesia can be supplemented with fentanyl (bolus dose of 5 to 15 µg/kg and maintained at an infusion rate of 0.03 to 0.1 µg/kg/min) or remifentanil (bolus dose of 0.5 to 0.1 µg/kg and maintained at an infusion rate of 0.1 to 0.4 µg/kg/min).

2. Sedation and Topical Anesthesia

Selected adult populations undergoing flexible fiberoptic laser excision can be managed with sedation and topical anesthesia. Topical anesthesia with sedation should be the first choice in adults who are cooperative and for quick endoscopy with a flexible bronchoscope. This is a favored method for lesions in the middle or lower third of the trachea. Complications are rare. Bleeding seems the most life-threatening complication.[149]

Sedative drugs can decrease ventilation and should be used judiciously in small children and elderly patients. Two distinct mechanisms are accountable for this reduction: decreased respiratory drive and upper airway obstruction. Sedatives alter normal respiratory responses to hypercarbia and hypoxia, thereby decreasing the respiratory drive. Brief hypercarbia and acidosis that may develop under such circumstances are ordinarily inconsequential. However, airway obstruction is a real and more dangerous outcome of sedation as it can quickly lead to oxygen desaturation. Hypoxemia from airway obstruction can have devastating consequences.[117] The exact mechanism of upper airway obstruction during sedation or anesthesia is not clear. It may be due to decreased muscular tone and increased collapsibility of the upper airway.[47] Midazolam induces upper airway obstruction during deep sedation. Flumazenil relieves this obstruction in addition to reversing the sedative effects of midazolam.[72]

Introduction of additional obstruction to a patient with an airway that is already narrowed by a fixed lesion is invariably fraught with danger. A perilous scenario can ensue with progressively increasing obstruction resulting in total loss of the airway. Prompt measures must be undertaken to relieve the obstruction. These include asking the patient to take deep breaths, jaw thrust, chin lift, and insertion of an oral or a nasal airway. Chin lift or jaw thrust may not always relieve the obstruction. However, when these two maneuvers are combined with positive airway pressure, the pharyngeal airway is widened, counteracting airway narrowing.[80] If a procedure being performed under sedation becomes prolonged, additional unplanned drugs have to be administered, increasing the risk of excessive intraoperative sedation and of postoperative somnolence.

D. SPECIAL ANESTHETIC CONSIDERATIONS IN LASER AIRWAY SURGERY

There are currently multiple options for anesthetic management for airway laser surgery. Selection of the ventilation method and type of laser depends upon the nature and location of the lesion, the condition of the patient, and the availability of equipment and expertise. Different anesthetic management techniques have been described in the treatment of recurrent respiratory papillomatosis using the carbon dioxide laser.[121] In a 1995 survey, 92% of otolaryngologists preferred using a CO_2 laser for removal of recurrent respiratory papillomas. However, there is no consensus with respect to anesthetic management. About 46% preferred using a laser-safe ET, 26% favored using jet ventilation, 16% preferred an apneic technique, and 12% preferred spontaneous ventilation.[38] Other options include awake with topical anesthesia, general anesthesia through an ET, rigid bronchoscopy with general anesthesia, and general anesthesia by a laryngeal mask. The possibility of complete airway collapse or inability to ventilate must be taken into consideration when deciding on spontaneous or positive-pressure ventilation.

When general anesthesia for laser airway surgery is conducted without an ET, special techniques are used. These techniques include Venturi jet ventilation, intermittent apneic technique, LMA, and insufflation, which are discussed later in this chapter.

If ventilation through an ET is proposed, prevention of an ET fire or explosion requires the use of special techniques and appropriate ETs (see Fig. 37-1). Surveys of otolaryngologists active in this type of surgery concerning the complications of carbon dioxide laryngeal surgery have found ET fires or explosions to be the most common major complication.[51,58] The reported incidence of airway fires has been estimated as 0.4% to 0.57% of the patients undergoing laser airway surgery.[25] The one or two deaths per year are usually secondary to airway fire. As reported by Cozine and colleagues, there have been patients' deaths resulting from the combustion of an ET during carbon dioxide laser surgery.[37]

For a fire, three components are needed:

1. *Fuel*—flammable material such as ET, drapes, ether, chloroform, and other older anesthetics
2. *Oxidant*—oxygen, nitrous oxide
3. *Source of ignition*—laser radiation, electrocautery

The influence of special equipment and anesthesia on airway fires is discussed in the following.

1. Flammability Limits of Potent Inhaled Anesthetics

In 1850 in Boston, Massachusetts, the first recorded fire occurring in the operating theater was reported during facial surgery. With the use of ether, acetylene, ethylene, and cyclopropane, many more reports followed.[74] The range of flammability of potent inhaled anesthetics used today is well above the alveolar concentrations that would be applied to patients in clinical practice.

Leonard,[70] in investigating the lower limits of flammability of halothane, enflurane, and isoflurane, noted that halogenation renders such compounds less flammable but may not prevent their combustion under all circumstances. He found that it was possible to ignite a mixture of 4.75% halothane in 30% oxygen with the remainder composed of nitrous oxide (Table 37-2). In 20% oxygen with the remainder nitrous oxide, halothane concentrations greater than 3.25% were combustible. In oxygen–nitrous oxide mixtures of 20% and 30% oxygen, enflurane could be ignited at concentrations greater than 4.25% and 5.75%, whereas isoflurane required 5.25% and 7.0%, respectively. These values were obtained under laboratory conditions designed to encourage flammability. A closed-combustion vessel was used that contained no water vapor, carbon dioxide, or nitrogen. Ignition was initiated with a 15-kV transformer that delivered a 60-mA current across a 0.25-inch gap. However, because the spark

Table 37-2   **Minimum Flammable Concentrations of Halothane, Enflurane, and Isoflurane**

N₂O	20% O₂/ Remainder N₂O (%)	30% O₂/ Remainder N₂O (%)
Halothane	3.25	4.75
Enflurane	4.25	5.75
Isoflurane	5.25	7.0

From Leonard PF: The lower limits of flammability of halothane, enflurane, and isoflurane. Anesth Analg 54:238, 1975.

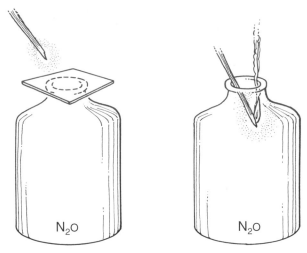

Figure 37-8 Glowing wooden splint thrust into nitrous oxide bursts into flame. (From Sosis MB: Adv Anesth 6:175, 1989.)

duration was not specified, the total energy delivered could not be calculated. The ignition power used (900 W) was, however, higher than the maximum power output delivered by most electrosurgical equipment. Leonard noted that the energy used in this experiment was much greater than that of a static discharge in the operating room. He concluded that even if the fraction of nitrous oxide administered to the patient exceeds 70%, the lowest flammable concentration of each of the three volatile halogenated anesthetic agents is above that which would be used clinically, except perhaps at the beginning of an inhalation induction.

A study by Pashayan and Gravenstein[100] showed that the addition of 2% halothane to a mixture of 40% oxygen and 60% helium significantly decreased the mean time to combustion of polyvinyl chloride (PVC) ET segments that were subjected to carbon dioxide laser radiation.

Ossoff and colleagues found that the addition of 2% halothane significantly retarded the ignition of Rusch red rubber ETs in atmospheres of 30%, 40%, and 50% oxygen–balance helium at power settings of 10, 15, and 20 W.[95]

The ratio (3.3) of the percentage of desflurane at the lower limits of flammability in 70% nitrous oxide to the minimum alveolar concentration 6% is not markedly different from what Leonard reported with enflurane (3.4), halothane (6.3), or isoflurane (6.1).[44,93] Sevoflurane is also considered to be nonflammable over the entire anesthetizing concentration range in the presence of air, oxygen, and nitrous oxide.[44,152]

2. Effect of Anesthetic Gases on Endotracheal Tube Flammability

The anesthetic gases used during airway laser surgery can profoundly influence combustibility. It cannot be stressed too strongly that nitrous oxide should not be considered an inert gas during laser airway surgery (Fig. 37-8). Although nitrous oxide cannot support life, it can readily decompose into oxygen, nitrogen, and energy according to the following equation:

$$N_2O = N_2 + \tfrac{1}{2} O_2 + energy$$

In an experiment analogous to one with oxygen, a glowing match thrust into a vessel containing nitrous oxide bursts into flames. In fact, it has been found that nitrous oxide supports combustion to approximately the same extent as oxygen.[75]

Chilcoat and coworkers stressed that the reduction in oxygen concentration on dilution with nitrous oxide did not provide any additional safety when performing laryngeal laser surgery. They recommended the use of either nitrogen, air, or helium when it was desired to reduce the oxygen concentration in anesthetic gas mixtures to levels of 30% or less for laser surgery.[31] Wolf and Simpson showed that nitrous oxide and oxygen are linearly additive in their ability to sustain combustion.[154] Therefore, nitrous oxide should not be considered safe and careful consideration is required before using it with laser surgery.

Helium and nitrogen are both inert gases and when added to oxygen could delay ET flammability (Table 37-3). Both Pashayan and Gravenstein[100] and Osoff[93] found that helium was more protective than nitrogen in retarding laser-ignited ET fires. The protective effect of helium is probably due to its high thermal diffusivity (quantity of heat passing through 1 cm² of cross-sectional area per unit of time) or thermal conductivity (time rate of transfer

Table 37-3   **Physical Properties of Helium and Nitrogen (26° C)**

Physical Properties	Helium	Nitrogen
Thermal conductivity (cal [sec-cm²⁰ C-cm⁻¹ − 10⁻⁶]⁻¹)	360.36	62.40
Thermal capacity (cal g⁻¹⁰ K⁻¹)	1.24	0.249
Density (g L⁻¹)	0.179	1.25
Thermal diffusivity (cm² sec⁻¹)	1.621	0.199

From Pashayan AG, Gravenstein JS: Helium retards endotracheal tube fires from carbon dioxide lasers. Anesthesiology 62:274, 1985.

of heat by conduction). Presumably, helium diffusivity prevents a rise in temperature around the site of laser exposure, thus preventing the laser-irradiated ET from reaching its temperature of spontaneous ignition.

Pashayan and Gravenstein[100] studied the carbon dioxide laser–induced combustibility of 2-cm segments of PVC ETs (National Catheter Corporation Division, Mallinckrodt, Glens Falls, NY). Each ET segment was placed in a 250-cm³ glass cylinder into which a catheter delivered known gas mixtures. Both the interior and exterior of the ETs were thus exposed to the gas mixtures. A carbon dioxide laser (Systems 450, Coherent Inc., Santa Clara, CA) with a beam diameter of 0.8 mm was aimed at the ET segment being studied through a hole drilled in the side of the glass cylinder and was actuated until combustion occurred or 60 seconds had elapsed. The mean time to ignition was determined. In the first part of this experiment with a laser power setting of 5 W, 10 ET segments were tested with concentrations of oxygen and helium from 20% oxygen–80% helium to 50% oxygen–50% helium. A second group of 10 ET segments was studied in an atmosphere of oxygen mixed with nitrogen, again in concentrations ranging from 20% oxygen–80% nitrogen to 50% oxygen–50% nitrogen. In another series of experiments, laser radiation at power settings of 7.5, 10, and 12.5 W was aimed at 10 ET segments in 40% oxygen–60% helium and 10 segments in 40% oxygen–60% nitrogen. Another part of the study examined 10 ET segments in 40% oxygen–60% helium and 2% halothane with a laser power of 10 W.

In the studies outlined thus far, the laser was aimed at a clear area of the PVC ET segment under study. Care was taken to avoid aiming the laser at the ET's radiopaque barium stripe. However, in a final part of the experiment, the laser beam was intentionally aimed at the barium stripe of 10 ET segments in an atmosphere of 40% oxygen–60% helium and 10 segments in an atmosphere of 40% oxygen–60% nitrogen.

Pashayan and Gravenstein[100] found that even when laser-induced ET combustion did not occur, laser exposure produced a hole in all the ETs studied. At a laser power setting of 5 W with 20% oxygen in either 80% nitrogen or helium, ET combustion did not occur after 60 seconds of laser actuation. At oxygen concentrations of 30% and 40%, the mean time to ignition with nitrogen was significantly shorter than the time for the same concentration of O_2 in He. An oxygen concentration of 50% resulted in a mean time to combustion in helium that was not statistically significantly different from that with nitrogen. Similarly, at 7.5 and 10 but not at 12 W, the mean time to ignition with O_2 in N was significantly shorter than that with O_2 in He. At a power setting of 10 W, adding 2% halothane to a mixture of 40% oxygen and 60% helium significantly shortened the mean time to combustion to 25.3 ± 1.9 seconds (mean $\pm$ SEM) from 43.1 ± 5.4 seconds. On directing the 10-W laser beam onto the radiopaque barium stripe on the PVC ETs, the mean times to combustion with both nitrogen and helium were significantly shorter than

occurred when the same gas mixture was used but the laser was aimed at the clear portions of the ETs.

Pashayan and Gravenstein[100] concluded that helium in concentrations at or above 60% delays carbon dioxide laser–induced combustion of PVC ETs if the laser power output is less than or equal to 10 W. They also conclude that the radiopaque barium stripe on the PVC ET is more combustible than the clear portions of the ET and it should be positioned away from the laser. It must be realized that reflected beams may reach a stripe that appears to be out of the direct line of sight, and using an ET without such stripes would be preferred.

Ossoff compared the incendiary characteristics of three ETs in various oxygen concentrations diluted with either helium or nitrogen using a carbon dioxide laser. First they were tested using the laser in the pulsed mode with 0.1-second exposures, then with same protocol but the laser in a continuous mode. An ET was suspended from a ring stand, and gases were delivered at a rate of 2.5 or 3 L/min through the circuit of a Vernitrol vaporizing system laboratory anesthesia machine (Ohmeda Products, Division of BOC Group, Inc., Murray Hill, NJ). A Sharplan model 730 carbon dioxide laser with maximum power output of 40 W was coupled with a Zeiss operating microscope. The lasers were powered at 10, 15, and 20 W in shuttered mode for a maximum of 60 pulses (each pulse lasting 0.1 second in 1-second intervals) and in combustion mode for a maximum of 180 seconds. The three tubes tested were the National catheter 6.0 mm internal diameter (ID) PVC ET, Rusch red rubber 6.0 mm ID ET, and Xomed Laser-Shield 6.0 mm ID ET.

Following the experiment with 100% oxygen, studies were run using 30%, 40%, 50% oxygen in nitrogen and 30%, 40%, 50% oxygen in helium. The endpoint was onset of an intraluminal fire that continued to burn between laser pulses or a full 60 pulses delivered or delivery of 180 seconds of continuous laser energy without an onset of fire. The data showed that helium was superior to nitrogen. They found that (1) 30% oxygen in helium was significantly better at retarding ignition than in nitrogen in the Rusch tube at 10 W ($P < .01$) and in the Xomed tube at 10 and 15 W ($P < .01$) and (2) 40% oxygen in helium was significantly better at retarding ignition than 40% oxygen in nitrogen in the Rusch tube at 15 W ($P < .01$) and 50% oxygen in helium was significantly better than 50% oxygen in nitrogen. Varying oxygen concentrations were calculated using oxygen in helium because of the superiority over nitrogen. With the Rusch tube 30% oxygen in helium at all three powers was significantly different ($P < .1$) from 40% and 50% oxygen in helium as well as 40% to 50% oxygen in helium only at 15 W. For the Xomed tube the results were for 30% versus 40% oxygen in helium at 10, 15, and 20 W. In summary, they found that helium was better than nitrogen as an inert mixture with use of the carbon dioxide laser to decrease flammability. They also showed that the safest anesthetic gas mixture was 30% oxygen in helium.[93]

Al Haddad and Brenner[4] studied the combustion of 1- to 2-inch PVC ET segments with the KTP laser and carbon dioxide laser in helium-oxygen and nitrogen-oxygen atmospheres. They compared these two lasers because of their different wavelengths and penetration characteristics that are commonly used in airway laser surgery. A 6 L/min flow of the gas mixture under study entered a hole at the base of a glass test cylinder. A 10-W KTP laser beam (Laserscope Microbeam II) or carbon dioxide beam was passed through a side hole in the cylinder at the ET segment until combustion occurred or 1 minute had elapsed. The gas mixtures studied were 21%, 30%, and 40% O_2 in N and 30% and 40% O_2 in He. A commercial oxygen analyzer was used to determine the oxygen concentration. The data were analyzed using analysis of variance and Kruskal-Wallis tests.

With the KTP laser, at oxygen concentrations of 21%, 30%, and 40% in nitrogen, the mean times to ignition were 17.44 ± 23.26, 15.6 ± 19.47, and 12.83 ± 19.14 seconds, respectively. For the 30% and 40% oxygen-helium mixtures, the times to combustion were 9.89 ± 5.33 and 11.04 ± 14.47 seconds, respectively. The differences in the times to combustion with oxygen-helium and oxygen-nitrogen mixtures at 30% and 40% oxygen were not statistically significant.

With the carbon dioxide laser at oxygen concentrations of 21%, 30%, and 54% in nitrogen the mean times to ignition were 51.29 ± 11.3, 41.28 ± 10.83, and 21.51 ± 6.42 seconds, respectively. For the 30% and 40% oxygen-helium mixtures the times to combustion was 60 ± 0 and 50.34 ± 10.96 seconds, respectively.

The carbon dioxide laser mean ignition time in helium was prolonged compared with nitrogen ($P < .001$), whereas increasing the oxygen concentration reduced the ignition time for both nitrogen and helium. With KTP, there was no significant difference for ignition between the five groups of oxygen concentrations or between nitrogen and helium. Al Haddad and Brenner reconfirmed that helium, as part of the mixture with 30% oxygen, is safest for the carbon dioxide laser but concluded that the use of helium instead of nitrogen confers no added safety during KTP laser surgery.

Simpson and colleagues[122] determined the flammability of four types of ETs in mixtures of helium and oxygen or nitrous oxide compared with mixtures of nitrogen and oxygen or nitrous oxide. The gases were metered with precision flowmeters and directed to a mixing chamber and then into a test cylinder 7.5 cm in diameter and 60 cm long. The ETs studied were (1) PVC (Portex, Wilmington, MA), (2) red rubber (Rusch, Waiblingen, Germany), (3) silicon (National Catheter, Argyle, NY), and (4) Xomed Laser-Shield I (Xomed, Jacksonville, FL). The gas flow rates were maintained at 30 to 35 L/min, and the gas concentrations were measured at the level of the clamp holding the ET in the test chamber. The oxygen concentration was measured by a paramagnetic technique and the nitrous oxide by an infrared technique. Unlike the other researchers, Simpson and colleagues did not use a

laser to ignite the ETs. The ignition of the ETs was accomplished with a propane torch. The ETs were initially ignited in oxygen and nitrogen, and the nitrogen was quickly discontinued and replaced with helium. The helium concentration was increased until the candle-like flame on the ET was extinguished. The oxygen concentrations just before the flame's extinction with helium were defined as the "oxygen/helium index of flammability." This procedure was repeated five times for each type of ET tested.

A similar experimental design was used with mixtures of nitrogen and oxygen until the propane torch–induced combustion of the four types of ETs was extinguished. This was defined as the "oxygen/nitrogen index of flammability." Next, the oxygen was replaced by nitrous oxide and the procedure was repeated to determine the "nitrous oxide/helium" and "nitrous oxide/nitrogen indices of flammability." The indices of flammability of each type of ET studied were averaged, and the results were compared using Bonferroni corrected t-tests.

The oxidant oxygen/helium indices for the PVC, red rubber, silicon, and Xomed ETs were, respectively, 0.274 ± 0.0055 (mean $\pm$ SD), 0.194 ± 0.0089, 0.194 ± 0.0055, and 0.256 ± 0.0055. The oxidant oxygen/nitrogen indices for the PVC, rubber, silicon, and Xomed ETs were 0.254 ± 0.0055, 0.182 ± 0.0045, 0.200 ± 0, and 0.230 ± 0, respectively. These results show that the PVC ET is flammable in 27.4% oxygen with the remainder consisting of helium and in 25.4% oxygen with the remainder nitrogen. In all cases, the oxidant oxygen/helium values were statistically significantly higher than the oxygen/nitrogen values for the same type of ET ($P < .05$). The oxidant nitrous oxide/helium indices for the PVC, red rubber, silicon, and Xomed ETs were (mean $\pm$ SD) 0.526 ± 0.0055, 0.434 ± 0.0114, 0.416 ± 0.0055, and 0.456 ± 0.0055, respectively. The values for the oxidant nitrous oxide/nitrogen indices were 0.472 ± 0.0084, 0.356 ± 0.0055, 0.392 ± 0.0045, and 0.0444 ± 0.0114 for the PVC, red rubber, silicon, and Xomed ETs, respectively. The oxidant nitrous oxide/helium indices were statistically higher than the nitrous oxide/nitrogen indices for all except the Xomed ET.

However, Simpson and colleagues noted that the differences between helium and nitrogen indices determined in this study are not clinically significant. For example, for a PVC ET, the difference between 27.4% O_2 in He and 25.4% O_2 in He needed for combustion is very small. Their study also showed that the PVC ETs were less flammable than the red rubber, silicon, and Xomed ETs.

3. The Use of Metallic Foil Tapes to Protect the Shafts of Combustible Endotracheal Tubes from Laser Radiation

Foil tapes were first suggested as a simple, inexpensive means of protecting the shafts of combustible ETs from laser beams by Strong and Jako in 1972 (Fig. 37-9).[145]

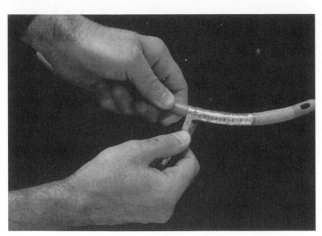

Figure 37-9 Technique of foil wrapping a rubber endotracheal tube is illustrated using 3M no. 425 aluminum foil tape. (From Sosis M: Anesthesia for laser surgery. Int Anesthesiol Clin 28:119, 1990.)

A problem related to the use of metallic foil tapes is that none are manufactured for medical applications, nor has the U.S. Food and Drug Administration sanctioned such use. One manufacturer, when questioned, cautioned against the use of its aluminum tape for medical purposes.[134] However, the use of protective metal tape during laser surgery is widely advocated in the literature[5,36,44,135] and is an inexpensive technique. Metallic foil tape provides protection only from the direct impact of the laser beam. Indirect combustion caused by sparks or heat from gaseous or tube combustion is still possible[60] because the ETs used are generally combustible and usually have an enriched concentration of oxygen flowing through them (Fig. 37-10). Furthermore, a case of an obstruction of the airway from metallic tape that came loose from a wrapped ET has been reported.[64]

In an experiment designed to evaluate the protection offered by metallic foil tapes to the shafts of combustible ETs from the carbon dioxide laser, 8-mm ID Mallinckrodt Hi-Lo PVC ETs were studied after wrapping them with five types of tape.[134] The ETs were wrapped with a continuous strip of ¼-inch (0.6-cm) self-adhesive foil tape.

Starting at the distal (cuffed) end, the ET was wrapped in a spiral fashion. The tape was applied in an overlapping manner so that bending the ET would not expose any unprotected area. The taping was begun at the cuffed end of the tube so that it would overlap in a way that would prevent laser radiation coming from above from striking the foil's adhesive. The tapes used were Minnesota Mining and Manufacturing (3M) (St. Paul, MN) nos. 425, 1430, and 433; Radio Shack (Tandy Corporation, Ft. Worth, TX) no. 44-1155; and 0.001-inch-thick copper foil tape (Venture Tape Corporation, Rockland, MA). During the trials, 5 L/min of 100% oxygen flowed through the ETs being tested as they rested horizontally on wet towels and were surrounded by air. A LaserSonics (Santa Clara, CA) model LS880 carbon dioxide laser and Zeiss (Jena, Germany) operating microscope with a 400-mm lens and 0.68-mm beam diameter were used. The laser beam was directed onto the shafts of the foil-wrapped ETs perpendicularly at the point of overlapping of the tape. A power of 70 W in the continuous mode of laser operation was used. The time until the appearance of smoke, flames, perforation, or "blowtorch" ignition was recorded. Finally, a segment of tape was wrapped adhesive side outward and the procedure repeated to determine whether unexpected contact of the laser with the adhesive would cause combustion.

The nonadhesive sides of the 3M tapes 425 and 433 and the Venture copper tape were unaffected by 25 seconds of laser impact and thus protected the ETs from the carbon dioxide laser. ET penetration and a blowtorch fire occurred at 7 and 14 seconds, respectively, with the Radio Shack 44-1155 (see Fig. 37-1) and 3M 1430 tapes.

On directing the laser onto the reverse (adhesive) side of the tapes, the adhesive backings of 3M tape 433 and Radio Shack tape 44-1155 were ignited and the tapes perforated within 0.1 second of the laser's impact. Flaming of the adhesive occurred at 1 second without penetration of 3M tape 1430 or the Venture copper tape. The adhesive side of 3M tape 425 started to smoke at 2 seconds, but no flames occurred and there was no perforation.

The results of this carbon dioxide laser study (see Table 37-4) show that the type of metallic tape used

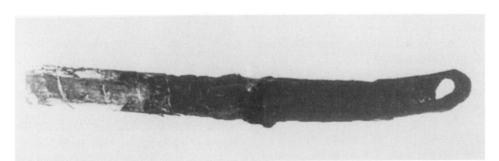

Figure 37-10 A foil-wrapped plastic endotracheal tube has undergone indirect combustion. (From Vourc'h G, Tannieres M, Freche G: Ignition of a tracheal tube during laryngeal laser surgery. Anaesthesia 34:685, 1979.)

Table 37-4 **The Effect of Carbon Dioxide Laser Radiation on Foil-Wrapped Endotracheal Tubes**

Tape Studied	Nonadhesive Side	Adhesive Side
Radio Shack no. 44-1155	7-sec tube penetration 14-sec combustion	Ignition and perforation <0.1 sec
3M no. 425	No effect by 25 sec	Smoking at 2 sec No flames or perforation
3M no. 433	No effect by 25 sec	Ignition and perforation >1 sec
3M no. 1430	7-sec tube penetration 14-sec combustion	Flaming of adhesive at 1 sec No penetration
Venture copper foil	No effect by 25 sec	Flaming of adhesive at 1 sec No penetration

From Sosis MB: Evaluation of five metallic tapes for protection of endotracheal tubes during CO_2 laser surgery. Anesth Analg 68:392, 1989.

to protect combustible ETs is critical. Radio Shack tape 44-1155 and 3M tapes 1430 and 433 offer inadequate protection of flammable ETs and should not be used for this purpose. Patel and Hicks[102] reported similar results for Radio Shack tape 44-1155. Venture copper foil tape and 3M 425 tape provided excellent protection of the shafts of the ETs. Therefore, Sosis and colleagues recommended their use during carbon dioxide laser surgery in proximity to the airway. However, a subsequent study has shown that if blood is applied to these tapes, laser-induced combustion may occur.[141] Therefore, caution is advised. The malleability of the Venture copper foil allows a smoother external contour than that of the 3M 425 aluminum tape.

The possibility of changes in the composition of any metallic foil tape requires that every batch of tape be evaluated for its incendiary characteristics before use.[36] In the evaluation of metallic foil tape for protecting combustible ETs, the laser beam must be directed at the adhesive side of the tape because some tapes, such as Radio Shack tape 44-1155, have an inner plastic layer that is highly flammable (Fig. 37-11). This plastic layer would not be detected if the laser beam was focused on the center of the tape. The impingement of the laser beam onto the edge of the tape, however, could cause an ET fire.

Sosis and colleagues[141] noted that ETs wrapped with 3M 425 tape and copper foil tape have been gas sterilized without affecting their ability to withstand the carbon dioxide laser impact, thus allowing a sterile ET to be used in clinical practice.

Sosis and Dillon[139] performed an evaluation of metallic foil tapes for the protection of combustible ETs from the Nd:YAG laser because a case report[27] of an ET fire with this type of laser has been published and no ET had been shown to provide adequate protection from the Nd:YAG laser.[53]

In part one of their study, five red rubber Rusch ETs were wrapped with ¼-inch-wide self-adhesive metallic tape (see later) in an overlapping spiral fashion beginning at the cuffed end of the ET. Red rubber ETs were used

because they are highly flammable when exposed to the Nd:YAG laser.[53] Five liters per minute of 100% oxygen flowed through the ETs so that ET perforation and combustion by the laser would be clearly seen. A second segment of each ET was wrapped with the same tape but with its adhesive side outward to determine the flammability of the adhesive because the laser might make contact with if aimed at the edge of the tape. The tapes used were (1) Radio Shack no. 44-1155 tape; (2) 3M no. 425 aluminum tape; (3) 3M no. 433 aluminum tape; (4) 3M no. 1430 aluminum tape; and (5) copper foil tape (0.001-inch thick) (Venture Tape Corporation). An unwrapped red rubber ET served as a control.

To study the effects of a high ambient oxygen concentration in part two of the study, red rubber ETs wrapped with 3M no. 425 and Venture copper foil tape were

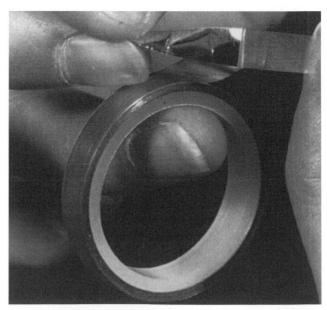

Figure 37-11 Radio Shack no. 44-1155 tape has been peeled apart to show a thin metallic layer and a plastic layer. (From Sosis M: Anesthesia for laser surgery. Int Anesthesiol Clin 28:119, 1990.)

placed in a cylindrical copper chamber that was flushed with oxygen. The concentration of oxygen was determined to be 98% both before and after laser discharge as measured on the tape with a catheter connected to a mass spectrometer. Each type of foil wrapping was evaluated five times. A LaserSonics model 1700 carbon dioxide/Nd:YAG laser, in the Nd:YAG mode with a handheld laser probe, was used in part one of this study. The laser's output was set at 50 W in the continuous mode, with a beam diameter of 0.68 mm. The beam was directed perpendicularly at the shafts of the foil-wrapped ETs and the laser's emission was continued until vigorous combustion was noted or up to a maximum of 60 seconds. A blowtorch fire, if observed, was noted. In part two, the laser was set to its maximum output of 110 W in the continuous mode of operation and was attached to a Zeiss operating microscope with a 400-mm lens. The laser beam was directed perpendicularly at the wrapped ETs in the test chamber. The Venture copper foil and 3M no. 425 tape were each evaluated five times. The laser was operated until combustion occurred or until 1 minute of discharge had elapsed.

The results of part one of this study are summarized in Table 37-5. The bare red rubber ET burned with a blowtorch effect after 13 seconds of Nd:YAG laser contact. Combustion and a blowtorch fire occurred in 6 and 15 seconds, respectively, after laser contact with Radio Shack no. 44-1155 tape. Its reverse side was not tested. 3M no. 425 aluminum tape withstood 60 seconds of laser emission without any effect to its nonadhesive side. When its adhesive side was struck by the laser, smoking was noted immediately. After 60 seconds of laser contact, ET combustion was noted beneath the tape. 3M no. 433 aluminum tape withstood 60 seconds of laser contact. When its adhesive side was exposed to the laser, it burned immediately, and a blowtorch fire was observed after 12 seconds. In the case of 3M no. 1430 aluminum tape, combustion occurred immediately after laser exposure to either side. The laser was discontinued after vigorous flames were observed, and the flames were extinguished, so that no blowtorch effect was noted. There was no effect after 60 seconds of laser contact with the nonadhesive side

of the Venture copper tape. Smoking was seen after 5 seconds of Nd:YAG laser contact with the reverse (adhesive) side. Flaming was noted after 15 seconds. The nonadhesive side of the 3M no. 425 tape and Venture tapes were retested three more times with no effect from the laser.

In part two of the investigation, no evidence of combustion was noted in all five trials of laser impingement onto red rubber ETs wrapped with 3M no. 425 or Venture copper foil tape in an atmosphere of 98% oxygen after 1 minute of Nd:YAG laser fire at a power of 110 W. The findings of Sosis and Dillon regarding the use of the 3M no. 425 tape for ET protection mark the first report of a method of providing adequate protection of the exterior aspect of a combustible ET from the Nd:YAG laser at 110 W and a duration of 1 minute. However, the presence of blood on these foil tapes is likely to impair their Nd:YAG laser resistance. The lumen of the ET remains unprotected when metallic foil taping is used, and therefore combustion could be initiated by a fiberoptic filament used during Nd:YAG endoscopic surgery if it is placed inside the tube.

4. Evaluation of the Laser-Guard Protective Coating for Protecting the Shafts of Combustible Endotracheal Tubes from Laser Radiation

The Merocel (Mystic, CT) Laser-Guard ET protective coating consists of a rectangular sheet of embossed silver foil covered with a thin absorbent Merocel sponge layer on one side and adhesive on the other (Fig. 37-12). It is available in four sizes for application to size 4.0 to 7.5 mm ID rubber and 5.0 to 8.5 mm ID plastic ETs (Table 37-6). The U.S. Food and Drug Administration has examined it for this application. After removing the protective backing from the adhesive layer of the Laser-Guard, the ET to be protected is pressed down along the centerline. The tube is then rolled until completely covered.

The Merocel Laser-Guard is designed to be an easy-to-use, highly resistant barrier to laser radiation and is moderately priced. Silver is used for the foil layer because this metal has high thermal conductivity. The thermal conductivity of a laser-protective ET coating is thought

Table 37-5   **Effect of Nd:YAG Laser Radiation on Foil-Wrapped Endotracheal Tubes**

Tape Studied	Nonadhesive Side	Adhesive Side
Radio Shack no. 44-1155	6-sec combustion; 15-sec blowtorch fire	Not tested
3M no. 425	No effect by 60 sec	Immediate smoking; tube combustion at 60 sec
3M no. 433	No effect by 60 sec	Immediate combustion and blowtorch fire after 12 sec
3M no. 1430	Immediate combustion	Immediate combustion
Venture copper foil	No effect by 60 sec	Smoking at 5 sec; flames at 15 sec

From Sosis M, Dillon F: What is the safest foil tape for endotracheal tube protection during Nd-YAG laser surgery? A comparative study. Anesthesiology 72:553, 1990.

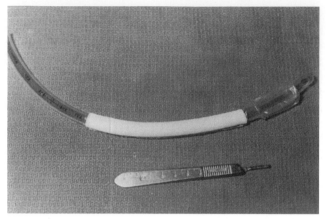

Figure 37-12 Polyvinyl chloride endotracheal tube wrapped with the Laser-Guard protective coating. (From Sosis M, Dillon F: Prevention of CO_2 laser–induced endotracheal tube fires with the laser-guard protective coating. J Clin Anesth 4:25, 1992.)

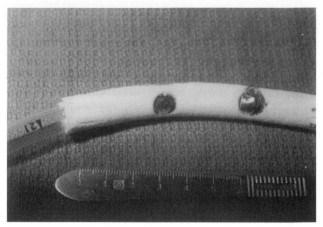

Figure 37-13 Two areas of laser contact with the Laser-Guard protective coating. The corrugated silver foil layer can be seen where the foam layer has been struck by the laser beam. (From Sosis M, Dillon F: Prevention of CO_2 laser-induced endotracheal tube fires with the laser-guard protective coating. J Clin Anesth 4:25, 1992.)

to be important because the incident laser beam's energy can be conducted away from the site of impact and thus dissipated without harm to the patient or the ET. The Merocel sponge layer, when wet, acts as a heat sink and gives the external aspect of a wrapped ET a smooth, nontraumatic contour. The sponge layer must be kept wet because in the dry state it is combustible. A solvent-soaked wipe is included with the Laser-Guard for cleaning the ET's shaft to improve adherence. Also included are strung pledgets for protecting the ET's cuff.

Sosis and Dillon[139] examined the efficacy of the Laser-Guard protective ET covering. They used a LaserSonics model LS880 carbon dioxide/Nd:YAG laser in the continuous carbon dioxide mode of operation with a Zeiss operating microscope, 400-mm lens, and "joystick" micromanipulator. The laser was directed perpendicularly at Mallinckrodt (St. Louis, Mo) size 8.0 mm ID Hi-Lo PVC ETs through which 5 L/min of oxygen was flowing. A bare Mallinckrodt PVC ET served as a control. Wrapping their shafts with the Laser-Guard protective coating protected five other identical ETs. The ETs to be tested were placed horizontally on wet towels and were surrounded by air during the study. Power settings of 10 and 70 W were used in this investigation. According to the manufacturer's directions, Sosis and Dillon wet the sponge layer of the Laser-Guard protective coating with

water after its application to the ET's shaft. The laser exposure was actuated until either combustion of the ET occurred or 60 seconds of laser fire had elapsed.

At a laser power setting of 10 W, the plain, unprotected PVC ET was penetrated after 50 seconds of laser exposure. Smoking and minor nonsustained combustion accompanied this trial; however, no blowtorch fire occurred. At 70 W of power, laser exposure of the bare PVC tube resulted in combustion and a blowtorch fire of the ET after only 3 seconds. The wet Laser-Guard–covered PVC ET shafts were not significantly damaged by 60 seconds of laser exposure at either 10 or 70 W. A small amount of smoke, but no flames, was seen when the laser was fired at it (Fig. 37-13). The Laser-Guard's sponge coating was missing, with minimal evidence of thermal decomposition of the sponge in a small area surrounding the site of laser impingement. The bare corrugated silver foil was noted to be intact.

In the study of Sosis and Dillon,[139] the Laser-Guard covering protected PVC ET shafts from laser-induced combustion during test conditions of continuous exposure to carbon dioxide laser radiation of 70 W for 60 seconds with 5 L/min of oxygen flowing through the ETs. The researchers stated that these settings are probably more severe than any that are encountered clinically so that safety in clinical use should be ensured.

Table 37-6 **Manufacturer's Specifications for the Merocel Laser-Guard Endotracheal Tube Protector**

Laser	Power (W)	Beam Diameter (mm)	Power Density (W/cm²)	Time (sec)
CO_2	70	0.68	19,275	60
Nd:YAG*	61	<1	9,588	60
KTP	18	0.4	14,324	60

*Noncontact, optically guided. Courtesy of Merocel Inc., Mystic, CT.

The control, a bare Mallinckrodt PVC ET, when exposed to the laser under the same conditions, burned like a blowtorch almost immediately after the laser was turned on. Sosis and Dillon stated that such rigorous testing of protective wrappings and special ETs manufactured for laser airway surgery is important because previous investigations by their group have shown that not all such products are efficacious.[36,131]

Sosis and Dillon concluded that the Laser-Guard protective coating was easier to apply to PVC ET shafts than the foil tapes their group had previously investigated. The Laser-Guard adhered well to the ETs tested. When its foam layer was moistened with water, it had a smoother surface than foil-wrapped ETs. Sosis and Dillon stated that this is important because laryngeal tissues are easily traumatized.

In a similar investigation comparing metallic foil tapes and the Laser-Guard for protecting the shafts of PVC ETs from the KTP laser, Sosis and Braverman[138] concluded that the Laser-Guard provided the best protection. A subsequent study determined that the presence of blood does not affect the Laser-Guard protection from the carbon dioxide laser.[141]

In common with foil wrapping, Laser-Guard–protected ETs have a slightly larger external diameter than unprotected ETs. However, whereas foil-wrapped ETs can be protected over virtually the entire shaft of the tube, Laser-Guard–protected ETs have a fixed length of protective covering. After applying the Laser-Guard coating to an ET, care must be taken to avoid flexing the tube excessively or the foil layer will fracture and its laser resistance will be compromised.

5. Prevention of Laser-Induced Polyvinyl Chloride Endotracheal Tube Cuff Fires by Filling the Cuff with Saline

During laser airway surgery, the high energy of the laser is often used in proximity to combustible ETs that may have anesthetic gases flowing through them that support or enhance combustion. Although the shafts of combustible ETs can be protected from the carbon dioxide and other types of lasers by techniques such as foil wrapping,[36] the cuff remains vulnerable to the laser's effects. LeJeune and colleagues[69] suggested that filling ET cuffs with saline during laser airway surgery would prevent their combustion; however, they did not evaluate this suggestion experimentally. Sosis and Dillon[140] designed the following controlled study to test this hypothesis.

A LaserSonics model LS8800 carbon dioxide laser with a beam diameter of 0.68 mm in the continuous mode of operation was used. The cuffs attached to size 8.0 mm ID PVC ETs (Mallinckrodt Hi-Lo; Argyle, NY) were each inserted into the neck of an empty 250-mL Pyrex Erlenmeyer flask. A circle anesthesia system attached to an anesthesia machine was then connected to the ET being tested. Five liters per minute of oxygen flowed through the ET and into the flask for 5 minutes. The ET cuff was

then inflated to just seal at a pressure of 20 cm H_2O, which was maintained within the ET, flask, and anesthesia circuit by adjusting the pressure relief (popoff) valve on the anesthesia machine. The laser beam was then directed perpendicularly at the part of the cuff that was protruding from the neck of the flask and that was, therefore, surrounded by air (Fig. 37-14). At a laser power setting of 5 W, the times to cuff perforation and loss of airway pressure were noted in 10 ET cuffs: 5 inflated with saline and 5 inflated with air. To evaluate further the combustibility of the ETs when their cuffs were inflated with saline or air, the laser's power was increased to 40 W; again, 10 ETs were studied, 5 with their cuffs filled with saline and 5 with air. In all cases, the laser was actuated until combustion occurred or 1 minute had elapsed.

Table 37-7 shows the times to cuff perforation and circuit deflation of ETs with cuffs that were filled with air or saline. The saline-filled cuffs exposed to 5 W of continuous laser radiation were perforated in 4.21 ± 3.91 seconds (mean ± SD). This was not statistically different from the times necessary to perforate the

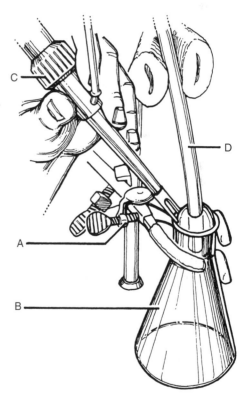

Figure 37-14 Diagram of the apparatus used to evaluate endotracheal tube (ET) cuff flammability. A ring stand and clamp (A) support the Erlenmeyer flask (B) used during the trial. The laser handpiece (C) delivers carbon dioxide laser radiation from its console (not shown) toward a polyvinyl chloride ET's cuff (D). The ET was connected to a circle anesthesia circuit and anesthesia machine, and the ET and flask had been flushed with oxygen for 5 minutes before inflation of the cuff with either saline or air. (From Sosis MB, Dillon F: Saline-filled cuffs help prevent laser-induced polyvinylchloride endotracheal tube fires. Anesth Analg 72:187, 1991.)

Table 37-7　**Time (sec) to Cuff Perforation and Circuit Deflation (Carbon Dioxide Laser Set to 5 W)**

Cuff	*n*	Perforation	Deflation
Air	5	1.00 ± 0.83	$2.59 \pm 1.9^{a*}$
Saline	5	$4.21 \pm 3.91^{\dagger}$	$104.6 \pm 67.5^{*\dagger}$

Values are mean ± SD.
$*P < .05$; paired Student's *t*-test, air versus saline.
$^{\dagger}P < .01$; paired Student's *t*-test perforation versus deflation.
From Sosis MB, Dillon FX: Saline-filled cuffs help prevent laser-induced polyvinylchloride endotracheal tube fires. Anesth Analg 72:187, 1991.

air-filled cuffs (1.00 ± 0.83 seconds). However, because of the greater viscosity of water, leakage from the saline-filled cuffs was significantly slower than that from the air-filled cuffs; therefore, a longer interval elapsed before cuff leakage caused circuit decompression. When they were struck by the laser, deflation occurred after 2.59 ± 1.97 seconds in the air-filled ET cuffs and after 104.60 ± 67.5 seconds in the ET cuffs filled with saline ($P < .05$). The deflation of the saline-filled cuffs was significantly slower than their times to perforation. No combustion occurred during the trials at 5 W.

Table 37-8 shows the incidence of combustion with the carbon dioxide laser set to 40 W. During all five trials with air-filled cuffs, combustion occurred after less than 1 second of laser discharge. Both the cuff and adjacent ET shaft were noted to be on fire (Fig. 37-15). The saline-filled cuffs prevented laser-induced ET explosions in all but one of the trails, during which the tube ignited in 5.19 seconds. The Mann-Whitney U test was used to compare the incidence of flammability in the saline-filled and air-filled ETs. It revealed a statistically significant difference at $P < .05$.

The shafts of combustible ETs can be protected from the carbon dioxide and other types of lasers by techniques such as careful foil wrapping of their shafts with the correct metallic tape. The cuffs of ETs, however, are thin and remain vulnerable to the effects of the laser beam, which may be directed at them during laryngologic surgery because they cannot be protected with foil tape. The fact that the laser beam is often aligned along

Table 37-8　**Incidence of Endotracheal Tube Combustion with Air- and Saline-Filled Cuffs (Carbon Dioxide Laser Set to 40 W)**

Cuff	*n*	Combustion (%)
Air	5	100*
Saline	5	20*

$*P < .05$, Mann-Whitney U test.
From Sosis MB, Dillon FX: Saline-filled cuffs help prevent laser-induced polyvinylchloride endotracheal tube fires. Anesth Analg 72:187, 1991.

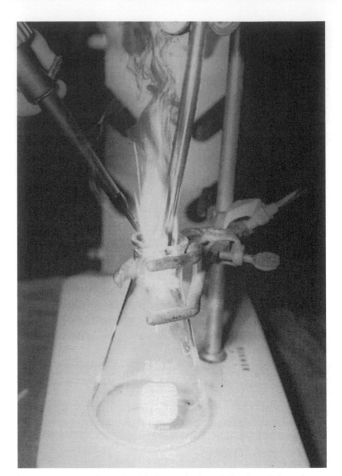

Figure 37-15 Carbon dioxide laser–induced fire involving the endotracheal tube cuff and adjacent shaft. (From Sosis MB, Dillon F: Saline-filled cuffs help prevent laser-induced polyvinylchloride endotracheal tube fires. Anesth Analg 72:187, 1991.)

the axis of an operating laryngoscope during laryngeal surgery predisposes to its impingement on the ET's cuff. Furthermore, the cuffs provide a large target because undersized ETs are often used during airway surgery to provide better exposure of the larynx for the surgeon; thus, a large cuff is necessary to ensure a seal for positive-pressure ventilation of the lungs.

It has been suggested by LeJeune and associates[69] that filling ET cuffs with saline would protect them from the carbon dioxide laser because impingement of the laser beam onto the cuff results in a jet of water that acts as a "built-in fire extinguisher" (Fig. 37-16). The saline should also act as a heat sink; however, this suggestion has not been previously tested experimentally. In this study, ET cuff perforation by the carbon dioxide laser set to 5 W (see Table 37-7) was not inhibited by saline filling. However, the saline-filled cuffs, although perforated by the laser beam as rapidly as air-filled cuffs, were significantly slower to deflate, allowing more time before reaching the point at which airway pressure could no longer be maintained. The use of saline-filled cuffs prevented ET ignition by the carbon dioxide laser set to 40 W (see Table 37-8) in a statistically significant

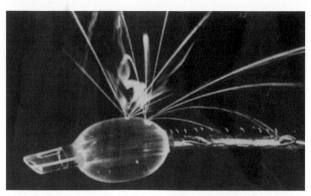

Figure 37-16 Polyvinyl chloride endotracheal tube cuff has been struck by a CO_2 laser after it was filled with saline. (From LeJeune FE Jr, Guice C, LeTard F, et al: Heat sink protection against lasering endotracheal cuffs. Ann Otol Rhinol Laryngol 91:606, 1982.)

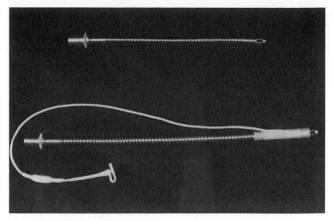

Figure 37-17 Two Norton endotracheal tubes are shown. The lower tube has been equipped with a separate rubber cuff. (From Sosis M: Anesthesia for laser surgery. Int Anesthesiol Clin 28:119, 1990.)

number of cases when compared with the control group of air-filled cuffs. Saline filling of ET cuffs is, therefore, recommended for laser airway surgery. It is also suggested that a small amount of dye, such as methylene blue, should be added to the saline so that laser-induced ET cuff perforation would become obvious to the surgeon, who can then immediately terminate operation of the laser. Further protection of the ET cuffs can be obtained by placing moistened pledgets above them and keeping the pledgets moist throughout the procedure.[137]

V. SPECIALLY MANUFACTURED ENDOTRACHEAL TUBES FOR LASER AIRWAY SURGERY

A. NORTON LASER ENDOTRACHEAL TUBE

The Norton laser ET (A. V. Mueller, Niles, IL) is constructed from spiral-wound stainless steel and is the only commercially constructed completely nonflammable ET (Fig. 37-17).[90] The Norton tube has no cuff; however, a separate latex cuff may be attached to it. Alternatively, the pharynx may be packed with wet gauze to seal the system and to allow positive-pressure ventilation of the lungs. The Norton ET has a matte or sandblasted finish, rather thick walls, and a somewhat rough exterior.[123] The matte finish acts to diffuse reflected laser beams.[90] A 4.8 mm ID Norton ET has a wall thickness of 1.4 mm (Table 37-9). The large wall thickness of this ET is considered a disadvantage because the tube would obscure the surgeon's view more than an ET with the same internal diameter but with thinner walls—an important consideration during laser airway surgery. This ET's large size and stiffness may make surgical exposure and laryngoscope positioning difficult. If an external cuff is added to this ET, the assembly is no longer completely nonflammable. Furthermore, the presence of

the pilot tube leading to the cuff for its inflation is inconvenient. The sponges or packs that may be used to make a seal if a cuff is not used are also potentially combustible if they are allowed to dry out. Therefore, they must be kept wet at all times. The Norton ET is not airtight (Fig. 37-18); a case of difficulty ventilating the lungs of a patient when this tube was used has been reported.

Even if ventilation of the patient's lungs is not compromised by leakage with the Norton ET, the presence of anesthetic gases in the oropharynx both increases the possibility of combustion in the surgical field and increases operating room pollution. The Norton ET is reusable and may be autoclaved but is expensive. It came in size 4.0, 4.8, and 6.4 mm IDs (see Table 37-9).

The Norton ET is no longer manufactured. However, it is still in use in many locations because it is reusable.

B. XOMED LASER-SHIELD I ENDOTRACHEAL TUBE

The Xomed Laser-Shield I ET (Xomed-Treace, Jacksonville, FL) is a silicon rubber tube that has been

Table 37-9 **Internal Diameter (ID), External Diameter (OD), and Wall Thickness for Norton Laser Endotracheal Tubes**

Endotracheal Tube Size (French)	ID (mm)	OD (mm)	Wall Thickness* (mm)
24	4.0	6.6	1.3
26	4.8	7.4	1.3
28	6.4	9.3	1.45

*Calculated.
Courtesy of A. V. Mueller, Niles, IL.

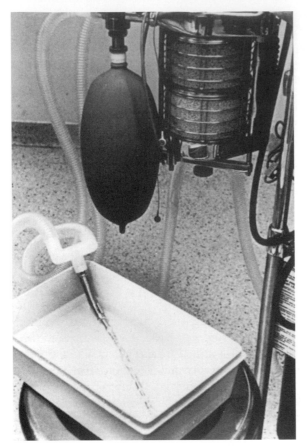

Figure 37-18 Norton endotracheal tube under 30 cm H$_2$O pressure immersed in water. (From Sosis MB: Anesth Rev 16:39, 1989.)

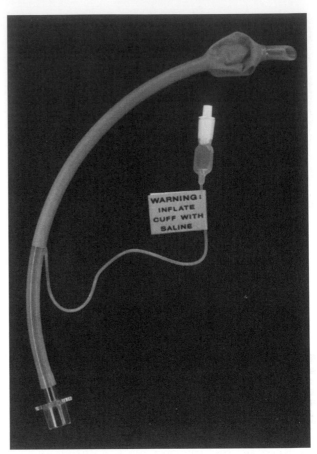

Figure 37-19 Xomed Laser-Shield I endotracheal tube. (From Sosis MB: Anesthesia for laser surgery. Int Anesthesiol Clin 28:119, 1990.)

coated with a silicon elastomer to which metallic particles have been added (Fig. 37-19). The manufacturer states that the Xomed ET should be used only with the carbon dioxide laser. No more than 25 W of carbon dioxide laser power in the pulsed mode with pulse durations of 0.1 to 0.5 sec/pulse and a beam diameter of more than 0.8 mm should be used with this ET. Furthermore, no more than 25% oxygen should be used with it. However, a higher concentration of oxygen may be required in some patients having laser surgery. At a laser power of 25 W, 25 pulses of 0.1 second duration or five impacts at 0.5 second duration perforated the ET according to the manufacturer. These recommendations apparently apply only to the shaft of the ET because the cuff has been shown to be easily punctured by the carbon dioxide laser.[61] Three sizes of this ET were manufactured (Table 37-10).

Sosis,[136] in evaluating the Xomed Laser-Shield I ET, noted that a blowtorch fire was started quickly when a high-powered carbon dioxide laser was directed perpendicularly at its shaft. He also noted that the burning Xomed Laser-Shield I ET was more difficult to extinguish than ET fires involving PVC or red rubber ETs (Figs. 37-20 and 37-21). As a result of its combustion, the Xomed Laser-Shield I ET fragmented into silica debris and gave

off a bright light after laser contact. Similar results were found in an Nd:YAG laser evaluation of this ET.[135] Sosis and associates do not recommend the Xomed Laser-Shield I ET for laser surgery because safer ETs are available even though this tube carries U.S. Food and Drug Administration approval.

Ossoff[93] noted that laser impingement onto the Xomed ET raised its temperature significantly. It was recommended therefore that the laser be used only in the pulsed (shuttered) mode when this ET is used so it can cool between firings. In an experiment with the

Table 37-10 **Internal Diameter (ID), External Diameter (OD), and Wall Thickness of Xomed Laser-Shield I Endotracheal Tubes**

ID (mm)	OD (mm)	Wall Thickness (mm)*
4.0	6.0	1.0
5.0	7.0	1.0
6.0	9.4	1.7

*Calculated.
Courtesy of Xomed-Surgical Products, Jacksonville, FL.

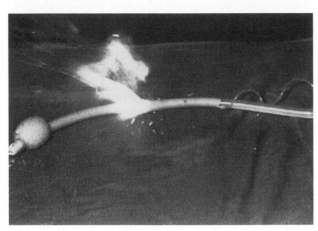

Figure 37-20 CO_2 laser–induced fire has been started on a Xomed Laser-Shield I endotracheal tube. (From Sosis MB: Which is the safest endotracheal tube for use with the CO_2 laser? A comparative study. J Clin Anesth 4:217, 1992.)

carbon dioxide laser comparing the combustibility of the Xomed, Rusch red rubber, and PVC ETs in 100% oxygen, the red rubber ET was found to be significantly more resistant to the laser than the PVC or Xomed Laser-Shield I ET.

The following case report of an ET fire in which the Xomed Laser-Shield I ET was ignited by a carbon dioxide laser serves to illustrate the unsafe nature of this ET.[129] The patient was a 56-year-old man of ASA physical status I weighing 79 kg who had hoarseness. A carbon dioxide laser excision of a vocal cord polyp was planned. Anesthesia was induced with 100 ∝g of fentanyl and 400 mg of thiopental administered intravenously. Endotracheal intubation was facilitated with succinylcholine, 100 mg, given intravenously. The patient underwent orotracheal intubation with a 6.0 mm ID Xomed Laser-Shield I ET. Its cuff was inflated with 5 mL of isotonic saline. No leakage of anesthetic gases was heard during positive-pressure

ventilation of the lungs. The carbon dioxide laser was set to a power of 20 W in the pulsed mode of operation, with a duration of 0.2 sec/pulse. Anesthesia was maintained with 4 L/min nitrous oxide and 2 L/min oxygen along with isoflurane at inspired concentrations up to 1.5% as delivered by a calibrated vaporizer. Intermittent intravenous boluses of atracurium provided paralysis.

Near the end of the resection, the surgeon noticed bleeding at the edge of one of the vocal cords. Actuation of the laser for hemostasis resulted in smoke emerging from the patient's mouth, with the surgeon noting flames coming from the ET. The anesthetist also noted flames in the disposable corrugated anesthesia circuit connected to the ET. The flames were doused with saline. Breath sounds were absent, and an obvious leak of anesthetic gases could be heard when the ventilator cycled. The patient's lungs were not being ventilated. The delivery of nitrous oxide and oxygen was terminated and the ventilator was turned off. After ventilation of the lungs by mask, the patient's trachea was reintubated with a PVC ET. FOB subsequently revealed extensive burns to the trachea and both bronchi. No fragments of the ET were seen in the respiratory tract. The Xomed ET was later noted to be intact, with a ruptured cuff and with evidence of combustion of the cuff and distal shaft. The patient had a long intensive care unit stay requiring positive-pressure ventilation of the lungs, antibiotics, and vigorous pulmonary toilet. He subsequently underwent a permanent tracheostomy and had several dilation procedures.

C. XOMED LASER-SHIELD II ENDOTRACHEAL TUBE

The Xomed Laser-Shield II ET (Medtronic Xomed Surgical Products) has a laser-resistant overwrap of aluminum foil tape and a Teflon cover. The proximal and distal ends of the silicon elastomer shaft and cuff are not protected and therefore are not laser resistant (Fig. 37-22). The metallic tape provides protection against laser impact. The Teflon tape gives the tube a smooth

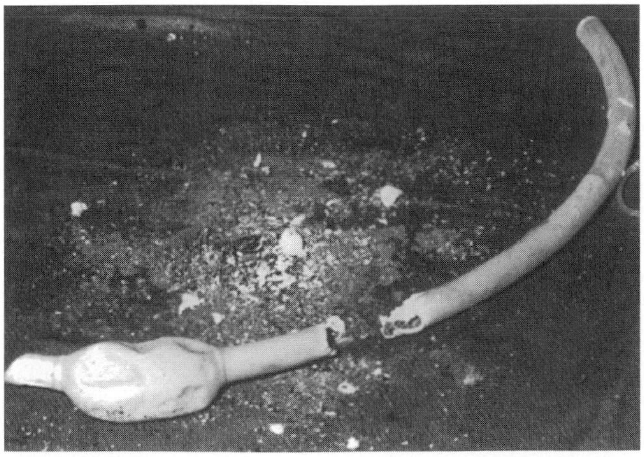

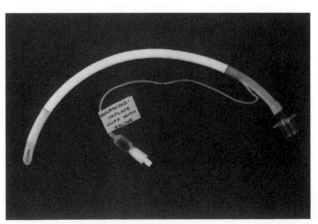

Figure 37-21 Results of CO_2 laser ignition of a Xomed Laser-Shield I endotracheal tube. (From Sosis MB: Adv Anesth 6:175, 1989.)

Figure 37-22 Xomed Laser-Shield II endotracheal tube. (From Sosis MB: Probl Anesth 7:157, 1993.)

surface to minimize mucosal injury from tube manipulation and tracts from a point of laser impact to expose the metallic wrap beneath. No adhesives are used because adhesives with metallic tape have been shown to increase the risk of ET fire.[60] Dry methylene blue dye has been placed in the cuff inflation valve to enable the detection of cuff rupture. The Xomed Laser-Shield comes packaged with neurosurgical cottonoid, which is used wet, to protect the distal shaft and cuff for an added margin of safety.

Dillon and associates evaluated the combustibility of the Xomed Laser-Shield II ET and compared it with 3M no. 425 aluminum foil–wrapped combustible PVC ETs with a carbon dioxide laser and an Nd:YAG laser.[39] Bare PVC ETs were also studied as controls.

A Cooper LaserSonics Z500 carbon dioxide laser equipped with a handheld probe was used for all carbon dioxide laser trials. A Cooper LaserSonics 8000 Nd:YAG laser with Zeiss optical microscope guidance was used for the Nd:YAG laser trials. Both lasers were set to a power of 50 W in the continuous mode of operation. All laser beams were directed perpendicularly at the shafts of ETs being tested. Oxygen (5 L/min) flowed through the ETs during laser exposure. The laser's output was continued until combustion occurred or 60 seconds had elapsed. Xomed Laser-Shield II ETs and foil-wrapped 7.5 mm ID Mallinckrodt (St. Louis, MO) PVC ETs were used for four series of 10 trials. Undamaged sections of the ET shafts were exposed to laser fire in each trial.

When the foil-covered shafts of either the Xomed Laser-Shield II or foil-wrapped PVC ETs were exposed to 50 W of carbon dioxide laser radiation for 60 seconds, no combustion occurred in 10 trials with each tube. When the foil-covered shafts of the Xomed Laser-Shield II ETs were exposed to 50 W of Nd:YAG laser radiation in 10 trials, the Teflon layer was noted to be missing at the site of laser impingement, exposing the aluminum foil beneath it. The foil was undamaged. In 1 trial out of 10, Nd:YAG laser exposure to the shafts of 3M no. 425 foil–covered PVC ETs resulted in combustion occurring after 53 seconds. In this case, evidence of combustion was seen at the site of overlap between two turns of the self-adhesive metallic foil tape.

Exposure of bare Mallinckrodt PVC ETs to the Nd:YAG and carbon dioxide lasers caused rapid combustion in 4.5 ± 3.6 seconds (mean ± SD) and in 0.8 ± 0.2 seconds, respectively ($P = .05$). Exposure of the bare silicon rubber shaft of the Laser Shield-II ET to carbon dioxide laser radiation resulted in combustion in 2.1 ± 0.7 seconds; Nd:YAG laser radiation–induced combustion occurred at 3.3 ± 4.5 seconds ($P = .05$). The silicon rubber burned with a bright flame and disintegrated. It was difficult to extinguish.

Dillon and colleagues[39] concluded that the foil-wrapped shaft of the Laser Shield-II ET provides adequate protection against high-power, continuous-mode Nd:YAG and carbon dioxide laser radiation, as did the shafts of 3M no. 425-wrapped PVC ETs. They stated that because

adhesives on foil tape have been shown to contribute to laser-induced ET combustion.[39]

Ossoff and colleagues also studied the Laser-Shield II for combustibility with carbon dioxide and KTP lasers. They evaluated the Laser-Shield II ET dry, with blood, with a blood/K-Y jelly mixture, and with K-Y jelly alone on the ET. Each tube was clamped and 100% oxygen at 3 L/min was delivered through it. All trials were performed with 3 minutes of continuous output. The maximum power output used was 40 W for the CO_2 laser and 15 W for the KTP laser. These settings far exceed the clinical settings used. With the KTP laser (13.5 to 15 W), no fires were observed, regardless of surface penetration. For the CO_2 laser, no fires were observed at 40 W for 3 minutes continuous mode with the dry ET. Blood, KY-jelly, or both decreased the resistance of the ET to CO_2 laser radiation. For the tube with blood alone, 25 W was the highest power that the tubes withstood without ignition. For the K-Y jelly/blood mixture the maximum power was reduced to 19 W. With K-Y jelly alone, no fire occurred at the maximum power setting of 40 W.[94]

The Xomed Laser-Shield II ET offers the potential advantage of an adhesive-free foil wrapping for ET protection. However, the choice of silicon for this ET's shaft is considered questionable because it disintegrates during combustion, whereas rubber and PVC tend to retain their integrity. Also, the use of Teflon to overwrap the foil raises questions because the pyrolysis of Teflon may liberate toxic fumes that can cause polymer fume fever.

Medtronic Xomed recommends only the Xomed Laser-Shield II for all surgical procedures involving the use of carbon dioxide or KTP lasers in either a normal pulsed or continuous mode of delivery that is noncontact. It is contraindicated for use with any Nd:YAG laser or argon laser or any laser other than CO_2 or KTP. It has been shown that when the laser beam hits the Laser-Shield II Teflon, the reflective aluminum wrapping may be exposed, and it is possible for the beam to be reflected into the patient's tissue.

The sizes of Xomed Laser-Shield II ETs available are given in Table 37-11.

D. BIVONA LASER ENDOTRACHEAL TUBE

The Bivona (Gary, IN) laser ET has a metallic core and a silicon covering (Fig. 37-23). It has a polyurethane foam cuff with a silicon envelope that must have the air or saline aspirated from it before its insertion into or removal from the larynx.[65] A large syringe is recommended for this purpose. When the ET has been inserted, the pilot tube need only be opened to air for the cuff to inflate passively. However, saline is recommended for filling ET cuffs for laser surgery.[69,140] The pilot tube runs along the exterior of the ET and is black so that it can be positioned away from the laser because damage to the pilot tube would make it impossible to deflate the cuff.

Table 37-11   Internal Diameter (ID), External Diameter (OD), and Wall Thickness for Xomed Laser-Shield II Endotracheal Tubes

ID (mm)	OD (mm)	Wall Thickness (mm)*
4.0	6.6	1.3
4.5	7.3	1.4
5.0	8.0	1.5
5.5	8.6	1.55
6.0	9.0	1.5
6.5	10.0	1.75
7.0	10.5	1.75
7.5	11.0	1.75
8.0	11.5	1.75

*Calculated.
Courtesy of Xomed-Surgical Products, Jacksonville, FL.

Table 37-12   External Diameter (OD), Internal Diameter (ID), and Wall Thickness for Bivona Laser Endotracheal Tubes

ID (mm)	OD (mm)	Wall Thickness (mm)*
3.0	5.5	1.25
4.0	6.5	1.25
5.0	7.5	1.25
6.0	8.5	1.25
7.0	9.5	1.25

*Calculated.
Courtesy of Bivona, Inc, Gary, IN.

Trauma to the vocal cords may result if the cuff cannot be deflated.[16] In addition, a high incidence of patients complaining of a sore throat postoperatively has been noted when this type of ET has been used for anesthesia.[73] The external location of the pilot tube and the necessity for active deflation of the cuff are additional disadvantages of this ET. The Bivona laser ET is nonreusable and is moderately expensive (Table 37-12). The manufacturer recommends that it be used only with the carbon dioxide laser. Sosis[136] noted that the Bivona ET ignited quickly when the carbon dioxide laser operating at high power was applied to it. A blowtorch fire occurred, and the ET disintegrated into several pieces (Fig. 37-24). Similar results and recommendations were noted by Sosis[135] with the Nd:YAG laser. Consequently, he did not recommend this ET for laser surgery.

E. MALLINCKRODT LASER-FLEX ENDOTRACHEAL TUBE

Mallinckrodt (Glens Falls, NY) Laser-Flex ETs have corrugated stainless steel shafts. They are designed as a single-use item and are expensive. The manufacturer states that this type of ET should be used only with the carbon dioxide and KTP lasers. The adult version of this ET incorporates two PVC cuffs. The manufacturer suggests that the distal cuff can be used if the laser damages the proximal one. The adult tube's distal end, including its Murphy eye and the proximal 15-mm connector, is also constructed from combustible PVC (Figs. 37-25 and 37-26). The Laser-Flex ET's cuffs are inflated by means of two separate 1-mm-diameter PVC pilot tubes that are located on the inside of the ET. An Nd:YAG or other laser fiber should never be inserted through this tube.

A case report by Heyman and colleagues[59] notes that prolonged laser impingement on the shaft of a Mallinckrodt Laser-Flex ET may prevent cuff deflation. A 64-year-old man with a history of laryngeal carcinoma was scheduled for microsuspension laryngoscopy and carbon dioxide laser debulking of his tumor. After intravenous

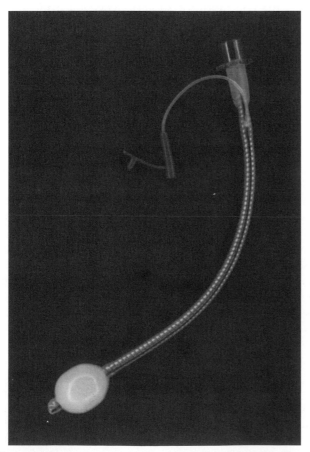

Figure 37-23 Bivona laser endotracheal tube. (From Sosis MB: Anesthesia for laser surgery. Int Anesthesiol Clin 28:119, 1990.)

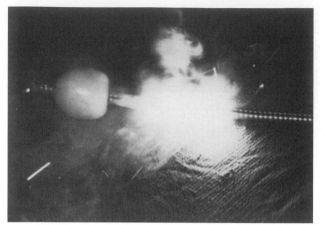

Figure 37-24 CO_2 laser–induced endotracheal tube (ET) fire involving the Bivona laser ET. (From Sosis MB: Which is the safest endotracheal tube for use with the CO_2 laser? A comparative study. J Clin Anesth 4:217, 1992.)

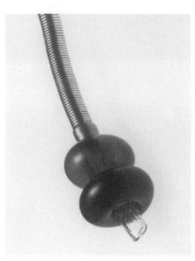

Figure 37-26 Detail of the two polyvinyl chloride cuffs on the Mallinckrodt Laser-Flex endotracheal tube. (From Sosis MB: Probl Anesth 7:157, 1993.)

anesthetic induction with propofol and succinylcholine, an unstyletted Laser-Flex ET (5.0 ID, 7.5 external diameter; lot ML02740) was advanced very slowly and gently through the narrowed glottic opening with mild resistance noted. The ET had been checked before use by injecting and then easily aspirating 5 cm^3 of air from each

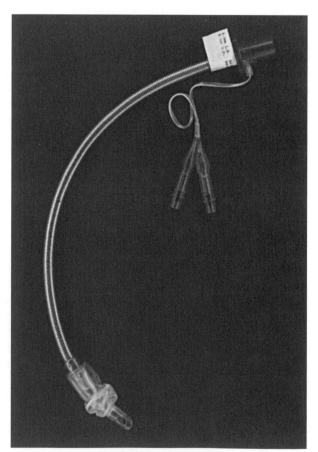

Figure 37-25 Mallinckrodt Laser-Flex endotracheal tube. (From Sosis MB: Probl Anesth 7:157, 1993.)

of the two cuffs, according to the manufacturer's instructions. The distal cuff was inflated with 15 mL of isotonic sterile saline, which was necessary to obliterate the air leak during manual ventilation of the lungs. The proximal cuff was then inflated with approximately 12 mL of isotonic sterile saline. At no time was a suction catheter passed through the ET.

At the conclusion of surgery, when the patient was ready for tracheal extubation, they readily aspirated the full volume of saline from the proximal cuff. However, they were unable to aspirate more than 1 mL from the distal cuff. They attempted to withdraw the ET slowly past the vocal cords without success. Inspection of the pilot balloon and valve revealed no obvious damage or disruptions. Repeated attempts were made using very slow aspirations with 3- and 10-mL syringes. The pilot balloon and inflating valve were cut off, assuming they might have been malfunctioning. They were still unable to force the saline out of the cuff by direct or indirect pressure.

The ear, nose, and throat surgeon inserted a Dedo laser microlaryngoscope, an anterior commissure scope, to a point just below the vocal cords. With cephalad traction on the ET and intensely bright fiberoptic lighting, the distal cuff was identified readily. The surgeon subsequently passed a Tucker mediastinoscope aspirating needle through the laryngoscope and punctured the cuff. After aspiration of a few milliliters of saline, the ET was removed easily, and the patient was allowed to awaken. His emergence from anesthesia was uneventful.

Heyman and colleagues[59] noted that in the case they reported the laser was used in the continuous mode of operation for 46 seconds at a power setting of 11 W with a spot size of 0.7 mm. They stressed the importance of aspirating the saline from the cuffs in a slow, gentle manner. Virag has reported that the stainless steel shaft of the Mallinckrodt Laser-Flex ET "becomes incandescent, perforates, and burns at power levels higher than 25 W when exposed to a single perpendicular 0.5-mm diameter carbon dioxide laser beam for more than 20 seconds in an environment of 98% O_2."[150] He stated that the PVC cuff inflation tube situated within the ET may be damaged by exposure to low levels of laser energy to the exterior of the tube's shaft. In the case reported, the 46-second period of laser contact with the tube's shaft makes the laser the likely cause for the failure of the cuff inflation tube. Virag stated that if difficult tracheal extubation owing to inability to deflate the cuff is encountered, it might be necessary to pierce the cuff with a spinal needle.

The adult sizes of Mallinckrodt Laser-Flex ETs available with the double-cuff system are 4.5, 5.0, 5.5, and 6.0 mm ID. Three pediatric sizes (3.0, 3.5, and 4.0 mm ID) of uncuffed Mallinckrodt Laser-Flex ETs are also available. They are all stainless steel except for a PVC 15-mm adapter. They are not equipped with Murphy eyes (Table 37-13).

Unlike the all-stainless-steel Norton ET, the Mallinckrodt Laser-Flex ET has an airtight shaft. However, the walls of both types of tubes are somewhat rough. In their product information for the uncuffed pediatric tubes, Mallinckrodt states, "due to the spiral design of the tube, the airflow resistance for a given size will be approximately equal to a PVC tube, which is 0.5 mm smaller." They add, "due to the bore size of the tube, patients should be monitored closely to guard against overinflation of the respiratory system and a build-up of expiratory gases."[87]

Sosis and coworkers[141] studied the resistance to CO_2 laser radiation of size 4.5 mm ID Mallinckrodt Laser-Flex ETs. The tubes were positioned horizontally on a stainless steel tabletop covered with a wet towel. An oxygen flow of 5 L/min passed through the tubes as a Sharplan (Tel Aviv, Israel) model 734 CO_2 laser was aimed at an ET's shaft. A laser power setting of 35 W with a beam

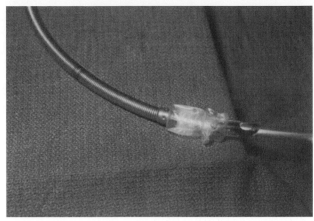

Figure 37-27 Nd:YAG laser–induced fire ignited in a Mallinckrodt Laser-Flex endotracheal tube. (From Sosis MB: Probl Anesth 7:157, 1993.)

diameter of 0.6 mm was used. This resulted in a power density of 13,400 W/cm. The laser, set to the continuous mode of operation, was activated for 90 seconds or until combustion occurred. Blowtorch combustion occurred in one of five Laser-Flex ETs studied. However, when human blood was applied to the shafts of four 4.5 mm ID Mallinckrodt Laser-Flex ETs, blowtorch combustion occurred in all cases.

In another study, Sosis and Dillon[130] noted that there is less danger of a reflected laser beam causing damage when the Mallinckrodt Laser-Flex ET is used compared with foil-wrapped ETs. In an evaluation of the Laser-Flex ET with the Nd:YAG laser, however, Sosis found that the shaft of the Laser-Flex ET could be ignited in all cases by the Nd:YAG laser when operated at high power (Fig. 37-27).[135] *Clinical Laser Monthly* reported the occurrence of an airway fire during a case in which a Mallinckrodt Laser-Flex ET was used during a laser excision of vocal cord polyps.[89] They stated that the patient had minor burns. They reported that at the time of the fire, the cuffs of the ET were not inflated with saline as recommended by the manufacturer.

Table 37-13 **Internal Diameter (ID), External Diameter (OD), and Wall Thickness for Mallinckrodt Laser-Flex Endotracheal Tubes**

Type	ID (mm)	OD (mm)	Wall Thickness* (mm)
Cuffed	4.5	7.0	1.25
	5.0	7.5	1.25
	5.5	7.9	1.20
	6.0	8.5	1.25
Uncuffed	3.0	5.2	1.10
	3.5	5.7	1.10
	4.0	6.1	1.05

*Calculated.
Courtesy of Mallinckrodt Medical, Inc., St. Louis, MO.

F. SHERIDAN LASER-TRACH ENDOTRACHEAL TUBE

The Sheridan (Argyle, NY) Laser-Trach ET c-Clamp tube is spiral wrapped with nonflammable, embossed copper foil from cuff to the proximal end of the tube. The copper foil is covered by an outer absorbent fabric that provides an atraumatic external surface. The company recommends saturating the outer layer with sterilized isotonic saline prior to use, and it must remain saturated during the procedure. The covering reduces heat buildup and must be vaporized before the copper foil is reached with the laser beam. The laser tube is recommended only for use with CO_2 and KTP lasers (Fig. 37-28).

Sosis and associates[132] compared 6.0-mm ID Sheridan Laser-Trach ETs with plain (bare) Rusch red rubber ETs

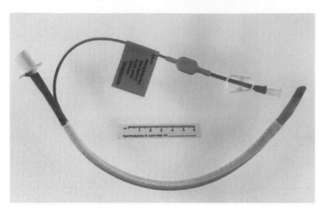

Figure 37-28 Sheridan Laser-Trach endotracheal tube.

of the same internal diameter. Five liters per minute of oxygen flowed through the tubes being studied. The tubes were subjected to either continuous radiation at 40 W from a Sharplan carbon dioxide laser or 40 W of continuous output from a Laserphotonics (Orlando, FL) Nd:YAG laser. The Nd:YAG laser radiation was propagated by a 600-μm fiber bundle. Each type of laser was directed perpendicularly at the ET to be studied. The laser's output was continued until a blowtorch fire occurred or 50 seconds elapsed. No ignition occurred after 60 seconds of carbon dioxide laser fire to the shafts of eight Sheridan Laser-Trach ETs tested. However, blowtorch ignition of all eight bare rubber ETs tested occurred after 0.87 ± 21 (mean $\pm$ SD) seconds of carbon dioxide laser fire. Nd:YAG laser contact with the Sheridan copper and fabric-covered rubber ETs resulted in perforation and blowtorch ignition in all tubes tested after 18.79 ± 7.83 seconds. This was significantly ($P < .05$) longer than the 5.45 ± 4.75 seconds required for blowtorch ignition of all eight plain red rubber ETs tested with the Nd:YAG laser.

It was concluded that under the conditions of the study, the Sheridan Laser-Trach ET was resistant to carbon dioxide laser radiation. It is not recommended for use with the Nd:YAG laser. Table 37-14 lists the sizes of the Sheridan Laser-Trach ETs available. These tubes are single-use items and are expensive.

Table 37-14 **Internal Diameter (ID), External Diameter (OD), and Wall Thickness of Sheridan Laser-Trach Endotracheal Tubes**

ID (mm)	OD (mm)	Wall Thickness*
4.0	8.2	2.10
5.0	9.5	2.25
6.0	10.6	2.30

*Calculated.
Courtesy of Sheridan Catheters, Argyle, NY.

G. LASERTUBUS ENDOTRACHEAL TUBE

Lasertubus (Rusch, Duluth, GA) is a laser-resistant ET with its shaft made of soft white rubber and a laser guard approximately 17 cm long, consisting of Merocel sponge and silver foil with a double cuff. According to the manufacturer, the Lasertubus offers resistance to all types of medical lasers such as argon, Nd:YAG, and carbon dioxide, with wavelengths ranging from 0.488 to 10.6 nm. Sosis and colleagues evaluated the Rusch Lasertubus in vitro.[133]

Jacobs and colleagues reported crimping of the Lasertubus resulting in hypoxemia in a patient. After placement of the Lasertubus, the surgeon extended the patient's head and neck and within 30 seconds, peak inspiratory pressures increased, oxygen saturation decreased, and no end-tidal CO_2 was evident. Immediate direct laryngoscopy confirmed that the ET was in correct placement. On inspection in situ no kinks or obvious obstruction was seen. Ultimately, the laser tube was removed and patient reintubated with a PVC ET. The patient's oxygen saturations returned to 100%. On inspection of the Lasertubus, the tube had crimped under the tape. Although this was a small defect not obvious to cursory inspection, it resulted in complete obstruction to airflow. They then experimented by bending unused laser tubes and found that a weakness within the wall of the tube remained, predisposing to crimping with minimal force and complete obstruction to airflow.[62]

VI. ANESTHETIC TECHNIQUES FOR LASER AIRWAY SURGERY

A. LARYNGEAL MASK AIRWAY AND AIRWAY LASER SURGERY

The LMA was first described in 1983.[19] It is used in routine anesthetic practice as well as for management of the difficult airway.[89] The LMA and reinforced laryngeal mask airway (RLMA) have been reported for both awake and anesthetized patients undergoing fiberoptic bronchoscopy for diagnostic and airway evaluation.[21,49] It has also been used for laser pharyngoplasty.[119] Carinal obstruction was managed using a combination of Nd:YAG laser therapy through an FOB inserted through an LMA and subsequent Nd:YAG through an FOB with a rigid bronchoscope.[124] Two other reports used LMA and high-frequency jet ventilation for resection in tracheal surgery.[41]

The LMA and RLMA are constructed from silicon rubber that contains silica filler, which provides high-temperature resistance and some flame retardation. The same material has been used to manufacture laser-resistant ETs.[19] Pennant and colleagues did a limited study of the incendiary characteristics of the LMA and RLMA, suggesting that they are resistant to CO_2 lasers at power densities below 1.25 to 2.35×10^3 W/cm^2, but 1.2×10^4 W/cm^2 produced immediate ignition.[103] Brimacombe looked at the incendiary characteristics of the LMA and RLMA with the CO_2 laser and compared them with two standard PVC ETs: Mallinckrodt reinforced armored tube and Mallinckrodt RAE tube. A Sharplan 1060 CO_2 laser with Zeiss operating microscope was used. Laser output was set at 6, 12, and 25 W with a spot diameter of 0.57 mm given a power density of 2.35, 4.7, and 9.8×10^8 W/cm^2, respectively. Each tube had either 6 L O_2 or mixture of 2 L O_2 and 4 L N_2O. The cuffs were filled with either air or O_2-N_2O. The tubes were surrounded by air. At the lowest power density (2.5×10^3 W/cm^2), pulses of 0.05 to 0.5 seconds did not penetrate the LMA or RLMA tube or cuff. Continuous firing led to light smoke production and penetration of the tube at 20 to 30 seconds. Both PVC tubes were penetrated at 0.5 to 2 seconds and ignition occurred at 2 to 6 seconds with 100% O_2 and 2 to 8 seconds with O_2-N_2O.[20]

At intermediate power density (4.7×10^3 W/cm^2), LMA and RLMA were penetrated at 0.5 to 2 seconds and ignited in 2 to 5 seconds with 100% O_2 and O_2-N_2O. At the highest power setting (9.8×10^3 W/cm^2), all four (LMA, RLMA, and two PVC ETs) ignited in 0.05 to 0.1 second with 100% O_2. The LMA and RLMA are more resistant to CO_2 laser fire than standard PVC tubing. The CO_2 laser at power densities below 2.35×10^3 W/cm^2 appears to be safe with the LMA and RLMA.

The RLMA was also assessed for resistance to the KTP laser beam. Gas flow through the RLMA was provided by a standard coaxial breathing system for a Boyle machine. With the RLMA freestanding in room air, not attached to the anesthetic system, no penetration was seen on the clear part of the shaft at power densities of 3.47 and 6.57 W/mm^2 at distances of 5 and 3 mm. At 10 W/mm^2, a small yellow green flare was noted after 7 seconds but no penetration of the shaft. On the black line of the RLMA an instant flare was seen and after 20 seconds produced a crater filled with silica ash. When 2 L O_2–4 L N_2O flowed through the tube at 3.47 W/mm^2, the shaft remained laser resistant. They showed that longer exposures to the laser strike had detrimental effects; a power density of 6.57 W/mm^2 for 20 seconds had no effect but a slightly higher power density of 6.94 W/mm^2 for 60 seconds caused shaft penetration. With a flow of 2 L O_2–4 L N_2O through the tube at a power density of 35.7 W/mm^2, a flame appeared at 10 seconds spreading along the laser fiber; after 60 seconds the crust of ash was removed from the shaft and the shaft underneath was penetrated and metal rings broken. At 71.4 W/mm^2 in 15 seconds an instant glow and flames spread over the surface of the shaft. At 71.4 W/mm^2 with a mixture of 2 L O_2 and 4 L air, smoke was observed on the shaft at 10 to 12 seconds. At 45 seconds the silica crust was removed and again the shaft was penetrated and metal rings broken. They also looked at the cuff and found the air-filled cuff ruptured at 6 seconds at power densities as low as 0.37 W/mm^2, but even with further continuous firing of the laser the ruptured cuff did not ignite. With saline

placed in the cuffs, even 60 seconds of continuous firing at a power density of 0.37 W/mm^2 had no effect. At higher power density, an explosive rupture of the air-filled cuff was seen within 3 seconds (1.22 W/mm^2). The saline-filled cuffs lasted between 5 and 11 seconds before penetration and only a small jet leak of saline occurred.

Pandit and colleagues showed that at laser outputs and distances of the KTP fiber tip from the RLMA normally encountered in clinical practice, the RLMA was not penetrated or ignited.[97] Keller and associates looked not only at the standard LMA (silicon based) and RLMA (silicon based with metal wire) but also at a disposable LMA (PVC based) and intubating LMA (silicon and steel based) and PVC-based ETs using KTP and Nd:YAG lasers at two power densities used commonly in airway surgery (570 and 1140 W/cm^2).[66] Each airway device was fixed to a table in room air and attached to closed circuit breathing system with 30% oxygen in air at 3 L/min. The laser was fired at the same distance of 3 mm. They also evaluated the marked and unmarked parts of the airway device and the unmarked device after application of 0.1 mL of unclotted fresh human blood. They evaluated the cuff with air or undiluted methylene blue dye.

There was no ignition of any airway devices. The impact sites of the silicon-based LMA for both lasers revealed a layer of silica ash just like that of Pandit and colleagues. The silicon-based device tubes were less easily penetrated the PVC-based tubes except for the intubating LMA, which flared sooner than with the KTP laser at both densities. The disposable LMA cuff was more resistant to penetration than the silicon LMA cuff or PVC ET. The cuffs filled with air were penetrated more rapidly than those with methylene blue.[64]

Pandit and Keller and their colleagues showed that the cuff is more vulnerable to a laser strike with the CO_2 and KTP lasers, especially when filled with air. Pandit filled the cuff with saline and Keller filled the cuff with nondilute methylene blue, both showing increased resistance to the laser strike. The disadvantage of using saline in the cuff is that the manufacturers recommend filling the cuff only with air. It has been reported that if not all the saline is withdrawn from the cuff after use in the standard reusable LMA, cuff rupture may occur during autoclaving.[7,17] Coorey and coauthors reported a technique in which they were able to empty the saline-inflated LMA reliably by a syringe without the plunger with the cuff held above the syringe to facilitate gravitational drainage. The cuff was then manually squeezed. The LMA with the syringe barrel attached was then placed in a warming cupboard at 60° C for 12 hours. They stated that filling the LMA cuff with saline is a viable option for laser surgery on the airway.[35]

The other option is the disposable LMA, for which filling the cuff with saline is not a concern because it is a one-time use. The only concern is that the disposable LMA shaft is more easily penetrated than the silicon-based LMA, but the disposable LMA cuff was more resistant to penetration than the silicon-based LMA or PVC ET cuffs. When filled with methylene blue dye with the Nd:YAG laser at 570 W/cm² , none of the cuffs were affected after 30 seconds.[66]

B. ANESTHETIC MANAGEMENT FOR TRACHEOBRONCHIAL TREE LASER SURGERY

Laser resection is the preferred method for removal of obstructive lesions from the trachea and bronchus. It is a safe and effective means of relieving central airway obstruction. With more than 4000 published interventions, the safety and efficacy of laser bronchoscopy have been well established.[41] Providing safe anesthesia for laser excision of lesions that are in the tracheobronchial tree is a daunting task. Maintaining unhampered views of the operative field, gaining free and safe access to the laser, and supplying adequate ventilation are essential in choosing a method of anesthetic management. These are not easy measures to provide with an obstructed airway. The challenge is to preserve adequate gas exchange while maintaining good visualization and surgical access to the lesion.

The primary advantage of using a laser for recurrent benign tumors is that multiple resections can be safely performed in outpatients. This is of immense benefit because it avoids the increased morbidity of open thoracotomy procedures. In cancer patients, endoscopic palliation helps in evaluation and staging of malignant tumors. These treatments reduce morbidity during chemotherapy without increasing surgical complications.[148] In cases of severe obstruction by unresectable tumors, a patent airway can be cored with a laser.[83,155] The combination of laser and rigid bronchoscopy is ideal for treating central airway obstruction.[144] Relief of acute ventilatory distress is one major benefit of bronchoscopic laser resections.[106] Therapeutic bronchoscopy should be considered even in individuals with cancer requiring intubation and mechanical ventilation. Often, mechanical ventilation is successfully discontinued and death by suffocation postponed.[33]

When anesthesiologists and surgeons simultaneously handle the airway, it is fundamental to have a predetermined plan for intraoperative and postoperative management. Good communication and cooperation are very important, and development of a team approach is necessary for successful results.[109] Devising such a plan is made easier if the current problems are conceptualized in two broad categories: mechanical and patient-related issues. Mechanical issues deal with attaining good surgical access while simultaneously providing adequate gas exchange and anesthesia. Distal lesions pose a greater challenge because they can cause complete airway obstruction and are difficult to reach with laser treatment. An ideal treatment modality for endoscopic ablation provides secure airway protection, excellent visualization of the lesion, and delivery of safe and effective method of treatment. Use of a contact Nd:YAG fiberoptic laser system through a rigid bronchoscope has performed well in meeting these criteria.[78] Patient-related topics such as age, size, pulmonary function, and the status of general health should be the basis for all final decisions. It is important first to decide on the type of laser therapy, type of scope, and technique of ventilation. An anesthesia management plan can then be formulated on the basis of patient-related factors, available equipment, and expertise.

1. Rigid Ventilating Bronchoscopy

Although the rigid bronchoscope is an old instrument, it continues to play a major role in newer therapies for access to the airway.[8] Rigid bronchoscopy is the standard technique for anesthesia management during laser resection of severely obstructing tracheal masses.[22] The main advantage of the rigid bronchoscope is complete control of the airway. The bronchoscope ultimately functions as a rigid ET. The area and clarity of the view of the surgical field with rigid scopes are superior to those with flexible scopes. However, the view is limited to the trachea, carina, and the main bronchi. Subglottic lesions are best visualized through a rigid bronchoscope. Rigid bronchoscopes, compared with flexible bronchoscopes, have large-diameter instrument side channels. A variety of baskets, forceps, and grabbers that are used for a wide range of therapeutic procedures can pass easily through these wide channels. In the event of significant bleeding or tenacious secretions, the telescope can be withdrawn and suction catheters passed directly down the bronchoscope while maintaining oxygenation and control of the airway. In addition, the rigid bronchoscope has a side port that can be attached to any conventional anesthesia delivery system. It substitutes for the ET during the procedure. A removable eyepiece allows surgical interventions when open and control of ventilation when in place. Usually there is a variable leak around the scope, which can easily be compensated for by increasing the fresh gas flow.

The rigid bronchoscope provides an excellent view of the larynx, similar to the view provided by the direct laryngoscope. Ventilation can be provided through the rigid bronchoscope. Eliminating the ET improves the access to the surgical field and reduces the risk of airway fire. Rigid bronchoscopy is simple to use, with low-cost equipment, and relatively safe when the proper precautions are observed.

Rigid bronchoscopy can be invaluable and lifesaving in cases of severe obstruction because the bronchoscope can be pushed past the obstruction.[14,124] It is unsurpassed in evaluation, control, and therapeutic manipulation of the tracheobronchial tree.[151] A retrospective review of 300 patients over a 12-year period concluded that the use of rigid bronchoscopy offers certain advantages in ventilation during general anesthesia. Rigid therapeutic bronchoscopic intervention is increasingly accepted to treat patients with central airway obstruction. Laser resection is applicable when the obstruction is caused by malignant exophytic tracheobronchial lesions, benign granulation tissue, or tracheobronchial stenosis with scar tissue formation.[33] In one study rigid bronchoscopy was preferred for proximal lesions and FOB used for distal lesions. Often both rigid and flexible bronchoscopes were used together to maximum advantage.[28]

There are some drawbacks in rigid bronchoscopy, including increased secretions and finite access to the distal airways and upper lobes. Conditions such as ankylosis of the jaw or rigid cervical spine that make direct visualization of the larynx difficult may preclude the use of a rigid bronchoscope. General anesthesia is often necessary for rigid bronchoscopy, whereas flexible bronchoscopy can be performed with sedation and topical anesthesia. Patients do not tolerate pressure on the soft tissues and significant neck extensions that are painful.[105]

2. Flexible Bronchoscopy

Flexible bronchoscopy is used to reach lesions in distal airways. Flexible fiberoptic scopes are more suited for procedures under sedation and local anesthesia.[34] Flexible bronchoscopes are built with bundles of optical fibers. The fibers deliver light to the tip and transmit pixels. An image is constituted when all the pixels are reassembled. However, the image formed is not as good as the view from direct laryngoscopy. It is possible to visualize the entire airway because the tip of the bronchoscope can be flexed through an arc of 220 degrees. In addition, there is usually a working channel, which can be used for suction and to pass instruments. In adults, 5.5- to 6.0-mm flexible bronchoscopes are used, and in children 3.6- and 2.2-mm scopes are popular. The disadvantage of the smaller scopes is that there is no instrument channel or, if present, it is too narrow. As technological improvements occur in the design of smaller instruments and improved forceps, the therapeutic and diagnostic role of flexible bronchoscopes will become more prevalent.[32]

3. Jet Ventilation Techniques

Jet ventilation has certain advantages in laser surgery of the tracheobronchial tree. Sanders first described ventilating attachments to rigid bronchoscopes in 1967.[113] Various improvements and modifications have been made on this original concept.[98] Jet ventilation can be accomplished in many different ways. There are different frequencies, driving pressures, and ventilatory techniques. A jet can be delivered to the larynx at the supraglottic region or infraglottically directly into the trachea. Hunsaker introduced a laser-safe subglottic monojet ventilation tube.[61,92] The frequency of ventilation and the location of the jet cannula should be selected according to the degree of airway obstruction and the location of the tumor. There are various specially designed catheters, laryngoscopes, bronchoscopes, and ventilators for the clinician to choose from. Many techniques have been described claiming different advantages over the other methods. There is no clear consensus about the ideal ventilation modes or the laser techniques. Selection, therefore, has to be done on basis of through understanding of the pathophysiology of airway obstruction and individual experience with use of these devices.

a. Low-Frequency Jet Ventilation

In low-frequency mode, a metal cannula positioned inside a laryngoscope or a rigid bronchoscope is connected to a source of oxygen. To prevent barotrauma, a reducing valve and a pressure regulator should be in line so that the oxygen pressure is limited to 50 psi for adults. In children, extreme caution should be used. One should start with much lower values and gradually increase the pressure while observing the chest movements. Holding down the handheld lever controls the duration and frequency of the jet of oxygen. The actual delivered tidal volume, concentration of oxygen, and inspiratory pressures depend on the amount of air entrapment by the jet, length of the cannula and its alignment to the trachea, size of the laryngoscope, and the lung compliance. These are hard to measure in a clinical situation with any great precision and at best are estimates. Adequate ventilation is accomplished in most patients who are anesthetized and given muscle relaxants.

The minimal possible pressure that can provide adequate ventilation should be used. The Venturi jet must be kept in perfect alignment with the trachea to achieve streaming of the flow into the lungs. Anesthesiologists should be watchful after any readjustment of the operating laryngoscope to which the jet is clamped, which may impair ventilation of the lungs. Oxygen saturation must be constantly monitored and chest movement continually observed. To minimize damage to normal tissue, the timing of each breath can be coordinated with the surgeon operating the laser. Intravenous agents such as propofol infusions are used maintain anesthesia. Short-acting muscle relaxants are used to prevent movements of the patient that are dangerous during a laser operation. An immobile surgical field may be difficult to achieve during Venturi jet ventilation of the lungs despite adequate paralysis of the patient with muscle relaxants because of the fluttering of the cords related to the Venturi jet. Even small movements are magnified under the operating microscope. Therefore, if possible, the Venturi jet should be triggered during pauses between the actuation of the surgical laser to keep the vocal cords from moving during surgery. A nasogastric tube is placed to prevent gastric distention. Adequate fluids are given intraoperatively, and gases are humidified in the postoperative period to prevent mucosal drying.

Jet ventilation is helpful in many situations in which a laser is not used. Intermittent jet ventilation has been applied through the instrument channel of the flexible FOB to expand atelectatic lungs and through the Hunsaker jet ventilation tube for one-lung ventilation for lobectomy.[111] However, extreme care should be taken to avoid pulmonary barotrauma.

Jet ventilation is not useful when the larynx is obstructed or when chest wall or lung compliance is poor. Pulmonary barotrauma is a real danger because of high oxygen pressure at the source. There are several reports of pneumopericardium, pneumothorax, and pneumomediastinum.[67,91,120] Tumors distal to the jetting opening can cause trapdoor or ball valve–like obstruction to expiration resulting in high lung volumes and barotrauma. High jet pressure also increases the risk of subcutaneous emphysema related to facial plane dissection in the neck, especially when there is disruption of the mucous membrane during surgery. If mucosal disruption is noticed, the jetting catheter should positioned away from the mucosal opening because pressure drops rapidly with distance from the jetting orifice. As there is no ET to protect the airway, vomitus, blood, smoke or debris, and seeding of papillomas down the tracheobronchial tree can occur. In addition, there is a possibility of polluting the operating room with infections agents or the anesthetic gases. Gastric distention, with possible regurgitation, may occur with a misaligned cannula.[29] Mucosal dehydration and inspissated secretions can result from dry jetting gases. End-tidal CO_2 cannot be easily measured. Volatile agents cannot be used, and scavenging of gases and production of combustion are problematic.

b. High-Frequency Jet Ventilation

In high-frequency jet ventilation (HFJV), small tidal volumes are delivered at a rate of 60 to 100 cycles per minute from a high-pressure source (5 to 50 psi) with inspiration taking 20% to 30% of each cycle. This is an effective ventilation method providing adequate gas exchange. This method has been used in rigid bronchoscopy. Hautmann and colleagues[56] described a technique of delivering HFJV through a noncompliant insufflation catheter. The catheter can be threaded through the sidearm of the bronchoscope and positioned either in the trachea or in the main stem bronchus. Medici and coworkers[79] used an insufflation catheter with a side hole in the contralateral main stem to deliver high-frequency positive-pressure ventilation during endobronchial surgery using an Nd:YAG laser. HFJV catheters can be placed transtracheally; however, in a prospective multicenter study the rate of subcutaneous emphysema was 8.4%.[18]

An advantage of HFJV is that it provides excellent views and access to the surgical site. Catheters are small and hence obstruct the surgical field less than larger conventional ETs. To-and-fro movements of the major airways that are invariably present during normal respiratory excursions are not present. Because a small tidal volume is used, there is less movement of larynx, trachea, and the lungs. This greatly facilitates the precise operation of the laser beam.

Although the reported incidence of pulmonary barotrauma in HFJV is low, it can lead to serious complications. Pulmonary barotrauma can result from high driving gas pressures and air trapping. Ventilators should initially be set at the lowest possible driving pressures and increased incrementally while carefully observing chest movements. There is a potential risk of barotrauma if the air pressures are not monitored. In addition to an injector catheter, Unzueta and associates[146] used a second identical catheter placed 7 cm distal to the injector site to measure airway pressure continually. Continuous monitoring of end-expired CO_2 and O_2 by conventional methods is difficult to interpret because of fast respiratory rates and high gas flows. However, there is a well-defined relationship between arterial CO_2 concentrations and end-tidal CO_2 concentration when expiratory gas is obtained by side-stream sampling during jet ventilation.[55] Observation of chest wall movements and blood gas analysis are reliable methods in assessing the adequacy of ventilation. Klein and coauthors[67] suggested the use of a double-lumen jet catheter for respiratory monitoring.

Air trapping and stacking of breaths are inherent problems in high-frequency ventilation because of short expiratory times.[142] In airways distal to the obstruction, injurious excess pressure can easily build up. Obstruction to gas outflow can easily occur not only because of the tumor but also because of the presence of surgical instruments, bleeding, and mucosal edema. In addition, light anesthesia or inadequate muscle relaxation can cause laryngospasm, closing the glottis and further obstructing the airflow. In order to prevent barotrauma, it is essential to ensure that there is adequate outflow by paying attention to the preceding details.

c. Combined Frequency Jet Ventilation

There is some evidence that there is improvement of oxygenation and CO_2 elimination by using low-frequency and high-frequency ventilation in combination. In this method the location of the gas inflow in the airway seems to influence the efficiency of jet ventilation. Supraglottic combined frequency ventilation seem to be superior to subglottic monofrequent jet ventilation in providing an unobstructed view and access to glottis.[10] With intratracheal jet ventilation, aspiration and air entrapment are virtually absent. There is no clear advantage of one ventilation technique over the other.[11] In a study of 37 adult patients, supraglottic combined frequency ventilation was more efficient than subglottic low-frequency or subglottic combined frequency ventilation.[9] However, in a bench model of laryngotracheal stenosis, supraglottic HFJV was associated with significantly larger end-expiratory pressures and peak inspiratory pressures.[85] There are two different risks that are built in because of the location of the jet cannula: aspiration at the supraglottic location and barotrauma at the subglottic location.

High-frequency ventilation should be reserved for patients with severe airway obstruction or severe pulmonary dysfunction. Most cases do well with a variety of simpler techniques that are well established. These include ventilation with a laser-resistant tube or microlaryngoscopy tube, supraglottic jet ventilation with a jet needle, and subglottic jet ventilation with a catheter.[101]

Table 37-15 Complications Associated with Jet Ventilation of the Lungs (49 Complications in 4151 Patients)

Ventilation Related	Ventilation Unrelated
Major	**Major**
Pneumothorax (9)	None
Hypoxemia during anesthesia (6)	
Mediastinal air (2)	
Tension pneumothorax (1)	
Minor	**Minor**
Carbon dioxide retention during anesthesia (3)	Prolonged mask support (10)
Subcutaneous emphysema (2)	Prolonged endotracheal intubation (5)
Gastric dilation (2)	Laryngospasm (5)
Airway bleeding (2)	Prolonged sleep or paralysis (2)
Recall of procedure (1)	

From Cozine K, Stone JG, Shulman S, et al: Ventilatory complications of carbon dioxide laser laryngeal surgery. J Clin Anesth 3:20, 1991.

There is no perfect mode of ventilation that suits all clinical conditions. Complications that have been associated with various ventilation techniques in laser resections have been reported (Table 37-15). Table 37-16 suggests a general schema that is used in the pediatric population.

d. The Intermittent Apneic Technique for Laser Laryngeal Surgery

Weisberger and Miner[153] described the use of an intermittent apneic technique for laser laryngeal surgery in the resection of juvenile papillomatosis of the larynx without the presence of an ET. The investigators stated that a clear, unobstructed view of the airway and complete immobility of the surgical field are essential for the surgeon during these cases. The presence of an ET is considered a hindrance (Fig. 37-29). They noted that the development of pulse oximetry allows the patient's state of oxygenation to be easily established, thus allowing the use of an apneic technique for anesthesia.

During a 2-year period, 51 procedures were performed by the investigators on nine patients who had juvenile laryngeal papillomatosis. Their average age was 10.5 years, with a range of 3.5 to 37 years. After the induction of general anesthesia, the patients were paralyzed with atracurium or vecuronium and the anesthesia maintained with halothane or enflurane in 100% oxygen. The patients' tracheas were intubated with small-caliber ETs wrapped with foil tape. In addition to standard monitoring equipment including an electrocardiogram, thermometer, and sphygmomanometer, oxygen saturation was continuously monitored by pulse oximetry. In cases of extensive papillomatosis, the resection was started with the ET in situ while the patients' lungs were ventilated with 40% oxygen. Otherwise, the ETs were removed and the surgery started. The surgery was interrupted when the oxygen saturation decreased. The patients' tracheas were then reintubated, and they were hyperventilated with 100% oxygen. This resulted in a rapid rise in the oxygen saturation so that repeated extubations and surgery could continue. The median number of apneic episodes required for each procedure was two, with a range of one to five. The duration of apneic episodes was 2.6 minutes, with a range of 1 to 4.5 minutes. A suspension laryngoscope and microscope, which provide excellent visualization of the larynx, were used in these cases so that endotracheal intubation could be readily accomplished without moving the laryngoscope. The apneic technique removes all the flammable material from the larynx during laser actuation and is thought to decrease greatly the possibility of an airway fire. Weisberger and Miner[153] stated that the apneic period should be shortened for small children because of their decreased functional residual capacity. This technique is contraindicated in patients in whom visualization of the larynx is difficult. At the end of the procedure, the patient's vocal cords were sprayed with 4% lidocaine (3 to 4 mg/kg) to prevent laryngospasm, and the patients received cool humidified air in the recovery room. They were given nebulized racemic epinephrine as needed.

Weisberger and Miner[153] reported that most of the patients undergoing the laryngologic procedures were outpatients. There were no major complications; however,

Table 37-16 Techniques for Pediatric Laser Bronchoscopy

Site	Scope	Laser	Ventilation Method
Supraglottic or immediate subglottic	Direct laryngoscope	CO_2	Venturi, safe ETs
Trachea, main stem bronchus	Rigid bronchoscope	Flexible KTP or argon laser	Manual ventilation via side arm $Fio_2 < 0.5$
Distal to main stem bronchus	Flexible bronchoscope through a standard ET	Flexible KTP or argon laser	Manual ventilation, via standard ET $Fio_2 < 0.5$

ET, endotracheal tube; Fio_2, fraction of inspired oxygen; KTP, potassium titanyl phosphate.

Figure 37-29 Additional pathologic condition noted in posterior larynx when the endotracheal tube is removed. (From Weisberger EC, Miner JD: Apneic anesthesia for improved endoscopic removal of laryngeal papillomata. Laryngoscope 98:693, 1988.)

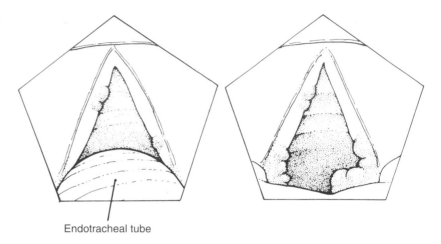

Endotracheal tube

reintubation of the trachea was difficult during two procedures because of inadequate paralysis. Nevertheless, the ETs were correctly placed within 20 seconds. One patient had a few short episodes of bigeminy at the onset of several of her procedures. These episodes were not associated with the apneic portion of the procedure and were resolved by substituting enflurane for halothane.

Weisberger and Miner[153] also reported that the apneic technique is especially useful in the surgical resection of lesions of the airway that are normally obscured by the presence of the ET. These include lesions of the vocal process of the arytenoid cartilage, the posterior commissure, the subglottis, and the upper trachea. Weisberger and Miner discussed a case in which it was thought that all the papillomas were removed after airway surgery with an ET in place. However, on inspection of the larynx after removing the ET, lesions were discovered in the posterior glottis and subglottis.

In comparing the intermittent apneic technique with the technique of jet ventilation of the lungs, Weisberger and Miner noted that with the former technique drying of the respiratory mucosa is avoided and the physical dissemination of virus-containing papilloma particles to the lower airway should be reduced. Furthermore, other complications of jet ventilation such as pneumomediastinum and pneumothorax do not occur. Also, there is no motion of the vocal cords with the apneic technique such as occurs with jet ventilation of the lungs.

e. Anesthesia by Insufflation for Laser Airway Surgery of Infants with Subglottic Stenosis

Rita and associates[110] have noted that the carbon dioxide laser has been used successfully to excise subglottic stenosis in infants, thus avoiding a tracheostomy. These cases present an anesthetic challenge because unobstructed exposure of the larynx and trachea is usually required to perform this procedure and the presence of an ET impedes the surgeon. Rita's group reported that their anesthetic approach for these cases also included a method for scavenging anesthetic gases for infants with subglottic stenosis undergoing carbon dioxide laser excision.

In a report of a case, a 7-week-old girl weighing 3.9 kg, whose trachea had been intubated transorally and who was receiving continuous positive airway pressure ventilatory support, was admitted to the intensive care unit. She had a history since birth of "noisy breathing," which had become progressively worse. Laryngoscopy at another hospital had provided the diagnosis of congenital subglottic stenosis. Within several hours of the endoscopic procedure, marked respiratory difficulty developed in the infant, necessitating intubation of the trachea. A 2.5-mm ID ET was inserted into the trachea transorally, and she was transferred to the institution of Rita and associates. During the initial physical examination, coarse rhonchi were auscultated in both lung fields. While the patient received continuous positive airway pressure with an inspired oxygen fraction of 40%, arterial blood gas analysis showed the pH_a was 7.37, the partial pressure of CO_2 in arterial blood ($PaCO_2$) was 45 mm Hg, and the PaO_2 was 88 mm Hg.

The patient was scheduled for an endoscopic evaluation. Atropine, 0.1 mg intramuscularly, was given 30 minutes before the induction of anesthesia with halothane and 50% nitrous oxide through the previously placed ET. When an adequate anesthetic depth had been achieved, the patient's trachea was extubated and the epiglottis, arytenoid cartilages, vocal cords, and trachea were sprayed with 1% lidocaine. An 8 Fr catheter attached to the anesthetic machine was introduced into the patient's nasopharynx through the right nostril. Direct observation confirmed its placement immediately above the laryngeal opening. Anesthetic gases were then insufflated with the infant breathing spontaneously. A suction catheter connected to the wall suction was taped to the proximal opening of the laryngoscope close to the patient's mouth to scavenge the anesthetic vapors.

Atmospheric nitrous oxide was measured at the head of the patient using a Foregger 410 nitrous oxide monitor. With the trachea intubated, atmospheric nitrous oxide was 5 to 7 ppm. When the ET was removed for the insufflation technique, the concentration rose to 75 ppm without scavenging. When suction was placed close to the infant's mouth for close scavenging, the concentration dropped to 7 to 10 ppm and remained steady throughout the procedure.

During the laryngoscopic examination, a small band of tissue between the arytenoid cartilages and anterior subglottic narrowing was seen. The surgeon was not able to pass a 3-mm Storz bronchoscope. The carbon dioxide laser was then used to excise the posterior commissure band and the excess subglottic soft tissues. Dexamethasone, 4 mg, was given intravenously and the infant was transferred to the postanesthesia care unit room awake, with the trachea extubated, but with some stridor. She was placed in a high-humidity environment, and after observation for 60 minutes she was discharged to the ward in satisfactory condition.

On the first postoperative day, progressive respiratory distress occurred with substernal and intercostal retractions. While the patient was breathing an inspired fraction of 40% oxygen, an analysis of arterial blood gas tensions noted that the pH_a was 7.44, the $PaCO_2$ was 50 mm Hg, and the PaO_2 was 80 mm Hg. Dexamethasone, 4 mg, was again given intravenously and racemic epinephrine (0.2 mL of 2.25% solution diluted in 2.5 mL of saline nebulized with 100% oxygen) was administered through a face mask. The infant's condition improved, and she was discharged from the hospital 2 days later. A normal airway was observed at bronchoscopy 3 months later, and she has remained asymptomatic.

Rita and associates[110] noted that three other infants with severe subglottic stenosis have undergone endoscopic treatment with the carbon dioxide laser using the spontaneous ventilation insufflation technique at their institution. One child had subglottic stenosis develop as a consequence of prolonged intubation of the trachea, whereas the other two had congenital subglottic stenosis. They noted that in the child with the acquired subglottic stenosis, the laser was used twice, whereas it was used three times in one case and seven times in the other case of congenital stenosis. They reported a favorable outcome for all cases without the need for a tracheostomy. Rita's group noted that the carbon dioxide laser has been used to treat both localized and circumferential stenosis. In the latter case, only one side is treated with the laser at each session.

Rita and associates[110] reported that they have been using the insufflation technique for microlaryngeal surgery, including carbon dioxide laser excision of laryngeal papillomas for 10 years. They pointed out that ETs of any size make surgery in these infants difficult or impossible because the operative field is obstructed. They stated that in some infants with subglottic stenosis, even a 2.5 mm ID ET is difficult to pass through the stenotic area.

Rita's group[110] have noted that the insufflation technique for administering anesthetics has several potential problems. In these cases, the anesthesiologist does not have complete control of the airway because no ET is used. The insufflation technique therefore requires very close cooperation between the anesthesiologist and the surgeon. The plane of anesthesia is very important in these cases. If the level of anesthesia is too deep, cardiac dysrhythmias or apnea may ensue. If the patient's anesthetic plane is too light, coughing or laryngospasm may occur. The patient must be carefully observed at all times to be sure that adequate unobstructed breathing is occurring. If the respirations are shallow, the concentration of the volatile anesthetic used (usually halothane) should be reduced. Rapid or deep respiratory efforts may signal the need for a higher level of inspired inhaled anesthetics. Rita's group reported that arterial blood gas samples that were randomly drawn from their patients showed carbon dioxide tensions in the range of 46 to 52 mm Hg.

When the insufflation technique is used to provide anesthesia, the position of the insufflation catheter must be carefully checked to ensure that it is close to the laryngeal opening. If the catheter is inadvertently inserted too far, it may enter the esophagus, causing marked gastric distention and possible regurgitation. In this case, a catheter should be placed in the stomach to decompress it, and the insufflation catheter should be repositioned near the glottic opening.

The conduct of anesthesia by insufflation is often associated with operating room pollution from volatile anesthetic agents because an open system is used. The pollution represents a distinct disadvantage of this technique. According to Rita and associates, this mode of anesthesia has resulted in higher blood levels of inhaled anesthetics among surgeons performing these endoscopic cases compared with surgeons doing cases with better pollution control. Rita's group placed a high-intensity suction catheter near the infant's mouth to scavenge the anesthetic gases during those cases. They reported that random determinations of nitrous oxide levels in the air of the operating room showed much lower levels when the suction scavenging technique was used.

Rita and associates[110] reported that movement of the vocal cords in their patients was minimal or absent even though spontaneous breathing was maintained, provided that an adequate level of anesthesia was provided.

Rita and associates[110] administered dexamethasone intravenously at the end of the laser resections of the subglottic stenosis to decrease edema of the airway because even a small degree of airway encroachment may result in stridor in infants. In the postanesthesia care unit, their patients were observed closely as they breathed humidified gases. In case of a significant respiratory obstruction, racemic epinephrine was administered by mask. After discharge from the postanesthesia care unit by the anesthesiologist, the patients continued to breathe humidified gases in their hospital rooms.

Rita and associates[110] concluded that although the insufflation technique is potentially hazardous, if it is done correctly, it provides an appropriate anesthetic technique for surgery on the larynges of infants.[45] They reported good results with this technique over the course of many years.

VII. MANAGEMENT OF AN AIRWAY FIRE

This chapter has thus far discussed the potential and prevention of an airway fire. Multiple factors must be considered when an airway fire occurs. All operating room personnel must be prepared for the possibility of an airway fire during laser endoscopic surgery. In the event an airway fire occurs, sterile isotonic saline or water should be immediately available in a 30- or 60-mL syringe. Another ET laser and PVC should be available. A plan of action should be rehearsed by operating room personnel so that rapid action can be taken if a fire occurs.

Schramm and colleagues discussed acute management of airway fire. The management protocol calls for immediate removal of the ET.[116] Sois wrote a laser airway fire protocol in which certain steps should be taken simultaneously by the anesthesiologists and surgeon (Box 37-1).[128] In the event of an airway fire, the protocol calls for immediate cessation of ventilation and turning off of all anesthetic gases, especially oxygen, by either disconnecting the hose from the common gas outlet, detaching the ET from the anesthetic circuit, or clamping the ET or turning off the flowmeters. At the same time, the flames should be extinguished with sterile saline or water solution. Presuming an easy airway, the protocol calls for the ET to be removed immediately because it no longer provides an airway and may be on fire. Once the ET has been removed and the fire completely extinguished, the patient's lungs should be ventilated with 100% oxygen by bag and mask.

Chee and Benumof[30] presented "a patient scheduled for an elective tracheostomy whose airway evaluation revealed an in situ 8.0 mm ID PVC ET, swollen lips, an edematous tongue protruding out of the mouth and an oropharynx filled with secretions." General anesthesia was induced with 300 mg of intravenous propofol and maintained with 0.4% inspired isoflurane (Forane) and 35% oxygen-air mixture. The vital signs remained stable. Electrocautery was used for coagulation by the surgeons.

The patient was administered 100% oxygen immediately before insertion of the tracheostomy tube. Suddenly the surgeons reported a blue flame shooting up vertically from the patient's neck. The breathing circuit was disconnected immediately from the ET; 20 mL of 0.9% saline was flushed in the ET. The fire was extinguished promptly. The ET was not removed because the ability to reintubate was uncertain. Despite a leak around the perforated cuff, the seal was sufficient to generate a peak inspiratory pressure of 20 cm H_2O. Meanwhile the surgeons were able to insert a tracheostomy tube into the trachea. Fiberoptic bronchoscopy was performed in the operating room and postoperatively revealed generalized upper airway edema consistent with prolonged intubation, no distal airway burn injury, and minimal burn injury to the proximal aspect of the tracheostomy site. The patient experienced no sequelae from the airway fire.

Each patient prior to laser surgery must be evaluated for risk of possible difficult intubation. If the patient is difficult to intubate or potentially a high risk for difficult intubation and an airway fire occurs, the patient will still be difficult to intubate. In these circumstances, the risk of removing the ET and not being able to reestablish an airway outweighs the risk of leaving the tube in after the airway fire is extinguished. Van Der Spek and coauthors[147] suggested that if the patient is not easy to intubate, a long stylet can be passed through the existing tube before removing it in order to facilitate the passage of a new one. Chee and Benomuf also suggested that the ET can serve as a conduit for a tube exchanger.[30] For reintubation, an airway exchange catheter is placed through the ET with the assistance of a laryngoscope, if possible, to facilitate the passage of a new ET over the airway exchange catheter. It has been suggested that to minimize the risk of failing to pass an ET over the airway exchange catheter, one should use a relatively small ET over a relatively large airway exchange catheter. The airway exchange catheter allows ventilation, which allows time for an alternative reintubation strategy such as a surgical airway or FOB.[15]

Once an airway is reestablished, the extent of the airway damage should be assessed. Foreign bodies (pieces of tube, metal foil, pledgets) should be removed. This may entail fiberoptic bronchoscopy through an ET or rigid bronchoscopy. Careful clinical judgment must be used to decide whether to extubate. Extensive burns should be managed with controlled ventilation of the lungs through an ET or tracheostomy. The use of antibiotic and steroids should be considered if burns are severe. All inhaled gasses should be humidified.

Box 37-1   Laser Airway Fire Protocol

- Cease ventilation and turn off all anesthetic gases, *including oxygen.**
- Extinguish flames with saline solution.*
- Remove endotracheal tube (ET) after deflating cuff.* Be certain entire ET has been removed.
- Ventilate the patient's lungs by mask after all burning material has been removed and extinguished.
- Examine airway for burns and foreign bodies such as fragments of the ET or packing materials.

*These steps should be taken simultaneously by the anesthesiologist and surgeon.

From Sosis MB: Probl Anesth 7: 1993.

ACKNOWLEDGMENT

We would like to acknowledge Michael Sois, MD, for parts of the chapter that are reused from the previous edition.

REFERENCES

1. Abramson AL, DiLorenzo TP, Steinberg BM: Is papillomavirus detectable in the plume of laser-treated laryngeal papilloma? Arch Otolaryngol Head Neck Surg 116:604, 1990.

2. Adelsmayr E, Keller C, Erd G, et al: The laryngeal mask and high-frequency jet ventilation for resection of high tracheal stenosis. Anesth Analg 86:907, 1998.

3. Alberti PW: The complications of CO_2 laser surgery in otolaryngology. Acta Otolaryngol 91:375, 1981.

4. Al Haddad S, Brenner J: The effect of helium on endotracheal tube flammability during KTP/532 laser use. Anesthesiology 73:A491, 1990.

5. Andrews AH Jr, Goldenberg RA, Moss HW, et al: Carbon dioxide laser for laryngeal surgery. Surg Annu 6:459, 1974.

6. APSF Newslett 47, 1999-2000.

7. Asai T, Koga K, Morris S: Damage to the laryngeal mask by residual fluid in the cuff. Anaesthesia 52:977, 1997.

8. Ayers ML, Beamis JF Jr: Rigid bronchoscopy in the twenty-first century. Clin Chest Med 22:355, 2001.

9. Bacher A, Lang T, Weber J, et al: Respiratory efficacy of subglottic low-frequency, subglottic combined-frequency, and supraglottic combined-frequency jet ventilation during microlaryngeal surgery. Anesth Analg 91:1506, 2000.

10. Bacher A, Pichler K, Aloy A: Supraglottic combined frequency jet ventilation versus subglottic monofrequent jet ventilation in patients undergoing microlaryngeal surgery. Anesth Analg 90:460, 2000.

11. Baer GA: No need for claims: Facts rule performance of jet ventilation. Anesth Analg 91:1040, 2000.

12. Baggish MS, Elbakry M: The effects of laser smoke on the lungs of rats. Am J Obstet Gynecol 156:1260, 1987.

13. Beamis JF Jr, Vergos K, Rebeiz EE, et al: Endoscopic laser therapy for obstructing tracheobronchial lesions. Ann Otol Rhinol Laryngol 100:413, 1991.

14. Benumof J: Anesthesia for Thoracic Surgery. Philadelphia, WB Saunders, 1987.

15. Benumof JL: Airway exchange catheters for safe extubation: The clinical and scientific details that make the concept work. Chest 111:1483, 1997.

16. Birkham HJ, Heifetz M: "Uninflatable" inflatable cuffs. Anesthesiology 26:578, 1965.

17. Biro P: Damage to laryngeal masks during sterilization. Anesth Analg 77:1079, 1993.

18. Bourgain JL, Desruennes E, Fischler M, et al: Transtracheal high frequency jet ventilation for endoscopic airway surgery: A multicentre study. Br J Anaesth 87:870, 2001.

19. Brain AI: The laryngeal mask—A new concept in airway management. Br J Anaesth 55:801, 1983.

20. Brimacombe J: The incendiary characteristics of the laryngeal and reinforced laryngeal mask airway to CO_2 laser strike—A comparison with two polyvinyl chloride tracheal tubes. Anaesth Intensive Care 22:694, 1994.

21. Brimacombe J, Tucker P, Simons S: The laryngeal mask airway for awake diagnostic bronchoscopy: A retrospective study of 200 consecutive patients. Eur J Anaesthiol 12(4):357-361, 1995.

22. Brownlee KG, Crabbe DC: Paediatric bronchoscopy. Arch Dis Child 77:272, 1997.

23. Brutinel WM, Cortese DA, McDougall JC: Bronchoscopic phototherapy with the neodymium-YAG laser. Chest 86:158, 1984.

24. Brutinel WM, McDougall JC, Cortese DA: Bronchoscopic therapy with neodymium-yttrium-aluminum-garnet laser during intravenous anesthesia. Effect on arterial blood gas levels, pH, hemoglobin saturation, and production of abnormal hemoglobin. Chest 84:518, 1983.

25. Burgess GE 3rd, LeJeune FE Jr: Endotracheal tube ignition during laser surgery of the larynx. Arch Otolaryngol 105:561, 1979.

26. Carruth JA, McKenzie AL, Wainwright AC: The carbon dioxide laser: Safety aspects. J Laryngol Otol 94:411, 1980.

27. Casey KR, Fairfax WR, Smith SJ, et al: Intratracheal fire ignited by the Nd-YAG laser during treatment of tracheal stenosis. Chest 84:295, 1983.

28. Chan AL, Tharratt RS, Siefkin AD, et al: Nd:YAG laser bronchoscopy. Rigid or fiberoptic mode? Chest 98:271, 1990.

29. Chang JL, Meeuwis H, Bleyaert A, et al: Severe abdominal distention following jet ventilation during general anesthesia. Anesthesiology 49:216, 1978.

30. Chee WK, Benumof JL: Airway fire during tracheostomy: Extubation may be contraindicated. Anesthesiology 89:1576, 1998.

31. Chilcoat RT, Byles PH, Kellman RM: The hazard of nitrous oxide during laser endoscopic surgery. Anesthesiology 59:258, 1983.

32. Cohen S, Pine H, Drake A: Use of rigid and flexible bronchoscopy among pediatric otolaryngologists. Arch Otolaryngol Head Neck Surg 127:505, 2001.

33. Colt HG, Harrell JH: Therapeutic rigid bronchoscopy allows level of care changes in patients with acute respiratory failure from central airways obstruction. Chest 112:202, 1997.

34. Conacher ID: Anaesthesia and tracheobronchial stenting for central airway obstruction in adults. Br J Anaesth 90:367, 2003.

35. Coorey A, Brimacombe J, Keller C: Saline as an alternative to air for filling the laryngeal mask airway cuff. Br J Anaesth 81:398, 1998.

36. Cork RC: Anesthesia for otolaryngologic surgery involving use of a laser. In Brown BR Jr (ed): Anesthesia and ENT Surgery. Philadelphia, FA Davis, 1987.

37. Cozine K, Stone JG, Shulman S, et al: Ventilatory complications of carbon dioxide laser laryngeal surgery. J Clinical Anesth 3:20, 1991.

38. Derkay CS: Task force on recurrent respiratory papillomas. A preliminary report. Arch Otolaryngol Head Neck Surg 121:1386, 1995.

39. Dillon F, Sosis M, Heller S: Evaluation of a new foil wrapped endotracheal tube for laser airway surgery. Anesthesiology 75:A392, 1991.

40. Divatia JV, Sareen R, Upadhye SM, et al: Anaesthetic management of tracheal surgery using the laryngeal mask airway. Anaesth Intensive Care 22:69, 1994.

41. Duhamel DR, Harrell JH 2nd: Laser bronchoscopy. Chest Surg Clin North Am 11:769, 2001.

42. Dumon JF, Shapshay S, Bourcereau J, et al: Principles for safety in application of neodymium-YAG laser in bronchology. Chest 86:163, 1984.

43. Eastwood PR, Szollosi I, Platt PR, et al: Collapsibility of the upper airway during anesthesia with isoflurane. Anesthesiology 97:786, 2002.

44. Edelist G: Anaesthesia for endoscopy and laser surgery. Can Anaesth Soc J 31:S1, 1984.

45. Eger E II, Weiskopf R, Eisendraft J: The pharmacology of inhaled anesthetics. 2002.

46. Einstein A: A Zar Quanten theorie der Strahlung. Physiol 18:121, 1917.

47. Ferenczy A, Bergeron C, Richart RM: Carbon dioxide laser energy disperses human papillomavirus deoxyribonucleic acid onto treatment fields. Am J Obstet Gynecol 163:1271, 1990.

48. Ferenczy A, Bergeron C, Richart RM: Human papillomavirus DNA in CO_2 laser–generated plume of smoke and its consequences to the surgeon. Obstet Gynecol 75:114, 1990.

49. Ferson DZ, Nesbitt JC, Nesbitt K, et al: The laryngeal mask airway: A new standard for airway evaluation in thoracic surgery. Ann Thorac Surg 63:768, 1997.

50. Freitag L, Eugene J: Chemical composition of laser tissue interaction smoke plume. J Laser Appl 20, 1989.

51. Fried MP: A survey of the complications of laser laryngoscopy. Arch Otolaryngol 110:31, 1984.

52. Fuller TA: The physics of surgical lasers. Lasers Surg Med 1:5, 1980.

53. Geffin B, Shapshay SM, Bellack GS, et al: Flammability of endotracheal tubes during Nd-YAG laser application in the airway. Anesthesiology 65:511, 1986.

54. George PJ, Garrett CP, Nixon C, et al: Laser treatment for tracheobronchial tumours: Local or general anaesthesia? Thorax 42:656, 1987.

55. Gottschalk A, Mirza N, Weinstein GS, et al: Capnography during jet ventilation for laryngoscopy. Anesth Analg 85:155, 1997.

56. Hautmann H, Gamarra F, Henke M, et al: High frequency jet ventilation in interventional fiberoptic bronchoscopy. Anesth Analg 90:1436, 2000.

57. Hayes DM, Gaba DM, Goode RL: Incendiary characteristics of a new laser-resistant endotracheal tube. Otolaryngol Head Neck Surg 95:37, 1986.

58. Healy GB, Strong MS, Shapshay S, et al: Complications of CO_2 laser surgery of the aerodigestive tract: Experience of 4416 cases. Otolaryngol Head Neck Surg 92:13, 1984.

59. Heyman DM, Greenfeld AL, Rogers JS, et al: Inability to deflate the distal cuff of the laser-flex tracheal tube preventing extubation after laser surgery of the larynx. Anesthesiology 80:236, 1994.

60. Hirshman CA, Smith J: Indirect ignition of the endotracheal tube during carbon dioxide laser surgery. Arch Otolaryngol 106:639, 1980.

61. Hunsaker DH: Anesthesia for microlaryngeal surgery: The case for subglottic jet ventilation. Laryngoscope 104:1, 1994.

62. Jacobs JS, Lewis MC, DeSouza GJ, et al: Crimping of a laser tube resulting in hypoxemia. Anesthesiology 91:898, 1999.

63. Janda P, Sroka R, Baumgartner R, et al: Laser treatment of hyperplastic inferior nasal turbinates: A review. Lasers Surg Med 28:404, 2001.

64. Kaeder CS, Hirshman CA: Acute airway obstruction: A complication of aluminum tape wrapping of tracheal tubes in laser surgery. Can Anaesth Soc J 26:138, 1979.

65. Kamen JM, Wilkinson CJ: A new low-pressure cuff for endotracheal tubes. Anesthesiology 34:482, 1971.

66. Keller C, Brimacombe J, Coorey A, et al: Liability of laryngeal mask airway devices to thermal damage from KTP and Nd:YAG lasers. Br J Anaesth 82:291, 1999.

67. Klein U, Karzai W, Gottschall R, et al: Respiratory gas monitoring during high-frequency jet ventilation for tracheal resection using a double-lumen jet catheter. Anesth Analg 88:224, 1999.

68. Leibowitz PG: Corneal injury produced by carbon dioxide laser radiation. Arch Ophthalmol 81:713, 1969.

69. LeJeune FE Jr, Guice C, LeTard F, et al: Heat sink protection against lasering endotracheal cuffs. Ann Otol Rhinol Laryngol 91:606, 1982.

70. Leonard PF: The lower limits of flammability of halothane, enflurane, and isoflurane. Anesth Analg 54:238, 1975.

71. Levine DL: More laser accidents: One state health department reacts. J Clin Laser Med Surg 8:8, 1990.

72. Litman RS, Hayes JL, Basco MG, et al: Use of dynamic negative airway pressure (DNAP) to assess sedative-induced upper airway obstruction. Anesthesiology 96:342, 2002.

73. Loeser EA, Machin R, Colley J, et al: Postoperative sore throat—Importance of endotracheal tube conformity versus cuff design. Anesthesiology 49:430, 1978.

74. MacDonald AG: A short history of fires and explosions caused by anaesthetic agents. Br J Anaesth 72:710, 1994.

75. Macintosh R, Mushin WW, Epstein HG: Physics for the Anaesthetist. Oxford, Blackwell, 1963.

76. Maiman T: Stimulated optical radiation in ruby. Nature 187:493, 1960.

77. McDougall JC, Cortese DA: Neodymium-YAG laser therapy of malignant airway obstruction. A preliminary report. Mayo Clin Proc 58:35, 1983.

78. McQueen CT, Cullen RD: Endoscopic ablation of distal tracheal lesions using Nd:YAG contact laser. Int J Pediatr Otorhinolaryngol 67:181, 2003.

79. Medici G, Mallios C, Custers WT, et al: Anesthesia for endobronchial laser surgery: A modified technique. Anesth Analg 88:298, 1999.

80. Meier S, Geiduschek J, Paganoni R, et al: The effect of chin lift, jaw thrust, and continuous positive airway pressure on the size of the glottic opening and on stridor score in anesthetized, spontaneously breathing children. Anesth Analg 94:494, 2002.

81. Meretoja OA, Taivainen T, Raiha L, et al: Sevoflurane–nitrous oxide or halothane–nitrous oxide for paediatric bronchoscopy and gastroscopy. Br J Anaesth 76:767, 1996.

82. Milliken RA, Bizzarri DV: Flammable surgical drapes—A patient and personnel hazard. Anesth Analg 64:54, 1985.

83. Morris CD, Budde JM, Godette KD, et al: Palliative management of malignant airway obstruction. Ann Thorac Surg 74:1928, 2002.

84. Nezhat C, Winer WK, Nezhat F, et al: Smoke from laser surgery: Is there a health hazard? Lasers Surg Med 7:376, 1987.

85. Ng A, Russell WC, Harvey N, et al: Comparing methods of administering high-frequency jet ventilation in a model of laryngotracheal stenosis. Anesth Analg 95:764, 2002.

86. Lasers in medicine and surgery. Council on Scientific Affairs. JAMA 256:900, 1986.

87. No author: Mallinckrodt Anesthesia Products. St Louis, 1990.

88. No author: Practice guidelines for management of the difficult airway. A report by the American Society of Anesthesiologists Task Force on Management of the Difficult Airway. Anesthesiology 78:597, 1993.

89. No author: Safety design can't eliminate endotracheal tube fires. Clin Laser Mon 8:148, 1990.

90. Norton ML, de Vos P: New endotracheal tube for laser surgery of the larynx. Ann Otol Rhinol Laryngol 87:554, 1978.

91. Oliverio R Jr, Ruder CB, Fermon C, et al: Pneumothorax secondary to ball-valve obstruction during jet ventilation. Anesthesiology 51:255, 1979.

92. Orloff LA, Parhizkar N, Ortiz E: The Hunsaker Mon-Jet ventilation tube for microlaryngeal surgery: Optimal laryngeal exposure. Ear Nose Throat J 81:390, 2002.

93. Ossoff RH: Laser safety in otolaryngology–head and neck surgery: Anesthetic and educational considerations for laryngeal surgery. Laryngoscope 99:1, 1989.

94. Ossoff RH, Aly A, Gonzales D, et al: A new endotracheal tube for carbon dioxide and KTP laser surgery of the aerodigestive tract. Otolaryngol Head Neck Surg 108:96, 1993.

95. Ossoff RH, Hotaling AJ, Karlan MS, et al: CO_2 laser in otolaryngology–head and neck surgery: A retrospective analysis of complications. Laryngoscope 93:1287, 1983.

96. Ott AE: Disposable surgical drapes—A potential fire hazard. Obstet Gynecol 61:667, 1983.

97. Pandit JJ, Chambers P, O'Malley S: KTP laser-resistant properties of the reinforced laryngeal mask airway. Br J Anaesth 78:594, 1997.

98. Parsons DS: Tracheoscope: An old instrument with new applications. Ann Otol Rhinol Laryngol 102:834, 1993.

99. Parsons RB, Milestone BN, Adler LP: Radiographic assessment of airway tumors. Chest Surg Clin North Am 13:63, 2003.

100. Pashayan AG, Gravenstein JS: Helium retards endotracheal tube fires from carbon dioxide lasers. Anesthesiology 62:274, 1985.

101. Patel A, Randhawa N, Semenov RA: Transtracheal high frequency jet ventilation and iatrogenic injury. Br J Anaesth 89:184, 2002.

102. Patel KF, Hicks JN: Prevention of fire hazards associated with use of carbon dioxide lasers. Anesth Analg 60:885, 1981.

103. Pennant JH, Gajraj NM, Miller JF: Resistance of the laryngeal mask airway to CO_2 laser. Anesthesiology 79:A1055, 1993.

104. Pinsonneault C, Fortier J, Donati F: Tracheal resection and reconstruction. Can J Anaesth 46:439, 1999.

105. Plummer S, Hartley M, Vaughan RS: Anaesthesia for telescopic procedures in the thorax. Br J Anaesth 80:223, 1998.

106. Prakash UB: Advances in bronchoscopic procedures. Chest 116:1403, 1999.

107. Quintal MC, Cunningham MJ, Ferrari LR: Tubeless spontaneous respiration technique for pediatric microlaryngeal surgery. Arch Otolaryngol Head Neck Surg 123:209, 1997.

108. Rampil I: Anesthetic considerations for laser surgery. Anesth Analg 74:424, 1992.

109. Rimell FL: Pediatric laser bronchoscopy. Int Anesthesiol Clin 35:107, 1997.

110. Rita L, Seleny F, Holinger LD: Anesthetic management and gas scavenging for laser surgery of infant subglottic stenosis. Anesthesiology 58:191, 1983.

111. Robinson RJ: One-lung ventilation for thoracotomy using a Hunsaker jet ventilation tube. Anesthesiology 87:1572, 1997.

112. Rontal M, Rontal E, Wenokur ME, et al: Anesthetic management for tracheobronchial laser surgery. Ann Otol Rhinol Laryngol 95:556, 1986.

113. Sanders RD: Two ventilating attachments for bronchoscopes. Del Med J 39:170, 1967.

114. Satoh M, Hirabayashi Y, Seo N: Spontaneous breathing combined with high frequency ventilation during bronchoscopic resection of a large tracheal tumour. Br J Anaesth 89:641, 2002.

115. Sawchuk WS, Weber PJ, Lowy DR, et al: Infectious papillomavirus in the vapor of warts treated with carbon dioxide laser or electrocoagulation: Detection and protection. J Am Acad Dermatol 21:41, 1989.

116. Schramm VL Jr, Mattox DE, Stool SE: Acute management of laser-ignited intratracheal explosion. Laryngoscope 91:1417, 1981.

117. Seijo LM, Sterman DH: Interventional pulmonology. N Engl J Med 344:740, 2001.

118. Shapshay SM, Beamis JF Jr: Safety precautions for bronchoscopic Nd-YAG laser surgery. Otolaryngol Head Neck Surg 94:175, 1986.

119. Sher M, Brimacombe J, Laing D: Anaesthesia for laser pharyngoplasty—A comparison of the tracheal tube with the reinforced laryngeal mask airway. Anaesth Intensive Care 23:149, 1995.

120. Shikowitz MJ, Abramson AL, Liberatore L: Endolaryngeal jet ventilation: A 10-year review. Laryngoscope 101:455, 1991.

121. Shykhon M, Kuo M, Pearman K: Recurrent respiratory papillomatosis. Clin Otolaryngol Allied Sci 27:237, 2002.

122. Simpson JI, Schiff GA, Wolf GL: The effect of helium on endotracheal tube flammability. Anesthesiology 73:538, 1990.

123. Skaredoff MN, Poppers PJ: Beware of sharp edges in metal endotracheal tubes. Anesthesiology 58:595, 1983.

124. Slinger P, Robinson R, Shennib H, et al: Case 6-1992. Alternative technique for laser resection of a carinal obstruction. J Cardiothorac Vasc Anesth 6:749, 1992.

125. Slonim AD, Ognibene FP: Amnestic agents in pediatric bronchoscopy. Chest 116:1802, 1999.

126. Smith JP, Moss CE, Bryant CJ, et al: Evaluation of a smoke evacuator used for laser surgery. Lasers Surg Med 9:276, 1989.

127. Smith JP, Topmiller JL, Shulman S: Factors affecting emission collection by surgical smoke evacuators. Lasers Surg Med 10:224, 1990.

128. Sosis MB: Problems in Anesthesia 7, 1993.

129. Sosis M: Airway fire during carbon dioxide laser surgery using a Xomed laser endotracheal tube. Anesthesiology 72:747, 1990.

130. Sosis M, Dillon F: Reflection of CO_2 laser radiation from laser-resistant endotracheal tubes. Anesth Analg 73:338, 1991.

131. Sosis M, Dillon F: What is the safest foil tape for endotracheal tube protection during Nd-YAG laser surgery? A comparative study. Anesthesiology 72:553, 1990.

132. Sosis M, Braverman B, Ivanovich AD: Evaluation of a new laser-resistant fabric and copper foil wrapped endotracheal tube. Anesthesiology 79:A536, 1993.

133. Sosis M, Kelanic S, Caldarelli DD: An in vitro evaluation of a new laser resistant endotracheal tube: The Rusch Lasertubus. Anesthesiology 87:A483, 1997.

134. Sosis MB: Evaluation of five metallic tapes for protection of endotracheal tubes during CO_2 laser surgery. Anesth Analg 68:392, 1989.

135. Sosis MB: What is the safest endotracheal tube for Nd-YAG laser surgery? A comparative study. Anesth Analg 69:802, 1989.

136. Sosis MB: Which is the safest endotracheal tube for use with the CO_2 laser? A comparative study. J Clin Anesth 4:217, 1992.

137. Sosis MB: Saline soaked pledgets prevent carbon dioxide laser–induced endotracheal tube cuff ignition. J Clin Anesth 7:395, 1995.

138. Sosis MB, Braverman B: Evaluation of foil coverings for protecting plastic endotracheal tubes from the potassium-titanyl-phosphate laser. Anesth Analg 77:589, 1993.

139. Sosis MB, Dillon F: Prevention of CO_2 laser–induced endotracheal tube fires with the laser-guard protective coating. J Clin Anesth 4:25, 1992.

140. Sosis MB, Dillon FX: Saline-filled cuffs help prevent laser-induced polyvinylchloride endotracheal tube fires. Anesth Analg 72:187, 1991.

141. Sosis MB, Pritikin JB, Caldarelli DD: The effect of blood on laser-resistant endotracheal tube combustion. Laryngoscope 104:829, 1994.

142. Spackman DR, Kellow N, White SA, et al: High frequency jet ventilation and gas trapping. Br J Anaesth 83:708, 1999.

143. Stacey S, Hurley E, Bush A: Sedation for pediatric bronchoscopy. Chest 119:316, 2001.

144. Stanopoulos IT, Beamis JF Jr, Martinez FJ, et al: Laser bronchoscopy in respiratory failure from malignant airway obstruction. Crit Care Med 21:386, 1993.

145. Strong MS, Jako GJ: Laser surgery in the larynx. Early clinical experience with continuous CO_2 laser. Ann Otol Rhinol Laryngol 81:791, 1972.

146. Unzueta MC, Casas I, Merten A, et al: Endobronchial high-frequency jet ventilation for endobronchial laser surgery: An alternative approach. Anesth Analg 96:298, 2003.

147. Van Der Spek AF, Spargo PM, Norton ML: The physics of lasers and implications for their use during airway surgery. Br J Anaesth 60:709, 1988.

148. Venuta F, Rendina EA, De Giacomo T, et al: Nd:YAG laser resection of lung cancer invading the airway as a bridge to surgery and palliative treatment. Ann Thorac Surg 74:995, 2002.

149. Vilaseca-González I, Bernal-Sprekelsen M, Blanch-Alejandro JL, et al: Complications in transoral CO_2 laser surgery for carcinoma of the larynx and hypopharynx. Head Neck 25:382, 2003.

150. Virag R: In reply. Anesthesiology 80:237, 1994.

151. Wain JC: Rigid bronchoscopy: The value of a venerable procedure. Chest Surg Clin North Am 11:691, 2001.

152. Wallin RF, Regan BM, Napoli MD, et al: Sevoflurane: A new inhalational anesthetic agent. Anesth Analg 54:758, 1975.

153. Weisberger EC, Miner JD: Apneic anesthesia for improved endoscopic removal of laryngeal papillomata. Laryngoscope 98:693, 1988.

154. Wolf GL, Simpson JI: Flammability of endotracheal tubes in oxygen and nitrous oxide enriched atmosphere. Anesthesiology 67:236, 1987.

155. Wood DE: Management of malignant tracheobronchial obstruction. Surg Clin North Am 82:621, 2002.

38

THE TRAUMATIZED AIRWAY

Ron M. Walls
Robert J. Vissers

I. DEFINING THE PROBLEM

A. THE CLINICAL CHALLENGE

Airway management in the trauma patient can be particularly challenging because of the coexistence of a difficult airway with the need for rapid action. The traumatized airway is often anatomically disrupted, presenting particular barriers to oral direct laryngoscopy, and the presence of blood in the upper airway confounds attempts at fiberoptic intubation. Manual in-line stabilization of the cervical spine is required in most cases of blunt trauma and many cases of penetrating trauma, compounding the airway difficulties. The patients are often intubated outside the operating room, usually in the emergency department resuscitation area, but can also present to the operating room requiring intubation for emergency surgery. In the emergency department, trauma patients are intubated primarily by emergency physicians, but patients with direct trauma to the airway are often handled by a team approach, with emergency physicians, anesthesiologists, and surgeons working in concert to achieve the desired result. In the operating room, or in other areas of the hospital, trauma airway management is usually the responsibility of the anesthesiologist, although surgeons may be called upon to assist when the airway is disrupted.

The need for prompt intervention to secure the airway requires rapid evaluation of potential difficult airway attributes, development of an airway management plan, including fallback techniques in the event of failure, and a willingness to act quickly, even if information is incomplete. In most cases, the need is apparent to intervene and secure the airway rapidly, but in certain situations there may be a misleading and incorrect perception that the airway is "stable," causing unnecessary delay and exposing the patient to additional risk. In many traumatized airway cases, although the patient is breathing spontaneously and maintaining an airway, delayed intervention can be hazardous because of the significant deterioration that can occur with little external warning. Swelling, hematoma, or subcutaneous air may cause dramatic and potentially lethal airway distortion, even though external examination findings remain fairly stable until the patient suddenly develops a crisis. Thus, the imperative with the traumatized airway is for early assessment and decisive action. Delay or observation, although often seeming the prudent course at first, can lead to catastrophic airway compromise and make airway intervention much more difficult (or impossible) than if it had been undertaken earlier.

The traumatized patient requires airway intervention primarily in two settings: prehospital and in-hospital, with the latter including both acute presentations (usually to the emergency department) and delayed need for intervention. This can be classified as follows.

1. Emergency Department/Trauma Resuscitation Room

Patients who have been subjected to acute trauma, either blunt or penetrating, present on a spectrum from minor, localized insults to catastrophic multisystem trauma. In the trauma room, indications for intubation may be related to direct trauma to the head, face, neck, or airway; compromise of pulmonary gas exchange by thoracic injury; or overall management and resuscitation of the critically injured patient in hypovolemic shock. In most cases, the usual paradigms of airway management that are used in elective anesthesia are not applicable. Care of the acute, high-grade trauma victim is generally best done using a team approach with a clearly identified and designated "captain" who controls the decision making, sequencing, and flow of the entire resuscitation. Airway management decisions are not driven simply by the need for operative intervention. Rather, airway intervention decisions are based on a complex series of considerations related to the patient's specific injuries, the risk of deterioration, the need for transport to locations in the hospital where resuscitation is not easily undertaken (e.g., angiography suite), and the patient's overall condition. This type of airway decision making may be more complicated than that related to elective surgery, and a unique approach to airway intervention is needed. In smaller hospitals, where a trauma team approach is not used, decisions regarding resource allocation and prioritization of interventions are even more challenging.

2. Early Hospital Care of the Traumatized Patient

Trauma and burn patients frequently undergo surgery that is not related to their acute resuscitation but is required during the first few days of their hospital stay. Burn débridement and grafting, fracture fixation, complex wound revision and repair, and other procedures are often required hours or days after the patient has been stabilized and more acute, life-threatening problems have been resolved. Decision making in this setting is easier with respect to airway management because the decision to intubate is driven by the need for surgery and anesthetic management; however, careful preoperative assessment is essential. In addition to the usual comorbidities that can make airway management difficult, trauma patients often have other complicating factors such as direct airway injury, pulmonary injury with anticipated rapid oxyhemoglobin desaturation, persistently tenuous hemodynamic status, cerebral injury with elevated intracranial pressure, or any one of a number of other complicating factors. In addition, patients with significant total body surface area burns, crush injuries, or spinal cord injuries develop acetylcholine receptor upregulation with its attendant risk of hyperkalemia if succinylcholine is administered.[31] Although classical teaching is that this vulnerability to succinylcholine-induced hyperkalemia begins on the seventh postinjury day, some effect is seen as early as 3 to 5 days.[32] In any case, this combination of considerations, specifically unresolved problems related to the injuries, the possibility of hyperkalemia, and preexisting comorbidity, can make airway management in this intermediate-term window anything but routine. A careful approach, including a detailed consideration of possible difficult airway management and relevant comorbidities, is essential.

3. Delayed Surgery

Traumatized patients frequently require multiple operative repairs or revisions before and during their rehabilitation phase. These delayed surgeries often occur between 1 and 6 months after injury and may involve many of the considerations outlined previously, particularly related to succinylcholine-induced hyperkalemia. In general, however, this population of patients is more stable and most have already undergone procedures that require endotracheal intubation, so airway difficulties have been elucidated.

Although the management of these patients raises important issues, this chapter focuses on the acutely traumatized patient and issues related to airway management in that setting.

B. THE DECISION TO INTUBATE

The decision to intubate the acute trauma patient is the most important resuscitative decision yet is often the one with which the provider struggles the most. There is a discomforting unpredictability related to resuscitation of the multiple-trauma patient. Although the risk of deterioration is substantial and such deterioration usually makes subsequent airway management both more urgent and more difficult, each contemplated airway intervention also carries its own set of risks. Because of this, an orderly approach is needed. Decision making must be based on a consistent, reproducible series of principles that accounts for the patient's current condition, likelihood of deterioration, planned diagnostic and therapeutic interventions (including transport), preinjury comorbidity, and the resources and expertise available in the resuscitation area. Although intubation decisions can be based upon the presence or absence of specific injuries, such as direct injury to the airway, the approach is most often dictated by an overall evaluation of the factors just enumerated. In addition, any difficulty in management of the airway itself must be considered just as for any other potentially difficult airway encountered in an elective setting. Thus, the approach to the airway requires two distinct evaluations, the first being the need for intubation and the second being a methodical evaluation of the likelihood of difficult laryngoscopy and intubation.

At its most basic level, the decision to undertake emergency intubation can be broken into three fundamental questions:

1. Is there a failure to maintain or protect the airway?
2. Is there a failure of oxygenation or ventilation?
3. Is there a need for intubation based on the anticipated clinical course?

Questions 1 and 2 are relatively straightforward in the setting of the trauma patient. Failure to maintain the airway is clinically obvious. Loss of the ability to protect the airway usually occurs in the setting of depressed mental status caused by head trauma, hypovolemic shock, or ingestion of drugs or alcohol and is a condition with which the emergency physician and anesthesiologist are very familiar. Airway protection is best tested by evaluation of the patient's ability to phonate (if this is possible). Phonation requires an unobstructed upper airway and the ability to execute complex, coordinated maneuvers. After phonation, the patient's ability to swallow and handle secretions is assessed. The ability to sense the pooling of secretions in the posterior pharynx and to perform the coordinated series of reflexive maneuvers to swallow requires a high degree of function and connotes airway protection. The gag reflex, which is often tested in the prehospital setting and has been advocated by the Advanced Trauma Life Support (ATLS) program as part of the evaluation of the patient's ability to protect the airway, is much less reliable, being absent in up to 25% of the normal adult population.[51] In addition, the presence of a gag reflex does not equate to airway protection, nor does its absence indicate a need to intubate. The presence or absence of the gag reflex is better thought of as a neurologic evaluation (cranial nerves IX and X) rather than as part of an airway evaluation. The wisdom of inserting a tongue blade or other device to stimulate the patient's posterior oral pharynx, when the patient is supine on a spine board and immobilized with tape

and sandbags, is also questionable, as vomiting is easily provoked and difficult to deal with.

The ability of a patient to maintain appropriate oxygenation and ventilation can be assessed clinically, anchored by pulse oximetry and capnography. Although arterial blood gas values are useful in the general evaluation of the trauma patient with respect to identification of occult acidosis that may represent more severe shock than is clinically apparent, they have little or no role in the decision to intubate the multiple-trauma patient. Thus, evaluations of the patient's respiratory effort and the overall sense of the patient's injuries, in the context of pulse oximetry readings, are more important to the intubation decision than arterial blood gas values. Patients with compromised ventilation or oxygenation should receive high-flow oxygen (at least through a nonrebreather mask) and any reversible issues should be addressed. Hemothorax, pneumothorax, flail chest, and opioid overdose are examples of reversible conditions that compromise oxygenation, ventilation, or both. In reality, the majority of cases of hypoxemia or hypoventilation in multitrauma patients are multifactorial and do not respond to simple interventions. In such cases, early intubation is almost always indicated.

The majority of multitrauma patients who require intubation meet neither criterion 1 nor criterion 2. Most trauma patients are able to maintain and protect their airways and exhibit adequate or correctable oxygenation and ventilation. In such cases, it is the anticipated clinical course that guides the decision to intubate. This is the most sophisticated and most important of the decisions facing the airway manager or trauma captain. A patient may be "stable" at the time of evaluation, but deterioration can be predicted as a natural course of their injuries. For example, the patient with burns from a closed space fire with significant smoke inhalation (see Chapter 41) may present with a somewhat hoarse voice or a simple cough but an otherwise patent airway. Failing to recognize the likelihood of progressive compromise of this airway, which has been subjected to both toxic and thermal insult, and to intervene in timely fashion, could lead to disaster. Although the patient may not meet the criteria for emergency intubation related to airway maintenance and protection, oxygenation, or ventilation, the likelihood of the deterioration is sufficient to warrant airway intervention on that basis alone.[79] Here, it is the predictability of the deterioration that determines the decision to intubate. Alternatively, the upper airway can be examined by fiberoptic laryngoscopy, thus informing the airway manager of the stability or fragility of airway patency.

Similarly, the patient with a stab wound to the neck with an obvious, but unchanging, hematoma may be thought to be secure because the airway appears fully patent and functional and the hematoma is not "expanding." The myth of the expanding hematoma is one of the most dangerous in trauma resuscitation. Many or most hematomas expand in the deep tissue planes of the neck, where expansion cannot be externally detected. The external appearance of the hematoma may remain unchanged while the patient's airway becomes progressively compromised. As is the case with the burn patient, the airway compromise may proceed insidiously to a critical state before either the patient or the clinician is aware of it.[27,69,81] At such a time, the patient is in need of immediate intubation but the deep space hemorrhage has distorted the upper airway anatomy sufficiently that intubation may be impossible. In more severe cases, the external anatomy may also be sufficiently distorted to confound surgical airway management. Again, early intervention, by securing the airway when the anatomy is reasonably normal, is the most prudent course.

A third scenario worth considering is that of the multi-trauma patient with shock. The patient with moderate head injury (e.g., Glasgow Coma Scale score of 12), unilateral pneumothorax (but with adequate oxygenation), intra-abdominal hemorrhage, and pelvic and long bone fractures should be intubated relatively early in order to facilitate resuscitation and prevent the respiratory failure related to persistent hypovolemic shock. This also facilitates the performance of any invasive procedures (tube thoracostomy, long tong fixation, pelvic fixation) that may be necessary. In addition, such patients frequently require prolonged stays in radiology for plain films and computed tomography (CT) scanning and may require angiography for embolization of pelvic vessels. Such trips outside the safety of the resuscitation room constitute a significant risk for the patient because facilities for emergency airway management are rarely, if ever, adequate in such locations. Again, it is the consideration of the patient as a whole, of the individual injuries and how they interact, of the effects of these injuries on the patient and on the patient's premorbid illnesses, and of the need for interventions (including transport) that frequently guides a prudent and rational decision to intubate, even though the patient does not have an "airway" problem and oxygenation and ventilation are both adequate.

Most issues identified with respect to trauma airway management and preventable morbidity or mortality relate to the failure to intubate when intubation was indicated rather than to a mishap related to the intubation itself. In other words, it is most often the delay in intubating a patient that leads to a poor outcome. When considering patients for intubation, it is therefore better to err on the side of intubating early and securing a potentially threatened airway rather than observing the patient with a false sense of security born of the fact that the patient has adequate oxygenation and ventilation. The purpose of such observation is to see whether obstruction or airway failure ensues, but if either occurs, the results may be disastrous. In circumstances in which one is tempted to observe the patient for the development of possible airway obstruction, it is almost always better simply to intubate the patient while the procedure is still fairly easily done

and there is sufficient time to do so, to prevent impending obstruction.

II. ANATOMY OF THE AIRWAY: TRAUMA CONSIDERATIONS

Although airway anatomy is thoroughly covered in Chapter 1, the following is a brief description of elements to consider, particularly in the trauma setting. The airway begins at the nares or lips and ends with the terminal bronchioles and alveoli of the lungs. The upper airway consists of the oral and nasal cavities and the pharynx, which provide a conduit for the movement of gases to the larynx, through the glottis, and into the trachea. The nasopharynx, oropharynx, and hypopharynx (Fig. 38-1) form a continuous space that conducts air from the outside world to the glottic aperture. The nasopharynx is protected anteriorly and laterally by the maxillary bones, the nasal bones, and nasal cartilage. Direct injury to the face, particularly from an impact with an object of high mass, high velocity, and low surface area (such as a baseball bat), can collapse the maxillary structures into the nasopharynx and cause extensive hemorrhage, both threatening the airway and complicating attempts to manage it. Similarly, the oropharynx is protected by the maxillary bones, alveolar ridges, and mandible but is subject to the same sort of intrusive injuries. Blows to the face producing Le Fort I, II, or III fractures (see Fig. 38-4) can also simultaneously threaten the airway and complicate airway management.

The larynx and trachea are essentially subcutaneous structures in the anterior neck. The larynx, in particular,

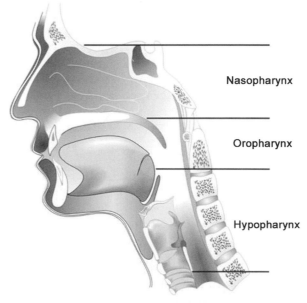

Figure 38-1 Pharynx divided into three segments: nasopharynx, oropharynx, and hypopharynx. (From Redden RJ: Anatomic considerations in anesthesia. In Hagberg CA [ed]: Handbook of Difficult Airway Management. Philadelphia, Churchill Livingstone, 2000, p 7.)

is separated from the skin only by subcutaneous fat and the anterior cervical fascia. It is for this reason that the thyroid notch, cricothyroid membrane, and cricoid cartilage can be easily palpated to provide the critical landmarks for surgical airway access (see Chapter 29 for further details). The airway is mobile in the neck but is fairly firmly anchored by the strap muscles and cervical fascia. Tracheal deviation as a result of pneumothorax or hemothorax occurs, if at all, in patients who are severely compromised.[37] Thus, tracheal deviation is not helpful as a sign of pneumothorax because it usually occurs only when the pneumothorax is at an advanced state and easily identifiable. Tracheal deviation can be seen with disruption of the neck anatomy itself caused by hemorrhage or extensive subcutaneous emphysema. It is also seen with chronic scarring, such as that related to previous radiotherapy. In any case, palpation of the trachea and larynx is a valuable exercise in the event that surgical airway management becomes necessary. It is also valuable to establish the position of the airway in the neck even if oral intubation is contemplated. Oral intubation can be extraordinarily difficult or impossible when the tracheal or larynx is displaced laterally.

Vascular structures in the neck, such as the carotid artery and jugular vein, do not have a direct bearing on the airway but can be the cause of significant airway compromise when vascular injury from blunt or penetrating trauma creates hemorrhage that displaces or otherwise changes the configuration of the airway. The nerves (Fig. 38-2) supplying the sensation to the supraglottic larynx and the remainder of the airway are rarely injured in trauma.

Knowledge of the anatomy of the upper airway is no more or less important in the management of the multitrauma patient than in any other setting in which emergency airway management is required. When specific trauma to the maxillofacial area or neck both threatens and disrupts the airway, however, anatomic knowledge and the ability to improvise one's approach may be key determinants of success.

III. SPECIFIC CLINICAL CONSIDERATIONS IN TRAUMA

A. DIRECT AIRWAY TRAUMA

Direct trauma to the airway can be classified into broad categories of blunt and penetrating trauma, and each of these can be considered in the context of direct injury to the airway itself versus compromise or threat to the airway caused by the proximity of the injury in the neck. Further, injury to the airway can occur at one or more levels. Maxillofacial trauma can compromise the upper airway, direct injury to the neck can compromise the airway from the hypopharynx to the trachea, and injuries to the chest can disrupt the lower trachea, main stem bronchi,

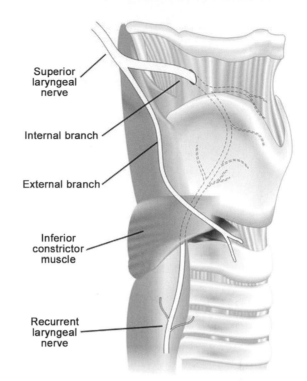

Figure 38-2 Oblique view of the larynx. Note that the internal branch of the superior laryngeal nerve pierces the thyrohyoid membrane midway between the hyoid bone and the superior border of the thyroid cartilage. (Redden RJ: Anatomic considerations in anesthesia. In Hagberg CA [ed]: Handbook of Difficult Airway Management. Philadelphia: Churchill Livingstone, 2000, p 11.)

or other lesser bronchi. The approach to airway management is dictated by the clinical presentation of the patient and the best judgment of the operator.

1. Penetrating Neck Trauma

Penetrating neck trauma ranges in scope from stab or puncture wounds through major lacerations to missile injures, both low velocity (BBs, pellets) and high velocity (crossbow, firearm). The consequences of these various mechanisms are vastly different. The overall mortality is 2% to 6%, with significantly lower mortality for low-velocity injuries.[7,42] The patient with a stab wound to the neck usually has identifiable anatomy and can undergo a planned airway evaluation and early intubation under controlled circumstances. Patients with high-velocity injuries, on the other hand, often have significant vascular and hollow structure injuries, and anatomic distortion can make airway management challenging.[70] These injuries mandate urgent airway management, but the approach is confounded by the myriad of injuries caused by the missile.[20]

For the purposes of classification of penetrating injury, the neck is divided into three zones (Fig. 38-3). Zone 1 extends from the clavicles inferiorly to the level of the cricoid cartilage superiorly. Zone 2 extends from the cricoid cartilage to a line drawn through the angles of

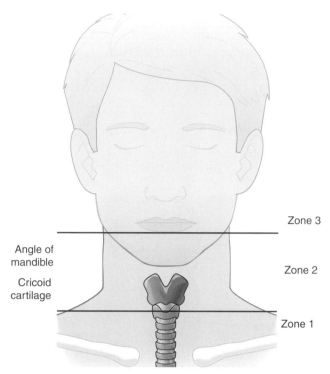

Angle of
mandible

Cricoid
cartilage

Zone 3

Zone 2

Zone 1

Figure 38-3 Zones of the neck.

the mandible, and zone 3 is the area above the angles of the mandible. This classification is most useful for low-velocity penetration, such as from a stab, low-velocity handgun, or long-distance birdshot, but has also been applied to high-velocity injuries, such as rifle wounds.[70] These zones were designated because of their unique anatomic characteristics.[4] Zone 1 is dominated by the major vascular structures of the root of the neck, specifically the carotid artery, internal jugular vein, subclavian artery and vein, and innominate artery and vein. In addition, the airway at this level is relatively inaccessible except by tracheotomy. Zone 1 injuries are relatively infrequent (less than 10% of penetrating neck injuries) but are often associated with major vascular injuries or injuries to the dome of the lung.[40] Thus, patients with zone 1 injuries often require emergency airway management because of threat to the airway by the hemorrhage related to the vascular injury. Early airway management can also be indicated on the basis of the profound shock that can ensue. There is little literature to guide the selection of airway management techniques for zone 1 penetrating injuries. Most information is limited to small case series of subsets of larger series that are dominated by zone 2 injuries. The approach to airway management is dictated more by the nature of the threat to the airway than by the actual location of the inciting wound. The overall approach to airway management in penetrating neck injuries is outlined subsequently.

Zone 2 is a most common location for penetrating neck injuries, accounting for the great majority of all reported cases.[5] Zone 2 injuries require emergency airway intervention in approximately one third of cases, with a large proportion of the remainder undergoing subsequent

intubation related to evaluation or surgical repair. The area of concern in zone 2 extends from the anterior margins of the paravertebral muscles bilaterally. In this area, major vascular structures (common carotid artery, internal jugular vein), sympathetic ganglia associated with the common carotid arteries, the hypopharynx, esophagus, larynx, and trachea are all at risk. The most common cause of airway compromise in zone 2 injuries is external distortion by a hemorrhage related to vascular injuries or direct injuries to the airway itself. The approach is outlined subsequently. Zone 3 injuries are uncommon (less than 10% of all penetrating neck injuries) because of the very small area involved and the protection provided by the mastoid process posteriorly, the mandible anteriorly, and the base of the skull superiorly. The area, however, is rich with major vascular structures (carotid artery and internal jugular vein) and provides easy access to the pharynx. Surgical repair of injuries in this area is very difficult and the majority of these patients undergo extensive evaluation by angiography, with stenting of vascular injuries often the intervention of choice. Because zone 1 injuries involve the pharynx, direct airway compromise is uncommon except by hemorrhage into the airway from a through-and-through injury to the carotid artery. In these rare circumstances, immediate airway intervention is required and may be difficult because of the torrential hemorrhage. Oral intubation is usually successful in these cases, particularly if the patient is positioned head down to prevent the blood from entering the operator's view. Once the airway is secure, the mouth can be packed tightly with gauze to control the hemorrhage from the inside, and direct pressure assists with control on the outside until the patient can be taken to the operating room.

Approach

The approach to the airway in the patient with penetrating neck trauma is guided by the same principles that were outlined earlier in this chapter. Compromised airway patency or protection because of hemorrhage, for example, is an indication for active airway management. Similarly, severe shock with overall obtundation of the patient and inability to protect the airway or ventilate and oxygenate adequately makes the intubation decision fairly straightforward. The difficulty lies in the patient who has evidence of injury to the neck but does not have an obviously compromised airway at the time of evaluation. It is in these cases that judgment is most important and that most tactical errors are made.

The best approach is to consider two specific issues:

1. Is there evidence of a direct injury to an air-containing structure in the neck?

The presence of subcutaneous air indicates injury to an air-filled structure in the neck.[30] This air-filled structure could be the airway (including the hypopharynx or pharynx) or the esophagus. In severe cases, particularly those with injury to both vascular and air-filled structures, airway obstruction can occur rapidly, requiring emergency cricothyrotomy.[29] In less precipitant cases, it is virtually impossible to tell whether the esophagus or airway is involved, and early direct or fiberoptic examination of the airway is indicated. Intubation, per se, is not mandatory, but fiberoptic examination under systemic sedation with topical anesthesia allows the operator to determine whether the injury is to the airway itself, its exact location, and its severity. A small to moderate-size endotracheal tube (ET) (e.g., 6.0 to 7.0 mm inside diameter) mounted on the scope prior to initiating endoscopy facilitates prompt intubation if the injury is significant. If the scope has been placed successfully distal to the injury, the patient can be gently intubated over the fiberscope. In general, if direct airway injury is identified, it is best to intubate the patient and secure the airway distal to the injury. At the very least, this ensures that the patient is safe until he or she can be transported to the operating room for further evaluation by an otolaryngologist or general surgeon. Tracheostomy is often necessary in these cases, but temporary oral endotracheal intubation over the fiberscope ensures airway control and minimizes the subsequent leakage of air into the tissues, facilitating later repair.[30] If no airway injury is identified and there is no evidence of increase in the subcutaneous emphysema in the neck during spontaneous or assisted ventilation, the injury can be presumed to be esophageal. If, however, circumstances change and the subcutaneous emphysema begins to increase, even slightly, intubation is recommended because development of large amounts of subcutaneous emphysema causes sufficient airway anatomy distortion that later intubation or even surgical airway management may become impossible. As with all penetrating neck injuries, early intubation, even if it does not appear obviously necessary at the time, is the most prudent course.

2. Is there evidence of significant vascular injury to the neck?

All penetrating neck wounds have some external bleeding, although this can be surprisingly modest. The issue with respect to airway management and initial management of the neck injury itself is whether injury has occurred to any of the major vascular structures in the neck (carotid arteries, jugular veins). Presence of a hematoma of any size, external hemorrhage, or any indication of displacement of the airway structures themselves is evidence of direct vascular injury to the neck. As soon as it has been established that direct vascular injury has occurred, active airway management is indicated.[25,81] Most of these patients present early in the course of their injury when anatomy is preserved and oral intubation is likely to be relatively easily achieved. Waiting to see whether the hematoma is expanding is perilous, as most of the hemorrhage into the neck occurs into the deep tissue planes, distorting and displacing the airway without external evidence until a crisis occurs. At this time, the patient obviously needs immediate airway management but anatomic distortion may be sufficient to make oral

intubation impossible and even compromise surgical airway management. The time-honored dictum that hematomas of the neck should be observed to see whether they are "expanding" is not rational, and any evidence of direct vascular injury to the neck is sufficient justification for intubation. Early intubation can proceed using a rapid sequence technique if a careful examination for difficult airway attributes fails to identify problems and there is a sound rescue strategy planned in the event of intubation failure.[78] This early intervention allows the operator to intubate in a controlled fashion rather than scrambling to secure an emergency airway later in the patient's course when airway obstruction is imminent or has occurred.

If there is significant doubt regarding oral access, three approaches can be considered.

1. The first option is to perform oral rapid sequence intubation under a double setup with preparations and personnel in place to perform immediate surgical cricothyrotomy if oral intubation is not possible. This approach should be undertaken only if the preintubation airway assessment indicates that oral intubation, although potentially difficult, is likely to be successful and therefore requires that anatomy be relatively preserved. Similarly, there has to be confidence that bag-mask ventilation will be successful in maintaining the patient's oxygenation, if required.
2. The second option is to perform fiberoptic intubation under sedation and topical anesthesia as described earlier. This allows the operator to use the fiberscope to identify and enter the airway, even if the anatomy has become distorted. If this is undertaken early in the patient's course, there are sufficient time and control to yield a high success rate.
3. The third option is to proceed directly with planned surgical cricothyrotomy. This requires that the airway be identifiable with clear landmarks to permit a surgical approach. Local anesthetic infiltration and transcricothyroid puncture or instillation of local anesthesia into the airway is likely to make the procedure easier to perform (see Chapter 29).

In all cases of penetrating neck trauma, early consultation with otolaryngology or general surgery is essential. Initially innocuous injuries may bear catastrophic consequences for the patient if not identified and managed early.[12] As is clear from the preceding discussion, early airway intervention permits a controlled resuscitation and evaluation and prevents the major morbidity related to penetrating neck injury, which is airway compromise with resultant hypoxia or anoxia.

2. Blunt Neck Trauma

Many of the issues related to penetrating neck trauma apply in analogous fashion to management of the patient with blunt neck trauma. The primary difference is related to the inability to localize injury precisely (there is no obvious skin penetration to identify the point of injury) and the fact that blunt injury is usually more diffuse. Initial evaluation of the patient with blunt neck trauma should include identification of any bruising or ecchymosis related to the external injury. The oropharynx should be inspected to ensure that there is no injury to the tongue or dentition. The external neck should then be palpated carefully from the mandible to the clavicle. Palpation is focused on three findings:

1. Identification of any swelling, hemorrhage, or subcutaneous emphysema
2. Evaluation for tenderness (if possible) of the neck and in particular of the airway structures
3. Evaluation of the anatomy of the upper airway both for direct airway injury and for the anatomic landmarks that are important if surgical airway intervention is required (see Chapter 29)

Subcutaneous emphysema may be occult and requires careful palpation. Gentle posterior pressure on the larynx itself accompanied by a side-to-side movement of the larynx should produce retrolaryngeal crepitus, a sort of fine "bumping" feeling as the larynx moves back and forth across the tissues behind it. The absence of such crepitus, especially if accompanied by pain during this maneuver, suggests retrolaryngeal hemorrhage. Extensive ecchymosis suggests blunt vascular injury with free hemorrhage (which is usually venous) or formation of a pseudoaneurysm. The presence of extensive ecchymosis or extensive swelling is strongly suggestive of impending airway compromise and urgent airway intervention is advisable.[43] Infrequently, direct blunt neck trauma can cause laryngeal fracture or tracheal transsection. Tracheal transsection in this setting is usually rapidly fatal, but patients may arrive in the trauma resuscitation area alive because of incomplete transsection.[26] In such cases, there is usually massive subcutaneous air, often accompanied by swelling, and pain is noted on palpation of the anterior airway. Although a trial of bag-mask ventilation may be tempting, it promptly produces profound subcutaneous emphysema and accelerates the patient's deterioration. The best approach when such an injury is identified is prompt transfer to the operating room for surgical exploration of the anterior neck and establishment of the airway by tracheostomy distal to the transsection. Often, however, airway management must be undertaken before the surgery. In such cases, awake careful fiberoptic intubation over a small fiberscope after inhalational induction may be the least of all evils. If the airway must be secured in the emergency department, for example, in preparation for transport to a level one trauma center, the same approach is used, substituting intravenous sedation and topical anesthesia for inhalational anesthesia because the latter is rarely available in the emergency department.

As with penetrating neck injury, the key error in the management of the patient with blunt neck trauma is observing an already distorted airway to see whether it becomes worse. If the patient exhibits evidence of significant neck injury, it can be assumed that the airway is threatened. When this threat advances to actual airway compromise, it both threatens the patient's life and thwarts subsequent attempts at airway management. As with penetrating trauma, therefore, early airway management is indicated when there is evidence of significant blunt injury to the neck.

Airway management is complicated by the fact that patients with blunt anterior neck trauma must be presumed to have cervical spine injury. Cervical spine injury has been reported in up to 50% of patients with blunt airway injury.[16] See the later discussion of airway management in the context of presumed cervical spine injury.

Special mention must be made of "clothesline" injuries in which the neck is struck, usually transversely, by a fence wire or similar object. In these cases, the central neck area may be significantly but occultly disrupted by the blunt trauma from the impact.[29] Although these injuries can be dramatic and often require immediate airway management, the airway itself is often intact, signified by identification of intact structures and the absence of air bubbling or gurgling during negative-pressure or positive-pressure ventilation. In such cases, early intubation from above, preferably over a fiberscope, is best. If the airway has been breached and gurgling or subcutaneous air is evident in the tissues of the neck, positive-pressure bag-mask ventilation is not likely to be successful in oxygenating the patient, and attempts at bag-mask ventilation may result in insufflation of large amounts of air into the soft tissues of the neck, further compromising both the airway and the attempts to secure it. The best approach in these cases is to attempt to secure the airway over a fiberscope using sedation and topical anesthesia, with a plan to progress directly to a cricothyrotomy or emergency tracheostomy if fiberoptic intubation is unsuccessful.

3. Maxillofacial Trauma

Mandibular fractures are usually isolated injuries but can occur in the setting of multiple trauma, particularly in unrestrained occupants of motor vehicles in crashes and victims of severe assault. The airway is rarely threatened by mandibular fractures unless the anterior mandible is fractured, allowing the tongue to fall back into the airway. Usually, the obstruction is easily relieved by pulling the anterior segment of the mandible forward. This maneuver also remedies any interference with endotracheal intubation by the posteriorly displaced tongue. Patients with fractures of the angle of the mandible or the mandibular condyles often have limited mouth opening. This restriction of mouth opening is related both to pain and to anatomic restriction and is not completely abolished by neuromuscular blockade. It is important to establish the extent of mouth opening and whether this is adequate to permit intubation prior to administering neuromuscular blocking agents to patients with mandibular fractures.

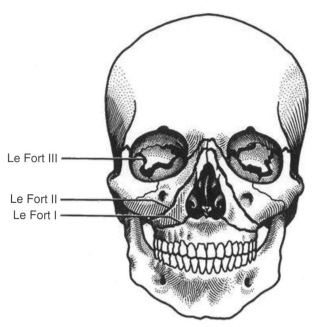

Figure 38-4 Le Fort classification of facial fractures. Le Fort I: palatofacial disjunction. Le Fort II: pyramidal disjunction. Le Fort III: craniofacial disjunction.

Maxillary fractures usually occur in one of the classically described Le Fort patterns. Although the precise location of the Le Fort fracture patterns is sometimes difficult to remember, the Le Fort I, II, and III fractures can be thought of as follows (Fig. 38-4). The Le Fort I fracture represents separation of the roof of the mouth from the face—the fracture extends through the alveolar ridge to the base of the nose, separating the alveolar ridge and hard palate from the rest of the face. The Le Fort II fracture is a separation of the central face from the rest of the face and cranium. Here the fractures extend from the base of the nasal bones through the medial orbits down through the maxilla to the posterior molars. This fracture effectively creates a free-floating central face fragment. The Le Fort III fracture is a separation of the face from the skull. This fracture extends from the base of the nasal bones through the orbits to the lateral orbital rims, then through the zygomatic arch and down through the pterygoid plate. This causes complete separation of the face from the base of the skull.

Le Fort I fractures rarely cause airway compromise. If the fracture fragment has displaced posteriorly, it can easily be pulled forward by gripping the upper incisors or alveolar ridge. Le Fort II fractures similarly do not compromise the airway unless extensive hemorrhage is present. The fracture fragment, although free floating, rarely displaces posteriorly sufficiently to compromise the airway. In the absence of hemorrhage, the mouth and oral pharynx are usually patent and functional. Le Fort III fractures can compromise the airway by posterior displacement of the entire central face, thus compromising the oral and nasal pharynx. Similarly, extensive swelling or hemorrhage related to the fractures may threaten the airway. In all cases, careful oral inspection and suctioning to determine the patency and adequacy of the oral cavity, followed by early intubation for airway protection and overall management of the patient, are advisable.

An unfortunately common presentation of maxillofacial injury occurs when an attempted suicide fails because the gun (usually a shotgun) is oriented in such a way as to have the mass of the shot pass upward through the face rather than on a posterior trajectory through the brain stem. This often happens when the patient places a rifle or shotgun under the chin and then tries to reach downward for the trigger. This naturally leads to extension of the neck and the trajectory of the missile is altered, causing it to pass upward through the face (Fig. 38-5). Although such

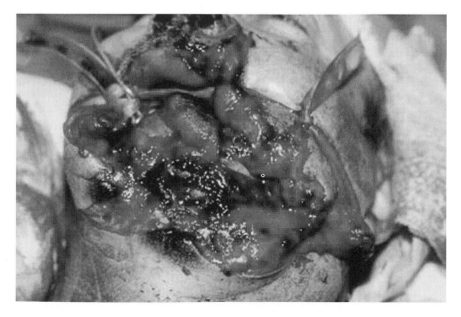

Figure 38-5 Self-inflicted gunshot wound in a 67-year-old man. (© 2006 The Airway Course, with permission)

injuries occur with massive facial distortion, airway management can range from easy to virtually impossible. Destruction of the mandible, tongue, palate, and nasopharynx often makes oral intubation impossible. In addition, hemorrhage is usually extensive. In such cases, primary surgical airway management is usually the method of choice. At other times, however, the injury can be predominantly anterior, sparing the airway, and the mandible and tongue can be displaced forward, permitting adequate oral access for oral intubation. Efficient suctioning is usually required because the hemorrhage can be significant.

B. CERVICAL SPINE INJURY

Unstable injury to the cervical spine presents a particular hazard with respect to airway management because of the potential to cause or exacerbate spinal cord injury. Cervical spine injury usually occurs when there is high energy transfer, such as in a motor vehicle collision, but can occur with relatively minor trauma in patients with significant degenerative disease of the cervical spine, such as rheumatoid arthritis or osteopenia. Motor vehicle collisions are the greatest cause of spinal injury, accounting for approximately 50%, followed by falls, athletic injury, and interpersonal violence.[13]

In the trauma resuscitation room, all patients who have been subjected to significant blunt trauma should be assumed to have a cervical spine injury until it has been excluded. Penetrating trauma can also cause spinal injury, but creation of an unstable spine injury without concomitant spinal cord injury is exceedingly rare. Thus, with penetrating injury, it is usually apparent whether spinal injury has occurred because the patient has neurologic disability.

One of the significant challenges related to airway management in patients with blunt trauma is the inability to determine definitively whether the patient does or does not have cervical spine injury before intubation is required. Fortunately, most patients with cervical spine injury do not require intubation during the acute phase of their resuscitation. However, it is precisely those with the most severe trauma who are likely to require intubation, and this is the same population at highest risk for spinal injury.[77] It has been estimated that 2% to 14% of all patients with serious blunt trauma have a significant cervical spine injury.[6,28] The decision whether to obtain portable cervical spine radiographs before intubation must account for the following principles:

1. *A single portable lateral cross-table cervical spine radiograph is highly insensitive for significant cervical spine injury.* At least 25% of lateral cervical spine radiographs fail to visualize the cervical-thoracic junction (C7-T1).[21] Even if the lateral radiograph is adequate, it should be considered no more than 80% sensitive for cervical spine injury.[73] In addition, a complete three-view

cervical spine series fails to identify approximately 15% of significant cervical spine injuries.[62] In consideration of this, no plain radiograph should be interpreted as indicating that the cervical spine is free of injury and that movement can be undertaken with impunity during intubation.

2. *The severe limitations of portable cervical spine radiographs question the value of even obtaining these prior to intubation.* Advocates argue that more information is always better and that, for example, if a cervical spine injury is identified, one can plan the intubation more carefully. The countervailing view is that because these radiographs are so insensitive, all patients should be presumed to have an unstable cervical spine injury and all should be handled as if one has just viewed a radiograph demonstrating a clearly unstable injury.

In light of the preceding discussion, it appears most prudent to obtain a lateral cervical spine radiograph or a three-view portable radiograph series in the trauma bay only when obtaining such radiographs does not delay airway management. In other words, if airway management is clearly indicated, the patient should be presumed to have a cervical spine injury and precautions should be taken accordingly (see later). If, on the other hand, intubation is considered necessary but there is not a need to perform it within the next few minutes, cervical radiographs can be obtained along with anterior-posterior radiographs of the chest and pelvis. In this case, however, only a positive cervical spine radiograph can be considered to provide additional information. The incidence of a negative radiograph, despite significant injury, is sufficiently high that no reassurance should be taken from a negative study. CT scanning is much more accurate than plain radiography in trauma, but a CT scan of the cervical spine is rarely obtained before airway intervention is required.

Airway management in the patient with cervical spine injury must be undertaken with strict attention to immobilization of the cervical spine. This is best done by a second operator whose sole function is to maintain the existing relationship between the head, neck, and torso. The best immobilization technique is one that allows the person performing the immobilization to have direct contact with both the head and the torso. Two common methods are described. In one method, the assistant approaches the head from the thorax, resting his or her forearms on the upper chest and clavicles and passing the wrists and hands up alongside the neck bilaterally so that the hands, with fingers spread, can grip and immobilize the occipital-parietal area of the head. This allows the assistant to both prevent and detect any change in the angle of the head on the neck or the neck on the body during laryngoscopy and intubation. It is vitally important that the assistant provide direct feedback to the intubator if any motion is felt. The second method requires the assistant to crouch below the operating table, usually to the intubator's right side. The assistant then reaches up over the head of the table and immobilizes the base of the occiput with the heels of both hands. The fingers extend down alongside the neck to the top of the patient's shoulders, again permitting the assistant to immobilize both the head and neck and to detect movement.

Although intubation often takes place with a cervical collar in situ, the cervical collar has not been demonstrated to reduce significant cervical spine movement during intubation and is not a substitute for manual in-line stabilization as described.[52] In addition, the cervical collar usually extends up above the patient's chin, thus holding the mouth shut. The anterior portion of the collar must therefore be removed to permit intubation. Cricothyrotomy can be performed through openings in the anterior collar, but this is often technically challenging, and it is preferable to remove the anterior half of the collar before undertaking surgical airway management. The debate regarding nasotracheal intubation versus various awake intubation (AI) techniques versus rapid sequence intubation in the trauma patient is discussed in the section on principles of airway management.

C. INTRACRANIAL INJURY

Intracranial injury commonly occurs with both blunt and penetrating trauma. In penetrating trauma, the injury is obvious because the penetration must occur proximate to the cranial vault. With blunt trauma, however, the presence of intracranial injury can be much more difficult to establish. Although the Glasgow Coma Scale score is widely used in trauma, it is at best a crude instrument. A Glasgow Coma Scale score of 8 or less, however, in the absence of a reversible cause (e.g., opioid overdose) indicates coma and mandates intubation, on the basis of both airway protection and anticipated deterioration. In general, any patient with a Glasgow Coma Scale score of 12 or less should be considered to have significant head injury until cranial CT scanning can prove otherwise. These patients may have elevated intracranial pressure (ICP), and all patients with a Glasgow Coma Scale score of 8 or less should be presumed to have elevated ICP with loss of cerebral autoregulation. This has some impact on the agents selected for intubation and, to a lesser degree, the method used (see later).

Airway management in the patient with intracranial injury is dictated by an often conflicting series of choices between optimizing the adverse responses in the brain related to intubation and maintaining overall management of the patient's hemodynamic status and resuscitation. In patients with elevated ICP, stimulation of the supraglottic airway by a laryngoscope or other device results in an increase in the ICP.[1] This increase in ICP appears to occur by two separate mechanisms:

1. A release of sympathetic adrenergic transmitters results in elevation in heart rate and blood pressure

(BP), which, in the non-autoregulated brain, translates to an elevation in ICP.[55]

2. A direct reflexive increase in ICP caused by laryngeal stimulation, although the mechanism is not precisely defined.[83]

In addition, succinylcholine, which is the drug of choice for rapid sequence intubation of the multitrauma patient (see later), is believed to cause an elevation in ICP, although this has been disputed.[11,46,72]

The mitigation of these potential elevations in ICP is an important theme in the airway management of the multiple-trauma patient with cranial injury. In addition, avoidance of hypoxia and hypercarbia and maintenance of adequate perfusion BP are vital to producing the best possible outcome for the patient.

Lidocaine has been studied in the context of prevention of the ICP response that is sympathetically mediated and also the ICP response that is considered reflexive. Although there is some evidence supporting the use of lidocaine, 1.5 mg/kg intravenously, to blunt the sympathetically mediated hemodynamic response that occurs during laryngoscopy and intubation, conflicting results have been obtained in patients both with and without cardiovascular disease.[16,35,49,59,71,75] On balance, it appears that there is insufficient evidence to recommend the use of lidocaine for the purpose of suppression of sympathetic discharge during intubation. There have been no studies evaluating the use of lidocaine to prevent the intracranial response to laryngoscopy in patients with traumatic brain injury. However, lidocaine, 1.5 mg/kg intravenously, has been shown to blunt the direct ICP response to tracheal suctioning and laryngeal stimulation in hypocarbic patients with elevated ICP.[22,83] On balance with lidocaine's wide therapeutic margin, familiarity, safety profile, and ready availability, it appears rational to administer lidocaine, 1.5 mg/kg intravenously, 3 minutes before the induction agent when undertaking rapid sequence intubation of a patient with elevated ICP. Lidocaine, used in this manner, can be presumed to have a beneficial effect on the direct ICP response to laryngoscopy and intubation.

The sympathetic response to intubation has been extensively studied, and both synthetic opioids and β-blockers have been shown to attenuate the reflex sympathetic response to laryngoscopy. Administration of a β-blocker to a trauma patient may worsen hemodynamic instability and is rarely desirable except in certain cases of isolated head trauma. Similarly, administration of full sympathetic blocking doses of the synthetic opioids, such as fentanyl, could also have adverse effects, particularly in patients with hypovolemia, who are dependent on sympathetic drive. Fentanyl, in a dose of 2 to 3 µg/kg as a pretreatment agent, has been shown to attenuate the reflex sympathetic response to laryngoscopy and should have minimal adverse cardiovascular effects.[71] Care must be used, however, to ensure that the fentanyl does not cause respiratory depression with resulting hypercarbia and that the patient has sufficient hemodynamic stability to tolerate even this small dose.

Competitive neuromuscular blocking agents, such as rocuronium, achieve intubating conditions almost as rapidly as succinylcholine but without the attendant rise in ICP.[60,66] The duration of paralysis when rocuronium 1.0 mg/kg is used for intubation, however, is 46 minutes.[45] Succinylcholine, with its ultrarapid onset and short duration of action, remains the drug of choice for emergency intubation of trauma patients, including those with elevated ICP. The exacerbation of the ICP elevation by succinylcholine, however, is clearly not desirable. There is evidence that a defasciculating dose of a competitive neuromuscular blocking agent, such as rocuronium 0.06 mg/kg or vecuronium 0.01 mg/kg, can mitigate the ICP response to succinylcholine.[56,72] Therefore, it is reasonable to administer a defasciculating dose of rocuronium or vecuronium 3 minutes before succinylcholine in patients with elevated ICP undergoing rapid sequence intubation.

Agent selection for induction for patients with ICP is discussed subsequently. When rapid sequence intubation is planned, however, and there is no contraindication, it is rational to administer lidocaine 1.5 mg/kg intravenously, fentanyl 3 µg/kg intravenously, and a defasciculating dose of rocuronium or vecuronium 3 minutes before the administration of the induction agent and succinylcholine for rapid sequence intubation.

Laryngoscopy and intubation should be as gentle and atraumatic as possible. There is evidence that minimizing laryngeal stimulation helps reduce the hemodynamic and ICP responses to laryngoscopy and intubation. Varying devices have been evaluated to see whether they are less traumatic than direct laryngoscopy. Intubations through the laryngeal mask airway (LMA) or using the Trachlight lighted stylet appear to be less stimulating in hypertensive patients than intubation by direct laryngoscopy.[44] Studies comparing intubation over a lighted stylet with direct laryngoscopy indicate that the placement of the ET into the trachea is more stimulating than the laryngoscopy itself.[74]

D. INTRAOCULAR INJURY

Fortunately, most patients with open globe injuries can be intubated in the operating room under maximal control. Penetrating globe injuries are usually isolated and are caused primarily by implements (sticks, children's toys) or by low-velocity missiles (BBs, pellets). On occasion, however, open globe injury occurs in the context of multitrauma requiring intubation in the trauma bay. In such cases, decisions related to overall management of the patient's multiple injuries take precedence over management of the eye injury per se. Whether the intubation occurs in the trauma resuscitation area or in the operating room, however, the concern related to open globe injuries is whether succinylcholine, which is known to cause a transient rise in intraocular pressure, could theoretically or

actually cause an extrusion of intraocular contents on that basis.[17] There has never been a single case report of vitreous extrusion following the use of succinylcholine in a patient with an open globe injury.[76] The paramount consideration, therefore, appears to be prevention of straining, coughing, or bucking during the intubation, arguing for a rapid sequence technique. It has been recommended that a defasciculating dose of a competitive neuromuscular blocking agent be given 3 minutes before administration of succinylcholine in patients with open globe injuries to mitigate the elevation of intraocular pressure, but this has never been subjected to study. On balance, it would appear that defasciculation is appropriate for patients with open globe injuries receiving succinylcholine unless there is a contraindication, such as severe respiratory compromise.

E. THORACIC INJURY

Both blunt and penetrating injuries can cause sufficient compromise of respirations or oxygenation to mandate intubation. Injuries associated with penetrating trauma vary greatly depending on the implement or missile used and the location and path of the injuring object. High-velocity gunshot wounds to the chest are often fatal, causing disruption of the major vasculature, main stem bronchi, or the heart itself. Lower velocity gunshot wounds, especially those more peripherally placed, often cause much less blast-type injury to the chest, resulting in minor pulmonary contusion and a surprisingly low incidence of hemopneumothorax requiring intervention beyond simple tube thoracostomy.[38] Pneumothorax is common in penetrating injury, whether caused by missile or implement, and cardiac injury with pericardial tamponade can occur. Blunt chest trauma tends to be more diffuse and is more often associated with pulmonary contusion, disruption of the chest wall with rib fractures, costochondral separation, hemopneumothorax, and, if severe, disruption of a main stem bronchus or of the aorta.

In addition to physical examination and a determination of vital signs including oxygen saturation, early portable anterior-posterior chest radiography is invaluable in assessing patients who are victims of thoracic trauma. Despite the value of the radiograph, however, obvious life-threatening conditions such as tension pneumothorax should be treated prior to radiographic confirmation. A patient presenting with external evidence of chest trauma (for example, a motor vehicle crash victim with multiple rib fractures and subcutaneous air) who has signs compatible with tension pneumothorax (hypotension, tachycardia, tachypnea, oxygen desaturation) should have immediate decompressive thoracostomy prior to any radiographic studies. As described earlier, the finding of tracheal deviation occurs only in the final stages of tension pneumothorax when the patient is in extremis, and the presence of a midline trachea should never be taken as evidence that tension pneumothorax is not present. If there are not sufficient personnel to manage all of the necessary tasks simultaneously, a needle thoracostomy can be done, pending insertion of the chest tube. Needle thoracostomy, however, is strictly a short-term temporizing measure and tube thoracostomy with at least a 34 Fr chest tube should be performed at the earliest opportunity. The objective is simply to release sufficient air that the tension phenomenon that is impairing venous return and cardiac contractility is mitigated, pending placement of the chest tube. Release of tension pneumothorax also facilitates choice of the induction agent for intubation because the BP generally improves significantly. In addition, mitigation of the intrathoracic pressure helps to avoid the hypotension that may occur when positive-pressure ventilation is instituted after intubation.

Overall, thoracic injury generally has three effects with respect to airway management:

1. The intrathoracic injuries themselves may be the primary reason for intubation. Pulmonary contusion, bilateral hemothorax, flail chest with respiratory compromise, and major life-threatening intrathoracic injury are all indications for early intubation.
2. The thoracic injuries may compromise preoxygenation and promote rapid oxyhemoglobin desaturation during intubation. Preoxygenation is essential when performing rapid sequence intubation, and patients with severe pulmonary injury may not preoxygenate well. It may be difficult to get the oxygen saturation above 90% even with high-flow oxygen. Rapid oxyhemoglobin desaturation can be anticipated, and these patients may require bag-mask ventilation throughout the intubation sequence (with Sellick's maneuver) in order to maintain adequate oxygenation. This is particularly important if the patient has concomitant head injury.
3. Hypotension related to the thoracic injuries may limit agent selection. Some induction agents, such as sodium thiopental, are potent venodilators and negative inotropes. When they are given to patients with hemodynamic compromise related to thoracic or multisystem injuries, the hypotension can be severe and prolonged. Therefore, thoracic trauma (along with other injuries) often precludes the use of such agents or requires significant reduction in dosage.

The intubation technique for patients with thoracic trauma is dictated by the overall status of the patient. Rarely does the thoracic trauma itself determine the technique. In general, rapid sequence intubation is preferred; this is usually performed with manual in-line stabilization because of the risk of spine injury (see earlier). Care must be taken to preoxygenate the patient adequately and to maintain adequate oxygenation throughout the intubation sequence. Once the patient is intubated, positive-pressure ventilation may further compromise venous return and mean arterial BP and the mechanical ventilation should be managed to maintain adequate oxygenation with the least effective tidal volume until the hemodynamic effects of the positive-pressure ventilation can be determined. Patients with pulmonary injury, such as pulmonary contusion, generally do better with modest amounts of positive end-expiratory pressure, such as 10 cm H_2O, but this has the potential to compromise venous return further and must be instituted with caution.

F. HEMORRHAGIC SHOCK

The patient with profound shock has significant metabolic debt, experiences rapid muscle fatigue, is susceptible to respiratory compromise and failure, and usually requires intubation with positive-pressure ventilation unless the shock process can be reversed. In addition to contributing to the indication for intubation, hemorrhagic shock greatly limits the choice of agents for intubation. Induction agents such as sodium thiopental and propofol have significant adverse hemodynamic consequences.[8] These agents should therefore be used in greatly reduced doses or preferably avoided altogether in patients with hemorrhagic shock. The most stable of the induction agents is ketamine, which can be used in a reduced dose of 1 mg/kg, even in patients with significant hemodynamic compromise. Ketamine is hemodynamically very stable and stimulates catecholamine release.[34,82] In frank shock, however, ketamine, like every other induction agent, depresses myocardial contractility and must be used with extreme caution.[34,82] It has been implicated in transient elevations of ICP, but the evidence in this regard is highly conflicted.[3] Overall, in the context of head injury with significant hypovolemia, ketamine's superior hemodynamic characteristics probably greatly outweigh its potential to cause small transient rises in ICP. Therefore, although caution is advised in administering ketamine to patients with head injury and to those in shock, it may be the least of evils if given in a reduced dose in such patients.

Etomidate, an imidazole derivative, also has remarkable hemodynamic stability.[50] In the induction dose of 0.3 mg/kg, it causes virtually no change in mean arterial BP in normal patients. In very large doses, two to three times the induction dose, however, etomidate consistently causes hypotension.[67] Even when patients are hypovolemic, however, etomidate in the standard induction dose maintains a high degree of hemodynamic stability. For patients with frank shock, the dose can be reduced to 0.15 to 0.2 mg/kg. Etomidate appears to have some cerebral protective effect and can significantly lower ICP without adverse effects on perfusion pressure.[57] It is therefore a rational agent for use in patients with multisystem trauma and hypovolemic shock. A recent review questioned the use of etomidate for intubation of patients with sepsis on the basis of the drug's ability to depress endogenous cortisol production.[39] This effect is minor, however, and is corrected by administration of exogenous corticosteroids. The hemodynamic benefits of etomidate outweigh the potential negative effects with respect to the adrenocortical axis, and it is not known whether there are any adverse effects in the trauma patient.

Midazolam is infrequently used as an induction agent in multiple-trauma patients and exhibits many of the same adverse hemodynamic effects as propofol and pentothal. If it is used, the dose should be greatly reduced to 0.1 mg/kg or as low as 0.05 mg/kg in patients in frank shock. At this dose, midazolam is a minimally effective induction agent and may not provide amnestic protection for the patient.[63]

In addition to influencing the decision to intubate and the choice of agents, hemorrhagic shock greatly complicates overall management of the patient. Drug circulation times can be longer and one may have to allow more time between the administration of succinylcholine and the first attempt at intubation. Succinylcholine itself is remarkably hemodynamically stable, and an increased dose or a repeated dose may be required because of poor drug distribution in patients who have hemorrhagic shock. Pretreatment agents are generally avoided in hemorrhagic shock with the exception of lidocaine for elevated ICP. Administration of fentanyl is contraindicated by its relative sympathetic blocking activity, and administration of a defasciculating agent is ill advised because of the patient's severe respiratory fatigue caused by the hypovolemia.

Overall resuscitation from the hypovolemic state must occur in parallel with preparation for intubation. The use of a high-flow blood infusing unit can provide warmed packed red blood cells at a rate as high as 500 mL/min.[24] Care must be taken not to "overshoot" the resuscitation, however, particularly in the presence of penetrating injuries and those believed to be associated with ongoing bleeding. Maintenance of an adequate perfusion pressure to support the brain and vital organs until surgical repair can be undertaken is the desirable goal. There is no evidence that restoration of the BP to a "normal" range is beneficial, and it may be harmful.[19] Crystalloid fluid can be used for the first 2 L of resuscitation but should be rapidly replaced with blood if shock is ongoing. A Foley catheter may be helpful to monitor urine output. Arterial blood gas values, with particular attention to the base deficit, can help monitor treatment of the shock. In cases in which the patient is not going to be transported promptly to the operating room, placement of an arterial line is highly advisable.

IV. PRINCIPLES OF AIRWAY MANAGEMENT IN THE TRAUMA PATIENT

A. CONTROL OF THE COMBATIVE PATIENT

Trauma patients, particularly those who are intoxicated or who have sustained head injury, are frequently agitated or combative upon arrival to the emergency department or trauma resuscitation room. In some cases, this agitation is a result of an overwhelming combination of confusing sensory inputs to the patient. The patient may be intoxicated, head injured, frightened, disoriented, or in severe pain. All of these factors may contribute to combative behavior. In addition, it is important to evaluate all patients early on for possible underlying medical conditions, especially hypoglycemia. This is especially true when the patient's mental status appears significantly altered, consistent with significant head injury, but emergency medical technicians report a fairly minor crash mechanism or "minimal vehicle damage." This suggests that a medical condition may have preceded the motor vehicle crash and thus most of the abnormal presentation may be due to the medical condition rather than to injury.

Initially, attempts should be made to reassure the patient and to help him or her orient to the otherwise chaotic environment of the resuscitation room. Patients are often in a traumatic, emotional "delirium" and may be helped by the physician placing his or her face relatively close to the patient's and speaking in a clear, firm, controlled, and reassuring voice. Usually, however, the combative behavior is multifactorial, as just described, and requires physical and chemical restraint. Physical restraint is, at best, temporizing, and these patients are often restrained on a long spine board with a cervical collar, tape, and sandbags. Despite this, the patient's ability to move and to exert significant forces on the potentially injured spine warrants further action.

The decision whether to sedate a patient or simply to intubate for behavioral control should be made on the basis of the patient's overall injuries. If the patient's injuries are such that intubation would be warranted in any case, even if the combative behavior were not present, early intubation is the best approach. Rapid sequence intubation allows protection of the cervical spine, complete control of the patient, and treatment of the multiple injuries without further disruption or pain to the patient. If, on the other hand, the patient's overall injuries are deemed to be relatively modest and intubation would not be indicated in the absence of the combative behavior, chemical restraint without intubation is the best approach. Administration of repeated, titrated doses of a butyrophenone, such as haloperidol, can rapidly achieve control of the patient without compromising respiration or significantly altering the neurologic examination. In the hemodynamically stable patient, haloperidol, 5 mg, can be given in repeated doses intravenously every 5 minutes with observation for effect.[23] Most patients calm rapidly under the influence of the haloperidol, and management can then proceed in a more orderly fashion. Haloperidol has been rumored to lower the seizure threshold and thus be contraindicated in patients with head trauma, but this is a trauma "myth," which originated from a single rat study in the early 1960s. There is no human evidence to support this oft-cited "contraindication." Droperidol was equally effective and commonly used for this purpose before the Food and Drug Administration issued a highly controversial "black box" warning about QT interval prolongation, greatly curtailing its use.[41]

Other agents, such as the benzodiazepines, are often used but have the potential for significantly more respiratory depression than does haloperidol. Benzodiazepines must therefore be used with great caution, particularly in patients with concomitant alcohol intoxication. The practice of using haloperidol in combination with benzodiazepines (e.g., 5 mg haloperidol plus 1 mg of lorazepam) simply complicates matters by giving two drugs when one drug would do. Although newer major tranquilizers are now approved, haloperidol has stood the test of time in trauma patients, is remarkably hemodynamically stable, and can be given in large doses when necessary. Haloperidol does not in any way alter the need to investigate the cause of the patient's combative behavior with CT scan, neurologic examination, and metabolic testing, but it does rapidly help achieve control of the patient and permit ongoing evaluation.

B. PREVENTION OF ASPIRATION

All trauma patients are considered at high risk for aspiration on the basis of their inability to protect their airways and the fact that they have sustained their trauma in a nonfasted state. Thus, all precautions should be taken to prevent aspiration, particularly of gastric contents, during overall management of the trauma patient and, in particular, during airway management. Choice of technique is discussed in the next section, but most patients are managed either by rapid sequence induction or by some awake technique (fiberoptic intubation, awake direct laryngoscopy). Regardless of the approach used, continuous vigilance to prevent aspiration is essential. If a rapid sequence technique is used, the early and proper application of Sellick's maneuver (as soon as consciousness is lost) and its continued application throughout laryngoscopy, intubation, and the initial few ventilations until tube placement is confirmed with end-tidal CO_2 reduce the likelihood of regurgitation and aspiration.[64] In addition, if bag-mask ventilation is necessary, application of Sellick's maneuver in the fully paralyzed patient results in only 1 to 2 cm^3 of air passing down the esophagus with each tidal volume breath.[48] Early and generous suction, particularly when hemorrhage is present, reduces the aspiration of blood, although this is not nearly as devastating as aspiration of low-pH gastric contents.

If the patient vomits while on the spine board, the patient and the board should be rolled together into the right lateral decubitus position to permit suctioning and evacuation of the vomitus from the mouth. Vomiting itself is an indication for early intubation in patients who require immobilization on a spine board. The patient may be relatively helpless with respect to being able to manage the vomitus once it is in the mouth. This is due to a combination of the injuries and possible obtunded state of the patient and the effect of being strapped in a supine position, unable to move. During awake intubation (AI) techniques, adequate sedation and topical anesthesia should be used to prevent gagging and emesis. If the patient vomits during AI, there is increased risk of aspiration because of the topical anesthesia of the supraglottic area and the vocal cords. Prompt suctioning and repositioning of the patient as necessary help reduce this risk. In addition, if the patient is sufficiently sedated, an assistant can apply Sellick's maneuver throughout the AI procedure. There is no evidence that one particular device or technique is more likely to prevent aspiration than any other with the exception of rapid sequence intubation, which minimizes the risk of aspiration of gastric contents in patients who have not fasted prior to induction of anesthesia.

C. CHOICE OF TECHNIQUE

The issues related to approach to the airway are discussed in detail in the individual sections earlier in this chapter. Overall, the choice of technique must balance the physiologic status of the patient, the nature of the injuries, the urgency of the airway intervention, and the availability of various devices and surgical backup. Historically, the ATLS course advocated blind nasotracheal intubation for most victims of blunt trauma on the basis that it was believed to be less likely to cause cervical spine movement. This belief turned out to be completely unfounded, and blind nasotracheal intubation has fallen out of favor as a method of airway management in the trauma patient.[68,77,78] This is principally because blind nasotracheal intubation has a lower success rate, takes longer to complete, causes greater oxygen desaturation, and has a higher complication rate than oral rapid sequence intubation. The original proscription of rapid sequence intubation was based on two premises:

1. Direct laryngoscopy, regardless of the technique used, would subject the cervical spine to movement. Cadaver studies and those done in living patients have failed to support this contention. In fact, there is no evidence that gentle laryngoscopy performed with in-line stabilization subjects the cervical spine to any risk. This is not to say that intubation should be forceful or prolonged. Rather, there is good evidence that manual in-line stabilization combined with a gentle oral intubation does not appear to pose any risk to the cervical spinal cord.[27,52,77]

2. The muscle tone of the nonparalyzed patient provides valuable splinting support for the potentially injured cervical spine. Again, this widespread belief arose without any evidence to support it. It is more likely that the potential for coughing, bucking, gagging, or other movement during "awake" intubation techniques poses far greater risk to the cervical spine from the contraction of these nonparalyzed muscles than any theoretical threat that might ensue when muscle tone is lost because of neuromuscular blockade.

As a result of these two fundamentally incorrect beliefs, trauma intubations through the 1970s and 1980s were largely performed awake. AI persisted as an operating technique into the mid-1990s, largely because of reticence to accept emerging information that oral rapid sequence intubation with manual in-line stabilization is safe. In fact, cadaver studies and other evidence support the use of rapid sequence intubation with in-line stabilization even when the cervical spine is known to be injured. In the National Emergency Airway Registry, a multicenter study of more than 15,000 emergency intubations, a phase two data analysis of trauma intubations showed that 80% of patients underwent rapid sequence intubation and 10% were intubated with no medications (these were largely patients in full arrest or nearly full arrest who were completely unresponsive on presentation and underwent immediate direct laryngoscopy with intubation and manual in-line stabilization). The remainder of the patients were intubated using nasotracheal intubation (5%) and other methods.[34]

D. THE DIFFICULT AIRWAY

Clearly, there are patients who have been subjected to trauma and who present with difficult airways (DAs). As discussed earlier, some of these patients have had their DA attributes before the trauma, others have acquired them as a result of the trauma, and others have both problems. An efficient but detailed DA assessment is necessary prior to embarking on paralysis in the multitrauma patient. The DA is discussed in detail elsewhere in this textbook, but conventional DA assessments such as might occur during a preoperative visit are not possible in the trauma bay. Specifically, it is rarely possible to obtain a prior surgical anesthetic history from the patient. The National Emergency Airway Course (the Airway Course) and The Difficult Airway Course-Anesthesia have developed a mnemonic for a rapid DA assessment tool.[58] The tool, which was derived from proven DA prediction instruments, was validated partially in one study and is currently subject to further validation in the National Emergency Airway Registry Phase III multicenter study.[61] The mnemonic is "LEMON" and is used as shown in Box 38-1. Identification of one or more DA attributes using the LEMON mnemonic requires consideration of management of the patient as a DA (see Box 38-1).

Evaluation of the DA using the LEMON tool or another similar approach identifies most patients with a difficult intubation. The tool is overly sensitive at the cost of specificity, but that is more desirable than the converse. If a difficult intubation is anticipated, the approach is dictated by how stable the patient is, in particular the oxygenation, as this dictates the time available to

---

Box 38-1   LEMON Mnemonic for Rapid DA Assessment

- **L**ook externally. This describes the initial gestalt impression of the patient. Gestalt is highly specific but insensitive for identifying a difficult airway. The rule "if it looks difficult, it is difficult" applies. Unfortunately, the converse is not true. At the time of initial inspection, it is also important to ascertain whether the patient may be difficult to ventilate with bag and mask. Facial disruption, absent dentition, hemorrhage of the upper airway, disruption of the airway itself, morbid obesity, late-term pregnancy, reactive airways disease, facial hair, and many other attributes can predict difficult bag-mask ventilation. These can be represented by the mnemonic MOANS (Box 38-2). This is also the time to perform a brief examination of the anterior neck, identifying the landmarks for possible surgical airway management and determining whether surgical airway management would probably be difficult. Here, the mnemonic is SHORT, as explained in Box 38-3.
- **E**valuate 3-3-2. This tool allows one to determine rapidly the geometry for direct laryngoscopy. In order to obtain a reasonable view of the cords, the mouth should open sufficiently to permit three *of the patient's* fingers to be placed between the incisors. Because the patient is rarely cooperative, it is necessary to compare the operator's fingers with the patient's fingers in order to estimate this three-finger mouth opening. Similarly, three fingers should be able to be placed along the floor of the mandible from the mentum extending posteriorly without encountering the hyoid bone. Finally, two fingers should be able to be placed in the patient's thyroid notch without hitting the floor of the mandible. This quick measure, 3-3-2, helps ensure that the relationship between mouth opening, mandibular size, and location of the larynx in the neck permits a view of the cords by direct laryngoscopy.
- **M**allampati. The Mallampati score is shown in Figure 38-6 and is described elsewhere in this book.
- **O**bstruction? If obstruction is identified in the upper airway, particularly as a result of direct trauma, intubation can be anticipated to be difficult. Presence of stridor, altered voice, subcutaneous air, neck hematoma, and direct penetrating or blunt injury are all associated with possible obstruction.
- **N**eck mobility. In many trauma patients, the neck is immobile because of appropriate cervical spine immobilization for prevention of possible cervical injury. In other patients, in whom cervical spine injury is not an issue (e.g., penetrating injury to the abdomen), the cervical spine should be assessed for proper extension and the ability to be placed in the sniffing position for intubation.

MALIAMPATI SIGNS AS INDICATORS OF DIFFICULT INTUBATION

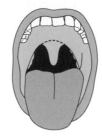

Class I: soft palate, uvula, fauces, pillars visible

No difficulty

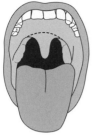

Class II: soft palate, uvula, fauces visible

No difficulty

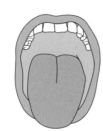

Class III: soft palate, base of uvula visible

Moderate difficulty

Class IV: hard palate, only visible

Severe difficulty

Figure 38-6 Mallampati scale for prediction of difficult airway intubation. (Adapted from Walls RM, Murphy MF, et al: Manual of Emergency Airway Management, 2nd ed. Philadelphia, Lippincott, Williams and Wilkins, 2005.)

consider alternative approaches. If the patient is well oxygenated and is reasonably stable (i.e., does not need to be intubated in the next 2 to 3 minutes), a methodical stepwise plan can be made.

If, on the other hand, the patient is critically desaturated and highly unstable, it is probably necessary to proceed directly with some form of airway intervention promptly without the luxury of a planned DA approach. Usually, this is a rapid sequence intubation with a double setup, prepared for immediate surgical cricothyrotomy.

Box 38-2 MOANS Mnemonic for Difficult Bag-Mask Ventilation

M – mask seal poor
O – obesity
A – aged (age > 55 years)
N – no teeth
S – "stiff" – i.e., resistance to ventilation, as in COPD, asthma

Adapted from Walls RM, Murphy MF, et al: Manual of Emergency Airway Management, 2nd ed. Philadelphia, Lippincott, Williams and Wilkins, 2004 and The Dificult Airway Course: Anesthesia (www.theairwaysite.com) with permission.

Box 38-3 SHORT Mnemonic for Difficult Cricothyrotomy

S – surgery (previous - remote or recent)
H – hematoma
O – obesity
R – radiation therapy (previous)
T – tumor

Adapted from Walls RM, Murphy MF, et al: Manual of Emergency Airway Management, 2nd ed. Philadelphia, Lippincott, Williams and Wilkins, 2005 and The Difficult Airway Course: Anesthesia (www.theairwaysite.com) with permission.

Alternatively, primary cricothyrotomy might be the method of choice, although the patient's combativeness or agitation often precludes this. Rarely, other devices, such as the fiberscope or intubating LMA (ILMA), are useful.

When there is sufficient time to plan the intubation approach carefully, the patient should be evaluated for the likelihood of successful rapid sequence intubation. This evaluation can be broken down into two component questions. First, is it likely that the patient can be successfully bag-mask ventilated? This is a necessary precursor to consideration of paralysis. If it is the judgment of the intubator that the patient cannot be bag-mask ventilated successfully, a technique using neuromuscular blockade is out of the question unless it is part of a double setup with immediate ability to move to a surgical airway should the first attempt at laryngoscopy be unsuccessful. Second, is intubation likely to be successful? Again, the judgment of the operator comes into play. If it is felt that the patient is likely to be successfully intubated by direct laryngoscopy despite the DA attributes, taking into consideration that the patient should be successfully bag-mask ventilated, rapid sequence intubation can be planned with a surgical backup as necessary.

In fact, in the majority of circumstances in trauma patients, DA attributes are identified but the operator can still be confident that both bag-mask ventilation and direct laryngoscopy will be successful, thus permitting rapid sequence intubation. If, however, in the opinion of the operator, either bag-mask ventilation or direct laryngoscopy is unlikely to be possible, it is better to proceed with an awake technique. This involves administration of sedation and use of topical anesthesia to permit awake laryngoscopy by either a direct or fiberoptic technique. This is described in detail in Chapter 10. Awake laryngoscopy has one of three possible outcomes: (1) the cords are well visualized and the patient is intubated; (2) the cords are well visualized and the decision is made that rapid sequence intubation is possible (in this case, the awake laryngoscopy is terminated and the patient undergoes rapid sequence intubation); or (3) awake laryngoscopy determines that oral intubation is impossible and an alternative approach is necessary.

If, after awake laryngoscopy, it is determined that the patient cannot be intubated orally, there are a number of alternative techniques. All of these are described in detail elsewhere in this book. In the trauma patient, the most useful of these is surgical cricothyrotomy, although rigid or flexible fiberoptic intubation, video laryngoscopy, the ILMA, or a lighted stylet technique may be useful in selected cases. Retrograde intubation is rarely performed in the emergency department and is generally not a good choice in the trauma patient. Use of supraglottic or retroglottic devices, such as the LMA, the pharyngotracheal lumen airway, the King LT, and others, is rarely advisable in trauma patients because of the uncertainty about their ability to protect against aspiration. The goal in the trauma patient, even with an identified DA, is to achieve a secure tube in the trachea with an inflated cuff to protect against aspiration. Placement of a device that does not achieve this is normally considered only in circumstances in which there has been a failed airway or the patient has precipitously arrested and definitive airway management is not possible. These devices are discussed in more detail in the failed airway section later in this chapter.

E. PHARMACOLOGIC CONSIDERATIONS

The trauma patient presents a number of important, but not unique, considerations with respect to choice of pharmacologic agents to assist intubation. Because rapid sequence intubation is the most common approach to the injured patient, considerations must include appropriate selection of the induction agent, neuromuscular blocking agent, and pretreatment agents to secure the airway as rapidly as possible with the least likelihood of adverse effect.

As discussed earlier, trauma patients are frequently hypovolemic, even if their initial mean arterial BP is normal. Agent selection, therefore, must go hand in hand with volume resuscitation and other appropriate interventions such as tube thoracostomy, control of external hemorrhage, and pelvic stabilization. The individual decisions related to choice of pretreatment and induction agents are covered in the various sections throughout this chapter; however, a few points bear restating here.

Induction agents should be chosen to provide the best possible intubating conditions (used in conjunction with succinylcholine) with the least likelihood for adverse hemodynamic consequences. Etomidate, in a dose of 0.3 mg/kg, is remarkably hemodynamically stable, appears to provide some degree of cerebral protection, and has an onset-duration profile similar to that of succinylcholine. Although etomidate has been associated with adrenal cortical suppression, this is not an issue when a single dose is used for induction for intubation.[65] Etomidate can cause myoclonic jerks during its onset, but use of a rapidly acting neuromuscular blocking agent, such as succinylcholine, mitigates this substantially. Ketamine is an appropriate induction agent for hypotensive trauma patients without head injury. Ketamine's role in head injury has been questioned because of its tendency to cause elevated ICP, but it is likely that the preservation of cerebral perfusion by maintenance of mean arterial BP is more important than any theoretical risk to the brain caused by ketamine's tendency to increase cerebral activity and ICP.[36,76] Other induction agents, such as propofol, pentothal, and midazolam, have much more tendency to cause hypotension and should be used in reduced doses and with caution in compromised patients. Pretreatment agents are discussed in various sections throughout this chapter.

The choice of agents for sedation and AI is also influenced by the patient's general status. It is advisable to use the agents with which the operator is most familiar for sedation. For example, if the operator typically sedates patients for painful procedures using propofol this might also be the best choice to sedate the trauma patient for awake laryngoscopy. In the absence of operator preference, ketamine may be ideally suited, especially when combined with an antisialagogue, because of its ability to preserve respirations and hemodynamic status.[34] Overall, familiarity with the drugs and the ability to titrate them carefully are probably more important than the individual pharmacodynamic characteristics of the drug.

F. THE FAILED AIRWAY

In the severely traumatized patient, as in other patients, it is important to have a clear a priori definition of airway failure and an action plan to follow when this occurs. The definition of a failed airway used in The Airway Course and The Difficult Airway Course-Anesthesia is as follows: a failed airway exists when (1) there have been three failed attempts by an experienced intubator or (2) there has been one failed attempt by an experienced intubator combined with an inability to maintain adequate oxygen saturation with a bag and mask.[80]

In either of these cases, it is necessary to recognize that oral intubation is not going to succeed in this particular patient and the operator must move on to a rescue technique (Fig. 38-7). In the "can't intubate, can't oxygenate" scenario, the most appropriate rescue device is surgical cricothyrotomy. Although other devices, such as the Combitube or LMA, could be rapidly inserted, neither of them provides a definitive airway, and if they, too, are unsuccessful, precious time has been lost prior to the initiation of the cricothyrotomy. It is therefore important that the operator always first consider cricothyrotomy when a can't intubate, can't oxygenate scenario arises; however, it is perfectly appropriate to attempt the rapid placement of a Combitube or an LMA *simultaneously* with preparations for cricothyrotomy. The attempted placement of the Combitube or LMA must not delay the initiation of the surgical airway and must be accomplished in parallel with the preparations for the surgical approach. The more common circumstance is

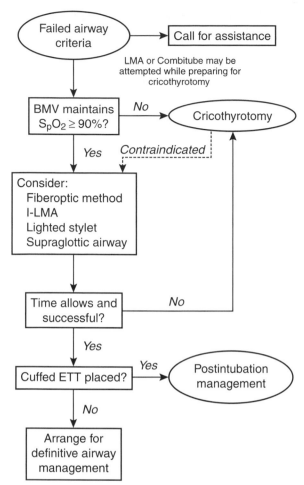

Figure 38-7 The failed airway algorithm. (From Walls RM [ed]: Manual of Emergency Airway Management, 2nd ed. Philadelphia, Lippincott Williams & Wilkins, 2004.)

one in which airway failure occurs because of inability to intubate on three attempts at direct laryngoscopy but bag-mask ventilation is adequate. In such cases, there are a number of rescue devices and techniques that can be used. These are discussed in detail in the next section. A failed airway algorithm has been developed for The Airway Course and The Difficult Airway Course-Anesthesia and is shown in Figure 38-7.[80] Note that the underlying theme in the algorithm is that decisions are driven by whether there is sufficient time to consider alternatives. If at any time a can't intubate, can't oxygenate scenario arises, the pathway leads to cricothyrotomy.

G. RESCUE TECHNIQUES

The ultimate rescue technique for a failed airway in the trauma patient is surgical cricothyrotomy, and this is covered in detail in Chapter 29. When intubation has failed but ventilation is possible, a number of devices warrant consideration. These appear in the central box of the algorithm (see Fig. 38-7).

The Combitube has been evaluated both as a primary airway management device and as a rescue device. Numerous studies have shown that emergency medical technicians can successfully insert Combitubes with a high likelihood of success.[18,84] When studied in a cadaver unstable cervical spine model, the Combitube produced more posterior cervical spine displacement than the LMA or fiberoptic methods. The meaning of this is not clear, but it suggests at the least that in-line stabilization is equally important during Combitube insertion as during direct laryngoscopy.[10] Insertion with a cervical collar in place, however, has yielded mixed results, with one study showing a high insertion success rate and another showing successful blind insertion in only one third of patients with a semirigid collar on.[53,54] Ventilation with the Combitube, however, is generally highly successful.[54] The primary use of the Combitube is as a rescue device in the "can't intubate but can ventilate" scenario in which other airway devices are thought unlikely to be successful. The Combitube is a less desirable choice because it does not place a cuffed ET in the trachea when located in the esophageal position, but it usually suffices for ventilation and oxygenation. Another role for the Combitube is as a temporizing measure during preparations for cricothyrotomy in a can't intubate, can't oxygenate patient. In this circumstance (described earlier), only a single expeditious attempt at placement is warranted.

Patients may arrive in the trauma bay with the Combitube inserted, inflated, and functioning. Because the Combitube does not provide a definitive airway (defined as a cuffed ET in the trachea), it is advisable, in most circumstances, to intubate the patient and remove the Combitube. Details of insertion and use of the Combitube are discussed elsewhere in this textbook (see Chapter 25), but there is a specific technique that must be used to intubate when the Combitube is in place. The Combitube has two cuffs, which are inflated through two separate channels. The proximal (pharyngeal) cuff is the larger of the two and is indicated by the blue filling valve. After assurance that the patient is stabilized and adequately preoxygenated, this proximal cuff should be deflated. The Combitube should then be moved over to the left corner of the patient's mouth to permit access from the right-hand side for laryngoscopy. Because the Combitube is almost always placed in the esophagus, it can remain in situ while laryngoscopy proceeds. Direct laryngoscopy proceeds pretty much as usual, and after the patient is intubated with the ET cuff inflated and tube position assured by end-tidal CO_2 detection, the distal cuff on the Combitube can be deflated and the Combitube can be removed. In the small number of cases in which the Combitube is inserted in the trachea, it can serve as a definitive airway, and tracheal placement is identified because successful ventilation and CO_2 detection are occurring through its no. 2 port. Although not mandatory, it has been recommended that a nasogastric tube be passed and the stomach decompressed prior to removal of the Combitube. It is quite possible for regurgitation to occur after removal of the Combitube, particularly if bag-mask ventilation occurred before placement of the Combitube in the prehospital setting.

In the emergency department and trauma resuscitation room, the ILMA is preferable to the standard LMA. It is equally or more easily inserted[14] and permits a conduit for subsequent intubation with a significantly higher success rate than the standard LMA.[47] The ILMA has also been used to facilitate fiberoptic and lighted stylet intubation.[2] It has primarily served as a DA device and has not been well studied in trauma. The standard LMA and the LMA ProSeal have reasonable insertion success rates in the context of cervical spine immobilization, but this has not been evaluated for the ILMA.[9] The ILMA has two main uses in the trauma patient. First, it can be used as the primary intubation method in a patient with an identified DA. In the trauma patient, however, particularly with an immobilized cervical spine, it would be an uncommon circumstance in which the ILMA would be the first device selected. More commonly, the ILMA would be used as a rescue device in a can't intubate but can oxygenate scenario. Here, placement of the ILMA allows ongoing ventilation with a very high success rate and facilitates endotracheal intubation. Like the Combitube, the ILMA can be placed as a temporizing measure during preparation for a cricothyrotomy in a can't intubate, can't oxygenate situation, as long as the placement and attempted ventilation through the ILMA do not delay the initiation of surgical cricothyrotomy (see earlier discussion).

The lighted stylet has not been studied specifically in trauma either as a primary intubating device or as a rescue device. Lighted stylet intubation has been thought to be somewhat less stimulating than direct laryngoscopy in terms of reflex sympathetic discharge, although this is controversial, and has been reported to have a high intubation success rate.[74] Excluding airways in which there is anatomic distortion or significant hemorrhage that would limit the use of the lighted stylet, it would appear a useful device in selected trauma cases. This device would be used in a can't intubate but can oxygenate scenario and has the benefit of placing a cuffed ET in the trachea, when successful. Success rates in routine intubation have mirrored those of conventional laryngoscopy.

V. CONCLUSIONS

Taken at its most fundamental level, the trauma airway is simply a subset of the DA. The difficulties are somewhat particular to the trauma patient in that there is often hemodynamic instability, and anatomic disruption or other confounding factors, such as brisk upper airway hemorrhage, may confound intubation in relatively specific ways. Nevertheless, the fundamental principles that are applied to the DA should be applied equally soundly to the trauma airway. An orderly approach, including prioritization of various resuscitation steps, careful evaluation of the specific DA attributes of the patient, careful selection of pharmacologic agents and techniques (on the basis of the patient's hemodynamic status and airway attributes), and coordination with other members of the resuscitation team, provides the foundation for success.

REFERENCES

1. Adachi YU, Satomoto M, Higuchi H, Watanabe K: Fentanyl attenuates the hemodynamic response to intubation more than the response to laryngoscopy. Anesth Analg 95:233-237, 2002.
2. Agro F, Brimacombe J, Carassiti M, et al: The intubating laryngeal mask—Clinical appraisal of ventilation and blind tracheal intubation in 110 patients. Anaesthesia 53:1084-1090, 1998.
3. Albanese J, Arnarud S, Rey M, et al: Ketamine decreases intracranial pressure and electroencephalographic activity in traumatic brain injury patients during propofol sedation. Anesthesiology 87:1328-1334, 1997.
4. Asensio JA, Valenziano CP, Falcone RE, Grosh JD: Management of penetrating neck injuries: The controversy surrounding zone II injuries. Surg Clin North Am 71:267-296, 1991.
5. Atta HM, Walker ML: Penetrating neck trauma: Lack of universal reporting guidelines. Am Surg 64:222-225, 1998.
6. Berne JD, Velmahos GC, El-Tawil Q, et al: Value of complete cervical helical computed tomographic scanning in identifying cervical spine injury in the unevaluable blunt trauma patient with multiple injuries: A prospective study. J Trauma 47:896-902, 1999.
7. Biffl WL, Moore EE, Rehse DH, et al: Selective management of penetrating neck trauma based on cervical level of injury. Am J Surg 174:678-682, 1997.
8. Billard V, Moulla F, Bourgain JL, et al: Hemodynamic response to induction and intubation. Propofol/fentanyl interaction. Anesthesiology 81:1384-1393, 1994.
9. Brain AI: Use of the LMA in the unstable cervical spine. Singapore Med J Suppl 1:46-4, 20018
10. Brimacombe J, Keller C, Kunzel KH, et al: Cervical spine motion during airway management: A cinefluoroscopic study of the posteriorly destabilized third cervical vertebrae in human cadavers. Anesth Analg 91:1274-1278, 2000.
11. Brown MM, Parr MJ, Manara AR: The effect of suxamethonium on intracranial pressure and cerebral perfusion pressure in patients with severe head injuries following blunt trauma. Eur J Anaesthesiol 13:474-477, 1996.
12. Bumpous JM, Whitt PD, Ganzel TM, McClane SD: Penetrating injuries of the visceral compartment of the neck. Am J Otolaryngol 21:190-194, 2000.
13. Burney RE, Maio RF, Maynard F, Karunas R: Incidence, characteristics and outcome of spinal cord injury at trauma centers in North America. Arch Surg 128:596-599, 1993.

14. Choyce A, Avidan MS, Shariff A: A comparison of the intubating and standard laryngeal mask airways for airway management by inexperienced personnel. Anaesthesia 56:357-360, 2001.

15. Chraemmer-Jorgensen B, Hoilund-Carlsen PF, Marvin J, Christensen V: Lack of effect of intravenous lidocaine on hemodynamic responses to rapid sequence induction of general anesthesia: A double-blind controlled clinical trial. Anesth Analg 65:1037-1041, 1986.

16. Crosby ET, Lui A: The adult cervical spine: Implications for airway management. Can J Anaesth 37:77-93, 1990.

17. Cunningham AJ, Barry P: Intraocular pressure—Physiology and implications for anaesthetic management. Can Anaesth Soc J 33:195-208, 1986.

18. Davis DP, Valentine C, Ochs M, et al: The Combitube as a salvage airway device for paramedic rapid sequence intubation. Ann Emerg Med 42:697-704, 2003.

19. de Guzman E, Shankar MN, Mattox K: Limited volume resuscitation in penetrating thoracoabdominal trauma. AACN Clin Issues 10:61-68, 1999.

20. Demetriades D, Asensio JA, Velmahos G, Thal E: Complex problems in penetrating neck trauma. Surg Clin North Am 76:661-683, 1996.

21. Domenicucci M, Preite R, Ramieri A, et al: Three-dimensional computed tomographic imaging in the diagnosis of vertebral column trauma: Experience based on 21 patients and review of the literature. J Trauma 42:254-259, 1997.

22. Dronegan MF, Bedford RF: Intravenously administered lidocaine prevents intracranial hypertension during endotracheal suctioning. Anesthesiology 52:516-518, 1980.

23. Durbin CGJ: Sedation of the agitated, critically ill patient without an artificial airway. Crit Care Clin 11:913-936, 1995.

24. Eaton MP, Dhillon AK: Relative performance of the Level 1 and Ranger pressure infusion devices. Anesth Analg 97:1074-1077, 2003.

25. Eggen JT, Jorden RC: Airway management in penetrating neck trauma. J Emerg Med 11:381-385, 1993.

26. Ford HR, Gardner MJ, Lynch JM: Laryngotracheal disruption from blunt pediatric neck injuries: Impact of early recognition and intervention on outcome. J Pediatr Surg 30:331-334, 1995.

27. Gerling MC, Davis DP, Hamilton RS, et al: Effects of cervical spine immobilization technique and laryngoscope blade selection on an unstable cervical spine in a cadaver model of intubation. Ann Emerg Med 36:293-300, 2000.

28. Gonzalez RP, Fried PO, Bukhalo M, et al: Role of clinical examination in screening for blunt cervical spine injury. J Am Coll Surg 189:152-157, 1999.

29. Goudy SL, Miller FB, Bumpous JM: Neck crepitance: Evaluation and management of suspected upper aerodigestive tract injury. Laryngoscope 112:791-795, 2002.

30. Grewal H, Rao PM, Mukerji S, Ivatury RR: Management of penetrating laryngotracheal injuries. Head Neck 17:494-502, 1995.

31. Gronert GA: Cardiac arrest after succinylcholine: Mortality greater with rhabdomyolysis than receptor upregulation. Anesthesiology 94:523-529, 2001.

32. Gronert GA: Succinylcholine hyperkalemia after burns. Anesthesiology 91:320-322, 1999.

33. Gurr DE, Kulkarni RG, Walls RM, et al: On behalf of the NEAR investigators: Trama airway management in the emergency department: Indications, methods, and success rates. Ann Emerg Med 35:S33, 2000.

34. Haas DA, Harper DG: Ketamine: A review of its pharmacologic properties and use in ambulatory anesthesia. Anesth Prog 39:61-68, 1992.

35. Helfman SM, Gold MI, DeLisser EA, Herrington CA: Which drug prevents tachycardia and hypertension associated with tracheal intubations: Lidocaine, fentanyl, or esmolol? Anesth Analg 72:482-486, 1991.

36. Himmelseher S, Durieux ME: Revising a dogma: Ketamine for patients with neurological injury? Anesth Analg 101:524-534, 2005.

37. Holloway VJ, Harris JK: Spontaneous pneumothorax: Is it under tension? J Accid Emerg Med 17:222-223, 2000.

38. Inci I, Ozcelik C, Tacyildiz I, et al: Penetrating chest injuries: Unusually high incidence of high-velocity gunshot wounds in civilian practice. World J Surg 22:438-442, 1998.

39. Jackson WL: Should we use etomidate as an induction agent for endotracheal intubation in patients with sepic shock: A critical appraisal. Chest 127:1031–1038, 2005.

40. Jurkovich GJ, Gussack GS, Luterman A: Laryngotracheal trauma: A protocol approach to a rare injury. Laryngoscope 96:660-665, 1986.

41. Kao LW, Kirk MA, Evers SJ, Rosenfeld SH: Droperidol, QT prolongation, and sudden death: What is the evidence? Ann Emerg Med 41:546-558, 2003.

42. Kendall JL, Anglin D, Demetriades D: Penetrating neck trauma. Emerg Med Clin North Am 16:85-105, 1998.

43. Keogh IJ, Rowley H, Russell J: Critical airway compromise caused by neck haematoma. Clin Otolaryngol Allied Sci 27:244-245, 2002.

44. Kihara S, Brimacombe J, Yaguchi Y, et al: Hemodynamic responses among three tracheal intubation devices in normotensive and hypertensive patients. Anesth Analg 96:890-895, 2003.

45. Kirkegaard-Nielsen H, Caldwell JE, Berry PD: Rapid tracheal intubation with rocuronium: A probability approach to determining dose. Anesthesiology 91: 131-136, 1999.

46. Kovarik WD, Mayberg TS, Lam AM, et al: Succinylcholine does not change intracranial pressure, cerebral blood flow velocity, or the electroencephalogram in patients with neurologic injury. Anesth Analg 78:469-473, 1994.

47. Langeron O, Semjen F, Bourgain JL, et al: Comparison of the intubating laryngeal mask airway with the fiberoptic intubation in anticipated difficult airway management. Anesthesiology 94:968-972, 2001.

48. Lawes EG, Campbell I, Mercer D: Inflation pressure, gastric insufflation and rapid sequence induction. Br J Anaesth 59:315-318, 1987.

49. Levitt M, Dresden G: The efficacy of esmolol versus lidocaine to attenuate the hemodynamic response to intubation in isolated head trauma patients. Acad Emerg Med 8:19-24, 2001.

50. Lindeburg T, Spotoft H, Bredgaard Sorensen M, Skovsted P: Cardiovascular effects of etomidate used for induction and in combination with fentanyl-pancuronium for maintenance of anaesthesia in patients with valvular heart disease. Acta Anaesthesiol Scand 26:205-208, 1982.

51. Mackway-Jones K, Moulton C: Towards evidence based emergency medicine: Best BETs from the Manchester Royal Infirmary. Gag reflex and intubation. J Accid Emerg Med 16:444-445, 1999.

52. Majernick TG, Bieniek R, Houston JB, Hughes HG: Cervical spine movement during orotracheal intubation. Ann Emerg Med 15:417-420, 1986.

53. Mercer MH, Gabbott DA: Insertion of the Combitube airway with the cervical spine immobilised in a rigid cervical collar. Anaesthesia 53:971-974, 1998.

54. Mercer MH, Gabbott DA: The influence of neck position on ventilation using the Combitube airway. Anaesthesia 53:146-150, 1998.

55. Miller CD, Warren SJ: IV lignocaine fails to attenuate the cardiovascular response to laryngoscopy and tracheal intubation. Br J Anaesth 65:216-219, 1990.

56. Minton MD, Grosslight K, Stirt JA, Bedford RF: Increases in intracranial pressure from succinylcholine: Prevention by prior nondepolarizing blockade. Anesthesiology 65:165-169, 1986.

57. Modica PA, Tempelhoff R: Intracranial pressure during induction of anaesthesia and tracheal intubation with etomidate-induced EEG burst suppression. Can J Anaesth 39:236-241, 1992.

58. Murphy MF, Walls RM: The difficult airway. In Walls RM (ed): Manual of Emergency Airway Management, 2nd ed. Philadelphia, Lippincott Williams & Wilkins, 2004.

59. Pathak D, Slater RM, Ping SS, From RP: Effects of alfentanil and lidocaine on the hemodynamic responses to laryngoscopy and tracheal intubation. J Clin Anesth 2:81-85, 1990.

60. Perry J, Lee J, Wells G: Rocuronium versus succinylcholine for rapid sequence induction intubation. Cochrane Database Syst Rev 1: CD002788, 2003.

61 Reed MJ, Dunn MJ, McKeown DW: Can an airway assessment score predict difficulty at intubation in the emergency department? Emerg Med J 22:99-102, 2005.

62. Ross SE, Schwab CW, David ET, et al: Clearing the cervical spine: Initial radiologic evaluation. J Trauma 27:1055-1060, 1987.

63. Sagarin MJ, Barton ED, Sakles JC, et al: Underdosing of midazolam in emergency endotracheal intubation. Acad Emerg Med 10:329-338, 2003.

64. Salem MR, Sellick BA, Elam JO: The historical background of cricoid pressure in anesthesia and resuscitation. Anesth Analg 53:230-232, 1974.

65. Schenarts CL, Burton JH, Riker RR: Adrenocortical dysfunction following etomidate induction in emergency department patients. Acad Emerg Med 8:1-7, 2001.

66. Schramm WM, Strasser K, Bartunek A, et al: Effects of rocuronium and vecuronium on intracranial pressure, mean arterial pressure and heart rate in neurosurgical patients. Br J Anaesth 77:607-611, 1996.

67. Shapiro BM, Wendling WW, Ammaturo FJ, et al: Vascular effects of etomidate administered for electroencephalographic burst suppression in humans. J Neurosurg Anesthesiol 10:231-236, 1998.

68. Shatney CH, Brunner RD, Nguyen TQ: The safety of orotracheal intubation in patients with unstable cervical spine fracture or high spinal cord injury. Am J Surg 170:676-679, 1995.

69. Shearer VE, Giesecke AH: Airway management for patients with penetrating neck trauma: A retrospective study. Anesth Analg 77:1135-1138, 1993.

70. Sofianos C, Degiannis E, Van den Aardweg MS, et al: Selective management of zone II gunshot injuries of the neck: A prospective study. Surgery 120:785-788, 1996.

71. Splinter WM, Cervenko F: Haemodynamic responses to laryngoscopy and tracheal intubation in geriatric patients: Effects of fentanyl, lidocaine and thiopentone. Can J Anaesth 36:370-376, 1989.

72. Stirt JA, Grosslight KR, Bedford RF, Vollmer D: "Defasciculation" with metocurine prevents succinylcholine-induced increases in intracranial pressure. Anesthesiology 67:50-53, 1987.

73. Streitwieser DR, Knopp R, Wales LR, et al: Accuracy of standard radiographic views in detecting cervical spine fractures. Ann Emerg Med 12:538-542, 1983.

74. Takahashi S, Mizutani T, Miyabe M, Toyooka H: Hemodynamic responses to tracheal intubation with the laryngoscope versus lightwand intubating device (Trachlight) in adults with normal airway. Anesth Analg 95:480-484, 2002.

75. Tam S: Intravenous lidocaine: Optimal time of injection before tracheal intubation. Anesth Analg 66:1036-1038, 1987.

76. Vachon CA, Warner DO, Bacon DR: Succinylcholine and the open globe: Tracing the teaching. Anesthesiology 99:220-224, 2003.

77. Walls RM: Airway management in the blunt trauma patient: How important is the cervical spine? Can J Surg 35:27-30, 1992.

78. Walls RM: Airway management. Emerg Med Clin North Am 11:53-60, 1993.

79. Walls RM: The decision to intubate. In Walls RM (ed): Manual of Emergency Airway Management. Philadelphia, Lippincott Williams & Wilkins, 2000, pp 1-8.

80. Walls RM: The emergency airway management algorithms. In Walls RM (ed): Manual of Emergency Airway Management, 2nd ed. Philadelphia, Lippincott Williams & Wilkins, 2004, pp 8-22.

81. Walls RM, Wolfe R, Rosen P: Fools rush in? Airway management in penetrating neck trauma. J Emerg Med 11:479-480, 1993.

82. Waxman K, Shoemaker WC, Lippmann M: Cardiovascular effects of anesthetic induction with ketamine. Anesth Analg 59:355-358, 1980.

83. Yano M, Nishiyama H, Yokota H, et al: Effect of lidocaine on ICP response to endotracheal suctioning. Anesthesiology 64:651-653, 1986.

84. Yardy N, Hancox D, Strang T: A comparison of two airway aids for emergency use by unskilled personnel. The Combitube and laryngeal mask. Anaesthesia 54: 181-183, 1999.

39

THE DIFFICULT AIRWAY IN NEUROSURGERY

Irene P. Osborn
David C. Kramer
Stephen R. Luney

"If the lips are blue, the brain is, too."

Elizabeth A.M. Frost

I. INTRODUCTION

Airway management in the neurosurgical patient is often a shared responsibility among emergency physicians, neurosurgeons, anesthesiologists, and critical care specialists. In achieving and maintaining a patent airway, it is important to consider its impact on the central nervous system and the well-being of the patient. This chapter represents the culmination of the authors' experiences anesthetizing neurosurgical patients in at least six different institutions in two countries. The 1990s were declared the "decade of the brain," yet since that time the variety of neurosurgical procedures, anesthetic techniques, and airway devices has increased dramatically. The evolution of neurosurgical practice and the performance of surgery in patients with complex disease provide a myriad of clinical challenges. In this chapter, we review the range of airway considerations faced daily by the neuroanesthesiologist. The goal is to address issues specific to the dedicated neuroanesthesiologist as well as those related to the neurosurgical patient who might be encountered by the generalist anesthesiologist. This discussion reflects the ever-changing considerations in airway management of the neurosurgical patient and offers solutions to common clinical problems that occur in this population of patients.

II. THE NEUROSURGICAL PATIENT

The American Academy of Neurological Surgeons (AANS) estimates that almost 1 million neurosurgical procedures are performed annually in the United States. Spine procedures are performed at three times the rate of cranial surgeries.[1] When considering the range of potential neurosurgical procedures, the variety of patients' pathophysiology is substantial. A patient presenting for neurosurgery may appear to be completely normal or can present with clinical symptoms of intracranial hypertension. The airway might be assessed as normal but the patient's head is fixed in a frame. Also, the patient may present with acromegaly for pituitary surgery or have a previous history of difficult intubation (DI). In addition, the unanticipated difficult airway (DA) becomes an even greater challenge in patients at risk for cerebral aneurysm rupture. Other challenges include the spine surgery patient in the prone position and considerations for extubation after prolonged surgery. Patients with central nervous system disease can be sensitive to the effects of hypnotic agents, which render them susceptible to apnea when premedication is given. Although neurosurgical procedures constitute only 7% of cases in the American Society of Anesthesiologists (ASA) closed claim database, they are associated with settlements that are 1.6 to 4 times more than those for general surgical procedures.[86] Understanding the patient's physiologic requirements, in addition to the surgeon's plan, is extremely important in this arena. It is wise to have a number of techniques for achieving, maintaining, and rescuing the neurosurgical airway.

A. INTRACRANIAL DYNAMICS AND THE AIRWAY

Intracranial pressure (ICP) is the pressure within the rigid skull. Airway management in the presence of intracranial hypertension is a frequent challenge for the neuroanesthesiologist as well as the emergency physician. The patient who does not require immediate airway control may benefit from the simple maneuver of elevating the head. The head-up position may have beneficial effects on ICP through changes in mean arterial pressure (MAP), airway pressure, central venous pressure, and cerebrospinal fluid displacement.[111] Cerebral perfusion pressure (CPP) is the effective perfusion pressure driving blood through the brain. It is defined as the difference between mean arterial and intracranial pressures ($CPP = MAP - ICP$). A frequent consideration in the neurosurgical patient is the need to balance and maintain intracranial dynamics, avoiding increases in ICP yet maintaining cerebral perfusion. Although head elevation may reduce ICP, raising the head above 30 degrees may place the patient at risk for a venous embolism, if performed intraoperatively.[4]

Ventilation is intimately related to cerebral blood flow (CBF) and is an integral part of neuroanesthesia management. The avoidance of hypercarbia is essential in management of patients with intracranial hypertension. Carbon dioxide dilates the cerebral blood vessels, increasing the volume of blood in the intracranial vault and therefore increasing ICP. Periarteriolar hydrogen ion concentration ($[H^+]$) powerfully influences cerebral arteriolar tone, and as the arterial carbon dioxide tension ($PaCO_2$) rises, $[H^+]$ increases, causing arteriolar dilatation. This leads to a concomitant decrease in cerebral vascular resistance, causing an increase in CBF and an increase in cerebral blood volume (CBV).[74] Difficult mask ventilation may quickly lead to hypercarbia, hypoxemia, and increased CBF. Hypoxia also remains one of the more potent arteriolar cerebrovascular dilators. Changes in the arterial oxygen tension (PaO_2) are associated with late increases in CBF. Hypoxia or ischemia leads to marked vasodilation, increased arterial vascular volume, and intracranial hypertension.[138]

Laryngoscopy and intubation, if performed with difficulty or improperly, can severely compromise intracranial dynamics and increase morbidity. Both the sympathetic and parasympathetic nervous systems mediate cardiovascular responses to endotracheal intubation.[156] Acute increases in ICP and MAP during laryngoscopy and endotracheal intubation have been well documented.[23,144] In 1975, Burney and Winn measured ICP in 12 patients undergoing craniotomy and 2 patients for carotid arteriogram. ICP did not change in response to the injection of contrast medium but rose significantly and dramatically in response to laryngoscopy and intubation. The increase appeared related to the initial ICP of these patients, possibly representing exhaustion of compensatory mechanisms.[29] Special attention must be given to this factor during manipulation of the larynx in neurosurgical patients with initial raised ICP or space-occupying intracranial lesions.

Techniques to blunt this sympathetic response have included (1) an additional dose of thiopental,[158] (2) use of β-blockers or other antihypertensive agents, and (3) use of intravenous lidocaine. Esmolol or lidocaine as an intravenous bolus of 1.5 mg/kg before laryngoscopy and intubation did not completely prevent the increase in MAP and ICP.[131] Etomidate has been shown to cause an early burst suppression pattern on electroencephalography, minimal changes in CPP, and a marked reduction in ICP. This decrease in ICP was maintained during the first 30 seconds and the following 60 seconds after intubation, as MAP and heart rate remained unchanged.[104] Although this is not a practical approach, it demonstrates the extent of efforts often made to obtund this response. Numerous methods have been advocated to prevent undesirable cardiovascular disturbances at intubation.[20] Whereas the cardiovascular response can be dramatic and substantial, the ICP response may lag behind and persist for a longer period of time. Once the patient is intubated, ventilation parameters may be adjusted to the clinical situation.

III. ISSUES IN MANAGEMENT OF PATIENTS

Airway assessment of the neurosurgical patient requires considerations similar to those described in other parts of this textbook. In particular, the patient who has undergone previous surgery and has a history of DI warrants particular attention. A review of the anesthetic record should reveal which techniques produced success or failure. Difficult mask ventilation is of particular concern because of the potential for causing hypercarbia and the detrimental changes described previously.

A. ELECTIVE CRANIOTOMY

Patients who are neurologically intact may demonstrate no evidence of intracranial pathology or alteration. Aside from history and physical examination, preoperative computed tomography (CT) or magnetic resonance imaging (MRI) scans of the head may give valuable information because lesions associated with a greater than 10 mm midline shift or cerebral edema usually indicate intracranial hypertension.[21] These patients should be appropriately managed to avoid undue increases in ICP and CBF. Such measures include proper head positioning, preoxygenation, and appropriate dosing of induction agents and relaxants to achieve a smooth intubation. The primary challenge in anesthetizing a patient with a supratentorial mass lesion is to avoid further increases in ICP when one has limited intracranial compliance. There is no "ideal anesthetic" for this group of patients, and the perioperative management should to be individualized. However, the anesthesiologist should be aware of the effects of anesthetic agents on intracranial dynamics.

The preoperative use of midazolam for anxiety in these patients should not cause harm if they are carefully observed. A 1- to 2-mg dose of intravenous midazolam in adult patients may facilitate the induction of anesthesia without altering intracranial dynamics.[53] Opioids, on the other hand, should be restricted to very small amounts and given under constant supervision because of possible hypercarbia and resultant effects. The efficacy of depth of anesthesia was recognized early as a technique for avoiding intracranial hypertension.[107] Deep inhalation anesthesia was replaced by a combination of intravenous induction agents, notably thiopental in combination with fentanyl. Thiopental produces a dose-dependent reduction in CBF and cerebral metabolic rate of oxygen consumption ($CMRO_2$). Other barbiturates, pentobarbital and methohexital, essentially have similar effects. ICP is reduced by barbiturates, probably because of the reduction in CBF and CBV. Propofol has largely replaced thiopental as the induction agent of choice for neuroanesthesia. Despite initial concerns about decreasing MAP and CPP, propofol provides a smooth transition to unconsciousness without an increase in heart rate, as observed with thiopental. This often produces less hypertension with laryngoscopy and intubation.[125,157]

Clinically used doses of most opioids have minimal to modest depressive effects on CBF and $CMRO_2$. Early studies demonstrate that ICP is either not elevated or slightly decreased with fentanyl alone or in combination with droperidol. Reported ICP increases in patients with space-occupying lesions have been attributed to hypercapnia.

The variability in response to opioids appears to be due to the background anesthetic. When vasodilating drugs are used as part of the anesthetic management, the effect of the opioid is consistently that of a vasoconstrictor. Sufentanil was thought to produce an increase in ICP in patients with an intracranial mass effect, but this was later attributed to a decrease in MAP.[167] Alfentanil produces little change or slight decreases in CBF.[147] The beneficial effect of synthetic opioids is in their ability to blunt the hemodynamic response to laryngoscopy and intubation without affecting intracranial dynamics. Remifentanil produces the most profound and consistent response with lack of hypertension, tachycardia, or increase in ICP.[38,59] A continuous infusion throughout induction may provide the most effective hemodynamic control while adequate ventilation is maintained.

The volatile agents, including nitrous oxide, can be considered dose-dependent cerebral vasodilators.[45] As a component of neuroanesthesia, volatile agents are commonly used in moderate doses in combination with opioids and hypnotic agents. The effects on cerebral circulation and metabolism of sevoflurane and desflurane are largely comparable to isoflurane. Both induce a direct vasodilation of the cerebral vessels, resulting in a less pronounced increase in CBF, compared with the decrease in cerebral metabolism.

Induction may be followed by hyperventilation with a volatile agent to deepen the anesthetic, decrease $CMRO_2$ (and CBF), and provide bronchodilation in patients with asthma or chronic obstructive pulmonary disease. Sevoflurane is useful in both pediatric and adult patients by allowing inhalation induction without the adverse effects of coughing or breath-holding.[50] A frequently employed technique in the cooperative patient is the use of active hyperventilation prior to induction. This initiates hypocapnia and decreases CBF as the patient loses consciousness. The use of topical anesthesia applied to the larynx and trachea can also prevent further response to laryngoscopy and intubation.[108] The large number of techniques recommended to suppress cardiovascular responses reflects the fact that no single method has gained widespread acceptance (Table 39-1).

The obtunded patient with symptoms of intracranial hypertension requires additional attention to detail, avoiding premedication and maneuvers that increase coughing. If a rapid sequence induction is not indicated and the patient's airway anatomy is adequate for laryngoscopy, anesthetic induction may proceed with voluntary hyperventilation with 100% oxygen by mask, if possible. Following loss of consciousness, manual hyperventilation should proceed both before and after administration of muscle relaxant. The administration of opioids may begin at this time to prevent the sympathetic response to laryngoscopy. Intravenous lidocaine (1 mg/kg) may be administered to blunt the hemodynamic and ICP response to laryngoscopy. Alternatively, a β-blocker or an additional dose of propofol may be given. Esmolol or lidocaine 1.5 mg/kg as an intravenous bolus before laryngoscopy

Table 39-1   **Anesthetic Techniques to Avoid Increased Intracranial Pressure**

	Precautions
Avoid hypercapnia	Be vigilant of patient's respiratory status
	Avoid undue sedation
Avoid hypoxia	Supplemental oxygen use mandatory
	Be vigilant of patient's respiratory status
	Take precautions to avoid aspiration
	Preoxygenation prior to induction of anesthesia/endotracheal intubation
Avoid marked hypertension	Be vigilant to changes in degree of painful stimulation
	Ensure adequate depth of anesthesia prior to intubation attempts/ surgical or procedural attempts
Avoid severe neck rotation	Attempt to maintain neck in neutral position
	Be vigilant to head positioning of patient during surgery
Avoid compression of jugular veins	Consider avoiding internal jugular neck lines when possible
Elevate head	If back-up position not possible, use reverse Trendelenburg position (avoid hypotension)
Decrease blood viscosity and intracerebral vascular volume	Avoid rapid infusion of mannitol, which may paradoxically increase intracranial pressure
Avoid sustained increases in intrathoracic pressure	Use maneuvers/pharmacology to avoid bucking, movement, vomiting
	Avoid high ventilatory pressures when possible
	Avoid positive end-expiratory pressure when possible
Avoid cerebral venodilators	Consider β-blocker use to treat hypertension
	Consider calcium channel blockers
	Avoid nitroglycerine, nitroprusside if possible

and intubation does not completely prevent the increase in MAP and ICP. Complete neuromuscular blockade should be verified prior to laryngoscopy to prevent cough and associated increases in ICP. Proper airway management is essential to avoid the twin insults of hypoxia and hypercarbia. An obstructed airway may also lead to a rise in intrathoracic pressure. This may produce an elevated venous pressure, increase in intracranial blood volume, and elevated ICP. If the patient can be mask ventilated but intubation is difficult, one may choose to proceed with an alternative device that may facilitate intubation.

The light wand can be useful in failed intubation, particularly in patients with a small chin or limited mouth opening. Because it is inserted without use of a laryngoscope, there is a potential for less hypertension and tachycardia. This finding was demonstrated by Nishikawa and colleagues in 60 patients undergoing awake intubation (AI) for emergency surgery.[113] Its successful use in the DA requires experience and practice.[4] Kihara and associates compared the hemodynamic responses of the light wand and intubating laryngeal mask airway (LMA Fastrach or ILMA) with direct

laryngoscopy in hypertensive and normotensive patients. In their series, both the ILMA and the light wand attenuated the hemodynamic stress response to endotracheal intubation compared with direct laryngoscopy in hypertensive, but not in normotensive, anesthetized paralyzed patients.[79] The ILMA is particularly useful in the failed intubation sequence, and the ability to ventilate is extremely important in neurosurgical patients. The success of the ILMA as a ventilatory device has been impressive, as demonstrated in several of the early evaluation studies.[17,43] It is also extremely useful in the setting of a failed fiberoptic intubation.[164]

The patient for aneurysm surgery who presents with a DA requires careful attention. If the airway is anticipated or known to be difficult, fiberoptic intubation is often the method of choice. This is assuming that one is skillful using the fiberoptic scope and is prepared to perform this technique in the awake, cooperative patient. See Chapter 10 regarding preparation for AI. Intravenous fentanyl and midazolam may be carefully administered if the patient does not exhibit signs of intracranial hypertension. An arterial line is generally placed prior to induction. Additional techniques include remifentanil infusion (0.05 µg/kg/min) and dexmedetomidine infusion.[57,129] Both techniques require careful monitoring of the patient and may be useful. Once the glottis is viewed, a dose of lidocaine may be given through the fiberoptic scope to prevent coughing and "bucking" with intubation.

Alternative techniques for failed sedation or topicalization include awake placement of the ILMA or other alternative techniques that do not produce excessive hemodynamic responses. The concomitant administration of β-blockers or vasodilators may be necessary for blood pressure (BP) control. Essentially, the ASA difficult airway management algorithm should be followed with close monitoring of BP and heart rate at all times until the airway is secured.

B. ACROMEGALY

Acromegaly is a rare condition afflicting three to four per million people.[97] Just a few years after Marie's 1882 description of the disease,[91] Chappel published a report of the death of an acromegalic patient secondary to airway obstruction.[33] Airway obstruction is one of several mechanisms that are associated with DI in these patients. The occurrence of the DA in acromegaly is well described, and the incidence of DI in these patients is reported to range from 10% to 30%.[43,101] This challenge has been attributed to prognathism, macroglossia, and thickening of pharyngeal and laryngeal soft tissue. In addition, thickening of the vocal cords, recurrent laryngeal nerve paralysis, decrease in width of the cricoid arch, and hypertrophy of arytenoepiglottic and ventricular folds have been described. Schmitt and coworkers found a 26% incidence of Cormack and Lehane grade III views on direct laryngoscopy in acromegalic patients[134] (Table 39-2).

Several case reports have described the inability to ventilate and intubate the acromegalic patient.[65,81] Preinduction airway assessment may not correlate with difficulty of intubation (Fig. 39-1). Although the Mallampati classification may be helpful, the thyromental distance is an insensitive indicator of difficulty of intubation. The lack of large prospective studies in this disease precludes an absolute statement regarding the predictive value of preoperative assessment for difficulty of intubation at this time.

Airway management in the acromegalic patient remains problematic. Several authors have advocated the use of awake fiberoptic intubation in patients with acromegaly[116,148,170] to avoid the creation of a surgical airway. In the patient with an anticipated DA, awake fiberoptic intubation remains the present standard of care.[48] When considering awake fiberoptic intubation in these patients, the increased incidence of coronary artery disease in patients with acromegaly should also be taken into account.[94] An anesthetic plan must be formulated to balance the risk of losing the airway and risk of precipitating myocardial ischemia. The plan should include (1) the presence of a second anesthesiologist if a DA is anticipated, (2) the presence of a DA cart, and (3) a surgeon who is skilled in performing a surgical airway.

In addition to difficulty with intubation of these patients, ventilation may be challenging. Various explanations have been given for the difficulty in ventilating these patients. The prognathic jaw may impede proper mask placement, the large tongue or redundancy of soft tissue may lead to airway obstruction with recumbence and the use of muscle relaxants, and the decreased range of neck motion secondary to cervical osteophyte formation may impede the attainment of proper sniffing position. There is a 16% to 30% incidence of upper airway obstruction diagnosed by spirometry in patients with acromegaly.[49,63] In addition, the incidence of sleep apnea is increased in these patients,[121]

Table 39-2   Airway Considerations in Patients with Acromegaly

Prognathic jaw
Macroglossia
Osteophyte formation of cervical spine and decreased range of motion of neck
Thickening of pharyngeal and laryngeal soft tissue
Thickening of vocal cords
Recurrent laryngeal nerve paralysis
Decrease in width of cricoid arch
Hypertrophy of arytenoepiglottic
Hypertrophy of ventricular folds
Central sleep apnea

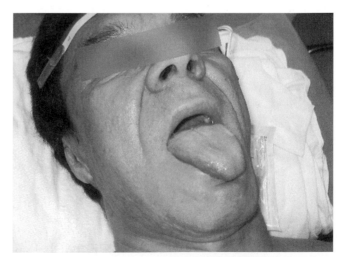

Figure 39-1 Patient with acromegaly. Note prognathic jaw and large facial features.

as well as stenosis of the cervical spine.[102] A history of obstructive sleep apnea, hoarseness, or stridor should alert the anesthesiologist to possible glottic and infraglottic involvement[106] and the potential for difficulty with intubation or ventilation, or both. This propensity toward airway obstruction must also be kept in mind in the immediate postoperative period, especially in the setting of bilateral nasal packing.[135,149] Postoperative negative-pressure pulmonary edema has been described in acromegalic patients because of partial obstruction following extubation.

The ILMA has been advocated as an adjunct for intubating patients with acromegaly, but the failure rate may be too high for its use as a primary tool. Law-Koune and associates reported a 47.4% first attempt failure rate with the ILMA in acromegalic patients induced with propofol.[85] The authors concluded, "The rate of failed blind intubation through the ILMA precludes its use as a first choice for elective airway management." Further research is required to determine whether the use of the ILMA as a conduit for light wand or fiberoptically assisted intubation would improve the success rate. As a rescue strategy in failed laryngoscopic or fiberoptic intubation, the ILMA may be an option if awakening the patient is not a realistic alternative. The technique of fiberoptic intubation through the LMA Classic (cLMA) (sizes 5 and 6) has been used by one of the authors in two patients with acromegaly when the ILMA did not allow successful intubation.

Use of video laryngoscopy may also be beneficial in this population of patients. Excellent results have been obtained at the author's institution using the GlideScope as a primary or secondary instrument for intubating patients with acromegaly (Fig. 39-2). The GlideScope's construction allows easy navigation around the large tongue and usually provides excellent visualization of the glottic opening.[152] Experience with the device is recommended in normal airways before attempting use in a potentially DA.

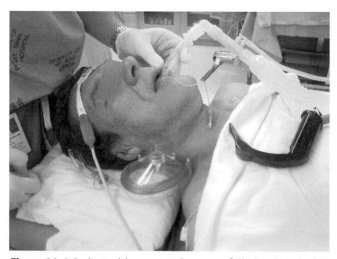

Figure 39-2 Patient with acromegaly successfully intubated with the GlideScope.

C. HEAD INJURY

Traumatic brain injury (TBI) is unfortunately a prevalent disease in the United States. The incidence of TBI is 175 to 300 per 100,000, and it accounts for 56,000 deaths per year in the United States.[19] With the increased use of seat belts, motor vehicle accidents are now secondary to gunshot wounds as the leading causes of TBI. Early intubation of the head-injured patient is critical and is often established in the field if providers are trained to do so. It is essential for optimal management of the patient as it (1) provides efficient ventilation and oxygenation, (2) helps to prevent aspiration of gastric contents, and (3) allows suction of the lungs and pulmonary toilet. However, patients who are unconscious and breathing adequately may be transported with oxygen by mask throughout their initial assessment. This is intuitive in the apneic and unresponsive patient with a Glasgow Coma Scale (GCS) score of 8 or less.

The GCS was introduced by Teasdale and Jennett in 1974.[153] The scale has remained a good predictor of neurologic outcome and has high degree of interobserver reproducibility. The GCS is divided into three components: eye opening, best motor response, and best verbal response. The highest obtainable scale is 15 and the lowest is 3. The scale may be qualified as minimal deficit (13 to 15), moderate deficit (9 to 12), severe deficit (3 to 8), and vegetative state (3). Uncooperative patients who require a CT scan or other radiologic studies usually require intubation because patients with suspected head injury should not be sedated without ensuring control of ventilation (i.e., endotracheal intubation).

The anesthesiologist caring for the patient with TBI must understand that although primary mechanisms of injury (*primary insults*) are a large determinant of the patient's outcome, attention to *secondary insults*, such as hypoxia, hypotension, intracranial hypertension, and decreased CPP, can dramatically affect morbidity, mortality, and quality of life of the TBI patient.[127] There is evidence to support this as mortality from TBI nationally has decreased over the past quarter century.[82,127] Mortality in severe head injury has fallen from about 36% in 1987[127] to 20% to 24% in a survey of head injury studies reported in 1997.[127] Hypoxia in TBI patients is a frequent occurrence, particularly in the prehospital setting. Interestingly, hypoxia was identified in 44% of patients with TBI on arrival in the emergency department.[142] Similarly, Jones and colleagues reported that hypoxia is one of three predictors of mortality in adult brain-injured patients.[76] Hypoxia dramatically impacts on morbidity and mortality in TBI. Miller and Becker found that hypoxia in TBI is associated with a doubling of mortality to 50% and that hypercapnia increased mortality to 67%.[103]

Hypotension is the secondary insult that has been most frequently cited as contributing to a poor outcome after TBI. Hypertension is independently related to mortality in multivariate analysis.[75] Information from the Traumatic Coma Data Bank illustrated that a systolic BP less than

80 mm Hg was one of five factors that worsened patients' outcome at 6 months.[92] Hypotension during any phase in the brain trauma patient's hospital course is associated with a greater likelihood of a severe disabled and vegetative state.[35,120] Hypotension, particularly early in the course of brain trauma and especially when combined with hypoxia, is devastating. Chestnut and colleagues showed that when hypotension and hypoxia occur together, mortality is 75%.[34] Furthermore, the frequency of hypotensive episodes in nonsurvivors of TBI is 150% that in survivors.

Techniques minimizing head movement should be utilized in TBI patients and by those who are the most skilled (Table 39-3). However, concern about a cervical fracture should never take precedence over relieving hypoxemia. It is of critical importance to ensure that appropriate monitoring is present throughout airway maneuvers. Nasal intubation should be avoided in head injury, particularly in patients with basilar skull fractures and sinus injuries. Alternative airway devices, such as the ILMA, any of the indirect rigid laryngoscopes, or light wand or fiberoptic stylets, may be useful in situations in which the head must remain immobilized.[136] As most emergency patients are assumed to have a "full stomach," it is important to weigh the risk of aspiration, which is a potential problem during laryngoscopy and intubation. If the situation warrants, surgeons should be prepared to perform a rapid cricothyroidotomy if intubation attempts fail and ventilation becomes impossible.

D. CERVICAL SPINE DISEASE

1. Acute Cervical Spine Injury

In the United States, cervical trauma has an incidence of approximately 5000 to 10,000 annually, making up 4% of all blunt trauma. The relative risk of cervical spinal injury (CSI) is increased in the presence of severe head injury by a factor greater than 8.[112] In trauma victims with a GCS of 13 to 15, the incidence of CSI is 1.4%, but the incidence rises dramatically to 10.2% if the GCS is less than 8. If a CSI is missed or its detection delayed, the incidence of secondary neurologic deficit increases from 1.4% to 10.5%.[58] Up to 4.3% of all cervical fractures may be missed, with two thirds of this group subsequently developing a neurologic deterioration. Where a diagnosis of CSI is delayed, almost one third of patients may develop permanent neurologic deficit.

One of the areas of controversy is how best to "clear" the cervical spine in the trauma patient. Detection of CSI requires a variety of modalities that vary in their sensitivity. These may include clinical evaluation, plain film radiographs, CT, MRI, and dynamic fluoroscopy.

a. Clinical Evaluation

In order to clear the cervical spine, the following criteria must be met:

1. GCS 15, with the patient alert and oriented
2. Absence of injuries that may draw attention away from a CSI
3. Absence of any drugs or intoxicants that may interfere with the patient's sensorium
4. Absence of signs or symptoms on examining the neck, specifically:
   a. No midline pain or tenderness
   b. Full range of active movement
   c. No neurologic deficit attributable to the cervical spine

Clearly, only a very small number of trauma patients fulfill these criteria.

i. Plain Radiographs The cross-table lateral view alone, even if technically adequate and interpreted by an expert, misses 15% of injuries. Of cross-table lateral films taken in emergency rooms, approximately a quarter are anatomically inadequate, necessitating further imaging modalities for evaluation, usually of the cervicothoracic junction. A three-view cervical series includes the cross-table lateral view, open mouth odontoid view, and anterior-posterior view. Using these views, the sensitivity increases to detect 90% of those with an actual injury. Again, from 25% to 50% of these series may be inadequate anatomically. In low-risk

Table 39-3 **Airway Techniques for the Unstable Cervical Spine**

Awake fiberoptic intubation
Nasal intubation
Indirect rigid laryngoscopy
Bullard, Wu, and Upsher scopes
GlideScope and DCI Video Laryngoscope
Direct laryngoscopy with in-line stabilization
Fiberoptic intubation using laryngeal mask airway (LMA) as conduit
LMA Classic
LMA-Fastrach
LMA C-Trach
Intubating laryngeal airway
Light wand or fiberoptic lighted stylets
Trachlight
Shikani Optical Stylet and Bonfils Retromolar Intubation Fiberscope
Retrograde intubation
Surgical airway
Cricothyrotomy
Tracheostomy

patients, plain radiography is an efficient diagnostic examination with a specificity of 100%. In high-risk patients, plain radiography is a good adjunctive screening examination in conjunction with CT scan, with a sensitivity of 93.3% and specificity of 95%[112] (Figs. 39-3 to 39-5).

ii. Computed Tomography CT scanning (either of the entire cervical spine or directed at areas missed by plain film radiographs), when used in addition to the three-view cervical series, enables a complementary approach and reduces the risk of missing a CSI to less than 1%. In the evaluation of the cervical spine, a helical CT scan has higher sensitivity and specificity than plain radiographs in the moderate- and high-risk trauma population, but it is more costly. In fact, helical CT scanning is the preferred initial screening test for detection of cervical spine fractures among moderate- to high-risk patients seen in urban trauma centers, reducing the incidence of paralysis resulting from false-negative imaging studies and institutional costs, when settlement costs are taken into account.[58]

It is not uncommon for the anesthesiologist to be confronted with a patient with a CSI who requires intubation. In one series, 26% of patients admitted to a large trauma center required intubation over the first day of admission. There is, furthermore, a growing body of literature indicating that any patient with a CSI above C5 should be intubated electively, early in the course of

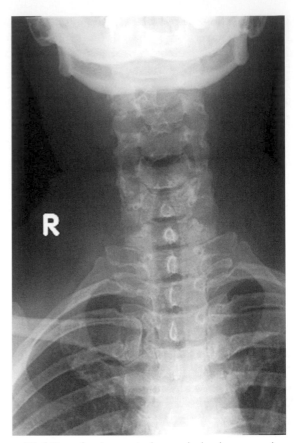

Figure 39-4 Normal anteroposterior cervical spine x-ray view. (Courtesy of Prasanna Vibhute, MD, Department of Radiology, Mount Sinai Medical Center.)

the presentation.[160] The following survey attempts to review airway devices and assign utility on the basis of the clinical presentation of cervical injury.

Direct laryngoscopy, if performed appropriately, is safe in the setting of CSI.[118,133,139,146,169] No neurologic sequelae were noted in a review of 73 patients with known

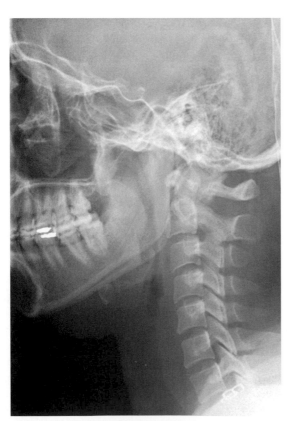

Figure 39-3 Normal lateral cervical spine x-ray view. (Courtesy of Prasanna Vibhute, MD, Department of Radiology, Mount Sinai Medical Center.)

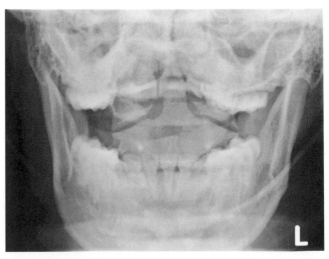

Figure 39-5 Normal odontoid cervical spine x-ray view. (Courtesy of Prasanna Vibhute, MD, Department of Radiology, Mount Sinai Medical Center.)

cervical spine fractures intubated after rapid sequence induction with the application of cricoid pressure and manual in-line stabilization of the head and neck and direct laryngoscopy.[42] Although potentially uncomfortable and despite concerns about undue head movement, awake direct laryngoscopy has been shown to be safe.[100] When intubating the patient with direct laryngoscopy, the anterior portion of the hard cervical collar can be removed to facilitate opening of the mouth at the time of intubation, yet in-line stabilization must be maintained.

b. Effects of Direct Laryngoscopy

The effects of direct laryngoscopy have been studied in a range of patients, including those with normal neck anatomy under anesthesia, as well as in cadavers with and without cervical lesions caused to simulate fractures at a variety of levels.[88] In the anesthetized paralyzed patient whose cervical anatomy is normal, a variety of movements may occur using a No. 3 Macintosh blade. On elevation of the blade to obtain a view of the larynx, there is superior rotation of the occiput and C1 in the sagittal plane, C2 remains near neutral, and there is mild inferior rotation of C3-C5.[87] The most significant movement is produced at the atlanto-occipital and atlantoaxial joints. In cadaveric models of unstable cervical segments (C1-C2) the movement associated with maneuvers such as chin lift and jaw thrust are greater than those produced by the intubation itself. The application of cricoid pressure produced no significant movement at the site of injury in this setting.

c. Immobilization

In view of the risk of secondary neurologic injury to the acutely injured, unstable cervical spine, it is widely viewed as the standard of care to immobilize the cervical spine in situations in which this is suspected. The most commonly practiced measures include manual in-line immobilization, immobilization of the head between two sandbags, and placement of a rigid cervical collar and spinal board. This latter management is far from benign and is itself associated with significant morbidity and mortality. It may increase the difficulty of intubation or increase the likelihood of airway compromise and risk of aspiration. Nonetheless, the use of manual in-line immobilization (not traction) is the best means to minimize movement of the cervical spine during airway manipulations and should always be practiced. It should be recognized, however, that the presence of a cervical collar does not necessarily protect against movement at the occipitocervical and cervicothoracic junctions.

In a cooperative patient, awake fiberoptic intubation allows the patient to be intubated without movement of the cervical spine. It may be performed with a hard collar in place, which is one of the benefits of this technique. The patient's airway may be topicalized, which may, in theory, increase the potential for aspiration in patients at risk for regurgitation and aspiration. Ovassapian and coauthors found, however, no evidence of aspiration in a review of 105 patients at risk.[117] Awake fiberoptic intubation may prove to be time consuming and unsuccessful in as many as 90% on the first attempt.[2] It is because of these issues (i.e., lack of assurance of expedient intubation and risk of aspiration) that we advocate that the fiberoptic bronchoscope be used in the cooperative patient in the urgent situation and in the nonurgent patient who is not at risk for aspiration. This recommendation is a general guideline, and expertise with any given airway device must be taken into account when utilizing an airway technique in a specific clinical situation.

Another alternative to direct laryngoscopy is the ILMA. Wahlen, Waltl, and colleagues claimed that the ILMA produced less extension of the upper cervical spine than direct laryngoscopy.[161,163] The ILMA has been shown to be an expedient method of securing the airway in patients with cervical collars and unstable necks.[136] Ferson and associates, in a series of 254 difficult-to-manage airways, reported 70 patients with acutely unstable necks who were all successfully intubated with the ILMA, 92.6% on first attempt and 7.4% on the second attempt.[51] There was no report of worsening neurologic outcome or aspiration as a result of this intervention.

This information has to be viewed, however, in light of cadaveric experiments in which the ILMA has been demonstrated to create posterior pressure on the midportion of the cervical spine.[26,126] This may be particularly relevant in cervical flexion injuries. If the ILMA is to be used in a patient in a hard cervical collar with cricoid pressure, one should be aware of difficulties, which have been described in this scenario. In one study in which intubation was attempted with the ILMA in patients who were in a cervical collar and receiving the Sellick maneuver, the failure rate was 80%.[162] Another study addressing the patient with cervical pathology and neurologic outcome was described by Brimacombe in which 106 patients were intubated using the ILMA. Almost all (99%) tolerated the procedure without neurologic sequelae, and one patient (1%) developed a new neurologic deficit (allegedly unrelated to airway management).[27] Wong and colleagues presented two cases in which the ILMA was used in awake topicalized patients with unstable cervical spines without difficulty.[168] In light of these studies indicating that the ILMA may produce cervical motion and excessive pressure on the cervical spine and the fact that it is difficult to place with application of cricoid pressure and the presence of a hard cervical collar, the authors feel that the ILMA cannot be recommended as a primary device in the setting of acute cervical injury. It should be viewed as a rescue device should direct or fiberoptic intubation fail.

Cricothyrotomy has been suggested as an alternative to direct laryngoscopy in patients with cervical neck trauma[47]; however, it has been demonstrated that cricothyrotomy may produce a small but significant movement of the cervical spine.[56] Although often suggested as a primary mode of intubation of the unstable patient with CSI, the procedure is associated with a high complication rate.[95,124]

In one study of long-term complications in emergency departments in the United Kingdom, only 41.5 % survived to hospital discharge. A mere 25.9% of these patients who survived experienced no long-term complications (10.9% of all patients receiving emergency cricothyroidotomy).[73] This high incidence of complications may be related to the decreasing number of cricothyroidotomies performed[32] and the unfamiliarity of many physicians with the procedure.[66] Emergency cricothyrotomy may be associated with infection, and it may interfere with the anterior repair of the cervical fracture.

The incidence of emergency surgical airway in the setting of trauma has decreased over the past several decades. In one review of procedures preformed by emergency medicine residents during their training, emergency cricothyrotomy was performed on an average of only once or twice over the course of an entire residency. It is therefore the view of the authors that emergency cricothyrotomy should be reserved as a rescue procedure in the management of the airway in patients with acute cervical spine injuries.

Another alternative for the patient with acute cervical trauma is the GlideScope. This relatively new device allows indirect laryngoscopy without alignment of the oral, pharyngeal, and tracheal axes.[152] It provides an excellent laryngoscopic view,[40] with 100% of patients having a Cormack-Lehane grade I or II view. In 45% of patients the view is improved by one or two grades over the direct laryngoscopic view.[122] Use of the GlideScope is promising in the intubation of the DA as a primary or a rescue device.[41] The authors have used the GlideScope for patients requiring rapid sequence induction who are unable to extend the neck fully. We have not encountered difficulty with this method and have not witnessed aspiration during this procedure. The DCI Video Laryngoscope (Karl Storz Endoscopy, Culver City, CA) was also proved to be useful in situations in which neck mobility is decreased or cervical motion minimized.[61]

Optimal airway management strategies in patients with an unstable CSI remain controversial. The light wand (Trachlight) or an intubating fiberoptic stylet, such as the Shikani Optical Stylet (Clarus Medical, Minneapolis, MN) or Bonfils Retromolar Intubation Fiberscope (Karl Storz Endoscopy), may avoid hyperextension of the neck. However, there are few objective data that guide us in selecting the appropriate devices. Inoue and colleagues conducted a prospective randomized study of 148 patients receiving general anesthesia for procedures related to clinical or radiographic evidence of cervical abnormality.[71] The Trachlight or ILMA was used for endotracheal intubation with the head and neck held in a neutral position. In the Trachlight group, intubation was successful at the first attempt in 67 of 74 (90.5%) cases and at the second attempt in 5 (6.8%) cases. In contrast, in the ILMA group, 54 of 74 (73.0%) patients were intubated within the protocol. The mean time for successful endotracheal intubation at the first attempt was significantly shorter in the Trachlight group than in the ILMA group. The Trachlight may be more advantageous for orotracheal intubation in patients with cervical spine disorders than the ILMA with respect to reliability, rapidity, and safety. Skill and experience with the device are essential to achieving this success.

d. Intubation of the Unstable Patient with a Cervical Spinal Injury

As appreciated from the preceding discussion, the problem with airway management in these settings is that the techniques that are normally employed to secure the airway have the potential to cause movement and thereby risk causing secondary neurologic injury. Although a strategy for clearing the cervical spine has been outlined, the emergent nature of management of these often multiply injured patients may mean that time does not permit this to be done. There therefore remains a group of patients whose cervical spinal integrity is uncertain and who must be managed as if their cervical spine is, in fact, injured. In addition, although it may be desirable on occasion to perform an awake fiberoptic intubation, in reality the patient may not be able to cooperate for reasons of intoxication, hypoxia, or head injury. As has been discussed, the need for the airway to be secured is often urgent as a consequence of the spinal injury or associated head or facial injury.

Another confounding problem is that cricoid pressure may either obstruct or occlude the airway even when appropriately applied.[141] Also, the presence of a rigid cervical collar may make airway management difficult. It may impede adequate mouth opening and make airway maneuvers more difficult. Application of cricoid pressure is also difficult to impossible with the collar in place. For these reasons, with manual in-line immobilization in place, we recommend that the front part of the collar be removed or opened prior to attempted intubation.

The Combitube is a supraglottic ventilatory device that is designed to function as an alternative to ventilation by mask and endotracheal intubation (see Chapter 25 for details).[5] As is the LMA, the Combitube is recommended as a primary rescue device in "cannot intubate, cannot ventilate" situations by the European Resuscitation Council, the American Heart Association, and the ASA.[8,155] It is considered an alternative to conventional airway management devices in difficult and emergency airway management.[16] Compared with conventional endotracheal intubation, (1) it can be easily and promptly inserted, (2) it may be inserted blindly, and (3) it provides adequate ventilation and oxygenation when situated in the esophageal or tracheal position.[83]

The Combitube allows application of positive pressures and is thought to minimize the risk of aspiration. It has also been used effectively in prehospital ventilatory management. It has been used in elective patients as well as in emergency situations.[55] Its use in conventional airway management may, however, be complicated by an unsatisfactory incidence of sore throat and dysphagia.[22]

In patients with cervical spine abnormalities, such as in patients with functional restriction (e.g., trauma)[46] or anatomic restriction (e.g., rheumatoid arthritis or prior cervical fixation) of cervical movement, it may be inserted with minimal realignment of the cervical spine.[99,139] It may be considered in patients who are in a halo with ventilatory failure after extubation.[98] Its use is contraindicated in patients with tracheal or esophageal trauma.

The Combitube is designed to isolate the lungs from the esophagus, and therefore it may be considered in patients at risk for aspiration (e.g., trauma, CSI). The Combitube is available in two sizes: 37 Fr SA (small to average height adults) and 41 Fr (patients taller than 72 inches).[6] A pediatric size is not commercially available at present.

2. Chronic Spine Disease with Myelopathy

Just as patients with ischemic heart disease present for noncardiac surgery, patients with cervical spine disease present for surgery for non-neurosurgical procedures. Thus, their airway management is of interest to all and not solely those providing anesthesia for complex spinal surgery (Fig. 39-6). One of the problems in relation to this group of patients is predicting difficulty with intubation, by both direct laryngoscopy and fiberoptic intubation.[136]

Regarding fiberoptic intubation, the traditional bedside tests commonly used to predict difficult direct laryngoscopy may not necessarily be predictive of difficulty in fiberoptic intubation. Difficulty with visualizing the vocal cords in fiberoptic intubation has been extensively documented and is most commonly due to secretions or blood or both in the airway, distortion of the upper airway, and, of particular relevance, resistance to passage of the endotracheal tube (ET) in a high proportion of cases. The last problem has been shown to relate to the size of the fiberscope in relation to the ET and indeed the design of the ET itself. Patients with rheumatoid arthritis may pose additional difficulty because of alteration in the plane of their vocal cords. Efforts at establishing which features of the patient influence difficulty in the passage of the ET, or impingement, have been directed at examining radiologically common features. Neither the Mallampati grade nor the thyromental distance correlated with the degree of impingement on passage of the tube. There was, however, a positive correlation with the size of the epiglottis and the size of the tongue. The thickness was more important than the length of the tongue, an issue of particular relevance in patients with acromegaly.

DI is well recognized as more common in patients with cervical spine disease. In particular, ankylosing spondylitis, rheumatoid arthritis, and Klippel-Feil abnormality, among others, are all conditions presenting additional difficulty. One of the problems with predicting DI is its incidence and the sensitivity and specificity of the tests used to detect it.[72] DI in the undifferentiated anesthesia community has an incidence of approximately 1%. The positive predictive value (PPV, the proportion of cases predicted to be difficult that actually were so) of the commonly used tests such as Mallampati or Wilson Risk Sum is about 8%, and the PPV of the tests used in combination is approximately 30%.[115] With tests predicting DI with a sensitivity of 95% and specificity of 99%, there is a 51% false-positive rate. However, if the prevalence of DI is theoretically 10%, the problem of false positives would decrease to 8.7% (with sensitivity of 95% and specificity of 99%). One might, therefore, expect prediction of DI to be more rewarding in a subgroup of patients with a high incidence of DI such as those with cervical spine disease. In an effort to improve prediction of DI, discriminant analysis has been employed to examine the PPV of tests in this population of patients, with an improvement of 68%.

A number of important correlates have emerged from this examination. As previously discussed, when performing direct laryngoscopy, most significant movement is produced at the atlanto-occipital and atlantoaxial joints.[133] It should come as no surprise, therefore, that patients with reduced mobility at this level present increased difficulty of intubation.[30] There is, however, a highly significant association between disease of the occipitoatlantoaxial complex and impaired mandibular protrusion. This is mainly, but not uniquely, due to rheumatoid disease. It should be noted that extension at the craniocervical junction is needed in order to open the mouth fully, yet another limiting factor when it comes to direct laryngoscopy.

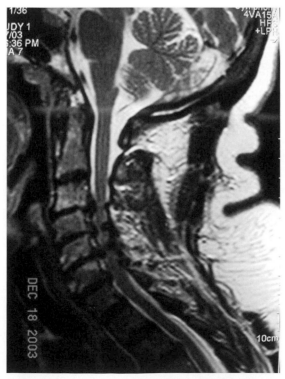

Figure 39-6 Cervical stenosis in an elderly patient.

a. Rheumatoid Arthritis

Three areas in which rheumatoid arthritis affects the airway and cervical spine are worthy of particular mention, namely cricoarytenoid arthritis, temporomandibular arthritis, and atlantoaxial instability.[15]

The presence of laryngeal involvement in rheumatoid arthritis is 45% to 88%. Depending on which investigations are used, 59% demonstrate laryngeal involvement on physical examination, 14% show extrathoracic airway obstruction on spirometry, and 69% show one or more signs of laryngeal involvement. Of those with laryngeal involvement, 75% have symptoms of breathing difficulties. For these, the greatest risk is after extubation. Intubation, even if of brief duration, can lead to sufficient mucosal edema to cause postextubation stridor and airway obstruction. Interestingly, the incidence of postextubation stridor is much lower following fiberoptic intubation (1%) than after direct laryngoscopy (14%).[62] Up to two thirds of patients with long-standing rheumatoid arthritis may have limited temporomandibular joint mobility with consequent limited mouth opening. Of those with severe temporomandibular joint destruction, up to 70% may undergo episodes of airway obstruction similar to that seen in patients with micrognathia or sleep apnea syndrome.[68]

Atlantoaxial instability is present in roughly 25% of all patients with rheumatoid arthritis and is more likely to be seen in patients with severe peripheral rheumatoid involvement. Symptoms correlate poorly with radiologic findings, and a worrying aspect of this is that some series have found atlantoaxial instability in approximately 5% of patients with rheumatoid arthritis presenting for elective orthopedic surgery. The direction of the instability is variable, and a significant percentage exhibit vertical subluxation or cranial "settling." This results in impingement of the odontoid peg on the brain stem[165] (Fig. 39-7).

The patient who presents for elective surgery with symptoms of cervical myelopathy deserves careful airway management to avoid further injury. Intubation techniques described for the CSI patient are appropriate and best performed by experienced practitioners. When possible, AI followed by demonstration of extremity movement is ideal and recommended. When this is not possible, a technique that produces minimal head movement and airway maintenance is acceptable. A thoughtful approach is based on the patient's anatomy, risk of intubation difficulty, and a rescue plan for intubation or ventilation failure.

IV. FAILED INTUBATION OR ANTICIPATED DIFFICULT AIRWAY

A. CERVICAL IMMOBILIZATION

1. Halo Devices

Early halo immobilization is a common practice in patients with potentially unstable cervical injuries and may facilitate the diagnostic work-up and treatment of

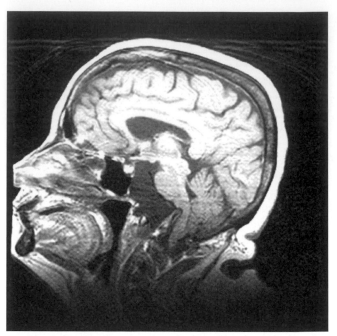

Figure 39-7 Patient with rheumatoid arthritis and migration of the odontoid peg.

trauma patients with multiple injuries.[67] The halo device provides the most rigid form of external cervical immobilization (Fig. 39-8). Although the halo is an effective form of cervical immobilization, complications with its use are periodically encountered. This cumbersome device prevents easy access to the patient's airway and also prevents extension of the head. Patients treated with halo fixation present unique challenges in terms of airway control. The halo prevents proper positioning for laryngoscopy by restricting atlanto-occipital extension. Oral intubation is often possible, but it is a function of other variables such as mouth opening, tongue size, upper dentition, and ability to protrude the lower jaw forward. In the nonemergent setting, fiberoptic bronchoscopy can overcome the

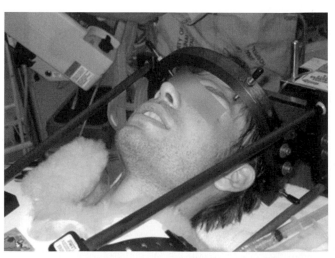

Figure 39-8 Young patient immobilized in a halo.

difficulties in intubating these patients,[77] but in an emergency setting, these intubations can be extremely difficult. Sims and Berger reported a retrospective survey of 105 patients managed with halo fixation at a level I trauma center. In this series, 14 of the patients (13%) required emergent or semiemergent airway control, with almost half the patients dying in the attempts or shortly after.[143] On the basis of their findings, the authors suggested that early tracheostomy be considered in hospitalized trauma patients requiring halo fixation who present with a high Injury Severity Score, a history of cardiac disease, or a condition requiring intubation on arrival. Patients who are intubated on arrival may be more likely to require emergent reintubation during their hospital stay. Older patients and those with a history of cardiac disease are more at risk for arrest-related death (Table 39-4).

Respiratory failure or airway obstruction in the patient wearing a halo frame becomes a serious emergency. If the airway needs to be secured and endotracheal intubation has failed, the use of adjuncts may be lifesaving. The halo frame immobilizes the head and neck and prevents use of the sniffing position for laryngoscopy or assisted ventilation. Case reports have described a variety of techniques for airway rescue in the patient wearing halo fixation. The Bullard laryngoscope was used after failed laryngoscopy in a patient who additionally had a DA.[37] The ILMA was successfully used in an awake patient when a fiberoptic scope was unavailable.[137] This device was also used by one of the authors after a failed intubation attempt following a respiratory arrest. A Combitube was utilized by Mercer in a 78-year-old patient suffering respiratory deterioration following extubation when LMA insertion proved impossible.[98]

Patients who present for elective surgery in halo fixation should be approached carefully with a plan for intubation. The techniques described earlier for the anticipated DA should be employed. It is imperative that clinicians involved have (1) skills and equipment for alternative intubation techniques, (2) a neurosurgeon or professional who can safely remove the halo if necessary, and (3) a rescue plan in case of failed ventilation in these challenging patients.

2. Stereotactic Head Frames

Stereotactic localization is widely used in neurosurgery and has revolutionized practice over the past 30 years. The term "stereotactic" originated from the Greek words *stereo* meaning three-dimensional and *tactos* meaning touched. Lars Leksell is best known as the neurosurgeon who brought stereotaxis into easy clinical use, although it was originally described by Horsley and Clarke in 1908.[119] In 1949, he designed the first instrument to be based on the arc-center principle, a system that provided precise mechanical three-dimensional control in intracranial space. It served to identify the target and to calculate the angles and distances to be used with the frame. The stereotactic system has undergone many refinements over the years. The early stereotactic frames produced by Leksell provided head fixation but significantly interfered with airway access. The later frames have a cross-bar that may (potentially) be directed cephalad for easier access to the nose and mouth. The cross-bar can be removed by unscrewing two screws with an Allen wrench (which should always be available). Despite moderate access to the airway, head positioning and fixation to the table can make proper positioning for airway management extremely difficult (Fig. 39-9).

Applications of stereotaxis are increasing, and it is presently used for biopsy, craniotomy, or procedures for movement disorders. Neuronavigational techniques require the acquisition of radiologic studies such as CT or MRI while the patient is wearing the stereotactic frame. Stereotactic neurosurgery may require general anesthesia or conscious sedation. Cooperative patients who are neurologically intact may easily tolerate frame placement under sedation with local anesthetic applied at the pin sites. Conscious sedation is desirable when patients must be transported for diagnostic radiologic procedures in the head frames. This is the anesthetic technique appropriate for intracranial biopsies and the surgical treatment of Parkinson's disease. The use of intravenous sedation must be carefully monitored, and the agents chosen should provide analgesia, sedation, and cardiovascular stability.[84]

Table 39-4 **Recommendations for Early Tracheostomy in Trauma Patients with Halo Fixation**

High cervical injury score
History of cardiac disease
Age older than 60 years
Intubated on arrival
Previous history of difficult intubation
Anticipated length of intubation greater than 1 week
Capability of surgical airway not available

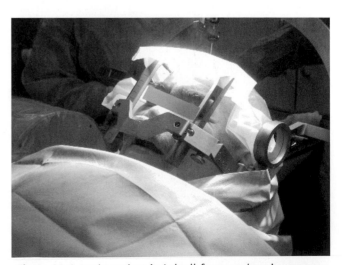

Figure 39-9 Awake patient in Leksell frame undergoing surgery.

Oxygen should be administered by nasal cannula, and monitoring of capnography is extremely useful. It is essential to monitor head positioning during frame fixation to the operating table. Excessive head flexion may lead to airway obstruction when sedative agents are given.[151]

Potential complications of the surgical procedure include bleeding and the potential for air entrainment. Air entrainment may occur from the surgical site if near the venous sinuses or from the pin sites if placed near diploic veins.[14] This is usually noted by the development of coughing, dyspnea, and decreased oxygen saturation. It is important to make the diagnosis and inform the surgeon, who must then flood the operative field to prevent further air entry. Another, and more serious, risk is internal bleeding. Postoperatively, patients usually undergo a CT scan to check for signs of hemorrhage or hematoma formation.

The patient's cooperation is an important factor in these procedures, and pediatric patients, obtunded patients, and those at risk for seizures present increased management challenges. The obese patient or the patient susceptible to airway obstruction requires careful consideration for this technique, which perhaps should be done under general anesthesia. When this decision is made, the patient is anesthetized and intubated before frame placement and must be ventilated, sedated, and monitored for transport to and from a diagnostic radiologic area. Alternatively, a cooperative patient may tolerate placement of the head frame and diagnostic radiology but the lesion is in the occipital region requiring prone positioning. This problem may be solved by AI in the head frame, followed by positioning after anesthesia is induced. If AI fails, an alternative technique may be utilized (Figs. 39-10 to 39-12). The LMA is extremely useful in this scenario and may be used as the sole airway in appropriate patients having the procedure in the supine position. It is important to be familiar with a number of airway techniques and to have a plan for alternative methods of airway management should these challenges occur[36] (Table 39-5).

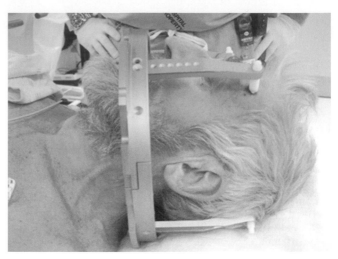

Figure 39-11 Lateral view of patient in stereotactic frame.

B. AWAKE CRANIOTOMY

Craniotomy in the awake state has been performed since ancient times. Present-day indications include resection of a lesion in the eloquent or speech center of the brain. Surgical procedures for the treatment of epilepsy, tumors, or arteriovenous malformation are sometimes performed in the awake patient. With refinement of neurophysiologic monitoring techniques, awake craniotomies are necessary in only a small percentage of patients. However, surgery for movement disorders has again increased the use of this technique. Intraoperative complications of awake craniotomy include restlessness and agitation.[10] This may occur when the patient is overly sedated yet experiences discomfort. More serious complications are hypoventilation, nausea, and seizures.[44] A change in the level of sedation often resolves these problems. It is important to maintain good rapport with the patient, which was ideally established preoperatively. Comfortable positioning of the patient to avoid discomfort, allowing surgical access, and avoidance of a claustrophobic atmosphere are essential

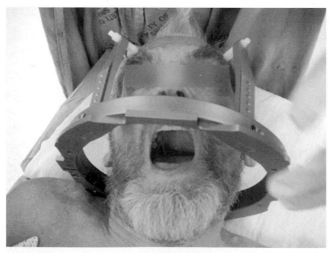

Figure 39-10 Patient for stereotactic biopsy; note limited airway access.

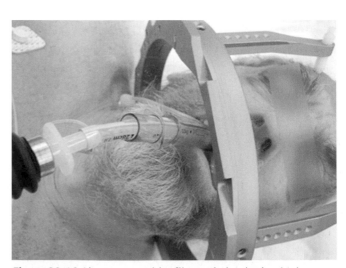

Figure 39-12 Airway secured by fiberoptic intubation by laryngeal mask.

Table 39-5   Airway Management Techniques for Stereotactic Surgery

Spontaneous ventilation with oxygen supplementation
Awake or asleep laryngeal mask airway (LMA)
Awake oral or nasal fiberoptic intubation
Spontaneous intubation and blind nasal intubation
Awake or asleep fiberoptic intubation by LMA
Awake or asleep lighted stylet intubation

and require cooperation of the entire operating room staff.

The evolution of anesthetic technique has progressed from fentanyl-droperidol to the current use of propofol infusion with alfentanil or remifentanil or dexmedetomidine.[128,168] Intraoperative nausea is rare with the use of propofol infusions. Dexmedetomidine is a selective α_2-adrenergic agonist that has been shown to produce sedation and analgesia without respiratory depression. The onset is slower than that of propofol, and it must be given by infusion. This may be beneficial for the older patient, pediatric patient, or potentially debilitated patient and has been used throughout intraoperative testing.[11] Seizure control is sometimes necessary; methohexital (1 mg/kg) or a benzodiazepine (midazolam) is effective. Terminating the seizure requires careful titration of sedatives to avoid apnea.

If necessary, general anesthesia may be required for an uncooperative or very young patient.[60] The "asleep-awake-asleep" technique has been utilized by some centers in an effort to minimize patients' discomfort and perhaps provide better operating conditions for the surgeon. The patient undergoes a light general anesthetic with additional local anesthesia and is awakened intraoperatively for testing at the appropriate time.

Airway management can be challenging, and several maneuvers have been reported. Huncke and colleagues utilized awake fiberoptic intubation, which was accomplished in 10 patients.[70] This effective but arduous technique required significant skill and a special catheter to deliver local airway anesthetic. Some clinicians have also utilized nasal airways and blind nasal intubation, assuming that one does not cause bleeding or significant discomfort. The most useful technique in recent years has been the LMA for control of the airway.[132] This has been described in several reports and can be achieved (with skill) without having to remove drapes or change the position of the patient.[140] In our experience using the cLMA and the LMA-ProSeal for adults, patients could be induced and asleep for the resection after the intraoperative testing was finished. This allowed the surgeon a "quiet field" as many patients become hypercarbic while awake and sedated (Fig. 39-13). The LMA-ProSeal is particularly advantageous for the ability to provide positive-pressure ventilation and entry into the gastric tract.[27]

C. EMBOLIZATION PROCEDURES

Endovascular treatment of intracranial aneurysms and arteriovenous malformations is now an option for many patients. This new therapy offers significant decreases in morbidity, mortality, and hospital stay compared with craniotomy.[89,171] In patients with acute subarachnoid hemorrhage, one must consider the likelihood of increased ICP, changes in transmural pressure, and cerebral ischemia. During endovascular treatment, the two most serious potential complications are cerebral infarction and hemorrhage. Endovascular coiling may be safely applied within hours of the aneurysm rupture with a low probability of aneurysm perforation. General anesthesia is preferred for patients who have acute subarachnoid hemorrhage. Despite concern for neurologic evaluation, most neuroradiologists now prefer general anesthesia for optimal imaging studies and techniques. Airway control through an ET or LMA allows improved oxygenation, anesthetic administration, and a motionless patient. Radiologic imaging methods include high-resolution fluoroscopy and high-speed digital subtraction angiography (DSA) with a "road mapping" function. The computer superimposes images onto live fluoroscopy so that the progress of the radiopaque catheter tip can be seen. Any motion during this stage of the procedure profoundly degrades the image. The anesthesiologist is typically off to the side of the patient and must

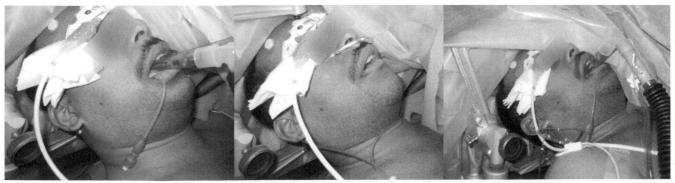

Figure 39-13 "Asleep-awake-asleep" technique utilizing the laryngeal mask airway ProSeal.

negotiate around the myriad of monitors and equipment, which are part of this terrain. One benefit of this environment is the ability to obtain fluoroscopic confirmation of ET positioning or make the diagnosis of atelectasis.

Although the radiology suite may be in a remote location, the patient with an anticipated DA should be approached in the same manner as in the operating room. A potential limiting factor is the flat table, which does not allow the patient's head to be raised. Supporting blankets should be utilized to produce the optimal position for laryngoscopy or AI, if necessary. The techniques described earlier apply in this setting, and the authors have utilized the fiberoptic bronchoscope, ILMA, light wand, and GlideScope in the radiology suite. Emergence from anesthesia should be smooth with avoidance of excessive coughing and bucking. Hypertension should be controlled to prevent potential cerebral edema and bleeding at the femoral cannulation site. There is minimal pain, and patients are required to remain supine for a period of time.

D. THE ROLE OF THE LARYNGEAL MASK AIRWAY IN NEUROSURGERY

Although use of both the LMA and ILMA for neurosurgical procedures has been previously described, this section addresses additional issues and further details of their use in this population of patients. The LMA can in no way be a substitute for the ET, but it can be used in a number of situations in which an ET would be difficult or impossible to insert. In addition, the beneficial effects on cardiovascular and intracranial reflexes make it a wise choice in certain neurosurgical procedures. This assumes that one is skilled in its placement and manages the anesthetic appropriately. Several case reports described LMA use in craniotomy, but these were scenarios of failed intubation and the necessity for an airway in fasted patients.[3,12] Although the ILMA has been discussed extensively as a device for airway management in patients with limited neck movement, its role in the failed intubation scenario was demonstrated by Combes and colleagues. In their prospective study of unanticipated DI, they concluded that the ILMA and the gum elastic bougie are effective to solve most problems occurring during unexpected DA management.[39] This is particularly important for the neurosurgical patient who may not easily tolerate repeated laryngoscopy attempts, inadequate ventilation, and excessive hypertension and tachycardia.

The cLMA can also be used as a conduit for fiberoptic intubation as a rescue airway technique and is preferred by some clinicians over the ILMA.[24] The cLMA, as well as the ILMA, can be inserted with the patient in a variety of positions. This becomes useful in the dreaded situation of extubation in the prone position as well as loss of the airway in a sedated patient fixed in a head frame.[123] Assuming the mouth opening is adequate, the device can easily be placed by facing the patient and using the thumb to insert along the hard palate. Elective use in the prone position is considered controversial by some but can be performed safely in appropriate patients with proper positioning.[171] A case report describes anesthetic induction and management in the prone position for a penetrating spine injury at C1-C2 using an LMA.[159] Hypertension, coughing, and bucking are preferably avoided in the neurosurgical patient. When this is particularly a consideration or the patient has severe asthma or chronic obstructive pulmonary disease, extubation may be facilitated by exchanging the ET for the LMA (i.e., using the LMA as "bridge to extubation").[150] This is performed while the patient is still deeply anesthetized, without airway reflexes. The exchange technique is also useful when an elaborate head draping is required and excessive neck movement is likely to provoke coughing and bucking. The LMA provides a number of airway options for the neurosurgical patient and should always be readily available.

V. POSTOPERATIVE CONSIDERATIONS

A. AIRWAY INJURY AND FUNCTION FOLLOWING NEUROSURGERY

A range of airway problems are possible in the patient who has undergone neurosurgery. There is potential risk from the surgical intervention, an intraoperative seizure, hypoxia, or hypoperfusion of an ischemic penumbral area that may produce an obtunded postoperative state. These factors, in addition to the residual effects of anesthetic drugs, may render patients unable to maintain their own airway safely. Patients undergo neurosurgery in a variety of positions other than supine, and the effects of gravity, venous pressure, and fluid administration may alter the integrity of the airway structures. Thus, although the airway itself may not be considered to be a DA, there are reasons why airway function may not automatically return immediately after neurosurgery. In addition to this global effect on the ability to maintain the airway, there are a variety of specific risks of alteration in airway function following neurosurgery.

1. Supratentorial Craniotomy

In addition to general issues to do with impaired level of consciousness as mentioned previously, patients may present with airway problems who have previously undergone temporoparietal or pterional craniotomy. When these patients subsequently present for surgery (either further neurosurgery or other non-neurosurgical procedures), they may now have a DA because of limited mouth opening not in evidence at the time of their original craniotomy. This is as a consequence of scar formation in the region of the temporalis muscle.[114] The likelihood of this having occurred is much greater in those who have had a period of sedation and ventilation in the intensive care unit after their original craniotomy, as they do not resume normal eating and talking activities. Even those who are extubated immediately after their craniotomy and do resume normal eating and talking are at risk for developing restricted mouth opening if, for reasons of excessive pain, they limit jaw movement and subsequently develop restrictive scarring. Kawaguchi and colleagues were able to characterize postcraniotomy changes in mouth opening that occurred in 92 patients following surgery.[78] The postoperative reduction in maximal mouth opening was greater in the group that underwent frontotemporal craniotomy (compared with parietal and occipital regions). Limited mouth opening resolved after 3 months in most patients. Supratentorial craniotomies separated by short intervals can increase the risk of limited mouth opening, which may result in a DI.[64]

There is a risk of the anesthesiologist being lulled into a false sense of security in this setting if the assessment of the airway is limited to reviewing the previous anesthesia chart. This describes only the grade of laryngoscopy at that time, and if the anesthesiologist does not perform a new postcraniotomy assessment of the airway, with particular reference to mouth opening, he or she may find a critical reduction in ease of laryngoscopy.

2. Cervical Spine Surgery

The intraoperative management of the patient scheduled for cervical spinal surgery was considered in detail earlier in this chapter. A significant number of problems, however, arise only on completion of the surgery. The surgery performed has goals of alleviating spinal cord compression, reduction of dislocation, or fixation of instability, and almost invariably these procedures result in a reduction of range of cervical movement. Consequently, on emergence, it may be difficult to maintain the airway in the presence of residual anesthesia, as airway maneuvers that were possible following induction of anesthesia are no longer possible.

Anterior cervical spinal surgery may result in recurrent laryngeal nerve injury or hematoma causing airway obstruction following extubation. The most common cause of vocal cord paralysis is compression of the recurrent laryngeal nerve within the endolarynx. Monitoring of ET cuff pressure and release after retractor placement may prevent injury to the recurrent laryngeal nerve.[9]

Edema may also develop in the tissues of the neck, as the esophagus and trachea are retracted during the course of these procedures in order to obtain access to the cervical spine. In contrast to problems associated with recurrent laryngeal nerve injury, angioedema, or hematoma, which tend to occur early, airway edema may not develop until 2 to 3 days after the procedure. If these patients require reintubation, it is often difficult to perform, with published series showing significant rates of death and hypoxic sequelae as a result. Consequently, attempts have been made to identify risks and strategies used to predict the at-risk groups and plan alternative management.

Sagi and associates reported that 19 (6.1%) patients had an airway complication, 6 (1.9%) patients required reintubation, and 1 patient died.[130] Symptoms developed on average 36 hours postoperatively. All complications except for two were attributable to pharyngeal edema. Variables that were found to be statistically associated with an airway complication were exposing more than three vertebral bodies; intraoperative blood loss greater than 300 mL; exposures involving C2, C3, or C4; and an operative time greater than 5 hours. A history of myelopathy, spinal cord injury, pulmonary problems, smoking, anesthetic risk factors, and the absence of a drain did not correlate with an airway complication. Thus, patients with prolonged procedures (5 hours); exposure of more than three vertebral levels that include C2, C3, or C4; and more than 300 mL of blood loss should remain intubated or be extubated over an airway exchange catheter and watched carefully for respiratory insufficiency.

Swallowing difficulties and dysphonia may occur in patients undergoing anterior cervical discectomy and fusion. The etiology and incidence of these abnormalities are not well defined. Once again, there is a tendency for patients undergoing multilevel surgery to demonstrate an increased incidence of swallowing abnormalities on postoperative radiographic studies.[54] Patients undergoing multilevel procedures are at an increased risk for these complications, in part because of soft tissue swelling in the neck. Although more rare, there is a risk of migration of the bone or synthetic graft or plate either into the airway or compressing the airway with resultant obstruction. In addition to necessitating reintubation, this has the added hazards of intubation being required in a patient with a potentially unstable cervical spine and the need for further surgery.[96,154]

The issues surrounding airway complications of *posterior* cervical spinal surgery, which are additional to those of *anterior* cervical spinal surgery, relate mainly to anesthesia conducted with the patient in the prone position, which is discussed next.

3. Posterior Fossa Surgery

Because of the position of the lower cranial nerves in relation to the posterior fossa, the patients' ability to maintain their airway may be compromised postoperatively. Careful history taking preoperatively may unmask subtle impairment of the gag reflex with increased episodes of choking on food, and family members may have noticed changes in the character of speech. Duration of surgery, proximity of the surgical site to the lower cranial nerves, and the presence of either edema or hematoma in relation to them may result in loss of the gag reflex and the ability to maintain and protect the airway following posterior fossa surgery. Because of the proximity of the brain stem, further hazards are presented postoperatively as central control of respiration may be jeopardized, and these factors dictate the safety of timing of extubation.[28,109]

Potential postoperative airway problems divide essentially into those of the prone and sitting position and those of surgery on the structures in the posterior fossa. On a simple level, patients are at risk even before the end of these surgeries because securing the ET in this setting is problematic as secretions and skin preparation solutions are ongoing threats to its security. Even if it is securely fastened to the skin, facial edema may result in the ET migrating out of the trachea, especially in children, in whom the distance between endobronchial intubation and extubation is small. Facial edema itself is not necessarily hazardous to the airway, but macroglossia and oropharyngeal edema clearly are problematic.[28]

A variety of mechanisms have been proposed to account for the macroglossia seen after posterior cervical spinal and posterior fossa surgery.[80] Clearly, if the tongue becomes inadvertently trapped between the teeth, lingual edema results. The venous drainage of the tongue may be obstructed by the presence of an oropharyngeal airway, and if an esophageal stethoscope is there along with an oral ET, these further risk impairing the venous and lymphatic drainage of the tongue in the prone position. Other factors that may contribute to the formation of edema are lateral rotation of the head and neck and flexion of the neck, as these two maneuvers may impair venous drainage of the head and neck.[64] The duration of surgery as well as blood loss and fluid replacement should also be taken into account concerning the likelihood of developing macroglossia.[69,145]

In all these settings, although macroglossia may be immediately apparent and preclude extubation, the oropharyngeal airway or the ET or both may be the only elements maintaining the airway, and it is only on their removal that the edema becomes apparent, risking airway compromise. A more rare neurologic complication affecting airway function after surgery in this position is quadriplegia. The putative mechanism for this is thought to be a combination of a prolonged period of hyperflexion, overstretching of the cord, and compromise of blood supply to the cord.[105,130] Clearly, extubation of the neurosurgical patient after prolonged surgery requires careful consideration, a review of the patient's intraoperative course, and assessment of airway and neurologic responses. Patients who appear to have obvious facial or airway swelling with a minimal response to the ET are best left intubated until they are fully recovered and meet all criteria for extubation.

B. STRATEGIES FOR EXTUBATION AFTER PROLONGED SURGERY OR BRAIN STEM INJURY

Prolonged surgery is a frequent scenario in the neurosurgical arena. Prompt awakening at the conclusion of surgery is often desired and expected for evaluation of neurologic function. It is assumed that most elective patients who are neurologically intact will remain the same and, barring no intraoperative problems, will be extubated almost immediately following surgery. The decision to extubate or not may sometimes be difficult and involve many factors. Modern anesthetic agents and techniques allow emergence from anesthesia despite many hours of surgical time. Monitoring of anesthetic depth is helpful, and careful

timing with neurosurgical closure allows anesthetics to be discontinued and reversed, if necessary. The main areas for consideration are neurologic function, length and ease of the case, patient's position, amount of intraoperative blood loss and intravenous fluid administration, and difficulty of intubation.

All patients' pulmonary function should be assessed (e.g., tidal volume, vital capacity, muscle strength) at the end of surgery. If loss of neurologic function related to the patient's pathology resulted in preoperative respiratory insufficiency, extubation is unwise in most cases. One particular operation in which this may be a problem is resection of an intramedullary spinal cord or lower medulla tumor. If neurophysiologic monitoring or hemodynamic changes indicate that brain stem manipulation or injury may have occurred, it is important to be cautious regarding extubation. These patients should be very carefully assessed for respiratory and upper extremity strength and respiratory drive. This is particularly important when the procedure is prolonged and performed in the prone position, as described earlier. Despite positioning of the patient, extensive traction on cranial nerves IX and X may result in a loss or impairment of the gag reflex postoperatively. A similar dangerous complication is impaired swallowing and coughing reflex postoperatively, which exposes the patient to the risk of aspiration pneumonia.

The decision to extubate after prolonged surgery also entails communication with the neurosurgeons and staff who are monitoring the patient postoperatively. As the patient is emerging from anesthesia, it may be possible to elicit the necessary movements that are reassuring to the surgeon, yet the patient may not be suitable for extubation. In this situation, it may be prudent to have the patient remain intubated until there is demonstration of a full cough response, adequate tidal volume, and response to commands. Patients who were difficult to intubate are most likely candidates for delayed extubation, especially when skilled anesthesia staff are unavailable. If a trial of extubation is requested for the patient's comfort and evaluation, a plan for reintubation, possibly utilizing an airway exchange catheter, must be considered.

VI. SUMMARY

The scope of airway considerations in the neurosurgical patient is vast. We have reviewed some of the general and specific concerns in management of patients, including airway assessment and emergency airway algorithms. These patients often present with a number of disease processes, which must be considered in relation to the anesthetic as well as to airway management. This task becomes more challenging as patients become older, live longer, and present with multiple medical problems. In addition, neurosurgical procedures, both in and out of the operating room, are becoming more complex with time. Some procedures take place in the prone, lateral, or sitting position.

Others require the patient to be awake temporarily and then asleep. The approach to airway control is a decision made by the anesthesiologist, often in collaboration with the surgeon.

It is important for the anesthesiologist to explore new airway devices and techniques and to gain skill in those that benefit this population of patients. A myriad of problems may occur in the neurosurgical patient following surgery; vigilance during the entire perioperative period is essential. Our role as perioperative physicians requires that we provide close observation of the patient throughout the perioperative period and render the safest of care.

REFERENCES

1. AANS National Neurosurgical Statistics Report—1999 Procedural Statistics.
2. Afilalo M, Guttman A, Stern E, et al: Fiberoptic intubation in the emergency department: A case series. J Emerg Med 11:387-391, 1993.
3. Agarwal A, Shobhana N: LMA in neurosurgery. Can J Anaesth 42:750, 1995.
4. Agro F, Barzoi G, Montecchia F: Tracheal intubation using a Macintosh laryngoscope or a GlideScope in 15 patients with cervical spine immobilization. Br J Anaesth 90:705-706, 2003.
5. Agro F, Frass M, Benumof J, et al: The esophageal tracheal combitube as a non-invasive alternative to endotracheal intubation. A review. Minerva Anestesiol 67:863-874, 2001.
6. Agro F, Frass M, Benumof JL, et al: Current status of the Combitube: A review of the literature. J Clin Anesth 14:307-314, 2002.
7. Agro F, Totonelli A, Gherardi S: Planned lightwand intubation in a patient with a known difficult airway. Can J Anaesth 51:1051-1052, 2004.
8. American Society of Anesthesiologists Task Force on Management of the Difficult Airway: Practice guidelines for management of the difficult airway. An updated report. Anesthesiology 95:1269-1277, 2003.
9. Apfelbaum RI, Kriskovich MD, Haller JR: On the incidence, cause and prevention of recurrent laryngeal nerve palsies during anterior cervical spine surgery. Spine 25:2906-2912, 2000.
10. Archer DP, Joycelyne MA: Conscious-sedation during craniotomy for intractable epilepsy: A review of 354 consecutive cases. Can J Anaesth 35:338-344, 1998.
11. Ard JL Jr, Bekker AY, Doyle WK: Dexmedetomidine in awake craniotomy: A technical note. Surg Neurol 63:114-116, 2005.
12. Audu P, Cooper H: Craniotomy performed with LMA. A case report. J Neurosurg Anesthesiol 12:112-113, 2000.
13. Avellino AM, Mann FA, Grady MS, et al: The misdiagnosis of acute cervical spine injuries and fractures in infants and children: The 12-year experience of a level I pediatric and adult trauma center. Childs Nerv Syst 21:122-127, 2005.
14. Balki M, Manninen PH, McGuire GP, et al: Venous air embolism during awake craniotomy in a supine patient. Can J Anaesth 50:835-838, 2003.
15. Bandi V, Munnur U, Braman SS: Airway problems in patients with rheumatologic disorders. Crit Care Clin 18:749-765, 2002.
16. Banyai M, Falger S, Roggla M, et al: Emergency intubation with the Combitube in a grossly obese patient with bull neck. Resuscitation 26:271-276, 1993.
17. Baskett PJ, Parr MJ, Nolan JP: The intubating laryngeal mask. Results of a multicentre trial with experience of 500 cases. Anaesthesia 53:1174-1179, 1998.
18. Bayless P, Ray VG: Incidence of cervical injuries in association with blunt head trauma. Am J Emerg Med 7:139-142, 1989.
19. Bedell E, Pough DS: Anesthetic management of traumatic brain injury. Anesthesiol Clin North Am 20:417-439, 2002.
20. Bedford RF, Marshall WK: Cardiovascular response to endotracheal intubation during four anesthetic techniques. Acta Anaesthesiol Scand 28:563, 1984.
21. Bedford RF, Morris L, Jane JA: Intracranial hypertension during surgery for supratentorial tumor: Correlation with preoperative tomography scans. Anesth Analg 61:430-433, 1982.
22. Bein B, Carstensen S, Gleim M, et al: A comparison of the proseal laryngeal mask airway, the laryngeal tube S and the oesophageal-tracheal combitube during routine surgical procedures. Eur J Anaesthesiol 22:341-346, 2005.
23. Bekker AY, Mistry A, Ritter AA, et al: Computer simulation of intracranial pressure changes during induction of anesthesia: Comparison of thiopental, propofol, and etomidate. J Neurosurg Anesthesiol 11:69-80, 1999.
24. Benumof JB: Laryngeal mask airway and the ASA difficult airway algorithm. Anesthesiology 84:686-699, 1996.
25. Brimacombe J, Keller C, Boehler M, et al: Positive pressure ventilation with the ProSeal versus classic laryngeal mask airway: A randomized, crossover study of health female patients. Anesth Analg 93:1351-1353, 2001.
26. Brimacombe J, Keller C, Kunzel, et al: Cervical spine motion during airway management: A cinefluoroscopic study of the posteriorly destabilized third cervical vertebrae in fresh cadavers. Anesth Analg 89:1296-1300, 1999.
27. Brimacombe JR: Intubating LMA for airway intubation. In Brimacombe JR (ed): Laryngeal Mask Anesthesia: Principles and Practice. Philadelphia, WB Saunders, 2005, pp 469-504.
28. Bruder N, Ravussin P: Recovery from anesthesia and postoperative extubation of neurosurgical patients: A review. J Neurosurg Anesth 11:282-293, 1999.
29. Burney RG, Winn R: Increased cerebrospinal fluid pressure during laryngoscopy and intubation for induction of anesthesia. Anesth Analg 54:687-690, 1975.
30. Calder I, Calder J, Crockard HA: Difficult direct laryngoscopy in patients with cervical spine disease. Anaesthesia 50:756-763, 1995.

31. Cattano D, Panicucci E, Paolicchi A, et al: Risk factors assessment of the difficult airway: An Italian survey of 1956 patients. Anesth Analg 99:1774-1779, 2004.

32. Chang RS, Hamilton RJ, Carter WA: Declining rate of cricothyrotomy in trauma patients with an emergency medicine residency: Implications for skills training. Acad Emerg Med 5:247-251, 1988.

33. Chappel WF: A case of acromegaly with laryngeal and pharyngeal symptoms. J Laryngol Otol 10:142, 1896.

34. Chestnut RM, Marshall SB, Piek J, et al: Early and late systemic hypotension as a frequent and fundamental source of cerebral ischemia following severe brain injury in the Traumatic Coma Data Bank. Acta Neurochir 59(Suppl):121-125, 1993.

35. Chestnut RM: Avoidance of hypotension: Condition sine qua non of successful severe head-injury management. J Trauma 42:S4-S9, 1997.

36. Chung YT, Wu HS, Lin YH, et al: Frequent use of alternative airway techniques makes difficult intubations less and easier. Acta Anaesthesiol Taiwan 42:141-145, 2004.

37. Cohn AI, Lau M, Leonard J: Emergent airway management at a remote hospital location in a patient wearing a halo traction device. Anesthesiology 89:845, 1998.

38. Coles JP, Leary TS, Monteiro JN, et al: Propofol anesthesia for craniotomy: A double-blind comparison of remifentanil, alfentanil, and fentanyl. J Neurosurg Anesthesiol 12:15-20, 2000.

39. Combes X, Le Roux B, Suen P, et al: Unanticipated difficult airway in anesthetized patients. Anesthesiology 100:1146-1150, 2004.

40. Cooper RM: Use of a new videolaryngoscope (GlideScope) in the management of a difficult airway. Can J Anaesth 50:611-613, 2003.

41. Cooper RM, Pacey JA, Bishop MJ, et al: Early clinical experience with a new videolaryngoscope (GlideScope) in 728 patients: Can J Anaesth 52:191-198, 2005.

42. Criswell JC, Parr MJ, Nolan JP: Emergency airway management in patients with cervical spine injuries. Anaesthesia 49:900-903, 1994.

43. Cros AM, Maigrot F, Esteben D: Fastrach laryngeal mask and difficult intubation. Ann Fr Anesth Reanim 18:1041-1046, 1999.

44. Danks RA, Rogers M, Agolio LS, et al: Patient tolerance of craniotomy performed with the patient under local anaesthesia with conscious sedation. Neurosurgery 42:28-34, 1998.

45. De Deyne C, Joly LM, Ravussin P: Newer inhalation anaesthetics and neuro-anaesthesia: What is the place for sevoflurane or desflurane? Ann Fr Anesth Reanim 23:367-374, 2004.

46. Deroy R, Ghoris M: The Combitube elective anesthetic airway management in a patient with cervical spine fracture. Anesth Analg 87:1441-1442, 1998.

47. Domino KB: Care of the acutely unstable patient. In Cortell JE, Smith DS (eds): Anesthesia and Neurosurgery. St. Louis, Mosby, 2001, pp 251-274.

48. Dougherty TB, Cronau LH Jr: Anesthetic implications for surgical patients with endocrine tumors. Int Anesthesiol Clin 36:31-44, 1998.

49. Evans CC, Hipkin LJ, Murray GM: Pulmonary function in acromegaly. Thorax 32:322-327, 1997.

50. Fairgrieve R, Rowney DA, Karsli C, Bissonnette B: The effect of sevoflurane on cerebral blood flow velocity in children. Acta Anaesthesiol Scand 47:1226-1230, 2003.

51. Ferson DZ, Rosenblatt WH, Johansen MJ, et al: Use of the intubating LMA-Fastrach in 254 patients with difficult-to-manage airways. Anesthesiology 95:1175-1181, 2001.

52. Figueredo-Gaspari E, Fredes-Kubrak R, Canosa-Ruiz L: Macroglossia after surgery of the posterior fossa. Rev Esp Anesthesiol Reanim 44:157-158, 1997.

53. Forster A, Juge O, Morel D: Effects of midazolam on cerebral blood flow in human volunteers. Anesthesiology 56:453-455, 1982.

54. Frempong-Boadu A, Houten JK, Osborn B, et al: Swallowing and speech dysfunction in patients following anterior cervical discectomy and fusion: A prospective objective preoperative and postoperative assessment. J Spinal Tech 15:362-368, 2002.

55. Gaitini LA, Vaida SJ, Mostafa S, et al: The Combitube in elective surgery: A report of 200 cases. Anesthesiology 94:79-82, 2001.

56. Gerling MC, Davis DP, Hamilton RS: Effect of surgical cricothyrotomy on the unstable cervical spine in a cadaver model of intubation. J Emerg Med 20:1-5, 2001.

57. Grant SA, Breslin DS, MacLeod DB, et al: Dexmedetomidine infusion for sedation during fiberoptic intubation: A report of three cases. J Clin Anesth 16:124-126, 2004.

58. Grogan EL, Morris JA Jr, Dittus RS, et al: Cervical spine evaluation in urban trauma centers: Lowering institutional costs and complications through helical CT scan. J Am Coll Surg 200:160-165, 2005.

59. Guy J, Hindman BJ, Baker KZ, et al: Comparison of remifentanil and fentanyl in patients undergoing craniotomy for supratentorial space-occupying lesions. Anesthesiology 86:514-524, 1997.

60. Hagberg C, Berry J, Hacque S: The laryngeal mask for awake craniotomy in pediatric patients. Anesthesiology 83:A184, 1995.

61. Hagberg CA, Iannucci DG, Goodrich AL: An evaluation of the Macintosh video™ laryngoscope in the intubation of potential difficult to intubate patients: A pilot study. Anesthesiology A-1500, 2003.

62. Hakala P, Randell T: Intubation difficulties in patients with rheumatoid arthritis. A retrospective analysis. Acta Anaesthesiol Scand 42:195-198, 1998.

63. Harrison BDU, Millhouse KA, Harrington M, et al: Lung function in acromegaly. Q J Med 67: 512-532, 1978.

64. Harrop JS, Vaccaro A, Przybylski GJ: Acute respiratory compromise associated with flexed cervical traction after C2 fractures. Spine 26:E50-E54, 2001.

65. Hassan SZ, Matz GJ, Lawrence AM, Collins PA: Laryngeal stenosis in acromegaly: A possible cause of airway difficulties associated with anesthesia. Anesth Analg 55:57-60, 1976.

66. Hayden SR, Panacek EA: Procedural competency in emergency medicine: The current range of resident experience. Acad Emerg Med 6:728-735, 1999.

67. Heary HF, Hunt CD, Kreiger AJ, et al: Acute stabilization of the cervical spine by halo/vest application facilitates evaluation and treatment of multiple trauma patients. J Trauma 33:445-451, 1992.

68. Horton WA, Fahy L, Charters P: Disposition of the cervical vertebrae, atlanto-axial joint, hyoid and mandible during x-ray laryngoscopy. Br J Anaesth 63:435-438, 1989.

69. Howard R, Mahoney A, Thurlow AC: Respiratory obstruction after posterior fossa surgery. Anaesthesia 45:222-224, 1990.

70. Huncke K, Van de Weile B, Fried I, Rubenstein EH: The asleep-awake-asleep anesthetic technique for intraoperative language mapping. Neurosurgery 42:1312-1316, 1998.

71. Inoue Y, Koga K, Shigematsu A. A comparison of two tracheal intubation techniques with trachlight and fastrach in patients with cervical spine disorders. Anesth Analg 94:667-671, 2002.

72. Iohom G, Ronayne M, Cunningham AJ: Prediction of difficult tracheal intubation. Eur J Anaesthesiol 20: 31-36, 2003.

73. Isaacs JH: Emergency cricothyrotomy: Long-term results. Am Surg 67:346-349, 2001.

74. Ito H, Kanno I, Ibaraki M, et al: Changes in cerebral blood flow and cerebral blood volume during hypercapnia and hypocapnia measured by positron emission tomography. J Cereb Blood Flow Metab 23:665-670, 2003.

75. Jeremitsky E, Omert L, Dunham MC, et al: Harbingers of poor outcome the day after severe brain injury: Hypothermia, hypoxia, and hypoperfusion. J Trauma 54:312-319, 2003.

76. Jones PA, Andrews PJ, Dearden NM, et al: The role of secondary insult during in head-injured patients during intensive care. J Neurosurg Anesthesiol 6:4-14, 1994.

77. Kang M, Vives MJ, Vaccaro AR: The halo vest: Principles of application and management of complications. J Spinal Cord Med 26:186-192, 2003.

78. Kawaguchi M, Sakamoto T, Furuya H, et al: Pseudoankylosis of the mandible after supratentorial craniotomy. Anesth Analg 83:731-734, 1996.

79. Kihara S, Brimacombe J, Yaguchi Y, et al: Hemodynamic responses among three tracheal intubation devices in normotensive and hypertensive patients. Anesth Analg 96:890-895, 2003.

80. Kimovec MA, Ambrose J: Predictors of airway and respiratory complications after posterior fossa craniotomies. J Neurosurg Anesthesiol 4:315, 1992.

81. Kitahata LM: Airway difficulties associated with anaesthesia in acromegaly: Three case reports. Br J Anaesth 43:1187-1190, 1971.

82. Klauber MR, Marshall LF, Toole BM, et al: Cause of decline in head-injury mortality rate in San Diego County, California. J Neurosurg 62:528-531, 1985.

83. Krafft, Schebesta K: Alternative management techniques for the difficult airway: Esophageal-tracheal Combitube. Curr Opin Anaesthesiol 17:499-504, 2004.

84. Lanier WL, Hool GL, Faust RJ, et al: Sedation for stereotactic headframe application: A randomized comparison of two techniques. Appl Neurophysiol 50:227-232, 1987.

85. Law-Koune JD, Liu N, Szekely B, et al: Using the intubating laryngeal mask airway for ventilation and endotracheal intubation in anesthetized and unparalyzed acromegalic patients. J Neurosurg Anesthesiol 16:11-13, 2004.

86. Lee LA, Posner KL, Cheney FW, et al: ASA closed claims project: An analysis of claims associated with neurosurgical anesthesia. Anesthesiology 99:A362, 2003.

87. Lennarson PJ, Smith D, Todd MM, et al: Segmental spine motion during orotracheal intubation of the intact and injured spine with and without external stabilization. J Neurosurg 92(2 Suppl):201-206, 2000.

88. Majernick TG, Bieniek R, Houston JB, et al: Cervical spine movement during orotracheal intubation. Ann Emerg Med 15:417-420, 1997.

89. Manninen PH, Gignac EM, Gelb AW, Lownie SP: Anesthesia for interventional neuroradiology. J Clin Anesth 7:44-52, 1995.

90. Manninen PH, Raman SK, Boyle K, el-Beheiry H: Early postoperative complications following neurosurgical procedures. Can J Anaesth 46:7-14, 1999.

91. Marie P: Sur deux d'acromégalie: Hypertrophie singulière non congénitale des extremités supérieures, inférieures et céphalique. Rev Med 6:297-333, 1986.

92. Marmarou A, Anderson RL, Ward JD, et al: Impact of ICP instability and hypotension on outcome in patients with severe head trauma. J Neurosurg 75: S59-S66, 1991.

93. Marshall LF, Gautille T, Klauber MR, et al: The outcome of severe head injury. J Neurosurg 75:528-536, 1991.

94. Matta MP, Caron P: Acromegalic cardiomyopathy: A review of the literature. Pituitary 6:203-207, 2003.

95. McGill J, Clinton JE, Ruiz E: Cricothyrotomy in the emergency department. Ann Emerg Med 11:361-364, 1982.

96. McLorinan GC, Choudhari KA, Cooke RS: Life threatening complication of biocompatible osteoconductive polymer graft after anterior cervical discectomy. Br J Neurosurg 15:363-365, 2001.

97. Melemed S: Acromegaly. N Engl J Med 322:966-975, 1990.

98. Mercer M: Respiratory failure after tracheal extubation in a patient with halo frame cervical spine immobilization—Rescue therapy using the Combitube airway. Br J Anaesth 86:886-891, 2001.

99. Mercer MH, Gabbott DA: The influence of neck position on ventilation using the Combitube airway. Anaesthesia 53:146-150, 1998.

100. Meschino A, Devitt JH, Koch JP, et al: The safety of awake tracheal intubation in cervical spine injury. Can J Anaesth 39:114-117, 1992.

101. Messick JM Jr, Cucchiara RF, Faust RJ: Airway management in patients with acromegaly [letter]. Anesthesiology 56:157, 1982.

102. Mikawa Y, Watanabe R, Nishishita Y: Cervical myelopathy in acromegaly. Report of a case. Spine 17:1542-1543, 1992.

103. Miller JD, Becker DP: Secondary insults to the injured brain. J R Coll Surg Edinb 27:292-298, 1982.

104. Modica PA, Tempelhoff R: Intracranial pressure during induction of anaesthesia and tracheal intubation with etomidate-induced EEG burst suppression. Can J Anaesth 39:236-241, 1992.

105. Morandi X, Riffaud L, Amlashi SF, Brassier G: Extensive spinal cord infarction in the sitting position: Case report. Neurosurgery 54:1512-1515, 2004.

106. Morewood DJW, Belchetz PE, Evans CC, et al: The extrathoracic airway in acromegaly. Clin Radiol 37: 243-246, 1986.

107. Moss E: Volatile anesthetic agents in neurosurgery. Br J Anaesth 63:4-6, 1989.

108. Mostafa SM, Murthy BV, Barrett PJ, McHugh P: Comparison of the effects of topical lignocaine spray applied before or after induction of anaesthesia on the pressor response to direct laryngoscopy and intubation. Eur J Anaesthesiol 16:7-10, 1999.

109. Narayan VB, Umamaheswara GS: Unilateral facial and neck swelling after infratentorial surgery in the lateral position. Anesth Analg 89:1290-1291, 1999.

110. Ng A, Raitt DG, Smith G: Induction of anesthesia and insertion of a laryngeal mask airway in the prone position for minor surgery. Anesth Analg 94:1194-1198, 2002.

111. Ng I, Lim J, Wong HB: Effects of head posture on cerebral hemodynamics: Its influences on intracranial pressure, cerebral perfusion pressure, and cerebral oxygenation. Neurosurgery 54:593-597, 2004.

112. Nguyen GK, Clark R: Adequacy of plain radiography in the diagnosis of cervical spine injuries. Emerg Radiol 11:158-161, 2005.

113. Nishikawa K, Kawana S, Namiki A: Comparison of the lightwand technique with direct laryngoscopy for awake endotracheal intubation in emergency cases. J Clin Anesth 13:259-263, 2001.

114. Nitzan DW, Azaz B, Constantini S: Severe limitation in mouth opening following transtemporal neurosurgical procedures. J Neurosurg 76:623-625, 1992.

115. Oates JD, Macleod AD, Oates PD, et al: Comparison of two methods for predicting difficult intubation. Br J Anaesth 66:305-309, 1991.

116. Ovassapian A, Doka JC, Romsa DE: Acromegaly—Use of fiberoptic laryngoscopy to avoid tracheostomy. Anesthesiology 54:429-430, 1981.

117. Ovassapian A, Krejcie TC, Yelich SJ, Dykes MH: Awake fiberoptic intubation in the patient at high risk of aspiration. Br J Anaesth 62:13-16, 1989.

118. Patterson H: Emergency department intubation of trauma patients with undiagnosed cervical spine injury. Emerg Med J 21:302-305, 2004.

119. Perkins WJ, Kelly PJ, Faust RJ: Stereotactic surgery. In Cucchiara RF, Michenfelder JD (eds): Clinical Neuroanesthesia. New York, Churchill Livingston, 1990, pp 379-420.

120. Pietropaoli JA, Rogers FB, Shackford SR, et al: The deleterious effects of intraoperative hypotension on outcome in patients with severe brain injuries. J Trauma 33:403-407, 1992.

121. Piper J, Dirks BA, Traynelis VC, et al: Perioperative management and surgical outcome of the acromegalic patient with sleep apnea. Neurosurgery 36:70-75, 1995.

122. Rai MR, Dering A, Verghese C: The Glidescope system: A clinical assessment of performance. Anaesthesia 60:60-64, 2005.

123. Raphael J, Rosenthal-Ganon T, Gozal Y: Emergency airway management in a patient placed in the prone position. J Clin Anesth 16:560-561, 2004.

124. Ratnayake B, Langford RM: A survey of emergency airway management in the United Kingdom. Anaesthesia 51:908-911, 1996.

125. Ravussin P, Guinard J, Ralley F, et al: Effect of propofol on cerebrospinal fluid pressure in patients undergoing craniotomy. Anaesthesia 43:37-41, 1988.

126. Reardon RF, Martel M: The intubating laryngeal mask airway, suggestions for use in the emergency department. Acad Emerg Med 8:833-838, 2001.

127. Reilly PL: Review Brain injury: the pathophysiology of the first hours. 'Talk and Die revisited'. J Clin Neurosci 8:398-403, 2001.

128. Remifentanil and propofol for awake craniotomy: Case report with pharmacokinetic simulations. J Neurosurg Anesthesiol 10:25-29, 1998.

129. Reusche MD, Egan TD: Remifentanil for conscious sedation and analgesia during awake fiberoptic tracheal intubation: A case report with pharmacokinetic simulations. J Clin Anesth. 11:64-68, 1999.

130. Sagi HC, Beutler W, Carroll E, Connolly PJ: Airway complications associated with surgery on the anterior spine. Spine 27:949-953, 2002.

131. Samaha T, Ravussin P, Claquin C, Ecoffey C: Prevention of increase of blood pressure and intracranial pressure during endotracheal intubation in neurosurgery: Esmolol versus lidocaine. Ann Fr Anesth Reanim 15:36-40, 1996.

132. Sarang A, Dinsmore J: Anaesthesia for awake craniotomy—Evolution of a technique that facilitates awake neurological testing. Br J Anaesth 90:161-165, 2003.

133. Sawin PD, Todd MM, Traynelis VC, et al: Cervical spine movement with direct laryngoscopy and orotracheal intubation. An in vivo cinefluoroscopic study of subjects without cervical abnormality. Anesthesiology 85:26-36, 1996.

134. Schmitt H, Buchfelder M, Radespiel-Tröger M: Difficult intubation in acromegalic patients: Incidence and predictability. Anesthesiology 93:110-114, 2000.

135. Scholtes FJ, Scholtes JL: Airway obstruction in acromegaly: A method of prevention. Anaesth Intensive Care 16:491-492, 1988.

136. Schuschnig C, Waltl B, Erlacher W, et al: Intubating laryngeal mask and rapid sequence induction in patients with cervical spine injury. Anaesthesia 54:793-797, 1999.

137. Sener EB, Sarihasan B, Ustun E, et al: Awake tracheal intubation through the intubating laryngeal mask airway in a patient with halo traction. Can J Anaesth 49:610-613, 2002.

138. Shapiro HM, Wyte SR, Harris AB, Galindo A: Acute intraoperative intracranial hypertension in neurosurgical patients: Mechanical and pharmacologic factors. Anesthesiology 37:399-405, 1972.

139. Shatney CH, Brunner RD, Nguyen TQ: The safety of orotracheal intubation in patients with unstable cervical spine fractures or high spinal cord injury. Am J Surg 53:676-680, 1995.

140. Shinokuma T, Shono S, Iwakiri S, et al: Awake craniotomy with propofol sedation and a laryngeal mask airway: A case report. Masui 51:529-531, 2002.

141. Shorten GD, Alfille PH, Giklich RE: Airway obstruction following application of cricoid pressure. J Clin Anesth 3:403-405, 1991.

142. Silverston P: Pulse oximetry at the roadside: A study of pulse oximetry in immediate care. BMJ 298: 711-713, 1989.

143. Sims CA, Berger DL: Airway risk in hospitalized trauma patients with cervical injuries requiring halo fixation. Ann Surg 225:280-284, 2002.

144. Singh NC, Kissoon N, Frewen T, Tiffin N: Physiologic responses to endotracheal and oral suctioning in paediatric patients: The influence of endotracheal tube sizes and suction pressures. Clin Intensive Care 2: 345-350, 1991.

145. Sinha A, Agarwal A, Gaur A, Pandey CK: Oropharyngeal swelling and macroglossia after cervical spine surgery in the prone position. J Neurosurg Anesthesiol 13:237-239, 2001.

146. Smith CE: Cervical spine injury and tracheal intubation: A never-ending conflict. Trauma Care 10:20-26, 2000.

147. Souter MJ, Andrew PJD, Piper IR, et al: Effects of alfentanil on cerebral hemodynamics in an experimental model of traumatic brain injury. Br J Anaesth 79:97-102, 1997.

148. Southwick JP, Katz J: Unusual airway difficulty in the acromegalic patient: Indications for tracheostomy. Anesthesiology 51:72-73, 1979.

149. Spiekermann BF, Stone D, Bogdonoff DL: Airway management in neuroanesthesia. Can J Anaesth 43: 820-834, 1996.

150. Stix MS, Borromeo CJ, Sciortino GJ, Teague PD: Learning to exchange an endotracheal tube for a laryngeal mask prior to emergence. Can J Anaesth 48:795-799, 2001.

151. Stokes MA, Soriano SG, Tarbell NJ, et al: Anesthesia for stereotactic radiosurgery in children. J Neurosurg Anesthesiol 7:100-108, 1995.

152. Sun DA, Warriner CB, Parsons DG: The GlideScope Video Laryngoscope: Randomized clinical trial in 200 patients Br J Anaesth 94:381-384, 2005.

153. Teasdale G, Jennett B: Assessment of coma and impaired consciousness: A practical scale. Lancet 2: 81-84, 1974.

154. Terao Y, Matsumoto S, Yamashita K, et al: Increased incidence of emergency airway management after combined anterior-posterior cervical spine surgery. J Neurosurg Anesthesiol 16:282-286, 2004.

155. The American Society of Anesthesiologists Task Force on Management of the Difficult Airway: A Report by the American Society of Anesthesiologists Task Force on Management of the Difficult Airway. Anesthesiology 78:597-602, 1993.

156. Traystman RJ, Fitzgerald RS, Loscutoff SC: Cerebral circulatory responses to arterial hypoxia in normal and chemodenervated dogs. Circ Res 42:649-657, 1978.

157. Tseitlin AM, Lubnin AIU, Baranov OA, Luk'ianov VI: The use of propofol (Diprivan) for inducing anesthesia in neurosurgical patients. II. Its effect on intracranial pressure and on cerebral perfusion pressure. Anesteziol Reanimatol (4):39-43, 1998.

158. Unni VK, Johnston RA, Young HS, McBride RJ: Prevention of intracranial hypertension during laryngoscopy and endotracheal intubation. Use of a second dose of thiopentone. Br J Anaesth 56:1219-1223, 1984.

159. Valero R, Serrano S, Adalia R, et al: Anesthetic management of a patient in prone position with a drill bit penetrating the spinal canal at C1-C2, using a laryngeal mask. Anesth Analg 98:1447-1450, 2004.

160. Velmahos GC, Toutouzas K, Chan L, et al: Intubation after cervical spinal cord injury: To be done selectively or routinely? Am Surg 69:891-894, 2003.

161. Wahlen BM, Gercek E: Three-dimensional cervical spine movement during intubation using the Macintosh and Bullard laryngoscopes, the Bonfils fiberscope and the intubating laryngeal mask airway. Eur J Anaesthesiol 21:907-913, 2004.

162. Wakeling HG, Nightingale J: The intubating laryngeal mask airway does not facilitate tracheal intubation in the presence of a neck collar in simulated trauma. Br J Anaesth 84:254-256, 2000.

163. Waltl B, Melischek M, Schuschnig C: Tracheal intubation and cervical spine excursion: Direct laryngoscopy vs. intubating laryngeal mask. Anaesthesia 56:221-226, 2001.

164. Watson NC, Hokanson M, Maltby JR, Todesco JM: The intubating laryngeal mask airway in failed fibreoptic intubation. Can J Anaesth 46:376-378, 1999.

165. Weisman BN, Aliabadi P, Weinfeld MS, et al: Prognostic features of atlantoaxial subluxation in rheumatoid arthritis patients. Radiology 144:745-751, 1982.

166. Welling EC, Donegan J: Neuroleptanalgesia using alfentanil for awake craniotomy. Anesth Analg 68:57-60, 1989.

167. Werner C, Kochs E, Bause H, et al: Effects of sufentanil on cerebral hemodynamics and intracranial pressure in patients with brain injury. Anesthesiology 83:721-726, 1995.

168. Wong JK, Tongier WK, Armbruster SC, White PF: Use of the intubating laryngeal mask airway to facilitate awake orotracheal intubation in patients with cervical spine disorders. J Clin Anesth 11:346-338, 1999.

169. Wright SW, Robinson GG II, Wright MB: Cervical spine injuries in blunt trauma patients requiring emergent endotracheal intubation. Am J Emerg Med 10:104-109, 1992.

170. Young ML, Hanson CW: An alternative to tracheostomy following transsphenoidal hypophysectomy in a patient with acromegaly and sleep apnea. Anesth Analg 76: 446-449, 1993.

171. Young WL, Pile-Spellman J: Anesthetic considerations for interventional neuroradiology. Anesthesiology 80:427-456, 1994.

172. Zwienenberg-Lee M, Muizalaar J: Clinical pathophysiology of traumatic brain injury. In Winn RH (ed): Youmans Neurological Surgery, 5th ed. Philadelphia, WB Saunders, 2004.

THE NEW AMERICAN ASSOCIATION OF ANESTHESIOLOGISTS OBSTRUCTIVE SLEEP APNEA GUIDELINE

Jonathan L. Benumof

I. INTRODUCTION

A. WHAT IS OBSTRUCTIVE SLEEP APNEA? WHY DOES IT HAPPEN? SYSTEMIC PATHOPHYSIOLOGY

There are three different pharynxes (Fig. 40-1, top). The nasopharynx (also called the velopharynx) is the airspace that is posterior to all of the soft palate (to the tip of the uvula). Therefore, the nasopharynx is a retropalatal pharynx. The oropharynx is the airspace that is posterior to the tip of the uvula to the tip of the epiglottis. Therefore, the oropharynx is a retroglossal pharynx. The laryngopharynx (also called the hypopharynx) is the airspace that is posterior to the tip of the epiglottis to the vocal cords. Therefore, the laryngopharynx is a retroepiglottic pharynx.

The adult human is essentially the only animal to have a space between the uvula and the epiglottis. All other mammals and the newborn human have an interlocking uvula and epiglottis (they touch one another). As the newborn human grows, the larynx descends and the space between the uvula and epiglottis increases. Thus, the adult human is the only animal to have an upper airway that is essentially a long, soft-walled tube that has no bony support anteriorly or laterally. The long, soft-walled tube gives the adult human the potential to have obstructive sleep apnea (OSA), and the adult human is essentially the only animal to have OSA.[2] The only reason the long, soft-walled tube remains open is the action of muscles.

The muscles that keep the upper airway open are as follows (Fig. 40-1, middle).[3] The tensor palatine retracts the soft palate away from the posterior pharyngeal wall, thereby maintaining the patency of the retropalatal nasopharynx. The genioglossus moves the tongue anteriorly to open the retroglossal oropharynx. The geniohyoid, sternohyoid, and thyrohyoid muscles move the epiglottis forward by tensing the hyoepiglottic ligament, thereby enlarging the retroepiglottic laryngopharynx.

When the human goes to sleep, loss of muscle tone occurs throughout the body, and the deeper the sleep (either natural or pharmacologically induced), the greater the relaxation. There are two major stages of sleep: nonrapid eye movement (NREM) and rapid eye movement (REM) sleep. Within NREM sleep, there are four substages of sleep, which simply represent progressive slowing of the waves on the electroencephalogram (EEG). Deep and restorative sleep occurs during the deeper NREM and REM sleep stages. It is nocturnal deep and restorative sleep that allows one to function the next day without requiring any diurnal sleep.

During deep and restorative sleep the pharyngeal muscles participate in the loss of muscle tone. The loss of pharyngeal muscle tone causes pharyngeal collapse, to some extent, in everyone. If the loss of pharyngeal muscle tone and pharyngeal collapse are partial, but still great enough to cause the inspired air to flutter around the uvula and/or the tongue and/or the epiglottis (Fig. 40-1, bottom), there will be snoring and hypopnea (formally defined as a decrease in airflow more than 50% of awake value for more than 10 seconds).[21] If the loss of pharyngeal muscle tone and pharyngeal collapse are great enough to cause complete obstruction, there will be silence and apnea (formally defined as no airflow for more than 10 seconds despite continuing ventilatory effort).[21] The presence of apnea and hypopnea during sleep is called sleep-disordered breathing (SDB) (Fig. 40-2).

In order to survive each obstructive episode, the patient has to have some sort of arousal. In the vast majority of instances the arousal is a mini-arousal. The mini-arousal is expressed internally as a burst of activity on the EEG and externally as either extremity movement and/or turning and/or vocalization. The mini-arousal activates the pharyngeal muscles, and this opens the pharyngeal airway (often accompanied by a snorting noise). The reopened airway allows the patient to go back into a deep sleep, which causes, in turn, pharyngeal muscle relaxation, pharyngeal collapse, and pharyngeal obstruction. Thus, the cycle of deep sleep, pharyngeal obstruction, arousal, deep sleep, and so forth recurs over and over again.

There are four mechanisms of arousal,[3] as follows. First and second, as the duration of the apnea or hypopnea progresses, the magnitude of arterial hypoxemia and hypercapnia increases. Third, these two chemical changes induce an increased ventilatory effort. Finally, the increased ventilatory effort against an obstructed airway causes increased negative pressure in the airway. Any one or all four mechanisms together can be responsible for increased neural traffic in the reticular activating system and arouse the individual.

Obviously the arousals are necessary for survival. However, each arousal causes sympathetic nervous system stimulation, which in turn causes systemic and pulmonary hypertension (Fig. 40-3).[3] Furthermore, patients with OSA have 5 to 9 times the risk of suffering from the metabolic syndrome and vice versa.[6,11] In time, the hypertension in one or both circulations becomes fixed, which in turn and in time causes hypertrophy in one or both of the respective ventricles. The hypoxemia can cause myocardial ischemia, which can cause myocardial dysrhythmias and sudden and unexpected death. The increased negative intrathoracic pressure can cause reflux from the positive-pressure stomach to the negative-pressure esophagus (increasing the incidence of gastroesophageal reflux disease), and data from studies in dogs suggest that mild degrees of nocturnal negative-pressure pulmonary edema (NPPE) may occur.[8] The repetitive arousals fragment the sleep and rob the patient of deep and restorative sleep. Therefore, these patients have somnolence during the quiet times of the day and are at high risk for motor vehicle accidents and personality, behavioral, and cognitive changes. Finally, because they make much noise and are moving during sleep, they make undesirable bed partners and suffer from nocturnal social isolation.

UPPER AIRWAY ANATOMY

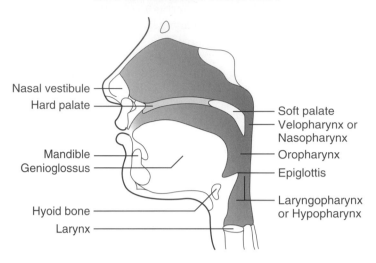

Nasal vestibule
Hard palate

Mandible
Genioglossus

Hyoid bone
Larynx

Soft palate
Velopharynx or Nasopharynx
Oropharynx
Epiglottis
Laryngopharynx or Hypopharynx

Figure 40-1 Upper airway anatomy (**top**); pharyngeal dilator muscles (**middle**); pharyngeal collapse with pharyngeal muscle relaxation (**bottom**).

ACTION OF THE UPPER AIRWAY DILATOR MUSCLES

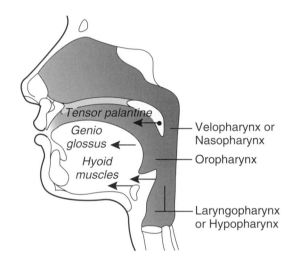

Tensor palantine
Genio glossus
Hyoid muscles

Velopharynx or Nasopharynx
Oropharynx
Laryngopharynx or Hypopharynx

SITES OF OBSTRUCTION DURING SLEEP APNEA

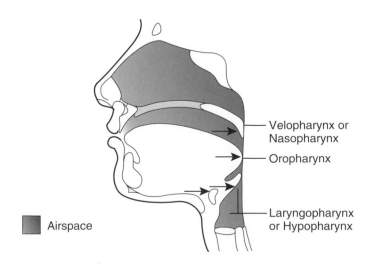

Velopharynx or Nasopharynx
Oropharynx
Laryngopharynx or Hypopharynx

Airspace

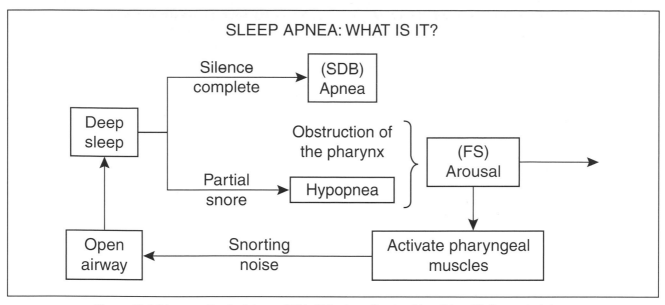

Figure 40-2 Primary pathophysiology of OSA. SDB, sleep-disordered breathing; FS, fragmented sleep.

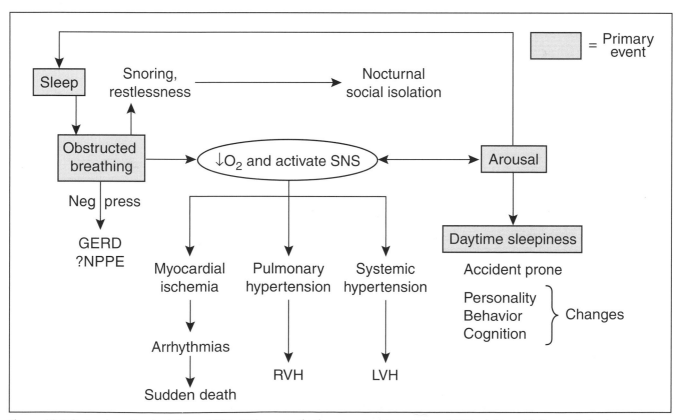

Figure 40-3 Systemic pathophysiology of OSA. SNS, sympathetic nervous system; RVH and LVH, right and left ventricular hypertrophy, respectively; Neg press, negative pressure; GERD, gastroesophageal reflux disease; NPPE, negative-pressure pulmonary edema.

B. OBSTRUCTIVE SLEEP APNEA AND ANESTHESIA CREATE A MULTIDIMENSIONAL PROBLEM

The literature indicates that at the present time disastrous respiratory outcomes during the perioperative management of patients with OSA are a major and increasing problem for the anesthesia community.[3,4,13,16] The disastrous outcomes are due to (1) failure to secure the airway during the induction of anesthesia, (2) respiratory obstruction soon after extubation, and (3) respiratory arrest after the administration of opioids and/or sedation to postoperative extubated patients. The growing OSA management problem is almost certainly fueled by the growing obesity epidemic; the large majority of these patients (70% to 90%) are obese (body mass index (BMI) >30).[5,20,23,24] The number of people with clinically significant OSA in 1993 was approximately 18 million[14] and is certainly much higher currently. The end point for failure to manage the intubation, extubation, and pain management problems is often brain damage or death (BD/D).

1. Brain Damage or Death Around the Time of Induction of Anesthesia

The latest report from the ASA Closed Claims database shows that the incidence of BD/D in lawsuits involving failure to secure the airway during the induction of anesthesia, in all types of patients, has decreased from 62% during 1985 to 1993 (1993 was the year the ASA difficult airway algorithm was published) to 35% from 1993 to 2001 ($P = 0.04$).[16] Thus, according to ASA Closed Claims data, there has been an improvement in the management of induction in cannot ventilate/cannot intubate situations, but it is still a significant problem. The specific data for OSA patients are not known, but it is likely the data are similar or worse in OSA patients, especially in obese OSA patients.

2. Brain Damage or Death Around the Time of Extubation

According to the ASA Closed Claims database, lawsuits involving losing the airway on the extubation side of airway management have a much higher incidence of BD/D compared to losing the airway on induction; during the 1985 to 1993 time period the incidence of BD/D in the lawsuits was 100%, and during the 1993 to 2001 time period the incidence of BD/D in the lawsuits was 83% (NS).[7] In 67% of the lawsuits wherein extubation failure led to BD/D, the patients were obese and/or had a history of OSA. I speculate that at least in some of these patients the extubation crisis developed after the monitors had been removed, the patient had been moved to the transport gurney, and the favorable airway management position that existed at the beginning of the case was no longer present.

3. Brain Damage or Death Associated with Pain Management

Finally, it is my opinion that at the present time there are many cases wherein postoperative obese patients with OSA are receiving opioids and/or sedatives in unmonitored beds and are found near death or dead in bed by some caregiver or friend. There are no data on the incidence of BD/D in these cases, but given the above definition of clinical context, the incidence must be very high.

II. THE SPECIFICS OF THE NEW AMERICAN SOCIETY OF ANESTHESIOLOGISTS OBSTRUCTIVE SLEEP APNEA GUIDELINE

A. THE LOGIC OF THE GUIDELINE

The ASA OSA Guideline[17] will be best understood if the underlying logic is well appreciated (Fig. 40-4). The logic is as follows. The causes of OSA must be known. If a cause or causes are present in a patient, questions to rule in or to rule out a presumptive clinical diagnosis of OSA should be asked. If a presumptive clinical diagnosis of OSA is made, the severity of the OSA must be decided upon or determined. The severity of OSA will then factor into determining perioperative risk along with the invasiveness of anesthesia and/or surgery and the anticipated postoperative opioid requirement. Perioperative risk will then determine perioperative management.

B. CAUSES OF OBSTRUCTIVE SLEEP APNEA

One must know the causes of OSA because it is unreasonable to ask all patients questions that allow a presumptive clinical diagnosis of OSA. If a cause of OSA is present, it is reasonable to investigate whether OSA exists. In the United States, obesity is by far the most important cause of OSA.

1. Obesity

Obesity is best expressed quantitatively as body mass index (BMI):

$$BMI = mass/height^2 = kg/m^2 \text{ or } 703 \times lb/inches^2$$

where underweight, normal, overweight, obesity, and morbid obesity equal < 19.0, 19.0 to 24.9, 25.0 to 29.9, 30.0 to 34.9, and > 35, respectively.[15]

Obese patients are uniquely susceptible to OSA because there is an inverse relationship between pharyngeal area and obesity.[22] Magnetic resonance imaging studies show that decreased pharyngeal area results from deposition of adipose tissue in the uvula, tonsils, tonsillar pillars, tongue, aryepiglottic folds, and the lateral pharyngeal walls[9] and the volume of fat deposited in these structures correlates well with the severity of OSA.[19] From the sites of fat deposition, it is obvious that

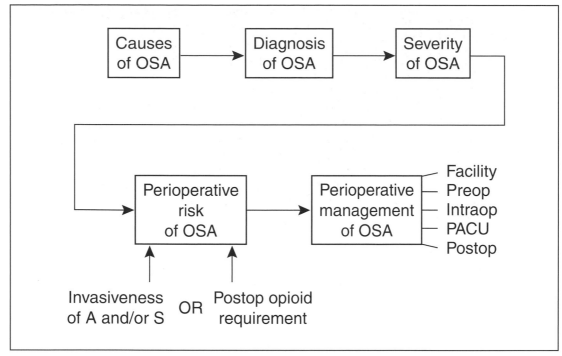

Figure 40-4 The logic of the ASA OSA Guideline.[17] A and/or S, anesthesia and/or surgery.

all three pharynxes are involved. The converse is also true; weight loss results in a very significant decrease in the severity of OSA.[18] Thus, when an obese patient goes into a deep sleep and there is a given degree of loss of pharyngeal muscle tone and pharyngeal collapse, the greater the amount of intraluminal fat, the greater the pharyngeal obstruction.

2. Thick/Fat Neck

The patency of the soft-walled collapsible pharynx is determined by the transmural pressure across the wall (the difference between extraluminal and intraluminal pressure). In obese patients, extraluminal pressure is increased by superficially located fat masses.[10] Thus, when an obese patient goes into a deep sleep and there is a given degree of loss of pharyngeal muscle tone and pharyngeal collapse, the greater the amount the airway is compressed externally, the greater the degree of the obstruction. Indeed, the incidence and severity of OSA correlate better with increased neck circumference (men, >17 inches; women, >16 inches) than with general obesity.[7]

3. Micrognathia and Retrognathia (Small Receding Mandible)

A small receding mandible often places the tongue in a relatively posterior position. For a given degree of loss of pharyngeal muscle tone and pharyngeal muscle collapse, the more posterior the tongue, the greater the degree of pharyngeal obstruction.

4. Large Tongue (High Oropharyngeal Classification)

For a given degree of loss of pharyngeal muscle tone and pharyngeal muscle collapse, the larger the tongue, the greater the degree of pharyngeal obstruction.

5. Large Tonsils

For a given degree of loss of pharyngeal muscle tone and pharyngeal muscle collapse, the larger the tonsils, the greater the degree of pharyngeal obstruction.

6. Nasal Obstruction (Any Etiology)

For a given degree of loss of pharyngeal muscle tone and pharyngeal muscle collapse, the greater the degree of nasal obstruction, the greater the degree of pharyngeal obstruction.

If a cause of OSA is known to be present, then the patient should be asked questions that will allow the anesthesiologist to rule in or to rule out a presumptive clinical diagnosis of OSA.

C. PRESUMPTIVE CLINICAL DIAGNOSIS OF OBSTRUCTIVE SLEEP APNEA

Three fundamental questions need to be asked in order to make a presumptive clinical diagnosis of OSA: (1) Is there a history or observation of apnea or snoring with hypopnea during sleep (sleep-disordered breathing)?

(2) Is there a history or observation of arousal from sleep (extremity movement, turning, vocalization, snorting)? (3) Is there a history or observation of daytime somnolence (easily falls asleep during the quiet times of the day)? Sleep-disordered breathing (SDB) plus arousals plus daytime somnolence make up the classic triad of signs and symptoms that make a presumptive clinical diagnosis of OSA. However, since the arousals may not be readily apparent, the diagnosis can and will have to be made on the basis of SDB and daytime somnolence.

Making a presumptive clinical diagnosis of OSA, even if it is just prior to taking the patient to the operating room for the induction of anesthesia, will likely have three benefits. First, it may improve immediate outcome because if it is known/suspected that a disease requires management, it is likely the management will be better; just as in all of medicine, proper diagnosis must precede proper treatment. Thus, the Guideline states "pre-procedure identification improves perioperative outcome."[17] Second, making a presumptive clinical diagnosis of OSA may inspire the caregivers to delay surgery and confirm and quantitate the diagnosis with a sleep study. Third, repetitively making a presumptive clinical diagnosis of OSA just before surgery may inspire the caregivers to set up protocols that will allow much earlier identification and evaluation of OSA and preparation of an appropriate perioperative management plan. If a preoperative presumptive clinical diagnosis of OSA is made, the caregiver should decide or determine the severity of OSA.

D. SEVERITY OF OBSTRUCTIVE SLEEP APNEA

The Guideline recommends that the anesthesiologist decide or determine the severity (grade) of OSA as mild, moderate, or severe (scored as 1, 2, or 3, respectively). As with any disease, in terms of providing proper perioperative management, it matters a great deal whether the OSA is mild, moderate, or severe. There are only two ways to determine the severity of OSA: by clinical impression and polysomnography.

1. Determining the Severity of Obstructive Sleep Apnea Based on Clinical Impression

The determination of the severity of OSA on the basis of clinical impression is best understood if the issue is first polarized between deciding whether it is mild or severe. A prototypical patient with mild OSA is obese, snores most of the time when asleep (but not necessarily all the time because the snoring may be position dependent; i.e., positive while supine and negative while in the lateral or prone positions), has not had definite observed apneas or arousals, and falls asleep during some of the quiet times that occur each day. Given the presence of obesity, the history of snoring during most of sleep, and

some diurnal sleeping, it would be reasonable, in the interest of being safe rather than sorry, to make an OSA severity judgment of mild and assign a severity score of 1. A prototypical patient with severe OSA is morbidly obese, snores virtually all the time while asleep, has definite observed apneas and frequent arousals but occasionally has an apnea that is unaccompanied by arousal and therefore becomes cyanotic (creating panic in observers), and falls asleep during most/many of the quiet times during the day. Given the presence of morbid obesity and the history of snoring during all sleep, occurrence of apneas, arousals, cyanotic episodes, and diurnal sleep during most quiet times, it would be reasonable to make a severity judgment of severe and assign a severity score of 3. Between these two extremes (severity moderate, severity score 2) the caregiver has to exercise judgment; admittedly, there is some imprecision in making a severity judgment of moderate OSA based on clinical impression. The only other way of determining severity of OSA is by a sleep study, and it is always desirable to determine severity with a sleep study.

2. Determining the Severity of Obstructive Sleep Apnea Based on a Sleep Study

A full polysomnography sleep study consists of monitoring the EEG (for stage of sleep and arousal), the electrooculogram (for NREM versus REM sleep), chest and abdominal pressure and movement (for breathing effort), oral and nasal airflow sensors and capnography (for actual movement of air), noise (for detecting snoring, vocalization, and snorting), submental and extremity electromyography (for pharyngeal muscle activity and extremity movement, respectively), oximetry for SpO_2, and electrocardiography (ECG) for heart function (Fig. 40-5).

The breathing effort monitors along with the actual air-flow monitors provide the raw data that allow a diagnosis of obstructive versus central sleep apnea, and oximetry determines their effect on oxygenation. Obstruction exists when a patient tries to breathe (generates negative pressure in the chest) but fails to breathe; after several progressively harder attempts to breathe, the airway opens with a few large breaths and then ordinary breathing resumes. In central apnea a patient does not try to breathe (does not generate negative pressure within the chest) and therefore does not breathe; after a variable pause, the patient begins to breathe with an ordinary effort and breath. In a mixed apnea a patient starts out with a central apnea, which is followed by an obstructive apnea, which terminates as described above. In a typical patient with moderate OSA, 85% to 95% of the apneas are obstructive, a few are central, and a few are mixed. With all three types of apneas, after a variable phase lag, SpO_2 decreases.

The raw sleep study data are gathered into a clinical report, which the anesthesiologist should be interested

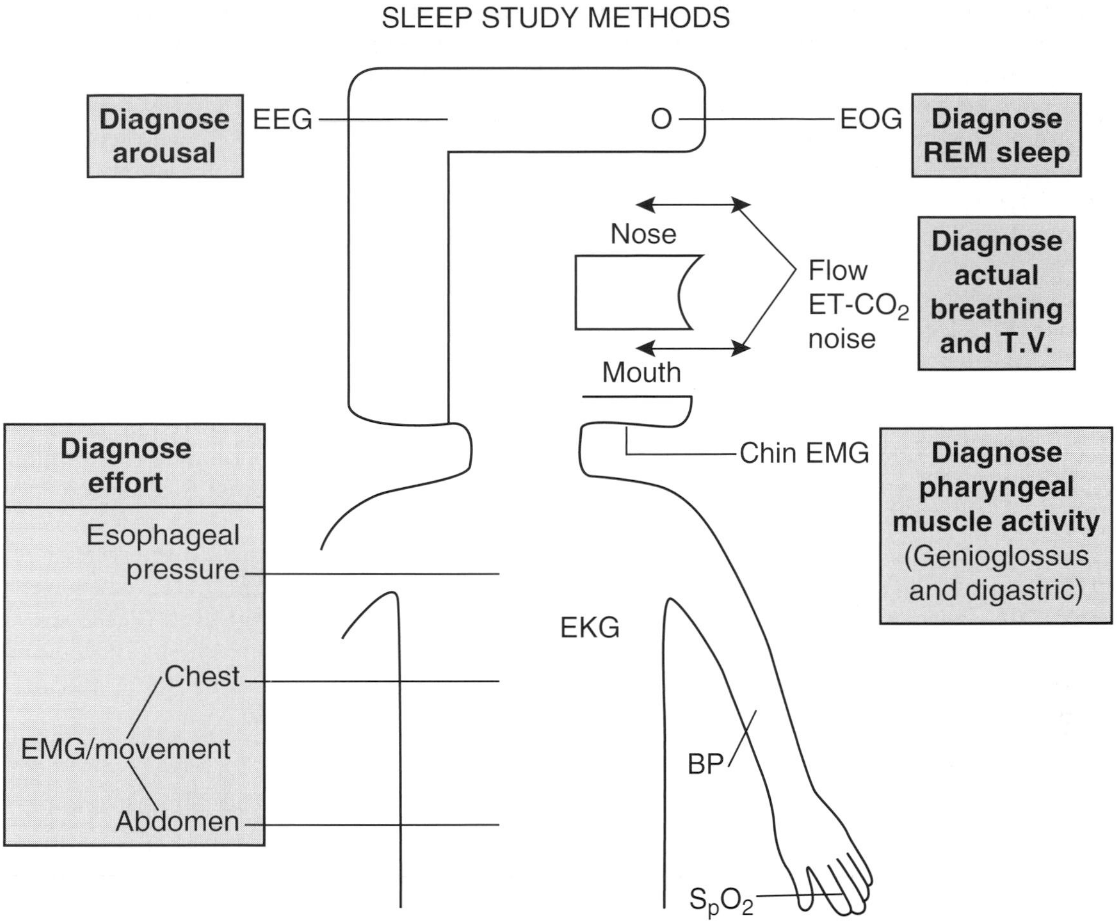

SLEEP STUDY METHODS

Figure 40-5 Schematic illustrating the methodology of polysomnography (sleep study). BP, blood pressure; EEG, electroencephalography; EKG, electrocardiography; EMG, electromyography; EOG, eletro-oculography; ET-CO$_2$, end-tidal CO$_2$; REM, rapid eye movement; Spo$_2$, oxygen saturation from pulse oximetry.

EVENTS	INDEXES
Apnea = no airflow >10 sec Hypopnea = TV <50% >10 sec Desaturation = SpO$_2$ ↓ >4% Arousal = clinical or EEG	Events/hour; AHI, ODI, AI Severity of sleep apnea is f(AHI): 6–20 = mild; 21–40 = moderate; >40 = severe

SpO$_2$ data also number of events per 60%–69%; 70%–79%; 80%–89%;
Extremes in heart rate and changes in ECG
are usually narrative descriptions

REPEAT THE ABOVE WITH CPAP TITRATION

Figure 40-6 Understanding the sleep study report. TV, tidal volume; AHI, apnea hypopnea index; ODI, oxygen desaturation index; AI, arousal index; M,M,S, mild, moderate, or severe.

in reading. Just as it would be unacceptable for an anesthesiologist to be informed that an ECG or chest x-ray is simply abnormal (everyone should want to know in what way and how much), the same should be true of a sleep study. Thus, it is important that the anesthesiologist know how to read a sleep study (Fig. 40-6).

The results of a sleep study are reported as events and indexes. An apnea event is no airflow for more than 10 seconds; a hypopnea event is a tidal volume less than 50% of the control awake value for more than 10 seconds; a desaturation event is a decrease in the SpO_2 greater than 4%; and an arousal event can be clinical (vocalization, turning, extremity movement) or a burst of waves on the EEG.[3] Indexes are events per hour; the apnea hypopnea index (AHI) is the number of times the patient was either apneic or hypopneic per hour; the oxygen desaturation index (ODI) is the number of times the patient had a decrease in SpO_2 greater than 4% per hour; and the arousal index (AI) is the number of times the patient aroused per hour. The severity of OSA is most universally expressed in terms of the AHI where 6 to 20 = mild, 21 to 40 = moderate, and >40 = severe; it is scored as 1, 2, or 3, respectively. The SpO_2 data will also be reported as the number of events per 10% epochs of SpO_2; that is, the number of times and the total time the patient was in the 60% to 69%, 70% to 79%, or 80% to 89% range. Extremes in heart rate and changes in ECG are usually narrative descriptions. If the patient has OSA, all of the above will be repeated with a continuous positive airway pressure (CPAP) titration either in the second half of the first night of the sleep study or on a second separate night of a sleep study in order to determine the level of CPAP that causes a significant decrease in the AHI. Thus, if an anesthesiologist reads a sleep study report, he or she will understand the severity of OSA not only in terms of AHI, but also in terms of how the patient arouses; the effect of OSA on oxygenation, heart rate, and heart rhythm; and the efficacy of CPAP.

E. PERIOPERATIVE RISK

Once the severity of OSA has been decided upon or determined, the severity of OSA will then factor into determining perioperative risk along with the invasiveness of anesthesia and/or surgery (I of A/S) and the postoperative opioid requirement (POR). The Guideline offers a methodology for determining perioperative risk from these three fundamental determinants (Fig. 40-7).

Perioperative risk is equal to the severity of OSA plus either the I of A/S or the POR, whichever is greater. The reason the I of A/S and POR are "either/or, whichever is greater" components of determining perioperative risk is that these two determinants largely or mainly occur sequentially.

1. Severity of Obstructive Sleep Apnea

The grading and scoring of severity of OSA are mild, moderate, or severe and 1, 2, or 3, respectively, and have already been discussed (see Section II. D). Now we will discuss grading and scoring of I of A/S and POR and then very simply illustrate how the perioperative risk is calculated.

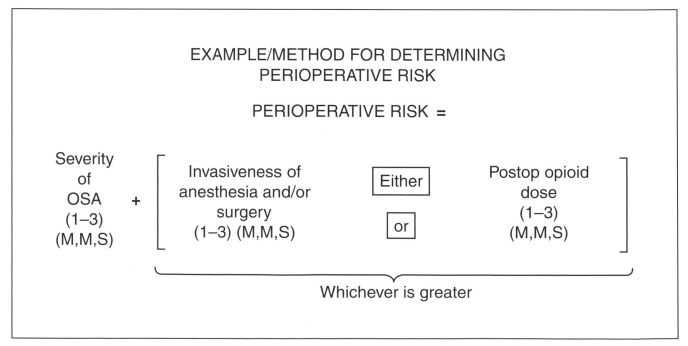

Figure 40-7 Calculating perioperative risk.

2. Invasiveness of Anesthesia and/or Surgery

The grading and scoring scales for I of A/S are the same as those for severity of OSA and are mild, moderate, or severe and 1, 2, or 3, respectively. The grading and scoring scales are best understood if the issue is approached in a stepwise manner. If the surgery performed is superficial and performed under local anesthesia or peripheral nerve block anesthesia, with no sedation, then neither the anesthesia nor surgery is invasive, and in terms of risk to the OSA patient, the invasive grade/score is 0. If the surgery performed remains superficial but moderate sedation is employed, then in terms of risk to an OSA patient, the invasiveness of the anesthesia has been increased and the invasive grade/score should be increased from zero to mild/1. If the surgery performed remains superficial but general anesthesia is employed, then in terms of risk to an OSA patient, the invasiveness of anesthesia has been increased, and the invasive grade/score should be increased from mild/1 to moderate/2. If the anesthesia is kept constant as a general anesthetic and the surgery is changed from superficial to either major cavitary or airway surgery, then in terms of risk to an OSA patient, the invasiveness of the surgery has been increased, and the invasive grade/score should be increased to moderate/2 to severe/3.

3. Postoperative Opioid Requirement

The grading/scoring scales for POR are the same as for severity of OSA and I of A/S and are mild, moderate, or severe and 1, 2, or 3, respectively. The grading/scoring scales for POR are best understood if approached in a stepwise manner. No POR has a grade/score of 0. A low-dose oral POR has a grade/score of mild/1. Moderate-dose oral POR has a grade/score of moderate/2. A high-dose oral or parenteral or neuraxial POR has a grade/score of severe/3.

4. Calculating Perioperative Risk

The ASA OSA Guideline defines "increased risk" as a risk score of 4 and "significantly increased risk" as a risk score of 5 or greater. Perioperative risk is either the sum of the severity of OSA score (1, 2, or 3) and the I of A/S score (1, 2, or 3) or the severity of OSA score (1, 2, or 3) plus the POR score (1, 2, or 3).[17] Using the sum of the severity of OSA score plus the I of A/S score formula (Table 40-1), "increased risk" (risk score of 4) is calculated with the combinations of moderate/2 + moderate/2 (2 + 2 = 4) or mild/1 + severe/3 (1 + 3 = 4) or severe/3 + mild/1 (3 + 1 = 4), and "significantly increased risk" (risk score of 5) is calculated with the combinations of moderate/2 + severe/3 (2 + 3 = 5) or severe/3 + moderate/2 (3 + 2 = 5). Once the anesthesiologist has a handle on perioperative risk and the factors that determine perioperative risk, perioperative risk then logically determines perioperative management.

F. PERIOPERATIVE MANAGEMENT

The ASA OSA Guideline makes a number of statements/recommendations regarding the capabilities of the facility in which the surgery is to be performed, preoperative management, intraoperative management, parameters for discharge from the postanesthesia care unit (PACU) to an unmonitored setting, and postoperative management.

1. Capabilities of the Facility in Which the Surgery Is to Be Performed

If it has been decided or determined that there is increased perioperative risk from OSA (risk score of 4; see section E, above), based on some combination of severity of OSA, the I of A/S, or the POR, then the Guideline states that any facility in which the surgery is to be performed should have emergency difficult airway equipment, respiratory care equipment (nebulizers, CPAP machines, ventilators), portable chest x-ray and ECG capability, a clinical laboratory for arterial blood gas (ABG) determination, electrolytes, hematocrit and hemoglobin, and a transfer arrangement to an inpatient facility. The above capability simply defines the care a patient with increased risk due to OSA deserves; the geographical location of the facility is irrelevant.

Table 40-1 **Calculating Perioperative Risk from Severity of Obstructive Sleep Apnea and Invasiveness of Anesthesia and/or Surgery**

OSA Severity	Invasiveness	OSA Risk
Moderate (2)	Moderate (2)	
Severe (3)	Mild (1)	Increased risk = 4
Mild (1)	Severe (3)	
Moderate (2)	Severe (3)	Significantly increased risk = 5
Severe (3)	Moderate (2)	

Finally, airway surgery (e.g., uvulopalatopharyngoplasty) in adults, tonsillectomy in children less than 3 years of age, and upper abdominal laparoscopy in adults should not be performed on an outpatient basis in OSA patients with increased risk (risk score of 4).

If it has been decided or determined that there is significantly increased risk from OSA (risk score of 5 or greater), based on some combination of severity of OSA, the I of A/S, or the POR, then the Guideline states that these patients are "generally not good candidates for surgery in a free standing facility."[17]

2. Preoperative Preparation

The Guideline states "that preoperative use of positive airway pressure (CPAP) or noninvasive positive pressure ventilation may improve the preoperative condition of patients who are at increased perioperative risk from OSA."[17] In fact, 3 months of CPAP treatment may reverse OSA-induced cardiovascular dysfunction and the metabolic syndrome.[12]

3. Intraoperative Management

For airway management in general, the ASA OSA Guideline defers to the ASA difficult airway Guideline.[1] In addition, the Guideline states that "general anesthesia with a secure airway is preferable to deep sedation without an airway for superficial procedures" and for "patients with OSA undergoing procedures involving the upper airway." For specific airway management, the ASA OSA Guideline recommends that patients at increased perioperative risk from OSA "be extubated when fully awake" in the nonsupine position (upright) when possible and only after verification of full reversal of neuromuscular blockade. With respect to anesthesia management, the Guideline states "respiratory CO_2 monitoring should be used during moderate or deep sedation" and "major conduction anesthesia (spinal/epidural) should be considered for peripheral procedures" in patients at increased risk from OSA.[17]

4. Discharge from the Postanesthesia Care Unit to an Unmonitored Bed/Environment

The Guideline states "patients with OSA should be monitored for a median of three hours longer than their non-OSA counterparts before discharge from the facility" and that "monitoring patients with OSA should continue for a median of seven hours after the last episode of airway obstruction or hypoxemia while breathing room air in an unstimulating environment."[17] In other words, these patients need to be watched carefully and for longer periods of time in the PACU, prior to discharge to an unmonitored setting.

5. Postoperative Management

The Guideline makes a number of statements about postoperative opioid use in OSA patients. If one agrees with the general proposition that decreasing and increasing exposure to opioids is good and bad, respectively, for respiratory function in OSA patients, then the following Guideline statements will make sense to the anesthesiologist. First, postoperative regional analgesia decreases adverse outcomes compared to the use of systemic opioids. Second, the Guideline states that exclusion of opioids from neuraxial analgesia reduces risk for OSA patients. Third, nonsteroidal anti-inflammatory drugs have an opioid-sparing effect and therefore their use (when acceptable) may result in less opioid use and a decrease in adverse outcomes. Finally, the Guideline points out that the literature in general suggests that use of basal patient-controlled analgesia rates will result in an increased incidence of hypoxemia.

With regard to postoperative respiratory care, the Guideline states that CPAP or noninvasive positive-pressure ventilation should be administered as soon as possible after surgery to patients with OSA who were receiving it preoperatively. In my opinion, feasible means when immediate post-extubation suctioning, nausea and vomiting, level of consciousness, communication, color of face and facial edema, and drug depression issues are resolved and the patient remains nonambulatory (i.e., he or she can go to sleep); in most OSA patients, this usually means that the CPAP should be applied toward the end of the PACU stay. In my opinion, waiting for the patient to be transferred to the floor in order to apply CPAP incurs unnecessary risk. The Guideline states that compliance with CPAP is increased when patients bring their own equipment to the hospital. It states that supplemental oxygen should be administered as needed to maintain "acceptable" SpO_2 and that "continuous SpO_2 in an intensive care unit (ICU), step down unit or by telemetry or by a dedicated professional observer in a private room, reduces the likelihood of perioperative complications among patients who they believe are at an increased perioperative risk from OSA." Importantly, "continuous bedside SpO_2 without continuous observation does not provide the same level of safety."[17]

G. COST OF IMPLEMENTATION OF THE GUIDELINE IN THE FIRST YEAR

The cost of implementation of the ASA OSA Guideline in the surgicenters and hospitals of the consultants to the Guideline is approximately \$100,000 to \$110,000 in the first year (Fig. 40-8). A relatively minor fraction of the cost is for additional sleep studies, CPAP machines, and portable ECG, chest x-ray, and ABG capability. The major fraction of cost is for increased

An ounce of prevention is better than a ton of treatment

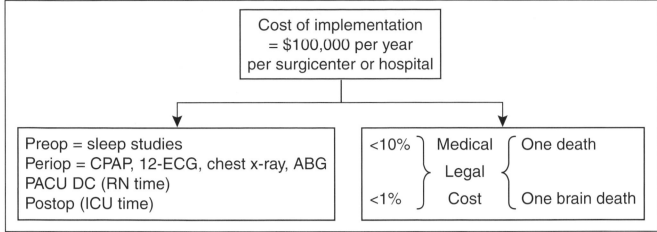

Figure 40-8 Cost of implementation of the ASA OSA Guideline. DC, discharge time.

PACU and ICU time. It is important to remind the reader that with a pretrial settlement or jury decision favorable to the plaintiff, $100,000 is approximately 10% of the average medical legal cost of an outright death and approximately 1% of the average medical legal cost of one severe brain death or damage. Thus, as is true in all medicine, an ounce of prevention is worth a ton of treatment.

REFERENCES

1. American Society of Anesthesiologists Task Force on Management of the Difficult Airway, Caplan RA, Benumof JL, Berry FA, et al: Practice Guidelines for Management of the Difficult Airway: An Updated Report by the American Society of Anesthesiologists Task Force on Management of the Difficult Airway. Anesthesiology 98:1269-1277, 2003.
2. Barsh CI: The origin of pharyngeal obstruction during sleep. Sleep Breathing 3:17-21, 1999.
3. Benumof JL: OSA in the adult obese patient: Implications for airway management. Clin Anesth 13:144-156, 2001.
4. Benumof JL: Policies and procedures needed for sleep apnea patients. Anesthesia Patient Safety Foundation Newsletter 17:57, 2002.
5. Bresnitz ER, Goldberg R, Kosinski RM: Epidemiology of obstructive sleep apnea. Epidemiol Rev 16:210-227, 1994.
6. Coughlin SR, Mawdsley L, Mugarza JA, et al: Obstructive sleep apnea is independently associated with an increased prevalence of metabolic syndrome. Eur Heart J 25:735-741, 2004.
7. Davies RJ, Ali NJ, Stradling JR: Neck circumference and other clinical features in the diagnosis of the obstructive sleep apnoea syndrome. Thorax 1992; 47: 101-105.
8. Fletcher EC, Proctor M, Yu J, Zhang J, et al: Pulmonary edema develops after recurrent obstructive apnea. Am J Respir Crit Care Med 160:1688-1696, 1999.
9. Horner RL, Mohiaddin RH, Lowell DG, et al: Sites and sizes of fat deposits around the pharynx in obese patients with obstructive sleep apnea and weight matched controls. Eur Respir J 2:613-622, 1989.
10. Koopmann CF, Field RA, Coulthard SW: Sleep apnea syndrome associated with a neck mass. Otolaryngol Head Neck Surg 89:949-952, 1981.
11. Lam JCM, Lam B, Lam CL, et al: Obstructive sleep apnea and the metabolic syndrome in community-based Chinese adults in Hong Kong. Respir Med 100:980-987, 2006.
12. Lattimore JL, Wilcox I, Skilton M, et al: Treatment of obstructive sleep apnea leads to improved microvascular endothelial function of the systemic circulation. Thorax 61:493-495, 2006.
13. Lofsky A: Sleep apnea and narcotic postoperative pain medication: A morbidity and mortality risk. Anesthesia Patient Safety Foundation Newsletter 17:24-25, 2002.
14. National Commission on Sleep Disorders Research: Wake Up America: A national alert. Washington, DC, Government Printing Office, 1993.
15. Obesity: Preventing and Managing the Global Epidemic: Report of a WHO Consultation on Obesity, Geneva, June 3-5, 1997. Geneva, World Health Organization, 1998.
16. Peterson GN, Domino KB, Caplan RA, et al: Management of the difficult airway: A closed claims analysis. Anesthesiology 103:33-39, 2005.
17. Practice Guidelines for the Perioperative Management of Patients with Obstructive Sleep Apnea. A Report by the American Society of Anesthesiologists Task Force on the Perioperative Management of Patients with Obstructive Sleep Apnea. Anesthesiology 104:1081-1093, 2006.

18. Rubinstein I, Colapinto N, Rotstein LE, et al: Improvement in upper airway function after weight loss in patients with obstructive sleep apnea. Am Rev Respir Dis 138:1192-1195, 1988.

19. Shelton KE, Gay SB, Woodson H, et al: Pharyngeal fat in obstructive sleep apnea. Am Rev Respir Dis 148:462-466, 1993.

20. Strohl KP, Redline S: Recognition of obstructive sleep apnea. Am J Respir Crit Care Med 154:279-289, 1996.

21. Strollo PJ, Rogers RM: Obstructive sleep apnea. N Engl J Med 334:99-104, 1996.

22. White DP, Lombard RM, Cadieux J, Zwillich CW: Pharyngeal resistance in normal humans: Influence of gender, age and obesity. J Appl Physiol 58:365-371, 1985.

23. Willet WC, Dietz WH, Colditz GA: Guidelines for healthy weight. N Engl J Med 341:427-434, 1999.

24. Young T, Palta M, Dempsey J, et al: The occurrence of sleep-disordered breathing among middle-aged adults. N Engl J Med 328:1230-1235, 1993.

41

AIRWAY MANAGEMENT IN BURN PATIENTS

Bettina U. Schmitz
Stephen M. Koch
Donald H. Parks

I. INTRODUCTION

The outcome, for both survival and quality of life, has improved dramatically for burn patients over the past 20 years. However, airway and respiratory complications remain a common cause of morbidity and mortality. The airway of the burn patient presents special problems and requires certain considerations, not only in the initial stage of the burn injury but also daily during the hospital course and, in some patients, even after the burn injury throughout their life.

II. AIRWAY MANAGEMENT IN THE ACUTELY BURNED PATIENT

A. EVALUATION OF THE PATIENT AFTER ACUTE BURN INJURY AND INDICATIONS FOR EARLY AIRWAY MANAGEMENT

1. History

Burns are a major cause of traumatic injury in all ages of the population. There were 25,000 burn patients admitted to burn units in the United States in 2001. Of these, approximately 50% required placement of an artificial airway and 4500 eventually succumbed to their initial injury or subsequent complications. Up to 10,000 patients die per year in the United States of burn-related infections, with pneumonia as the most common etiology.[38] However, other publications highlight the significant risk of immediate death from toxic gases, which account for the largest proportion of fire deaths.[7,30]

The first priority at the scene of the injury is the establishment of an adequate airway. In evaluating any burn patient for early airway management, several factors need to be addressed. Burn patients are often intubated in the field, the most common indications being loss of consciousness and severe facial burn or injury. After transport and admission to the emergency department, these patients are intubated for airway protection secondary to either continued or progressive change in mental status or clinical suspicion of impending airway compromise such as dyspnea, tachypnea, progressive hoarseness, or stridor. As soon as the patient arrives in the emergency area, all important information should be gathered. If the patient is unable to communicate, the rescue team and, if possible, the family should be questioned. It is imperative to know (1) the location and type of injury (e.g., explosion, flame, fluid, steam, chemicals, high voltage), (2) the circumstances (e.g., open space, confined space, duration of exposure), (3) the type of accidents (e.g., car, motorbike, jump to escape, fall), (4) the level of consciousness, and (5) evidence of aspiration. Furthermore, it is important to ascertain past medical history.[6,18,47]

The blast of an explosion can cause additional injuries related to the pressure, such as pneumothorax or ear drum perforation, or injuries related to a fall, if it should occur. Inhalation of hot steam is rare but can rapidly progress to severe edema of the upper airway, as can accidentally ingested hot fluid. The extension of a thermal injury with hot fluid is often more difficult to estimate in the initial phase after the injury in comparison with an injury caused by fire. This kind of injury is more common in smaller children, making the fluid management even more challenging. Certain chemicals continue to destroy tissue after the visible fire has stopped.

High-voltage injuries can cause specific problems in addition to the burn injury. Depending on the pathway of the current, brain edema, cardiac dysrhythmias, extensive necrosis of muscles, compartment syndrome, rhabdomyolysis with or without renal failure, and fractures can occur and are commonly seen problems after high-voltage accidents.

The circumstances of an injury—open space versus confined space, household or industrial fire—and the duration of exposure are relevant to know to estimate the probability and the possible degree of a superimposed inhalation injury, such as carbon monoxide (CO) or cyanide poisoning and inhalation of other toxic substances.

Additional injuries need to be ruled out in burn victims involved in a motor vehicle or motor cycle accident or when the patient tried to escape from a fire by jumping out a window. Finally, information about signs of impaired airway reflexes (i.e., aspiration) and the initial mental status should be obtained.

2. Altered Mental Status

An isolated burn injury itself usually does not alter the mental status in the initial stage. A patient who is disoriented, stuporous, or unconscious after a burn injury is suspected to have an additional injury. Coexisting conditions that are related to the burn injury include inhalation injury with hypoxemia, CO and cyanide intoxication, or direct injury, such as high-voltage electric shock. Other reasons for an altered mental state are trauma, intoxication with alcohol or other drugs, hyper- and hypoglycemia, postictal state, and acute psychotic reaction. Semiconscious and unconscious patients after a burn injury need to be intubated to secure the airway and ventilated with 100% oxygen, which treats two likely causes, CO intoxication and hypoxemia. When an injury of the cervical spine is likely, for example, after a fall or jump to escape a fire or car accident, intubation should be performed under cervical spine injury precautions.[6,16,18,24,57]

3. Cardiovascular Abnormalities

Cardiovascular instability, dysrhythmia, and cardiac arrest can be the consequences of severe CO intoxication, caused by a preexisting cardiac disease, or a combination of both. Hypotension can be caused by the massive fluid loss that occurs with a burn injury and responds to fluid therapy in most patients. Additional injuries that can contribute to hypovolemic shock, such as a fall, a jump, or an accident, should be considered. Intubation and ventilation with 100% oxygen are performed when the patient does not respond to fluid resuscitation in the presence of severe cardiovascular instability or dysrhythmia.[6,17,57] The management of the patient is much easier and safer if the cardiovascular status is stable.

4. Respiratory Insufficiency

The diagnosis of respiration damage is often suggested by history and physical examination of the burn patient upon presentation to the hospital. Pulmonary damage is much more likely to occur if burns take place in a closed-space fire. For instance, respiratory insufficiency and apnea are most often seen in patients with severe inhalation trauma and CO intoxication. Obstruction of the upper airway after hot fluid or steam exposure is an acute life-threatening condition. Less common causes are drug overdose and intoxication or conditions unrelated to burn injury that cause respiratory failure, such as head injury and shock.[6,24,34,57]

5. Burns to Neck and Face

Extensive burns of the face and the neck can result in often gross edema formation that makes a translaryngeal intubation difficult or impossible. These patients often have an inhalation injury with edema formation in the pharynx and larynx further complicating the intubation. Any delay in performing the intubation can result in a "cannot ventilate, cannot intubate" (CICV) situation. Emergency surgical airway, cricothyrotomy, and tracheostomy are then the only possibilities left for access to the airway.[6,24,34,57]

6. Extensive Burns

Patients with an extensively burned body surface area often have concomitant inhalation injury, which usually requires ventilator support. The generalized edema formation can make intubation difficult after a few hours of resuscitation. The cardiovascular changes related to the massive fluid loss after a major burn injury can make ventilator support necessary. After the initial phase of the burn injury, the patients develop a hypermetabolic state with high oxygen demand and increased CO_2 production and often require ventilator support. In most burn centers, patients with burns of 60% or more of their body surface area undergo prophylactic intubation and ventilation.[6,17]

7. Additional Injuries

Burn injury can result as an aftermath of any other kind of accident, trauma, or metabolic disorder. For instance, the burn injury itself can lead to additional injuries when the victim tries to escape the fire by jumping out a window. Consequently, all patients should be evaluated for additional trauma, metabolic conditions, and intoxication as a cause or a consequence of the burn injury. Because cervical spine injuries can change the airway management plan, cervical spine injury should be considered and ruled out when possible in all patients with an unknown or unclear history of injury.

B. SURGERY IN THE INITIAL STATE OF BURN INJURY

The early surgical treatment of burn injuries has become very common. The anesthesiologist should consider that most of the patients are probably not fasted. A burned patient, like any trauma victim, may have a full stomach at the time of injury; hence, the possibility of regurgitation and aspiration is ever present. The high level of stress hormones in combination with opioid-based pain management prolongs gastric emptying.

Another concern is the unpredictable course of edema formation. Aggressive fluid resuscitation for the initial trauma, high demands for further fluid administration during surgery, and fluid shifts because of the primary burn trauma and the surgical intervention cause massive edema within a short time. Securing the airway with an endotracheal tube (ET) is the safest way to avoid hazardous problems.

C. INHALATION INJURY

Approximately 20% of patients admitted to regional burn centers have some degree of inhalation injury. It has adverse effects on both gas exchange and hemodynamics, but the severity of individual injuries is predictable only on the basis of history, physical examination, and currently available diagnostic tests. Understanding of the distinct pathophysiology of the different types of inhalation injury has enabled the physician to better assess and treat such injuries. Inhalation injury is defined as the sequela of aspiration of the following gases or products.

• Toxic gases and heat/airway-lung interface in fire victims
• Intoxicant gases
• Irritants
• Thermal damage to the airways from smoke

Inhalation injuries are caused both by the heat of inhaled smoke and by toxic chemicals inhaled into the respiratory tract. Heat and inhaled chemicals cause injury in different fashions. In an enclosed environment burn, temperatures exceeding 800° C may be achieved with reduced oxygen content as low as 10% concurrently with CO concentrations exceeding 0.5%.[54,55] The hallmarks of smoke inhalation injury are hypoxia and hypercapnia. There are two distinct mechanisms of pulmonary injury following inhalation: smoke toxicity and CO intoxication. Direct thermal injuries are described in Table 41-1.

The nature of toxic gases that cause death from smoke inhalation is not well described. In addition to CO, hydrogen cyanide inhalation from residential fires has been demonstrated, and an elevated plasma lactate concentration is a useful indicator of cyanide toxicity without severe burn.[4] Predictive factors for smoke inhalation in patients are (1) soot deposits in the oropharynx, (2) dysphonia, (3) rhonchi, (4) loss of consciousness (higher CO level), (5) bronchospasm, and (6) a positive sputum culture. A chest radiograph is usually normal and is not required for diagnosis. In a study involving patients, Masanes and colleagues used bronchoscopy and biopsy to diagnose early inhalation injury.[29] Their findings are summarized in Table 41-2. In burned patients, airway mucosal injury remains the primary pathology, increasing the risks for airway management. The key pathologic signs are depicted in Table 41-3.

Table 41-1   **Direct Thermal Inhalation Injuries**

Present in one third of burn patients
Leading cause of death in fires is smoke inhalation and not burns
Mortality from smoke inhalation alone is 5% to 8%
Soot deposition
Heat injury usually confined to above the cords
Gas injury: chemical tracheobronchitis—severity depends on the type of inhaled fumes and the duration of the exposure
Loss of surfactant
Pneumonia (aspiration or nosocomial or both)
Pulmonary congestion
Chemical pulmonary edema: alveolar injury or retrograde flow of bronchorrhea
Acute respiratory distress syndrome: delayed presentation— may be relatively asymptomatic for the first 3 to 5 days
Atelectasis
Pulmonary emboli

Nieman and associates demonstrated in animals that smoke inhalation produces a significant but brief (15 minutes) increase in the pressure drop across the pulmonary veins that may accelerate the formation of pulmonary edema, which is not associated with changes in thromboxane B_2 or prostaglandin $F_{1\alpha}$.[40] Using an ovine model of severe smoke inhalation injury, Cox and coauthors reported that heparin decreased tracheobronchial cast formation, improved oxygenation, minimized barotrauma, and reduced pulmonary edema.[12] Inhalation injury of the airway is a result of steam (heat), carbenoids, and chemical and toxic products of fire or combustion. The injury can be described anatomically or in terms of

Table 41-2   **Bronchoscopy and Biopsy to Diagnose Early Inhalation Injury[29]**

130 consecutive burn patients underwent bronchoscopy at admission
Bronchoscopy or biopsy positive in 46 cases
23 of 44 (52%) with chemical inhalation developed acute respiratory distress syndrome (ARDS)
Of 83 negative cases, only 6 developed ARDS (7%)
Absence of bronchial edema was a poor prognostic sign indicating deep mucosal damage

Table 41-3   **Key Pathologic Signs of Airway Mucosal Injury**

Soot present: macroscopic soot deposits always associated with histologic signs of inhalation injury even if the rest of the bronchi are normal
Erythema, edema, ulceration
Mucosal fragility (hemorrhage on contact with the bronchoscope)
Increase in bronchial secretions
Loss of cough reflex a poor prognostic sign signaling greater depth of mucosal injury
Mucosal breakdown and sloughing into the endobronchial tree
Mucosal necrosis
Sloughing of scar tissue

the inhaled agent. In most patients, the entire airway is involved to various degrees and several chemical or toxic agents are inhaled. The upper airway can be described as the area of the vocal cords and above and the major airway described as the tracheobronchial tree and the parenchyma such as the terminal bronchi and alveoli.[35]

1. Upper Airway Injury

Direct injury of the upper airway with steam, super-heated air, or liquid is rare. The heat-conducting capacity of air is low; hot air cools down rapidly in the oro- and nasopharynx. Reflex closure of the glottis usually protects the structures below the vocal cords. Although uncommon, this injury can be life threatening within a short period of time because of the rapidly developing massive edema with complete obstruction of the upper airway. Consequently, early airway management is mandatory in these patients.[17,24,27,28] In a study involving 18 patients, Gaissert and coworkers reported that strictures of the upper airway related to inhalation injury were associated with prolonged inflammation and involved larynx and trachea in a majority of patients. These complex injuries respond to prolonged tracheal stenting and resection or stenting of subglottic stenoses with recovery of a functional airway and voice in most patients.[16]

2. Major Airway Injury

Most injuries of the upper and major airway result from chemical toxins from the fire or combustion, such as ammonia, nitrogen dioxide, sulfate, and chlorine. These agents cause edema of the mucosa and impair ciliary function. Patients should undergo early intubation to avoid airway difficulties and respiratory deterioration.[17,24,28,47]

3. Lung Parenchymal Injury

Distal propagation of chemicals adherent to fine particles, such as aldehydes, phosgene, hydrochloric acid, and nitrogen acids, causes injury of the parenchyma, usually in combination with injury of the upper and major airways by damaging the alveolar membrane. Aldehydes denature membrane proteins and nitrogen alters the membrane lipids, reducing surfactant production and impairing local defenses. Consequences are obstruction of the airway with sloughed endobronchial debris, accumulated secretions, and reduced production of surfactant with atelectasis and air trapping. The higher capillary permeability contributes to edema formation.[8,24,28,39,47]

4. Symptoms

In 90% of patients with burns to the face and neck, an airway injury is present. Absence of facial burns does not rule out significant airway injury. Singed nasal hairs, swelling of the tongue, hoarseness (present in 50% of patients with inhalation injury), and stridor (present in about 20% of patients) are not seen in all patients but are serious symptoms indicating injury of the laryngeal structures with edema formation. Progressive symptoms may be followed by partial or complete loss of the airway; therefore, early intubation is mandatory. Cough, bronchospasm with wheezing, and respiratory distress with labored breathing and use of accessory muscles indicate injury of the smaller airways. Carbonated sputum does not necessarily indicate injury below the vocal cords; it can be of nasal origin.[6,18,24,27,34,47,57]

5. Diagnosis

The "gold standard" for diagnosis of an inhalation injury is direct inspection of the airway by laryngoscopy and fiberoptic bronchoscopy. This can be performed at the bedside, avoiding the necessity to transport the patient and interrupt the resuscitation. It should initially be performed to document the presence and extent of the injury and should be frequently repeated in the following days and weeks to follow the course of the injury and remove debris, thereby reducing the rate of further complications, such as obstruction and atelectasis.[6,8,18,27,33,35,47,57] Flow-volume curves are often difficult to obtain and depend on the cooperation of the patient.[6,47] Arterial blood gas analysis should be obtained early to rule out or confirm CO intoxication. An isolated inhalation injury does not necessarily change the arterial blood gases in the early phase.[6,47] The chest radiograph is often normal in the early phase of inhalation injury but can show signs of previously existing problems or additional injuries.[6,47] Injuries of the smaller airways and the parenchyma can be diagnosed with radioisotope evaluation. After intravenous injection of xenon 133 or inhalation of technetium 99, the healthy lung rapidly clears the isotopes. In the presence of an inhalation injury, the clearance is delayed and asymmetric.

Unfortunately, it cannot be performed at the bedside and is therefore not practical for all patients.[28,35,47,57]

D. CARBON MONOXIDE POISONING

Carbon monoxide is a product of combustion and fire; it is colorless, odorless, and tasteless. Victims of fire are suspected of having and evaluated for carbon monoxide poisoning, especially when the accident happened in a confined space. CO binds to the iron-containing enzymes hemoglobin and cytochrome. The affinity of CO for hemoglobin is 200-fold greater than the affinity of oxygen for hemoglobin. Replacing the oxygen molecule on hemoglobin, CO reduces the oxygen available to the patient. Carboxyhemoglobin shifts the oxygen dissociation curve to the left, further impairing oxygen delivery to the tissue. Binding to cytochrome oxidase in the mitochondria, CO impairs oxygen utilization on the cellular level with the consequence of tissue hypoxia and metabolic acidosis.[6,24,27,28,47]

Carbon monoxide poisoning is the leading cause of death by either accidental or intentional poisoning in the United States.[1] The diagnosis is frequently overlooked because of the nonspecific nature of the most common symptoms: fatigue, headache, weakness, dizziness, confusion, and transient loss of consciousness.[3,6] Patients arriving at an acute care facility with these symptoms have no specific clinical findings to suggest CO poisoning. The diagnosis must be made by laboratory evaluation as follows.

1. Diagnosis

a. History
- Circumstances of the burn injury (i.e., fire or smoke exposure)
- Time of exposure
- Sources (internal combustion engines, smoke inhalation, stoves, furnaces, tobacco, industrial, exacerbated in enclosed areas or those with poor ventilation)[14,32,41]

b. Pathophysiology
- CO combining with hemoglobin with an affinity 240 times that of O_2
- Reduction of the total O_2 carrying capacity of blood
- Tissue hypoxia[32]
- Oxyhemoglobin curve shifted to left (hemoglobin saturated at a much lower partial pressure of oxygen with decreased oxygen delivery)
- Release of the remaining O_2 on hemoglobin diminished
- Pulmonary excretion directly related to minute ventilation

c. Laboratory (Table 41-4)
- Partial pressure of oxygen in arterial blood, pulse oximetry, and arterial oxygen saturation do not reflect CO poisoning and can be normal.[6,27,57]

Table 41-4   **Symptoms, Signs, and Neurologic Disorders following Carbon Monoxide Poisoning**

Symptoms	Signs	Neurologic Findings
Fatigue	Tachycardia	Tinnitus
Headache	Increased minute ventilation (13)	Loss of hearing
Dizziness	Tachypnea	Nystagmus
Confusion	± hypertension	Ataxia
Nausea		Cerebral edema
Dyspnea		Delayed sequelae [32,36,41]
Weakness		3 days to 3 weeks
Diarrhea		Intellectual deterioration
Abdominal pain		Memory impairment
Visual changes		Personality changes
Angina		Irritability
		Violence
		Aggressiveness
		Moodiness

- Normally carboxyhemoglobin is less than 2 in nonsmokers.[23]
- It is slightly higher in pregnancy because of fetal CO production.
- In smokers it is chronically 3% to 8%, immediately after smoking 10% to 15%.
- When exposure is not recognized, an influenza-like viral illness is the most common presentation[19,32]
- Pets have a similar presentation.

d. Symptoms (Table 41-5)
- Few or no symptoms are observed with a CO-hemoglobin less than 10%.
- Headache, nausea, fatigue, and dizziness are seen with CO-hemoglobin levels of 10% to 20%.
- Disorientation and confusion are present with a CO of 20% to 40% and hallucination, combativeness, stupor, and coma when levels reach 40% to 60%. Also, dysrhythmias may occur in these patients.
- CO-hemoglobin levels higher than 60% usually result in death.[6,8,27,28,57]

2. Treatment

Oxygen at 100% accelerates the dissociation of CO-hemoglobin by 50% every 30 minutes and should be administered initially to every burned patient. Patients with carbon monoxide levels higher than 20% to 25% or central nervous or cardiovascular system signs of carbon monoxide poisoning, or both, should undergo intubation.

Table 41-5   **Correlation of Symptoms with Measured Blood Levels**

Blood Level (Carboxyhemoglobin %)	Symptoms
0-10	Decreased exercise ability in pulmonary disease patients, decreased anginal threshold
10-20	Headache, dyspnea with mild exertion, angina, dilation of cutaneous vessels
20-30	Headache, nausea ± vomiting, easy fatigue, irritable, difficulty concentrating
30-40	Severe headache, dizziness, fatigue, weakness, syncope with exertion, impaired thought processes
40-50	Tachypnea, tachycardia, syncope, confusion
50-60	Respiratory failure, collapse, seizures, coma
60-70	Respiratory failure, severe hypotension, coma, frequently fatal
>70	Coma, rapidly fatal

Elective bilateral myringotomies should be performed and all air-filled devices (ET cuffs) should have the air replaced by water prior to pressurization in the hyperbaric chamber. Common protocols place the patient in a hyperbaric chamber at 2 to 3 atmospheres for about 90 minutes with two to three short interruptions. The data are inconclusive about whether hyperbaric oxygen treatment prevents a long-term aftermath of CO poisoning, but hyperbaric oxygen therapy for unconscious patients or patients with high CO levels is recommended in several reports.[8,17,27,28] Challenges of hyperbaric oxygen therapy include limited availability and difficulty continuing the initial fluid resuscitation with the usually limited space and access to the patient in a hyperbaric chamber.[6,8,27,28]

3. Long-Term Aftermath

Delayed neurologic symptoms such as ataxia, mental deterioration, and incontinence are seen in about 12.5% of patients with higher initial CO-hemoglobin levels. The computed tomography scans of these patients show bilateral areas of decreased density in the globus pallidus.[6,8,24,27,47,57] Therapy in this setting should be directed at minimizing intracranial pressure, utilizing such modalities as hyperventilation, elevation of the head of the bed, avoidance of excess fluids, and possibly corticosteroid administration.

E. CYANIDE POISONING

Cyanide is a product of burning plastic containing high amounts of nitrogen such as polyurethane, polyacrylonitrite, and acrocyanate. Cyanide causes asphyxia on the cellular level by inhibiting intracellular cytochrome oxidase activity and impairing mitochondrial oxygen consumption. Lactate acidosis is a result of an interruption of the tricarboxylic acid cycle. Adenosine triphosphate production in the involved cells becomes anaerobic.[6,8,27,47]

1. Diagnosis

Inhalation injury in a confined space and longer exposure make cyanide intoxication possible. With a high CO-hemoglobin concentration, the probability of cyanide poisoning is higher. The symptoms of cyanide intoxication are comparable to those of CO poisoning. Although no specific diagnosis exists, lactate levels in the blood correlate with the cyanide levels.[27]

2. Treatment

Although some authors consider specific treatment not necessary, others recommend treatment with sodium thiosulfate, sodium nitrite, or hydroxycobalamin. Sodium sulfate enforces the hepatic metabolism of cyanide. Thiosulfate is the substrate in the metabolism of cyanide by hepatic rhodanase. Cyanide binds to methemoglobin.

As a result, methemoglobinemia is induced by intravenous administration of sodium nitrite. Methemoglobin and hydroxycobalamin bind with cyanide and thereby neutralize its effects on patients. However, this therapy offers some difficulties. The amount of medication necessary is not known, and methemoglobinemia may further contribute to reduced oxygen availability.[8,16,27,47]

F. AIRWAY MANAGEMENT

1. General Considerations

Airway assessment is best done clinically on the basis of the history and physical examination, supplemented with laryngoscopy and bronchoscopy in selected patients. Patients with stridor or hoarseness are susceptible to edema formation in the laryngeal structures. If one waits until edema is advanced, intubation can be very difficult. Because edema formation is progressive over time, these patients need to be evaluated with a fiberoptic bronchoscope (FOB), and an ET should be placed if edema is present. Patients with injury of the upper airway need to be intubated as soon as possible; a delay in performing the intubation can result in total obstruction of the upper airway. An FOB intubation, performed either nasally or orally, is advantageous in that the patient stays awake, breathes spontaneously, and keeps the airway open. The degree of pathologic change is difficult to judge without examination. The FOB approach allows evaluation of the upper airway, laryngeal structures, trachea, main stem bronchi, and smaller airways.

When the FOB approach is not successful, the intubation can be performed by direct laryngoscopy with a regular laryngoscope, Bullard laryngoscope, intubation stylet, or FOB through an LMA-Fastrach (intubating laryngeal mask airway [ILMA]). Because mask ventilation is often difficult or impossible in the presence of facial burns and the fasting status of the patient is often unknown or questionable, a rapid sequence intubation should be performed. Succinylcholine is considered safe to administer in the first 24 hours after a burn injury. After this initial period, the use of succinylcholine is contraindicated because of the development of atypical acetylcholine receptors over the entire muscle membrane, causing massive release of potassium with possible lethal potassium levels. Consequently, it is recommended to avoid the use of succinylcholine for up to 2 years after the burn injury. Although no contraindication exists for the use of certain hypnotics, the cardiovascular status and the presence of dysrhythmia should be taken into account when choosing the hypnotic agent.* The airway in a burn patient can offer a variety of expected and unexpected difficulties. The immediate availability of ETs of different sizes, supraglottic ventilatory devices (SVDs), a variety of laryngoscopes, an FOB, and a set for emergency

---

*References 6, 8, 15, 18, 24, 27, 28, 34, 47, 51-53, 57.

Figure 41-1 Carbonaceous sputum, singed nasal hairs, and facial burns indicate possible upper airway thermal injury.

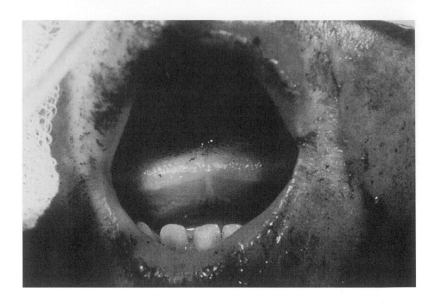

cricothyrotomy and tracheostomy in a difficult airway cart can avoid stressful and potentially dangerous situations (Figs. 41-1 and 41-2).

In patient with third- to fourth-degree burns of the neck, laryngoscopy can be impossible because of the rigidity of the cervical tissue, and a vertical incision from the sternal notch to the chin can facilitate laryngoscopy. Extensive or circumferential third- to fourth-degree burns to the chest wall can cause severe restrictive insufficiency and may require immediate escharotomy of the anterior chest wall (Fig. 41-3).

2. Urgent Airway Management

Rapidly progressive upper airway obstruction or accidental extubation can be a serious, life-threatening event in the burn patient. The worst, but not uncommon, consequence is the CICV situation. The edema formation in a burned patient is progressive in the first 72 hours; it is generalized and not only present in the burned areas. Dressings further restrict access to the airway. Placing a face mask and establishing sufficient mask ventilation can be impossible. Positioning a laryngoscope and visualizing the epiglottis and the vocal cords may be difficult or impossible because of edema of the face, neck, and laryngeal structures. In the spontaneously breathing patient, an FOB intubation can be attempted. The size of an ET should be reduced by half or even a full size smaller than the previous ET. An experienced physician may attempt intubating the nonbreathing patient with an FOB; otherwise, an attempt to intubate the patient with direct laryngoscopy with a Macintosh or Miller blade, a Bullard laryngoscope, a light wand, or an ILMA should be performed. At the same time, preparation to perform a surgical airway, cricothyrotomy, or tracheostomy should be initiated. The decision to provide surgical airway access should not be delayed by multiple attempts to intubate translaryngeally because the same obstacles that make the conventional intubation difficult also complicate the surgical approach. Identification of the anatomic landmarks can be impossible. Exposure of larynx and trachea with a longitudinal incision and placing the tube under direct vision may be the fastest approach in very difficult cases. To bridge the time in establishing a definite airway, an LMA or Combitube can maintain oxygenation and ventilation of the patient.[47]

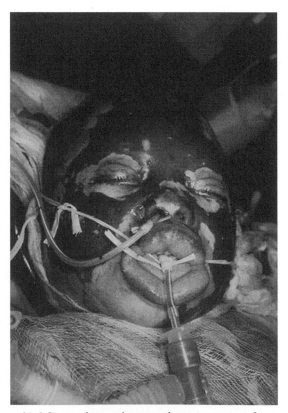

Figure 41-2 Severe airway edema continues to progress for several days after initial injury and intubation.

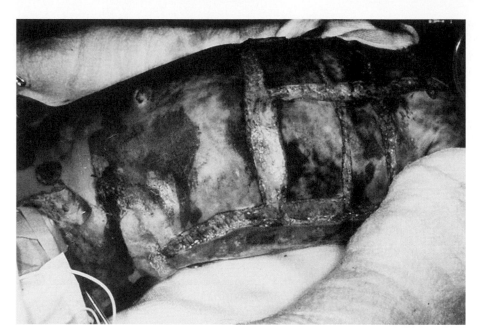

Figure 41-3 Escharotomy of the chest.

3. Special Considerations in Children

Because of the smaller airway diameter in children, even a modest degree of airway edema can result in total airway obstruction. Because resistance to flow is inversely proportional to the fourth power of the radius of the tube, decreasing the radius by half increases resistance to flow 16 times. When symptoms of upper airway injury such as hoarseness and stridor are present, the intubation needs to be performed as soon as possible. Although an awake FOB intubation is sometimes not possible, the intubation can be performed under deep inhalation anesthesia maintaining spontaneous ventilation or after induction with a sedative hypnotic and muscle relaxant with a Macintosh laryngoscope, a pediatric Bullard laryngoscope, or an LMA.[6,24,27,34,47,53] In addition, a straight Miller blade can be used to good effect in infants and small children because of the high position of the larynx and allows the ability to lift the epiglottis. The risk of subsequent loss of airway patency is particularly acute in small children, in whom moderate mucosal edema can lead to complete airway occlusion. The use of heliox has been proposed as a way to avoid intubation in such children.[44]

4. Tracheostomy

Tracheostomy is frequently performed in burn patients when a translaryngeal intubation fails. Elective tracheostomy for burn patients who need longer intubation and ventilation has been considered controversial.[1,6,27,43] Older reports found more frequent complications of strictures and stenosis in patients after tracheostomy. Most of these studies were not prospective and randomized, and the durations of intubation and ventilation were longer in the patients who underwent tracheostomy.[26,35] Most of the more recent reports do not confirm this higher incidence of complications of tracheostomies in burn patients,

whether performed in the operating room or at the bedside or by a surgical or dilative approach.[9,25] Studies in children reach the same conclusion.[3,11,42] One study documented no significantly higher incidence of complications following tracheostomy.[20] These findings were confirmed by Palmieri and colleagues, who reported that early tracheostomy in severely burned children is safe and effective.[42] It provides a secure airway and may result in improvement in ventilator management for these children. Another report could not document any advantage in the outcome in patients with tracheostomy versus patients with translaryngeal intubation.[45] Whether the tracheostomies were performed through burned or intact skin has not been reported. At this time, it seems to be safe to perform an elective tracheostomy in burn patients without a significantly higher risk of airway complications.[5]

The lack of studies with larger numbers of patients and long-term follow-up of patients after translaryngeal intubation and tracheostomy makes it impossible to give a recommendation whether to prefer the prolonged translaryngeal intubation or to perform a tracheostomy when a longer period of respiratory support is expected. A retrospective analysis of 36 patients with burn injuries was conducted to compare conventional tracheostomy with percutaneous dilational tracheostomy.[9] The authors concluded that percutaneous dilatational tracheostomy allows a shorter duration of mechanical ventilation, thereby decreasing patients' morbidity, hospital stay, and cost.

5. Extubation of the Burned Patient

After a burn injury and inhalation trauma, special consideration should be given to the patient's airway patency in preparation for extubation. Tracheal stenosis and tracheal strictures are well-described complications after long-term intubation and traumatic intubation. Although reports of severe airway stenosis after inhalation injury are infrequent, the consequences are severe and must be anticipated. In patients with an inhalation injury of the airway, the inflammation response further contributes to the development of complications. Changes of the larynx are vocal cord granuloma, vocal cord palsy, and complete or partial vocal cord fusion.[10] Changes of the major airway include granuloma, subglottic stenosis, and stenosis on various levels of the trachea and the main stem bronchi. Patients can be symptomatic immediately after extubation or in the following weeks or months as a result of a progressive scar formation. Initial leading symptoms are stridor and hoarseness; later, respiratory distress and use of the auxiliary breathing muscles ensue.

The patency of the upper airway has to be confirmed before extubation. Inspection of the laryngeal structures and the major airways prior to extubation may rule out severe pathologic changes that may lead to an early extubation failure. Working suction devices, pulse oximetry monitors, reintubation supplies and standard intubating medications, a respiratory therapist, the patient's nurse, and the clinician who approved the extubation should be at the bedside for timely reintubation should acute respiratory distress, stridor, or desaturation occur. As burn patients are usually intubated preoperatively, they should receive appropriate therapy before extubation for such conditions as cardiac disease, pulmonary disease such as inhalation injury or edema, nosocomial infections, acute electrolyte disturbances (severe hypokalemia or hypophosphatemia), severe hypo- or hyperthermia, profound anemia, acute adrenal insufficiency, or altered mental status.

Before extubation the entire gastrointestinal tract should be assessed, including dentition, a history of epistaxis, herpes stomatitis, recent upper gastrointestinal bleeding, or postoperative ileus. Gastric tube feedings are typically discontinued at least 4 hours before extubation, but naso- or orogastric tubes are left in place to decompress the stomach and guide correct tube placement should reintubation be required.

Iatrogenic limitations to extubation include procedures that require additional sedation or analgesia, including new line placement, transport out of the intensive care unit for imaging studies, and emergent reoperation. Generally accepted pulmonary mechanics can be applied to burn patients. Extubation is delayed if the patient requires a fraction of inspired oxygen greater than 40%, positive end-expiratory pressure greater than 5 cm H_2O to maintain oxygen saturation 94% or higher, and pressure support ventilation greater than 10 cm H_2O to achieve an appropriate spontaneous tidal volume.

In the first days after extubation, the patient should be monitored closely for the development of airway stenosis. Because stenosis can become relevant weeks or months after the initial trauma, a follow-up should be considered in patients with a history of severe airway injuries and in patients who show scars and granuloma

after extubation.[10,16,26,28,33,47,49,50,56] When extubation is performed, reintubation is assumed to be difficult because of restricted mouth opening, limited range of motion of the neck, residual edema, and scar formation. A Cook catheter can be placed in the trachea before extubation and left in place for the next hours after extubation. These catheters have been left in place for 72 hours. Should the extubation attempt fail, the Cook catheter can be used as a guide for reintubation.

Patients in stable condition without airway difficulties can be extubated after surgery. When the airway access was difficult or after extensive procedures with the possibility of a fluid shift and edema formation, it is safer to delay the extubation until the patient is stable. The same criteria for extubation of the burn airway as detailed earlier apply in this clinical situation. A Cook catheter placed in the trachea prior to extubation is recommendable in patients with very difficult airways.[22,27,47]

6. Tube Fixation

The fixation of the ET is a challenge in the burned patient. The importance of securing the tube cannot be overemphasized; establishing an airway and then losing it a few hours later when the edema is at its peak jeopardizes the life of the patient. The ideal fixation secures the tube safely without additional injury to the tissue of the face and is flexible enough to adjust to edema formation, especially in the first hours and after surgery. Unfortunately, no fixation meets all of these demands. Individual solutions, depending on the sites of burns, grafts, and edema, which are checked regularly, are the best possibility. Suturing the tube to the gums, wiring the tube around a tooth, and circumferential fixation or devices that allow frequent adjustment are examples. The usual forms of adhesive tape are not effective in the burned patient because they do not adhere adequately even to nonburned skin. Usually, a soft sling ribbon (Harrington or umbilical tape) is used. It is tied at the back of the head (not the neck), and gauze padding should be added to avoid constriction of soft tissues. Its tightness must be checked frequently because swelling may cause the ribbon to cut into the tissues. The position of the ET should be confirmed with a chest radiograph. The fixation of the tube has to be checked especially before changes in position and before transporting the patient to avoid accidental extubation.[47]

III. AIRWAY MANAGEMENT IN THE LATER STAGES OF BURN INJURY

During the clinical course and after the initial hospital stay, patients with a burn injury return to the operating room frequently for skin grafts, scar release, and other reconstructive procedures. Regional anesthesia offers an alternative to general anesthesia when the site of surgery is limited to one extremity, but in most patients multiple sites of surgery make general anesthesia necessary. SVDs can be considered as an alternative to intubation of the trachea when the anatomy of the upper airway is normal or nearly normal and the operation can be performed in a supine or lateral position. Although reports of safe usage of the LMA in the prone position in children and adults exist, most anesthesiologists probably prefer to intubate patients who have to undergo prone positioning.[31] A variety of airway devices including SVDs, different laryngoscope blades, the Bullard laryngoscope or light wand and an ILMA, as well as a cricotomy set, an FOB, and tubes of different sizes should be available. All patients are considered to have possible difficult airways even when previous intubation offered no problems.

Before surgery, the anesthesiologist and surgeon should discuss the planned site of surgery, the expected extent of surgery, and the position of the patient during surgery. In patients with dressings or skin grafts of the face, the possibility of removing the dressing and the stability of the skin grafts should be discussed. In certain patients, the positioning of a tight-fitting face mask may not be possible. The mouth opening and the mobility of the neck may be limited because of dressings, edema, scars, or skin grafts. Inhalation injury predisposes to scars, webs, and stenosis of the airway. These changes may occur rapidly and early or may be delayed and are sometimes not symptomatic in the spontaneously breathing patient. Possible symptoms are hoarseness and stridor. After a burn injury of the neck, the underlying structures are often unidentifiable under edema and scar tissue. Previous anesthetic records can be useful in anticipating difficulties. The anesthetic plan should be discussed with patient and surgeon. The intubation can be performed with an FOB in the sedated spontaneously breathing patient or in the anesthetized patient with direct laryngoscopy, Bullard laryngoscope, or ILMA. For the expected difficult airway, the FOB approach is preferable. An evaluation of the larynx and the subglottic area can be performed during the procedure. When intubation of the trachea is planned under general anesthesia, the airway can be briefly evaluated before administration of a nondepolarizing muscle relaxant to rule out unexpected difficulties. In patients with a face dressing or other conditions that make mask ventilation impossible, use of an SVD can maintain oxygenation and ventilation until the muscle relaxation is appropriate for intubation. The reason for the airway access chosen, the difficulties faced, the pathologic findings, and their management should be documented meticulously on the anesthesia record for further anesthetics.

IV. CONCLUSION

The burn patient presents unique problems in both airway and pulmonary management to the anesthesiologist. Careful consideration of concurrent medical conditions and planned diagnostic and therapeutic procedures is critical in determining the need for ventilatory support. As a practical matter, we consider all burn patients to have difficult airways, and our airway management is designed to limit complications.

REFERENCES

1. Ames WA: Management of the major burn. Update Anesth 10:10, 1999.
2. Aub JC, Pittman H, Brues AM: The pulmonary complications: A clinical description. Ann Surg 117:834-840, 1943.
3. Barret JP, Desai MH, Herndon DN: Effects of tracheostomies on infection and airway complications in pediatric burn patient. Burns 26:190-193, 2000.
4. Baud FJ, Barriot P, Toffis V, et al: Elevated blood cyanide concentrations in victims of smoke inhalation. N Engl J Med 325:1761-1766, 1991.
5. Beeley JM, Clark RJ: Respiratory problems in fire victims. In Settle JAD (ed): Principles and Practice of Burns Management. New York, Churchill Livingstone, 1996, pp 117-127.
6. Blanding R, Stiff J: Perioperative anesthetic management of patients with burns. Anesth Clin North Am 17: 237-249, 1999.
7. Brough MD: The King's Cross fire. Part I: The physical injuries. Burns 17:6-9, 1991.
8. Cahalane M, Demling RH: Early respiratory abnormalities from smoke inhalation. JAMA 251:771-773, 1984.
9. Caruso DM, Al-Kasspooles MF, Matthews MR, et al: Rationale for 'early' percutaneous dilatational tracheostomy in patients with burn injuries. J Burn Care Rehabil 18: 424-428, 1997.
10. Cobley TDD, Hart WJ, Baldwin DL, et al: Complete fusion of the vocal cords; an unusual case. Burns 25: 361-363, 1999.
11. Coln CE, Purdue GF, Hunt JL: Tracheostomy in the young pediatric burn patient. Arch Surg 133:537-540, 1998.
12. Cox CS Jr, Zwischenberger JB, Traber DL, et al: Heparin improves oxygenation and minimizes barotrauma after severe smoke inhalation in an ovine model. Surg Gynecol Obstet 176:339-349, 1993.
13. Demling RH: Smoke inhalation injury. New Horiz 1:422-434, 1993.
14. Dolan MC: Carbon monoxide poisoning. CMAJ 133: 392-399, 1985.
15. Evan: Awake fiberoptic intubation for airway burns. J R Army Med Corps 144:105-106, 1998.
16. Gaissert HA, Lofgren RH, Grillo HC: Upper airway compromise after inhalation injury. Ann Surg 218672-678, 1993.
17. Gueugniaud PY, Carsin H, Bertin-Maghit M, Petit P: Current advances in the initial management of major thermal burns. Intensive Care Med 26:848-856, 2000.
18. Herndon DN, Spies M: Modern burn care. Semin Pediatr Surg 10:28-31, 2001.

19. Ilano AL, Raffin TA: Management of carbon monoxide poisoning. Chest 97:165-169, 1990.

20. Jones WG, Madden M, Finkelstein J, et al: Tracheotomies in burn patients. Ann Surg 209:471-474, 1989.

21. Judkins KC: Anaesthesia. In Settle JAD (ed): Principles and Practice of Burns Management. New York, Churchill Livingstone, 1996, pp 305-327.

22. Karam R, Ibrahim G, Tohme H, et al: Severe neck burns and laryngeal mask airway for frequent general anesthetics. Middle East J Anesthesiol 13:527-535, 1996.

23. Kirkpatrick JN: Acute carbon monoxide poisoning. West J Med 146:52-56, 1987.

24. Kohn D: [Burn trauma. Preclinical and clinical care from an anesthesiologist's point of view]. Anaesthesist 49: 359-370, 2000.

25. Lujan HJ, Dries DJ, Gamelli RL: Comparative analysis of bedside and operating room tracheostomies in critically ill patients with burns. J Burn Care Rehabil 16:258-261, 1995.

26. Lund T, Goodwin CW, McManus WF, et al: Upper airway sequelae in burn patients requiring endotracheal intubation or tracheostomy. Ann Surg 201:374-382, 1985.

27. MacLennan N, Heimbach DM, Cullen BF: Anesthesia for major thermal injury. Anesthesiology 89:749-770, 1998.

28. Madden MR, Finkelstein JL, Goodwin CW: Respiratory care of the burn patient. Clin Plast Surg 13:29-38, 1986.

29. Masanes MJ, Legendre C, Lioret N, et al: Using bronchoscopy and biopsy to diagnose early inhalation injury: Macroscopic and histologic findings. Chest 107: 1365-1369, 1995.

30. Mayes RW: The toxicological examination of the victims of the British Air Tours Boeing 737 accident at Manchester in 1985. J Forensic Sci 36:179-184, 1991.

31. McCall JE, Fischer CG, Schomaker E, Young JM: Laryngeal mask airway use in children with acute burns: Intraoperative airway management. Paediatr Anaesth 9:515-520, 1999.

32. Meredith TJ, Vale JA: Carbon monoxide poisoning. Br Med J 296:77-79, 1988.

33. Minamihaba O, Nakamura H, Sata M, et al: Progressive bronchial obstruction associated with toxic epidermal necrolysis. Respirology 4:93-95, 1999.

34. Mlcak R, Cortiella J, Desai MH, et al: Emergency management of pediatric burn victims. Pediatr Emerg Care 14:51-54, 1998.

35. Moylan JA, Chan C-K: Inhalation injury—An increasing problem. Ann Surg 188:34-37, 1978.

36. Myers RAM, Snyder SK, Emhoff TA: Subacute sequelae of carbon monoxide poisoning. Ann Emerg Med 14:1163-1167, 1985.

37. Nakae H, Tanaka H, Inaba H: Failure to clear casts and secretions following inhalation injury can be dangerous: Report of a case. Burns 27:189-191, 2001.

38. National Institutes of General Medical Sciences: Fact Sheets—Trauma, Burn, Shock, and Injury: Facts and Figures. www.nigms.nih.gov/news/trauma/facts/ figures.html.

39. Nguyen TT, Gilpin A, Meyer N, et al: Current treatment of severely burned patients. Ann Surg 223:14-25, 1996.

40. Nieman GF, Clark WR, Paskanik A, Feldbaum D: Segmental pulmonary vascular resistance following wood smoke inhalation. Crit Care Med 23:1264-1271, 1995.

41. Olson KR: Carbon monoxide poisoning: Mechanisms, presentation, and controversies in management. J Emerg Med 1:233-243, 1984.

42. Palmieri TL, Jackson WRRT, Greenhalgh DG: Benefits of early tracheostomy in severely burned children. Crit Care Med 30:922-924, 2002.

43. Prater ME, Deskin RW: Bronchoscopy and laryngoscopy findings as indications for tracheostomy in the burned child. Arch Otolaryngol Head Neck Surg 124:1115-1117, 1998.

44. Rodeberg DA, Maschinot NE, Housinger TA, Warden GD: Decreased pulmonary barotraumas with the use of volumetric diffusive respiration in pediatric patients with burns: The 1992 Moyer Award. J Burn Care Rehabil 13:506-511, 1992.

45. Saffle JR, Morris SE, Edelmann L: Early tracheostomy does not improve outcome in burn patient. J Burn Care Rehabil 23:431-438, 2002.

46. Settle JAD: General management. In Settle JAD (ed): Principles and Practice of Burns Management. New York, Churchill Livingstone, 1996, pp 223-241.

47. Sheridan RL: Airway management and respiratory care of the burn patient. Int Anesthesiol Clin 38:129-145, 2000.

48. Tan KK, Lee JK, Tan I, Sarvesvaran R: Acquired tracheo-oesophageal fistula following tracheal intubation in a burned patient. Burns 19:360-361, 1993.

49. Timon CI, McShane D, McGovern E, et al: Treatment of combined subglottic and critically low tracheal stenoses secondary to burn inhalation injury. J Laryngol Otol 1083-1086, 1989.

50. Valova M, Konigova R, Broz L, et al: Early and late fatal complications of inhalational injury. Acta Chir Plast 44: 51-54, 2002.

51. Venus B, Matsuda T, Copiozo JB, et al: Prophylactic intubation and continuous positive airway pressure in the management of inhalation injury in burn victims. Crit Care Med 9:519-523, 1981.

52. Wagner A, Roeggla M, Roeggla G, et al: Emergency intubation with the combitube in a case of severe facial burn. Am J Emerg Med 13:681-683, 1995.

53. Watts AMI, McCallum MID: Acute airway obstruction following facial scalding: Differential diagnosis between a thermal and infective cause. Burns 22:570-573, 1996.

54. Woolley WD, Ames SA, Smith PG: The Manchester Woolworths store fire, May 1979: Burning characteristics of the furniture. Fire Saf J 3:55-65, 1980.

55. Woolley WD, Smith PG, Fardell PJ, et al: The Stardust Disco fire, Dublin 1981. Studies of combustion products during simulated experiments. Fire Saf J 7:267, 1984.

56. Yang JY, Yang WG, Chang LY, et al: Symptomatic tracheal stenosis in burns. Burns 25:72-80, 1999.

57. Yowler CJ, Fratienne RB: Current status of burn resuscitation. Clin Plast Surg 27:1-10, 2000.

42

REGIONAL ANESTHESIA AND THE DIFFICULT AIRWAY

Jacques E. Chelly

I. INTRODUCTION

Regional anesthesia (RA) is recognized as an effective alternative to general anesthesia and is included in the American Society of Anesthesiologists (ASA) difficult airway algorithm as such (Fig. 42-1).[4] The anesthesiologist should carefully balance the risks and benefits when considering the use of RA versus securing the airway prior to the administration of any anesthesia in a patient with an established difficult airway (DA). Indeed, the anesthesiologist has a responsibility to provide safe anesthetic care, including maintaining appropriate conditions to manage the airway effectively during the perioperative period. It is well established that morbidity and mortality as a consequence of mismanagement or lack of proper management of the airway represent a major cause of concern to anesthesiologists worldwide. Although management of the airway is most often easily performed prior to surgery, serious consideration should be given to the increased difficulty associated with the need to control the airway during the course of surgery, especially in a patient with an established DA. The anesthesiologist needs to determine on an individual basis what is most appropriate, whether it be preoperative management of a DA or the use of RA, and the risks associated with management of the airway during the course of surgery. This represents a complex decision requiring the consideration of many different factors.

II. PRACTICE GUIDELINES FOR MANAGEMENT OF THE DIFFICULT AIRWAY

Irrespective of the final decision, an appropriate assessment of the patient's airway represents the first step. Although the ability to predict accurately a DA preoperatively would be of great value, it is evident from the literature that no single airway assessment can reliably predict a DA.[13] Nevertheless, a preoperative airway history and physical examination should be performed in order to facilitate the choice and management of the DA as well as reduce the likelihood of adverse outcomes (see Chapter 8).[25]

Langeron and colleagues have also established five factors that are frequently associated with DA management.[19] In addition, it is well established that airway management may be more difficult in trauma cases and patients with comorbidity such as severe rheumatoid arthritis, morbid obesity, metabolic diseases, deformities, or pregnancy. In fact, Rocke and coauthors demonstrated that the incidence of DA is 10 times higher during

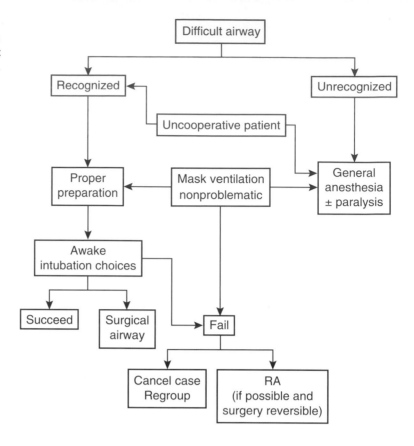

Figure 42-1 In the present airway algorithm, regional anesthesia (RA) represents an acknowledged alternative to a failed intubation. (From Hagberg CA [ed]: Handbook of Difficult Airway Management. Philadelphia, Churchill Livingstone, 2000.)

pregnancy than in the general population. In addition, they documented the potential risk factors for DA in the obstetric patient.[26] These risk factors included short neck, missing protruding incisors, receding mandible, facial edema, and high Mallampati scores. The relative risk of experiencing a difficult intubation (DI) in comparison with an uncomplicated class I airway assessment has been established as follows: class II, 3.23; class III, 7.58; class IV, 11.3; short neck, 5.01; receding mandible, 9.71; and protruding maxillary incisors, 8.0. Using the probability index or a combination of risk factors, or both, showed that a combination of either class III or IV plus protruding incisors, short neck, or receding mandible, the probability of difficult laryngoscopy to be greater than 90%.

It is also important to recognize that the concept of DA has different meanings for different individuals. Although most anesthesiologists agree that a patient with very limited mouth opening, Mallampati IV, and a very short neck has a DA, there is more controversy related to the relative difficulty of managing the airway in a patient with cervical trauma or obesity. This is in part due to the increase in expertise in airway management that anesthesiologists have acquired and continue to acquire and also to the increase in number of airway devices designed to facilitate airway management. For example, Hagberg and colleagues demonstrated that Cormack-Lehane grade III airways on "laryngoscopy" were reduced to grade II and even grade I when using the video laryngoscope.[14,15]

Therefore, the relative experience of the anesthesiologist with DA management and access to certain airway management devices represent important factors in establishing the relative difficulty of managing the airway of a given patient.

III. FACTORS INFLUENCING THE CHOICE BETWEEN THE USE OF REGIONAL ANESTHESIA AND THE PREOPERATIVE MANAGEMENT OF THE AIRWAY

In the past few years, there has been increased interest in using regional anesthesia as the primary anesthesia technique, especially in patients undergoing gynecologic or obstetric; plastic; ear, nose, throat; trauma; and orthopedic surgery. Consequently, anesthesiologists have become better experienced at these techniques (e.g., higher success rate and lower frequency of complications). However, no regional technique provides a 100% success rate or is completely free of complications. RA complications include hematoma, nerve injury, and local anesthetic–associated complications such as cardiac arrest, seizures, and death. When deciding whether to perform a regional technique in lieu of securing the airway preoperatively, these complications need to be taken into consideration as they may lead to the requirement for immediate and urgent control of the airway, either because of the sudden loss of respiratory function (total spinal) or because of the development of local anesthesia–related complications (cardiac arrest and seizures). It is also important to recognize that the occurrence of these complications may be delayed, even if in most cases these complications occur within minutes after the performance of a block. This leads to the need to be prepared to control the airway during the entire perioperative period. Although any regional technique intrinsically carries the risk of such complications, the relative risk is different for each regional technique. For example, the use of an ulnar block at the wrist for an open reduction and internal fixation of the fifth finger performed using 5 to 6 mL of 0.5% ropivacaine is associated with a much lower risk of local anesthetic toxicity than the use of a transarterial axillary block performed with 40 mL of 0.5% bupivacaine. Clearly, the specific type of approach, technique (transarterial versus neurostimulator versus paresthesia), volume of local anesthetic, and relative proximity of the injection site to either a vessel or the central nervous system represent some of the factors associated with the risks of toxicity associated with the use of RA. Therefore, it is important to take into account the following considerations before making the decision to use RA in a patient with an established DA (Table 42-1).

A. SELECTION OF PATIENTS

Not all patients are necessarily good candidates for RA, especially in the context of an established DA. The use of RA as the plan of anesthetic management rather than securing the airway may be considered in adult patients who are calm and possess good communication skills as well as understand and accept the risks and benefits of a regional technique over general anesthesia. The consent for RA should also include consent for the perioperative management of the airway in the case of a failed block or other uncertainty arising in the context of surgery. It is therefore important to consider the patient's psychological status and not perform RA in a patient who (1) consents to RA in order to avoid an awake fiberoptic intubation (negative previous experience); (2) has a history of claustrophobia, a condition that may be exacerbated by the need to place a surgical sheet over the face of the patient; (3) is unable to remain still, especially in the context of minimal sedation use, because of preexisting medical or surgical conditions (e.g., severe rheumatoid arthritis, back pain, prostate hypertrophy, hyperactive bladder, poor peripheral circulation); or (4) has a psychiatric condition, such as severe depression, hysteria, psychosis, or Alzheimer's disease.

B. ANESTHETIC ENVIRONMENT

1. Anesthesiologist's Expertise

The use of RA as an alternative to the preoperative management of the airway in a patient with a known DA can be considered only if the anesthesiologist has appropriate

Table 42-1 Factors Influencing the Choice of RA versus Control of the Airway in Patients with Established DAs

Patient
Informed consent
Cooperative and calm
Hemodynamically stable
Ability to tolerate sedation, if required
Ability to communicate with anesthesiologist throughout procedure
No history of claustrophobia
Adequate intravenous access
Anesthesiologist
Expertise in both RA and DA management
Enough preoperative time to perform RA technique
Appropriate RA technique for surgical procedure
Prepared for alternative plans for DA
Surgeon
Dependable and reliable
Willing and able to supplement RA with local anesthetics, if necessary
Cooperative with primary and alternative plans for DA management
Types of Surgery
Nonemergent (exception cesarean section)
Short duration
Patient's position allows good airway access
Can be interrupted for DA management
Limited or moderate blood loss
Support
Availability of appropriate equipment for RA and DA management
Staff (anesthesiologists, operating room nurses)

DA, difficult airway; RA, regional anesthesia.

expertise with regional techniques and DA management. Peripheral nerve blocks can be classified according to the degree of difficulty (Table 42-2).

a. Regional Anesthesia

Before considering the use of RA in patients with an established DA, it is necessary to verify that RA is not contraindicated. General contraindications for the use of

Table 42-2   Peripheral Nerve Block Classification According to Difficulty

Basic
Femoral
Axillary
Superficial cervical
Intravenous
Posterior sciatic
Posterior popliteal sciatic
Intermediary
Interscalene
Lateral sciatic
Infraclavicular
Anterior sciatic
Continuous femoral
Continuous axillary
Lumbar plexus
Parasacral
Paravertebral
Complex
Continuous paravertebral
Continuous infraclavicular
Continuous lumbar plexus
Continuous anterior
Parasacral sciatic block
Pediatric blocks

RA include coagulopathy and infection. Specific contraindications must also be considered, such as chronic obstructive pulmonary disease for interscalene block. Although it is well established that the use of RA is associated with intrinsic risks, evidence also supports the concept that appropriate expertise in RA represents an important determinant not only of the success but also of reducing the risk of complications. The relevant expertise includes proper experience in the chosen technique, appropriate knowledge of the relevant anatomy and innervation, knowledge of equipment, and knowledge of the pharmacology of local anesthetics and any medications either added to a local anesthetic mixture or given for sedation.

The use of neurostimulator and ultrasound techniques should be preferred to the use of paresthesia or transarterial techniques, or both, in the performance of RA to increase the likelihood of success and minimize

the required dose of local anesthetics, thus minimizing the risk of seizures related to an intravascular injection. Consideration should also be given to the use of the smallest needle possible to avoid an intrathecal placement of the needle when performing an interscalene or a lumbar plexus block. Table 42-3 shows the needle sizes related to the practice of the most common peripheral nerve blocks.

Although the literature provides information related to the relative success rate of each technique for a given surgical procedure, the anesthesiologist's personal experience is more important in the consideration of which RA technique is most appropriate. Thus, to optimize the success rate and minimize the risk of complications associated with the use of RA in the context of an established DA, the anesthesiologist should favor the techniques that he or she is most comfortable with for a given surgical procedure rather than base the choice on the literature. For example, it is established that most shoulder or knee surgeries can be performed using an interscalene or a combined sciatic and femoral nerve block, respectively. However, if the anesthesiologist responsible for the care of the patient does not routinely use peripheral nerve blocks for these types of surgery, the preoperative management of the airway is clearly preferable.

i. Regional Anesthesia Complications. In the case of a patient with an established DA, the complications of interest are those that would lead to the immediate need to secure the airway because of a total spinal, cardiac arrest, or seizure. In this respect, neuraxial blocks are the regional techniques with an established higher rate of complications.[2,5,7,12,17,20] Closed claim studies have demonstrated that young healthy patients undergoing surgery during spinal anesthesia can experience sudden cardiac arrest.[6] In obstetrics, 70% of the RA-related deaths occurred among women who had epidural anesthesia and the remaining 30% were associated with spinal anesthesia. These deaths resulted when the block became

Table 42-3   Needle Length for Most Common Peripheral Nerve Blocks

Type of Block	Length (cm)
Interscalene and supraclavicular blocks at the elbow and the wrist	2.5
Axillary, high humeral, posterior popliteal	
Infraclavicular(coracoid) and femoral blocks	5.0
Lumbar plexus, lateral sciatic, gluteal, and infragluteal	10.0
Posterior sciatic, anterior sciatic, and high lateral sciatic blocks	15.0

high for adequate ventilation and the airway could not be secured, leading to hypoxia or aspiration, or both.[16,27]

The ASA study of closed claims in obstetrics also showed that about 25% of the anesthesia-related maternal deaths were associated with RA. Ananthanarayan and associates presented a case of DI with brain stem anesthesia after retrobulbar block.[1] Following failed endotracheal intubation, the airway was secured using a laryngeal mask airway.[1] Among the peripheral nerve blocks, lumbar plexus block,[21,23,24] interscalene and axillary brachial plexus block,[3,8-11,18,22,28] intercostal block, and retrobulbar block[1] represent the blocks most often associated with complications requiring immediate control of the airway. However, such a possibility also exists with the performance of any peripheral nerve blocks, especially when relatively large volumes of local anesthetic are injected relatively quickly or when there is a vein or artery located in proximity to the nerve.

ii. Local Anesthetics. The choice of the local anesthetic mixture, its volume and concentration, and the mode of administration deserve serious consideration. Although these choices are clearly dictated by the technique (major conduction blockade versus peripheral nerve blocks), the choice of the local anesthetic mixture should be based even more on the safety of patients with a DA, with special focus on complications requiring immediate airway intervention. Local anesthetics that have the highest safety profile and provide adequate anesthesia covering the entire surgical period are most suitable. Furthermore, the maximum dose of local anesthetics should be determined to decrease the risk of toxicity. Table 42-4 shows the different local anesthetics along with the maximum accepted doses.

b. Expertise in Management of the Difficult Airway

Because perioperative management of the airway may be required during the course of the procedure in a patient undergoing surgery under RA, the anesthesiologist should also be appropriately trained in DA management. The use of RA in a patient with an established DA cannot be considered an appropriate alternative for the anesthesiologist inexperienced in or unprepared for DA management. Therefore, the anesthesiologist should also be knowledgeable and experienced in this area.

Table 42-4 Maximum Dose of Commonly Used Local Anesthetics

Anesthetic	Maximum Dose (mg)	pH
Lidocaine	300	6.5
Mepivacaine	500	4.5
Bupivacaine	150	4.5-6
Ropivacaine	225-300	4.6

c. Proper Anesthetic Environment

In addition to proper expertise in both RA and DA management, it is critical that the proper equipment allowing DA management be in good order and readily accessible during the entire perioperative period. Proper support should be available because calling for help is one of the first steps according to the revised version of the airway algorithm.[25] Furthermore, the time commitment to manage the airway appropriately should be weighed against the relative availability of the anesthesiologist during the entire perioperative period because management of the airway may be required intraoperatively. This is especially important when the anesthesiologist supervises more than one location. Certainly, the anesthesiologist supervising residents or certified registered nurse anesthetists or on call is not as available as when he or she supervises one location.

C. SURGICAL ENVIRONMENT

1. Type of Surgery

The use of a RA technique is not appropriate for all types of surgeries. Furthermore, in the context of a patient with an established DA, a successful block does not represent a guarantee that the airway will not require intraoperative management because the patient becomes uncomfortable or there are major hemodynamic changes or bleeding. Therefore, RA should be considered for shorter procedures with minimum expected blood loss. For example, a short abdominal procedure may benefit from a spinal, epidural, or in some cases bilateral paravertebral blocks. It is important to recognize that the diaphragmatic function is not blocked by a spinal or epidural, which explains why most anesthesiologists favor the use of neuraxial blocks for low rather than high abdominal procedures. In orthopedics, it is important to take into consideration all surgical requirements, especially those related to the use of a tourniquet. Although in surgical procedures of less than 30 minutes duration, tourniquet pain is usually not an issue, the mechanism of tourniquet pain should be well understood and managed because it usually requires sedation or analgesics, or both, that are often contraindicated in patients with an unsecured DA (Table 42-5).

2. Cooperation between Surgeon and Anesthesiologist

Especially in the case of a patient with an established DA, it is necessary that both the anesthesiologist and the surgeon agree that the surgery can be performed using RA alone or with supplementation of the block by local anesthesia during the procedure. The anesthesiologist also needs to be familiar with the surgeon, the surgical procedure, and the surgical environment, including the availability of surgical equipment and support staff. For example, in the case of joint replacements, many

Table 42-5   **Examples of Surgeries That Might Be Performed Using a Regional Anesthetic and Those More Suitable for the Preoperative Management of the Airway in Patients with an Established Difficult Airway**

Examples of Surgeries That Might Be Performed Using Regional Anesthesia
Peripheral nerve blocks
Minor orthopedic trauma of the upper and lower extremity
Open reduction with internal fixation of the small finger, elbow, and ankle and wrist fracture
Minor arthroscopy surgery (shoulder, knee, and ankle)
Neuraxial blocks
Gynecologic surgery and cesarean sections
Examples of Surgeries More Suitable for Preoperative Airway Management
Long surgeries associated with major blood loss
Major or multiple trauma, major abdominal surgery, revised total hip surgery, and major orthopedic oncology surgery
Long surgeries performed in the prone position
Spine surgery and Achilles' tendon surgery
Blocks unlikely to provide adequate anesthesia
Interscalene for high humeral fracture, lumbar plexus for hip surgery

hospitals and surgery centers depend upon the presence of a prosthesis representative. The availability of such representatives may involve significant time delays, creating significant limitations for the use of RA. Furthermore, in a patient with an established DA, the use of RA requires that the surgical procedure be well defined because prolonged surgical time or hemodynamic instability or blood loss can lead to significant problems. If RA is preferred, the surgeon should proceed only after careful determination that the patient is properly anesthetized and that inflation of a tourniquet, if utilized, is well tolerated. Because there is a relationship between cuff inflation pressure and tourniquet pain, it is important to minimize the pressure level at which the tourniquet is inflated. Although it is well established that pain associated with a tourniquet can be either immediate at the time of the inflation or delayed, it is critically important to verify that the tourniquet is tolerated at the time of inflation. In short procedures, delayed tourniquet pain represents a lesser concern.

3. Positioning of the Patient

The patient's position during surgery also represents a critical element of choice between the preoperative management of the airway and the use of RA. Prone and lateral positions are more likely to make management of the airway during surgery more difficult. The sitting position is also an unfavorable position for the use of RA unless it is possible to convert quickly to the supine position (i.e., a patient undergoing shoulder surgery in a beach chair position under an interscalene block). Although it is always possible to change to the supine position urgently, it is far from optimum medical management. Of all the positions, the supine position allows the best access to the airway. When considering the patient's positioning for a surgical procedure, it is also important to take into consideration the relationship between the surgical preparation and patient's positioning even when supine. For example, in the case of an open reduction and fixation of an elbow fracture, the elbow is often elevated and flexed over the patient, then draped. In the case of pediatric or claustrophobic patients, this surgical positioning may be associated with significant stress and anxiety, favoring preoperative management of the airway rather than RA.

If RA is found to be an appropriate alternative to the preoperative management of the airway, it is possible to proceed with the performance of RA. The chosen technique can be physically performed either outside or inside the operating room, depending on the specific block and the facility's preference. Enough time should be available for the performance of the block and evaluation of its effects. Because complications can and do occur, it is necessary to be prepared for cardiovascular and central nervous system resuscitation.

IV. CONCLUSION

The use of RA in patients with an established DA remains the exception rather than the rule in our current practice. RA represents an acceptable alternative to the preoperative management of the airway assuming that certain conditions are met: (1) establishment of proper indications for the use of RA, (2) appropriate consent by the patient is obtained, (3) the anesthesiologist is experienced in both RA and DA management and is readily available during the entire perioperative period, and finally (4) equipment and support are readily available during the entire perioperative period.

REFERENCES

1. Ananthanarayan C, Cole AF, Kazdan M: Difficult intubation and brain-stem anaesthesia. Can J Anaesth 44: 658-661, 1997.
2. Auroy Y, Narchi P, Messiah A, et al: Serious complications related to regional anesthesia: Results of a prospective survey in France. Anesthesiology 87:479-486, 1997.
3. Baraka A, Hanna M, Hammoud R: Unconsciousness and apnea complicating parascalene brachial plexus block: Possible subarachnoid block. Anesthesiology 77: 1046-1047, 1992.
4. Benumof JL: ASA Difficult Airway Algorithm: New thoughts and considerations. In Hagberg CA (ed): Handbook of Difficult Airway Management. Philadelphia, Churchill Livingstone, 2004, pp 31-48.
5. Caplan RA, Ward RJ, Posner K, Cheney FW: Unexpected cardiac arrest during spinal anesthesia: A closed claims analysis of predisposing factors. Anesthesiology 68:5-11, 1988.
6. Cheney FW: The American Society of Anesthesiologists Closed Claims Project: What have we learned, how has it affected practice, and how will it affect practice in the future? Anesthesiology 91:552-556, 1999.
7. Chester WL: Spinal anesthesia, complete heart block, and the precordial chest thump: An unusual complication and a unique resuscitation. Anesthesiology 69:600-602, 1988.
8. Cook LB: Unsuspected extradural catheterization in an interscalene block. Br J Anaesth 67:473-475, 1991.
9. Durrani Z, Winnie AP: Brainstem toxicity with reversible lock-in syndrome after intrascalene brachial plexus block. Anesth Analg 72:249-252, 1991.
10. Dutton RP, Eckhardt WF III, Sunder N: Total spinal anesthesia after interscalene blockade of the brachial plexus. Anesthesiology 80:939-941, 1994.
11. Edde RR, Deutsch S: Cardiac arrest after interscalene brachial-plexus block. Anesth Analg 56:446-447, 1977.
12. Frerichs RL, Campbell J, Bassell GM: Psychogenic cardiac arrest during extensive sympathetic blockade. Anesthesiology 68:943-944, 1988.
13. Hagberg CA, Ghatge S: Does the airway examination predict difficult intubation? In Fleisher L (ed): Evidence-Based Practice of Anesthesiology. Philadelphia, WB Saunders, 2004, pp 34-46.
14. Hagberg CA, Iannucci DG, Goodrich AL: An evaluation of endotracheal intubation using the Macintosh video laryngoscopy. Anesth Analg 96(2S):157, 2003.
15. Hagberg CA, Kaplan MB, Lazada L, et al: The experience of four American clinics with the Macintosh video laryngoscopy. Eur J Anaesthesiol 20:A-164, 2003.
16. Hawkins JL: Anesthesia-related maternal mortality. Clin Obstet Gynecol 46:679-687, 2003.
17. Hodgkinson R: Total spinal block after epidural injection into an interspace adjacent to an inadvertent dural perforation. Anesthesiology 55:593-595, 1981.
18. Kumar A, Battit GE, Froese AB, Long MC: Bilateral cervical and thoracic epidural blockade complicating interscalene branchial plexus block: Report of two cases. Anesthesiology 35:650-652, 1971.
19. Langeron O, Masso E, Huraux C, et al: Prediction of difficult mask ventilation. Anesthesiology. 92:1229-1236, 2000.
20. Liguori GA, Sharrock NE: Asystole and severe bradycardia during epidural anesthesia in orthopedic patients. Anesthesiology 86:250-257, 1997.
21. Lonnqvist PA, MacKenzie J, Soni AK, Conacher ID: Paravertebral blockade. Failure rate and complications. Anaesthesia 50:813-815, 1995.
22. McGlade DP: Extensive central neural blockade following interscalene brachial plexus blockade. Anaesth Intensive Care 20:514-516, 1992.
23. Muravchick S, Owens WD: An unusual complication of lumbosacral plexus block: A case report. Anesth Analg 55:350-352, 1976.
24. Pousman RM, Mansoor Z, Sciard D: Total spinal anesthetic after continuous posterior lumbar plexus block. Anesthesiology 98:1281-1282, 2003.
25. Practice Guidelines for Management of the Difficult Airway: An updated report by the American Society of Anesthesiologists Task Force on Management of the Difficult Airway. Anesthesiology 98:1269-1277, 2003.
26. Rocke DA, Murray WB, Rout CC, Gouws E: Relative risk analysis of factors associated with difficult intubation in obstetric anesthesia. Anesthesiology 77:67-73, 1992.
27. Ross BK: ASA closed claims in obstetrics: Lessons learned. Anesthesiol Clin North Am 21:183-197, 2003.
28. Ross S, Scarsborough CD: Total spinal anesthesia following brachial-plexus block. Anesthesiology 39:458, 1973.

43

AIRWAY MANAGEMENT IN INTENSIVE CARE MEDICINE

Peter Krafft
Michael Frass

I. INTRODUCTION

A major responsibility of the anesthesiologist or critical care physician is the maintenance of adequate ventilation and pulmonary gas exchange in critically ill patients. In the operating room (OR) the incidence of airway catastrophes resulting in emergency tracheostomy, brain damage, or death is in the range of 0.01 to 2 cases per 10,000 procedures. Emergency airway management is often even more challenging in the intensive care unit (ICU) setting. The increasing demand for critical care medicine makes it necessary to focus on specific airway problems encountered in ICU patients.

Major differences exist between airway management in a controlled setting such as the OR and airway management in the ICU. Difficult laryngoscopy and endotracheal intubation are often successful after multiple attempts in the OR because of adequate preparation and positioning of the patient. To the contrary, endotracheal intubation of the "crashing" critically ill patient with poor cardiopulmonary reserve in a relatively uncontrolled environment requires a different approach in order to prevent deleterious consequences.

This chapter briefly describes noninvasive and "invasive" airway management with special consideration of the recommendations of the Task Force on Management of the Difficult Airway of the American Society of Anesthesiologists (i.e., ASA algorithm) first presented in 1991.[20] The basic principles of the ASA algorithm are meticulous evaluation of the patient before sedation or anesthesia induction, awake intubation if problems are suspected, and preparation of an alternative approach in case of failure (see respective chapter).

Those recommendations are at least in part valuable for the management of ICU patients, also. The population treated in the ICU consists of postoperative surgical patients, neurologic patients, septic patients, and patients presenting with single- or multiple-organ failure or other rare diseases. Besides normal airway anatomy, this heterogeneous set of patients comprises a variety of airway abnormalities, requiring special airway management considerations and techniques. Unfortunately, the ASA algorithm has a number of characteristics that prevent direct application to the ICU situation.

Airway management in ICU patients is usually urgent or emergent, often depriving the physician of the time necessary to evaluate the patients and plan the lifesaving intervention. The patient is presumed to have a full stomach and must therefore undergo awake airway management or rapid sequence induction (RSI). The option of reemergence from anesthesia to resume spontaneous ventilation if difficulty is encountered is mostly unfeasible. However, at least part of the algorithm is of major importance for ICU airway management and is therefore presented in detail (see "Difficult Airway Management in Intensive Care").

ICU airway management is a complex topic that is difficult to cover in a single chapter. Therefore, we concentrated on the most important topics of ICU airway management in order to provide the reader with the majority of information necessary for daily ICU practice. The chapter begins with a brief overview of noninvasive airway management (including continuous positive airway pressure by mask or helmet) and proceeds with prelaryngoscopic airway assessment. This special aspect is extensively addressed because many airway catastrophes can be prevented solely by adequate evaluation and preparation of the patient prior to the administration of sedatives. Thereafter, the "gold standard" techniques for the performance of direct laryngoscopy and oral or nasal endotracheal intubation are presented. Alternatives to direct laryngoscopy (especially awake endotracheal intubation) are discussed, and the control of the patient's airway in emergency situations is presented. One of the four following emergency techniques must be chosen immediately in order to prevent deleterious cerebral hypoxia: laryngeal mask airway (LMA), esophageal-tracheal Combitube (ETC), transtracheal jet ventilation (TTJV), or the performance of a surgical airway. For planned as well as emergency ICU airway management, those alternative methods or techniques must be readily available before sedation and must be practiced in routine cases.

Long-term translaryngeal intubation may result in serious laryngeal damage, such as ulcer formation or tracheal stenosis. Therefore, indication, timing, and recent techniques of tracheostomy are discussed and individual advantages and drawbacks of every technical approach are presented. Airway management in ICU patients is a matter of ongoing research and discussion. For example, the percentage of patients undergoing tracheostomy and the timing of tracheostomy underwent dramatic changes after the introduction of percutaneous dilational tracheostomy (PDT) in the 1980s. Irrespective of the individual technique used, PDT can be performed quickly at the bedside, has a relatively low incidence of complications in trained hands, is inexpensive, and cosmetic results are excellent (see later).

Last, routine airway care maneuvers such as tracheal suctioning are presented (Section VIII). The chapter closes with an often overlooked problem in ICU airway management, namely difficult extubation (Section IX). Difficult extubation is commonly encountered in patients after ear, nose, and throat (ENT) procedures or those with other reasons for pharyngeal-laryngeal swelling or distortion. Close interaction with the attending ENT specialist is necessary, and coping strategies for the prevention of catastrophes during extubation are presented.

Several aspects of this chapter are also presented in detail elsewhere in this book, and we advise the reader to check the index for further information on special topics of ICU airway management.

II. NONINVASIVE AIRWAY MANAGEMENT

It has become widely accepted to use noninvasive ventilation, especially in patients suffering from chronic obstructive lung disease and patients with cardiac failure, because weaning from respirator and cannula may become extremely difficult. In selected patients with respiratory failure, noninvasive positive-pressure ventilation (NPPV) helps to reduce the work of breathing. Noninvasive airway management is a promising approach to ventilatory support of ICU patients and may become even more important in the near future. Carlucci and colleagues[36] evaluated the changes in the practice of noninvasive ventilation for the treatment of patients with chronic obstructive pulmonary disease (COPD) between 1992 and 1999. In this special patients' collective, the failure rate of NPPV was constant over the years (17%). Although the severity of acute respiratory failure (ARF) episodes increased (defined by pH and Acute Physiology and Chronic Health Evaluation [APACHE] II at admission), the risk of failure for a patient with a pH less than 7.25 was threefold lower in the period 1997 to 1999 compared with 1992 to 1996. Furthermore, a significantly higher percentage of patients (pH > 7.28) were treated in the normal ward and not in the ICU, which allowed a significant cost reduction. The future will show whether this trend away from invasive toward noninvasive ventilatory support in routine care of patients is sustained.

Over the past decade, NPPV has increased in popularity in the setting of acute exacerbations of COPD. Keenan and associates[121] performed a systematic review of the literature to assess the effect of NPPV on rate of endotracheal intubation, length of hospital stay, and in-hospital mortality in patients with an acute exacerbation of COPD. The addition of NPPV to standard care in patients with an acute exacerbation of COPD decreased the rate of endotracheal intubation (risk reduction, 28% [95% confidence interval, 15% to 40%]), length of hospital stay (absolute reduction, 4.57 days [CI, 2.30 to 6.83 days]), and in-hospital mortality rate (risk reduction, 10% [CI, 5% to 15%]). However, subgroup analysis showed that these beneficial effects occurred only in patients with severe exacerbations, not in those with milder exacerbations.

A similar approach was used by the Cochrane Database group, presenting a systematic review of the effectiveness of NPPV in management of acute COPD exacerbations.[172] Only randomized controlled trials were selected by two independent reviewers. NPPV not only decreased mortality (relative risk [RR] 0.41; 95% CI: 0.26, 0.64) but also decreased the need for intubation (RR 0.42; 95% CI 0.31, 0.59) and treatment failures (RR 0.51; 95% CI 0.39, 0.67). In addition, complications associated with treatment (RR 0.32; 95% CI 0.18, 0.56) and length of hospital stay (−3.24 days; 95% CI −4.42, −2.06) were reduced in the NPPV group. The reviewers concluded that NPPV should be used as the first-line intervention in all patients with respiratory failure secondary to an acute exacerbation of COPD. Trying NPPV should be considered early in the course of respiratory failure in order to avoid endotracheal intubation and reduce mortality and treatment failure.

A. NONINVASIVE POSITIVE AIRWAY PRESSURE VENTILATION BY MASK

NPPV can be administered by either face or nasal mask. The technique includes a mask that is pressed against the patient's face with the help of an elastic band (e.g., Classen band). The patient may now be supported by either continuous positive airway pressure, pressure support ventilation, or volume- or pressure-cycled systems (e.g., bilevel positive airway pressure). However, dyspneic ARF patients often breathe through the mouth, causing air leakage and reducing the efficacy of nasal NPPV. The face mask is preferable in these patients. As a disadvantage, the pressure of the face mask against the patient's face and especially against the root of the nose causes significant mask discomfort and skin lesions, and several patients refuse prolonged application.[92,149]

B. NONINVASIVE POSITIVE AIRWAY PRESSURE VENTILATION BY HELMET

The helmet consists of a cylindrically shaped transparent part, which is drawn over the patient's head (e.g., CaStar, Starmed, Italy). When the helmet is closed, the lower part contains an elastic ring that allows a tight seal at the patient's neck (Figs. 43-1 and 43-2). There are two fittings opening sideways to ventilatory tubing, allowing supportive ventilation such as continuous flow or pressure support ventilation. The helmet provides several advantages. It is a noninvasive means of ventilation, and the patient has a free view through the transparent helmet and can even wear glasses, which do not fog up because of the circulating air. A new model of the CaStar helmet includes an additional round opening with a diameter of about 10 cm for care of the patient's face. This new helmet was used as first-line intervention to treat patients with hypoxemic ARF, in comparison with NPPV by standard facial mask.[9] Thirty-three consecutive patients without COPD and with hypoxemic ARF (defined as severe dyspnea at rest, respiratory rate >30 breaths/min, ratio of arterial oxygen tension to fraction of inspired oxygen [PaO_2:FIO_2] < 200, and active contraction of the accessory muscles of respiration) were enrolled. The 33 patients and the 66 control subjects had similar characteristics at baseline. Eight patients (24%) in the helmet group and 21 patients (32%) in the facial mask group ($P = .3$) failed NPPV and were intubated. No patients failed NPPV because of intolerance of the technique in the helmet group in comparison with eight patients (38%) in the mask group ($P = .047$). Complications related to the technique (skin necrosis, gastric distention, and eye irritation) were fewer in the helmet group than

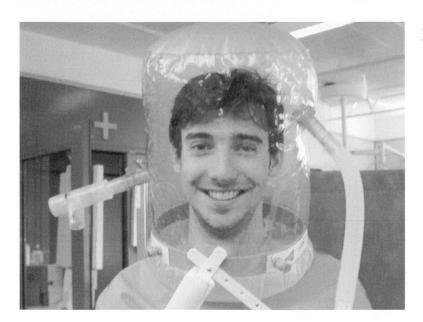

Figure 43-1 Application of CaStar helmet in a healthy volunteer.

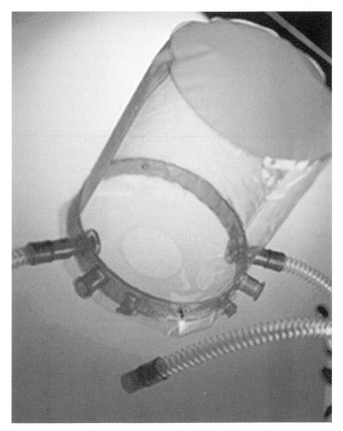

Figure 43-2 Rüsch 4Vent helmet. (Courtesy of Rüsch, Vienna, Austria.)

the mask group (no patients versus 14 patients [21%], $P = .002$). The helmet allowed continuous application of NPPV for a longer period of time ($P = .05$). NPPV by helmet successfully treated hypoxemic ARF, with better tolerance and fewer complications than facial mask NPPV.

In another prospective, clinical investigation in a general ICU, the feasibility and safety of fiberoptic bronchoscopy (FOB) with bronchoalveolar lavage (BAL) were tested during NPPV delivered by helmet in patients with ARF and suspected pneumonia.[10] Four adult patients with ARF underwent NPPV through the helmet and required fiber-optic BAL for suspected pneumonia. NPPV was delivered through the helmet in the pressure support ventilation mode. The specific seal connector placed in the plastic ring of the helmet allowed passage of the bronchoscope, maintaining assisted ventilation. Arterial blood gas levels, pH, oxygen saturation, respiratory rate, heart rate, and mean arterial blood pressure were monitored during the study. Helmet NPPV avoided gas exchange deterioration during FOB and BAL, with good tolerance. During the procedure heart rate increased by 5% and mean arterial blood pressure by 7% over baseline; these levels returned to prebronchoscopic values immediately after withdrawal of the bronchoscope. Endotracheal intubation was never required during the 24 hours after the procedure. BAL yielded diagnostic information in three of four patients. NPPV through the helmet allows safe diagnostic FOB with BAL in patients with hypoxemic ARF, avoiding gas exchange deterioration and endotracheal intubation.

Several special aspects of the helmet, such as the effects of direct exposure of external and middle ear to positive airway pressure, remain to be determined. Cavaliere and coauthors[38] recommended the use of ear plugs in selected NPPV patients treated with the helmet, especially during long-term support at high airway pressures. NPPV has become an integral part of daily ICU care for many patients suffering from acute and chronic respiratory failure. However, the potential effectiveness of NPPV varies among different populations of patients. The greatest benefit is seen in patients with pure hypercapnic respiratory failure such as COPD patients. The more severe hypoxemia becomes, the fewer beneficial effects are observed. Clearly, further studies are necessary to identify the patients with hypoxemic respiratory failure who might benefit from NPPV.[120]

A new design of the helmet offers further advantages. The Rüsch 4Vent (Teleflex Rüsch, Kernen, Germany) allows an unrestricted field of view and minimum level of noise. Tubing and accessories are connected to the rigid ring of the 4Vent. Diffusers prevent the stream of gas from blowing directly into the patient's face. By using filters, the noise inside the helmet is considerably reduced. As with the CaStar helmet, the patient is able to speak and take liquid food and drinks. Because of the supple material, the helmet can also be worn lying down (Fig. 43-2).

III. ENDOTRACHEAL INTUBATION IN INTENSIVE CARE

A. ORAL VERSUS NASAL ENDOTRACHEAL INTUBATION

Oral intubation and especially nasal intubation are characterized by special advantages and complications, with orotracheal intubation being currently favored by most authors. The contraindications for nasal intubation in critically ill patients are shown in Table 43-1.

The most common complication of *nasotracheal intubation* is nasal bleeding, occurring in roughly 45% of patients.[56] The incidence of bleeding can be reduced with adequate preparation (vasoconstrictors). In most cases,

Table 43-1 **Contraindications for Nasal Intubation**

Severe coagulopathy
High-dose systemic anticoagulation
Known nasal or paranasal pathologies
Infection of paranasal sinuses
Basilar skull fractures
Traumatic brain injury with liquor leakage

bleeding is self-limited and no further intervention is needed. Other complications are necrosis of the tip or wing of the nose (reported in up to 4% of patients[11]) and complications induced by the impaired drainage of paranasal sinus secretions. Nasotracheal intubation impairs the drainage of the maxillary sinus, resulting in congestion of secretions, followed within a few days by bacterial overgrowth and sinusitis. This typical complication of intensive care occurs within 8 days in 25% to 100% of transnasally intubated patients.[12,94] The incidence is closely related to the duration of endotracheal intubation, from 37% after 3 days to 100% after 1 week, with the majority resolving within 1 week after extubation.[72] Therefore, in all ICU patients presenting with fever of unknown origin, a high index of suspicion for sinusitis must be maintained. Radiologic or ultrasound studies, including computed tomography (CT) studies, may be necessary and demonstrate the presence of fluid or inflammation. Bacterial sinus infection may ultimately lead to bacteremia and a systemic inflammatory response. These infections tend to be polymicrobial but often display a predominance of gram-negative bacilli (particularly *Pseudomonas aeruginosa*), *Staphylococcus aureus*, or fungi. Treatment includes removal of all nasal tubes and institution of appropriate antibiotic therapy, along with decongestant therapy. In some cases, surgical drainage may be necessary.

Oral intubation, on the other hand, markedly interferes with oral and pharyngeal hygiene, and even small lesions of oral soft tissues may result in extensive bacterial or viral soft tissue infections (e.g., herpetic lesions[198]). Most authors admit that all complications typically seen with nasal intubation may also occur during orotracheal intubation but with a significantly lower incidence. Therefore, oral endotracheal intubation is the preferred route of tube passage and nasal intubation is reserved for special indications, mainly for short-term ventilatory support in oral surgery. For patients requiring intubation for more than 7 days, the nasotracheal route should always be avoided.[190]

B. CHOOSING THE CORRECT ENDOTRACHEAL TUBE SIZE

According to the literature, there is a clear association between endotracheal tube (ET) diameter and the incidence of laryngeal complications. Injury is located mainly in the posterior part of the glottis, where pressures up to 200 or 400 mm Hg are exerted by poorly deformable ETs.[225] This pressure is reduced by the use of softer ETs with a smaller diameter. It has been clearly demonstrated in routine anesthesia patients that the use of a smaller ET reduces the incidence of postoperative sore throat, presumably because of the decreased pressure at the ET-mucosal interface. Stout and colleagues[201] studied 101 patients randomly assigned to either larger ETs (9 mm for men and 8.5 mm for women) or smaller ETs (7 mm for men and 6.5 mm for women); the incidence of postoperative sore throat was 48% (large ET) versus 22% (small ET), respectively. No ventilatory difficulties were observed in either group.

The limiting factor for minimizing ET diameter is the increased flow resistance and work of breathing. The pressure gradient required to generate gas flow can be calculated according to the Hagen-Poiseuille relationship, where the rapidity of gas flow is directly proportional to the square of the ET diameter (D) and the pressure (P) and indirectly to the ET length and gas viscosity (valid only in laminar flow conditions). In other words, the pressure gradient through the airways proportionally rises with flow, viscosity, and ET length but increases exponentially when ET radius decreases. Viscosity of the gas administered is not without clinical consequence; with lower viscosity, a lower pressure gradient necessarily results in a lower airflow resistance. For example, gas mixtures consisting of a high percentage of helium are commonly used to overcome upper airway obstruction[107] (e.g., related to tracheal compression or stenosis) and for the treatment of most severe status asthmaticus.[108]

In all patients, endotracheal intubation artificially increases airway resistance because the ET inner diameter (ID) is smaller than the tracheal diameter. Usually, the ET length exceeds the length of the natural airway. Resistance is further increased by the curved design of the tubes necessary to resemble the patients' airway. Resistance measured with curved tubes is about 3% higher than with straight tubes.[218] Therefore, the pressure gradient to generate gas flow is minimized by using an ET with a larger diameter, short length, and straight design.[156] Flow resistance can be translated into work of breathing, which is inversely proportional to ET diameter (Fig. 43-3). The nonelastic work of breathing is increased twofold by using a 7.0 mm ID ET and onefold by using an 8.0 mm ID ET compared with a 9.0 mm ID ET.[164] With respect to gas flow, it is warranted to use as large an ET as is practical for patients presenting with respiratory dysfunction (best is a short tracheal cannula with a 9.0 to 10 mm ID).

The clinical implication is that using a smaller ET seems to reduce laryngeal damage. The use of an ET with an ID less than 6.0 mm does not present a problem in anesthetized patients without spontaneous ventilation because relatively low gas flow velocities are necessary to maintain

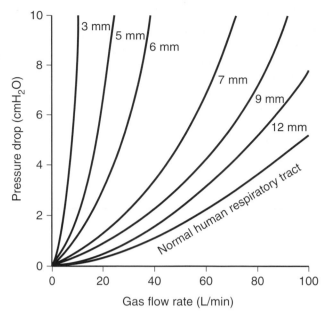

Figure 43-3 Pressure drop across endotracheal tubes of various sizes at flow rates of 0 to 100 L/min. Note wide disparity between 6-mm and 7-mm tubes as flow rate increases to the range typically seen in patients with respiratory failure. (From Nunn JF: Applied Respiratory Physiology, 3rd ed. Boston, Butterworth-Heinemann, 1987.)

adequate ventilation. However, gas flow resistance drastically increases especially in spontaneously breathing patients in respiratory distress, who benefit from larger ETs. Therefore, ETs of 7.0 to 8 mm ID seem appropriate for women and 8.0 to 9.0 mm ID for men.

An interesting aspect of ET selection is airway management for professional singers. Powner[168] sent a written survey to all physician members of the Voice Foundation concerning their opinions on airway management in professional singers. A strong consensus (76%) favored a smaller ET for singers (6 to 7 mm ID for males and 6.0 mm ID for females) by the oral (46%) versus nasal (36%) route. Intubation-extubation by the most expert or experienced personnel was emphasized to minimize laryngeal trauma. Preferences for an early tracheostomy (6 days) versus the usual time (10 days) were approximately equal (44% versus 50%, respectively).

The tracheal cuff has also been implicated as a cause of tracheal damage following long-term ventilatory support. Red rubber ETs equipped with low residual volume, high-pressure cuffs exert high pressures on the tracheal mucosa and are thought to be damaging.[148] Using an experimental study design in rabbits, Nordin and colleagues[154] investigated tracheal mucosal perfusion and cuff–tracheal wall pressures exerted by low residual volume, high-pressure cuffs and compared the results with those obtained with high-volume, low-pressure cuffs. Blood flow to the tracheal mucosa adjacent to the high-pressure cuff ceased at greater than 30 mm Hg. Using high-volume cuffs, mucosal blood flow did not cease up to intracuff pressures in the range of 80 to 120 mm Hg. However, cautious recommendations were made and cuff pressure should be maintained below 30 cm H_2O.[148]

Conditions in ICU patients differ from those in routine anesthesia patients. ICU patients are mainly breathing spontaneously or with partial ventilatory support. Spontaneous breathing results in cuff pressure changes, namely cuff pressure decreases during inspiration and increases during expiration. Active changes in pleural pressure by forced inspiratory efforts combined with direct modulation of tracheal musculature result in marked increases of tracheal diameter and a fall in cuff pressure even toward 0 cm H_2O.

Prolonged airway support using an ET or tracheal cannula may result in severe damage to the tracheal mucosa and an increased incidence of late complications such as tracheal stenosis. Tracheal stenosis may be induced by direct trauma or by the pressure exerted by the ET cuff. The presence of an ET sutured to canine tracheal mucosa induced laryngeal erythematous mucosa within less than 1 day, proceeding to mucosal ulceration and loss of airway architecture in less than 1 week.[24] Although damage was generally severe after 1 week, no further tendency to worsen after 1 week was observed.

The tracheal vascular supply to the tracheal submucosa is oriented in a circumferential direction anteriorly and longitudinally in the posterior part of the trachea. Seegobin and van Hasselt[189] investigated tracheal mucosal blood flow in 40 routine surgery patients using an endoscopic photographic technique while varying cuff inflation pressure. They suggested that tracheal blood flow is nearly normal at 25 cm H_2O. Increasing cuff pressure resulted in a pale appearance of the tracheal mucosa at 40 cm H_2O and a blanched appearance at 50 cm H_2O; flow was completely absent at 60 cm H_2O. Hence, it was recommended that a cuff inflation pressure of 30 cm H_2O (22 mm Hg) should not be exceeded.

Similar results were observed by Joh and coworkers.[115] They measured tracheal mucosal blood flow in an experimental model using the hydrogen clearance method. No significant depression in mucosal blood flow was observed with the cuff inflated to a maximum of 20 mm Hg. Increasing cuff pressures to 30 or even 45 mm Hg resulted in a significant reduction in mucosal blood flow, and they concluded from the data that cuff pressures should be kept at or below 20 mm Hg.[115] Incorrect cuff pressure settings may result in tracheomalacia and subglottic stenosis (too high pressures) or late-onset nosocomial pneumonia (insufficient pressures). Several authors suggested that microaspirations might thereby be facilitated and recommended the use of automatic cuff pressure regulators.[71,167] In a randomized study involving 130 patients, Pothmann and colleagues[167] reported a significant reduction in late-onset pneumonias when a microprocessor-controlled automatic cuff pressure regulator was used. However, no major randomized studies have been published as full papers, and the devices described can currently not be recommended for routine care of patients.

C. DRUGS USED FOR SEDATION AND ANALGESIA

In general, less is more in conscious sedation for airway management. Drugs must be administered in dosages that do not interfere with protective reflexes and patients' cooperation. Therefore, short-acting drugs with a potential antidote should be used. We prefer the combination of low-dose midazolam (i.e., 1 to 4 mg) and an opioid such as fentanyl (50 to 100 μg). Both substances can be immediately antagonized using flumazenil and naloxone, respectively. Several studies have focused on the use of remifentanil as a sole sedative and analgesic agent in this setting. Puchner and associates[169] prospectively studied remifentanil (0.1 to 0.5 μg/kg/min) alone versus fentanyl plus midazolam for the performance of fiberoptic intubation. Fiberoptic nasal intubation was possible in all patients, with a better suppressed hemodynamic response and tolerance of ET advance in the remifentanil group. Recall was significantly more common in the remifentanil group. A combination of remifentanil and midazolam is a valuable approach.[116] Promising alternative drugs are S(+)-ketamine and propofol.[59] Both have special disadvantages (e.g., increased salivation induced by ketamine and a small therapeutic range with propofol).

The presumption that the patient has a full stomach in emergency intubations dictates the use of an RSI technique. Cricoid pressure and laryngoscopy at the earliest possible moment place increased demands on the physician preparing to intubate the patient.[158] The ICU patient presents with even more risk factors than the routine OR patient; with facial distortion, swelling, secretions, and mandibular or cervical spine injury, these patients present the most challenging airway management problems.

Concerning the use of muscle relaxants in emergency airway management, several points have to be considered. Especially in the ICU setting, the choice of the appropriate muscle relaxant and the use of a muscle relaxant at all have to be discussed.[64] If endotracheal intubation fails, the merits of preserving spontaneous ventilation versus the optimized intubating conditions using nondepolarizing muscle relaxants should be considered. The distinct advantages and drawbacks of available substances are shown in Table 43-2.

Concerning succinylcholine, Benumof and colleagues[21] clearly demonstrated that even the short duration of action of this drug is too long and that critical hemoglobin desaturation occurs before return to an unparalyzed state even after a dose of 1 mg/kg body weight.

In the crashing patient, we waive administering muscle relaxants at all in order to preserve at least a minimum of spontaneous ventilatory efforts.

Table 43-2   **Distinct Advantages and Drawbacks of Available Muscle Relaxants**

Relaxant	Advantages	Disadvantages
Succinylcholine	Permits the option of early awakening	Requires repeated dosing to maintain optimal mask ventilation and transition to alternative plan for TI
Nondepolarizing agent of moderate duration (e.g., rocuronium or vecuronium)	Good mask ventilation for extended period of time, facilitating smooth transition to alternative TI plans	Does not permit early awakening
Nondepolarizing agent of short duration (e.g., rapacuronium)	Rapid onset of action	Does not permit early awakening

From El-Ganzouri AR: Management of the patient with difficult airway: 25 years' experience. Semin Anesth Periop Med Pain 20:134-143, 2001.

D. AWAKE ENDOTRACHEAL INTUBATION

Successful awake intubation is closely dependent upon proper preparation of the patient. Extensive psychological support and a clear explanation of the reason for and management of awake intubation are necessary and helpful in the ICU setting.

The airway has to be topically anesthetized with 5% to 10% lignocaine, which is sprayed with a flexible nozzle into the posterior pharynx in order to reduce coughing and buckling during intubation. If a fiberscope is used, the larynx is then sprayed with 2 mL of 2% lignocaine administered through the working channel of the fiberscope, after which the fiberscope is advanced into the trachea. Thereafter, a second spray is applied to the trachea before the ET is advanced. Alternative approaches, such as blockade of a superior laryngeal nerve or lingual nerve and transtracheal anesthesia, are presented in detail elsewhere.

Once the patient is properly prepared, any of the intubation techniques listed in Table 43-3 can be chosen according to the operator's preferences.

If the first attempt at awake endotracheal intubation fails because of equipment or operator failure or poor cooperation of the patient, the following options should be considered: a modified method for awake tracheal intubation (e.g., change from blind nasal to fiberoptic approach),

Table 43-3   **Nonsurgical Techniques for Awake Endotracheal Intubation**

Fiberoptic intubation (oral, nasal)
Intubation using rigid fiberoptic scopes
Blind intubation through laryngeal mask airway (Fastrach)
Direct rigid laryngoscopy
Retrograde techniques (± fiberoptic scope)
Trachlight or other lighted stylets
Blind nasal intubation

induction of general anesthesia, and transition to a fiberoptic-guided intubation method.[140,195] In our opinion, the first choice for awake airway management is fiberoptic oral or nasal intubation. If oral intubation is performed, a conduit (i.e., Ovassapian fiberoptic intubating airway[159]) facilitates fiberscope and ET insertion.

A valuable alternative approach is the insertion of the LMA Fastrach under local anesthesia and light sedation.[191] Intubation may then be performed either blindly or by the use of a fiberscope inserted through the LMA. Langeron and associates[130] prospectively compared LMA Fastrach intubation with fiberoptic intubation in patients with a difficult airway and reported similar success rates (beyond 90%) and durations for both techniques. Another interesting approach is the combination of Fastrach and lighted stylet. Dimitriou and colleagues[58] studied 44 of 11,621 patients in whom three attempts of direct laryngoscopy failed. In all those patients, an LMA Fastrach was inserted and sufficient ventilation was possible in all patients after a maximum of two attempts. Thereafter, a well-lubricated silicon ET loaded with a flexible light wand was introduced.[4] Light wand intubation was successful on the first attempt in 38 of 44 patients, on the second attempt in 3 of 44 patients, and on the third to fifth attempt in 2 of 44 patients. Intubation failed in only one patient. Finally, if all these alternatives fail, the establishment of a surgical airway should be considered.

E. ASSESSMENT OF CORRECT ENDOTRACHEAL TUBE PLACEMENT

Esophageal intubation is a major complication of airway management and can result in severe brain damage or even the patient's death. Evaluating the U.S.-American closed claims database (5480 closed claims), Cheney[41] reported the changing trends in anesthesia-related death and permanent brain damage. In the 1980s, 11% of claims associated with death or brain damage involved esophageal intubation, and this percentage decreased to 3% in the 1990s. This reduction was attributed to the introduction

Figure 43-4 Most common respiratory damaging events associated with brain damage by monitoring group. Sp_{O_2}, oxygen saturation from pulse oximetry. (From Cheney FW: Changing trends in anesthesia-related death and permanent brain damage. ASA Newslett 66:6-8, 2002.)

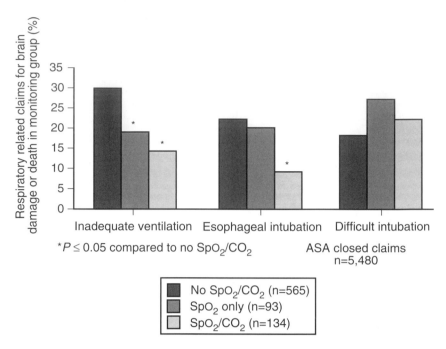

*P ≤ 0.05 compared to no SpO_2/CO_2

ASA closed claims n=5,480

No SpO_2/CO_2 (n=565)
SpO_2 only (n=93)
SpO_2/CO_2 (n=134)

of end-tidal CO_2 (ETCO$_2$) monitoring in the 1990s (Fig. 43-4).

Esophageal intubation is an issue even in sufficiently equipped ICUs. Schwartz and coauthors[188] studied nearly 300 emergency intubations in an ICU setting and reported an incidence of esophageal intubation in 8% of cases (ET misplacement was corrected in all patients before the onset of hypoxemia).

Techniques for clinical evaluation of ET position include direct visualization of the ET between the vocal cords,[95,166] ventilation bag compliance,[111] auscultation of breath sounds over lungs and epigastrium,[77] observation of symmetrical chest excursions, ET condensation,[8] lighted stylet,[138] esophageal detector device and self-inflating bulb,[27,203,217] acoustic reflectometry,[173,174] FOB,[159] chest radiography,[183] colorimetric ETCO$_2$ detector, and ETCO$_2$ measurement.[23,217]

Radiographic investigation is of limited value because of the delay in diagnosis. Fiberoptic evaluation requires special equipment and preparation and is time consuming. Acoustic reflectometry is a promising new approach giving excellent results at least in experienced hands. Raphael and colleagues[174] studied acoustic reflectometry in 200 adult intubated patients and reported a 99% correct tracheal and a 100% correct esophageal identification rate. Currently, CO_2 monitoring comes closest to the ideal monitor of correct ET positioning. CO_2 monitoring can be performed either colorimetrically with relatively inexpensive single-use CO_2 detectors (e.g., Easy Cap [Tyco Healthcare] or Colibri [ICOR AB, Bromma, Sweden])[171] or by capnography using infrared absorption.[23] Ventilation is assessed as ETCO$_2$ approximates Pa_{CO_2} within 2 to 6 mm Hg in normal lungs. Unfortunately, in many disease states, this discrepancy increases significantly. The concentration of CO_2 expired is determined by CO_2 production (e.g., body temperature and muscle tone), CO_2 transport (e.g.,

circulation and pulmonary perfusion), and CO_2 elimination (pulmonary and airway integrity). Therefore, absence of ETCO$_2$ indicates esophageal intubation, circuit disconnection, cardiac arrest, or airway obstruction.[216] A false-positive result may be obtained after gastric inflation with CO_2-containing gas or digestion of carbohydrate-enriched beverages. ET misplacement can be excluded by observing a normal ETCO$_2$ waveform for three to six consecutive breaths.[183]

Knapp and coworkers[123] investigated four different methods (auscultation, capnographic ETCO$_2$ determination, self-inflating bulb, and transillumination using Trachlight) for the verification of correct ET positioning in 152 examinations in an ICU setting. Only ETCO$_2$ monitoring was reliable for the verification of tracheal ET placement (Fig. 43-5). Poorer performance was reported only for patients with prehospital and in-hospital cardiac arrest. However, ETCO$_2$ concentrations are closely correlated with resuscitation outcome in this special setting.[96]

In conclusion, correct tracheal ET placement can be ensured unequivocally only by a physiologic ETCO$_2$ signal for several consecutive breaths (eventually combined with an esophageal detector device in the prehospital setting), by direct visualization of the ET between the vocal cords, or by fiberoptic visualization of tracheal cartilaginous rings and carina.[216] All other techniques may provide useful additional information but are susceptible to errors and misinterpretation.

IV. DIFFICULT AIRWAY MANAGEMENT IN INTENSIVE CARE

In critically ill patients, emergency endotracheal intubation is associated with a significant frequency of major complications. Airway management in intensive care

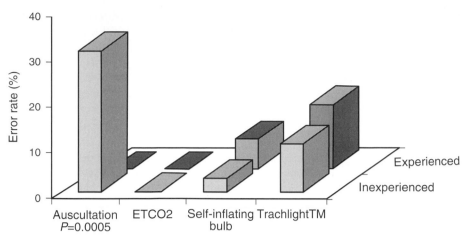

Figure 43-5 Error rates of experienced and inexperienced examiners obtained by evaluating endotracheal tube placement using one of the four methods. ETCO2, end-tidal CO_2. (From Knapp S, Kofler J, Stoiser B, et al: The assessment of four different methods to verify tracheal tube placement in the critical care setting. Anesth Analg 88:766-770, 1999.)

patients differs significantly from endotracheal intubation carried out for routine surgical procedures in the OR. Airway management in the ICU is often carried out in deteriorating patients suffering from respiratory failure, shock, or cardiopulmonary arrest, and little time may be available for evaluation, examination and preparation of the patient.

Therefore, the intensive care physician should approach the patient keeping four definitive questions in mind[160]:

1. Is mask ventilation likely to be successful when general anesthesia is induced before securing the airway?
2. Is endotracheal intubation likely to be successful when general anesthesia is induced before securing the airway?
3. Are there any obstacles that make awake fiberoptic intubation difficult?
4. If troubles are encountered, what is plan B?

Many studies focus on the incidence of difficult airways in patients with routine anesthesia. Primarily we have to consider the possibility of difficult face mask ventilation, difficult laryngoscopy, and difficult intubation. Langeron and colleagues[129] prospectively studied 1502 patients and observed difficulties in mask ventilation (DMV) in 75 patients (5%). DMV was anticipated by the anesthesiologist in only 13 patients (17% of the DMV cases). Using a multivariate analysis, five criteria were recognized as independent factors for DMV (age older than 55 years, body mass index > 26 kg/m², beard, lack of teeth, and history of snoring), the presence of two indicating a high likelihood of DMV (sensitivity, 0.72; specificity, 0.73). The implication for clinical practice is to avoid the administration of intravenous induction agents in patients with a high chance of difficult mask ventilation and secure the airway awake.

Difficult laryngoscopy or intubation, or both, is a common phenomenon even during routine care of patients in the OR.[82] Several investigations clearly demonstrated that minor problems necessitating a second intubation attempt are encountered in up to 8% of patients.[83,126,161]

Grade 3 laryngoscopy, requiring multiple attempts at intubation, occurs in 1% to 4% of all patients.[46,136,226] Inability to intubate because of grade 3 or 4 laryngoscopic views is present in 0.05% to 0.35% of routine anesthesia cases.[46,179,184] Fortunately, the cannot ventilate, cannot intubate situation is rare in the OR and occurs in approximately 2 of 10,000 cases.[18,22]

Management of the difficult airway in the emergency department (ED) and in the ICU has not been studied as well as in the OR. Sakles and coauthors[181] performed a 1-year study involving 610 patients requiring airway control in the ED. RSI was used in 84%, and 98.9% were successfully intubated. In 33 patients (5.4%), inadvertent esophageal intubation occurred. Seven (1.2%) patients could not be intubated and underwent cricothyrotomy. Three patients experienced sustained cardiac arrest after intubation. Bair and colleagues[13] published a prospective observational study on failed intubation attempts in the ER. They identified 7712 patients undergoing emergency intubation. In seven patients a definitive airway could never be established. A total of 207 patients (2.7%) with failed endotracheal intubation were then included in the study. The majority of the failed intubations occurred when RSI was not used as the first choice (i.e., oral intubation under sedation, oral intubation without sedation, or blind nasotracheal intubation). Among them, the most common rescue technique was RSI (49%). The second most common rescue technique was a surgical airway (21%). The authors concluded that invasive airway techniques are still important and rescue airway techniques should be emphasized in ongoing medical education.

Concerning endotracheal intubation in the ICU, Schwartz and associates[188] investigated the complications of 297 consecutive intubations in 238 adult critically ill patients studied prospectively over a period of 10 months. Eighty-nine percent of intubations were accomplished at the first attempt, and 8% of patients met criteria for difficult intubation. Four percent of intubations were possible only after four or more attempts. Esophageal intubation was observed in 8% of intubations, but all were recognized before any adverse sequelae resulted. New or unexplained pulmonary infiltrates were regarded as indicative of pulmonary aspiration of gastric contents and occurred in 4% of patients. Seven patients (3%) died during or within 30 minutes of the procedure.

To reduce the incidence of severe or catastrophic events during airway management (especially for anesthesia patients), the ASA task force on managing the difficult airway presented the difficult airway algorithm (ASA algorithm) in 1991.[20] The basic principles of this approach are meticulous evaluation of the patient before anesthesia induction, awake intubation if problems are suspected, and preparation of an alternative approach in case of failure (Fig. 43-6). Those recommendations are also

valuable for the management of critically ill patients. Unfortunately, the ASA algorithm has a number of characteristics that prevent direct application to the practice of ICU airway management. Airway management in the ICU is usually urgent or emergent, often depriving the physician of the time necessary to evaluate the patient and plan the lifesaving intervention. The patient is presumed to have a full stomach and therefore must undergo awake airway management or RSI. The option of reemergence from anesthesia to resume spontaneous ventilation if difficulty is encountered is often impossible. Therefore, modified algorithms with more specific considerations of the special circumstances encountered in ICU and emergency

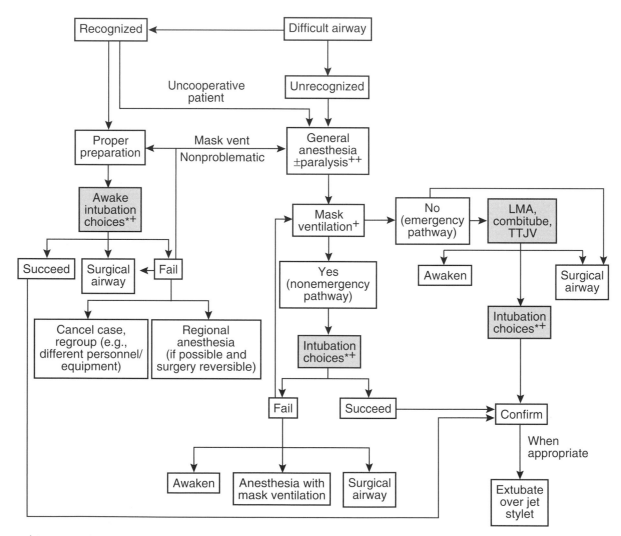

[+]Always consider calling for help (e.g., technical, medical, surgical etc.) when difficulty with mask ventilation and/or tracheal intubation is encountered

[++]Consider the need to preserve spontaneous ventilation

[*]Nonsurgical tracheal intubation choices consist of laryngoscopy with a rigid laryngoscope blade (many types), blind orotracheal or nasotracheal technique, fiberoptic/stylet technique, retrograde technique, illuminating stylet, rigid bronchoscope, percutaneous dilational tracheal entry. Reprinted with Permission.[20]

Figure 43-6 The American Society of Anesthesiologists difficult airway algorithm. LMA, laryngeal mask airway; TTJV, transtracheal jet ventilation. (From Benumof JL: Laryngeal mask airway and the ASA difficult airway algorithm. Anesthesiology 84:686-699, 1996.)

patients have been suggested (crash airway algorithm, failed airway algorithm).[219] Although these guidelines lack prospective evaluation, they may represent a more appropriate application of principles and constraints to airway management in the ED setting.[158]

The best means for coping with the problem of a failed airway is to prevent its occurrence. This requires optimization of the initial attempt of laryngoscopy in order to prevent multiple attempts causing bleeding and swelling. The net result may be a vicious circle with each attempt leading to a greater likelihood of failed intubation and ventilation with potentially disastrous consequences. Optimizing laryngoscopy requires appropriate positioning of the patient, use of a laryngoscope blade best fitting the situation, optimal external laryngeal pressure (BURP maneuver, i.e., backward, upward, rightward pressure on the cricoid cartilage), and eventually effective muscle relaxation.[158] When all these factors are taken into account, the first attempt of laryngoscopy is likely to be the best attempt.

According to the ASA difficult airway algorithm[20] and most other recommendations, there are only four appropriate options for the management of cannot-mask ventilate, cannot-intubate situations (see Fig 43-6): immediate insertion of LMA or ETC, manual TTJV, or surgical access to the patient's airway (tracheostomy or cricothyrotomy).

A. ESOPHAGEAL-TRACHEAL DOUBLE-LUMEN AIRWAY (COMBITUBE)

The ETC is a double-lumen airway (pharyngeal and distal lumen) invented by Frass and colleagues,[79] equipped with a pharyngeal balloon and a distal cuff (Tyco Healthcare, Mansfield, MA). The ETC is designed for blind insertion into the patient's esophagus or trachea. In more than 95% of all *blind* insertions the ETC enters the esophagus. After insertion, the pharyngeal balloon is inflated (maximum 85/100 mL air) and seals against the oral cavity, while the distal cuff (5 to 12/15 mL air) prevents gastric inflation. Test ventilation is started through the pharyngeal lumen (i.e., supraglottic ventilation). Absence of breath sounds or gastric inflation, or both, indicates one of the rare cases in which the ETC has blindly entered the trachea. In this case, ventilation is attempted through the distal lumen, the distal cuff blocked with the minimum amount of air providing an adequate seal, and the ETC is used like a conventional ET. Currently, the manufacturer produces two different ETC sizes: a small adult model (37 Fr, Combitube SA) for use in women and men ranging in height from 120 to 200 cm and a 41 Fr model for use in taller patients.[99,207]

The ETC has been used extensively in emergency situations as well as during routine surgery.[2,99,100,109] The authors recommend sufficient training during elective surgery before using the airway in emergency situations.[3,88,207] In routine cases, the ETC may be inserted using a standard laryngoscope to reduce the risk of tissue injury.[125,127] Contraindications for the use of the ETC are esophageal pathologies, ingestion of caustic substances, and central airway pathologies. Disadvantages are the lack of access to patients' airways (suctioning of tracheal secretions impossible), the lack of a pediatric ETC, and the risk of venous stasis and soft tissue (tongue) swelling after prolonged use. The former limitations will be eliminated by the introduction of a redesigned ETC enabling fiberoptic access to the patients' airways and the presentation of a pediatric version of the ETC.[106,128,187]

A major advantage of the Combitube is the protection against aspiration of gastric contents[157] and the applicability of high airway pressures. The ETC may stay in place for up to 8 hours, allowing time for further decision making.[78] Change of the ETC for a definitive airway (regular ET or tracheal cannula) may be performed by an attempt at direct laryngoscopy, fiberoptically,[89,128] or surgically (elective tracheostomy or cricothyrotomy).

B. LARYNGEAL MASK AIRWAY

The LMA (LMA North America, San Diego, CA) was presented in 1983,[29] gained widespread popularity, and is currently used extensively during general anesthesia.[19,29,213] The LMA may be placed for three different reasons: as a routine airway and ventilatory device; as an emergency airway in cannot intubate, cannot ventilate situations; or as a conduit for endotracheal intubation. Concerning use of the LMA as a routine airway, advantages over conventional face mask ventilation have been demonstrated clearly. Tidal volumes administered were higher and problems associated with airway management (difficulties in maintaining the airway or maintaining oxygen saturation from pulse oximetry [SpO_2] >95%) were less frequently encountered during LMA use compared with a regular face mask.[196] The LMA works well under these circumstances because exact positioning is not crucial for a clinically acceptable patent airway.

Furthermore, the potential use of this airway in respiratory emergency situations has been recognized.[28] Use of the LMA as the immediate airway in cardiopulmonary resuscitation has been described by Leach and coworkers,[132] and their findings were confirmed by a larger investigation.[206] A multicenter study was undertaken to assess the potential value of the LMA when inserted by ward nurses during resuscitation as a method of airway management prior to the arrival of the advanced life support team with endotracheal intubation capability. One hundred thirty nurses were trained and 164 cases of cardiac arrest were studied. The LMA was inserted at the first attempt in 71% and at the second attempt in 26% of cases. Satisfactory chest expansion occurred in 86% of cases. The mean interval between cardiac arrest and LMA insertion was 2.4 minutes. Regurgitation of gastric contents occurred before airway insertion in 20 cases (12%) and during insertion in 3 cases (2%).[206]

Therefore, the LMA has been incorporated into the ASA difficult airway algorithm[19] and may be inserted as a conduit for fiberoptic endotracheal intubation in the awake or anesthetized patient who cannot be conventionally intubated (mask ventilation may or may not be possible) and as a nonemergency or emergency airway in the anesthetized patient (Fig. 43-7).

Especially for patients with supraglottic pathologies and unfavorable anatomy for face mask ventilation or endotracheal intubation, an early LMA insertion should be considered. Drawbacks of the LMA include lack of access to the patients' central airways, risk of aspiration, limited positive airway pressures because of the often inadequate seal, and the need for training.[31] Moreover, the LMA is a supraglottic ventilatory device and thereby unable to establish adequate gas exchange in patients with central airway obstruction.

Several modifications of the LMA have been proposed and have been or will be introduced into clinical routine, such as the intubating LMA (Fastrach, the Laryngeal Mask Company). The so-called Fastrach differs from conventional LMAs by having a wider, shorter stainless steel tube, a handle to steady the device, and an epiglottic elevating bar (a movable flap fixed to the upper rim of the mask). The Fastrach accepts cuffed ETs up to an ID of 8.5 mm, enabling blind or fiberoptic intubation using the correctly placed Fastrach as a conduit. Success rates for blind Fastrach intubation in the range of 75% to more than 90% have been shown by several invstigators.[68,74,130]

The Fastrach has therefore been recommended as a rescue device for emergency airway management. Ferson and associates[74] used the Fastrach in 254 patients with different types of difficult airways. Insertion of the LMA Fastrach was accomplished in three attempts or fewer in all patients. The overall success rates for blind and fiberoptically guided intubations through the LMA Fastrach were 96.5% and 100.0%, respectively. Repeated blind intubation attempts with the LMA Fastrach resulted in esophageal perforation in one elderly patient.[30] Therefore, for blind Fastrach intubation the specially designed silicon tube with rounded bevel should be preferred because success rates exceed those encountered with standard reinforced tubes.[212] Muscle relaxation is not an absolute must for blind Fastrach intubation but increases success rates.[212]

LMA and LMA Fastrach versus Combitube: Sealing capacities and protection against regurgitation of gastric contents of LMA Fastrach seem to be inferior to those of the ETC[152,228]; for example, average leak fractions of the

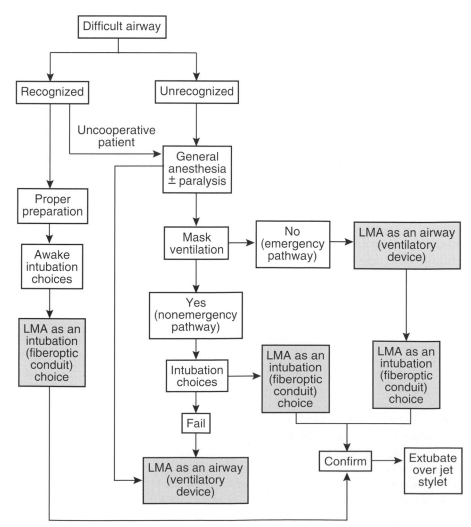

Figure 43-7 Laryngeal mask airway (LMA) and the American Society of Anesthesiologists difficult airway algorithm. (From Benumof JL: Laryngeal mask airway and the ASA difficult airway algorithm. Anesthesiology 84:686-699, 1996.)

LMA are in the range of 20% to 25% during positive-pressure ventilation with airway pressures ranging from 20 to 30 cm H_2O.[57] Use of the ETC offers higher peak airway pressures and permits PEEP ventilation, thereby enabling higher tidal ventilation[81] and maintenance of adequate gas exchange even in patients with severe underlying pulmonary pathology (e.g., aspiration of gastric contents). In contrast to findings with the ETC, blind or fiberoptic intubation is possible through the LMA lumen (using conventional ETs up to an ID of 6.5 mm) and especially through the Fastrach (up to 8.5 mm). With the currently available ETC model, no blind or fiberoptic access to the patient's airway is necessary. Krafft and colleagues[128] modified the standard ETC model and created a larger ventilation hole, which can be used for fiberoptic intubation or tracheal toilet. However, the redesigned model is currently not available and it is uncertain whether it will be produced in the near future.

C. TRANSTRACHEAL JET VENTILATION

In brief, TTJV is performed using a 16- or 14-gauge catheter and a 1.5- to 3.5-bar oxygen source (equipped with a pressure regulator) in combination with noncompliant tubing. The TTJV catheter is inserted through a cricothyroid puncture and correct tracheal placement is verified by the aspiration of 20 mL of free air. Noncompliant tubing is then connected and manual oxygen inflation started at an inspiratory time of less than 1 second (approximately 0.5 second) and an inspiratory/expiratory time ratio of 1:3 (to ensure enough time for passive exhalation). Alveolar ventilation is achieved by bulk flow of oxygen through the cannula as well as translaryngeal entrainment of room air (Venturi effect). For example, use of a 16-gauge cannula and a driving pressure of 3.5 bar results in a gas flow of approximately 500 mL/sec.[114] Facilitation of passive exhalation by maintaining patency of natural airways is of major importance to avoid overinflation and pulmonary barotrauma. Therefore, nasopharyngeal and oropharyngeal airways are inserted, maximum jaw thrust is well maintained throughout the entire procedure, and expiratory chest movements are observed continuously.

TTJV can be performed in elective as well as emergency situations with the major indications being lack of equipment for conventional airway management; the cannot ventilate, cannot intubate situation; and ventilatory support during upper airway surgery or during endotracheal intubation of the trachea by other techniques (e.g., ventilation during prolonged fiberoptic intubation).

Complications of TTJV are rare during *elective* application but are observed frequently during *emergency* TTJV (mainly limited to tissue emphysema). Monnier and colleagues[153] used high-frequency TTJV for ventilatory support during elective laser surgery for laryngeal and subglottic lesions and observed only one complication in 65 patients (mediastinal emphysema). To the contrary, Smith and coworkers[194] reported a 29% complication rate

in 28 emergency TTJV patients (exhalation difficulty in 14%, subcutaneous emphysema in 7%, mediastinal emphysema in 4%, and arterial perforation in 4%). Other complications of TTJV such as esophageal puncture, bleeding, or hematoma formation have been reported but occur only in rare instances.

D. EMERGENCY SURGICAL AIRWAY

RSI is the standard for emergency airway management in ICUs and EDs. Reported success rates of RSI are in the range of 97% to 99%, and an emergency surgical airway is necessary in only 0.5% to 2%.[182,204] Sakles and coauthors[182] evaluated a total of 610 patients requiring emergency airway management in the ED during a 1-year period. RSI was used in 515 (84%). A total of 603 patients (98.9%) were successfully intubated, and only 7 patients could not be intubated and underwent cricothyrotomy. Therefore, anesthesiologists and intensive care physicians have only limited experience with surgical airway management.[219,220] The ASA algorithm has proved to be an invaluable tool but only briefly addresses the circumstances in which a patient must be intubated immediately regardless of the difficulties presented. Because performance of a surgical airway is the final pathway of all airway algorithms, cricothyrotomy must be mastered by all clinicians involved in emergency airway management.

Surgical airway management comprises (1) percutaneous dilational cricothyrotomy or tracheostomy using the Seldinger technique,[150] (2) surgical cricothyrotomy, and (3) surgical tracheostomy. In emergency situations and in cases of unexpected intubation failure in the ICU, surgical or percutaneous cricothyrotomy using the Seldinger technique is preferred over tracheostomy and enables rapid and easy airway access and restoration of adequate gas exchange and ventilation.[47]

1. Percutaneous Cricothyrotomy

Several commercial kits are available, implying easy insertion and high success rates (e.g., Melker emergency cricothyrotomy catheter set and Arndt emergency cricothyrotomy set, both from Cook Critical Care, Bloomington, IN). Seldinger technique cricothyrotomy is achieved by performing cricothyroid puncture with a medium-sized needle, passing a wire through the needle, and then passing a dilator and airway over the wire (analogous to the insertion of a central venous line). Advertisement and promotion claim that percutaneous cricothyrotomy is a quick and easy procedure; in fact, after identification of the cricothyroid membrane (CTM), the Seldinger approach is not faster than open cricothyrotomy.[40] Furthermore, none of the percutaneous techniques provide a cuffed tube within the trachea.

Eisenburger and colleagues[63] compared Seldinger technique emergency cricothyrotomy with a conventional surgical approach in human cadavers. Tracheal placement of the tube was achieved in 60% ($n = 14$) in the Seldinger group compared with 70% ($n = 12$) in the open group (P = not significant). Furthermore, five attempts in the Seldinger group had to be aborted because of kinking of the guidewire. No differences in the time necessary to perform the procedures were registered.

Chan and associates[40] performed a similar study in cadavers but observed higher success rates: airway placement was accurate in 13 of 15 cases for the standard technique (87%) and 14 of 15 cases for the wire-guided technique (93%). Comparing wire-guided versus standard techniques, no differences in complication rates or performance times were observed. However, one has to keep in mind that all those results were obtained in an unstressed elective situation in the morgue. We assume that results in true emergency situations might be poorer.

2. Surgical Cricothyrotomy

Overlying vasculature is rich over the cervical trachea and strikingly absent over the CTM. Surgical cricothyrotomy can be performed only after correct identification of the CTM between thyroid and cricoid cartilage (the vertical length of the membrane is about 0.7 to 1.0 mm).

The set of instruments used should be simple: a scalpel with a no. 11 blade, a tracheal hook, a Trousseau dilator, and a cuffed tracheostomy tube.

The most commonly used approach is the "no-drop" technique, in which the larynx and trachea are immobilized by the operator's hand throughout the entire procedure (Fig. 43-8). Other techniques have been proposed (e.g., four-step technique), but the no-drop technique stood the test of time.[48]

Step 1: Identification of the CTM. Key landmark is the laryngeal prominence (Adam's apple), which is easier to palpate in men than in women. It can be identified in the midline at the junction of upper and middle thirds of the anterior neck. Thumb and long finger stabilize the larynx while the index finger is run down the anterior surface of the thyroid cartilage until the concavity of the CTM is reached.

Step 2: The larynx is immobilized by holding the superior horns of the thyroid between thumb and long finger and the skin is incised *vertically* (a vertical incision 2 to 3 cm long provides maximum flexibility and minimum trauma). Skin incision should be made through skin and subcutaneous tissues and not into the airway. Thereafter, the CTM is once again identified by using the index finger. Several authors prefer to leave the index finger in the wound even during the dissection of the membrane (enables membrane incision directly caudal to the index finger).

Step 3: The membrane is incised transversely in the distal third of the membrane whenever possible (avoiding the superior thyroid artery). The incision should be wide enough to permit easy insertion of the cannula (1.5 to 2 cm).

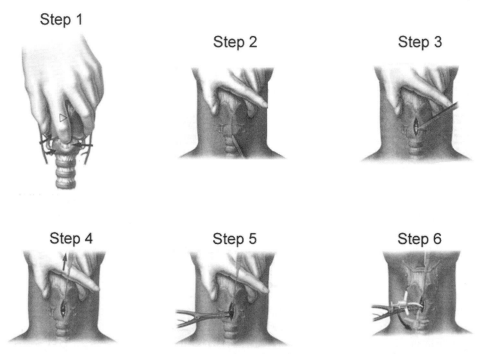

Figure 43-8 The "no-drop" technique for performing surgical cricothyrotomy. See text for details. (From Walls RM, Gibbs MA: Surgical Airway. Semin Anesth Periop Med Pain 20:183-192, 2001.)

Step 4: The tracheal hook is inserted transversely into the incised membrane and is then rotated 90 degrees to the midline (some authors waive the use of a tracheal hook for the performance of open cricothyrotomy). The hook strictly immobilizes the larynx and brings the opening within the membrane closer into the field of view.

Step 5: Next, the Trousseau dilator is inserted into the airway for just several millimeters and then opened in order to dilate the airway. Opening the branches in a rostrocaudal direction is preferred by several authors[219] because most resistance to cannulation is encountered between thyroid and cricoid. However, transverse dilation is also possible.

Step 6: The respective tracheal cannula is inserted with the right hand between the prongs opened with the operator's left hand. Sometimes, a slight twisting of the cannula of a 90-degree rotation of the Trousseau dilator is necessary to advance the tracheal cannula safely.

As mentioned, Seldinger cricothyrotomy and open cricothyrotomy are characterized by several pitfalls. Both techniques have to be trained in the manikin or better in human cadavers, and the individual operator has to choose the preferred technique. Several authors prefer the open approach because a cuffed cannula can be used and endotracheal suctioning or bronchoscopy is possible.

In conclusion, the ASA difficult airway algorithm was approved by the ASA House of Delegates on October 21, 1992 and became effective on July 1, 1993.[20] Every patient has to be screened for a difficult airway prior to anesthesia induction, and when difficulties are expected, airways have to be secured with the patient still awake (using the fiberoptic scope in most instances). If difficulties are encountered with the patient already anesthetized, one should refrain from repeated and forceful attempts at direct laryngoscopy but consider alternative methods. If a detrimental cannot ventilate, cannot intubate situation is encountered, either an LMA or Combitube must be inserted immediately. Further alternatives are institution of TTJV and immediate surgical access to the patient's airway. The most important point is to be alert and have plans B and C prepared in case troubles are encountered.

V. COMPLICATIONS OF TRANSLARYNGEAL INTUBATION

Hoarseness is a common complication after translaryngeal intubation and is reported to occur in 20% to 42% of patients.[148,199] Jones and coworkers[117] prospectively studied the incidence of hoarseness in 167 patients undergoing anesthesia, endotracheal intubation, and surgery. Fifty-four (32%) patients complained about postoperative hoarseness, with all but five returning to normal within 7 days. Vocal cord granuloma was observed in two patients.

The site of granuloma is typically at the tip of the vocal processes of the arytenoid cartilages because of their incessant movement.[112]

Stauffer and colleagues[198] prospectively studied 226 endotracheal intubations in 143 adult patients and reported that 62% of all patients developed at least one complication of long-term translaryngeal intubation (Fig. 43-9). The main complications in anatomic order are nasal and paranasal as well as laryngeal and tracheal injuries. Laryngeal injury is a common complication even after short-term translaryngeal intubation. Kambic and Radsel[118] examined 1000 patients at the end of anesthesia. Severe intubation lesions were registered in 6.2% of patients, with most injuries resolving within few days. However, 1% of patients suffered from sustained vocal cord dysfunction even after short-term translaryngeal intubation (Table 43-4 and Fig. 43-10).

In approximately 4% to 10% of patients, severe damage to the vocal apparatus is encountered (e.g., vocal cord paralysis, granuloma, or subluxation of the arytenoid cartilage).[55,119] Most severe complications are observed within the trachea itself (e.g., ulcerations, hematomas, up to necrosis and tracheomalacia).[11,198] These complications occur seldomly but may require extensive surgical interventions (i.e., resection of the trachea).

Laryngeal or tracheal trauma is even more common during acute airway management in emergency situations. Maxeiner[146] performed postmortem examinations in 294 cases involving emergency intubation. Acute macroscopic sequelae (mucosal hemorrhage or injury, deeper tissue hemorrhage in the [false] vocal cords) were observed in 18% of those resuscitated outside the hospital and in 16.9% of in-hospital patients. The majority of soft tissue hematomas were observed at the laryngeal opening (31%), vocal cords (37%), laryngeal opening and vocal cords (17%), subglottic region (17%), and hypopharynx (29%). Lesions at the laryngeal aperture were mainly located at the right part of the larynx.[146]

Other serious complications of translaryngeal intubation have also been reported. Lim and coauthors[137] reported three cases of recurrent laryngeal nerve palsy occurring in three patients after short-term intubation for surgery unrelated to the neck. As a main cause, pressure neuropraxia arising from an overinflated ET cuff compressing the peripheral anterior branches of the (right) recurrent laryngeal nerve was discussed. Frink and Pattison[86] and Castella and colleagues[37] reported posterior arytenoid dislocation after uneventful endotracheal intubation and anesthesia. Furthermore, both pharyngeal and esophageal perforations have been reported following repeated attempts at intubation, especially using a rigid stylet.[157] The tip of the rigid stylet should therefore never ever protrude from the distal tip of the ET.

Finally, endotracheal intubation may result in reduced clearance and retention of mucous secretions, bacterial colonization, and ventilator-associated pneumonia (VAP).[145] In a survey of 9080 ventilated patients, VAP

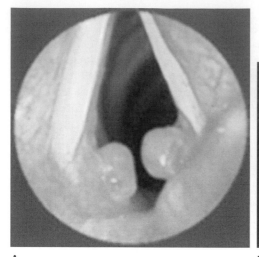

A

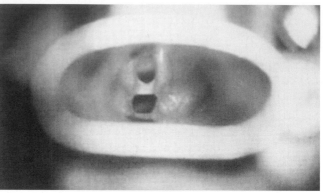

B

Figure 43-9 Laryngeal damage induced by long-term translaryngeal intubation: papilloma (**A**), synechia (**B**), and subglottic stenosis (**C**) after long-term tracheal intubation. (From Denk DM, Swoboda H, Neuwirth-Riedl K, Klepetko W: Glottic bridge synechia following intubation. Otorhinolaryngol Nova 3:41-44, 1993.)

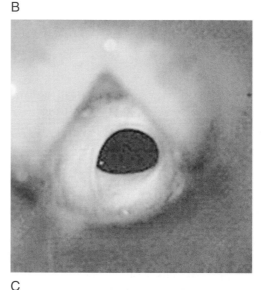

C

developed in 842 patients (9.3%).[176] The mean time interval between ICU admission and the diagnosis of VAP was 4.5 ± 7.5 days, and independent risk factors for the development of VAP were male gender and trauma admission. However, VAP seems to be a complication of endotracheal intubation and not of ventilatory support per se because studies show a reduced incidence in patients undergoing noninvasive mechanical ventilation.[103]

VI. AIRWAY MANAGEMENT FOR PROLONGED MECHANICAL VENTILATION

Tracheostomy is one of the oldest surgical procedures in history. Transcutaneous insertion of a cannula into the patient's trachea was first described in Egyptian and Hindu literature between 2000 and 1000 BC.[73] The first description of tracheostomy in modern times was by

Table 43-4 Outcome of Laryngeal Injury 3 Months after Short-Term Intubation

	Total	Cured	Cicatrix	Synechia
Vocal cord hematoma	45	38	7	—
Hematoma of supraglottic region	7	7	—	—
Laceration of vocal cord mucosa	8	7	—	1
Laceration of vocal muscle	1	—	1	—
Subluxation of arytenoid	1	1	—	—
Total	62	53	8	1

From Kambic V, Radsel Z: Intubation lesion of the larynx. Br J Anaesth 50:587-590, 1978.

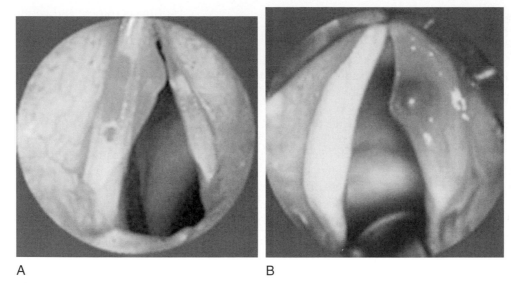

A   B

Figure 43-10 **A** and **B,** Acute laryngeal damage during airway management (hematoma of the true vocal cords after traumatic intubation attempts).

the Italian surgeon Fabricius of Aquapendente in the 17th century using a tracheal cannula.[67] Development proceeded as many case reports on alternative techniques were published in the following centuries.[54,102] The currently used technique for "conventional" surgical tracheostomy was first described by Jackson in 1909.[113] Until several years ago, "open" surgical tracheostomy was the only method and therefore gold standard for long-term airway management in intensive care medicine. However, the conventional approach has several disadvantages, such as need to transfer the patient to the OR and early and late complications such as bleeding or stoma infection. Shelden and colleagues reported a percutaneous access to the trachea. However, this procedure was relatively complicated and followed by deadly complications.[192,197] In 1985, Ciaglia and associates[43] proposed a percutaneous approach using the Seldinger technique and increasingly sized dilators for progressive tracheal dilation, as supposed by Sanctorius in the 17th century.[185]

Note the following definitions:

Tracheotomy: surgical incision of the upper third of the anterior tracheal wall to insert a cannula

Tracheostoma: artificial opening of the trachea to the outside created by tracheotomy or tracheostomy

Tracheostomy: surgical technique to create a permanent epithelialized tracheostoma

Cricothyrotomy: surgical incision of the CTM for the insertion of a cannula

Coniotomy: percutaneous emergency cricothyrotomy using special single-use sets

To improve clarity, we use only the term *tracheostomy* in this chapter.

A. TIMING OF TRACHEOSTOMY

The question of long-term translaryngeal intubation versus tracheostomy is now elucidated and favors secondary tracheostomy (Table 43-5).

In 1989, at the Consensus Conference on Artificial Airways in patients receiving mechanical ventilation,[165] the indications for nasal or oral ETs and tracheostomy tubes were forged. The consensus conference stated that "if the need for an artificial airway is anticipated to be greater than 21 days, a tracheostomy should be preferred."[165] With the introduction of percutaneous methods, the question of translaryngeal intubation versus tracheostomy has been

Table 43-5 Advantages of Tracheostomy over Translaryngeal Intubation

Reduced incidence of laryngeal or tracheal damage
Facilitation of nursing care, clearance of secretions
Shorter cannulas with greater diameter and reduced dead space
Reduced airway resistance, decreased work of breathing
Weaning facilitated
Improved tolerance by the patient
Swallowing and oral feeding facilitated
Possibility of communication (special tracheal cannulas)
Better fixation of the tube (especially during mobilization)
Reduced need for analgesics and sedatives

shifted to the question concerning the best time point at which to perform tracheostomy.

Data convincingly demonstrating an advantage of early tracheostomy (within the first week of critical illness) with respect to duration of ventilatory support, rate of complications, or length of hospital stay are still lacking. Rodriguez and colleagues[178] demonstrated in a prospective study involving 106 multiple-trauma patients that early tracheostomy within post-traumatic days 1 to 7 resulted in a shorter duration of ventilation and shorter length of ICU stay than in patients tracheotomized after day 8. However, the majority of the published studies could not demonstrate definitive advantages of early (day 3 to 5) versus later (day 10 to 14) tracheostomy.[62,202] In a systematic review (including the Rodriguez trial), Maziak and associates[147] performed a literature search yielding 8153 citations. From this list the authors identified 48 articles that might be relevant. Ultimately, 5 of the 48 articles met the inclusion criteria. After data review, the authors found no significant advantages of early (day 2 to 7) versus late (>day 4 to 14) tracheostomy. The authors concluded that there is insufficient evidence to support the concept that the timing of tracheostomy alters the duration of mechanical ventilation or extent of airway injury.

In a questionnaire study answered by 48 Swiss ICUs (1995 to 1996: 90, 412 patients and 243, 921 ventilator days), 10% of all patients ventilated more than 24 hours underwent tracheostomy.[76] The majority of tracheostomies (35%) were performed in the second week of critical illness. However, 68% of all interviewed physicians would also perform an early (<day 7) tracheostomy if indicated (expected longer ICU course). The authors concluded that tracheostomy in Swiss ICUs is far from being standardized with regard to indication, timing, and choice of technique.

A randomized, prospective study is required to examine the need for and the timing of tracheostomy in patients requiring prolonged mechanical ventilation. The findings of such a study would have an impact on clinical practice and hospital costs.[147]

Until that time, the following recommendations of the Consensus Conference of 1989[165] are still valid:

- Patients with an estimated duration of intubation of less than 7 to 10 days are managed by translaryngeal intubation.
- Reevaluation of the patient at day 7: extubation possible within the next 7 days? If yes, continue translaryngeal intubation (cumulative duration of translaryngeal intubation < 14 days).
- All patients with slow recovery or deterioration with an estimated duration of intubation of more than 14 days should undergo tracheostomy.
- Early elective tracheostomy (day 3 to 5) in patients with an estimated duration of intubation more than 21 days.
- Patients for whom estimation of ventilator days is difficult should undergo daily evaluation of the pros and cons of tracheostomy and continued translaryngeal intubation.[101]

VII. TRACHEOSTOMY TECHNIQUES

A. CONVENTIONAL SURGICAL TRACHEOSTOMY

Tracheal dissection to provide relief from airway obstruction resurfaced in the diphtheria epidemic in the 19th century. The currently used technique for "conventional" surgical tracheostomy was first described by Jackson in 1909.[113] Many variations exist in the technique used for surgical tracheostomy. In brief, the surgical tracheostomy is performed as follows.[216]

Surgical tracheostomy is preferably performed in the OR. In critically ill patients for whom transport seems too risky, tracheostomy can also be performed in the ICU bed, although mainly under inferior surgical conditions. The procedure is described briefly; a more detailed description is given in the respective chapter.

Positioning of the patient with head and neck extended and a small pillow under the patient's shoulders is a main part of a successful procedure. Overextension of the head should be avoided because the airway may be narrowed further and the tracheostomy site may be erroneously too low (near the innominate artery). The operating field should be prepared according to aseptic conditions. For patients who do not tolerate this position, a sitting or semirecumbent position is possible.

After proper preparation, the landmarks (e.g., thyroid and sternal notch, cricoid cartilage) are palpated and a 3-cm vertical skin incision extending inferior to the cricoid cartilage is performed. Several authors advocate a horizontal incision because of the better cosmetic results.

Subcutaneous fat can be resected using electrocautery, and the inferior limit of the surgical field should be screened for the proximity of the innominate artery. Platysma is dissected until the midline raphe between the strap muscles is identified. One must strictly adhere to the midline in order to avoid bleeding and paratracheal structures. After retraction of the strap muscles laterally, the pretracheal fascia and the thyroid isthmus are exposed. The thyroid may be retracted out of field, but a resection is recommended because of the reduced incidence of postoperative bleeding complications.

Securing the cricoid cartilage with a hook and superior traction improves control of the tracheal entry. Tracheal incision should be performed between the second and third or the third and fourth tracheal rings. The first tracheal ring should always be left intact in order to protect the cricoid cartilage.

Several options for a semipermanent tracheostomy exist: either a T-, U-, or H-shaped tracheal opening can be made, with the tracheal flaps sutured to the neck skin. Creation of a U-shaped flap (i.e., Björk flap) is not recommended because of the increased risk of flap necrosis. No tracheal cartilage should be resected, thereby minimizing the risk of tracheal stenosis.

A permanent tracheostoma is necessary for patients who indefinitely require secure transluminal access (e.g., patients with head injury). For the creation of a permanent stoma, a small portion of the anterior tracheal wall is resected and skin flaps are sutured to the rectangular tracheal opening (Fig. 43-11).

B. PERCUTANEOUS DILATIONAL TRACHEOSTOMY

During the last decade of the 20th century a dramatic change in airway management for long-term ventilatory support occurred with the introduction of percutaneous approaches to the trachea. The first description of a percutaneous tracheostomy was published by Shelden and coauthors in 1955[192]; the method never became popular because of severe complications.[197] With the introduction of a Seldinger technique by Ciaglia and colleagues,[43] a triumphant advance of percutaneous tracheostomy started because of presumed advantages (Table 43-6).

Simpson and associates[193] showed that the number of critically ill patients at their facility undergoing tracheostomy had increased from 8.5% to 16.8% of all critically ill patients since the introduction of PDT. This represents a doubling of the proportion of ICU patients undergoing tracheostomy. Tracheostomy was also performed significantly earlier, at a median of 4 days versus 8 days of mechanical ventilation.

Approximately 31,000 tracheostomies are performed in Germany (~80 million inhabitants), and more than 50% of them are PDTs.[222] The question concerning the best technique for tracheostomy (surgical approach versus percutaneous access) cannot be answered definitively.

1. Percutaneous Dilational Tracheostomy According to Ciaglia

PDT was introduced by Pasquale Ciaglia in 1985 as an alternative approach to conventional surgical tracheostomy (Cook Critical Care, Bloomington, IN).[43] Using the original Ciaglia technique, the correct puncture site in

Table 43-6   Major Advantages of the Percutaneous Approach

Bedside procedure, easy to learn
Reduced personnel required
Reduced incidence of wound infection

the midline between first and third tracheal rings is identified, the trachea is punctured (free aspiration of 20 mL of air possible), and a guidewire is inserted. Over this guidewire special dilators are introduced and the anterior wall of the trachea is dilated until an opening with a diameter of approximately 36 Fr is achieved (Fig. 43-12).

Advantages of this method are short duration of the procedure and bedside performability. However, contraindications have to be kept in mind (Table 43-7).

To enhance the patient's safety, the entire procedure should be monitored fiberoptically, as proposed by Marelli and others.[143] The use of a bronchoscope prevents endotracheal insertion out of the anterior midline and injury to the posterior tracheal wall, particularly during dilatation. A drawback of FOB control is that the insertion of the bronchoscope into the airway results in partial obstruction of the ventilatory path, thereby compromising ventilation.[175]

For performing PDT, the anesthetized patient is positioned with the head and neck extended. The anterior part of the neck is cleaned and draped in accordance with

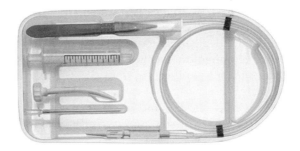

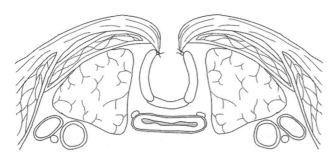

Figure 43-11 Permanent epithelialized tracheostoma. (From Hartung HJ, Osswald PM, Petroianu G [eds]: Die Atemwege. Stuttgart, Wissenschaftliche Verlagsgesellschaft, 2001, p 159.)

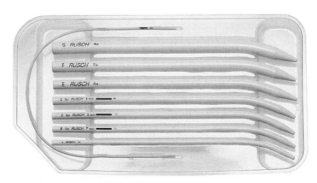

Figure 43-12 PercuQuick set for percutaneous tracheostomy. (Courtesy of Rüsch, Vienna, Austria.)

Table 43-7 **Contraindications for the Performance of Percutaneous Dilational Tracheostomy**

Trauma or infection in the region of the presumed stoma
Inability to localize the trachea
Palpable vessels at the puncture site
Coagulation disorders (platelet count < 30,000/µL, partial thromboplastin time > 50 seconds
Fraction of inspired oxygen > 0.8
Known or suspected difficult airway

the guidelines used for thyroid surgery. The fiberoptic bronchoscope is then introduced through the ET in place and the correct puncture site is identified. For this purpose the ET must be drawn back toward the glottic opening and the FOB must be inside the ET to prevent erroneous puncture of the scope (after the procedure, the scope must undergo a complete evaluation to prevent water intrusion).[105]

After puncturing the trachea in the midline between the first and third tracheal rings, a guidewire is inserted under fiberoptic vision (Fig. 43-13). Puncture has to be performed in the midline between the tracheal cartilages. Puncture near a tracheal ring has to be avoided because cartilage damage or fractures are associated with late complications such as tracheal stenosis.

Thereafter, a guidance cannula is slid over the guidewire and a 1.5-cm skin incision is performed. The puncture site is then dilated with seven (hydrophilic) plastic dilators up to a diameter of 36 Fr (12 mm). Last, the tracheal cannula (maximum ID 9.0 mm) is inserted guided by a medium-sized dilator. Slight resistance is commonly encountered during cannula insertion, which is overcome by using sufficient lubricating fluid and rotating movements during insertion. After cannula insertion, the FOB is removed from the ET and inserted into the tracheal cannula in order to verify correct placement, optimize cannula insertion depth, and remove bloody secretions from trachea and bronchi.

A modification of the system is the single-step dilational tracheostomy, that is, the Ciaglia Blue Rhino (Ciaglia Blue Rhino, Cook Critical Care), introduced in 1999. This development has only a single hydrophilic dilator, which is shaped similarly to the horn of a rhinoceros (Fig. 43-14). The dilation process can be performed in a single step, without the need to change dilators (Fig. 43-15). Therefore, the risk of injury to the posterior tracheal wall, of bleeding episodes, and of impaired oxygenation by repeated airway obstruction during the dilation process may be reduced.

Byhahn and colleagues[34] performed a prospective, randomized study comparing the classical PDT and Blue Rhino in 50 critically ill patients. This small randomized study reported a relatively high incidence of cartilage damage (33%) but no life-threatening complications with either method. Fikkers and associates[75] assessed perioperative, early, and late complications in 100 consecutive Blue Rhino tracheostomies. The success rate was 98%, with minor and major complications observed in 30% and 12%, respectively. Tracheal stenosis was observed in one patient (observation period 6 to 12 months). Whether the Blue Rhino equipment represents a major advance in clinical routine has to be evaluated in larger series of patients.

2. Percutaneous Dilational Tracheostomy According to Griggs

In 1989, Schachner and colleagues[186] presented a method using a single dilation tracheostomy forceps over a guidewire (Rapitrach; Fresenius, Runcom, Cheshire, UK), which carries a relatively high incidence of injury of the posterior tracheal wall. In 1990, Griggs and associates[93] developed another guidewire dilating forceps (Portex, Kent, England) with a smooth rounded tip (modified Howard-Kelly forceps with a blunt edge). The procedure (Fig. 43-16) is characterized by an approach similar to the Ciaglia technique with diaphanoscopy, puncturing of the trachea (18-gauge needle), guidewire insertion, and skin incision. Thereafter, all structures of the neck

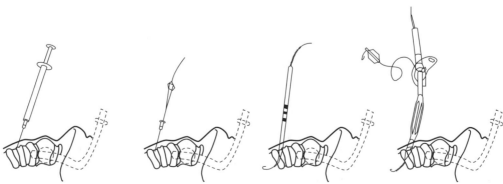

Figure 43-13 Percutaneous tracheostomy according to Ciaglia and colleagues.[43] (Courtesy of Rüsch, Vienna, Austria.)

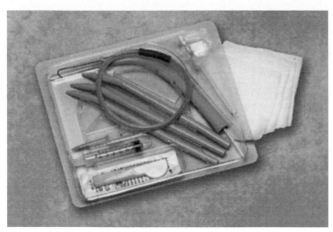

Figure 43-14 Single-step Ciaglia method—Blue Rhino. (Courtesy of Rüsch, Vienna, Austria.)

are slightly dilated by one small dilator. Next, the specially designed forceps is inserted via the guidewire until the trachea is reached and the skin and pretracheal tissues are dilated by opening the blades. The forceps is then carefully advanced into the trachea under fiberoptic control, with the tip of the forceps pointing toward the carina. By pulling both branches of the forceps apart, the trachea is also dilated. According to the Ciaglia technique, the tracheal cannula chosen is then inserted by means of an adequate dilator over the guidewire.

3. Translaryngeal Tracheostomy According to Fantoni

The translaryngeal approach for tracheostomy (TLT) was introduced by Fantoni and coauthors in 1996.[69,70] In contrast to all other percutaneous techniques, the initial puncture of the trachea is directed cranially (Fig. 43-17).

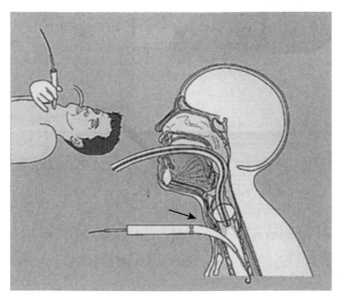

Figure 43-15 Performance of single-step Blue Rhino technique. (Courtesy of Rüsch, Vienna, Austria.)

After tracheal puncture, a guidewire is passed through the needle and passed toward the oropharynx alongside or inside the ET. The patient is then reintubated with the kit's 5 mm ID tube and the wire is connected with the tracheal cannula. The cannula is advanced through the pharynx into the trachea by constantly pulling on the guidewire. The pointed head is then pulled out the anterior tracheal wall and soft tissues of the neck. Next, the pointed head is cut off and the cannula is rotated 180 degrees downward using a plastic obturator. Thereafter, the fiberoptic scope is inserted through the cannula in order to check correct positioning in the trachea.

The major advantage of this approach is that no or hardly any skin incision is necessary and the bleeding risk is therefore minimized. Typical problems encountered with this technique are: difficulties with the intratracheal rotation of the cannula, the need to change the ET, and potential contamination of the tube during oropharyngeal passage.

Byhahn and colleagues[32] investigated the practicability and early complications of Fantoni's translaryngeal tracheostomy technique in 47 ICU patients. No severe complications (aspiration or bleeding) were observed, but oxygenation deteriorated in about one fourth of the patients. The authors concluded that translaryngeal tracheostomy is a valuable alternative to Ciaglia's approach but should be performed only in patients requiring an FIO_2 of less than 0.8.

Westphal and coauthors[223] compared TLT with the Ciaglia approach in a prospective study of 90 patients. Although success and complication rates were similar between the groups, problems during the procedure were far more common with the TLT technique (especially in positioning the guidewire correctly). Cantais and associates[35] prospectively compared the forceps dilational and translaryngeal techniques in 100 adult critically ill patients. Fantoni's translaryngeal technique took twice as long as forceps dilation (13 versus 7 minutes, respectively). Although there were fewer minor bleeding episodes in the Fantoni group, major complications were more common and unsolvable technical problems were encountered in 23% of patients. Nevertheless, the authors concluded that both techniques are safe and each physician should be able to choose the technique he or she prefers.

4. Rotating Dilational Tracheostomy (PercuTwist)

A new method of tracheal access by controlled rotating dilation has been reported.[87,224] The PercuTwist technique (PercuTwist, Teleflex Rüsch) offers an alternative real single-step percutaneous tracheostomy approach (Figs. 43-18 and 43-19). Preparation, puncturing of the trachea, and guidewire insertion are performed in accordance with the Ciaglia and Griggs techniques. After needle removal, an 8- to 10-mm skin incision is made and a special hydrophilic dilation screw (suited for either 8 or 9 mm ID tracheal cannulas) is slid over the guidewire until the skin incision is reached. Using slight pressure,

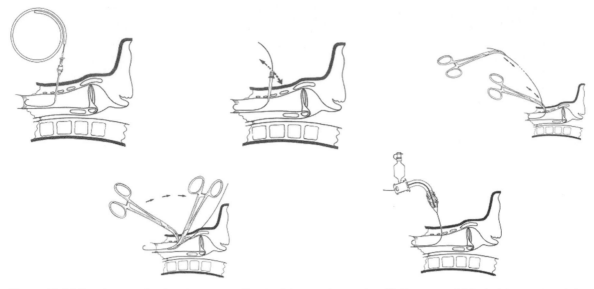

Figure 43-16 Percutaneous tracheostomy according to Griggs and coworkers.[93] (Courtesy of Rüsch, Vienna, Austria.)

the dilator is turned clockwise until the first threads are advanced into the pretracheal soft tissues. Thereafter, the PercuTwist is carefully advanced without pushing until the tip of the screw is fiberoptically visualized inside the trachea (Fig. 43-20). The screw is then advanced into the trachea twist by twist under gentle elevation of the anterior tracheal wall. Then the dilator is removed by counterclockwise rotation and the tracheal cannula is inserted using an insertion dilator guided by the in situ guidewire.

Frova and Quintel[87] reported the use of the PercuTwist system in 50 consecutive ICU patients with a 100% success rate without serious complications. Tracheal ring fractures were observed in 4 of 50 patients (8%), but no case of posterior tracheal wall injury was observed. Westphal and colleagues[224] studied 10 consecutive patients and did not

observe any early complications besides minor bleeding (<20 mL) in two patients. In a prospective randomized study in 70 consecutive patients, Byhahn and coworkers[33] compared the safety and efficacy of PercuTwist and Blue Rhino tracheostomy. Stoma dilatation was possible in all patients of both groups. Whereas cannula insertion was uneventful in all but one patient in the Blue Rhino group, it was difficult or impossible in eight patients in the PercuTwist group. Posterior tracheal wall injury was observed in two PercuTwist patients. However, no statistically significant differences in minor and overall complications were observed between the two techniques. Kinking of the guidewire seems to be a common complication when using the PercuTwist system and was observed in 8 of 50 patients in the Frova study[87] and

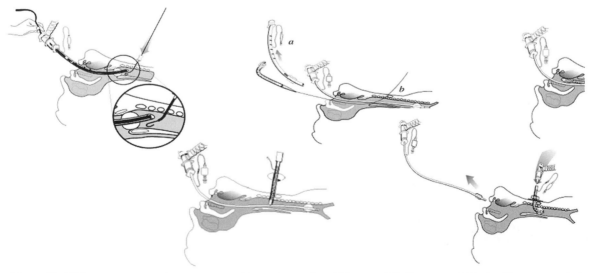

Figure 43-17 Percutaneous tracheostomy according to Fantoni and Ripamonti.[69] (Courtesy of Rüsch, Vienna, Austria.)

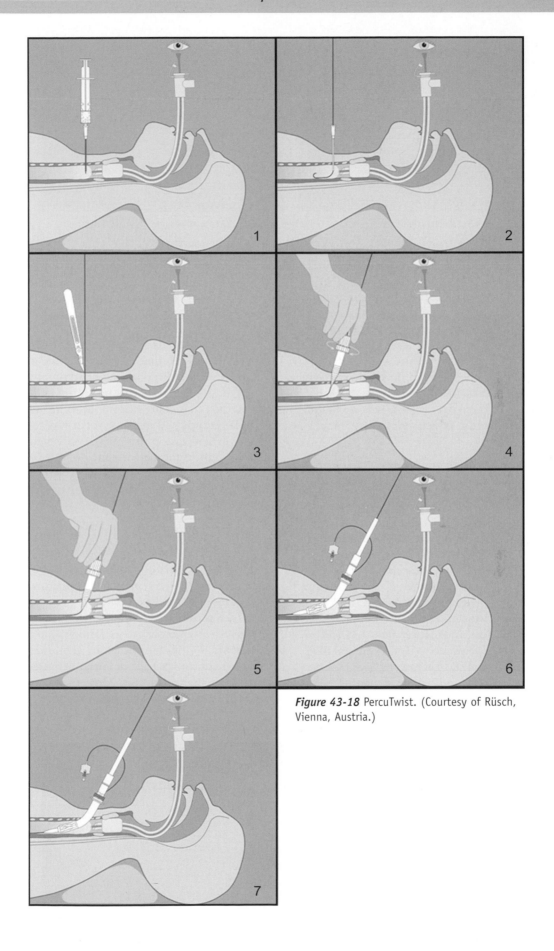

Figure 43-18 PercuTwist. (Courtesy of Rüsch, Vienna, Austria.)

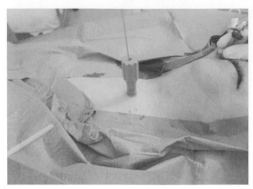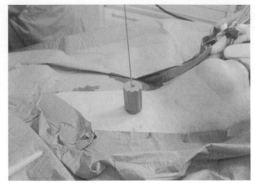

Figure 43-19 Performance of PercuTwist tracheostomy. (Courtesy of Rüsch, Vienna, Austria.)

in 2 of 35 patients in the Byhahn report.[33] A distinct advantage of the PercuTwist technique over all other percutaneous approaches may be that the stoma remains open after removal of the screw and immediate emergency intubation of the stoma with a small ET is possible. With all other devices, the dilated stoma closes under tissue pressure immediately after removal of the dilators. Whether the difficulties encountered during PercuTwist tracheostomy reflect drawbacks of the technique or represent the normal learning curve with a new technique remains to be determined in larger series of patients.

C. AIRWAY MANAGEMENT DURING PERCUTANEOUS DILATIONAL TRACHEOSTOMY

During puncturing of the trachea and the entire dilatation process, the ET has to be pulled back into the larynx in order to protect the bronchoscope and tube cuff. Therefore, alternative approaches such as ventilatory support using an LMA[97,139] or a Fastrach[214] have been suggested. Dosemeci and colleagues[60] performed a randomized controlled investigation studying LMA as an alternative airway for airway management during PDT in 60 patients. The authors concluded that LMA is an effective and successful ventilatory device during PDT. It improves visualization of the trachea and larynx during fiberoptically assisted PDT and prevents the difficulties associated with the use of an ET such as cuff puncture,

tube transsection by the needle, and accidental extubation. However, Ambesh and associates[7] demonstrated that changing the ET to an LMA may result in potentially life-threatening complications such as loss of the airway during PDT. In a prospective randomized study, the authors compared the safety and efficacy of ET versus LMA ventilation during PDT in 60 critically ill patients. Whereas the complication rate was low in the ET group (7% ET impalement, 7% cuff puncture, and 3% accidental extubation), a high rate of complications was observed in the LMA group (33% incidence of airway loss, inadequate ventilation, and gastric distention). A change of the ET for an LMA during the performance of PDT can therefore not be recommended and may be an alternative method only for patients not intubated prior to the procedure.

D. PERIOPERATIVE AND EARLY COMPLICATIONS OF PERCUTANEOUS DILATIONAL TRACHEOSTOMY

A number of potential complications during or immediately after PDT have been reported in the literature (Table 43-8).

Bleeding is the most common perioperative complication and was observed with an incidence of 0% to 4%.[162] The incidences of other complications such as emphysema and tracheal lesions are shown in Table 43-9.

Numerous studies have reported bedside PDT complications with an incidence similar to those observed during conventional surgical tracheostomy; others have proposed

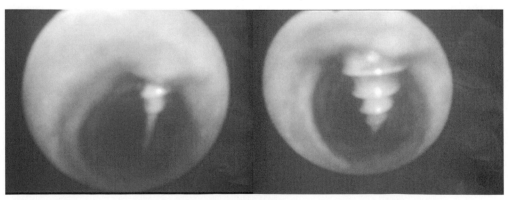

Figure 43-20 Fiberoptic control of the PercuTwist technique. (Courtesy of Rüsch, Vienna, Austria.)

Table 43-8 **Complications of Tracheostomy**

Early
Bleeding
Wound infection
Pneumothorax, pneumomediastinum
Tracheoesophageal fistula
Malpositioning of the cannula
Damage of the tracheal cartilages
Late
Infection
Granulation tissue
Tracheal stenosis
Persisting fistula after decannulation

a learning curve and a significantly lower complication rate thereafter.

Petros[162] demonstrated a learning curve in performing dilational tracheostomy after prospectively evaluating 234 PDTs (Fig. 43-21).

Massick and coauthors[144] performed a prospective analysis of the incidence of complications in the first 100 PDTs (Ciaglia) performed in a local community hospital. The authors clearly demonstrated a learning curve, with the first 20 patients exhibiting a significantly higher incidence of perioperative as well as late complications. Furthermore, patients with suboptimal anatomy were found to have significantly increased complication rates independent of operator and institutional experience. PDT involves a steep learning curve, with most perioperative, postoperative, and late complications occurring with the first 20 patients.

Beiderlinden and associates[17] assessed the incidence of early complications of fiberoptically guided PDT beyond the learning curve (all investigators personally performed > 100 PDTs). A total of 133 consecutive patients underwent 136 PDTs (conventional Ciaglia technique $n = 114$ and Blue Rhino $n = 22$); tubes were fixed at the patients' skin and no routine tube exchanges were performed. Insertion of the ET was easy or modestly difficult in 87%, and no procedure-related deaths were observed. The incidence of tube-related complications (e.g., tracheal wall lesion, bleeding, cannula misplacement) was low at 0.7%. Fracture of tracheal rings was observed in 24%. Despite this finding, the authors concluded that with experience in performing PDT, fixation of the tracheal cannula, and omission of routine tube changes, the complication rate of PDT is low.

Ambesh and colleagues[6] compared two percutaneous single dilation techniques, using the Blue Rhino and Griggs dilating forceps in 60 consecutive patients. Percutaneous access to the trachea was possible in all patients, with significantly more difficult cannulations in the Griggs group (30% versus 7%). Although overdilatation of the stoma occurred more frequently in the Griggs group (23% versus 0%), the Blue Rhino technique was commonly associated with tracheal ring fractures (30% versus 0%, respectively).

E. LATE COMPLICATIONS OF DILATIONAL PERCUTANEOUS TRACHEOSTOMY

The technique of PDT was introduced by Ciaglia and colleagues[43] in 1985. Many investigators have since published their experience with the technique and have concluded that the procedure is safe and cost effective. The perioperative complications of PDT are well described and are considered less frequent than those of open surgical tracheostomy.

Vigliaroli and associates[215] reported their clinical experience with Ciaglia's dilational tracheostomy during a 6-year period in 304 cases, with 41 of those being evaluated for late complications. There was no perioperative

Table 43-9 **Perioperative Complications (%) during Percutaneous Dilational Tracheostomy**

Author	n	Major Bleeding	Subcutaneous Emphysema	Pneumothorax	Tracheal Lesions	Death
Marelli et al[143]	61	1.6	0	0	0	1.6
Ciaglia and Graniero[44]	170	0	1.2	0	0	0
Friedman and Mayer[85]	100	4.0	2.0	0	?	1.0
Manara[142]	77	2.6	0	0	0	0
Fernandez et al[73]	162	0.6	0	0.6	2.5	0
Hill et al[104]	356	1.4	0	0.6	0	0.3
Van Heurn et al[211]	150	3.3	1.3	0	0	0
Petros and Engelmann[163]	137	0.7	2.2	0	2.9	0
Walz et al[221]	326	0.6	0.6	0	0.9	0.3

From Petros S: Percutaneous tracheostomy. Crit Care 3:R5-R10, 1999.

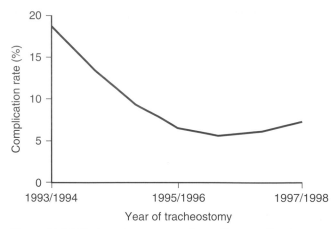

Figure 43-21 The learning curve: perioperative complications during percutaneous dilational tracheostomy. (From Petros S: Percutaneous tracheostomy. Crit Care 3:R5-R10, 1999.)

death, and the early complication rate was in the range of 5%. No late complications such as tracheal stenosis were observed in any of the fiberoptically investigated patients during a follow-up of up to 180 days.

Escarment and coauthors[66] evaluated the safety and complication rates of the Griggs technique in a consecutive series of 162 ICU patients. Early intraoperative complications occurred in 17% and were minor technical difficulties without morbidity (e.g., inadvertent extubation, difficult cannulation, hemorrhage). Average cannulation duration was 25 days, and stoma closure was effective in all patients after about 3 to 4 days. Follow-up was available for 81 patients, and endoscopic evaluation of the airways 3 months after decannulation was performed in 73 patients. Sixty-two patients (85%) were normal, seven (10%) had granulation tissue at the stoma site, and four (5%) had tracheal stenosis with dyspnea in two patients (3%).

Norwood and coworkers[155] determined the incidence of tracheal stenosis and other late complications after PDT in 422 patients undergoing tracheostomy between 1992 and 1999 (Ciaglia approach). There were 340 survivors, and 100 of them were interviewed and further evaluated by fiberoptic laryngotracheoscopy and tracheal CT scan. CT scans identified mild stenosis (11% to 25%) in 21% of patients (all of them asymptomatic), moderate stenosis (26% to 50%) in 8%, and severe stenosis (>50%) in 2% of patients (Fig. 43-22).

Hotchkiss and McCaffrey[110] performed a cadaver study in order to evaluate the stoma and surrounding insertion site for laryngotracheal injury in six fixed cadaver specimens. Puncture and dilation were performed using the Blue Rhino technique, and no fiberoptic control of the

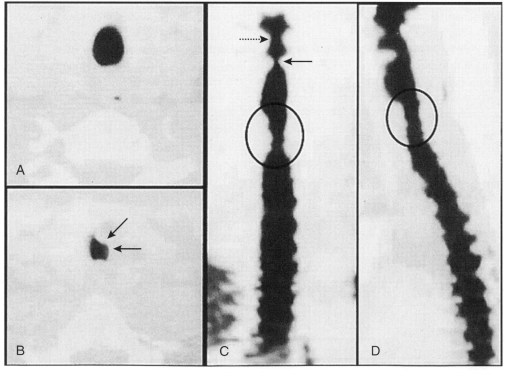

Figure 43-22 Patient with 45% tracheal stenosis. **A,** Axial view of normal trachea just above stoma level. **B,** Axial view of stoma level. *Arrows* denote areas of anterior and lateral stenosis. **C,** Coronal view with circled area of stenosis. *Dotted arrow* denotes false vocal cords. *Solid arrow* indicates true vocal cords. **D,** Sagittal view with circle denoting area of stenosis. (From Norwood S, Vallina VL, Short K, et al: Incidence of tracheal stenosis and other late complications after percutaneous tracheostomy. Ann Surg 232:233-241, 2000.)

procedure was used. Accurate prediction of the puncture level was achieved in only 50% of cadavers. Anterior tracheal internal wall mucosal injury was observed in all cadavers. Cartilaginous injury was severe in five of six specimens that sustained multiple comminuted injuries to two or more adjacent tracheal rings. The authors concluded that the injuries observed may significantly contribute to the development of tracheal stenosis. However, no data were presented concerning the potential impact of bronchoscopic guidance on the incidence of these complications.

Leonard and colleagues[134] assessed the late outcome following forceps tracheostomy in a prospective observational study of 49 patients. Tracheal stenosis was observed in one patient (2%), and other minor complications such as change in voice (49%) were observed frequently. However, whether this was due to preceding translaryngeal intubation or to the technique of tracheostomy could not be determined.

The main problem of PDT leading to tracheal stenosis is that tracheal rings are forced into a position that creates the opening for the cannula. This maneuver is capable of deforming the tracheal cartilage so that it protrudes into the airway (Fig. 43-23).

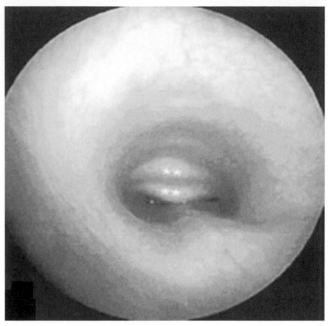

Figure 43-24 Endotracheal view revealing invagination of the cartilage rings. (From Koitschev A, Graumueller S, Zenner HP, et al: Tracheal stenosis and obliteration above the tracheostoma after percutaneous dilational tracheostomy. Crit Care Med 31:1574-1576, 2003.)

Koitschev and coauthors[124] reported on three patients with severe tracheal stenosis or obliteration after the PDT procedure (Figs. 43-24 and 43-25). In all patients, tracheal narrowing occurred above the level of the stoma. The authors speculated on a procedure-related mechanism (i.e., tracheal ring invagination and consecutive development of granulation tissue) rather than a mechanism based on the duration of cannulation (normally producing stenosis below the stoma).

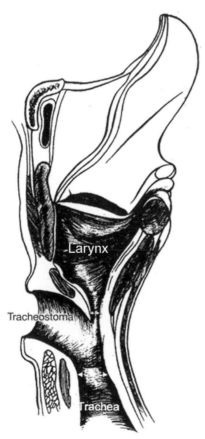

Figure 43-23 Suprastomal stenosis (anterior tracheal wall is invaginated into the lumen). (From Koitschev A, Graumueller S, Zenner HP, et al: Tracheal stenosis and obliteration above the tracheostoma after percutaneous dilational tracheostomy. Crit Care Med 31:1574-1576, 2003.)

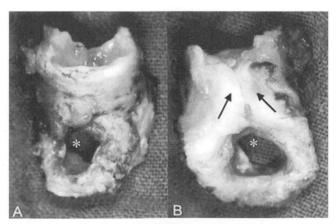

Figure 43-25 Anatomic specimen of a resected trachea. Front (**A**) and back (**B**) views. *Arrows* indicate scar tissue above the stoma. (From Koitschev A, Graumueller S, Zenner HP, et al: Tracheal stenosis and obliteration above the tracheostoma after percutaneous dilational tracheostomy. Crit Care Med 31: 1574-1576, 2003.)

In conclusion, PDT seems to be a safe, relatively simple, and quick procedure that can easily be performed at the bedside. The early complications and infection rate (~ 2%) may be lower and cosmetic results better than with surgical tracheostomy. However, several factors have to be adhered to strictly: PDT must be performed by an experienced operator at the correct puncture site, straight in the midline between two tracheal rings, and cannot be performed without fiberoptic guidance.[227] All the techniques proposed are characterized by special drawbacks or complications. For example, the Blue Rhino technique is associated with a relatively high incidence of tracheal ring fractures (in the range of 30%), and the PercuTwist approach seems to carry a higher risk of posterior tracheal wall injury. It is therefore difficult to compare PDT with the conventional surgical approach as they are completely different techniques with different success and complication rates. Much larger studies over a longer period of time studying clearly defined patients and techniques are necessary to answer the questions on the incidence of late complications after PDT. Currently, it is too early to draw a definitive conclusion about the question concerning the best percutaneous technique.

F. COMPARISON OF CONVENTIONAL VERSUS PERCUTANEOUS TRACHEOSTOMY

Comparing PDT with historical data on complications of surgical tracheostomy is erroneous and may give a biased picture. Moreover, varying definitions and different techniques used by the authors make interpretation of the data difficult. Complication rates for surgical tracheostomy vary widely in the literature between 6% and 66% with a mortality rate of 2%.[170] In order to reduce this incidence of complications and to perform a bedside procedure, the different percutaneous techniques have been proposed.

Several studies compared surgical and percutaneous access, and most of them reported lower complication rates with the individual percutaneous technique used (Table 43-10).[221,227] Dulguerov and colleagues[61] performed a meta-analysis comparing surgical and percutaneous access to the trachea. After a meticulous Medline

Table 43-10   **Complication and Mortality Rates for Surgical and Percutaneous Tracheostomy**

Study	Tracheostomy Type	n	Operative Mortality	Stenosis Rate[a]	Overall Complications
Dayal and el Masri	Open	50	0% (0/50)	0% (0/6)	38% (19/50)
Stauffer et al.[198]	Open	51	2% (1/51)	11% (2/18)[b]	63% (32/51)
Miller and Kapp	Open	84	1.2% (1/84)	8% (4/51)	45% (40/84)
Skaggs and Cogbill	Open	147	5% (7/147)	0% (0/57)	48% (71/147)
Schusterman et al.	Open	214	0.5% (1/214)	(>4% (9/?))	26% (56/214)
Mulder and Rubush	Open	428	5.1% (22/428)	8% (20/261)	45% (193/428)
Average complication rates for open tracheostomy			3.2% (31/974)	6.6% (26/393)	42% (411/974)
Hazard et al.	PDT	55	0% (0/55)	0% (0/14)	10.9% (6/55)
Marelli et al.[143]	PDT	61	1.6% (1/61)[c]	0% (0/13)	11.5% (7/61)
Winkler et al.[227]	PDT	71	0% (0/71)	0% (0/12)	5.5% (4/72)
Friedman and Mayer[85]	PDT	100	1.0% (1/100)[d]	3% (1/37)	19% (19/100)
McFarlane et al.	PDT	121	0% (0/121)	5% (4/77)	
Ciaglia and Graniero[44]	PDT	170	0% (0/170)	0% (0/30)	11% (19/170)
Present study	PDT	356	0.3% (1/356)	3.7% (8/214)	19% (69/356)
Average complication rates for PDT			0.3% (3/934)	3.3% (13/397)	15% (124/814)

[a]Percentage represents clinically symptomatic tracheal stenosis or radiographic evidence of >50% stenosis without clinical symptoms (total number of patients with stenosis/total number of patient with cannulas removed).
[b]Death caused by cardiac arrhythmia in one patient.
[c]One patient died because of tracheoinnominate artery fistula 6 days after PDT.
[d]Nine of 18 patients who had cannulas removed in this series had tracheal stenosis of >11% as determined by follow-up tomography studies i.e., 65% overall stenosis rate. One patient had obstructive symptoms caused by a 60% stenosis and died. One patient had >50% stenosis without symptoms.
From Hill BB, Zweng TN, Maley RH, et al: Percutaneous dilational tracheostomy. Report of 356 cases. J Trauma 41:238-244, 1996 with permission.

search, the authors grouped the study patients in the categories of surgical tracheostomy in the years 1960 to 1984 ($n = 17$ investigations in 4185 patients), surgical tracheostomy in 1985 to 1996 ($n = 21$ studies in 3512 patients), and PDT ($n = 27$ studies in 1817 patients). The highest perioperative and postoperative complication rates were observed in the "older" surgical studies (9% and 33%, respectively). Although perioperative complication rates were higher in the percutaneous studies (10% versus 3%), postoperative complications were lower than with the surgical approach (7% versus 10%). However, this meta-analysis was criticized because studies involving percutaneous tracheostomy without fiberoptic control were also included. Furthermore, it is difficult to perform a meta-analysis on this topic because the comparison involves not only the percutaneous approach versus surgical approaches. The percutaneous group is a mix of several different procedures and techniques used (i.e., with and without fiberoptic control, Ciaglia or Griggs technique). Ultimately, a major randomized controlled study is necessary to prove that percutaneous techniques represent a major advance not only with respect to the time needed but also with respect to perioperative morbidity and late postoperative complications, such as tracheal stenosis.[210]

Nevertheless, comparative studies have demonstrated that percutaneous techniques have certain advantages. Friedman and associates[84] published a relatively small randomized study comparing PDT ($n = 26$) with conventional surgical tracheostomy ($n = 27$). The authors concluded that PDT is superior to surgical tracheostomy logistically and can be quickly performed at the bedside. PDT is the faster procedure (8 versus 34 minutes, respectively) and involves fewer postprocedural complications (e.g., wound infection: 0% versus 15%). No late results were presented by the authors.

Melloni and coauthors[151] compared the late complications of surgical tracheostomy with PDT in a prospective randomized study involving 50 consecutive patients. Although no intraoperative complications were observed in the surgical group, two cases of minor hemorrhage occurred in the PDT group. Early postoperative complications were significantly higher in the surgical group (seven stoma infections), and only one case of minor bleeding was observed in the PDT group. No late tracheal pathology was observed in the conventional group, but two late tracheal complications (one segmental malacia and one stenosis at the stoma level) were observed in the PDT group.

Law and coworkers[131] examined 81 patients undergoing long-term ventilatory support after tracheostomy (mean duration, 4.9 months). All patients were examined fiberoptically prior to decannulation. Obstructive airway lesions were observed in 54 patients (67%). All tracheal lesions were anatomically located proximal to the stoma. No cuff lesions were observed. The two most commonly observed lesions were tracheal granuloma (60%) and tracheomalacia (29%). Less frequently observed lesions were tracheostenosis (14%) and vocal cord and laryngeal dysfunction (8%). As a result of the high frequency of tracheal abnormalities, the authors recommended that all decannulation candidates should undergo anatomic examination of the airways.

Despite the low perioperative complication rate and other perceived benefits of PDT (short duration, bedside procedure), long-term follow-up of both symptomatic and asymptomatic patients indicates a significant incidence of tracheal stenosis. Rates of moderate to severe stenosis range from 6% to 26%.[210,221]

Cost evaluations for PDT and surgical tracheostomy are difficult to perform because of varying reimbursement systems and hospital structures; most available studies show that PDT is considerably cheaper than the surgical route.[84,104,162,180] Fewer personnel and no OR time are required, and the patient does not need to be moved.

In conclusion, all studies clearly show that adequate training and teaching are the major factors reducing complications with PCT. Until those issues are settled, PDT can be recommended with some exceptions. Especially in patients presenting with a short, thick neck, goiter, or difficult airways,[207] PDT should be performed only by an experienced physician, with a physician prepared for a surgical tracheostomy present.[209] The most important factor is fiberoptic control of the entire procedure because erroneous punctures and direct trauma to the esophagus or tracheal wall are prevented or recognized early.[14]

VIII. ROUTINE AIRWAY CARE IN THE MECHANICALLY VENTILATED PATIENT

Tracheal suctioning is an intervention to remove accumulated mucus from ET, trachea, and lower airways in patients requiring intubation for mechanical ventilation. Intubation, ventilation, and especially sedation impair the transport of mucus in the airways. Furthermore, coughing is impaired because of the interference of the ET with glottic closure.

Tracheal suctioning, an essential aspect of airway management, is a potentially life-threatening procedure that can lead to hypoxia, cardiac dysrhythmias, trauma, and atelectasis.[49,50] Traditionally, tracheal suctioning is performed by disconnecting the patient from the respirator, applying manual hyperinflation ("bagging"), inserting a suctioning catheter into the patient's airways, and applying negative pressure to remove secretions.[135] Saline may be instilled to dilute secretions and facilitate suctioning. Tracheal suctioning is supposed to be a beneficial procedure, although only a few studies have been performed on this topic. Several investigations reported undesired adverse effects.[1,200] For example, Stone and colleagues[200] reported cardiac dysrhythmias in patients after cardiac surgery and Adlkofer and Powaser[1] reported a decrease in oxygen tension of 20 mm Hg.

Therefore, tracheal suctioning should be performed on an on-demand basis, and the need for suctioning as well as effectiveness of the procedure must be determined by chest auscultation.[49] Suctioning on a routine schedule (e.g., every 4 to 6 hours) should be abandoned. Before the procedure, the patients should be properly informed. Explanations should be given because tracheal suctioning is a frightening and unpleasant experience (for many patients tracheal suctioning is the only remembrance of their ICU stay).

In order to prevent hypoxemia and consequent complications, preoxygenation at an FIO_2 of 1 should be started 1 minute before suctioning. Suctioning is an invasive procedure, and sterile gloves should be worn during the process. Catheter selection is also an important issue; the external diameter of the suction catheter should not exceed one half of the ET ID.[229] Larger catheters are traumatic, and smaller catheters are often insufficient at removing viscous secretions. There has been much confusion and discussion about the instillation of normal saline for facilitating tracheal suctioning. Normal saline instillation (NSI) is purported to be beneficial in removing thick and tenacious secretions for patients receiving mechanical ventilation. Currently, no data confirming beneficial effects of saline irrigation exist. To the contrary, an increasing amount of literature focuses on harmful effects of routine tracheal saline instillation.[25,122] Despite the use of NSI for a period of 25 years, many questions remain to be answered, such as the volume of saline instilled. Volumes instilled in adult patients vary between 2 and 5 mL, 5 and 10 mL, and up to 40 mL.[25] Volume of saline used has never been evaluated in controlled research studies. Also, what happens to unretrieved saline? Hanley and coworkers[98] performed a very small study involving two humans and instilled saline tagged with technetium 99m. Only 20% of the saline instilled was retrieved by suctioning, and they concluded that NSI at the proximal end of the ET only sprinkles the trachea. It may be suggested that part of the remaining saline is "blown out" during brisk coughing, and several authors suggested that instillation at the distal end of the ET might minimize this risk.

Furthermore, NSI has a major impact on physiologic parameters. Gray and others[91] assessed minute volume and forced vital capacity in 15 patients suctioned with or without NSI. No statistically significant differences were found between the groups. However, Kinloch[122] showed that oxygenation status (i.e., mixed venous oxygen saturation) of patients suctioned with the use of 5 mL of normal saline was poorer than that of patients suctioned without saline instillation. In a systematic review, Blackwood concluded that after 25 years of inconsistent practice in trying to remove tenacious secretions, it is time to focus on techniques to prevent thick and tenacious secretions.[25]

Suctioning should be performed with continuous negative pressure at 80 to 150 mm Hg applied only during catheter withdrawal.[50,90] Higher pressures have been shown to cause hypoxemia, atelectasis, or catheter adherence to the tracheal mucosa. Duration of a single suctioning pass should not exceed 10 to 15 seconds, and the number of suctioning passes should not exceed three during one suctioning episode.[5] To minimize the risk of postsuctioning desaturation, the patients should be reconnected to the oxygen supply immediately (maximum 10 seconds) after suctioning. In order to evaluate the effectiveness of suctioning, it is recommended that a comprehensive respiratory assessment take place after suctioning.[90]

"Minimally invasive" endotracheal suctioning has been recommended as an alternative approach. Minimally invasive means that the suction catheter never reaches the trachea, no saline is instilled, no bagging is performed, and suctioning is performed only when clinically indicated. Leur and associates[135] performed a randomized controlled study of 383 ICU patients comparing routine suctioning ($n = 197$) with the proposed minimally invasive approach ($n = 186$). No differences were found in duration of intubation, ICU stay, pulmonary infection, and mortality. However, suctioning-related adverse effects such as desaturation, blood pressure elevation, and blood on mucus were significantly less in the minimally invasive group. In a further study, the same group[208] evaluated patients' recollection of the suctioning procedure. A total of 208 patients were interviewed within 3 days after ICU discharge, and the level of discomfort was quantified using a visual analog scale. A significantly lower prevalence of recollection of airway suctioning was found in the patients treated by the minimally invasive approach. Further studies are needed to prove those findings, but reconsidering the individual suctioning techniques seems to be valuable.

Furthermore, closed suctioning systems have been recommended. A reduced incidence of VAP was reported.[45] "Classical" open suctioning is routinely performed by disconnecting the patient from the ventilator and introducing a regular suctioning catheter through the ET into the upper airways.[141] Alternatively, suctioning can be accomplished with a closed suctioning system attached between the ET and ventilatory tubing, allowing introduction of the suctioning catheter into the airways without disconnecting the patient from the ventilator.[16,39] Closed suctioning has some advantages compared with the conventional open suctioning technique. It can be helpful in limiting environmental, personnel, and patients' contamination and in preventing the loss of lung volume and the alveolar derecruitment associated with standard suctioning in severely hypoxemic patients. However, the impact of closed suctioning on the incidence of VAP and its cost-effectiveness remain to be determined.[141]

An interesting approach using a visualized ET has been suggested by Frass and colleagues.[80] The so-called visualized endotracheal tube (VETT system; Pulmonx, Palo Alto, CA) corresponds to a standard ET with incorporated fiberoptic fibers, continuously displaying a view of the patient's trachea and carina. The device worked perfectly until extubation (mean duration of 137 hours), although the lens had to be rinsed approximately four times a day. On-line monitoring of ET position and amount of retained secretions is possible. Furthermore, targeted suctioning of right or left lung can be performed under visual control. Frass and colleagues[80] assumed that the frequency of suctioning maneuvers can be reduced by using this new technique. However, the VETT system is currently commercially not available.

IX. DIFFICULT EXTUBATION IN CRITICALLY ILL PATIENTS

Extubation of the trachea of ICU patients represents a special challenge to the attending physician. Every routine extubation (difficult airway absent) can be associated with severe complications including hemodynamic decompensation and cardiac failure, breath holding, laryngospasm, aspiration, or increased intracranial pressure. Several factors result in a relatively high incidence of difficult extubations in intensive care: special surgical procedures (i.e., head and neck surgery), swelling of laryngeal or pharyngeal tissues, limited airway access (i.e., maxillomandibular fixation, cervical immobilization, tracheal resection), and long-term ventilatory support with ventilatory muscle fatigue.

In patients with preexisting difficult airways, one should be aware that emergent reintubation is an entirely different situation. Extubation of those patients may result in airway catastrophes.

However, few articles focused on this integral part of difficult airway management, and there is insufficient literature to permit critical evaluation of extubation strategies. The ASA task force on difficult airway management recommended that each anesthesiologist and critical care physician has a preformulated strategy for extubation of patients with difficult airways.[177]

The preformulated strategy should include:

1. Evaluation for general clinical factors that may produce an adverse impact on postextubation ventilation
2. Formulation of an airway management plan that can be implemented if the patient is not able to maintain adequate ventilation after extubation
3. Consideration of short-term use of a guide that can serve as a guide for reintubation

By decreasing upper airway tract diameter, laryngeal edema increases airway resistance and manifests itself as stridor and respiratory distress. Reintubation may be required if the patient is unable to sustain the increased respiratory work. To discern patients with and without significant laryngeal edema, the cuff leak test has been described by De Bast and coauthors.[51] Leak was evaluated immediately prior to extubation in 76 patients and was expressed as the difference between expired tidal volume (assisted control mode) measured with the ET cuff inflated and deflated. The authors concluded that a cuff leak of more than 15.5% can be used as a screening test to limit the risk of reintubation in laryngeal edema.

Reintubation under emergency conditions in the ICU bed is an entirely different situation from the controlled circumstances in the OR. In these cases, the use of so-called endotracheal tube exchangers (e.g., Cook Critical Care)

may be indicated. This type of device is lubricated and then inserted through the lumen of the ET into the trachea before the ET is removed. Oxygen may be delivered continuously through the hollow lumen of an ET exchanger using the by-packed adapter. If severe respiratory insufficiency occurs, another ET may be slid over this guiding bar into the trachea (blindly or under direct laryngoscopy). Alternatively, extubation may be performed with the help of a fiberoptic bronchoscope left inside the trachea (in addition to a bite block). This procedure enables directed suctioning of tracheal secretions, especially during the sensible postextubation phase. Fiberoptically controlled reintubation is possible at any time point (this approach may be advantageous in ENT and maxillofacial patients).

Not only the extubation procedure per se but also the entire postextubation period (approximately 48 hours) is of utmost importance for patients' outcome. It is well known that the receptors associated with swallowing are altered by the presence of an ET.[52] The reason for swallowing dysfunction after extubation of the trachea seems to be a combination of "muscle freezing" because of nonuse and loss of proprioception related to superficial mucosal lesions. Leder and associates[133] investigated the incidence of aspiration following extubation in 20 consecutive trauma patients. All subjects underwent a bedside transnasal fiberoptic endoscopic evaluation of swallowing 24 ± 2 hours after extubation to determine objectively aspiration status. Aspiration was identified in 9 of 20 (45%) subjects, and 4 of these 9 (44%) were silent aspirators. The authors concluded that trauma patients have an increased risk for aspiration after orotracheal intubation and prolonged mechanical ventilation.

Moreover, it was suggested that silent aspiration may be an occult cause of postextubation pneumonia. This high incidence of aspirations could not be verified by a consecutive prospective study of the same group. Barquist and colleagues[15] found an aspiration rate of only 10% and delayed enteral nutrition in those patients. However, no beneficial effect of fiberoptic postextubation monitoring was observed in this small prospective study involving 70 patients.

Another important factor is the impact of accidental extubation with or without reintubation on patients' pneumonia risk and patients' outcome. Unplanned extubation (UEX) accounts for about 10% of extubations and requires reintubation in 60% of cases.[26,42] Boulain[26] performed a prospective multicenter study trial on predisposing factors and complications of UEX in more than 400 patients. An incidence of UEX of 10.8% was observed, which means 1.6 UEX per 100 ventilated days. By use of multivariate analysis, four factors contributing to UEX were determined: chronic respiratory failure, ET fixation with only thin adhesive tape, orotracheal intubation, and lack of intravenous sedation. The rates of mortality, laryngeal complications, and length of mechanical ventilation were similar in UEX and non-UEX patients. Patients were more often reintubated after UEX (every 2nd compared with every tenth non-UEX patient). It was hypothesized that easy measures such as strong fixation of the ET, adequate sedation, and particular attention to orally intubated patients should minimize the incidence of UEX.

Reintubation has been identified as a major risk factor for nosocomial pneumonia.[205] By means of a case-control study, Epstein and colleagues[65] found that either form of UEX (i.e., successfully tolerated or failed UEX during weaning or ventilatory support) was associated with a longer ICU stay but did not increase patients' mortality. De Lassence and coworkers[53] prospectively evaluated a 2-year database including 750 mechanically ventilated patients from six ICUs. They showed that accidental extubation but not self-extubation or reintubation after weaning increased the risk of nosocomial pneumonia. It is of utmost importance to recognize that the difficult airway has not been successfully managed until the trachea is safely extubated and reintubation is prevented for at least 48 hours.

X. CONCLUSIONS

Critical care physicians manage the airway with great efficacy for the vast majority of patients. However, in a certain percentage of patients (up to 10%) difficulties in laryngoscopy occur, caused by unfavorable anatomy of face, airway, or cervical spine. Failed intubation may potentially result in life-threatening hypoxia and has to be prevented by strict adherence to recommendations (see the ASA difficult airway algorithm). The main factors for successful emergency airway management are to be prepared, have a plan B ready, and secure the airway awake when trouble is suspected. Awake airway management using the fiberoptic scope is the most secure technique, leaving the patient's protective reflexes intact, and exerts only minor effects on the cardiocirculatory system.

Recognizing the difficult airway situation only after anesthesia induction may result in potentially dangerous cannot-intubate, cannnot-ventilate or catastrophic cannot-intubate, cannot-ventilate situations. Especially the last situation requires immediate intervention using either LMA, Combitube, or TTJV or performing a surgical airway (mainly emergency cricothyrotomy). All those techniques must be practiced in routine cases so that they can be performed successfully in emergency situations.

Concerning airway management for long-term ventilatory support, tracheostomy is currently receiving attention because of the introduction of percutaneous dilational tracheostomy into clinical routine. Long-term translaryngeal intubation may result in severe damage to the laryngeal apparatus and trachea (i.e., granuloma formation, stenosis). In patients requiring long-term ventilatory support, we recommend tracheostomy between the first and second week of using the ventilator in order to reduce the incidence of severe long-term damage to the laryngeal structures. Which technique of tracheostomy is used depends upon personal preferences and experience. However, one should be aware that both conventional surgical tracheostomy and PDT require training and knowledge and are characterized by distinct learning curves. PDT should be performed only by experienced operators and under continuous fiberoptic control (best using a television screen enabling the operator to observe the entire procedure). Complications of long-term airway management are common and associated with discernible morbidity.

Therefore, from the decision to intubate until extubation of the patient, we should always keep in mind: *first, do no harm.*

REFERENCES

1. Adlkofer RM, Powaser MM: The effect of endotracheal suctioning on arterial blood gases in patients after cardiac surgery. Heart Lung 7:1011-1014, 1978.
2. Agro F, Frass M, Benumof JL, Krafft P: Current status of the Combitube: A review of the literature. J Clin Anesth 14:307-314, 2002.
3. Agro F, Frass M, Benumof JL, et al: The esophageal tracheal Combitube as a non-invasive alternative to endotracheal intubation. Minerva Anestesiol 67:863-874, 2001.
4. Agro F, Hung OR, Cataldo R, et al: Lightwand intubation using the Trachlight: A brief review of current knowledge. Can J Anaesth 48:592-599, 2001.
5. Allen D: Making sense of suctioning. Nurs Times 84: 46-47, 1988.
6. Ambesh SP, Pandey CK, Srivastava S, et al: Percutaneous tracheostomy with single dilatation technique: A prospective, randomized comparison of Ciaglia blue rhino versus Griggs' guidewire dilating forceps. Anesth Analg 95: 1739-1745, 2002.
7. Ambesh SP, Sinha PK, Tripathi M, Matreja P: Laryngeal mask airway vs endotracheal tube to facilitate bedside percutaneous tracheostomy in critically ill patients: A prospective comparative study. J Postgrad Med 48: 11-15, 2002.
8. Andersen KH, Hald A: Assessing the position of the tracheal tube. The reliability of different methods. Anaesthesia 44:984-985, 1989.
9. Antonelli M, Conti G, Pelosi P, et al: New treatment of acute hypoxemic respiratory failure: Noninvasive pressure support ventilation delivered by helmet— A pilot controlled trial. Crit Care Med 30:602-608, 2002.
10. Antonelli M, Pennisi MA, Conti G, et al: Fiberoptic bronchoscopy during noninvasive positive pressure ventilation delivered by helmet. Intensive Care Med 29: 126-129, 2003.
11. Astrachan DI, Kirchner JC, Goodwin WJ Jr: Prolonged intubation vs tracheostomy: Complications, practical and

psychological considerations. Laryngoscope 98:1165-1169, 1988.

12. Bach A, Boehrer H, Schmidt H, Geiss HK: Nosocomial sinusitis in ventilated patients: Nasotracheal versus orotracheal intubation. Anaesthesia 47:335-339, 1992.

13. Bair AE, Filbin MR, Kulkarni RG, Walls RM: The failed intubation attempt in the emergency department: Analysis of prevalence, rescue techniques, and personnel. J Emerg Med 23:131-140, 2002.

14. Barba CA, Angood PB, Kauder DR, et al: Bronchoscopic guidance makes percutaneous tracheostomy a safe, cost-effective and easy-to-teach procedure. Surgery 118:879-883, 1995.

15. Barquist E, Brown M, Cohn S, et al: Postextubation fiberoptic endoscopic evaluation of swallowing after prolonged endotracheal intubation: A randomized, prospective trial. Crit Care Med 29:1710-1713, 2001.

16. Baun MM, Stone KS, Rogge JA: Endotracheal suctioning: Open versus closed with and without positive end-expiratory pressure. Crit Care Nurs Q 25:13-26, 2002.

17. Beiderlinden M, Walz MK, Sander A, et al: Complications of bronchoscopically guided percutaneous dilational tracheostomy: Beyond the learning curve. Intensive Care Med 28:59-62, 2002.

18. Bellhouse CP, Dore C: Criteria for estimating likelihood of difficulty of endotracheal intubation with the Macintosh laryngoscope. Anaesth Intensive Care 16:329-337, 1988.

19. Benumof JL: Laryngeal mask airway and the ASA difficult airway algorithm. Anesthesiology 84:686-699, 1996.

20. Benumof JL: Management of the difficult adult airway. With special emphasis on awake tracheal intubation. Anesthesiology 75:1087-1110, 1991.

21. Benumof JL, Dagg R, Benumof R: Critical hemoglobin desaturation will occur before return to an unparalyzed state following 1mg/kg intravenous succinylcholine. Anesthesiology 87:979-982, 1997.

22. Benumof JL, Scheller MS: The importance of transtracheal jet ventilation in the management of the difficult airway. Anesthesiology 71:769-778, 1989.

23. Birmingham PK, Cheney FW, Ward RJ: Esophageal intubation: A review of detection techniques. Anesth Analg 65:886-891, 1986.

24. Bishop MJ, Hibbard AJ, Fink BR, et al: Laryngeal injury in a dog model of prolonged endotracheal intubation. Anesthesiology 62:770-773, 1985.

25. Blackwood B: Normal saline instillation with endotracheal suctioning: Primum non nocere (first do no harm). J Adv Nurs 29:928-934, 1999.

26. Boulain T: Unplanned extubations in the adult intensive care unit: A prospective multicenter study. Association des Reanimateurs du Centre-Ouest. Am J Respir Crit Care Med 157:1131-1137, 1998.

27. Bozeman WP, Hexter D, Liang HK, Kelen GD: Esophageal detector device versus detection of end-tidal carbon dioxide level in emergency intubation. Ann Emerg Med 27:595-599, 1996.

28. Brain AI: Three cases of difficult intubation overcome by the laryngeal mask airway. Anaesthesia 40:353-355, 1985.

29. Brain AIJ: The laryngeal mask: A new concept in airway management. Br J Anaesth 55:801, 1983.

30. Branthwaite MA: An unexpected complication of the intubating laryngeal mask. Anaesthesia 54:166-167, 1999.

31. Brimacombe JR, Brain AIJ, Berry AM: The Laryngeal Mask Airway. A Review and Practical Guide. Philadelphia, WB Saunders, 1997.

32. Byhahn C, Lischke V, Westphal K: Percutaneous tracheostomy in intensive care. Practicability and early complications of the translaryngeal Fantoni technique. Anaesthesist 48:310-316, 1999.

33. Byhahn C, Westphal K, Meininger D, et al: Single-dilator percutaneous tracheostomy: A comparison of PercuTwist and Ciaglia Blue Rhino techniques. Intensive Care Med 28:1262-1266, 2002.

34. Byhahn C, Wilke HJ, Halbig S, et al: Percutaneous tracheostomy: Ciaglia blue rhino versus the basic Ciaglia technique of percutaneous dilational tracheostomy. Anesth Analg 91:882-886, 2000.

35. Cantais E, Kaiser E, Le-Goff Y, Palmier B: Percutaneous tracheostomy: Prospective comparison of the translaryngeal technique versus the forceps-dilational technique in 100 critically ill adults. Crit Care Med 30:815-819, 2002.

36. Carlucci A, Delmastro M, Rubini F, et al: Changes in the practice of non-invasive ventilation in treating COPD patients over 8 years. Intensive Care Med 29:419-425, 2003.

37. Castella X, Gilabert J, Perez C: Arytenoid dislocation after tracheal intubation: An unusual cause of acute respiratory failure? Anesthesiology 74:613-615, 1991.

38. Cavaliere F, Masieri S, Conti G, et al: Effects of non-invasive ventilation on middle ear function in healthy volunteers. Intensive Care Med 29:611-614, 2003.

39. Cereda M, Villa F, Colombo E, et al: Closed system endotracheal suctioning maintains lung volume during volume-controlled mechanical ventilation. Intensive Care Med 27:648-654, 2001.

40. Chan TC, Vilke GM, Bramwell KJ, et al: Comparison of wire-guided cricothyrotomy versus standard surgical cricothyrotomy technique. J Emerg Med 17:957-962, 1999.

41. Cheney FW: Changing trends in anesthesia-related death and permanent brain damage. ASA Newslett 66:6-8, 2002.

42. Christie JM, Dethlefsen M, Cane RD: Unplanned endotracheal extubation in the intensive care unit. J Clin Anesth 8:289-293, 1996.

43. Ciaglia P, Firsching R, Syniec C: Elective percutaneous dilatational tracheostomy. A new simple bedside procedure; preliminary report. Chest 87:715-719, 1985.

44. Ciaglia P, Graniero KD: Percutaneous dilatational tracheostomy. Results and long-term follow-up. Chest 101:464-467, 1992,

45. Combes P, Fauvage B, Oleyer C: Nosocomial pneumonia in mechanically ventilated patients, a prospective randomised evaluation of the Stericath closed suctioning system. Intensive Care Med 26:878-882, 2000.

46. Cormack RS, Lehane J: Difficult tracheal intubation in obstetrics. Anaesthesia 39:1105-1111, 1984.

47. Davidson TM, Magit AE: Surgical airway. In Benumof JL (ed): Airway Management. Principles and Practice. St. Louis, Mosby, 1996, pp 513-530.

48. Davis DP, Bramwell KJ, Vilke GM, et al: Cricothyrotomy technique: Standard versus the Rapid Four-Step Technique. J Emerg Med 17:17-21, 1999.

49. Day T: Tracheal suctioning: When, why and how. Nurs Times 96:13-15, 2000.

50. Day T, Farnell S, Haynes S, et al: Tracheal suctioning: An exploration of nurses' knowledge and competence in acute and high dependency ward areas. J Adv Nurs 39:35-45, 2002.

51. De Bast Y, De Backer D, Moraine JJ, et al: The cuff leak test to predict failure of tracheal extubation for laryngeal edema. Intensive Care Med 28:1267-1272, 2002.

52. de Larminat V, Montravers P, Dureuil B, Desmonts JM: Alteration in swallowing reflex after extubation in intensive care unit patients. Crit Care Med 23:486-490, 1995.

53. de Lassence A, Alberti C, Azoulay E, et al: Impact of unplanned extubation and reintubation after weaning on nosocomial pneumonia risk in the intensive care unit: A prospective multicenter study. Anesthesiology 97: 148-156, 2002.

54. Dekkers F: Exercitationes Practicae. Leiden, Luchtmans & Boutesteyn, Lugdunum Batavorum, 1695, pp 238-245.

55. Denk DM, Swoboda H, Neuwirth-Riedl K, Klepetko W: Glottic bridge synechia following intubation. Otorhinolaryngol Nova 3:41-44, 1993.

56. Depoix JP, Malbezin S, Videcoq M, et al: Oral intubation v. nasal intubation in adult cardiac surgery. Br J Anaesth 59:167-169, 1987.

57. Devitt JH, Wenstone R, Noel AG, O'Donell MP: The laryngeal mask airway and positive-pressure ventilation. Anesthesiology 80:550-555, 1994.

58. Dimitriou V, Voyagis GS, Brimacombe JR: Flexible light-wand-guided tracheal intubation with the intubating laryngeal mask Fastrach in adults after unpredicted failed laryngoscope-guided tracheal intubation. Anesthesiology 96:296-299, 2002.

59. Donaldson AB, Meyer-Witting M, Roux A: Awake fibre-optic intubation under remifentanil and propofol target-controlled infusion. Anaesth Intensive Care 30:93-95, 2002.

60. Dosemeci L, Yilmaz M, Gurpinar F, Ramazanoglu A: The use of the laryngeal mask airway as an alternative to the endotracheal tube during percutaneous dilatational tracheostomy. Intensive Care Med 28:63-67, 2002.

61. Dulguerov P, Gysin C, Perneger TV, Chevrolet JC: Percutaneous or surgical tracheostomy: A meta-analysis. Crit Care Med 27:1617-1625, 1999.

62. Dunham CM, LaMonica C: Prolonged tracheal intubation in the trauma patient. J Trauma 24:120-124, 1984.

63. Eisenburger P, Laczika K, List M, et al: Comparison of conventional surgical versus Seldinger technique emergency performed by inexperienced clinicians. Anesthesiology 92:687-690, 2000.

64. El-Ganzouri AR: Management of the patient with difficult airway: 25 years' experience. Semin Anesth Periop Med Pain 20:134-143, 2001.

65. Epstein SK, Nevins ML, Chung J: Effect of unplanned extubation on outcome of mechanical ventilation. Am J Respir Crit Care Med 161:1912-1916, 2000.

66. Escarment J, Suppini A, Sallaberry M, et al: Percutaneous tracheostomy by forceps dilation: Report of 162 cases. Anaesthesia 55:125-130, 2000.

67. Fabricius H: Opera Chirurgica. Boutesteniana. Leiden, Lugdunum Batavorum, 1617, pp 475-483.

68. Fan KH, Hung OR, Agro F: A comparative study of tracheal intubation using an intubating laryngeal mask (Fastrach) alone or together with a lightwand (Trachlight). J Clin Anesth 12:581-585, 2000.

69. Fantoni A, Ripamonti D: A non-derivative, non-surgical tracheostomy: The translaryngeal method. Intensive Care Med 23:386-392, 1997.

70. Fantoni A, Ripamonti D, Lesmo A, Zanoni CI: Translaryngeal tracheostomy. A new era? Minerva Anestesiol 62:313-325, 1996.

71. Farre R, Rotger M, Ferre M, et al: Automatic regulation of the cuff pressure in endotracheally-intubated patients. Eur Respir J 20:1010-1013, 2002.

72. Fassoulaki A, Pamouktsoglou P: Prolonged nasotracheal intubation and its association with inflammation of paranasal sinuses. Anesth Analg 69:50-52, 1989.

73. Fernandez L, Norwood S, Roettger R, et al: Bedside percutaneous tracheostomy with bronchoscopic guidance in critically ill patients. Arch Surg 131:129-132, 1996.

74. Ferson DZ, Rosenblatt WH, Johansen MJ, et al: Use of the intubating LMA-Fastrach in 254 patients with difficult-to-manage airways. Anesthesiology 95: 1175-1181, 2001.

75. Fikkers BG, Briede IS, Verwiel JM, Van Den Hoogen FJ: Percutaneous tracheostomy with the Blue Rhino trade mark technique: Presentation of 100 consecutive patients. Anaesthesia 57:1094-1097, 2002.

76. Fischler L, Erhart S, Kleger GR, Frutiger A: Prevalence of tracheostomy in ICU patients. A nation-wide survey in Switzerland. Intensive Care Med 26:1428-1433, 2000.

77. Forgacs P: The functional basis of pulmonary sounds. Chest 73:399-405, 1978.

78. Frass M, Agro F, Rich JM, Krafft P: Combitube: The all-in-one concept for securing the airway and adequate ventilation. Semin Anesth Periop Med Pain 20:201-212, 2001.

79. Frass M, Frenzer R, Zdrahal F, et al: The esophageal tracheal combitube: Preliminary results with a new airway for CPR. Ann Emerg Med 16:768-772, 1987.

80. Frass M, Kofler J, Thalhammer F, et al: Clinical evaluation of a new visualized endotracheal tube (VETT). Anesthesiology 87:1262-1263, 1997.

81. Frass M, Staudinger T, Losert H, Krafft P: Airway management during cardiopulmonary resuscitation—A comparative study of bag-valve-mask, laryngeal mask airway and Combitube in a bench model. Resuscitation 43:80-81, 1999.

82. Frerk CM: Predicting difficult intubation. Anaesthesia 46:1005-1008, 1991.

83. Fridrich P, Frass M, Krenn CG, et al: The UpsherScope in routine and difficult airway management: A randomized, controlled clinical trial. Anesth Analg 85:1377-1381, 1997.

84. Friedman Y, Fildes J, Mizock B, et al: Comparison of percutaneous and surgical tracheostomies. Chest 110:480-485, 1996.

85. Friedman Y, Mayer AD: Bedside percutaneous tracheostomy in critically ill patients. Chest 104:532-535, 1993.

86. Frink EJ, Pattison BD: Posterior arytenoid dislocation following uneventful endotracheal intubation and anesthesia. Anesthesiology 70:358-360, 1989.

87. Frova G, Quintel M: A new simple method for percutaneous tracheostomy: Controlled rotating dilation. A preliminary report. Intensive Care Med 28:299-303, 2002.

88. Gaitini LA, Vaida SJ, Mostafa S, et al: The Combitube in elective surgery: A report of 200 cases. Anesthesiology 94:79-82, 2001.

89. Gaitini LA, Vaida SJ, Somri M, et al: Fiberoptic-guided airway exchange of the esophageal-tracheal Combitube in spontaneously breathing versus mechanically ventilated patients. Anesth Analg 88:193-196, 1999.

90. Glass CA, Grap MJ: Ten tips for safer suctioning. Am J Nurs 95:51-53, 1995.

91. Gray JE, MacIntyre NR, Kronenberger WG: The effects of bolus normal-saline instillation in conjunction with endotracheal suctioning. Respir Care 35:758-790, 1990.

92. Gregoretti C, Confalonieri M, Navalesi P, et al: Evaluation of patient skin breakdown and comfort with a new face mask for non-invasive ventilation: A multicenter study. Intensive Care Med 28:278-284, 2002.

93. Griggs WM, Worthley LI, Gilligan JE, et al: A simple percutaneous tracheostomy technique. Surg Gynecol Obstet 170:543-545, 1990.

94. Grindlinger GA, Niehoff J, Hughes SL, et al: Acute paranasal sinusitis related to nasotracheal intubation of head-injured patients. Crit Care Med 15:214-217, 1987.

95. Grmec S: Comparison of three different methods to confirm tracheal tube placement in emergency intubation. Intensive Care Med 28:701-704, 2002.

96. Grmec S, Klemen P: Does the end-tidal carbon dioxide (Et CO$_2$) concentration have prognostic value during out-of-hospital cardiac arrest? Eur J Emerg Med 8: 263-269, 2001.

97. Grundling M, Kuhn SO, Riedel T, et al: Application of the laryngeal mask for elective percutaneous dilatation tracheostomy. Anaesthesiol Reanim 23:32-36, 1998.

98. Hanley MV, Rudd T, Butler J: What happens to endotracheal instillations? Am Rev Respir Dis (Suppl 124): 117, 1978.

99. Hartmann T, Krenn CG, Zoeggeler A, et al: The oesophageal-tracheal Combitube small adult. Anaesthesia 55:670-675, 2000.

100. Hartmann T, Zoeggeler A, Krenn CG, et al: The esophageal-tracheal Combitube: An appropriate alternative airway for laparoscopic surgery? Anaesthesia 55:670-675, 2000.

101. Heffner JE, Casey K, Hoffman C: Care of the mechanically ventilated patient with a tracheostomy. In Tobin MJ (ed): Principles and Practice of Mechanical Ventilation. New York, McGraw-Hill, 1994, pp 749-774.

102. Heister L: Institutiones Chirurgicae. Amstekaedam, Janssonis-Waesberge, 1750, pp 674-678.

103. Heyland DK, Cook DJ, Dodek PM: Prevention of ventilator-associated pneumonia: Current practice in Canadian intensive care units. J Crit Care 17:161-167, 2002.

104. Hill BB, Zweng TN, Maley RH, et al: Percutaneous dilational tracheostomy. Report of 356 cases. J Trauma 41:238-244, 1996.

105. Hinerman R, Alvarez F, Keller CA: Outcome of bedside percutaneous tracheostomy with bronchoscopic guidance. Intensive Care Med 26:1850-1856, 2000.

106. Hinterer I, Wurmitzer H, Wanzl O, et al: Use of a pediatric Combitube. Acta Anaesthesiol Scand 40 (Suppl 109):144, 1996.

107. Ho AM, Dion PW, Karmakar MK, et al: Use of heliox in critical upper airway obstruction. Physical and physiologic considerations in choosing the optimal helium:oxygen mix. Resuscitation 52:297-300, 2002.

108. Ho AM, Lee A, Karmakar MK, et al: Heliox vs air-oxygen mixtures for the treatment of patients with acute asthma: A systematic overview. Chest 123: 882-890, 2003.

109. Hoerauf KH, Hartmann T, Acimovic S, et al: Waste gas exposure to sevoflurane and nitrous oxide during anaesthesia using the oesophageal-tracheal Combitube small adult. Br J Anaesth 86:124-126, 2001.

110. Hotchkiss KS, McCaffrey JC: Laryngotracheal injury after percutaneous dilational tracheostomy in cadaver specimens. Laryngoscope 113:16-20, 2003.

111. Howells TH, Riethmuller RJ: Signs of endotracheal intubation. Anaesthesia 35:984-986, 1980.

112. Jackson C. Contact ulcer granuloma and other laryngeal complications of endotracheal anesthesia. Anesthesiology 14:425-436, 1953.

113. Jackson C: Tracheostomy. Laryngoscope 19:285-287, 1909.

114. Jacobs HB: Needle-catheter brings oxygen to the trachea. JAMA 222:1231-1233, 1972.

115. Joh S, Matsuura H, Kotani Y, et al: Change in tracheal blood flow during endotracheal intubation. Acta Anaesthesiol Scand 31:300-304, 1987.

116. Johnson KB, Swenson JD, Egan TD, et al: Midazolam and remifentanil by bolus injection for intensely stimulating procedures of brief duration: Experience with awake laryngoscopy. Anesth Analg 94:1241-1243, 2002.

117. Jones MW, Catling S, Evans E, et al: Hoarseness after tracheal intubation. Anaesthesia 47:213-216, 1992.

118. Kambic V, Radsel Z: Intubation lesion of the larynx. Br J Anaesth 50:587-590, 1978.

119. Kastanos N, Estopa MR, Marin PA, et al: Laryngotracheal injury due to endotracheal intubation: Incidence, evolution, and predisposing factors: A prospective long-term study. Crit Care Med 11:362-367, 1983.

120. Keenan SP: Noninvasive positive pressure ventilation in acute respiratory failure. JAMA 284:2376-2378, 2000.

121. Keenan SP, Sinuff T, Cook DJ, Hill NS: Which patients with acute exacerbation of chronic obstructive pulmonary disease benefit from noninvasive positive-pressure ventilation? A systematic review of the literature. Ann Intern Med 138:861-870, 2003.

122. Kinloch D: Instillation of normal saline during endotracheal suctioning: Effects on mixed venous oxygen saturation. Am J Crit Care 8:231-240, 1999.

123. Knapp S, Kofler J, Stoiser B, et al: The assessment of four different methods to verify tracheal tube placement in the critical care setting. Anesth Analg 88:766-770, 1999.

124. Koitschev A, Graumueller S, Zenner HP, et al: Tracheal stenosis and obliteration above the tracheostoma after percutaneous dilational tracheostomy. Crit Care Med 31:1574-1576, 2003.

125. Krafft P, Hartann T, Agro F, et al: Is it unethical to use the Combitube in elective patients? Anesthesiology 98:1022, 2003.

126. Krafft P, Krenn CG, Fitzgerald RD, et al: Clinical trial of a new device for fiberoptic orotracheal intubation (Augustine Scope). Anesth Analg 84:606-610, 1997.

127. Krafft P, Nikolic A, Frass M: Esophageal rupture associated with the use of the Combitube. Anesth Analg 87:1457, 1998.

128. Krafft P, Roeggla M, Fridrich P, et al: Bronchoscopy via a redesigned Combitube in the esophageal position. A clinical evaluation. Anesthesiology 86:1041-1045, 1997.

129. Langeron O, Masso E, Huraux C, et al: Prediction of difficult mask ventilation. Anesthesiology 92:1229-1236, 2000.

130. Langeron O, Semjen F, Bourgain JL, et al: Comparison of the intubating laryngeal mask airway with the fiberoptic intubation in anticipated difficult airway management. Anesthesiology 94:968-972, 2001.

131. Law JH, Barnhart K, Rowlett W, et al: Increased frequency of obstructive airway abnormalities with long-term tracheostomy. Chest 104:136-138, 1993.

132. Leach A, Alexander CA, Stone B: The laryngeal mask in cardiopulmonary resuscitation in a district general hospital: A preliminary communication. Resuscitation 25:245-248, 1993.

133. Leder SB, Cohn SM, Moller BA: Fiberoptic endoscopic documentation of the high incidence of aspiration following extubation in critically ill trauma patients. Dysphagia 13:208-212, 1998.

134. Leonard RC, Lewis RH, Singh B, van Heerden PV: Late outcome from percutaneous tracheostomy using the Portex kit. Chest 115:1070-1075, 1999.

135. Leur JP, Zwaveling JH, Loef BG, Van Der Schans CP: Endotracheal suctioning versus minimally invasive airway suctioning in intubated patients: A prospective randomised controlled trial. Intensive Care Med 29:426-432, 2003.

136. Levitan RM, Ochroch EA, Kush S, et al: Assessment of airway visualization: Validation of the percentage of glottic opening (POGO) scale. Acad Emerg Med 5:919-923, 1998.

137. Lim EK, Chia KS, Ng BK: Recurrent laryngeal nerve palsy following endotracheal intubation. Anaesth Intensive Care 15:342-345, 1987.

138. Locker GJ, Staudinger T, Knapp S, et al: Assessment of the proper depth of endotracheal tube placement with the Trachlight. J Clin Anesth 10:389-393, 1998.

139. Lyons BJ, Flynn CG: The laryngeal mask simplifies airway management during percutaneous dilational tracheostomy. Acta Anaesthesiol Scand 39:414-415, 1995.

140. MacQuarrie K, Hung OR, Law JA: Tracheal intubation using Bullard laryngoscope for patients with a simulated difficult airway. Can J Anaesth 46:760-765, 1999.

141. Maggiore SM, Iacobone E, Zito G, et al: Closed versus open suctioning techniques. Minerva Anestesiol 68:360-364, 2002.

142. Manara AR: Experience with percutaneous tracheostomy in intensive care: The technique of choice? Br J Oral Maxillofac Surg 32:155-160, 1994.

143. Marelli D, Paul A, Manolidis S, et al: Endoscopic guided percutaneous tracheostomy: Early results of a consecutive trial. J Trauma 30:433-435, 1990.

144. Massick DD, Powell DM, Price PD, et al: Quantification of the learning curve for percutaneous dilatational tracheostomy. Laryngoscope 110:222-228, 2000.

145. Mathews PJ, Mathews LM: Reducing the risks of ventilator-associated infections. Dimens Crit Care Nurs 19:17-21, 2000.

146. Maxeiner H: Soft-tissue damage in the larynx during emergency intubations. Anaesthesiol Intensivmed 29:42-47, 1988.

147. Maziak DE, Meade MO, Todd TR: The timing of tracheostomy: A systemic review. Chest 114:605-609, 1998.

148. McHardy FE, Chung F: Postoperative sore throat: Cause, prevention and treatment. Anaesthesia 54:444-453, 1999.

149. Meduri GU, Turner RE, Abou-Shala N, et al: Non invasive positive pressure ventilation via face mask. First line intervention in patients with acute hypercapnic and hypoxemic respiratory failure. Chest 109:179-193, 1996.

150. Melker JR, Florete OG: Percutaneous dilational and tracheostomy. In Benumof JL (ed): Airway Management. Principles and Practice. St. Louis, Mosby–Year Book, 1996, pp 484-512.

151. Melloni G, Muttini S, Gallioli G, et al: Surgical tracheostomy versus percutaneous dilatational tracheostomy. A prospective-randomized study with long-term follow-up. J Cardiovasc Surg 43:113-121, 2002.

152. Mercer MH: An assessment of protection of the airway from aspiration of oropharyngeal contents using the Combitube airway. Resuscitation 51:135-138, 2001.

153. Monnier PH, Ravussin P, Savary M, Freeman J: Percutaneous transtracheal ventilation for laser endoscopic treatment of laryngeal and subglottic lesions. Clin Otolaryngol 13:209-217, 1988.

154. Nordin U, Lindholm CE, Wolgast M: Blood flow in the rabbit tracheal mucosa under normal conditions and under the influence of tracheal intubation. Acta Anaesthesiol Scand 21:81-94, 1977.

155. Norwood S, Vallina VL, Short K, et al: Incidence of tracheal stenosis and other late complications after percutaneous tracheostomy. Ann Surg 232:233-241, 2000.

156. Nunn JF: Applied Respiratory Physiology, 3rd ed. Boston, Butterworth, 1987.

157. O'Neill JE, Giffin JP, Cottrell JE: Pharyngeal and esophageal perforation following endotracheal intubation. Anesthesiology 60:487-488, 1984.

158. Orebaugh SL: Difficult airway management in the emergency department. J Emerg Med 22:31-48, 2002.

159. Ovassapian A: Fiberoptic tracheal intubation in adults. In Ovassapian A (ed): Fiberoptic Endoscopy and the Difficult Airway. Philadelphia, Lippincott-Raven, 1996, pp 71-103.

160. Pandit JJ, Popat M: Difficult airway management in maxillofacial trauma. Semin Anesth Periop Med Pain 20:144-153, 2001.

161. Pernerstorfer T, Krafft P, Fitzgerald RD, et al: Stress response to tracheal intubation: Direct laryngoscopy compared with blind oral intubation. Anaesthesia 50:17-22, 1995.

162. Petros S: Percutaneous tracheostomy. Crit Care 3:R5-R10, 1999.

163. Petros S, Engelmann L: Percutaneous dilatational tracheostomy in a medical ICU. Intensive Care Med 23:630-634, 1997,

164. Plost GN, Campbell SC, Vagedes RT, Shon BY: The measurement of nonelastic work of breathing using a commercially available respiratory integrator. Biomed Instrum Technol 24:119-121, 1990.

165. Plummer AL, Gracey DR: Consensus conference on artificial airways in patients receiving mechanical ventilation. Chest 96:178-180, 1989.

166. Pollard BJ, Junius F: Accidental intubation of the oesophagus. Anaesth Intensive Care 8:183-186, 1980.

167. Pothmann W, Reissmann H, Bartling K, Nierhaus A: Decrease of nosocomial pneumonia by automatical cuff-pressure regulation. Intensive Care Med 23 (Suppl 1): S150, 1997.

168. Powner DJ: Airway considerations for professional singers—A survey of expert opinion. Voice 16:488-494, 2002.

169. Puchner W, Egger P, Puhringer F, et al: Evaluation of remifentanil as single drug for awake fiberoptic intubation. Acta Anaesthesiol Scand 46:350-354, 2002.

170. Quintel M, Roth H: Tracheostomy in the critically ill: Clinical impact of new procedures. Intensive Care Med 25:326-328, 1999.

171. Rabitsch W, Nikolic A, Schellongowski P, et al: Evaluation of an end-tidal portable ETCO$_2$ colorimetric breath indicator (COLIBRI). Am J Emerg Med 22:4-9, 2004.

172. Ram FS, Lightowler JV, Wedzicha JA: Non-invasive positive pressure ventilation for treatment of respiratory failure due to exacerbations of chronic obstructive pulmonary disease. Cochrane Database Syst Rev (1): CD004104, 2003.

173. Raphael DT: Acoustic reflectometry profiles of endotracheal and esophageal intubation. Anesthesiology 92:1293-1299, 2000.

174. Raphael DT, Benbassat M, Arnaudov D, et al: Validation study of two-microphone acoustic reflectometry for determination of breathing tube placement in 200 adult patients. Anesthesiology 97:1371-1377, 2002.

175. Reilly PM, Sing RF, Giberson FA, et al: Hypercarbia during tracheostomy: A comparison of percutaneous endoscopic, percutaneous Doppler, and standard surgical tracheostomy. Intensive Care Med 23:859-864, 1997.

176. Rello J, Ollendorf DA, Oster G, et al: Epidemiology and outcomes of ventilator-associated pneumonia in a large US database. Chest 122:2115-2121, 2002.

177. Report by the American Society of Anesthesiologists Task Force for the Management of the Difficult Airway: Practice guidelines for management of the difficult airway. Anesthesiology 78:597-602, 1993.

178. Rodriguez JL, Steinberg SM, Luchetti FA, et al: Early tracheostomy for primary airway management in the surgical critical care setting. Surgery 108:655-659, 1990.

179. Rose DK, Cohen MM: The airway: Problems and predictions in 18,500 patients. Can J Anaesth 41: 372-383, 1994.

180. Rosenbower TJ, Morris JA Jr, Eddy VA, Ries WR: The long-term complications of percutaneous dilatational tracheostomy. Am Surg 64:82-86, 1998.

181. Sakles JC, Laurin EG, Rantapaa AA, Panacek EA: Airway management in the emergency department: A one-year study of 610 tracheal intubations. Ann Emerg Med 31:325-332, 1998.

182. Sakles JC, Laurin EG, Rantapaa AA, Panacek EA: Airway management in the emergency department: A one-year study of 610 tracheal intubations. Ann Emerg Med 31:398-400, 1998.

183. Salem MR, Baraka A: Confirmation of tracheal intubation. In Benumof JL (ed): Difficult Airway Management. Principles and Practice. Mosby–Year Book, 1996, pp 531-560.

184. Samsoon GL, Young JR: Difficult tracheal intubation: A retrospective study. Anaesthesia 42:487-490, 1987.

185. Sanctorius S: Commentaria in primam fen primi libri canonis avicennae. Venetiis, Iacobum Sarcinam, 1626, pp 507-512.

186. Schachner A, Ovil Y, Sidi J, et al: Percutaneous tracheostomy—A new method. Crit Care Med 17: 1052-1056, 1989.

187. Schreier H, Papousek A, Aram L, et al: Use of the esophageal-tracheal Combitube in children. Acta Anaesth Scand 40(Suppl 109):149, 1996.

188. Schwartz DE, Matthay MA, Cohen NH: Death and other complications of emergency airway management in critically ill adults: A prospective investigation of 297 tracheal intubations. Anesthesiology 82:367-376, 1995.

189. Seegobin RD, van Hasselt GL: Endotracheal cuff pressure and tracheal mucosal blood flow: Endoscopic study of effects of four large volume cuffs. Br Med J (Clin Res Ed) 288:965-968, 1984.

190. Seiden AM: Sinusitis in the critical care patient. New Horiz 1:261-270, 1993.

191. Sener EB, Sarihasan B, Ustun E, et al: Awake tracheal intubation through the intubating laryngeal mask airway in a patient with halo traction. Can J Anaesth 49:610-613, 2002.

192. Shelden CH, Pudenz RH, Freshwater DB, Crue BL: A new method for tracheostomy. J Neurosurg 12: 428-431, 1955.

193. Simpson TP, Day CJ, Jewkes CF, Manara AR: The impact of percutaneous tracheostomy on intensive care unit practice and training. Anaesthesia 54:186-189, 1999.

194. Smith BR, Babinski M, Klain M: Percutaneous transtracheal ventilation. J Am Coll Emerg Physicians 5: 765-768, 1976.

195. Smith CE, Pinchak AB, Sidhu TS, et al: Evaluation of tracheal intubation difficulty in patients with cervical spine immobilization: Fiberoptic (WuScope) versus conventional laryngoscopy. Anesthesiology 91: 1253-1259, 1999.

196. Smith I, White PF: Use of the laryngeal mask airway as an alternative to a face mask during outpatient arthroscopy. Anesthesiology 77:850-855, 1992.

197. Smith VM: Perforation of trachea during tracheostomy performed with Shelden tracheotome. JAMA 165:2074-2076, 1957.

198. Stauffer JL, Olson DE, Petty TL: Complications and consequences of endotracheal intubation and tracheostomy: A prospective study of 150 critically ill adult patients. Am J Med 70:65-76, 1981.

199. Stock MC, Downs JB: Lubrication of tracheal tubes to prevent sore throat from intubation. Anesthesiology 57:418-420, 1982.

200. Stone KS, Talaganis SA, Preusser B, Gonyon DS: Effect of lung hyperinflation and endotracheal suctioning on heart rate and rhythm in patients after coronary artery bypass graft surgery. Heart Lung 20:443-450, 1991.

201. Stout DM, Bishop MJ, Dwersteg JF, Cullen BF: Correlation of endotracheal tube size with sore throat and hoarseness following general anesthesia. Anesthesiology 67:419-421, 1987.

202. Sugerman HJ, Wolfe L, Pasquale MD, et al: Multicenter, randomized, prospective trial of early tracheostomy. J Trauma 43:741-747, 1997.

203. Tanigawa K, Takeda T, Goto E, Tanaka K: Accuracy and reliability of the self-inflating bulb to verify tracheal intubation in out-of-hospital cardiac arrest patients. Anesthesiology 93:1432-1436, 2000.

204. Tayal VS, Riggs RW, Marx JA, et al: Rapid-sequence intubation at an emergency medicine residency: Success rate and adverse events during a two-year period. Acad Emerg Med 6:31-37, 1999.

205. Torres A, Gatell JM, Aznar E, et al: Re-intubation increases the risk of nosocomial pneumonia in patients needing mechanical ventilation. Am J Respir Crit Care Med 152:137-141, 1995.

206. UK Multi-centre trial: The use of the laryngeal mask airway by nurses during cardiopulmonary resuscitation: Results of a multicentre trial. Anaesthesia 49:3-7, 1994.

207. Urtubia RM, Aguila CM, Cumsille MA: Combitube: A study for proper use. Anesth Analg 90:958-962, 2000.

208. Van De Leur JP, Zwaveling JH, Loef BG, Van Der Schans CP: Patient recollection of airway suctioning in the ICU: Routine versus a minimally invasive procedure. Intensive Care Med 29:433-436, 2003.

209. Van Heerden PV, Weeb SA, Power BM, Thompson WR: Percutaneous dilational tracheostomy—A clinical study evaluating two systems. Anaesth Intensive Care 24:56-59, 1996.

210. Van Heurn LW, Goei R, de Ploeg I, et al: Late complications of percutaneous dilational tracheostomy. Chest 110:1572-1576, 1996.

211. Van Heurn LW, van Geffen GJ, Brink PRG: Clinical experience with percutaneous dilatational tracheostomy: Report of 150 cases. Eur J Surg 162:531-535, 1996.

212. Van Vlymen JM, Coloma M, Tongier WK, White PF: Use of the intubation laryngeal mask airway: Are muscle relaxants necessary? Anesthesiology 93:340-345, 2000.

213. Verghese C, Brimacombe JR: Survey of laryngeal mask airway usage in 11,910 patients: Safety and efficacy for conventional and nonconventional usage. Anesth Analg 82:129-133, 1996.

214. Verghese C, Rangasami J, Kapila A, Parke T: Airway control during percutaneous dilatational tracheostomy: Pilot study with the intubating laryngeal mask airway. Br J Anaesth 81:608-609, 1998.

215. Vigliaroli L, De Vivo P, Mione C, Pretto G: Clinical experience with Ciaglia's percutaneous tracheostomy. Eur Arch Otorhinolaryngol 256:426-428, 1999.

216. Vukmir RB (ed): Airway Management in the Critically Ill. New York, Parthenon Publishing Group, 2001.

217. Wafai Y, Salem MR, Baraka A, et al: Effectiveness of the self-inflating bulb for verification of proper placement of the esophageal tracheal Combitube. Anesth Analg 80:122-126, 1995.

218. Wall MA: Infant endotracheal tube resistance: Effects of changing length, diameter, and gas density. Crit Care Med 8:38-40, 1980.

219. Walls RM: The emergency airway algorithms. In Walls RM (ed): Manual of Airway Management. Philadelphia, Lippincott Williams & Wilkins, 2000, pp 16-25.

220. Walls RM, Gibbs MA: Surgical airway. Semin Anesth Periop Med Pain 20:183-192, 2001.

221. Walz MK, Peitgen K, Thürauf N, et al: Percutaneous dilatational tracheostomy—Early results and longterm outcome of 326 critically ill patients. Intensive Care Med 24:685-690, 1998.

222. Westphal K, Byhahn C: Update 2000: Tracheostomy on German intensive care units. Anaesth Intensivmed 42:70-74, 2001.

223. Westphal K, Byhahn C, Wilke HJ, Lischke V: Percutaneous tracheostomy: A clinical comparison of dilational (Ciaglia) and translaryngeal (Fantoni) techniques. Anesth Analg 89:938-943, 1999.

224. Westphal K, Maeser D, Scheifler G, et al: PercuTwist: A new single-dilator technique for percutaneous tracheostomy. Anesth Analg 96:229-232, 2003.

225. Weymuller EA Jr, Bishop MJ, Fink BR, et al: Quantification of intralaryngeal pressure exerted by endotracheal tubes. Ann Otol Rhinol Laryngol 92:444-447, 1983.

226. Williams KN, Carli F, Cormack RS: Unexpected, difficult laryngoscopy: A prospective survey in routine general surgery. Br J Anaesth 66:38-44, 1991.

227. Winkler WB, Karnik R, Seelmann O, et al: Bedside percutaneous dilational tracheostomy with endoscopic guidance: Experience in 71 ICU patients. Intensive Care Med 20:476-479, 1994.

228. Wissler RN: The esophageal-tracheal Combitube. Anesth Rev 20:147-152, 1993.

229. Wood CJ: Endotracheal suctioning: A literature review. Intensive Crit Care Nurs 14:124-136, 1998.

POSTINTUBATION PROCEDURES

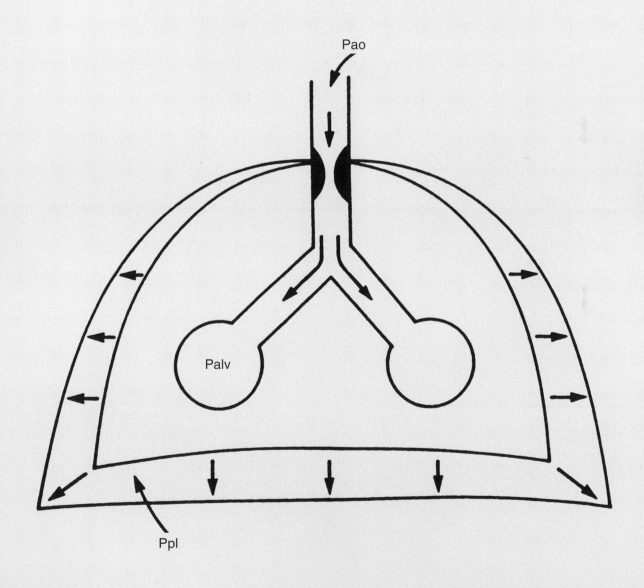

44

ENDOTRACHEAL TUBE AND RESPIRATORY CARE

Robert M. Pousman
C. Lee Parmley

I. INTRODUCTION

It could be argued that no single contribution to medicine has yielded as much benefit as the development and subsequent refinements of the endotracheal tube (ET). These refinements have proved invaluable in the realm of resuscitation and airway management as well as in the administration and delivery of general anesthesia. This chapter focuses on the brief history and development of the ET; describes the various ETs available with their indications and limitations; and reviews basic airway anatomy, proper positioning and stabilization of the ET, complications attributed to its use, and finally respiratory care of both the nonintubated and intubated and mechanically ventilated patient.

II. HISTORY

A. HISTORY OF THE ENDOTRACHEAL TUBE

The earliest recorded use of airway manipulation with an artificial device dates back to approximately the early Roman period when Asclepiades performed a tracheostomy for laryngeal edema. Over centuries, evolution of the procedure, as well as its indication, provided the incentive for a less invasive means to secure the airway. In fact, the evolved ETs were intended for assistance with resuscitation of near-drowning victims rather than administering inhalation anesthetics, which would be realized much later in time.[7] These original tubes were rigid, difficult implements to work with and not very forgiving. Trendelenburg greatly improved the devices when he described a tracheostomy tube with an inflatable rubber balloon in 1871.[158] However, anesthetic applications would not be realized until 1878, when William Macewen, a Scottish surgeon, performed an awake intubation with a brass tube for a patient having oral surgery. He filed a report in 1880 in the *British Medical Journal*.[7,91] Chloroform was then administered by "a few whiffs." Other pioneers such as American Joseph O'Dwyer and Franz Kuhn of Germany provided great advances. Perhaps best known are the contributions of British anesthetists Sir Ivan Magill and Stanley Rowbotham. In 1917 Magill and Rowbotham were using rubber ETs for gas introduction with a nasopharyngeal tube inserted for gas removal, and by 1928 they had developed a single catheter fashioned of rubber to intubate the trachea solely.[30] From this simplification, modern ET has evolved. Further modification by Guedel and Waters added a rubber cuff to Magill and Rowbotham's tube.

Up to this point ETs were manufactured from rubber. Rubber has limitations, such as its stiffness increasing with rising temperature, and adhesion properties of different polymers limit the cuffs to be manufactured from the same polymer as the tube.[158] This led to the search for alternative materials. In 1967, polyvinyl chloride (PVC) was popularized by Dr. S.A. Leader, and it has since been the material most commonly used. One property that makes PVC attractive is that it provides stiffness of an ET at room temperature to assist with intubation, yet softening occurs with an increase in temperature while in situ. Other properties are the ability to employ radiopaque lines to assist with positioning, the addition of an inflation line to connect the pilot balloon to the cuff, and its low cost.[158]

B. DEVELOPMENT AND PROPERTIES OF THE ENDOTRACHEAL TUBE CUFF

The cuffs employed on the early ETs were, like the tubes themselves, composed of rubber. These rubber ETs had limitations such as elevated inflation pressures required to fill the cuffs. The high inflation pressure translates to high lateral pressure transmitted to the tracheal wall in order to maintain a seal. Thus, the cuffs are described as low volume, high pressure. The clinical implication is related to the fact that the trachea is not circular but arched like the letter D; thus, in order to provide an adequate seal, high pressure is exerted on the tracheal wall, impairing capillary pressure and possibly resulting in mucosal ischemia.[90,158] (See later for a further discussion.)

The introduction of PVC as the cuff material mostly eliminated this problem. By virtue of making PVC inflatable and thinner walled, the ET cuff could now be high volume, low pressure and thus provide an adequate seal with lower lateral wall pressures.[90,132,158] Although some modifications have been made to assist with cuff function, the high-volume, low-pressure characteristic remains.

III. ENDOTRACHEAL TUBE (SINGLE-LUMEN) CARE

A. CHOICE OF ENDOTRACHEAL TUBE SIZE

In selecting an ET, consideration of appropriate size must take into account the function for which the ET is being placed. The size of tube chosen may be different in the case of short-term placement for anesthesia and surgery than for patients who require prolonged support with mechanical ventilation and perhaps fiberoptic bronchoscopy. ETs are manufactured in sizes according to internal diameter in increments of 0.5 mm, ranging between 2.5 and 10.0 mm. In general, the trachea of adult females accepts a tube of 7.5 to 8.0 mm and that of males 8.5 to 9.0 mm. For routine use, a tube of 7.0 to 7.5 mm for females and 7.5 to 8.0 mm for males is appropriate, but potential benefits of larger or smaller tubes should be considered in certain circumstances. An appropriately sized ET for children older than 1 year can be selected using the following formula: ET size (mm) = 4 + [age (in years)/4].[135]

1. Small Tubes and Airway Resistance

The physics of laminar gas flow through a conduit is described in the Hagen-Poiseuille equation, which reflects the relationship of resistance varying inversely with the fourth power of tube radius. Despite the fact that gas flow through ETs is often turbulent rather than laminar, the effect on resistance to gas flow represented by each millimeter decrease in tube size is considerable, ranging from 25% to 100%.[19] Airway resistance is affected by more than tube diameter, as the presence of secretion within the tube and positioning of the head and neck can also increase the tendency for turbulent flow.[16,57] The fundamental principle of which to be mindful is that airway resistance induced by an ET is inversely proportional to the tube size.[39]

As airway resistance increases, which occurs with decreasing ET diameter, work of breathing increases.[19] Although the increase in work of breathing associated with a 1-mm reduction in ET diameter varies in accordance with the tidal volume and respiratory rate at a given minute ventilation, the increase may be from 34% to 154%.[19] When ventilation is provided mechanically this increase in work of breathing related to ET resistance is seldom of consequence, although it may make weaning from ventilatory support difficult.[127,146] In fact, it has been suggested that an inability to ventilate adequately because of the work of breathing imposed by a 7-mm ET might indicate that a patient being weaned from mechanical ventilation will fail extubation regardless of tube size.[143]

Increased airway resistance associated with a small-diameter ET may also be associated with inadvertent positive end-expiratory pressure (PEEP). Some patients with high oxygen consumption, increased carbon dioxide production, or ventilation-perfusion relationships that produce high dead space ventilation require high minute ventilation. The gas flows necessary to maintain such minute ventilation are quite high, and the resistance imposed by a small-diameter ET may prohibit the completion of expiratory flow prior to the initiation of the subsequent inspiration. This results in air trapping and inadvertent PEEP, often called auto-PEEP, which increases the risk of barotrauma and circulatory compromise.[131]

The restriction to gas flow through an ET of any size increases dramatically when devices such as a fiberoptic bronchoscope are passed through it. The cross-sectional area of the tube is then effectively reduced in an amount equal to the cross-sectional area of the device inserted into the tube. The limitations of gas flow can have consequences for both the inspiratory and expiratory phases, where inspiratory flow may be inadequate to maintain ventilation during the procedure or expiratory flow may be limited to the point at which volume accumulates in the lungs and results in barotrauma or circulatory compromise.[101]

2. Large Tubes and Trauma

Whereas small-diameter ETs have disadvantages largely related to gas flow and airway resistance, larger tubes are more frequently associated with trauma to both the laryngeal structures and the tracheal mucosa.[23,73] Larger ETs are associated with a higher incidence of sore throat following general anesthesia than smaller diameter tubes.[144] With prolonged intubation, laryngeal trauma is more likely,[69] and women, because of the smaller size of their airway, are more susceptible than men.[70]

Laryngeal structures at particular risk are the vocal process of the arytenoid cartilages and the cricoid cartilage. Trauma results not only from the shape discrepancy between the round ET and the glottic opening[18] but also from direct contact and pressure on structures and tube movement, which causes erosion.[142] Mucosal injury can also occur because of irregular surfaces created by wrinkling and folding of the ET cuff. This is more likely to occur when large tubes are used and little cuff volume is required to seal the airway.[141]

B. ALTERNATIVE ENDOTRACHEAL TUBES

Rather than compensate for the resistance produced by the ET, a newly designed ET utilizes technology that allows production of an ultrathin-walled tube made of polyurethane rather than PVC that is wire reinforced to resist collapsing and kinking. The wire used to reinforce the tube is unique in that it has an elastic shape memory preventing deformation. The internal diameter is increased without compromising the rigid shape of the ET. The result is a tube with a resistance similar to that of the upper airway that is lighter, offers less airflow resistance, and when compressed forms an egg shape rather than an oval.[85] Experimentally, this new design was shown to decrease inspiratory and expiratory resistance by 60% each and inspiratory, expiratory, and total work of breathing by 70%, 47%, and 45%, respectively.[1,25]

1. Preformed and Reinforced Tubes

The use with proven safety of ETs in the operating room setting has been accompanied by efforts on the part of industry to develop and produce devices that further reduce risks and complications that are known to exist. Remote access to patients' airways has been associated with tube kinking and partial occlusion with devastating consequences, especially before development of more sophisticated anesthesia monitoring. In response to this and other interests, a variety of tubes were developed to maintain their shape and patency despite their need to be in locations where their shape and distortion might cause kinking and occlusion.

Rigid, preformed tubes such as those developed for long-term use in tracheostomy were known to maintain their patency despite the need for angulation. Preformed tubes have been developed for specific application in anesthesia practice as well. The Ring-Adair-Elwyn (RAE) tubes were designed to maintain a contour with the facial profile and facilitate safe positioning of the anesthetic circuit away from the anesthesia machine during head and neck surgery with less risk of kinking. Their contour also reduces the risk of pressure injury to the posterior pharynx. They are designed to have an intra-airway length that has the tube tip at an appropriate depth based on the size of a patient for whom the tube might be selected. Although originally developed for pediatrics, RAE tubes for either the nasal or oral route, with and without tracheal cuffs, are available in sizes appropriate for most adults and children[124] (Fig. 44-1).

An anode or armored tube with an embedded wire coil is designed to minimize kinking even with quite severe position-induced angulation. Armored tubes are popular for use in head and neck surgery where remote airway access and the potential for kinking of the ET are concerns. Placement of an armored tube through a tracheostomy for procedures such as laryngectomy is a common practice because it allows placement during surgical procedures where the tube can be mobilized or the circuit draped away from the field without high risk of tube kinking (Fig. 44-2).

The embedded wire concept of the armored ET has also been developed for long-term tracheostomy use. Although armored tracheostomy tubes are not free of risks, one advantage of this type of tracheostomy tube is that its flexibility allows its length and intratracheal depth to be adjusted, which may be beneficial when tracheomalacia at the level of the cuff develops.[106] These tracheostomy tubes are also popular for use in morbidly obese patients, in whom, because of the depth of tissue, preformed tracheostomy tubes may not have the shape necessary to fit individual patients.

2. Laser Tubes

Since the 1970s, progress in laser technology has advanced surgical capabilities especially for airway surgery. In order to protect patients and health care providers from laser-induced injury to eyes and airways, special precautions are required. Fire is the most serious danger associated with the use of lasers in the operating room, especially when a laser is used in airway surgery.[139] A major complication related to the use of lasers for laryngeal surgery is ignition of the ET, which may result in severe airway damage.[36] The laser beam may ignite the tube by direct penetration or indirectly if burning tissue is inhaled into the tube,[74] and the ease with which ignition may occur is related to the particular material from which the tube is constructed.[71] Most ETs are constructed of PVC, which is highly flammable. Ideally, PVC tubes should not be used for airways where a laser is employed.[134,138]

Special precautions to prevent airway fires and injuries include development of techniques to provide ventilation without an endotracheal airway as well as methods to prevent ignition of the tube. Tubes can be laser-proofed or protected from the laser beam by wrapping them with

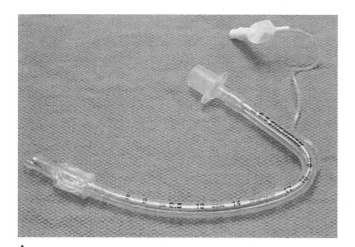

A

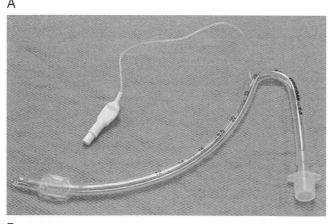

B

Figure 44-1 A, Cuffed nasal Ring-Adair-Elwyn (RAE) tube.
B, Cuffed oral RAE tube.

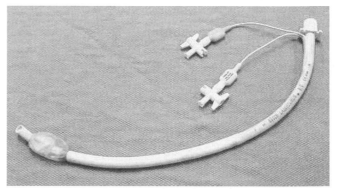

A

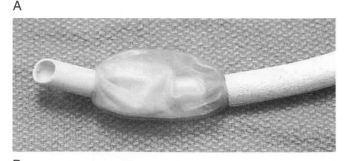

B

Figure 44-2 A, Armored endotracheal tube. **B,** Embedded wire reinforcement in armored endotracheal tube.

either reflective metal tape or muslin, or they can be constructed of noncombustible materials. In particular, the ET cuff is vulnerable to puncture by the laser beam and should be filled with saline or water, which allows more energy to be absorbed before disruption. Protecting the tube from the laser beam by wrapping with a foil tape has proved effective.[136] Tubes made of materials such as metal and silicone and having special double cuffs have also reduced the risk of airway fires and injury during laser airway surgery (Fig. 44-3).[59,136]

3. Evac Tubes

Hospitalized patients who require mechanical ventilation are susceptible to the development of pneumonia. Ventilator-associated pneumonia (VAP) is know to increase hospital length of stay, health care costs, and mortality.[11] Organisms that grow in pooled subglottic secretions above the cuff of the ET are known to leak into the lungs and are associated with an increased incidence of VAP. Measures to reduce the incidence of VAP caused by this route have focused on improved oral care, reduction of the biofilm and bacterial load associated with endotracheal airways, and evacuation of secretions pooled above the cuff of the ET. Drainage of subglottic secretions has been shown to prevent VAP.[14,42,82,96] Currently available are tubes that have a suction lumen that opens to the surface of the ET just above the cuff (Fig. 44-4). This lumen is attached to constant or intermittent suction and, in conjunction with aggressive oral hygiene, can be part of a program to reduce VAP. Current interest is focused on reduction of biofilm by impregnating ETs

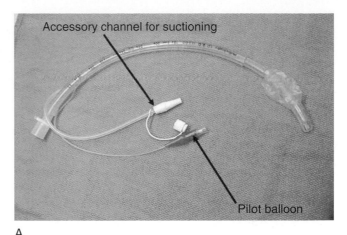

A

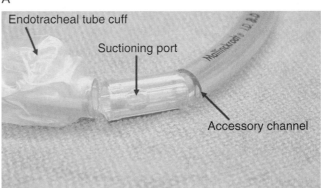

B

Figure 44-4 A, Mallinckrodt Hi-Lo Evac endotracheal tube. **B,** Cross section of Mallinckrodt Hi-Lo Evac endotracheal tube displaying suction port with accessory channel.

with antimicrobial agents.[15,109] The ability of such developments to affect the incidence of VAP has not yet been proved.

IV. PROPER POSITIONING AND STABILIZATION OF ENDOTRACHEAL TUBES

A. IDENTIFYING PROPER POSITION OF THE ENDOTRACHEAL TUBE

1. Detection of Esophageal Intubation

Once the clinician has deemed intubation necessary and has provided the intervention, confirmation of proper ET placement must be provided expeditiously. The malpositioned ET can produce adverse effects, especially in an apneic patient. Unrecognized esophageal intubation can have disastrous consequences with a reported incidence of 8% in critical patients.[130] Therefore, a brief discussion of verification of ET placement is warranted.

If intubation is necessary in a spontaneously breathing patient, confirmation of proper placement of the ET in the trachea can be achieved by the detection of end-tidal carbon dioxide (ETCO$_2$) in expired gases by using capnography or other colorimetric methods. Additional methods

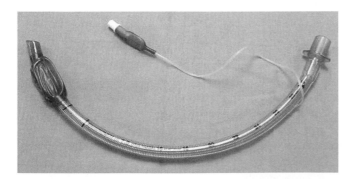

A

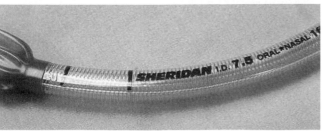

B

Figure 44-3 A, Silicone endotracheal tube for laser airway surgery. **B,** Double-cuff system for saline inflation.

Figure 44-5 **A,** Beck Airway Flow Monitor (BAAM). **B,** Beck Airway Flow Monitor (BAAM) attached to endotracheal tube. (Courtesy of Life-Assist, Inc., Rancho Cordova, CA.)

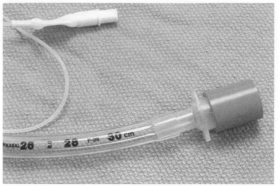
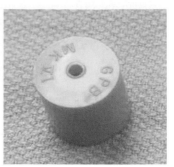

A   B

of confirmation include confirmation of the reservoir bag inflating and deflating with the patient's respiratory effort and the use of auditory cues of gas flow through the ET. Indeed this modality is employed in "blind" nasal intubation and may be augmented with devices (i.e., Beck Airway Flow Monitor [BAAM], Life-Assist, Inc., Rancho Cordova, CA) placed at the proximal end of the ET to assist with confirmation (Fig. 44-5).[31-33]

If intubation is to occur in the apneic patient with the use of either pharmacologic induction agents or skeletal muscle relaxants, these modalities are inadequate. Many methods exist to verify correct placement (Table 44-1), but not one is without limitations.[128] Direct visualization of the ET entering the glottis and traversing the vocal cords by the clinician is the first and most immediate method. Condensation from expired gas found in the ET has also been used but may be present in esophageal intubations

Table 44-1   Methods Used to Verify Endotracheal Tube Placement

Direct visualization between vocal cords
Condensation in endotracheal tube
Auscultation over lungs, axillae, epigastrium
Visualization of chest wall movement or reservoir bag synchrony, or both, with spontaneous efforts
Auditory flow perception with spontaneous efforts
Palpation of cuff at neck
Chest roentgenogram
Fiberoptic visualization
Transtracheal illumination
Self-inflating bulb or bulb syringe
Exhaled CO_2 by capnography or colorimetric methods
Pulse oximetry
Acoustic reflectometry

as well,[128] yet the "gold standard" utilized today is the presence of $ETCO_2$ in expired gases using capnography or other colorimetric techniques.

Capnography not only yields quantified measurements of inspired and expired gas but also provides a waveform visualized on a breath-to-breath basis. Although not without limitations (lack of portability, need for a power source), capnography reliably identifies proper placement of the ET. If esophageal intubation has occurred, a gradual reduction in height of the capnograph waveforms occurs with successive breaths. False-positive results during esophageal intubations may occur in situations of ingested CO_2 containing or liberating substances prior to intubation, bag-mask ventilation with entrainment of expired air into the stomach, and intubation of the pharynx.[3] Inappropriate extubations may occur with false-negative situations of proper placement and lack of an $ETCO_2$ waveform. This may occur with unrecognized circuit disconnections, an obstructed or kinked ET or gas sampling line or both, gas sampling line condensation or leaks, equipment failure, or severe bronchospasm. Unquestionably, capnography is dependent on pulmonary blood flow. In the absence of perfusion as in cardiac arrest, capnography's utility is limited, but it is vital in low-flow states. Ornato and colleagues used an animal model to evaluate the relationship between cardiac output (CO) and $ETCO_2$. Through manipulation of CO with inotropes or with controlled hemorrhage, a logarithmic relationship between CO and $ETCO_2$ was found.[106] This finding demonstrated that capnography is useful in cardiac resuscitation to assist with evaluation of low-flow states and adequacy of perfusion.

To alleviate the logistical concerns with capnography in emergency situations, mainly the lack of portability and need for a power source, a portable and reliable means of detecting $ETCO_2$ was developed. Colorimetric $ETCO_2$ utilizes a detector impregnated with metacresol purple. This indicator is pH sensitive and changes color, purple to yellow, in the presence of CO_2. The devices are disposable, attach between the ET and circuit or bag (Easy Cap $ETCO_2$ Detector, Nellcor, Inc., New York, NY), and provide indication of carbon dioxide on a gradation scale of A (purple) with a CO_2 level of 0.5%, B (tan) corresponding to a level of 0.5% to 2%, and C (yellow) corresponding to a level of greater than 2% of CO_2 rapidly and reliably (Fig. 44-6).[60,128] Limitations of this method are exposure to humidified gas, which makes it ineffective, and in cases of cardiac arrest or low-perfusion states. False-positive results can occur, as in capnography. Delays in recognition of esophageal intubation with the Easy Cap have been reported in patients ventilated with CO_2-containing gas prior to intubation, suggesting that capnography is the best method of detection of esophageal intubation.[116]

Another method advocated for the detection of an esophageal intubation capitalizes on the physical characteristics of the esophagus, which, unlike the trachea, collapses when negative pressure is applied. One such device consists of a syringe that attaches to the end of the ET. When the plunger is withdrawn, resistance is felt when an esophageal intubation occurs as the walls of the esophagus collapse around the ET, as opposed to free aspiration of the plunger with proper tracheal placement. A modification of this method is the use of a self-inflating bulb. This device replaces the syringe with the self-inflating bulb, which, when compressed prior to attachment to the ET, remains deflated when an esophageal intubation occurs and with proper tracheal placement.

These devices are reported to be reliable and effective, with one study reporting a sensitivity and specificity of 100% and 99%, respectively.[78] However, other studies reported limitations and false-negative results in patients with copious or aspirated secretions, vomitus in the airway, morbid obesity or reduced functional residual capacity, and gastric distention.[4,88,147,148]

One author described the use of acoustic reflectometry to create a one-dimensional profile between the patent's trachea and the collapsed esophagus. Although it is promising, further validation is required and impractical limitations hinder its use.[119]

2. Confirmation of Appropriate Depth of Insertion of Endotracheal Tubes

After verifying correct tracheal placement of the ET, identifying the correct depth of the ET is imperative. Before addressing the various methods that assist in confirmation of appropriate ET depth, a brief discussion of what is considered the correct depth of the ET is warranted. Malpositioning of the ET occurs frequently, with unrecognized right main stem intubation occurring in approximately 4% of chest radiographs.[130] The generally accepted depth of insertion of the ET is between 2 and 7 cm above the carina, optimally between 4 and 7 cm above the carina with the head and neck in a neutral position.[64,66,119,128] It is important to realize this as flexion-extension movements of the neck can displace the ET upward or downward with resultant extubation or main stem intubation occurring, respectively. Typically, the right main stem bronchus is entered, and if endobronchial intubation remains undetected, resultant hyperinflation of the lung may occur with subsequent pneumothorax and concomitant atelectasis of the unventilated left lung. Indeed, it has been reported that up to 15% of chest radiographs reveal malpositioned ETs in intubated patients.[72,129]

The use of chest radiography to verify proper positioning of the ET is common in the intensive care setting. Proper position can be confirmed by locating the carina and the distal tip of the ET. The carina can be visualized by following the left main stem bronchus proximally,[119] locating the T5-T7 vertebrae as the carina overlies this location in more than 90% of patients, and locating the ET tip at the T2-T4 vertebral levels.[64] In underexposed chest radiographs, the aortic arch or knob can be located and a tangential line can be drawn from the inferior portion of the aorta across to the right side of the patient, which 95% of the time approximates a location 2 cm above the carina. The ET tip should be located 3 to 5 cm above this line.[113]

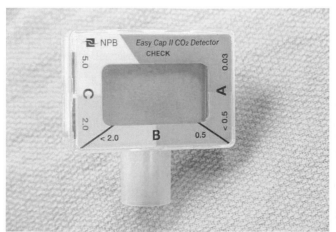
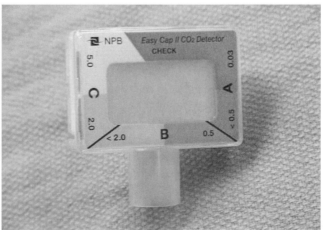

A   B

Figure 44-6 Easy Cap end-tidal CO_2 detector. **A,** Before CO_2 detection (note purple colorization of indicator). **B,** After CO_2 detection (note yellow colorization of indicator). (Courtesy of Nellcor, Inc., New York, NY.)

Typically, locating the tip of the ET distal to the heads of the clavicles situated approximately midmanubrium is generally adequate. The acquisition of immediate chest radiographs to confirm proper position has been challenged with the recommendation that routine films should suffice when intubation was performed by experienced personnel.[92]

In the operating room, chest radiographs are not used to confirm proper position; rather, clinical assessment (i.e., auscultation of bilateral breath sounds, visualization of equal chest expansion, and direct visualization of ET tip placed just below the vocal cords) is utilized. The ET is also manufactured with centimeter markings to aid in gauging the depth of insertion. It has been advocated that in orally intubated patients, a depth of 23 cm at the teeth or corner of the mouth be used for men and 21 to 22 cm for women.[110,126] In nasotracheal intubations, a depth of 26 cm at the nares in women and 28 cm in men should be sufficient for proper tracheal position.[121] Other methods utilized include direct visualization of the ET tip in reference to the carina with a fiberoptic scope or catheter,[130] transtracheal illumination,[102] and ballottement of the ET cuff at the suprasternal notch.[114]

B. STABILIZATION OF ENDOTRACHEAL TUBES

When verification and confirmation of proper tracheal placement and position have been achieved, care should be focused on securing the ET in its proper position and, if prolonged mechanical ventilation is necessary, daily assessments should be made to recognize malposition.

At the most basic level, recording and confirming the depth of the ET at either the patient's teeth or lips in centimeters should be routine. This should be documented on the anesthetic record or the respiratory care flow sheet, or both, in the intensive care unit. In patients requiring prolonged mechanical ventilation, this depth should be assessed and documented daily along with clinical assessments of bilateral chest expansion and equal bilateral breath sounds.

Proper securing and surveillance of the ET are important not only to ensure proper depth and positioning but also to reduce the incidence of inadvertent extubation of patients. Unplanned extubation is primarily a problem in the intensive care unit. It has a reported incidence of approximately 2% to 16%[24,34,151] with 80% requiring reintubation, contributing to a higher mortality rate.[24,26] Although much attention has been paid to inadequate sedation of mechanically ventilated patients, a few studies specifically address techniques utilized in securing ETs. In a study comparing four techniques of securing ETs, Levy and Griego[89] concluded that the technique of using simple adhesive tape split at both ends and secured to both the ET and patient's face was most effective compared with proprietary methods as it also allowed more effective nursing care, improved oral hygiene, and comfort of the patient. The use of twill tape was reported to provide

less skin breakdown and was recommended when skin integrity is an issue. In a similar study comparing two methods of securing an ET, adhesive versus twill tape, Barnason and colleagues[9] found no statistical difference in preventing unplanned extubation, allowing oral hygiene, or facial integrity between the methods. Another study addressed the use of a knot tied around the ET versus a bow; one issue evaluated was the necessity of cutting the knot and the implied complications (i.e., accidental pilot balloon damage) along with malposition, skin integrity, and inadvertent extubation.[28] The authors found no difference in complications; however, the nursing staff preferred the bow method for patients' comfort and skin integrity even though the perception was that the knot-tying method was more secure.

Attention to proper ET stabilization primarily focuses on the reduction of malpositioning and dislodgement as it pertains to extubation, improved comfort of the patient, and ease of nursing care. One study addressed massive air leaks and attributing factors.[79] The authors defined a massive air leak as one that requires extubation. Over a 2-year period, 18 ETs were removed for massive air leaks, of which 61% were found to be free of mechanical defects (i.e., cuff intact). Fourteen of the 18 patients required reintubation, of whom 2 aspirated gastric contents and 1 suffered severe epistaxis from a nasal reintubation, thus a 21% complication rate. The authors concluded that malposition was the most plausible explanation for the apparent air leaks. This study reinforces the importance of securing the ET and daily vigilance to ensure that the proper depth and positioning are confirmed and maintained.

Despite these studies, no consensus exists about the "best" method of securing the ET. We prefer a method we describe as a "barber's pole" technique for operating room intubations (Fig. 44-7) and a more secure "four-point" technique for intubations anticipated for 24 hours or longer (Figs. 44-8 and 44-9).

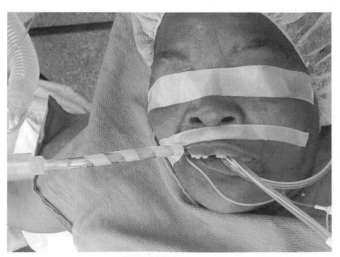

Figure 44-7 Barber's pole technique of securing endotracheal tube.

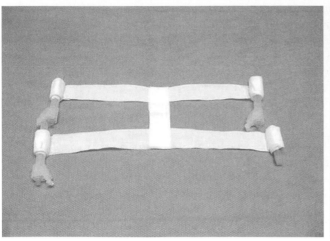
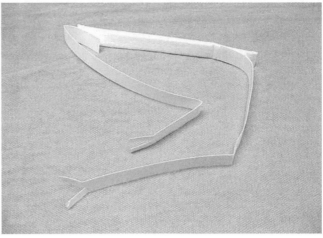

A   B

Figure 44-8 Four-point securing tapes prior to application. **A,** Self-made. **B,** Proprietary.

V. RESPIRATORY CARE OF THE INTUBATED–MECHANICALLY VENTILATED PATIENT

In an effort to reduce or eliminate the potential long-term complications associated with intubation, it is prudent that every attempt to liberate the patient from mechanical ventilation be made. Indeed, providing a noninvasive means of airway support (i.e., nasal or face mask continuous positive airway pressure [CPAP] or bilevel PAP) in certain selected patients may circumvent the problems associated with prolonged intubation. As soon as the etiology of the patient's respiratory compromise or need for a definitive airway has been realized and the underlying process corrected or stabilized, the removal from assisted ventilation or weaning process should begin. Many factors can impede this process. The presence of the ET bypasses the host defenses of the upper airway, eliminates the humidification of inspired gases, increases the work of breathing, and limits the administration of medications and oral hygiene, all of which promote bacterial colonization, inflammation, and sputum production. Inability to clear these secretions actively because of the patients' inability to mount an effective cough as well as difficulty with passive removal by health care personnel can lead to plugging of proximal and distal airways, not to mention the ET. These retained secretions can result in the formation of atelectasis, shunt, hypoxemia, and increased respiratory load, all of which can prolong the duration of mechanical ventilation. Therefore, aggressive respiratory care must be provided for the intubated patient in order to avoid complications and further morbidity.

A. HUMIDIFICATION OF INSPIRED GAS

The insertion of an ET, whether it is nasal or oral, effectively bypasses the upper airway and the ability to heat and humidify inspired gas is lost. The result is a dry, cool gas

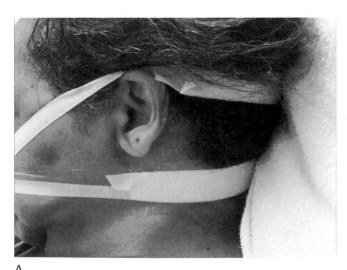
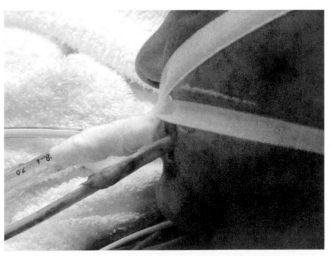

A   B

Figure 44-9 Application of four-point securing technique. **A,** Posterior view. **B,** Anterior view.

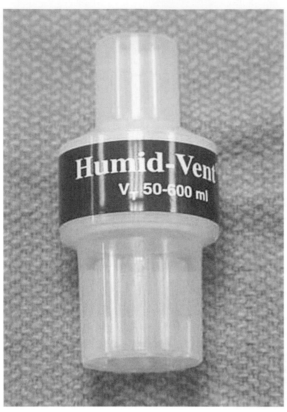

A

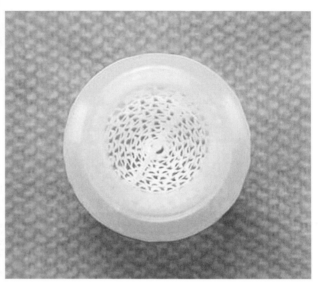

B

Figure 44-10 A, Heat and moisture exchanger (HME). **B,** HME demonstrating internal hydrophobic and hygroscopic material.

that is damaging to the respiratory tract and impedes mucociliary function. Secretions may become dry and inspissated with possible occlusion of the ET occurring. If left unrecognized, this may lead to barotrauma and death.[100] The most common method to protect against this is the use of heated humidifiers (HHs) or heat and moisture exchangers (HMEs).

1. Heat and Moisture Exchangers and Heated Humidifiers

HMEs are typically cylindrical devices that are fitted to the ventilator circuit usually just proximal to the ET connector and the Y-connector (Figs. 44-10 and 44-11). They are composed of either hydrophobic material only or both hydrophobic and hygroscopic materials. The materials provide heat, humidification, and filtering properties, which earned the nickname "artificial nose." They are lightweight, inexpensive, require no power source, and reduce circuit condensation, making them attractive alternatives to the more expensive HHs.

The use of HHs is associated with the production of nearly 100% humidity of the inspiratory gas and is thus more effective than HMEs. This creates substantially greater condensate in ventilator tubing and requires more labor at the bedside to ensure proper removal of collected water vapor. These units also require an external power source and additional circuitry, further contributing to

their increased cost. Although proper humidification is important, overhumidification can be just as detrimental to the mucociliary apparatus. Accidental overheating can occur and create additional damage to the airway if temperatures are not frequently monitored.

The efficacies of the various HMEs have been compared. The purely hydrophobic HMEs perform less efficiently than hydrophobic and hygroscopic HMEs, especially at minute volumes greater than 10 L/min, and are therefore

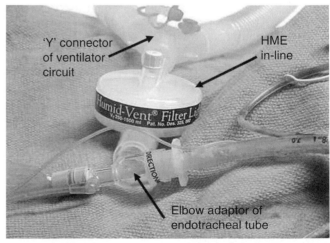

Figure 44-11 Heat and moisture exchanger E connected in line to ventilator circuit.

not universally recommended.[99] The recommended minimum amount of absolute humidity that the HME should deliver is between 24 and 30 mg H_2O/L to avoid ET occlusion.[52] Effective ET diameter has been better preserved with hygroscopic HMEs and HHs than with hydrophobic HMEs in patients requiring prolonged mechanical ventilation, suggesting better humidification with the former devices.[155] The efficiency of delivered humidification with HMEs can be confirmed by visually inspecting for condensate in the circuit; if condensate is not present, it is recommended to replace the HME or switch to an HH.[125] One downside of HMEs is the resistance to gas flow that can be created, especially if they become contaminated with secretions or blood.[27]

A common concern regarding the degree of humidification and condensation produced in ventilator circuits with HHs is the potential for bacterial colonization and subsequent nosocomial infection. There is no consensus about the proper duration of use of these implements. Some clinicians advocate daily changes of HMEs, HHs, or the ventilator circuit because they contend that extended use increases VAP incidence. Multiple studies have failed to show a correlation of an increased incidence of pneumonia with HHs versus HMEs, and frequent changes of HMEs or HHs as well as ventilator circuits, unless they are visually soiled or less than every 7 days, is not cost effective or efficacious.[48,83,84,123,145]

B. SECRETION CLEARANCE AND CONTROL THERAPIES

After the discussion of the effects of bypassing the upper airway's means to heat, humidify, and filter inspired air, it should be clear that secretion clearance and control are of major importance to the care of the intubated patient. The use of HMEs and HHs helps circumvent some of the problems encountered when an ET is in place and adds protection against the inherent drying of secretions that can occur if insufficient ambient humidity is applied. However, they do not eliminate the problem altogether, as mucociliary function is complex and proper function beyond merely supplying appropriate humidity is required. Many therapies and modalities have been offered to patients to assist in this regard, and this section discusses those more commonly used in both nonintubated and intubated patients.

1. Mucolytic Agents

Although providing adequate hydration and nutrition assists with the physical characteristics of mucus and promotes proper ciliary function and muscle strength, additional pharmacotherapy is available. Agents to decrease the viscosity of tracheobronchial secretions and assist with their production and clearance have been employed for decades. The primary agent used is *N*-acetylcysteine (NAC) or Mucomyst. NAC is a sulfhydryl-containing compound; thus, it is classified as a thiol. It has extensive first-pass metabolism in the gastrointestinal tract and liver when administered orally and is virtually completely absorbed as minimal amounts are excreted in the feces. The plasma half-life is approximately 2 hours, with a terminal effect at approximately 12 hours.

The majority of NAC's biochemical effects appear to be from its sulfhydryl group, enabling it to reduce cystine to cysteine and promote glutathione synthesis, which in turn acts to detoxify and reduce the production of potent oxygen and hydroxyl radicals.[41] These effects have provided many uses for NAC beyond a mucolytic agent, such as for hepatic protection in acetaminophen overdose[137] and renal protection from contrast-induced nephropathy.[150] NAC's effects on mucus viscosity result from its ability to disrupt the disulfide bridges and render them more liquid, thus affecting the rheologic properties.[80] NAC is usually delivered by nebulizer in combination with a β-agonist as it can induce bronchospasm.[118] Clinically, its effects have been variable in patients with chronic bronchitis, a population susceptible to excessive mucus production, in which orally administered NAC is used to assist with exacerbations and daily symptomatic relief.[21,103,120] Another mucolytic agent, *N*-acetylcysteine L-lysinate (L-NAC, Nacystelyn), appears to have better efficacy in disturbing the mucoelastic properties of mucus and when compared with NAC experimentally.[152,153]

Although mucus viscosity may be an important factor in its clearance, other factors such as DNA content may be more significant. DNA contributes to the viscosity of secretions as it accumulates from the degradation of bacteria and neutrophils that chronically inhabit the airways of patients with persistent inflammatory disorders. An agent that can be considered mostly a mucokinetic agent, recombinant deoxyribonuclease (DNase, Pulmozyme), has been used in nebulized form in patients with bronchiectasis caused by cystic fibrosis with good results; however, it is expensive and its use beyond this population of patients is not indicated.[8]

One interesting therapy that the authors employ in burn patients with a documented inhalation injury is nebulized heparin combined with daily toilet bronchoscopy. Heparin assists with decreasing and removing bronchial casts that form with inhalation injury. Mucosal sloughing along with proteinaceous material from inflammation adds adhesiveness to the secretions. Plugging of airways and ETs can occur with fatal results. Heparin's anticoagulant effects assist with removal of casts, and it may act as a free radical scavenger that has anti-inflammatory effects as well. Although studies have not consistently shown a significant change in pulmonary function, cast formation and removal are favorably altered.[35,149]

2. Chest Physiotherapy

Providing chest physiotherapy encompasses a variety of techniques that include changing position, percussion of the chest wall, vibration of the chest wall, and inducing coughing. These are dogmatic approaches that have historically provided poor results, not to mention burdening many a respiratory therapist and patient. Newer, alternative techniques have shown promising results.

a. Percussion and Postural Drainage

Used extensively in patients with cystic fibrosis, the technique of percussion with postural drainage (P & PD) utilizes external percussion of the chest wall overlying the affected lung region. Percussion can be applied manually with a cupped hand or by automated, usually pneumatic, devices. Vibration along with percussion is frequently coadministered as well. The application of percussion or vibration, or both, to the chest wall functions to loosen the secretions in the bronchi and facilitate their mobilization. This is traditionally performed while exploiting the extremes of position that the patient can tolerate. A steep Trendelenburg position of 25 degrees or more is employed, less if the patient cannot tolerate this angle, to facilitate the gravitational effects on mucus clearance.[115,160] The benefits of this therapy are drainage of secretions from the affected lung regions into the central airways with further lung expansion.[133] Relative contraindications to the postural component of this therapy are the presence of increased intracranial pressure; unprotected airway with aspiration potential; recent esophageal, ophthalmic, or intracranial surgery; congestive heart failure; and uncontrolled hypertension.[2] As for percussion or vibration, application over recent surgical sites such as split-thickness skin grafts, presence of rib fractures or chest trauma, pulmonary contusions, burns, unstable spine fractures, coagulopathy, subcutaneous emphysema, and bronchospasm are relative contraindications.[115] Hazards include hypoxemia and accidental extubation in the intubated patient.

Clinically and experimentally, the use of P & PD in cystic fibrosis patients is supported,[122] with one report showing a fall in forced expiratory flows and vital capacity after 3 weeks when the therapy was withheld and a return to their baseline when the therapy was reinstituted.[40] However, patients' compliance remains a concern, as it is burdensome not only for patients but also for the caregivers.

b. Positive End-Expiratory Pressure Therapy

PEEP therapy as a secretion clearance technique utilizes a restriction to expiratory flow by means of a face mask or mouthpiece. The resistance is adjusted to 10 to 20 cm H_2O of back pressure during expiration, which allows airflow to move into distal airways and lung units, past secretions, and mobilize them toward the larger airways. The maneuver is utilized with gentle and forceful coughs lasting up to 20 minutes, and aerosolized medications can be administered concomitantly. Patients with an increased work of breathing and dyspnea may have difficulty performing this technique and thus be unable to participate. Studies show that PEEP therapy is at least as, if not more, effective at secretion clearance as P & PD; however, patients' satisfaction is markedly more favorable.[97,104,107]

c. Flutter Valve

The flutter valve is a hand-held device that incorporates PEEP therapy with airway oscillation. Oscillations are produced by a steel ball that is housed in a cone-shaped encasement within the cylindrical device. As the patient expires through the cylinder pressure builds in both the airways and the device, moving the ball until it begins to vibrate and oscillate, which is transmitted down the airways. Intermittent PEEP up to 35 cm H_2O can be generated with forceful expirations.[89] The patient performs about 5 to 15 breaths followed by 2 forceful breaths, and a session lasts approximately 15 minutes. Results have demonstrated improved pulmonary function and secretion clearance compared with standard chest physiotherapy for cystic fibrosis patients.[62,86]

d. Intrapulmonary Percussive Ventilation

A unique device that can be controlled by the patient provides an oscillating pressure that is pneumatically powered to the patient's airway. Intrapulmonary percussive ventilation (IPV) can be delivered through a mouthpiece or to the end of the ET. Its high-frequency oscillations function to loosen retained secretions, expand airways and lungs, and reduce atelectasis. Conceptualized and designed by Dr. Forrest Bird, IPV uses a phasetron, which is a sliding Venturi providing 5 to 35 cm H_2O during oscillations of 2 to 5 Hz.[159] Aerosolized medications may be delivered during IPV treatments. IPV has been reported on favorably for secretion clearance and lung expansion in patients with cystic fibrosis and other disorders.[17,75] It offers advantages in patients who lack the ability to perform the previously described techniques.

e. High-Frequency Chest Wall Compression

An inflatable vest is applied around the chest, hoses are attached that deliver air, and the air is then rapidly withdrawn. The high-frequency oscillations that are produced range from 5 to 25 Hz and can generate pressures up to 50 cm H_2O. This creates a gentle "squeezing" of the patient's chest mimicking small coughs. The frequency of the oscillations can be adjusted, and sensors in the vest reduce the pressure delivered when the patient's chest expands as in a deep cough or breath.[89] Secretion clearance and improvement in mucus rheology have been reported.[154,157] Perhaps the biggest drawback of this method is its cost, U.S.$15,900.

3. Suctioning

Perhaps the simplest and most logical means to assist with secretion clearance is direct suctioning. This is a safe modality, but when it is performed carelessly complications may occur such as soft tissue or airway trauma, aspiration, laryngospasm, increased intracranial pressure, bronchospasm, hypoxemia, and cardiac dysrhythmias.[38] Airway suctioning can be performed in the presence of an ET or tracheostomy as well as without an artificial airway in place. Hypoxemia can be minimized if preoxygenation with a fraction of inspired oxygen (FIO_2) of 100% is performed. In patients with intracranial hypertension, mild hyperventilation with manual breaths delivered through an Ambu bag or blunting the cough reflex with instilled lidocaine just prior to suctioning may reduce the risks of additional rises in intracranial pressure. The procedure should be brief and the vacuum applied only after the suction catheter has been advanced. Suction should be applied intermittently rather than continuously upon withdrawal of the catheter. Following each pass of the catheter, lung reexpansion with a few gentle manual breaths should be administered. Suctioning can be applied by a single-use open system in which the catheter is left unprotected from the patient or a closed system (Fig. 44-12) that sheathes the catheter in a sterile protective covering.

Closed systems are usually incorporated into the ventilator breathing circuit at the junction of Y connector and the ET or tracheostomy tube, allowing continued ventilation while suctioning with no need to disconnect from the circuit. This is important as patients requiring aggressive ventilator management as in high PEEP therapy are less susceptible to alveolar derecruitment compared with open suctioning. Because the system is part of the circuit, there is no need to provide preoxygenation or additional ventilation, as this can be accomplished by increasing the FIO_2 or the minute volume on the ventilator. The catheter is completely retractable and does not add any additional restriction to airflow. It is intended for single-patient use but multiple uses in patients when concern about infection and cross-contamination is an issue. There are concerns that colonization of these devices with aspiration of bacterial particles and cross-contamination may predispose to VAP.[140] Such concerns have led to different opinions on the appropriate timing of changing the systems. Kollef and colleagues performed a study in 521 patients randomly assigned to scheduled changes every 24 hours or no

routine change except when there is a malfunction or visible soiling with blood or gastric secretions.[81] Of patients who developed VAP, 15% were in both groups. The only difference found was in total cost; $11,016 in the group with scheduled changes versus U.S. $837 in the group with no scheduled changes.

The use of fiberoptic bronchoscopy for routine secretion management is not advocated. It is expensive, requires proficient training, and may produce complications of barotrauma secondary to a marked reduction to cessation of expiratory airflow, depending on the airway caliber, in intubated patients. In our practice, it is reserved for assisting with lobar collapse not amenable to conventional treatments, "toilet" bronchoscopy as may be needed in an inhalation injury to evaluate for tracheobronchial injury, diagnosis of significant hemoptysis, and to assist with specimen procurement when there is suspicion of VAP.

4. Positioning of the Patient

The appropriate position in which to maintain the patient requiring mechanical ventilation has been debated. Current recommendations from the Centers for Disease Control and Prevention state that elevating the head 30 to 40 degrees reduces the risk of VAP. A study examining the rate of VAP in semirecumbent versus supine patients concluded early after interim analysis showed an incidence of microbiologically confirmed pneumonias of 5% versus 23%, respectively.[47] The semirecumbent position has also been supported with regard to nursing care and gastric reflux with aspiration and shown to have no effect on the hemodynamic status of the patient, a common theoretical concern.[65]

Special beds such as those that provide continuous lateral rotation have been used for patients who cannot be positioned, such as those with severe head or traumatic brain injury, or who are pharmacologically paralyzed, such as patients with acute respiratory distress syndrome. These beds are promoted to enhance skin care, reduce thrombotic events, and improve pulmonary function. Their use is proposed to reduce atelectasis and pneumonia formation; however, studies have remained conflicting.[5,29]

5. Inhaled Bronchodilators

Airway reactivity continues to be a considerable process that hinders respiratory function and prolongs the duration of mechanical ventilation. Additional morbidity can be attributed to persistent bronchospastic disease as the inflammation that persists promotes further mucus production, airway hyperemia and edema, and narrowing of small airways with an increase in closing volume. These processes adversely affect oxygenation as functional residual capacity is decreased, not to mention CO_2 elimination as expiratory flow is limited. At extremes of expiratory flow limitation, generous amounts of intrinsic PEEP (auto-PEEP) are

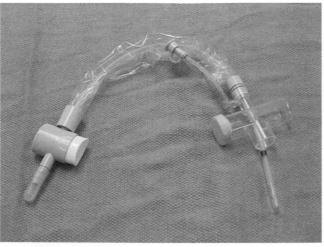

Figure 44-12 Multiple-use closed suctioning system.

generated; this can impede cardiac filling by reducing preload and hypotension and cardiac arrest may result. The physical effects of auto-PEEP are not limited to the cardiovascular system; the obvious effects of alveolar overdistention can lead to increased dead space and barotrauma, especially when mechanical ventilation is being instituted. Pneumothorax, pneumomediastinum, and pneumoperitoneum may all occur as well as ventilator dyssynchrony.

There are many maneuvers to alleviate or reduce the effects of bronchospasm, including decreasing the respiratory rate, prolonging the expiratory time, decreasing tidal volume, and increasing inspiratory flow rate. Pharmacologically, the use of β-adrenergic agonists, specifically β$_2$-agonists such as albuterol, is the mainstay therapy. Systemic methylxanthines such as theophylline do not add much benefit in the acute stage of treating bronchospasm and reactive airways as they have a narrow therapeutic window, which increases the potential for toxicities. β$_2$-Receptors on bronchial smooth muscle promote relaxation and dilation of the airway diameter when stimulated.

β$_2$-Agonists also have a beneficial effect on respiratory cilia, causing an increase in the beat frequency.[156] This is mediated by β-adrenergic receptors and the effect can be blocked with β-blocking agents. The increase in the frequency of ciliary beating promotes mucus clearance over the epithelium. Other effects are increased water secretion onto the airway surface, facilitating mucus clearance.[37] Indeed, the beneficial effects of β-agonists on bronchial reactivity and mucociliary clearance are evident; however, there are data suggesting a more robust effect in healthier airways than in chronically diseased airways such as in chronic bronchitis.[13]

Although inhaled β-agonists are pivotal in the reduction of airway reactivity, the use of inhaled anticholinergics such as ipratropium bromide needs to be emphasized. It is well appreciated that many of the mechanisms of airway reactivity and inflammation associated with bronchospastic disease are cholinergically mediated. In patients suffering from chronic obstructive pulmonary disease, their use alone or in combination with β-agonists is the foundation of maintenance therapy and in acute exacerbations.[54]

6. Inhaled Antibiotics

Inhaled antibiotics have been used for decades, falling in and out of favor over the years. They are used primarily for treatment and suppression of chronic airway bacterial colonization as in cystic fibrosis patients; the theoretical advantages are better drug delivery and concentrations at the site of infection, improved efficacy, and better bacterial eradication when compared with systemic administration.[76] The primary concern with this therapy is the potential to develop resistant bacteria.

Results differ on the efficacy. The airways of patients with cystic fibrosis are commonly colonized with bacteria, namely *Pseudomonas aeruginosa*. Inhaled antibiotics, mainly aminoglycosides, have been used extensively in cystic fibrosis patients with good results.[56,111] Palmer and colleagues[110] reported a marked reduction in volume of airway secretions and a decrease in laboratory markers of inflammation in a prospective study of mechanically ventilated patients with chronic respiratory failure. The study, however, was not randomized.

Other studies fail to show the same benefits and show poor, unpredictable drug delivery.[105] Uneven ventilation, atelectasis, lobar collapse, and consolidation impair the even distribution of drug. Bronchospasm with chest tightness has been reported.[95] Use of inhaled antibiotics should be limited to selected patients such as those with cystic fibrosis. Routine use to assist with secretion production and clearance in the mechanically ventilated patient is not recommended.

C. VOLUME EXPANSION THERAPY

Designed to mimic the normal physiologic sighs that occur involuntarily to overcome small airway collapse, volume expansion therapies are used to promote maximal inspiratory efforts and thus maintain normal lung volume. Lung volumes can be decreased or at risk of reduction for many reasons in both nonintubated and intubated patients. Patients unable or reluctant to exhibit a strong, effective cough are at risk for retained secretions. Reduced lung volumes from decreased tidal breathing not only can impair oxygenation and predispose to hypercarbia if minute ventilation is not increased but also can lead to atelectasis. Left uncorrected, atelectasis may develop into lobar collapse, pneumonitis, and subsequent pneumonia. Common causes include recent chest or abdominal surgery or trauma, residual anesthetics or narcotic analgesics, neuromuscular disorders, and poor effort. Patients who are susceptible to atelectasis such as those with poor pain control who have sustained multiple rib fractures or undergone upper abdominal surgery and who demonstrate reduced lung volumes can be treated prophylactically or therapeutically with volume expansion therapy.

1. Incentive Spirometry

The incentive spirometer (IS) (Fig. 44-13) is designed to promote lung expansion by having the patient achieve a maximal inspiratory effort and, more important, one that is sustained. There are many techniques, but most commonly it is used with some visual feedback system incorporated into the device, such as raising a disc or a ball that the patient's effort controls. The greater and more sustained the effort, the higher and longer the ball is raised. The patient makes a maximal inspiratory effort through a mouthpiece connected to a chamber. For IS to be

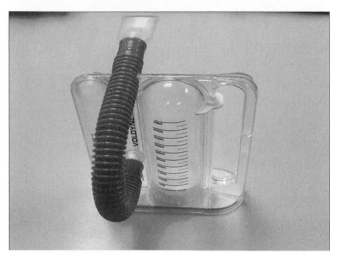

Figure 44-13 Typical incentive spirometer.

effective, proper teaching must take place. The patient must be coherent and cooperative as well as motivated. An inspiratory capacity of greater than 12 mL/kg or vital capacity greater than 14 mL/kg is a goal.[115] It is inexpensive, portable, and convenient to use as it can be used at the patient's bedside or taken on transport. When used 10 times every hour while the patient is awake, it has been shown to reduce pulmonary complications after abdominal surgery.[10] We commonly instruct patients to use the device during every commercial while watching television.

2. Intermittent Positive Pressure Breathing

Intermittent positive pressure breathing (IPPB) is generally performed by applying a face mask to the patient; when an inspiratory effort is sensed, a positive-pressure breath is delivered and lung expansion occurs. IPPB is indicated when the patient's vital capacity is less than 15 mL/kg, when other modalities such as IS have failed, or when the patient cannot or will not cooperate. Proper technique should produce results that increase the vital capacity by 100%.[115] Concerns about aerophagia, gastrointestinal insufflation, and risk of aspiration are theoretically valid in patients with altered mental status, and a more definitive means of therapy may be warranted if volume expansion cannot be achieved. IPPB is used routinely and not always justified as its utility has not been rigorously examined clinically. It is labor intensive, expensive, and usually poorly tolerated by patients.

D. INHALATION DRUG DELIVERY

The presence of an ET does not limit drug delivery to the lungs but actually may enhance it; thus, some clinicians take advantage of this route. The predominant methods used to deliver agents are with metered-dose inhalers (MDIs) or nebulizers, and the drugs they deliver are most commonly bronchodilators, mucolytics, corticosteroids, and antibiotics. Inhaled drugs achieve efficacy comparable to that of systemically delivered drugs with a smaller dose.[49,50] Administering medications by inhalation has advantages over systemic administration. Systemic side effects can be reduced as systemic absorption is minimized. Penetration and distribution of aerosol to the lower tract have been variably reported as 0% to 42% with nebulizers and 0.3% to 98% with MDIs; however, when the delivery method is standardized, the amount delivered is similar at about 15%.[46,55,58] A host of factors contribute to the overall deposition of drug in intubated patients, such as the physical characteristics of the aerosol-delivering device, ventilator settings, chemical and physical properties of medication such as particle size, humidity of inspired gas, position of the device in relation to the circuit and ET, and the anatomy of the airway.[49]

The internal diameter of the ET influences resistance to airflow and promotes turbulent flow, as discussed earlier. The smaller the diameter, the greater the resistance and the more turbulence created, especially at high airflow rates. This influences the deposition of aerosol; however, the effects can be overcome by utilizing proper technique and with different devices.[45]

Particle size plays another important role in delivery. The larger the particle, the less likely it is to be delivered to the lungs. Aerosol particles ranging between 1 and 5 μm are optimal for proper deposition to occur.[44,49,50]

The density of the gas carrying the aerosol also influences the delivery in an inverse relationship. Improvement in delivery has been reported when a mixture of helium-oxygen was used in the ventilator circuits for both MDIs and nebulizers.[63]

1. Nebulizers

The performance of a nebulizer depends on multiple factors including the model, operating pressure, flow rate, and volume of diluent utilized. Nebulizers are capable of generating aerosols with a particle size of 1 to 3 μm and the size produced is inversely influenced by the flow rate or pressure used; the greater the flow rate, the smaller the particle.[49,50] Nebulizers may be used continuously or intermittently. Intermittent use appears to be more efficient than continuous delivery with less waste of aerosol.[43] Placing the nebulizer upstream from the Y connector and ET also increases delivery.[43-45] The use of continuous nebulization may also impair the ability of the patient to initiate a negative-pressure breath in the pressure support mode of ventilation, leading to hypoventilation.[12]

2. Metered-Dose Inhalers

The medication delivered by an MDI is delivered in combination with a mixture of pressurized propellants, preservatives, flavoring agents, and surfactants. The final concentration of active drug constitutes about 1% of the total volume in the canister.[49] When the stem on the MDI canister is depressed, a finite amount of drug is released at a certain velocity and a spray cloud develops. Various adapters are available that fit in line with the ventilator circuit, such as a collapsible holding chamber (Fig. 44-14); a rigid, noncollapsible holding chamber (Fig. 44-15); or on the end of the ET, "elbow adapters." These holding chambers or spacers appear to provide better delivery or aerosol compared with the more commonly used elbow adapters.[98] MDIs cause more aerosol deposition on the ET than nebulizers. Particles can adhere in the ET. This may be alleviated by utilizing a spacer and performing the maneuver with meticulous attention to timing of the administration; it is most effective during inspiration and when synchronized with the patient's spontaneous effort. Dhand and Tobin have reported on their technique of MDI delivery with excellent results.[43]

In comparing the overall efficacy of nebulizers versus MDIs, several factors favor the use of MDIs in mechanically ventilated patients. Nebulizers may become colonized with bacteria and aerosolized inoculums. There is variability in the efficiency of the delivery systems used as well as the amount of drug delivered; thus, ventilator adjustments in inspiratory flow and tidal volume must be made to adjust for the additional nebulized flow, and they are more expensive. Indeed, Bowton and colleagues reported a potential saving of U.S. $300,000 annually when MDIs were used over nebulizers.[20]

E. OVERCOMING THE WORK OF BREATHING IMPOSED BY ENDOTRACHEAL TUBES, TRACHEOSTOMY TUBES, AND VENTILATOR CIRCUITS

As discussed previously, the ET and its characteristics place a certain physical burden on the patient that must

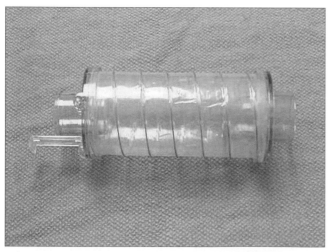

Figure 44-14 Metered-dose inhaler with collapsible holding chamber.

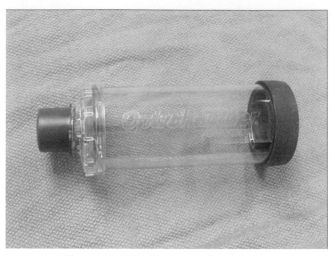

Figure 44-15 Rigid metered-dose inhaler.

be overcome. Even though the upper airway is bypassed with translaryngeal intubation and thus the resistance it imparts removed, there is still a substantial amount of work performed by the patient. The work of breathing (WOB) encompasses the efficiency of the respiratory system with regard to oxygen consumption. The greater the work, the higher the oxygen cost. WOB is minimal during normal, quiet breathing, accounting for about 5% of the oxygen consumption at rest. With increases in WOB, oxygen consumption can be markedly increased to 30% or more. This may not be tolerated in the critically ill patient. In addition to the respiratory fatigue that can result, the additional WOB (WOB_{add}) imposed by the artificial airway and ventilator apparatus not only hinders weaning and liberation from mechanical ventilation but also impairs tissue oxygenation and alters critical blood flow, which can lead to worsened organ dysfunction. In order to initiate a "breath" from the ventilator, a pressure differential across the ET, circuit, and connectors must be produced. The patient must overcome this resistance in order to initiate the demand flow needed for ventilation to occur. It has been shown experimentally that the ET, ventilator circuit, and ventilator itself all add varying degrees of additional work for the patient to overcome despite the underlying disorder that required intubation and mechanical ventilation.[16]

1. Pressure Support

Various modalities have been designed to overcome the WOB_{add} imposed by the artificial airways and ventilator. One such mode is the use of pressure support (PS) as either an adjunct or a mode of ventilation (PSV). PS is designed to aid the spontaneously breathing patient on mechanical ventilation with overcoming the resistance and thus WOB_{add} that the artificial airway and ventilator impose. It is a preset pressure chosen by the clinician that is added to the airway opening pressure when inspiration is triggered. It is flow cycled and allows the patient to control the duration and depth of inspiration as the PS ceases when some preset gas flow has diminished, usually 25% of the peak flow achieved.[94] Moreover, the patient controls his or her own ventilation as each breath is initiated by the patient and so is the minute ventilation. PS has been shown to decrease WOB_{add} with normal lungs[94,152]; however, in patients with obstructive pulmonary disease and expiratory flow limitation or auto-PEEP, flow may not decelerate quickly enough and active exhalation may be necessary to terminate the PS, creating additional WOB.[77] It is usually added as 4 to 10 cm H_2O, and it is recommended that PS be added to all spontaneously breathing patients to assist with overcoming the resistance of the ET or tracheostomy alone.[22] Additional PS may be necessary if tidal volumes or respiratory rates, or both, are not adequate. We "titrate" the PS to a certain exhaled tidal volume desired, usually 5 mL/kg of ideal body weight. Most patients tolerate PS well, but decreased tolerance in patients susceptible to expiratory flow limitation must be appreciated.

2. Continuous Positive Airway Pressure

CPAP is applied at end exhalation in spontaneously breathing patients. CPAP circuitry must initiate rapidly at the end of inhalation to maintain circuit pressure without creating additional resistance to exhalation. Much like PEEP, CPAP is designed to offset the degree of atelectasis that occurs inherently in the intubated, supine patient. CPAP should be provided for all spontaneously breathing patients, usually in 3 to 10 cm H_2O increments to compensate for this loss of expiratory lung volume and promote oxygenation. The reduction in WOB seen with CPAP alone has been appreciated primarily in the setting of expiratory airflow reduction as CPAP counters the auto-PEEP, reducing the work required to generate the next inspiration.[117] The type of flow-triggered mechanism and where the flow differential is measured, at the tracheal end of the ET, have been shown experimentally to decrease the inspiratory WOB as well.[6] CPAP is usually applied along with PS added for further benefits.

3. Automatic Tube Compensation

The ET imposes a substantial degree of resistance to inspiration, and the modalities described thus far assist with decreasing some of the work needed to overcome this burden. PS and PSV assist with compensating for the resistance primarily encountered during inhalation but not during exhalation and are not consistently provided because of the varying flow across the ET during normal breathing.[67] Much resistance is produced by the ET to exhalation. Indeed, the internal diameter of the ET greatly reduces this, but other factors such as gas flow characteristics play a role as well, not to mention secretions adherent to the ET wall. Automatic tube compensation (ATC) is a feature on some newer ventilators. It is designed to assist with the resistance imposed by the ET or tracheostomy tube during both inspiratory and expiratory phases of the respiratory cycle. By altering the PS delivered, raising it during inspiration and lowering it during expiration according to the pressure-flow characteristics of the ET, ATC adjusts for the resistance and the pressure drop across the ET during spontaneous breathing. A computer assists by calculating the pressure difference across the ET (ΔP_{ET}) after the ET size is entered into the computer, measuring gas flow and airway pressure and selecting the resistive properties of the ET.[67] ATC cannot be utilized as a ventilatory mode like PSV; it is an adjunct component to mechanical ventilation.

One drawback with ATC is its inability to correct for reductions in the airway diameter that can occur with secretions or kinking. This limitation results in an inaccurate measurement of ΔP_{ET} and ATC undercompensates for the pressure difference across the airway. A high index of suspicion is necessary to monitor for this possibility.

Clinically, ATC has been shown to decrease the WOB_{add} encountered with ETs and tracheostomy tubes.[53,68] When used to assist with weaning and extubation in patients in a T-piece trial, there was no difference in the workload encountered with ATC and T piece alone, whereas adding PS to the T-piece trial at 7 cm H_2O unloaded this additional work.[87]

REFERENCES

1. Adair CG, Gorman SP, O'Neill FB, et al: Selective decontamination of the digestive tract (SDD) does not prevent the formation of microbial biofilms on the endotracheal tubes. J Antimicrob Chemother 31:689-697, 1993.
2. American Association for Respiratory Care: AARC clinical practice guideline: Postural drainage therapy. Respir Care 36:1418-1425, 1991.
3. Andersen KH, Hald A: Assessing the position of the tracheal tube: The reliability of different methods. Anaesthesia 44:984-985, 1989.
4. Andres AH, Langenstein H: The esophageal detector device is unreliable when the stomach has been ventilated. Anesthesiology 91:566-568, 1999.
5. Anzueto A, Peters JI, Seidner SR, et al: Effects of continuous bed rotation and prolonged mechanical ventilation on healthy, adult baboons. Crit Care Med 25:1560-1564, 1997.
6. Banner MJ, Blanch PB, Kerby RR: Imposed work of breathing and methods of triggering a demand-flow, continuous positive airway pressure system. Crit Care Med 21:183-190, 1993.
7. Barash PG, Cullen BF, Stoelting RK (eds): Clinical Anesthesia, 3rd ed. Philadelphia, Lippincott-Raven, 1997.
8. Barker AF: Bronchiectasis. N Engl J Med 346:1383-1393, 2002.

9. Barnason S, Graham J, Wild MC, et al: Comparison of two endotracheal tube securement techniques on unplanned extubation, oral mucosa, and facial skin integrity. Heart Lung 27:409-417, 1998.

10. Bartlett RH: Postoperative pulmonary prophylaxis: Breathe deeply and read carefully. Chest 81:1-3, 1982.

11. Baughman RP: Diagnosis of ventilator-associated pneumonia. Microbes Infect January 4, 2005 [Epub ahead of print].

12. Beaty CD, Ritz RH, Benson MS: Continuous in-line nebulizers complicate pressure support ventilation. Chest 96:1360-1363, 1989.

13. Bennett WD: Effect of β-adrenergic agonists on mucociliary clearance. J Allergy Clin Immunol 110: S291-S297, 2002.

14. Berra L, De Marchi L, Panigada M, et al: Evaluation of continuous aspiration of subglottic secretion in an in vivo study. Crit Care Med 32:2071-2078, 2004.

15. Berra L, De Marchi L, Yu ZX, et al: Endotracheal tubes coated with antiseptics decrease bacterial colonization of the ventilator circuits, lungs, and endotracheal tube. Anesthesiology 100:1446-1456, 2004.

16. Bersten AD, Rutten AJ, Vedig AE, et al: Additional work of breathing imposed by endotracheal tubes, breathing circuits, and intensive care ventilators. Crit Care Med 17:671-677, 1989.

17. Birnkrant D, Pope J, Lewarski J, et al: Persistent pulmonary consolidation treated with intrapulmonary percussive ventilation: A preliminary report. Pediatr Pulmonol 21:246-249, 1996.

18. Bishop MJ, Weymuller EA, Fink BR: Laryngeal effects of prolonged intubation. Anesth Analg 63:335, 1984.

19. Bolder PM, Healy TE, Bolder AR, et al: The extra work of breathing through adult endotracheal tubes. Anesth Analg 65:853, 1986.

20. Bowton DL, Goldsmith WM, Haponik EF: Substitution of metered-dose inhalers for hand-held nebulizers: Success and cost savings in a large, acute-care hospital. Chest 101:305-308, 1992.

21. British Thoracic Society Research Committee: Oral N-acetylcysteine and exacerbation rates in patients with chronic bronchitis and severe airway obstruction. Thorax 40:832-835, 1985.

22. Brochard L, Rua F, Lorino H, et al: Inspiratory pressure support compensates for the additional work of breathing caused by the endotracheal tube. Anesthesiology 75: 739-745, 1991.

23. Bryce DP, Briant TD, Pearson FG: Laryngeal and tracheal complications of intubation. Ann Otol Rhinol Laryngol 77:442, 1968.

24. Carrion MI, Ayuso D, Marcos M, et al: Accidental removal of endotracheal and nasogastric tubes and intravascular catheters. Crit Care Med 28:63-66, 2000.

25. Chastre J, Fagon JY: Ventilator-associated pneumonia. Am J Respir Crit Care Med 165:867-903, 2002.

26. Chevron V, Menard JF, Richard JC, et al: Unplanned extubation: Risk factors of development and predictive criteria for reintubation. Crit Care Med 26:1049-1053, 1998.

27. Chiaranda M, Verona L, Pinamonti O, et al: Use of heat and moisture exchangers filters in mechanically ventilated ICU patients: Influence on airway flow resistance. Intensive Care Med 19:462-466, 1993.

28. Clarke T, Evans S, Way P, et al: A comparison of two methods of securing an endotracheal tube. Aust Crit Care 11:45-50, 1998.

29. Clemmer RP, Green S, Ziegler B: Effectiveness of the kinetic treatment table for preventing and treating pulmonary complications in severely head-injured patients. Crit Care Med 18:614-617, 1990.

30. Condon HA, Gilchrist E: Stanley Rowbotham: Twentieth century pioneer anaesthetist. Anaesthesia 41:46-52, 1986.

31. Cook RT, Moglia BB, Consevage NW, et al: The use of the Beck Airway Airflows Monitor for verifying intratracheal endotracheal tube placement in patients in the pediatric emergency department and intensive care unit. Pediatr Emerg Care 12:331-332, 1996.

32. Cook RT, Stene JK, Marcolina B: Use of a Beck Airway Airflow Monitor and controllable-tip endotracheal tube in two cases on nonlaryngoscopic oral intubation. Am J Emerg Med 13:180-183, 1995.

33. Cook RT, Stene JK: The BAAM and endotrol endotracheal tube for blind oral intubation. Beck Airway Air Flow Monitor. J Clin Anesth 5:431-432, 1993.

34. Coppolo DP, May JJ: Self-extubations: A 12-month experience. Chest 98:165-169, 1990.

35. Cox CS, Zwischenberger JB, Traber DL, et al: Heparin improves oxygenation and minimizes barotraumas after severe smoke inhalation in an ovine model. Surg Gynecol Obstet 176:339-349, 1993.

36. Cozine K, Rosenbaum LM, Askanazi J, Rosenbaum SH: Laser-induced endotracheal tube fire. Anesthesiology 55:553-583, 1981.

37. Davis B, Marin MG, Yee JW, et al: Effect of terbutaline on movement of Cl⁻ and Na⁺ across the trachea of the dog. Am Rev Respir Dis 120:547-552, 1979.

38. Demers RR: Complications of endotracheal suctioning procedures. Respir Care 27:453-435, 1982.

39. Demers RR, Sullivan MJ, Paliotta J: Airflow resistance of endotracheal tubes. JAMA 237:1362, 1977.

40. Desmond K, Schwenk F, Thomas E, et al: Immediate and long term effects of chest physiotherapy in cystic fibrosis. J Pediatr 103:538-542, 1983.

41. DeVries N, DeFlora S: N-Acetyl-1-cysteine. J Cell Biochem 17F:S270-S277, 1993.

42. Dezfulian C, Shojania K, Collard HR, et al: Subglottic secretion drainage for preventing ventilatory-associated pneumonia: A meta-analysis. Am J Med 118:11-18, 2005.

43. Dhand R, Tobin MJ: Bronchodilator delivery with metered-dose inhalers in mechanically-ventilated patients. Eur Respir J 9:585-595, 1996.

44. Dhand R, Tobin MJ: Inhaled bronchodilator therapy in mechanically ventilated patients. Am J Respir Crit Care Med 156:3-10, 1997.

45. Dhand R: Special problems in aerosol delivery: Artificial airways. Respir Care 45:636-645, 2000.

46. Diot P, Morra L, Smaldone GC: Albuterol delivery in a model of mechanical ventilation: Comparison of metered-dose inhaler and nebulizer efficiency. Am J Respir Crit Care Med 152:1391-1394, 1995.

47. Drakulovic MB, Torres A, Bauer TT, et al: Supine position as a risk factor for nosocomial pneumonia in

mechanically ventilated patients: A randomized trial. Lancet 354:1851-1858, 1999.

48. Dreyfuss D, Djedaini K, Gros I, et al: Mechanical ventilation with heated humidifiers or heat and moisture exchanges: Effects on patient colonization and incidence of nosocomial pneumonia. Am J Respir Crit Care Med 151:986-992, 1995.

49. Duarte AG, Dhand R, Reid R, et al: Serum albuterol levels in mechanically ventilated patients and healthy subjects after metered-dose inhaler administration. Am J Respir Crit Care Med 154:1658-1663, 1996.

50. Duarte AG, Fink JB, Dhand R: Inhalation therapy during mechanical ventilation. Respir Care Clin North Am 7:233-260, 2001.

51. Emergency Care Research Institute: Heat and moisture exchangers. Health Devices 12:155, 1983.

52. Fabry B, Hapeerthur C, Zappe, et al: Breathing pattern and additional work of breathing in spontaneously breathing patients with different ventilatory demands during inspiratory pressure support and automatic tube compensation. Intensive Care Med 23:545-552, 1997.

53. Fernandez A, Lazaro A, Garcia A, et al: Bronchodilators in patients with chronic obstructive pulmonary disease on mechanical ventilation: Utilization of metered-dose inhalers. Am Rev Respir Dis 141:164-168, 1990.

54. Fink JB, Dhand R, Duarte AG, et al: Deposition of aerosol from metered-dose inhaler during mechanical ventilation: An in vitro model. Am J Respir Crit Care Med 154:382-387, 1996.

55. Frederiksen B, Koch C, Hoiby N: Antibiotic treatment of initial colonization with *Pseudomonas aeruginosa* postpones chronic infection and prevents deterioration of pulmonary function in cystic fibrosis patients. Pediatr Pulmonol 23:330-335, 1997.

56. Fuller HD, Dolovich MB, Posmituck G, et al: Pressurized aerosol versus jet aerosol delivery to mechanically ventilated patients: Comparison of dose to the lungs. Am Rev Respir Dis 141:440-444, 1990.

57. Gal TJ, Suratt PM: Resistance to breathing in healthy subjects following endotracheal intubation under topical anesthesia. Anesth Analg 59:270, 1980.

58. Gelman JJ, Aro M, Weiss SM: Tracheo-innominate artery fistula. J Am Coll Surg 179:626-634, 1994.

59. Goldberg JS, Rawle PR, Zehnder JL, et al: Colorimetric end-tidal carbon dioxide monitoring for tracheal intubation. Anesth Analg 70:191-194, 1990.

60. Gondor M, Nixon PA, Mutich R, et al: Comparison of Flutter device and chest physical therapy in the treatment of cystic fibrosis pulmonary exacerbation. Pediatr Pulmonol 28:255-260, 1999.

61. Goode ML, Fink JB, Dhand R, et al: Improvement in aerosol delivery with helium-oxygen mixtures in mechanical ventilation. Am J Respir Crit Care Med 163:109-114, 2001.

62. Goodman LR, Conrardy PA, Laing F, et al: Radiographic evaluation of endotracheal tube position. AJR Am J Roentgenol 127:433-434, 1976.

63. Grap MJ, Cantley M, Munro CL, et al: Use of backrest elevation in critical care: A pilot study. Am J Crit Care 8:475-480, 1999.

64. Grenvik A, Ayres SM, Holbrook PR, Shoemaker WC (eds): Textbook of Critical Care, 4th ed. Philadelphia, WB Saunders, 2000.

65. Guttman J, Haberthur C, Mois G: Automatic tube compensation. Respir Care Clin North Am 7:475-471, 2001.

66. Haberthur C, Fabry B, Stocker R, et al: Additional inspiratory work of breathing imposed by tracheostomy tubes and non-ideal ventilator properties in critically ill patients. Intensive Care Med 25:514-519, 1999.

67. Harrison GA, Tonkin JP: Prolonged endotracheal intubation. Br J Anaesth 40:241, 1968.

68. Hawkins DB: Glottic and subglottic stenosis from endotracheal intubation. Laryngoscope 87:339, 1977.

69. Henschke CI, Yankelevitz DF, Wand A, et al: Accuracy and efficacy of chest radiography in the intensive care unit. Radiol Clin North Am 34:21-31, 1996.

70. Hermens JM, Bennett MJ, Hirschman CA: Anesthesia for laser surgery. Anesth Analg 62:218-229, 1983.

71. Hilding AC: Laryngotracheal damage during intratracheal anesthesia. Ann Otol Rhinol Laryngol 80:565, 1971.

72. Hill BB, Zweng TN, Maley RH, et al: Percutaneous dilational tracheostomy. J Trauma 41:238-244, 1996.

73. Homnick D, Shite F, deCatro C: Comparison of effects of an intrapulmonary percussive ventilator to standard aerosol and chest physiotherapy in treatment of cystic fibrosis. Pediatr Pulmonol 20:50-55, 1995.

74. Itokazu GS, Weinstein RA: Aerosolized antibiotics: Another look. Crit Care Med 26:5-6, 1998.

75. Jubran A, Van de Graaff WB, Tobin MJ: Variability of patient-ventilator interaction with pressure support ventilation in patients with chronic obstructive pulmonary disease. Am J Respir Crit Care Med 152:129-136, 1995.

76. Kasper CL, Deem S: The self-inflating bulb to detect esophageal intubation during emergency airway management. Anesthesiology 88:898-902, 1998.

77. Kearl RA, Hooper RG: Massive airway leaks: An analysis of the role of endotracheal tubes. Crit Care Med 21:518-521, 1993.

78. Kelly GS: Clinical applications of N-acetylcysteine. Altern Med Rev 3:114-127, 1998.

79. Kollef MH, Prentice D, Shapiro SD, et al: Mechanical ventilation with or without daily changes of in-line suction catheters. Am J Respir Crit Care Mcd 156:466-472, 1997.

80. Kollef MH, Shapiro SD, Fraser VJ, et al: Mechanical ventilation with or without 7-day circuit changes. Ann Intern Med 123:168-174, 1995.

81. Kollef MH, Skubas NJ, Sundt TM: A randomized clinical trial of continuous aspiration of subglottic secretions in cardiac surgery patients. Chest 116:1155-1156, 1999.

82. Kollef MH, Shapiro SD, Boyd V, et al: A randomized clinical trial comparing an extended-use hygroscopic condenser humidifier with heated-water humidification in mechanically ventilated patients. Chest 113:759-767, 1998.

83. Kolobow T, Tsuno K, Rossi N, et al: Design and development of ultrathin-walled, nonkinking endotracheal tubes of a new "no-pressure" laryngeal seal design—A preliminary report. Anesthesiology 81:1061-1067, 1994.

84. Konstan M, Stern R, Doershuk C: Efficacy of the Flutter device for airway mucus clearance in patients with cystic fibrosis. J Pediatr 124:689-693, 1994.

85. Kuhlen R, Max M, Dembinski R, et al: Breathing pattern and workload during automatic tube compensation, pressure support and T-piece trials in weaning patients. Eur J Anaesthesiol 20:10-16, 2003.

86. Lang DJ, Wafai Y, Salem MR, et al.: Efficacy of the self-inflating bulb in confirming tracheal intubation in the morbidly obese. Anesthesiology 85:246-253, 1996.

87. Langenderfer B: Alternatives to percussion and postural drainage. J Cardiopulm Rehabil 18:283-289, 1998.

88. Leigh JM, Maynard JP: Pressure on the tracheal mucosa from cuffed tubes. Br Med J 1:1173-1174, 1979.

89. Levy H, Griego L: A comparative study of oral endotracheal tube securing methods. Chest 104:1537-1540, 1993.

90. Lotano R, Gerber D, Aseron C, et al: Utility of postintubation radiographs in the intensive care unit. Crit Care 4:50-53, 2000.

91. Macewen W: Report. Br Med J 2:122, 1880.

92. MacIntyre NR: Respiratory function during pressure support ventilation. Chest 89:677-683, 1986.

93. Maddison J, Dodd M, Webb AK: Nebulized colistin causes chest tightness in adults with cystic fibrosis. Respir Med 88:145-147, 1994.

94. Mahlmeister M, Fink J, Hoffman G, et al: Positive-expiratory-pressure mask therapy: Theoretical and practical considerations and a review of the literature. Respir Care 36:1218-1229, 1991.

95. Mahul P, Auboyer C, Jospe R, et al: Prevention of nosocomial pneumonia in intubated patients: Respective role of mechanical subglottic secretions drainage and stress ulcer prophylaxis. Intensive Care Med 18:20-25, 1992.

96. Manthous CA, Chatila W, Schmidt GA, et al: Treatment of bronchospasm by a metered-dose inhaler albuterol in mechanically ventilated patients. Chest 107:210-213, 1995.

97. Martin C, Papazian L, Perrin G, et al: Performance evaluation of three vaporizing humidifiers and two heat and moisture exchangers in patients with minute ventilation > 10L/min. Chest 102:1347-1350, 1992.

98. Martin C, Perrin G, Gevaudan M, et al: Heat and moisture exchangers in the intensive care unit. Chest 97:144-149, 1990.

99. Matsushima Y, Jones R, King E, et al: Alterations in pulmonary mechanics and gas exchange during routine fiberoptic bronchoscopy. Chest 86:184, 1984.

100. Mehta S: Transtracheal illumination for optimal tracheal tube placement: A clinical study. Anaesthesia 44:970-972, 1989.

101. Miller AB, Pavia D, Agnew JE, et al: Effect of oral N-acetylcysteine on mucus clearance. Br J Dis Chest 79:262-266, 1985.

102. Mortensen J, Falk M, Groth S, et al: Effects of postural drainage and positive expiratory pressure physiotherapy on tracheobronchial clearance in cystic fibrosis. Chest 100:1350-1357, 1991.

103. Mukhopadhyay S, Staddon GE, Eastman C, et al: The quantitative distribution of nebulized antibiotic in the lung in cystic fibrosis. Respir Med 88:203-211, 1994.

104. Muzzi DA, Losasso TJ, Cucchiara RF: Complication from a nasopharyngeal airway in a patient with a basilar skull fracture. Anesthesiology 74:366-368, 1991.

105. Oberwalder B, Evans JC, Zach MS: Forced expirations against a variable resistance: A new chest physiotherapy method in cystic fibrosis. Pediatr Pulmonol 2:358-367, 1986.

106. Ornato JP, Garnett AR, Glauser FL: Relationship between cardiac output and the end-tidal carbon dioxide tension. Ann Emerg Med 19:1104-1106, 1990.

107. Owens RL, Cheney F: Endobronchial intubation: A preventable complication. Anesthesiology 67:255-257, 1987.

108. Pacheco-Fowler V, Gaonkar T, Wyer PC, Modak S: Antiseptic impregnated endotracheal tubes for the prevention of bacterial colonization. J Hosp Infect 57:170-174, 2004.

109. Pai VB, Nahata MC: Efficacy and safety of aerosolized tobramycin in cystic fibrosis. Pediatr Pulmonol 32:314-327, 2001.

110. Palmer LB, Smaldone GC, Simon SR, et al: Aerosolized antibiotics in mechanically ventilated patients: Delivery and response. Crit Care Med 26:31-39, 1998.

111. Pappas JN, Goodman PC: Predicting proper endotracheal tube placement in underexposed radiographs: Tangent line of the aortic arch. AJR Am J Roentgenol 173:1357-1359, 1999.

112. Pattnaik SK, Bodra R: Ballotability of cuff to confirm the correct intratracheal position of the endotracheal tube in the intensive care unit. Eur J Anaesthesiol 17:587-590, 2000.

113. Peruzzi WT, Smith B: Bronchial hygiene therapy. Crit Care Clin 11:79-96, 1995.

114. Puntervoll SA, Søreide E, Jacewicz W, et al: Rapid detection of oesophageal intubation: Take care when using colorimetric capnometry. Acta Anaesthesiol Scand 46:455-457, 2002.

115. Ranieri VM, Grasso S, Fiore T, et al: Auto-positive end-expiratory pressure and dynamic hyperinflation. Clin Chest Med 17:379-395, 1996.

116. Rao S, Wilson DW, Brooks RA: Acute effects of nebulization of N-acetylcysteine on pulmonary mechanics and gas exchange. Am Rev Respir Dis 102:17-22, 1970.

117. Raphael, DT: Acoustic reflectometry profiles of endotracheal and esophageal intubation. Anesthesiology 92:1293-1299, 2000.

118. Rasmussen JB, Glennow C: Reduction in days of illness after long-term treatment with N-acetylcysteine controlled-release tablets in patients with chronic bronchitis. Eur Respir J 1:351-355, 1988.

119. Reed DB, Clinton JE: Proper depth of placement of nasotracheal tubes in adults prior to radiographic confirmation. Acad Emerg Med 4:1111-1114, 1997.

120. Reisman J, Rivington-Law B, Corey M, et al: Role of conventional therapy in cystic fibrosis. J Pediatr 113:632-636, 1988.

121. Ricard JD, Le Miere E, Markowicz P, et al: Efficiency and safety of mechanical ventilation with a heat and moisture exchanger changed only once a week. Am J Respir Crit Care Med 161:104-109, 2000.

122. Ricard JD, Markowicz P, Djedaini K, et al: Bedside evaluation of efficient airway humidification during mechanical ventilation of the critically ill. Chest 115:1646-1652, 1999.

123. Ring WH, Adair JC, Elwyn RA: A new pediatric endotracheal tube. Anesth Analg 54:273-274, 1975

124. Roberts JR, Spadafora M, Cone DC: Proper depth placement of oral endotracheal tubes in adults prior to radiographic confirmation. Acad Emerg Med 2:20-24, 1995.

125. Sahn SA, Lakshminarayan S, Petty TL: Weaning from mechanical ventilation. JAMA 235:2208, 1976.

126. Salem MR: Verification of endotracheal tube position. Anesthesiol Clin North Am 19:813-839, 2001.

127. Schwartz DE, Lieberman JA, Cohen NH: Women are at a greater risk than men for malpositioning of the endotracheal tube after emergent intubation. Crit Care Med 22:1127-1131, 1994.

128. Schwartz DE, Matthay MA, Cohen NH: Death and other complications of emergency airway management in critically ill adults: A prospective investigation of 297 tracheal intubations. Anesthesiology 82:367-376, 1995.

129. Scott LR, Benson MS, Bishop MJ: Relationship of endotracheal tube size to auto-PEEP at high minute ventilation. Respir Care 31:1080, 1986.

130. Seegobin RD, van Hasselt GL: Endotracheal cuff pressure and tracheal mucosal blood flow: Endoscopic study of effects of four large volume cuffs. Br Med J 288:965-968, 1984.

131. Shapiro BA: Chest physical therapy administered by respiratory therapists. Respir Care 26:655-656, 1981.

132. Sim WS, Chung IS, Chin JU, et al: Risk factors for epistaxis during nasotracheal intubation. Anaesth Intensive Care 30:449-452, 2002.

133. Skinner MW, Waldron, RJ, Anderson MB: Normal laryngoscopy and intubation. In Hanowell LH, Waldron RJ (eds): Airway Management. Philadelphia, Lippincott-Raven, 1996, pp 81-96.

134. Smilkstein MJ, Knapp GL, Kulig KW, et al: Efficacy of oral N-acetylcysteine in the treatment of acetaminophen overdose. Analysis of the national multicenter study (1976-1985). N Engl J Med 319:1557-1562, 1988.

135. Sois M, Dillon F: What is the safest foil tape for endotracheal tube protection during Nd-YAG laser surgery? A comparative study. Anesthesiology 72:553, 1990

136. Sole ML, Poalillo FE, Byers JF, et al: Bacterial growth in secretions and on suctioning equipment of orally intubated patients: A pilot study. Am J Crit Care 11:141-149, 2002.

137. Sosis MB, Dillon FX: Saline-filled cuffs help prevent laser-induced polyvinylchloride endotracheal tube fires. Anesth Analg 72:187, 1991

138. Sosis MB: Hazards of laser surgery. Semin Anesth 9:90, 1990

139. Stamm AM: Ventilator-associated pneumonia and frequency of circuit changes. Am J Infect Control 26:71-73, 1998.

140. Steen JA: Impact of tube design and materials on complications of tracheal intubation. In Bishop MJ (ed): Physiology and Consequences of Tracheal Intubation: Problems in Anesthesia, vol 2(2). Philadelphia, JB Lippincott, 1988, pp 211-223.

141. Stenqvist O, Sonander H, Nilsson K: Small endotracheal tubes: Ventilator and intratracheal pressures during controlled ventilation. Br J Anaesth 51:375, 1979.

142. Stone DJ, Bogdonoff DL: Airway considerations in the management of patients requiring long-term endotracheal intubation. Anesth Analg 74:276, 1992.

143. Stout DM, Bishop MJH, Dwersteg JF, et al: Correlation of endotracheal tube size with sore throat and hoarseness following general anesthesia. Anesthesiology 67:419, 1987.

144. Sullivan M, Paliotta J, Saklad M: Endotracheal tube as a factor in measurement of respiratory mechanics. J Appl Physiol 41:590, 1976.

145. Tanigawa K, Takeda T, Goto E, et al: Accuracy and reliability of the self-inflating bulb to verify tracheal intubation in out-of-hospital cardiac arrest patients. Anesthesiology 93:1432-1436, 2000.

146. Tanigawa K, Takeda T, Goto E, et al: The efficacy of esophageal detector devices in verifying tracheal tube placement: A randomized cross-over study of out-of-hospital cardiac arrest patients. Anesth Analg 92:375-378, 2001.

147. Tasaki O, Mozingo DW, Dubick MA, et al: Effects of heparin and lisofylline on pulmonary function after smoke inhalation injury in an ovine model. Crit Care Med 30:637-643, 2002.

148. Tepel M, Van Der Giet M, Schwarzfeld C, et al: Prevention of radiographic-contrast-agent-induced reductions in renal function by acetylcysteine. N Engl J Med 343:180-184, 2000.

149. Tindol GA, DiBenedetto RJ, Kosciuk L: Unplanned extubation. Chest 105:1804-1807, 1994.

150. Tomkiewicz RP, App EM, Coffiner M, et al: Mucolytic treatment with N-acetylcysteine L-lysinate metered dose inhaler in dogs: Airway epithelial changes. Eur Respir J 7:81-87, 1994.

151. Tomkiewicz RP, App EM, De Sanctis GT, et al: A comparison of a new mucolytic N-acetylcysteine L-lysinate with N-acetylcysteine: Airway epithelial changes and mucus changes in dog. Pulm Pharmacol 8:259-265, 1995.

152. Tomkiewicz RP, Biviji A, King M: Rheologic studies regarding high-frequency chest compressions (HFCC) and improvement of mucus clearance in cystic fibrosis [abstract]. Am J Respir Crit Care Med 149:A669, 1994.

153. Villafane MC, Cinnella G, Lofaso F, et al: Gradual reduction of endotracheal tube diameter during mechanical ventilation via different humidification devices. Anesthesiology 85:1341-1349, 1996.

154. Wanner A, Salathe M, O'Riordan TG: Mucociliary clearance in the airways. Am J Respir Crit Care Med 154:1868-1902, 1996.

155. Warwick W, Hansen L: Long-term effect of high-frequency chest compression therapy on pulmonary complications of cystic fibrosis. Pediatr Pulmonol 11:265-271, 1991.

156. Watson WF: Development of the PVC endotracheal tube. Biomaterials 1:41-46, 1980.

157. White G: Equipment Theory for Respiratory Care. Albany, NY, Delmar, 1996.

158. Wong J, Keens T, Wannamaker E, et al: Effects of gravity in tracheal transport rates in normal subjects and in patients with cystic fibrosis. Pediatrics 60:146-152, 1977.

159. Wright PE, Marini JJ, Bernard GR: In vitro versus in vivo comparison of endotracheal airflow resistance. Am Rev Respir Dis 140:10, 1989.

45

MECHANICAL VENTILATION

Atul Malhotra
Robert M. Kacmarek

I. INTRODUCTION

Support of cardiopulmonary function with mechanical ventilation has traditionally involved intermittent application of positive pressure to the patient's airway. With early ventilatory support techniques, the patient was essentially a passive recipient. Patients often tried to breathe against the ventilator, leading to the well-known phrase "fighting the ventilator." As a result, patients frequently required substantial sedation and neuromuscular relaxation. Subsequent developments in mechanical ventilatory support in the past 20 to 30 years have allowed a more active role for the patient. Although newer techniques reflect important differences in the interaction between patient and ventilator, they still involve manipulation of airway pressure depending on respiratory mechanics. Also of note, in the past 10 years, there has been mounting evidence that the ventilator itself can be injurious to the lung if not applied carefully. Thus, a number of strategies have evolved to maximize patient-ventilator synchrony and to minimize ventilator-induced lung injury (VILI).

Safe application of mechanical ventilatory support depends on the knowledge of normal and abnormal lung mechanics and cardiopulmonary relationships in health and disease and an understanding of the mechanisms and limitations of modes of ventilation provided by modern ventilators.

II. PHYSIOLOGIC CONSIDERATIONS

A. MECHANICS OF BREATHING (Fig. 45-1)

Inspiration occurs when a pressure differential is created between the airway opening and alveolus. During spontaneous inspiration, diaphragmatic contraction decreases pleural pressure, thereby creating a pressure differential by dropping alveolar pressure below airway opening pressure. During passive mechanical ventilation, a pressure differential is created by application of positive pressure at the airway opening. In either case, the distending or transpulmonary pressure (PTP)

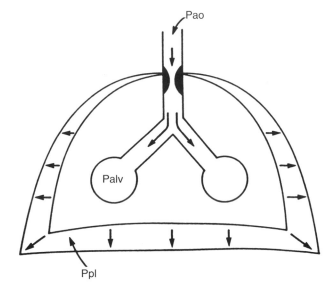

Figure 45-1 Pressures relevant to inflation of the chest and lung during passive positive-pressure ventilation. Inspiration occurs as a result of difference in airway opening pressure P_{ao} minus visceral pleural surface pressure P_{pl}. (From Perel A, Stock C: Handbook of Mechanical Ventilatory Support. Baltimore, Williams & Wilkins, 1992.)

(pressure at the airway opening [P_{ao}] minus pleural pressure [P_{pl}])

$$PTP = P_{ao} - P_{pl}$$

is increased.[94] The magnitude of change in PTP and the rate of the change determine both tidal volume (V_T) and inspiratory gas flow ($\dot{V}$). For a given PTP, the resultant V_T depends on the respiratory system compliance and resistance. Distensibility of the respiratory system can be quantified by calculating compliance (C), the change in volume (ΔV) divided by the change in pressure (ΔP):

$$C = \Delta V / \Delta P$$

The reciprocal of compliance is elastance ($\Delta P / \Delta V$). The sum of 1 over the compliance of the lungs (C_L) and 1 over the compliance of the thorax (C_T) equals 1 over the compliance of the respiratory system (C_{RS}). In other words, the elastances of the chest wall and lung sum to be the elastance of the respiratory system because the changes in volume of the lung and chest wall (in the denominator of the elastance equation) are equal. Each of the three compliances can be calculated by measuring the change in distending or transstructural pressure and the associated change in volume:

$$C_L = \Delta V / \Delta P_{(ao-pl)}$$

$$C_L = \Delta V / \Delta P_{(pl-bs)}$$

$$C_{RS} = \Delta V / \Delta P_{(ao-bs)}$$

where P_{bs} is the pressure at the surface of the thorax (body surface pressure).[94]

Under quasistatic conditions (i.e., negligible airflow resistance), pressure is required only to oppose the elastic recoil of the respiratory system. During inspiration, pressure must also be generated to overcome frictional or viscous forces. The ratio of this additional pressure (P) to the rate of airway flow that it produces ($\dot{V}$) is defined as the airway resistance (R_{aw}).

$$R_{aw} = \Delta P / \dot{V}$$

Resistance to gas flow increases when laminar flow becomes turbulent or airway diameter decreases.[94] The ΔPTP required to produce a given V_T is similar whether generated by spontaneous breathing or mechanical ventilation. However, the distribution of inspired gas varies. The regional distribution of P_{pl} is primarily the result of gravitational forces and is influenced by the effect of gravity on both the lung and the thorax and by the relative compliance of each structure.[124] Pleural pressure and alveolar pressure are determined by the static recoil of the lung. Regional inequalities in the distribution of inspired gas between dependent and nondependent regions can be explained as the combined effect of the curvilinear volume-pressure (compliance) curve and the existence of a pleural pressure gradient (Fig. 45-2).[124]

At functional residual capacity (FRC), PTP in dependent alveoli is low, and they operate on the steep portion of the volume-pressure curve. During inspiration, the proportional change in PTP is greater in the dependent than the nondependent regions of the lung; thus, these alveoli receive the bulk of ventilation. Blood flow is greatest in the dependent regions, thus allowing optimal matching of perfusion to ventilation (Fig. 45-3).[124] When inspiration occurs from a lung volume less than FRC, preferential ventilation of nondependent alveoli occurs because of a functional shift of the compliance curve. As FRC declines, dependent alveoli assume lower compliance characteristics. This model is commonly employed to illustrate regional inhomogeneities of ventilation, but it assumes that the entire lung is isoelastic and the magnitude of pleural pressure swings during inspiration is uniform.

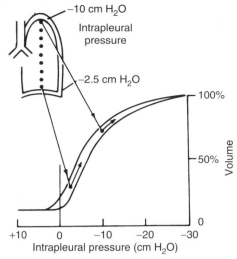

Figure 45-2 An explanation of the regional differences of ventilation down the lung. Because of the weight of the lung, intrapleural pressure is less negative at the base than at the apex. As a consequence, the basal lung is relatively compressed in its resting state but expands better on inspiration than the apex. (From West JB: Ventilation/Blood Flow and Gas Exchange, 4th ed. Oxford, Blackwell, 1985.)

Although these assumptions may not always be valid, the model provides a useful description of inspiration.

During spontaneous ventilation in the supine position, there is greater displacement of the dependent (posterior) portion of the diaphragm, resulting in greater swings in pleural pressure over dependent regions than over the nondependent zones (Fig. 45-4).[102] Therefore, preferential distribution of inspired gas to dependent lung regions results not only from a more favorable

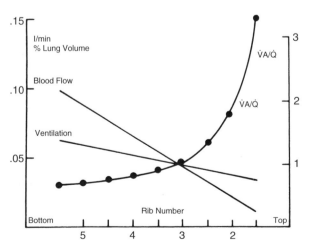

Figure 45-3 Distribution of ventilation and blood flow down the upright lung. Note that greatest blood flow and ventilation are located at bottom of lung. Note that ventilation-perfusion ratio ($\dot{V}A/\dot{Q}$) decreases down the lung. (From West JB: Ventilation/Blood Flow and Gas Exchange, 4th ed. Oxford, Blackwell, 1985.)

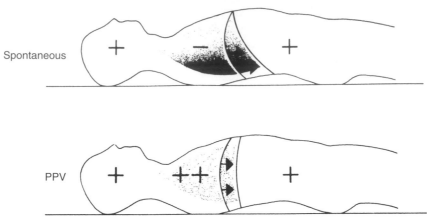

Figure 45-4 Spontaneous ventilation provides optimal distribution of ventilation in relation to perfusion because of mechanics of spontaneously contracting diaphragm. In addition, venous return is optimized because intra-abdominal and intracranial pressures are more positive than intrathoracic pressures. Positive-pressure ventilation (PPV) results in greater air distribution to non–gravity-dependent portions of lung and potentially hinders venous return because intrathoracic pressure is more positive than intra-abdominal or intracranial pressure. (From Shapiro BA, Kacmarek RM, Cane RD, et al: Clinical Application of Respiratory Care, 4th ed. Baltimore, Mosby–Year Book, 1991.)

pulmonary compliance but also from a more subatmospheric pleural pressure.[102] During positive-pressure ventilation (PPV), the nondependent (anterior) part of the diaphragm is displaced more than the posterior portion, favoring gas distribution primarily to nondependent lung regions. This redistribution of inspired gas appears to be unrelated to the rate of gas flow. As a consequence of altered gas distribution with mechanical ventilation, ventilation and perfusion are less well matched than during spontaneous ventilation.

B. ALVEOLAR TIME CONSTANTS (Fig. 45-5)

Alveolar time constants (τ), the product of compliance and resistance, describe the time required for alveolar filling or emptying to occur. Alveolar ventilation follows a wash-in/wash-out exponential function; one time constant (1τ) is associated with an exchange of 63% of the alveolar volume, 2τ with 86.5% exchange, 3τ with 95% exchange, and 4τ with 98% exchange.[89]

In pathologic lung states, gas distribution is altered to a greater extent than in normal lungs as a result of compliance inhomogeneity. To improve distribution of ventilation, a slow sustained inflation permits gas to distribute to slow alveoli and so tends to distribute gas in relation to the compliance of the different functional units.[89] Distribution of inspired gas depends on the rate, duration, and frequency of inspiration. As the respiratory rate increases, the inspiratory and expiratory times become increasingly shorter. Slower filling alveoli may not fill or empty properly, leading to uneven distribution of ventilation.[89]

C. CARDIOPULMONARY COUPLING (Fig. 45-6)

The pulmonary system affects cardiovascular function primarily by variation in venous return. In steady state, conservation of mass requires that venous return is equivalent to cardiac output. Venous return to the right atrium depends on the transthoracic vascular pressure, that is, the difference between mean circulatory filling pressure and transmural right atrial pressure. Transmural right atrial pressure is the difference between atrial pressure and pericardial (cardiac surface) pressure. When the pericardium does not limit diastolic filling, pleural pressure can be used to estimate pericardial pressure.[94] Pleural pressure is normally subatmospheric at FRC because of the balance of forces between chest wall recoil outward and lung recoil inward. Any change in these forces alters the intrapleural pressure and the transthoracic vascular pressure.

During spontaneous inhalation, intrapleural pressure decreases from an average of −3 cm H_2O to −6 to −10 cm H_2O in reference to atmospheric pressure, resulting in dilatation of the intrathoracic vasculature. This dilatation produces an immediate decrease in intrathoracic vena caval, pulmonary arterial, and aortic pressures. Left ventricular output and the systemic arterial pressure decrease because of the increased left ventricular afterload. As transthoracic vascular pressure increases, venous return increases, and right ventricular stroke volume increases through Frank-Starling mechanisms. At end inspiration, the pulmonary arterial and aortic pressures and the cardiac output decline as venous blood flow increases and fills the expanded pulmonary vasculature. During spontaneous exhalation, intrapleural pressure and pulmonary artery blood flow return to baseline, cardiac output and systemic

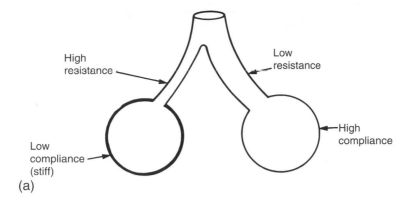

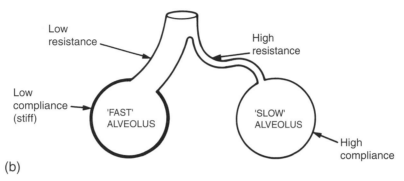

Figure 45-5 Schematic diagrams of alveoli illustrate conditions under which static and dynamic compliances may differ. In idealized state (a) that is probably not realized even in the healthy subject, the reciprocal relationship between resistance and compliance results in gas flow that is preferentially delivered to the most compliant regions regardless of rate of inflation. Static and dynamic compliances are equal. In a state that is typical of many patients with respiratory disease (b), alveoli can conveniently be divided into fast and slow groups. A direct relationship between compliance and resistance results in inspired gas being preferentially delivered to stiff alveoli if the rate of inflation is rapid. An end-inspiratory pause then permits redistribution from fast alveoli to slow alveoli. (From Nunn JF: Nunn's Applied Respiratory Physiology, 4th ed. Oxford, Butterworth-Heinemann, 1993).

arterial pressure increase, and pulmonary vascular capacitance diminishes.[94] Thus, cardiac output and systemic arterial pressure fluctuate with breathing pattern, reflecting phasic alterations in blood flow to and from the thorax. This process is reversed during positive-pressure breathing. Overall, positive-pressure breathing decreases the transthoracic vascular pressure, venous inflow, right ventricular stroke volume, left ventricular stroke volume, and cardiac output.[94] The magnitude of the impact of positive airway pressure on cardiovascular function depends on the degree of airway pressure transmission to the visceral pleura, which is determined by lung (C_L) and thoracic compliance (C_T):

$$C_L = VT/\Delta P_L = VT/\Delta P_{(ao-pl)}$$

ΔP_L is the change in pressure within the lung; it measures the difference between airway opening pressure and pleural pressure. Whenever lung volume changes, there must be an equivalent alteration in the volume of the thorax.

Therefore:

$$VT = C_L \Delta P_{(ao-pl)} = c_{pl}^{t\Delta P}$$

The fractional transmission of airway pressure to the pleural space ($\Delta P_{pl}/\Delta P_{ao}$) can be determined in the following way:

$$C_L \Delta P_{ao} = (C_T + C_L)P_{pl}/\Delta P_{ao} = C_L(C_T + C_L)$$

If $C_L = C_T$, about 50% of the change in airway pressure is transmitted to the pleural space.[94] If C_L decreases, fractional transmission is less than 50%. A reduction in C_T leads to an increase in pressure transmission to the intrathoracic organs.

Figure 45-6 The effect of a positive-pressure breath on preloads of right **(A)** and left **(B)** ventricles. Changes in left ventricular stroke output are reflected in arterial pressure, which increases during early inspiration and later decreases as a result of inspiratory decrease in venous return. AO, aorta; LA, left atrium; LV, left ventricle; PA, pulmonary artery; RA, right atrium; RV, right ventricle. (From Perel A, Stock C: Handbook of Mechanical Ventilatory Support. Baltimore, Williams & Wilkins, 1992.)

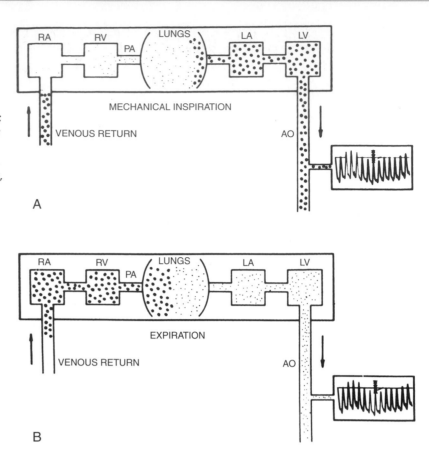

Patients with acute respiratory failure characterized by low CL usually tolerate positive-pressure breathing without deleterious cardiovascular consequences because of reduced transmission of positive airway pressure to the pleural space.[94] Patients with abdominal distention or decreased lung volume following operative procedures often have reduced thoracic compliance and increased airway pressure transmission.[94] Chronic obstructive pulmonary disease (COPD) is associated with decreased CT and increased CL, both of which result in increased transmission of the positive airway pressure to the visceral pleura. Therefore, COPD patients often manifest cardiovascular depression with PPV and are more susceptible to hemodynamic compromise from intrinsic PEEP, which tends to develop in areas of slow time constants (high compliance, high resistance).

Measurements of thoracic vascular pressures are frequently used to evaluate cardiac filling and function.[94] When airway pressure increases, all or part of the change in pleural pressure is transmitted to the lumen of the intrathoracic vessels. Thus, evaluation of cardiac function may be difficult without accurate estimation of true intravascular filling pressure. Intravascular filling pressure is determined by subtraction of the intrapleural from the intravascular pressure. Therefore, precise knowledge of the pleural pressure may be valuable. At present, the measurement of pleural pressure is difficult, requiring the placement of a

catheter between the visceral and parietal pleura. Attempts to estimate pleural pressure with an esophageal balloon have been made, but interpretation of esophageal pressure is difficult because great pressure variations occur within the esophagus. In addition, when esophageal pressure exceeds atmospheric pressure, compliance of the esophageal balloon may limit accuracy of the measurement. Such inaccuracy may influence calculated filling pressures and lead to important errors. Examining the variability in the pulmonary artery waveform can provide information regarding filling pressure. Similarly, fluctuations in central venous pressure with tidal inspiration have been used as an index of volume sensitivity. Therefore, clinicians should consider the impact of pleural pressure on vascular pressures, even if direct measurements of pleural pressures are not available.

Expiratory pleural pressure varies little with different respiratory patterns as long as expiration is passive. Therefore, the most important determinant of mean airway, pleural, and vascular filling pressures is the inspiratory airway pressure pattern.[94] During passive mechanical inspiration, transmural filling pressures decrease because airway and pleural pressures are increased. When transmural filling pressure is lowered, cardiac output is likely to decrease. This is not the case during spontaneous breathing, even with continuous positive airway pressure (CPAP). During spontaneous exhalation with CPAP, pleural and filling pressures are equivalent to those recorded during mechanical ventilation with the same end-expiratory pressure level. However, during inspiration with CPAP, pleural pressure decreases, increasing cardiac filling. The effect of spontaneous inspiration on filling pressures of the heart and cardiac output depends on the change in airway pressure rather than the absolute pressure.

Airway pressure and lung volume are the major pulmonary factors that affect pulmonary vascular resistance (PVR), pulmonary blood flow, and its distribution.[94] When end-expiratory lung volume (FRC) is normal, PVR is at its nadir. Variation in lung volume above or below normal FRC increases PVR. Therefore, normal FRC should be maintained whenever possible. Even though FRC may be independent of the inspiratory airway pressure pattern, the mode of inspiration can affect PVR. During mechanical inspiration with large tidal volumes, PVR may increase if some alveoli become overdistended. Increased PVR and decreased venous return from elevated pleural pressure combine to depress cardiac output.

In a specific individual, the impact of respiration on cardiovascular function can be somewhat unpredictable. Factors such as volume status, magnitude of respiratory efforts, lung versus chest wall compliance, and underlying cardiac function can all influence the effects of pleural pressure changes on cardiac preload and afterload. Therefore, we recommend consideration of the preceding concepts accompanied by customization of these principles to the individual patient's characteristics.

D. VENTILATION-PERFUSION RELATIONSHIPS
(Fig. 45-7)

The relationship between alveolar ventilation ($\dot{V}A$) and perfusion ($\dot{Q}$) plays a major role in determining arterial blood gas values. The gas values in venous blood passing through unventilated, perfused alveoli (e.g., $\dot{V}A/< 0.00001$), or shunt units, remain unchanged. In lung regions with very low but finite $\dot{V}A/\dot{Q}$ (e.g., <0.1), end-capillary blood gas tensions are only slightly altered from those in venous blood; such $\dot{V}A/\dot{Q}$ ratios are functionally like those of shunt units.[89] As $\dot{V}A/\dot{Q}$ increases above 0.1, end-capillary blood gas tensions approximate alveolar gas tensions. Efficient gas exchange occurs when $\dot{V}A/\dot{Q}$ is nearly equal to 0.8. As previously discussed, spontaneous inspiration directs the majority of ventilation toward dependent regions of the lung. Gravitational effects ensure a similar distribution of blood flow. Under healthy conditions, the $\dot{V}A/\dot{Q}$ normally approaches unity in all lung regions.[89] Mechanical ventilation is associated

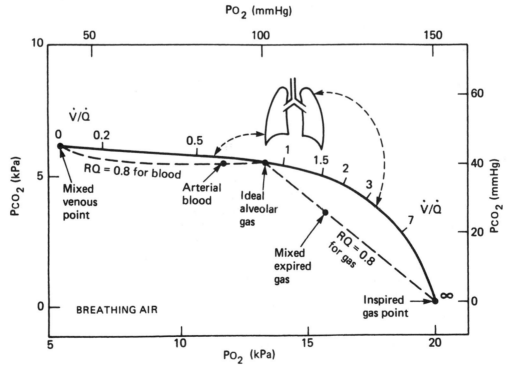

Figure 45-7 Heavy line indicates all possible values for P_{O_2} and P_{CO_2} of alveoli with ventilation/perfusion ($\dot{V}/\dot{Q}$) ratios ranging from zero to infinity (subject breathing air). Values for normal alveoli are distributed as shown in accord with their vertical distance up the lung field. Mixed expired gas may be considered as a mixture of ideal alveolar and inspired gas (dead space). Arterial blood may be considered as a mixture of blood with same gas tensions as ideal alveolar gas and mixed venous blood (the shunt). (From Nunn JF: Nunn's Applied Respiratory Physiology, 4th ed. Oxford, Butterworth-Heinemann, 1993).

with an increase in ventilation to the nondependent lung without a concomitant change in the distribution of pulmonary blood flow. This leads to an increase in lung units with $\dot{V}A/\dot{Q}$ greater than 1 in the nondependent lung and with low but finite $\dot{V}A/\dot{Q}$ (<1, >0.1) in the dependent lung.[89]

III. PATHOLOGIC CONSIDERATIONS

A. ACUTE RESPIRATORY FAILURE

Respiratory failure is invariably associated with abnormal $\dot{V}A/\dot{Q}$ that usually necessitates supportive intervention. An increased $\dot{V}A/\dot{Q}$ associated with a decreased VT results in an increase in the ratio of physiologic dead space (VD) to VT (VD/VT), which may require mechanical ventilation if spontaneous breathing cannot provide adequate alveolar ventilation to sustain carbon dioxide elimination. Both anatomic and alveolar compartments contribute to the total physiologic dead space. When patients are weaned from mechanical ventilation, VD returns to predicted normal values. Because VD increases during mechanical ventilation, minute ventilation during ventilatory support usually exceeds that during spontaneous breathing.

A decrease in $\dot{V}A/\dot{Q}$ results in hypoxemia (Figs. 45-8 and 45-9). Because the majority of gas exchange occurs during the expiratory phase of the ventilatory cycle, improvement in overall $\dot{V}A/\dot{Q}$ must occur primarily during exhalation.[124] Mechanical ventilation alone is usually not effective in improving hypoxemia associated with low but finite $\dot{V}A/\dot{Q}$ because the ratio increases only during the inspiratory phase of the ventilatory cycle.[124] Positive pressure applied during exhalation can improve low $\dot{V}A/\dot{Q}$. However, positive end-expiratory pressure (PEEP) may increase VD and decrease $\dot{V}A$, especially in conjunction with mechanical ventilation. Maintaining near-normal FRC with PEEP frequently improves $\dot{V}A/\dot{Q}$ and reduces hypoxemia.[124]

Acute respiratory failure is often characterized by a decrease in FRC and an increase in intrapulmonary shunt

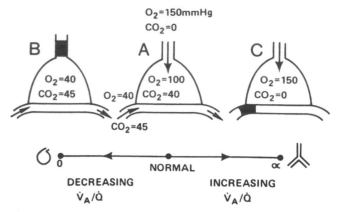

Figure 45-8 Effect of altering ventilation-perfusion ratio on P_{O_2} and P_{CO_2} in a lung unit. (From West JB: Ventilation/Blood Flow and Gas Exchange, 4th ed. Oxford, Blackwell, 1985.)

($\dot{Q}_{va}/\dot{Q}_t$), for example, in acute lung injury or acute respiratory distress syndrome. Intrapulmonary shunt refers to the degree of admixture of mixed venous blood with pulmonary end-capillary blood that would be required to produce the observed difference between the arterial and pulmonary end-capillary P_{O_2}. Therapy for acute respiratory failure should include applying PEEP to increase FRC, improving pulmonary gas exchange, increasing arterial oxygen tension, and decreasing PVR.

B. WORK OF BREATHING

If patients with acute lung injury are to maintain effective gas exchange and patient-ventilator synchrony, the work of breathing must be appropriately decreased. Few clinical studies have attempted to quantify the work of breathing in patients with respiratory failure, perhaps because quantification of work requires techniques not readily available in the clinical setting. Any alteration in the pressure-volume (P-V) relationship of the lung alters the work of breathing. A normal P-V curve for the lung-thorax system is shown in Figure 45-10. As a result of a small pressure change, normal tidal breathing from FRC

Figure 45-9 O_2-CO_2 diagram showing a ventilation-perfusion ratio line. P_{O_2} and P_{CO_2} of a lung unit move along this line from the mixed venous point to the inspired gas point I as its ventilation-perfusion ratio is increased. (From West JB: Ventilation/Blood Flow and Gas Exchange, 4th ed. Oxford, Blackwell, 1985.)

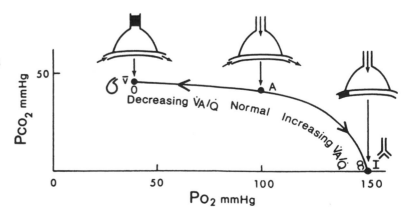

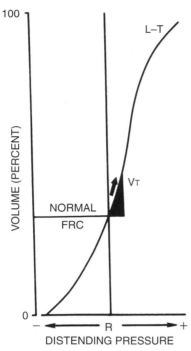

Figure 45-10 Normal pressure-volume curve of the lung-thorax (L-T). Volume as a percentage of total lung capacity is plotted as a function of distending pressure (R). At ambient airway pressure, R equals zero. During inspiration, R is increased and lung volume (VT) increases from normal functional residual capacity (FRC). As a result of a small pressure change, normal tidal breathing from FRC occurs along the pressure-volume curve, as indicated by the *arrow*. The elastic work of inspiration can be estimated from the black area under the curve. (From Downs JB, Douglas ME: Physiologic effects of respiratory therapy. In Shoemaker W, Ayers S, Grenvik A, et al [eds]: Textbook of Critical Care, 2nd ed. Philadelphia, WB Saunders, 1989.)

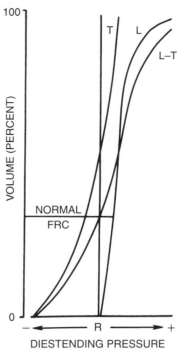

Figure 45-11 Normal pressure-volume curves of the thorax (T), lung (L), and lung-thorax (L-T). Volume as a percentage of total lung capacity is plotted as a function of distending pressure (R). Lung-thorax R is zero when airway pressure is ambient; distending pressure of lung is, therefore, equal but opposite to that of thorax. These equal counterforces determine and maintain functional residual capacity (FRC). (From Downs JB, Douglas ME: Physiologic effects of respiratory therapy. In Shoemaker W, Ayers S, Grenvik A, et al [eds]: Textbook of Critical Care, 2nd ed. Philadelphia, WB Saunders, 1989.)

occurs along the P-V curve as indicated by the arrow.[21] The elastic work of inspiration can be estimated by the black area under the curve. Figure 45-11 shows the P-V curves for normal lung, thorax, and lung-thorax. At FRC, the distending pressure of the lung is equal but opposite to that of the thorax. Any alteration in the P-V relationships for the lung or the thorax, or both, alters the lung-thorax curve and changes FRC.

The likely alteration of the lung P-V curve associated with acute lung injury is shown in Figure 45-12.[21] Because the P-V relationships of the lung and thorax can be altered in multiple ways by acute respiratory failure, a family of right-shifted lung-thorax curves can result. Each has a reduced FRC (Fig. 45-13). A shift in the P-V curve not only decreases FRC but also can increase the work of breathing. When FRC is decreased, the required pressure change to achieve a given VT is increased, and the area within the curve representing work is also increased (Fig. 45-14). If this occurs, the patient decreases tidal volume and increases respiratory rate in an effort to minimize work.[21] Because of these changes, the work of breathing is partially or completely assumed by the ventilator

during mechanical ventilation. However, restoration of FRC accomplished by instituting PEEP may assist in decreasing the work of breathing. Restoration of FRC can be accomplished with the application of PEEP in mechanically ventilated patients and CPAP in spontaneously breathing patients (Fig. 45-15).[21] Because severity of injury may vary from patient to patient, PEEP must be individualized, titrated for each patient, and reassessed frequently.

C. CARDIAC FAILURE

Left ventricular failure causes an increase in left atrial and pulmonary venous pressure. The increased pulmonary venous pressure can precipitate gas exchange abnormalities by altering the distribution of pulmonary blood flow or increasing extravascular lung water, or both. Increased pulmonary venous pressure initially produces a redistribution of perfusion to nondependent lung regions. However, as pulmonary venous pressure continues to rise, the transvascular flux of fluid increases, the interstitial space becomes maximally expanded, the lymphatic clearance mechanism is overwhelmed, alveoli become

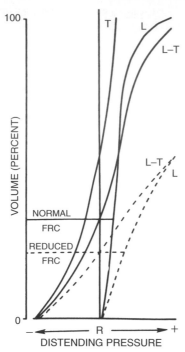

Figure 45-12 Normal *(solid lines)* and abnormal *(dotted lines)* pressure-volume curves of thorax (T), lung (L), and lung-thorax (L-T). Distending pressure (R) is zero when airway pressure is ambient. Abnormally right-shifted pressure-volume curve of lung, which is characteristic of respiratory failure, results in a new L-T pressure-volume curve and a reduction in functional residual capacity (FRC). (From Downs JB, Douglas ME: Physiologic effects of respiratory therapy. In Shoemaker W, Ayers S, Grenvik A, et al [eds]: Textbook of Critical Care, 2nd ed. Philadelphia, WB Saunders, 1989.)

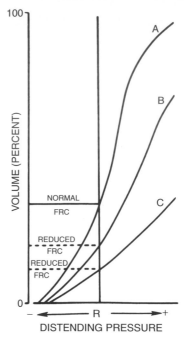

Figure 45-13 Volume as a percentage of total lung capacity is plotted as a function of distending pressure (R). R is zero when airway pressure is ambient. Curve A represents normal pressure-volume relationship for lung-thorax. Curves B and C are shifted to the right. Each curve results in reduced functional residual capacity (FRC). Pressure-volume relationships of lung and thorax can be altered in an infinite number of ways during respiratory failure, resulting in a family of right-shifted lung-thorax curves. Each curve has a lower FRC than the curve on its left. (From Downs JB, Douglas ME: Physiologic effects of respiratory therapy. In Shoemaker W, Ayers S, Grenvik A, et al [eds]: Textbook of Critical Care, 2nd ed. Philadelphia, WB Saunders, 1989.)

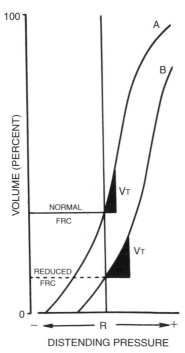

Figure 45-14 Pressure-volume curves of lung-thorax. Volume as a percentage of total lung capacity is plotted as a function of distending pressure (R). R is zero when airway pressure is ambient. Curve A represents normal pressure-volume relationship. Curve B represents a right-shifted curve. (From Downs JB, Douglas ME: Physiologic effects of respiratory therapy. In Shoemaker W, Ayers S, Grenvik A, et al [eds]: Textbook of Critical Care, 2nd ed. Philadelphia, WB Saunders, 1989.)

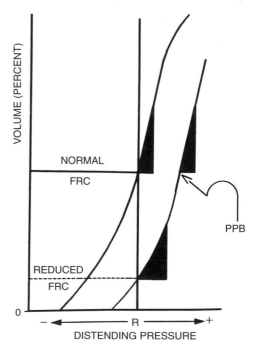

Figure 45-15 These pressure-volume curves of lung-thorax are equivalent to those in Figure 45-14. When distending pressure (R) is increased by positive airway pressure, functional residual capacity (FRC) can be normalized. When FRC is increased, work of breathing may be reduced to nearly normal. PPB, positive-pressure breathing. (From Downs JB, Douglas ME: Physiologic effects of respiratory therapy. In Shoemaker W, Ayers S, Grenvik A, et al [eds]: Textbook of Critical Care, 2nd ed. Philadelphia, WB Saunders, 1989.)

flooded, FRC and C_{RS} decrease, and $\dot{V}_A/\dot{Q}$ mismatching increases.[94]

Patients in left-sided heart failure typically exhibit a characteristic breathing pattern characterized by tachypnea and inspiratory intercostal or epigastric retractions caused by large reductions in pleural pressure. Alterations in pleural pressure may alter left ventricular function as described earlier. Marked reductions in pleural pressure may impede left ventricular ejection (because of increased aortic transmural pressure or afterload), whereas increases in pleural pressure may facilitate left ventricular ejection (because of decreased aortic transmural pressure or afterload). In left-sided heart failure, in which left ventricular contractility is reduced and relatively unresponsive to changes in preload, decreasing left ventricular afterload increases stroke volume.[94] Because increased intrapleural pressure reduces left ventricular afterload, the application of mask CPAP improves cardiac performance and lung function in patients suffering from congestive heart failure. In addition, forced expiratory maneuvers have been observed in patients with congestive heart failure. The associated pleural pressure elevations may serve to improve cardiac output.

IV. PATHOPHYSIOLOGIC EFFECTS AND COMPLICATIONS OF POSITIVE AIRWAY PRESSURE THERAPY

A. VENTILATOR-INDUCED LUNG INJURY (VILI)

Laboratory data have defined two primary settings in which the mechanical ventilator can induce lung injury, overdistention of lung at end inspiration and collapse and reexpansion of unstable lung during ventilation.

1. Overdistention

Figure 45-16 depicts the impact of a large tidal volume without PEEP on a rat lung compared with a rat lung ventilated with a small tidal volume and one with 10 cm H_2O PEEP and a large tidal volume.[123] As noted, within 1 hour the large tidal volume ventilation with zero PEEP caused marked hemorrhagic edema. This type of injury has been termed volutrauma by Dreyfuss and colleagues because it is believed that the injury is caused primarily by excessive tidal volume.[28] However, as described previously, increased tidal volume is accompanied by an excess of PTP, making such distinctions between pressure and volume injury somewhat semantic. VILI results in an increase in the permeability of the alveolar capillary membrane, the development of pulmonary edema, the accumulation of neutrophils and protein within the lung parenchyma, the disruption of surfactant production, the development of hyaline membranes, and a decrease in compliance.[28] VILI is indistinguishable from human acute respiratory distress syndrome (ARDS) and can be produced in rats within minutes during large tidal volume ventilation (Fig. 45-17).[26] Indeed, VILI caused by the

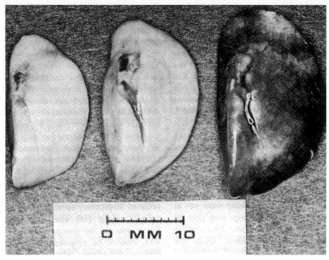

Figure 45-16 Comparison of lungs excised from rats ventilated with peak pressure of 14 cm H_2O, zero positive end-expiratory pressure (PEEP), peak pressure 45 cm H_2O, 10 cm H_2O PEEP, and peak pressure 45 cm H_2O, zero PEEP (left to right). The perivascular groove is distended with edema in the lungs from rats ventilated with peak pressures of 45 cm H_2O, 10 cm H_2O PEEP. The lung ventilated at 45 cm H_2O zero PEEP is grossly hemorrhaged. (From Webb HH, Tierney D: Experimental pulmonary edema due to intermittent positive pressure ventilation, with high inflation pressure protection by positive end expiratory pressure. Am Rev Respir Dis 110:556-565, 1974.)

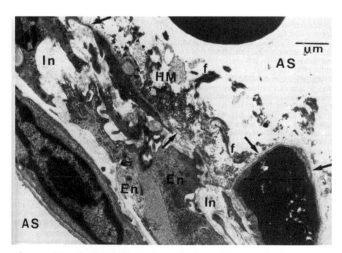

Figure 45-17 Electron microscopic view of the cross-action of the alveolar-capillary complex of a rat ventilated with large tidal volumes at a peak pressure of 45 cm H_2O with zero positive end-expiratory pressure. Markedly altered alveolar septum with three capillaries. At the right side, the epithelial lining is destroyed, denuding the basement membrane *(arrows)*. Hyaline membrane (HM) composed of cell debris and fibrin (f) is present. Two endothelial cells (En) of another capillary are visible inside the interstitium (In). At the lower left side, a monocyte fills the lumen of a third capillary with a normal blood-air barrier. (From Dreyfuss D, Basset G, Soler P, Saumon G: Intermittent positive pressure hyperventilation with high inflation pressures produces pulmonary microvascular injury in rats. Am Rev Respir Dis 132:880-884, 1985.)

use of large tidal volumes has been demonstrated in many small and large animal models. Parker and coworkers[90] demonstrated in isolated perfused dog lungs that ventilating pressures beyond 30 cm H_2O peak alveolar pressure result in VILI. Hernandez and colleagues,[49] Egan,[29] and Kolobow and associates[65] demonstrated similar injuries in large animal models. Ventilation of all species evaluated with large tidal volumes results in the development of VILI and an increase in the severity of an already existent lung injury.

The single factor most responsible for the development of VILI appears to be the PTP across the lung (pressure inside minus pressure outside).[27] In a now classical experiment, Dreyfuss and colleagues[27] demonstrated that rats with their chest walls strapped were protected from VILI compared with those ventilated with the same peak pressure but without chest wall binding. In fact, injury was similar regardless of the use of positive- or negative-pressure ventilation provided high PTPs were established. As a result, higher ventilating pressures can be used in the presence of a decreased chest wall compliance without the development of VILI because the decreased chest wall compliance decreases PTP at a specific peak pressure and results in lower tidal volumes.

2. Recruitment/Derecruitment Injury

As noted in Figure 45-16, the application of 10 cm H_2O PEEP in spite of a peak airway pressure of 45 cm H_2O decreased the level of VILI compared with that in similar animals with the same peak pressure but zero PEEP.[123] Only mild interstitial edema developed in the animals with 10 cm H_2O PEEP. Similar findings have been reported by

Corbridge and coauthors in dogs with hydrochloric acid–induced lung injury.[17] Dogs ventilated with 12.5 cm H_2O PEEP and a VT of 15 mL/kg after lung injury had much lower ratios of wet lung weight and dry lung weight to body weight at autopsy than dogs ventilated with 3.2 cm H_2O PEEP and 30 mL/kg tidal volumes, in spite of the fact that peak alveolar pressure (33 cm H_2O) was the same during the 5 hours of ventilation (Fig. 45-18).

Other groups have also shown in various animal models that PEEP has a protective effect on the development or extension of lung injury. Dreyfuss and colleagues, in healthy rats, showed that the beneficial effects of PEEP on reducing the extent of lung injury could be minimized by the administration of dopamine.[27] They argued that part of the reduction of edema formation with PEEP was a direct result of cardiac output reduction and decreased pulmonary perfusion. Data from Broccard and associates also point to a relationship between pulmonary vascular flow and VILI.[8] This group studied the effects of three levels of constant intravenous infusion and two levels of end-inspiratory plateau pressure (P_{PLAT}) at zero PEEP. Isolated rabbit lungs receiving 900 mL/min of perfusion at a P_{PLAT} of 30 cm H_2O demonstrated the greatest decrease in lung compliance, the highest level of alveolar hemorrhage, and the greatest weight gain as compared with animals receiving 300 mL/min perfusion at a P_{PLAT} of 30 cm H_2O or 500 mL/min perfusion at a P_{PLAT} of 15 cm H_2O. These data support the suggestion that PEEP protects the lung by decreasing vascular flow.

Although vascular flow may affect the level of VILI, the data from Muscedere and coauthors support the independent effect of PEEP on the development of VILI (Fig. 45-19).[83] This group studied the effect of PEEP on

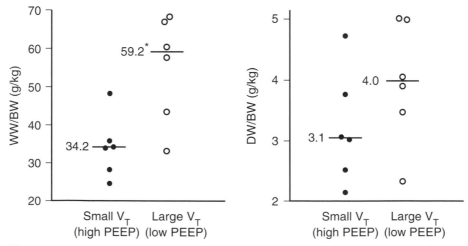

Figure 45-18 Gravimetric estimates of edema. Wet weight/body weight ratios (WW/BW) (g/kg) and dry weight/body weight ratios (DW/BW) (g/kg) with median values are shown for all animals in both groups. *Median WW/BW was statistically higher in the large VT–low positive end-expiratory pressure (PEEP) group (P =.041). Median DW/BW was not significantly different between groups. (From Corbridge TC, Wood DH, Crawford GP: Adverse effects of large tidal volume and low PEEP in canine acid aspiration. Am Rev Respir Dis 142:311-314, 1990.)

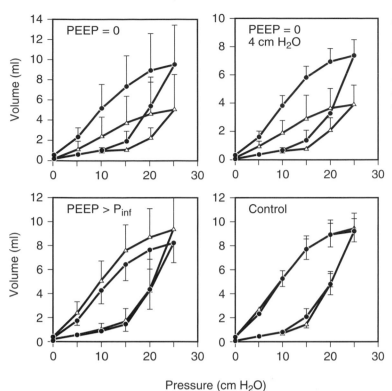

Figure 45-19 Composite pressure-volume curves before *(circles)* and after *(triangles)* ventilation with different levels of positive end-expiratory pressure (PEEP) in an ex vivo rat lung. See text for detail. (From Muscedere JF, Mullen BM, Gan K, Slutsky AS: Tidal ventilation at low airway pressure can augment lung injury. Am J Respir Crit Care Med 149:1327-1334, 1994.)

the development of VILI in an ex vivo rat lung model. Four groups were compared: PEEP of 0 cm H_2O (peak pressure 30 cm H_2O), PEEP less than P_{flex} (4 cm H_2O, peak pressure 26 cm H_2O), PEEP greater than P_{flex} (15 cm H_2O, peak pressure 32 cm H_2O), and PEEP of 4 cm H_2O (control, no ventilation), where P_{flex} is the "inflection point" on the inspiratory P-V curve of the lung. Following a 2-hour ventilation period, animals in the PEEP greater than P_{flex} group demonstrated no change in compliance (similar to control animals), whereas the PEEP of 0 cm H_2O and PEEP less than P_{flex} groups showed a marked decrease in compliance (consistent with the development of lung injury).

The benefit of setting PEEP above P_{flex} was also demonstrated by Takeuchi[111] and Herrera[50] and their associates. Takeuchi[111] showed in a lavage lung-injured sheep model that PEEP above P_{flex} resulted in less activation of pulmonary inflammatory mediators and histologic injury than PEEP set on the basis of an oxygenation target (Fig. 45-20). Herrera[50] showed that PEEP greater than P_{flex} in a sepsis-induced lung injury rat model modulated the pulmonary and systemic inflammatory responses and decreased mortality.

Several points are noteworthy regarding the so-called P_{flex}. First, P_{flex} is measured on the inflation limb of the volume-pressure curve, whereas collapse tends to occur *during exhalation*, leading some investigators to question the rationale for the inflation limb P_{flex}. The deflation limb P_{flex} may be the more relevant value with regard to setting PEEP to prevent derecruitment. Second, an inflection point is technically defined as a change in slope

(e.g., positive to negative) of a curve rather than a change in shape. Thus, the P_{flex} to which investigators have referred is perhaps better called a "point of maximum curvature" or "point of maximal compliance change" rather than P_{flex}. Third, the assumption underlying the use of P_{flex} was that the initially collapsed lung experiences a sudden increase in volume for a small change in pressure analogous to "opening the lung." Several studies have now demonstrated that the inflation limb P_{flex} represents the start of recruitment and that ongoing recruitment takes place throughout the inflation limb. Thus, the use of the volume-pressure curve is complex, and the utility of the inflation limb P_{flex} to set the ventilator is encouraging but questionable.

Although the precise mechanism by which PEEP protects against the VILI is unclear, Mead and colleagues,[76] using mathematical and mechanical models, have provided the most reasonable explanation. As illustrated in Figure 45-21, a collapsed lung unit lying next to an expanded lung unit experiences marked stress and strain on the common wall between these units during expansion of the already inflated lung unit. The effective stress pressure (P_{eff}) across the alveolar wall can be quantified by the following equation:

$$P_{eff} = P_{appl}(V/Vo)^{2/3}$$

where P_{appl} is applied alveolar pressure, V is the final alveolar volume, and Vo is the initial alveolar volume. On the basis of this equation, Mead and colleagues[76] predicted that the stress on the wall of a collapsed lung unit would

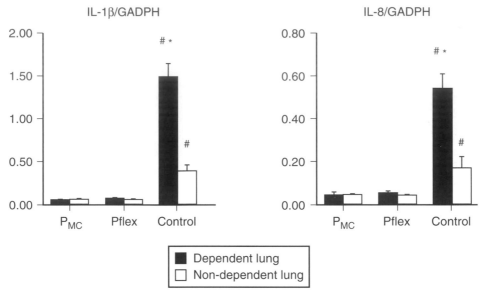

Figure 45-20 Messenger RNA levels of interleukin-1β-GADPH and interleukin-8-GADPH in the cells of lung lavage fluid in the three groups: $P < .01$ versus *nondependent lung of the same group and the point of maximum curvature group (P_{MC}) and above the lower inflection point group (P_{flex}). See text for detail. (From Takeuchi M, Goddon S, Kacmarek RM, et al: Set positive end-expiratory pressure during protective ventilation affects lung injury. Anesthesiology 97:682-692, 2002.)

be about 140 cm H_2O if the peak alveolar pressure was about 30 cm H_2O. Thus, heterogeneity within the lung can lead to substantial local shear forces and contribute to further lung injury.

3. Translocation of Cells

Fu and coworkers[40] have clearly demonstrated that high alveolar distending volumes and low PEEP not only disrupt the alveolar epithelium but also can cause tears in capillary endothelium (Fig. 45-22). As a result, cells and other substances are able to move across the alveolar-capillary wall when lung injury is present. This process has been clearly demonstrated in animal models.[84,120] Nahum and others[84] showed that, after instillation of *Escherichia coli* into the lungs of dogs, injurious mechanical ventilation strategies were linked to the subsequent dissemination of *E. coli* into the systemic circulation.

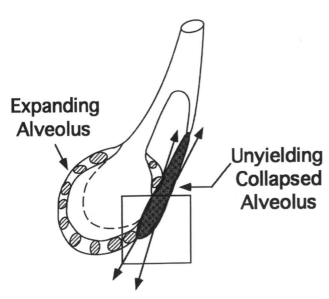

Figure 45-21 Illustration of a collapsed and expanded alveolus showing area *(box)* where high shear stress can develop during inflation of the expanded alveolus. (Courtesy of John Marini.)

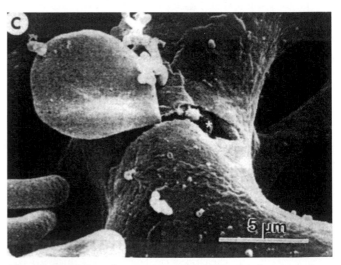

Figure 45-22 Scanning electron micrograph showing examples of disruptions of blood-gas barrier in rabbit lungs ventilated with large volumes, showing complete rupture of blood-gas barrier with a red blood cell protruding into opening and others underneath (*). (From Fu Z, Costello ML, Tsukimoto K, et al: High lung volume increases stress failure in pulmonary capillaries. J Appl Physiol 73:123-133, 1992.)

Animals ventilated with a low tidal volume and high PEEP were protected, but almost all animals ventilated with a large tidal volume and no PEEP developed bacteremia. Similar findings in pigs were demonstrated by Verbrugge and coworkers.[120]

4. Biotrauma

Slutsky and Tremblay[104] referred to the activation of pulmonary and systemic inflammatory mediators by an inappropriate ventilatory pattern as "biotrauma." Increasing data from both animal and clinical studies indicate that ventilatory strategy does affect the level of pulmonary and systemic inflammatory response. Tremblay and colleagues[115] demonstrated in an ex vivo healthy and injured rat lung model that both pro- and anti-inflammatory mediators are activated by ventilatory patterns associated with high peak alveolar pressure and zero PEEP (Fig. 45-23). In the animals in which PEEP was set greater than P_{flex} and overdistention was avoided, minimal mediator activation was observed. Similar data were reported by Bethmann and coauthors in an ex vivo perfused mouse lung model.[5] Hyperventilation at 2.5 times normal PTP using either positive- or negative-pressure ventilation resulted in a 1.75-fold increased expression of tumor necrosis factor α (TNF-α) and interleukin 6 messenger RNA (mRNA). Imai[58] and Takata[110] and their coworkers noted greater TNF-α mRNA expression with conventional ventilation at low peak pressure (30 cm H_2O) and low PEEP (5 cm H_2O) compared with high-frequency oscillation at a mean airway pressure of 15 cm H_2O (same as with conventional ventilation). Ranieri and associates showed the same effect of ventilatory pattern on pulmonary lavage and serum TNF-α level in ARDS patients.[100] In a randomized comparison, patients ventilated with PEEP set greater than P_{flex} and peak alveolar pressure kept below the upper inflection point of the pressure-volume curve had a decrease in lung lavage and serum TNF-α levels after 36 hours. Patients randomly assigned to PEEP on the basis of oxygenation and V_T set to produce eucapnia had increased TNF-α levels after 36 hours. In addition, the ARDSnet[21] demonstrated a lower systemic proinflammatory mediator response in a low tidal group than a high tidal volume group.

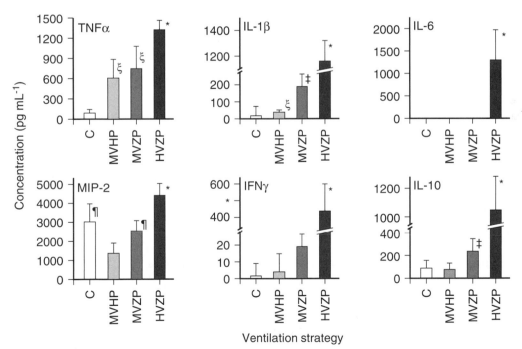

Figure 45-23 Effect of ventilation strategy on absolute lung lavage cytokine concentration for animals previously lung injured with lipopolysaccharide injection. C, control; MVHP, moderate volume, high positive end-expiratory pressure (PEEP); MVZP, moderate volume, zero PEEP; HVZP, high volume, zero PEEP; TNFα, tumor necrosis factor α; IL-1β, interleukin-1β; MIP-2 IFNγ, immune interferon. The pattern of lavage cytokines seen in response to ventilation strategy was similar to that of the saline-treated groups except for MIP-2, in which the control group (C) has levels comparable to those of the MVZP group (both increased significantly versus the MVHP group). *$P < .05$ versus C, MVHP, MVZP; ‡$P < .05$ versus C, MVHP; CP < 0.05 versus C; ¶$P < .05$ versus MVHP. (From Tremblay L, Valenza F, Riberiro S, et al: Injurious ventilatory strategies increase cytokines and c-fos mRNA expression in an isolated rat lung model. J Clin Invest 99:944-952, 1997.)

Chu and coworkers[16] demonstrated that lung maintained at high lung volume by CPAP or ventilated at the same high peak pressure as CPAP had the same marked activation of inflammatory mediators.

On the basis of these data, both Slutsky and Tremblay[104] and Dreyfuss and Saumon[24] proposed that the lung was the engine that drives the development of multisystem organ failure in ARDS patients. The injury as a result of inappropriate mechanical ventilation causes the movement of inflammatory mediators into the systemic circulation, increasing systemic production of mediators and influencing the function of distal organs. In support of this hypothesis is the correlation between interleukin 6 (released by the injured lung) and renal failure in a prior report. In addition, renal cellular apoptosis has been associated with injurious mechanical ventilation strategies. These data provide suggestive evidence that in both animals and humans mechanical ventilation strategy can affect systemic organ function.

As a result, it seems reasonable to conclude, as discussed by Marini,[72] that "excessive mechanical forces produce lung damage by at least three mechanisms: (1) the signaling of proinflammatory mediator release by mechanical stress, (2) trauma to the epithelium of the lung parenchyma by repetitive opening at high pressures and subsequent closing with each breath, and (3) physical stress on the parenchyma by high peak alveolar pressures." Marini also pointed out that there is some evidence that ventilatory frequency[56] (higher frequency, greater injury), high pre- and postalveolar microvascular pressures,[10] decreased surfactant production,[91] supine body position,[9] high body temperature,[109] and immune suppression[62] all enhance the development and severity of VILI.

B. PATIENT-VENTILATOR SYNCHRONY

Patient-ventilator synchrony is important for every patient breathing spontaneously and triggering the ventilator. A lack of synchrony increases ventilatory effort, respiratory rate, and work of breathing. Pressure-targeted modes of ventilation are recommended over volume-targeted modes to reduce the likelihood of dyssynchrony because pressure ventilation allows ventilator-delivered flow to vary each breath on the basis of the patient's inspiratory demand.[75] In addition, most ventilators now allow an adjustment of the slope of the increase in flow delivery (rise time) to ensure that gas delivery is matched to the patient's inspiratory flow demand.[13] Patient-ventilator synchrony is also affected by inspiratory time. The ventilator inspiratory time and the patient's neuroinspiratory time should be equal. It is rare to find a stressed, spontaneously breathing patient with an inspiratory time greater than 1.0 second. In fact, some stressed adult patients desire inspiratory times as short as 0.6 second. As a result, inspiratory time should be set to ensure that the patient and ventilator begin exhalation at the same time.

Sensitivity should always be set as high as possible without causing autotriggering, and, in general, flow triggering is recommended over pressure triggering.[45] A final factor affecting patient-ventilation synchrony is auto-PEEP,[93] normally a problem only in patients with airways obstruction but a potential concern in all patients. If a patient's inspiratory efforts fail to trigger the ventilator, the issue is almost always auto-PEEP.[105]

C. MALDISTRIBUTION OF VENTILATION

Acute respiratory failure results in nonhomogeneous changes in compliance and resistance. PPV results in further maldistribution of ventilation to nondependent lung. The combination of these effects commonly results in a need for elevated minute ventilation to maintain $PaCO_2$. As discussed, arterial oxygenation may be impaired by changes in $\dot{V}A/\dot{Q}$ consequent to pathology and positive pressure and require oxygen, PEEP, and vascular volume.

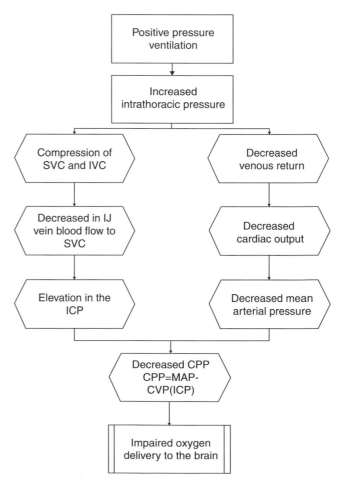

Figure 45-24 Positive-pressure ventilation effects on the central nervous system. CPP, cerebral perfusion pressure; CVP, central venous pressure; ICP, intracranial pressure; IJ, internal jugular; IVC, inferior vena cava; MAP, mean arterial pressure; SVC, superior vena cava.

D. ORGAN SYSTEM DYSFUNCTION

PPV affects not only intrathoracic organs but practically every major organ system. By understanding the physiologic consequences of PPV, clinicians may minimize or at least anticipate the undesirable effects.

1. Central Nervous System (Fig. 45-24 and Box 45-1)

PPV may result in an increase in intracranial pressure (ICP) because of elevated mean airway pressure. Impaired venous return can result from increased intrathoracic pressure.[102] However, in patients with elevated ICP, there exists a Starling resistor at the junction of the intracranial and extracranial veins. As a result, venous return from the head in these patients is relatively independent of the downstream pressure influences of intrathoracic pressure. Cerebral perfusion pressure (CPP) may be impaired in patients receiving PPV as a result of impaired cardiac output, decreased mean arterial pressure, and increased ICP. Effects of PPV on the central nervous system are greatest in patients with decreased thoracic or increased pulmonary compliance.

2. Cardiac (Fig. 45-25 and Box 45-2)

Hemodynamic instability on initiation of PPV is predictable in the critically ill.[91] As a rule, there is a decrease in cardiac output secondary to a decrease to right ventricular preload, an increase in right ventricular afterload, and a decrease in left ventricular preload. As a result, there is an observed decrease in mean arterial pressure. Patients with compromised intravascular volume may be more susceptible to these effects. A large-bore intravenous catheter is usually indicated prior to commencing PPV in case aggressive fluid resuscitation is needed.

A decrease in sympathetic tone following initiation of mechanical support because of decreased work of breathing and improved gas exchange may lead to vasodilatation, further exacerbating a drop in mean arterial pressure.

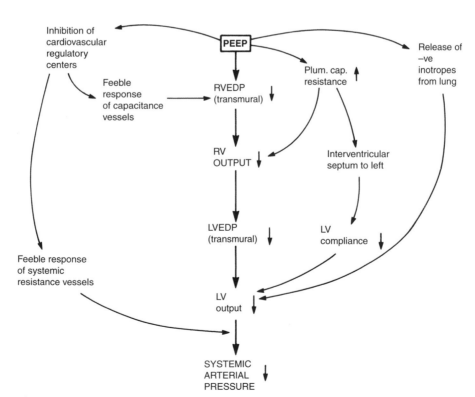

Figure 45-25 Cardiovascular effects of positive end-expiratory pressure (PEEP). LV, left ventricle; LVEDP, left ventricular end-diastolic pressure; RV, right ventricle; RVEDP, right ventricular end-diastolic pressure. (From Nunn JF: Nunn's Applied Respiratory Physiology, 4th ed. Oxford, Butterworth-Heinemann, 1993.)

Box 45-2   Positive-Pressure Ventilation Causes Decreased Cardiac Output

1. Decreased venous return to right ventricle
2. Right ventricular dysfunction secondary to elevated pulmonary vascular resistance and decreased preload
3. Alterations of left ventricular distensibility

In addition, sedative-anesthetic medications are frequently provided before intubation, which can further compromise hemodynamics. In patients who are intubated in the operating room, blood pressure (BP) frequently increases because of the catecholamine surge associated with intubation. However, in the critically ill, who have preexisting elevations in catecholamines, the initiation of mechanical ventilation frequently leads to a fall in catecholamine levels. Thus, hemodynamic compromise from intubation is more of an issue in the intensive care unit (ICU) than in the operating room.

Another potential problem is the increase in PVR leading to impaired right ventricular ejection. Patients with right ventricular dysfunction tend to do poorly with PPV. Increased PVR may also increase right-to-left shunting in patients with an atrial septal defect or ventricular septal defect.[124] These patients may be at higher risk for an embolus passing to the systemic circulation.

3. Pulmonary (Box 45-3)

Most complications of PPV in the pulmonary system have been previously discussed. Other complications associated with PPV are pneumonia and risks associated with endotracheal intubation.[124] The incidence of pneumonia is increased in endotracheally intubated patients, with the risk of infection increasing with ongoing mechanical ventilation. The actuarial risk of ventilator-associated pneumonia has been reported to be 6.5% at 10 days, 19% at 20 days, and 28% at 30 days.[34] This risk of infection from prolonged mechanical ventilation must be balanced against the risk of premature extubation. The risk of endotracheal intubation can be divided into complications associated with the placement and those seen as a result of long-term presence of a foreign body in the trachea. Patients with elevated mean airway pressure and those requiring high levels of PEEP or with compromised perfusion may be at increased risk for tracheal injury.

Box 45-3   The Most Common Pulmonary Complications Associated with Positive-Pressure Ventilation

1. Ventilator-induced lung injury
2. Pneumothorax/barotrauma
3. Nosocomial pneumonia

Box 45-4   Positive-Pressure Ventilation May Impair Hepatic and Gastrointestinal Function in the Following Ways

1. Decreased cardiac output
2. Increased hepatic vascular resistance
   a. Elevated venous pressure
   b. Elevated intra-abdominal pressure
   c. Diaphragmatic compression
3. Elevated bile duct pressure

---

4. Hepatic (Box 45-4)

PPV increases intrathoracic pressures and results in impaired venous return leading to congestion of the hepatic sinusoids. Diaphragmatic compression leads to an increase in intra-abdominal pressure, further impairing hepatic blood flow. Worsening this situation is the drop in cardiac output and oxygen delivery to the liver. This is particularly a problem in patients with liver disease who have altered parenchymal architecture.

An increase in resistance in the flow of bile through the common bile duct may influence liver function. Elevated bile duct pressure has been described in animal studies, with the proposed mechanism being vascular engorgement of the duct.[60]

5. Splanchnic and Gastrointestinal Tract (Box 45-5)

The deleterious effects of PPV on the splanchnic circulation are due to venous engorgement and decreased perfusion. Elevation in intrathoracic pressure limits venous return from the inferior vena cava and the portal vein. Decreases in cardiac output, in addition, limit perfusion pressure. This dual effect of poor perfusion and venous engorgement may lead to an increased risk for intestinal anastomosis breakdown, increased bacterial translocation from the gut, and an increase in upper gastrointestinal hemorrhage.[124] Bacterial translocation is presently considered the possible source for the initiation of the sepsis syndrome. Tied in with this problem is nutrition, which is usually limited because of endotracheal intubation. Early enteral feeding may improve the viability of gastrointestinal mucosa, limiting this complication. However, some data support increased risk of aspiration with early enteral nutrition, highlighting the need for further research in this area.

Box 45-5   Positive-Pressure Ventilation Effects on Splanchnic Circulation

1. Increase in intestinal anastomosis breakdown
2. Possible increase in bacterial translocation
3. Increase in upper gastrointestinal hemorrhage
4. Ileus and gastric dilation

Upper gastrointestinal hemorrhage has been observed in approximately 40% of patients receiving PPV for more than 3 days.[44] Prophylaxis to elevate the stomach pH ameliorates this problem but may increase the risk of nosocomial pneumonia.

Patients with full ventilatory support require sedation and occasionally neuromuscular blockade. This may lead to an ileus and gastric dilation, both of which can contribute to aspiration risk and limit the feasibility of enteral nutrition.

6. Renal (Fig. 45-26 and Box 45-6)

Renal impairment upon initiating mechanical ventilation is multifactorial. Proposed causes can be subdivided into direct and indirect effects. Impaired renal function is usually due to decreased cardiac output and altered venous return to the heart. Redistribution of renal blood flow from the cortex to the juxtamedullary regions leads to decreased urine volume and decreased sodium excretion. Also involved, although indirectly, are the sympathetic and endocrine systems. Decreased levels of carotid sinus baroreceptor simulation lead to an increase in renal sympathetic stimulation, which leads to decreased renal blood flow and a decrease in urinary sodium excretion. The liberation of increasing levels of antidiuretic hormone and up-modulation of the renin-angiotensin-aldosterone system again lead to water retention and renal impairment. Another component is atrial natriuretic factor, released as a result of cardiac distention. Its release is greatly reduced in patients with PPV. Atrial natriuretic factor has potent diuretic and natriuretic effects. Elevations in interleukin 6 released by the lung and renal

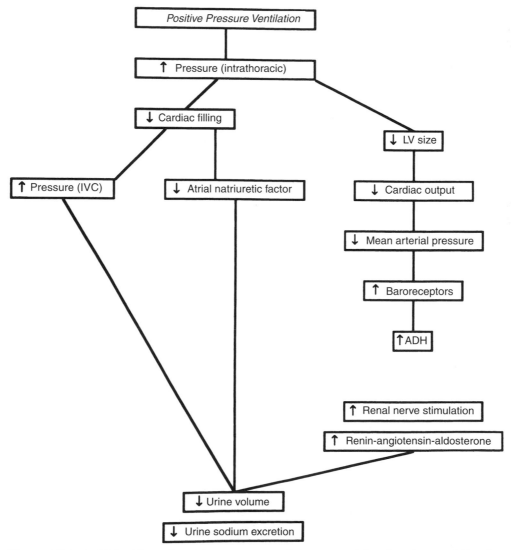

Figure 45-26 Multiple effects of positive-pressure ventilation on renal function. ADH, antidiuretic hormone; IVC, inferior vena cava; LV, left ventricular. (Modified from Perel A, Stock C: Handbook of Mechanical Ventilatory Support. Baltimore, Williams & Wilkins, 1992.)

Box 45-6   Positive-Pressure Ventilation May Impair Renal Function in the Following Ways

1. Direct
   a. Decreased cardiac output
   b. Redistribution of renal blood flow from cortical to intramedullary zones, which in turn leads to the following:
      (1) Decreased urine volume
      (2) Decreased sodium excretion
   c. Increased intrathoracic pressures resulting in elevated portal and inferior vena cava pressures
2. Indirect
   a. Sympathetic stimulation
      (1) Increased epinephrine levels
   b. Hormonal changes
      (1) Decreased atrial natriuretic factor
      (2) Increased renin-angiotensin-aldosterone
      (3) Increased antidiuretic hormone

cellular apoptosis have been reported to contribute to renal dysfunction in the context of mechanical ventilation.

V. APPLICATION OF MECHANICAL VENTILATION

A. BASIC VENTILATOR SETTINGS

Regardless of the mode of ventilation selected, a number of variables are either set or are a result of other settings that must be considered by the clinician each time mechanical ventilation is initiated. These include tidal volume, plateau pressure, peak flow and flow waveform, inspiratory time, expiratory time, inspiratory-to-expiratory (I:E) ratio, ventilatory rate, fraction of inspired oxygen (FIO_2), and PEEP/ CPAP.

1. Tidal Volume

Over the past 10 years, emphasis has been placed on the relationship between tidal volume and VILI.[25] Epidemiologic studies indicate that the most common tidal volume used to manage patients in acute respiratory failure is about 10 mL/kg of predicted body weight (PBW).[12] However, it is also important to emphasis that all healthy, relaxed mammals breathe with a tidal volume of about 6 to 7 mL/kg PBW.[113] There is no evidence to indicate that tidal volumes greater than 10 mL/kg PBW are ever indicated in the management of critically ill patients. In fact, evidence from a retrospective review indicates that the development of acute lung injury is linked to large tidal volumes (>10 mL/kg PBW).[42] As a rule, all critically ill patients should be ventilated with less than 10 mL/kg PBW VT regardless of the cause of acute ventilatory failure. Patients with acute lung injury or ARDS ideally should be ventilated with VT 4 to 8 mL/kg PBW.[114]

2. Plateau Pressure

As discussed earlier, the plateau pressure (end-inspiratory equilibration pressure) is a reflection of the mean peak alveolar pressure and is reflective of the PTP. As with VT, it is unknown whether there is a specific plateau pressure that is safe. Because of the high shear forces associated with the ventilation of heterogeneous lung, mechanical lung injury is theoretically possible even with PTP values below 30 cm H_2O. However, most would agree that a plateau pressure less than 25 cm H_2O probably does not reflect an injurious level of overdistention and that provided plateau pressures are in this range, tidal volumes less than 10 mL/kg PBW are acceptable. However, as plateau pressure increases, the delivered tidal volume should be decreased. VT should be less than 8 mL/kg PBW if the plateau pressure is 25 to 30 cm H_2O and less than 6 mL/kg PBW if plateau pressures are above 30 cm H_2O. Ideally, all patients should be managed with a plateau pressure less than 30 cm H_2O unless there is a marked decrease in chest wall compliance. If the chest wall compliance is decreased, the PTP is decreased and the risk of overdistention is reduced. In patients with stiff chest walls and abdomens because of sepsis, abdominal distention, fluid resuscitation, and so forth, a plateau pressure higher than 30 cm H_2O may be necessary and not associated with an increased risk of VILI.[72] However, in all patients plateau pressure should ideally be maintained below 40 cm H_2O. Alternatively, some have advocated the use of an esophageal balloon to estimate pleural pressure and guide mechanical ventilation strategies to limit PTP.

3. Peak Flow and Flow Waveform

Precisely how gas is delivered is critical during patient-triggered approaches to ventilatory support to ensure patient-ventilator synchrony and minimize patients' work of breathing. If a patient is spontaneously triggering the ventilator, peak flow delivery should at least match the patient's inspiratory demand.[73] Most patients with a moderate to strong ventilatory demand require a peak flow greater than 80 L/min. As clearly demonstrated by Marini and colleagues (Fig. 45-27), if the peak flow does not meet the patient's inspiratory demand, the work performed by the patient increases. The efficiency of the work may be greater than during spontaneous breathing, but the patient's overall work may be similar.[73]

It is important to remember that if the patient is triggering the positive-pressure breaths, the work of breathing is shared between the patient and the ventilator. It is for this reason that patients originally receiving assisted ventilation demonstrate altered gas delivery patterns when sedated to apnea. With the transition to controlled ventilation, peak airway and plateau pressures usually increase in volume ventilation and tidal volumes decrease in pressure ventilation.[51] Because the patient is no longer performing a portion of the work of breathing, the work performed by the ventilator must increase.

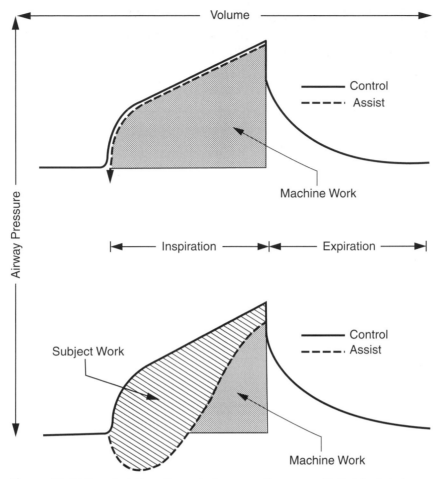

Figure 45-27 Top, depiction of an actual pressure-time curve *(dotted line)* during volume control ventilation superimposed on the ideal curve reflecting total work of breathing. **Bottom**, Note the scooped-out actual pressure waveform when patient's demand increases. The hatched area reflects the work performed by the patient during assisted volume-targeted ventilation. (From Marini JJ, Rodrigues RM, Lamb V: The inspiratory workload of patient-initiated mechanical ventilation. Am Rev Respir Dis 134:902-909, 1986.)

Most ventilators during volume ventilation can deliver gas flow in a decelerating or square wave flow pattern. If patients are triggering inspiration, we recommend the use of a decelerating flow pattern, especially when a small V_T is delivered. A decelerating flow pattern allows a high peak flow to be delivered but also ensures that inspiratory time can be adequately set.

In patients who are sedated and not triggering the ventilator, the choice of flow waveform is academic and the setting of peak flow is dependent on the clinician-selected inspiratory time and tidal volume.

4. Inspiratory Time

In patients triggering each breath, the set inspiratory time should equal the patient's neural inspiratory time.[36] As illustrated in Figure 45-28, when inspiratory time is decreased to equal the patient's desired inspiratory time and peak flow is increased to match the patient's demand,

the patient's work of breathing and effort correspondingly decrease. It is rare that a stressed patient desires an inspiratory time greater than 1 second.[36] In fact, many stressed adults desire an inspiratory time between 0.6 and 0.9 second. Carefully matching the patient's inspiratory time generally markedly improves patient-ventilator synchrony.

In patients receiving controlled ventilation, inspiratory time is set on the basis of tidal volume and the clinician's perceived optimal time. In most settings an inspiratory time of about 1.0 second is ideal. There are clearly groups who prefer to lengthen inspiratory time is ARDS or acute lung injury to inverse the I:E ratio; however, there are no data to indicate that long inspiratory times result in better oxygenation or better outcomes than appropriately set PEEP.[70,81] Prolongation of inspiratory time can have a minor effect on CO_2 elimination by allowing time for inspired gas to travel from lung units with fast time constants to adjacent units with slow time constants

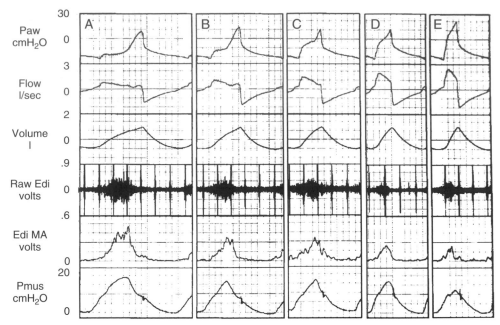

Figure 45-28 Representative example of the effect of alternations in peak flow and inspiratory time on airway pressure (P_{aw}), the raw diaphragmatic electromyography (EMG) signal (R_{aw} Edi), the diaphragmatic EMG signal after removal of the electrocardiographic interference and rectification, and the calculated pressure output of the inspiratory muscles (P_{mus}). As flow increases, note the reduction in EMG activity and muscle output. (From Fernandez R, Mendez M, Younes M: Effect of ventilator flow rate on respiratory timing in normal humans. Am J Respir Crit Care Med 159:710-719, 1999.)

(so-called pendelluft). In patients with severe asthma, inspiratory time may need to be increased to 1.2 to 1.5 seconds to ensure distribution of ventilation past severely obstructed airways.[51] It should be remembered that in asthma, airway resistance is increased not only during exhalation but also during inspiration.

5. Respiratory Rate

In most settings, the respiratory rate provided by the ventilator is selected by the patient. The specific rate may vary considerably depending on pathophysiology; patients with neuromuscular disease or postoperative respiratory failure without marked ventilatory demand may choose a rate in the 12 to 20/min range. Patients with COPD may choose a rate in the 20s, and patients with ARDS or acute lung injury may require rates in the low 30s. The only factor that truly needs to be considered other than why the ventilatory demand is so high and what can be done to reduce it is auto-PEEP. The greater the rate in any patient, the more likely auto-PEEP is to develop.[93] Auto-PEEP is a problem in any ventilated patient because auto-PEEP in volume ventilation increases peak and plateau pressure and in pressure ventilation decreases tidal volume.[51] Auto-PEEP is a particular problem in patients triggering the ventilator because increases in auto-PEEP result in greater effort and work of breathing to trigger the ventilator,

increasing ventilatory demand and further increasing the rate.[93] The application of extrinsic PEEP can be helpful in the spontaneously breathing patient with auto-PEEP to help reduce this inspiratory threshold load. Careful monitoring of end-expiratory flow identifies the presence of auto-PEEP (Fig. 45-29).

In patients requiring controlled ventilation, the rate should be set to maintain an acceptable $Paco_2$. VT should not be the primary variable adjusted to achieve the $Paco_2$; rate should always be optimized first. As with assisted ventilation, the only factor limiting rate is auto-PEEP.

6. Expiratory Time and Inspiratory-to-Expiratory Ratio

Expiratory time, like respiratory rate, is limited only by auto-PEEP. Ideally, the expiratory time should be long enough to ensure that auto-PEEP does not develop or limit the development of auto-PEEP in patients with airway obstruction. Setting the I:E ratio is not a concern during the ventilation of acutely ill patients. If care is taken to ensure that inspiratory and expiratory times are properly set, I:E ratio is simply the resultant (i.e., dependent variable). As stated earlier, there are no data to indicate that inverse ratio ventilation (a prolonged inspiratory time resulting in an inverse I:E ratio) is of benefit in the management of ARDS or acute lung injury.[70,81]

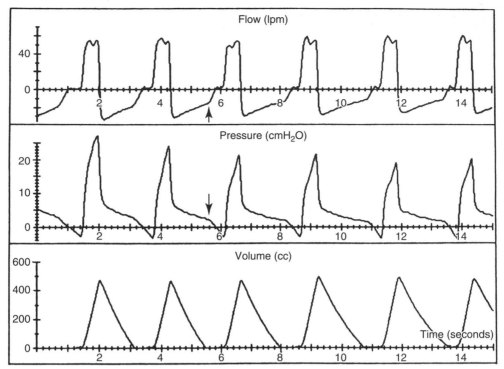

Figure 45-29 Flow, pressure, and volume waveforms in a patient dyssynchronous with the mechanical ventilator (variable airway pressure curves) and with auto-PEEP present and an insensitive trigger. The *arrow* on the pressure and flow curves indicates end of exhalation. Note the considerable expiratory flow at this transition. Whenever expiratory flow does not return to zero, air trapping and auto-PEEP are present. Also note the notching of inspiratory flow, suggestive of asynchrony. PEEP, positive end-expiratory pressure. (From Kacmarek RM, Hess D, Stoller J: Monitoring in Respiratory Care. St. Louis, Mosby, 1993, p 511.)

7. Positive End-Expiratory Pressure/Continuous Positive Airway Pressure

PEEP is set to prevent unstable lung units from collapsing at end expiration. It is important to understand that PEEP does not recruit lung; peak inspiratory pressure (PIP) recruits lung. However, an increase in PEEP results in an increase in PIP (if tidal volume is held constant), but it is the increase in PIP and not PEEP that overcomes the opening pressure of collapsed lung units. In all settings, the least PEEP necessary to maintain unstable lung open at end exhalation should be set.[51]

A number of methods are used to set PEEP: (1) by an algorithm, either defined or intuitive, that relates PEEP and FIO_2 to PaO_2 as used by the ARDSnet (Fig. 45-30)[11,114]; (2) by the use of the patient's measured P-V curve of the total respiratory system, specifically the lower inflection point on the P-V curve (P_{flex}) (Fig. 45-31); (3) by the use of an increasing PEEP trial[22]; and (4) by the use of a decremental PEEP trial.[53,116]

The ARDSnet has demonstrated in two studies that their PEEP/FIO_2 table can be used to set PEEP.[11,114] In the ARDSnet Hi/Low PEEP trial, the use of either the low-PEEP or high-PEEP table had a similar impact on outcome.[11] However, the table does not take into consideration the unique lung mechanics of the individual patient. In addition, on the basis of reports evaluating the response of ARDS patients to standard ventilator settings[35,121] and the ARDS mortality in epidemiologic studies,[12,25] it can be argued that the vast majority of patients studied in both ARDSnet trials had acute lung injury, not ARDS. More severe illness may be required to realize the benefits of PEEP because the sickest patients are the ones likely to have the highest surface tensions, yielding high closing pressures promoting derecruitment. In addition, the ARDSnet Hi/Low PEEP study neglected the potential hemodynamic effects of PEEP on gut perfusion because the high-PEEP patients may require more aggressive volume resuscitation than lower PEEP patients. Excessive PEEP can promote increased pulmonary dead space, which has been associated with a poor outcome in ARDS.

Amato[1] and Ranieri[99] and their colleagues, as well as numerous animal studies,[50,90,111] have demonstrated that setting PEEP above P_{flex} on the P-V curve of the total respiratory system results in a better outcome than the use of oxygenation as the targeted endpoint for setting PEEP. However, there are many problems with obtaining and interpreting P-V curves that make them impractical

Lower-PEEP group													
FIO$_2$	0.3	0.4	0.4	0.5	0.5	0.6	0.7	0.7	0.7	0.8	0.9	0.9	0.9	1.0
PEEP	5	5	8	8	10	10	10	12	14	14	14	16	18	18–24

Higher-PEEP group (before protocol changed to use higher levels of PEEP)												
FIO$_2$	0.3	0.3	0.3	0.3	0.3	0.4	0.4	0.5	0.5	0.5–0.8	0.8	0.9	1.0
PEEP	5	8	10	12	14	14	16	16	18	20	22	22	22–24

Higher-PEEP group (after protocol changed to use higher levels of PEEP)									
FIO$_2$	0.3	0.3	0.4	0.4	0.5	0.5	0.5–0.8	0.8	0.9	1.0
PEEP	12	14	14	16	16	18	20	22	22	22–24

Figure 45-30 PEEP-FIO$_2$ tables for the ARDSnet low-PEEP group and high-PEEP group. ARDS, acute respiratory distress syndrome; FIO$_2$, fraction of inspired oxygen; PEEP, positive end-expiratory pressure. (From Brower RG, Lanken PN, MacIntyre N, et al: Higher versus lower positive end-expiratory pressures in patients with the acute respiratory distress syndrome. N Engl J Med 351:327-336, 2004.)

for use in everyday clinical practice.[87,112] Until the ventilator manufacturers make it simple to use the ICU ventilator to obtain a P-V curve and provide analysis of the curve, the use of P-V curves for setting PEEP will mostly remain a research tool.

An increasing PEEP trial has been used as a method of setting PEEP for more than 30 years.[22] This approach should always be used with all other ventilation settings held constant because altering VT can affect the level of PEEP that appears most optimal.[107] During an increasing PEEP trial, PaO$_2$, shunt fraction, PaCO$_2$, compliance, cardiac output, and oxygen delivery have been used as endpoints for the best PEEP level.[102] In the absence of a lung recruitment maneuver this approach works well; however, if a lung recruitment maneuver is performed starting at a low level of PEEP, titrating up allows initial derecruitment, negating the effect of the lung recruitment maneuver.

If a lung recruitment maneuver is performed, the best method of identifying the minimal PEEP level that sustains the benefits of the lung recruitment maneuver is a decremental PEEP trial.[53] In this approach, after completion of the recruitment maneuver, PEEP is set at a level above that considered necessary (in adults 18 to 20 cm H$_2$O), and the FIO$_2$ is then decreased until the PaO$_2$ is within the target range. PEEP is then slowly decreased in 1 to

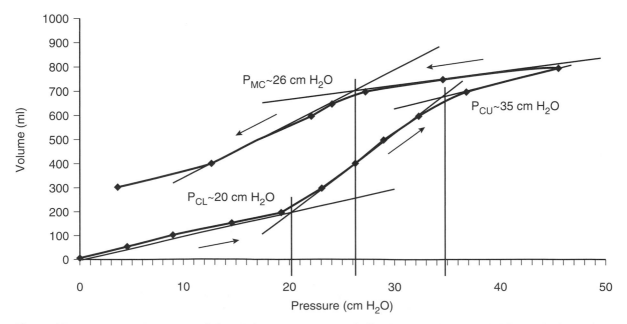

Figure 45-31 Pressure-volume curve of the total respiratory system indicating the inflation and deflation limb. *Arrows* indicate direction of flow. P$_{CL}$, lower inflection point-P$_{flex}$; P$_{CU}$ upper inflection point; P$_{MC}$ point of maximum compliance charge on deflation limb. (From Kacmarek RM, et al: Essentials of Respiratory Care, 4th ed. St. Louis, Mosby, 2005, p 753.)

2 cm H_2O steps every 15 to 20 minutes until the PaO_2 drops 10% below the highest level observed during the decremental trial.[101,116] Generally, PaO_2 first increases and then decreases as the trial proceeds. The PEEP level preceding the 10% drop in PaO_2 is the ideal level. The lung is rerecruited and PEEP and FIO_2 are set at the identified levels.

Regardless of the approach, sufficient PEEP should always be set to eliminate end-expiratory collapse. If this is done carefully, the highest PEEP level applied to a patient should occur on the first day of ventilation for ARDS or acute lung injury and then decrease over time as the disease improves.[1] Although the optimal amount of PEEP must be individualized to the specific patient, we found that the majority of patients with acute lung injury require about 8 to 15 cm H_2O PEEP and ARDS patients require about 12 to 20 cm H_2O PEEP. However, in either group a patient may rarely need more than 20 cm H_2O PEEP.

Postoperative hypoxemia has been managed for years with the use of mask CPAP.[57] Levels from 8 to 12 cm H_2O seem most appropriate in these patients. However, care should be exercised to avoid continuing mask CPAP in the event that the respiratory failure progresses.[18] Continuous CPAP or intermittent CPAP in this setting has been shown to avoid intubation.

In COPD patients, PEEP is applied to offset the impact of auto-PEEP on work of breathing and triggering the ventilator.[95] In this setting PEEP should be slowly titrated in 1 cm H_2O steps until the patient's respiratory rate and the ventilator response rate are equal.

8. Fraction of Inspired Oxygen

With all patients requiring ventilatory support, the FIO_2 is adjusted to maintain a PaO_2 greater than 60 mm Hg, although in severe ARDS a PaO_2 greater than 50 mm Hg may be acceptable.[51] Ideally, the lowest FIO_2 achieving the target should be set. Most prefer maintaining the FIO_2 below some defined level to avoid the potential of oxygen toxicity and nitrogen washout atelectasis.[102] We generally prefer FIO_2 less than 0.6 on the basis of older data suggesting that FIO_2 above this value may predict residual lung disease following ARDS. Some authors have suggested that high levels of FIO_2 in prior studies may in fact be a marker of inadequate PEEP. Therefore, the FIO_2 should be minimized before the PEEP level is markedly adjusted downward.

B. LUNG RECRUITMENT

As noted in Figure 45-31, lung volume at any PEEP level is greater if ventilation occurs on the deflation as opposed to the inflation limb of the pressure-volume curve of the respiratory system. The goal of lung recruitment maneuvers is to move lung volume to the deflation limb by opening collapsed lung. Proponents of lung recruitment cite the fact that the recruited lung requires less pressure to ventilate, less FIO_2 to oxygenate, is less likely to develop pneumonia, and has more normal surfactant production than the collapsed lung.[51] On the other hand, opponents of lung recruitment cite the fact that in a number of studies improved oxygenation early in the course of ARDS did not translate into improved outcome.[19,43,114] However, the question should not be whether a better PaO_2 is important when managing ARDS or acute lung injury but whether it is important to open lung that is recruitable to avoid the development of VILI. The answer to this question is yes in animal models,[41,119] but data are lacking for patients.

A number of approaches to recruiting the lung have been studied: the use of periodic sighs,[92] the use of high pressure control levels for short periods,[77] and the use of high CPAP levels for short periods.[1] A number of groups have demonstrated short-term improvement in PaO_2 when using periodic sighs achieved by either increasing the tidal volume for a few breaths or increasing the PEEP level for a few breaths each minute.[68,92] Of concern with this approach is the potential long-term impact on lung injury from achieving a peak airway pressure of 40 to 45 cm H_2O repetitively over several days. No data are currently available to address this concern.

The use of high-level pressure control ventilation for a few minutes does recruit lungs. Generally, with this approach PEEP is set to 20 to 25 cm H_2O and PIP to 40 to 50 cm H_2O with inspiratory time set about 2 to 3 seconds and the rate decreased to 8 to 12/min. Ventilation at this level is maintained for 1 to 3 minutes, and then a decremental PEEP trial is used to identify the optimal PEEP. During the PEEP trial, PIP, inspiratory time, and rate are readjusted to the level achieving the desired VT and respiratory rate.

The approach to lung recruitment that has received the most study is the use of a CPAP of 40 to 50 cm H_2O for more than 30 to 40 seconds.[1,46,67,116] After the maneuver, normal ventilation is resumed and a decremental PEEP trial performed. Recruitment maneuvers do not improve oxygenation and lung mechanics in all patients with ARDS or acute lung injury. They are most likely to work if performed on the first or second day of ARDS or acute lung injury in patients with secondary ARDS whose chest walls are not stiffer than normal and who are cardiovascularly stable.[46,67] In fact, the data seem to indicate that if recruitment maneuvers are performed later in the course of ARDS, the maneuvers are unlikely to be successful and there is an increased likelihood of cardiovascular compromise.[46]

Lung recruitment maneuvers should not be performed in patients who are hemodynamically unstable, and patients should be adequately sedated during the maneuver to avoid fighting the ventilator and increased hemodynamic instability. Ideally, patients should be stabilized with 100% oxygen before the recruitment maneuver. During the maneuver, oxygen saturation from pulse oximetry, heart rate, BP, and cardiac rhythm should be carefully monitored and the maneuver immediately aborted if instability develops. If patients are carefully selected, little hemodynamic compromise has been reported, and barotrauma is a rarity if peak alveolar pressures are kept below 50 cm H_2O. However, clinicians should be alert to the fact that barotrauma may occur during a recruitment maneuver. Of note, heavy sedation or paralysis is required during recruitment maneuvers because any drop in pleural pressure is potentially dangerous if alveolar pressure is maintained above 40 cm H_2O.

C. PRESSURE VERSUS VOLUME VENTILATION

Regardless of the ventilator selected or mode of ventilation employed, gas delivery is provided in one of two basic formats: volume ventilation and pressure ventilation (Table 45-1). With volume ventilation a specific tidal volume is set as well as a flow waveform and peak flow or inspiratory time. What is allowed to vary on a breath-to-breath basis is airway and alveolar pressure. The opposite is true with pressure ventilation. Here a peak pressure and as a result a maximum alveolar pressure are set along with inspiratory time. What varies on a breath-to-breath basis is tidal volume. If the clinician's preference is to maintain V_T, volume preset ventilation is the approach, whereas if the desire is to maintain peak alveolar pressure, pressure preset ventilation is the approach. The discussion of which is preferred is academic in the patient who is not triggering the ventilator. However, in spontaneously breathing patients actively triggering the ventilator, patients' inspiratory demand is better met with pressure ventilation and the likelihood of patient-ventilator synchrony is increased with pressure ventilation.[75]

The impact of changes in lung mechanics and as a result monitoring of patients with volume versus pressure ventilation also varies considerably. Any factor that alters lung mechanics in volume ventilation results in an alteration in peak and plateau pressures. As a result, it is critical to monitor changes in pressure during volume ventilation. However, with pressure ventilation changes in lung mechanics alter V_T and require careful monitoring of delivered volume (Table 45-2).

Table 45-1 Pressure versus Volume Ventilation

	Volume	Pressure
Peak flow	Constant	Variable
Flow pattern	Preset	Decelerating
Inspiratory time	Preset	Preset
Minimum rate	Preset	Preset
Peak airway pressure	Variable	Constant
Peak alveolar pressure	Variable	Constant
Tidal volume	Constant	Variable

Table 45-2 Ventilator Response and Monitoring during Pressure and Volume Ventilation

	Volume	Pressure
Decreased compliance	↑ Pressure	↓ Volume
Increased compliance	↓ Pressure	↑ Volume
Increased auto-PEEP	↑ Pressure	↓ Volume
Decreased auto-PEEP	↓ Pressure	↑ Volume
Pneumothorax	↑ Pressure	↓ Volume
Bronchospasm	↑ Pressure	↓ Volume
Mucosal edema	↑ Pressure	↓ Volume
Secretions	↑ Pressure	↓ Volume
Pleural effusion	↑ Pressure	↓ Volume
Increased effort by patient	↓ Pressure	↑ Volume
Decreased effort by patient	↑ Pressure	↓ Volume

PEEP, positive end-expiratory pressure.

It is clear that there are advantages to the use of both pressure and volume ventilation. As a result, some manufacturers have attempted to develop modes of ventilatory support that combine the beneficial aspects of each of these approaches to ventilatory support. These new modes of ventilation are frequently referred to as mixed modes of ventilation.

D. NONINVASIVE POSITIVE-PRESSURE VENTILATION

It has become increasingly evident over the past 10 years that many patients with acute respiratory failure can be adequately maintained with noninvasive positive-pressure ventilation (NPPV). The evidence supporting the benefits of NPPV is overwhelming in patients with an acute exacerbation of COPD.[63] Numerous randomized controlled trials indicate that the use of NPPV avoids intubation, decreases the length of mechanical ventilation, decreases ICU and hospital length of stay, decreases the incidence of nosocomial pneumonia, and decreases mortality.[63] It is clear that NPPV should be the first-line therapy for COPD patients with an acute exacerbation.

The use of mask CPAP in acute cardiogenic pulmonary edema has also been shown to avoid intubation and improve gas exchange better than standard therapy.[4] CPAP is indicated provided the patient can still adequately ventilate. However, if CO_2 levels are increased, noninvasive mask ventilation is the treatment of choice.[85] There are also data indicating that if the patient in acute pulmonary edema also presents with a myocardial infarction, intubation and conventional ventilation should be initiated to avoid further risk.[79]

NPPV has been used in many other settings: immunosuppressed patients,[3] patients awaiting lung transplantation,[2] patients having difficulty weaning,[37] patients in whom extubation failed,[64] patients with asthma,[78] those with cystic fibrosis,[55] and those with acute lung injury.[38] The data for these groups are limited and somewhat controversial. For immunosuppressed patients and those awaiting transplantation, the data, although limited, are good and NPPV should be used in these settings. In all other applications, care should be exercised when using NPPV and intubation provided if clinical status does not rapidly improve with the use of NPPV. For example, poor outcomes have been observed among patients with hypoxemic respiratory failure when noninvasive ventilation is provided for several days without resolution of the underlying etiology of respiratory disease.

To improve the likelihood of successful application of NPPV, careful and attentive monitoring of patients is required for at least the first hour. Having a knowledgeable and experienced clinician at the bedside continuously during this period clearly increases the likelihood of success. In addition, careful selection of both the mask and ventilator is critical. For acute respiratory failure, we have found an oronasal mask to be ideal when used with a ventilator designed to provide NPPV in the ICU. The ventilator should provide appropriate monitoring and alarms including airway pressure, flow, and volume waveforms so that patient-ventilator synchrony can be carefully assessed. Finally, peak airway pressures should be maintained less than 20 cm H_2O. The greater the peak pressure, the greater the leak problem, the greater the likelihood of clinically significant gastric distention, and the greater the likelihood that intubation is indicated. If peak pressures are maintained less than 20 cm H_2O, a nasogastric tube is rarely indicated. In addition, humidity should be added to the circuit during all acute applications of NPPV. Without the use of passover humidity heated to about 28° to 30° C, the probability of retained secretions causing the need for intubation is markedly increased.

E. CLASSICAL MODES OF VENTILATION

On today's mechanical ventilators there are numerous modes of ventilatory support available. All ventilators today provide what can be referred to as the four classical modes of ventilatory support: control, assist/control, assist (pressure support), and synchronized intermittent mandatory ventilation (SIMV) (Table 45-3). All of these modes except pressure support are available in either a pressure or volume ventilation format. Pressure support is available only in a pressure ventilation gas delivery format. These four are the basic modes of ventilation that are used in the vast majority of patients.

1. Control Mode

This is the original mode of ventilatory support. With this mode the ventilator is programmed to deliver a positive-pressure breath at a set rate and the patient is a

Table 45-3   Modes of Ventilatory Support

Classical Modes
Control ventilation
Assist/control ventilation
Pressure support ventilation
Intermittent synchronized mandatory ventilation
New Modes of Ventilation
Pressure-regulated volume control
Volume support
Airway pressure release ventilation
Bilevel ventilation
Automatic tube compensation

passive recipient of the breath (Fig. 45-32). The patient has no ability to influence gas delivery. With today's ventilators the mode is modified. Setting the sensitivity to the most insensitive setting is the only way to minimize the patient's ability to trigger a breath. However, even at the most insensitive setting, patients with a strong ventilatory drive are able to trigger the ventilator. True control ventilation with modern ventilators is achieved only by sedation to apnea and is rarely used outside of the operating room.

2. Assist/Control Mode

With this mode the patient can trigger the positive-pressure breath by appropriate setting of the sensitivity (Fig. 45-33). If the patient does not trigger the breath, a control breath is delivered at the preset backup or minimal rate. As with control ventilation, assist/control (A/C) can be provided with volume ventilation (VA/C) or pressure ventilation (PA/C). During VA/C, V_T, flow waveform, peak flow or inspiratory time, backup rate, PEEP, F_{IO_2}, and sensitivity must be set. With PA/C, pressure control level, inspiratory time, backup rate, PEEP, F_{IO_2}, and sensitivity must be set.

3. Pressure Support

This is a true assisted mode of ventilation without a backup rate (Fig. 45-34). However, all modern ventilators have an apnea ventilation mode that takes over if the patient becomes apneic for a period of about 20 to 60 seconds. During pressure support, pressure level, sensitivity, F_{IO_2}, and PEEP are set. The patient controls the inspiratory time. With all ventilators the primary factor that terminates the pressure support breath is flow. When flow decreases to a percentage of peak flow, usually 25%, the breath ends. If the patient chooses to end the breath before flow decreases to the termination level, an increase in pressure above the set level after about 300 milliseconds

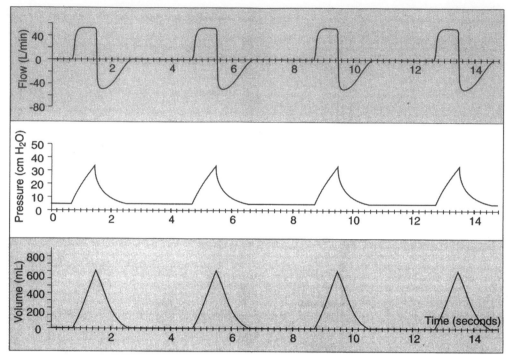

Figure 45-32 Flow, airway pressure, and volume waveforms during volume-targeted square wave flow, control mode ventilation. Note that there are no negative airway pressure deflections indicating patient's effort. (From Hess DR, MacIntyre NR, Mishoe SC, et al: Respiratory Care: Principles and Practice. Philadelphia, WB Saunders, 2002, p 790.)

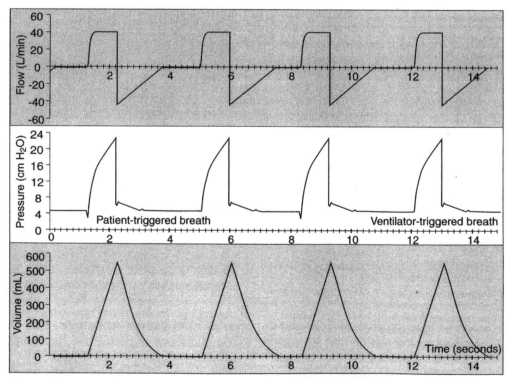

Figure 45-33 Airway pressure, flow, and volume waveforms during volume-targeted, square wave flow, assist/control ventilation. Note the negative airway pressure deflection at the start of each breath. (From Hess DR, MacIntyre NR, Mishoe SC, et al: Respiratory Care: Principles and Practice. Philadelphia, WB Saunders, 2002, p 786.)

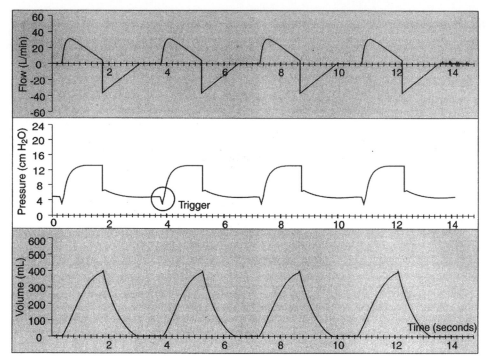

Figure 45-34 Airway pressure, flow, and volume waveforms during pressure support ventilation. Note that every breath is patient triggered. (From Hess DR, MacIntyre NR, Mishoe SC, et al: Respiratory Care: Principles and Practice. Philadelphia, WB Saunders, 2002, p 787.)

into the breath (by expiratory muscle effort) also terminates the breath. A third criterion ending a pressure support breath is time. If inspiratory time is greater than about 2 to 5 seconds (dependent upon the ventilator), the breath ends. This is typically an issue in the setting of leak (e.g., endotracheal tube cuff leak or bronchopleural fistula) but can occasionally be an issue in severe emphysema with slow time constant lung units.

Pressure support is a mode of ventilation that gives the patient control over the process of ventilatory support. It is a reasonable mode to utilize in all patients with an intact ventilatory drive who can maintain a normal ventilatory pattern. However, problems can exist at both the onset and termination of a pressure-supported breath (Fig. 45-35).[33] Two controls now available on many ventilators, rise time and inspiratory termination criteria,

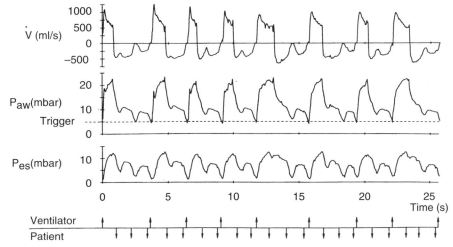

Figure 45-35 Gas flow, airway pressure, and esophageal pressure during pressure-supported ventilation with marked patient-ventilator dyssynchrony. Pressure spikes at the onset and termination of the breath indicate dyssynchrony as well as the difference between the patient's inspiratory efforts *(arrows)* and the ventilator response *(arrows)*. (From Fabry BE, Guttmann J, Eberhard LE, et al: An analysis of dys-synchrony between the spontaneously breathing patient and ventilator during inspiratory pressure support. Chest 1995; 107:1387-1394, 1995.)

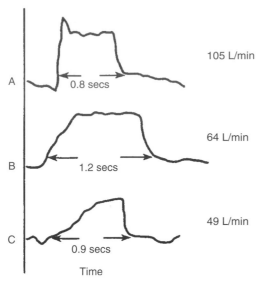

Figure 45-36 Effect of changing rise time in a patient preferring a midrange rise time. **A**, Rise time is in excess of patient's demand and the pressure spike is seen. As rise time is decreased (**B**), inspiratory time lengthens and the pressure spike is absent—machine output matches patient's demand. When rise time is further reduced (**C**), patient's demand exceeds machine flow rate and inspiratory time falls. Deformation of the pressure waveform during the rise to the set pressure support ventilation level is seen in **C**. (From Branson RD, Campbell RS, Davis K, et al: Altering flowrate during maximum pressure support ventilation (PSV$_{max}$): Effects on cardiorespiratory function. Respir Care 35:1056-1064, 1990.)

are designed to improve synchrony at the onset (rise time) and termination of a pressure support breath.[51]

As illustrated in Figure 45-36, rise time varies the slope of the airway pressure rise by varying the time it takes flow to reach its peak level.[7] A rapid rise time (attack rate) results in an almost immediate rise to peak flow.

In most patients with a high ventilatory demand, a rapid rise time is indicated, whereas those with a more limited demand prefer a moderate rise time.[69] A slow rise time is almost never indicated.

Inspiratory termination criteria vary the percentage of peak flow that ends the pressure support breath.[6] Ideally, at the end of the breath there should be a smooth transition from set pressure to exhalation (Fig. 45-37). If the peak pressure increases above the set level at the termination of the breath, the patient is activating muscles at the end of the ventilator's inspiratory phase to force exhalation.[61] This increases ventilatory drive and ventilatory rate. Increasing the percentage of the peak flow terminating the breath improves synchronous cycling to exhalation. The termination criteria should be slowly increased until the spike in pressure at the end of the breath is eliminated.

4. Synchronized Intermittent Mandatory Ventilation

This approach to ventilatory support provides a clinician a selected but fixed number of mandatory positive-pressure patient-triggered breaths. In between the mandatory patient-triggered breaths, unassisted spontaneous breathing around the PEEP/CPAP level is allowed (Fig. 45-38). If the patient does not trigger a positive-pressure breath within a defined assist window of time, a control breath is provided. In all of today's ventilators, pressure support can be applied to the spontaneous breaths in between the mandatory breaths (Fig. 45-39).

The advantages of SIMV are improved distribution of ventilation and cardiac output because of the negative intrathoracic pressure generated in between mandatory breaths. The disadvantages are the high work of breathing and patient's effort along with dyssynchrony in

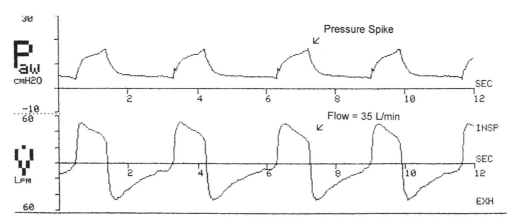

Figure 45-37 Airway pressure and flow waveforms during pressure support ventilation with the Nelcor Puritan Bennett 7200 demonstrating pressure cycling to exhalation. The spike in the airway pressure at the end of the breath is a result of the patient beginning exhalation before the ventilator is ready to make the transition to exhalation. The increase in pressure causes the breath to end. (From Branson RD, Campbell RS: Pressure support ventilation, patient-ventilator synchrony, and ventilator algorithms. Respir Care 43:1045-1047, 1998.)

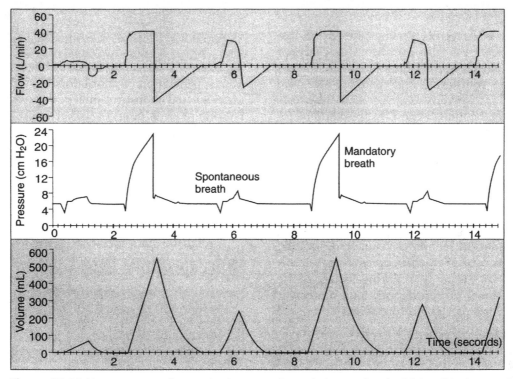

Figure 45-38 Airway pressure, flow, and volume waveforms during synchronized intermittent mandatory ventilation. (From Hess DR, MacIntyre NR, Mishoe SC, et al: Respiratory Care: Principles and Practice. Philadelphia, WB Saunders, 2002, p 786.)

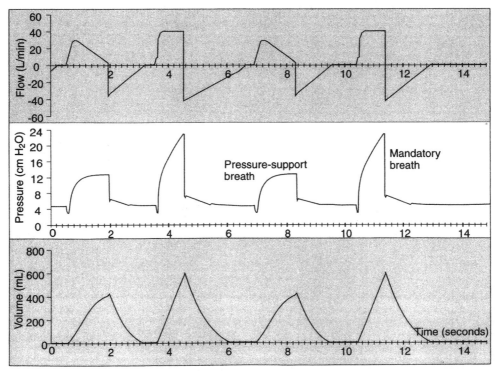

Figure 45-39 Airway pressure, flow, and volume waveforms during synchronized intermittent mandatory ventilation with pressure support applied to the nonmandatory breaths. (From Hess DR, MacIntyre NR, Mishoe SC, et al: Respiratory Care: Principles and Practice. Philadelphia, WB Saunders, 2002, p 788.)

patients with a high ventilatory demand.[74] As observed by Marini and colleagues (Fig. 45-40) more than 15 years ago, as the mandatory rate decreases, the work of breathing increases not only for the spontaneous unassisted breaths but also for the mandatory breaths. Note in Figure 45-41 that the diaphragmatic electromyographic activity as well as esophageal pressure swings are as great during the mandatory breaths as during the spontaneous unassisted breaths.[59] As the mandatory rate decreases, the respiratory center has a difficult time altering its output between the high load during unassisted breaths and the low load during the mandatory breaths.

F. NEW MODES OF VENTILATORY SUPPORT

The newest generation of mechanical ventilators have included a number of new modes of ventilatory support, some of which incorporate features of the classical modes of ventilatory support while others are unique. The three modes that have the widest distribution in the newest generation of mechanical ventilators are pressure-regulated volume control (PRVC) and volume support (VS), airway pressure release ventilation (APRV) and bilevel ventilation, and automatic tube composition.

1. Pressure-Regulated Volume Control

PRVC and VS are true dual modes of ventilatory support. Each targets both a maximum pressure and V_T

and each readjusts gas delivery on the basis of the previously delivered breath.

PRVC is essentially PA/C with a volume target. That is, the clinician sets a maximum peak pressure, the targeted V_T, inspiratory time, sensitivity, FIO_2, PEEP, and rise time. VS is essentially pressure support in which the clinician sets a maximum peak pressure, the targeted V_T, sensitivity, FIO_2, PEEP, rise time, and in some ventilators inspiratory termination criteria. In both of these modes, the ventilator initially provides a test breath at a low pressure, then calculates the peak pressure necessary to deliver the tidal volume. Subsequently, the necessary pressure level is delivered either in a single jump to the calculated pressure or by a second test breath and then a jump to the calculated pressure.

A notable feature of these modes is that if the targeted V_T is not provided on a given breath the peak pressure is adjusted on the next breath from 1 to 3 cm H_2O to achieve the targeted V_T. Theoretically, the peak pressure could be adjusted every breath if the V_T is not on target. Airway pressure can increase to the maximum level set or can decrease to baseline (PEEP/CPAP). That is, positive

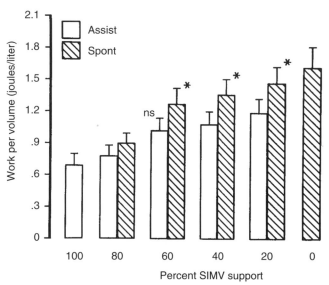

Figure 45-40 Inspiratory work per unit volume (work per liter, Wp/L) done by the patient during assisted cycles *(open bars)* and spontaneous cycles *(reverse crosshatched bars)*. Wp/L increased monotonically with decreasing synchronized intermittent mandatory ventilation (SIMV) percentage for both types of breath. Wp/L for spontaneous breaths tended to exceed Wp/L for machine-assisted breaths. Asterisk indicates $P < .01$. (From Marini JJ, Smith TC, Lamb VJ: External work output and force generation during synchronized intermittent mechanical ventilation. Am Rev Respir Dis 138:1169-1179, 1988.)

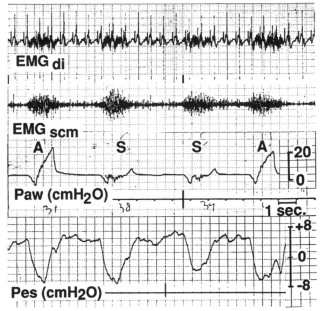

Figure 45-41 Electromyograms of the diaphragm (EMG$_{di}$) and of the sternocleidomastoid muscles (EMG$_{scm}$) in a representative patient, showing similar intensity and duration of electrical activity in successive assisted (A) and spontaneous (S) cycles. Note the contamination of EMG$_{di}$ by the QRS wave of the electrocardiogram signal regularly sensed by the esophageal electrodes. Apparent variations in the amplitude of QRS waves represent a photocopy artifact and not displacement of the esophageal electrodes. Paw, airway pressure; Pes, esophageal pressure. (From Imsand C, Feihl F, Perret C, et al: Regulation of inspiratory neuromuscular output during synchronized intermittent mechanical ventilation. Anesthesiology 80:13-22, 1994.)

pressure could be eliminated if the patient were capable of inspiring spontaneously the delivered VT without ventilatory support.

There are limited data indicating the effectiveness of PRVC and VS. Two randomized controlled trials in children have evaluated the ability with these modes to wean patients from ventilatory support. In one study weaning was more rapid but the control group protocol was poorly designed, whereas in the other no difference in weaning rate was noted.[96,98]

PRVC can be applied without concern in patients not triggering the ventilator. With this controlled setting, PRVC very adequately adjusts gas delivery to maintain both targeted volume and pressure. Of potential concern with both PRVC and VS is the patient with a strong ventilatory demand. If a patient's ventilatory demand is increased by fever, hypoxemia, or anxiety and the patient can exceed the targeted VT, the ventilating pressure may be reduced inappropriately to zero. In this setting, both modes should be cautiously applied. Unique terms are used by some ventilator manufacturers to describe these modes of ventilation.

2. Airway Pressure Release Ventilation

APRV and bilevel ventilation are modes of ventilation that are a unique mix of SIMV and inverse ratio pressure control ventilation. APRV was first described by Stock and coauthors as the application of two levels of CPAP (Fig. 45-42).[106] At both levels the patient is allowed to breath spontaneously. Some authors recommend limiting the time at the low CPAP level to avoid complete exhalation by the patient causing air trapping and auto-PEEP as well as avoidance of spontaneous breathing at this level.[15] Others allow complete exhalation with the lower CPAP level set as one would set PEEP.[97] Essentially, the low CPAP level is set to treat hypoxemia and the higher CPAP level to assist the patient's spontaneous breathing in CO_2 elimination. As with other modes, the VT created by movement from a high to low CPAP level should be limited.

The advantages of APRV are better distribution of ventilation and improved cardiac output because the patient is spontaneously breathing and creating a large decrease in intrathoracic pressure with each breath. The disadvantages are patient-ventilator dyssynchrony and increased work of breathing.[86] Dyssynchrony is observed primarily when the patient is trying to exhale and the ventilator moves from the lower to the higher CPAP level or when the patient is inhaling and the ventilator goes from the high to the low CPAP level. As illustrated in Figure 45-43, spontaneous breathing during APRV can result in markedly high pleural pressure changes with each breath, exceeding 10 cm H_2O.[86] This indicates high effort and work by the patient. This increased work is in part responsible for the increase in cardiac output observed with APRV.

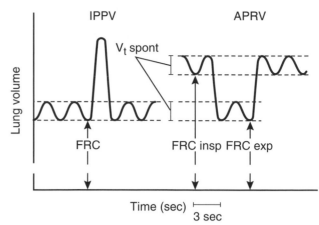

Figure 45-42 Theoretical spirometric tracing depicting change in lung volume that would occur in a patient with a mechanical IPPV breath compared with the change that would occur with an APRV breath. IPPV, intermittent positive pressure ventilation; APRV, airway pressure release ventilation. Inspiratory lung volume is the lung volume during spontaneous inspiration with continuous positive airway pressure during APRV. Expiratory lung volume is the lung volume during release of Paw during APRV, that is, lung volume after mechanical expiration. Expiratory lung volume is similar to functional residual capacity (FRC) during IPPV. FRC is the passive expiratory lung volume during APRV and is greater than FRC during IPPV. (From Stock MC, Downs JB, Frolicher DA: Airway pressure release ventilation. Crit Care Med 15:462-467, 1987.)

Bilevel ventilation, available on some ventilators, is a modification of APRV. Two additional features improve synchrony and work of breathing. First, the transition from high to low and low to high CPAP level is coordinated with the patient's effort to reduce dyssynchrony, and second, pressure support can be applied to the spontaneous breaths at the low or the high CPAP level or both levels. These additions modify the disadvantages of APRV but also minimize the advantages of APRV because unassisted spontaneous breathing is eliminated.

Both of these approaches have been used primarily in hypoxemic respiratory failure in postoperative patients or patients with acute lung injury. They should be avoided in patients with airway obstruction because of the air trapping that is associated with the short expiratory time and the lack of uniform ventilatory support for each breath. No data are currently available to indicate that these modes are preferable to assist/control in the management of ARDS or acute lung injury, but there are data to indicate that less sedation is required with APRV/ bilevel than assist/control ventilation.[97]

3. Automatic Tube Compensation

This mode of ventilation has been referred to as electronic extubation. Essentially, the ventilator determines the amount of pressure needed to overcome the resistance to gas flow through the endotracheal tube.[48] In order to do this, resistive features of various types and sizes of artificial airways are programmed into the ventilator. The clinician

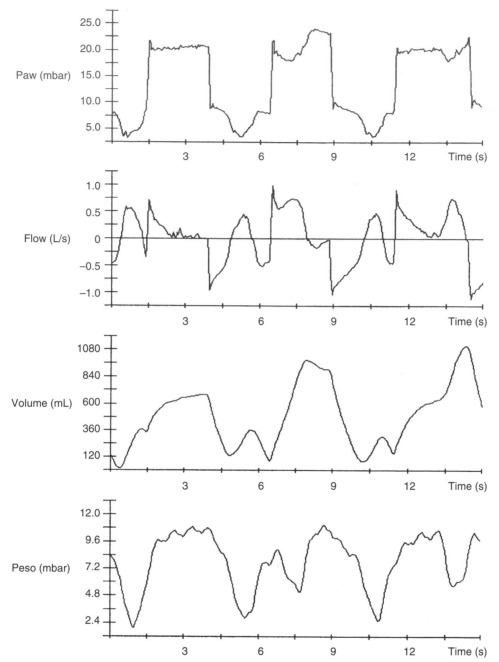

Figure 45-43 Airway pressure release ventilation original tracing. Airway pressure (Paw), flow, volume, and esophageal pressure (Peso) are shown for time intervals of the upper (P$_{high}$) and lower airway pressure (P$_{low}$) set to 2.5 seconds each. Note that spontaneous breathing occurs on the upper and lower airway pressure and that tidal volumes vary considerably depending on the pressure level from which an inspiration was started. Breaths were classified as type A, spontaneous breath on the lower pressure level; type B, spontaneous breath on the upper pressure level; type C, the pressure increase from the lower to the upper pressure level was triggered by an inspiratory effort of the patient; type D, mechanical breath; type E, combined mechanical and spontaneous inspiration without a triggered pressure increase from P$_{low}$ to P$_{high}$. (From Neumann P, Golisch W, Strohmeyer A, et al: Influence of different release times on spontaneous breathing pattern during airway pressure release ventilation. Intensive Care Med 28:1742-1749, 2002.)

must indicate the airway type and size. During inspiration, the ventilator can instantaneously monitor the flow demand of the patient. Knowing these two factors, the ventilator can calculate the amount of pressure (pressure = resistance × flow) needed to overcome the resistance of the artificial airway at any flow rate. As noted in Figure 45-44, the airway pressure waveform is similar to pressure support but can vary considerably from pressure support. With this mode, pressure is applied only when inspiratory flow is generated, that is, high flow, high pressure and low flow, low pressure. At the end of the breath the pressure decreases if the patient's inspiratory flow demand decreases. As a result, automatic tube compensation (ATC) is less likely to cause overdistention than pressure support because it does not force a ventilatory pattern. ATC gives control of ventilatory support to the patient. If the patient's ventilatory demand decreases, the applied pressure decreases. There is no set variable except the percentage of ATC. That is, the clinician sets the percentage of the resistance that is to be overcome during inspiration, 100% or a lower level. Thus, the patient may choose a ventilatory pattern with 200 mL VT and a rate of 40/min or 600 mL VT and a rate of 15/min.

Few data on the application of ATC are available. It does work as described, but it is difficult to identify the clinical setting in which it is most useful. Theoretically, if patients are maintained only with ATC and require a low level of pressure, 5 to 7 cm H_2O, they may be ready for extubation. In the patient with a strong ventilatory demand, ATC can be used to identify the pressure support level needed to meet the patient's demand.[32] This is a mode of ventilation requiring greater research before its use can be recommended.

VI. VENTILATORY MANAGEMENT OF ASTHMA, CHRONIC OBSTRUCTIVE PULMONARY DISEASE, AND ACUTE RESPIRATORY DISTRESS SYNDROME

A. ASTHMA

Asthma is a chronic eosinophilic inflammatory airway disease associated with bronchospasm, mucosal edema, and mucous plugging and characterized by reversible airflow obstruction.[23] Although the mortality associated with

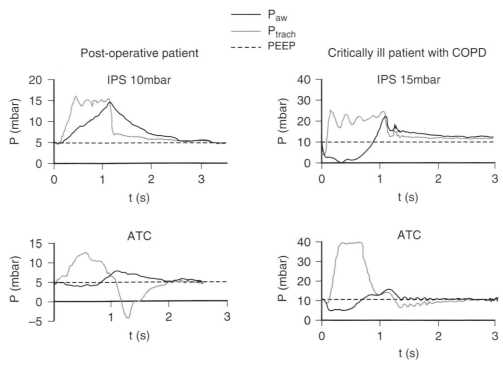

Figure 45-44 Airway pressure and tracheal pressure curves under inspiratory pressure support (IPS) and automatic tube compensation (ATC) in a patient after open heart surgery and a critically ill patient with chronic obstructive pulmonary disease (COPD). Note that although the ventilator lowers P_{aw} during expiration to subatmospheric pressure (bottom left), controlling the expiratory valve ensures that P_{trach} is above or equal to positive end-expiratory pressure (PEEP). The patient with acute respiratory insufficiency under ATC generates an inspiratory gas flow of greater than 21/s bottom right, which accounts for part of the deviation between P_{trach} and PEEP. (From Fabry B, Haberthür C, Zappe D, et al: Breathing pattern and additional work of breathing in spontaneously breathing patients with different ventilatory demands during inspiratory pressure support and automatic tube compensation. Intensive Care Med 23:545-552, 1997.)

asthma is rising for the population overall, the outcome for critically ill patients with status asthmaticus is now remarkably good. In fact, some authors have reported 0% mortality among patients mechanically ventilated for status asthmaticus in the modern era. However, a thorough understanding of the principles of mechanical ventilation related to asthma is required to achieve these excellent outcomes.

1. Assessment of Airflow Obstruction

a. Measurement of End-Expiratory Airflow

Modern mechanical ventilators have waveform displays that allow the assessment of airflow versus time. The shape of the expiratory airflow curve has been used by some to estimate the presence or absence of auto-PEEP. The presence of ongoing airflow at the end of exhalation is indeed indicative of alveolar pressure in excess of applied PEEP. However, caution must be exercised in assessing the degree of auto-PEEP from the quantity of expiratory airflow. Because high expiratory airflow resistance can yield low flow rates in the presence of high alveolar pressures, the estimation of the degree of auto-PEEP based on the quantity of expiratory airflow can be problematic. On the other hand, the absence of expiratory airflow at end exhalation does provide reasonable evidence of alveolar pressure equal to airway opening pressure, assuming airway patency.

b. Measurement of Auto-PEEP

A specialized nomenclature has been developed to characterize the airflow abnormalities of patients with severe airflow obstruction.[117] Auto-PEEP, also known as occult PEEP, is defined as an alveolar pressure above airway opening pressure and can be caused by flow limitation, dynamic hyperinflation, high minute ventilation, expiratory muscle activity, or high intra-abdominal pressure. Occult-occult PEEP is a term that has been defined to describe lung units with trapped gas that do not communicate with the airway opening, even after a prolonged end-expiratory pause. Occult-occult PEEP is probably a function of airway closure or occlusion secondary to mucous plugging and can be difficult to detect clinically. The performance of an end-expiratory occlusion maneuver can be helpful clinically to estimate auto-PEEP if the patient is not making expiratory muscle efforts. However, the absence of auto-PEEP with this technique should not be completely reassuring because occult-occult PEEP may still be present. In severe asthma, it is frequently better to monitor plateau pressure, which increases or decreases as occult-occult PEEP increases or decreases.

c. Measurement of Volume at End Inspiration

One measure of hyperinflation that has been employed by some investigators is the volume at end inspiration (VEI).[118] This value is determined by the collection of gas during a prolonged exhalation following a tidal inspiration. This can be achieved with many ventilators by setting a respiratory rate of 1 so that adequate time is allowed for full exhalation. Retrospective studies have suggested that an elevated value of VEI is associated with a poor outcome. Thus, some anesthesiologists have titrated mechanical ventilator settings according to this parameter. However, prospective studies are needed to define the optimal use of this metric.

d. Measurement of Inspiratory Airflow Resistance

The calculation of inspiratory airflow resistance is based on the peak minus plateau pressure divided by the inspiratory airflow. The basis for this calculation is that a plateau pressure (end-inspiratory pause) estimates mean peak alveolar pressure. Because the peak pressure and the plateau pressure are measured at the same lung volume, the difference in these pressures is a function of airflow resistance rather than respiratory system compliance. The major caveat with this technique is that the value derived is an inspiratory resistance, whereas the major issue with the ventilation of these patients is a result of expiratory flow limitation. However, the inspiratory resistance is easy to obtain and is commonly used clinically.

e. Measurement of Pulsus Paradoxus

Pulsus paradoxus is defined as an exaggeration of the normal phenomenon of an inspiratory fall in BP. A number of mechanisms have been reported to explain this finding, including an increase in left ventricular transmural pressure (yielding higher afterload), a shift of the interventricular septum toward the left ventricle, and pericardial constraint with right ventricular dilation. Nevertheless, in the spontaneously breathing patient, a measurement of the inspiratory fall in BP can be a useful method to quantify the severity of airflow obstruction. Placement of an arterial line can make this measurement more accurate than use of a manual cuff.

2. Selection of Ventilator Settings

Because the principal abnormality in asthmatic patients is a result of expiratory airflow obstruction, many practitioners have focused on increased exhalation time to minimize dynamic hyperinflation and auto-PEEP. However, there exists substantial complexity in this area, making bedside titration of an individual's ventilator settings imperative to optimize care. A number of strategies have been employed with regard to the ventilator settings in addition to the maximization of bronchodilator and anti-inflammatory therapy.

a. Increased Inspiratory Flow Rate

As stated, increases in inspiratory flow rate are commonly used to allow greater time for exhalation. In so doing, the goal is to alleviate dynamic hyperinflation by providing adequate time for the establishment of resting lung volume. However, such a strategy can be a "double-edged sword" because high inspiratory flow rates can trigger neural reflexes that affect breathing pattern. On volume ventilation, a high inspiratory flow rate has been associated with respiratory alkalosis, whereas on pressure ventilation high inspiratory flow leads to tachypnea. In spontaneously breathing patients with asthma, high inspiratory flow rates can either improve or worsen clinical status.

b. Permissive Hypercapnia

Permissive hypercapnia refers to the ventilator strategy that allows the P_{CO_2} to rise in a controlled fashion in an effort to reduce lung injury and the burden of gas exchange. Although a P_{CO_2} value of 40 mm Hg is considered normal in healthy humans, higher values may well be adaptive in disease.[54] Permissive hypercapnia can be achieved by reductions in respiratory rate or tidal volume, or both. The resulting reduction in minute ventilation leads to higher P_{CO_2} values and reduces the propensity for auto-PEEP. As a result of expiratory flow limitation, the amount of gas that can exit the lung in a given amount of time is fixed; therefore, reductions in inspired tidal volume lead to less gas trapping. Although no randomized trials have been performed demonstrating the efficacy of permissive hypercapnia, both clinical experience and case series suggest that this strategy is effective in status asthmaticus.

c. Increased Inspiratory Time

Inspiratory time in asthma must be sufficient to allow adequate distribution. Frequently, inspiratory time must be set between 1.0 and 1.5 seconds. In addition to gas exchange, one of the goals of the mechanical ventilator strategy is to optimize the delivery of bronchodilator medications. Because of issues of particle nebulization, very brief inspiratory times do not allow adequate medication delivery.[52] Therefore, during the nebulizer treatments, some advocate slow inspiratory flow rates to allow adequate inspiratory time to deliver bronchodilator therapy. This approach, however, must be used cautiously because auto-PEEP may worsen if inadequate expiratory time is allocated.

d. Heliox Therapy

Heliox is a mixture of helium and oxygen that has low gas density.[71] Heliox is often used to treat upper airway obstruction, including use in children with croup. By reducing gas density and increasing gas viscosity, heliox leads to a reduced Reynolds number. The Reynolds number is a dimensionless constant that is the principal determinant of flow turbulence; a lower Reynolds number favors laminar rather than turbulent flow. As a result, heliox tends to change turbulent flow into laminar flow and reduces the pressure required to achieve a given flow rate. The use of heliox in asthma has been somewhat controversial as clinical trials have been primarily small and uncontrolled. In addition, the delivery of heliox through a mechanical ventilator is problematic. Despite these issues, we have had good clinical experience with the use of heliox in

critically ill patients who are mechanically ventilated for status asthmaticus.

e. Avoidance of Paralysis

Because of the issues regarding the need to control breathing pattern, neuromuscular paralysis is frequently used to promote patient-ventilator synchrony. More recently, there has been recognition of the syndromes of critical illness polyneuropathy and critical illness myopathy plus prolonged neuromuscular blockade that have substantial morbidity associated with them. The combination of glucocorticoid therapy and paralytic agents is thought to be particularly hazardous from the standpoint of the risk of neuromuscular weakness. Thus, in status asthmaticus patients who require systemic glucocorticoid therapy, we favor the avoidance of paralysis if at all possible. These patients can usually be managed with heavy sedation alone.

In summary, we recommend individualized therapy for status asthmaticus patients requiring mechanical ventilation. We generally follow pulsus paradoxus in spontaneously breathing patients and VEI in passively ventilated patients. We generally use permissive hypercapnia to deliver a relatively low minute ventilation (small V_T) and adjust inspiratory time to minimize auto-PEEP and maximize gas delivery during inspiration.

B. CHRONIC OBSTRUCTIVE PULMONARY DISEASE

COPD is a smoking-related disease characterized by chronic productive cough (chronic bronchitis) or dilation and destruction of lung parenchyma leading to reduced lung elastic recoil (emphysema).[108] The principles of mechanical ventilation are similar to those for asthma, although a few distinctions are noteworthy.

1. Noninvasive Ventilation

Noninvasive ventilation is the treatment of choice for exacerbations of COPD.[108] Therefore, it has become more common than invasive mechanical ventilation for this population of patients. There are also some data to suggest that when these patients are invasively mechanically ventilated they can be extubated to noninvasive ventilation, even if they do not meet conventional spontaneous breathing criteria. However, some controversy exists regarding the applicability of these clinical trial data to clinical practice. The use of noninvasive ventilation has been independently associated with improvements in mortality for patients with acute exacerbations of COPD.

2. Applied Positive End-Expiratory Pressure

When airflow obstruction is caused by dynamic airflow limitation as in COPD, applied PEEP reduces the patient's effort to trigger the ventilator. That is, applied PEEP can be titrated up to about 80% of the measured auto-PEEP without increasing overall air trapping. Applying PEEP in this setting increases central airway pressure so that the pressure change needed to trigger the ventilator is reduced, increasing patient-ventilator synchrony. From a practical perspective, because the auto-PEEP level is difficult to measure in the spontaneously breathing patient, applied PEEP is increased in 1 to 2 cm H_2O steps until every inspiratory effort made by the patient triggers the ventilator. In some patients this may be over 10 cm H_2O applied PEEP. During controlled ventilation, controversy exists over the benefit of applying PEEP to balance the auto-PEEP because no spontaneous efforts are present.

3. Antimicrobial Therapy

Antimicrobial therapy has clearly been shown to provide mortality benefit for the intubated COPD patient. Although it is not the focus of this chapter, randomized trials performed in intubated patients with COPD exacerbations have demonstrated the efficacy of antimicrobial therapy. The use of ofloxacin led to reduced mortality compared with placebo in this population. No such data have been reported for asthma patients.

C. ACUTE RESPIRATORY DISTRESS SYNDROME

ARDS is a severe disease characterized by the acute onset of a substantial gas exchange impairment (PaO_2/ FiO_2 < 200), bilateral alveolar-interstitial infiltrates, and the absence of congestive heart failure. Multiple etiologies exist for ARDS, including trauma, sepsis, aspiration, medication reactions, inhalational exposures, and pancreatitis.[122] There has been substantial controversy regarding the optimal strategy for the mechanical ventilation of these patients. Although several positive clinical trials have been published, it is likely that the optimal ventilatory therapy for ARDS has yet to be defined. We offer the following therapeutic principles based on the available data.

1. Avoid Overdistention

High PTPs can lead to overdistention injury. The most compelling data are from the ARDS Network,[114] which reported a mortality benefit of 6 mL/kg PBW tidal volume as compared with 12 mL/kg PBW. Overdistention injury can lead to overt damage to the lung in the form of pneumothorax ("barotrauma") and VILI.

2. Apply Positive End-Expiratory Pressure

Low levels of end-expiratory PTP can promote cyclical opening and closing of lung units with resulting lung injury. High levels of shear forces can occur at junctions of heterogeneity within injured lung. The implication of this is that even at relatively modest applied peak alveolar pressures, lung injury may occur as a result of shear stress. Even in the spontaneously breathing patient, lung

injury can be perpetuated by diaphragmatically generated PTPs. Thus, lobar pneumonia may progress to ARDS at least in part as a result of mechanical stress on the lung.

As a result, the ideal strategy for mechanical ventilation in ARDS includes the promotion of homogeneity by avoiding areas of atelectasis and keeping the lung at a relatively uniform level of aeration. One strategy to minimize shear forces, therefore, would involve the use of recruitment maneuvers to minimize atelectasis, followed by high PEEP to prevent the collapse of alveoli at end exhalation.[1]

3. Manage Physiologic Dead Space

High pulmonary dead space is associated with increased mortality in ARDS patients. Dead space is defined as areas of the lung that are ventilated without perfusion. Nuckton and colleagues[88] demonstrated that elevated pulmonary dead space has excellent prognostic utility in ARDS patients. The authors postulated that microcirculatory thrombosis can contribute to reduced perfusion of lung units and thus lead to elevations to pulmonary dead space. They have subsequently begun a phase II study to examine the impact of activated protein C on pulmonary dead space in ARDS patients. However, a number of factors can contribute to elevations in pulmonary dead space, including excessive PEEP (intrinsic or extrinsic), low cardiac stroke volume, hypovolemia, and pulmonary embolism. Thus, in some cases elevated pulmonary dead space may be caused by inadequate hemodynamic resuscitation. In addition, because PEEP requirements are highly variable, excessive PEEP may have contributed to high dead space in some patients. We believe that elevations in pulmonary dead space should prompt a search for an underlying etiology. Specific therapies are available for most of the underlying etiologies; for example, excessive extrinsic PEEP should lead to lower applied PEEP, excessive intrinsic PEEP can be managed with bronchodilation and permissive hypercapnia, low cardiac output with inotropes, hypovolemia with crystalloid resuscitation, and pulmonary embolism with anticoagulation.

4. High-Frequency Oscillation

High-frequency oscillation (HFO) is a technique of applying very small tidal volumes rapidly in order to avoid overdistention injury while maintaining a relatively constant airway pressure to prevent derecruitment. In adults, tidal volumes about equal to anatomic dead space are delivered at rates of 4 to 6 Hz. There have been clinical case series[39,80] supporting the potential benefits of this therapy compared with conventional mechanical ventilation strategies in ARDS. However, in the one randomized controlled trial,[20] no difference in mortality was observed in spite of the use of large tidal volumes and high plateau pressures in the control group. This may have led to harm from the inappropriate ventilation in the control group rather than benefit from HFO. However, ongoing efforts may help demonstrate the potential utility of HFO over conventional mechanical ventilation strategies.

5. Prone Positioning

Prospective case series have demonstrated that use of the prone position in acute lung injury or ARDS improves oxygenation in 60% to 80% of patients to a degree enabling a reduction in FIO_2.[14,82] The ability of prone ventilation to improve patients' survival, however, is less clear. Two large randomized controlled trials involving patients with ARDS or acute lung injury have failed to demonstrate decreased mortality among those treated with prone ventilation.[43,47] The larger of these trials enrolled 791 patients with acute hypoxemic respiratory failure and a PaO_2/FIO_2 ratio less than 300.[47] Patients were randomly assigned to prone positioning for at least 8 hours a day or standard (supine) positioning throughout mechanical ventilation. Although prone positioning was associated with a significant increase in PaO_2/FIO_2 ratio, the groups did not differ with respect to 28-day all-cause mortality, the primary endpoint of the trial. The duration of mechanical ventilation and 90-day mortality were also similar in both groups. However, there was a trend toward increased iatrogenic complications, including ET obstruction, bronchial intubation, and pressure sores, among patients receiving prone ventilation. Of note in this trial, the duration of pronation was modest (8 hours/day) and the mechanical ventilator settings were not ideal (large tidal volumes).

Similar findings were noted in a smaller multicenter, prospective trial in which 304 ICU patients were randomly assigned to standard (supine) ventilation or 6 hours of prone ventilation daily for 10 days.[43] All patients met criteria for ARDS or acute lung injury at the time of study inclusion. In this trial, prone ventilation was associated with improvements in PaO_2/FIO_2 ratio similar to those found in previous series. Nonpulmonary organ failure was not decreased with a prone ventilatory strategy, and the rate of iatrogenic complications was similar in both groups. Mortality at 10 days, ICU discharge, and 6 months was similar for both groups (23%, 49%, and 61%, respectively). Post hoc subgroup analysis did suggest decreased 10-day mortality with prone ventilation in the sickest patients, specifically those with PaO_2/FIO_2 less than 88 or Simplified Acute Physiology Score greater than 49. However, the study was not powered to stratify outcome in this way. One possible explanation for the negative results of this study with respect to patients' mortality was the relatively short duration of prone ventilation used in the experimental protocol. In addition, the ventilatory strategy employed relatively low levels of applied PEEP and high tidal volumes (>10 mL/kg), a strategy that could independently propagate lung injury. One could argue that if pronation does serve to recruit lung, excess tidal volume and inadequate PEEP may be serious flaws with these studies because the recruited lung would be predicted to undergo repetitive collapse. An additional study is needed before conclusions on the impact of prone positioning on mortality in ARDS can be fully defined. In the interim, we would recommend prone positioning in patients with optimized ventilator settings still requiring an FIO_2 greater than 0.6 and evidence of dependent atelectasis and consolidation. In addition, for optimal benefit, prone positioning should be maintained for more than 20 hours a day.

6. Acute Respiratory Distress Syndrome Ventilatory Strategy

On the basis of the preceding discussion, we advocate the following strategy for the treatment of ARDS patients. First, we advocate recruitment maneuvers (sustained high-pressure inflations) to open the atelectatic lung units. Second, high levels of PEEP are probably required to prevent alveolar collapse at end exhalation. The combination of recruitment maneuvers and high PEEP is necessary to create lung homogeneity, that is, relatively uniformly open alveoli. Third, the measurement of pulmonary dead space can be helpful prognostically. In cases of high dead space, the underlying physiologic cause should be considered, including the possibility of excessive PEEP (intrinsic or extrinsic) or low pulmonary blood flow (related to inadequate resuscitation or low cardiac stroke volume). Therapies targeting the underlying cause of the increased dead space are likely to be beneficial. Fourth, tidal volume should be maintained in the 4 to 8 mL/kg PBW range to avoid overdistention. Fifth, plateau pressure should be maintained as low as possible, ideally less than 30 cm H_2O. Sixth, prone positioning should be used if, after optimization, FIO_2 values are still excessive.

VII. WEANING FROM MECHANICAL VENTILATION

There has been considerable research regarding the optimal strategy to liberate critically ill patients from mechanical ventilation. We would offer the following principles to summarize the existing literature[31]: Strategies to minimize the duration of mechanical ventilation prevent ventilator-associated pneumonia. Thus, one of the fundamental principles of mechanical ventilation is to minimize the duration of mechanical ventilation.

Daily spontaneous breathing trials reduce the duration of mechanical ventilation compared with conventional therapy. Ely and colleagues demonstrated that a respiratory therapist–driven protocol to attempt liberation from mechanical ventilation on a daily basis reduces the duration of mechanical ventilation compared with usual care.[30] Thus, we advocate a daily trial of spontaneous breathing in essentially all mechanically ventilated patients capable of spontaneous ventilation to assess the patient's readiness for spontaneous breathing.

The rapid shallow breathing index (RR/VT) is probably the best of the physiologic parameters to predict a patient's readiness to breathe spontaneously. Yang and Tobin[125] examined a number of variables, and the RR/VT provided the best metric to predict a patient's readiness to be extubated. A value of RR/VT in excess of 100 provided a reliable index that the patient was not yet ready for extubation. On the other hand, patients with RR/VT less than 100 are typically ready for extubation. This metric is difficult to validate in prospective studies because breathing pattern is typically one of the variables that is assessed as an inclusion criterion in clinical studies. In addition, the predictive value of RR/VT has been questioned in elderly patients and in women. Nevertheless, the RR/VT does provide a simple and useful variable to assess a patient's appropriateness for extubation.

Daily reduction of sedation can help reduce the risk of oversedation and the potential for prolonged mechanical ventilation. Kress and coworkers[66] studied daily reduction of sedation in critically ill patients who were mechanically ventilated. This strategy did lead to improvements in outcome compared with usual care. The relevance of these findings has been questioned with the widespread use of propofol, which has a short half-life, even after prolonged infusions. Nevertheless, a sedation strategy should be employed that does not unnecessarily prolong the duration of mechanical ventilation. This can be achieved by use of short-acting medications or by minimizing the dose and duration of longer acting medicines.

VIII. SUMMARY

Much progress has been made in the area of mechanical ventilation over the past several decades. A thorough understanding of the physiologic principles is important in management of patients because in many cases optimal therapy requires customized care. Clinical trials have shown benefits to limiting overdistention, and ongoing trials will be required to define further the role of other ventilatory strategies and techniques.

REFERENCES

1. Amato MBP, Barbas CSV, Medeiros DM, et al: Effect of a protective-ventilation strategy on mortality in the acute respiratory distress syndrome. N Engl J Med 338: 347-354, 1998.
2. Antonelli M, Conti G, Bufi M, et al: Noninvasive ventilation for treatment of acute respiratory failure in patients undergoing solid organ transplantation. JAMA 283:235-241, 2000.
3. Antonelli M, Conti G, Rocco M, et al: A comparison of noninvasive positive-pressure ventilation and conventional mechanical ventilation in patients with acute respiratory failure. N Engl J Med 339:429-435, 1998.
4. Bersten AD, Holt AW, Vedig AE, et al: Treatment of severe cardiogenic pulmonary edema with continuous positive airway pressure delivered by face mask. N Engl J Med 325:1825-1830, 1991.
5. Bethmann AN, Brasch F, Nusing R, et al: Hyperventilation induces release of cytokines from perfused mouse lung. Am J Respir Crit Care Med 157:263-272, 1998.
6. Branson RD, Campbell RS: Pressure support ventilation, patient-ventilator synchrony, and ventilator algorithms. Respir Care 43:1045-1047, 1998.
7. Branson RD, Campbell RS, Davis K, et al: Altering flowrate during maximum pressure support ventilation (PSV$_{max}$): Effects on cardiorespiratory function. Respir Care 35:1056-1064, 1990.
8. Broccard AF, Hotchkiss JR, Kuwayama N, et al: Consequences of vascular flow on lung injury induced by mechanical ventilation. Am J Respir Crit Care Med 1935-1942, 1998.
9. Broccard A, Shapiro R, Schmitz L, et al: Prone positioning attenuates and redistributes ventilator-induced lung injury in dogs. Crit Care Med 28:2295-2303, 2000.
10. Broccard A, Vannay C, Feihl F, et al: Impact of low pulmonary vascular pressure on ventilator-induced lung injury. Crit Care Med 30:2183-2190. 2002.
11. Brower RG, Lanken PN, MacIntyre N, et al: Higher versus lower positive end-expiratory pressures in patients with the acute respiratory distress syndrome. N Engl J Med 351:327-336, 2004.
12. Brun-Buisson C, Minelli C, Bertolini G, et al: Epidemiology and outcome of acute lung injury in European intensive care units. Results from the ALIVE Study. Intensive Care Med 30:51-61, 2004.
13. Chatburn RL: Mechanical ventilators. In Branson RD, Hess DR, Chatburn RL (eds): Respiratory Care Equipment, 2nd ed. St. Louis, Lippincott, 1999.
14. Chatte G, Sab JM, Dubois JM, et al: Prone position in mechanically ventilated patients with severe acute respiratory failure. Am J Respir Crit Care Med 155: 473-478, 1997.
15. Chiang AA, Steinfeld A, Gropper C, et al: Demand-flow airway pressure release ventilation as a partial ventilatory support mode: Comparison with synchronized intermittent mandatory ventilation and pressure support ventilation. Crit Care Med 22:1431-1437, 1994.
16. Chu EK, Whitehead T, Slutsky AS: Effects of cyclic opening and closing, and low and high volume ventilation on bronchoalveolar lavage cytokines. Crit Care Med 32:168-174, 2004.
17. Corbridge TC, Wood LD, Crawford GP, et al: Adverse effects of large tidal volume and low PEEP in canine acid aspiration. Am Rev Respir Dis 142:311-315, 1990.
18. Delclaux C, L'Her E, Alberti C, et al: Treatment of acute hypoxemic nonhypercapnic respiratory insufficiency with continuous positive airway pressure delivered by a

face mask: A randomized controlled trial. JAMA 284: 2352-2360, 2000.

19. Dellinger RP, Zimmerman JL, Taylor RW, et al: Effects of inhaled nitric oxide in patients with acute respiratory distress syndrome: Results of a randomized phase II trial. Inhaled Nitric Oxide in ARDS Study Group. Crit Care Med 26:15-23, 1998.

20. Derdak S, Mehta S, Stewart TE et al: High-frequency oscillatory ventilation for acute respiratory distress syndrome in adults: A randomized, controlled trial. Am J Respir Crit Care Med 166:801-808, 2002.

21. Downs JB, Douglas MI: Physiologic effects of respiratory therapy. In Shoemaker W, Ayers S, Grenvik A, et al (eds): Textbook of Critical Care, 2nd ed. Philadelphia, WB Saunders, 1989.

22. Downs JB, Klein EF, Modell JH: The effect of incremental PEEP on PaO_2 in patients with respiratory failure. Anesth Analg 52:210-215, 1973.

23. Drazen JM, Israel E, O'Byrne PM: Treatment of asthma with drugs modifying the leukotriene pathway. N Engl J Med 340:197-206, 1999.

24. Dreyfuss D, Saumon G: From ventilator-induced lung injury to multiple organ dysfunction? Intensive Care Med 24:102-104, 1998.

25. Dreyfuss D, Saumon G: Ventilator induced lung injury: Lessons from experimental studies. Am J Respir Crit Care Med 157:294-323, 1998.

26. Dreyfuss D, Basset G, Soler P, Saumon G: Intermittent positive-pressure hyperventilation with high inflation pressures produces pulmonary microvascular injury in rats. Am Rev Respir Dis 132:880-884, 1985.

27. Dreyfuss D, Soler P, Basset G, Saumon G: High inflation pressure pulmonary edema: Respective effects of high airway pressure, high tidal volume, and positive end-expiratory pressure. Am Rev Respir Dis 137:1159-1164, 1988.

28. Dreyfuss D, Soler P, Saumon G: Mechanical ventilation-induced pulmonary edema: Interaction with previous lung alterations. Am J Respir Crit Care Med 151:1568-1575, 1995.

29. Egan A: Lung inflation, lung solute permeability, and alveolar edema. J Appl Physiol 53:121-125, 1982.

30. Ely EW, Baker AM, Dunagan DP, et al: Effect on the duration of mechanical ventilation of identifying patients capable of breathing spontaneously. N Engl J Med 335:1864-1869, 1996.

31. Evidence-Based Guidelines for Weaning and Discontinuing Ventilatory Support: A collective task force facilitated by the American College of Chest Physicians; the American Association for Respiratory Care; and the American College of Critical Care Medicine. Chest 120:S375-S395, 2001.

32. Fabry B, Haberth,r C, Zappe D, et al: Breathing pattern and additional work of breathing in spontaneously breathing patients with different ventilatory demands during inspiratory pressure support and automatic tube compensation. Intensive Care Med 23:545-552, 1997.

33. Fabry BE, Guttmann J, Eberhard LE, et al: An analysis of dys-synchrony between the spontaneously breathing patient and ventilator during inspiratory pressure support. Chest 107:1387-1394, 1995.

34. Fagon J, Chastre J, Domart Y, et al: Nosocomial pneumonia in patients receiving continuous mechanical ventilation. Am Rev Respir Dis 139:877, 1989.

35. Ferguson ND, Kacmarek RM, Chicke JD, et al: Screening of ARDS patients using standardized ventilator settings: Influence on enrolment in a clinical trial. Intensive Care Med 30:1111-1116, 2004.

36. Fernandez R, Mendez M, Younes M: Effect of ventilator flow rate on respiratory timing in normal humans. Am J Respir Crit Care Med 159:710-719, 1999.

37. Ferrer M, Esquinas A, Arancibia F, et al: Noninvasive ventilation during persistent weaning failure: A randomized controlled trial. Am J Respir Crit Care Med 168:70-76, 2003.

38. Ferrer M, Esquinas A, Leon M, et al: Noninvasive ventilation in severe hypoxemic respiratory failure: A randomized clinical trial. Am J Respir Crit Care Med 168:1438-1444, 2003.

39. Fort P, Farmer C, Westerman J, et al: High-frequency oscillatory ventilation for adult respiratory distress syndrome—A pilot study. Crit Care Med 25:937-947, 1997.

40. Fu Z, Costello ML, Tsukimoto K, et al: High lung volume increases stress failure in pulmonary capillaries. J Appl Physiol 73:123-133, 1992.

41. Fujino Y, Goddon S, Dolhnikoff M, et al: Repetitive high-pressure recruitment maneuvers required to maximally recruit lung in a sheep model of acute respiratory distress syndrome. Crit Care Med 29:1579-1586, 2001.

42. Gajic O, Dara SI, Mendez JL, et al: Ventilator associated lung injury in patients without acute lung injury at the onset of mechanical ventilation. Crit Care Med 32:1817-1824, 2004.

43. Gattinioni L, Tognoni G, Pesenti A, et al: The Prone-Supine Study Group. Effect of prone positioning on the survival of patients with acute respiratory failure. N Engl J Med 345:568-573, 2001.

44. Geiger K, Georgieff M, Lutz H: Side effects of positive pressure ventilation on hepatic function and splanchnic circulation. Int J Clin Monit Comput 12:103-111, 1986.

45. Goulet R, Hess D, Kacmarek RM: Pressure vs. flow triggering during pressure support ventilation. Chest 111:1649-1654, 1997.

46. Grasso S, Mascia L, Del Turco M, et al: Effects of recruiting maneuvers in patients with acute respiratory syndrome ventilated with protective ventilatory strategy. Anesthesiology 96:795-802, 2002.

47. Guerin C, Gaillard S, Lemasson S: Effects of systematic prone positioning in hypoxemic acute respiratory failure: A randomized controlled trial. JAMA 292:2379-2387, 2004.

48. Guttmann J, Eberhard L, Fabry B, et al: Continuous calculation of intratracheal pressure in tracheally intubated patients. Anesthesiology 79:503-513, 1993.

49. Hernandez LA, Coker PJ, May S: Mechanical ventilation increases microvascular permeability in oleic acid-injured lungs. J Appl Physiol 69:2057-2061, 1990.

50. Herrera MT, Toledo C, Villar J, et al: Positive end-expiratory pressures modulates local and systemic inflammatory responses in a sepsis-induced lung injury model. Intensive Care Med 29:1345-1353, 2003.

51. Hess D, Kacmarek RM: Essentials of Mechanical Ventilation, 2nd ed. New York, McGraw-Hill, 2002.

52. Hess DR, Dillman C, Kacmarek RM: In vitro evaluation of aerosol bronchodilator delivery during mechanical ventilation: Pressure-control vs. volume control ventilation. Intensive Care Med 29:1145-1150, 2003.

53. Hickling KG: Reinterpreting the pressure-volume curve in patients with acute respiratory distress syndrome. Curr Opin Crit Care 8:832-838, 2002.

54. Hickling KG, Town IG, Epton M, et al: Pressure-limited ventilation with permissive hypercapnia and minimum PEEP in saline-lavaged rabbits allows progressive improvement in oxygenation, but does not avoid ventilator-induced lung injury. Intensive Care Med 22:1445-1452, 1996.

55. Hodson ME, Madden BP, Steven MH, et al: Noninvasive mechanical ventilation for cystic fibrosis patients—A potential bridge to transplantation. Eur Respir J 4:524-527, 1991.

56. Hotchkiss JR, Blanch LL, Murias G, et al: Effects of increased respiratory frequency on ventilator induced lung injury. Am J Resp Crit Care Med 161:463-468, 2000.

57. Hurst JM, DeHaven CB, Branson RD: Use of CPAP mask as the sole mode of ventilatory support in trauma patients with mild to moderate respiratory insufficiency. J Trauma 25:1065-1068, 1985.

58. Imai Y, Kawawo T, Miyasaka K, et al: Inflammatory chemical mediators during conventional ventilation and during high frequency oscillatory ventilation. Am J Respir Crit Care Med 180:1550-1554, 1994.

59. Imsand C, Feihl F, Perret C, et al: Regulation of inspiratory neuromuscular output during synchronized intermittent mechanical ventilation. Anesthesiology 80:13-22, 1994.

60. Johnson E, Hedley-Whyte J: Continuous positive-pressure ventilation and choledochoduodenal flow resistance. J Appl Physiol 19:937, 1985.

61. Jubran A, Van de Graaff WB, Tobin MJ: Variability of patient-ventilator interaction with pressure support ventilation in patients with chronic obstructive pulmonary disease. Am J Respir Crit Care Med 152:129-136, 1995.

62. Kawano T, Mori S, Cybulsky M, et al: Effect of granulocyte depletion in a ventilated surfactant-depleted lung. J Appl Physiol 62:27-33, 1987.

63. Keenen SP: Noninvasive positive-pressure ventilation for severe worsening of chronic obstructive pulmonary disease. Ann Intern Med 138:127-135, 2003.

64. Keenan SP, Powers C, McCormack DG, Block G: Noninvasive positive-pressure ventilation for postextubation respiratory distress. JAMA 287:3238-3244, 2002.

65. Kolobow T, Moretti MP, Fumagalli R, et al: Severe impairment in lung function induced by high peak airway pressure during mechanical ventilation. Am Rev Respir Dis 135:312-315, 1987.

66. Kress JP, Pohlman AS, O'Connor MF, et al: Daily interruption of sedative infusions in critically ill patients undergoing mechanical ventilation. N Eng J Med 342:1471-1477, 2000.

67. Lapinsky SE, Aubin M, Mehta S, et al: Safety and efficacy of a sustained inflation for alveolar recruitment in adults with respiratory failure. Intensive Care Med 25:1297-1301, 1999.

68. Lim CM, Kohy Y, Park W, et al: Mechanistic scheme and effect of "extended sigh" as a recruitment maneuver in patients with acute respiratory distress syndrome: A preliminary report. Crit Care Med 29:1255-1260, 2001.

69. MacIntyre NB, Ho L: Effects of initial flow rate and breath termination criteria on pressure support ventilation. Chest 99:134-138, 1991.

70. Mang H, Kacmarek RM, Ritz R, et al: Cardiorespiratory effects of volume- and pressure-controlled ventilation at various I/E ratios in an acute lung injury model. Am J Respir Crit Care Med 151:731-736, 1995.

71. Manthous CA, Hall JB, Caputo MA, et al: Heliox improves pulsus paradoxus and peak expiratory flow in nonintubated patients with severe asthma. Am Respir Crit Care Med 151:310-314, 1995.

72. Marini J: Relative importance of stretch and shear in ventilator-induced lung injury. Crit Care Med 32:302-304, 2004.

73. Marini JJ, Rodrigues RM, Lamb V: The inspiratory workload of patient-initiated mechanical ventilation. Am Rev Respir Dis 134:902-909, 1986.

74. Marini JJ, Smith TC, Lamb VJ: External work output and force generation during synchronized intermittent mechanical ventilation. Effect of machine assistance on breathing effort. Am Rev Respir Dis 138:1169-1179, 1988.

75. McIntyre NR, McConnell R, Cheng KC, Sane A: Patient-ventilator flow dyssynchrony: Flow-limited versus pressure-limited breaths. Crit Care Med 25:1671-1677, 1997.

76. Mead J, Takishima T, Leith D: Stress distribution in lungs: A model of pulmonary elasticity. J Appl Physiol 28:596-608, 1970.

77. Medoff BD, Harris RS, Kesselman H, et al: Use of recruitment maneuvers and high positive end-expiratory pressure in a patient with acute respiratory distress syndrome. Crit Care Med 28:1210-1216, 2002.

78. Meduri GU, Cook TR, Turner RE, et al: Noninvasive positive pressure ventilation in status asthmaticus. Chest 110:767-774, 1996.

79. Mehta S, Jay GD, Woolard RH, et al: Randomized, prospective trial of bilevel versus continuous positive airway pressure in acute pulmonary edema. Crit Care Med 25:620-628, 1997.

80. Mehta S, Lapinsky SE, Hallett DC, et al: Prospective trial of high-frequency oscillation in adults with acute respiratory distress syndrome. Crit Care Med 29:1360-1369, 2001.

81. Munoz J, Guerrero JE, Escalante JL, et al: Pressure-controlled ventilation versus controlled mechanical ventilation with decelerating inspiratory flow. Crit Care Med 21:1143-1148, 1993.

82. Mure M, Martling C-R, Lindahl SGE: Dramatic effect on oxygenation in patients with severe acute lung insufficiency treated in the prone position. Crit Care Med 25:1539-1544, 1997.

83. Muscedere JF, Mullen BM, Gan K, Slutsky AS: Tidal ventilation at low airway pressures can augment lung injury. Am J Respir Crit Care Med 149:1327-1334, 1994.

84. Nahum A, Hoyt J, Schmitz L, et al: Effect of mechanical ventilation strategy on dissemination of intratracheally instilled Escherichia coli in dogs. Crit Care Med 25:1733-1743, 1997.

85. Nava S, Carbone G, DiBattista N, et al: Noninvasive ventilation in cardiogenic pulmonary edema. Am J Respir Crit Care Med 168:1432-1437, 2003.

86. Neumann P, Golisch W, Strohmeyer A, et al: Influence of different release times on spontaneous breathing pattern during airway pressure release ventilation. Intensive Care Med 28:1742-1749, 2002.

87. Nishida T, Suchodolski K, Schettino GPP, et al: Peak volume history and peak P-V curve pressures independently affect the shape of the P-V curve of the respiratory system. Crit Care Med 32:1358-1364, 2004.

88. Nuckton TJ, Eisner, MD, Matthay MA: Pulmonary dead space and survival [letter]. N Engl J Med 347:850-852, 2002.

89. Nunn JF: Nunn's Applied Respiratory Physiology, 4th ed. Baltimore, Butterworth-Heinemann, 1993.

90. Parker JC, Hennandez LA, Longenecker GL, et al: Lung edema caused by high peak inspiratory pressures in dogs. Am Rev Respir Dis 142:321-328, 1990.

91. Parker JC, Hernandez LA, Peevy KJ: Mechanisms of ventilator-induced lung injury. Crit Care Med 21:131-143, 1993.

92. Pelosi P, Cadringher P, Bottino N, et al: Sigh in acute respiratory distress syndrome. Am J Respir Crit Care Med 165:165-170, 1999.

93. Pepe PE, Marini JJ: Occult positive end-expiratory pressure in mechanically ventilated patients with airflow obstruction: The auto-PEEP effect. Am Rev Respir Dis 126:166-170, 1982.

94. Perel A, Stock C: Handbook of Mechanical Ventilatory Support. Baltimore, Williams & Wilkins, 1992.

95. Petrof BJ, Legare M, Goldberg P, et al: Continuous positive airway pressure reduces work of breathing and dyspnea during weaning from mechanical ventilation in severe COPD. Am Rev Respir Dis 141:281-285, 1990.

96. Piotrowski A, Sobala W, Kawczynski P: Patient-initiated, pressure-regulated, volume-controlled ventilation compared with intermittent mandatory ventilation in neonates: A prospective, randomized study. Intensive Care Med 23:975-981, 1997.

97. Putensen C, Sech S, Hermann W, et al: Long-term effects of spontaneous breathing during ventilatory support in patients with acute lung injury. Am J Respir Crit Care Med 164:43-49, 2001.

98. Randolph AG, Wypij D, Venkataraman ST, et al: Effect of mechanical ventilator weaning protocols on respiratory outcomes in infants and children. JAMA 288:2561-2568, 2002.

99. Ranieri VM, Suter PM, Tortorella C, et al: Effect of mechanical ventilation on inflammatory mediators in patients with acute respiratory distress syndrome: A randomized controlled trial. JAMA 282:54-61, 1999.

100. Ranieri VM, Tortorella D, DeTullio R, et al: Limitation of mechanical lung stress decreased BAL cytokines in patients with ARDS. JAMA 282:54-61, 1999.

101. Sedeek KA, Takeuchi M, Suchodolski K, et al: Open lung protective ventilation with PCV, HFO, and ITPV results in similar gas exchange, hemodynamics and lung mechanics. Anesthesiology 99:1102-1111, 2003.

102. Shapiro BA, Kacmarek RM, Cane RD, et al: Clinical Application of Respiratory Care, 4th ed. St. Louis, Mosby–Year Book, 1991.

103. Sinclair SE, Kregenow DA, Lamm WJ, et al: Hypercapnic acidosis is protective in an in vivo model of ventilator-induced lung injury. Am J Respir Crit Care Med 166:403-408, 2002.

104. Slutsky A, Tremblay L: Multiple organ system failure: Is mechanical ventilation a contributing factor? Am Rev Resp Crit Care Med 157:1721-1725, 1998.

105. Smith TC, Marini JJ: Impact of PEEP on lung mechanics and work of breathing in severe airflow obstruction. J Appl Physiol 64:1488-1496, 1988.

106. Stock MC, Downs JB, Frolicher DA: Airway pressure release ventilation. Crit Care Med 15:462-469, 1987.

107. Suter PM, Fairley HB, Isenbert MD: Optimum end expiratory airway pressure in patients with acute pulmonary failure. N Engl J Med 292:284-289, 1975.

108. Sutherland ER, Cherniack RM: Management of chronic obstructive pulmonary disease. N Engl J Med 350:2689-2697, 2004.

109. Suzuki S, Hotchkiss JR, Marini JJ, et al: Effect of body temperature on ventilator-induced lung injury. Crit Care Med 161:463-468, 2000.

110. Takata M, Abe J, Tanaka H, et al: Intraalveolar expression of tumor necrosis factor alpha gene during conventional and high-frequency ventilation. Am J Respir Crit Care Med 156:272-279, 1997.

111. Takeuchi M, Goddon S, Kacmarek RM, et al: Set positive end-expiratory pressure during protective ventilation affects lung injury. Anesthesiology 97:682-692, 2002.

112. Takeuchi M, Sedeek KA, Schettino GPP, et al: Peak pressure during volume history and pressure-volume curve measurements affects analysis. Am J Respir Crit Care Med 32:1358-1364, 2004.

113. Tenney SM, Remmers JE: Comparative quantitative morphology of the mammalian lung: Diffusing area. Nature 197:54-56, 1963.

114. The Acute Respiratory Distress Syndrome Network: Ventilation with lower tidal volumes as compared with traditional tidal volumes for acute lung injury and the acute respiratory distress syndrome. N Engl J Med 342:1301-1308, 2000.

115. Tremblay L, Valenza F, Riberiro S, et al: Injurious ventilatory strategies increase cytokines and c-fos mRNA expression in an isolated rat lung model. J Clin Invest 99:944-952, 1997.

116. Tugrul S, Akinci O, Ozcan PE, et al: Effects of sustained inflation and post-inflation positive end expiratory pressure in acute respiratory distress syndrome: Focusing on pulmonary and extrapulmonary forms. Crit Care Med 31:738-744, 2003.

117. Tuxen D: Detrimental effects of positive end-expiratory pressure during controlled mechanical ventilation of patients with severe airflow obstruction. Am Rev Respir Dis 140:5-9, 1989.

118. Tuxen DV, Williams TJ, Scheinkestel CD, et al: Use of a measurement of pulmonary hyperinflation to control the level of mechanical ventilation in patients with acute severe asthma. Am Rev Respir Dis 146:1136-1142, 1992.

119. Van der Kloot TE, Blanch L, Youngblood AM, et al: Recruitment maneuvers in three experimental models of acute lung injury. Am J Respir Crit Care Med 161:1485-1494, 2000.

120. Verbrugge SJC, Sorm V, Veen A, et al: Lung overinflation without positive end-expiratory pressure promotes bacteremia after experimental *Klebsiella pneumoniae* inoculation. Intensive Care Med 24:172-177, 1998.

121. Villar J, Perez-Mendez L, Kacmarek RM: Current definitions of acute lung injury and the acute respiratory distress syndrome do not reflect their true severity and outcome. Intensive Care Med 25:930-935, 1999.

122. Ware LB, Matthay MA: The acute respiratory distress syndrome. N Engl J Med 342:1334-1349, 2000.

123. Webb HH, Tierney D: Experimental pulmonary edema due to intermittent positive pressure ventilation, with high inflation pressures, protection by positive end-expiratory pressure. Am Rev Respir Dis 110: 556-565, 1974.

124. West JB: Ventilation/Blood Flow and Gas Exchange, 4th ed. Oxford, Blackwell, 1985.

125. Yang KL, Tobin MJ: A prospective study of indexes predicting the outcome of trials of weaning from mechanical ventilation. N Engl J Med 324:1445-1450, 1991.

46

MONITORING THE AIRWAY AND PULMONARY FUNCTION

Neal H. Cohen
David E. Schwartz

I. INTRODUCTION

The patient with respiratory failure or tenuous respiratory function presents a number of challenges. First, the patient requires ongoing and careful assessment of the current respiratory status, gas exchange, and the potential need for intervention. Second, once the decision is made to provide either airway management or respiratory support, the clinician must have a clear understanding of the reason for the intervention and the potential complications that might result from manipulation of the airway, delivery of noninvasive ventilatory support, or mechanical ventilation through an artificial airway. The assessment and management have become more complicated as the therapeutic options have become more diverse. For example, the patient who presents with respiratory failure but is able to maintain a clear airway may not require tracheal intubation but may need some level of noninvasive ventilatory support. If the patient's condition deteriorates, however, urgent or emergent airway management may be required. The assessment of the patient therefore requires an understanding of the airway anatomy, the patient's mental status, the underlying physiologic abnormalities, and the patient's respiratory reserve. In addition, the underlying clinical conditions often dictate the need for respiratory interventions, not specifically because of compromised pulmonary function but to optimize gas exchange, acid-base status, or work of breathing in an otherwise tenuous clinical situation. As a result, the patient who requires airway management or assisted ventilation must be carefully evaluated and the respiratory status closely monitored. The evaluation must be ongoing to ensure that the therapeutic and supportive interventions are appropriate or to determine when additional therapies should be instituted.

A wide variety of monitoring techniques are available to evaluate the patient's airway, gas exchange, acid-base status, and pulmonary function. In order to select the correct monitoring technique, the clinician must understand which monitoring techniques are available, which are most appropriate for the clinical situation, and what information the monitor provides *and* what it does not provide.

The monitoring options have expanded and improved, as have the respiratory support devices. Unfortunately, the extension of technology into monitoring of respiratory function has created challenges for the clinician. Obviously, the most useful monitors are those that are easily applied, simple to use, and have few, if any, contraindications or complications associated with their use. These monitors can provide data that allow the clinician to optimize care in the most cost-effective way.[30,133] Most of the currently available monitoring techniques fulfill these requirements. Many have also been demonstrated to improve patients' care or reduce costs.[29,35,85,88] At the same time, the increasing use of technology to assist in monitoring respiratory status has created a barrier between the physician and the patient. In order to understand the value of the clinical evaluation and the most appropriate use of monitors of respiratory status, this chapter describes techniques for monitoring the patient's airway, ensuring that ventilatory support is appropriate to the clinical needs of the patient, and initiating weaning from mechanical ventilation on the basis of physiologic response. It defines the clinical applications for and identifies the limitations of each monitor. The chapter is divided into sections describing techniques for monitoring the airway, monitoring respiratory function and gas exchange, and evaluating respiratory status during administration of and weaning from mechanical ventilatory support.

II. MONITORING THE AIRWAY

A. PRIOR TO TRACHEAL INTUBATION

Monitoring of the patient's airway is a critical component of respiratory monitoring for any patient. As a result of underlying anatomic abnormalities, physiologic alterations in level of consciousness or edema of the airway, or administration of respiratory depressants, a patient can develop upper airway dysfunction with life-threatening consequences. The assessment of the airway should include the clinical evaluation that is routinely performed by the anesthesiologist prior to initiating anesthesia. The evaluation includes history and physical examination. The patient should be asked about snoring or episodes of airway obstruction during sleep, previous experiences with tracheal intubation including difficulty with intubation, hoarseness after airway manipulation, hoarseness with exercise, previous lengthy tracheal intubation, or history of tracheostomy or tracheal abnormalities, including stenosis or tracheomalacia. Patients with rheumatoid arthritis should be questioned about upper airway problems, particularly related to potential arthritic changes in the cricoarytenoid joints. Patients who have had previous neck or mediastinal surgery should be carefully evaluated for evidence of unilateral or bilateral vocal cord dysfunction.

The examination of the airway for any patient presenting with respiratory insufficiency should include thorough assessment of the upper airway, including evaluation of mobility of the jaw, chin, and neck as well as estimation of the potential ease or difficulty of tracheal intubation based on the size of the mandible and visualization of the airway (Mallampati classification). For patients who have airway abnormalities, alternative methods to secure the airway should be considered and the appropriate equipment should be readily available to allow rapid control using a standard laryngoscope, laryngeal mask airway (LMA), fiberoptic technique, light wand, or, in emergent situations, cricothyroidotomy or tracheostomy.

B. DURING AND AFTER TRACHEAL INTUBATION

Although there are a number of situations in which the airway can be monitored and noninvasive ventilatory support provided, most patients who receive general anesthesia or are critically ill require placement of an artificial airway. For some surgical patients, the LMA is sufficient to allow spontaneous ventilation during inhalational anesthesia. Direct visualization of LMA placement is rarely required, and positioning is determined on the basis of clinical signs. If the patient is breathing comfortably without evidence of obstruction, the LMA is usually in good position. In some situations, positive-pressure ventilation may be desired for the patient with an LMA in place. Although ventilatory support is possible for some patients, positive-pressure ventilation may cause a leak around the LMA, compromising the ability to provide ventilatory support. More important, ventilation through the LMA does not prevent entrainment of gas into the stomach, and the risk of regurgitation and aspiration must be considered.

Although a variety of masks and other devices are available to facilitate ventilatory support without tracheal instrumentation, most often the patient requiring airway protection or positive-pressure ventilation undergoes tracheal intubation, either transoral, transnasal, or through a surgical airway (for more details about tracheal intubation, see Chapter 16). The most reliable method to assess the location of an artificial airway within the trachea is direct visualization of the tube passing through the vocal cords at the time of intubation. Physical examination is also important to ensure that after placement of the airway, both lungs are being ventilated. Auscultation over the lung fields (particularly the apices of the lungs) and stomach should routinely be performed to assess endotracheal tube (ET) placement. When the ET is within the trachea, equal breath sounds should be heard over both lung fields while listening over the apices. Auscultation over the upper lung fields minimizes the likelihood of hearing sounds transmitted from the stomach. For most adult patients, if the ET is located within the trachea, no breath sounds should be heard over the stomach. Unfortunately, auscultation can be misleading. Occasionally, particularly in children, breath sounds are transmitted to the stomach even when the ET is in proper position. For patients with extensive parenchymal lung disease, effusions, or endobronchial lesions, breath sounds may not be heard equally over both lung fields even when the ET is in proper position within the trachea. Other clinical signs can be useful in determining whether the ET is within the trachea. These include identifying mist within the lumen of the ET during exhalation, palpation of the cuff of the ET in the suprasternal notch, and the normal "feel" of a reservoir bag during manual ventilation. Despite the clinical usefulness of these methods, none is infallible, and false-positive and false-negative evaluations have been reported.[9]

Another more reliable monitor to confirm that the artificial airway is within the trachea is the identification of carbon dioxide (CO_2) in exhaled gas. If the airway is within the trachea and the patient is either ventilating spontaneously or receiving positive-pressure ventilation, CO_2 should be eliminated by the lungs. The presence of CO_2 or measurement of CO_2 concentration can be used to determine the location of the ET. A number of devices are currently available to monitor CO_2 in expired gases. In the operating room, CO_2 can be measured using an infrared device,[129] Raman effect scattering, or mass spectrometry. In the intensive care unit (ICU), emergency department, or other settings including out-of-hospital locations, colorimetric techniques[49,78,99] that estimate CO_2 concentration or infrared devices that accurately measure CO_2 concentration in expired gases have been used successfully. As a result of the ease of use and widespread availability of these devices, the documentation of CO_2 in exhaled gas following placement of an artificial airway (capnography) has become the standard of care in anesthesia practice and is now routinely used during emergency airway management in many hospitals and emergency settings. A detailed description of capnography is provided in Chapter 30. Unfortunately, even these devices can provide misleading information and the information they provide is not foolproof.[32,47]

Capnography can be misleading when the patient has been ventilated by mask prior to intubation and there is CO_2-containing gas in the stomach. This problem is even more common when capnography is used to monitor the patient who has recently received bicarbonate-containing solutions or has been drinking CO_2-containing beverages before placement of the artificial airway. In these situations, CO_2 is eliminated from the stomach during the first few breaths provided through the ET. The presence of CO_2 from exhaled gas, therefore, should be monitored for at least a few breaths. If CO_2 continues to be eliminated through the ET after four or five breaths, endotracheal placement of the tube can be assured.[47] Another problem with capnography when used to confirm ET placement is that CO_2 elimination occurs only if the patient has sufficient cardiac output to deliver CO_2 to

the lungs. If the patient has suffered a cardiac arrest and cardiac output is very low or absent, no CO_2 is delivered to the lung. The capnogram reveals neither a digital display of CO_2 from exhaled gas nor, if the CO_2 waveform is being monitored, a capnographic display, even when the ET is within the trachea.[39,58,72,115] Sometimes, even when cardiac output is inadequate, chest compressions are effective at eliminating enough CO_2 from the lungs to confirm ET placement.

When the position of the ET within the trachea has been confirmed, it is also important to assess the location of the tube within the trachea to avoid placement too proximal (increasing the risk of accidental extubation) or too distal (endobronchial). Incorrect positioning of the ET has been associated with a number of complications, including pneumothorax and death.[157] The location of the ET should not only be confirmed at the time of placement but also be regularly assessed while the artificial airway remains in place because the ET position can change even after it is secured. Flexion of the neck moves the ET toward the carina, and extension moves the tube up toward the vocal cords. In adult patients, flexion and extension of the head change the position of the ET tip by ± 2 cm.[23] In addition, as the ET softens or the patient manipulates the ET with the tongue, the tube position changes. As a result of these changes in ET position, patients are at risk for self-extubation even when the tube is secured at the mouth and the extremities are restrained.

A number of techniques can be used to assess the positioning of the ET within the trachea. Placement of the ET to a predetermined distance has been suggested as a way to minimize the likelihood of endobronchial intubation. Owen and Cheney suggested that if the tube is placed to a depth of 21 cm in women and 23 cm in men when referenced to the anterior alveolar ridge or the front teeth, endobronchial intubation can be avoided.[101] Subsequent studies have not confirmed that this technique prevents endobronchial intubation in critically ill adults[14,52,120] or that it is predictive of the relationship between the position of the ET at the teeth and the tube's position relative to the carina.[120]

Fiberoptic bronchoscopy has also been used to determine proper positioning of the ET.[50] The technique is useful although it is not without some risk, particularly for the recently intubated critically ill patient. Insertion of the bronchoscope reduces the effective cross-sectional area of the ET, potentially compromising ventilation and oxygenation.[75] Peak inspiratory pressure increases. In addition, the partial obstruction of the ET results in an increase in airway resistance, which may lead to the development of occult end-expiratory pressure and increase the risk of pneumothorax or cause hemodynamic compromise.[107] The routine use of this technique is also costly as it requires sterilization between uses. Nonetheless, flexible fiberoptic bronchoscopy can be useful to provide a rapid confirmation of ET positioning.

Capnography can also be used to identify endobronchial migration of an ET.[46] With distal migration of the tube, the end-tidal CO_2 falls. The change is usually associated with an increase in peak inspiratory pressure. These changes, although not always reliable, can provide early evidence of ET migration because the CO_2 changes precede a change in arterial blood gases or other signs of displacement.

Probably the most commonly used method to assess the location of the ET within the trachea is the routine postintubation chest x-ray (CXR). The distance of the ET from the carina can be measured from a portable anteroposterior film obtained at the bedside. Although many clinicians have questioned whether the cost of the CXR warrants routine use for documentation of ET placement, it still remains the most useful and reliable method to determine the appropriate depth of the ET within the trachea.[14,52,120]

There is one special clinical situation that warrants additional monitoring of the artificial airway. Some patients require placement of a double-lumen ET to facilitate a unilateral surgical procedure of the lung, to provide differential lung ventilation, or to protect one lung from contamination with blood or infected secretions from the other lung. In these cases, the proper placement of the double-lumen ET must be assured. Physical examination alone and other monitoring techniques are usually insufficient to confirm proper positioning of these tubes. Fiberoptic evaluation is most often required, not only to confirm the ET positioning after initial placement but also to reevaluate the placement after the patient is repositioned for a surgical procedure[59] or while in place in the ICU. Direct visualization of the tip of the double-lumen tube and the relationship between the tracheal and bronchial lumens ensures that the tube is providing the support needed and that the two lungs are isolated. Other techniques can be used to diagnose malpositioning of double-lumen tubes, although there are few studies that confirm their value. Capnography, which has been shown to be useful in identifying endobronchial migration of a single-lumen ET,[46] might provide information about the location of a double-lumen tube. Spirometry, which can be obtained from in-line monitoring devices added to the anesthesia circuit or monitoring techniques provided by critical care ventilators, can also provide early detection of double-lumen tube malpositioning.[126] As the ET migrates, expiratory flow obstruction can be detected as a change in the shape of the expiratory limb of the flow-volume loop. Inspiratory obstruction is best diagnosed by a change in the pressure-volume loop.

C. DURING WEANING

Careful evaluation and monitoring of the patient's airway are also required before and immediately after endotracheal extubation. After the patient is weaned from ventilatory support and is being prepared for extubation, the patient's ability to protect and maintain the airway after endotracheal extubation must be assessed. A variety of clinical criteria have been used to determine whether the patient can protect the airway. The most common criteria are presence of a normal gag and a strong cough. If the patient has a gag when the back of the throat is stimulated and a cough during suctioning, most clinicians feel confident that the patient will be able to prevent aspiration after extubation. These criteria, however, have never been subjected to scientific evaluation. Some patients who have a poor gag or cough with the ET in place are able to handle secretions and cough effectively after endotracheal extubation. Others who seem to have a satisfactory cough or gag prior to extubation are still unable to protect their airway when extubated. The problem with airway protection may become clinically apparent only when the patient begins to eat because pharyngeal function may remain abnormal for a number of hours to days after endotracheal intubation.[54] Nonetheless, these criteria continue to be the most commonly used to determine whether the patient can be extubated safely.

Once a decision is made that the patient can protect the airway, some assessment of the airway size and vocal cord function must be made *prior to* ET removal. Most commonly, for patients intubated for a straightforward surgical procedure, routine clinical evaluation is sufficient; no formal assessment of airway size is required before extubation. If the patient develops significant edema of the head and neck during surgery or has a surgical procedure of the head or neck that might compromise the airway, a more thorough assessment is required. One of the common techniques used to assess airway size is to determine whether the patient can breathe around the ET when the ET cuff is deflated or whether there is a leak around the cuff when positive pressure is applied through the ET.[109] Some clinicians require that a leak occur when the airway pressure is low, usually below 15 cm H_2O prior to extubation, although studies have documented neither the value of the leak test at all nor a specific "leak pressure" above which extubation would be contraindicated. If the airway pressure required to identify a leak during positive-pressure inspiration is high, probably over 20 to 25 cm H_2O, the patient *may* have sufficient upper airway edema to warrant leaving the ET in place until the edema resolves.

D. AFTER TRACHEAL DECANNULATION

After the ET is removed from either the surgical patient or the ICU patient, the airway must continue to be closely monitored. For most surgical patients, the risk of airway compromise after ET intubation is small. Occasionally, airway edema can be a problem. Less commonly, vocal cord dysfunction or cricoarytenoid dislocation can cause hoarseness or airway obstruction.

The patients at risk for upper airway edema include those who have required large amounts of fluid or blood products for resuscitation in the operating room or ICU and patients who were cared for in the prone position. Most of these patients do not have the ET removed until the edema resolves. However, sometimes the assessment of the edema of the airway is difficult or the ET acts as a stent, keeping the airway patent until the tube is removed. In these cases, upper airway edema may compromise the airway after extubation. In these situations emergent intubation may be required. Special equipment, including fiberoptic intubation equipment and cricothyroidotomy kits, should be readily available. When upper airway edema compromises the patient's airway after extubation but does not necessitate immediate reintubation, vaso-constrictors can be used to reduce airway swelling. Nebulized racemic epinephrine has been used success-fully, although it must be administered with caution. The vasoconstrictive effects of the epinephrine reduce the edema and improve the cross-sectional area of the airway. After discontinuation of the epinephrine, however, particularly when treatment is repeated over an extended period, rebound hyperemia can occur. If repeated epineph-rine treatments are required, the epinephrine dose and frequency of treatment should be tapered (in frequency or dose) rather than abruptly withdrawn. Systemic steroids can also be used to reduce upper airway edema. The onset of action of the steroids is slow. If upper airway edema is suspected and steroids are to be administered, the steroids should be administered 6 to 8 hours *before* the anticipated extubation.

Vocal cord function can also be impaired after surgery. Postoperative vocal cord dysfunction can be caused by direct trauma at the time of endotracheal intubation or edema. Recurrent laryngeal nerve dysfunction can also occur, most commonly from nerve retraction or transec-tion during surgery or from direct trauma caused by high intratracheal pressure transmitted from the ET cuff.[16] With the ET in place, vocal cord function is difficult to assess. The evaluation usually requires that the ET be removed (see Chapter 47). Fiberoptic evaluation is the most common method to assess laryngeal and vocal cord function. After removal of the ET, the fiberoptic laryn-goscope or bronchoscope can be used to assess the airway. Although the assessment can be performed in the ICU, the more common approach is to perform the evaluation under more controlled conditions in the oper-ating room, where all of the emergency airway and surgical equipment is available to secure the airway. The extuba-tion can be performed after the patient is anesthetized with a volatile anesthetic agent and breathing spontaneously. If severe stridor or airway obstruction develops, the patient can be reintubated or have a tracheostomy performed for long-term airway maintenance. (See also Chapter 29.) In most cases, unilateral vocal cord palsies are tolerated well without evidence of upper airway compromise unless the patient's inspiratory flows are excessive. The greatest risk for upper airway obstruction occurs for the patient who suffers bilateral vocal cord palsies after surgery.

Initially, while still sedated, the patient may not have stridor or evidence of airway obstruction. However, as the patient awakens and inspiratory flows increase, the stridor becomes obvious and usually requires emergent tracheal intubation or, more commonly, tracheostomy.

Stridor can also occur as a result of dislocation of the cricoarytenoid joint. The risk of cricoarytenoid disloca-tion is greatest in patients with rheumatoid arthritis, in whom the joint may be affected. However, dislocation should be suspected in any patient for whom tracheal intubation is difficult and requires multiple attempts and extensive manipulation of the airway.

III. MONITORING RESPIRATORY FUNCTION

A. CLINICAL ASSESSMENT

The clinical examination remains one of the most important and valuable methods to monitor a patient's respiratory status. Too often, attention is placed on technologically sophisticated monitoring devices and the physical exami-nation is not performed or the clinical signs and symptoms are ignored. Nonetheless, a great deal of useful informa-tion about actual or potential airway problems and abnormalities in pulmonary mechanical function or gas exchange can be obtained from a carefully performed and thorough examination. Many of the early signs of respiratory failure are apparent first on physical assess-ment (see Chapter 8) before the abnormalities are apparent by other means. For example, the respiratory rate provides important information about respiratory reserve, dead space, and respiratory drive, particularly when interpreted in conjunction with arterial carbon dioxide tension (Pa_{CO_2}). Tachypnea is frequently the earliest sign of impending respiratory failure. In addition to the respiratory rate, the patient's pattern of breathing should be evaluated. Subtle changes in the rate, tidal volume, and pattern of breathing may provide an early indication of increased work of breathing (as might occur with reduced lung compliance, increased airway resistance, or phrenic nerve dysfunction) or altered ventilatory drive. Although inspiratory flow is difficult to assess by clinical examination, respiratory distress is often manifest as the patient attempts to increase alveolar ventilation by taking larger, more rapid inspirations.

The presence of upper airway obstruction, as might occur after manipulation of the airway, in association with epiglottitis or a mass in or around the airway can be assessed by careful clinical evaluation. Nasal flaring, stridor, and chest wall movement in the absence of airflow suggest upper airway obstruction. If the patient is making respi-ratory efforts and has abdominal expansion during inspi-ration without chest excursions, the patient has upper airway obstruction and may require manipulation of the upper airway and a jaw thrust, initiation of positive-pressure ventilation with either continuous positive airway pressure (CPAP) or biphasic positive airway pressure, or endotracheal intubation. When the patient presents with stridor, the physical evaluation can facilitate diagnosis of the location of the airway compromise. When the stridor occurs primarily during inspiration, it is due to extrathoracic obstruction; when it occurs during exhalation, it reflects an intrathoracic obstruction. If the stridor occurs during both inspiration and exhalation, the obstruction is fixed. The fixed obstruction is rarely amenable to conservative treatment; endotracheal intubation is most likely to be required until a more definitive therapy can be provided.

Respiratory dyssynchrony is an early and critical indicator of respiratory muscle fatigue and impending respiratory failure.[21,115] Respiratory dyssynchrony (when the patient has no evidence of upper airway obstruction) is identified by assessing chest wall and abdominal movement during normal tidal breathing. A paradoxical respiratory pattern suggests that the patient may have inadequate muscle strength to sustain spontaneous respiration and that positive-pressure ventilatory support may be required. Tobin and colleagues found that respiratory muscle dyssynchrony can occur before the development of fatigue,[134,135] although fatigue of the respiratory muscles does not always result in the development of dyssynchrony.[79]

The clinical observation of the patient should include careful assessment of the respiratory muscles in large part to evaluate respiratory reserve. Use of accessory muscles, including the sternocleidomastoid and scalene muscles, is commonly seen in patients with long-standing respiratory failure associated with chronic obstructive pulmonary disease.[114] The position of the diaphragm and diaphragmatic motion are also affected in patients with severe chronic obstructive pulmonary disease. The patient who relies on accessory muscles and has minimal diaphragmatic excursion does not have any respiratory reserve. The patient is at risk for recurrent respiratory failure and presents a significant challenge during weaning when mechanical ventilatory support is required.

The routine physical examination of the lungs is an essential monitoring technique and should not be forgotten. The examination can provide evidence of parenchymal lung abnormalities and cardiopulmonary pathology. Palpation of the chest and auscultation of the lungs can provide useful information about the presence of pleural effusions, pneumothorax, or other extrapulmonary air as well as assess the location of the diaphragms. The examination can provide information about potential physiologic abnormalities and guide in the selection of other monitoring techniques including arterial blood gases, CXR, and other monitors.

Although the physical examination is very useful and should be performed regularly, some of the physical signs and symptoms of respiratory failure do not appear early enough to provide adequate warning, nor do they change quickly enough to determine whether an intervention was appropriate. The greatest value of the physical examination is that it provides an ongoing assessment of pulmonary function when used in conjunction with other monitors of the respiratory system.

B. RADIOLOGIC EVALUATION

The chest radiograph is an important monitor of the respiratory status and one that is commonly obtained in the ICU setting. It is occasionally also a useful monitor for the unstable patient undergoing surgery, providing information that influences clinical management, including the need for prolonged ventilatory support postoperatively (see Chapter 2). The CXR provides confirmation of proper ET placement after endotracheal intubation.[52,120] It is helpful in differentiating the causes of abnormal physical findings and can be used to determine the presence of atelectasis, consolidation, or pulmonary edema. The radiographic findings consistent with pulmonary edema include bronchial cuffing, perihilar pulmonary infiltrates, and Kerley's B lines. The CXR can identify abnormalities in the larger airways, including tracheal stenosis, dilatation (as might occur when the ET cuff is overinflated), or tracheomalacia, although tracheomalacia may require more sophisticated studies that assess the dynamic nature of the abnormality, including cine studies or magnetic resonance imaging (MRI).

As is true of all monitors, the routine CXR has limitations when used as a monitor of respiratory status. Radiographic findings do not always correlate with other clinical and physiologic monitors because the radiologic changes can be delayed in onset and resolution. The radiologic technique also influences the value of the CXR as a monitor. Most commonly, a portable anteroposterior film is obtained with the patient in the supine position. When it is performed in this manner, interpretation of heart size and differentiation of atelectasis and pleural effusions and the presence of pneumothoraces may be difficult. When trying to identify any of these abnormalities, other views, including upright or lateral decubitus films, should be requested, depending on the suspected pathology. Occasionally, an ultrasound or computed tomography (CT) scan of the chest may be required to confirm the presence of pleural effusions, pulmonary abscesses, or other abnormalities.

Other radiologic evaluations can be useful for further evaluation of abnormalities noted on the CXR or physical examination. Ventilation and perfusion scans have been used to detect pulmonary emboli, although the $\dot{V}/\dot{Q}$ scans are often inadequate for assessing critically ill patients. For the ICU patient with suspected pulmonary emboli, bedside ventilation scans are difficult to perform, but perfusion scans are often sufficient, particularly when perfusion defects are correlated with abnormalities on portable chest films. More commonly, however, pulmonary arteriograms or spiral CT scans are now performed because they can be completed quickly and provide better diagnostic information than the $\dot{V}/\dot{Q}$ scan alone.

CT and MRI scans can provide important information about the airway and pulmonary parenchyma.

They can define the location, extent, and character of upper airway abnormalities, including mass lesions, pulmonary intraparenchymal lesions, pleural effusions, and other pulmonary and extrapulmonary abnormalities.

C. GAS EXCHANGE

One of the most important goals in monitoring pulmonary function is to determine whether the lung is able to sustain satisfactory oxygenation and ventilation. Both invasive and noninvasive monitors of gas exchange are now used routinely. Although noninvasive devices are useful and provide important information about oxygenation and ventilation, the arterial blood gas remains the most frequently used monitor of oxygenation, ventilation, and acid-base abnormalities.[143]

1. Arterial Blood Gas Monitoring

Arterial blood gas measurement remains an essential component of respiratory monitoring. The arterial blood gas provides direct measurement of arterial oxygen tension (PaO_2), $PaCO_2$, and pH. From these measured data, bicarbonate concentration (HCO_3^-), oxygen saturation (SaO_2), and base excess (BE) or base deficit are calculated. The measured and calculated parameters define adequacy of gas exchange, acid-base balance, and overall cardiorespiratory status.

PaO_2, $PaCO_2$, and pH are used routinely in the operating room, ICU, emergency room, and occasionally other clinical settings to evaluate gas exchange and respiratory reserve. Direct measurement of PaO_2 from a sample of arterial blood obtained either from a direct arterial puncture or from an indwelling arterial catheter has been the traditional method for assessing oxygenation. To interpret PaO_2 accurately requires an understanding of normal pulmonary physiology and the influences of alterations in ventilation and perfusion on the *predicted* arterial oxygen tension. Normal PaO_2 declines with age. PaO_2 can vary over time by as much as ±10%, and the PaO_2 measured by a blood gas machine can vary by ±10%. Hypoxemia can result from a number of factors, including inadequate inspired oxygen (low alveolar oxygen tension), ventilation-perfusion mismatch, shunt, or inadequate cardiac output (low mixed venous oxygen tension). The confirmation of an acceptable PaO_2 is reassuring, although it does not confirm that oxygen delivery is sufficient. In order to assess the adequacy of oxygen delivery, additional studies are necessary, including evaluation of acid-base status, measurement of serum lactate and mixed venous oxygen content, and cardiac output measurement.

The $PaCO_2$ is measured to monitor ventilation. The $PaCO_2$ can differentiate whether ventilation is normal or abnormal. The normal $PaCO_2$ is 40 mm Hg; however, the $PaCO_2$ must be interpreted in relation to the pH. In response to changes in pH, ventilatory drive changes. When a patient develops a metabolic alkalosis, as might occur after a bicarbonate infusion or the administration of large quantities of citrated bank blood, the ventilatory drive is decreased. The $PaCO_2$ rises, but the decrease in minute ventilation is appropriate and is not an indication of respiratory failure. Similarly, the patient who has a significant metabolic acidosis should increase minute ventilation to normalize the pH. If the $PaCO_2$ is 40 mm Hg with a low pH, the ventilatory effort is inadequate, suggesting respiratory failure despite the normal $PaCO_2$.

When arterial blood cannot be obtained, venous blood sampling (either peripheral or central) has been used to *estimate* arterial PCO_2. In some clinical situations, the difference between $PaCO_2$ and mixed venous CO_2 tension ($PvCO_2$) is small, and $PvCO_2$ can be used as an estimate of $PaCO_2$. However, the exact relationship between arterial and venous PCO_2 is not consistent from patient to patient or within a single patient as the clinical condition changes. $PvCO_2$ cannot be used as a substitute for $PaCO_2$.

Although monitoring gas exchange using arterial blood gas measurements is important, the technique has some limitations. Blood gas monitoring is invasive; samples must be drawn from an indwelling arterial catheter or an arterial puncture. Frequent blood gas sampling can result in significant blood loss, which may be a clinical problem for any unstable patient, particularly the pediatric patient or anemic adult. The placement and maintenance of an arterial catheter also have associated risks, including hemorrhage, hand ischemia, arterial thrombosis and embolism, infection,[3,77] and development of a radial artery aneurysm.[151]

Blood gas monitoring is generally obtained by intermittent sampling from an arterial puncture or indwelling arterial catheter. When a patient's respiratory status is unstable, is rapidly evolving, or when frequent adjustments in ventilatory support are required, intermittent monitoring might be insufficient. In these clinical situations, continuous monitoring would be preferable. Continuous intra-arterial blood gas monitors can provide useful real-time data regarding gas exchange and acid-base status,[60,82] although the clinical utility of these monitors has not yet been validated and the technology is not widely available.[8,138] The continuous monitors utilize fluorescence-based probes placed through an arterial catheter to provide a continuous assessment of PaO_2, $PaCO_2$, and pH. The information obtained from these instruments should provide more immediate information about changes in gas exchange or acid-base balance. However, the probes and monitors are more expensive than intermittent blood gas analysis and have not yet become routine monitors.

2. Noninvasive Monitoring of Gas Exchange

Assessment of gas exchange using noninvasive techniques has revolutionized clinical care, particularly for anesthesiologists and intensive care providers. Because clinical evaluation of gas exchange is unreliable[22] and often a late sign of deterioration, noninvasive, continuous devices that monitor oxygenation and ventilation are valuable tools. A number of noninvasive methods are available for evaluating oxygenation and ventilation. The most commonly used devices include the pulse oximeter for monitoring oxygenation and the capnograph for evaluating ventilation.

a. Pulse Oximetry

Pulse oximetry provides a rapid, continuous, and non-invasive estimation of the oxygen saturation of hemoglobin in arterial blood[83,155] and is used routinely to monitor clinical care involving airway management in the operating room, emergency department, and the ICU.[15,50] In addition, it has become the standard monitor of oxygenation during administration of sedation for procedures as well as during general medical care.[28,36,119,122] With routine use of this monitor, a high prevalence of clinically unde-tected hypoxemia in both adults and children has been demonstrated.[26,83,86,89,122] These episodes of desaturation may affect morbidity and mortality.[12,48] With severe and sustained hypoxemia (oxygen saturation from pulse oximetry [SpO_2] less than 85% for more than 5 minutes), patients with known cardiac disease were twice as likely to have perioperative ischemia following noncardiac surgery.[48] In medical patients, those who experienced episodes of hypoxemia within the first 24 hours of hospi-talization were three times as likely to die 4 to 7 months following discharge.[12]

It is logical to assume that the routine use of pulse oximetry has made caring for patients safer by increasing the detection of hypoxemia, better understanding its causes, and allowing more rapid and effective interventions to correct the pathophysiologic causes. Some authors have suggested that the early detection of arterial oxygen desaturation with the use of pulse oximetry may improve outcome.[29,35,85] Although clinical studies do not confirm this belief, they do not negate the presumed benefit of

this monitoring tool.[34,88,98,99,105] A systematic review of the Cochrane database found no evidence of an outcome benefit of the use of pulse oximetry in anesthesia practice.[104]

To measure the oxygen saturation of hemoglobin in arterial blood, pulse oximetry utilizes two fundamental principles: (1) the differential light absorption of oxyhe-moglobin (O_2Hb) and reduced hemoglobin (Hb) and (2) the increase in light absorption produced by pulsatile blood flow compared with that of a background of connective tissue, skin, bone, and venous blood.[119,131] The spectrophotometric principle that forms the basis for oximetry is the Lambert-Beer law (equation 1), which allows the determination of the concentration of an unknown solute in a solvent by light absorption.

$$I_1/I_0 = e^{-\alpha lc} \qquad (1)$$

where I_1 is the intensity of the light out of the sample, I_0 is the intensity of the incident light, α is the absorp-tion coefficient of the substance, l is the distance the light travels through the material (the path length), c is the concentration of the absorbing species, and e is the base of the natural logarithm.

The use of the Lambert-Beer law allows the determina-tion of the concentration of a solute in a solvent as long as the extinction coefficient is known. It also follows that for a solution with multiple solutes, a separate wavelength of light is needed for differentiation of the solutes. That is, for a solution with four solutes, four separate wave-lengths of light are required.

The commercially available pulse oximeters use light-emitting diodes (LEDs) that transmit light at specific, known wavelengths, 660 nm (red) and 940 nm (infrared). These wavelengths were selected because the absorption characteristics of O_2Hb and reduced Hb are sufficiently different at these wavelengths to allow differentiation of O_2Hb and Hb (Fig. 46-1).

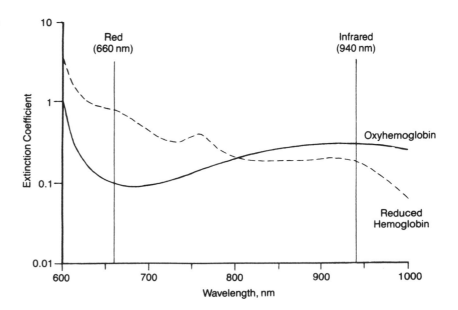

Figure 46-1 Absorption (extinction) character-istics of oxyhemoglobin and reduced hemoglo-bin are shown. There are marked differences between the two at light wavelengths 660 nm (red) and 940 nm (infrared). (From Tobin MJ: Respiratory monitoring. JAMA 264:244, 1990.)

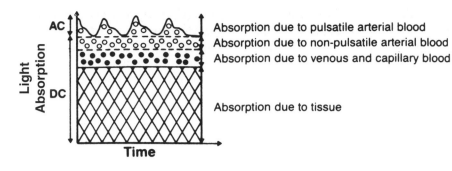

Figure 46-2 Schematic representation of light absorption through living tissue. Note that the AC signal is due to pulsatile component of arterial blood, and the DC signal comprises all the nonpulsatile absorbers of light in the tissue including nonpulsatile blood in the veins and capillaries and nonpulsatile blood in all other tissues. (From Tremper KK, Barker SJ: Pulse oximetry. Anesthesiology 70:98, 1989.)

The pulse oximeter determines arterial saturation by timing the measurement to pulsations in the arterial system. During pulsatile flow, the vascular bed expands and contracts, creating a change in the light path length.[155] These pulsations alter the quantity of light transmitted to the sensor and provide a plethysmographic waveform.[64] This timing of the signal allows the pulse oximeter to differentiate arterial oxygen saturation from venous saturation on the basis of the ratio of pulsatile and baseline absorption of red and infrared light (Fig. 46-2).

The pulse oximeter displays the oxygen saturation based on a ratio (R) of pulsatile and baseline absorption at the two wavelengths transmitted (660 nm, 940 nm) in the tissue bed. The relationship is represented by the following equation:

$$R = \frac{\text{pulsatile absorbance at 660 nm/nonpulsatile absorbance at 660 nm}}{\text{pulsatile absorbance at 940 nm/nonpulsatile absorbance at 940 nm}} \quad (2)$$

The oxygen saturation displayed by the pulse oximeter is empirically related to this calculated value on the basis of calibration curves derived for healthy nonsmoking adult males breathing oxygen at varying concentrations.

Most commercially available pulse oximeters are calibrated over the range 70% to 100%. The accuracy of pulse oximetry in determining the arterial oxygen saturation of Hb has been shown to be excellent over this range,[155] with an error of less than ±3% to 4%.[122,133]

Although pulse oximetry has become a ubiquitous monitoring device, particularly to confirm adequacy of oxygenation during airway management, it has a number of limitations. First, the measurement of oxygen saturation does not provide a direct assessment of oxygen tension. Because of the shape of the oxygen-hemoglobin dissociation curve, at higher levels of oxygenation measurements of SpO_2 are insensitive in detecting significant changes in PaO_2 (Fig. 46-3). Second, the pulse oximeter is not accurate when oxygen saturation is below 70%. The inaccuracy is due to both the limited range of oxygen saturation used in the calibration process and the difficulty in obtaining reliable human data at these low oxygen saturations.[132]

The accuracy of pulse oximeters during hypoxemia has been extensively studied and reviewed.[18,55,62,123,124,134] Most of these studies have been performed on healthy volunteers who had desaturation induced by breathing hypoxic gas mixtures for short periods of time.

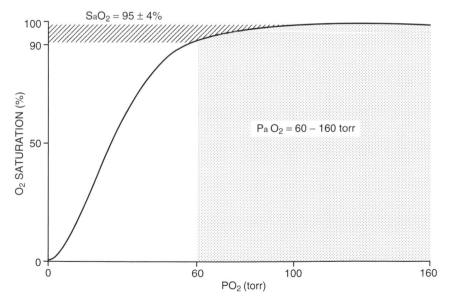

Figure 46-3 Oxygen dissociation curve. Because pulse oximeters have 95% confidence limits for oxygen saturation (SaO_2) of ±3% to 4%, an oximeter reading 95% could represent an arterial oxygen tension (PaO_2) of 60 (saturation 91%) or 160 mm Hg (saturation of 99%). (From Tobin MJ: Respiratory monitoring in the intensive care unit. Am Rev Respir Dis 138:1625, 1988.)

Pulse oximeters from various manufacturers varied in their accuracy during hypoxemia; the direction of error differs among these devices, with some overestimating and some underestimating true arterial oxygen saturation. The results of some of these studies documented problems with the calibration curves and resulted in the revision of the algorithms by the manufacturers.[18,55,62,123,124,132,136] These modifications to the algorithms have resulted in improved performance of the oximeters.[122]

A number of other factors affect the performance of pulse oximeters. The response characteristics of pulse oximeters are clinically important, particularly in situations in which the saturation may be changing rapidly, as can occur during management of the difficult airway. A number of investigators have studied the response characteristics of pulse oximetry in clinical practice.[18,55,62,123,134,136,146] West and colleagues studied five obese, nonsmoking males with the sleep apnea syndrome.[146] During spontaneous desaturation, the pulse oximeter underestimated the minimum SaO_2, and during spontaneous resaturation there was an overshoot of the maximum SpO_2. The location of the probe also influences the response time for the pulse oximeter. Probes placed on the ear respond more quickly to sudden decrease in SaO_2 than probes placed on a digit.[62,123] The response time to changes in oxygen saturation of the pulse oximeter also depends on heart rate. For fingertip sensors, as heart rate increases, the response to an acute change in saturation is faster; for ear or nasal probes, the relationship is reversed so that, as heart rate increases, the response to changes in SaO_2 is slower.[146]

There are a number of clinical situations in which the accuracy of the pulse oximeter is altered (Table 46-1).

Table 46-1   Conditions Affecting the Accuracy of Pulse Oximetry

External light sources
Electrocautery
Motion of the probe

Dyshemoglobinemias
  Carboxyhemoglobin
  Methemoglobin

Dyes and pigments
  Indocyanine green
  Methylene blue
  Indigo carmine

Nail polish
Severe anemia
Low perfusion
Excessive venous pulsations

Excessive light, such as fluorescent or xenon arc surgical lights, bilirubin lights, and heating lamps, can cause falsely low or high SpO_2 values.[110,122,131] Covering the probe with an opaque material helps to eliminate this problem. Electrocautery devices can produce significant electrical interference, which results in improper functioning of the pulse oximeter.[119] Motion of the probe, such as when a patient or caregiver moves the digit on which the oximeter probe is placed, can cause artifactual readings from the pulse oximeter. Vibration of the sensor delays the detection time for hypoxemia and causes spurious decreases in SpO_2.[68] Movement can result in errors of as much as 20%.[108] In a large prospective study, patients' motion was the major reason for abandoning the use of a pulse oximeter in the postanesthesia care unit.[87] In pediatric patients, 71% of all alarms were false.[69] Attempts have been made to minimize the effect of motion by timing the measurement of SpO_2 to the electrocardiogram (ECG). Pulse oximeters that possess ECG linkage and time the measurement of arterial saturation to the ECG have been shown to perform better during vibration than those without this feature.[68] Although this ECG interface is helpful, it has not completely eliminated motion as a problem, particularly in very active or agitated patients. Another approach to decreasing the effect of patients' motion on the accuracy of oximetric data has been to reject motion artifact retrospectively using changes in the plethysmographic waveform that immediately preceded the questionable event.[108] This results in fewer "detected" episodes of false oxygen desaturation but at the price of missing true events.[141]

More recently, a number of manufacturers have added technology designed to minimize motion artifact and to extract a more accurate (true) signal. As introduced by Masimo Corporation, Masimo Signal Extraction Technology (Masimo SET) uses unique sensor designs and software algorithms to reduce the incidence of false alarms. When the performance of oximeters using this technology was compared in volunteers with that of the Nellcor N-3000 Symphony (OXISMART) with improved low-signal performance and the older Nellcor N-200, the oximeters using Masimo SET were superior in both error and signal dropout rate.[5] Baker and colleagues compared the functioning and accuracy of 20 pulse oximeter models in volunteers with hypoxemia during motion and found that the Masimo SET had the best overall performance.[2] When used in the neonatal ICU, Masimo SET resulted in dramatically fewer false alarms and captured more true events than the Nellcor N-200.[57] Oximeters using Masimo SET were found to be more reliable in detecting bradycardia and hypoxemic episodes in patients in the neonatal ICU than the N-3000.[10] This is evidence that more reliable data from oximetry can improve the process of care in a cost-effective manner. In adults following cardiac surgery, the use of more reliable oximeters (those with Masimo SET) compared with conventional oximeters resulted in a more rapid reduction in fraction of inspired oxygen (FIO_2) with the need for fewer arterial blood gases during mechanical ventilation.[33]

Another problem with the pulse oximeter is related to its inability to differentiate oxyhemoglobin from other hemoglobins, such as methemoglobin and carboxyhemoglobin. An oximeter is able to differentiate only as many substances as the number of wavelengths of light it emits.[119,136] Therefore, commercially available oximeters can detect only two types of hemoglobin, reduced and oxygenated (Hb and O_2Hb). Pulse oximeters derive a "functional saturation" of hemoglobin, which is defined as:

$$\text{Functional saturation} = \frac{O_2Hb}{O_2Hb + Hb} \times 100\% \qquad (3)$$

This functional saturation does not account for other hemoglobins, such as methemoglobin (MetHb) or carboxyhemoglobin (COHb). In order to assess the presence of these other hemoglobin species, two additional wavelengths of light must be incorporated into the measuring device. Spectrophotometric heme-oximeters (co-oximeters) that utilize at least four wavelengths of light are able to measure other hemoglobin species and calculate the "fractional saturation" using the following equation:

$$\text{Fractional saturation} =$$
$$\frac{O_2Hb}{O_2Hb + Hb + MetHb + COHb} \times 100\% \qquad (4)$$

When COHb or MetHb is present, the pulse oximeter does not provide a true measurement of *oxygen* saturation.[6,7] The presence of COHb causes a false elevation in the SpO_2 measurement.[6] As shown in Figure 46-4, COHb has minimal light absorption at 940 nm, and at 660 nm its absorption coefficient is nearly identical to that of O_2Hb. The pulse oximeter cannot differentiate COHb from O_2Hb; it overestimates the O_2Hb.[6] The SpO_2 displayed by the pulse oximeter approximates the sums of COHb and O_2Hb. This problem with pulse

oximeters is important to consider when assessing oxygenation in patients who have sustained smoke inhalation or patients who have smoked just prior to proposed airway management. COHb can also be present in long-term ICU patients because carbon monoxide (CO) is a metabolic product of heme metabolism.[113,127] The influence of this potential endogenous source of CO on the accuracy of SpO_2 in the critically ill patient requires further evaluation. In any case, when high CO levels are suspected, oxygen saturation should be measured using a co-oximeter rather than a pulse oximeter.

MetHb also interferes with pulse oximeter measurements.[7,37] As MetHb levels exceed 30% to 35%, SpO_2 becomes independent of MetHb level, approaching 85%. This occurs because the MetHb absorption coefficient at 660 nm is almost identical to that of reduced hemoglobin, whereas at 940 nm it is greater than that of other hemoglobins (see Fig. 46-4). The pulse oximeter therefore overestimates or underestimates the true SaO_2, depending on the level of MetHb.[136] Some causes of high MetHb levels include administration of nitrates, local anesthetics (lidocaine, benzocaine), metoclopramide, sulfa-containing drugs, ethylenediaminetetraacetic acid (EDTA), and diaminodiphenylsulfone (DDS) (Dapsone) and primaquine phosphate used to treat patients with acquired immunodeficiency syndrome (AIDS). Some patients can also have congenitally high MetHb levels. Fetal Hb has not been shown to affect the accuracy of the pulse oximeter.[110,119,122] The effect of other dyshemoglobinemias, such as sulfhemoglobin, on the accuracy of pulse oximetry has not been investigated.[110]

Other pigments interfere with the accuracy of pulse oximeter measurements, including indocyanine green, methylene blue, and indigo carmine.[110] These dyes cause transient artifactual falls in saturation; the extent of the problem depends on the absorption characteristics of the dye. Skin pigmentation has a minimal effect on pulse oximeter readings, although very dark pigmentation can

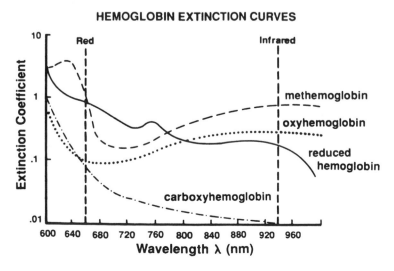

Figure 46-4 Transmitted light absorbance spectra of four hemoglobin species: oxyhemoglobin, reduced hemoglobin, carboxyhemoglobin, and methemoglobin. (From Tremper KK, Barker SJ: Pulse oximetry. Anesthesiology 70:98, 1989.)

to diagnose rebreathing of CO_2; with rebreathing, as can occur when fresh gas flow is inadequate, the baseline (inspired) CO_2 concentration increases.

Capnography has significant limitations as a monitor of ventilation for patients with impaired pulmonary function or hemodynamic instability. The biggest problem is that the correlation between $PaCO_2$ and $P_{ET}CO_2$ is variable and sometimes poor in patients with low cardiac output or altered ventilation-perfusion relationships. More important, the correlation varies as the patient's clinical condition changes, making interpretations of ventilation from $P_{ET}CO_2$ measurements alone unreliable.

IV. MONITORING RESPIRATORY FUNCTION DURING MECHANICAL VENTILATORY SUPPORT

The assessment of pulmonary mechanical function can be performed using a variety of monitoring techniques for the patient who is breathing spontaneously as well as the mechanically ventilated patient.[63,80,106,128] The techniques are useful for optimizing ventilatory support in the critically ill patient, determining the extent to which the patient can initiate spontaneous ventilation, guiding the use of supportive modes of ventilation such as pressure support ventilation, and determining when and how to initiate weaning from mechanical ventilatory support. With a number of new modes of ventilation and supportive techniques to augment patient-initiated breaths, these monitoring techniques have become an essential component of respiratory management.

A. ASSESSMENT OF PULMONARY MECHANICAL FUNCTION

Assessment of dead space ventilation is critical to understanding the nature of a patient's respiratory dysfunction and defining the ventilatory needs of the patient. The dead space ventilation represents "wasted" ventilation in that it increases the work of breathing without contributing to gas exchange.

In general, most clinicians measure $PaCO_2$ to determine whether the patient has adequate ventilation, defined as effective removal of CO_2 by the lungs. $PaCO_2$ is a critical and useful monitor of respiratory function and cardiorespiratory relationships, although interpretation of $PaCO_2$ requires an understanding not only of respiratory function but also of acid-base status and compensatory mechanisms by which the patient may adjust to decreased alveolar ventilation. To evaluate adequacy of ventilation, therefore, requires an understanding of both alveolar and dead space ventilation.

The determinants of $PaCO_2$ are represented in equation (5):

$$PaCO_2 = kVCO_2/V_A \qquad (5)$$

where $k = 0.863$, VCO_2 = carbon dioxide production (mL/min), and V_A = alveolar ventilation (L/min).

The equation assumes that inspired CO_2 is zero. Carbon dioxide elimination through the lung is dependent solely on the ventilation of alveoli (V_A), the area within the lung where gas exchange occurs.[128] The remainder of the lung and large airways represent dead space, the volume of gas that does not participate in gas exchange; ventilation of dead space (V_D) has no effect on CO_2 elimination.

The required minute ventilation to maintain CO_2 homeostasis depends on the relationship between alveolar and dead space ventilation. As the dead space increases, the work of breathing (either respiratory rate or tidal volume) must increase in order to compensate for the wasted ventilation and maintain a normal $PaCO_2$. For the clinician caring for the patient with respiratory failure, having knowledge of a patient's dead space provides important information about the minute ventilation that is required to maintain a normal $PaCO_2$ and therefore whether the patient is a candidate for weaning from mechanical ventilatory support.

Minute ventilation (V_E) is the sum of V_A and V_D and can be represented by equation (6):

$$V_E = V_D + V_A \qquad (6)$$

Dead space is composed of anatomic dead space, alveolar dead space, and dead space imposed by equipment used to maintain the airway and ensure ventilation. The anatomic dead space is the volume of gas within the conducting airways; in the normal, 70-kg man, it averages approximately 156 mL (about 1 mL per pound).[44] The volume of the anatomic dead space increases with increases in lung volume and decreases in the supine position.[4] Intubation of the airway with an ET decreases the anatomic dead space by approximately 50% because of the elimination of the extrathoracic airway (the nose and mouth, which do not contribute to gas exchange).[96,97] Depending on the intraluminal volume of the ET and any additional added apparatus dead space, the actual reduction of the anatomic dead space that occurs after endotracheal intubation may be inconsequential. Alveolar dead space is defined as the amount of gas that penetrates to the alveolar level but does not participate in gas exchange. In healthy individuals, this volume is minimal; however, alveolar dead space is increased in patients with ventilation-perfusion inequalities, such as those with pulmonary emboli or severe lung injury. The physiologic dead space is the sum of the anatomic and alveolar dead spaces and is represented by the total volume of gas in each breath that does not participate in gas exchange.

The portion of each breath that is dead space can be determined by calculating the ratio of dead space to tidal volume (V_D/V_T). The V_D/V_T is a useful clinical monitor of the overall work of breathing. It can be estimated using the Bohr equation:

$$V_D/V_T = PACO_2 - PECO_2/PACO_2 - PICO_2 \qquad (7)$$

where $PACO_2$ refers to alveolar carbon dioxide tension, $PECO_2$ the carbon dioxide tension in mixed expired gas, and $PICO_2$ the inspired carbon dioxide tension. The V_D/V_T can be estimated more easily by assuming that $PICO_2$ is zero and estimating alveolar CO_2 as arterial CO_2. This simplified formula represents the Enghoff modification of the Bohr equation[56,98,131,132]:

$$V_D/V_T = PaCO_2 - PECO_2/PaCO_2 \qquad (8)$$

The normal V_D/V_T is 0.3 at rest; it decreases during exercise primarily as a result of an increase in tidal volume, a more efficient way to increase alveolar ventilation with increasing oxygen consumption and CO_2 production.[45,56,157] Patients with severe respiratory failure may have a V_D/V_T as high as 0.75 even with an ET in place. In this situation, the patient's work of breathing is so high that discontinuation of some level of ventilatory support is not possible, although modes of ventilation that increase tidal volume without an accompanying increase in work of breathing, such as pressure support ventilation, may facilitate spontaneous ventilatory work.

From a measurement of $PECO_2$ and $PaCO_2$, the V_D/V_T can be calculated. $PECO_2$ can be measured by collecting expired gas in a large-volume reservoir (Douglas bag or meteorologic balloon)[142] for 3 to 5 minutes and measuring the CO_2 tension of a sample of this gas. $PaCO_2$ is measured from blood gas obtained simultaneously during the collection of the expired gas.

Some technical factors must be taken into account when measuring V_D/V_T in mechanically ventilated patients. A correction must be made for gas compression within the ventilator, connecting tubing, and any additional dead space from the apparatus.[28] If the compression volume is ignored, the true physiologic dead space is underestimated by as much as 16%. In addition, physiologic dead space was found to increase markedly when the duration of inspiration during mechanical ventilation was decreased from 1 to 0.5 second in paralyzed patients.[144] A nomogram of the relationship between minute ventilation, V_D/V_T, and arterial CO_2 tension in mechanically ventilated patients was developed to aid in the titration of ventilatory support, assess the response to medical therapy, and increase the precision of the therapeutic management of critically ill patients.[121]

A simpler method for estimating V_D/V_T has been described. Measurement of the carbon dioxide pressure (PCO_2) in the condensate of expired gas in the collection bottle from the expiratory limb of the mechanical ventilator has been shown to be equivalent to the cumbersome technique of collecting the mixed expired gas.[142] This PCO_2 value can be substituted for $PECO_2$, greatly simplifying the measurement of physiologic dead space in mechanically ventilated patients.

Another approach to the noninvasive assessment of the physiologic dead space/tidal volume ratio substitutes $P_{ET}CO_2$ for $PaCO_2$. For normal subjects, the relationship between $P_{ET}CO_2$ and $PaCO_2$ is well established.[61,112]

At rest, $P_{ET}CO_2$ underestimates $PaCO_2$ by 2 to 3 mm Hg.[112] However, with exercise, $P_{ET}CO_2$ can overestimate $PaCO_2$.[61,112] The difference between $P_{ET}CO_2$ and $PaCO_2$ varies directly with tidal volume and cardiac output and inversely with respiratory rate.[61]

For patients undergoing general anesthesia or with respiratory failure, the gradient between arterial and end-tidal CO_2 ($P[a\text{-}_{ET}]CO_2$) increases.[97,152] This increase reflects more ventilation to lung units with high ventilation/perfusion ($\dot{V}/\dot{Q}$) relationships. For patients with normal pulmonary function who are mechanically ventilated during general anesthesia, the $P[a\text{-}_{ET}]CO_2$ averages 5 mm Hg; the $P[a\text{-}_{ET}]CO_2$ can be as high as 15 mm Hg in the supine position.[103] The average $P[a\text{-}_{ET}]CO_2$ increases to 8 mm Hg when these patients are placed in the lateral decubitus position. In patients with respiratory failure, the $P[a\text{-}_{ET}]CO_2$ can be even greater.[152] In patients with respiratory failure, there is a close correlation between $P[a\text{-}_{ET}]CO_2$ and V_D/V_T.[152] The $P[a\text{-}_{ET}]CO_2$ can therefore be used as an indicator of the efficiency of ventilation.

A number of techniques can be used to assess pulmonary function in the patient who requires ventilatory support. Assessments of airway resistance, lung and thorax compliance, and other aspects of lung function are useful guides to differentiating physiologic problems with the patient from problems imposed by the equipment used to support the patient.[63,128]

1. Airway Resistance and Lung-Thorax Compliance

In the intubated ventilated patient, airway resistance and lung-thorax compliance can be differentiated by evaluating peak and plateau pressures and the difference between them (Fig. 46-7). The peak airway pressure generated by the ventilator reflects the pressure necessary to overcome airway resistance and compliance of the lung and chest wall. The peak pressure is elevated when airway resistance

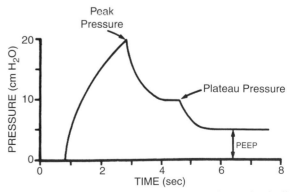

Figure 46-7 Graphic display of airway pressure in mechanically ventilated patient. Peak inspiratory pressure is achieved during gas flow into lung. Plateau pressure is achieved by temporary occlusion of expiratory tubing. From these pressures, dynamic and static compliance can be calculated. PEEP, positive end-expiratory pressure.

is increased, as might occur with increased pulmonary secretions or a kinked ET[53] *or* when lung-thorax compliance is reduced. The peak pressure is influenced by a number of other factors, however, including ventilator parameters such as inspiratory flow rate and pattern, tidal volume, and the size of the ET. The ratio of the tidal volume delivered divided by the pressure change, the difference between the peak inspiratory pressure and positive end-expiratory pressure (PEEP), is the dynamic compliance. Dynamic compliance is reduced when airway resistance is increased *or* lung-thorax compliance is reduced.

To differentiate the cause for reduced dynamic compliance and increased peak airway pressure, the static compliance must be calculated. Static compliance can be assessed by determining the plateau pressure, the pressure achieved in the airways when the lung is inflated to a specific tidal volume under conditions of zero gas flow. Static compliance is measured when inspiration is complete and the lung remains inflated with no further gas flow. Most mechanical ventilators have the capability to provide an inspiratory pause (hold) that allows measurement of the plateau pressure. The pressure generated in the lung during the inspiratory pause is the pressure required to overcome lung and chest wall compliance. Because there is no gas flow at the time of measurement, airway resistance does not contribute to the measured pressure. The static compliance can be estimated by dividing the tidal volume by the difference between the plateau pressure and PEEP. The normal static compliance measured using this method is 60 to 100 mL/cm H_2O. The static compliance is reduced in patients with an extensive pulmonary infiltrate, pulmonary edema, atelectasis, endobronchial intubation, pneumothorax, or any decrease in chest wall compliance as might occur with chest wall edema or subcutaneous emphysema.

2. Intrinsic Positive End-Expiratory Pressure

Hyperinflation (overdistention) of the lung occurs in some mechanically ventilated patients because of air trapping. Gas can be trapped within the lung during the expiratory phase because of dynamic airflow limitation (e.g., associated with asthma) or inadequate expiratory time, as might occur when the inspiratory flow is so low that it causes a high inspiratory/expiratory ratio. The hyperinflation that results has been termed auto-PEEP, intrinsic PEEP (PEEPi), or occult PEEP.[41,107] The presence of auto-PEEP increases the risk of barotrauma, compromises hemodynamics by reducing venous return, increases the patient's work of breathing, and can result in unilateral lung hyperinflation.[28,41,107]

The identification of PEEPi is difficult. PEEPi is not reflected in the pressure measured on the manometer of the ventilator at the end of exhalation because at end expiration the exhalation valve is either open to atmospheric pressure (PEEP = 0) or reflects the level of PEEP provided by the ventilator (Fig. 46-8). The presence of PEEPi can be quantitated by occluding the expiratory port of the ventilator circuit at the end of exhalation immediately before the next breath is delivered. The pressure in the lungs and ventilator circuit equilibrates. The level of PEEPi is then displayed on the manometer. Another method to determine whether PEEPi is present, but not to quantitate it, uses evaluation of the expiratory flow waveform. If expiratory flow does not fall to zero before the next inspiration, gas is trapped within the lung, creating PEEPi (Fig. 46-9). When PEEPi is identified

Figure 46-8 A, Presence of auto-positive end-expiratory pressure (auto-PEEP) is detected by occlusion of the end-expiratory port just prior to initiation of the next ventilator inflation cycle. *B,* The ventilator's manometer measures alveolar pressure (auto-PEEP) only when pressures are allowed to equilibrate by occlusion of the expiratory port and end exhalation. (From Pepe PE, Marini JJ: Occult positive end-expiratory pressure in mechanically ventilated patients with airflow obstruction: The auto-PEEP effect. Am Rev Respir Dis 126:166, 1982.)

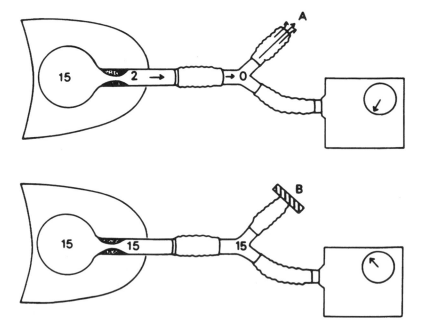

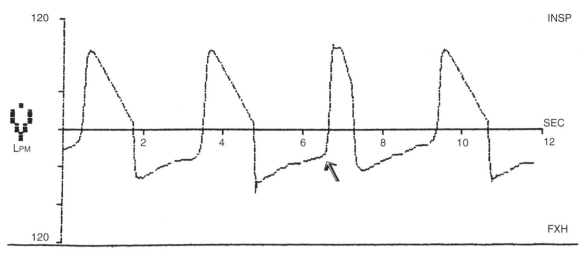

Figure 46-9 Flow-time curve demonstrating expiratory flow continuing until initiation of inspiration *(arrow)*. In normal patient, expiratory flow falls to zero, indicating complete emptying to functional residual capacity. Continued expiratory flow indicates gas trapping.

using this method, the flow waveform can be monitored while adjusting ventilator parameters to minimize PEEPi.

3. Ventilatory Waveform Analysis

Ventilatory waveform analysis is also a useful method to assess airway patency, pulmonary function, and the patient-ventilator interface. Most critical care ventilators now have waveform monitoring capabilities; other independent monitors are available for use in the operating room or ICU to assess waveform and work of breathing. The waveforms provide a visual display of the inspiratory and expiratory flow patterns and pressure-volume and flow-volume loops. The waveforms allow assessment of the appropriateness of ventilator parameters, such as inspiratory gas flow and sensitivity to the patient's need. Figure 46-10 illustrates waveforms that identify excessive work of breathing during patient-initiated breaths. While monitoring the waveforms, adjustments can be made in ventilator parameters to optimize flow patterns and minimize airway pressures, PEEPi, and work of breathing.

4. Work of Breathing

The work of breathing required of a critically ill patient (WOBp) can be assessed by clinical evaluation at the bedside[73] or calculated utilizing data obtained from an esophageal balloon and flow transducer at the airway.[4] The clinical evaluation of WOBp, although useful, can be misleading. Some patients who appear to have excessive WOBp indicate that they are comfortable. Others with a low minute ventilation and slow respiratory rate are already working maximally and, although they appear comfortable at the current level of ventilatory support, will not tolerate any further increase in their WOBp. To better assess the WOBp and monitor the patient's efforts more closely while adjusting the level of ventilatory support, the WOBp can be measured directly using bedside monitors. The monitors require placement of an esophageal balloon to measure esophageal pressure as an estimate of intrapleural pressure. The WOBp is calculated by integrating the area under the pressure-volume loop. With an understanding of each of the components of WOBp, flow-resistive, elastic, and apparatus-induced modifications can be made in ventilator parameters to minimize the patient's WOBp. This monitoring technique has been recommended as a way to adjust pressure support

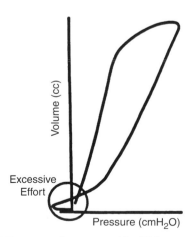

Figure 46-10 Pressure-volume curve identifying excessive effort by the patient to initiate a patient-triggered breath. Excessive effort would be required to initiate a breath for either assist-control ventilation or pressure support ventilation. (From Bedside Respiratory Mechanics Monitoring. Wallingford, Conn, Novametrix Medical Systems.)

ventilation to optimize gas exchange while minimizing WOBp. Although the additional information about the patient-ventilator interface has resulted in modifications of methods of ventilating critically ill patients, no studies to date have documented which parameters are most useful to monitor and which modifications to ventilator management result in the best outcome.

B. ASSESSMENT OF PULMONARY FUNCTION DURING WEANING

A number of measures of pulmonary mechanical function are used to evaluate the likelihood of weaning success in the mechanically ventilated ICU patient.[30,31,66,84,118,133,154] Vital capacity (VC) and maximum inspiratory pressure (MIP or P_i^{max}) are commonly employed to evaluate pulmonary mechanical function. A VC of 10 mL/kg and P_i^{max} more negative than −20 cm H_2O have been shown to be useful predictors of weaning success in some patients. Other measures of mechanical function that have been used to predict weaning success include maximum voluntary ventilation (MVV) greater than two times the resting level and minute ventilation (V_E) less than 10 L/min. A dead space/tidal volume ratio (V_D/V_T) greater than 0.6 has been shown to predict weaning failure consistently. Unfortunately, although each of these parameters can be used to assess pulmonary mechanical function, a number of studies have demonstrated that none predicts weaning success.

A number of other monitoring techniques have been employed to predict weaning success, including continuous measurement of oxygen consumption.[31,84] Although many studies have attempted to define key factors in predicting weaning success, changes in mechanical ventilatory capabilities and our understanding of the risks and benefits of mechanical ventilatory support have had a major impact on methods for assessment and monitoring of patients. The use of pressure support ventilation and noninvasive modes of ventilatory support have made interpretation of the studies and recommendations difficult. In fact, one of the key components in the decision-making process about weaning and discontinuation of mechanical ventilatory support is now related to the patient's ability to protect the airway and the need for intensive respiratory care rather than specific respiratory mechanical parameters. Many patients previously thought to be unweanable can now be weaned from mandatory ventilatory support and provided with ventilatory assistance either using pressure support ventilation through an ET or using noninvasive ventilation, bilevel positive-pressure ventilation by mask, or mask CPAP. As a result, the traditional methods for assessing weaning may no longer apply. Nonetheless, an understanding of the various methods that have been used to assess weaning potential is critical to defining the most effective way to have a patient make the transition from positive-pressure ventilation to spontaneous ventilation.

1. Weaning Indices

A number of indices have been developed to predict when a patient can be successfully weaned from mechanical ventilatory support. These indices combine multiple individual parameters to predict weaning success; some incorporate indices of gas exchange. One study evaluated multiparameter indices, including the rapid shallow breathing (RSB) index, the ratio of respiratory frequency divided by tidal volume in liters, and the CROP index (CROP abbreviated from thoracic *c*ompliance, respiratory *r*ate, arterial *o*xygenation, P_i^{max}), which incorporates measures of dynamic lung compliance, respiratory rate, gas exchange, and inspiratory pressure.[154] An RSB index less than 105 was shown to have a high predictive value of weaning success, whereas the CROP index and more traditional indices had poor predictive value. A study could not confirm these findings and demonstrated that an RSB index below 105 did not predict failed weaning.[70]

2. Breathing Pattern Analysis

Respiratory impedance plethysmography (RIP) can be used to assess breathing pattern by measuring tidal volume, respiratory frequency, inspiratory time, and the contribution of the rib cage and abdomen to lung volume changes.[134,135] Using RIP, the relationship between rib cage and abdominal contributions to tidal volume (respiratory muscle dyssynchrony) has been quantitated. RIP is useful for evaluating changes in functional residual capacity and level of PEEPi as ventilator parameters are adjusted. As a method for predicting weaning success, the technique has had variable success.

3. Airway Occlusion Pressure

The airway occlusion pressure has been used as an index of respiratory drive. Airway occlusion pressure is the pressure generated 0.1 second ($P_{0.1}$) after initiating an inspiratory effort against an occluded airway. The $P_{0.1}$ in normal subjects is generally less than 2 cm H_2O. Some studies suggest that $P_{0.1}$ greater than 6 cm H_2O is incompatible with successful weaning for patients with chronic obstructive pulmonary disease.[99,153] Few studies have not confirmed the value of airway occlusion pressure as a predictor of successful weaning success,[42,90] and its clinical utility remains unclear.

V. CONCLUSION

Assessments of the airway and respiratory function are critical components of the management of any patient for whom mechanical ventilatory support is required and for all patients with respiratory failure. A variety of methods are available to monitor the patient, including clinical assessment, monitors of gas exchange, and various methods to evaluate pulmonary mechanical function. The selection of the most appropriate monitor or monitors for each patient depends upon an understanding of the clinical situation, the available monitoring techniques and standards for their use, the information each monitor provides, and the limitations of each monitor. The challenge for the physician is to identify and appropriately utilize the monitoring techniques that actually optimize clinical management and reduce morbidity and mortality rather than using any monitor simply because it is available. As respiratory care and airway management techniques continue to improve, the selection and proper use of the monitors will become even more critical to patients' safety and outcomes.

REFERENCES

1. Awad AA, Ghosbashy AM, Stout RG, et al: How does the plethysmogram derived from the pulse oximeter relate to arterial blood pressure in coronary artery bypass graft patients? Anesth Analg 93:1466, 2001.
2. Baker SJ: Motion-resistant pulse oximetry: A comparison of new and old models. Anesth Analg 95:967, 2002.
3. Band JD, Maki DG: Infections caused by arterial catheters used for hemodynamic monitoring. Am J Med 67:735, 1979.
4. Banner MJ, Jaeger MJ, Kirby RR: Components of the work of breathing and implication for monitoring ventilator-dependent patients. Crit Care Med 22:515, 1994.
5. Barker SJ, Shah NK: The effects of motion on the performance of pulse oximeters in volunteers. Anesthesiology 86:101, 1997.
6. Barker SJ, Tremper KK: The effect of carbon monoxide inhalation on pulse oximetry and transcutaneous PO_2. Anesthesiology 66:677, 1987.
7. Barker SJ, Tremper KK, Hyatt J: Effects of methemoglobinemia on pulse oximetry and mixed venous oximetry, Anesthesiology 70:112, 1989.
8. Bearden E, Lopez JA, Solis RT: Evaluation of a continuous intraarterial blood gas sensor in critically ill patients. Crit Care Med 22:A25, 1994.
9. Birmingham PK, Cheney FW, Ward RJ: Esophageal intubation: A review of detection techniques. Anesth Analg 65:886, 1986.
10. Bohnhorst B, Peter CS, Poets CF: Pulse oximeter's reliability in detecting hypoxemia and bradycardia: Comparison between a conventional and two new generation oximeters. Crit Care Med 28:1565, 2000.
11. Borum S: Transesophageal pulse oximetry for monitoring patients with extensive burn injury. Anesthesiology 88:1416, 1998.
12. Bowton DL, Scuderi PE, Haponik EF: The incidence and effect on outcome of hypoxemia in hospitalized medical patients. Am J Med 97:38, 1994.
13. Brunel W, Cohen NH: Evaluation of the accuracy of pulse oximetry in critically ill patients. Crit Care Med 16:432, 1988.
14. Brunel W, Coleman DL, Schwartz DE, et al: Assessment of routine chest roentgenograms and the physical examination to confirm endotracheal tube position. Chest 96:1043, 1989.
15. Caples SN, Hubmayr RD: Respiratory monitoring tools in the intensive care unit. Curr Opin Crit Care 9:230, 2003.
16. Cavo JW: True vocal cord paralysis following intubation. Laryngoscope 95:1352, 1985.
17. Chelluri L, Snyder JV, Bird JR: Accuracy of pulse oximetry in patients with hyperbilirubinemia. Respir Care 36:1383, 1991.
18. Choe H, Tasiro C, Fukumitsu K, et al: Comparison of recorded values from six pulse oximeters. Crit Care Med 17:678, 1989.
19. Clayton DG, Webb RK, Ralston AC, et al: A comparison of the performance of 20 pulse oximeters under conditions of poor perfusion. Anaesthesia 46:3, 1991.
20. Clayton DG, Webb RK, Ralston AC, et al: Pulse oximeter probes. Anaesthesia 46:260, 1991.
21. Cohen CA, Zagelbaum G, Gross D, et al: Clinical manifestations of inspiratory muscle fatigue. Am J Med 73:308, 1982.
22. Comroe JH, Botelho S: The unreliability of cyanosis in the recognition of arterial anoxemia. Am J Med Sci 214:1, 1947.
23. Conrardy PA, Goodman LR, Lainge F, et al: Alteration of endotracheal tube position. Crit Care Med 4:8, 1976.
24. Cook LB: Extracting arterial flow waveforms from pulse oximeter waveforms. Anaesthesia 56:551, 2001.
25. Cote CJ, Goldstein EA, Cote MA, et al: A single-blind study of pulse oximetry in children. Anesthesiology 68:184, 1988.
26. Cote CJ, Goldstein EA, Fuchsman WH, et al: The effect of nail polish on pulse oximetry. Anesth Analg 67:683, 1988.
27. Council on Scientific Affairs, AMA: The use of pulse oximetry during conscious sedation. JAMA 270:1463, 1993.
28. Crossman PF, Bushnell LS, Hedley-Whyte J: Dead space during artificial ventilation: Gas compression and mechanical dead space. J Appl Physiol 28:94, 1970.
29. Cullen DJ, Nemeskal AR, Cooper JB, et al: Effect of pulse oximetry, age, and ASA physical status on the frequency of patients admitted unexpectedly to a postoperative intensive care unit and the severity of their anesthesia-related complications. Anesth Analg 74:181, 1992.
30. de Chazal I, Hubmayr RD: Novel aspects of pulmonary mechanics in intensive care. Br J Anaesth 91:81, 2003.
31. Donaldson L, Dodds S, Walsh TS: Clinical evaluation of a continuous oxygen consumption monitor in mechanically ventilated patients. Anaesthesia 2003;58:455.
32. Dunn SM, Mushlin PS, Lind LJ, et al: Tracheal intubation is not invariably confirmed by capnography. Anesthesiology 73:1285, 1990.
33. Durbin CG, Rostow SK: More reliable oximetry reduces the frequency of arterial blood gas analyses and hastens

oxygen weaning after cardiac surgery: A prospective, randomized trial of the clinical impact of a new technology. Crit Care Med 30:1735, 2002.

34. Eichhorn JH: Effect of monitoring standards on anesthesia outcome. Int Anesthesiol Clin 31:181, 1993.

35. Eichhorn JH: Prevention of intraoperative anesthesia accidents and related severe injury through safety monitoring. Anesthesiology 70:572, 1989.

36. Eichhorn JH, Cooper JB, Cullen DJ, et al: Standards for patient monitoring during anesthesia at Harvard Medical School. JAMA 256:1017, 1986.

37. Eisenkraft JB: Pulse oximeter desaturation due to methemoglobinemia. Anesthesiology 68:279, 1988.

38. Eveloff SE, Rounds S, Braman SS: Unilateral lung hyperinflation and herniation as a manifestation of intrinsic PEEP. Chest 98:228, 1990.

39. Falk JL, Rackow EC, Weil MH: End-tidal carbon dioxide concentration during cardiopulmonary resuscitation. N Engl J Med 318:607, 1988.

40. Farber NE, McNeely J, Rosner D: Skin burn associated with pulse oximetry during perioperative photodynamic therapy. Anesthesiology 84:983, 1996.

41. Fernandez R, Benito S, Blanch LI, et al: Intrinsic PEEP: A cause of inspiratory muscle ineffectivity. Intensive Care Med 15:51, 1988.

42. Fernandez R, Raurich JM, Mut T, et al: Extubation failure: Diagnostic value of occlusion pressure (P0.1) and P0.1-derived parameters. Intensive Care Med 30:234, 2004.

43. Fitzgerald RK, Johnson A: Pulse oximetry in sickle cell anemia. Crit Care Med 29:1803, 2001.

44. Fowler WS: Lung function studies. II. The respiratory dead space. J Appl Physiol 154:405, 1948.

45. Fowler WS: Lung function studies. IV. Postural changes in respiratory dead space and functional residual capacity. J Clin Invest 29:1437, 1950.

46. Gandhi SK, Munshi CA, Coon R, et al: Capnography for detection of endobronchial migration of an endotracheal tube. J Clin Monit 7:35, 1991.

47. Garnett AR, Gervin CA, Gervin AS: Capnographic waveforms in esophageal intubation: Effect of carbonated beverages. Ann Emerg Med 18:387, 1989.

48. Gil NP, Wright B, Reilly CS: Relationship between hypoxaemic and cardiac ischaemic events in the perioperative period. Br J Anaesth 68:471, 1992.

49. Goldberg JS, Rawle PR, Zehnder JL, et al: Colorimetric end-tidal carbon dioxide monitoring for tracheal intubation. Anesth Analg 70:191, 1990.

50. Golden JA, Schwartz DE, Gamsu G, et al: Sheathed FOB for assessing endotracheal tube position. Chest 100:20S, 1991.

51. Golparvar M, Naddafnia H, Saghaei M: Evaluating the relationship between arterial blood pressure changes and indices of pulse oximetric plethysmography. Anesth Analg 95:1681, 2002.

52. Gray P, Sullivan G, Ostryniuk P: Value of postprocedural chest radiographs in the adult intensive care unit. Crit Care Med 20:1513, 1992.

53. Haberthur C, Lichtwarck-Aschoff M, Guttmann J: Continuous monitoring of tracheal pressure including spot-check of endotracheal tube resistance. Technol Health Care 11:413, 2003.

54. Habib MP: Physiologic implications of artificial airways. Chest 96:180, 1989.

55. Hannhart B, Haberer JP, Saunier C, Laxenaire MC: Accuracy and precision of fourteen pulse oximeters. Eur Respir J 4:115, 1991.

56. Harris EA, Seelye ER, Whitlock RML: Revised standards for normal resting dead-space volume and venous admixture in men and women. Clin Sci Mol Med 55:125, 1978.

57. Hay WW, Rodden DJ, Collins SM, et al: Pulse oximetry in the NICU: Conventional vs Masimo SET. Pediatr Res 45:304A, 1999.

58. Higgins D, Hayes M, Denman W, et al: Effectiveness of using end-tidal carbon dioxide concentration to monitor cardiopulmonary resuscitation. BMJ 300:581, 1990.

59. Hurford WE, Alfille PH, Bailin MT, et al: Placement and complications of double-lumen endotracheal tubes. Anesth Analg 74:S141, 1992.

60. Ishikawa S, Ohmi S, Nakazawa K, Makita K: Continuous intra-arterial blood gas monitoring during thoracic surgery. J Anesth 14:119, 2000.

61. Jones NL, Robertson DG, Kane JW: Difference between end-tidal and arterial PCO_2 in exercise. J Appl Physiol 47:954, 1979.

62. Kagle DM, Alexander CM, Berko RS, et al: Evaluation of the Ohmeda 3700 pulse oximeter: Steady-state and transient response characteristics. Anesthesiology 66:276, 1987.

63. Kallet RH, Katz JA: Respiratory system mechanics in acute respiratory distress syndrome. Respir Care Clin N Am 9:297, 2003.

64. Kidd JF, Vickers MD: Pulse oximeters: Essential monitors with limitations. Br J Anaesth 62:355, 1989.

65. Kober A, Scheck T, Lieba F, et al: The influence of active warming on signal quality of pulse oximetry in prehospital trauma care. Anesth Analg 95:961, 2002.

66. Krieger BG, Ershowsky PF, Becker DA, et al: Evaluation of conventional criteria for predicting successful weaning from mechanical ventilatory support in elderly patients. Crit Care Med 17:858, 1989.

67. Kyriacou PA, Powell SL, Jones DP, Langford RM: Evaluation of oesophageal pulse oximetry in patients undergoing cardiothoracic surgery. Anaesthesia 58:422, 2003.

68. Langton JA, Hanning CD: Effect of motion artefact on pulse oximeters: Evaluation of four instruments and finger probes. Br J Anaesth 65:564, 1990.

69. Lawless ST: Crying wolf: False alarms in a pediatric intensive care unit. Crit Care Med 22:981, 1994.

70. Lee KH, Hui KP, Chan TB, et al: Rapid shallow breathing (frequency-tidal volume ratio) did not predict extubation outcome. Chest 105:540, 1994.

71. Lee S, Tremper KK, Barker SJ: Effects of anemia on pulse oximetry and continuous mixed venous hemoglobin saturation monitoring in dogs. Anesthesiology 75:118, 1991.

72. Lepilin MG, Vasilyev AV, Bildinov OA, et al: End-tidal carbon dioxide as a noninvasive monitor of circulatory status during cardiopulmonary resuscitation: A preliminary clinical study. Crit Care Med 15:958, 1987.

73. Lewis WD, Chwals W, Benotti PN, et al: Bedside assessment of work of breathing. Crit Care Med 16: 117, 1988.

74. Lima AP, Beelen P, Bakker J: Use of a peripheral perfusion index derived from the pulse oximetry signal as a noninvasive indicator of perfusion. Crit Care Med 30:12:1210, 2002.

75. Lindholm CE, Ollman B, Snyder JV, et al: Cardiorespiratory effects of flexible fiberoptic bronchoscopy in critically ill patients. Chest 74:362, 1978.

76. Lindo D, Browne D, Lindo J: Toe deformity from prolonged pulse oximetry. Arch Dis Child 87:533, 2002.

77. Lindsay SL, Kerridge R, Collett BJ: Abscess following cannulation of the radial artery. Anaesthesia 42:654, 1987.

78. MacLeod BA, Heller MB, Yealy DM, et al: Verification of endotracheal tube placement with colorimetric end-tidal CO_2 detection. Ann Emerg Med 20:267, 1991.

79. Mandor MJ: Respiratory muscle fatigue and breathing pattern. Chest 100:1430, 1991.

80. Marini JJ: Monitoring during mechanical ventilation. Clin Chest Med 9:734, 1988.

81. Mendelson Y, Yocum BL: Noninvasive measurement of arterial oxyhemoglobin saturation with a heated and a non-heated skin reflectance pulse oximeter sensor. Biomed Instrum Technol 25:472, 1991.

82. Menzel M, Soukup J, Henze D, et al: Experiences with continuous intra-arterial blood gas monitoring: Precision and drift of a pure optode-system. Intensive Care Med 29:2180, 2003.

83. Mihm FG, Halperin BD: Noninvasive detection of profound atrial desaturations using a pulse oximetry device. Anesthesiology 62:85, 1985.

84. Miwa K, Mitsuoka M, Takamori S, et al: Continuous monitoring of oxygen consumption in patients undergoing weaning from mechanical ventilation. Respiration 70:623, 2003.

85. Moller JT, Jensen PF, Johannessen NW, et al: Hypoxaemia is reduced by pulse oximetry monitoring in the operating theatre and in the recovery room. Br J Anaesth 68:146, 1992.

86. Moller JT, Johannessen NW, Berg H, et al: Hypoxaemia during anesthesia: An observer study. Br J Anaesth 66:437, 1991.

87. Moller JT, Johannessen NW, Espersen K, et al: Randomized evaluation of pulse oximetry in 20,802 patients: II. Perioperative events and postoperative complications. Anesthesiology 50:445, 1993.

88. Moller JT, Pedersen T, Rasmussen LS, et al: Randomized evaluation of pulse oximetry in 20,802 patients: I. Design, demography, pulse oximetry failure rate, and overall complication rate. Anesthesiology 78:436, 1993.

89. Moller JT, Wittrup M, Johansen SH: Hypoxemia in the post-anesthesia care unit: An observer study. Anesthesiology 73:890, 1990.

90. Montgomery AB, Holle RHO, Neagley SR, et al: Prediction of successful ventilatory weaning using airway occlusion pressure and hypercapnic challenge. Chest 91:496, 1987.

91. Morley TF: Capnography in the intensive care unit. J Intensive Care Med 5:209, 1990.

92. Murciano D, Boczkowski J: Tracheal occlusion pressure: A simple index to monitor respiratory fatigue during acute respiratory failure in patients with chronic obstructive pulmonary disease. Ann Intern Med 108:800, 1988.

93. Murphy KG, Secunda JA, Rockhoff MA: Severe burns from pulse oximeter. Anesthesiology 73:350, 1990.,

94. Niehoff J, DelGuercio C, LaMorte W, et al: Efficacy of pulse oximetry and capnometry in postoperative ventilatory weaning. Crit Care Med 16:701, 1988.

95. Nunn JF, Campbell EJM, Peckett BW: Anatomical subdivisions of the volume of respiratory dead space and effect of position of the jaw. J Appl Physiol 14: 174, 1959.

96. Nunn JF, Hill DW: Respiratory dead space and arterial to end-tidal CO_2 tension difference in anesthetized man. J Appl Physiol 15:383, 1960.

97. Nunn JF: Nunn's Applied Respiratory Physiology. Oxford, Butterworth-Heinemann, 1993.

98. Orkin FK: Practice standards: The Midas touch or the emperor's new clothes? Anesthesiology 70:567, 1989.

99. Orkin FK, Cohen MM, Duncan PG: The quest for meaningful outcomes. Anesthesiology 78:417, 1993.

100. Ornato JP, Shipley JB, Racht EM, et al: Multicenter study of a portable, hand-size, colorimetric end-tidal carbon dioxide detection device. Ann Emerg Med 21:518, 1992.

101. Owen RL, Cheney FW: Endobronchial intubation: A preventable complication. Anesthesiology 67:255, 1987.

102. Palve H, Vuori A: Accuracy of three pulse oximeters at low cardiac index and peripheral temperature. Crit Care Med 19:560, 1991.

103. Pansard JL, Cholley B, Devilliers C, et al: Variation in arterial to end-tidal CO_2 tension differences during anesthesia in the "kidney rest" lateral decubitus position. Anesth Analg 75:506, 1992.

104. Pedersen T, Dyrlund Pedersen B, Moller AM: Pulse oximetry for perioperative monitoring. Cochrane Database Syst Rev 3:CD002013, 2003.

105. Pedersen T, Moller AM, Pedersen BD: Pulse oximetry for perioperative monitoring: Systematic review of randomized, controlled trials. Anesth Analg 96:426, 2003.

106. Pedersen T, Viby-Mogensen, Ringsted C: Anaesthetic practice and postoperative pulmonary complications. Acta Anaesthesiol Scand 36:812, 1992.

107. Pepe PE, Marini JJ: Occult positive end-expiratory pressure in mechanically ventilated patients with airflow obstruction: The auto-PEEP effect. Am Rev Respir Dis 126:166, 1982.

108. Plummer JL, Ilsley AH, Fronsko RRL, Owen H: Identification of movement artifact by the Nellcor N-200 and N-3000 pulse oximeters. J Clin Monit 13:109, 1997.

109. Potgieter PD, Hammond JMJ: "Cuff" test for safe extubation following laryngeal edema. Crit Care Med 16:818, 1988.

110. Ralston AC, Webb RK, Runciman WB: Potential errors in pulse oximetry. Anaesthesia 46:291, 1991.

111. Ries AL, Prewitt LM, Johnson JJ: Skin color and ear oximetry. Chest 96:287, 1989.

112. Robbins PA, Conway J, Cunningham DA, et al: A comparison of indirect methods for continuous estimation of arterial PCO_2 in men. J Appl Physiol 68:1727, 1990.

113. Rodgers PA, Vreman HJ, Dennery PA, et al: Sources of carbon monoxide (CO) in biological systems and applications of CO detection technologies. Semin Perinatol 18:2, 1994.

114. Roussos C: Function and fatigue of respiratory muscles. Chest 88:124S, 1985.

115. Roussos C, Macklem PT: The respiratory muscles. N Engl J Med 307:786, 1982.

116. Sanders AB, Kern KB, Otto CW, et al: End-tidal carbon dioxide monitoring during cardiopulmonary resuscitation: A prognostic indicator for survival. JAMA 262:1347, 1989.

117. Sassoon CS, Te TT, Mahutte CK, et al: Airway occlusion pressure: An important indicator for successful weaning in patients with chronic obstructive pulmonary disease. Am Rev Respir Dis 135:107, 1987.

118. Scheinhorn DJ, Artinian BM, Catlin JL: Weaning from prolonged mechanical ventilation: The experience at a regional weaning center. Chest 105:534, 1994.

119. Schnapp LM, Cohen NH: Pulse oximetry: Uses and abuses. Chest 105:534, 1990.

120. Schwartz DE, Lieberman JA, Cohen NH: Women are at greater risk than men for malpositioning of the endotracheal tube after emergent intubation. Crit Care Med 22:1127, 1994.

121. Selecky PA, Wasserman K, Klein M, et al: A graphic approach to assessing interrelationships among minute ventilation, arterial carbon dioxide tension, and ratio of physiologic deadspace to tidal volume in patients on respirators. Am Rev Respir Dis 117:181, 1978.

122. Severinghaus JW, Kelleher JF: Recent developments in pulse oximetry. Anesthesiology 76:1018, 1992.

123. Severinghaus JW, Naifeh KH: Accuracy of response of six pulse oximeters to profound hypoxia. Anesthesiology 67:551, 1987.

124. Severinghaus JW, Naifeh KH, Koh SO: Errors in 14 pulse oximeters during profound hypoxemia. J Clin Monit 5:72, 1989.

125. Shamir M, Eidelman LA, Floman Y, et al: Pulse oximetry plethysmographic waveform changes in blood volume. Br J Anaesth 82:178, 1999.

126. Simon BA, Hurford WE, Alfille PH, et al: An aid in the diagnosis of malpositioned double-lumen tubes. Anesthesiology 76:862, 1992.

127. Sjöstrand T: Endogenous formation of carbon monoxide in man under normal and pathological conditions. Scand J Clin Lab Invest 1:201, 1949.

128. Stenqvist O: Practical assessment of respiratory mechanics. Br J Anaesth 91:92, 2003.

129. Stewart KG, Rowbottom SJ: Inaccuracy of pulse oximetry in patients with severe tricuspid regurgitation. Anaesthesia 46:668, 1991.

130. Szaflarski NL, Cohen NH: Use of capnography in critically ill adults. Heart Lung 20:363, 1991.

131. Tobin MJ: Respiratory monitoring during mechanical ventilation. Crit Care Clin 6:679, 1990.

132. Tobin MJ: Respiratory monitoring in the intensive care unit. Am Rev Respir Dis 138:1625, 1988.

133. Tobin MJ: Respiratory monitoring. JAMA 264:244, 1990.

134. Tobin MJ, Guenther SM, Perez W, et al: Konno-Mead analysis of ribcage-abdominal motion during successful and unsuccessful trials of weaning from mechanical ventilation. Am Rev Respir Dis 135:1320, 1987.

135. Tobin MJ, Perez W, Guenther SM, et al: Does ribcage-abdominal paradox signify respiratory muscle fatigue? J Appl Physiol 63:851, 1987.

136. Tremper KK, Barker SJ: Pulse oximetry. Anesthesiology 70:98, 1989.

137. Vegfors M, Lindberg LG, Oberg PA, et al: The accuracy of pulse oximetry at two haematocrit levels. Acta Anaesthesiol Scand 36:454, 1992.

138. Venkatesh B, Clutton-Brock T, Hendry S: Intraoperative use of the Paratrend 7 intravascular blood gas sensor. Crit Care Med 22:A21, 1994.

139. Veyckemans F, Baele P, Guillaume JE, et al: Hyperbilirubinemia does not interfere with hemoglobin saturation measured by pulse oximetry. Anesthesiology 70:118, 1989.

140. Vicenzi, M, Gombotz H, Krenn H, et al: Transesophageal versus surface pulse oximetry in intensive care unit patients. Crit Care Med 28:2268, 2000.

141. Visram AR, Jones RDM, Irwin MG, Bacon-Shone J: Use of two oximeters to investigate a method of movement artifact rejection using plethysmographic signals. Br J Anaesth 72:388, 1994.

142. Von Pohle WR, Anholm JD, McMillan J: Carbon dioxide and oxygen partial pressure in expiratory water condensate are equivalent to mixed expired carbon dioxide and oxygen. Chest 101:1601, 1992.

143. Walsh TS: Recent advances in gas exchange measurement in intensive care patients. Br J Anaesth 91;120, 2003.

144. Watson WE: Observations on physiological deadspace during intermittent positive pressure respiration. Br J Anaesth 34:502, 1962.

145. Weinberger SE, Schwartzstein RM, Weiss JW: Hypercapnia. N Engl J Med 321:1223, 1989.

146. West P, George CF, Kryger MH: Dynamic in vivo response characteristics of three oximeters: Hewlett-Packard 47201A, Biox III, and Nellcor N-100. Sleep 10:263, 1987.

147. White PF, Boyle WA: Nail polish and oximetry. Anesth Analg 68:546, 1989.

148. Wille J, Braams R, van Haren WH, van der Werken C: Pulse oximeter-induced digital injury: Frequency rate and possible causative factors. Crit Care Med 28:3555, 2000.

149. Wisely NA, Cook LB: Arterial flow waveforms from pulse oximetry compared with measured Doppler flow waveforms. Anaesthesia 56:556, 2001.

150. Woehlck H, Herrmann D, Kaslow O: Safe use of pulse oximetry during verteporfin therapy. Anesth Analg 96:177, 2003.

151. Wolf S, Mangano DT: Pseudoaneurysm, a late complication of radial-artery catheterization. Anesthesiology 52:80, 1980.

152. Yamanaka MK, Sue DY: Comparison of arterial-end-tidal PCO_2 difference and dead space/tidal volume ratio in respiratory failure. Chest 92:832, 1987.

153. Yang KL: Reproducibility of weaning parameters—A nced for standardization. Chest 102:1829, 1992.

154. Yang KL, Tobin MJ: A prospective study of indexes predicting the outcome of trials of weaning from mechanical ventilation. N Engl J Med 324:1445, 1991.

155. Yelderman M, New W: Evaluation of pulse oximetry. Anesthesiology 59:349, 1983.

156. Zeballos RJ, Weisman IM: Reliability of noninvasive oximetry in black subjects during exercise and hypoxia. Am Rev Respir Dis 144:1240, 1991.

157. Zimmerman MI, Brown LK, Sloane MF: Estimated vs. actual values for dead space/tidal volume ratios during incremental exercise in patients evaluated for dyspnea. Chest 106:131, 1994.

158. Zwillich CW, Pierson DJ, Creagh CE, et al: Complications of assisted ventilation. Am J Med 57:161, 1974.

47

EXTUBATION AND CHANGING ENDOTRACHEAL TUBES

Richard M. Cooper

I. INTRODUCTION

Tracheal extubation has received relatively limited critical scrutiny compared with attention to the identification and management of the potentially difficult intubation (DI). Textbooks, reviews, and conferences focusing on the airway frequently ignore this facet of management despite the observation that airway complications are significantly more likely to be associated with extubation than intubation.[14] Many of these "complications" are relatively minor, such as coughing and transient breath-holding, and have little or no impact upon outcome. Some, however, are life threatening. Moreover, some can be predicted and, with proper preparation, morbidity and mortality can be reduced.

The American Society of Anesthesiologists (ASA) Task Force on Management of the Difficult Airway[4,5] and the Canadian Airway Focus Group[67] recommended that each anesthesiologist have a preformulated strategy for extubation of the difficult airway (DA) and an airway management plan for dealing with postextubation hypoventilation. This chapter classifies the complications associated with tracheal extubation (and the exchange of endotracheal tubes), attempts to stratify the risk of extubation (and tube exchange) in various clinical settings, and proposes strategies that may prove helpful in reducing serious complications or death. Low-risk or routine extubation has been reviewed elsewhere[124,192] and is discussed in less detail. It is important to point out that neither the proposed stratification nor the strategies recommended in dealing with intermediate- and high-risk extubations have been validated by controlled, prospective trials. Such trials would be helpful, but it may not be prudent to await their conclusion.

II. RESPIRATORY COMPLICATIONS DURING OR AFTER EXTUBATION

An extubation fails when an attempt to remove a endotracheal tube (ET) is unsuccessful. An ET exchange is unsuccessful when an attempt to replace an ET is unsuccessful. There is no agreed upon time frame; therefore, the reported incidence varies widely. It is reasonable to consider the failed extubation in two different clinical settings: the intensive care unit (ICU), where such failures are relatively common, and the operating room (OR) or postanesthesia care unit (PACU), where they are less frequent.

In the ICU, the ability to predict readiness for endotracheal extubation is imprecise despite a host of predictive criteria.[75,111,183] To minimize the risks, discomfort, and expense of prolonged intubation, a "trial of extubation" is often attempted, not infrequently followed by reintubation. The incidence of required reintubation is on the order of 6% to 25%,[183] depending upon the clinical mix of patients, their critical acuity, pressures stemming from limitations of critical care resources, and the threshold levels for extubation. Compared with routine postoperative patients, intensive care patients are more likely to have failed extubation because neurologic obtundation may leave them unable to protect their airways. In addition, debilitation and impaired mucociliary clearance may interfere with pulmonary toilet, and diminished strength, altered pulmonary mechanics, increased dead space, and venous admixture may result in hypercapnic or hypoxemic respiratory failure.

Although the complications associated with the extubation of postoperative patients may be more frequent than those associated with intubation, they rarely require reintubation. Retrospective studies involving a wide case mix of postsurgical patients show a high degree of concordance regarding the incidence of required reintubation. Combining the results of three large studies involving nearly 50,000 patients, the incidence ranged from 0.09% to 0.19%.[130,186,221] The reintubation rate is significantly higher (1% to 3%) following selected surgical procedures such as panendoscopy[130] and a variety of head and neck procedures.[91,160,173,254,256]

Postoperative reintubation, although infrequent, may represent a considerable challenge for the anesthesiologist. Anatomic distortion may conspire with physiologic instability, incomplete information concerning the patient, or lack of essential equipment, personnel, or expertise, converting a previously easily managed airway to a disaster. As well, a DA adequately managed during a controlled induction is completely different from the DA in an agitated, hypoxemic, and hypotensive patient.

III. CLASSIFICATIONS

A. ROUTINE EXTUBATIONS

The complications of "routine" extubation" are summarized in Table 47-1. Extubation failures for the most part fall into one or more of the following categories: (1) failure of oxygenation, (2) failure of ventilation, (3) inadequate clearance of pulmonary secretions, or (4) loss of airway patency. These are discussed first in general terms, followed by consideration of complications that do not necessarily require reintubation. Lastly, we discuss specific clinical situations in which these problems are more likely to occur. When these occur with a higher frequency, they have been termed intermediate-risk extubations; when reintubation may be problematic, they have been termed high-risk extubations.

1. Hypoventilation Syndromes

One of the first reports from the ASA closed claims study noted that 4% of 1175 closed claims resulted from critical respiratory events in the PACU, the highest proportion being due to inadequate ventilation, in which a large

Table 47-1 **Complications of Routine Extubations**

Failed extubation
Hypoxia
Hypoventilation
Pulmonary toilet
Obstruction
Unintended extubation
Tube entrapment
Hemodynamic changes
Tachycardia or other dysrhythmias
Hypertension
Increased intraocular pressure
Increased intracranial pressure
Coughing, breath-holding
Laryngospasm
Negative-pressure pulmonary edema
Tracheal or laryngeal trauma
Laryngeal edema
Arytenoid dislocation
Vocal fold paralysis
Laryngeal incompetence
Pulmonary aspiration

proportion of the patients died or suffered brain damage.[268]

A wide variety of clinical conditions may give rise to postoperative ventilatory failure. In a large French multicenter prospective survey conducted between 1978 and 1982, involving nearly 200,000 patients, postoperative respiratory depression accounted for 27 of 85 respiratory complications that were life threatening or resulted in serious sequelae. Such complications were responsible for seven deaths and five cases of hypoxic encephalopathy.[248] Rose and colleagues found that 0.2% of 24,000 patients had a respiratory rate of less than 8 breaths/min, as detected by PACU nurses following general anesthesia.[221,222]

Hypoventilation may be mediated centrally at the level of the upper motor neuron, the anterior horn cell, the lower motor neuron, the neuromuscular junction, or the respiratory muscles. Clinical correlates include central sleep apnea, carotid endarterectomy,[259] medullary injuries, demyelinating disorders, direct injury to peripheral nerves, poliomyelitis, Guillain-Barré syndrome, motor neuron disease, myasthenia gravis, and botulism. As well, hypoventilation may result from the loss of lung or pleural elasticity, diaphragmatic splinting caused by abdominal pain or distention, thoracic deformities such as kyphoscoliosis, or multifactorial entities such as morbid obesity and severe chronic obstructive pulmonary disease.

Rarely, hypercapnia results from an excess of carbon dioxide production or a marked increase in physiologic dead space.

The residual effects of anesthetic drugs contribute to inadequate postoperative ventilation.[153,116,197] This may be exacerbated by incomplete reversal of neuromuscular blockers,[94] hypocalcemia or hypermagnesemia, or the administration of other drugs, including antibiotics, local anesthetics, diuretics, and calcium channel blockers, which may potentiate neuromuscular blockade.

2. Hypoxemic Respiratory Failure

There are many causes of postoperative hypoxemia, a review of which is beyond the scope of this chapter. Generally, these might occur as a result of hypoventilation, a low inspired oxygen concentration, ventilation-perfusion mismatch, right-to-left shunting, increased oxygen consumption, diminished oxygen transport, or rarely an impairment of oxygen diffusion. Clearly, there are clinical situations in which such events are more likely because of preexisting medical conditions or anesthetic and surgical interventions. If the situation is sufficiently severe, there may be a requirement for continuous positive airway pressure (CPAP) or reintubation and mechanical ventilation.

3. Inability to Protect Airway

ICU or postoperative patients may be unable to protect their airway because of preexisting obtundation, neurologic injury, or the effects of residual anesthesia. Patients may be at an equally high risk for pulmonary aspiration at extubation as they are during intubation. Extubation of patients at increased risk for regurgitation should be delayed if the risks can be lessened by such postponement. Alternatively, turning them on their side, placing them head up (or head down), or reversing residual medications with antagonists should be considered. These measures may not restore airway competence, and lack of resolution may necessitate reintubation.

4. Failure of Pulmonary Toilet

Inadequate clearance of pulmonary secretions may be due to a depressed level of consciousness with impaired airway reflexes, overproduction of secretions, an alteration of sputum consistency leading to inspissation and plugging, impaired mucociliary clearance, or inadequate neuromuscular reserve. These may result in atelectasis or pneumonia with attendant hypoxemic respiratory failure. Alterations in pulmonary mechanics may also lead to hypercapnia, necessitating reintubation.

5. Inadvertent Extubations

Inadvertent extubations may result from movement of or by the patient with an inadequately secured ET.

Intraoperatively, this may occur in prone positioning, when the airway is shared with the surgeon, when the head and neck are extended, when draping obscures the view, or when drapes adherent to the ET or circuit are carelessly removed. In the ICU, this may occur when the patient is repositioned for radiographs or routine nursing care. Fastidious attention to securing the tube, providing support for the circuit, and, when necessary, moving the patient and the tube as an integral unit should help to reduce the frequency of this complication. Self-extubations may occur during emergence from anesthesia when the patient is confused, agitated, or distressed, prompting premature extubation. In the ICU, it may not be possible to know whether a self-extubation is accidental or deliberate, but many of these patients require reintubation[33] and are more likely to exhibit postextubation stridor,[193] and the situation may involve multiple intubation attempts, esophageal intubation, and death.[194,255]

6. Entrapment

The ET may also become entrapped because of an inability to deflate the cuff[161,246] or difficulties with the pilot tube.[129,238] This can occur as a consequence of a crimped pilot tube or defective pilot valve. Fixation of the ET by Kirschner wires,[169] screws,[165] or ligatures[3] and entanglement with other devices[99,132] have been described. Entrapment can also occur during the performance of a percutaneous tracheostomy.[56] Mechanical obstruction of an entrapped tube is a life-threatening complication. As well, partial transection of the ET by an osteotome during a maxillary osteotomy has resulted in the partially cut tube forming a "barb" that caught on the posterior aspect of the hard palate.[229] One report of entrapment had fatal consequences. This involved a Carlens tube that was inadvertently sutured to the pulmonary artery.[83] Lang and coauthors[165] have recommended routine intraoperative testing for ET movement when fixation devices are used in proximity to the airway. Uncertainty about tube movement should prompt fiberoptic examination prior to emergence from general anesthesia.[165]

7. Hypertension and Tachycardia

Transient hemodynamic disturbances accompany extubation in most adults. These responses may be prevented by deep extubation[147] or insertion of a laryngeal mask airway (LMA) prior to emergence[15,198] or attenuated by concurrent medication. Most healthy patients not receiving antihypertensives or other cardioactive drugs exhibit increases in heart rate and systolic blood pressure (BP) of more than 20%.[86] Following coronary artery bypass surgery, these changes tend to be transient, lasting 5 to 10 minutes, and are generally not associated with electrocardiographic evidence of myocardial ischemia.[208] Coronary sinus lactate extraction measurements, however, indicate that among patients with poor cardiac function,

extubation can be associated with myocardial ischemia.[264] Patients with inadequately controlled hypertension, carcinoid, pheochromocytoma, hypertension associated with pregnancy, or hyperthyroidism might be expected to display even more marked increases in BP in response to tracheal extubation. The need for specific strategies to attenuate these generally transient changes is dictated by the clinical context. Such strategies, not universally effective, include the use of intracuff,[98,97] intratracheal[245] or intravenous lidocaine,[139,208,239] β-blockers,[86,196,203] and nitrates.

8. Intracranial Hypertension

Endotracheal intubation and suctioning is associated with a rise in intracranial pressure (ICP). It is probable that extubation is associated with comparable or even more marked rises in ICP. There is evidence, albeit contradictory, that intravenous lidocaine[22] and endotracheal lidocaine[42] attenuate this effect.

9. Intraocular Pressure

Madan and colleagues compared the intraocular pressure (IOP) changes of endotracheal intubation and extubation in children with and without glaucoma.[180] They observed significantly greater increases 30 seconds and 2 minutes following *deep* extubation compared with the corresponding times following uncomplicated intubations. These differences were seen in both groups of children. If significant increases in IOP were noted following deep extubation, it is likely that these would have been even higher had extubation occurred following recovery of consciousness. Lamb and coworkers observed similar effects of extubation on IOP in adults, noting that this increase could be prevented by using an LMA rather than an ET.[163]

10. Coughing

Coughing on emergence from general anesthesia is virtually ubiquitous,[151] particularly when an ET is utilized. Surprisingly, Kim and Bishop did not detect a difference between smokers and nonsmokers.[151] In some clinical settings, coughing can be particularly troublesome and may result in serious morbidity. Coughing at extubation may be particularly troublesome in the setting of ophthalmologic, neurologic, tonsil, thyroid, and vascular surgery.

A variety of strategies have been proposed to minimize coughing, including deep endotracheal extubation, the primary use of or conversion to an LMA,[12,154,198] the intravenous or topical application of a local anesthetic to the vocal folds,[239] and the use of intracuff lidocaine.[97,98]

Apart from the aforementioned settings, coughing upon emergence is both common and relatively benign for most patients. As this chapter is being prepared, a respiratory illness (severe acute respiratory syndrome [SARS]) has emerged with significant transmission to health care workers, particularly those involved with airway management. Currently, there is no specific treatment for SARS and it is associated with considerable morbidity and mortality. This has resulted in a reevaluation of the risks of coughing, at least in a subset of patients. It is premature to speculate upon the long-term and geographic implications of this illness; however, from the perspective of an anesthesiologist in the North American epicenter for SARS, Toronto, Canada,[38,215] coughing upon emergence potentially disperses infected respiratory droplets on those in the patient's vicinity. Currently, this has necessitated a "new normal" protective strategy including appropriate apparel (goggles and/or visor, N95 particulate respirator, gloves, gown, and an air-powered protective respirator hood when SARS is suspected or diagnosed) for those in the patient's vicinity.

11. Glottic Edema

Several of the complications of endotracheal intubation do not become apparent until after extubation occurs. Laryngeal or tracheal trauma may occur despite a good laryngeal view[189] or during awake fiberoptic intubation.[182] Anatomic or functional laryngeal problems are more likely to develop as a consequence of difficult or prolonged intubation attempts.[221] Possible airway injuries include laryngeal edema, laceration, hematoma, granuloma formation, vocal fold immobility, and dislocation of the arytenoid cartilages.[249]

Glottic edema has been classified as supraglottic, retroarytenoidal, and subglottic.[36] Supraglottic edema results in posterior displacement of the epiglottis reducing the laryngeal inlet and causing inspiratory obstruction. Retroarytenoidal edema restricts movement of the arytenoid cartilages, limiting vocal cord abduction during inspiration. Subglottic edema, a particular problem in neonates and infants, results in swelling of the loose submucosal connective tissue, confined by the nonexpandable cricoid cartilage. In neonates and small children, this is the narrowest part of the upper airway and small reductions in diameter result in a significant increase in airway resistance. In children, laryngeal edema is promoted by a tight-fitting ET, traumatic intubation, duration of intubation greater than 1 hour, coughing on the ET, and intraoperative alterations of head position.[156] These investigators found an incidence of 1% in children younger than 17 years. Laryngeal edema should be suspected when inspiratory stridor develops within 6 hours of extubation. Management of laryngeal edema depends upon its severity. Treatment options include head-up positioning, supplemental humidified oxygen, racemic epinephrine, helium-oxygen administration, reintubation, and tracheostomy.

Clinical studies in children and adults, evaluating the role of prophylactic corticosteroids in the prevention of postextubation stridor, have yielded contradictory findings, although the majority fail to identify a benefit from dexamethasone or methylprednisolone administration.[8,70,114,133] It is possible that the benefits of steroids are restricted to high-risk populations and require the administration of multiple doses.[233] In addition, questions remain about the methodology of some of the studies.[174]

An alternative classification has been proposed for laryngotracheal injury following prolonged intubation.[25] Immediate postextubation airway obstruction results from glottic and subglottic granulation tissue, which may swell upon removal of the ET. Posterior glottic and subglottic stenosis related to contracting scar tissue results in increasing obstruction weeks or months following extubation. Benjamin found that fiberoptic evaluation or laryngoscopy with the tube in situ was of limited value. An ET obscures the view of the posterior glottis and subglottis. These lesions were best identified using rigid telescopes with image magnification during general anesthesia. This permitted the anticipation of problems and the development of a management strategy.[25]

12. Laryngospasm

Laryngospasm is a common cause of postextubation airway obstruction, particularly in children.[205] Even in adults, Rose and colleagues found that it accounted for 23.3% of critical postoperative respiratory events.[222] Olsson and Hallen observed an increased incidence among patients presenting for emergency surgery, those requiring nasogastric tubes, and those undergoing tonsillectomy, cervical dilation, hypospadias correction, oral endoscopy, or excision of skin lesions.[205] A variety of triggers are recognized, including vagal, trigeminal, auditory, phrenic, sciatic, splanchnic nerve stimulation, cervical flexion or extension with an indwelling ET, or vocal cord irritation from blood, vomitus, or oral secretions.[217] Laryngospasm involves bilateral adduction of the true vocal folds, the vestibular folds, and the aryepiglottic folds that outlasts the duration of the stimulus. This is protective to the extent that it prevents aspiration of solids and liquids. It becomes maladaptive when it restricts ventilation and oxygenation. The intrinsic laryngeal muscles are the main mediators of laryngospasm. These include the cricothyroids, lateral cricoarytenoids, and the thyroarytenoid muscles. The cricothyroid muscles are the vocal cord tensors, an action mediated by the superior laryngeal nerve. Management of laryngospasm consists of prevention by either extubating at a sufficiently deep plane of anesthesia[147] or awaiting recovery of consciousness. Potential airway irritants should be removed and painful stimulation should be discontinued. If laryngospasm occurs, oxygen by sustained positive pressure may be helpful, although this may push the aryepiglottic folds more tightly together.[228] Very small doses of a short-acting neuromuscular blocker[55,164] with or without reintubation may be necessary.

13. Macroglossia

Massive tongue swelling may complicate prolonged posterior fossa surgery[82,158,162,237] performed in the sitting, prone, or "park bench" position. It may result from arterial, venous, or mechanical compression; have a neurogenic origin; or possibly result from angioneurotic edema. In the ICU setting, it may be seen as a complication of severe volume overload or tongue trauma, particularly when this is further complicated by a coagulopathic state. If this occurs or progresses after extubation, it can lead to partial or complete airway obstruction making reintubation necessary but difficult or impossible.[158] Lam and Vavilala postulated that in most cases, positioning results in venous compression leading to arterial insufficiency and a subsequent reperfusion injury.[162] Alternatively, local compression may cause venous or lymphatic obstruction with resultant immediate but generally milder tongue swelling. The latter form is less severe but more apparent, and extubation is likely to be postponed.

14. Laryngeal or Tracheal Injury

Laryngeal injuries accounted for 33% of all airway injury claims and 6% of all claims in the ASA closed claims database.[80] These range from transient hoarseness to vocal fold paralysis. Even when direct laryngoscopy results in a satisfactory glottic view[189] or intubation is facilitated by fiberoptic instrumentation,[182] airway injury may occur and go unsuspected until the ET is removed. Although airway injuries may be less likely if intubation is easy, this provides no assurance that such injury has not occurred. Indeed, the ASA closed claims analysis revealed that 58% of *airway* trauma and 80% of the *laryngeal* injuries were associated with "nondifficult" intubations.[51,80] (Judging from the closed claims analysis, DIs were more likely to result in *pharyngeal* and *esophageal* injuries.) Tracheal and laryngeal trauma may, however, produce dislocation of the arytenoid cartilages.[249]

Tolley and others described three cases involving two adults and one child.[249] A prematurely born male had required prolonged ventilation for infantile respiratory distress syndrome. At 6 years of age, he came to medical attention for investigation of a weak voice. A unilateral prolapsed arytenoid was noted and was managed with speech therapy. The adults had had difficult and unsuccessful intubations, whereas the child had not. Removal of the ET in one case and the tracheostomy tube in the other case was followed by stridor requiring immediate reintubation or recannulation. Laryngoscopy revealed a unilateral dislocated arytenoid in one case and contralateral vocal cord palsy in the other case. In both cases, an arytenoidectomy was performed. The authors suggested that this complication could be more common than the literature would have us believe. Persistent postextubation hoarseness, a breathy voice, and an ineffective cough should prompt an assessment by an otolaryngologist.

The diagnosis is confirmed by endoscopic visualization of an immobile vocal cord associated with a rotated arytenoid cartilage.[177] If the diagnosis is made early, before the onset of ankylosis, it may be possible to manipulate the arytenoid back into position.

Vocal fold paralysis results from injury to the vagus or one of its branches (recurrent laryngeal [RLN] or external division of the superior laryngeal nerves [ex-SLN]) and may resemble arytenoid dislocation or ankylosis. Differentiation may require palpation of the cricoarytenoid joints under anesthesia or laryngeal electromyography.[177] When vocal fold paralysis occurs as a surgical complication, it is usually associated with head and neck, thyroid, or thoracic surgery. The left RLN can also be compressed by thoracic tumors, aortic aneurysmal dilation, left atrial enlargement, or during closure of a patent ductus arteriosus. Occasionally, a surgical cause cannot be implicated. Cavo postulated that an overinflated ET cuff may result in injury to the anterior divisions of the RLN.[47]

The ex-SLN supplies the cricothyroid muscle and is a true vocal cord tensor. The RLN supplies all of the intrinsic laryngeal muscles except the cricothyroid. *Unilateral ex-SLN* results in the retention of adduction but the affected vocal fold is shorter with a shift of the epiglottis and the anterior larynx toward the affected side. This results in a breathy voice but produces no obstruction. *Bilateral ex-SLN* injury causes the epiglottis to overhang, making the vocal folds difficult to visualize. If seen, they are bowed. This produces hoarseness with reduction in volume and range but no obstruction. *Unilateral RLN injury* causes the vocal fold to assume a fixed paramedian position with a hoarse voice. There may be a marginal airway with a weak cough. *Bilateral RLN* results in both vocal folds being fixed in the paramedian position with inspiratory stridor, often necessitating a tracheostomy.[179]

Pharyngeal, nasopharyngeal, and esophageal injuries including perforation, lacerations, contusions, and infections may be associated with difficult laryngoscopy or intubation but may also result from the blind passage of a gum elastic bougie, nasogastric[117] or nasotracheal tube,[230] suction catheter, or transesophageal echo[150] or temperature probe. Unfortunately, recognition of pharyngeal perforation may be delayed, resulting in mediastinitis, retropharyngeal abscess, and death.[263] Following a brief intubation, soft tissue injury resulting in airway obstruction is more likely to result from edema or hematoma than infection. Most of the preceding injuries do not significantly complicate extubation per se. Likewise, laryngeal and tracheal stenoses are serious complications but they are rarely evident at the time of extubation.

15. Airway Injury

Burn patients may have both "intrinsic" and "extrinsic" airway injuries. Circumferential neck involvement is an example of an extrinsic injury. Smoke inhalation or thermal injuries are examples of intrinsic injuries. Burn patients are at particular risk for requiring reintubation. They are known to exhibit bronchorrhea and have impairment of mucociliary clearance and local defenses, laryngeal and supraglottic edema, increased carbon dioxide production, and progressive acute respiratory distress syndrome (ARDS). Carbon monoxide may also diminish their level of consciousness and thus their ability to protect their airway. Kemper and associates reported on the management of 13 burn patients younger than 15 years, 7 of whom exhibited postextubation stridor. Treatments with helium and oxygen resulted in lower stridor scores than those of patients treated with an air-oxygen mixture.[149] They found that 11 of 30 extubated burn victims required treatment for stridor after extubation, consisting of racemic epinephrine, helium-oxygen, reintubation ($n = 5$), or tracheostomy ($n = 1$). The absence of a cuff leak was considered to be the best predictor of failure, with a sensitivity of 100% and a positive predictive value of 79%.[149]

A variety of conditions may lead to airway edema severe enough to encroach on the ET, preventing leakage of expired gas around the deflated cuff. If tissue swelling is sufficiently severe, it may result in airway obstruction following extubation. These conditions include generalized edema, angioneurotic edema, anaphylaxis, deep neck infections, pemphigus, and epidermolysis bullosa. The most common situation probably occurs in the ICU after prolonged intubation. Adderley and Mullins described the cuff leak test to evaluate children with croup.[1] This was performed by deflating the ET cuff, occluding the tube, and assessing air movement around the tube. Kemper and coworkers concluded that the cuff leak test was the best predictor of successful extubation in a pediatric burn and trauma unit.[148] Fisher and Raper found the test to be sensitive but not specific for predicting stridor, necessitating reintubation.[103] Others have measured the cuff leak volume as the difference between inspiratory and expiratory tidal volumes during assist-control ventilation, following cuff deflation.[88,193] Both studies found the cuff leak volume to be predictive of postextubation stridor. Efferen and Elsakr found that 8 of 45 patients exhibited stridor, 4 of whom required reintubation.[88] In another study involving 88 adult medical ICU patients (100 intubations), 6 patients exhibited stridor, 3 of whom required reintubation. They observed a significantly lower cuff leak in patients who subsequently developed stridor, concluding that this measurement was the best predictor of the presence or absence of stridor.[193]

Using the same protocol as Miller and Cole, Engoren evaluated 561 consecutive patients following cardiothoracic surgery.[92] The majority of their patients (79%) were extubated within 24 (median 12) hours. Only three patients exhibited stridor, two of whom were managed medically with racemic epinephrine. All three patients had cuff leak volumes much higher than the threshold of 110 mL proposed by Miller and Cole. None of the patients with cuff leak volumes less than 110 developed stridor, leading Engoren to conclude that this test was not reliable in his population.

Using absolute cuff leak volumes and determining the percentage of tidal volume leaked, Sandhu and colleagues[226] observed that adult trauma patients who developed stridor or needed reintubation had been intubated for a significantly greater length of time. This was confirmed in another study involving adult patients in a combined medical-surgical ICU.[72] Cuff leaks of less than 10%[226] or 15.5% of tidal volume[72] identified patients at risk for developing stridor or requiring reintubation with a specificity of 72% to 96%. Sandhu and colleagues observed stridor in nearly 12% of their patients, 6 of 13 of whom required reintubation. De Bast and coauthors found that a low leak volume and intubation greater than 48 hours had a positive predictive value of 37%. They also found that patients with a high cuff leak had a very high probability of not developing laryngeal edema.[72]

Jaber and coworkers[141] prospectively studied the extubations of 112 consecutive adult medical-surgical ICU patients. The extubation failure rate was 10% and the incidence of postextubation stridor was 12%. They identified a threshold cuff leak volume of 130 mL and 12% of the inspiratory tidal volume with an associated specificity of 85% and 95%, respectively.

All of these studies have identified a group of patients with a small cuff leak who can be successfully extubated, although there may be a greater probably of requiring reintubation. The optimal strategy to manage this relatively common problem has not been determined. Persistence with endotracheal intubation may worsen laryngotracheal injury, subject the patient to greater discomfort, and have considerable economic or resource implications. Tracheostomy, on the other hand, may be unnecessary in a significant proportion of patients. Reintubation in the ICU is associated with significant morbidity and mortality,[75,194] particularly if it cannot be achieved easily. The following approach seems reasonable regarding patients in an intensive care setting: if the previous intubation is known to have been easy, no new factors have intervened to complicate laryngoscopy, and experienced personnel are and will remain immediately available, it may be sound to extubate a patient in the absence of a large cuff volume leak. If there is any doubt about the ease of reintubation, either a tube exchanger may be employed (see later) or a tracheostomy should be performed. Patients with little or no cuff leak prior to extubation should be monitored very closely.

In view of the discrepant findings of Engoren[92] versus Sandhu[226] and De Bast,[72] it would be helpful to know the significance of the absence of a cuff leak in the immediate postoperative period. Venna and Rowbottom[256] described 180 patients who had undergone upper cervical spinal surgery, deemed by the surgeon to be at high risk for postoperative swelling. They elected not to extubate patients if they failed (unspecified) extubation criteria, which included demonstration of a cuff leak and the absence of significant upper airway edema on laryngoscopy. This strategy resulted in an average extubation time of 33.5 hours, with 12 patients (6.6%) developing postextubation stridor and breathing problems, 5 of whom required reintubation. Interestingly, the average time from extubation to required reintubation was 14.6 hours and the resultant duration was 6 days. Two deaths occurred as a result of an inability to reintubate. This suggests that such patients warrant careful postoperative monitoring if they fulfill criteria for extubation. Furthermore, reliance on these criteria alone may fail to identify patients who require but cannot be successfully reintubated.

16. Postobstructive Pulmonary Edema

Severe airway obstruction from any cause may complicate extubation and lead to postobstructive or negative-pressure pulmonary edema.[207] This occurs when a forceful inspiratory effort is made against a closed glottis, generating large negative intrapleural pressures promoting venous return. It may also result in a rightward shift of the interatrial and interventricular septa, raising left atrial and ventricular pressures. In turn, this can promote transudation of fluids into the pulmonary interstitial and alveolar spaces. In some instances, there may also be a permeability defect with exudative fluid and inflammatory cells.[79,107,121,135,168]

In adults, this generally occurs in patients with upper airway tumors, severe laryngospasm, or rarely bilateral vocal cord palsy,[78] whereas in children it occurs most commonly as a complication of croup or epiglottitis.[166] The onset may be within minutes of the development of airway obstruction. It generally resolves with relief of obstruction and supportive treatment for pulmonary edema.

B. INTERMEDIATE- AND HIGH-RISK EXTUBATIONS

Although the preceding complications may follow a routine extubation, the need to reintubate is more likely to occur with intermediate-risk extubations. In contrast to the high-risk extubations, they are more easily dealt with. Bag-mask ventilation or reintubation, if required, should not pose a particular challenge. The intermediate-risk patient, for example, may have a preexisting medical condition[172] such as Wegener's granulomatosis or sarcoidosis that results in airway obstruction. They may undergo surgical procedures that are associated with an increased risk of postoperative airway obstruction. Chronic pulmonary or cardiac disease may compromise spontaneous ventilation and necessitate intubation. The patient with an ineffective cough or increased secretions may have a need for pulmonary toilet. An obtunded patient may be unable to protect his or her airway. A more complete list of intermediate- and high-risk extubations is provided in Table 47-2.

As previously mentioned, the high-risk designation applies to settings in which replacement of a removed ET

Table 47-2 Intermediate- and High-Risk Extubations

Inability to Tolerate Extubation
Hypoxemia
Low F_{IO_2}
Ventilation-perfusion abnormality
Right-to-left shunt
Increased oxygen consumption
Decreased oxygen delivery
Impaired pulmonary diffusion
Hypoventilation
Central sleep apnea
Severe chronic obstructive pulmonary disease
Residual volatile anesthesia
Residual neuromuscular blockade
Preexisting neuromuscular disorders
Diaphragmatic splinting
Relative hypoventilation
Excess CO_2 production
Increased dead space
Failure of pulmonary toilet
Obtundation
Pulmonary secretions
Bronchorrhea
Tenacious secretions
Impaired mucociliary clearance
Loss of airway patency (see Table 47-3)
Obstructive sleep apnea
Tongue
Tumor
Swelling (macroglossia)
Hematoma
Paradoxical vocal cord motion
Laryngeal edema
Bilateral RLN paralysis
Intrinsic airway swelling
Extrinsic airway compression
Tracheomalacia or bronchomalacia
Difficulty Reestablishing Airway
Known difficult airway
Multiple attempts required
Need for alternative airway adjunct (e.g., FOB)
Limited access
Cervical immobility (or instability)
Intermaxillary fixation
"Guardian suture"
Limited resources
Personnel or expertise
Equipment
Airway injury
Thermal or inhalation injury

FOB, fiberoptic bronchoscope; RLN, recurrent laryngeal nerve.

may be reasonably expected to be difficult, complicated, or unsuccessful. *Reintubation is potentially and fundamentally different from the original intubation* because it is likely to occur in an urgent or emergent setting, with limited information and equipment. The patient is more likely to be hypoxic, acidemic, agitated, or hemodynamically unstable, and the procedure may be done in haste. A preemptive strategy is appropriate in the management of such patients.

1. Clinical Settings (Table 47-3)

a. Paradoxical Vocal Cord Motion

Perhaps the most interesting and quintessential example of intermediate-risk extubation is paradoxical vocal cord motion (PVCM). The probable need for reintubation is very high, although it is not necessarily difficult to accomplish. This is an uncommon (or rarely diagnosed[191]) and poorly understood condition, frequently mistaken for refractory asthma[126] or recurrent laryngospasm.[115,190] Endoscopy reveals the cause of upper airway obstruction to be vocal fold adduction on inspiration.[10,54,242,251]

Table 47-3 **Clinical Settings for Intermediate- and High-Risk Extubations**

Paradoxical vocal cord motion
Airway instrumentation (diagnostic laryngoscopy or rigid bronchoscopy)
Thyroid surgery Hematoma or swelling Nerve injury (RLN or ex-SLN) Tracheomalacia
Maxillofacial surgery
Deep neck infections
Cervical spine surgery
Carotid endarterectomy
Posterior fossa surgery
Tracheal resection
Preexisting airway obstruction Parkinson's syndrome Rheumatoid arthritis Epidermolysis bullosa Pemphigus
Tracheomalacia or bronchomalacia

Ex-SLN, external branch of the superior laryngeal nerve; RLN, recurrent laryngeal nerve.

Hammer and colleagues[122] described a 32-year-old woman with recurrent episodes of stridor, sometimes associated with cyanosis, despite normal flow-volume loops and pulmonary function tests. The diagnosis of PVCM was made endoscopically and managed with "relaxation techniques." Following preoperative sedation, topical lidocaine, and bilateral SLN blocks, she underwent an awake fiberoptic intubation. At the conclusion of her surgery, extubation was performed when she was fully awake; however, sustained inspiratory stridor ensued, resulting in reintubation. A subsequent attempt the following day confirmed inspiratory vocal fold adduction and a tracheostomy was required for 58 more days. Michelsen and Vanderspek[191] described recurrent postextubation stridor complicating a cesarean section. General anesthesia was reestablished and laryngoscopic examination showed appropriate vocal fold motion until consciousness resumed.

PVCM, in and of itself, imposes no special requirements for intubation. The abnormality is functional rather than anatomic. Most authors have advised that speech therapy, psychotherapy, hypnosis, and calm reassurance are helpful, but such is not always the case.[126] Some reports have recommended electromyographically guided botulinum toxin injection into the thyroarytenoid muscle for recalcitrant cases. The optimal anesthetic management of these patients is not known. Regional anesthesia avoids airway intervention but does not ensure that a condition that may be stress related will not occur. Familiarity with this condition, calm reassurance when there is prior suspicion, and perhaps deep extubation seem prudent. This author has cared for a patient precisely fitting the description of the typical patient—a young, female, health care worker with a prior history of postextubation stridor requiring repeated reintubations.[126] Extubation was performed under deep propofol sedation, an LMA was inserted, and the upper airway was observed endoscopically with spontaneous respiration. The airway was widely patent and normal, functionally and anatomically. As the sedation was reduced and consciousness was regained, the false and true vocal folds increasingly constricted, obstructing the laryngeal inlet and resulting in stridor. Tracheal extubation was accomplished by very gradually reducing the propofol infusion.

b. Laryngoscopic Surgery

Mathew and colleagues[186] looked at 13,593 consecutive PACU admissions between 1986 and 1989. Twenty-six of these patients (0.19%) required reintubation while in the PACU; 7 of the 26 had undergone ear, nose, and throat (ENT) procedures. All these patients required reintubation related to airway obstruction.

Patients undergoing laryngoscopy and panendoscopy (laryngoscopy, fiberoptic bronchoscopy, and esophagoscopy) are at an increased postoperative risk for airway obstruction and are approximately 20 times as likely to require reintubation as those having a wide variety of other surgical procedures.[130] Reviewing the records of 324 diagnostic laryngoscopies and 302 panendoscopies, Hill and coauthors found that patients who had undergone laryngeal biopsy were at the greatest postoperative airway risk. Thirteen of 252 (5%) patients required reintubation, most within 1 hour of extubation. Twelve of 13 had undergone laryngeal biopsy. Most of these patients had chronic obstructive pulmonary disease, and their need for reintubation was attributed largely to this. They did not state whether their patients had received topical anesthesia or vasoconstrictors. They had not received prophylactic steroids, although the value of this adjunct is not well established.[130]

Robinson prospectively studied 183 patients having 204 endoscopic laryngeal procedures.[219] Seven patients had tracheostomies prior to or subsequent to their surgery because of "high-risk" airways. Two of the remaining patients developed postoperative stridor, one of whom required reintubation and the other a delayed tracheostomy. Indirect laryngoscopy, carried out 4 to 6 hours following surgery, revealed mucosal hemorrhage or laryngopharyngeal swelling in 32% of cases. The patients undergoing tracheostomy were not described, and it is possible that the low incidence of reintubation resulted from an aggressive approach to preemptive tracheostomy.[186]

c. Thyroid Surgery

A variety of injuries following thyroidectomies have been described. Lacoste and colleagues retrospectively reviewed the records of 3008 patients who underwent thyroidectomies between 1968 and 1988.[160] The RLN had been identified intraoperatively in 2427 of these patients. Indirect laryngoscopy was performed on the third or fifth postoperative day. Postoperatively, the RLN was found to be damaged in 0.5% of patients with benign goiters and 10.6% of patients with thyroid cancer. *Unilateral recurrent laryngeal nerve palsy* was observed in 1.1% of patients. Three patients had bilateral RLN palsy and required tracheostomy. Six of a total of 16 deaths during the first 30 postoperative days were attributed to respiratory complications. One death occurred following failed intubation related to a deviated, constricted trachea. A second death was due to difficulties performing a tracheostomy. Two deaths resulted from aspiration or pneumonia, possibly related to RLN dysfunction.

These authors reviewed published reports with at least 1000 patients in which postoperative laryngoscopy was performed. The incidence of permanent nerve palsies with benign goiters was 0.5 per 100 operations. This was more common in substernal goiters (4%) and thyroid cancer (9%). In the latter group, it is sometimes necessary to sacrifice the nerve to achieve an adequate resection. It remains to be determined whether methods of intraoperative RLN monitoring will reduce this complication.[128,131] Although bilateral RLN palsy is rare,

thyroidectomy is the leading cause of this injury. The external branch of the superior laryngeal nerve, supplying the cricothyroid muscle that tenses the vocal folds, is believed to be vulnerable during thyroid dissection; however, the frequency of this injury is unknown.[160]

Local *hemorrhage* or *hematoma* occurred postoperatively in 0.1% to 1.1% of the patients in the literature review and in 0.36% of the patients cared for by Lacoste and colleagues.[160] These occurred from 5 minutes to 3 days postoperatively. Reexploration within the first day was required only twice. Airway obstruction may result from significant laryngeal and pharyngeal edema and wound evacuation may be of limited value in the relief of airway obstruction.[34] The prophylactic placement of surgical drains probably reduces the incidence of this complication. Rarely, wound evacuation may result in a significant improvement of the airway obstruction.[43]

d. Carotid Endarterectomy

Neck swelling or hematoma formation after carotid endarterectomy may be relatively common. When defined radiographically, it occurs frequently and to an alarming degree.[46] When defined by a need for postoperative reintubation or exploration, the incidence is 1% to 3%.[232] Kunkel and others described 15 patients who developed *wound hematomas* following carotid endarterectomy.[159] Eight of these were evacuated under local anesthesia. In six of seven cases in which general anesthesia was induced, difficulties arose with airway management, resulting in two deaths and one patient with severe neurologic impairment.

O'Sullivan and coauthors described six patients with airway obstruction after carotid endarterectomy.[204] Five of these patients had been taking antiplatelet drugs preoperatively. They found that stridor was not relieved by wound evacuation. Of particular importance, the administration of muscle relaxants made manual mask ventilation virtually impossible and intubation was complicated by marked glottic or supraglottic edema. Cyanosis and extreme bradydysrhythmias or asystole occurred in four patients. Although the authors endorsed Kunkel's recommendation of the use of local anesthetic infiltration for wound evacuation, they felt that much of the airway compromise was related to edema from venous or lymphatic congestion. They emphasized that the degree of external swelling may lead one to underestimate the internal oropharyngeal edema.

Munro and coworkers described four patients with post–carotid endarterectomy airway obstruction.[195] The early signs (voice changes) were relatively subtle with rapid clinical deterioration when stridor developed. Two patients suffered respiratory arrest and were intubated blindly. These authors argued that the time course favored venous and lymphatic congestion as the mechanism of injury. Carmichael and associates compared pre– and post–carotid endarterectomy computed tomography (CT) scans in 19 patients.[46] These demonstrated significant swelling of the retropharyngeal space and a reduction of the anteroposterior and transverse airway diameter, particularly at the level of the hyoid. Compared with preoperative CT scans, the calculated volume reduction averaged 32% ± 7% for extubated patients. Patients requiring postoperative endotracheal intubation showed a significantly greater volume reduction of 62% ± 9% ($P < .025$). A subsequent study by this group failed to demonstrate any clinical benefit from the prophylactic administration of dexamethasone.[138]

Accelerated carotid atherosclerosis may occur after cervical irradiation. Airway obstruction after carotid surgery occurred in two of five such patients described by Francfort and colleagues.[106] The mechanisms of obstruction included supraglottic and glottic edema in one patient and periglottic trauma in the other patient. Cervical irradiation may further complicate reintubation if the tissues are indurated and noncompliant.

Bilateral vocal cord[254] and bilateral *hypoglossal nerve palsies*[173] have been described after staged bilateral carotid endarterectomies. In the latter case, the first procedure, performed under regional anesthesia, had been complicated by a wound hematoma resulting in numbness over the anterior neck and diminished sensation in the C2 and C3 distribution. The subsequent endarterectomy, done 4 weeks later under deep cervical plexus block with subcutaneous infiltration, caused intraoperative airway obstruction and asystole. The airway was secured, but recurrent attempts at extubation resulted in persistent obstruction related to bilateral hypoglossal nerve palsy.

e. Maxillofacial Surgery and Trauma

Maxillary and mandibular surgery produces conspicuous and often worrisome swelling. Anxiety regarding postoperative care may be heightened by limited airway access, fear that airway intervention may disrupt the surgical repair, and anecdotal reports of near misses or actual fatalities. As many of these patients are young and otherwise healthy, undergoing elective surgery for functional or cosmetic improvement, there may also be anxiety and fear of litigation. It is speculative whether this results in more or less aggressive care.

Although clearly all of these concerns mandate special care (see later), deaths rarely occur. Beed and Devitt reviewed the charts of 461 perioperative deaths reported to the coroner between 1986 and 1995 in Ontario, Canada.[24] They found only one death associated with orthognathic surgery, although they were unable to determine how many such cases had been performed. They were unable to determine the frequency or to identify nonlethal complications. Meisami and others performed postoperative magnetic resonance imaging (MRI) scans approximately 24 hours following maxillary or mandibular surgery, or both, in 40 patients.[188] Despite the significant facial swelling seen in almost all the patients, none exhibited soft tissue swelling from the base of the tongue to the glottis.

Complete airway obstruction following elective orthognathic surgery, although rare, has been reported. Dark and Armstrong described a single case involving a young woman who underwent seemingly uneventful mandibular and maxillary osteotomies with submental liposuction.[69] Immediately following extubation, she developed airway obstruction requiring reintubation. Repeated fiberoptic examination and CT imaging showed severe and extensive edema from the tongue to the trachea, maximal at the level of the hyoid. By the fourth postoperative day, a cuff leak was detected and the patient was successfully extubated over a tube exchanger.

Maxillofacial injuries are generally the result of unrestrained occupants of motor vehicles encountering an unyielding dashboard, windshield, or steering wheel. Gunshot wounds or physical altercations also cause maxillofacial injury. Airway obstruction is a primary cause of morbidity and mortality in these patients.[211] These patients may have a fractured larynx or tracheal disruption and not survive to admission to hospital. Those with less life-threatening injuries are likely to present with a full stomach, and many have associated head and neck injuries such as lacerations, loose or avulsed teeth, intraoral fractures, or fractures extending into the paranasal sinuses, the orbit, or through the cribriform plate. As well, there may be instability of the cervical spine or damage to the neural axis. Injuries to the lower face raise the possibility of a laryngeal fracture.

Intermaxillary fixation may be part of the surgical plan, necessitating a nasal intubation or a surgical airway. Timing of tracheal extubation is complex. It must take into consideration such factors as the patient's level of consciousness, the patient's ability to maintain satisfactory gas exchange, and the integrity of protective airway reflexes. In addition, consideration must be paid to the difficulties originally encountered in securing the airway and an evaluation of whether reintubation would be easier or more difficult as a consequence of surgery and resuscitation. The lack of guidance from the literature makes communication between anesthesiologist, surgeon, and intensivist essential. Intermaxillary fixation requires that wire cutters be immediately available and that personnel know which wires to cut, should this prove necessary. A fiberoptic bronchoscope, provisions for an emergency surgical airway, and the required expertise should be immediately available at the time of extubation. Many would advocate that fiberoptic airway evaluation be performed prior to extubation, although assessment may be limited to supraglottic structures and exclusion of tube entrapment. Ideally, extubation should be accomplished in a "reversible" manner, permitting oxygenation, ventilation, and reintubation should this prove necessary (see "Extubation Strategies" in Section IV of this Chapter).

f. Deep Neck Infections

Infections involving the submandibular, sublingual, submental, and retropharyngeal fascial spaces present a significant airway management challenge, whether intubation is achieved for surgical drainage or for protection during medical management. The literature is unclear about the indications for preoperative or postdrainage tracheostomy, although clearly a surgical airway is required if efforts to intubate are unsuccessful or constitute a serious risk of rupturing the abscess. Potter and colleagues retrospectively compared the outcomes of 34 patients in whom a tracheostomy was performed and 51 patients who remained intubated following surgical drainage.[214] All patients had undergone surgical drainage for impending airway compromise and required airway support postoperatively. It was not always evident to the investigators why a particular strategy was chosen. Airway loss occurred more commonly in the intubated patients, but this was not statistically significant. Two deaths occurred, one resulting from an unplanned extubation and the other from postextubation laryngeal edema and inability to reestablish the airway. Interestingly, the latter patient was noted to have a cuff leak prior to extubation and developed signs of obstruction 30 minutes after the ET was removed. If a decision is made to manage the patient without a tracheostomy, great care must be taken to ensure proper timing of extubation and the immediate provision of equipment and expertise to attend to potential complications. It is improbable that drainage will result in immediate airway improvement, and reintubation or an emergent surgical airway, if required, may be complicated by edema, tissue distortion, and urgency.

g. Cervical Surgery

Lehmann and coauthors described a patient with advanced rheumatoid arthritis (RA) who underwent a posterior occipitocervical fusion.[170] Complete airway obstruction occurred immediately following extubation, and neither bag-mask ventilation nor attempts at reintubation were successful. Following a successful surgical airway, fiberoptic examination revealed massive hypopharyngeal edema. The patient succumbed to hypoxic encephalopathy.

Emery and associates studied the records of 133 patients who underwent cervical corpectomies.[91] Seven (5.3%) required postoperative reintubation. Three had had DIs because of limited access or cervical immobility. The patients had undergone an anterior approach to achieve a three-level vertebral body and disc resection with bone grafting. This surgical approach requires tracheal and esophageal retraction to permit exposure. Drains were placed and all patients were immobilized by halo vest or a rigid head-cervical-thoracic orthosis. Three of the patients were extubated in the OR and four were extubated at 12 to 91 hours postoperatively. Reintubation was immediately necessary in one case, within 30 minutes in two cases, and within 2 to 23 hours in four cases. Reintubation was required because of severe hypopharyngeal and supraglottic edema in four patients, but the indication was not specified in the other three. Five of the reintubations had no serious sequelae; these patients

were extubated within 2 to 8 days. One patient required a cricothyrotomy, but delay resulted in hypoxic encephalopathy and death. The other patient was reintubated but developed and succumbed to severe adult respiratory distress syndrome. The risk factors identified by Emery and colleagues included a smoking history, moderate or severe preoperative myelopathy, extensive multilevel decompression with prolonged surgery, and tissue retraction.[91] The authors recommend 1 to 3 days of elective intubation postoperatively, determination of the presence of a cuff leak, and direct laryngoscopy at extubation.

Sagi and coworkers conducted a retrospective chart review of 311 anterior cervical procedures.[224] In this series, 6.1% of patients had airway complications, but only six (1.9%) required reintubation. Most of these complications were attributed to pharyngeal edema. Risk factors included increased intraoperative bleeding, prolonged surgery (more than 5 hours), and exposure of more than three vertebral bodies, particularly when these included C2, C3, or C4. Reviewing the literature, these workers identified an airway complication rate of 2.4% (from 1615 cases), with 35 patients requiring reintubation or tracheostomy. On average, those requiring reintubation did so at 24 hours.

Venna and Rowbottom reviewed the records of 180 patients who had undergone a variety of cervical surgical procedures.[256] On the basis of the Emery study, they had made the decision to keep high-risk patients intubated until they met specified criteria including a demonstrable cuff leak and absence of significant airway edema on laryngoscopy. The average time to extubation was 33.5 hours. Despite the delay and the aforementioned criteria, 12 patients (6.6%) demonstrated postextubation stridor and breathing difficulties and 5 (2.7%) required reintubation. Two patients required tracheostomy, and two deaths occurred related to airway obstruction and unsuccessful reintubation.

Epstein and coworkers developed a collaborative protocol involving the neurosurgeon and anesthesiologist, with the specific intention of avoiding reintubations.[93] Although their study involved only 58 patients, these were high-risk, lengthy procedures involving several cervical levels and significant blood loss. All patients remained electively intubated overnight and underwent fiberoptic airway examination prior to considering extubation. The majority of patients were extubated the day following surgery; however, three remained intubated until day 7. Only one patient required reintubation. This reintubation rate was essentially the same as that observed by Emery and colleagues, but it appears that Epstein's cohort underwent higher risk surgery.

Wattenmaker and others studied patients with RA (see later) undergoing posterior cervical spine procedures.[262] Their primary objective was to compare direct laryngoscopic and flexible fiberoptic intubation with respect to perioperative airway complications. This study retrospectively reviewed 128 consecutive posterior cervical procedures in patients with RA, comparing the methods of securing the airway. Overall, upper airway obstruction, characterized by stridor, occurred in 9 of 128 patients, 1 of 70 patients intubated fiberoptically, and 8 of 58 patients intubated "nonfiberoptically" (direct laryngoscopy or blind nasotracheal technique). Five patients (all in the nonfiberoptic group) required emergency reintubation, which proved very difficult, with two near fatalities and one death. Although the two groups were similar with regard to age, gender, American Rheumatology Association classification, ASA physical status, the duration of surgery and anesthesia, fluid balance, and postoperative immobilization, there were significant differences in time to extubation. Seven of the patients could not be intubated fiberoptically and were therefore intubated by a nonfiberoptic technique. The patients were not randomly assigned to different methods, criteria for the method of intubation and techniques were not described, all patients were intubated awake, and the study was carried out over an 11-year period.[60] Although it is not possible to draw firm conclusions from this study, there was a high incidence (7%) of postextubation stridor and difficult or failed reintubations, regardless of the intubation technique.

h. Posterior Fossa Surgery

Posterior fossa surgery can cause injury to cranial nerves, bilateral vocal cord paralysis, brain stem[237] or respiratory control center injury,[11] and macroglossia. Howard and colleagues described a patient with a recurrent choroid plexus papilloma involving the fourth ventricle.[136] Preoperatively, the patient displayed bulbar dysfunction. His extubation on the first postoperative day was complicated by complete airway obstruction, hypoxia, and a seizure. Following neuromuscular blockade, laryngoscopy revealed mildly edematous, abducted vocal cords. Following reintubation and elective tracheostomy, fiberoptic examination showed the vocal folds in a neutral position. For the following month, the tracheostomy was retained because of periodic breathing. This patient demonstrated central apnea and bulbar dysfunction with hypoglossal paralysis and unopposed vocal fold adduction. Artru and others described a patient with a cerebellar mass, severe papilledema, and bulbar signs.[11] Postoperatively, despite recovery of consciousness and strength, the patient remained apneic and ventilatory support was required for 7 days. The authors cautioned that the dorsal pons and medulla are the sites of the cardiovascular and respiratory centers that control hemodynamics and ventilation. They are also host to several of the cranial nerve nuclei. Damage to these areas can result from edema, disruption, ischemia, or compression and may result in a loss of respiratory drive or airway obstruction.

Dohi and coworkers described a patient who developed bulbar signs including bilateral vocal cord paralysis following excision of a recurrent cerebellopontine angle tumor.[78] Negative-pressure pulmonary edema developed as a consequence of a bilateral, presumably central RLN injury and a tracheostomy was required until recovery, 3 months later. During the initial intubation, the glottis could not be seen by direct laryngoscopy and blind intubation was performed. There were three unsuccessful extubations requiring reintubation, the details of which were not described. However, 5 minutes *following* the first reintubation, the arterial partial pressure of oxygen (PaO_2) was 36 and the $PaCO_2$ was 64. Such "trials of extubation" are life threatening and unjustifiable.

i. Stereotactic Surgery/Cervical Immobilization

Stereotactic neurosurgery is finding increasing applications. The head frames may prevent proper positioning for laryngoscopy and physically interfere with the insertion of the laryngoscope. Patients in cervical immobilization devices for spinal cord protection may also be undergoing high-risk surgical procedures. Careful planning for their extubation is critical because reintubation may be difficult and surgical access may be virtually impossible. Full recovery of strength and consciousness, persistence of respiratory drive, the presence of a cuff leak, and the absence of significant tongue swelling are the prerequisites for extubation. Several of the strategies described subsequently (LMA with or without fiberoptic laryngeal examination or extubation over a tube exchanger) should be given serious consideration.

j. Tracheal Resections

Patients with moderate or severe tracheal stenosis may come for surgical tracheal resection. These patients generally have tracheal stenosis, frequently secondary to prolonged intubation. Some may have compromised preoperative respiratory function. Following an end-to-end anastomosis, the surgeon may elect to place a "guardian suture" from the chin to the chest, maintaining the head and neck in flexion and thereby minimizing traction on the suture lines[209,212] (Fig. 47-1). The preference is for early extubation to avoid positive pressure and the presence of a foreign body in the airway. A cough-free extubation is highly desirable, as is avoidance of a need for reintubation, which, if required, could prove very challenging. Strategies are discussed in the following sections.

k. Airway Obstruction—Preexisting Medical Conditions

Parkinson's syndrome. Susceptibility to aspiration is common among patients with Parkinson's disease (PD) and is the most common cause of death. Dysphonia, most frequently hypophonia, is also common and occurs in approximately 90% of patients with PD. Several neurodegenerative diseases have some features in common with PD, which include dysphonia, and these patients may exhibit bilateral abductor vocal fold paresis. Typically, their symptoms progress insidiously, are not

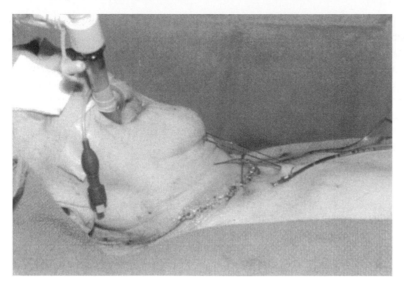

Figure 47-1 This patient has undergone a cricotracheal resection. Cervical extension is restricted by a chin-to-chest guardian suture. The patient has been extubated and a laryngeal mask airway has been introduced, prior to reversal of neuromuscular blockade or awakening. This reduces coughing on emergence, allowing the gradual recovery and assessment of spontaneous respiratory while minimizing cough and the potential distraction of the surgical anastomosis.

recognized by the patient, and may be associated with nocturnal stridor. These features resemble obstructive sleep apnea by polysomnography. Interestingly, many such patients may benefit from nocturnal CPAP or bilevel positive airway pressure.[37] Blumin and Berke described seven patients, only one of whom presented for surgery. This patient underwent a transurethral prostate resection under general anesthesia and 2 weeks after surgery returned with biphasic stridor necessitating an emergent tracheostomy. It is unclear that there was any relationship between the surgery or anesthesia and subsequent airway obstruction.

Vincken and coworkers studied 27 patients with extrapyramidal disorders.[258] Twenty-four had flow-volume loops, many of which demonstrated saw-toothed oscillations. Fiberoptically, they observed oscillations with rhythmic (4 to 8 Hz) or irregular movements of the glottis and supraglottic structures. Ten patients exhibited intermittent upper airway obstruction. Four patients had stridor or dyspnea. The authors believed that the upper airway was the primary site of involvement. In a subsequent report, they observed symptomatic improvement with levodopa, despite persistence of the oscillatory pattern on flow-volume loops.[257]

Easdown and colleagues described a patient with PD who had a respiratory arrest 60 hours following surgery.[87] Prior to that event, the patient had episodic desaturation, labored breathing, and progressive hypercapnia in the absence of tremor or rigidity. His condition improved following intubation. This patient's antiparkinsonian medications had not been resumed postoperatively, and the authors speculated that upper airway obstruction secondary to withdrawal from levodopa/carbidopa was either causative of or contributory to this event. Fitzpatrick described a patient who developed airway obstruction and acute respiratory acidosis requiring intubation *preoperatively* because of withholding his antiparkinsonian medications while he was being fasted.[105] The authors

emphasized the importance of continuing with these medications throughout the perioperative period.

Liu and others described airway obstruction during induction of anesthesia.[175] Despite being unable to visualize the larynx, they attributed this to laryngospasm. Nonetheless, the obstruction resolved with awake, blind nasal intubation but recurred 24 hours later upon extubation. At that point, fiberoptic examination showed inspiratory vocal fold adduction, necessitating reintubation. It is unclear whether they were observing manifestations of PD or PVCM; however, extubation was uneventful 24 hours later after increasing the dosage of levodopa/carbidopa.

Backus and coauthors described a patient who became aphonic, developed stridor, and suffered a respiratory arrest shortly after taking cough medication.[19] After being weaned from mechanical ventilation, she was extubated and upper airway obstruction recurred with vocal fold apposition. Four days later, the patient extubated herself with no further complications. The authors interpreted this "spontaneous" laryngospasm as a manifestation of PD. Others have noted upper airway dysfunction, airflow limitation, and bilateral abductor vocal cord paralysis in association with PD. The first episode may not have been spontaneous but rather a consequence of aspiration of the cough medicine. Nonetheless, there remains a possibility that such patients are more susceptible to laryngospasm, whether spontaneous or induced by glottic stimulation.

Rheumatoid arthritis. Autopsy studies suggest that 30% to 50% of patients with RA have significant cervical spine involvement. *Cervical subluxation* has been reported to occur clinically in 43% to 86% of such patients[119] and may represent a serious neurologic risk during intubation.[117,201] In addition, these patients may have a restricted range of cervical motion, narrowed glottic aperture, limited mouth opening because of involvement of their temporomandibular joints (TMJs), micrognathism, laryngeal deviation, and cricoarytenoid and cricothyroid involvement.[262,155] Kohjitani and colleagues retrospectively described four patients undergoing bilateral TMJ replacement, three of whom had glottic erythema and swelling at endoscopy, three had obstructive sleep apnea, and three experienced laryngospasm at intubation and following extubation.[155] *TMJ involvement* may result in loss of ramal height and micrognathia with or without ankylosis and associated obstructive sleep apnea.

Cricoarytenoid arthritis. Its consequences have long been recognized in the anesthesia and general medical literature.[48,109,146,176,235] Although RA is the most common cause of this condition, it may also be seen in association with bacterial infections, mumps, diphtheria, syphilis, tuberculosis, Reiter's syndrome, ankylosing spondylitis, systemic lupus erythematosus, gout, progressive systemic sclerosis, and others.[171] Cricoarytenoid involvement is often unsuspected until airway obstruction occurs during induction or following extubation. Indeed, Bamshad and coauthors described airway obstruction from neck manipulation alone, severe enough to necessitate tracheostomy.[20] They described another patient in whom attempts at intubation were unsuccessful, resulting in the surgery being aborted. Four hours later, the patient "suddenly" experienced a respiratory arrest requiring a cricothyroidotomy.

Keenan and coworkers described tracheal deviation, laryngeal rotation, and anterior angulation as well as vocal fold adduction seen fiberoptically and on CT scans.[146] This "tracheal scoliosis" was presumed to be due to loss of vertical height and asymmetric bone erosions.

Dysphonia, dyspnea, or stridor may be misinterpreted or obscured by other features of the disease. Kolman and Morris described a patient who developed severe recurrent airway obstruction following extubation, despite an easy atraumatic intubation performed by direct laryngoscopy.[157] At laryngoscopy, the vocal folds appeared white, thickened, and poorly mobile despite complete reversal of neuromuscular blockade. An urgent ENT consultation confirmed the diagnosis of paramedian vocal cord fixation secondary to cricoarytenoid arthritis. The glottic inlet was severely narrowed, necessitating a tracheostomy under local anesthesia. Decannulation was achieved after 1 month. Complete airway obstruction is a well-described but fortunately an infrequent complication, despite involvement of the cricoarytenoids in 26% to 86% of patients with RA.[155,157] This disarticular joint can be affected like any other joint with inflammation, pannus formation, cartilaginous or ligamentous erosion, joint space obliteration, ankylosis, and fibrosis. Chronic cricoarytenoid arthritis may be mistaken for asthma or chronic bronchitis, with symptoms of dyspnea, hoarseness, or stridor. At laryngoscopy, the mucosa may be rough and thick and the vocal chink is narrowed. Although airway obstruction occurs most commonly in patients with long-standing RA having polyarticular and systemic involvement, laryngeal stridor has been described as the sole manifestation of this disease.[118]

The combination of a potentially unstable cervical spine, difficult direct laryngoscopy, and the risk of postextubation airway obstruction makes the patient with RA the prototype of the high-risk extubation. Several authors have recommended postponing extubation until the patient is wide awake. Unfortunately, this provides increased protection against nothing other than laryngospasm and aspiration. In addition, the prevailing wisdom is that patients with limited mouth opening and a potentially unstable cervical spine should be intubated with a flexible fiberscope.[262] This method involves the blind passage of the ET through the cords, which may be traumatic,[60,182] particularly in the presence of preexisting cricoarytenoid arthritis. Regional anesthesia should be considered as an alternative to general anesthesia when appropriate. When intubation cannot be avoided, proposed extubation strategies include a preemptive tracheostomy or a method that increases the "reversibility" of extubation. Neither strategy has been prospectively evaluated in this population. These are discussed in detail under "Extubation Strategies."

Epidermolysis bullosa. This rare condition, with more than 25 described variations, results in separation of layers of skin and mucous membranes with fluid accumulation caused by a deficiency in intercellular bridges.[266] Shearing forces are particularly damaging and may result in separation, bullous formation, hemorrhage and healing by scar formation, and subsequent tissue contraction. Laryngeal involvement is extremely rare, and tracheal bullae have never been reported.[41] A retrospective report involving 33 patients undergoing 329 surgical procedures identified no postoperative airway problems, although microstomia was noted in 13 of the patients.[142] Giant oropharyngeal bullae and profuse bleeding from a ruptured oral bulla and a large fibrosing supraglottic bulla have, however, been reported to cause airway obstruction.[102]

Pemphigus. Pemphigus embraces a group of rare immunologically mediated vesiculobullous diseases (vulgaris, foliaceus, pemphigoid, and others), which frequently involve mucous membranes. Ninety percent of patients with vulgaris have oromucosal involvement at some point.[266] Most lesions heal without scarring unless they become secondarily infected. Microstomia is not a feature. Management of such patients is similar to that of patients with epidermolysis bullosa. Severe upper airway obstruction secondary to cicatricial laryngeal pemphigoid has been reported,[81,90,267] although this complication appears to be uncommon.[181]

Tracheomalacia. Tracheomalacia is a dynamic airway obstruction resulting from loss of the cartilaginous tracheal support. Clinically, it should be considered when unexpected inspiratory obstruction is identified. The diagnosis may be confirmed fiberoptically during spontaneous breathing. The negative intrathoracic pressure of inspiration results in partial collapse of the affected segment. Diagnosis may also be confirmed by CT[9] or MRI scans.[100] This may be congenital[185] or result from vascular compression,[252] be caused by an intrathoracic goiter (see later), or develop as a consequence of prolonged intubation. The latter is presumably related to cuff-induced erosion of the tracheal cartilage with or without extension to the membranous trachea. The severity of the dynamic obstruction is proportional to the inspiratory force. Thus, a distressed patient is more likely to exhibit severe symptoms. Positive pressure or bypassing the lesion with an ET provides relief while further management options are considered. These might include medical management, surgical resection, or placement of a stent.[265] Additional suggestions for the extubation of a patient with suspected tracheomalacia are proposed later.

Relapsing polychondritis. Relapsing polychondritis is a rare, multisystem disease characterized by episodic inflammation of cartilaginous structures resulting in tissue destruction.[134] Laryngeal and tracheal tract involvement occurs in approximately half of the patients. This usually occurs early in the course of the disease and may be manifested by complaints of hoarseness, nonproductive cough, shortness of breath, and stridor. Upper airway obstruction is usually diffuse and may progress to involvement of the glottis, subglottic area, trachea, and bronchial cartilages. Histologically, there is evidence of perichondral inflammation and replacement of cartilage by fibrous tissue, manifesting in inflammatory swelling and progressive destruction of cartilage. The clinical manifestations range from bronchorrhea and recurrent pneumonia to airway collapse. Medical management consists of steroids, nonsteroidal anti-inflammatory drugs, and immunosuppressants, but these are of variable benefit. Surgical management consists of external airway splinting or self-expanding metallic stents. These patients may present for fiberoptic bronchoscopy, tracheostomy, tracheal or nasal reconstruction, aortic valve replacement, or stent placement.[35,44,104,127,252] Airway collapse following extubation should be anticipated and may be effectively dealt with by CPAP.[2,253]

Obstructive sleep apnea syndrome. Obstructive sleep apnea (OSA) correlates positively with age and obesity, both of which are becoming increasingly prevalent. It has been estimated that 80% to 95% of patients with OSA are undiagnosed.[28] OSA syndrome also appears to be associated with difficulty in mask ventilation,[167] laryngoscopic intubation,[53,96,218] and accelerated arterial oxygen desaturation.[29] The risk of airway obstruction following surgery has been noted to be increased for patients with OSA,[216] with an incidence of life-threatening postextubation obstruction of 7 of 135 (5%) patients.[96] Rapid desaturation,

difficult mask ventilation, and difficult direct laryngoscopy[144] make this a particularly high-risk setting. It is essential that such a patient be fully awake, recovered from neuromuscular blockade, and have a sustained spontaneous respiratory rate; that nasal CPAP be available or routinely implemented[143,216,218]; and that consideration be given to extubation over a tube exchanger.[28] (These strategies have been associated with better outcomes, and anecdotal comparisons are very compelling but they have not been subjected to controlled, randomized trials.)

A variety of surgical procedures have been employed to treat OSA including uvulopalatopharyngoplasty (UPPP), midline glossectomy, mandibular advancement, limited mandibular osteotomies with genioglossal advancement, and hyoid bone suspension.[244] Pepin and colleagues published a critical analysis of the literature related to the risks and benefits of surgical treatment of snoring and OSA.[210] They identified "at least five deaths" following UPPP and drew attention to the fact that few studies have adequate numbers to allow conclusions to be drawn regarding their outcome. In addition, fewer than half of the studies commented on the frequency of complications. Haavisto and Suonpaa retrospectively reviewed 101 UPPP procedures and found an early postoperative respiratory complication rate of 10%.[120] Ten of 11 patients required reintubation, with one death resulting from airway obstruction.

UPPP surgery was introduced to deal with retropalatine collapse. However, in approximately half of the adult patients with OSA, obstruction occurs at the retrolingual pharynx. Tongue suspension is one of several approaches introduced to manage the latter group of patients.[57] This involves the placement of an anchoring screw in the geniotubercle and the attachment of a suture through the base of the tongue. Szokol and associates described a morbidly obese patient with OSA in whom such a procedure was performed.[244] Both laryngoscopy and bag-mask ventilation had been difficult. At the conclusion of the procedure, the patient was fully awake, able to sustain a head lift for 5 seconds, demonstrated a negative inspiratory pressure of 40 cm H_2O, and was extubated. Stridor was noted immediately, and bag-mask and LMA ventilation was ineffective. Attempts to reintubate the patient were unsuccessful, necessitating a cricothyrotomy. Subsequent direct laryngoscopy showed a markedly swollen epiglottis and grossly edematous laryngeal and hypopharyngeal tissue. The patient developed negative-pressure pulmonary edema and a tracheostomy was performed 2 days later because of persistent swelling. Tracheal decannulation occurred uneventfully 2 weeks later. The authors speculated that airway manipulation during the surgery was the cause of this patient's swelling. They did not consider that the swelling may have resulted from or at least been worsened by repeated attempts at laryngoscopy.

Laryngeal incompetence. Laryngeal function may be disturbed for at least 4 hours after tracheal extubation.[45]

Immediately following extubation, 8 of 24 (33%) patients aspirated swallowed radiopaque dye; five showed radiologic evidence of massive aspiration. Four hours following extubation, 4 of 20 (20%) patients aspirated, 3 massively. At 24 hours, the rate was reduced to 5%. In this study, patients had been intubated for 8 to 28 hours during and following cardiac surgery. Although the authors did not observe a relationship with duration of intubation (8 to 28 hours), it is unclear whether the presumed laryngeal incompetence occurs with a brief duration of intubation or is more severe or common with more prolonged intubation. The mechanism of laryngeal incompetence was postulated to be primarily sensory because patients who aspirated dye did not cough.

Residual neuromuscular paralysis is a common problem in postoperative patients and may result in hypoventilation, hypoxemia, and pharyngeal and laryngeal dysfunction or increase the risk of pulmonary aspiration.[71,252] Pharyngeal function was impaired in conscious volunteers receiving a continuous infusion of vecuronium and resulted in laryngeal penetration of contrast medium proportional to the degree of blockade.[95] Relaxation of the upper esophageal sphincter was also noted. None of the volunteers coughed or demonstrated respiratory symptoms. Berg and colleagues noted a higher incidence of postoperative pulmonary complications (pulmonary infiltrate or atelectasis, or both, associated with cough, sputum, or shortness of breath) among patients randomly assigned to receive a long-acting versus intermediate-acting neuromuscular blocker.[32] It is intriguing to speculate on how residual neuromuscular blockade may contribute to "laryngeal incompetence."

Pulmonary aspiration of gastric contents. Although gastroesophageal reflux (GER) is increasingly diagnosed, the recognition of perioperative pulmonary aspiration has not changed in recent decades.[200,260] Many factors in addition to GER may predispose a patient to aspiration, including emergency surgery, pain, obesity, narcotics, nausea, ileus, pregnancy, some surgical positions, depressed level of consciousness, inadequate depth of anesthesia, postoperative drowsiness, and residual neuromuscular blockade, yet clinically important aspiration is uncommonly identified. Prior to intubation, difficult bag-mask ventilation may result in gastric distention. This may be further complicated if laryngoscopy proves difficult because this may delay securing the airway and repeated laryngoscopic attempts may cause edema, thereby decreasing the glottic opening. Clearly, aspiration can cause serious morbidity and death.[200,206,260] In a multicenter, prospective study looking at major complications associated with anesthesia, aspiration was identified in 27 of 198,103 general anesthetics resulting in 4 deaths and 2 cases of anoxic encephalopathy.[248] Aspiration may also result from obtundation or conditions that impair vocal cord apposition (e.g., vocal cord paralysis, residual neuromuscular blockade, and granulomata).

Although the majority of incidents of aspiration seem to occur at induction, a significant number occur during maintenance and recovery periods.[152] Numerous strategies have been described to reduce the risk at induction, but relatively little information is available on how best to prevent this later on. Postoperative nausea, delayed gastric emptying, residual neuromuscular blockade, relaxation of the esophageal sphincters, decreased level of consciousness, gagging on an ET, and impaired laryngeal competence may all make emergence from anesthesia and tracheal extubation as problematic as induction. At present, it is not possible to offer evidence-based recommendations on an extubation strategy to reduce aspiration. It would seem logical to minimize the preceding contributing factors—postoperative nausea and vomiting, residual neuromuscular blockade, decreased level of consciousness and associated diminished protective airway reflexes, and perhaps gastric evacuation. We do not know whether gastric decompression reduces aspiration, although a well-seated ProSeal LMA (PLMA) may[61,184] or may not[63] offer some protection from aspiration. Nonetheless, with the present body of information, it is not appropriate to recommend specifically the use of this device in a patient recognized to be at increased risk for aspiration.

2. Previous Difficulties Encountered

Multiple attempts at laryngoscopy by experienced personnel, a need for alternative airway management techniques because of failure of direct laryngoscopy, and a history of prior difficulty prompting the primary use of such an alternative technique represent settings in which the need for reintubation may be problematic. Under urgent or emergent circumstances, methods that had previously been successful may not be available or appropriate. The required equipment, necessary skills, or time required to perform alternative techniques may not be available. Uncertainty regarding the probable success of laryngoscopy may appropriately result in reluctance to administer paralytic and sedating drugs that may actually make laryngoscopy easier, yet result in an apneic patient who can be neither ventilated nor intubated. Thus, knowledge of prior difficulties may result in intubation conditions that are less favorable to success. Awake flexible fiberoptic bronchoscopy generally requires a dry field for visualization and adequate topical anesthesia. Blood and secretions in the airway or an agitated, hypoxic patient makes such a technique less likely to be successful.

3. Limited Access

Limited access to the airway is exemplified by (1) intermaxillary fixation; (2) severe cervical restriction, instability, or immobilization; and (3) the chin-to-chest guardian suture to prevent traction tracheal resection. In each case, there may be additional risks related to oxygenation, ventilation, airway obstruction, or pulmonary toilet. For example, following cervical fixation, the patient may also have macroglossia or supraglottic edema. A patient requiring tracheal resection may be unable to clear blood or secretions from the airway.

C. HIGH-RISK EXTUBATIONS

We have previously defined a high-risk extubation as a situation wherein reestablishing a lost airway, be it due to failure of oxygenation, ventilation, pulmonary toilet, or loss of patency, is likely to be difficult or impossible without significant risk. Many of the preceding clinical examples (e.g., OSA, RA, anterior cervical surgery, inter-maxillary fixation) represent a high risk because reintubation may be challenging. In addition, the clinical "playing field" may not be level at all hours of the day. The immediate availability of highly trained primary and support personnel, equipment, and the relevant clinical information may be problematic at night or during periods of intense activity. As previously mentioned, the consultants of the ASA Task Force on Management of the Difficult Airway[5] and the Canadian Airway Focus Group[66] both recommended a preformulated strategy for extubation of the DA. Patients at risk for hypoventilation, hypoxemia, and loss of airway patency have been discussed at length. The remainder of this chapter is related to specific extubation strategies.

IV. EXTUBATION STRATEGIES

To the extent that any of the high-risk extubation conditions exist or are anticipated, it behooves the clinician to consider a strategy that does not cut off access to the airway (Table 47-4). Ideally, such a strategy should permit the continued administration of oxygen or the ability to ventilate a failing patient even while the airway is being reestablished. Such objectives are consistent with the ASA Task Force[5] and Canadian Airway Focus Group[67] recommendations.

The extubation risk stratification is largely based upon intuition, anecdotal reports, and limited clinical series. It is hoped that the proposed classification and strategies will become broader and deeper with time. Because the majority of patients—even those at high risk—are successfully extubated, it is essential that any proposed strategy entail less risk than simply removing the ET and hoping for the best. It should also involve minimal discomfort, at an acceptable cost; and facilitate oxygenation, ventilation, and reintubation.

A. DEEP VERSUS AWAKE EXTUBATION?

Extubations may be performed before or after recovery of consciousness. Deep extubation ordinarily would involve the prior reversal of neuromuscular blockade and

Table 47-4   Extubation Strategies

Deep (versus awake) extubation
Substitution of an LMA
Extubation over FOB
Substitution of and LMA combined with FOB
Use of gum elastic bougie or Mizus obturator
Jet stylet
TTX or JETTX (Sheridan-RCI)
CAEC (Cook Critical Care)
ETVC (CardioMed Supplies)
Double-lumen tube exchanges
Nasal-oral conversions

CAEC, Cook airway exchange catheter; ETVC, endotracheal ventilation catheter; FOB, fiberoptic bronchoscope; JETTX, jet ventilation/tracheal tube exchanger; LMA, laryngeal mask airway; TTX, tracheal tube exchanger.

resumption of spontaneous ventilation. Its purported advantage is the avoidance of the adverse reflexes associated with extubation, such as hypertension, dysrhythmias, coughing, laryngospasm, and increased IOP or ICP. The fundamental disadvantage of deep extubation is the patient's inability to protect the airway against obstruction and aspiration. If it is improperly executed, laryngospasm and its attendant complications are more likely to occur. Although not having to await the recovery of consciousness may accelerate OR turnover, the exhalation of unscavenged volatile anesthetic agents may result in occupational health and safety issues. A significant proportion of American anesthesiologists practice the technique, at least some of the time, yet there are very few data in adults comparing the safety of deep versus awake extubation.[68] Koga and colleagues compared three small groups of adult patients, extubated deep, awake, or extubated deep following the insertion of an LMA.[154] Straining occurred in a high (but comparable) proportion of patients whether the ET was removed prior or subsequent to recovery of consciousness. Deep extubation followed by LMA insertion (isoflurane 2% to 3%) is discussed subsequently. Deep extubation is contraindicated when mask ventilation was found or is likely to have become difficult, the risk of aspiration is increased, endotracheal intubation had been difficult, or airway edema is likely.

B. EXTUBATION WITH LARYNGEAL MASK AIRWAY

Upon emergence from general anesthesia, most patients tolerate an LMA with less coughing and changes in IOC, ICP, and BP (see Fig. 47-1).[40,108,154,163] Silva and Brimacombe substituted an LMA for the ET in a small series of patients while they were still asleep and paralyzed following completion of neurosurgical procedures.[234] Muscle relaxation was then reversed and the anesthetic was discontinued. The LMAs were removed when the patients resumed spontaneous ventilation and obeyed commands. None of the 10 patients coughed, and changes in the rate-pressure product were minimal. The authors concluded that the technique might prove useful in patients undergoing other types of surgical procedures. They stressed that this substitution should be performed only by those skilled in LMA insertion. Patients must be at a sufficient depth of anesthesia or coughing, breath holding, laryngospasm, and the very pressor responses this substitution is intended to avoid may occur. Bailey and others recommended that the LMA be inserted prior to removal of the ET, with the purported advantage of not risking loss of the airway following tracheal extubation.[77,154] Compared with deep tracheal extubation followed by Guedel airway insertion, there was a lower incidence of coughing and requirement for airway manipulation.[77] Koga and coworkers compared this technique with deep and awake tracheal extubation. As previously mentioned, they observed no difference in recovery conditions between patients in whom the ET was removed either deep or awake; however, they noted a significant improvement in recovery conditions when the LMA substitution was performed. This technique might be useful in patients undergoing procedures in which coughing, straining, and intraocular, intracranial, and BP changes could be particularly detrimental. Patients at risk for aspiration are not protected. Furthermore, patients difficult to intubate by laryngoscopy are probably poor candidates for this technique because airway patency cannot be guaranteed after the LMA substitution.

ET exchange using an LMA has also been described. Asai described a patient who had had a difficult endotracheal intubation further complicated by rupture of the ET cuff.[13] He introduced a 7.0-mm ET over a fiberoptic bronchoscope and passed these through an unmodified size 5 LMA Classic, extending the length of the ET with a second ET inserted into the proximal end of the replacement tube. A smaller LMA would have necessitated cutting of the aperture bars or use of a smaller ET. Stix and coworkers modified an intubating LMA (ILMA) by removing the epiglottic elevator bar.[241] They used this to convert from a double-lumen tube (DLT) to a single-lumen ET. In addition, they employed a 14 Fr jet ventilation tube exchanger (type unspecified) through the tracheal lumen of the DLT. Had the intubation through the ILMA proved unsuccessful, this would have provided a means of oxygenating and ventilating that could be used as a stylet for the replacement ET.

Matioc and Arndt proposed another approach.[187] They wished to substitute an ET for a No. 5 PLMA, despite a grade II view as seen through the LMA.[39] Using an Arndt Airway Exchange Catheter Set (Cook Critical Care, Bloomington, IN), they introduced a fiberoptic bronchoscope through the PLMA into the trachea. A 144-cm

guidewire (Amplatz extra stiff) was passed through the fiberoptic bronchoscope and the latter was removed. A No. 11 Fr 70-cm Cook airway exchange catheter (see later) was introduced over the guidewire and the PLMA was removed. The replacement ET was then advanced over the exchange catheter.

A simpler approach using a ventilation/exchange bougie (Aintree Intubation Catheter, Cook Critical Care) has been described. This can be used with a COPA (cuffed oropharyngeal airway, Mallinckrodt)[125] or an LMA Classic.[213] There are several advantages of this technique. It can be used to facilitate conversion from an unmodified LMA to an oral ET of adequate size. It affords sufficient length that the LMA can be removed with minimal risk of losing the airway. The Aintree Intubation Catheter fits tightly to the insertion cord of the fiberoptic bronchoscope and in turn to the ET, thereby reducing the size discrepancy that often results in difficult glottic passage. The catheter can be used as a conduit for manual or jet ventilation during an exchange. An LMA Classic, inserted as a rescue device (cannot intubate, cannot ventilate), can facilitate safe tube exchange without the need for an ILMA.

C. EXTUBATION OR REINTUBATION OVER FIBEROPTIC BRONCHOSCOPE OR LARYNGOSCOPE

In situations with the possibility of tube entrapment, extubation over a fiberoptic bronchoscope (FOB) can detect and potentially avert a disastrous outcome. With a spontaneously breathing patient, extubation over a bronchoscope provides the opportunity of visually assessing the trachea and laryngeal anatomy and function. This can be very helpful in the patient suspected of having tracheomalacia, vocal cord paresis, or PVCM. It also permits the assessment of supraglottic structures.[74] In this author's experience, such opportunities are maximized by reassuring the patient, judicious sedation, an antisialagogue, and the use of an auxiliary Yankauer sucker for oral secretions. The FOB is placed above the carina and the cuff is slowly deflated to minimize coughing. The ET is slowly withdrawn into the oropharynx with subsequent, very gradual withdrawal of the FOB to the supraglottic region. Once the patient is comfortable, the FOB is further withdrawn to a position just above the vocal cords. Even with such a deliberate technique, the exercise is frequently frustrated by excessive secretions, coughing, swallowing, or poor tolerance with insufficient opportunity to visualize the structures of interest.

If the technique is successful, it may enable the anticipation of complications. When significant abnormalities are noted, a decision must be made whether to reinsert the ET or withdraw the FOB immediately and manage the patient with agents such as corticosteroids (see earlier), racemic epinephrine, or helium-oxygen.[148,149] This technique is not a practical way of performing a trial of extubation, in part because such a trial lasts only seconds or minutes.

Hudes and coauthors described two patients who had had DIs and required tube exchange.[137] This was accomplished by the prior removal of the plastic connector on the original tube, mounting the new tube over a bronchoscope, advancement of the FOB, and withdrawal of the original tube. This tube was then filleted with a scalpel blade and peeled off to allow the replacement tube to be advanced. They claimed to have achieved this in 20 and 30 seconds. In this author's opinion, such a technique is awkward and places the patient, the FOB, and the operator's fingers in jeopardy.

Others have used the FOB to change ETs. Rosenbaum and colleagues placed a bronchoscope through the opposite nostril of a patient with an existing but inadequate nasotracheal tube.[223] Watson endorsed the use of an FOB to exchange ETs, citing the advantages of minimal sedation, risk of aspiration, hemodynamic embarrassment, and uncertainty about tube placement.[261] His technique involved passing the "loaded" FOB alongside the existing ET. He had used such a technique successfully in 13 of 15 attempts. Dellinger considered the FOB to offer the least likelihood of reintubation failure, suggesting a "cumbersome" technique that places the preloaded bronchoscope alongside the ET to be replaced and subsequent advancement of the FOB.[74] The existing tube is removed and the new tube is advanced. He suggested that if the bronchoscope could not be advanced, it should be positioned just above the vocal folds and the existing tube withdrawn from the trachea followed by reintubation. Admittedly, this risks loss of the airway.

There can be no more certain means of exchanging an ET than performing this operation with continuous visual control. Andrews and Mabey described the use of a WuScope (Achi Corporation, Fremont, CA and Asahi Optical, Tokyo, Japan) to perform a tube exchange.[6] Their patient had previously had a DI related to morbid obesity and limited head extension. He was also suffering from severe ARDS. A WuScope allowed successful glottic visualization, permitting the insertion of a suction catheter anterior to the existing nasotracheal tube. The latter was withdrawn and the replacement oral ET was easily advanced over the suction catheter with minimal interruption of mechanical ventilation. In this author's opinion, the visual control possible with a WuScope (or presumably a Bullard Scope [Circon, Santa Barbara, CA], Upsher UltraScope [Mercury Medical, Clearwater, FL], or videolaryngoscope) is preferable to the blind passage of an ET over an FOB or tube exchanger. A hollow tube exchanger, however, would have permitted jet ventilation if desaturation or difficulties with tube advancement had occurred. The author has had personal experience performing tube exchanges under direct vision using the Bullard laryngoscope and the GlideScope (Saturn Biomedical, Burnaby, BC).

D. EXTUBATION WITH LARYNGEAL MASK AIRWAY ± BRONCHOSCOPE

Extubation of a DA over an FOB or with an LMA has the limitations referred to previously. The combination of these devices, however, offers significant advantages. Replacement of an ET with an LMA provides an excellent means of performing a fiberoptic assessment of glottic and subglottic anatomy and function. After the substitution is performed and with the patient under anesthesia or a suitable degree of sedation, muscle relaxation can be reversed and spontaneous ventilation be allowed to resume. An FOB is then be passed through an LMA, and dynamic vocal fold movement and appearance can be assessed while concentrations of oxygen and volatile agents (if necessary) can be controlled. The view is also protected from oral secretions and inadequate ventilation can be supplemented. The presence of PVCM or tracheomalacia can be evaluated, although both may be minimal if the patient is deeply anesthetized.

This technique is useful in patients with recurrent postextubation stridor or those at risk for static or dynamic tracheal stenosis. The author frequently employs this technique in patients undergoing thyroidectomies when either tracheomalacia or vocal fold paralysis is suspected.

E. EXTUBATION OVER GUM ELASTIC BOUGIE/METTRO-MIZUS OBTURATOR

Finucane and Kupshik described an awake blind nasal intubation in a patient with cervical instability.[101] After confirming correct placement and neurologic integrity, anesthesia was induced, at which point they discovered that the nasotracheal tube cuff had been damaged. They used the 63-cm-long, 4-mm outer diameter (OD) plastic sleeve from a brachial central venous catheter as a stylet and performed a tube exchange without difficulty. Others have used a gum elastic bougie to achieve similar objectives.[21,76,220,250]

Cook Critical Care has designed the METTRO (Mizus ET replacement obturator) for the replacement of endotracheal and tracheostomy tubes (Fig. 47-2). It is available in two sizes, 70 cm (7.0 Fr) for replacement of ETs as small as 3 mm and 80 cm long (19 Fr) to pass through tubes 7 mm or larger. It is a single-use, flexible, radiopaque, solid device with a tapered tip. It bears distance markings. Early package inserts had instructed the user to advance this until resistance is encountered. Such a recommendation can result in coughing, discomfort, hypertension, and tachycardia. (Tracheal perforation has been reported using different devices but following similar recommendations.[73,231])

The smaller airway obturator has been used to maintain airway access during 22 tracheostomies and for "tentative extubations" in seven patients.[18] The authors preferred the smaller caliber device because there was minimal discomfort of the patient during tube exchanges and it was "unobtrusive" during surgical tracheostomies.

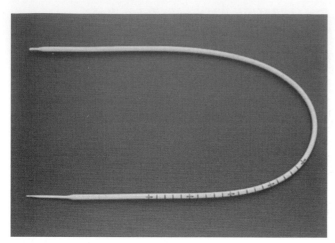

Figure 47-2 The METTRO (Mizus endotracheal tube replacement obturator, Cook Critical Care) is a solid device, tapered at the end. It is available in two diameters (7 and 19 Fr) and two lengths (70 and 80 cm). (Courtesy of Cook Critical Care.)

The obturator was removed when it was apparent that the patient was unlikely to require reintubation. In their experience, the 19 Fr obturator was not conducive to spontaneous breathing. Chipley and colleagues used a METTRO in an obese patient with a fractured occipital condyle recovering from respiratory failure.[52] They left this in place for 48 hours, removing it when extubation appeared to be successful. They also described the use of the obturator to stimulate coughing, although this may have been ill advised given the previously cited complication of tracheal perforation.

F. CONCEPT OF JET STYLET

The ubiquitous nasogastric tube has been used as an exchange catheter,[240] but these devices are specifically formulated to become softer as they are warmed. Such thermolability is not likely to be a desirable attribute for a tube exchanger.

Bedger and Chang coined the term "jet stylet" to refer to a self-fashioned long (65 cm) plastic catheter with a removable 15-mm adapter for connection to an anesthesia machine or jet injector.[23] They created three side ports cut into the distal 5 cm to minimize catheter whip during jet ventilation. They used their stylet for the extubation or reintubation of 59 patients. It also functioned "adequately" in the patients in whom it was used for jet ventilation and oxygen insufflation. Although no complications were encountered in this series, the same authors, in an earlier report, described tension pneumothoraces in 3 of 600 patients ventilated at 15 pounds per square inch through a 3.5-mm (OD) pediatric chest tube.[50] This "stylet" had been used to provide airway access and ventilation during direct laryngoscopy. They speculated that the pneumothoraces might have resulted from endobronchial migration of the catheter. They did not consider the possibility that barotrauma occurred as a result of jet ventilation against apposed vocal cords as their patients were recovering from neuromuscular blockade.

G. COMMERCIAL TUBE EXCHANGERS

There are now a number of commercial products that incorporate many of the features described by Bedger and Chang.[23] These are long, hollow catheters that may include connectors for jet or manual ventilation, or both. Most have distance and radiopaque markers. They also have end or distal side holes, or both. They can be introduced through an existing ET, permitting its withdrawal. Oxygen insufflation or jet ventilation can be provided through the tube exchanger. Respiratory monitoring can also be achieved by connection to a capnograph. Spontaneous breathing may take place around the device. In most reports, these have been tolerated well enough that they can be left in situ until it is probable that reintubation will not be required. Even with the catheter in place, most patients are able to talk or cough. If reintubation or a tube exchange is required, this can be facilitated with gentle laryngoscopy, not necessarily to reveal the glottis but to retract the tongue. Reintubation using a tube exchanger is similar to intubation over an FOB, and the difference of diameters between the tube exchanger and the advancing ET may predict the relative ease of tube advancement. If resistance is encountered, ET rotation may successfully release the tube from the pyriform fossa or arytenoid cartilage.

These devices are consistent with the ASA Task Force[5] and Canadian Airway Focus Group[67] recommendations regarding the extubation of the DA. They increase the probability that a reintubation will succeed; should difficulty be encountered, the device provides a means whereby oxygen by insufflation or ventilation, if necessary, can be accomplished while alternative techniques are explored. This may be thought of as a reversible extubation. With the device in place, other options can be pursued, including an evaluation of the benefits of helium-oxygen or the inhalation of racemic epinephrine. Knowing that the patient is satisfactorily oxygenated (and ventilated), additional information, equipment, or expertise can be recruited. There are differences between these commercial products—and such differences may be important—but they are far less important than the concept of the reversible extubation. In this author's opinion, reintubation of the high-risk patient may have a low likelihood of being required, but it must have a high probability of being successful. The differences between the devices are now detailed.

1. Tracheal Tube Exchanger

The most basic commercial tube exchanger is the Sheridan TTX (Hudson Respiratory Care Incorporated, Temulca, CA) (Fig. 47-3). These are available in four

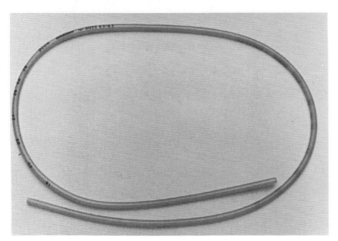

Figure 47-3 The tracheal tube exchanger (Sheridan TTX, Hudson, RCI) is a simple catheter with no proximal or distal modifications. These devices are available in four diameters and two lengths. If the device is to be used for ventilation, it must be adapted by the user. There are no distal side ports, which makes jet injection potentially hazardous. (From Cooper RM: The difficult airway—II. Anesthesiol Clin North Am 13:683-707, 1995.)

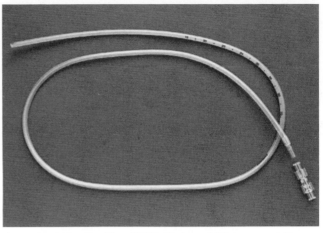

Figure 47-4 The Sheridan JETTX (Hudson, RCI) is essentially a modification of the tracheal tube exchanger (TTX), being 100 cm in length, featuring a proximal adapter for jet ventilation, and having a single distal end hole. As with the TTX, this is likely to result in catheter whip and might increase the risk of jet injection injury. (From Cooper RM: Extubation and changing endotracheal tubes. In Benumof JL [ed]: Airway Management: Principles and Practice, 1st ed. St. Louis, Mosby, 1996, pp 864-885.)

diameters (2.0, 3.3, 4.8, and 5.8 mm OD) and two lengths (56 and 81 cm). The smallest can be inserted into ETs as small as 2.5 mm inner diameter (ID). They are firm (durometry of 85 shore) although thermolabile and therefore subject to softening with heat. They are frosted to minimize drag and have a radiopaque stripe and distance markings. There are no side holes, nor are there connectors.

Benumof has described the combined use of a TTX and FOB in replacing a 7.0-mm nasotracheal tube with a 8.0-mm orotracheal tube in a patient with halo fixation.[26] Benumof has also described modifications of the TTX to enable jet ventilation, although these must be prepared in advance and may be somewhat difficult to disassemble when the original ET is being off-loaded. Consequently, the manufacturer has produced an alternative product referred to as the Sheridan JETTX exchanger (Fig. 47-4). This is a longer device (100 cm) but available in only a single size, suitable for ETs greater than 6.5 mm ID. It incorporates a proximal slip-fit connector that can be Luer-locked to a jet ventilator. As with the TTX, there is only a single distal end hole.

2. Cook Airway Exchange Catheters*

Cook Critical Care has developed a family of hollow stylets, known as airway exchange catheters (CAECs) (Fig. 47-5). These are available in French sizes 8.0, 11, 14, and 19 mm corresponding to 2.7, 3.7, 4.7, and 6.33 mm ODs, respectively. The 8 Fr CAEC is 45 cm in length and

the others are 83 cm long. The smallest can be used with a 3 mm ID ET. These devices are radiopaque and have distance markings between 15 and 30 cm from the distal end. There are two distal side holes and an end hole. Proximally, there are two types of connectors, secured and released by a patented Rapi-Fit adapter. These were designed for easy adapter removal as the ET is being off-loaded and subsequent reattachment for ventilation while the new tube is being introduced. A secure

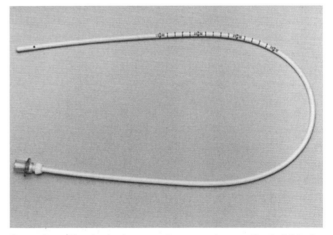

Figure 47-5 The Cook airway exchange catheters (Cook Critical Care) are available in four diameters and two lengths. They are radiopaque and have distance markings at each centimeter throughout the working length. Proximally, there is a Rapi-Fit adapter that can be easily and securely added or removed. They are packaged with both 15-mm and jet ventilation connectors. Distally, there are an end hole and two side holes. (Courtesy of Cook Critical Care.)

---

*The author served as a consultant to Cook in the development of this product.

Luer-Lok fitting is available for jet ventilation and a 15-mm connector for manual ventilation. The length and inner diameters (1.6 to 3.4 mm) make manual ventilation with a resuscitation bag possible but impractical because resistance is so high. The 15-mm Rapi-Fit connector serves primarily as a means of connecting the exchange catheter to an oxygen source. During jet ventilation, the paucity of distal side holes potentially increases catheter whip and the risk of barotrauma.[89] Loudermilk and others used the 11 Fr, 83 cm CAEC in 40 high-risk adult extubations, 3 of which required reintubation. This was easily performed with each attempt. The exchange catheters were also used for oxygen insufflation. All but one patient tolerated the device, and dislodgement occurred in one patient.[178]

Atlas and Mort examined the relationship between the diameter of the two larger CAECs and tolerance as well as the ability to phonate and cough.[17] It is unclear whether their patients were randomly assigned to specific sizes of catheters. Phonation and discomfort were similar in both groups with only 3 of 101 patients experiencing significant discomfort. Cough effort tended to be reduced in the larger sized CAEC, but this did not achieve significance. Atlas also looked at a larger tube exchanger (JEM 400 ET Changer, Instrumentation Industries, Bethel Park, PA), which it was reasoned would have a higher degree of success as a tube exchanger. This device has an OD of 6.35 mm and is said to be stiffer. Atlas adapted the JEM 400 using the Rapi-Fit connector from the CAEC 19-83 to enable jet ventilation.[16] This device, however, has only a single end hole and is not recommended for jet ventilation (see later).

As previously mentioned (see METTRO-Mizus obturator), the manufacturer originally had recommended insertion of the CAEC until resistance was encountered, presumably at the carina. Such a recommendation was ill advised as it could result in tracheal injury or barotrauma, particularly if used for ventilation. The instructions now clearly state that the distal end of the CAEC should be aligned with the distal end of the ET or preferably 2 to 3 cm proximal to the carina.

3. Endotracheal Ventilation Catheter*

This device is manufactured by CardioMed Supplies (Gormley, ON, Canada) of a hybrid plastic (Fig. 47-6). It is 85 cm in length and has an OD and ID of 4 and 3 mm, respectively. It has a radiopaque stripe along its entire length and distance markings at 4-cm intervals. Proximally, it has a male hose barb with a threaded adapter welded into the catheter. These attachments have been constructed so as not to restrict the catheter's

---

*This device was designed by the author, who has no financial interest in CardioMed Supplies Inc. but has received limited royalties from sales of the ETVC.

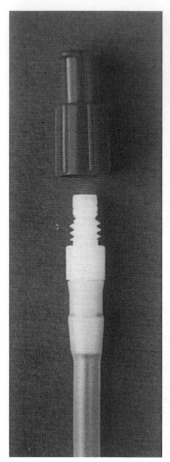
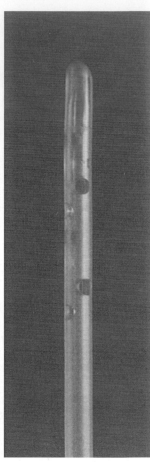

Figure 47-6 The endotracheal ventilation catheter (ETVC, CardioMed Supplies) is available in one length (85 cm) with an outer diameter of 4 mm. It is nonthermolabile and has a radiopaque stripe along its length. There are distance markings every 4 cm. Proximally, there is a welded plastic adapter with a threaded Luer-Lok adapter for jet ventilation **(A)**. Distally, there are an end hole and eight helically arranged side holes **(B)**. These minimize catheter whip and reduce the jet injection pressure. A removable metal stylet is available for additional stiffening. (From Cooper RM, Cohen DR: The use of an endotracheal ventilation catheter for jet ventilation during a difficult intubation. Can J Anaesth 41:1198, 1994.)

inner diameter. The threaded adapter connects to an easily removed Luer-Lok adapter. Distally, it is blunt ended with one end hole and eight helically arranged side holes to minimize catheter whip and jet ventilation pressures (see later). Studies by the manufacturer indicate no significant softening over time at body temperature. This is desirable for a product that may remain in situ and be required to serve as a stylet. A metal guidewire is available to provide additional stiffness, but the author has not found this to be necessary.

The endotracheal ventilation catheter (ETVC) was designed to facilitate reversible extubation.[65] It has been used by the author in at least 500 patients, the first 202 of whom have been reported.[62] Although the ETVC had been used to facilitate reintubation, in the majority of cases this was not required. In the original series, reintubation or tube exchange was performed in 32 of 202 uses (16%), a figure very similar to that reported by Loudermilk and coworkers.[178] In both series, the ETVC[62] and the CAEC,[178] respectively, had been used mostly to maintain airway access. The ETVC was also used for oxygen insufflation (31 patients), jet ventilation (45), and postextubation capnography (54).

Reintubation was successful in 20 of 22 attempts. One failure occurred with a softer prototype. The second failure resulted when an inexperienced and unsupervised operator attempted a tube exchange. Difficulty was occasionally encountered advancing the ET through the glottis, similar to that experienced when using an FOB to intubate.[145] Rotation of the ET usually remedied this situation. Many of the early patients in whom the ETVC was used had undergone orthognathic surgery or had been difficult to intubate. Early in our experience, the majority of the orthognathic surgery patients had postoperative intermaxillary fixation. In some cases, tube exchanges were necessitated by damaged cuffs or inadequate tube length.

Oxygen insufflation was achieved by connecting the male component of the ETVC to an oxygen flow meter with 2 to 4 L/min flow, titrated to the arterial saturation. *Jet ventilation* is discussed later. The ETVC has also been used to facilitate intubation when the glottis could be seen only through a rigid bronchoscope.

Complications included barotrauma, intolerance, unintended dislodgment, and tracheal penetration. Barotrauma is discussed in the next section. *Intolerance* occurred in 2 of 202 patients (generally because of carinal irritation) and in 1 patient recently recovered from status asthmaticus. Patients' intolerance should prompt a reassessment of the depth of insertion. If the depth is clinically or radiographically appropriate and the ETVC continues to be required, tolerance can generally be achieved by instilling lidocaine through the ETVC. Most patients, including those with reactive airways, have tolerated the ETVC without difficulty. *Dislodgment* occurred when the ETVC was inadequately secured or the patient "tongued" the catheter out. Tracheal or bronchial *perforation* with different instrumentation has been described previously.[73,231] In our case, it occurred in a patient with obstructing, proliferative tracheal papillomatosis and a chronic tracheostomy. A rigid prototype catheter was inserted alongside the tracheostomy, penetrating the posterior tracheal wall. Jet ventilation resulted in fatal barotrauma. *Aspiration* and *laryngospasm* have not been observed.

H. EXCHANGE OF DOUBLE-LUMEN TUBES

Generally, DLTs are selected for procedures requiring lung isolation. Although the resistance through a larger sized DLT does not preclude postoperative ventilation or weaning, it may be desirable to replace this with a single-lumen tube, particularly if care is to be transferred to an area where familiarity is lacking. The DLT may also have to be changed because of damage to a cuff or because the initial tube was of an inappropriate size. Such a substitution can often be achieved by direct laryngoscopy. While the larynx is in view, the DLT is withdrawn and immediately replaced with a single-lumen tube. Occasionally, this cannot be accomplished.[27] Whether tube substitution is single-to-double, double-to-single, or double-to-double lumen tube, the requirements are similar and the previously mentioned tube exchangers may not be sufficiently long or firm.[64,123]

Hudson RCI manufactures a DLT exchanger known as the Sheridan ETX Exchanger (catalog number 5-24105). This device is 100 cm in length and was designed for use with the Sheri-Bronch 35 to 41 Fr DLT. It has one distal end hole. There are distance markings and "tracheal" and "bronchial" markings to indicate when the distal tip of the ETX is at the opening of the distal lumen. This device lacks a connector for manual ventilation and the manufacturer recommends against the use of jet ventilation.

Cook Critical Care provides "extra firm" tube exchangers in 11 and 14 Fr sizes, which are 100 cm long and were designed primarily for the exchange of double-lumen ETs (designation C-CAE-11.0-100-DLT-EF and CAE-14.0-100-DLT-EF). These devices have ODs of 3.7 and 6.3 mm, respectively.

I. CONVERSION FROM NASAL TO ORAL

Blind or fiberoptically assisted nasal intubation is sometimes performed when oral approaches are difficult or not possible. The nasal tube may have to be converted to an oral one because of complications or intended surgery. Unless circumstances have changed making laryngoscopy now feasible, it is unlikely that conversion from nasal to oral can be achieved under direct visual control. Fiberoptic conversion, flexible[247] or rigid[7] may be possible as described previously (see "Extubation or Reintubation over Fiberoptic Bronchoscope or Laryngoscope" in Section IV. C). Occasionally, the required equipment is not available, the glottis cannot be visualized, or the patient must be ventilated throughout the exchange. This has been achieved using a variety of techniques.

Gabriel and Azocar described a patient in halo fixation in whom the connector was detached and the nasotracheal tube was advanced deeper into the trachea.[110] The tube was then grasped close to the uvula with forceps and digitally extracted through the mouth. Novella used a Sheridan TTX to perform a nasal-to-oral conversion in a patient with Klippel-Feil syndrome who first underwent orthognathic surgery and a subsequent septorhinoplasty.[202] Following the completion of the orthognathic surgery, the TTX was inserted into the nasal ET and the latter was withdrawn. The TTX was then grasped with two Magill forceps, the caudal one used to stabilize the catheter and the cephalad one to withdraw the proximal end out of the mouth. An oral tube was then "railroaded" over the TTX. Cooper described a similar maneuver in a patient in whom oral fiberoptic intubation could not be accomplished; however, fiberoptic nasal intubation was achieved.[58] He passed an ETVC through the existing nasal tube and removed the latter. The ETVC was then stabilized with caudal Magill forceps and withdrawn through the mouth with the cephalad forceps. Oxygen insufflation was provided through the ETVC, which was then used to thread an oral tube into the trachea. In the latter case, oxygen desaturation was thereby avoided, although the procedure was easily and quickly accomplished.

J. CONVERSION FROM ORAL TO NASAL

During efforts to convert from an oral to a nasal ET, Sumiyoshi and coworkers used negative-pressure ventilation during the tube exchange.[243] Their patient was in a halo and chest cast because of a cervical injury and laryngoscopy had been unsuccessful. An attempt to introduce a 4.8-mm FOB adjacent to the existing tube (with a tube exchanger through it) was unsuccessful. A subsequent effort involved a 3.5-mm FOB and a 7 Fr Mizus obturator using negative pressure to achieve ventilation. A smaller hollow tube exchanger might have been successful and could have avoided the risk of negative-pressure pulmonary edema resulting from both an ET and FOB occupying a small glottic opening.[59] Smith and Fenner performed an oral-to-nasal conversion using a 4.0-mm (OD) FOB, which they inserted through the glottis, anterior to an oral tube.[236] The latter was withdrawn and a nasal tube was advanced over the FOB.

Dutta and colleagues had been unable to intubate a sedated child orally or nasally using a flexible FOB.[84] Oral intubation was achieved by direct laryngoscopy assisted by a stylet, but nasal placement was required for the intended surgical procedure. An FOB was inserted through the nose and retrieved through the mouth. Its distal end was threaded through the oral ET to the level of the carina. The bronchoscope was retroflexed and both were withdrawn through the naris. Such a maneuver seems fraught with danger to both patient and equipment. Salibian and coworkers, facing a similar problem, advanced a CAEC (11-83) through the nose, retrieving it from the mouth.[225] They then inserted this into the existing oral ET, providing oxygen insufflation. The oral ET was then withdrawn into the mouth, where it was filleted with a scalpel and torn away. A nasal tube was then successfully advanced over the CAEC. This, too, was a high-risk maneuver for patient, bronchoscope, and the operator's fingers. Interestingly, the authors did not mention whether any special precautions were taken at the time of extubation.

A far simpler technique was described by Nakata and Niimi employing a Patil two-part intubation catheter (Cook Critical Care).[199] This intubation-extubation device

consists of two components that can be screwed together at its midpoint (see Fig. 47-6). The distal segment was introduced into the existing oral ET. The proximal part was introduced through the nose and retrieved through the mouth. The oral tube was then removed, the two parts were connected, and the Rapi-Fit jet adapter was connected. Jet ventilation was provided. The entire assembly was then used as a stylet and the replacement nasal tube was successfully advanced.

V. JET VENTILATION THROUGH STYLETS

The preceding sections stressed the importance of being able to supplement oxygenation during a tube exchange. In most circumstances, a patient's oxygen content can be adequately sustained with insufflation, obviating the need for high-pressure jet ventilation. If oxygen requirements are high prior to a tube exchange, equipment should be immediately available to provide jet ventilation. In its simplest form, this equipment consists of a manually cycled, Venturi-type jet ventilator with a Luer-Lok adapter and an in-line pressure-reducing valve (Fig. 47-7).[30] The objective of jet ventilation is to correct life-threatening hypoxemia, not to normalize arterial blood gases. Although the achievement of normal $Paco_2$ may be attainable, the risks probably exceed the benefits. Barotrauma, in some cases fatal, has occurred through such misguided objectives.

A. IN VITRO STUDIES

Transtracheal jet ventilation by means of an intravenous catheter or intratracheal ventilation using a stylet or tube exchanger has been advocated in the management of the cannot intubate, cannot ventilate patient.[5,31] In general, the *inspiratory volume* depends upon the driving pressure, injection time, the respiratory compliance and resistance, and the resistance of the tube exchanger. The latter is determined by the device's inner diameter and length. The *expiratory volume* depends on the exhalation time, the elastic recoil of the lungs, and the airway resistance.[30,85] Mismatch between inspiratory and expiratory volumes can have serious consequences.

In vitro studies using jet stylets have been conducted to determine flow, pressure, and entrainment characteristics. Using an in vitro model, with three sizes of Sheridan TTX catheters, Dworkin and colleagues measured the inspiratory and expiratory flows resulting from 50 psi injection as the simulated upper airway resistance, lung compliance, gas flow rate, and injection times were varied.[85] The upper airway resistance was determined by the effective tracheal diameter, which they defined as a computed difference between the OD of the TTX and tracheal diameter. They simulated upper airway obstruction by using various sizes of ET adapters, ranging from 11 to 3.5 mm ID, in the proximal airway. The gas flows

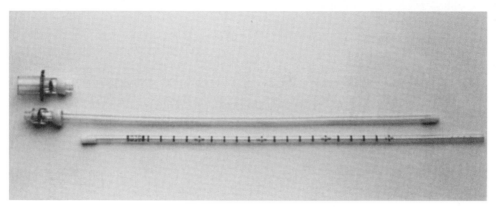

Figure 47-7 The Patil two-part intubation catheter (Cook Critical Care, Bloomington, IN). It is 63 cm in length with an outer diameter of 6.0 mm (18 Fr) and an inner diameter of 3.4 mm. Proximally, it accommodates a Rapi-Fit adapter with both a 15-mm connector and a Luer-Lok jet adapter. Distally, there is a total of eight side holes. At its midpoint, there is threading to enable the two halves to be separated or assembled to achieve its full length. (From Cooper RM: The difficult airway—II. Anesthesiol Clin North Am 13:683-707, 1995.)

through the large, medium, and small tube exchangers, when connected to a pressure source of 50 psi, were 63, 33, and 12 L/min, respectively. In their model, if the difference between the tracheal and TTX diameters resulted in an effective tracheal diameter that was greater than 4 to 4.5 mm, air trapping did not occur. Because increased upper airway resistance and reduced effective tracheal diameter resulted in larger tidal volumes, they concluded that jet ventilation through a long catheter, positioned close to the carina, caused little Venturi effect. Such ventilation was not greatly dependent upon air entrainment. Placement of the catheter close to the carina may ensure a higher oxygen concentration (by reducing room air entrainment), but it also increases the risk of distal catheter migration and barotrauma.

In another in vitro model, calculations based on oxygen dilution and direct measurement using a pneumotachograph revealed that air entrainment accounted for 0% to 31% of the inspired volume.[112] The largest TTX and "lung compliance" resulted in the greatest entrainment. These authors used a high driving pressure (50 psi), long inspiratory time (1 second), and brief expiratory time (1 second). Even within a low-compliance system, the large TTX was associated with excessive tidal volumes.

Prolonging expiratory time reduces the minute ventilation by reducing the respiratory rate. This technique still exposes the lungs to potentially injurious tidal volumes. An alternative approach would be to reduce the driving pressure. Gaughan and others assessed the tidal volumes and air entrainment in a model lung with a range of compliance sets, ventilated by high and low flow regulators through 14 and 16 g intravenous catheters.[113] Their high-flow regulator, at steady state, produced flow rates of 320 L/min at 100 psi, whereas the low-flow regulator produced flows up to 15 L/min at 9 to 5 psi. Intravenous catheters, because of their short length, offer considerably less resistance to flow. Their proximity to

the upper airway also results in greater air entrainment (15% to 74%). Both high- and low-flow regulators allowed adequate minute ventilation in the setting of normal tracheal and bronchial diameters and normal compliance. The authors recommended that during transtracheal jet ventilation, when low-flow regulators were used, an inspiratory/expiratory ratio of 1:1 should be used because it yields the greatest minute ventilation. Although this observation is undoubtedly true, it remains to be determined whether such minute volumes are either clinically necessary or safe.[30,64]

B. IN VIVO STUDIES

Chang and coworkers provided intraoperative jet ventilation using a 3.5-mm chest tube as a jet catheter.[50] Ventilating with 15 psi at 10 to 16 breaths/min, they continued until spontaneous ventilation was deemed adequate. The patient was recovered and was noted to have a left pneumothorax that the authors attributed to catheter migration and unilateral ventilation. They mentioned that they had encountered three cases of pneumothoraces and one pneumoperitoneum in approximately 600 such procedures. The authors drew attention to the importance of catheter placement and advised that even brief airway obstruction can result in barotrauma. However, they failed to mention that vocal fold apposition as recovery occurs may promote such a complication. In a subsequent paper, the same authors stated that the "jet stylet" had been used for the ventilation of six patients resulting in normocarbia and adequate ventilation.[23]

Egol and associates described pneumothoraces or a pneumoperitoneum in three patients using a variety of delivery devices and driving pressures.[89] These included an 18 Fr suction catheter at 50 psi, a nasogastric sump tube at 20 psi (inspiratory time = 30%), and a fiberoptic

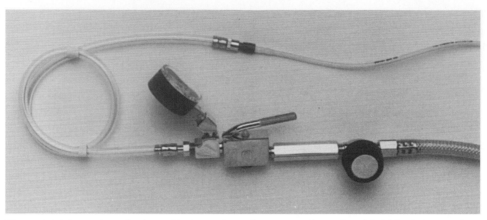

Figure 47-8 An endotracheal ventilation catheter is connected to a hand-held jet injector. The Rapi-Fit adapter or the JETTX device could be similarly attached. A pressure-reducing valve enables the operator to select a driving pressure that yields adequate chest expansion while minimizing the risk of barotrauma. (From Cooper RM, Cohen DR: The use of an endotracheal ventilation catheter for jet ventilation during a difficult intubation. Can J Anaesth 41:1196-1199, 1994.)

laryngoscope at 40 psi. They attributed the barotrauma observed to incorrect catheter placement, ventilation during phonation, and possible direct mucosal penetration from jet injection. They examined the relationship between the number of distal side holes in the tube exchanger and the pressure at the catheter tip. The more side holes at a given driving pressure, the lower the pressure at the catheter tip. They recommended vigilance regarding the location of the catheter tip (avoidance of direct mucosal contact, insertion into orifices where exhalation may be restricted, and securing the catheter to minimize migration); advocated for catheters with multiple side holes, the use of small-diameter jet catheters to minimize the resistance to exhalation, and the use of the minimal effective driving pressure; and encouraged the development and use of an effective pressure sensor and pressure cutoff device.

As previously mentioned, the ETVC has an end hole and eight distal side holes. Its use to provide jet ventilation during general anesthesia with muscle relaxation on 45 occasions was described.[62] Its attachment to a hand-held jet ventilator with a pressure-reducing valve is illustrated in Figure 47-8. Between 1991 and 1993, Irish and colleagues used this device with a driving pressure of 50 psi in anesthetized and paralyzed patients undergoing percutaneous tracheostomies.[140] They observed barotrauma in one patient. Arterial blood gases in 12 consecutive critically ill patients revealed (mean ± SD) a pH of 7.37 ± 0.09, $Paco_2$ 45.5 ± 10.8, and Pao_2 256 ± 126. In a subsequent report, a patient ventilated for 90 minutes at only 20 psi developed a pneumothorax.[64] Chan and Manninen also described the use of the ETVC to provide jet ventilation.[49] After performing a fiberoptic intubation in a patient with an unstable cervical spine, they discovered that the cuff of the ET had been damaged. They inserted an FOB through the other nostril and advanced this through the cords, anterior to the original ET. They then passed an ETVC through the original ET and provided three breaths of jet ventilation at 50 psi. The patient developed a pneumothorax. Unfortunately, they used a high driving pressure through an exchange catheter that may have been too deeply inserted in the setting of a significantly reduced effective tracheal diameter (partial cuff deflation, 6-mm ET, and FOB passing through the vocal cords).

These cases reinforce the general principles previously stated. The need for jet ventilation should always be weighed against its possible risks. It should be immediately available and used when there is evidence of a deterioration in a patient's oxygenation. An in-line pressure-reducing valve should be used and ventilation should begin with the lowest pressure capable of producing adequate chest expansion. The duration of inspiration should be minimized while the duration of exhalation is determined by observing the return of the thoracic diameter to its preinspiratory position. The depth of catheter insertion should be far enough from the carina that distal migration does not occur but not so proximal that jet ventilation results in the catheter's ejection from the glottis. Multiple distal side holes reduce both catheter whip and the distal catheter pressure during jet ventilation. Finally, every effort must be taken to minimize expiratory resistance.

VI. SUMMARY

Successful airway management does not end with endotracheal intubation. Although respiratory complications are more common at extubation than during intubation, the majority of these are relatively minor and do not result in a need for reintubation. However, such a need cannot always be predicted. Reintubation could prove to be difficult and dangerous in a variety of circumstances, discussed in detail. Accordingly, the ASA Task Force and the Canadian Airway Focus Group have recommended that each anesthesiologist have a preformulated strategy for extubation of the DA. This chapter proposes a risk stratification scheme in an effort to identify patients in whom special extubation precautions might be of benefit. A variety of strategies are presented, although generally the benefits of these have not been subjected to rigorous evaluation. The concept of a reversible extubation using a tube exchanger has been presented. When such a device is used as a stylet, it does not provide a guarantee that reintubation will succeed. Carefully used, however, it should enhance patients' safety by providing oxygen insufflation and jet ventilation while other avenues are explored.

REFERENCES

1. Adderley RJ, Mullins GC: When to extubate the croup patient: The "leak" test. Can J Anaesth 34:304-306, 1987.
2. Adliff M, Ngato D, Keshavjee S, et al: Treatment of diffuse tracheomalacia secondary to relapsing polychondritis with continuous positive airway pressure. Chest 112:1701-1704, 1997.
3. Akers JA, Riley RH: Failed extubation due to 'sutured' double-lumen tube. Anaesth Intensive Care 18:577, 1990.
4. American Society of Anesthesiologists: Practice guidelines for management of the difficult airway. A report by the American Society of Anesthesiologists Task Force on Management of the Difficult Airway. Anesthesiology 78:597-602, 1993.
5. American Society of Anesthesiologists: Practice Guidelines for Management of the Difficult Airway: An updated report by the American Society of Anesthesiologists Task Force on Management of the Difficult Airway. Anesthesiology 98:1269-1277, 2003.
6. Andrews SR, Mabey MF: Tubular fiberoptic laryngoscope (WuScope) and lingual tonsil airway obstruction. Anesthesiology 93:904-905, 2000.
7. Andrews SR, Norcross SD, Mabey MF, Siegel JB: The WuScope technique for endotracheal tube exchange. Anesthesiology 90:929-930, 1999.
8. Anene O, Meert KL, Uy H, et al: Dexamethasone for the prevention of postextubation airway obstruction: A prospective, randomized, double-blind, placebo-controlled trial. Crit Care Med 24:1666-1669, 1996.
9. Aquino SL, Shepard JA, Ginns LC, et al: Acquired tracheomalacia: Detection by expiratory CT scan. J Comput Assist Tomogr 25:394-399, 2001.
10. Arndt GA, Voth BR: Paradoxical vocal cord motion in the recovery room: A masquerader of pulmonary dysfunction. Can J Anaesth 43:1249-1251, 1996.
11. Artru AA, Cucchiara RF, Messick JM: Cardiorespiratory and cranial-nerve sequelae of surgical procedures involving the posterior fossa. Anesthesiology 52:83-86, 1980.
12. Asai T: Use of the laryngeal mask after tracheal extubation. Can J Anaesth 46:997-998, 1999.
13. Asai T: Use of the laryngeal mask for exchange of orotracheal tubes. Anesthesiology 91:1167-1168, 1999.
14. Asai T, Koga K, Vaughan RS: Respiratory complications associated with tracheal intubation and extubation. Br J Anaesth 80:767-775, 1998.
15. Asai T, Shingu K: Use of the during emergence from anesthesia in a patient with an unstable neck. Anesth Analg 88:469-470, 1999.
16. Atlas G: A high-risk endotracheal tube exchanger. Anesth Analg 95:785, 2002.
17. Atlas G, Mort TC: Extubation of the difficult airway over an airway exchange catheter: Relationship of catheter size and patient tolerance. Crit Care Med 27:A57-1999.
18. Audenaert SM, Montgomery CL, Slayton D, Berger R: Application of the Mizus endotracheal obturator in tracheostomy and tentative extubation. J Clin Anesth 3:418-421, 1991.
19. Backus WW, Ward RR, Vitkun SA, et al: Postextubation laryngeal spasm in an unanesthetized patient with Parkinson's disease. J Clin Anesth 3:314-316, 1991.
20. Bamshad M, Rosa U, Padda G, Luce M: Acute upper airway obstruction in rheumatoid arthritis of the cricoarytenoid joints. South Med J 82:507-511, 1989.
21. Baraka A, Louis F, Sibai AN, Usta N: A simple manoeuvre for changing the tracheal tube. Intensive Care Med 13:216-217, 1987.
22. Bedford RF, Persing JA, Pobereskin L, Butler A: Lidocaine or thiopental for rapid control of intracranial hypertension. Anesth Analg 59:435-437, 1980.
23. Bedger RC Jr, Chang JL: A jet-stylet endotracheal catheter for difficult airway management. Anesthesiology 66:221-223, 1987.
24. Beed SD, Devitt JH: Mortality associated with orthognathic surgery. Can J Anaesth 43A:40, 1996.
25. Benjamin B: Prolonged intubation injuries of the larynx: Endoscopic diagnosis, classification, and treatment. Ann Otol Rhinol Laryngol Suppl 160:1-15, 1993.
26. Benumof JL: Additional safety measures when changing endotracheal tubes. Anesthesiology 75:921-922, 1991.
27. Benumof JL: Difficult tubes and difficult airways. J Cardiothorac Vasc Anesth 12:131-132, 1998.
28. Benumof JL: Obstructive sleep apnea in the adult obese patient: Implications for airway management. Anesthesiol Clin North Am 20:789-811, 2002.
29. Benumof JL, Dagg R, Benumof R: Critical hemoglobin desaturation will occur before return to an unparalyzed state following 1 mg/kg intravenous succinylcholine. Anesthesiology 87:979-982, 1997.
30. Benumof JL, Gaughan SD: Concerns regarding barotrauma during jet ventilation. Anesthesiology 76:1072-1073, 1992.
31. Benumof JL, Scheller MS: The importance of transtracheal jet ventilation in the management of the difficult airway. Anesthesiology 71:769-778, 1989.
32. Berg H, Roed J, Viby-Mogensen J, et al: Residual neuromuscular block is a risk factor for postoperative pulmonary complications. A prospective, randomised, and blinded study of postoperative pulmonary complications after atracurium, vecuronium and pancuronium. Acta Anaesthesiol Scand 41:1095-1103, 1997.

33. Betbese AJ, Perez M, Bak E, et al: A prospective study of unplanned endotracheal extubation in intensive care unit patients. Crit Care Med 26:1180-1186, 1998.

34. Bexton MD, Radford R: An unusual cause of respiratory obstruction after thyroidectomy. Anaesthesia 37:596, 1982.

35. Biro P, Rohling R, Schmid S, et al: Anesthesia in a patient with acute respiratory insufficiency due to relapsing polychondritis. J Clin Anesth 6:59-62, 1994.

36. Blanc VF, Tremblay NA: The complications of tracheal intubation: A new classification with a review of the literature. Anesth Analg 53:202-213, 1974.

37. Blumin JH, Berke GS: Bilateral vocal fold paresis and multiple system atrophy. Arch Otolaryngol Head Neck Surg 128:1404-1407, 2002.

38. Booth CM, Matukas LM, Tomlinson GA, et al: Clinical features and short-term outcomes of 144 patients with SARS in the greater Toronto area. JAMA 289: 2801-2809, 2003.

39. Brain AI, Verghese C, Strube PJ: The LMA 'ProSeal'— A laryngeal mask with an oesophageal vent. Br J Anaesth 84:650-654, 2000.

40. Brimacombe J: The advantages of the LMA over the tracheal tube or facemask: A meta-analysis. Can J Anaesth 42:1017-1023, 1995.

41. Broster T, Placek R, Eggers GW Jr: Epidermolysis bullosa: Anesthetic management for cesarean section. Anesth Analg 66:341-343, 1987.

42. Brucia JJ, Owen DC, Rudy EB: The effects of lidocaine on intracranial hypertension. J Neurosci Nurs 24:205-214, 1992.

43. Bukht D, Langford RM: Airway obstruction after surgery in the neck. Anaesthesia 38:389-390, 1983.

44. Burgess FW, Whitlock W, Davis MJ, Patane PS: Anesthetic implications of relapsing polychondritis: A case report. Anesthesiology 73:570-572, 1990.

45. Burgess GE III, Cooper JR Jr, Marino RJ, et al: Laryngeal competence after tracheal extubation. Anesthesiology 51:73-77, 1979.

46. Carmichael FJ, McGuire GP, Wong DT, et al: Computed tomographic analysis of airway dimensions after carotid endarterectomy. Anesth Analg 83:12-17, 1996.

47. Cavo JW Jr: True vocal cord paralysis following intubation. Laryngoscope 95:1352-1359, 1985.

48. Chalmers A, Traynor JA: Cricoarytenoid arthritis as a cause of acute upper airway obstruction. J Rheumatol 6:541-542, 1979.

49. Chan AS, Manninen PH: Bronchoscopic findings of a tension pneumothorax. Anesth Analg 80:628-629, 1995.

50. Chang JL, Bleyaert A, Bedger R: Unilateral pneumothorax following jet ventilation during general anesthesia. Anesthesiology 53:244-246, 1980.

51. Cheney FW, Posner KL, Caplan RA: Adverse respiratory events infrequently leading to malpractice suits. A closed claims analysis. Anesthesiology 75:932-939, 1991.

52. Chipley PS, Castresana M, Bridges MT, Catchings TT: Prolonged use of an endotracheal tube changer in a pediatric patient with a potentially compromised airway. Chest 105:961-962, 1994.

53. Chou HC, Wu TL: Large hypopharyngeal tongue: A shared anatomic abnormality for difficult mask ventilation, difficult intubation, and obstructive sleep apnea? Anesthesiology 94:936-937, 2001.

54. Christopher KL, Wood RP, Eckert RC, et al: Vocal-cord dysfunction presenting as asthma. N Engl J Med 308:1566-1570, 1983.

55. Chung DC, Rowbottom SJ: A very small dose of suxamethonium relieves laryngospasm. Anaesthesia 48:229-230, 1993.

56. Ciaglia P, Firsching R, Syniec C: Elective percutaneous dilatational tracheostomy. A new simple bedside procedure; preliminary report. Chest 87:715-719, 1985.

57. Coleman J, Bick PA: Suspension sutures for the treatment of obstructive sleep apnea and snoring. Otolaryngol Clin North Am 32:277-285, 1999.

58. Cooper RM: Conversion of a nasal to an orotracheal intubation using an endotracheal tube exchanger. Anesthesiology 87:717-718, 1997.

59. Cooper RM: Negative pressure ventilation during tracheal tube exchange. Anesthesiology 82:1533-1534, 1995.

60. Cooper RM: Rheumatoid arthritis is a common disease with clinically important implications for the airway. J Bone Joint Surg Am 77:1463-1465, 1995.

61. Cooper RM: The LMA, laparoscopic surgery and the obese patient—Can vs should. Can J Anaesth 50:5-10, 2003.

62. Cooper RM: The use of an endotracheal ventilation catheter in the management of difficult extubations. Can J Anaesth 43:90-93, 1996.

63. Cooper RM: Use of a new videolaryngoscope (GlideScope) in the management of a difficult airway. [L'usage d'un nouveau videolaryngoscope (GlideScope) pour une intubation difficile]. Can J Anaesth 50: 611-613, 2003.

64. Cooper RM, Cohen DR: The use of an endotracheal ventilation catheter for jet ventilation during a difficult intubation. Can J Anaesth 41:1196-1199, 1994.

65. Cooper RM, Levytam S: Use of an endotracheal ventilation catheter for difficult extubations. Anesthesiology 77A:1110, 1992.

66. Crosby ET: Modifications to the Bullard laryngoscope; when time is short [letter]. Can J Anaesth 45:94-95, 1998.

67. Crosby ET, Cooper RM, Douglas MJ, et al: The unanticipated difficult airway with recommendations for management. Can J Anaesth 45:757-776, 1998.

68. Daley MD, Norman PH, Coveler LA: Tracheal extubation of adult surgical patients while deeply anesthetized: A survey of United States anesthesiologists. J Clin Anesth 11:445-452, 1999.

69. Dark A, Armstrong T: Severe postoperative laryngeal oedema causing total airway obstruction immediately on extubation. Br J Anaesth 82:644-646, 1999.

70. Darmon JY, Rauss A, Dreyfuss D, et al: Evaluation of risk factors for laryngeal edema after tracheal extubation in adults and its prevention by dexamethasone. A placebo-controlled, double-blind, multicenter study. Anesthesiology 77:245-251, 1992.

71. Debaene B, Plaud B, Dilly MP, Donati F: Residual paralysis in the PACU after a single intubating dose of nondepolarizing muscle relaxant with an intermediate duration of action. Anesthesiology 98:1042-1048, 2003.

72. De Bast Y, De Backer D, Moraine JJ, et al: The cuff leak test to predict failure of tracheal extubation for laryngeal edema. Intensive Care Med 28:1267-1272, 2002.

73. DeLima LG, Bishop MJ: Lung laceration after tracheal extubation over a plastic tube changer. Anesth Analg 73:350-351, 1991.

74. Dellinger RP: Fiberoptic bronchoscopy in adult airway management. Crit Care Med 18:882-887, 1990.

75. Demling RH, Read T, Lind LJ, Flanagan HL: Incidence and morbidity of extubation failure in surgical intensive care patients. Crit Care Med 16:573-577, 1988.

76. Desai SP, Fencl V: A safe technique for changing endotracheal tubes. Anesthesiology 53:267-1980.

77. Dob DP, Shannon CN, Bailey PM: Efficacy and safety of the laryngeal mask airway vs Guedel airway following tracheal extubation. Can J Anaesth 46:179-181, 1999.

78. Dohi S, Okubo N, Kondo Y: Pulmonary oedema after airway obstruction due to bilateral vocal cord paralysis. Can J Anaesth 38:492-195, 1991.

79. Dolinski SY, MacGregor DA, Scuderi PE: Pulmonary hemorrhage associated with negative-pressure pulmonary edema. Anesthesiology 93:888-890, 2000.

80. Domino KB, Posner KL, Caplan RA, Cheney FW: Airway injury during anesthesia: A closed claims analysis. Anesthesiology 91:1703-1711, 1999.

81. Drenger B, Zidenbaum M, Reifen E, Leitersdorf E: Severe upper airway obstruction and difficult intubation in cicatricial pemphigoid. Anaesthesia 41:1029-1031, 1986.

82. Drummond JC: Macroglossia. Déjà vu. Anesth Analg 89:534, 1999.

83. Dryden GE: Circulatory collapse after pneumonectomy (an unusual complication from the use of a Carlens catheter): Case report. Anesth Analg 56:451-452, 1977.

84. Dutta A, Chari P, Mohan RA, Manhas Y: Oral to nasal endotracheal tube exchange in a difficult airway: A novel method. Anesthesiology 97:1324-1325, 2002.

85. Dworkin R, Benumof JL, Benumof R, Karagianes TG: The effective tracheal diameter that causes air trapping during jet ventilation. J Cardiothorac Anesth 4:731-736, 1990.

86. Dyson A, Isaac PA, Pennant JH, et al: Esmolol attenuates cardiovascular responses to extubation. Anesth Analg 71:675-678, 1990.

87. Easdown LJ, Tessler MJ, Minuk J: Upper airway involvement in Parkinson's disease resulting in postoperative respiratory failure. Can J Anaesth 42:344-347, 1995.

88. Efferen LS, Elsakr A: Post-extubation stridor: Risk factors and outcome. J Assoc Acad Minor Phys 9:65-68, 1998.

89. Egol A, Culpepper JA, Snyder JV: Barotrauma and hypotension resulting from jet ventilation in critically ill patients. Chest 88:98-102, 1985.

90. el Sayed Y, al Muhaimeed H: Cicatricial pemphigoid of the larynx: A case report of surgical treatment. Ear Nose Throat J 75:658-660, 665, 668, 1996.

91. Emery SE, Smith MD, Bohlman HH: Upper-airway obstruction after multilevel cervical corpectomy for myelopathy. J Bone Joint Surg Am 73:544-551, 1991.

92. Engoren M: Evaluation of the cuff-leak test in a cardiac surgery population. Chest 116:1029-1031, 1999.

93. Epstein NE, Hollingsworth R, Nardi D, Singer J: Can airway complications following multilevel anterior cervical surgery be avoided? J Neurosurg 94(2 Suppl): 185-188, 2001.

94. Eriksson LI: Evidence-based practice and neuromuscular monitoring: It's time for routine quantitative assessment. Anesthesiology 98:1037-1039, 2003.

95. Eriksson LI, Sundman E, Olsson R, et al: Functional assessment of the pharynx at rest and during swallowing in partially paralyzed humans: Simultaneous videomanometry and mechanomyography of awake human volunteers. Anesthesiology 87:1035-1043, 1997.

96. Esclamado RM, Glenn MG, McCulloch TM, Cummings CW: Perioperative complications and risk factors in the surgical treatment of obstructive sleep apnea syndrome. Laryngoscope 99:1125-1129, 1989.

97. Estebe JP, Dollo G, Le Corre P, et al: Alkalinization of intracuff lidocaine improves endotracheal tube-induced emergence phenomena. Anesth Analg 94:227-230, table, 2002.

98. Fagan C, Frizelle HP, Laffey J, et al: The effects of intracuff lidocaine on endotracheal-tube-induced emergence phenomena after general anesthesia. Anesth Analg 91:201-205, 2000.

99. Fagraeus L: Difficult extubation following nasotracheal intubation. Anesthesiology 49:43-44, 1978.

100. Faust RA, Rimell FL, Remley KB: Cine magnetic resonance imaging for evaluation of focal tracheomalacia: Innominate artery compression syndrome. Int J Pediatr Otorhinolaryngol 65:27-33, 2002.

101. Finucane BT, Kupshik HL: A flexible stilette for replacing damaged tracheal tubes. Can Anaesth Soc J 25:153-154, 1978.

102. Fisher GC, Ray DA: Airway obstruction in epidermolysis bullosa. Anaesthesia 44:449-1989.

103. Fisher MM, Raper RF: The 'cuff-leak' test for extubation. Anaesthesia 47:10-12, 1992.

104. Fitzmaurice BG, Brodsky JB, Kee ST, et al: Anesthetic management of a patient with relapsing polychondritis. J Cardiothorac Vasc Anesth 13:309-311, 1999.

105. Fitzpatrick AJ: Upper airway obstruction in Parkinson's disease. Anaesth Intensive Care 23:367-369, 1995.

106. Francfort JW, Smullens SN, Gallagher JF, Fairman RM: Airway compromise after carotid surgery in patients with cervical irradiation. J Cardiovasc Surg (Torino) 30:877-881, 1989.

107. Frank LP, Schreiber GC: Pulmonary edema following acute upper airway obstruction. Anesthesiology 65:106, 1986.

108. Fujii Y, Toyooka H, Tanaka H: Cardiovascular responses to tracheal extubation or LMA removal in normotensive and hypertensive patients. Can J Anaesth 44:1082-1086, 1997.

109. Funk D, Raymon F: Rheumatoid arthritis of the cricoarytenoid joints: An airway hazard. Anesth Analg 54:742-745, 1975.

110. Gabriel DM, Azocar RJ: A novel technique for conversion of nasotracheal tube to orotracheal. Anesthesiology 93:911, 2000.

111. Gandia F, Blanco J: Evaluation of indexes predicting the outcome of ventilator weaning and value of adding supplemental inspiratory load. Intensive Care Med 18:327-333, 1992.

112. Gaughan SD, Benumof JL, Ozaki GT: Quantification of the jet function of a jet stylet. Anesth Analg 74:580-585, 1992.

113. Gaughan SD, Ozaki GT, Benumof JL: A comparison in a lung model of low- and high-flow regulators for transtracheal jet ventilation. Anesthesiology 77:189-199, 1992.

114. Gaussorgues P, Boyer F, Piperno D, et al: [Laryngeal edema after extubation. Do corticosteroids play a role in its prevention?]. Presse Med 16:1531-1532, 1987.

115. Golden SE: The management and treatment of recurrent postoperative laryngospasm. Anesth Analg 84:1392, 1997.

116. Goodman NW: Volatile agents and the ventilatory response to hypoxia. Br J Anaesth 72:503-505, 1994.

117. Gruen R, Cade R, Vellar D: Perforation during nasogastric and orogastric tube insertion. Aust N Z J Surg 68:809-811, 1998.

118. Guerra LG, Lau KY, Marwah R: Upper airway obstruction as the sole manifestation of rheumatoid arthritis. J Rheumatol 19:974-976, 1992.

119. Gurley JP, Bell GR: The surgical management of patients with rheumatoid cervical spine disease. Rheum Dis Clin North Am 23:317-332, 1997.

120. Haavisto L, Suonpaa J: Complications of uvulopalatopharyngoplasty. Clin Otolaryngol 19:243-247, 1994.

121. Halow KD, Ford EG: Pulmonary edema following post-operative laryngospasm: A case report and review of the literature. Am Surg 59:443-447, 1993.

122. Hammer G, Schwinn D, Wollman H: Postoperative complications due to paradoxical vocal cord motion. Anesthesiology 66:686-687, 1987.

123. Hannallah M: Evaluation of Tracheal Tube Exchangers for replacement of double-lumen endobronchial tubes. Anesthesiology 77:609-610, 1992.

124. Hartley M, Vaughan RS: Problems associated with tracheal extubation. Br J Anaesth 71:561-568, 1993.

125. Hawkins M, Roberts EA: Use of a cuffed oropharyngeal airway and Aintree catheter in a difficult airway. Anaesthesia 54:909-910, 1999.

126. Hayes JP, Nolan MT, Brennan N, FitzGerald MX: Three cases of paradoxical vocal cord adduction followed up over a 10-year period. Chest 104:678-680, 1993.

127. Hayward AW, al Shaikh B: Relapsing polychondritis and the anaesthetist. Anaesthesia 43:573-577, 1988.

128. Hemmerling TM, Schmidt J, Bosert C, et al: Intraoperative monitoring of the recurrent laryngeal nerve in 151 consecutive patients undergoing thyroid surgery. Anesth Analg 93:396-399, 2001.

129. Heyman DM, Greenfeld AL, Rogers JS, et al: Inability to deflate the distal cuff of the laser-flex tracheal tube preventing extubation after laser surgery of the larynx. Anesthesiology 80:236-238, 1994.

130. Hill RS, Koltai PJ, Parnes SM: Airway complications from laryngoscopy and panendoscopy. Ann Otol Rhinol Laryngol 96:691-694, 1987.

131. Hillermann CL, Tarpey J, Phillips DE: Laryngeal nerve identification during thyroid surgery—Feasibility of a novel approach. [L'identification du nerf larynge pendant l'opération de la thyroide—La faisabilité d'une nouvelle approche]. Can J Anaesth 50:189-192, 2003.

132. Hilley MD, Henderson RB, Giesecke AH: Difficult extubation of the trachea. Anesthesiology 59:149-150, 1983.

133. Ho LI, Harn HJ, Lien TC, et al: Postextubation laryngeal edema in adults. Risk factor evaluation and prevention by hydrocortisone. Intensive Care Med 22:933-936, 1996.

134. Hochberg MC: Relapsing polychondritis. In Ruddy S, Harris ED, Sledge CB (eds): Kelley's Textbook of Rheumatology, 6th ed. Philadelphia, WB Saunders, 2001, pp 1463-1468.

135. Holmes JR, Hensinger RN, Wojtys EW: Postoperative pulmonary edema in young, athletic adults. Am J Sports Med 19:365-371, 1991.

136. Howard R, Mahoney A, Thurlow AC: Respiratory obstruction after posterior fossa surgery. Anaesthesia 45:222-224, 1990.

137. Hudes ET, Fisher JA, Guslitz B: Difficult endotracheal reintubations: A simple technique. Anesthesiology 64:515-517, 1986.

138. Hughes R, McGuire G, Montanera W, et al: Upper airway edema after carotid endarterectomy: The effect of steroid administration. Anesth Analg 84:475-478, 1997.

139. Hung O: Understanding hemodynamic responses to tracheal intubation. Can J Anaesth 48:723-726, 2001.

140. Irish JC, Brown DH, Cooper RM: Airway control during percutaneous tracheotomy. Laryngoscope 104:1178-1180, 1994.

141. Jaber S, Chanques G, Matecki S, et al: Post-extubation stridor in intensive care unit patients. Risk factors evaluation and importance of the cuff-leak test. Intensive Care Med 29:69-74, 2003.

142. James I, Wark H: Airway management during anesthesia in patients with epidermolysis bullosa dystrophica. Anesthesiology 56:323-326, 1982.

143. Johnson JT, Braun TW: Preoperative, intraoperative, and postoperative management of patients with obstructive sleep apnea syndrome. Otolaryngol Clin North Am 31:1025-1030, 1998.

144. Juvin P, Lavaut E, Dupont H, et al: Difficult tracheal intubation is more common in obese than in lean patients. Anesth Analg 97:595-600, 2003.

145. Katsnelson T, Frost EA, Farcon E, Goldiner PL: When the endotracheal tube will not pass over the flexible fiberoptic bronchoscope. Anesthesiology 76:151-152, 1992.

146. Keenan MA, Stiles CM, Kaufman RL: Acquired laryngeal deviation associated with cervical spine disease in erosive polyarticular arthritis. Use of the fiberoptic bronchoscope in rheumatoid disease. Anesthesiology 58:441-449, 1983.

147. Kempen P: Extubation in adult patients: Who, what, when, where, how, and why? J Clin Anesth 11:441-444, 1999.

148. Kemper KJ, Izenberg S, Marvin JA, Heimbach DM: Treatment of postextubation stridor in a pediatric patient with burns: The role of heliox. J Burn Care Rehabil 11:337-339, 1990.

149. Kemper KJ, Ritz RH, Benson MS, Bishop MS: Helium-oxygen mixture in the treatment of postextubation stridor in pediatric trauma patients. Crit Care Med 19:356-359, 1991.

150. Kharasch ED, Sivarajan M: Gastroesophageal perforation after intraoperative transesophageal echocardiography. Anesthesiology 85:426-428, 1996.

151. Kim ES, Bishop MJ: Cough during emergence from isoflurane anesthesia. Anesth Analg 87:1170-1174, 1998.

152. Kluger MT, Short TG: Aspiration during anaesthesia: A review of 133 cases from the Australian Anaesthetic Incident Monitoring Study (AIMS). Anaesthesia 54: 19-26, 1999.

153. Knill RL, Gelb AW: Ventilatory responses to hypoxia and hypercapnia during halothane sedation and anesthesia in man. Anesthesiology 49:244-251, 1978.

154. Koga K, Asai T, Vaughan RS, Latto IP: Respiratory complications associated with tracheal extubation. Timing of tracheal extubation and use of the laryngeal mask during emergence from anaesthesia. Anaesthesia 53:540-544, 1998.

155. Kohjitani A, Miyawaki T, Kasuya K, et al: Anesthetic management for advanced rheumatoid arthritis patients with acquired micrognathia undergoing temporo-mandibular joint replacement. J Oral Maxillofac Surg 60:559-566, 2002.

156. Koka BV, Jeon IS, Andre JM, et al: Postintubation croup in children. Anesth Analg 56:501-505, 1977.

157. Kolman J, Morris I: Cricoarytenoid arthritis: A cause of acute upper airway obstruction in rheumatoid arthritis. Can J Anaesth 49:729-732, 2002.

158. Kuhnert S, Faust RJ, Berge KHM, Piepgras DG: Postoperative macroglossia: Report of a case with rapid resolution after extubation of the trachea. Anesth Analg 88:220-223, 1999.

159. Kunkel JM, Gomez ER, Spebar MJ, et al: Wound hematomas after carotid endarterectomy. Am J Surg 148:844-847, 1984.

160. Lacoste L, Gineste D, Karayan J, et al: Airway complications in thyroid surgery. Ann Otol Rhinol Laryngol 102:441-446, 1993.

161. Lall NG: Difficult extubation. A fold in the endotracheal cuff. Anaesthesia 35:500-501, 1980.

162. Lam AM, Vavilala MS: Macroglossia: Compartment syndrome of the tongue? Anesthesiology 92:1832-1835, 2000.

163. Lamb K, James MF, Janicki PK: The laryngeal mask airway for intraocular surgery: Effects on intraocular pressure and stress responses. Br J Anaesth 69:143-147, 1992.

164. Landsman IS: Mechanisms and treatment of laryngospasm. Int Anesthesiol Clin 35:67-73, 1997.

165. Lang S, Johnson DH, Lanigan DT, Ha H: Difficult tracheal extubation. Can J Anaesth 36: 340-342, 1989.

166. Lang SA, Duncan PG, Shephard DAE, Ha HC: Pulmonary oedema associated with airway obstruction. Can J Anaesth 37:210-218, 1990.

167. Langeron O, Masso E, Huraux C, et al: Prediction of difficult mask ventilation. Anesthesiology 92:1229-1236, 2000.

168. Lathan SR, Silverman ME, Thomas BL, Waters WC: Postoperative pulmonary edema. South Med J 92: 313-315, 1999.

169. Lee C, Schwartz S, Mok MS: Difficult extubation due to transfixation of a nasotracheal tube by a Kirschner wire. Anesthesiology 46:427, 1977.

170. Lehmann T, Nef W, Stalder B, et al: Fatal postoperative airway obstruction in a patient with rheumatoid arthritis. Ann Rheum Dis 56:512-513, 1997.

171. Leicht MJ, Harrington TM, Davis DE: Cricoarytenoid arthritis: A cause of laryngeal obstruction. Ann Emerg Med 16:885-888, 1987.

172. Lerner DM, Deeb Z: Acute upper airway obstruction resulting from systemic diseases. South Med J 86: 623-627, 1993.

173. Levelle JP, Martinez OA: Airway obstruction after bilateral carotid endarterectomy. Anesthesiology 63: 220-222, 1985.

174. Lewis IH: Required sample size for randomized clinical trials. Anesthesiology 78:609-610, 1993.

175. Liu EH, Choy J, Dhara SS: Persistent perioperative laryngospasm in a patient with Parkinson's disease. Can J Anesth 45:495, 1998.

176. Lofgren RH, Montgomery WW: Incidence of laryngeal involvement in rheumatoid arthritis. N Engl J Med 267:193-195, 1962.

177. Loh KS, Irish JC: Traumatic complications of intubation and other airway management procedures. Anesthesiol Clin North Am 20:953-969, 2002.

178. Loudermilk EP, Hartmannsgruber M, Stoltzfus DP, Langevin PB: A prospective study of the safety of tracheal extubation using a pediatric airway exchange catheter for patients with a known difficult airway. Chest 111:1660-1665, 1997.

179. Ludlow CL, Gracco C, Sasaki CT, et al.: Neurogenic and functional disorders of the larynx. In Ballenger JJ, Snow JB (eds): Otorhinolaryngology: Head and Neck Surgery, 15th ed. Philadelphia, Williams & Wilkins, 1996, pp 556-584.

180. Madan R, Tamilselvan P, Sadhasivam S, et al: Intra-ocular pressure and haemodynamic changes after tracheal intubation and extubation: A comparative study in glaucomatous and nonglaucomatous children. Anaesthesia 55:380-384, 2000.

181. Mahalingam TG, Kathirvel S, Sodhi P: Anaesthetic management of a patient with pemphigus vulgaris for emergency laparotomy. Anaesthesia 55:160-162, 2000.

182. Maktabi MA, Hoffman H, Funk G, From RP: Laryngeal trauma during awake fiberoptic intubation. Anesth Analg 95:1112-1114, 2002.

183. Marini JJ, Wheeler AP: Weaning from mechanical ventilation. In Marini JJ, Wheeler AP (eds): Critical Care Medicine: The Essentials, 1st ed. Baltimore, Williams & Wilkins, 1997, pp 173-195.

184. Mark DA: Protection from aspiration with the LMA-ProSeal after vomiting: A case report. [La protection contre l'aspiration avec le ML-ProSeal après des vomissements: Une étude de cas]. Can J Anesth 50: 78-80, 2003.

185. Masters IB, Chang AB, Patterson L, et al: Series of laryngomalacia, tracheomalacia, and bronchomalacia disorders and their associations with other conditions in children. Pediatr Pulmonol 34:189-195, 2002.

186. Mathew JP, Rosenbaum SH, O'Connor T, Barash PG: Emergency tracheal intubation in the postanesthesia care unit: Physician error or patient disease? Anesth Analg 71:691-697, 1990.

187. Matioc A, Arndt GA: Intubation using the ProSeal laryngeal mask airway and a Cook airway exchange catheter set. Can J Anesth 48:932, 2001.

188. Meisami T, Musa M, Keller AM, et al: Postoperative evaluation of airway compromise using MRI following orthognathic surgery. 2006.

189. Mencke T, Echternach M, Kleinschmidt S, et al: Laryngeal morbidity and quality of tracheal intubation: A randomized controlled trial. Anesthesiology 98: 1049-1056, 2003.

190. Mevorach DL: The management and treatment of recurrent postoperative laryngospasm. Anesth Analg 83:1110-1111, 1996.

191. Michelsen LG, Vanderspek AF: An unexpected functional cause of upper airway obstruction. Anaesthesia 43:1028-1030, 1988.

192. Miller KA, Harkin CP, Bailey PL: Postoperative tracheal extubation. Anesth Analg 80:149-172, 1995.

193. Miller RL, Cole RP: Association between reduced cuff leak volume and postextubation stridor. Chest 110:1035-1040, 1996.

194. Mort TC: Unplanned tracheal extubation outside the operating room: A quality improvement audit of hemodynamic and tracheal airway complications associated with emergency tracheal reintubation. Anesth Analg 86:1171-1176, 1998.

195. Munro FJ, Makin AP, Reid J: Airway problems after carotid endarterectomy. Br J Anaesth 76:156-159, 1996.

196. Muzzi DA, Black S, Losasso TJ, Cucchiara RF: Labetalol and esmolol in the control of hypertension after intracranial surgery. Anesth Analg 70:68-71, 1990.

197. Nagyova B, Dorrington KL, Robbins PA: Effect of low-dose enflurane on the ventilatory response to hypoxia in humans. Br J Anaesth 72:509-514, 1994.

198. Nair I, Bailey PM: Use of the laryngeal mask for airway maintenance following tracheal extubation. Anaesthesia 50:174-175, 1995.

199. Nakata Y, Niimi Y: Oral-to-nasal endotracheal tube exchange in patients with bleeding esophageal varices. Anesthesiology 83:1380-1381, 1995.

200. Ng A, Smith G: Gastroesophageal reflux and aspiration of gastric contents in anesthetic practice. Anesth Analg 93:494-513, 2001.

201. Norton ML, Ghanma MA: Atlantoaxial instability revisited. An alert for endoscopists. Ann Otol Rhinol Laryngol 91:567-570, 1982.

202. Novella J: Intraoperative nasotracheal to orotracheal tube change in a patient with Klippel-Feil syndrome. Anaesth Intensive Care 23:402-403, 1995.

203. O'Dwyer JP, Yorukoglu D, Harris MN: The use of esmolol to attenuate the haemodynamic response when extubating patients following cardiac surgery—A double-blind controlled study. Eur Heart J 14:701-704, 1993.

204. O'Sullivan JC, Wells DG, Wells GR: Difficult airway management with neck swelling after carotid endarterectomy. Anaesth Intensive Care 14:460-464, 1986.

205. Olsson GL, Hallen B: Laryngospasm during anaesthesia. A computer-aided incidence study in 136,929 patients. Acta Anaesthesiol Scand 28:567-575, 1984.

206. Olsson GL, Hallen B, Hambraeus-Jonzon K: Aspiration during anaesthesia: A computer-aided study of 185,358 anaesthetics. Acta Anaesthesiol Scand 30:84-92, 1986.

207. Oswalt CE, Gates GA, Holmstrom MG: Pulmonary edema as a complication of acute airway obstruction. JAMA 238:1833-1835, 1977.

208. Paulissian R, Salem MR, Joseph NJ, et al: Hemodynamic responses to endotracheal extubation after coronary artery bypass grafting. Anesth Analg 73:10-15, 1991.

209. Pearson FG, Gullane P: Subglottic resection with primary tracheal anastomosis: Including synchronous laryngotracheal reconstructions. Semin Thorac Cardiovasc Surg 8:381-391, 1996.

210. Pepin JL, Veale D, Mayer P, et al: Critical analysis of the result of surgery in the treatment of snoring, upper airway resistance syndrome (UARS), and obstructive sleep apnea (OSA). Sleep 19(9 Suppl): S90-S100, 1996.

211. Phero JC, Weaver JM, Peskin RM: Anesthesia for maxillofacial/mandibular trauma. Anesthesiol Clin North Am 11:509-523, 1993.

212. Pinsonneault C, Fortier J, Donati F: Tracheal resection and reconstruction. Can J Anaesth 46:439-455, 1999.

213. Popat M: Practical Fibreoptic Intubation. Oxford, Butterworth-Heinemann, 2001.

214. Potter JK, Herford AS, Ellis E III: Tracheotomy versus endotracheal intubation for airway management in deep neck space infections. J Oral Maxillofac Surg 60: 349-354, 2002.

215. Poutanen SM, Low DE, Henry B, et al: Identification of severe acute respiratory syndrome in Canada. N Engl J Med 348:1995-2005, 2003.

216. Rennotte MT, Baele P, Aubert G, Rodenstein DO: Nasal continuous positive airway pressure in the perioperative management of patients with obstructive sleep apnea submitted to surgery. Chest 107:367-374, 1995.

217. Rex MAE: A review of the structural and functional basis of laryngospasm and a discussion of nerve pathways involved in reflexes and its clinical significance in man and animals. Br J Anaesth 42:891-899, 1970.

218. Riley RW, Powell NB, Guilleminault C, et al: Obstructive sleep apnea surgery: Risk management and complications. Otolaryngol Head Neck Surg 117: 648-652, 1997.

219. Robinson PM: Prospective study of the complications of endoscopic laryngeal surgery. J Laryngol Otol 105:356-358, 1991.

220. Robles B, Hester J, Brock-Utne JG: Remember the gum-elastic bougie at extubation. J Clin Anesth 5: 329-331, 1993.

221. Rose DK, Cohen MM: The airway: Problems and predictions in 18,500 patients. Can J Anaesth 41: 372-383, 1994.

222. Rose DK, Cohen MM, Wigglesworth DF, DeBoer DP: Critical respiratory events in the postanesthesia care unit. Patient, surgical, and anesthetic factors. Anesthesiology 81:410-418, 1994.

223. Rosenbaum SH, Rosenbaum LM, Cole RP, et al: Use of the flexible fiberoptic bronchoscope to change endotracheal tubes in critically ill patients. Anesthesiology 54:169-170, 1981.

224. Sagi HC, Beutler W, Carroll E, Connolly PJ: Airway complications associated with surgery on the anterior cervical spine. Spine 27:949-953, 2002.

225. Salibian H, Jain S, Gabriel D, Azocar RJ: Conversion of an oral to nasal orotracheal intubation using an endotracheal tube exchanger. Anesth Analg 95:1822-2002.

226. Sandhu RS, Pasquale MD, Miller K, Wasser TE: Measurement of endotracheal tube cuff leak to predict postextubation stridor and need for reintubation. J Am Coll Surg 190:682-687, 2000.

227. Sarodia BD, Dasgupta A, Mehta AC: Management of airway manifestations of relapsing polychondritis: Case reports and review of literature. Chest 116:1669-1675, 1999.

228. Sasaki CT, Isaacson G: Functional anatomy of the larynx. Otolaryngol Clin North Am 21:595-612, 1988.

229. Schwartz LB, Sordill WC, Liebers RM: Difficulty in removal of accidentally cut endotracheal tube. J Oral Maxillofac Surg 40:518-519, 1982.

230. Seaman M, Ballinger P, Sturgill TD, Maertins M: Mediastinitis following nasal intubation in the emergency department. Am J Emerg Med 9:37-39, 1991.

231. Seitz PA, Gravenstein N: Endobronchial rupture from endotracheal reintubation with an endotracheal tube guide. J Clin Anesth 1:214-217, 1989.

232. Self DD, Bryson GL, Sullivan PJ: Risk factors for post-carotid endarterectomy hematoma formation. Can J Anaesth 46:635-640, 1999.

233. Shemie S: Steroids for anything that swells: Dexamethasone and postextubation airway obstruction. Crit Care Med 24:1613-1614, 1996.

234. Silva LCE, Brimacombe JR: Tracheal tube/laryngeal mask exchange for emergence. Anesthesiology 85:218, 1996.

235. Skues MA, Welchew EA: Anaesthesia and rheumatoid arthritis. Anaesthesia 48:989-997, 1993.

236. Smith JE, Fenner SG: Conversion of orotracheal to nasotracheal intubation with the aid of the fibreoptic laryngoscope. Anaesthesia 48:1016-1993.

237. Spiekermann BF, Stone DJ, Bogdonoff DL, Yemen TA: Airway management in neuroanaesthesia. Can J Anaesth 43:820-834, 1996.

238. Sprung J, Conley SF, Brown M: Unusual cause of difficult extubation. Anesthesiology 74:796-797, 1991.

239. Staffel JG, Weissler MC, Tyler EP, Drake AF: The prevention of postoperative stridor and laryngospasm with topical lidocaine. Arch Otolaryngol Head Neck Surg 117:1123-1128, 1991.

240. Steinberg MJ, Chmiel RA: Use of a nasogastric tube as a guide for endotracheal reintubation. J Oral Maxillofac Surg 47:1232-1233, 1989.

241. Stix MS, Borromeo CJ, Ata S, Teague PD: A modified intubating laryngeal mask for endotracheal tube exchange. Anesth Analg 91:1021-1023, 2000.

242. Sukhani R, Barclay J, Chow J: Paradoxical vocal cord motion: An unusual cause of stridor in the recovery room. Anesthesiology 79:177-180, 1993.

243. Sumiyoshi R, Kai T, Takahashi S: Application of negative-pressure ventilation when changing endotracheal tubes. Anesthesiology 81:1551-1552, 1994.

244. Szokol JW, Wenig BL, Murphy GS, Drezek E: Life-threatening upper airway obstruction after tongue base surgery. Anesthesiology 94:532-534, 2001.

245. Takita K, Morimoto Y, Kemmotsu O: Tracheal lidocaine attenuates the cardiovascular response to endotracheal intubation. Can J Anesth 48:732-736, 2001.

246. Tanski J, James RH: Difficult extubation due to a kinked pilot tube. Anaesthesia 41:1060-1986.

247. Tapnio RU, Viegas OJ: An alternative method for conversion of a nasal to an orotracheal intubation. Anesthesiology 88:1683-1684, 1998.

248. Tiret L, Desmonts JM, Hatton F, Vourc'h G: Complications associated with anaesthesia—A prospective survey in France. Can Anaesth Soc J 33:336-344, 1986.

249. Tolley NS, Cheesman TD, Morgan D, Brookes GB: Dislocated arytenoid: An intubation-induced injury. Ann R Coll Surg Engl 72:353-356, 1990.

250. Tomlinson AA: Difficult tracheal intubation. Anaesthesia 40:496-497, 1985.

251. Tousignant G, Kleiman SJ: Functional stridor diagnosed by the anaesthetist. Can J Anaesth 39:286-289, 1992.

252. Triglia JM, Nicollas R, Roman S, Kreitman B: Tracheomalacia associated with compressive cardiovascular anomalies in children. Pediatr Pulmonol Suppl 23:8-9, 2001.

253. Tso AS, Chung HS, Wu CY, et al: Anesthetic management of a patient with relapsing polychondritis— A case report. Acta Anaesthesiol Sin 39:189-194, 2001.

254. Tyers MR, Cronin K: Airway obstruction following second operation for carotid endarterectomy. Anaesth Intensive Care 14:314-316, 1986.

255. Vassal T, Anh NG, Gabillet JM, et al: Prospective evaluation of self-extubations in a medical intensive care unit. Intensive Care Med 19:340-342, 1993.

256. Venna RP, Rowbottom JR: A nine year retrospective review of post operative airway related problems in patients following multilevel anterior cervical corpectomy. Anesthesiology 95A:1171, 2002.

257. Vincken WG, Darauay CM, Cosio MG: Reversibility of upper airway obstruction after levodopa therapy in Parkinson's disease. Chest 96:210-212, 1989.

258. Vincken WG, Gauthier SG, Dollfuss RE, et al: Involvement of upper-airway muscles in extrapyramidal disorders. A cause of airflow limitation. N Engl J Med 311:438-442, 1984.

259. Wade JG, Larson CP Jr, Hickey RF, et al: Effect of carotid endarterectomy on carotid chemoreceptor and baroreceptor function in man. N Engl J Med 282:823-829, 1970.

260. Warner MA, Warner ME, Weber JG: Clinical significance of pulmonary aspiration during the perioperative period. Anesthesiology 78:56-62, 1993.

261. Watson CB: Use of fiberoptic bronchoscope to change endotracheal tube endorsed. Anesthesiology 55:476-477, 1981.

262. Wattenmaker I, Concepcion M, Hibberd P, Lipson S: Upper-airway obstruction and perioperative management of the airway in patients managed with posterior operations on the cervical spine for

rheumatoid arthritis. J Bone Joint Surg Am 76:360-365, 1994.

263. Weber S: Traumatic complications of airway management. Anesthesiol Clin North Am 20:265-274, 2002.

264. Wellwood M, Aylmer A, Teasdale S, et al: Extubation and myocardial ischemia. Anesthesiology 61:A132, 1984.

265. Wright CD: Tracheomalacia. Chest Surg Clin N Am 13:349-357, viii, 2003.

266. Yancey KB, Lawley TJ: Immunologically mediated skin diseases. In Fauci AS, Braunwald E, Isselbacher KJ et al (eds): Harrison's Principles of Internal Medicine, 14th ed. New York, McGraw-Hill, 1998, pp 1869-1874.

267. Yong AS, Elborn JS, Stanford CF: Cicatricial pemphigoid presenting as upper airways obstruction. Br J Clin Pract 48:47-48, 1994.

268. Zeitlin GA: Recovery room mishaps in the ASA closed claims study. ASA Newslett 53:28-30, 1989.

48

COMPLICATIONS OF MANAGING THE AIRWAY

Carin A. Hagberg
Rainer Georgi
Claude Krier

use electrocautery during the surgical procedure. This lack of communication between the anesthesiologist and the surgeon led to the patient having a burn injury to his face as a result of the high concentration of oxygen under the drapes.[208]

C. PLANNING AND SCHEDULING

A high number of complications in airway management result from insufficient communication between the members of the medical team and improper coordination of the patients in the daily OR schedule. A patient with a known difficult airway should be scheduled at a time when the most experienced personnel (anesthesiologists and surgeons) are available. Good communication of the entire staff is absolutely necessary to create optimal conditions for patient's safety.

Insufficient documentation of the results of the preoperative examination is a further source of difficulties. This is of greater concern when the anesthesiologist who is scheduled to secure the airway is not the same anesthesiologist who performed the preanesthetic examination.

Finally, a delay in the recognition of complications may lead to delayed therapy. Inadequate monitoring, nonfunctional equipment, and untrained staff are also important reasons for potential airway catastrophes. For optimal airway management, especially when unexpected difficulties arise, a difficult airway cart should be readily available and include additional devices and special equipment for managing airway problems at all anatomic levels.

II. COMPLICATIONS WITH SUPRAGLOTTIC DEVICES

A. MASK VENTILATION

The maximum risk of airway problems arises in the "cannot intubate and cannot ventilate" situation.[2] Difficult mask ventilation is an underestimated aspect of the difficult airway. The ability to ventilate and oxygenate the patient sufficiently using a bag-mask breathing system is an essential job of the anesthesiologist, and achieving proficiency in this task is essential. Mask ventilation is commonly performed at the onset of administration of almost all general anesthetics. As benign as both the technique and the mask may seem, each has its own potential set of problems.

1. Sterilization Process

Before any reusable mask is applied to a patient's face, it should be checked for leaks or pinhole defects in its air-filled bladder. If air or fluid is expressed from the bladder, the mask should be discarded immediately. A case report was published in which sterilizing solutions found access to the bladder of a reusable mask while it was being cleaned. Subsequent application of the mask to a patient's face resulted in extravasation of the cleaning fluid onto his cheeks. Some of that fluid leaked into his eyes, causing severe burning and irritation.[97] Another report identified a patient who contracted chemical conjunctivitis from glutaraldehyde on an anesthesia mask.[241] All reusable items applied to the skin of a patient should be free of residual cleansing agents. If the common cleaning solution, ethylene oxide, is not completely rinsed and aerated from reusable surfaces, it can cause serious mucosal injury. Water added to ethylene oxide forms ethylene glycol, an irritant. The presence of residual glutaraldehyde on an improperly rinsed laryngoscope blade has been implicated in causing massive tongue swelling and life-threatening allergic glossitis during an otherwise uncomplicated administration of general anesthesia.[143] Care must also be taken to rinse thoroughly the suction channel of a fiberoptic bronchoscope after cleaning. Residual agents may drip out of the bronchoscope port into the larynx or trachea, causing severe chemical burns.

2. Mechanical Difficulties

A mask is typically applied to a patient's face *before* induction of general anesthesia. Preoxygenation of the patient is the first and vital step in securing the airway. It should be performed almost immediately when the patient is on the OR table. The mask should be applied during spontaneous ventilation, prior to the administration of any pharmacologic agents. During such placement, the air-filled bladder of the mask should be inspected to ensure that when gentle pressure is applied, no rigid parts of the mask are in direct contact with the bridge of the nose or mandible. Bruising and soft tissue damage may occur in these regions if they are subjected to excessive pressure. Care must be taken to avoid contact with the eyes to prevent corneal abrasions, retinal artery occlusions, or blindness. As induction proceeds, both firmer mask pressure and stronger lifting pressure on the angle of the mandible are necessary to maintain a tight mask fit and secure an adequate airway. Pressure on the soft tissue of the submandibular region may obstruct the airway, especially in small children. In addition, excessive pressure on the mandible may damage the mandibular branch of the facial nerve, resulting in transient facial nerve paralysis.[133] Pressure from the rim of the mask on the mental nerves as they exit from the foramina has been implicated in causing lower lip numbness in two patients.[14]

Occasionally, the base of the tongue may fall back into the oropharynx during induction and obstruct the airway. Oropharyngeal airways must be gently inserted into the mouth to avoid injury, such as broken teeth or mucosal tears. Improper placement may cause worsened airway obstruction by forcing the tongue backward. Equal care should be given to the placement of nasopharyngeal airways to avoid nosebleeds and epistaxis.

Before insertion of an oropharyngeal or nasopharyngeal airway, optimal enlargement of the oropharyngeal space should be achieved. During conventional mask ventilation, the mandible is pressed against the maxilla. This maneuver generates a block in the condylar process. This phenomenon hinders sufficient mouth opening and maximal extension of the base of the tongue. Opening the mouth as a first step and drawing the mandible forward and upward as a second step avoid this unfavorable situation. Thus, the base of the tongue is displaced at a ventral position and the oropharyngeal space is increased.

During the course of induction, the lifting pressure applied to the angle of the mandible is sometimes sufficient to subluxate the temporomandibular joint (TMJ). Patients may experience persistent pain or bruising at these points and may even have chronic dislocation of the jaw, which may cause severe discomfort to the patient. These problems are not typical in small children but may be pronounced in adults.

Positive airway pressure can force air into the stomach instead of the trachea. This may result in an exaggerated condition of gastric distention, causing more difficult ventilation and an increased propensity for regurgitation. For these reasons, mask ventilation should not be performed in nonfasted or morbidly obese patients and patients with intestinal obstruction, Trendelenburg position, tracheoesophageal fistula, or massive oropharyngeal bleeding. Cricoid pressure can help reduce the amount of air being forced into the stomach and limit the likelihood of vomiting.

Langeron and coauthors[204] published an excellent paper regarding the prediction of difficult mask ventilation. Independent risk factors for difficulties with mask ventilation included the presence of a beard, body mass index greater than 26 kg/m^2, lack of teeth, age older than 55 years, and history of snoring. They determined that the presence of two of these factors was the best indicator of a difficult mask ventilation. Numerous factors can make mask ventilation difficult or impossible, such as patients with large tongues; heavy jaw muscles that resist mandibular subluxation; poor atlanto-occipital extension; uncertain pharyngeal pathology, especially masses; and facial burns or deformities such as nasal polyposis and receding mandible. In such cases, it may be best to avoid mask ventilation and perform awake fiberoptic intubation.

Patients with trauma to the pharyngeal mucosa may be at risk for subcutaneous emphysema. Patients who play wind instruments are also at risk because sufficiently high intrapharyngeal pressures can cause weakened soft tissue and laryngoceles in the lateral pharynx. The authors personally experienced difficulty with mask ventilation in a patient with an inner laryngocele, scheduled for its surgical removal. During mask ventilation, a valve mechanism developed at the base of the laryngocele. When positive-pressure ventilation with the bag-mask system was performed, the anesthetic gases filled the laryngocele, increasing it to a large balloon. Thus, further

mask ventilation and oxygenation were impossible. Routine direct laryngoscopy did not succeed, and endotracheal intubation was finally accomplished using a rigid bronchoscope.

Adequate monitoring during mask ventilation is necessary, such as observation of chest movement, pulse oximetry, measurement of end-tidal CO_2, and pressure control of ventilation. A precordial stethoscope is also recommended, especially in infants.

3. Prolonged Mask Ventilation

When a mask has been used for a prolonged amount of time, vulnerable parts of the face should be inspected for skin and soft tissue injury. The bridge of the nose and the area along the mandible are at particular risk for compromised blood flow.[307] Because mask ventilation offers no protection against silent regurgitation, the anesthesiologist should always be vigilant for any questionable airway noise, coughing, or bucking. Unlike opaque masks, transparent masks allow visualization of the mouth and early identification of vomitus, if it should occur.

As previously mentioned, extra care should be taken to avoid undue pressure on the eyes or the orbits to avoid abrasions or injuries to the retinal artery. Whenever continuous positive airway pressure is applied to patients with basilar skull fractures, pneumocephalus may occur.[172,194] At least one published case report identified positive airway pressure as the cause of bilateral otorrhagia.[353]

B. LARYNGEAL MASK AIRWAY

The laryngeal mask airway (LMA), a device designed for upper airway management, serves as a cross between a face mask and an ET. Thus far, the LMA has been used in millions of patients and is accepted as a safe technique in a large variety of surgical procedures. With use of the LMA, muscle relaxation is unnecessary, laryngoscopy is avoided, and hemodynamic changes are minimized during insertion. Because the LMA is tolerated at a lighter depth of anesthesia than an ET, its use may promote more rapid awakening and earlier discharge from the postanesthesia care unit.[358] The LMA has a clear advantage when laryngeal trauma must be minimized (e.g., in opera singers); when a standard mask fit is impossible because of facial burns, delicate skin, or a full beard; and when light planes of anesthesia are desired. It has also proved valuable in situations in which mask ventilation is unexpectedly difficult and direct laryngoscopy is impossible,[270] and it may be used as a conduit for a fiberoptic intubation with a standard ET. The device has been included in modified ASA difficult airway algorithm since 1996.[22]

Placing the LMA correctly can be difficult in some patients. The mask may fold on itself either under or over its main axis. Pressure on the epiglottis can push the device down into the glottic opening or entrap it within the laryngeal inlet of the mask. In the worst case, the tip of the epiglottis can be folded into the vocal cords, inducing increased work of breathing, coughing, laryngospasm, and sometimes complete airway obstruction.[37] Excess lubricant can leak into the trachea, also promoting coughing or laryngospasm.[37] Regardless of the problems encountered in placing the LMA, airway patency is usually maintained. Inadequate mouth opening (less than 1.5 cm), inadequate anesthetic depth, insertion with the cuff partially inflated, using an inappropriately sized LMA, inadequate force during insertion, and inadequate volumes for cuff inflation are some of the reasons for malpositioning the LMA.

Numerous complications are associated with the LMA. A known disadvantage of the device is its inability to protect against pulmonary aspiration and regurgitation of gastric contents. Because the LMA does not isolate the trachea from the esophagus, its use is risky when the patient has a full stomach or when high airway pressures are necessary for positive-pressure ventilation. Furthermore, the pressure in the lower esophageal sphincter is much lower in patients breathing spontaneously with an LMA than in those breathing through a face mask or a Guedel airway.[279] In one series, the incidence of regurgitation of small amounts of gastric contents was as high as 25% in patients breathing spontaneously with an LMA.[18] Fortunately, most of the reported patients had favorable outcomes because the regurgitated material was not aspirated or because the aspiration was relatively mild.[178] The overall risk of aspiration and regurgitation using the LMA is in the same low range as that with endotracheal intubation when the indications and contraindications of LMA usage are respected.[199] The potential risk of aspiration, which is due to the typical design of the airway device, has to be weighed against the advantages of the LMA in cases of difficult intubation and ventilation, in which the LMA is able to solve the problem immediately in many situations.

Several other complications of varying severity have been reported with use of the LMA. They are dependent upon the user's skill and experience, depth of anesthesia, and anatomic or pathologic factors related to the patient.[44] Failure to insert the LMA often results from inadequate anesthesia, suboptimal head and neck position, incorrect mask deflation, failure to follow the palatopharyngeal curve during insertion, inadequate depth of insertion, cricoid pressure, and enoral pathology such as large tonsils. Laryngospasm and coughing may result from inadequate anesthesia, tip impaction against the glottis, or aspiration. Mask leaks or inability to ventilate the lungs may also result from inadequate anesthesia, malpositioning or inappropriate mask size, and high airway pressures. Hypoventilation related to deep anesthesia may lead to a high end-tidal carbon dioxide concentration. Displacement of the LMA after insertion may be caused by inadequate anesthetic depth, a pulled or twisted tube, and inadequate mask size. Problems during emergence include laryngospasm and coughing when oral secretions enter the larynx following cuff deflation

or removal of the LMA at an inappropriate anesthetic depth, tube occlusion by biting, and regurgitation. Effects of pharyngolaryngeal reflexes such as laryngospasm, coughing, gagging, bronchospasm, breath holding, and retching may also be associated with usage of an LMA.

The incidence of sore throat with this device is reported to be 7% to 12%, an incidence similar to that seen with oral airways.[5,303] The incidence of failed placement is 1% to 5%, although this tends to decrease with increasing operator experience.[343] The LMA cuff is permeable to nitrous oxide and carbon dioxide, which results in substantial increases in cuff pressure and volume during prolonged procedures.[222] Increased intracuff pressures may increase the incidence of postoperative sore throat or cause transient dysarthria. Several published case reports mention edema of the epiglottis, uvula, and posterior pharyngeal wall; at the worst, these conditions have led to airway obstruction.[210,222,235] Hypoglossal nerve paralysis,[192] postobstructive pulmonary edema,[109] tongue cyanosis,[370] and transient dysarthria[214] have also been reported. Cuff pressure control is absolutely necessary to prevent these complications. Other problems with the LMA include dislodgment, kinking, and foreign bodies in the tube, leading to airway obstruction.[70] A case of complete separation of the tube from the LMA-Unique during removal of the mask was reported.[313]

New designs of the LMA have been developed in order to expand its comfort or safety in special situations. To minimize the risk of aspiration and regurgitation, the LMA ProSeal, a laryngeal mask with an esophageal vent, was developed.[38] Studies involving the LMA ProSeal show that it isolates the glottis from the upper esophagus when it is in correct position, with possible implications for further airway protection.[46,186] Cases of gastric insufflation and aspiration have been reported when this device was malpositioned.[48,111] Thus, testing the patency of the drain tube after each insertion is recommended.[45]

The intubating laryngeal mask airway (ILMA) was designed for difficult airway management to overcome unexpected difficult laryngoscopic intubation. Successful use of the ILMA in patients with difficult airways has been reported.[113,175] Tracheal intubation through the ILMA using its special silicone ETs is easier than using the LMA Classic as a conduit. Blind insertion of an ET through the standard laryngeal mask is associated with a low success rate.[23] The success rate of blind insertion of an ET through the ILMA is greater than 90%.[217] Branthwaite reported a case of laryngeal perforation leading to mediastinitis and the patient's death with this method of intubation.[40] The highest success rate of inserting an ET through any LMA is with fiberoptic guidance, which also has the lowest rate of damage of any laryngeal structures.

Contraindications to using an LMA include nonfasted patients, morbid obesity, necessity of high inspiratory pressures greater than 20 to 25 cm H_2O in the presence of low pulmonary compliance or chronic obstructive pulmonary disease, acute abdomen, hiatal hernia,

Zenker's diverticulum, trauma, intoxication, airway problems at the glottic or infraglottic level, and thoracic trauma.

C. ESOPHAGEAL-TRACHEAL COMBITUBE

The esophageal-tracheal Combitube is an esophagotracheal double-lumen airway designed for emergency use when standard airway management measures have failed.[116,117] Use in elective surgery has been reported.[120,149,161,338] The device is inserted blindly into the mouth and advanced to preset markings. The distal portion of the device is usually positioned within the esophagus. A distal cuff is inflated within the esophagus, and a large-volume proximal cuff is inflated inside the pharynx. Ventilation is first attempted through the esophageal lumen because esophageal intubation occurs in approximately 96% of insertions. If ventilation through this lumen fails, ventilation is attempted through the tracheal lumen. Although the device is designed for single use only, a study involving multiple reuse of the Combitube indicated no problems with reprocessing.[213] Another study warned against reuse because insufficient cleaning may lead to transmission of iatrogenic infections.[237]

The Combitube 37 Fr small adult (SA) is not recommended for patients below 120 cm in height, and the Combitube 41 Fr is not recommended for patients below 150 cm. Disregarding these recommendations may induce injury to the esophagus. Further contraindications to using a Combitube are intact gag reflexes, ingestion of caustic substances, known esophageal disease, airway problems at the glottic or infraglottic level,[116] and latex allergy.

There are some disadvantages of the Combitube because of its special design: maximal 8 hours of application (tracheobronchial care is difficult through the Combitube), inability to suction the trachea with the Combitube in the esophageal position (which may become a problem in patients with copious tracheal secretions), possible injuries of pharyngeal and esophageal soft tissues, and the fact that no pediatric sizes are available.

Few complications have been reported with use of the Combitube. In two patients, the device was inserted too far, causing the large pharyngeal cuff to lie directly over the glottis and obstruct the upper airway.[139] Consequently, no ventilation through either of the two lumens was possible. This problem was easily resolved by partially withdrawing the Combitube until breath sounds were auscultated. Although tongue discoloration has been reported while the pharyngeal cuff was inflated, it usually resolves immediately without further adverse sequelae when the cuff is deflated. Subcutaneous emphysema, pneumomediastinum, and pneumoperitoneum have been reported during resuscitation settings.[345] Two esophageal lacerations were reported in the study by Vézina and colleagues, but in both cases the distal cuff was overinflated with 20 to 40 mL instead of the recommended 12 mL and the larger Combitube (41 Fr) was used in a small patient. A 16% to 48% incidence of sore throat with the use of this device has been reported.[149,251,338]

The Combitube is widely accepted as a device for managing the difficult airway. It is included in the algorithm of the "Practice guidelines for management of the difficult airway" of the ASA,[8] "Guidelines for cardiopulmonary resuscitation and emergency cardiac care" of the American Heart Association,[7] and "Guidelines for the advanced management of the airway and ventilation during resuscitation" of the European Resuscitation Council.[108]

D. OTHER SUPRAGLOTTIC AIRWAY DEVICES

Many other devices are available for managing the airway at the supraglottic level: SoftSeal laryngeal mask (Smiths Medical, Keene, NH), Ambu AuraOnce (Ambu, Inc, Glen Burnie, MD), laryngeal tube (LT; King Systems, Noblesville, IN),[93] laryngeal tube suction (LTS; King Systems),[290] EasyTube (Teleflex Medical Ruesch, Bannockburn, IL),[329] perilaryngeal airway (CobraPLA; Engineered Medical Systems, Indianapolis, IN)[322] and SLIPA (SLIPA Medical Ltd, London, UK),[236] none of which are listed in the ASA Difficult Airway Algorithm. The EasyTube and SLIPA are only available in the UK. Like the LMA, the SoftSeal and the other devices do not efficiently protect the airway from regurgitation and aspiration, and are therefore contraindicated in nonfasting patients or in those who may have a full stomach. The ProSeal, LT, LTS, and EasyTube may provide better protection. All of these airway tools are cuffed devices designed for separating the airway from the esophagus. They have several advantages and disadvantages, and the main contraindications in routine use are similar to those of the LMA.

Most complications result from dislodgement, overfilling of cuffs, and insufficient depth of anesthesia. Most of the devices were developed in the last few years, and their acceptance is variable in routine practice. Although there is now a wide variety of alternative supraglottic devices, the practitioner should keep in mind that it is difficult to become proficient in all of them. These devices should first be utilized in the routine setting with "normal airways" as evidence that they can be used in difficult airways is being collected.

III. COMPLICATIONS WITH INTUBATION

A. ENDOTRACHEAL INTUBATION

1. Anatomic Considerations

Successful oral intubation requires four anatomic traits: adequate mouth opening, sufficient pharyngeal space (determined by visualization of the hypopharynx), compliant submandibular tissue (determined by measuring the thyromental distance), and adequate atlanto-occipital extension.[287] If the patient's anatomy is compromised in any of these factors, intubation is difficult at the very least. For optimal conditions, a free view to the vocal cords is necessary and the introduction of an ET can be easily performed.

The opening to the airway may be inadequate because of facial scars, TMJ disease, macroglossia, or dental disease. Nasal intubation techniques, such as blind or especially fiberoptic approaches, may overcome this problem. Blind techniques are associated with a higher incidence of complications and should be used cautiously.

The pharyngeal space may be limited by tumors, abscesses, edema, and surgical or traumatic disruption. Awake intubation may be necessary and should be considered whenever the pharyngeal space is limited by these conditions. If direct laryngoscopy is performed, the patient should be placed in the proper "sniffing" position and a styletted ET strongly considered. Every effort—backward upward rightward pressure (BURP)[324] or optimal external laryngeal manipulation (OELM)[25]—should be made to optimize visualization and identification of the laryngeal and pharyngeal structures.

The compliance of the submandibular space is critical to ensuring that the tongue is easily displaced in order to view the glottis. Compliance may be decreased by scarring, changes caused by radiation, or localized infections. Awake intubation or fiberoptic techniques should be strongly considered in these instances.

Extension of the atlanto-occipital region is critical in lifting the epiglottis off the posterior pharyngeal wall during direct laryngoscopy. A fused, fixed, or unstable spine may be rigid enough to impede visualization of the glottic structures. Again, fiberoptic techniques should be strongly considered.

2. Laryngoscope Modifications and Rigid Optical Instruments

Traditional laryngoscopes are designed for endotracheal intubation by direct vision of the vocal cords. In general, there are two types: the curved Macintosh blade and the straight blade (Miller with a curved tip and Wisconsin or Foregger with a straight tip). Most blade types are available in different sizes for all ages. The main injury in using laryngoscopes is damage to the teeth. In situations in which the glottis cannot be directly visualized, changing the patient's head position may lead to success. In some cases, a blade of inadequate size may be responsible for intubation failure. External laryngeal manipulation (BURP, OELM) may move the vocal cords into the line of vision and thus facilitate intubation. Unless performed with adequate topical anesthesia, laryngoscopy usually requires deep anesthesia because it causes stimulation of physiologic reflexes, and negative respiratory, cardiovascular, and neurologic adverse effects are possible (Table 48-3).[196] Patients with history of hypertension, pregnancy-induced hypertension, and ischemic heart disease are at additional risk. Deep anesthesia, application of topical anesthetics, drug prevention of the sympathoadrenal response using atropine or intravenous lidocaine, and minimizing mechanical stimulation attenuate these adverse effects.

Table 48-3 **Pathophysiologic Effects and Complications of Laryngoscopy and Endotracheal Intubation**

Cardiovascular system
Dysrhythmia
Hypertension
Myocardial ischemia and infarction
Respiratory system
Hypoxia
Hypercarbia
Laryngeal spasm
Bronchospasm
Central nervous system
Increased intracranial pressure
Eye
Increased intraocular pressure
Miscellaneous
Toxic and adverse effects of drugs related to laryngoscopy and intubation

Modified from Shang Ng W: In Latto IP, Vaughan RS: Difficulties in Tracheal Intubation. London, Saunders, 1997.

In order to optimize the sight of the vocal cords during laryngoscopy, many modifications of the classical laryngoscopes have been developed. The flexible tip blade from Corazelli-London or McCoy and Mirakhur may achieve a better view to the glottis by upright drawing of the epiglottis.[244]

Rigid optical instruments such as the Bonfils retromolar intubation fiberscope; the Bullard (ACMI, Southborough, MA), Upsher (Mercury Medical, Clearwater, FL) and WuScope (Achi Corp, San Jose, CA) laryngoscopes and the rigid bronchoscope are not common in all anesthesiology departments. In addition, they require more skill in handling and therefore should be used in routine cases in order to gain experience. The disadvantages of these instruments include a relative closed sight through the tube, injury potential of the laryngeal structures, possible perforation of the hypopharynx, and risk of damage to the teeth.

3. Difficult Intubation

Despite optimal positioning of the head and neck, the glottis is sometimes impossible to visualize, even in patients without any obvious predisposing features.[23,57,357] Risk factors for difficult tracheal intubation include male sex, age 40 to 59 years, and obesity.[287] Summarizing the literature regarding direct measurements of osseous structures, anesthesiologists should be aware of a potential difficult intubation in the following circumstances:

- long maxilla with protruding teeth
- anterior depth of mandible > 4.8 cm
- posterior depth of mandible > 2.7 cm (which limits submandibular displacement of the soft tissues)

- correlation between effective length of the mandible to posterior depth < 3.6
- rostral positioned angle of the mandible (i.e., a phenotypical receding mandible)
- caudally positioned hyoid bone (i.e., increasing of the mandible-hyoid distance)
- distance between the occiput and spinous process of C1 ~ 2.6 mm
- distance between spinous process of C1 and C2 ~ 2.6 mm (which narrows the limits of head extension)
- large neck circumference > 50 cm[21,57,65,166,246,357]

A chin-to-thyroid cartilage distance of less than three fingerbreadths (about 7 cm) hampers visualization of the glottis.[118] This is most likely because the soft tissues cannot be displaced into the submandibular space during direct laryngoscopy. In the absence of jaw measurements, the degree of difficulty of intubation may be predicted by performing a test described by Mallampati and associates[221] and modified by Samsoon and Young.[293] Miscellaneous causes of difficult securing of the airway are shown in Table 48-4.[199,289] Patients who prove difficult to intubate should be informed so that they may notify future anesthesiologists. In addition, patients should be registered with the Medic Alert system, as recommended by the ASA Task Force on the Difficult Airway.[8]

4. Traumatic Intubation

There is a close relationship between difficult intubation and traumatic intubation. In case of difficult intubation (poor view of the vocal cords), the practitioner tends to increase the lifting forces of the laryngoscope blade, which may lead to damage of the intraoral tissues and osseous structures. A vicious circle begins if the operator makes repeated attempts to intubate the patient without changing the length or type of blade or improving technique (positioning, OELM). A difficult intubation, thus, may become a traumatic intubation. Use of increasing forces may induce swelling, bleeding, or perforation as the intubation becomes more and more difficult and lead to a "cannot intubate" and possibly even a "cannot ventilate" situation. If intubation fails after multiple attempts, another technique should be used in accordance with the airway management algorithm.[8]

a. Lip Trauma

Lip injuries, which are typically found on the right upper lip, include lacerations, hematomas, edema, and teeth abrasions. They are usually secondary to inattentive laryngoscopy performed by inexperienced practitioners, the laryngoscope blade, and the teeth. Although these lesions are annoying to the patient, they are usually self-limited.

b. Dental Trauma

The incidence of dental injuries associated with anesthesia is greater than 1 in 4500.[350] Maxillary central incisors are at most risk. Fifty percent of dental trauma happens

Table 48-4 Miscellaneous Causes of Difficult Securing of the Airway

Symptoms
Dumpling voice
Hoarseness
Pathologic respiratory sound
Foreign body feeling
Odynophagia
Constitutional factors
Mouth opening < 3 cm
Microstomia
Dental abnormalities
Macroglossia
Receding mandible
Obesity
Buffalo neck
Moon face
Beard
Diseases
Limited temporomandibular joint mobility
Limited atlanto-occipital and atlantoaxial joint mobility
Unstable cervical spine
Limited laryngeal mobility
Postoperative or post-traumatic rigidity of the soft tissue of mouth and neck
Congenital, postoperative, post-traumatic anomalies of face and neck
Abscesses and tumors in face and neck
Paradontosis
Phlegmon of the floor of the mouth and of the neck
Epiglottitis
Mediastinitis
Stenosis of the upper airway
Enlarged goiter

Modified from Krier C, Georgi R: Airway management—Is there more than one "gold standard"? Anasthesiol Intensivmed Notfallmed Schmerzther 36:193-194, 2001.

during laryngoscopy, 23% following extubation, 8% during emergence, and 5% in context with regional anesthesia. Dental injuries are also associated with LMA devices and oropharyngeal airways. Dental injuries are most common in small children, patients with periodontal disease (in which structural support is poor) or fixed dental work (such as bridges and capped teeth), and patients in whom intubation is difficult. Preexisting dental pathology should be thoroughly explored before the induction of anesthesia. All loose, diseased, chipped, or capped teeth must be noted in the anesthetic preoperative assessment before intubation,[60] and the patient must be advised of the risk of dental damage. Protrusion of the upper incisors (overbite), carious teeth, paradentosis (degenerative process), and periodontitis (inflammatory process) are causes for dental injuries during laryngoscopy. Although tooth guards may be awkward and possibly obstruct vision,[11] their use may be indicated in certain situations and the time for intubation is not significantly longer.[52]

If a tooth is chipped or partially broken, the fragment should be located and retrieved. Unfortunately, it cannot be reaffixed to the original tooth. In the event that an entire tooth is avulsed, it should be retrieved and saved in a moist gauze or in normal saline without cleansing. Great care should be taken to ensure that any dislodged teeth or tooth fragments do not slip into the pharynx to become lodged later into the esophagus or larynx. Tooth aspiration may induce serious complications requiring rigid or flexible bronchoscopy for removal. With a rapid response from an oral surgeon or dentist, an intact tooth can often be reimplanted and saved,[278] but only when performed within 1 hour.

c. Tongue Injury

Massive tongue swelling, or macroglossia, has been reported in numerous instances. This condition occurs in both adult and pediatric patients.[226,326] Although macroglossia (occasionally to a life-threatening degree) is associated with angiotensin-converting enzyme inhibitors,[190] some cases have occurred while a bite block was in place, some with an oral airway, some with soft tissue compression of the chin, and some with no protective device at all. The common denominator was that they all occurred when there was substantial neck flexion during endotracheal intubation and surgery was prolonged. Macroglossia is thought to be secondary to obstructed venous and lymphatic drainage of the tongue. In each case, it was thought that the ET may have severely compromised the circulation on the affected side of the tongue. There has also been a report of sudden onset of tongue swelling after the surgical repair of a cleft palate.[267] During this surgery, the tongue was retracted extensively, which may have led to postoperative swelling. Obstruction of the submandibular duct by an ET may also lead to massive tongue swelling.[156] Loss of tongue sensation is possible after a compression injury to the lingual nerve during forceful laryngoscopy or after LMA placement with an overinflated or malpositioned cuff.[354] Reduced sense of taste and cyanosis of the tongue caused by lingual artery compression are additional injuries that may be caused by an oversized, malpositioned, or overinflated LMA.

d. Damage to the Uvula

The uvula can be traumatized by anything that is placed in the oral cavity. It is usually associated with an ET, oropharyngeal and nasopharyngeal airways, an LMA,[84] or an alternative supraglottic airway device or by overzealous use of a suction catheter.[36] The results of damaging the uvula are edema and necrosis.[84,197] Sore throat, odynophagia, painful swallowing, coughing, foreign body sensation, and serious life-threatening airway obstruction have been reported.[150]

e. Pharyngeal Mucosal Damage

The incidence of sore throat after intubation is approximately 40% and is greater than 65% when blood is noted on the airway instruments.[239] The incidence of macroscopic blood on the LMA varies between 1% and 22%, depending on the insertion technique.[44] The incidence of sore throat following LMA placement is 20% to 42%, depending on cuff inflation, and 8% with face mask ventilation.[47] Sore throat, hoarse voice, and epiglottic edema have been reported following ILMA usage.[56] The incidence of sore throat associated with use of the Combitube is 16% to 48%.[149,251,338] Aggressive suctioning of the posterior pharynx should be discouraged. The incidence of a sore throat is substantially higher in women and in patients after thyroid surgery. No correlation has been made with such factors as age, use of muscle relaxants, type of narcotic, number of intubation attempts, or duration of intubation. Fortunately, pain on swallowing usually lasts no more than 24 to 48 hours and can be relieved in part by having the patient breathe humidified air. Topical anesthesia, such as lidocaine jelly, applied to the ET does not lessen the incidence of this problem and may actually worsen it.

f. Laryngeal Trauma and Damage to the Vocal Cords

Trauma to the larynx is not uncommon following endotracheal intubation. It depends on the experience and the skill of the intubator as well as the degree of difficulty. In one large study, 6.2% of patients sustained severe lesions, 4.5% developed a hematoma of the vocal cords, 1% developed a hematoma of the supraglottic region, and 1% sustained lacerations and scars of the vocal cord mucosa.[181] Recovery is generally prompt with conservative therapy,[271] although hoarseness may appear even after a 2-week interval.[284]

Granulations usually occur as a complication of long-term intubation but have been reported with short-term intubation as well.[94] Intubation can result in varying degrees of laryngeal trauma, such as thickening, edema, erythema, hematoma, and granuloma of the vocal folds.[5,233] Injuries of the laryngeal muscles and suspensory ligaments are also possible. It is recommended that the larynx be inspected for injury before insertion of the ET to document and treat any preexistent lesions. Anesthesiologists should be vigilant in all cases of hoarseness. These patients should be examined by an ear, nose, and throat (ENT) specialist preoperatively. A small but significant number of patients sustain laryngeal injuries during short-term intubation.[94] Damage to the larynx is possible by direct traumatization during an intubation procedure (leads to anterior arytenoid luxation) and also by the pressure of the ET (leads to posterior arytenoid luxation).

Arytenoid dislocation and subluxation have been reported as rare complications.[83,119,137,158] Mitigating factors include traumatic and difficult intubations, repeated attempts at intubation, and attempted intubation using blind techniques such as light-guided intubation,[9] retrograde intubation, and use of the McCoy laryngoscope.[339] Yet these complications have been reported following easy intubations as well.[125] Early diagnosis and operative reposition of arytenoid dislocation are necessary because fibrosation with consecutive malposition and ankylosis may occur after 48 hours.

The vocal process of the arytenoid is the most common site of injury caused by the ET, as it is positioned between the vocal cords. Granuloma formation most commonly occurs at this site. The degree of injury worsens as the size of the tube[34] and the duration of intubation increase.

Numerous investigators have reported vocal cord paralysis (VCP) after intubation with no other obvious source of injury.[39,59,212,249] One report associated VCP with the use of ethylene oxide to sterilize ETs.[174] VCP may be more prominent after certain surgical procedures, including ENT procedures, carotid endarterectomy and anterior cervical fusions. Interestingly, VCP after cardiovascular surgery has been reported to occur at the rate of 2% to 32%.[86,171] Paralysis may be unilateral or bilateral. Hoarseness occurs with unilateral paralysis, whereas respiratory obstruction occurs with bilateral problems. The most likely source of injury is an ET cuff, malpositioned in the subglottic larynx, that presses on the recurrent laryngeal nerve as it passes between the thyroid cartilage and the vocal process of the arytenoid cartilage.[59,212] Recently, Itagaki et al demonstrated that aortic procedures and prolonged operation increase the risk of VCP and that most poor outcomes were found in aortic rather than non-aortic procedures, such as coronary artery bypass.

Itagaki suggested that the use of deep hypothermia and double lumen tubes, as well as surgical invasion to the recurrent laryngeal nerve may be associated with a relatively high risk of VCP. Permanent voice change after intubation because of external laryngeal nerve trauma has been reported in up to 3% of patients undergoing surgery in sites other than the head or neck. However, vocal cord paralysis after intubation is usually temporary. Its incidence may be decreased by avoiding overinflation of the ET cuff and by placing the ET at least 15 mm below the vocal cords.[59] Vocal cord paralysis may also have a central origin. One case was reported in which an infant with a Dandy-Walker cyst sustained left vocal cord paralysis after placement of a cystoperitoneal shunt.[226]

Eroded vocal cords may adhere together, eventually forming synechiae. This is a potential problem whenever airflow between the vocal cords has been compromised as a result of tracheostomy.[193] Surgical correction is usually necessary.

g. Tracheobronchial Trauma

Tracheal trauma is caused by various sources.[341] Injury may result from an overinflated ET cuff, inadequate tube size, malpositioned tube tip, laryngoscope, stylet, tube exchanger, or related equipment. Predisposing factors include anatomic difficulties, blind or hurried intubation, inadequate positioning, poor visualization, or, most commonly, inexperience on the part of the intubator. The presence of an ET may lead to edema, desquamation, inflammation, and ulceration of the airway.[184] The severity of the injury may be related to the duration of intubation, although this relation is not well established.[314] Any irritating stimulus, such as pressure from an oversized ET, dry inhaled gases, allergic reactions to inhaled sprays, or chemical irritation from residual cleaning solutions, can initiate an inflammatory response and cause mucosal edema in the larynx or trachea. Edema after extubation limits the lumen diameter and increases airway resistance. Small children are most susceptible to this problem, in which a sudden increase in airway resistance results from laryngotracheobronchitis or croup. Almost 4% of children 1 to 3 years of age develop croup following endotracheal intubation.[177,269] In addition, mechanical trauma may result from sharp objects within the trachea, such as a stylet tip that extends beyond the length of the ET. Tracheal rupture, especially after emergency intubation, has been reported,[224,347] as well as a bronchial rupture secondary to use of an ET exchanger.[299]

ET cuffs inflated to a pressure greater than that of the capillary perfusion may devitalize the tracheal mucosa, leading to ulceration, necrosis, and loss of structural integrity.[253] Ulceration occurs at even lower pressures in hypotensive patients. The need for increasing cuff volumes to maintain a seal is an ominous sign of tracheomalacia.[147] Massive gastric distention in an intubated patient may signal the presence of a tracheoesophageal fistula as the cuff progressively erodes into the esophagus.[328] Likewise, any patient with more than 10 mL of blood in the ET without a known cause should be suspected of having a tracheocarotid fistula.[215] The various nerves in this region of the neck are also at risk. Erosion of the ET into the paratracheal nerves may result in dysphonia, hoarseness, and laryngeal incompetence. Tracheomalacia results from erosion confined to the tracheal cartilages. It is imperative that the anesthesiologist inflate the cuff of the ET only as much as necessary to ensure an adequate airway seal. If using nitrous oxide during a lengthy surgical procedure, the pressure in the ET cuff should be checked by a cuff pressure control device. In the presence of 70% nitrous oxide, intracuff pressures take an average of 12 minutes to increase to levels that are potentially high enough to cause tracheal ischemia.[253] The cuff pressure should not exceed 25 cm H_2O. Increasing cuff pressure by surgical manipulations can also be observed and prevented by using a cuff pressure control device.

A potential adverse consequence of the ET is erosion of the tracheal mucosa. Denuded tissue is eventually replaced with scar tissue, which ultimately retracts and leads to stenoses of the trachea, larynx, or nares. The incidence of granulomas has been reported to range from 1 in 800[167] to 1 in 20,000.[308] They are more common in women than in men and occur only rarely in children. The most common site of erosion is along the posterior laryngeal wall, where granulation tissue easily overgrows. Side effects of granulomas include cough, hoarseness, and sore throat pain. The growths may be prevented by minimizing the trauma associated with laryngoscopy and intubation. When granulomas do occur, surgical excision is usually required.

Membranes and webs may eventually replace tracheal and laryngeal ulcers. These growths are commonly thick and gray. Care should be taken while intubating patients with such lesions because inadvertent detachment may result in respiratory obstruction or bleeding into the airway. With time, the inflammatory process associated with laryngeal ulcers may extend to the laryngeal cartilage. Should this occur, the cartilage may become inflamed (chondritis) or softened (chondromalacia).

Several months after prolonged endotracheal intubation, tracheal stenosis and fibrosis may occur. This usually represents the end stage of a progression from tracheal wall erosion to cartilaginous weakening to healing with fibrosis formation.[341] Stenoses typically occur at the site of an inflated cuff, although they may occur at the location of the ET tip. Symptoms include a nonproductive cough, dyspnea, and signs of respiratory obstruction. Dilation of the stenosis is curative if the stenosis is caught in its early stages. However, surgical correction may be necessary when the tracheal lumen has been reduced to 4 to 5 mm.[127,229]

Supraglottic complications induced by long-term intubation may be prevented by early tracheostomy. There is no evidence about the ideal time of tracheostomy in long-term ventilated patients.

h. Barotrauma

Barotrauma results from high-pressure distention of intrapulmonary structures. High-flow insufflation techniques in which small catheters are used distal to the larynx are most often associated with barotrauma. Such problems are common in microlaryngeal surgery in which jet ventilation is used.[15,61,101,260,356] Direct impingement of the catheter tip on the tracheal mucosa may also cause barotrauma.[101] Edema or hematoma may occur if the jet of air strikes the mucosa of the larynx or the vocal cords, leading to laryngospasm.[216] Whenever air leaks into the peribronchial tissues, it can traverse into the subcutaneous space, the lung interstitium, or the pleural and pericardial cavities. Pneumomediastinum or tension pneumothorax is the result. The progressive accumulation of air may cause loss of pulmonary compliance, loss of ventilatory volume, or, if the accumulation is large enough, pericardial and pulmonary tamponade. Safety mechanisms should be in place to prevent high-pressure airflow in the event that intrapulmonary pressures become excessive. For diseased pulmonary tissue, the least possible airway pressure should be used to prevent parenchymal blowout. This advice also applies to patients with blunt thoracic trauma who have subcutaneous emphysema. Such patients should be presumed to have a bronchial leak until proved otherwise, and only low-pressure ventilation should be used until the lesions are located. In the presence of pneumothorax, chest tubes help relieve the problem until it is corrected surgically.

i. Nerve Injuries

Laryngoscopy and cuffed supraglottic airway devices may cause periodic or permanent nerve injury. Transient weakness, numbness, or paralysis of the tongue can occur after laryngoscopy, presumably because of pressure on the laryngeal and hypoglossal nerves.[318] One patient experienced a loss of sensation in the tongue for 1 month because of lingual nerve compression during a difficult intubation.[327] Damage to the internal branch of the superior laryngeal nerve during difficult intubation leading to anesthesia of the upper surface of the larynx has been reported in two patients.[12] Fortunately, the latter complication usually does not persist.

Transient palsies were described when using an LMA device by affecting the hypoglossal[243] and lingual[207] nerves. Malposition of the cuff or tube may be one reason for these rare injuries. Ahmad and Yentis postulated that the lingual nerve injury may occur where the nerve distal to its gingival branch is compressed by the shaft of the LMA tube against the side of the tongue.[3] Overinflation of the cuff is another reason for nerve damage. This practice can also lead to tongue cyanosis and trauma to the uvula, tonsils, posterior pharyngeal wall, and larynx.

The authors personally observed five cases of uncomplicated nasotracheal intubation for head and neck surgery (augmentation of the mandible or the maxillary sinus for teeth implantation) resulting in a hyposmia and in one case an anosmia. We used preformed nasotracheal tubes, presoaked in warm water and well lubricated with lidocaine jelly. Males were intubated with a tube inner diameter of 7.5 mm, females with 6.5 mm. The hyposmias completely recovered in 3 to 6 months, whereas the anosmia became permanent. Consultations were made with ENT surgeons, neurologists, pharmacologists, and other anesthesia colleagues, but no explanation for this phenomenon could be ascertained.

j. Spinal Cord and Vertebral Column Injury

Airway management techniques such as chin lift, jaw thrust, and direct laryngoscopy transmit movement to the cervical spine and may disturb the spine to some degree. When a patient's neck is fused as a result of ankylosing spondylitis, adequate neck extension may be impossible to obtain. Attempts to hyperextend the necks of these patients may result in cervical fractures and quadriplegia.[291] Fixation of a head in a cervical collar or halo does not allow neck extension and may limit the successful use of direct laryngoscopy. A fiberoptic intubation or an intubation with an indirect rigid fiberoptic laryngoscope or stylet may be considered in these cases. However, in emergency settings fiberoptic intubation is often impractical.[333] In urgently required intubations, sufficient manual in-line stabilization should be performed during direct laryngoscopy for orotracheal intubation.[78]

This might reduce the risk of secondary injury induced by movement, but this has not been proved, and it does not completely prevent spinal movement.

Special attention should be given to patients with C1 or C2 fractures because any degree of extension might compromise spinal cord function. Ten percent to 25% of spinal cord injuries occur secondary to improper immobilization of the vertebral column after trauma.[69,272,285] Hastings and Kelley[157] reported neurologic deterioration associated with direct laryngoscopy in a patient with a cervical spine injury. They found a 1% to 3% incidence of neurologic deterioration after elective surgery with tracheal intubation. Inadequate airway management may result in the disaster of permanent spinal cord injury. A case of quadriplegia after bag-mask ventilation, direct laryngoscopy, and cricothyroidotomy in an unrecognized cervical spine–injured patient has been reported.[157]

Several conditions, such as Down syndrome and rheumatoid arthritis, are associated with atlantoaxial instability.[77,362] Twenty-five percent of all Down patients have a flabby atlantoaxial joint. Excessive neck extension in a patient with an undiagnosed Arnold-Chiari malformation may cause worsening of cerebellar tonsil herniation.[91] Also, elderly patients and those with pathologic fragility, such as connective tissue disorders, lytic bone tumors, and osteoporosis, should be intubated with caution. Extreme extension should be avoided in every patient because of loss of muscle tone with curarizing drugs. Whenever reasonable doubt about the degree of neck extension exists (regardless of the cause), a range-of-motion test and an assessment of neck extension should be performed before inducing anesthesia. To prevent neurologic deterioration, awake fiberoptic intubation should be considered in all cases when time is not crucial.

k. Eye Injuries

Corneal abrasions are reported to be the most common eye complication that occurs during general anesthesia.[132] They are primarily caused by a face mask being placed on an open eye[19,309] or by the eyelids not being completely closed during anesthesia. Jewelry, identification cards, and loose-fitting watch bands have been implicated in scratching the eye.[344] In addition, a stethoscope hanging from the neck of a clinician can fall forward and strike the patient's eyes or forehead. Prevention consists of vigilance on the part of the anesthesiologist and application of adhesive tape over the closed eyelids. Especially during head and neck surgery, the eyelids should be closed by tape and covered carefully with soft eye pads. Some clinicians routinely apply lubricating ointment, such as petroleum, mineral oil, and lanolin (Lacri-Lube), to the inside of the eyelids, yet this has not been proved to increase efficacy. Although these injuries typically heal within 24 hours, they are usually painful and can lead to corneal ulceration. An immediate ophthalmologic consultation is recommended. Local anesthetics should not be applied because they can delay regeneration of the epithelium and may promote keratitis. Treatment consists of allowing the injured eye to rest by use of an eye patch and applying an antibiotic ointment.

In the presence of a penetrating eye injury, anesthesia should be induced without coughing and bucking and, if succinylcholine is used, a nondepolarizing relaxant should be used for precurarization in order to avoid increasing intraocular pressure.

l. Temporomandibular Joint Injuries

The anatomy of the TMJ is special: one side cannot be moved without the other side. Both joints represent a functional unit, and injuries to one TMJ concern the opposite side. Opening the mouth is a combination of rotary and translational movement in the joint. The rotary movement allows a mouth opening of approximately 25 mm. Maximal opening is achieved by the translational movement. Pathologic changes such as bone cysts and atrophy of the mandible related to age can reduce joint mobility, which may lead to fractures.

Rupture of the lateral ligament is possible. TMJ injuries are caused by increasing forces during laryngoscopy to optimize the view of the glottis. As a result, limited mouth opening, pain in the joint, lateral deviation of the mandible (in case of unilateral luxation), protrusion of the mandible (in case of bilateral luxation), and lockjaw (in case of fixation after joint luxation) may occur. Most of the cases of TMJ injury have not been associated with difficult airway management.[63] In the ASA closed claims database, only 17% of the claims had documented preexisting TMJ disorders, such as pain.[90] The presence of predisposing factors as described previously is more probable.

4. Nasotracheal Intubation

a. Cranial Intubation

Nasotracheal intubations are potentially hazardous. In the presence of basilar skull fractures or certain facial fractures (such as Le Fort II or III fractures), the ET may be inadvertently introduced into the cranial vault (Fig. 48-1).[164] Green and colleagues[138] reported a case of an uncomplicated nasotracheal intubation in which asystole occurred after the tube was introduced into the orbit. Substantial facial trauma and evidence of basilar skull fractures are usually considered to be contraindications for this technique. However, Bähr and Stoll[16] argued that if special care is taken, the complication rates of oral and nasal intubation do not differ. Nevertheless, if nasal intubation is going to be attempted in a patient with a known or suspected skull fracture, it should be performed only by using fiberoptic bronchoscopy and with extreme caution in the inferior nasal meatus. The middle turbinate bone is part of the frontal base of the skull. In case of midfacial fractures with primary intact dura mater, it is possible to open the dura by manipulation during nasotracheal intubation. Nasotracheal tubes may also dissect backward and run behind the posterior pharyngeal wall. Patients with an obstructed nasal passage secondary to convoluted turbinates are at increased risk for this complication.

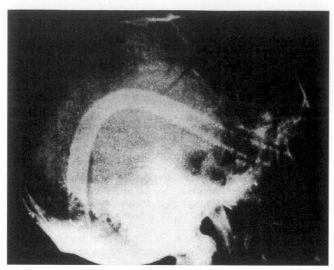

Figure 48-1 Intracranial nasotracheal tube (computer enhanced). (From Horellou MF, Mathe D, Feiss P: A hazard of naso-tracheal intubation [letter]. Anaesthesia 33:73-74, 1978.)

b. Nasal Injury

Although problems with nasotracheal intubation are more likely to occur in the presence of hypertrophic turbinates, extreme deviation of the nasal septum, prominences of the nasal septum, chronic infections in the nasal cavity, and nasal polyposis, nasal injury can occur during the performance of any nasotracheal intubation.

Nasal intubation may cause lacerations of the nasal mucosa, hemorrhage, and epistaxis. Nosebleeds are common but are relatively easy to prevent. It is paramount that the nasal mucosa be vasoconstricted before instrumentation. Some agents used for this purpose are 0.5% phenylephrine in 4% lidocaine or 0.1% xylometazoline.[254] Cocaine 4% may be associated with severe adverse effects and caution should be exercised with its use.[199] To minimize the chance of nasal injury, a small ET that has been lubricated well and presoaked in warm water (to increase its pliability) should be used. Minor bruising occurs in 54% of nasal intubations and most commonly involves the mucosa overlying the inferior turbinate and the adjacent septum.[250] Should epistaxis occur, it is recommended that the ET cuff be inflated and remain in the nostril to tamponade the bleeding.

Additional complications caused by nasotracheal intubation include dislodgement of nasal polyps[32] or of a nasal turbinate,[273,360] adenoidectomy, injury of the nasal septum, and perforation of the piriform recess or epiglottic vallecula. In case of injury to the piriform recess, damage of the internal branch of superior laryngeal nerve (which supplies the epiglottis and soft tissue of pharynx and larynx) or superior laryngeal vessels may occur. Rents in the pharyngeal mucosa can mature into retropharyngeal abscesses.[146] One case of external compression of the nasotracheal tube related to the displaced bone fragments of multiple Le Fort fractures has been reported.[175]

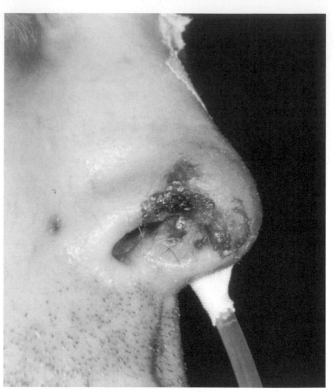

Figure 48-2 Necrosis of right nasal wing after a 3 days of intubation with an anatomic preformed tube.

Delayed complications of nasotracheal intubation are pharyngitis, rhinitis, and synechia between the nasal septum and inferior turbinate bone. When the tube is secured in the trachea, care should be taken to ensure that it is also secured properly at the level of the nostril. Distortion of the nares can lead to ischemia, skin necrosis, or nasal adhesion. Some injuries to the nose and endonasal structures have already been described. Using anatomically preformed tubes for head and neck surgery may also lead to pressure necrosis (Fig. 48-2). Wrapping the tube with foam material at the entrance to the nares and careful nursing in long-term intubation may reduce or avoid this complication.

Even in the absence of gross trauma, the mechanical damage to the superficial epithelial layers caused by nasal intubation results in mucociliary slowing in 65% of patients[106] and bacteremia in another 5.5%.[87] The most common organisms introduced into the blood are nasopharyngeal commensal organisms (e.g., *Streptococcus viridans*), which are known to cause endocarditis and systemic infection. Even short-term intubation has been reported to cause nasal septal and retropharyngeal abscesses. Acute otitis media has been reported to occur in 13% of nasally intubated neonates.[144] Paranasal sinusitis has also been reported, most commonly with nasal intubation for more than 5 days.[257,359] Infection may be related to sustained edema and occlusion of the sinus drainage pathways. Prompt diagnosis is critical, and paranasal sinusitis should be suspected in any patient with facial tenderness, pain, or purulent nasal discharge or in any nasally intubated patient who develops sepsis with no other obvious source.

Fractures of the frontal part of the skull base with cerebrospinal rhinorrhea, intranasal abscesses or abscesses with intranasal expansion, choanal atresia, hyperplastic tonsils, tendency to uncontrollable nasal bleeding, and coagulopathies are contraindications for nasotracheal intubation.

A careful examination of the patient is absolutely necessary. Hypertonia, coagulopathies, and post-traumatic and postoperative conditions of the nasal structures should be ascertained in the patient's history. Any history of previous trauma or surgery involving the nasal structures should also be noted.

c. Foreign Bodies

The nostrils are common sites for entry of foreign bodies. Small children, who are known for placing small objects into their orifices, find that the nostrils are some of the most accessible sites. Over 80% of patients with aspiration of a foreign body are children,[101] with a mean age between 1 and 3 years.[115,302] Foreign body aspiration is the cause of death in 7% of the children younger than 4 years.

Smith and coworkers reported a rhinolith that became dislodged during nasotracheal intubation.[306] The mass was formed around the rubber tire of a toy car that the patient had placed in his nose 30 years earlier. Fortunately, the rhinolith caused no problems. However, during nasotracheal intubation, great potential exists to dislodge any similar foreign bodies, after which they may obstruct the ET, pharynx, or trachea. If a nasal foreign body is known or suspected, it should be gingerly dislodged and advanced into the oropharynx, if possible, where it can be retrieved before intubation. Mask ventilation may also dislodge foreign bodies into the lower parts of the airway.

6. Esophageal Intubation

a. Endotracheal Tube Placement

When visualization of the glottis is difficult, the ET may inadvertently be introduced into the esophagus. Esophageal intubation is more common with inexperienced practitioners, but it may also occur in experienced hands. Intubating the esophagus is not disastrous, but failing to detect and correct the condition is. Recognition of this error must be rapid to avoid the adverse effects of prolonged hypoxia. A closed claims analysis of adverse anesthetic events reported that 18% of respiration-related claims involved esophageal intubation.[55] Preoxygenation can help alleviate this problem by allowing a longer apneic period before intubation and by delaying the onset of hypoxemia for up to 6 to 9 minutes after nitrogen elimination.[234]

End-tidal CO_2 monitoring is essential in confirming endotracheal placement of the ET. Capnography should be available wherever intubation is performed.

In out-of-hospital practice and emergency medicine, where capnography may not be available, calorimetric single-use CO_2 detectors or the esophageal detector device has been reported to be successful in detecting failed intubation 94.6% of the time.[325] Fiberoptic bronchoscopy is another safe method to confirm the proper position of an ET. All other signs, such as equal bilateral breath sounds, symmetric bilateral chest wall movement, epigastric auscultation, and observation of tube condensation, are potentially misleading.[33] Esophageal intubation can briefly produce an end-tidal CO_2 capnogram (for example, in the presence of CO_2-containing drinks in the stomach),[373] but the waveform diminishes rapidly after three to five breaths.[320] Excessive distention of the stomach with gas containing CO_2 may follow vigorous manual inflation while testing for correct tube placement. The use of video laryngoscopy, in which endotracheal intubation can be visualized on a monitor, may prove efficacious in the prevention of inadvertent esophageal intubation.

It is recommended that a misplaced tube remain in place while the trachea is correctly intubated. This not only helps identify the correct orifice for intubation but also protects the trachea from invasion by regurgitated stomach contents. Once proper endotracheal intubation is achieved after an esophageal intubation, the stomach should be suctioned to minimize vomiting, gastric perforation, or compromise of ventilation.

b. Esophageal Perforation and Retropharyngeal Abscess

Perforation of the esophagus has been reported on several occasions.[13,103,122,173,198,211,219,248,372] It is most likely to occur when inexperienced clinicians handle emergency situations, when intubation is difficult, or in the presence of esophageal pathology. Perforation occurs most commonly over the cricopharyngeus muscle on the posterior esophageal wall, where the esophagus is narrowed and thin. Subcutaneous emphysema, pneumothorax, fever, cellulitis, cyanosis, sore throat, mediastinitis, empyema, pericarditis, and death can occur. Early detection and treatment of the condition are critical because the mortality rate of mediastinitis is greater than 50%. An esophageal perforation should be suspected in any patient with a fever, sore throat, and subcutaneous emphysema following a history of difficult intubation.

A published case report identified a traumatic tracheal perforation through the esophagus in a patient with difficult intubation.[283] As previously mentioned, two cases of esophageal perforation were reported with the use of a Combitube in emergency situations, either in the presence of esophageal pathology or using an inappropriate size of the device.[345]

7. Bronchial Intubation

a. Standard Endotracheal Tube Placement

Bronchial intubation often occurs and is sometimes difficult to identify. Asymmetric chest expansion, unilateral absence of breath sounds (usually on the left side), and eventual arterial blood gas abnormalities are diagnostic features. Bronchial intubation (most commonly right sided) is more common in infants and children because of the small distance between the carina and the glottis. The position of the tip of the tube should be carefully monitored in children. If bronchial intubation goes undetected, it may lead to atelectasis, hypoxia, and pulmonary edema.[196] Transillumination of the neck with a light wand[231] can assist in ET location, but not in patients with a large amount of soft tissue in the anterior neck, such as obese patients and those with large goiters. Fiberoptic bronchoscopy is the best method to detect proper position of the ET. Also, the ET may be deliberately advanced into a main stem bronchus and withdrawn until bilateral breath sounds are auscultated.

The tip of the ET may be moved during flexion or extension of the patient's head as the patient is positioned for surgery. Conrardy and colleagues[71] showed that the tip of the ET moved an average of 3.8 cm toward the carina when the neck was moved from full extension to full flexion. In some patients, this change was as great as 6.4 cm (Fig. 48-3).[71] It is easy to remember that the tip of the ET moves in the same direction as the patient's nose. If the patient's neck is flexed, the nose is pointed downward and the ET advances farther into the trachea. In addition, the tube moves away from the carina an average of 0.7 cm during lateral rotation of the head. Care should be taken in cases where the surgeon shares the airway during surgery, such as cleft palate surgery or tonsillectomy. Special blades used by the surgeon to achieve a free sight may move the ET forward during positioning of the blade. A stethoscope placed on the left chest is helpful to identify an endobronchial displacement of the ET.

When inadvertent bronchial intubation is discovered, the ET should be withdrawn several centimeters and the lungs hyperinflated sufficiently to expand any atelectatic areas. In cases of chronic atelectasis, bronchoscopy may be required to remove the mucous plugs. This problem can be avoided by measuring the length of the ET alongside the patient before intubation. The tip of the ET should ideally be at least 2 cm above the carina, which may be approximated at the sternal angle (of Louis) adjacent to the junction of the sternum with the second rib. In general, approximate orotracheal tube depths are 21 cm from the teeth in adult women and 23 cm in adult men[262] and nasotracheal tube depths 25 cm from the nares in women and 27 cm in men.

b. Double-Lumen Tube Placement

Safe limits for the placement of double-lumen tubes have been outlined by Benumof and associates.[27] Modern fiberoptic bronchoscopes have removed the guesswork surrounding ET tip location. The double-lumen tube may be inserted blindly into the appropriate bronchus and followed by bronchoscopic confirmation of its position, or the bronchoscope may be inserted initially and used as a stylet over which the double-lumen tube is advanced. Fiberoptic bronchoscopy significantly reduces malposition of the double-lumen tube and its routine use is recommended after intubation, changing the patient's position, increasing ventilation pressures, and irregular auscultation. However, even in the best of hands, tracheobronchial injuries occur.[165] Bronchial rupture is a serious complication that requires immediate attention. Using too large double-lumen tubes may cause bronchial trauma.[348] Size recommendations for double-lumen tubes are 35 to 37 Fr for women and smaller men and 39 to 41 for larger men.

B. MAINTENANCE OF THE ENDOTRACHEAL TUBE

1. Airway Obstruction

A patent airway is an absolute requirement for safe anesthesia. Airway obstruction can occur at any time during administration of a general anesthetic, particularly in prolonged surgeries or in patients with predisposing anatomic abnormalities. Airway obstruction should be considered whenever an intubated patient has diminished breath sounds associated with increasing peak inspiratory pressures. Such obstruction can result from diverse factors,[35] including a sharp bend or kink in the ET or a tube that is obstructed with mucus, blood, foreign bodies, or lubricant.[102,288] The ET may become warm with continued use during prolonged procedures; under these circumstances, the ET may kink and cause an obstruction. Reinforced wire tubes may avoid these problems, and their use is recommended in prolonged procedures, in enoral surgery, or during surgery associated with special positioning

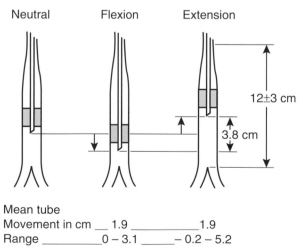

Figure 48-3 The mean movement of an endotracheal tube with flexion and extension of the neck from a neutral position. The mean tube movement between flexion and extension is one third to one fourth the length of a normal adult trachea (12 ± 3 cm). (From Conrardy PA, Goodman LR, Lainge F, et al: Alteration of endotracheal tube position: Flexion and extension of the neck. Crit Care Med 4:8, 1976.)

of the patient. When kinking of an ET occurs, a decrease in compliance usually occurs, which may be accompanied by wheezing. Many clinicians mistakenly treat the patient for bronchospasm when, in fact, the turbulent air movement comes from the ET and not from the patient. At least two cases have been reported in which the plastic coating on a stylet sheared off and occluded the lumen of an ET.[71,374] In another case, an ET was obstructed by the prominent knuckle of an aortic arch.[295] Nitrous oxide can cause expansion of gas bubbles trapped in the walls of an ET, leading to airway obstruction.[275]

Even a reinforced anode wire tube is susceptible to problems. The anode tube can kink at the area between the end of the plastic adapter and the beginning of the support wire. In addition, the soft distal tip can fold backward into the tube and cause obstruction. Finally, although wire tubes have added reinforcement, patients can bite them and cause occlusion of the tube.[128,230,300] Therefore, the use of an oral airway is recommended upon emergence.

The cuff of an ET can also cause airway obstruction. An overinflated cuff may compress the bevel of the ET against the tracheal wall, occluding its tip.[369] The cuff may also herniate over the tip of the ET and cause an obstruction.[336] When faced with any of these problems, the best solution is to pass a suction catheter or a fiberoptic bronchoscope down the lumen of the ET and attempt to clear it. If the ET is totally obstructed, passage of a stylet should be attempted. Total obstruction that cannot be remedied quickly requires removal of the ET, and the patient should be reintubated as rapidly as possible. It is recommended that the ET and connecting hoses be supported and, if necessary, taped to prevent kinking caused by their own weight. Inspiratory gases should be humidified during long anesthesia to prevent ET obstruction from dried secretions.

Unusual causes of airway obstruction have been reported. In two patients, complete airway obstruction occurred secondary to achalasia and esophageal dilation.[188,355] Two cases of tension hydrothorax that caused airway obstruction during laparoscopic surgery have been reported. In the first case, the patient had malignant ascites that, when combined with a pneumoperitoneum, led to such a rapid accumulation of pleural fluid that severe respiratory and cardiovascular compromise resulted.[228] The second case occurred during operative hysteroscopy when a large volume of glycine was absorbed through opened myometrial vessels under high intraabdominal pressure.[121] In each case, more than 1.5 L of clear fluid was drained when chest tubes were placed.

2. Disconnection and Dislodgment

A common and serious complication of endotracheal intubation is disconnection of the ET from the remainder of the anesthesia circuit. This was identified as the most common critical incident in a study of anesthesia-related human errors and equipment failures.[73] A trained anesthesiologist usually identifies this problem immediately. The low-pressure alarm sounds first, and the patient's breath sounds become absent. However, if the ventilator continues to function normally, the physician may be unaware of the nature of the problem. Disconnections are most likely to occur if the connections are made of dissimilar materials, if the patient's head is turned away from the anesthesiologist, or if the airway connections are hidden beneath the surgical drapes. Alarms to signal airway disconnection are included on all modern anesthesia machines, and their signals should be taken seriously. It is recommended that connections between the ET and the breathing circuit be checked and reinforced at the outset, before the anesthesiologist loses visual "control" of the airway. There should be no tension on the connections from the weight of the corrugated tubing or the drapes. Furthermore, members of the surgical team should be discouraged from inadvertently leaning on any portion of the breathing circuit. The exact site of disconnection should be ascertained rapidly by checking each connection, beginning at the patient's airway and moving proximally back to the machine.[281] Nonetheless, it is imperative that the anesthesiologist have a prearranged plan in mind in the event that an airway is inadvertently disconnected or dislodged during surgery.

3. Circuit Leaks

Leaks in an air delivery circuit can cause hypoventilation and dilution of the inspired gases by entry of room air into the system. With an ascending bellows system, such as that found in newer models of anesthesia machines, the bellows do not rise completely during exhalation. This situation indicates that the circuit leak exceeds the inflow of fresh gas. Older machines with a descending bellows system do not provide such a visual clue and appear to function normally. The anesthesiologist should be vigilant at all times for signs of a potential circuit leak. The inspired oxygen concentration measured at the gas sampling port is reduced because of dilution with room air, and the partial pressure of end-tidal CO_2 increases. Cyanosis, a decrease in the oxygen saturation (SpO_2), or hypertension and tachycardia associated with hypercapnia may be the presenting signs, although each of these is typically a late finding.

4. Laser Fires

Lasers are frequently used in the OR to ablate benign and neoplastic tissues in the airway. The use of special laser guarded or metal tubes is recommended, and all inflammatory materials such as dentures and nasogastric tubes should be removed. One of the most catastrophic events associated with their use is an airway fire, which occurs when the laser ignites the ET.[159,258,310] The risk that a laser beam will come in contact with the wall of an

ET is 1:2.[264] Perforation of the tube with a blowtorch-like flame may occur. Oxygen-rich inspired gas concentrations fuel brisk ignition of the plastic in the ET and can fuel a fire in both directions. In essence, the ET acts as a blowtorch; the fire is fed by the combustible walls of the ET and is intensified by the high rate of oxygen flow. The heat and fumes of the burning plastic may cause severe damage to the airway. Treatment consists of immediately disconnecting the circuit from the ET and removing the burning tube from the airway. The fire should be extinguished with saline, and the patient should be supported by face mask ventilation. The airway should be evaluated for damage with bronchoscopy, and the appropriate supportive respiratory care should be given. If the ET is not burning, leaving the tube in situ should be considered because complete loss of the airway may occur with removal of the tube.

Numerous precautions can reduce the risk of an airway fire. If possible, placement of an ET may be avoided altogether if air can be delivered through a ventilating laryngoscope, a jet ventilation system, or intermittent apneic ventilation.[152] If a tracheostomy tube is in place, ventilation may occur distal to the site of laser surgery. ETs may be protected by wrapping them in noncombustible tapes; alternatively, red rubber or metal noncombustible ETs may be used. However, these techniques increase the potential for airway trauma or obstruction.[160,179] Most modern protective tapes are not 100% effective in the prevention of airway fires.[311] Cuff ignition can be minimized by filling the cuff with saline solution instead of air. Furthermore, should the cuff ignite and rupture, the saline helps extinguish the fire. Placing a dye in the saline, such as methylene blue, further alerts the anesthesiologist in the event of a fire, as steam that is the color of the dye is emitted. Nitrous oxide should not be used in laser surgery because it easily supports combustion.[367] On the basis of laboratory simulations, it is recommended that inert gases, such as helium or nitrogen, be used instead of nitrous oxide and that concentrations of oxygen do not exceed 40%.[265] Five centimeters of positive end-expiratory pressure with forced inspiratory oxygen no greater than 40% prevents ignition of polyvinyl chloride components.[266]

C. SPECIAL TECHNIQUES

1. Fiberoptic Intubation

Fiberoptic intubation is one of the most common methods utilized in cases of anticipated difficult intubation. It combines direct vision with the flexibility to view the pharynx when direct laryngoscopy is considered difficult or impossible. Flexible fiberoptic bronchoscopy is not a quick technique, and it probably should not be considered when speed is required unless the anesthesiologist is very skilled in this technique. Although the flexible fiberoptic bronchoscope (FOB) can be used in many different situations involving airway management and preoperative evaluation of critical patients, it also has several limitations and potential complications.

Intubation with FOB should not be attempted when the pharynx is filled with blood or saliva, when inadequate space exists within the oral cavity to identify pharyngeal structures, or when time is critical and creating a surgical airway is the priority. *Relative* contraindications include marked tissue edema, distortion of the oropharyngeal anatomy, blood in the airway, soft tissue traction, or a severe cervical flexion deformity. The FOB may be difficult to use if the operator is inexperienced, if topical anesthesia is inadequate, if light is not sufficient or the focus is not correct, if the lens is markedly fogged, or if an ET cannot be passed over the bronchoscope,[261] if it displaces out of the trachea during "railroading" the tube (because the introduction depth is suboptimal), and if it cannot be physically removed out of the ET.

Potential complications associated with the FOB include bleeding, epistaxis (especially if a nasal airway is attempted), laryngotracheal trauma (especially when multiple attempts at threading the ET into the trachea are made), laryngospasm, bronchospasm, and aspiration of blood, saliva, or gastric contents. Another possible hazard is associated with the practice of insufflating oxygen through the suction channel. Although this technique can help to keep the tip of the bronchoscope clean and provide for a high volume of forced inspiratory oxygen, it can also result in high-pressure submucosal injection of oxygen should the tip cut into the pharyngeal mucosa. If this sequence occurs, the result may be pronounced subcutaneous emphysema of the pharynx, face, and periorbital regions.[17] A case of gastric rupture has also been reported with prolonged oxygen insufflation; thus, continuous anatomic identification is necessary with this technique.[155]

2. Lighted Stylets

The lighted stylet may be used to facilitate intubation under both local and general anesthesia. A light at the tip of a flexible stylet is used to transilluminate the soft tissues of the pharynx. The device can be used blindly or as an aid when direct laryngoscopy is difficult. It may also serve to confirm that the tip of an ET is still within the cervical trachea and to establish that the tube has not been advanced too far.[232]

Because use of the lighted stylet is a blind technique, the pharyngeal pathologic condition cannot be visualized or avoided. This method should not be used in patients with suspected abnormalities of the upper airway, such as tumors, polyps, infections (e.g., epiglottitis or retropharyngeal abscess), trauma, or foreign bodies. The lighted stylet should also be used with caution in patients in whom transillumination of the anterior neck will be limited, such those with dark skin pigmentation, morbid obesity, limited neck mobility, large tongue, and long epiglottis.[168] If placement of the stylet is difficult, the anesthesiologist should consider abandoning the technique for fear of worsening a pathologic process.

Several real and potential complications have been reported with the use of this device. Sore throat, hoarseness, and mucosal damage are possible.[168] Several cases have been reported in which the light fell off of the end of the stylet.[104,317,363] In another instance, the protective tubing was not removed from the stylet and thus had the potential to become dislodged within the trachea.[240] Finally, several cases of arytenoid subluxation have been reported with the use of this device.[137,321] Heat damage to the tracheal mucosa in prolonged intubation is a potential risk with inappropriate handling.[81] To avoid heat damage, the Trachlight bulb flashes on and off after 30 seconds.

Recommendation for use in emergency cases cannot be given because the risk of regurgitation is high, cricoid pressure may affect the ease of intubation, and more than one attempt is often necessary.[4] The transillumination technique is not suitable for verification of the ET position because of misinterpretations.

IV. COMPLICATIONS WITH INFRAGLOTTIC PROCEDURES

Infraglottic airway access is the last step in the ASA airway management algorithm.[8] In cases in which endotracheal intubation is impossible and the patient's condition deteriorates into a cannot ventilate, cannot intubate situation, lifesaving steps must be immediately undertaken. Although these procedures are associated with complications, they are not usually as fatal as the complications resulting from cannot ventilate, cannot intubate situations, that is, brain damage and death. There are no contraindications for infraglottic procedures in these critical situations. The most severe complication is failure to establish an airway before brain damage or death results. These conditions occur either because the decision to progress to a surgical airway is not made soon enough or because the procedure is performed too slowly. In all cases of possible difficult airway management, the anesthesiologist should evaluate the possibility of infraglottic airway access. Difficult anatomic situations, marked scars, abscesses, or morbid obesity may limit infraglottic access techniques.

Infraglottic airway techniques are not only suitable for emergency situations, they are also indicated for both oxygenation and ventilation of anesthetized patients. Surgical procedures of the upper airway, laryngeal surgery, and diagnostic procedures have been successfully managed with this technique.

A. TRANSLARYNGEAL AIRWAY

1. Retrograde Wire Intubation

Retrograde wire intubation is an excellent technique for securing a difficult airway. It can be used whenever anatomic limitations obscure the glottic opening. Because the technique is blind, it is important to exercise caution so as not to worsen any preexisting conditions. There are many variations of this technique, such as using the FOB by passing the wire through the suction channel or through a tube exchanger, that are discussed in Chapter 19.

Although simple in concept, the basic technique has numerous problems and potential complications. The procedure takes some time to perform and should not be considered under emergency circumstances unless the anesthesiologist is very experienced. The tip of the ET has been known to become caught on the glottic structures and fail to enter the larynx. The problem may be alleviated somewhat by using a tapered dilator inside the ET or by using an epidural catheter as the wire to assist with passing the ET through the glottis. Bleeding may occur at the site of the tracheal puncture in quantities sufficient to cause a tracheal clot or airway obstruction. Cases of severe hemoptysis with resultant hypoxia, cardiopulmonary arrest, dysrhythmias, and death following retrograde wire intubation have been reported.[180,297,312,337] Subcutaneous emphysema localized to the area of the transtracheal needle puncture is common but self-limited. In severe cases, the air may track back through the fascial planes of the neck, leading to tracheal compression with resultant airway compromise, pneumomediastinum, and pneumothorax.[224,274] Laryngospasm may result from irritation by the retrograde wire unless the vocal cords are anesthetized or relaxed. Other, less common complications include esophageal perforation, tracheal hematoma, laryngeal edema, infection, tracheitis, tracheal fistula, trigeminal nerve injury, and vocal cord damage.[111,294] The complications reported previously with retrograde wire intubation were mostly associated with multiple attempts, large-gauge needles, and untrained personnel in emergency settings.[263]

2. Cricothyroidotomy

In both surgical cricothyroidotomy (using a scalpel) and needle cricothyroidotomy (using a needle set) procedures, the cricothyroid membrane requires penetration. Acute complications are bleeding (especially during surgical cricothyroidotomy) and misplacement of the tube (especially after needle cricothyroidotomy). When cricothyroidotomy is performed in case of totally upper airway obstruction, barotrauma may occur because of expiratory blockade. Subcutaneous emphysema, pneumothorax, pneumomediastinum, and pneumopericardium may occur during this technique. Additional acute complications are tube malposition or failure of airway access, bleeding, wound infection, displaced cartilage fractures, and laryngotracheal separation.[136,170] Granulation tissue around the tracheostomy site, subglottic stenosis, massive laryngeal mucosa trauma, endolaryngeal hematoma and laceration, vocal cord paralysis, hoarseness, and thyroid cartilage fracture with dysphasia are direct long-term complications. Indirect long-term complications are brain damage or mental impairment related to hypoxia when the cricothyroidotomy takes more than 2 to 3 minutes.[136,170] All emergency translaryngeal airways should be eventually changed to a formal tracheostomy. Subglottic stenosis is a delayed complication, especially in children.

B. TRANSTRACHEAL AIRWAY

1. Transtracheal Jet Ventilation

Transtracheal jet ventilation (TTJV) is accomplished by introducing a small percutaneous catheter into the trachea and insufflating the respiratory tract with high-pressure oxygen over a jet ventilator or a hand jet device (Manujet, VBM). Although this technique may be helpful in critical situations, life-threatening problems are associated with its use.

To accomplish TTJV, a long, large-bore catheter is advanced through the cricothyroid membrane into the trachea. If this catheter is displaced from the trachea, subcutaneous emphysema, hypoventilation, pneumomediastinum, pneumothorax, severe abdominal distention, or death may result.[101] In a study of 28 emergency patients managed with TTJV, 2 developed subcutaneous emphysema and 1 developed mediastinal emphysema.[304] On the basis of normal skin compliance, a 4-inch catheter could be pulled from an intratracheal position into the subcutaneous space simply by applying traction to its proximal end. Thus, the hub of the TTJV catheter must be continuously pressed firmly against the skin line.

Barotrauma is another potential complication of this technique.[76,298] Oxygen delivered through a transtracheal catheter must be able to escape the lungs freely or overdistention and pulmonary rupture may occur.[255,305] It is imperative that any change in breath sounds, chest wall expansion, or hemodynamics be suspected as secondary to pneumothorax. In cases of total airway obstruction, the risk for pneumothorax is greatly increased because gas cannot escape from the lungs. Strong consideration should be given to placing a second transtracheal "egress" catheter or performing a cricothyrotomy in these circumstances. Laryngospasm can also impede the outward flow of oxygen from the trachea. This should be prevented by providing adequate local anesthesia to the neighboring structures or by relaxing the patient.[298] If the larynx is obstructed by a foreign body, only low-flow oxygen should be delivered until safe egress of gas is established.

Inadvertent placement of a gas delivery line into the gastrointestinal tract may also result in complications. In one case report, gas delivery introduced inadvertently into the stomach caused gastric rupture.[41] Other gastrointestinal complications include esophageal perforations, bleeding, hematoma, and hemoptysis.[26]

Damage to the tracheal mucosa may occur in patients who are managed with long-term TTJV, especially if the gas is not humidified.[330] The possibility of tracheal mucosal ulceration should be considered in any patient if nonhumidified TTJV is attempted through single-orifice catheters for a prolonged period of time.

2. Percutaneous Dilatational Tracheostomy

Although this technique is not usually recommended for emergency use, it appears to be suitable for emergency situations in skilled hands, and different sets are available. Insertion techniques have been further developed.[67,112,142]

Bleeding, subcutaneous and mediastinal emphysema, pneumothorax, airway obstruction, aspiration, infection, and death are early complications. Accidental extubation is a serious complication and, unfortunately, replacement of the cannula may be impossible. In this situation, an orotracheal intubation or a translaryngeal oxygenation is required.[28] Delayed complications are tracheal stenosis, scars, hoarseness, and tracheoesophageal and tracheocutaneous fistula. The incidence of injury for percutaneous dilatational tracheostomy is 2%,[218] which is lower than that for a formal tracheostomy.

3. Formal Tracheostomy

A formal tracheostomy is never recommended in emergency situations. Various instruments, assistance, and sterile conditions are required, and it should be performed by a trained surgeon.

Bleeding is a complication of any surgical procedure, including airway access procedures. Minitracheostomy occasionally results in excess bleeding into the airway, necessitating progression to a full surgical tracheostomy.[348] The inflated cuff of the formal tracheostomy prevents pulmonary aspiration of blood. In rare cases, the innominate artery can rupture into the trachea because of excessive pressure from the tracheostomy tube, with resultant massive hemorrhage into the airway. Air embolism during the operative procedure is also possible.

If an air leak occurs and the cervical skin has healed around the tracheostomy tube, air can escape into the subcutaneous spaces of the neck, resulting in subcutaneous emphysema. If the condition goes unrecognized and the patient is maintained with high-pressure mechanical ventilation, the air may track to other locations. Air escaping into the paratracheal spaces can result in a pneumomediastinum. Furthermore, air released into the pleural cavity can result in a tension pneumothorax.

Subglottic stenosis is a complication of long-term intubation. It usually results when the decision to progress to a tracheostomy is delayed too long. On the other hand, tracheal stenosis is a complication of long-term tracheostomy. Subglottic stenoses are much more difficult to repair and frequently result in permanent speech impairment or laryngeal damage. If either of these types of stenoses are left untreated, they may eventually progress to granulomas, which require surgical excision.

A tracheostomy tube can cause tracheal erosion, particularly into the esophagus (tracheoesophageal fistula) or the brachiocephalic artery. These tubes typically sit low in the trachea and are designed with a fixed curve. Furthermore, tube pressure can damage the skin at the insertion site.

Accidental extubation and dislodgement of the cannula occur occasionally, most commonly in the early postoperative period. If the cannula is inadvertently removed from a fresh tracheostomy, it should be replaced as quickly as possible. Infection, mediastinal sepsis, tracheal stenosis, and tracheomalacia are rare late complications.

V. RESPONSES TO INTUBATION

The larynx has the greatest afferent nerve supply of the airway. Airway reflexes are important in protection of the airway. They require suppression for stress-free airway management, especially for endotracheal intubation. Intensive autonomic response may occur during placement, maintenance, and removal of all airway management devices.

A. HEMODYNAMIC CHANGES

Direct laryngoscopy and endotracheal intubation are both potent stimuli that may instigate an intense autonomic response.[20,205] Tachycardia, hypertension, dysrhythmias, bronchospasm, and bronchorrhea are common; hypotension and bradycardia occur less often. Patients with preexisting hypertension are even more at risk when they are under stress.

Oczenski and colleagues have shown that the insertion of a Combitube was associated with higher and longer lasting increases in systolic, diastolic, and mean arterial pressure; heart rate; and plasma catecholamine concentration compared with insertion of an LMA and laryngoscopic endotracheal intubation (Fig. 48-4).[251] Hemodynamic and catecholamine responses to insertion of an LMA are minimal.[365,368] Under sevoflurane anesthesia, hemodynamic responses to endotracheal intubation with the Trachlight do not differ from those with a direct laryngoscope.[323] This contrasts with the results from Nishikawa's study, in which the use of a light wand device was accompanied by a smaller increase in systolic blood pressure compared with the laryngoscopic technique.[247]

The sympathetically mediated responses to mechanical stimulation of the larynx, trachea-carina, and bronchi may be completely blocked by topical and partially blocked by intravenous lidocaine.[145] The magnitude of stimuli to the upper airway depends on the number and duration of intubation attempts. In cases of difficult airway situations, a greater increase of hemodynamic responses is anticipated. The hemodynamic response may also be blocked by giving opioids or short-acting selective α_1-blockers[163] before laryngoscopy and intubation. A dose of 2 µg/kg of fentanyl attenuates the autonomic changes, and 6 µg/kg completely abolishes them.[61,181] Remifentanil (4 µg/kg) combined with thiopental (5 mg/kg) provided satisfactory intubation conditions and acceptable hemodynamic changes, as shown by Durmus and coauthors. This technique may be appropriate when a neuromuscular block is undesirable.[98]

Because many patients have coexisting cardiovascular disease and cannot meet increased myocardial oxygen demands, it is imperative that large hemodynamic responses be prevented. More than 11% of patients with myocardial disease develop some degree of myocardial ischemia during intubation.[100] The key element is to provide an adequate depth of anesthesia with either intravenous or inhalation agents before instrumentation of the airway.

Fiberoptic intubation performed under sufficient local anesthesia and conscious sedation is an appropriate technique to prevent major hemodynamic changes during intubation. Minor hemodynamic changes and minor increase of plasma catecholamine concentration are nevertheless apparent in this technique. Fiberoptic intubation using a special mask adapter is associated with less hemodynamic changes than laryngoscopy after induction of anesthesia. The lowest cardiovascular responses were registered in patients after insertion of an LMA.[169]

B. LARYNGOSPASM

Reflex responses to stage II of anesthesia during intubation or extubation can be problematic. Laryngospasm can occur, in which the patient makes respiratory efforts but cannot perform any air exchange. If direct laryngoscopy was performed, the vocal cords would be completely adducted. However, laryngospasm involves more than spastic closure of the vocal cords. An infolding of the arytenoids and the aryepiglottic folds occurs; these structures are subsequently covered by the epiglottis.[114] This explains why a firm jaw thrust can sometimes break the spasm—the hyoid is elevated, thereby stretching the epiglottis and aryepiglottic folds to open the forced closure. Malpositioning related to incorrect insertion techniques, as well as inadequate depth of anesthesia during LMA insertion, may induce laryngospasm. It may also occur during fiberoptic intubation performed in nonanesthetized or subanesthetized laryngeal structures.

Positive mask pressure may help by distending the pharynx or vocal cords, but this technique is not always adequate. Treatment with a short-acting muscle relaxant, such as 10 to 20 mg of succinylcholine, may be necessary to break the spasm.

C. BRONCHOSPASM

Tracheal irritation from the ET can cause bronchospasm that is sufficiently severe to prevent air movement

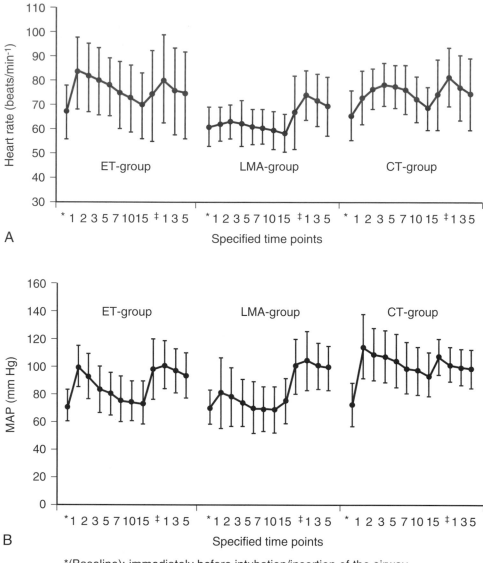

*(Baseline): immediately before intubation/insertion of the airway
‡Immediately before extubation/removal of the airway

Figure 48-4 Heart rate **(A)** and mean arterial blood pressure (MAP) **(B)** at specified time points (mean ± SD; $n = 73$) during insertion of endotracheal tube (ET), laryngeal mask airway (LMA), and Combitube (CT). (Modified from Oczenski W, Krenn H, Dahaba AA, et al: Hemodynamic and catecholamine stress responses to insertion of the combitube, laryngeal mask airway or tracheal intubation. Anesth Analg 88:1389, 1999.)

throughout the lungs.[88] Approximately 80% of the measurable resistance to airflow occurs in the large central airways; the remaining 20% occurs in the smaller peripheral bronchioles.[219] The incidence of intraoperative bronchospasm is almost 9% with endotracheal intubation and 0.13% with an LMA but is close to 0% with mask ventilation.[42,200] Poor correlation is seen with age, sex, duration or severity of reactive airway disease, duration of anesthesia, or the forced expiratory volume in 1 second (FEV_1).[200] Other factors that may contribute to bronchospasm include inhaled stimulants, release of allergic mediators, viral infections, exercise, or pharmacologic factors (including α-blockers, prostaglandin inhibitors, and anticholinesterases). Bronchospasm may occur during fiberoptic intubation if parts of the subglottic airway are insufficiently anesthetized.

The spasm can be treated with inhalation of epinephrine or isoproterenol or a α_2-agonist (such as albuterol, metaproterenol, or terbutaline) or by deepening the level of a volatile anesthetic.

D. COUGHING AND BUCKING

Two additional adverse responses to intubation are coughing and bucking on the ET.[135] Such responses are potentially hazardous in cases of increased intracranial pressure,[361] intracranial vascular anomalies, open-globe injuries, and ophthalmologic surgery[92] or in cases in which increased intra abdominal pressure could rupture an abdominal incision. Performing endotracheal intubation only when an adequate depth of anesthesia has been achieved helps to prevent this reflex.

Coughing and bucking occur less frequently with the LMA; however, in the presence of lubricant globules on the anterior surface of the cuff, light anesthesia, or malpositioning, these adverse reactions may be observed. The incidence of coughing, gagging, and retching has been reported as 0.8% using an LMA with a fentanyl-propfol-O_2-N_2O-isoflurane technique.[42]

E. VOMITING, REGURGITATION, AND ASPIRATION

The overall incidence of aspiration during general anesthesia varies and has been reported as 1 in 2,131 (in Sweden) to 1 in 14,150 (in France) and 1 in 3,216 in the United States, with an associated mortality of 1 in 71,829 in the United States.[107]

A meta-analysis of publications concerning the LMA (547 publications) suggested that the overall incidence of pulmonary aspiration was approximately 2 in 10,000.[43] The ET and Combitube are most effective to prevent pulmonary aspiration. To reduce the risk of pulmonary aspiration, some new designs of airway management devices were developed, the ProSeal LMA and the Laryngeal Tube Suction as previously mentioned.

In any patient considered to have a full stomach, the likelihood of vomiting in response to irritation of the airway is increased, and aspiration of stomach contents is a constant concern. Aspiration leads to coughing, laryngospasm, and bronchospasm, assuming that protective reflexes are intact. In consequence of these reactions, hypertonia, bradycardia, asystole, and hypoxia may occur. The magnitude of pulmonary reactions depends on the type and quantity of the aspirated material.[276]

The Sellick maneuver, or cricoid pressure, has removed much of the fear of emergency intubation. Cricoid pressure is effective in raising the pressure in the upper esophageal sphincter to a value greater than that found at rest, provided that at least 40 N of force (equivalent to 4.1 kg or 9 lb) is used.[342] Cricoid pressure has proved to be effective even in the presence of a nasogastric tube.[292] It is critical that the ease of intubation be assessed before inducing any patient with a potentially full stomach. Should any doubt exist about the success of endotracheal intubation, awake techniques should be considered. It is possible to obstruct the airway completely with cricoid pressure. Furthermore, reports have been published of airway obstruction during cricoid pressure as a result of lingual tonsils, lingual thyroid glands,[129] and undiagnosed laryngeal trauma.[301]

F. INTRAOCULAR PRESSURE

With thiopental, etomidate, and halothane anesthesia, an increase of intraocular pressure to 25% was observed during laryngoscopy and to 5% to 10% during LMA use.[167,202,351] Intraocular pressure increases during extubation but not during LMA insertion or endotracheal intubation with total intravenous anesthesia without the use of muscle relaxants[191] or with remifentanil and sevoflurane.[105] Decreases in intraocular pressures were observed with endotracheal intubation during general anesthesia with propofol and sevoflurane, both combined with remifentanil.[296]

It has been demonstrated that insertion of an LMA does not increase intraocular pressure in children after sevoflurane induction.[96] Sufentanil is also effective in preventing an intraocular pressure increase caused by rapid sequence induction with succinylcholine.[130] It is extremely important to avoid an increase of intraocular pressure in patients with penetrating eye injury.

G. INTRACRANIAL PRESSURE

Intracranial pressure rises markedly and transiently during laryngoscopy and endotracheal intubation. Patients with head injury are at higher risk from this increase as it reduces cerebral perfusion and thus may increase secondary brain damage.[286] Although fiberoptic bronchoscopy has been shown to produce a substantial but transient increase of intracranial pressure,[189] deep anesthesia during induction can prevent these adverse effects.

H. APNEA

Apnea may be seen as a reflex response of tracheal irritation caused by the ET or other airway techniques. Extraneous reasons for the apnea—for example, the patient is a premature or full-term neonate,[131] has had induction drugs or excessive narcotics, or has a reflux response to light levels of anesthesia—should be ruled out initially. If no central reason exists for the patient's lack of respiratory effort, mechanical ventilation can be initiated and spontaneous ventilation can be attempted later.

I. LATEX ALLERGY

Almost 17% of overall anaphylaxis in surgical procedures is related to latex anaphylaxis.[344] To prevent anaphylaxis in patients during anesthesia and surgery, the patient's history has to be evaluated preoperatively. There is currently no therapy for latex allergy, and avoidance of latex-containing products is mandatory for predisposed individuals.[154] Latex allergy is present in 8% of the general U.S. population, with a prevalence of 30% in health care workers.[123,201] There was an increased incidence of type I and type IV latex sensitivity in the general population from 1% in 1980 to 8% in 1996.[280] The prevalence of latex sensitivity among anesthesiologists is approximately 12.5% and of allergy 2.4%.[53]

Patients with spina bifida, rubber industry workers, atopic patients, and patients with a multiple surgery history are most at risk.[187] Patients with certain exotic food allergies may have a coexisting latex allergy,[85] in one study reported as 86%.[124]

Patients with type I hypersensitivity are at risk for developing anaphylaxis with hypotension, rash, and bronchospasm. Type I hypersensitivity symptoms are localized contact urticaria with pruritus and edema. Generalized reactions are rash or hives, tearing, rhinitis, hoarseness, dyspnea, nausea, vomiting, bronchospasm, abdominal cramping, and diarrhea.

Contamination with latex in anesthesia is possible through *direct contact* by face mask, endotracheal and gastric tubes, gloves, syringes, and electrodes; through *inhalation* from contaminated circuits and room air; and through the *parenteral path* with latex-containing intravenous administration sets.

Considerations for anesthesiologists handling patients with latex allergy are available at the website of the ASA (http://www.asahq.org/publicationsandservices/latexallergy.html), and all anesthesiology departments should have a special "latex safe cart" with all medical supplies and devices. Anesthesiologists should always be prepared for this type of reaction. There was a report of sudden bronchospasm 5 minutes after intubation in a patient with latex allergy.[153] In a pediatric study, Nakamura and colleagues found that a high percentage of children with home mechanical ventilation have undiagnosed latex allergy.[245] Another study, evaluating generalized allergic reactions during anesthesia, showed that in 1 of 28 patients the immunoglobulin E latex radioallergosorbent test was positive.[31] Most airway management devices are available as latex-free products. Because the oropharyngeal cuff of the Combitube contains latex, it is contraindicated in patients with known latex allergy.

VI. COMPLICATIONS WITH EXTUBATION

Primary and secondary responses to extubation are possible. The primary effects are local and systemic responses (Table 48-5). The same responses that occur after intubation may be observed at extubation. During intubation, the patient is more protected by anesthesia induction than during extubation; therefore, the cardiovascular responses may be more exaggerated. The most serious complication after extubation is the occurrence of acute airway obstruction. Decrease of consciousness, central respiratory depression, decrease of muscle tone, and tongue obstruction may lead to inspiratory or expiratory stridor, dyspnea, cyanosis, tachycardia, hypertension, agitation, and sweating. Urgent treatment is necessary to prevent hypoxia, brain damage, and death. Other complications following extubation are not caused by the removal of the tube itself; they are consequences of the previous intubation and the duration of the tube placement, such as laryngitis, edema, ulcerations, granuloma, or synechia of the vocal cords. The quality of endotracheal intubation

Table 48-5 Pathophysiologic Effects of Tracheal Extubation

Primary Local Effects
Airway
Obstruction
Coughing
Breath holding
Damage to the vocal cords
Arytenoid dislocation/luxation
Primary Systemic Effects
Cardiovascular system
Tachycardia
Increased systemic arterial pressure
Increased pulmonary arterial pressure
Secondary Effects
Central nervous system
Increased intracranial pressure
Eye
Increased intraocular pressure

Modified from Hartley M: Difficulties in tracheal extubation. In Latto IP, Vaughan R (eds): Difficulties in Tracheal Intubation. London, Saunders, 1997.

contributes to laryngeal morbidity, and excellent conditions are less frequently associated with postoperative hoarseness and vocal cord sequelae.[233]

A. HEMODYNAMIC CHANGES

Hemodynamic changes, including a 20% increase in heart rate and blood pressure, occur in most patients at the time of extubation.[30,366] Increases of heart rate, systemic arterial pressure, pulmonary arterial pressure, pulmonary arterial occlusion pressure, and myocardial contractility are caused by increased sympathoadrenal activity. Such changes, which are thought to result from catecholamine release in response to stimulation by the ET, are usually transient and rarely require treatment. Although most patients tolerate these hemodynamic responses well, patients with cardiac disease,[100] pregnancy-induced hypertension,[73] and increased intracranial pressure[241] may be at particular risk for life-threatening ischemic myocardial episodes. Patients with cardiac disease have shown decreased ejection fractions at the time of extubation.[75] Management consists of deep extubation or pharmacologic therapy. Deep extubation is appropriate for some patients but is inappropriate for patients with a difficult airway, those at high risk for aspiration, and those with compromised airway access. Pharmacologic strategies emphasize the importance of decreasing the heart rate, which is more likely than an increase in blood pressure to cause left ventricular failure followed by pulmonary edema. Cerebral hemorrhage is possible.

Removal of an LMA may be associated with significantly reduced local and cardiovascular responses if the cuff pressure is minimized to avoid overstimulation of the patient.[44]

B. LARYNGOSPASM

Laryngospasm, the most frequent cause of postextubation airway obstruction, is a protective reflex mediated by the vagus nerve. This reflex is an attempt to prevent aspiration of foreign bodies into the trachea. It may be provoked by movement of the cervical spine, pain, vocal cord irritation by secretions, or sudden stimulation while the patient is still in a light plane of anesthesia.[282] In a large computer-aided study involving 136,929 patients, the incidence of laryngospasm was 50 in 1000 in children with bronchial asthma and airway infection and 25 in 1000 in children in the age group 1 to 3 months when endotracheal intubation had been performed.[256]

The optimal course for treating laryngospasm is to avoid it in the first place. It is imperative that no saliva, blood, or gastric contents touch the glottis while the patient is lightly anesthetized. In cases in which laryngospasm is anticipated, the patient may undergo a deep extubation. The back of the oropharynx should be suctioned before emergence to remove any suspicious material from the posterior pharynx. A patient undergoing deep extubation should be placed in the lateral position with the head down to keep the vocal cords clear of secretions during emergence. Because suctioning of the oropharynx does not adequately remove secretions around the vocal cords, it is best to extubate patients during a positive-pressure breath. The vigorous exhalation after extubation helps to remove any remaining secretions. Also, extubation during a positive-pressure breath is the procedure of choice in children. Valley and coworkers showed that children could be safely extubated in deep anesthesia with 1.5 times the minimum effective alveolar anesthetic concentration of either sevoflurane or desflurane.[340]

A survey of U.S. anesthesiologists[79] showed that deep extubation is performed by 64% of the interviewed practitioners. The most common reasons for deep extubation were unclipped intracranial aneurysm, reactive airway disease, and open-globe eye surgery. The most common reason for not performing deep extubation was concern regarding potential laryngospasm and aspiration. Koga and coauthors showed that the rate of airway obstruction in patients extubated during deep anesthesia (17 of 20) was not higher than that in patients extubated after regaining consciousness (18 of 20).[195]

C. LARYNGEAL EDEMA

Laryngeal edema is an important cause of postextubation obstruction, especially in neonates and infants. This condition has various causes and is classified as supraglottic, retroarytenoidal, and subglottic.[148] Supraglottic edema most commonly results from surgical manipulation, positioning, hematoma formation, overaggressive fluid management, impaired venous drainage, or coexisting conditions (such as preeclampsia or angioneurotic edema). Retroarytenoidal edema typically results from local trauma or irritation. Subglottic edema occurs most often in children, particularly neonates and infants. Factors associated with the development of subglottic edema include traumatic intubation, intubation lasting longer than 1 hour, bucking on the ET, changes in head position, and tight-fitting ETs. Laryngeal edema usually arises as stridor within 30 to 60 minutes after extubation, although it may start as late as 6 hours after extubation.[80] Regardless of the cause of laryngeal edema, management depends on the severity of the condition. Therapy consists of humidified oxygen, racemic epinephrine, head-up positioning, and, occasionally, reintubation with a smaller ET. The practice of administering parenteral steroids with the goal of preventing or reducing edema is controversial.[80]

D. LARYNGOTRACHEAL TRAUMA

Unlike trauma during intubation, airway trauma at the time of extubation is not well described. Arytenoid cartilage dislocation has been reported after both difficult and routine intubations.[271,334] Symptoms become apparent soon after extubation and may be mild (difficulty swallowing and voice changes) or major (complete airway obstruction). Management depends on the severity of the condition. Options include reintubation, arytenoid reduction, or tracheostomy. If laryngotracheal trauma is suspected, an otolaryngology consultation is warranted.

E. BRONCHOSPASM

In patients at risk for bronchospasm, the timing of extubation is of equal concern. These patients may be extubated either during deep anesthesia (if this approach can be used safely) or when they are fully awake and their own airway reflexes are present. Although the degree of spasm in this condition may be severe, it is usually self-limited and short lived.

F. NEGATIVE-PRESSURE PULMONARY EDEMA

When airway obstruction occurs after extubation, such as in case of laryngospasm, negative-pressure pulmonary edema may occur in the spontaneously breathing patient. As a result of inspiratory effort against the closed glottis, these patients generate negative intrapleural pressures greater than 100 cm H_2O. Rib retraction with poor air movement, laryngospasm, and stridor may lead to this condition. Increases in left ventricular preload and afterload, altered pulmonary vascular resistance, increased adrenergic state, right ventricle dilatation, intraventricular septum shift to the left, left ventricular diastolic dysfunction, increased left heart loading conditions, enhanced microvascular intramural hydrostatic pressure, negative pleural pressure, and transmission to the lung interstitium may result in a marked increase in transmural pressure, fluid filtration into the lung, and development of pulmonary edema.[50]

The condition is seen within minutes after extubation. Hemoptysis and alveolar hemorrhage are rare symptoms. Management involves removing the obstruction, supporting the patient with oxygen, monitoring the patient closely, and reducing the afterload. Reintubation is rarely necessary; most cases resolve spontaneously without further complications.

G. ASPIRATION

Pulmonary aspiration of gastric contents is a constant threat for any patient who has a full stomach or is at risk for postoperative vomiting. Laryngeal function is altered for at least 4 hours after tracheal extubation.[54] Coughing is a physiologic response to protect the airway from aspiration. Depression of reflexes, along with the presence of residual anesthetic agents, places almost all recently extubated patients at risk. Aspiration is probably more prevalent than is currently thought. Most cases are so minor that they do not affect the patient's postoperative course. Reducing gastric contents by suctioning through a gastric tube and extubation with the patient placed in the lateral position with a head-down tilt provide the greatest protection against aspiration. Perioperative problems, if they do occur, are usually attributed to such factors as atelectasis. Management consists of supportive measures. Depending on the extent of the aspiration, measures include supportive care, ranging from administration of oxygen through a nasal cannula to reintubation with mechanical ventilation and positive end-expiratory pressure.

H. AIRWAY COMPRESSION

External compression of the airway after extubation may lead to obstruction. An excessively tight postsurgical neck dressing is a cause of external compression that is easily resolved. A more ominous situation is a rapidly expanding hematoma in close proximity to the airway. This may occur after certain surgeries, such as carotid endarterectomy, and must be quickly diagnosed and treated before total airway obstruction occurs.[259] Immediate surgical reexploration is indicated, although the airway concerns in these patients should be approached with extreme caution. To minimize airway distortion, general anesthesia should be avoided until the wound is evacuated under local anesthesia. However, even after surgical drainage, airway obstruction may occur as the result of venous or lymphatic congestion. Any use of muscle relaxants during anesthesia induction in these patients may result in catastrophe regardless of whether the wound was

previously drained. Conservative options for managing the airway in this situation include awake fiberoptic intubation, surgical airway, or inhalation induction. Muscle relaxants should be avoided until the airway is secured.

External compression of the neck, such as chronic compression of a goiter, may also result from tracheomalacia.[126] This condition is usually seen after the goiter has been removed, although one case was reported in which the airway collapsed as soon as muscle relaxants were administered for induction.[346] Airway obstruction in these patients becomes apparent soon after extubation. Management includes reintubation, surgical tracheal support (stenting), or tracheostomy below the level of obstruction.

I. DIFFICULT EXTUBATION

Occasionally, ETs are difficult to remove. Possible causes are failure to deflate the cuff, use of an oversized tube,[148] adhesion of the tube to the tracheal wall,[82] and transfixation of the tube by an inadvertent suture to a nearby organ,[49,95] a wire,[157,209] a screw in oromaxillofacial surgery, or a broken drill.[203] Possible sequelae of these complications include airway leak, aspiration, tube obstruction, and trauma from attempts at forceful extubation. One case was reported in which a nasogastric tube made a loop around the ET.[110] In most cases, the problem arises from an inability to deflate the cuff, commonly as a result of failure in the cuff-deflating mechanism. Should this problem occur, the cuff should be punctured with a transtracheal needle. When tube fixation is suspected, it is recommended to check the passage of the tube with a suction catheter or to use a fiberscope. Forceful removal of an ET with the cuff inflated may result in damage to the vocal cords and arytenoid dislocation.

Airway exchange catheters (AECs) may also be used as a bridge to extubation in patients with a known difficult airway or there is a question of successful extubation. These catheters have a dual function: (1) oxygenation/ventilation, and (2) use as an intubation stylet. The literature suggests four potential risks associated with the use of these devices: catheter misplacement, bronchial or lung trauma, laryngeal trauma, and barotraumas related to either oxygenation or jet ventilation via these catheters.[54-56] These complications may be avoided by proper placement of these catheters, which ensures appropriate length of placement (22 to 25 cm for oral placement and 27 to 30 cm for nasal placement in adults), confirmation of endotracheal placement (direct laryngoscopy, fiberoptic laryngoscopy, end-tidal CO_2 monitoring), and proper use of oxygenation and ventilation techniques.

J. ACCIDENTAL EXTUBATION

Accidental extubation during anesthesia was reported with disposable tonsillectomy instruments,[370] change of the patient's head position,[319] and neurosurgery in the knee-elbow position.

Most accidental extubations were reported in intensive care unit patients. In these patients, self-extubation was the most common incident (77% to 85%).[29,66,182] The need for reintubation was 37% to 57%.[29,66] The requirement for reintubation is higher in patients with full ventilatory support than in patients during the weaning phase.

Patients at risk for accidental extubation are characterized by oral intubation and insufficient sedation.[64] Achauer and colleagues reported a higher accidental extubation rate in burn patients (66%) in conjunction with painful and invasive procedures.[1]

Complications after accidental extubation may be hypoxia, hypercarbic respiratory failure, aspiration, retention of pulmonary secretion, arrhythmia, and tachycardia. Techniques to avoid unplanned extubation include securing the tube with special tube holders[183] or with waterproof tape[135] and fixation with a knot or a bow.[68] Reintubation may be very difficult, especially after a difficult intubation. Use of the Combitube or the LMA[134] is required in some cases of inadequate access to the patient's head in the intensive care setting.

VII. CONCLUSION

This chapter has identified many of the challenges and complications that anesthesiologists may face when managing an airway. Errors may be technical or judgmental. By learning from the mistakes of the past, we may avoid them in the future. To minimize problems, we should anticipate them and devise a safe plan (as well as a backup plan) for every patient, maintain vigilance throughout all operative procedures, and use common sense at all times.

REFERENCES

1. Achauer BM, Mueller G, Vanderkam VM: Prevention of accidental extubation in burn patients. Ann Plast Surg 38:280-282, 1997.
2. Adnet F: Difficult mask ventilation. Anesthesiology 92:1217-1218, 2000.
3. Ahmad NS, Yentis SM: Laryngeal mask airway and lingual nerve injury. Anaesthesia 51:707-708, 1996.
4. Ainswoth QP, Howells TH: Transilluminated tracheal intubation. Br J Anaesth 62:494-497, 1989.
5. Alessi DM, Hanson DG, Berci G: Bedside videolaryngoscopic assessment of intubation trauma. Ann Otol Rhinol Laryngol 98:586-590, 1989.
6. Alexander CA, Leach AB: Incidence of sore throats with the laryngeal mask [letter]. Anaesthesia 44:791, 1989.
7. American Heart Association: Combination esophageal-tracheal tube. In Guidelines for Cardiopulmonary Resuscitation and Emergency Cardiac Care—Recommendations of the 1992 National Conference of the American Heart Association. JAMA 268:2203, 1992.
8. American Society of Anesthesiologists Task Force on Management of the Difficult Airway: Practice guidelines for management of the difficult airway: An updated report by the American Society of Anesthesiologists Task Force on Management of the Difficult Airway. Anesthesiology 98:1269-1277, 2003.
9. Aoyanma K, Takenaka I, Nagaoka E, et al: Potential damage to the larynx associated with light-guided intubation: A case and series of fiberoptic examinations. Anesthesiology 94:165-166, 2001.
10. Arné J, Descoins P, Fusciardi J, et al: Preoperative assessment for difficult intubation in general and ENT surgery. Predictive value of a clinical multivariate risk index. Br J Anaesth 80:140-146, 1998.
11. Aromaa U, Pesonen P, Linko K, et al: Difficulties with tooth protectors in endotracheal intubation. Acta Anaesthesiol Scand 32:304-307, 1988.
12. Aucott W, Prinsley P, Madden G: Laryngeal anaesthesia with aspiration following intubation. Anaesthesia 44:230-231, 1989.
13. a' Wengen DF: Piriform fossa perforation during attempted tracheal intubation. Anaesthesia 42:519-521, 1987.
14. Azar I, Lear E: Lower lip numbness following general anesthesia [letter]. Anesthesiology 65:450-451, 1986.
15. Badran I, Jamal M: Pneumomediastinum due to Venturi system during microlaryngoscopy. Middle East J Anesthesiol 9:561-564, 1988.
16. Bähr W, Stoll P: Nasal intubation in the presence of frontobasal fractures: A retrospective study. J Oral Maxillofac Surg 50:445-447, 1992.
17. Bainton CR: Complications of managing the airway. In Benumof JL (ed): Airway Management: Principles and Practice. St. Louis, Mosby, 1996, pp 886-899.
18. Barker P, Langton JA, Murphy PJ: Regurgitation of gastric contents during general anaesthesia using the laryngeal mask airway. Br J Anaesth 69:314-315, 1992.
19. Batra YK, Bali IM: Corneal abrasions during general anesthesia. Anesth Analg 56:363-365, 1977.
20. Bedford RF: Circulatory responses to tracheal intubation. Probl Anesth 2:201, 1998.
21. Bellhouse CP, Doré C: Criteria for estimating likelihood of difficulty of endotracheal intubation with the Macintosh laryngoscope. Anaesth Intensive Care 16:329-337, 1988.
22. Benumof JL: Laryngeal mask airway and the ASA difficult airway algorithm. Anesthesiology 84:686-699, 1996.
23. Benumof JL: Management of the difficult adult airway: With special emphasis on awake tracheal intubation. Anesthesiology 75:1087-1110, 1991.
24. Benumof JL: The glottic aperture seal airway: A new ventilatory device. Anesthesiology 88:1219-1226, 1998.
25. Benumof JL, Cooper SD: Quantitative improvement in laryngoscopic view by optimal external laryngeal manipulation. J Clin Anesth 8:136-140, 1996.
26. Benumof JL, Scheller MS: The importance of transtracheal jet ventilation in the management of the difficult airway. Anesthesiology 71:769-778, 1989.

27. Benumof JL, Partridge BL, Salvatierra C, et al: Margin of safety in positioning modern double-lumen endotracheal tubes. Anesthesiology 67:729-738, 1987.

28. Berrouschot J, Oeken J, Steiniger L, et al: Perioperative complications of percutaneous dilational tracheostomy. Laryngoscope 107:1538-1544, 1997.

29. Betbese AJ, Perez M, Bak E, et al: A prospective study of unplanned endotracheal extubation in intensive care unit patients. Crit Care Med 26:1180-1186, 1998.

30. Bidwai AV, Bidwai VA, Rogers CR, et al: Blood pressure and pulse-rate responses to endotracheal extubation with and without prior injection of lidocaine. Anesthesiology 51:171-173, 1979.

31. Binkley K, Cheema A, Sussman G: Generalized allergic reactions during anesthesia. J Allergy Clin Immunol 89:768-774, 1992.

32. Binning R: A hazard of blind nasal intubation [letter]. Anaesthesia 29:366-367, 1974.

33. Birmingham PK, Cheney FW, Ward RJ: Esophageal intubation: A review of detection techniques. Anesth Analg 65:886-891, 1986.

34. Bishop MJ, Weymuller EA Jr, Fink BR: Laryngeal effects of prolonged intubation. Anesth Analg 63:335-342, 1984.

35. Blanc VF, Tremblay NAG: The complications of tracheal intubation: A new classification with a review of the literature. Anesth Analg 53:202-213, 1974.

36. Bogetz MS, Tupper BJ, Vigil AC: Too much of a good thing: Uvular trauma caused by overzealous suctioning. Anesth Analg 72:125-126, 1991.

37. Brain AIJ: The Intravent Laryngeal Mask Instruction Manual, 2nd ed. Berkshire, UK, Brain Medical, 1992.

38. Brain AIJ, Verghese C, Strube PJ: The LMA "ProSeal"—A laryngeal mask with an oesophageal vent. Br J Anaesth 84:650-654, 2000.

39. Brandwein M, Abramson AL, Shikowitz MJ: Bilateral vocal cord paralysis following endotracheal intubation. Arch Otolaryngol Head Neck Surg 112:877-882, 1986.

40. Branthwaite MA: An unexpected complication of the intubating laryngeal mask. Anaesthesia 54:166-167, 1999.

41. Braverman I, Sichel JY, Halimi P, et al: Complication of jet ventilation during microlaryngeal surgery. Ann Otol Rhinol Laryngol 103:624-627, 1994.

42. Brimacombe JR: Analysis of 1500 laryngeal mask uses by one anaesthetist in adults undergoing routine anaesthesia. Anaesthesia 51:76-80, 1996.

43. Brimacombe J, Berry A: The incidence of aspiration associated with the laryngeal mask airway—A meta-analysis of published literature. J Clin Anesth 7:297-305, 1993.

44. Brimacombe JR, Brain AIJ: The Laryngeal Mask Airway. Philadelphia, WB Saunders, 1997.

45. Brimacombe J, Keller C: Aspiration of gastric contents during use of a ProSeal laryngeal mask airway secondary to unidentified foldover malposition. Anesth Analg 97:1192-1194, 2003.

46. Brimacombe J, Keller CH: The ProSeal laryngeal mask airway. Anesthesiology 93:104-109, 2000.

47. Brimacombe J, Holyoake L, Keller C, et al: Pharyngolaryngeal, neck, and jaw discomfort after anesthesia with the face mask and laryngeal mask airway at high and low cuff volumes in males and females. Anesthesiology 93:26-31, 2000.

48. Brimacombe J, Keller CH, Berry A: Gastric insufflation with the ProSeal laryngeal mask. Anesth Analg 92:1614-1615, 2001.

49. Brisson H, Welter J, Wiel E, et al: Complication inhabituelle de l'extubation. Ann Fr Anesth Reanim 20:573-574, 2001.

50. Broccard AF, Liaudet L, Aubert JD, et al: Negative pressure post-tracheal extubation alveolar hemorrhage. Anesth Analg 92:273-275, 2001.

51. Brodsky JB, Lemmens HJM, Brock-Utne JG, Vierra M, Saidman LJ: Morbid obesity and tracheal intubation. Anesth Analg 94:732-736, 2002.

52. Brosnan C, Radford P: The effect of a toothguard on the difficulty of intubation. Anaesthesia 52:1011-1014, 1999.

53. Brown RH, Schauble JF, Hamilton RG: Prevalence of latex allergy among anesthesiologists: Identification of sensitized but asymptomatic individuals. Anesthesiology 89:287-288, 1998.

54. Burgess GE III, Cooper JR Jr, Marino RJ, et al: Laryngeal competence after tracheal extubation. Anesthesiology 51:73-77, 1979.

55. Caplan RA, Posner KL, Ward RJ, et al: Adverse respiratory events in anesthesia: A closed claims analysis. Anesthesiology 72:828-833, 1990.

56. Caponas G: Intubating laryngeal mask airway. Anaesth Intensive Care 30:551-569, 2002.

57. Cass NM, James NR, Lines V: Intubation under direct laryngoscopy. Br Med J 2:488, 1956.

58. Cataneo AJM, Reibscheid SM, Ruiz RL Jr, et al: Foreign bodies in the tracheobronchial tree. Clin Pediatr 36:701-706, 1997.

59. Cavo JW Jr: True vocal cord paralysis following intubation. Laryngoscope 95:1352-1359, 1985.

60. Chadwick RG, Lindsay SM: Dental injuries during general anaesthesia. Br Dent J 180:255-258, 1996.

61. Chang JL, Bleyaert A, Bedger R: Unilateral pneumothorax following jet ventilation during general anesthesia. Anesthesiology 53:244-246, 1980.

62. Chen CT, Toung TJK, Donham RT, et al: Fentanyl dosage for suppression of circulatory response to laryngoscopy and endotracheal intubation. Anesthesiol Rev 13:37, 1986.

63. Cheney FW, Posner KL, Caplan RA: Adverse respiratory events infrequently leading to malpractice suits. Anesthesiology 75:932-939, 1991.

64. Chevron V, Menard JF, Richard JC, et al: Unplanned extubation: Risk factors of development and predictive criteria for reintubation. Crit Care Med 26:1049-1053, 1998.

65. Chou HC, Wu TL: Mandibulohyoid distance in difficult laryngoscopy. Br J Anaesth 71:335-339,1993.

66. Christie JM, Dethlefsen M, Cane RD: Unplanned endotracheal extubation in the intensive care unit. J Clin Anesth 8:289-293, 1996.

67. Ciaglia P, Firsching R, Syniec C: Elective percutaneous dilatational tracheostomy. A new simple bedside procedure; preliminary report. Chest 87:715-719, 1985.

68. Clarke T, Evans S, Way P, et al: A comparison of two methods of securing an endotracheal tube. Aust Crit Care 11:45-50, 1998.

69. Cloward RB: Acute cervical spine injuries. Clin Symp 32:1-32, 1980.
70. Conacher ID: Foreign body in a laryngeal mask airway [letter]. Anaesthesia 46:164, 1991.
71. Conrardy PA, Goodman LR, Lainge F, et al: Alteration of endotracheal tube position: Flexion and extension of the neck. Crit Care Med 4:7-12, 1976.
72. Cook WP, Schultetus RR: Obstruction of an endotracheal tube by the plastic coating sheared from a stylet. Anesthesiology 62:803-804, 1985.
73. Cooper JB, Newbower RS, Kitz RJ: An analysis of major errors and equipment failures in anesthesia management: Considerations for prevention and detection. Anesthesiology 60:34-42, 1984.
74. Cooper RM: Extubation and changing endotracheal tubes. In Benumof JL (ed): Airway Management: Principles and Practice. St. Louis, Mosby, 1996, p 866.
75. Coriat P, Mundler O, Bousseau D, et al: Response of left ventricular ejection fraction to recovery from general anesthesia: Measurement by gated radionuclide angiography. Anesth Analg 65:593-600,1986.
76. Craft TM, Chambers PH, Ward ME, et al: Two cases of barotrauma associated with transtracheal jet ventilation. Br J Anaesth 64:524-527, 1990.
77. Crosby ET, Lui A: The adult cervical spine: Implications for airway management. Can J Anaesth 37:77-93, 1990.
78. Crosby F: Airway management after upper cervical spine injury: What have we learned? Can J Anaesth 49:733-744, 2002.
79. Daley MD, Norman PH, Coveler LA: Tracheal extubation of adult surgical patients while deeply anesthetized: A survey of United States anesthesiologists. J Clin Anesth 11:445-452, 1999.
80. Darmon JY, Rauss A, Dreyfuss D, et al: Evaluation of risk factors for laryngeal edema after tracheal extubation in adults and its prevention by dexamethasone: A placebo-controlled, double-blind, multi-center study. Anesthesiology 78:609-610, 1993
81. Davis L, Cook-Sather SD, Schreiner MS: Lighted stylet tracheal intubation: A review. Anesth Analg 90:745-756, 2000.
82. Debain JJ, Le Brigand H, Binet JP: Quelques incidents et accidents de l'intubation trachéale prolongué. Ann Otolaryngol Chir Cervicofac 85:379-386, 1968.
83. Debo RF, Colonna D, Deward G, et al: Cricoarytenoid subluxation: Complication of blind intubation with a lighted stylet. Ear Nose Throat J 68:517-520, 1989.
84. Diaz JH: Is uvular edema a complication of endotracheal intubation? Anesth Analg 76:1139-1141, 1993.
85. Diaz-Perales A, Collada C, Blanco C, et al: Cross-reactions in the latex-fruit syndrome: A relevant role of chitinases but not of complex asparagine-linked glycans. J Allergy Clin Immunol 104:681-687, 1999.
86. Dimarakis I, Protopapas AD: Vocal cord palsy as a complication of adult cardian surgery: Surgical correlations and analysis. Eur J Cardiothorac Surg 26:773-775, 2004.
87. Dinner M, Tjeuw M, Artusio JF Jr: Bacteremia as a complication of nasotracheal intubation. Anesth Analg 66:460-462, 1987.
88. Dohi S, Gold MI: Pulmonary mechanics during general anaesthesia: The influence of mechanical irritation on the airway. Br J Anaesth 51:205-214, 1979.
89. Domino KB: Closed malpractice claims for airway trauma during anesthesia. Am Soc Anesthesiol Newslett June 1968.
90. Domino KB, Posner KL, Caplan RA, et al: Airway injury during anesthesia: A closed claims analysis. Anesthesiology 91:1703-1711, 1999.
91. Dong ML: Arnold-Chiari malformation type I appearing after tonsillectomy. Anesthesiology 67:120-122, 1987.
92. Donlon JV: Anesthesia and eye, ear, nose, and throat surgery. In Miller RD (ed): Anesthesia, 3rd ed. New York, Churchill Livingstone, 1990, p 2004.
93. Dörges V, Ocker H, Wenzel V, et al: The laryngeal tube: A new simple airway device. Anesth Analg 90:1220-1222, 2000.
94. Drosnes DL, Zwillenberg DA: Laryngeal granulomatous polyp after short-term intubation of a child. Ann Otol Rhinol Laryngol 99:183-186, 1990.
95. Dryden GE: Circulatory collapse after pneumonectomy (an unusual complication from the use of a Carlens catheter): Case report. Anesth Analg 56:451-452, 1977.
96. Duman A, Ogun CO, Okesli S: The effect on intraocular pressure of tracheal intubation or laryngeal mask insertion during sevoflurane anaesthesia in children without the use of muscle relaxants. Paediatr Anaesth 11:421-424, 2001.
97. Durkan W, Fleming N: Potential eye damage from reusable masks [letter]. Anesthesiology 67:444, 1987.
98. Durmus M, Ender G, Kadir BA, et al: Remifentanil with thiopental for tracheal intubation without muscle relaxants. Anesth Analg 96:1336-1339, 2003.
99. Eberhart LHJ, Arndt C, Cierpka T, et al: The reliability and validity of the upper lip bite test compared with the Mallampati classification to predict difficult laryngoscopy: An external prospective evaluation. Anesth Analg 101:284-289, 2005.
100. Edwards ND, Alford AM, Dobson PM, et al: Myocardial ischaemia during tracheal intubation and extubation. Br J Anaesth 73:537-539, 1994.
101. Egol A, Culpepper JA, Snyder JV: Barotrauma and hypotension resulting from jet ventilation in critically ill patients. Chest 88:98-102, 1985.
102. Ehrenpreis MB, Oliverio RM Jr: Endotracheal tube obstruction secondary to oral preoperative medication. Anesth Analg 63:867-868, 1984.
103. Eldor J, Ofek B, Abramowitz HB: Perforation of oesophagus by tracheal tube during resuscitation. Anaesthesia 45:70-71, 1990.
104. Ellis DG, Jakymec A, Kaplan RM, et al: Guided orotracheal intubation in the operating room using a lighted stylet: A comparison with direct laryngoscopic technique. Anesthesiology 64:823-826, 1986.
105. Eltzschig HK, Darsow R, Schroeder TH, et al: Effect of tracheal intubation or laryngeal mask airway insertion on intraocular pressure using balanced anesthesia with sevoflurane and remifentanil. J Clin Anesth 13:264-267, 2001.

106. Elwany S, Mekhamer A: Effect of nasotracheal intubation on nasal mucociliary clearance. Br J Anaesth 59:755-759, 1987.

107. Engelhardt T, Webster NR: Pulmonary aspiration of gastric contents in anaesthesia. Br J Anaesth 83:453-460, 1999.

108. European Resuscitation Council Writing subcommittee; Baskett PJF, Bossaert L, Carli P, et al: Guidelines for the advanced management of the airway and ventilation during resuscitation. Resuscitation 31:201-230, 1996.

109. Ezri T, Priscu V, Szmuk P: Laryngeal mask and pulmonary edema [letter]. Anesthesiology 78:219, 1993.

110. Fagraeus L: Difficult extubation following nasotracheal intubation. Anesthesiology 49:43-44, 1978.

111. Faithfull NS: Injury to terminal branches of the trigeminal nerve following tracheal intubation. Br J Anaesth 57:535-537, 1985.

112. Fantoni A, Ripamonti D: A non-derivative, non-surgical tracheostomy: The translaryngeal method. Intensive Care Med 23:386-392, 1997.

113. Ferson DZ, Rosenblatt WH, Johansen MJ, et al: Use of the intubating LMA-Fastrach in 254 patients with difficult-to-manage airways. Anesthesiology 95:1175-1181, 2001.

114. Fink BR: Laryngeal complications of general anesthesia. In Orkin FK, Cooperman LH (eds): Complications in Anesthesiology. Philadelphia, JB Lippincott, 1983, pp 141-151.

115. Fitzpatrick PC, Guarisco JL: Pediatric airway foreign bodies. J La State Med Soc 150:138-141, 1998.

116. Frass M: The Combitube: Esophageal/tracheal double-lumen airway. In Benumof JL (ed): Airway Management: Principles and Practice. St. Louis, Mosby, 1996, p 444.

117. Frass M, Frenzer R, Zdrahal F: The esophageal tracheal combitube: Preliminary results with a new airway for CPR. Ann Emerg Med 16:768-772, 1987.

118. Frerk CM: Predicting difficult intubation. Anaesthesia 46:1005-1008, 1991.

119. Frink EJ, Pattison BD: Posterior arytenoid dislocation following uneventful endotracheal intubation and anesthesia. Anesthesiology 70:358-360, 1989.

120. Gaitini LA, Vaida SJ, Mostafa S, et al: The combitube in elective surgery. Anesthesiology 94:79-82, 2001.

121. Gallagher ML, Roberts-Fox M: Respiratory and circulatory compromise associated with acute hydrothorax during operative hysteroscopy. Anesthesiology 79:1129-1131, 1993.

122. Gamlin F, Caldicott LD, Shah MV: Mediastinitis and sepsis syndrome following intubation. Anaesthesia 49:883-885, 1994.

123. Garabrant DH, Schweitzer S: Epidemiology of latex sensitization and allergies in health care workers. J Allergy Clin Immunol 110:S82-S95, 2002.

124. Garcia Ortiz JC, Moyano JC, Alvarez M, et al: Latex allergy in fruit allergic patients. Allergy 53:532-536, 1999.

125. Gauss A, Treiber HS, Haehnel J, et al: Spontaneous reposition of dislocated arytenoid cartilage. Br J Anaesth 70:591-592, 1993.

126. Geelhoed GW: Tracheomalacia from compressing goiter: Management after thyroidectomy. Surgery 104:1100-1108, 1988.

127. Geffin B, Bland J, Grillo HC: Anesthetic management of tracheal resection and reconstruction. Anesth Analg 48:884-890, 1969.

128. Gemma M, Ferrazza C: "Dental trauma" to oral airways [letter]. Can J Anaesth 37:951, 1990.

129. Georgescu A, Miller JN, Lecklitner ML: The Sellick maneuver causing complete airway obstruction. Anesth Analg 74:457-459, 1992.

130. Georgiou M, Parlapani A, Argiriadou H, et al: Sufentanil or clonidine for blunting the increase in intraocular pressure during rapid-sequence induction. Eur J Anaesthesiol 19:819-822, 2002.

131. Gerhardt T, Bancalari E: Apnea of prematurity. I. Lung function and regulation of breathing. Pediatrics 74:58-62, 1984.

132. Gild WM, Posner KL, Caplan RA, et al: Eye injuries associated with anesthesia: A closed claims analysis. Anesthesiology 76:204-208, 1992.

133. Glauber DT: Facial paralysis after general anesthesia. Anesthesiology 65:516-517, 1986.

134. Goldik Z, Mecz Y, Bornstein J, et al: LMA insertion after accidental extubation. Can J Anaesth 42:1065, 1995.

135. Gonzalez RM, Bjerke RJ, Drobycki T, et al: Prevention of endotracheal tube-induced coughing during emergence from general anesthesia. Anesth Analg 79:792-795, 1994.

136. Granholm T, Farmer DL: The surgical airway. Respir Care Clin N Am 7:13-23, 2001.

137. Gray B, Huggins NJ, Hirsch N: An unusual complication of tracheal intubation. Anaesthesia 45:558-560, 1990.

138. Green JG, Wood JM, Davis LF: Asystole after inadvertent intubation of the orbit. J Oral Maxillofac Surg 55:856-859, Aug 1997.

139. Green KS, Beger TH: Proper use of the Combitube [letter]. Anesthesiology 81:513-514, 1994.

140. Greenberg RS, Toung T: The cuffed oro-pharyngeal airway—A pilot study. Anesthesiology 77:558, 1992.

141. Greenberg RS, Brimacombe JR, Berry A: A randomized controlled trial comparing the cuffed oropharyngeal airway and the laryngeal mask airway in spontaneously breathing anesthetized adults. Anesthesiology 88:970-977, 1998.

142. Griggs WM, Worthley LIG, Gilligan JE, et al: A simple percutaneous tracheostomy technique. Surg Gynecol Obstet 170:543-545, 1990.

143. Grigsby EJ, Lennon RL, Didier EP: Massive tongue swelling after uncomplicated general anaesthesia. Can J Anaesth 37:825-826, 1990.

144. Halac E, Indiveri DR, Obregon RJ: Complication of nasal endotracheal intubation [letter]. J Pediatr 103:166, 1983.

145. Hamaya Y, Dohi S: Differences in cardiovascular response to airway stimulation at different sites and blockade of the responses by lidocaine. Anesthesiology 93:95-103, 2000.

146. Hariri MA, Duncan PW: Infective complications of brief nasotracheal intubation. J Laryngol Otol 103:1217-1218, 1989.

147. Harris R, Joseph A: Acute tracheal rupture related to endotracheal intubation: Case report. J Emerg Med 18:35-39, 2000.

148. Hartley M, Vaughan RS: Problems associated with tracheal extubation. Br J Anaesth 71:561-568, 1993.

149. Hartmann T, Hoerauf KH, Benumof JL, et al: The esophageal-tracheal Combitube small adult. An alternative airway for ventilatory support during gynaecological laparoscopy. Anaesthesia 55:670-675, 2000.

150. Haselby KA, McNiece WL: Respiratory obstruction from uvular edema in a pediatric patient. Anesth Analg 62:1127-1128, 1983.

151. Hastings RH, Kelley SD: Neurologic deterioration associated with airway management in a cervical spine-injured patient. Anesthesiology 78:580-583, 1993.

152. Henn-Beilharz A, Hagen R: Besonderheiten der Atemwegssicherung in der Hals-Nasen-Ohren-Heilkunde. In Krier C, Georgi R (eds): Airway Management. Stuttgart, Thieme, 2001, pp 336-347.

153. Hepner DL: Sudden bronchospasm on intubation: Latex anaphylaxis? J Clin Anesth 12:162-166, 2000.

154. Hepner DL, Castells MC: Latex allergy: An update. Anesth Analg 96:1219-1229, 2003.

155. Hershey MD, Hannenberg AA: Gastric distention and rupture from oxygen insufflation during fiberoptic intubation. Anesthesiology 1996;85:1479-80.

156. Heuhns TY, Yentis SM, Cumberworth V: Apparent massive tongue swelling. Anaesthesia 49:414-416, 1994.

157. Hilley MD, Henderson RB, Giesecke AH: Difficult extubation of the trachea. Anesthesiology 59:149-150, 1983.

158. Hiong YT, Fung CF, Sudhaman DA: Arytenoid subluxation: Implications for the anaesthetist. Anaesth Intensive Care 24:609-610, 1996.

159. Hirshman CA, Smith J: Indirect ignition of the endotracheal tube during carbon dioxide laser surgery. Arch Otolaryngol 106:639-641, 1980.

160. Hirshman CA, Leon D, Porch D, et al: Improved metal endotracheal tube for laser surgery of the airway. Anesth Analg 59:789-791, 1980.

161. Hoerauf KH, Hartmann T, Acimovic S: Waste gas exposure to sevoflurane and nitrous oxide during anaesthesia using the oesophageal-tracheal Combitube small adult. Br J Anaesth 86:124-126, 2001.

162. Holden R, Morsman CD, Butler J, et al: Intra-ocular pressure changes using the laryngeal mask airway and tracheal tube. Anaesthesia 46:922-824, 1991.

163. Horak J, Weiss S: Emergent management of the airway. New pharmacology and control of comorbidities in cardiac disease, ischemia and valvular heart disease. Crit Care Clin 16:411-427, 2000.

164. Horellou MF, Mathe D, Feiss P: A hazard of naso-tracheal intubation [letter]. Anaesthesia 33:73-74, 1978.

165. Horie T, Higa K, Ken-Mizaki Y, et al: Tracheal rupture in a patient intubated with a double-lumen endobronchial tube. Masui 43:1366-1369, 1994.

166. Horton WA, Fahy L, Charters P: Disposition of cervical vertebrae, atlanto-axial joint, hyoid and mandible during x-ray laryngoscopy. Br J Anaesth 63:435-438, 1989.

167. Howland WS, Lewis JS: Postintubation granulomas of the larynx. Cancer 9:1244, 1956.

168. Hung OR, Pytka S, Morris I, et al: Clinical trial of a new lightwand device (Trachlight) to intubate the trachea. Anesthesiology 83:509-514, 1995.

169. Imai M, Matsumara C, Hanoka Y, et al: Comparison of cardiovascular responses to airway management: Fiberoptic intubation using a new adapter, laryngeal mask insertion, or conventional laryngoscopic intubation. J Clin Anesth 7:14-18, 1995.

170. Isaacs JH, Pedersen AD: Emergency cricothyroidotomy. Am Surg 63:346-349, 1997.

171. Ishimoto S, Ito K, Toyama M, et al. Vocal cord paralysis after surgery for thoracic aortic aneurysm. Chest 121:1911-1915, 2002.

172. Jarjour NN, Wilson P: Pneumocephalus associated with nasal continuous positive airway pressure in a patient with sleep apnea syndrome. Chest 96:1425-1426, 1989.

173. Johnson KG, Hood DD: Esophageal perforation associated with endotracheal intubation. Anesthesiology 64:281-283, 1986.

174. Jones GOM, Hale DE, Wasmuth CE, et al: A survey of acute complications associated with endotracheal intubation. Cleve Clin Q 35:23-31, 1968.

175. Joo DT, Orser BA: External compression of a nasotracheal tube due to the displaced bony fragments of multiple LeFort fractures. Anesthesiology 92:1830-1831, 2000.

176. Joo HS, Kapoor S, Rose DK, et al: The intubating laryngeal mask after induction of general anesthesia versus awake fiberoptic intubation in patients with difficult airway. Anesth Analg 92:1342-1346, 2001.

177. Jordon WS, Graves CL, Elwyn RA: New therapy for postintubation laryngeal edema and tracheitis in children. JAMA 212:585-588, 1970.

178. Joshi GP, Smith I, White PF: Laryngeal mask airway. In Benumof JL (ed): Airway Management: Principles and Practice. St. Louis, Mosby, 1996, p 368.

179. Kaeder CS, Hirshman CA: Acute airway obstruction: A complication of aluminum tape wrapping of tracheal tubes in laser surgery. Can Anaesth Soc J 26:138-139, 1979.

180. Kalinske RW, Parker RH, Brandt D: Diagnostic usefulness and safety of transtracheal aspiration. N Engl J Med 276:604-608, 1967.

181. Kambic V, Radsel Z: Intubation lesions of the larynx. Br J Anaesth 50:587-590, 1978.

182. Kapadia FN, Bajan KB, Raje KV: Airway accidents in intubated intensive care unit patients: An epidemiological study. Crit Care Med 28:659-664, 2000.

183. Kaplow R, Bookbinder M: A comparison of four endotracheal tube holders. Heart Lung 23:59-66, 1994.

184. Kastanos N, Miro RE, Perez AM, et al: Laryngotracheal injury due to endotracheal intubation: Incidence, evolution, and predisposing factors. A prospective long-term study. Crit Care Med 11:362-367, 1983.

185. Kautto UM: Attenuation of the circulatory response to laryngoscopy and intubation by fentanyl. Acta Anaesthesiol Scand 26:217-221, 1982.

186. Keller CH, Brimacombe J, Kleinsasser A, et al: Does the ProSeal laryngeal mask airway prevent aspiration of regurgitated fluid? Anesth Analg 91:1017-1020, 2000.

187. Kelly KJ, Kurup VP, Reijula KE, Fink JN: The diagnosis of natural rubber latex allergy. J Allergy Clin Immunol 93:813-816, 1994.

188. Kendall AP, Lin E: Respiratory failure as presentation of achalasia of the esophagus. Anaesthesia 46:1039-1040, 1991.

189. Kerwin AJ, Croce MA, Timmons SD, et al: Effects of fiberoptic bronchoscopy on intracranial pressure in patients with brain injury: A prospective clinical study. J Trauma 48:878-882, 2000.

190. Kharasch ED: Angiotensin-converting enzyme inhibitor-induced angioedema associated with endotracheal intubation. Anesth Analg 74:602-604, 1992.

191. Kilickan L, Baykara N, Gurkan Y, et al: The effect on intraocular pressure of endotracheal intubation or laryngeal mask use during TIVA without the use of muscle relaxants. Acta Anaesthesiol Scand 43:343-346, 1999.

192. King C, Street MK: Twelfth cranial nerve paralysis following use of a laryngeal mask airway. Anaesthesia 49:786-787, 1994.

193. Kirchner JA, Sasaki CT: Fusion of the vocal cords following intubation and tracheostomy. Trans Am Acad Ophthalmol Otolaryngol 77:ORL88-ORL91, 1973.

194. Klopfenstein CE, Forster A, Suter PM: Pneumocephalus: A complication of continuous positive airway pressure after trauma. Chest 78:656-657, 1980.

195. Koga K, Asai T, Vaughan RS, Latto IP: Respiratory complications associated with tracheal extubation. Anaesthesia 53:540-544, 1998.

196. Kramer MR, Melzer E, Sprung CL: Unilateral pulmonary edema after intubation of the right mainstem bronchus. Crit Care Med 17:472-474, 1989.

197. Krantz MA, Solomon DL, Poulos JC: Uvular necrosis following endotracheal intubation. J Clin Anesth 6:139-141, 1994.

198. Kras JF, Marchmont-Robinson H: Pharyngeal perforation during intubation in a patient with Crohn's disease. J Oral Maxillofac Surg 47:405-407, 1989.

199. Krier C, Georgi R: Airway management—Is there more than one "gold standard"? Anasthesiol Intensivmed Notfallmed Schmerzther 36:193-194, 2001.

200. Kumeta Y, Hattori A, Mimura M, et al: A survey of perioperative bronchospasm in 105 patients with reactive airway disease. Masui 44:396-401, 1995.

201. Kurup VP, Fink JN: The spectrum of immunologic sensitisation in latex allergy. Allergy 56:2-12, 2001.

202. Lamb K, James MFM, Janicki PK: The laryngeal mask airway for intraocular surgery: Effects on intraocular pressure and stress responses. Br J Anaesth 69:143-147, 1992.

203. Lang S, Johnson DH, Lanigan DT, Ha H: Difficult tracheal extubation. Can J Anaesth 36:340-342, 1989.

204. Langeron O, Masso E, Huraux C, et al: Prediction of difficult mask ventilation. Anesthesiology 92:1229-1236, 2000.

205. Latorre F, Hofmann M, Kleemann PP, et al: Fiberoptic intubation and stress. Anaesthesist 42:423-426, 1993.

206. Latto IP, Vaughan RS: Difficulties in Tracheal Intubation. London, Saunders, 1997.

207. Laxton CH, Kipling R: Lingual nerve paralysis following the use of the laryngeal mask airway. Anaesthesia 51:869-870, 1996.

208. Lederman IR: Fire hazard during ophthalmic surgery. Ophthalmic Surg 16:577-578, 1985.

209. Lee C, Schwartz S, Mok MS: Difficult extubation due to transfixation of a nasotracheal tube by a Kirschner wire. Anesthesiology 46:427, 1977.

210. Lee JJ: Laryngeal mask and trauma to uvula [letter]. Anaesthesia 44:1014-1015, 1989.

211. Levine PA: Hypopharyngeal perforation: An untoward complication of endotracheal intubation. Arch Otolaryngol 106:578-580, 1980.

212. Lim EK, Chia KS, Ng BK: Recurrent laryngeal nerve palsy following endotracheal intubation. Anaesth Intensive Care 15:342-345, 1987.

213. Lipp MDW, Jaehnichen G, Golecki N, et al: Microbiological, microstructure and material science examinations of reprocessed Combitubes after multiple reuse. Anesth Analg 91:693-697, 2000.

214. Lloyd JFR, Hegab A: Recurrent laryngeal nerve palsy after laryngeal mask airway insertion. Anaesthesia 51:171-172, 1996.

215. LoCicero J III: Tracheo-carotid artery erosion following endotracheal intubation. J Trauma 24:907-909, 1984.

216. Loh KS, Irish JC: Traumatic complications of intubation and other airway management procedures. Anesthesiol Clin North Am 20:953-969, 2002.

217. Lu PP, Yang CH, Ho AC, et al: The intubating LMA: A comparison of insertion techniques with conventional tracheal tubes. Can J Anaesth 47:849-853, 2000.

218. Lukaschewski T: Besonderheiten der Atemwegssicherung in der Intensivmedizin. In Krier C, Georgi R (eds): Airway Management. Stuttgart, Thieme, 2001, pp 362-374.

219. Macklem PT, Mead J: Resistance of central and peripheral airways measured by a retrograde catheter. J Appl Physiol 22:395-401, 1967.

220. Majumdar B, Stevens RW, Obara LG: Retropharyngeal abscess following tracheal intubation. Anaesthesia 37:67-70, 1982.

221. Mallampati SR, Gatt SP, Gugino LD: A clinical sign to predict difficult tracheal intubation: A prospective study. Can Anaesth Soc J 32:429-434, 1985.

222. Marjot R: Pressure exerted by the laryngeal mask airway cuff upon the pharyngeal mucosa. Br J Anaesth 70:25-29, 1993.

223. Marjot R: Trauma to the posterior pharyngeal wall caused by a laryngeal mask airway [letter]. Anaesthesia 46:589-590, 1991.

224. Marty-Ane CH, Picard E, Jonquet O, et al: Membranous tracheal rupture after endotracheal intubation. Ann Thorac Surg 60:1367-1371, 1995.

225. Massey JY: Complications of transtracheal aspiration: A case report. J Ark Med Soc 67:254-256, 1971.

226. Mayhew JF, Miner ME, Denneny J: Upper airway obstruction following cyst-to-peritoneal shunt in a child with a Dandy-Walker cyst. Anesthesiology 62:183-184 1985.

227. Mayhew JF, Miner M, Katz J: Macroglossia in a 16-month-old child after a craniotomy. Anesthesiology 62:683-684, 1985.

228. McConnell MS, Finn JC, Feeley TW: Tension hydrothorax during laparoscopy in a patient with ascites. Anesthesiology 80:1390-1393, 1994.

229. McEnery JT: Surgical management of tracheal stenosis. Ann Surg 179:819-824, 1974.

230. McTaggart RA, Shustack A, Noseworth T, et al: Another cause of obstruction in an armoured endotracheal tube [letter]. Anesthesiology 59:164, 1983.

231. Mehta S: Guided orotracheal intubation in the operating room using a lighted stylet [letter]. Anesthesiology 66:105, 1987.

232. Mehta S: Transtracheal illumination for optimal tracheal tube placement: A clinical study. Anaesthesia 44:970-972, 1989.

233. Mencke T, Echternach M, Kleinschmidt S, et al: Laryngeal morbidity and quality of tracheal intubation. Anesthesiology 98:1049-1056, 2003.

234. Mertzlufft F, Zander R: Optimale O_2-Applikation über den nasoralen Weg. Anasthesiol Intensivmed Notfallmed Schmerzther 32:381-385, 1996.

235. Miller AC, Bickler P: The laryngeal mask airway: An unusual complication. Anaesthesia 46:659-660, 1991.

236. Miller DM, Camporota L: Advantages of ProSeal™ and SLIPA™ airway over tracheal tubes for gynecological laparoscopies. Can J Anesth 53:188-193, 2006.

237. Miller DM, Youkhana I, Karunaratne WU, et al: Presence of protein deposits on "cleaned" re-usable anesthetic equipment. Anaesthesia 56:1069-1072, 2001.

238. Mondello E, Casati A; Italian PAXpress Group: A prospective, observational evaluation of a new supraglottic airway: The PAXpress. Minerva Anestesiol 69:517-25, 2003.

239. Monroe MC, Gravenstein N, Saga-Rumley S: Postoperative sore throat: Effect of oropharyngeal airway in orotracheally intubated patients. Anesth Analg 70:512-516, 1990.

240. Moukabary K, Peterson CJ, Kingsley CP: A potential complication with the lightwand [letter]. Anesthesiology 81:523-524, 1994.

241. Murray WJ, Ruddy MP: Toxic eye injury during induction of anesthesia. South Med J 78:1012-1013, 1985.

242. Muzzi DA, Black S, Losasso TJ, et al: Labetalol and esmolol in the control of hypertension after intracranial surgery. Anesth Analg 70:68-71, 1990.

243. Nagai K, Sakuramoto C, Goto F: Unilateral hypoglossal nerve paralysis following the use of the laryngeal mask airway. Anaesthesia 49:603-604, 1994.

244. Nagaoka E, Takenaka I, Kadoya T: The McCoy laryngoscope expands the laryngeal aperture in patients with difficult intubation. Anesthesiology 92:1855-1856, 2000.

245. Nakamura CT, Ferdman RM, Keens TG, et al: Latex allergy on home mechanical ventilation. Chest 118:1000-1003, 2000.

246. Nichol HC, Zuck D: Difficult laryngoscopy—The "anterior" larynx and the atlanto-occipital gap. Br J Anaesth 55:141-144, 1983.

247. Nishikawa K, Omote K, Kawana S, et al: A comparison of hemodynamic changes after endotracheal intubation by using the lightwand device and the laryngoscope in normotensive and hypertensive patients. Anesth Analg 90:1203-1207, 2000.

248. Norman EA, Sosis M: Iatrogenic oesophageal perforation due to tracheal or nasogastric intubation. Can Anaesth Soc J 33:222-226, 1986.

249. Nuutinen J, Karja J: Bilateral vocal cord paralysis following general anesthesia. Laryngoscope 91:83-86, 1981.

250. O'Connell JE, Stevenson DS, Stokes MA: Pathological changes associated with short-term nasal intubation. Anaesthesia 51:347-350, 1996.

251. Oczenski W, Krenn H, Dahaba AA, et al: Complications following the use of the Combitube, tracheal tube and laryngeal mask airway. Anaesthesia 54:1161-1165, 1999.

252. Oczenski W, Krenn H, Dahaba AA, et al: Hemodynamic and catecholamine stress responses to insertion of the combitube, laryngeal mask airway or tracheal intubation. Anesth Analg 88:1389, 1999.

253. O'Donnell JM: Orotracheal tube intracuff pressure initially and during anesthesia including nitrous oxide. CRNA 6:79-85, 1995.

254. O'Hanlon J, Harper KW: Epistaxis and nasotracheal intubation: Prevention with vasoconstrictor spray. Ir J Med Sci 163:58-60, 1994.

255. Oliverio R Jr, Ruder CB, Fermon C, et al: Pneumothorax secondary to ball-valve obstruction during jet ventilation. Anesthesiology 51:255-256, 1979.

256. Olsson GL, Hallen B: Laryngospasm during anaesthesia. A computer-aided incidence study in 136,929 patients. Acta Anaesthesiol Scand 28:567-575, 1984.

257. O'Reilly MJ, Reddick EJ, Black W: Sepsis from sinusitis in nasotracheally intubated patients: A diagnostic dilemma. Am J Surg 147:601-604, 1984.

258. Ossoff ARG: Laser safety in otolaryngology: Head and neck surgery—Anesthetic and educational considerations for laryngeal surgery. Laryngoscope 99(Suppl 48):1-26, 1989.

259. O'Sullivan JC, Wells DG, Wells GR: Difficult airway management with neck swelling after carotid endarterectomy. Anaesth Intensive Care 14:460-464, 1986.

260. O'Sullivan TJ, Healy GB: Complications of Venturi jet ventilation during microlaryngeal surgery. Arch Otolaryngol 111:127-131, 1985.

261. Ovassapian A: Fiberoptic tracheal intubation. In Fiberoptic Airway Endoscopy in Anaesthesia and Critical Care. New York, Raven Press, 1990.

262. Owen RL, Cheney FW: Endobronchial intubation: A preventable complication. Anesthesiology 67:255-257, 1987.

263. Parmet JL, Metz S: Anesthesiology issues in general surgery: Retrograde endotracheal intubation: An underutilized tool for management of the difficult airway. Contemp Surg 49(5), 1996, pp 300-306.

264. Pashayan AG, Gravenstein N: High incidence of CO_2 laser beam contact with the tracheal tube during operations on the upper airway. J Clin Anesth 1:354-357, 1989.

265. Pashayan AG, Gravenstein JS, Cassisi NJ, et al: The helium protocol for laryngotracheal operations with CO_2 laser: A retrospective review of 523 cases. Anesthesiology 68:801-804, 1988.

266. Pashayan AG, SanGiovanni C, Davis LE: Positive end-expiratory pressure lowers the risk of laser-induced polyvinyl chloride tracheal-tube fires. Anesthesiology 79:83-87, 1993.

267. Patane PS, White SE: Macroglossia causing airway obstruction following cleft palate repair. Anesthesiology 71:995-996, 1989.

268. Patil VU, Stehling LC, Zauder HL: Predicting the difficulty of intubation utilizing an intubation guide. Anesthesiol Rev 10:32, 1983.

269. Pender JW: Endotracheal intubation in children: Advantages and disadvantages. Anesthesiology 15:495, 1954.

270. Pennant JH, White PF: The laryngeal mask airway: Its use in anesthesiology. Anesthesiology 79:144-163, 1993.

271. Peppard SB, Dickens JH: Laryngeal injury following short-term intubation. Ann Otol Rhinol Laryngol 92: 327-330, 1983.

272. Podolsky S, Baraff LJ, Simon RR, et al: Efficacy of cervical spine immobilization methods. J Trauma 23: 461-465, 1983.

273. Politis C, Schiepers JP, Heylen R: Complete obstruction of a naso-endotracheal tube: A case report. Acta Stomatol Belg 93:13-16, 1996.

274. Poon YK: Case history number 89: A life-threatening complication of cricothyroid membrane puncture. Anesth Analg 55:298-301, 1976.

275. Populaire C, Robard S, Souron R: An armoured endotracheal tube obstruction in a child. Can J Anaesth 36:331-332, 1989.

276. Pothmann W: Der nicht nüchterne Patient. In Krier C, Georgi R (eds): Airway Management. Stuttgart, Thieme, 2001, pp 304-311.

277. Practice guidelines for management of the difficult airway: A report by the American Society of Anesthesiologists Task Force on Management of the Difficult Airway. Anesthesiology 78:597-602, 1993.

278. Quartararo C, Bishop MJ: Complications of tracheal intubation: Prevention and treatment. Semin Anesth 9:119, 1990.

279. Rabey PG, Murphy PJ, Langton JA, et al: Effect of the laryngeal mask airway on lower oesophageal sphincter pressure in patients during general anaesthesia. Br J Anaesth 69:346-348, 1992.

280. Randel GI: Latex allergy: Who is next? ASA Newslett 61(5), 1997.

281. Raphael DT, Weller RS, Doran DJ: A response algorithm for the low-pressure alarm condition. Anesth Analg 67:876-883, 1988.

282. Rex MAE: A review of the structural and functional basis of laryngospasm and a discussion of the nerve pathways involved in the reflex and its clinical significance in man and animals. Br J Anaesth 42:891-899, 1970.

283. Reyes G, Galvis AG, Thompson JW: Esophagotracheal perforation during emergency intubation. Am J Emerg Med 10:223-225, 1992.

284. Rieger A: Intubationsschäden: Inzidenz, Komplikationen, Konsequenzen. In Krier C, Georgi R (eds): Airway Management. Stuttgart, Thieme, 2001, pp 138-153.

285. Riggins RS, Kraus JF: The risk of neurologic damage with fractures of the vertebrae. J Trauma 17:126-133, 1977.

286. Robinson N, Clancy M: In patients with head injury undergoing rapid sequence intubation, does pretreatment with intravenous lignocaine/lidocaine lead to an improved neurological outcome? A review of the literature. Emerg Med J 18:453-457, 2001.

287. Rose DK, Cohen MM: The airway: Problems and predictions in 18,500 patients. Can J Anaesth 41: 372-383, 1994.

288. Rosenberg H, Rosenberg HK: Airway obstruction and causes of difficult intubation. In Orkin FK, Cooperman LH (eds): Complications in Anesthesiology. Philadelphia, JB Lippincott, 1983, p 125.

289. Rosenberg H, Rosenberg HK: Airway obstruction and tracheal intubation. In Gravenstein N, Kirby RR (eds): Complications in Anesthesiology. Philadelphia, Lippincott-Raven, 1996, p 219.

290. Roth H, Genzwuerker HV, Rothhaas A, et al: The ProSeal™ laryngeal mask airway and the Laryngeal Tube Suction™ for ventilation in gynaecological patients undergoing laparoscopic surgery. Eur J Anaesth 22:117-122, 2005.

291. Salathé M, Johr M: Unsuspected cervical fractures: A common problem in ankylosing spondylitis. Anesthesiology 70:869-870, 1989.

292. Salem MR, Joseph MJ, Heymann HJ, et al: Cricoid compression is effective in obliterating the esophageal lumen in the presence of a nasogastric tube. Anesthesiology 63:443-446, 1985.

293. Samsoon GLT, Young JRB: Difficult tracheal intubation: A retrospective study. Anaesthesia 42:487-490, 1987.

294. Sanchez A: Retrograde intubation technique. In Benumof JL (ed): Airway Management: Principles and Practice. St. Louis, Mosby, 1996, pp 320-341.

295. Sapsford DJ, Snowdon SL: If in doubt, take it out: Obstruction of tracheal tube by prominent aortic knuckle. Anaesthesia 40:552-554, 1985.

296. Schafer R, Klett J, Auffarth G, et al: Intraocular pressure more reduced during anesthesia with propofol than with sevoflurane: Both combined with remifentanil. Acta Anaesthesiol Scand 46:703-706, 2002.

297. Schillaci CR, Iacovoni VF, Conte RS, et al: Transtracheal aspiration complicated by fatal endotracheal hemorrhage. N Engl J Med 295:488-490, 1976.

298. Schumacher P, Stotz G, Schneider M, et al: Laryngospasm during transtracheal high frequency jet ventilation. Anaesthesia 47:855-856, 1992.

299. Seitz PA, Gravenstein N: Endobronchial rupture from endotracheal reintubation with an endotracheal tube guide. J Clin Anesth 1:214-217, 1989.

300. Sekerci S, Bilgin S, Tastan S: Endotracheal tube breaking during extubation. Eur J Anaesth 14:201-202, 1997.

301. Shorten GD, Alfille PH, Gliklich RE: Airway obstruction following application of cricoid pressure. J Clin Anesth 3:403-405, 1991.

302. Silva AB, Muntz HR, Clary R: Utility of conventional radiography in the diagnosis and management of pediatric airway foreign bodies. Ann Otol Rhinol Laryngol 107:834-838, 1998.

303. Smith I, White PF: Use of the laryngeal mask airway as an alternative to a face mask during outpatient arthroscopy. Anesthesiology 77:850-855, 1992.

304. Smith RB, Babinski M, Klain M, et al: Percutaneous transtracheal ventilation. JACEP 5:765-770, 1976.

305. Smith RB, Schaer WB, Pfaeffle H: Percutaneous transtracheal ventilation for anesthesia: A review and report of complications. Can J Anaesth 22:607-612, 1975.

306. Smith WD, Timms MS, Sutcliffe H: Unusual complication of nasopharyngeal intubation [letter]. Anaesthesia 44:615-616, 1989.

307. Smurthwaite GJ, Ford P: Skin necrosis following continuous positive airway pressure with a face mask. Anaesthesia 48:147-148, 1993.

308. Snow JC, Harano M, Balough K: Postintubation granuloma of the larynx. Anesth Analg 45:425, 1966.

309. Snow JC, Kripke BJ, Norton ML, et al: Corneal injuries during general anesthesia. Anesth Analg 54:465-467, 1975.

310. Snow JC, Norton ML, Saluja TS, et al: Fire hazard during CO_2 laser microsurgery on the larynx and trachea. Anesth Analg 55:146-147, 1976.

311. Sosis M, Dillon F: What is the safest foil tape for endotracheal tube protection during Nd-YAG laser surgery? A comparative study. Anesthesiology 72:553-555, 1990.

312. Spencer CD, Beaty HN: Complications of transtracheal aspiration. N Engl J Med 286:304-306, 1972.

313. Spielman FJ: Complete separation of the tube from the mask during removal of a disposable laryngeal mask airway. Can J Anaesth 49:990-992, 2002.

314. Stauffer JL, Olson DE, Petty TL: Complications and consequences of endotracheal intubation and tracheotomy. A prospective study of 150 critically ill adult patients. Am J Med 70:65-76, 1981.

315. Stemp LI: "Quick look" direct laryngoscopy to avoid cannot intubate/cannot ventilate induction [letter]. Anesth Analg 98:1815, 2004.

316. Stix MS, Borromeo CJ, O'Connor CJ Jr: Esophageal insufflation with normal fiberoptic positioning of the ProSeal laryngeal mask airway. Anesth Analg 94:1036-1039, 2002.

317. Stone DJ, Stirt JA, Kaplan MJ, et al: A complication of lightwand-guided nasotracheal intubation. Anesthesiology 61:780-781, 1984.

318. Streppel M, Bachmann G, Stennert E: Hypoglossal nerve palsy as a complication of transoral intubation for general anesthesia. Anesthesiology 86:1007, 1997.

319. Sugiyama K, Yokoyama K: Displacement of the endotracheal tube caused by change of head position in pediatric anesthesia: Evaluation by fiberoptic bronchoscopy. Anesth Analg 82:251-253, 1996.

320. Sum-Ping ST, Mehta MP, Anderton JM: A comparative study of methods of detection of esophageal intubation. Anesth Analg 69:627-632, 1989.

321. Szigeti CL, Baeuerle JJ, Mongan PD, et al: Arytenoid dislocation with lighted stylet intubation: Case report and retrospective review. Anesth Analg 78:185-186, 1994.

322. Szmuk P, Ezri T, Akca O, Alfery DD: Use of a new supraglottic airway device – the CobraPLA – in a 'difficult to intubate/difficult to ventilate' scenario. Acta Anaesthesiol Scand 49:421-423, 2005.

323. Takahashi S, Mizutani T, Miyabe M, et al: Hemodynamic responses to tracheal intubation with laryngoscope versus lightwand device (Trachlight) in adults with normal airway. Anesth Analg 95:480-484, 2002.

324. Takahata O, Kubota M, Mamiya K, et al: The efficacy of the "BURP" maneuver during a difficult laryngoscopy. Anesth Analg 84:419-421, 1997.

325. Takeda T, Tanigawa K, Tanaka H, et al: The assessment of three methods to verify tracheal tube placement in the emergency setting. Resuscitation 56:153-157, 2003.

326. Teeple E, Maroon J, Rueger R: Hemimacroglossia and unilateral ischemic necrosis of the tongue in a long-duration neurosurgical procedure [letter]. Anesthesiology 64:845-846, 1986.

327. Teichner RL: Lingual nerve injury: A complication of orotracheal intubation. Case report. Br J Anaesth 43:413-414, 1971.

328. Tessler S, Kupfer Y, Lerman A, et al: Massive gastric distention in the intubated patient: A marker for a defective airway. Arch Intern Med 150:318-320, 1990.

329. Thierbach AR, Piepho T, Maybauer MO: A new device for emergency airway management: The EasyTube™. Resuscitation 60:347, 2004.

330. Thomas T, Zornow M, Scheller MS, et al: The efficacy of three different modes of transtracheal ventilation in hypoxic hypercarbic swine. Can J Anaesth 35(Suppl):61, 1988.

331. Thomas TA, Cooper GM: Maternal deaths from anaesthesia. An extract from Why mothers die 1997-1999, the Confidential Enquiries into Maternal Deaths in the United Kingdom. Br J Anaesth 89:499-508, 2002.

332. Tiret L, Desmonts JM, Hatton F, et al: Complications associated with anaesthesia—A prospective survey in France. Can Anaesth Soc J 33:336-344, 1986.

333. Todd MM, Traynelis VC: Experimental cervical spine injury and airway management methods. Anesth Analg 93:799-801, 2001.

334. Tolley NS, Cheesman TD, Morgan D, et al: Dislocated arytenoid: An intubation-induced injury. Ann R Coll Surg Engl 72:353-356, 1990.

335. Tominaga GT, Rudzwick H, Scannell G, et al: Decreasing unplanned extubations in the surgical intensive care unit. Am J Surg 170:586-589, 1995.

336. Treffers R, de Lange JJ: An unusual case of cuff herniation. Acta Anaesthesiol Belg 40:87-90, 1989.

337. Unger KM, Moser KM: Fatal complication of transtracheal aspiration: A report of two cases. Arch Intern Med 132:437, 1973.

338. Urtubia RM, Aguila CM, Cumsille MA: Combitube: A study for proper use. Anesth Analg 90:958-962, 2000.

339. Usui T, Sato S, Goto F: Arytenoid dislocation while using a McCoy laryngoscope. Anesth Analg 92:1347-1348, 2001.

340. Valley RD, Freid EB, Bailey AG, et al: Tracheal extubation of deeply anesthetized pediatric patients: A comparison of desflurane and sevoflurane. Anesth Analg 96:1320-1324, 2003.

341. van Klarenbosch J, Meyer J, de Lange JJ: Tracheal rupture after tracheal intubation. Br J Anaesth 73:550-551, 1994.

342. Vanner RG, O'Dwyer JP, Pryle BJ, et al: Upper oesophageal sphincter pressure and the effect of cricoid pressure. Anaesthesia 47:95-100, 1992.

343. Verghese C, Smith TG, Young E: Prospective survey of the use of the laryngeal mask in 2359 patients. Anaesthesia 48:58-60, 1993.

344. Vervloet D, Magnan A, Birnbaum J, et al: Allergic emergencies seen in surgical suites. Clin Rev Allergy Immunol 17:459-467, 1999.

345. Vézina D, Lessard MR, Bussières J, et al: Complications associated with the use of the esophageal-tracheal Combitube. Can J Anaesth 45:76-80, 1998.

346. Wade JS: Cecil Joll lecture, 1979: Respiratory obstruction in thyroid surgery. Ann R Coll Surg Engl 62:15-24, 1980.

347. Wagner A, Roeggla M, Hirschl MM, et al: Tracheal rupture after emergency intubation during cardiopulmonary resuscitation. Resuscitation 30:263-266, 1995.

348. Wagner DL, Gammage GW, Wong ML: Tracheal rupture following the insertion of a disposable double-lumen endotracheal tube. Anesthesiology 63:698-700, 1985.

349. Wain JC, Wilson DJ, Mathieon DJ: Clinical experience with minitracheostomy. Ann Thorac Surg 49:881-885, 1990.

350. Warner ME, Benefeld SM, Warner MA, et al: Perianesthetic dental injuries. Anesthesiology 90:1302-1305, 1999.

351. Watcha MF, White PF, Tychsen L, et al: Comparative effects of laryngeal mask airway and endotracheal tube insertion on intraocular pressure in children. Anesth Analg 75:355-360, 1992.

352. Watson WJ, Moran RL: Corneal abrasion during induction [letter]. Anesthesiology 66:440, 1987.

353. Weaver LK, Fairfax WR, Greenway L: Bilateral otorrhagia associated with continuous positive airway pressure. Chest 93:878-879, 1988.

354. Weber S: Traumatic complications of airway management. Anesthesiology 20:265-274, 2002.

355. Westbrook JL: Oesophageal achalasia causing respiratory obstruction. Anaesthesia 47:38-40, 1992.

356. Wetmore SJ, Key JM, Suen JY: Complications of laser surgery for laryngeal papillomatosis. Laryngoscope 95:798-801, 1985.

357. White A, Kander PL: Anatomical factors in difficult direct laryngoscopy. Br J Anaesth 47:468-474, 1975.

358. Wilkins CJ, Cramp PG, Staples J, et al: Comparison of the anesthetic requirement for tolerance of laryngeal mask airway and endotracheal tube. Anesth Analg 75:794-797, 1992.

359. Willatts SM, Cochrane DF: Paranasal sinusitis: A complication of nasotracheal intubation: Two case reports. Br J Anaesth 57:1026-1028, 1985.

360. Williams AR, Burt N, Warren T: Accidental middle turbinectomy: A complication of nasal intubation. Anesthesiology 90:1782-1783, 1999.

361. Williams B: Cerebrospinal fluid pressure changes in response to coughing. Brain 99:331-346, 1976.

362. Williams JP, Somerville GM, Miner ME, et al: Atlanto-axial subluxation and trisomy-21: Another perioperative complication. Anesthesiology 67:253-254, 1987.

363. Williams RT, Stewart RD: Transillumination of the trachea with a lighted stylet [letter]. Anesth Analg 65:542-543, 1986.

364. Williamson JA, Webb RK, Cockings J, et al: The Australian Incident Monitoring Study. The capnograph: Applications and limitations—An analysis of 2000 incident reports. Anaesth Intensive Care 21:626-637, 1993.

365. Wilson IG, Fell D, Robinson SL, et al: Cardiovascular responses to insertion of the laryngeal mask. Anaesthesia 47:300-302, 1992.

366. Wohlner EC, Usubiaga LJ, Jacoby RM, et al: Cardiovascular effects of extubation [abstract]. Anesthesiology 51:S194, 1979.

367. Wolf GL, Simpson JI: Flammability of endotracheal tubes in oxygen and nitrous oxide enriched atmosphere. Anesthesiology 67:236-239, 1987.

368. Wood ML, Forrest ET: The haemodynamic response to the insertion of the laryngeal mask airway: A comparison with laryngoscopy and tracheal intubation. Acta Anaesthesiol Scand 38:510-513, 1994.

369. Wright PJ, Mundy JVB, Mansfield CJ: Obstruction of armoured tracheal tubes: Case report and discussion. Can J Anaesth 35:195-197, 1988.

370. Wynn JM, Jones KL: Tongue cyanosis after laryngeal mask airway insertion. Anesthesiology 80:1403, 1994.

371. Wynne DM, Marshall JN: Risk of accidental extubation with disposable tonsillectomy instruments. Br J Anaesth 89:659, 2002.

372. Young PN, Robinson JM: Cellulitis as a complication of difficult tracheal intubation [letter]. Anesthesia 42:569, 1987.

373. Zbinden S, Schupfer G: Detection of oesophageal intubation: The cola complication [letter]. Anaesthesia 44:81, 1989.

374. Zmyslowski WP, Kam D, Simpson GT: An unusual cause of endotracheal tube obstruction [letter]. Anesthesiology 70:883, 1989.

SOCIETAL CONSIDERATIONS

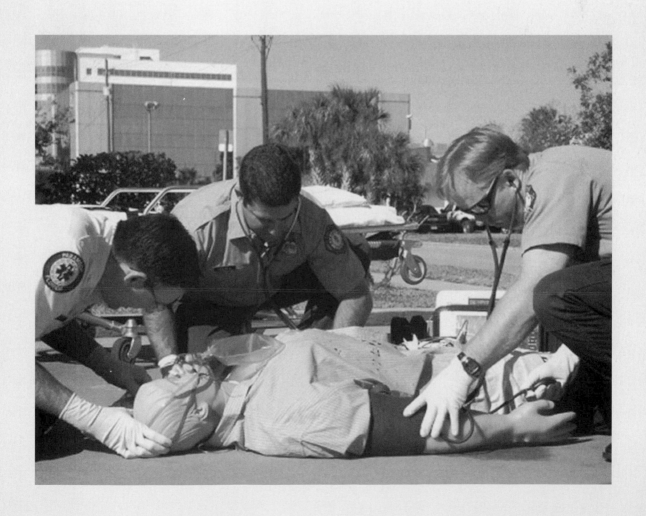

49

TEACHING AIRWAY MANAGEMENT OUTSIDE THE OPERATING ROOM: USE OF COMPUTERS AND INTERACTIVE TOOLS

George J. Sheplock
Stephen F. Dierdorf

I. BACKGROUND

II. LEARNING SKILLS FOR MANAGEMENT OF THE DIFFICULT AIRWAY

III. COMPUTER-ASSISTED INSTRUCTION

IV. THE INTERACTIVE AIRWAY MANAGEMENT INSTRUCTIONAL PROGRAM

V. THE ANESTHESIOLOGY ACADEMIC COMPUTER LABORATORY

VI. CONCLUSION

I. BACKGROUND

In 1985, the American Society of Anesthesiologists (ASA) Committee on Professional Liability began to analyze closed claim malpractice cases to assess objectively adverse outcomes from anesthesia. Respiratory events accounted for 37% of the claims (762 of 2046 cases). Eighty-five percent of the respiratory events resulted in permanent neurologic injury or death.[4] Three mechanisms of adverse outcome from respiratory events accounted for 75% of the adverse respiratory events: inadequate ventilation (38%), esophageal intubation (18%), and difficult endotracheal intubation (17%).[6] The reviewers concluded that 90% of the cases of inadequate ventilation and esophageal intubation could have been prevented if monitoring with capnography and pulse oximetry had been employed. It was also concluded that only 36% of the cases of difficult endotracheal intubation were preventable.

Because of the disproportionately high incidence of adverse outcomes from respiratory events and the finding that most cases of difficult endotracheal intubation were not easily preventable, the Task Force on Guidelines for Management of the Difficult Airway (DA) was convened. After an exhaustive search and evaluation of the medical literature concerning airway management published between 1973 and 1991, the task force published "Practice guidelines for management of the difficult airway" in March 1993.[1] These guidelines included recommendations for evaluation of the airway, basic preparation for DA management, strategy for intubation of the DA, strategy for extubation of the DA, and postoperative care. The task force also developed an algorithm for management of the DA. The purpose of the guidelines was to reduce the likelihood of adverse outcomes from untoward respiratory events.

A review of the closed claims database in 1999 revealed a decline in claims for adverse respiratory events, primarily related to a reduction in claims for inadequate ventilation and esophageal intubation.[5] Claims for adverse events secondary to difficult endotracheal intubation remained relatively constant, and an increase in claims for trauma to the upper airway was noted. The claims for pharyngeal and esophageal trauma were almost always associated with difficult endotracheal intubation. Updated guidelines, based on information accrued since 1993, were published in 2003.[14] The primary focus of the revised DA guidelines and algorithm is on important decision points that may be encountered during the process of airway management. The updated algorithm does, however, contain a specific device recommendation: the laryngeal mask airway (LMA). It is clear that today's anesthesiologist must have a broad and deep range of airway skills. Educational programs must be directed at developing the initial skills in anesthesiology residents during training and supplementing the skills of experienced anesthesiologists.

Although respiratory events are more likely to result in an adverse outcome, the incidence of patients with a DA in clinical practice is, in actuality, very low. The incidence of failure to intubate the trachea in a large series of surgical patients was only 0.3%.[17] As the incidence of patients with a DA is so low, how can an anesthesiologist in clinical practice learn and practice new airway management techniques? How can the ramifications of the critical decision points in airway management be learned? There is evidence that performance during critical clinical events is improved by regular simulated practice.[18] New developments in computers and software have provided the necessary tools for producing interactive programs directed at learning the algorithm and evaluating the merits of different airway management techniques. The interactive programs can be used frequently and repeatedly at relatively low cost. Today, increased computing power of personal computers and easy access to the Internet permit rapid availability of new information and updating of existing educational programs.

II. LEARNING SKILLS FOR MANAGEMENT OF THE DIFFICULT AIRWAY

Airway management at the level of expertise expected of an anesthesiologist is not an easy skill to learn, and educators must give careful consideration to the complexity of airway management. A comprehensive airway management curriculum must include didactic material that details the theory and use of different ventilation and endotracheal intubation techniques, demonstration of correct technique and instruction of students with specially designed mannequins, simulated use in dynamic simulators, and guided use by the learner in patients. Most clinical anesthesiologists, with proper instruction, develop the skill to use new airway devices in mannequins quickly and without difficulty. There may, however, be considerable reticence to transfer these newly learned skills to use in patients. Insertion of airway devices in mannequins may be considerably different from insertion and use in patients for a variety of reasons.

The other aspect of learning techniques for management of the DA is the development of an understanding of the critical decision points in the course of airway management. There are times when the clinical situation demands a rapid decision about airway management. That decision may result in successful resolution of the airway problem or may produce severe hypoventilation, hypoxemia, neurologic injury, or death. Traditional teaching techniques such as lecture and mannequin practice cannot convey the sense of time limitation that occurs during a true airway emergency.

III. COMPUTER-ASSISTED INSTRUCTION

The use of computer-assisted instruction in education has increased dramatically and continues to accelerate at a rapid pace. Early computer-assisted instruction consisted of little more than placing a text file into a word processor for the user to read. These computer presentations consisted of drills and tutorials and offered little more than a textbook. The results of this type of instruction could not be demonstrated to be any more effective than those of reading printed material. By the 1970s, however, it could be demonstrated that computer-assisted instruction did have positive and lasting educational benefits for secondary education students.[12] Computer-assisted instruction markedly reduced the time to learn as well as the effectiveness of learning. Despite a slow start during the mid-1980s and early 1990s, medical schools have now incorporated self-paced computer-assisted learning programs into most curricula. Hypermedia computer-assisted instruction is extremely popular with students at all educational levels and is an efficient means of disseminating new information and clinical techniques.[21]

Multimedia devices such as slides, video, audio, and overhead projectors have been used for educational purposes for many years. These devices certainly enhanced learning but in the past could not be linked to each other. Personal computers provide the technological capability for the instructor to acquire data in many different formats and integrate the information into a single system (hypermedia).[22] Patterns of learning are known to vary among individuals, and hypermedia can be organized by the instructor or the student in different ways to accommodate different learning methods.

New developments in software permit the assembly of interactive programs based on real situations from clinical practice by anesthesiologists with airway expertise. The combination of text material with imported photographs and diagrams can be used to explain concepts and techniques in considerable detail. After these aspects of the material have been learned, imported videos and internal algorithms can be used to present a true clinical situation with different management options in real time. This allows the student to explore different management options with accurate clinical information and time constraints as they would occur in clinical practice. The design of the teaching program provides rapid feedback of the results of the learner's decision. After an evaluation of the clinical scenario, making a management decision, and seeing the consequences of that decision, the learner can review didactic material germane to the clinical scenario. The objective of practicing these clinical decision-making processes in real time is to reduce reaction time and minimize the sense of panic that often accompanies the true airway emergency.

The capabilities of current personal computers allow the storage of large amounts of information in different formats in a self-contained medium. The student can progress at his or her own pace but have the advantage of mimicking real situations. Interactive programs are relatively inexpensive to develop, require only a personal computer for operation, require no instructor input, and can be used at any time that is convenient for the user. Technological advances that have improved the capabilities of personal computers include more powerful microprocessors, increased storage capacity, and high-resolution graphics. Images and video can easily be imported into programs and stored on high-capacity media (compact disk [CD], digital video disk [DVD]). In the late 1990s, inexpensive high-speed broadband Internet access became available to the consumer. Broadband access allows higher broadband content such as digital video to be delivered simultaneously to multiple computers connected by a local area network as well as by the Internet. New authoring languages permit nontechnical anesthesia educators to produce high-quality, interactive multimedia teaching programs. Interactive computer-assisted instructional programs are well established for regional anesthesia (RA).[7,9,19] Learning anatomy for RA is enhanced by cadaver dissection; however, cadaver dissection is not readily available to all anesthesiologists. Anatomic cadaver photographs at different dissection levels can be scanned, digitized, and imported into the personal computer. Once imported into the computer, the image can be enhanced, sharpened, and resized. The same format can be used for developing an interactive airway management program.

The use of human patient simulators for resident and postgraduate physician instruction has increased dramatically in the past decade.[13] The human patient simulator is relatively expensive and requires considerable instructor input to maximize the learning experience. Mastery of interactive programs is excellent preparation for educational sessions with a human patient simulator. Efficiency of learning with the human patient simulator can be enhanced by introductory material presented by an interactive computer program. Preliminary scientific validation of the effectiveness of interactive computer and patient simulator instruction has been attained, but additional research is certainly needed.[3,86] A comprehensive educational plan should be developed for airway instruction that employs different types of instructional techniques. It is important to define clearly the educational objective of each learning tool and match the method to the task that best achieves the desired goal.[11,15]

IV. THE INTERACTIVE AIRWAY MANAGEMENT INSTRUCTIONAL PROGRAM

There are several aspects of the Interactive Airway Management Instructional Program. The first part of the program is devoted to the ASA DA algorithm.[10] The entire algorithm is initially reviewed, and the user may explore the different branches of the algorithm (Fig. 49-1). The goal of this section is to focus the user's attention on making a critical airway management decision in real time. The first critical decision in the algorithm occurs after preoperative evaluation of the patient's airway. If the evaluation indicates an airway abnormality and difficult ventilation is anticipated, an awake intubation (AI) is mandated (Fig. 49-2).[2] If an AI cannot be achieved, the next decision to make is whether an airway must be established by an invasive method.

The next branch of the algorithm concerns the unrecognized DA. If the preoperative airway evaluation indicates that the airway is normal, induction of general anesthesia may proceed. If, after induction of general anesthesia, it is discovered that endotracheal intubation is difficult but positive-pressure ventilation can be administered, alternative intubation techniques may be employed. Should ventilation also become difficult, a rapid decision must be made concerning how ventilation can be achieved (e.g., supralaryngeal airway, invasive technique). The importance of this decision point must be appreciated because the inability to provide adequate ventilation very quickly leads to hypoxemia and neurologic injury or death.

Each branch of the airway algorithm may be isolated and displayed. Accompanying the display of each branch is text material that provides the user with an explanation of the purpose of the branch and the likelihood that the intervention will be successful. The text material also contains information about confirmation of ventilation and the consequences of inappropriate intervention techniques. Each branch may be reviewed until the critical decision points in DA management are thoroughly understood.

After an understanding of the algorithm is achieved, the user is presented with a clinical scenario mimicking an airway situation. Pulse oximetry data and audio signals are provided. A clock is set into motion so that the user must respond within an appropriate interval. Total elapsed time and apnea time are continually displayed (Fig. 49-3). As the user selects a management option, he or she receives information about the patient's response to the intervention. If the intervention is successful, the problem is resolved. If, however, the intervention is unsuccessful or inappropriate, the patient's condition may deteriorate and another technique must be selected (Fig. 49-4). After completion of the interactive scenario, it is displayed for further study (Fig. 49-5). Intervention techniques may also introduce other complicating factors into the scenario. The designer of the program can feature or

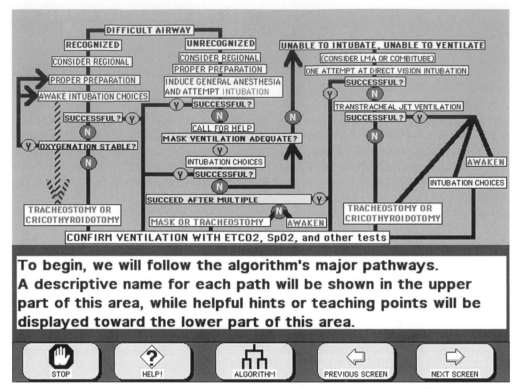

Figure 49-1 Interactive Airway Management Instructional Program: Exploring the Difficult Airway Algorithm of the American Society of Anesthesiologists. This first part consists of an initial review of the algorithm. The user may explore the different branches of the algorithm.

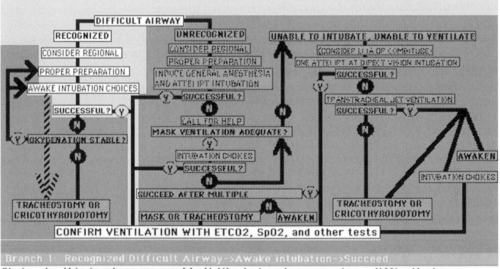

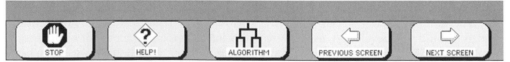

Figure 49-2 The goal of the section is to focus the user's attention on making critical airway management decision in real time. If the evaluation indicates an airway abnormality and difficult ventilation is anticipated, an awake intubation is mandated. If it cannot be achieved, the next decision to make is whether an airway must be established by an invasive method.

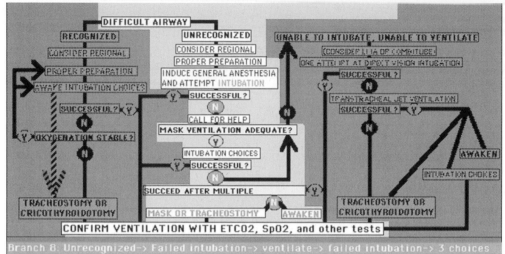

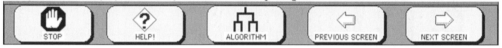

Branch 8: Unrecognized-> Failed intubation-> ventilate-> failed intubation-> 3 choices

After induction, you have failed to intubate the trachea. HELP! You are able to ventilate the patient, but after several attempts, you still cannot intubate the patient. If you persist indefinitely with attempts at intubation, you risk losing your patent airway due to edema, blood, secretions, laryngospasm, etc. The best course at this point is to choose one of the following: Awaken pt (if procedure elective); continue with mask (?aspiration risk; ?procedure); or tracheostomy (urgent/non-mask case).

Figure 49-3 The next step is to present the user with a clinical scenario mimicking an airway situation. Pulse oximetry data and audio signals are provided. A clock is set into motion so that the user must respond within an appropriate interval. Total elapsed time and apnea time are continually displayed.

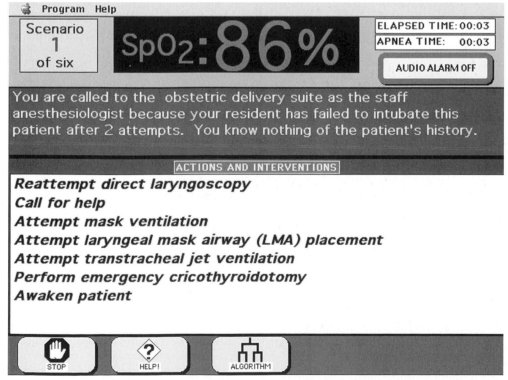

Figure 49-4 If the intervention is unsuccessful or inappropriate, the patient's condition may deteriorate and another technique must be selected.

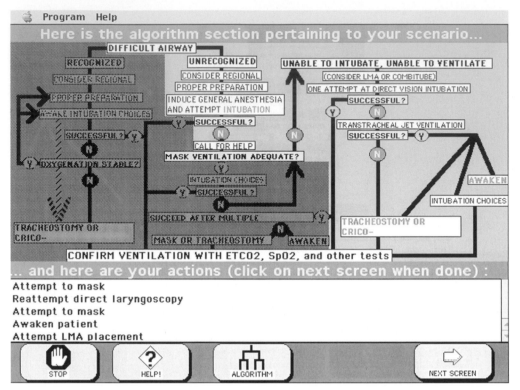

Figure 49-5 After completion, the interactive scenario is displayed for further study.

highlight any clinical situation or response that he or she feels should be emphasized. If the educator would like to emphasize use of the LMA, the clinical scenarios can be designed to direct the student to that conclusion.

The second part of the program is directed at fiberoptic-assisted endotracheal intubation.[20] The flexible fiberoptic laryngoscope is the most versatile of DA management techniques and has become an integral part of these techniques. The program initially presents the structure and mechanics of the fiberscope (Fig. 49-6). A thorough knowledge of the operational aspects of the fiberoptic laryngoscope increases the rapidity with which the user masters fiberscope manipulation skills. After the beginning endoscopist learns how to manipulate the fiberscope, navigation of the fiberscope through an abnormal airway becomes relatively easy. Imported photographs of the fiberscope in conjunction with text material are used to identify the different parts of the fiberscope and explain each part's function. Adjuncts designed to facilitate fiberoptic-assisted endotracheal intubation, such as intubating airways, are also shown and described. After the fiberscope has been described and its function explained, techniques for preparation of the patient, including management of secretions, sedation, positioning, and anesthesia, are presented (Fig. 49-7). A video sequence of a fiberoptic-assisted endotracheal intubation is shown (Fig. 49-8).

The next part of the interactive program is designed to display upper airway anatomy with special reference to sensory innervation in preparation for providing adequate topical anesthesia. The importance of learning techniques for producing airway anesthesia in the awake patient cannot be overemphasized.[16] Fiberoptic laryngoscopy becomes extremely difficult when the patient is poorly anesthetized, gagging, and coughing. The program displays the anatomy of the upper airway and color codes different sensory zones. The user quickly appreciates the fact that multiple sensory nerves supply the upper airway and can reach the information in two ways. When the cursor is placed on a colored area, the program reveals the name of the nerve supplying sensation to that area. Conversely, when the cursor is placed on the name of the nerve, the area the nerve supplies is highlighted in color.

The next section of the tutorial contains video clips that demonstrate clinical use of the fiberoptic laryngoscope (Fig. 49-9). Real-time video clips are powerful educational additions to any computer-assisted teaching program. Students at all levels quickly focus their attention on the video sequences. The user can halt the video clips at any time for further inspection of the still picture.

The third section of the tutorial is a series of videos that were recorded in the clinical practice of the diagnostic fiberoptic examination of the airway in fiberoptic-assisted endotracheal intubation. These videos demonstrate normal upper airway anatomy and upper airway disease. Pathologic conditions include laryngeal tumors, vocal cord polyps, superior vena cava syndrome, and rheumatoid arthritis. Newer generation videobronchoscopes produce high-resolution, wide-angle images of the upper airway. The videobronchoscope has a color charge-coupled

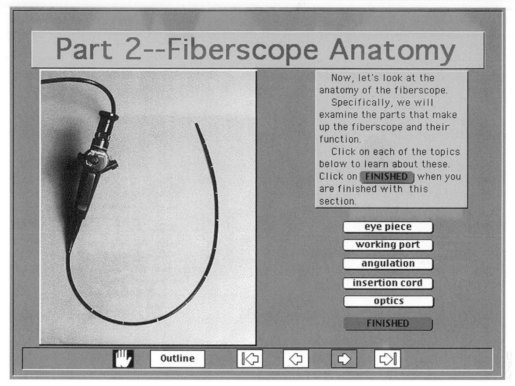

Figure 49-6 The second part of the program is directed at fiberoptic-assisted endotracheal intubation. The program initially presents the structure and mechanics of the fiberscope.

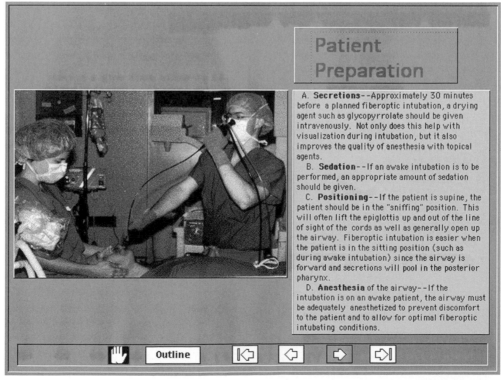

Figure 49-7 Techniques for preparation of the patient, including management of secretions, sedation, positioning, and anesthesia, are presented.

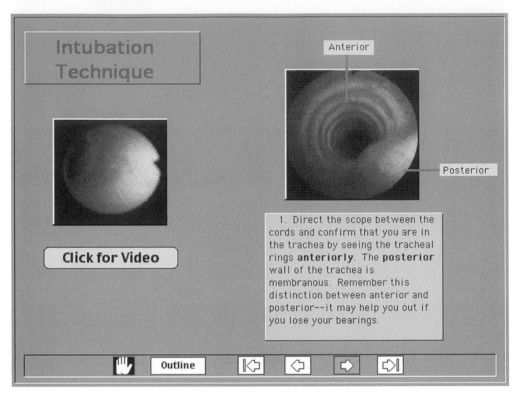

Figure 49-8 A video sequence of a fiberoptic-assisted endotracheal intubation is shown.

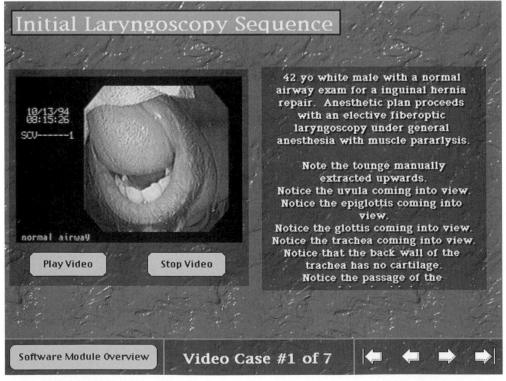

Figure 49-9 The next section of the tutorial contains video clips that demonstrate clinical use of the fiberoptic laryngoscope.

device (CCD) at the distal end of the fiberscope. The CCD chip converts light signals to electrical signals that are relayed to a microprocessor. The image is digitally constructed and displayed on a video monitor. Because there are no fiberoptic imaging bundles, the images are very high resolution as the optical distortion inherent in the long fiberoptic imaging bundles of conventional fiberscopes is not present. The video sequences can be imported into the computer through the tape deck for compilation and editing. Text material is added to the video material, and the program is tailored by the educator to emphasize important airway management concepts.

V. THE ANESTHESIOLOGY ACADEMIC COMPUTER LABORATORY

The primary purpose of an academic computer laboratory is to develop computer-assisted multimedia presentations and interactive educational software. Input is derived from multiple media sources including digitized sound, digitized color images from flatbed scanners and 35-mm slide scanners, and digitized video from camcorders or video cassette recorders (VCRs) (Fig. 49-10). Animation and three-dimensional modeling can also be included. Available computer and audiovisual hardware for the production station of an anesthesia interactive computer-assisted learning laboratory is listed in Table 49-1, and the production software and manufacturers for computer-assisted learning laboratory are listed in Table 49-2. Once the format is developed, this instructional software can be used to teach any facet of anesthesiology (Fig. 49-11). Educators preparing these programs use basic computer literacy skills acquired from using software for word processing, spreadsheets, animation, painting and drawing, slide making, scanning, and digitizing audio and video inputs. It is not, however, necessary that all anesthesiologists participating in the development process be facile with all aspects of the

Table 49-1 Computer and Audio-Visual Hardware for Production Station of an Anesthesia Interactive Computer-Assisted Leaning Laboratory

Computer Workstation
CPU: 1 gigahertz or greater
RAM: 1 gigabyte or greater
Internal hard drive: 100 gigabyte/7200 RPM
DVD/CD rewritable drive
Firewire, iLink (IEEE 1394) connectivity
10/100 Base-T Ethernet network adapter
External high-speed disk array (RAID) through ultra SCSI/fiber channel
DV editing acceleration PCI card-dual monitor/NTSC support
Accessory Hardware
Digital video tape deck (dual SVHS pro-DC deck)
NTSC monitor: visualize output for TV
DV camcorder
Digital camera
Medial converter for IN/OUT composite AV/S video and DV
USB jog/shuttle controller
DV disk recorder

computer techniques. One or two faculty members with the necessary computer expertise can effectively educate other faculty members. An important benefit of the academic computer laboratory is an increase in the computer literacy skills of the residents and faculty.

After selecting the subject to be presented and establishing the instructional goals, a database must be

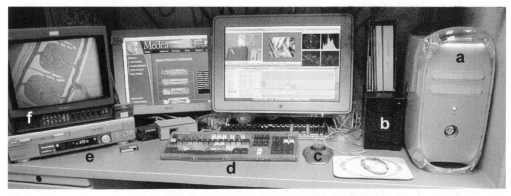

Figure 49-10 The goal of an academic computer laboratory is to develop computer-assisted multimedia presentations and interactive educational software, deriving input from multiple media sources including digitized sound, digitized color images from flatbed scanners and 35-mm slide scanners, and digitized video from camcorders or video cassette recorders.

Table 49-2 **Production Software for Computer-Assisted Learning Laboratory**

Image Processing	Authorware (Macromedia)
Photoshop (Adobe)*	Supercard (Solutions Etcetera)
Painter (Corel)	**DVD Production**
Digital Video Processing	iDVD (Apple)
Premiere and After Effects (Adobe)	Easy CD and DVD creator (Roxio)
Final Cut Pro (Apple)	Studio (Pinnacle)
Combustion (Discreet)	DVD Studio Pro (Apple)
Cleaner (Discreet)	**Data Acquisition, Systems Modeling and Control**
Three-Dimensional Modeling/Animation	Lab View (National Instruments) Database solutions
Lightwave (Newtek)	4th Dimension (4D)
3DS Max (Discreet)	Filemaker Pro (FileMaker)
Poser (Curious Labs)	**Support Software**
Development Software for Interactive Digital Media	Norton Antivirus (Symantec)
Studio MD (Macromedia)	Retrospect (Dantz)
Director MX (Macromedia)	Microsoft Office Suite (Microsoft)

*Manufacturer in parentheses.

acquired that contains material to be imported into the program and all necessary reference information. The database should be dynamic and allow updates and revisions. Interactive basic science software models that demonstrate the application of physiology and pharmacology to the understanding and management of pathologic processes are extremely valuable for the learner. Computer-assisted instruction can demonstrate many of these basic principles in new formats that enhance learning.

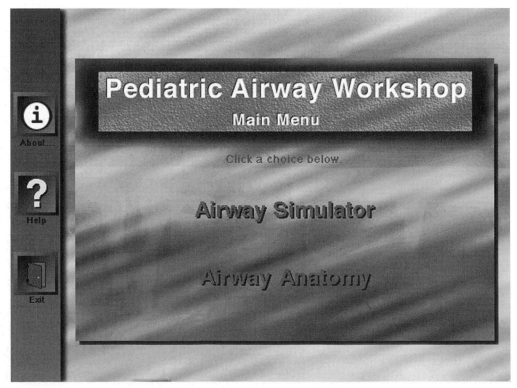

Figure 49-11 Once the format is developed, this instructional software can be used to teach any facet of anesthesiology.

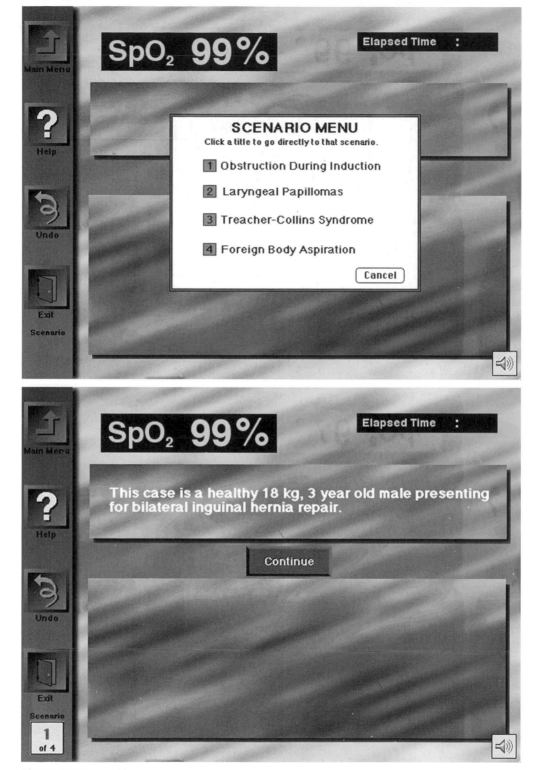

Figure 49-11, cont'd

Functional models of anesthesia equipment, including anesthesia delivery systems and monitoring devices, can be introduced. These models, with the aid of animation, can effectively teach operational principles, equipment limitations, and diagnosis of malfunctions. Computer-derived equipment models have proved to be pivotal in anesthesia equipment education projects. Past generations of anesthesiology residents were able to disassemble, examine, and reassemble anesthesia machines. Such exercises resulted in an exceptional understanding of how the devices functioned. As anesthesia equipment became more complex, disassembly and reassembly were no longer practical or safe. The computer model is a perfect substitute and may provide a better understanding of equipment function than more traditional methods of teaching. Animation can be used to demonstrate gas flow through the delivery system, vaporizer, valves, and breathing circuit. Interactive features permit the user to see how changing the position of the valves, components, or gas inlet lines may affect the function of the system.

When the basic format of the instructional program has been established, other specialized modules such as RA and transesophageal echocardiography can be added to the program. Faculty, organized into small groups, can produce a comprehensive educational program with a series of instructional modules.

There is considerable benefit for a teaching program to develop computer-assisted instructional presentations by incorporating images and videos from its own clinical practice. Anesthesiology residents are able to learn procedures and techniques exactly as they are taught by the faculty. The programs can be studied and completed by the resident prior to actual performance of the procedure. The capability to design the instructional material specifically results in a product that is superior to commercially prepared programs, which may present different techniques and introduce confusion into the teaching program. To enhance further the educational opportunities and computer literacy of the residents, electives can be offered during the CA-3yr that permit the resident to construct an interactive program.

Resources and personnel from outside the anesthesiology department can provide technical consultation with program development and networking. Most universities have active information technology services that provide expertise not found within the department. The computer laboratory provides noneducational capabilities such as data collection for quality assurance, clinical research, and statistical analyses.

VI. CONCLUSION

The development of powerful personal computers and the introduction of software that permits construction of interactive programs with little expertise in software management revolutionized medical education for students, residents, and anesthesiologists. The ability to import and integrate images and video sequences into an instructional interactive program enhances presentation. Programs can be specifically designed to demonstrate actual clinical events in the programmer's practice. The user can gain access to the information and interactive sequences in many different ways and can tailor the program that is most suitable for the individual techniques of the individual. Critical clinical events can be learned and practiced repeatedly at the user's own pace until the concepts are thoroughly understood. As computer capability and software power are continually updated, instructional effectiveness of interactive teaching programs will increase.

REFERENCES

1. American Society of Anesthesiologists Task Force on Management of the Difficult Airway: Practice guidelines for management of the difficult airway. Anesthesiology 78:597, 1993.
2. Benumof JL: Management of the difficult adult airway. Anesthesiology 75:1087, 1991.
3. Byrne AJ, Jones JG: Responses to simulated anaesthetic emergencies by anaesthetists with different durations of clinical experience. Br J Anaesth 78:553, 1997.
4. Caplan RA, Posner KL, Ward RJ, et al: Adverse respiratory events in anesthesia: A closed claims analysis. Anesthesiology 72:828, 1990.
5. Cheney FW: The American Society of Anesthesiologists closed claims project. Anesthesiology 91:552, 1999.
6. Cheney FW, Posner KL, Caplan RA: Adverse respiratory events infrequently leading to malpractice suits. Anesthesiology 75:932, 1991.
7. Fernandez O, Galindo A, Galindo P: Interactive Regional Anesthesia. New York, Churchill Livingstone, 1995.
8. Girard M, Drolet P: Anesthesiology simulators: Networking is the key. Can J Anaesth 49:647, 2002.
9. Hahn MB, McQuillan PM, Sheplock GJ: Regional Anesthesia. St. Louis, Mosby, 1995.
10. Jones R, Sheplock G, Goldstoff M: Airway algorithm program: Scientific exhibit. Presented at the annual meeting of the American Society of Anesthesiologists, San Francisco, Oct 1994.
11. Kneebone R: Simulation in surgical training: Educational issues and practical implications. Med Educ 37:267, 2003.
12. Kulik JA, Bangert RL, Williams GW: Effects of computer-based teaching on secondary school students. J Educ Psychol 75:19, 1983.
13. Morgan PJ, Cleave-Hogg D: A worldwide survey of the use of simulation in anesthesia. Can J Anaesth 49:659, 2002.
14. Practice guidelines for management of the difficult airway. An updated report by the American Society of

Anesthesiologists Task Force on Management of the Difficult Airway. Anesthesiology 98:1269, 2003.

15. Prideaux D: Curriculum design. BMJ 326:268, 2003.

16. Reed AP: Preparation of the patient for awake flexible fiberoptic bronchoscopy. Chest 101:844, 1992.

17. Rose DK, Cohen MM: The airway: Problems and predictions in 18,500 patients. Can J Anaesth 41:372, 1994.

18. Schwid HA, O'Donnell DO: Anesthesiologists' management of simulated critical events. Anesthesiology 76:495, 1992.

19. Sheplock GJ, Thomas PS, Camporesi EM: An interactive computer program for teaching regional anesthesia. Anesthesiol Rev 20:53, 1993.

20. Start R, Sheplock G, Goldstoff M, et al: Fiberscope training program: Scientific exhibit. Presented at the annual meeting of the American Society of Anesthesiologists, Washington, DC, Oct 1993.

21. Sultana CJ, Levy J, Rogers R: Video vs. CD-ROM for teaching pelvic anatomy to third-year medical students. J Reprod Med 46:675, 2001.

22. Wishnietsky DH: Hypermedia: The Integrated Learning Environment. Bloomington, Ind, Phi Kappa Delta Educational Foundation, 1992.

50

TEACHING AIRWAY MANAGEMENT OUTSIDE THE OPERATING ROOM: SIMULATOR TRAINING

John J. Schaefer III

I. THE NEED FOR DIFFICULT AIRWAY MANAGEMENT TRAINING

Over the past decade, significant strides in difficult airway (DA) management have been made, including improvements in monitoring of adequacy of ventilation with pulse oximetry and capnography, the development of a range of DA management techniques such as fiberoptic-guided intubation, the laryngeal mask airway (LMA), and emergent percutaneous cricothyrotomy, to name only a few, and the development of evidence-based guidelines for DA management such as the American Society of Anesthesiologists (ASA) DA algorithm. One of the implications of these developments is the need for comprehensive training to develop competence in the clinical application of these techniques and guidelines. Competence in DA management involves a specific, yet broad, range of knowledge, skills, and judgment. The inherent nature of the management of the DA includes uncertainty, time pressure, complexity, high risk, and high costs for failure, which can occur in both anticipated and unanticipated situations. The need to apply competence in this area is relatively infrequent for any average individual anesthesiologist, yet the severe implications of failure in management for the patient and the penalties an anesthesiologist may face for failure in successful management of the DA suggest that society is becoming more knowledgeable of "best practices" and less tolerant of failure.[4,6,33] Another indicator that DA management in anesthesiology may become a more significant issue is the known association between the incidence of a DA in the morbidly obese patient and the almost epidemic rise of morbid obesity in adults and children worldwide.[15,20,32]

As with any other discipline in the broad practice of anesthesia, competence in DA management can be achieved only through a dedicated, focused program of training combined with the appropriate balance of experience and maintenance of skills. In this chapter, we discuss the various barriers to training and review the current state of training in DA management in order to understand how to set up an effective training program. This chapter focuses on DA management training outside the clinical environment, focusing on educational best practices, training tools and methods, and integration with clinical training. Discussion includes continuing medical education considerations. The goal of this chapter is to provide the reader with an understanding of how to assemble a DA management training program utilizing tools and training methods that are available at this time.

II. BARRIERS TO TRAINING AND REVIEW OF CURRENT TRENDS IN DIFFICULT AIRWAY MANAGEMENT TRAINING

A. BARRIERS TO TRAINING

There are a number of barriers to effective training in DA management. Understanding these barriers is important in designing efficient, effective, and practical training programs that take these barriers into consideration. Obstacles vary from those of training in the clinical environment to those of setting up programs for resident training and continuing medical education programs.

The clinical environment is ideally the best environment for learning. Practicing techniques on patients such as direct laryngoscopy, fiberoptic bronchoscopy (FOB), and LMA placement as well as allowing trainees to assess airways or manage DA cases is ideal. However, there are a number of barriers to practical or effective, exclusive training in this environment, as listed in Table 50-1. Any training program that hopes to achieve true competence in an airway management technique or guidelines practice ultimately requires some training component that includes practice in the clinical environment. The opportunity for training outside the clinical environment is to focus on the elements that present barriers in the clinical environment, such as inadvertent risks associated with the early learning curve training of DA management techniques; inefficiencies of training in time-pressured, expensive environments; and appropriate matching of qualified and interested instructors with trainees. There are multiple opportunities for DA management training outside the clinical environment (Table 50-2) that are discussed in more detail.

Table 50-1 Barriers to Training Difficult Airway Management in the Clinical Environment

Infrequent training opportunities for certain skills in the clinical environment (e.g., retrograde intubation, transtracheal jet ventilation, percutaneous cricothyrotomy)
Time pressures in the clinical environment (e.g., taking an additional 15 minutes to allow training of fiberoptic bronchoscopy in the busy and expensive operating room)
Difficulty in matching dedicated and knowledgeable teachers with trainees with the right patient in the clinical environment
Perceived risks of practicing on patients when otherwise not indicated
High risk/cost for failure in managing DA inhibits allowing trainee to manage fully a DA situation, particularly an emergent one

DA, difficult airway.

Training of residents in DA management represents its own unique challenges (Table 50-3). In today's environment of strict clinical work hour limits and high labor costs, departments face the dual liability of increased clinical labor costs and reduced clinical time experience for competing educational interests. The inherent nature of DA management training includes significant direct costs (e.g., equipment, mannequins, simulators) and indirect costs (faculty and resident time values). Continuing medical education training in DA management faces the primary challenges of providing meaningful training to large numbers of people in expensive and time-compressed settings with trainers brought in from multiple locations, as well as the limited time for and perceived need to train by experienced anesthesiologists (Table 50-4).

B. REVIEW OF CURRENT DIFFICULT AIRWAY MANAGEMENT TRAINING TRENDS

It is instructive to review the current trends in DA management training as it is highly variable and arguably

Table 50-2 Opportunities for Training Difficult Airway Management Outside the Clinical Environment

Self-directed learning (e.g., reading assignments, interactive programs, Internet-based learning modules)
Lecture-based instruction
Problem-based learning instruction
Workshop-based training (e.g., skills stations, simulation training, and animal models)

Table 50-3 **Barriers to Developing Residency Training Programs in Difficult Airway Management**

Clinical workload time pressures (e.g., expensive to replace residents in the clinical setting and the presence of time limits on resident work hours)
The lack of detailed requirements or syllabus for DA management training
The lack of competence evaluations in DA management
The lack of validated "best practices" for DA management training
The costs of setting up dedicated training programs (e.g., DA management equipment, mannequins, simulators, and faculty labor costs)

DA, difficult airway.

does not meet the needs, as suggested by closed claims data, or keep up with the advances in either DA management guidelines or new airway equipment and techniques. In surveys of training programs in the United States, Koppel and Reed[19] in 1995 found that only 27% of training programs required residents to complete a dedicated airway rotation. In 2000, Hagberg[13] found that of the 60% of the programs that responded, only 33% had a DA rotation, 18% included mannequins or lung models, and 14% included the use of patient simulators in DA management training. The most frequent use of instruction included practice on patients, videotapes, and written instruction. Only 4% of the programs responding included written achievement tests in DA management. In 2003, Kiyama and colleagues[17] reported a survey in which only 28% of the responding Japanese anesthesiology

Table 50-4 **Barriers in Continuing Medical Education Difficult Airway Management Training**

Limited availability of time for CME training or instruction away from clinical practice
The lack of validated "best practices" for DA management training
The costs of setting up dedicated training programs (e.g., facility rental, DA management equipment, mannequins, simulators, and faculty labor costs)
Coordinating competent DA management instruction by trainers
The lack of competence evaluations in DA management
Indifferent attitudes to DA management training by experienced anesthesiologists

CME, continuing medical education; DA, difficult airway.

programs and 20% of the United Kingdom programs included a training module for DA management.

Although most resident training programs in anesthesiology throughout the world do not include comprehensive DA management training, even though DA management represents the highest anesthetic risk for mortality and significant morbidity, most bodies overseeing licensure in anesthesiology do not specify or require comprehensive DA management training. In the United States, the American Board of Anesthesiologists airway management training recommendation is less than one paragraph. In the United Kingdom, requirements for training have been expanded with regard to DA management training.[34-36] There are numerous continuing medical opportunities for training in DA management. An international and interdisciplinary society that focuses on airway management, the Society for Airway Management, was founded in 1993. A typical continuing medical education course in DA management training consists of a mix of lectures and workshops with various skill stations where instructors with some expertise in a technique are present to coach individuals or answer questions. In these settings, individuals rarely obtain extensive individual skill training and lectures do not facilitate skill training or allow individuals to practice cases or develop judgment.[18]

Given the lack of general availability of training or emphasis on DA management training, it is not surprising that Ezri and coauthors[8] reported that although most (86%) practicing anesthesiologists were comfortable using an LMA Classic and transtracheal jet ventilation, 74% were not comfortable with several of the airway management techniques recommended in the ASA DA guidelines (intubating LMA 61%, Combitube 43%, gum elastic bougie 24%, ventilating tube exchangers 28%, and fiberoptic intubation 59%).

III. TRAINING TOOLS AVAILABLE OUTSIDE THE OPERATING ROOM

Numerous training tools are available for training DA management outside the clinical domain. The range of training tools or resources includes texts, multimedia, teaching programs, airway models, mannequins, animal models, computer-based airway management training software programs, and simulators.

It is useful to categorize medical trainers in terms of their ability to teach all aspects of an educational task including affective, cognitive, and psychomotor objectives (knowledge, judgment, skill). This leads to the logical classification taxonomy of "whole task trainers" or "partial task trainers." A whole task trainer supports all components of knowledge, skill, and judgment of a given educational task, whereas a partial task trainer does not. This is not to state that partial task trainers are not useful. In fact, most training tools are partial task trainers. A simulation classification taxonomy would include the terms "microsimulator" and "macrosimulator." A medical macrosimulator is one that is approximately the same size as the subject being simulated (i.e., a mannequin-based simulator or IV arm). A microsimulator is a personal computer (PC)-based software product that includes medical simulation. A "virtual reality simulator" is a microsimulator with sensory feedback (sight, sound, and touch) interfaces. Note that the designation of a simulator as a partial or whole task trainer may vary with the training goals. For example, a simple airway mannequin could be considered a whole task trainer for laryngoscopy training but a partial task trainer for learning FOB. Many partial or whole task trainers also include some type of feedback or performance assessment functionality. As there are currently very few formal or academic validated feedback or assessment simulation training devices, it is incumbent upon the user of a device to assess the validity and reliability in the context of the training goals of any feedback or performance assessment component of a training device.

It is important to distinguish between the ability of a training device to provide the opportunity for partial or whole task training and the other components necessary for teachers to help students learn the goals and objectives that are the point of training. To make this point, a "learning system" is defined as the organized essential elements of: curriculum, training tools, performance assessment tools, and feedback tools that offer the opportunity for trainees to achieve specified training goals and objectives. Inherent in this concept is that with an ideal learning system, educational performance data can be collected and reported by course directors to the bodies who sponsored the training program. With this in mind and the preferred goal of competence in a given technique or set of guidelines, none of the current training tools can be thought of as a complete self-contained educational learning system. The critical implication of this is that it is incumbent upon the group or individual purchasing and using these training tools to take the time and resources to develop the elements of curriculum, performance evaluation and feedback tools, and data collection methods.

In the following sections, the range and general considerations of airway management partial and whole task training tools are presented and then reorganized by general task as a guide to those seeking information to create a specific training program. Table 50-5 provides an Internet list of websites that may be used to obtain specific information.

IV. RANGE AND CONSIDERATIONS OF AIRWAY MANAGEMENT TRAINING DEVICES

A. MODELS AND MANNEQUINS

Several airway models and mannequins are commercially available to supplement DA management training outside the clinical domain. Useful models can also be

Table 50-5 Websites of Partial and Whole Task Trainers

Anatomic models and mannequins	www.laerdal.com
	www.armstrongmedical.com
	www.gaumard.com
	www.simulaids.com
	www.global-technologies.net
	www.drmass.com
	www.ambu.com
Mannequin-based simulators	www.laerdal.com
	www.meti.com
	www.ux.his.no/tn/medtek/patsim.htm
	www.math-tech.dk
	www.ambu.com
Virtual reality/ PC-based trainers	www.laerdal.com
	www.anesoft.com
	www.immersion.com
Miscellaneous resources	www.wiser.edu
	www.hmc.psu.edu/simulation
	www.crme.med.miami.edu
	www.manbit.com

PC, personal computer.

made or adapted from commercially available models (Fig. 50-1). Airway models can generally be separated by whether or not they are interactive and further subdivided by what they can be used for. Static models in general are most useful as an aid to understanding three-dimensional anatomy as it relates to performing DA techniques.

The usefulness of mannequins or interactive models most likely depends on what skill is taught, what level of training it is being taught to (i.e., novice level versus

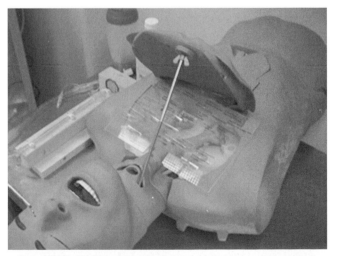

Figure 50-1 A homemade partial task trainer to teach psychomotor skills needed for fiberoptic bronchoscopy. The system consists of a commercial mannequin simulator with a transparent overlay outlining the anatomy of the airway down to the segmental level.

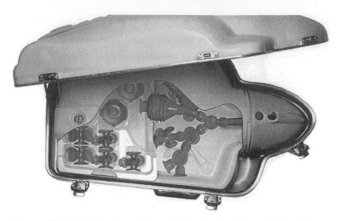

Figure 50-2 The Dexter endoscopic dexterity fiberoptic training system. (Reproduced with permission of Replicant Medical Simulators.)

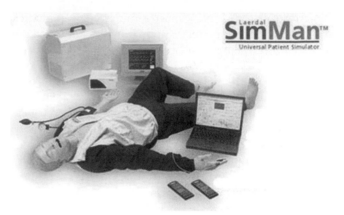

Figure 50-3 A virtual reality partial-task trainer to facilitate cognitive and psychomotor skills training in endoscopy. (Reproduced with permission of Immersion Medical Corp.)

expert level), and which mannequin training device is being used (Fig. 50-2). Plummer and Owen[26] found that in training endotracheal intubation to medical students and new anesthesiology residents, not only was there a significant difference among different airway mannequins but also training did not fully translate from one mannequin to another. Naik and coworkers[23] showed a benefit to fiberoptic skills training going from a simple model to anesthetized patients. The effectiveness of mannequins for LMA training has also been reported.[30] Cricothyrotomy models and mannequins have also been shown to improve both speed and success in performing cricothyrotomy.[27] The interactive mannequins and models should be considered partial task trainers appropriate for early learning curve training for the novice that needs supplementation by additional clinical, animal, or high-fidelity simulator training. Most programs do not provide full task training, problem solving training, or case practice. Certainly, these devices can play a significant role in any DA management training program and may overcome some of the barriers to clinical training (see Tables 50-1, 50-3, and 50-4).

B. PERSONAL COMPUTER–BASED SOFTWARE PROGRAM TRAINERS (PARTIAL TASK TRAINERS)

There are a number of PC-based software programs that support airway management training. They can generally be classified as primarily information oriented or simulation oriented. Their focus on airway management can be either primary or secondary (airway management as part of a larger subject). They are useful for conveying didactic information and, when simulation based, allow the opportunity to develop clinical judgment skills related to airway management through guided, experiential learning exercises. Excellent examples of information-oriented, primarily airway management–focused, PC programs are Management of the Difficult Airway (Cook Inc., Bloomington, IN) and Adult Airway

Management Principles and Techniques (SilverPlatter Education, Inc., Boston, MA). Two examples of simulation-oriented trainers in which airway management is a secondary focus include the Anesthesia Simulator 2001 (Anesoft, Issaquah, WA) and Resus Sim (Sophus Medical ApS, Copenhagen, Denmark). Although they are not specific to airway management, there is some evidence that programs such as Anesthesia Simulator 2001 improve performance more than mannequin-based simulators.[39]

C. VIRTUAL REALITY TRAINING DEVICES

Virtual reality training devices are PC-based devices that emulate the training environment and include an input and output device with visual and audio feedback. They may be further classified as either partial or whole task trainers. This is important to understand and assess critically when determining the utility of a simulator for training. The only virtual reality airway management training system currently available is the Immersion AccuTouch Endoscopy Simulator (Immersion Medical, Gaithersburg, MD). This is an example of a high-end virtual reality partial task trainer that delivers realistic, procedure-based content for cognitive and psychomotor skills training. The system (Fig. 50-3) consists of a PC, an interface device with interchangeable anatomy, proxy endoscopes, and software modules for a wide range of training scenarios. The bronchoscope looks, feels, and basically handles like a real scope, although placement of endotracheal tubes cannot actually be simulated (therefore the classification as a partial task trainer). The anatomy appears real (Fig. 50-4), and the "patient" reacts physiologically to the user's actions. The curriculum supplied with this training system covers the basics of endoscopy, airway anatomy, and a modest range of training scenarios including a pediatric DA training module. An attractive feature of this system is that it supports reports of the user's performance. The results of research into the usefulness of this device suggest that it leads to clinically

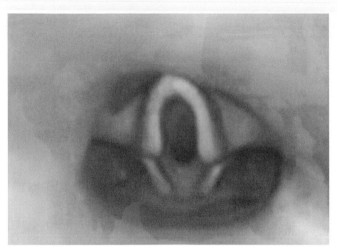

Figure 50-4 An airway image as seen through the endoscopy simulation training device shown in Figure 50-2.

significant improvement in novices' bronchoscopic skills.[25] In addition to providing virtual training in didactic, psychomotor, and judgment skills associated with fiberoptic intubation, this device can be used for colonoscopy training. Thus, it is a useful, albeit expensive (at a cost of more than U.S. $30,000) training system.

D. FULL-SCALE SIMULATORS (MANNEQUIN BASED)

Several full-scale airway management simulators are available from Laerdal (Laerdal, Inc., New York) or Medical Education Technologies (METI, Sarasota, FL).

1. Laerdal SimMan

At the University of Pittsburgh, Peter M. Winter Institute for Simulation, Education and Research, the Laerdal SimMan (about U.S. $25,000) for full-scale DA management patient simulation is used. The key features of this simulator are (1) relative affordability, (2) simplicity of operation by instructors (scenarios and evaluations can be preprogrammed), (3) portability, (4) high fidelity, and (5) ability to capture performance data (as labeled XML). Audio feedback can be provided to the trainee with this simulator by either the instructor's voice or activation of prerecorded sounds. Carotid, radial, and femoral pulses are palpable. The simulator's breathing rate and carbon dioxide concentration of "exhaled" air change according to trainee intervention with the simulator. In addition, the anatomy of the airway and lung compliance can be varied dynamically to facilitate training in management of DAs. The simulator can be used to train students in the use of all major airway devices and techniques and advanced life support skills. The bronchial tree is accurate down to the segmental level to facilitate fiberoptic intubation training. Breath sounds can be auscultated and present a variety of abnormalities. Heart sounds and bowel sounds can also be auscultated

and can be altered to represent abnormalities. Blood pressure can be obtained either manually or automatically. Invasive and noninvasive hemodynamic and capnographic values are displayed on a flat-screen monitor with touch-screen features. More than 1000 cardiac rhythms can be displayed and utilized in training sessions. In addition, the SimMan can be used to practice external defibrillation or external pacing.

The software necessary to operate SimMan can be run on a standard laptop and features an intuitive, Microsoft Windows–based operating system that has a short learning curve. The simulator can be operated from the computer with feedback from sensors located within the simulator that record and inform the operator of the results of the trainee's activity. The system can also be operated through intuitive, remote, wireless control units that support a number of programmable features. Physiologic responses can either be controlled directly or preprogrammed as a series of nonlinear trends. Open-ended programming of complicated clinical scenarios is supported through a simple rules-based programming system that is modestly difficult to learn. Performance decision points can be assigned within the scenario, programming a binary grade and associated with a feedback comment. Recorded data are recorded in a standard XML data language for later analysis if desired.

This system has some disadvantages: (1) it does not come with many predesigned scenarios or curriculum, (2) it is necessary to use the monitor that comes with it, (3) there is no drug recognition system (although this feature is reported to be available in the next version), and (4) there is a limited range for modifying lung compliance.

2. Laerdal AirMan

The Laerdal AirMan (Fig. 50-5) provides high-quality simulation of DA management situations in a simple, portable, lower cost platform (about U.S. $10,000). This simulator allows the instructor to present the following situations: restricted mouth opening, restricted neck

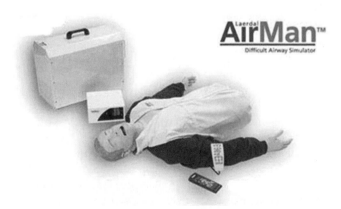

Figure 50-5 The Laerdal AirMan. (Reproduced with permission of Laerdal Medical Corporation.)

mobility, tongue swelling, pharyngeal swelling, laryngospasm of the vocal cords, and poor unilateral or bilateral pulmonary compliance. AirMan also comes with several sets of teeth of varying design, an anatomically correct cricothyroid membrane made of replaceable polymer tape that can be punctured and cannulated, inflatable lungs to allow training with conventional or transtracheal jet ventilation, treatment of pneumothorax (which reverses if the trainee performs needle decompression correctly), a realistic tracheobronchial tree to allow training in fiberoptic intubation and insertion of double-lumen tubes and bronchial blockers, a mechanism for spontaneous respiration that allows the instructor to control the respiratory rate and pattern and to produce apnea or coughing, a simulated pulse oximeter monitor that is directly controlled by the instructor and provides additional realistic visual and auditory feedback for the trainee, a source of carbon dioxide gas so that exhaled CO_2 can be detected during proper ventilation, and subcutaneous silicon rubber veins to allow intravenous cannulation and administration of medications.

A speaker can be concealed in the head pillow that allows the simulated patient to "speak" or "cough." The AirMan whole task airway management training system can be used for training in basic airway management techniques (i.e., bag-mask ventilation, insertion of oral or nasal pharyngeal airways, and endotracheal intubation by the oral or nasal route). Alternatively, by activating a handheld remote control, which is concealed from the trainee, the instructor can alter the clinical status of the simulated patient to present the trainee with one or more DA scenarios listed in the ASA airway algorithm.[3] For example, one could start with the "cannot intubate, can ventilate" situation, which can then be advanced to the "cannot intubate, cannot ventilate (emergency pathway)" situation. Scenarios can be presented either uninterrupted in "real time" or paused or suspended to emphasize teaching points and then restarted. Unlike the situation with the SimMan, these scenarios are manually controlled and there is no computer (PC); therefore, scenarios cannot be fully standardized and performance information is not recorded. This platform is particularly useful for training without formal evaluation.

3. Medical Education Technologies Simulators

Medical Education Technologies offers a variety of advanced full-scale (whole task) simulators with varying degrees of functionality for DA management. (1) The HPS-010 (Fig. 50-6) is METI's most advanced simulator (about U.S. $150,000 to $200,000), designed specifically for use in anesthesia training programs. It can present complex clinical scenarios. (2) The PediaSim (Fig. 50-7) (about U.S. $35,000) can be used to simulate basic and DA management situations in the pediatric patient. This simulator incorporates the same technology used in the adult HPS models. (3) The METI Emergency Care

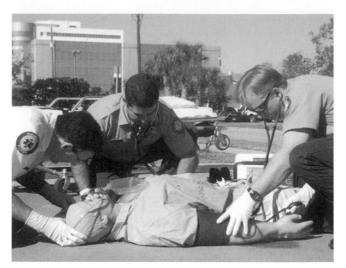

Figure 50-6 The METI Emergency Care Simulator (ECS) for use in teaching fundamental airway management techniques. (Reproduced with permission of Medical Education Technologies.)

Simulator (ECS) simulates entry-level airway management problems and is, therefore, useful in the education of all providers of airway care, including emergency medical technicians and technologists. A PC control rack and self-contained gas system are available for remote use. In contrast to those of the Laerdal simulators, the lungs offer a range of pulmonary compliance settings, and a drug recognition system is available. The system is based on a fixed modeled system that can be somewhat modified through access to parameters within the model. It does not support performance evaluation inherently, and the airway is accurate to the main stem bronchi. Lastly, these are modestly complicated systems to master and maintain.

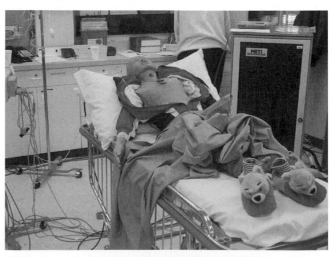

Figure 50-7 The PediaSim pediatric patient simulator. (Reproduced with permission of Medical Education Technologies.)

4. Other Full-Scale Simulators

A number of other full-scale simulators are available that are most likely classified as partial task trainers when used for DA management training, although they can be used for whole task training in other areas. Of note is the Danish Sima System (Math-Tech, Copenhagen), which consists of an interface box to which monitoring equipment, a PC running the simulation software, and a mannequin are connected.

5. Advantages, Opportunities, and Current Limitations of Simulators

Simulators as educational training tools should not be confused with "simulation" as an educational method. Simulation as an educational methodology is the representation of the functioning of one system or process by means of another[22] and has been used for thousands of years. With the advent of low-cost PCs and improvements in technology, software (PC-based) instruction, virtual reality and mannequin-based simulators are now commercially available for use in medical education. Some characteristics of an ideal DA management simulation learning system are shown in Table 50-6.

Whole task simulation, from an educational perspective, holds the promise of creating a learning environment that supports experiential and reflective learning. When this type of educational tool is used with the appropriate curriculum evaluation and feedback methods, a student has the opportunity to develop integrated emotional, cognitive, and psychomotor abilities, ultimately leading to a change in behavior and performance in the clinical setting. When applied to large groups of trainees, this may lead to cultural changes in clinical practice, as exemplified by cultural improvements in safety practices in the aviation industry.[14] Operational advantages of simulation training over traditional medical training methods include (1) provision of a safe (to both the patient and student) environment for training in risky procedures, (2) unlimited exposure to rare clinical events, (3) ability to plan and shape training opportunities rather than wait for a suitable situation to arise clinically, (4) the opportunity for team training, and (5) lower cost, both direct (i.e., more efficient use of expensive clinical training time such as in the operating theater) and indirect (i.e., decreased malpractice insurance claims).

Disadvantages of the current generation of medical simulators include high initial capital investment costs for equipment and training space, significant operational costs, lack of validated curriculum, and lack of validated performance evaluation. There are also challenges to broad application to large numbers of trainees and standardized data collection. The clinical challenges of DA management can include imprecise ability to predict a DA[7]; infrequent opportunities to practice the skills and judgment intrinsic in DA management; the critical time pressures associated with arterial desaturation[1]; the high morbidity, mortality, and personal costs associated with failure to manage; and the innate uncertainty with crisis situations.[9] Simulation has been used for decades to address analogous training problems in other high-risk disciplines (i.e., the aviation industry and the military).[10,11,16,24,29,31,40,41] Although medical simulation for DA management training is generally in its infancy and there is much work to be done before it offers a broad, practical, valid, and reliable solution to training,[2] it certainly has the promise and can be used now for valuable training with understood limitations.

Table 50-6   Characteristics of an Ideal Difficult Airway Management Simulation Training System

Trainee curriculum and instructor curriculum are included as part of the learning system.
Simulator simulates a wide variety of common and uncommon clinical airway scenarios.
Supports the accurate, "high-fidelity," clinical use of a wide variety of airway management techniques and devices.
Allows the trainee to experience reflective problem solving.
Provides valid high-fidelity interaction with a simulated patient
Is easy for facilitators to operate.
Is practically transportable for use in a variety of training environments (e.g., to run simulations at a CME meeting).
Includes valid performance evaluation and feedback tools.
Is affordable and reliable to allow widespread use and to support standardization of training.

CME, continuing medical education.

V. EDUCATIONAL METHODS AND BEST PRACTICES APPLIED TO DIFFICULT AIRWAY MANAGEMENT TRAINING

Designing, building, applying, and measuring the effect of a training course do not begin with the purchase of a mannequin or simulator; rather, they begin with applied educational best practices. This process starts with the establishment of the goals and objectives of training, followed by consideration of how to achieve these goals. In DA management training of residents, there are many different ways in which this can be approached. When considering the barriers to training from Tables 50-1 and 50-3 and the range of training opportunities listed in Table 50-2, some integrated combination of the following is needed: (1) didactic instruction, (2) workshops that offer skills training and reflective case-based problem solving, (3) organized clinical experience (i.e., airway rotation and a monitored procedure log system), and, finally, (4) a method of evaluation and feedback. The organization of training outside the clinical environment can be framed within the creation of a DA management learning system.

A. UNDERSTANDING ADULT LEARNERS

In order to create an effective DA management learning system, educational best practices suggest that it is important that one have a basic understanding of how adults approach learning. Although there are many theories about adult learning, one of the useful models for professional students is pictured in Figure 50-8. In this model, adult learners tend to fall into one of three categories: superficial (surface) learner, deep learner, or strategic learner. The superficial learner typically wants to do just the minimum necessary to get by. Characteristics of a superficial learner include fear of failure, memorization of facts without context of understanding concepts, and inability to relate facts. The deep learner understands the vocational relevance of the subject and wants to understand concepts as they relate to facts. The strategic learner is predominantly interested in achieving high grades and uses an approach to achieve these goals while doing the least amount of work.

One also needs to be sensitive to cultural differences in students, their communication skills, and reaction to authority. For example, an apparently passively learning student may actually reflect a different cultural norm in which the student normally does not question authority or may not be confident in his or her communication skills in a foreign language. Most residents or medical students tend to be strategic learners, given clinical or academic workload pressures. They are often a diverse group in whom cultural differences are present. Also, the typical continuing medical education adult trainee approaches airway training as either a superficial or deep learner. With these approaches to learning in mind, one can motivate residents by assigning grade values to important objectives, where they tend to study as needed to pass a test or perform 50 fiberoptic intubations if it is required as part of their residency. In designing a continuing medical education course, it is necessary to convey the training value early if one hopes to capture the attention of a superficial learner.

B. CREATING EDUCATIONAL GOALS AND OBJECTIVES

There are a number of methodologies for arranging educational goals and objectives. One of the most practical of these is that outlined by Gronlund[12] (Table 50-7). For example, to train residents in how to use a Combitube, a didactic lecture or computer-based software program would, at best, achieve the objective of "knowledge" in the cognitive domain, would achieve none of the objectives in the psychomotor domain, and might achieve the "receiving" objective in the affective domain. Training with a mannequin might achieve the objectives

of "comprehension" in the cognitive domain, "mechanism" in the psychomotor domain, and "valuing" in the affective domain. With a training program based on use of a good virtual reality or full-scale simulator, it is conceivable to set, reach, and measure educational objectives of "evaluation" in the cognitive domain, "adaptation" in the psychomotor domain, and "value complex" in the affective domain.

In the simulation-based training experience, the resident has the opportunity to compare and contrast the clinical appropriateness of the various types of airway management equipment and practice psychomotor skills, including troubleshooting problems, in a "real-time" clinical setting. Compared with a lecture, video, or practice session on a static mannequin, full-scale simulation provides a superior learning opportunity. By using simulators that allow flexibility and simulate a range of DA management clinical scenarios, the instructor is better able to evaluate objectively the trainee's potential clinical performance.[37] For example, a simulation can be run such that a patient undergoing general anesthesia develops an "unanticipated, cannot intubate, cannot ventilate" clinical situation that would result in death from hypoxia in 6 minutes unless an LMA is used properly to establish ventilation. Measurements of performance comparing the trainee's actions with a set of airway management guidelines can be determined, such as the trainee's knowledge of the guidelines, skill in placement of the LMA, and judgment in calling for help. With simulation, the instructor can standardize the clinical test.

If competence in the application of the ASA DA guidelines is the goal of training, competence in understanding and applying the concepts underlying these guidelines with the associated range of airway management techniques and devices is necessary (Table 50-8). Table 50-8 is not an all-inclusive list of the numerous devices and techniques currently available but simply shows the devices or techniques for which the ASA DA management guidelines task force found sufficient published evidence for including in its recommendations. Over time, these recommendations may change, and they were revised in 2003.[28] It is also noteworthy that for each technique or device, there are significant product variants, with each necessitating specific training needs.

Skill training does not involve just psychomotor training, as each technique includes its own set of knowledge and judgment that must be combined with skills to create meaningful competence. Beyond solely teaching airway management techniques, training is required to apply these techniques in the context of DA management guidelines. Table 50-9 offers a limited example of the cognitive domain objectives that can be covered in a comprehensive training program. The vast majority of academic and clinical educators responsible for creating and implementing anesthesia training programs have little, if any, formal training in the profession of adult education. Ideally, any formal training program in DA management

MODEL OF STUDENTS' APPROACHES TO LEARNING

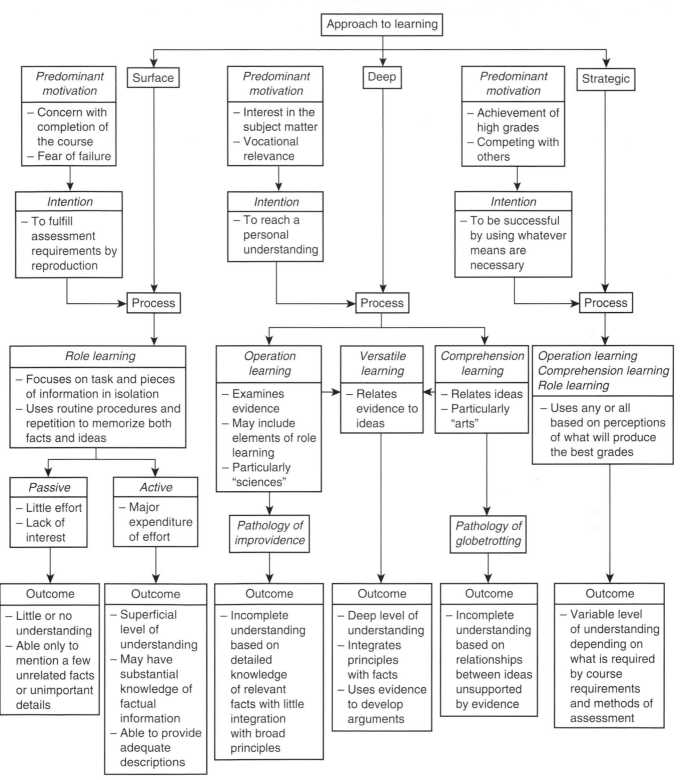

Figure 50-8 Model of students' approaches to learning.

Table 50-7   **Taxonomy of Educational Objectives**

Cognitive Domain	Psychomotor Domain	Affective Domain
Knowledge	Perception	Receiving
Remembering previously learned material	Using the sensory organs to obtain cues and guide motor activity	The student's willingness to pay attention
Comprehension	Set	Responding
The ability to grasp the meaning of the material	The readiness to take a particular action	Active participation by the student
Application	Guided response	Valuing
The ability to use learned material in new situations	Repeating a skill demonstrated by an instructor	The worth or value a student attaches to an educational objective
Analysis	Mechanism	Organization
The ability to break down material into its component parts	The learned responses have become habitual	The student compares, relates, and synthesizes values
Synthesis	Complex overt response	Value complex
The ability to put parts together to form a new whole	Skillful performance of motor acts	Internationalization of a value system
Evaluation	Adaptation	
The ability to judge the value of material	The student can modify motor acts to meet a need	
	Origination	
	Creates new movement patterns creatively based on highly developed skills	

Table 50-8   **Airway Management Techniques and Devices Included in the American Society of Anesthesiologists Difficult Airway Guidelines**

Optimal mask ventilation
Direct laryngoscopy
Elastic gum bougie
Fiberoptic-guided intubation
Laryngeal mask airway
Intubating laryngeal mask airway
Combitube
Lighted stylet
Retrograde intubation
Transtracheal jet ventilation
Cricothyrotomy
Tube exchangers

Table 50-9   **Examples of Cognitive Concepts Inherent in the American Society of Anesthesiologists Difficult Airway Management Guidelines***

Incidence, morbidity, mortality, and clinical associations surrounding the DA
Pertinent definitions within the guidelines (i.e., "difficult ventilation")
The basic concepts underlying the recommended approach to the DA
Methods, value, and limitations of airway assessment
Nonlinear Hg desaturation time for different types of patients
The value of preoxygenation
Issues in when, why, and what is meant by calling for help
Concepts differentiating airway management technique selection in the nonemergent and emergent pathways
Indications, contraindications, and complications associated with airway management technique choice
Concepts in applying the guidelines during extubation

*This is not an all-inclusive list.
DA, difficult airway.

would need to include consideration of how to train the trainers. The more formal the process and extensive the faculty support materials are, the greater the likelihood of interinstructor consistency in allowing trainees to achieve the desired goals and objectives.

VI. DIFFICULT AIRWAY MANAGEMENT TRAINING AT THE UNIVERSITY OF PITTSBURGH MEDICAL CENTER

A. COMPETENCE-BASED DIFFICULT AIRWAY MANAGEMENT SIMULATION TRAINING PROGRAM

The University of Pittsburgh Health System incorporates 20 hospitals and is affiliated with the University of Pittsburgh School of Medicine. As part of its commitment to quality assurance and patients' safety, training in DA management is required of all faculty, fellows, and residents in the departments of anesthesiology, critical care medicine, and emergency medicine. The Peter M. Winter Institute for Simulation, Education and Research (WISER) offers this training program in the University of Pittsburgh School of Medicine. WISER is a 10,000 square foot training facility supporting large-volume high-fidelity simulation training programs using multiple modalities of training including up to 16 mannequin-based simulators. The airway management training program described here is offered as an example of a mature (developed over 10 years) program incorporating multiple training methodologies applied to complement clinical training and experience. It incorporates advanced instructional technology, but other less expensive training tools could be substituted as means allow.

The goal of DA training in anesthesia is a measurable (as tested on mannequin-based simulators with a battery of simulated, real-time cases) competence in applying the ASA DA guidelines. A derivative of these guidelines has been developed through departmental consensus in the departments of emergency and critical care medicine and serves as the analogous goal of training in their courses. The learning system designed for these courses uses a separate intranet-based curriculum for participants and facilitators. The course includes 4 hours of independent intranet-based study followed by approximately 8 hours of workshop instruction in which 75% of the time is spent in hands-on, simulation-based training at a ratio of one facilitator to two trainees to one simulator. Two weeks prior to the course, each resident is required to review didactic material, including the ASA DA algorithm and videotaped examples of airway management techniques on the Internet. The workshop training includes a didactic session of concepts related to DA management and specifically those related to the guidelines. This is followed by focused instruction on individual techniques and multiple simulated case practice sessions. Evaluation throughout this training includes (1) a written pretest based on

the didactic material in the trainee's web-based preworkshop curriculum, (2) an individual simulation-based pretest at the beginning of the workshop that includes a battery of four simulations, (3) a similar (although different case stem) post-test, and (4) quality assurance surveys and a retest for those failing the post-test after additional focused instruction. Scoring and standard setting are reflective of all elements of the guidelines as developed by local expert consensus.

This course is an example of a competence-based learning system. Descriptive XML data from the simulator are collected automatically within a database and processed into an evaluation form with structured feedback. This standardized formative and summative feedback is immediately available to the facilitator to guide feedback and focused additional training. This intranet evaluation form is linked to digital video recording of the assessment, which can then be contextually accessed to enhance feedback.[21] Research into the validity, retention, and practical value of this type of training is ongoing. All anesthesiology residents attend this course once a year starting in their first year. Attendees take the course and are recertified every 2 years on the basis of successful management of simulated DA cases. To date, less than one third of the board-certified anesthesiologists have achieved a passing score prior to training, with a 25% mortality rate in the emergent pathway simulated evaluation arm. At the end of training, over 95% of the course attendees are able to demonstrate competence (as defined by strictly applying the ASA guidelines) with the first post-test.[38] This type of training outside the clinical environment complements, as a precursor, a clinical DA rotation and monitoring of procedure logs.

The ability to offer and run such a program is dependent on the support of WISER as a health system–medical school resource to share costs efficiently and the health system's commitment to patients' safety as a self-insured entity. Although few programs or departments currently have access to these types of training facilities, much can be accomplished with a smaller facility and alternative teaching aides (i.e., PowerPoint-based curriculum rather than intranet based). A similar course design with an Internet-based curriculum is offered for training in fiberoptic intubation.

B. ROLE OF CLINICAL TRAINING

The use of educational tools, whether they are partial task or whole task trainers, should be coupled wherever feasible with a structured clinical experience in airway management. This can best be achieved through a dedicated airway management rotation facilitated by competent, interested facilitators and monitored procedure logs.[5] Ideally, for safety reasons, experience should be gained first in managing DA problems in adults before seeking to manage these problems in the pediatric population. Similarly, fiberoptic intubation is ideally first mastered in the adult population. The use of simulation in the training of airway management does not replace clinical teaching; rather, it makes clinical teaching safer for the patient and makes the clinical learning experience more comfortable for the trainee.

REFERENCES

1. Benumof MD, Dagg R, Benumof R: Critical hemoglobin desaturation will occur before return to an unanalyzed state following 1 mg/kg intravenous succinylcholine. Anesthesiology 87:979-982, 1997.
2. Byrne AJ, Greaves JD: Assessment instruments used during anesthetic simulation: Review of published studies. Br J Anaesth 86:445-450, 2001.
3. Caplan R, Benumof J, Berry F: Practice guidelines for management of the difficult airway: A report by the American Society of Anesthesiologists Task Force on Management of the Difficult Airway. Anesthesiology 78:597-602, 1993.
4. Caplan RA, Posner KL, Ward RJ, Cheney FW: Adverse respiratory events in anesthesia: A closed claims analysis. Anesthesiology 72:828-833, 1990.
5. Cooper SD, Benumof JL: Teaching management of the airway: The UCSD airway rotation. In Benumof JL (ed): Airway Management, Principles and Practice. St. Louis, Mosby–Year Book, 1996, pp 903-910.
6. Domino KB, Posener KL, Caplan RL, Cheney FW: Airway injury during anesthesia: A closed claims analysis. Anesthesiology 91:1703-1711, 1999.
7. El-Ganzouri AR, McCarthy RJ, Tunman KJ, et al: Preoperative airway assessment: Predictive value of a multivariate risk index. Anesth Analg 82:1197, 1996.
8. Ezri T, Szmuk P, Warters RD, et al: Difficult airway management practice patterns among anesthesiologists practicing in the United States: Have we made any progress? J Clin Anesth 15:418-422, 2003.
9. Gaba D, Fish KJ, Howard SK: Crisis Management in Anesthesiology. New York, Churchill Livingstone, 1994.
10. Garrison P: Flying without Wings. Blue Ridge Summit, Penn, TAB Books, 1985, pp 1-31, 102-106.
11. Goodman W: The world of civil simulators. Flight Int Mag 18:435, 1978.
12. Gronlund NE: In Miller R (ed): How to Write and Use Instructional Objectives. New York, Macmillan, 1991.
13. Hagberg CA: Instruction and learning of airway management skills. Anesthesiology 93:1208A, 2000.
14. Helmreich RL, Merritt AC, Wilhelm JA: The evolution of crew resource management training in commercial aviation. Int J Aviat Psychol 9:19-32, 1999.
15. Hood DD, Dewan DM: Anesthetic and obstetric outcome in morbidly obese parturients. Anesthesiology 79:1210-1218, 1993.
16. Keys B, Wolfe J: The role of management games and simulations in education and research. J Manage 16:307-336, 1990.
17. Kiyama S, Muthuswamy D, Latto IP, Asai T: Prevalence of a training module for difficult airway management: A comparison between Japan and the United Kingdom. Anaesthesia 58:571-574, 2003.
18. Koppel JN, Reed AP: Are postgraduate fiberoptic-guided intubation workshops accomplishing their goals? Anesth Analg 78:S216, 1994.
19. Koppel JN, Reed AP: Formal instruction in difficult airway management. A survey of anesthesiology residency programs. Anesthesiology 83:1343-1346, 1995.
20. Lobstein T, Baur L, Uauy R: Obesity in children and young people: A crisis in public health. The International Association for the Study of Obesity. Obes Rev 5(Suppl 1): 4-85, 2004.
21. Lutz J, Schaefer J: The integration of performance logs with digital video for review of simulation training sessions. Anesth Analg 98(5S), 2004.
22. Merriam-Webster's Collegiate Dictionary, 11th ed. Springfield, Mass, Merriam-Webster, 2004.
23. Naik VN, Matsumoto ED, Houston PL, et al: Fiberoptic orotracheal intubation on anesthetized patients. Do manipulation skills learned on a simple model transfer into the operating room? Anesthesiology 95:343-348, 2001.
24. Office of Naval Research: Visual Elements in Flight Simulation. Washington, DC, National Council of the National Academy of Science, 1973.
25. Ost D, Rosiers A, Britt EJ, et al: Assessment of a bronchoscopy simulator. Am J Respir Crit Care Med 164:2248-2255, 2001.
26. Plummer JL, Owen H: Learning endotracheal intubation in a clinical skills learning center: A quantitative study. Anesth Analg 93:656-662, 2001.
27. Prabhu AJ, Wong DT, Correa RK, et al: Training improves cricothyrotomy success rate. Presented at the Difficult Airway Society Annual Meeting Annual Meeting, Oxford, 2001.
28. Practice guidelines for management of the difficult airway: An updated report by the American Society of Anesthesiologists Task Force on Management of the Difficult Airway. Anesthesiology 98:1269-1277, 2003.
29. Ressler EK, Armstrong JE, Forsythe GB: Military mission rehearsal. In Tekian A, McGuire C, McGaghie WC (eds): Innovative Simulations for Assessing Professional Competence. Chicago, Department of Medical Education, University of Illinois Medical Center, 1999, pp 157-174.
30. Roberts I, Allsop P, Dickinson M, et al: Airway management training using the laryngeal mask airway: A comparison of two different training programmes. Resuscitation 33:211-214, 1997.
31. Rolfe JM, Staples KJ: Flight Simulation. Cambridge, Cambridge University Press, 1986, pp 232-249.
32. Rose DK, Cohen MM: The airway: Problems and predictions in 18,500 patients. Can J Anaesth 41:372-383, 1994.
33. Rosenstock C, Moller J, Hauberg A: Complaints related to respiratory events in anaesthesia and intensive care medicine from 1994 to 1998 in Denmark. Acta Anaesthesiol Scand 45:53-58, 2001.
34. Royal College of Anaesthetists: Primary and Final Examinations for the FRCA. Syllabus. London, Royal College of Anaesthetists, 1997.
35. Royal College of Anaesthetists: The CCST in Anaesthesia II. Competency Based Senior House Officer Training and Assessment. A Manual for Trainees

and Trainers. London, Royal College of Anaesthetists, 2000.

36. Royal College of Anaesthetists: The CCST in Anaesthesia III. Competency Based Specialist Registrar Years 1 and 2 Training and Assessment. A Manual for Trainees and Trainers. London, Royal College of Anaesthetists, 2002.

37. Schaefer J: Mandatory competency-based difficult airway management training at the University of Pittsburgh Department of Anesthesiology—Preliminary findings. Anesth Analg 98:5S, 2004.

38. Schaefer JJ, Dongilli T, Gonzalez RM: Results of systematic psychomotor difficult airway training of residents using the ASA Difficult Airway Algorithm and dynamic simulation. Anesthesiology 89:60A, 1998.

39. Schwid HA, O'Donnell D: Anesthesiologists management of simulated critical incidents. Anesthesiology 76:495-501, 1992.

40. Streufert S, Pogash R, Piasecki M: Simulation based assessment of managerial competence: Reliability and validity. Personality Psychol 41:537-557, 1988.

41. Watchtel J: The future of nuclear power plant simulation in the United States. In Walton DG (ed): Simulation for Nuclear Reactor Technology. Cambridge, Cambridge University Press, 1985, pp 339-349.

51

THE INSTRUCTION OF AIRWAY MANAGEMENT IN THE OPERATING ROOM

Elizabeth C. Behringer

I. INTRODUCTION

Airway management of either the routine or difficult airway (DA) remains a critical aspect of both anesthesiology training and lifelong anesthetic practice. Anesthesiologists remain the most recognized "airway management specialists" and are routinely involved in elective and emergency procedures involving securing the airway throughout the hospital. Anesthesiologists may be asked to provide a secure airway as an application of advanced cardiac life support during cardiorespiratory arrest, as part of an elective or emergency surgical or radiologic procedure, or in the intensive care unit (ICU) in the care of the critically ill patient, for example.

The American Society of Anesthesiologists (ASA) closed claims analyses are a series of publications that review closed malpractice claims against anesthesiologists gleaned from the databases of 35 medical liability insurance carriers. The initial report was published in 1990.[7] This study reviewed adverse respiratory events associated with anesthesia care during the 1970s and 1980s. In the 1970s, 55% of all claims of death or brain damage were due to anesthetic-associated adverse respiratory events. Respiratory events during anesthetic care leading to adverse outcomes were the largest group of injuries resulting in malpractice litigation in this landmark study. This study highlighted the three mechanisms associated with adverse outcomes—inadequate ventilation, unrecognized esophageal intubation, and difficult endotracheal intubation. Other events noted in a subsequent study by the same authors included airway trauma, pneumothorax, aspiration of orogastric contents, and bronchospasm. These less common adverse respiratory events can be associated with anesthetic care as well.[8]

In 1998, a follow-up study noted a significant change in airway-related closed claims during the 1990s.[6] During this decade, a 10% decrease in the incidence of anesthetic-related adverse respiratory events was noted. This dramatic decline can be attributed to several factors, the routine use of pulse oximetry, capnography, and the advent and widespread use of the ASA DA management algorithm in continuing education.[34,35] In addition, the vital roles of residency training specifically focused on airway management, continuing education concerning airway management, and the scientific literature pertaining to the management of the DA are undeniable.[16]

II. THE IMPORTANCE OF LIFELONG LEARNING IN AIRWAY MANAGEMENT

The importance of clinical education in airway management during residency training and in the postgraduate setting can be underscored by a brief review of some of the literature concerning airway management in the ICU. Anesthesiologists are often consulted for airway management in the ICU during both residency training and postgraduate practice.[3] Nayyar and Lisbon surveyed anesthesiology residency training programs with regard to emergency airway management practices outside the operating room (OR).[32] In the vast majority of programs surveyed, anesthesiologists performed most of the intubations on the hospital ward, including the ICU. This study supports the importance of tailoring airway practice to the patients' environment as supported by the scientific literature.

Mort reviewed the incidence of hemodynamic and airway complications associated with tracheal reintubation after unplanned extubation in the ICU.[30] Fifty-seven patients who were reintubated after self-extubation were analyzed over a 27-month period; 93% of reintubations occurred within 2 hours of self-extubation. Of these patients, 72% had hemodynamic compromise or airway-related complications such as hypotension (35%), tachycardia (30%), hypertension (14%), multiple laryngoscopic attempts (22%), difficult laryngoscopy (16%), difficult intubation (DI) (14%), hypoxemia (14%), and esophageal intubation (14%). One patient required a surgical airway. One case of "cannot ventilate, cannot intubate" leading to cardiac arrest and death occurred. Less than one third of the patients studied had a "mishap-free" reintubation in the ICU.[30] Thus, it was recommended that individual ICUs develop strategies to decrease the rate of self-extubation based on patients' safety and the impact of emergency airway management.

Two additional studies of airway management in remote settings pertinent to clinical practice have been published by Mort.[28,29] The first study utilized an emergency intubation database from 1990 to 2002 in support of the ASA guidelines for management of the difficult airway, which suggests that when conventional intubation techniques fail after three attempts, advanced airway devices should be utilized and immediately available.[29] The database was divided into two periods. Period A (1990 to 1995) included 340 intubations in which accessory airway devices, such as the laryngeal mask airway (LMA), bougie, Combitube, or fiberoptic bronchoscope (FOB), were not routinely available. Period B (1995 to 2002) included 437 patients for whom these devices were readily available. The relationship between the use of any accessory airway devices and airway and hemodynamic complications, including number of intubation attempts, hypoxemia, regurgitation, aspiration, bradycardia, and dysrhythmia, was determined. Intubations were performed in the surgical ICU, medical ICU, hospital ward, neurosurgical or trauma ICU, coronary care ICU, emergency department, and postanesthetic care unit. The study found a 33% reduction in hypoxemic episodes (oxygen saturation [SpO_2] < 90%) and a 50% reduction in severe hypoxemic episodes (SpO_2 < 70%) in group B patients, for whom accessory airway devices were readily available. Regurgitation was reduced from 4% to 1.7%, aspiration from 2.1% to 0.2%,

bradycardia from 5% to 2%, dysrhythmia from 9.1% to 3.7%, and multiple intubation attempts from 30% to 15% in group A and B patients, respectively. The use of accessory airway devices increased from 5% in group A patients to 42% in group B patients. Notably, LMA use increased 21-fold. The aggressive approach of incorporating the ASA DA management guidelines by early intervention with accessory airway devices led to a remarkable reduction in multiple attempts at laryngoscopy and a decreased incidence of airway and hemodynamic complications. This study confirms the importance of application of the ASA DA management algorithm outside the OR setting and also justifies the immediate availability of a well-stocked DA cart in all hospital locations where emergency airway management is performed, especially the ICU setting. It also illustrates the importance of familiarity with and experience in the use of accessory airway devices as a mandatory part of the standard of care in routine anesthetic practice.

The second study reviewed the utility of exchanging an endotracheal tube (ET) in the ICU by two methods: direct laryngoscopy (DL) or airway exchange catheters (AECs).[28] ET exchanges from an 8-year quality improvement database were reviewed. Patients with an uncompromised glottic view (Cormack-Lehane view 1 and 2) were divided by method of exchange: DL ($n = 99$) versus AEC—Cook 14 or 19 Fr ($n = 34$). Hypoxemia, intubation attempts, esophageal intubation, bradycardia, cardiac arrest, and the need for a surgical airway were compared. Successful ET exchange on the first attempt was higher with use of an AEC (95% AEC versus 62% DL). The need for multiple attempts at laryngoscopy was higher in the DL group (26% DL versus 2.9% AEC). In addition, rescue airway techniques were utilized more frequently in the DL group (16 of 99 cases; a surgical airway was necessary in 5 of the 16 DL rescued airways). No rescue maneuvers were necessary in the AEC group. Hypoxemia and severe hypoxemia, esophageal intubation, bradyarrhythmias, and cardiac arrest during DL for ET exchange were also more frequent in the DL group. It was determined that use of an AEC during ET exchange in the ICU lowered the risk of complications considerably even in the presence of a previously uncompromised view of the glottic inlet. This study also highlights the importance of familiarity with alternative techniques to DL as part of safe airway management and anesthetic practice.

Mort also published a study highlighting the hazards of repeated attempts at laryngoscopy in critically ill patients.[27] Two thousand eight hundred and thirty-three critically ill patients were entered in an emergency intubation quality improvement database. Patients suffered from cardiovascular, pulmonary, metabolic, neurologic, or traumatic injuries. In this retrospective review, the practice analysis documented in the database was evaluated for both airway and hemodynamic complications.

These variables were correlated with the number of laryngoscopic attempts required for successful intubation. All of the patients required emergency intubation outside the OR setting. The author noted a statistically significant increase in airway-related complications when the number of laryngoscopic attempts increased to two or more intubation attempts. The incidences of hypoxemia, regurgitation of gastric contents, aspiration of gastric contents, bradycardia, and cardiac arrest were significantly higher when the number of attempts at conventional laryngoscopy increased. This study supports the recommendation of the ASA Task Force on Management of the Difficult Airway guidelines to limit the number of laryngoscopic attempts and be facile and familiar with alternative techniques of DA management.[27]

These studies serve to highlight the importance of the commitment to lifelong learning in a variety of techniques in advanced airway management available to the anesthesiologist. The purpose of this chapter is to focus on the means available to accomplish this goal by review of pertinent supporting literature.

III. TEACHING AIRWAY MANAGEMENT— THE COMPONENTS

The topic of teaching airway management skills can be divided into several components including anatomy, evaluation of the airway, and teaching materials, including airway simulators (see Chapters 49 and 50). In addition, the scientific literature supports teaching techniques in mask airway management, DL, fiberoptic intubation, LMA ventilation or assisted intubation, and surgical airway management. Finally, the scientific literature highlights the utility of instruction in airway management during anesthesiology residency training and postgraduate courses.

Several authors advocate review of basic anatomy as essential groundwork for mastery of DA management. Gaiser published a review of teaching airway management skills,[16] and he advocates the use of an anatomy textbook as a valuable teaching tool. Review of basic airway anatomy can be achieved in lecture format[9,16,24] or self-study.[16] Katz and colleagues used videotapes to review basic airway anatomy as a part of their learning module in fiberoptic intubation.[22] Haponik and associates utilized a computer software program to teach tracheobronchial anatomy as a preparation for a virtual training course on FOB.[20]

Evaluation of the airway for potential difficulty is an integral part of DA management. The second iteration of the ASA Task Force on Management of the Difficult Airway practice guidelines stress the importance of a thorough history and physical examination of each patient for anticipated difficulty.[35] This evidence-based guideline incorporates 11 physical examination points

related to the airway that provide a succinct set of predictors of potential airway difficulty. These findings are discussed in Chapter 9. The current guidelines for management of the difficult airway may also be found at the ASA website: www.asahq.org.

Although practicing anesthesiologists and anesthesiology residents have unlimited access to techniques for evaluation of potential difficulty in airway management, other physicians do not. The American College of Obstetricians and Gynecologists (ACOG) have emphasized the importance of identifying parturients at risk for possible DI during emergency delivery.[2] ACOG states that "The obstetric care team should be alert to the presence of risk factors that place the parturient at risk for complications from general anesthesia." Gaiser and his group at the Hospital of the University of Pennsylvania studied the ability of obstetricians to recognize parturients at risk for DI in light of the ACOG policy statement.[17] In Gaiser's study, 160 parturients had an airway examination conducted by four separate physicians, an attending and resident obstetrician, as well as an attending and resident anesthesiologist. The physicians were asked to complete a questionnaire about DI, use of antepartum consultation, and the choice of labor analgesia following each patient's examination. During the first 80 airway examinations, the obstetricians did not receive any guidance or education on recognition of the DA and complications associated with it. For the following 80 airway examinations, the obstetricians received a 30-minute tutorial concerning methods to examine the airway for potential difficulty, as well as the complications of DI.[17] The anesthesiologists' responses were used as the standard. The sensitivity, specificity, and positive and negative predictive values were calculated for the responses of the other physicians. Unfortunately, brief 30-minute tutorials did not affect the results of the obstetricians' ability to assess the airway. Instruction did not affect the number of consultations requested by either resident or attending obstetricians for possible DI. However, attending obstetricians were significantly more likely to utilize epidural analgesia for 2 cm cervical dilation in women with a possible DA in this study.[17] This study highlights the importance of discussing airway management and its potential complications with surgical colleagues because it can affect clinical judgment, in this case a change in the choice and timing of labor analgesia in parturients with a suspected DA.

IV. INSTRUCTION IN SPECIFIC TECHNIQUES OR DEVICES

The scientific literature is replete with studies pertaining to mastery of specific devices and techniques of airway management, and a brief review of several of these techniques (LMA, fiberoptic intubation, and surgical airway) is warranted.

Table 51-1 **Phases of Education for Incorporation of the Laryngeal Mask Airway (LMA) into Clinical Practice**

Phase one: Reading and viewing instructional material to gain an understanding of basic concepts of the use of the LMA
Phase two: Mannequin or cadaver training to develop basic motor skills for LMA use
Phase three: Use of the LMA clinically in simple, elective cases to acquire basic clinical skills
Phase four: Use of the LMA in more complex cases to acquire advanced clinical skills.

A. LARYNGEAL MASK AIRWAY

Brimacombe published an excellent chapter entirely devoted to educational considerations concerning the LMA.[5] This chapter aptly summarized the myriad of publications concerning the acquisition of skill using the various versions of the LMA. Gurman and coauthors[18] compared retention of airway management skills in a group of 47 medical students. The students were instructed in the use of DL, LMA, and Combitube placement during a 2-week rotation in anesthesiology. Mannequins were utilized for teaching and testing. The authors noted no diminution in skill with any device over a 6-month period following training.

Dickinson and Curry[11] studied the efficacy of mannequin training for proper LMA insertion in paramedics attending an advanced cardiac life support training course. A high success rate in the use of the LMA led to the conclusion that this was a suitable alternative to live training in patients.

Ferson and coworkers[15] studied 20 anesthesiologists over 2 months. They examined the efficacy of instruction in the use of the LMA, comparing manual or videotape training with hands-on training by an experienced anesthesiologist using a mannequin. More than 90% of participants in the hands-on training group achieved passing scores for LMA insertion technique after 17 insertions. Less than 30% of the group utilizing manual-videotape training achieved this score.

Brimacombe suggested that there are four phases of education in order to incorporate the LMA into clinical practice (Table 51-1). He further suggested that phases 2 to 4 are enhanced when a mentor (e.g., an experienced LMA user) is available to the novice for individualized training.[5]

B. FIBEROPTIC INTUBATION

Johnson and Roberts published an early study of clinical competence in the performance of fiberoptic laryngoscopy and endotracheal intubation.[21] The hypothesis of their study was that an acceptable level of technical expertise in fiberoptic intubation could be acquired within 10 intubations while maintaining patients' safety. The learning objectives included an intubation time of 2 minutes or less and greater than 90% success on the first intubation attempt. Ninety-one ASA I-II patients with normal laryngeal anatomy undergoing general anesthesia were intubated orally with an Olympus LF-1 fiberoptic scope after induction. The mean time for intubation was 1.92 ± 1.45 minutes. Four anesthesiology residents without prior fiberoptic experience intubated at least 15 patients each. A learning curve was generated using logarithmic analysis of the mean $\pm$ SD time for intubation of patients 1 to 15 for all residents combined. The learning curve noted that the mean intubation time decreased from 4.00 ± 2.91 minutes to 1.52 ± 0.76 minutes within the first 10 intubations. Following the 10th asleep fiberoptic intubation, the mean intubation time was 1.53 minutes with a greater than 95% success rate for the first attempt. No clinically significant changes in oxygen saturation, mean arterial pressure, or heart rate were noted during asleep fiberoptic intubation in this study. This study highlights that an acceptable level of technical expertise in fiberoptic intubation can be achieved safely by performing at least 10 elective asleep fiberoptic intubations by novice anesthesiologists.[21]

Erb also evaluated teaching orotracheal fiberoptic intubation in 100 anesthetized, spontaneously breathing patients.[14] Five anesthesia residents without prior experience in fiberoptic intubation participated in this study. Each resident randomly tracheally intubated 10 spontaneously breathing patients (group A) and 10 paralyzed patients (group B). An overall success rate of 96% was defined as successful endotracheal intubation in two or fewer attempts, which was not different between the two groups. During fiberoptic intubation, oxygen saturation remained greater than 95% in group A, whereas 2 of 10 patients in group B had oxygen saturation fall below 95% during fiberoptic attempts. The authors noted that fiberoptic intubation under conditions of spontaneous respiration is a well-established, standard of care technique of DA management. This study demonstrated a feasible and safe method to train novices in the skill of fiberoptic intubation under conditions of general anesthesia and spontaneous ventilation.[14]

Wheeler and colleagues[36] at the Children's Memorial Hospital at Northwestern University published an interesting study of teaching residents pediatric fiberoptic intubation of the trachea. Twenty clinical anesthesia year 2 (CA-2) residents were randomly assigned to either the traditional teaching group (fiberoptic intubation with standard eyepiece) or the video-assisted group (fiberoptic intubation using an integrated camera and video screen). All residents were novices in pediatric fiberoptic intubation. One of two attending anesthesiologists supervised each resident during the elective fiberoptic intubation of 15 healthy children, aged 1 to 6 years old. Variables measured included time from mask removal to confirmation of successful endotracheal intubation by end-tidal carbon dioxide detection and fiberoptic intubation attempts up to 3 minutes or three attempts. The primary outcome of time to success or failure was compared between the two groups. Failure rates, as well as the number of attempts, were also compared.

Three hundred intubations of patients were attempted; eight of these failed. On average, the group utilizing video-assisted fiberoptic intubation as a training tool was faster and three times more likely to achieve successful fiberoptic intubation. The video-assisted group also had significantly fewer attempts at intubation than the residents in the traditional group.[36] The authors concluded that a video-assisted system, where the attending anesthesiologist is able to provide real-time feedback during fiberoptic intubation of pediatric patients, was superior as a teaching method to the traditional teaching model.

Ovassapian provided a succinct review of learning fiberoptic intubation techniques[33] in which several points are emphasized in order to encourage the more frequent use of the fiberscope in anesthesia and critical care practices.

1. The techniques of fiberoptic endotracheal intubation are not difficult to learn. Mastery of the art of fiberoptic airway management readily develops with time and experience.

2. The technique of fiberoptic intubation is different from rigid laryngoscopy. Without formal training, the anesthesiologist should not expect immediate and successful use of the fiberscope for endotracheal intubation.

3. No anesthesiologist should perform a new technical task without studying and developing the required base of knowledge involved in its performance (Table 51-2).

Table 51-2   Information Necessary for Fiberoptic Intubation

How the fiberscope functions
How to avoid damaging the fiberscope
Indications for fiberoptic intubation
Limitations of fiberoptic intubation
How to recognize abnormal airway anatomy
Appropriate preparation of the patient
How to provide safe conscious sedation
How to provide good topical anesthesia of the airway
How to monitor the patient adequately
Causes of failure of fiberoptic intubation
Complications of fiberoptic airway endoscopy

Table 51-3   Essential Steps for Successful Fiberoptic Intubation

Organize a functional fiberoptic cart
Maintain a functional fiberscope
Follow a checklist prior to each use
Skillfully manipulate the fiberscope
Follow approaches and steps of fiberoptic intubation

4. The fiberscope is a simple but sophisticated airway management tool. It should be utilized to its full diagnostic and therapeutic potentials in airway management. The greater the experience of the anesthesiologist in using the fiberscope under a variety of clinical circumstances, the greater degree of skill that develops with time.

5. The essential steps for successful use of the fiberscope include organizing and maintaining a functional fiberoptic cart, setting up an instrument and intubation checklist, and practicing on models to develop the skills necessary for fiberoptic maneuvering (Table 51-3).

Naik and coauthors[31] published an interesting study to determine whether fiberoptic intubation skills learned outside the OR on a simple model could be transferred to the clinical setting. Twenty-four first-year anesthesiology and second-year internal medicine residents were recruited for this study. Residents were randomly allocated to a didactic teaching group ($n = 12$) or a model-training group ($n = 12$). The didactic teaching group received a detailed lecture from an expert in fiberoptic intubation. The model-training group was expertly guided through the tasks performed on a simple model designed to refine fiberoptic manipulation skills. After the training session, residents performed a fiberoptic orotracheal intubation on healthy, consenting, anesthetized, paralyzed female patients who were undergoing elective surgery and predicted to be easy laryngoscopic intubations. Two "blinded" anesthesiologists evaluated each patient.

The authors found that the model-training group outperformed the didactic group in the OR when evaluated with a global rating scale, as well as a preparatory checklist. The model-trained residents completed fiberoptic orotracheal intubation significantly faster and more successfully than didactic-trained residents. The authors concluded that training fiberoptic orotracheal intubation skills using a simple model is more effective than conventional didactic instruction when incorporating skills in the clinical setting. They suggested that incorporation of model-based training in fiberoptic intubation may greatly reduce the time accompanying subsequent training in the OR.[31]

Marsland and colleagues published a study of an educational resource specific to the acquisition and maintenance of endoscopic skills.[25] The authors describe the use of DEXTER, a nonanatomic, endoscopic dexterity training system designed to encourage practice in fiberoptic endoscopy as well as establish and maintain a state of procedural readiness. They determined that educational training systems such as DEXTER help to maintain these skills even if the anesthesiologists' clinical exposure to DA management is sporadic.[25]

The pulmonary literature also addresses the issue of training in fiberoptic bronchoscopy. Colt and colleagues[9] published a study of virtual reality bronchoscopic training. The authors hypothesized that novice trainees in the procedure of flexible FOB could rapidly acquire basic skills using a virtual reality skill center. They further hypothesized that they would compare favorably with senior colleagues who had been conventionally trained on live patients.[9]

Five novice bronchoscopists entering a pulmonary–critical care training program were studied prospectively. Flexible fiberoptic bronchoscopic inspection of the tracheobronchial tree was taught utilizing a virtual reality bronchoscopic skill center (a proxy flexible bronchoscope, robotic interface device, and personal computer with monitor and simulation software [PreOp Endoscopy Simulator; Immersion Medical, Gaithersburg, MD]). The proxy bronchoscope, modeled after a conventional FOB, provides realistic images to the users as they navigate through virtual tracheobronchial anatomy.[9] The authors measured dexterity, speed, and accuracy using the skill center as well as an inanimate airway model before and after 4 hours of group instruction and 4 hours of individual unsupervised practice. The results of this group were compared with those of a control group of four skilled physicians. Each of these pulmonologists had performed at least 200 bronchoscopies during 2 years of training. They found that novice bronchoscopists significantly improved dexterity and accuracy using either the virtual reality or inanimate airway model. After training, fewer bronchial segments were missed and fewer contacts with the tracheobronchial wall occurred. Speed and total time spent with unvisualized bronchial anatomy did not change. Following training, novice performance equaled or surpassed that of skilled physicians. Novices tended to perform more thorough examinations of the tracheobronchial tree. They missed significantly fewer bronchial segments in both the inanimate and virtual simulation models.[9]

Thus, it was concluded that a short, focused course of instruction and unsupervised practice using a virtual bronchoscopy simulator enabled novices to achieve a level of technical skill similar to that of colleagues with several years of experience. These skills were reproduced in an inanimate airway training model that mimics direct care of patients.[9]

C. SURGICAL AIRWAY

Correct and safe performance of a cricothyrotomy is lifesaving in patients who cannot be ventilated or intubated successfully. Eisenburger and coauthors[13] published a study comparing conventional surgical versus Seldinger technique emergency cricothyrotomy as performed by inexperienced clinicians.[13] The authors compared first-time performance of cricothyrotomy in adult human cadavers in two groups: group 1 (surgical technique) and group 2 (Seldinger technique). The ease of use and times to locate the cricothyroid membrane, to tracheal puncture, and to first lung ventilation were compared. Participants were allowed a single attempt at the procedure. A pathologist dissected the neck of each cadaver to assess the correct position of the tube and any injury to the airway. Subjective assessment of the technique on a visual analog scale (1 = easiest to 5 = hardest) was conducted. The age, height, and weight of the cadavers used in this study were uniform. Subjective assessment of each method as well as anatomy of the cadavers was not statistically different between the two groups. Correct tracheal placement of the tube was achieved in 70% of surgical cricothyrotomies ($n = 14$) and 60% of cricothyrotomy by the Seldinger technique ($n = 12$). Five attempts in group 2 (Seldinger) were aborted because of kinking of the guidewire. Time intervals between start of the procedure and location of the cricothyroid membrane, tracheal puncture, and first ventilation were not statistically different. Thus, in this limited study, each method showed equally poor performance and suggested that further study be undertaken to define the learning curve of this lifesaving procedure.[13]

McCarthy and colleagues[26] attempted to define the accuracy of cricothyrotomy performed in canine versus human cadaver models during surgical skills training. Thirty-three advanced trauma life support (ATLS) physician students performed cricothyroidotomy in canine models. Ten flight nurses performed a bimonthly surgical skills practicum on similarly prepared animals. Neck specimens of the euthanized animals were excised, fixed, and mapped by the authors. Subsequent courses in ATLS utilized human cadavers and similarly prepared trainees. In these models, cricothyrotomy sites were mapped in situ.

In canine models, 47 neck specimens of 52 attempted cricothyrotomies were inspected and mapped. Four specimens were excluded from the final analysis because of multiple attempts at cricothyrotomy. Thirteen of the 43 analyzed canine models had a misplaced cricothyrotomy (30.2%). Cricothyrotomy attempts were correct 27 of 28 times in the human cadaver model (96.4%). The authors concluded that placement accuracy in the canine model was low and that human cadaver models were superior for realistic training.[26]

Wong and associates[37] attempted to determine the minimum training experience required to perform surgical cricothyroidotomy in 40 seconds or less in mannequins.

Participants in this study were shown a video demonstrating the Seldinger technique of cricothyrotomy. The study participants were then asked to perform 10 consecutive cricothyrotomy procedures on a mannequin utilizing a preassembled percutaneous dilational cricothyrotomy set (Melker emergency percutaneous dilational set; Cook, Bloomington, IN). Each attempted procedure was timed from initial palpation of the skin to successful lung insufflation. Cricothyrotomy was considered successful if it was performed in 40 seconds or less. Cricothyrotomy time was considered to have reached a plateau when there was no significant reduction in time in three consecutive attempts.[37]

One hundred and two anesthesiologists participated in this study. A significant reduction in time for successful cricothyrotomy was found over the 10 attempts. The cricothyrotomy time reached a plateau by the fourth attempt. Success rate reached a plateau by the fifth attempt. The authors concluded that mannequin practice for percutaneous dilational cricothyrotomy led to a reduction in cricothyrotomy time and improved success rates of this procedure. By the fifth attempt, 96% of participants were able to perform a cricothyrotomy successfully in 40 seconds or less. The authors recommended that anyone providing emergency airway management be trained on mannequins for at least five attempts or until performance times of 40 seconds or less are achieved. The authors noted that clinical correlation and optimal retraining intervals for this procedure have yet to be determined.[37]

V. RESIDENT TRAINING IN ADVANCED AIRWAY MANAGEMENT

In 1995, a survey concerning formal training in advanced airway management techniques was sent to the program directors of 169 anesthesiology residency training programs in the United States.[23] One hundred and forty-three program directors responded to the survey. The authors found that formal rotations in advanced airway management were brief and often limited to didactic lectures. Only 27% of responding programs had a formal advanced airway course in their curriculum. Sixty percent of these courses were less than 2 weeks in duration.

Subsequently, a number of academic anesthesiology departments published accounts of their specific rotations in advanced airway management. Cooper and Benumof published a chapter concerning the University of California, San Diego Department of Anesthesiology's advanced airway rotation.[10] The goal of this rotation is to create nonurgent, nonstressful learning situations where a number of actual airway management techniques can be mastered in actual patients. The authors detail their rotation, including the administrative portion of setting up an airway rotation. Administrative aspects include (1) approval of the residency program director,

the departmental education committee, or both; (2) selecting experienced faculty to serve as instructors; (3) careful scheduling; (4) formulating the didactic program; and (5) having the appropriate equipment available (e.g., a dedicated DA cart). Residents receive a syllabus containing classic and current articles on both airway management devices and techniques prior to the rotation. The syllabus is the foundation for both formal didactic teaching and informal teaching in the OR.[10] Prior to its use in any patient, any new or unfamiliar airway device or technique is discussed thoroughly with regard to theory, description, insertion technique, and current clinical practice. Subsequently, the device is used in models, mannequins, or both. When invasive techniques are introduced (e.g., retrograde intubation, transtracheal jet ventilation, or percutaneous cricothyrotomy), a special workshop is held at the anatomy laboratory of the medical school. Human cadavers serve as models for instruction in the necessary technical skills involved in the procedure.

Selection of patients is critical during this rotation. According to the authors, relatively straightforward patients (e.g., ASA I-II patients undergoing elective general anesthesia without the need for extensive monitoring or setup) are ideal. Patients undergoing surgery in the supine position with ready access to the airway are desirable. Head and neck cases in which there is competition for the airway are generally avoided unless the patient requires an awake intubation (AI) technique. Patients with a known or suspected DA are prioritized to the resident on the airway management rotation. The goal of this rotation is to care for approximately 40 to 50 patients during the 1-month rotation.[10] Didactic teaching in this rotation includes performing a thorough evaluation of the airway based on the current recommendations of the ASA Task Force on Management of the Difficult Airway.[35] The findings of every airway examination are discussed with the supervising faculty. Residents are instructed in proper preparation of the patient for AI. In addition, they garner experience in devices such as the LMA, Combitube, lighted stylets, and advanced rigid fiberoptic laryngoscopes (e.g., Bullard scope, Wu Scope). The adjunct use of the FOB is encouraged. Once a patent airway is established, the resident is encouraged to identify all pertinent tracheobronchial anatomy by inserting an FOB through a bronchoscopy adapter.[10]

Dunn and his colleagues at Baystate Medical Center in Springfield, Massachusetts, published a description of their resident training in advanced airway management.[12] They developed a formal advanced airway management program consisting of two separate 1-month rotations. Each rotation has a separate focus. One month occurs during the later half of the CA-1 year. The second month occurs during the CA-2 year. Residents are given a set of objectives, a required reading list, and a required number of procedures unique to advanced airway management.

These procedures must be performed during the course of the rotation. This rotation consists of a core faculty group with expertise in airway management. According to the authors, five issues must be addressed in order to implement an airway rotation: (1) equipment, (2) core faculty, (3) curriculum, (4) time commitment, and (5) faculty development.

The Baystate Medical Center rotation utilizes seven DA carts distributed in five anesthetizing locations. The carts are uniformly set up and stocked. The authors feel that uniformity of equipment enhances physician performance of emergent airway management. Each cart and its contents cost approximately $30,000.[12] The contents of the DA carts include a variety of face masks, different sizes of the LMA Classic, Combitube, and transtracheal puncture equipment. The authors state that each of their DA carts is equipped with the three modalities of DA management that they feel are most helpful: flexible FOB, intubating LMA (Fastrach; LMA North America, San Diego, CA), and a variety of rigid fiberoptic laryngoscopes (Bullard scope, Circon Acmi, Stamford, CT; Wu Scope, Achi Corp., Fremont, CA; and the Upsher scope, Mercury Medical, Clearwater, FL). Each cart incorporates a video system, which the authors state improves teaching and is an integral part of their program.

The core faculty of the Baystate Medical Center program are proficient in all modalities of airway management. The size of the core faculty group is sufficient to ensure coverage during vacations, other clinical commitments, and so forth. At least one faculty member is available each day of the rotation. Contact with a core group of faculty ensures that residents master each technique in an adequately supervised fashion.[12]

The curriculum for this rotation includes a required reading list. Each of these publications requires discussion with a core faculty member in order to demonstrate adequate knowledge of the contents. The first month rotation for CA-1 residents focuses on the ASA DA management algorithm as well as techniques of flexible fiberoptic bronchoscopy. The second month rotation for CA-2 residents has a separate reading list and focuses on alternative techniques of advanced airway management as well as the complications of airway management.[12]

Requirements for successful completion of the first month of the Baystate Medical Center rotation include no fewer than 10 fiberoptic intubations, 10 Bullard scope intubations, and 6 LMA Fastrach intubations. In the second month of the airway rotation, the resident is required to perform at least 10 additional fiberoptic intubations (at least 2 pediatric fiberoptic intubations), 10 Bullard intubations, and 6 LMA Fastrach intubations. Residents in both months of the rotation are encouraged to seek out "known difficult airway" cases on the elective schedule as well as participate in the preoperative consultation of these patients. A worksheet detailing each DA case is kept by the resident and "signed off" by the core faculty.[12]

The authors detail the importance of departmental commitment to advanced airway management training as well as the development of faculty interested in advanced airway management.[12]

Hagberg and her colleagues at the University of Texas-Houston Medical School published a review of instruction of airway management skills during anesthesiology residency training.[19] This study was in follow-up of Koppel and Reed's study[23] and was conducted 3 years following the mandate made by the Accreditation Council for Graduate Medical Education (ACGME), which requires that residents have significant experience in specialized techniques of airway management such as fiberoptic intubation, double-lumen tube placement, and LMA use.[19] A survey of all directors of anesthesiology residency programs listed in the Graduate Medical Education Directory for the years 1998 to 1999 was conducted. The survey was sent by both email and fax to each program director. A second copy was sent to nonresponders 4 weeks following the initial mailing.

Of the 132 program directors surveyed, 79 (60%) replied. Of the 79 respondents, 26 reported programs (33%) that had a DA rotation. Interestingly, this number had increased only slightly since prior publications and the ACGME mandate.[23] An advanced airway management rotation was offered throughout the clinical base years of training in 13 (49%) programs of respondents. The rotation was 1 week in duration in 16 (61%) of the cases offering a program. Formal instruction was given prior to the start of the rotation in 18 (69%) programs. Instruction usually occurred using surgical patients (in 22 or 85% of programs), using ASA I or II patients (in 20 or 77% of programs), and was conducted by selected faculty (in 20 or 78% of programs).

The most commonly taught airway management modalities included the flexible FOB and the LMA. Invasive techniques such as percutaneous cricothyrotomy or tracheostomy were taught infrequently. There was a time limitation of 2 to 5 minutes or a maximum number of attempts in device-specific airway management in five programs (19%). A required case number for each device was found in five of the programs surveyed (19%). In this survey, instruction in advanced techniques of airway management occurred most commonly in the form of videotapes, written instruction, and practice on actual patients undergoing surgical procedures. Nontraditional methods of instruction such as computer-assisted instruction or patient simulators were used infrequently. Residents received both skills and written evaluation in 63% of the programs with a specific rotation in advanced airway management.[19]

Several interesting questions concerning the area of teaching advanced airway management were raised by this study. It was also suggested that further study needs to be undertaken concerning the efficacy of different training techniques. The authors are proponents of a future clinical certification process for training in advanced airway management for all anesthesiologists and suggest that the residency review committee for anesthesiology and the ACGME should establish number requirements for specific airway-related procedures in order to ensure standardization of resident training in this area. Lastly, follow-up studies are warranted when such mandates are in place, and establishment of these concepts may further decrease airway-related morbidity and mortality.[19]

Allen and Murray wrote a provocative letter concerning the issue of patients' consent when teaching airway management skills.[1] The authors suggested that any procedure that deviates significantly from the standard of care should invoke patients' consent. In the authors' practice, substitution of laryngoscope blades or use of the LMA or light wand does not require specific patients' consent. However, use of the Combitube, fiberoptic intubation, any retrograde technique, or elective repeated instrumentation with several different devices requires patients' consent. Most important, the authors stress that constant supervision of residents by experienced faculty is of paramount importance in order to minimize patients' risk. The authors also suggest that initial experience in advanced airway management in a simulated environment may further reduce patients' risk.[1]

Benumof and Cooper's reply to this letter suggested that special consent was not necessary for well-established and accepted airway management techniques, especially in the mandatory presence of experienced faculty.[4] Constant supervision by experienced faculty ensures against undue force or rough handling of the airway and ensures the ability to abort or change an initial airway management technique as needed. In Benumof and Cooper's published experience of approximately 1000 faculty–airway rotation resident cases, only three adverse outcomes occurred. In two cases, intubation through the self-sealing FOB adapter on an intubating anesthesia mask caused a piece of the blue diaphragm to be inadvertently carried into the trachea; thus, these adapters are no longer utilized. In each case, the complication was recognized immediately by the supervising faculty. Bronchoscopy forceps were utilized in both cases through the FOB's working channel to retrieve the piece of plastic without incident. The third event occurred when an improperly sterilized LMA was used. The LMA was inadvertently cleaned in glutaral (Cidex) and perilaryngeal edema ensued in the patient. The patient was tracheally intubated and, fortunately, suffered no long-term morbidity. The cleaning impropriety was corrected. The authors stress that careful use of accepted methods under strict and expert supervision does not mandate patients' consent.[4]

VI. CONCLUSION

Anesthesiologists are recognized as the airway management specialists in most aspects of modern medical practice. With this recognition comes responsibility. Anesthesiologists should make a career-long commitment to foster expertise in the recognition and management of the DA through proficient examination of the patient, communication of airway management concerns with physician colleagues, and appropriate application of specialized techniques of advanced airway management, when applicable. Fortunately, a variety of different methods are available for training and experience in advanced airway management. The key to learning and skill acquisition remains the interest and commitment of the individual.

REFERENCES

1. Allen G, Murray WB: Teaching airway management skills: What about patient consent? Anesthesiology 85:437, 1996.
2. American College of Obstetricians and Gynecologists: Anesthesia for Emergency Deliveries. ACOG Committee Opinion No. 104. Washington, DC, American College of Obstetricians and Gynecologists, 1992.
3. Behringer EC, Thaler ER: Airways and emergency airway management. In Lanken PN, Manaker S, Hanson CW (eds): The Intensive Care Unit Manual. Philadelphia, WB Saunders, 2001, pp 323-332.
4. Benumof JL, Cooper SD: Reply. Anesthesiology 85:438, 1996.
5. Brimacombe JR: Educational considerations. In Brimacombe JR (ed): Laryngeal Mask Anesthesia: Principles and Practice. Philadelphia, WB Saunders, 2005, pp 539-549.
6. Caplan RA: The ASA closed claims project: Lessons learned. In Annual Refresher Course Lectures No. 221, 1998.
7. Caplan RA, Posner KI, Ward RJ, et al: Adverse respiratory events in anesthesia: A closed claims analysis. Anesthesiology 72:828, 1990.
8. Cheney FW, Posner KI, Caplan RA: Adverse respiratory events infrequently leading to malpractice suits. A closed claims analysis. Anesthesiology 75:932, 1991.
9. Colt HG, Crawford SW, Galbraith O 3rd: Virtual reality bronchoscopy simulation: A revolution in procedural training. Chest 120:1333, 2001.
10. Cooper SD, Benumof JL: Teaching management of the airway: The UCSD airway rotation. In Benumof JL (ed): Airway Management: Principles and Practice. St. Louis, Mosby, 1996, pp 903-910.
11. Dickinson M, Curry P: Training for the use of the laryngeal mask in emergency and resuscitation situations. Resuscitation 28:111, 1995.
12. Dunn S, Connelly NR, Robbins L: Resident training in advanced airway management. J Clin Anesth 16:472, 2004.

13. Eisenburger P, Laczika K, List M, et al: Comparison of conventional surgical versus Seldinger technique emergency cricothyrotomy performed by inexperienced clinicians. Anesthesiology 92:687, 2000.

14. Erb T: Teaching the use of fiberoptic intubation in anesthetized, spontaneously breathing patients. Anesth Analg 89:1292, 1999.

15. Ferson DZ, Bui TP, Arens JF: Evaluation of the effectiveness of two methods of training for the insertion of the laryngeal mask airway. Anesthesiology 93:A558, 2000.

16. Gaiser RR: Managing the airway in critically ill patients: Teaching airway management skills—How and what to learn and teach. Crit Care Clin 16:515, 2000.

17. Gaiser RR, McGonigal ET, Litts P, et al: Obstetricians' ability to assess the airway. Obstet Gynecol 93:648, 1999.

18. Gurman GM, Tarnopolsky A, Weklser N, et al: Retention of airway management skills by medical students: A comparison between insertion of endotracheal tube (ET), laryngeal mask (LMA) and oesophageal combitube (OCT). Anesthesiology 91:A1139, 1999.

19. Hagberg CA, Greger J, Chelly JE, et al: Instruction of airway management skills during anesthesiology residency training. J Clin Anesth 15:149, 2003.

20. Haponik EF, Aquino SL, Vining DJ: Virtual bronchoscopy. Clin Chest Med 20:201, 1999.

21. Johnson C, Roberts JT: Clinical competence in the performance of fiberoptic laryngoscopy and endotracheal intubation: A study of resident instruction. J Clin Anesth 1:344, 1989.

22. Katz DB, Pearlman JD, Popitz M, et al: The development of a multimedia teaching program for fiberoptic intubation. J Clin Monit 13:287, 1997.

23. Koppel JN, Reed AP: Formal instruction in difficult airway management: A survey of anesthesiology residency programs. Anesthesiology 83:1343, 1995.

24. Larmon B, Schriger DL, Snelling R, et al: Results of a 4 hour endotracheal intubation class for EMT-basics. Ann Emerg Med 31:224, 1998.

25. Marsland CP, Robinson BJ, Chitty CH, et al: Acquisition and maintenance of endoscopic skills: Developing an endoscopic dexterity training system for anesthesiologists. J Clin Anesth 14:615, 2002.

26. McCarthy MC, Ranzinger MR, Nolan DJ, et al: Accuracy of cricothyroidotomy performed in canine and human cadaver models during surgical skills training. J Am Coll Surg 195:627, 2002.

27. Mort TC: Emergency tracheal intubation: Complications associated with repeated laryngoscopic attempts. Anesth Analg 99:607, 2004.

28. Mort TC: Exchanging an ET in the presence of an uncompromised view: Direct laryngoscopy vs. the airway exchange catheter. Crit Care Med 30: 2003.

29. Mort TC: Incorporating the ASA guidelines into emergency airway management: Benefit for patient care? Crit Care Med 30:A87, 2003.

30. Mort TC: Unplanned tracheal extubation outside the operating room: A quality improvement audit of hemodynamic and tracheal airway complications associated with emergency tracheal reintubation. Anesth Analg 86:1171, 1998.

31. Naik VN, Matsumoto ED, Houston PL, et al: Fiberoptic orotracheal intubation on anesthetized patients: Do manipulation skills learned on a simple model transfer into the operating room? Anesthesiology 95:343, 2001.

32. Nayyar P, Lisbon A: Non-operating room emergency airway management and endotracheal intubation practices: A survey of anesthesiology program directors. Anesth Analg 85:62, 1997.

33. Ovassapian A: Learning fiberoptic intubation techniques. In Ovassapian A (ed): Fiberoptic Endoscopy and the Difficult Airway, 2nd ed. Philadelphia, Lippincott-Raven, 1996, pp 263-271.

34. Practice guidelines for management of the difficult airway: A report by the American Society of Anesthesiology Task Force on Management of the Difficult Airway. Anesthesiology 78:597, 1993.

35. Practice guidelines for management of the difficult airway: An updated report by the ASA Task Force on Management of the Difficult Airway. Anesthesiology 98:1269, 2003.

36. Wheeler M, Roth AG, Dsida RM, et al: Teaching residents pediatric fiberoptic intubation of the trachea. Traditional fiberscope with an eyepiece versus video-assisted technique using a fiberscope with an integrated camera. Anesthesiology 101:842, 2004.

37. Wong DT, Prabhu AF, Coloma M, et al: What is the minimum training required for successful cricothyroidotomy? A study in mannequins. Anesthesiology 98:349, 2003.

52

EFFECTIVE DISSEMINATION OF CRITICAL AIRWAY INFORMATION: THE MEDIC ALERT* NATIONAL DIFFICULT AIRWAY/INTUBATION REGISTRY

Lynette Mark
Lorraine J. Foley
James Michelson

*Medic Alert is a federally registered trademark and service mark of the nonprofit, tax-exempt Medic Alert Foundation.

I. OVERVIEW

Communication of critical airway information traditionally has been accomplished by brief notes in the medical record, by letter, by verbal communication to patients and physicians, or by a combination of these. Significant shortcomings of these types of communication include questionable understanding by the patient or future provider of the significance of the airway difficulty and potential implications for future airway management, nonuniformity in documentation, and an inability to regain access to legible hard copy of these communications in a timely way. The Medic Alert National Difficult Airway/Intubation Registry was established in 1992 to facilitate uniform documentation and effective dissemination of standardized critical information related to complex airway management. The registry was created by the Anesthesia Advisory Council, a volunteer multidisciplinary team of anesthesiologists, otolaryngologists, and experts in quality assurance and risk management. The registry is expected, through dissemination of critical airway information and maintenance of a research database, to accomplish the goals of improving patients' safety and practitioners' security and to facilitate long-term tracking and outcome studies of patients. Such outcome studies may allow refinement of airway techniques, allow better anticipation of complex airway problems, and reduce future adverse outcomes.

The core of the registry is the nonprofit Medic Alert Foundation, the oldest and foremost international personal emergency medical information system. To create the registry, the Medic Alert Foundation system, which includes a 24-hour computerized emergency response center (with telephone access nationally and internationally without charge to the caller), wallet card, and identification emblem, was expanded to accommodate a more extensive database and a fax service for hard copy. Medic Alert Foundation has been endorsed by more than 50 organizations including the American Society of Anesthesiologists (ASA) in 1979, the World Federation of Societies of Anesthesiologists in 1992, and the American Academy of Otolaryngology-Head and Neck Surgery Foundation in 1993. Medic Alert Foundation International is currently organized in more than 35 countries. International expansion of the registry can be encouraged and promoted by Medic Alert Foundation and facilitated by the World Federation of Societies of Anesthesiologists.

This chapter discusses the Medic Alert Foundation and the registry, specifically addressing issues of documentation and dissemination of critical, standardized, clinically appropriate airway information. Objectives, components, and benefits of the registry are presented, as well as future plans for a comprehensive and integrated system on national and international levels. Strategies for implementation of the registry into clinical practice, including enrollment of patients and subsequent practitioner access to the registry, are discussed. Information on how to contact Medic Alert Foundation, receive Difficult Airway/Intubation Registry enrollment forms, or query the registry appears in Appendix A.

II. DIFFICULT AIRWAY/INTUBATION: A MULTIFACETED PROBLEM

Complex airway management is a multifaceted problem involving health care providers in a variety of clinical settings. The consequences of failed airway maintenance or endotracheal intubation, or both, can be devastating to the patient, the practitioner, and the health care system. Critical issues include identification of difficult airway/intubation patients, documentation of airway management techniques, dissemination of critical airway information to future health care providers, and medicolegal considerations.

A. IDENTIFICATION OF PATIENTS

Controversies regarding predictors and definitions of "difficult" exist, both intra- and interspecialty and dependent on and independent of practitioner skill, related to specific techniques and complicated by changing pathophysiology.[3] Historically, the anesthesiology literature cites an incidence of 1% to 3% of unanticipated difficult airway/intubation in patients undergoing general endotracheal anesthesia.[2,5,12,23] The airway management technique used to define difficult in this literature was conventional rigid laryngoscopy (Macintosh or Miller blades). Despite advances in airway management techniques and refinement of difficulty predictors, the 1% to 3% incidence of unanticipated difficulty cited has not changed and is still defined by conventional laryngoscopy.[2,19,21]

In an institution with approximately 25,000 general endotracheal anesthetic procedures annually, there are potentially 250 to 750 unanticipated difficult airway/intubations per year. On the basis of an ASA membership, which represents 90% of practicing anesthesiologists, and assuming that a full-time practicing anesthesiologist would encounter one unanticipated difficult intubation per year, there are potentially 30,000 to 90,000 unanticipated difficult airway/intubations annually in the United States. However, these numbers may underestimate the true incidence because anesthesiologists may not recall many near misses as vividly as a smaller number of difficult intubations in which, despite the effort, the result was suboptimal. On a national and international level, the scope of this problem and its impact on patients, practitioners, and the health care system are sufficient to warrant vigorous efforts to identify solutions.

In addition to patients who have unanticipated difficult airways on initial presentation, cohorts of patients have anticipated complex airway management, which can be successfully managed by a variety of innovative and specialty-specific techniques employed by other airway specialists (e.g., otolaryngology-head and neck surgeons, pulmonologists, emergency department physicians). Some of these techniques (laryngeal mask airway and Combitube) are readily available, require minimal practitioner education or training, and are inexpensive; whereas others may be available primarily in specialty centers, may require extensive practitioner skill, and may be relatively expensive (fiberoptic bronchoscope, surgical airway, specialized rigid laryngoscopes, and fluoroscopy-assisted intubation).

Some patients may have undergone head and neck surgery and have visible or hidden implants (e.g., laryngeal stents, thyroplasties). For these patients, specific considerations for airway management may be unknown to future providers (e.g., thyroplasty patients might require smaller endotracheal tubes than anticipated), compromising patients' safety and increasing practitioners' risk for preventable adverse events.

Successful future management of previously unanticipated difficult airway/intubations may be facilitated by identification of patients and by documentation and dissemination of information detailing successful and unsuccessful airway management techniques and primary difficulty encountered. For anticipated difficult airway patients, availability of this information promotes quality of care.

B. DOCUMENTATION AND DISSEMINATION OF CRITICAL INFORMATION

Written documentation of airway events is institution specific and specialty variable. No standardized, uniform, readily available document exists to record precisely airway events and summarize salient issues.

When patients with complex airway management are discharged, information about critical airway events may be inadvertently not communicated or miscommunicated. Verbal communication of difficult airway information by the provider to the patient is unreliable. Communication may be hindered by the patient's intubation or sedation, or both. The patient may be expeditiously discharged from the health care facility or discharged by personnel other than the primary health care provider before airway events have been fully communicated. Miscommunication may arise because of patients' lack of medical knowledge or overriding anxiety related to their primary medical condition. In addition, providers may underrepresent the severity of difficulty, attempting to allay patients' anxiety or fearing liability exposure. Written communication of difficult airway information by the provider to the patient may be a more effective strategy, but the patient may fail to convey this information accurately and comprehensively to future health care providers. Patients may lose the anesthesiologist's letter or memo or fail to give a copy of it to their primary care provider, and in an emergency the information will most likely be inaccessible.

When difficult airway/intubation patients reenter the health care system electively or emergently, they may relate vague verbal histories, deny any difficult airway history, or be physically unable to communicate. Attempts to retrieve prior anesthesia records and documentation should be initiated but may be unsuccessful because of constraints of time or availability. When available, written documentation may be incomplete and difficult for other health care providers to decipher. These situations create confusion about the exact nature of the airway difficulty encountered and airway management employed, potentially delaying or compromising patients' care.

Even when written documentation is adequate, dissemination of critical information is usually limited to the patient's medical record. Subsequent elective or emergent retrieval of records by future health care providers, separated by geography or time, may be untimely or impossible.

C. CONSEQUENCES OF DIFFICULT AIRWAY MANAGEMENT

The consequences of a difficult airway/intubation with or without adverse outcomes may be as unsettling as the event itself. There may be a patient-perceived threat to future anesthetic safety or lack of understanding of the significance of the difficulty. There may be a practitioner-perceived threat to professional security. The impact in direct and indirect costs to the health care system for complex airway management–related events is far-reaching.

Three studies specifically demonstrated the consequences of difficult airway management on liability exposure (L. Morlock, personal communication to L. M., July 17, 1994).[1,14] In an analysis of approximately 5000 claims filed in the Maryland legal system over a 15-year period that named one or more anesthesiologists as a defendant, insertion of an endotracheal tube was the sixth most common medical procedure leading to a liability claim. The great majority of these claims also included as defendants other members of the operating room team (e.g., general surgeons, nurse anesthetists, orthopedic surgeons, otolaryngologists, plastic surgeons, cardiac surgeons, dentists, nurses). Forty-five claims were resolved as of 1994; one resulted in a jury award of $5 million (L. Morlock, personal communication to L. M., July 17, 1994).

In a 1992 loss analysis study conducted by the Physicians Insurers Association of America, files retrieved from an aggregate of 43 physician-owned malpractice insurance companies (representing approximately 2000 anesthesiologists nationally) ranked "intubation problems" as the third most prevalent misadventure (behind "tooth injury" and "no medical misadventures"). The average paid indemnity for 175 of 339 files was $196,958.[14]

The ASA Committee on Professional Liability closed claims study found that respiratory events were the most common cause of brain damage and death during anesthesia, with difficult intubation being the likeliest category for risk reduction. The median payment for respiratory claims was $200,000.[1]

To put these statistics in perspective, the following must be considered: (1) the number of malpractice claims reported represents only a small fraction (one eighth) of all adverse outcomes,[4] with one malpractice claim filed for every 7.5 patient injuries from difficult airway events and adverse outcomes that are not the subject of a claim (L. Morlock, personal communication to L. M., July 17, 1994); (2) claims may often be aborted by good physician-patient communication; and (3) claims are often initiated against physicians because of poor communication and inadequate records (R. Kidwell, personal communication to L. M., July 17, 1994).

III. DIFFICULT AIRWAY/INTUBATION: RESPONSES TO THE PROBLEM

A. AMERICAN SOCIETY OF ANESTHESIOLOGISTS GUIDELINES

In response to the previously mentioned issues, the ASA developed and published "Practice guidelines for management of the difficult airway." These guidelines heightened practitioners' awareness of the scope and magnitude of problems related to complex airway management. They encouraged familiarity with a standardized clinical airway algorithm and stressed availability of technologies in addition to conventional rigid laryngoscopy for difficult airway management. The guidelines recommended that the anesthesiologist document in the medical record the presence and nature of airway difficulties, the various airway management techniques employed, and whether they were beneficial or detrimental in managing the difficult airway. Recommendations for dissemination of critical information included informing the patient (or responsible person) of the presence of a difficult airway, apparent reasons for difficulty, and implications for future care.[2]

B. ANESTHESIA ADVISORY COUNCIL

Coincident with the development of these guidelines, an Anesthesia Advisory Council (Appendix B) representing anesthesiologists, otolaryngologists, and experts in risk management joined together to create a comprehensive system for uniform documentation and effective dissemination of critical airway information. Specifically, they addressed the following questions: (1) When an airway event happens, is there a consistency in documentation and easy access to a central internationally accessible database? (2) Is there a uniform way that patients and health care personnel can be informed of critical airway information? The council identified and investigated two existing systems that were successful in documentation and dissemination of critical airway information: The University of Michigan Airway Clinic and the Medic Alert Foundation.

C. THE UNIVERSITY OF MICHIGAN AIRWAY CLINIC[17]

Martin L. Norton and colleagues at the University of Michigan pioneered efforts to evaluate more fully patients with complex airway management problems and to disseminate effectively critical information to patients and future health care providers. The University of Michigan Airway Clinic was established in 1987 as a multidisciplinary, national and international referral center. The core of its clinical documentation consisted of a handwritten airway consultation record, photodocumentation, and an information response center. As the clinic grew in size, it became increasingly apparent to house staff that the existing Medic Alert Foundation could more readily accommodate 24-hour emergency requests for information, and selected clinic patients were enrolled.

D. MEDIC ALERT FOUNDATION

Medic Alert Foundation is a 501(c)3 nonprofit organization that has 40 years of experience with information exchange. Its stated mission is to protect and save lives by disseminating critical information on patients immediately and accurately while maintaining patients' confidentiality and privacy. This service comprises a three-part system: a 24-hour emergency response center, a visible alert emblem worn by the patient (Fig. 52-1), and a wallet card (Fig. 52-2). Medic Alert reliably tracks patients and updates their medical information. An initial enrollment fee of $35 to $75 (depending on the type of metal selected for the emblem) is waived for patients who are unable to pay if enrollment is accompanied by a letter from the health care provider. Contact is made with patients yearly to update medical information, and

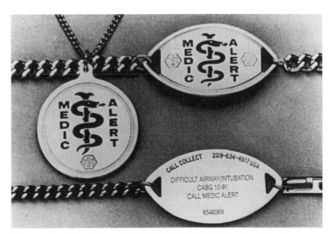

Figure 52-1 Clockwise from left, The Medic Alert emblem as a necklace, the Medic Alert emblem as a bracelet, and the reverse side of the Medic Alert emblem, which shows the Medic Alert collect phone number (accessible nationally and internationally without charge to the caller), the Difficult Airway/Intubation Registry designation, and the patient's unique identification number for the Medic Alert system.

Figure 52-2 The Medic Alert wallet card.

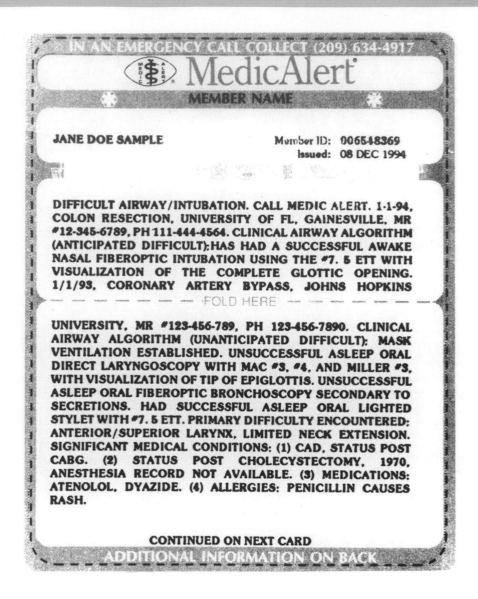

a $15 annual fee is requested. In 1979, Medic Alert Foundation was endorsed by the ASA House of Delegates. In 1992, the Anesthesia Advisory Council recommended the creation of the National Difficult Airway/Intubation Registry within the Medic Alert Foundation.

For years anesthesiologists have recognized the value of the Medic Alert emergency response system for patients with malignant hyperthermia (INDEX ZERO hotline) and have enrolled patients with difficult airways in a nonuniform way. The establishment of the National Difficult Airway/Intubation Registry within Medic Alert has promoted a standardization of terminology and an expanded database specifically for airway patients.

E. INSTITUTIONAL: IN-HOSPITAL REGISTRY

In response to the ASA Difficult Airway Task Force guidelines and the Anesthesia Advisory Counsel and Medic Alert Foundation, an In-Hospital Computerized Difficult Airway Registry at Beth Israel Deaconess Medical Center,

Boston, was initiated. This was developed to avoid delays in obtaining information on previous airway management and to enhance patients' compliance with registration in the National Medic Alert Registry. Many patients return to the same institution. Therefore, if patients are registered in the hospital, anesthesiologists do not have to rely completely on patients' compliance with registering into Medic Alert. As with Johns Hopkins Medical Institutions, once the patient has been identified in the operating room or another location within the hospital, a fluorescent orange bracelet labeled "Difficult Airway/Intubation" is placed on the wrist. A "Difficult Airway/Intubation" notice is placed on the patient's medical record. Another step was added, however; information about the management of the airway is also entered in the Clinical Computing Center System (CCCS) for access throughout the hospital.

The CCCS is an integrated hospital information system through which clinicians obtain patients' information. The anesthesiologists enter or edit information on the patient's airway management of difficult intubations into

CCCS with a key authorization. Throughout the hospital, CCCS terminals for entry and retrieval are available. Once the information is entered, only health care personnel can gain access to the airway status of the patient for viewing. Therefore, any patients admitted directly to the medical-surgical floors and through the emergency room receive a Difficulty Airway Intubation bracelet who have been identified through CCCS located in Nurse's Assessment under Airway Status. This allows immediate action for emergency or nonemergency intubation situations in which proper equipment, that is, a difficult airway cart and a standby surgeon, is required. This system ensures that any patient previously identified as having a difficult airway is recognized as such during the patient's hospital stay.[7]

Leveraging the electronic patient record at Johns Hopkins, a template for dictating a note for a difficult airway patient by the anesthesiologist has been developed and implemented. The note is labeled on the overview of the medical record so that subsequent care providers are aware of this specific issue.

IV. THE MEDIC ALERT NATIONAL DIFFICULT AIRWAY/INTUBATION REGISTRY

A. OBJECTIVES OF THE REGISTRY

The major objectives of the Medic Alert Anesthesia Advisory Council for this registry are (1) to develop and implement mechanisms for uniform documentation and dissemination of critical information, (2) to establish a central data bank of airway management information for research purposes, (3) to analyze and refine predictors of difficulty, (4) to develop innovative airway management technologies based on analysis of successful and unsuccessful techniques employed, (5) to analyze and refine difficult airway management based on clinical practices, (6) to conduct long-term tracking of patients to assess implications of adverse outcomes for future management, (7) to create a multidisciplinary concept of difficult airway/intubation, and (8) to determine whether rapid and economical dissemination of currently unavailable critical airway information has a positive impact on future care of patients and overall cost to the health care system.

B. DIFFICULT AIRWAY/INTUBATION CATEGORY AND IDENTIFICATION OF PATIENTS

The council established the uniform category difficult airway/intubation to provide standard nomenclature on the Medic Alert identification emblem. Patients are identified for enrollment in the registry after their surgery and medical management or by documented airway difficulty on their medical record, or both. They can be divided into at least three distinct groups: (1) anticipated difficult airway based on accepted predictors (genetic, disease specific, anatomic or physiologic, and patients' experience),

(2) previously unanticipated difficult airway, and (3) otolaryngology-head and neck surgery patients (with or without airway implants).

In an effort to circumvent controversies regarding the definition of difficult, patients are enrolled by providers who have medicolegal responsibility for them, enabling primary providers to use their own definition of difficult. To facilitate a common orientation for difficult airway management by various specialists, the following concept, adopted by the council, is useful:

Knowing what you now know about this patient's airway and successful/unsuccessful airway management techniques employed, if this patient required emergency surgery and endotracheal intubation, would you do a rapid sequence induction? If your answer is no—and you documented on the patient's medical record difficult airway/intubation—that is a difficult airway/intubation.

C. COMPONENTS OF THE REGISTRY

The core of the registry is the Medic Alert emergency response service: 24-hour emergency response center with phone and fax capability, identification emblem, and wallet card. The Medic Alert phone number (209-634-4917) is imprinted on the emblem. Callers are instructed to call collect. The number is accessible nationally and internationally, unlike an 800 number, which cannot be reached outside the United States.

The basic Medic Alert service was expanded to include the following components.

1. Specialized Enrollment Brochure

Enrollment in the registry is facilitated by a brochure specifically designed to address the concerns of health care providers and patients (Fig. 52-3). It consists of the following:

a. Health Care Provider Information Panel

Questions frequently asked by providers are addressed, such as the following:

> *Why the Medic Alert National Difficult Airway/Intubation Registry?*

Up to 3% of all patients undergoing anesthesia have unanticipated difficult airway/intubations. Knowledge of your experiences with these patients may facilitate future uncomplicated airway management. Medic Alert provides immediate access to this critical information with an alerting emblem, 24-hour emergency response center and database, and wallet card.

> *What is a difficult airway/intubation?*

Most practitioners use an intuitive definition to qualify a difficult airway/intubation. If your response to the question, "If this patient returned for emergency surgery requiring general endotracheal anesthesia in the middle of the night, would you do a rapid sequence induction?" is no—that is a difficult intubation.

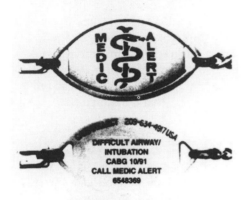

Medic Alert
National Registry
for Difficult
Airway/Intubation

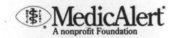

**Protect Your Patients,
Inform Your Colleagues.**

MedicAlert
A nonprofit Foundation

*Endorsed by the American Society of Anesthesiologists,
World Federation of Societies of Anaesthesiologists,
American Academy of Otolaryngology
Head and Neck Surgery*

Figure 52-3 The cover of the Medic Alert National Difficult Airway/Intubation Registry enrollment brochure.

I've never had an airway that I could not ultimately manage.

In urgent and emergency situations, medical personnel with less daily airway experience than you may be the first to manage this patient's airway. Give them the benefit of your experiences.

I already provide letters of explanation for patients with difficult airway/intubations.

Medic Alert provides a uniform document to disseminate critical information. Incorporating Medic Alert into your practice for selected patients may save you time and money and will protect them.

Should I enroll patients with airways that are anticipated to be difficult—either by examination or by history, or both?

Any patient who requires special techniques for airway management may benefit from enrollment in the registry.

I just encountered a registry patient and had no difficulty with airway management. Now what?

The registry provides a chronology of patients' events. Medic Alert invites review by members and their

physicians and regularly updates patients' files and wallet cards.

How detailed should I be in completing this application?

Please complete and sign the airway data bank section, especially the medical record number, and obtain the patient's signature. Give the form to a patient or family member to mail with the enrollment fee.

How do I enroll patients who are unable to pay for membership?

Medic Alert is a nonprofit foundation and provides membership without charge for an indigent patient if the completed enrollment form is accompanied by a statement of the financial need, written on official letterhead, and signed by the practitioner.

b. Patients' Information Panel

Many health care providers use candid questions and responses to facilitate perioperative discussion with patients. Questions most often asked by patients include the following:

What is difficult airway/intubation?

During general anesthesia, a specially trained professional assists your breathing. For the majority of patients, this is easily done by placing a mask over the nose and mouth or inserting a breathing tube into the windpipe, or both. Individual differences in jaw structure, mouth opening and dentition, and neck movement may make some patients more difficult to manage than others. If the physician can anticipate or is alerted to previous airway difficulty, he or she can implement special techniques that are safe and comfortable.

How can Medic Alert help?

Medic Alert can provide readily available information regarding your history of difficult airway/intubation for future elective and emergency medical situations. This is important, particularly in emergency situations, when someone other than your primary physician may provide you with emergency health care. The Medic Alert emblem immediately alerts the health care provider to vital information that is critical to your safety.

How can I enroll in Medic Alert?

If your physician noted airway difficulty and thinks you should be enrolled in the Medic Alert program, he or she will provide information about your airway management on this form. You must provide personal data and other significant medical conditions. When it is completed, please sign the form and mail with the enrollment fee.

c. Medic Alert Service

A visual and written description of the Medic Alert service is included for education of practitioners and patients, including information on updating patients' information and Medic Alert's 24-hour emergency response number (209-634-4917), a collect number for access nationally and internationally without charge to the caller.

d. Medic Alert Anesthesia Advisory Council

A list of names and affiliations of members of this voluntary council serves as a resource for questions, comments, or concerns that may arise regarding the registry (see Appendix B).

e. Legal Statement

A legal statement, designed to address practitioner and institutional liability exposure and facilitate research, must be signed by all patients prior to enrollment in the registry. The statement is as follows:

The member agrees not to wear the emblem or carry the wallet card until the emergency record has been carefully checked by the member for correctness and agrees to inform Medic Alert in writing of any error found. The member authorizes Medic Alert to relay information in response to emergency telephone calls. The member agrees to notify Medic Alert immediately whenever his or her medical condition or address changes.

Enrolling hospital/physician's sole responsibility is to provide information to Medic Alert. How information is used is the sole responsibility of provider and, therefore, member hereby holds harmless the enrolling institution, physician, and Medic Alert for actions taken based on information provided.

Member agrees to permit any information on this form to be collected and used anonymously for scientific and educational research.

f. Enrollment Section

Information requested for enrollment in Medic Alert includes patient's demographics, emergency contacts, medical information to be engraved on the emblem, and other emergency medical information. Specific registry information that is supplied by the practitioner includes hospital name, medical record number, surgical procedure, date of procedure, clinical anesthesia profile, nature of difficulty encountered, reason or reasons for difficulty, successful and unsuccessful techniques, best visualization of airway anatomy, clinically applied algorithm, and clinical outcome. This section of the brochure is scannable and faxable (Fig. 52-4). The enrolling health care provider's signature facilitates verification, and anonymity is honored, if requested. Selected information from this database is compiled in paragraph form, printed on the patient's wallet card, and sent by fax when requested. With the exception of specific airway requirements (related to tracheal surgery, stenosis, or other conditions requiring specific size of endotracheal tubes), recommendations for future airway management are *not* made, thereby avoiding

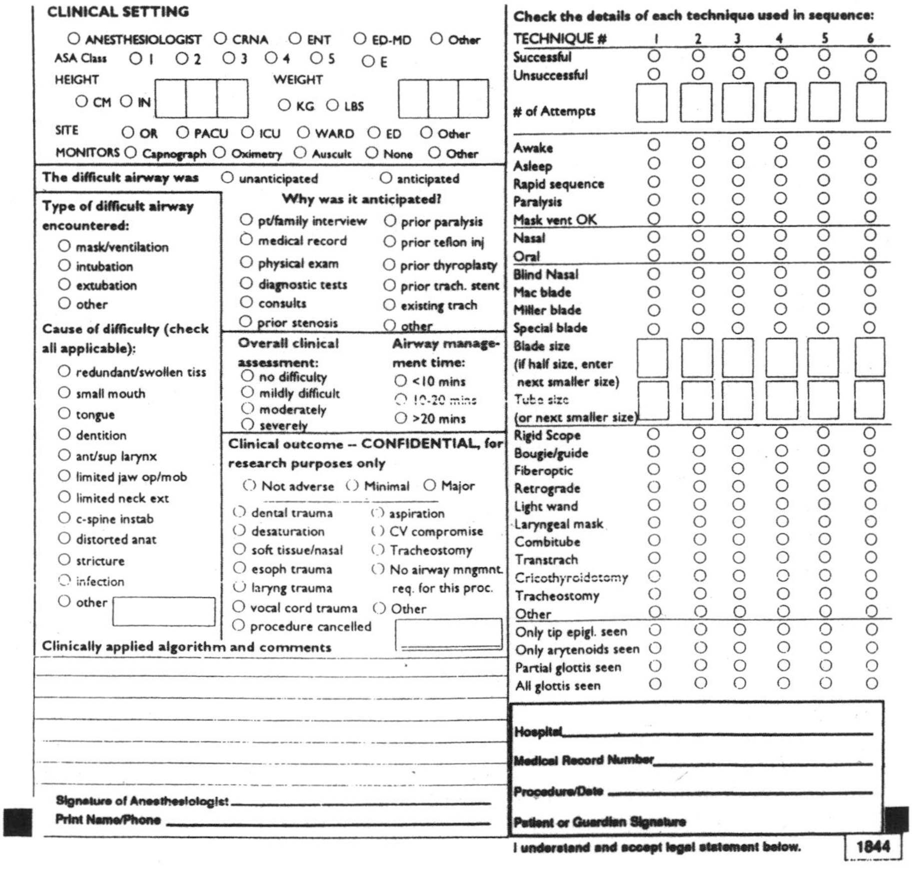

CLINICAL SETTING
O ANESTHESIOLOGIST O CRNA O ENT O ED-MD O Other
ASA Class O 1 O 2 O 3 O 4 O 5 O E
HEIGHT O CM O IN
WEIGHT O KG O LBS
SITE O OR O PACU O ICU O WARD O ED O Other
MONITORS O Capnograph O Oximetry O Auscult O None O Other

The difficult airway was O unanticipated O anticipated

Type of difficult airway encountered:
O mask/ventilation
O intubation
O extubation
O other

Why was it anticipated?
O pt/family interview O prior paralysis
O medical record O prior teflon inj
O physical exam O prior thyroplasty
O diagnostic tests O prior trach. stent
O consults O existing trach
O prior stenosis O other

Cause of difficulty (check all applicable):
O redundant/swollen tiss
O small mouth
O tongue
O dentition
O ant/sup larynx
O limited jaw op/mob
O limited neck ext
O c-spine instab
O distorted anat
O stricture
O infection
O other

Overall clinical assessment:
O no difficulty
O mildly difficult
O moderately
O severely

Airway management time:
O <10 mins
O 10-20 mins
O >20 mins

Clinical outcome -- CONFIDENTIAL, for research purposes only
O Not adverse O Minimal O Major
O dental trauma O aspiration
O desaturation O CV compromise
O soft tissue/nasal O Tracheostomy
O esoph trauma O No airway mngmnt. req. for this proc.
O laryng trauma
O vocal cord trauma O Other
O procedure cancelled

Clinically applied algorithm and comments

Signature of Anesthesiologist ____
Print Name/Phone ____

Check the details of each technique used in sequence:

TECHNIQUE #	1	2	3	4	5	6
Successful	O	O	O	O	O	O
Unsuccessful	O	O	O	O	O	O
# of Attempts						
Awake	O	O	O	O	O	O
Asleep	O	O	O	O	O	O
Rapid sequence	O	O	O	O	O	O
Paralysis	O	O	O	O	O	O
Mask vent OK	O	O	O	O	O	O
Nasal	O	O	O	O	O	O
Oral	O	O	O	O	O	O
Blind Nasal	O	O	O	O	O	O
Mac blade	O	O	O	O	O	O
Miller blade	O	O	O	O	O	O
Special blade	O	O	O	O	O	O
Blade size (if half size, enter next smaller size)						
Tube size (or next smaller size)						
Rigid Scope	O	O	O	O	O	O
Bougie/guide	O	O	O	O	O	O
Fiberoptic	O	O	O	O	O	O
Retrograde	O	O	O	O	O	O
Light wand	O	O	O	O	O	O
Laryngeal mask	O	O	O	O	O	O
Combitube	O	O	O	O	O	O
Transtrach	O	O	O	O	O	O
Cricothyroidotomy	O	O	O	O	O	O
Tracheostomy	O	O	O	O	O	O
Other	O	O	O	O	O	O
Only tip epigl. seen	O	O	O	O	O	O
Only arytenoids seen	O	O	O	O	O	O
Partial glottis seen	O	O	O	O	O	O
All glottis seen	O	O	O	O	O	O

Hospital ____
Medical Record Number ____
Procedure/Date ____
Patient or Guardian Signature
I understand and accept legal statement below.
1844

Figure 52-4 Airway management database section of the Medic Alert National Airway/Intubation Registry enrollment form. It can be scanned and faxed to facilitate rapid dissemination of critical airway information.

conflicts with other practitioners' choices for future airway management techniques. Clinical outcome information is confidential, collected for research purposes only, and not disseminated to the patient or future health care providers.

g. Patient's Signature
Informed consent must be obtained for enrollment.

2. Patient's Confidentiality

For more than 40 years there have been no claims against Medic Alert for breach of confidentiality or dissemination of incorrect medical information. Information contained in the registry is available from the patient's medical record. When patients sign the informed consent for enrollment in Medic Alert, they are agreeing to confidential exchange of physician-verified medical information.

Although Medic Alert is not defined as a "Covered Entity" under Health Insurance Portability and Accountability Act of 1996 (HIPAA) regulations, it follows rigid patients' information privacy standards that are consistent with the HIPAA rules. The data contained in its database of patients' information are kept confidential, being shared only with medical providers in the course of their caring for the patient. It also complies with the retention, collection, and safeguarding of data principles defined by the European Union SafeHarbor framework (www.export.cov/safeharbor/).

3. Physician Education Service

Primary or specialty physicians, or both, who are identified by the patient on the registry enrollment form are notified of the patient's difficult airway/intubation by first-class mail. The notification is intended to be placed in the patient's file for future reference.

4. Long-Term Tracking

In addition to the initial enrollment fee, a nominal annual fee enables Medic Alert to maintain current medical information and track patients on a long-term basis. Medic Alert sends updating forms (by first-class mail) to all members and encourages them to review and update their medical information. Unopened returned envelopes are address searched through the U.S. Postal Service and Social Security Administration. In this way, a current accounting of active members is maintained. In addition to this annual updating initiated by Medic Alert, patients are encouraged to update their medical information as often as necessary. Long-term tracking by Medic Alert allows the registry to compile a chronology of patients' airway events. This reflects changing patients' pathophysiology, which may have been manifest as complex airway management on one occasion and uncomplicated airway management on another (different techniques

and algorithms used). By providing a chronology of events, any concerns of permanently labeling a patient as difficult are negated.

5. Research Database

When patients sign the informed consent for enrollment, they agree to allow information in the registry database to be used anonymously for educational and research purposes. Patient information updates are automatically reflected in the registry database. Inquiries to the registry database by researchers are reviewed by the Anesthesia Advisory Council and granted by the Medic Alert Foundation board.

D. BENEFITS OF THE REGISTRY

1. Patients' Safety

Knowledge of prior airway events, as provided by the registry emergency response system, may significantly improve patients' safety by detailing for future care providers unsuccessful and successful airway techniques used in the past.

Lack of definitive predictors of airway difficulty,[18,20,22] changing patients' pathophysiology, and the use of conventional laryngoscopy as the first choice for airway management contribute to an unchanged incidence of 1% to 3% for unanticipated difficult airway/intubation. Until more accurate and comprehensive predictors of airway difficulty are identified, relatively healthy patients are at continued risk during anesthetic events—risk that cannot be completely addressed by improved monitoring techniques or through increased practitioner vigilance.

Identification of various combinations of anatomic abnormalities (as noted on the registry enrollment form) may contribute to the development of a difficult airway/intubation profile that is more accurate than any single predictor.

With enrollment in the registry, the patient's primary physician and specialist (as noted on the enrollment form) are notified of the patient's difficult airway/intubation status, thus providing for continuity of care.

2. Practitioner Security

Practitioner security could be increased by the registry in two ways: (1) by improving provider-patient communication and (2) by documenting and disseminating critical airway information for future health care providers.

Malpractice claims are often initiated because of poor communication (R. Kidwell, personal communication to L. M., July 17, 1994). Enrollment in the registry gives providers an opportunity to inform patients of their airway difficulties and adverse events while offering a way to protect them in the future. A survey of registry patients showed that, despite experiencing adverse outcomes (cancellation of surgery, dental trauma, soft tissue trauma, desaturation, cardiovascular compromise, and cricothy-rotomy or tracheostomy), 100% were satisfied with enrollment in the registry and had a sense of comfort that future health care providers would understand the significance of their difficult airway/intubation and the concept of Medic Alert.[6]

Patients may also favorably respond, after a difficult experience, to their anesthesiologists' knowledgeable presentation of organized efforts to register their problem and reduce the risk of recurrence.

Malpractice claims are often initiated because of poor documentation.[11] For future events, the intraoperative anesthesia record does not provide information in a standardized, easily readable form and is not readily accessible. Information from the registry is standardized and detailed and can be obtained by telephone or fax within 5 minutes of the request.

Enrollment in the registry, as documented in patients' charts, is a positive reflection on the providers' concern for the patient's future safety.

3. Cost Savings

The cost of initial enrollment in the registry may be justified by future savings realized by the patient and provider or institution. A preliminary study of selective patients' charges for anesthesia preparation time (i.e., anesthesiologist's professional fee, anesthesia resident's charge, drug and supply charges, and operating room time charges) was done for all 690 patients undergoing coronary artery bypass graft surgery as the first procedure of the day at the Johns Hopkins Hospital during a 10-month period. Of these patients, 684 had no airway difficulty (control group); 6 had difficult airway/intubation and were subsequently enrolled in the Medic Alert National Difficult Airway/Intubation Registry. The results showed that the mean selective patients' charge for anesthesia preparation time for the registry group was $1578.24; this represented a 59% increase over the control group mean selective patients' charge of $990.71.[16] Knowledge of difficulties previously encountered and techniques used could promote cost-effective use of equipment and operating room time.

Anticipation and preparation for a difficult airway/intubation patient, as identified by the registry, may decrease the incidence of cancellations, adverse outcomes, and malpractice claims. Even one settlement can cost the provider or institution significantly more than the time, effort, and cost of enrolling many patients in the registry.

4. Outcome Studies

The database of the registry is accessible for educational and research purposes by request to the Anesthesia Advisory Council. It is anticipated that these data will be used to improve anesthetic practice by refining airway techniques, identifying difficult airway/intubation patients more accurately, and decreasing the incidence of adverse outcomes.

At Beth Israel Deaconess Medical Center, anesthetic and medical records were reviewed of all patients registered in the in-hospital registry and returning for surgery in a 2-year period from 1995 to 1997. Of the 119 patients entered into the registry, 31 patients returned to the operating room one or more times after initial identification as a difficult airway. Only 3 of the 31 patients had conventional laryngoscopy, and 2 of the 3 again encountered airway difficulty. All but one of the seven patients who were induced before the establishment of an artificial airway had been known as a patient who was easy to mask ventilate. The remaining one patient had an inhalation induction and conventional laryngoscopy. All those who had been identified as difficult to mask ventilate had an awake fiberoptic intubation or nongeneral anesthesia. Although statistics could not be computed, there appears to be a trend away from general anesthesia when amenable and awake general fiberoptic intubation is required. There were no airway complications.[8]

Communication of a known difficult airway is one of the best predictors because there is no one good predictor for identifying patients with a difficult airway. This study shows that other alternatives for airway management can decrease or eliminate airway complications for difficult intubations. Knowing past experiences of a patient's airway management, especially if they are a difficult mask ventilation, can prevent negative outcomes.

E. CHARACTERISTICS OF REGISTRY PATIENTS

Between 1992 and 1994, more than 250 adult and pediatric patients throughout the United States were enrolled in the Medic Alert National Difficult Airway/Intubation Registry. Approximately 50% were in ASA classes I to II, and 50% were in ASA classes III to IV. Enrolled patients required general anesthesia, had difficulty, or did not require airway management at the time of enrollment but had a documented history of prior airway management. Patients were enrolled from private and academic institutions, outpatient surgical centers, and by self-referral. In a preliminary report of 111 of these patients, a variety of airway techniques were used and adverse outcomes were reported (Tables 52-1, 52-2, and 52-3).[15] To ensure patients' safety, providers encouraged these patients to enroll when there were minor or major adverse outcomes, despite concerns about liability exposure.

F. CLINICAL PRACTICES: IMPLEMENTATION OF THE MEDIC ALERT REGISTRY

1. Institutional Level

Patients presenting for surgery may have a history or physical features that suggest difficult airway management with conventional laryngoscopy, as identified by the provider. For these patients the provider may suggest

Table 52-1 **Characteristics of Patients Enrolled in the Medic Alert National Difficult Airway/Intubation Registry (*n* = 111)**

Characteristic	Cases (%)
Adult (age > 18 years)	99
Emergency	1
ASA classes I and II	54
ASA classes III and IV	46
ASA class V	0
Anticipated difficult	44
Unanticipated difficult	56
Difficult mask airway	10
Difficult intubation	97

ASA, American Society of Anesthesiologists.

enrollment in the registry during the preoperative interview. For all patients a simple, direct statement included as part of the anesthesia consent, mentioning the potential for unanticipated airway difficulty and the registry, may be appropriate. An institutional team approach has been instrumental in successful identification and enrollment of patients in the registry.

At the Johns Hopkins Medical Institutions, the following system has been implemented. The anesthesiologist identifies the difficult airway/intubation patient on the basis of clinical experiences and completes an in-hospital quality assurance scan form similar to the Medic Alert Registry scan form or simply uses the Medic Alert form. Medic Alert is the first registry to use a scan form system, which will allow reductions in costs of registry data entry.[10] The form can be submitted by fax to the registry within minutes or mailed. The nursing critical pathway, a key element in the successful education and enrollment of difficult airway/intubation patients, prompts nursing

Table 52-2 **Airway Management Techniques Used for Patients in the Medic Alert National Difficult Airway/Intubation Registry**

Technique	Outcome	
	Successful (*n* = 110)	Unsuccessful (*n* = 200)
Conventional laryngoscopy	20	170
Fiberoptic bronchoscopy	66	13
Lighted stylet	1	1
Surgical airway	11	3
Specialized others	12	13

Table 52-3 **Adverse Outcomes for Patients in the Medic Alert National Difficult Airway/Intubation Registry**

Type	Frequency (*n* = 31)
Cancellation	9
Dental trauma	3
Desaturation	7
Soft tissue or nasal trauma	8
Tracheal trauma	3
Cardiovascular compromise	2
Other	7

personnel to query specifically a difficult airway preoperatively and on arrival in the recovery room. If the condition is present, the critical pathway initiates implementation of a specific protocol that includes in-hospital identification, patient-family teaching, and enrollment in the registry (E. Krenzischek, personal communication to L. M., November 1, 1994). Difficult airway/intubation patient identification also includes a green identification wristband and a patient's chart airway alert label (Fig. 52-5). The wristband contains the Medic Alert insignia with the word "Temporary." This facilitates physician-patient communication and transition from a temporary in-hospital registry to the permanent Medic Alert Registry. Like an allergy alert band, the green difficult airway/intubation band provides continued identification and safety of the patient during hospitalization. The Joint Committee on Clinical Investigations at Johns Hopkins Medical Institutions issued a waiver to written informed consent to place wristbands on identified difficult airway/intubation patients. Health care personnel and patients recognize the tremendous implications for patients' safety (versus breach of confidentiality) as modeled in existing in-hospital allergy alert temporary wristbands and out-of-hospital permanent medical alert bracelets.[13] As mentioned earlier, a dictated difficult airway note is also placed into the patient's electronic medical record for future medical providers.

The registry database information in the Medic Alert enrollment brochure is filled out by the anesthesiologist, and the patient's informed consent and signature are obtained to initiate Medic Alert Foundation personnel completing registry enrollment. Issues of payment are discussed at this time. (See Notes to Practitioner in brochure description IV.C.1.a.)

Implementation at the institutional level should include physicians, nurses, and other health care providers from all areas who identify and treat difficult airway/intubation patients (e.g., anesthesiology, otolaryngology-head and neck surgery, pulmonology, emergency department).

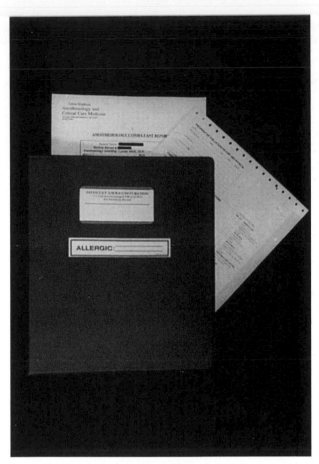

Figure 52-5 Institutional difficult airway/intubation alert label for patient's record.

use of the computerized patient record. In January 1994, the Computer-Based Patient Record Institute announced that it would seek major funding to finalize the development of standards for health care informatics. It seems inevitable, given the current interest and effort by government and private sectors, that a national computerized patient record will become a reality. However, because of the complexity and scope of issues involved, the time frame for accomplishing this goal remains far from certain. The objectives of the registry are in agreement with the organizations supporting development of the computerized patient record. The Medic Alert system (with its centralized and computerized database of medical information accessible by telephone or fax within 5 minutes and with Internet access in development) already embodies many of the concepts of the computerized patient record. Proposals are being developed to allow electronic data transfers while accommodating patients' confidentiality and medical records security through appropriate documentation and encryption techniques. When these safety mechanisms are in place, automated queries of the registry will become possible, obviating the need for telephone calls that interrupt the flow of evaluation of patients in busy outpatient practices. As computerized medical records become more common in preanesthetic evaluation,[9] such automated queries of the registry will become commonplace. Future developments could include supplementary photodocumentation. As development of the computerized patient record continues, Medic Alert's goals and information format will easily mesh with the infrastructure of an emerging computerized patient record.

2. National Level

National implementation of a comprehensive and integrated system for registry enrollment will involve identification of difficult airway/intubation patients at the point of entry into the health care system—physician's office, clinic, ambulatory surgery center, emergency department, or hospital—or during the episode of care (intraoperatively). All enrolled patients will then be readily identified upon reentry into the health care system, independent of time or place.

National availability of registry enrollment forms will be accomplished through distribution by airway equipment manufacturers (Laerdal and others) who have agreed to include registry forms in each box of equipment they ship and through printing the Medic Alert collect phone number on the malignant hyperthermia posters distributed to all anesthesia departments. (Medic Alert is the Malignant Hyperthermia INDEX ZERO hotline.)

Interest has been high for several years in the concept of a national computerized record of patients. In 1991 the Institute of Medicine set a goal of 10 years for widespread

3. International Level

The technologic development of an internationally accessible registry is now quite feasible and can be realized through the cooperative efforts of the Medic Alert Foundation, the World Federation of Societies of Anesthesiologists, and the Society for Technology in Anesthesia. Encryption techniques now easily allow the Internet or alternative commercial packet-switched networks to be used for extremely fast data transmission throughout most of the world. The prodigious advance of technology now makes the required equipment both inexpensive and plentiful. Even where computer technology is lacking, however, enrollment can be accomplished using a telephone, the mail, or the fax machine, and queries can be accomplished by telephone. By 1994, Medic Alert Foundation International existed in more than 35 countries. Attention must be given to disparities in availability of technology. Many countries will be able to implement technically and support a comprehensive system as described earlier; other countries may not. Enrollment can be facilitated with only a pencil and the registry enrollment form (or regular Medic Alert enrollment form).

V. CONCLUSION

There should be three levels of a difficult airway/intubation registry. The first is an in-hospital registry at the hospital where most patients will return for subsequent surgery. The second is Medic Alert National Difficult Airway/Intubation Registry. Both of these will document and disseminate critical airway information about difficult airway/intubation patients in a timely and standardized way to future health care providers. The third level would ultimately be an international level. Implementation of the registry on a national and international scale may improve patients' safety, increase practitioners' security, and facilitate refinement of airway predictors and techniques.

APPENDIX A

ADDRESSES

Completed registry enrollment forms should be mailed to the Medic Alert Foundation, 2323 Colorado Ave., Turlock, CA 95382.

Requests for additional registry enrollment forms should be directed to the Medic Alert Foundation, 2323 Colorado Ave., Turlock, CA 95382.
Phone: 1-800-432-5378
Fax: 1-209-669-2450
Internet: www.medicalert.com

For more information regarding this database:
Lynette Mark, MD, Association Professor, Department of Anesthesiology/Critical Care Medicine, The Johns Hopkins Hospital, 600 N Wolfe St., Tower 711, Baltimore, MD 21287.
Phone: 410-955-0631
Fax: 410-955-0994
lmark@jhmi.edu

James Michelson, M.D., Director of Clinical Informatics, Professor, Orthopaedic Surgery, George Washington University School of Medicine & Health Sciences, Washington, DC 20037
jmichel@jhmi.edu

Lorraine Foley, M.D., Clinical Assistant Professor, Winchester Anesthesia Associates, Winchester Hospital, Tufts School of Medicine, Boston, Massachusetts
ljfoley@comcast.net
phone: 781-729-7243
Fax: 781-756-7135

APPENDIX B

ANESTHESIA ADVISORY COUNCIL OF THE MEDIC ALERT FOUNDATION—1992 TO 1997

Lynette Mark, MD
Charles Beattie, PhD, MD
Charles W. Cummings, MD

Paul W. Flint, MD
Robert Forbes, MD
Gordon Gibby, MD
Paul Goldiner, MD
J.S. Gravenstein, Sr, MD
Martin L. Norton, MD, JD
Andranik Ovassapian, MD, FAC
A. Thomas Pedroni, Jr, Esq
Ellison C. Pierce, Jr, MD
J.G. Reves, MD
James Roberts, MD
Mark C. Rogers, MD
Henry Rosenberg, MD
James F. Schauble, MD
Alan Jay Schwartz, MD, MS Ed
Richard S. Wilbur, MD, JD
John F. Williams, Jr, MD

REFERENCES

1. American Society of Anesthesiologists Committee on Professional Liability: Preliminary study of closed claims. ASA Newslett 52:8, 1988.
2. American Society of Anesthesiologists Task Force on Guidelines for Management of the Difficult Airway: Practice guidelines for management of the difficult airway. Anesthesiology 78:597, 1993.
3. Benumof JL: Management of the difficult adult airway. Anesthesiology 75:1087, 1991.
4. Caplan RA: Anesthetic liability: What it is and what it isn't. In 1992 Review Course Lectures. Cleveland, International Anesthesia Research Society, 1994.
5. Caplan RA, Posner K, Ward RJ, et al: Adverse respiratory events in anesthesia: A closed claims analysis. Anesthesiology 72:828, 1990.
6. Cherian M, Mark L, Schauble J, et al: The National Medic Alert Difficult Airway/Intubation Registry: Patient safety and patient satisfaction [abstract]. Presented at the Annual Meeting of the American Society of Anesthesiologists, San Francisco, Oct 1994.
7. Foley L, Feinstein D, et al: Computerized in-hospital immediate access difficult airway/intubation registry [abstract]. Anesthesiology 83:A1124, 1995.
8. Foley L, Sands D, et al: Effect of difficult airway (DA) registry on subsequent airway management: Experience in the first two years of the DA registry [abstract]. Anesthesiology 89:A1220, 1998.
9. Gibby GL, Jackson KI, Gravenstein JS, et al: Development of problem categories for computerized preanesthesia evaluation of outpatients [abstract]. J Clin Monit 8:156, 1992.
10. Gibby GL, Mark L, Drake J: Effectiveness of Teleforms scanbased input tool for difficult airway registry: Preliminary results [abstract]. Presented at the Annual Meeting of the Society for Technology in Anesthesia, 1995.
11. How to avoid small complaints about quality of care [editorial]. Maryland BPQA (Maryland Board of Physician Quality Assurance) Newslett 1:1, 1993.
12. Mallampati SR, Gatt SP, Gugino LD, et al: A clinical sign to predict difficult intubation: A prospective study. Can Anaesth Soc J 32:429, 1985.

13. Mark L, Beattie C, Ferrell C, et al: The difficult airway: Mechanisms for effective dissemination of critical information. J Clin Anesth 4:247, 1992.

14. Mark L, Drake J: Professional liability and patient safety: The Medic Alert National Difficult Airway/Intubation Registry. Anesthesiol Alert 3:1, 1994.

15. Mark L, Gibby G, Fleisher L, et al: Practice guidelines to clinical practices: Medic Alert Difficult Airway/Intubation Registry [abstract]. Presented at the Annual Meeting of the American Society of Anesthesiologists, 1994.

16. Mark L, Schauble J, Turley S, et al: The Medic Alert National Difficult Airway/Intubation Registry: Technology that pays for itself [abstract]. Presented at the Annual Meeting of the Society for Technology in Anesthesia, 1995.

17. Norton ML (ed): Atlas of the Difficult Airway. St. Louis, Mosby, 1991.

18. Ovassapian A, Krejcie TC, Yelch SJ, et al: Awake fiberoptic intubation in the patient at high risk of aspiration. Br J Anaesth 62:13, 1989.

19. Rose DK, Cohen MM: The airway problem and predictors in 18,500 patients. Can J Anaesth 41:372, 1994.

20. Vaughan RS: Airways revisited. Br J Anaesth 62:1, 1989.

21. Williamson JA, Webb RK, Szekely S, et al: Difficult intubation: An analysis of 2000 incident reports. Anaesth Intensive Care 21:602, 1993.

22. Wilson ME, John R: Problems with the Mallampati sign. Anaesthesia 45:486, 1990.

23. Wilson ME, Spiegelhalter D, Robertson JA, et al: Predicting difficult intubation. Br J Anaesth 61:211, 1988.

53

MEDICAL-LEGAL CONSIDERATIONS: THE ASA CLOSED CLAIMS PROJECT

Karen L. Posner
Robert A. Caplan

I. HISTORICAL PERSPECTIVE

Anesthesiologists have a long-standing appreciation for risks associated with airway management. During the past six decades, a variety of studies have demonstrated that events involving the respiratory system are a prominent cause of adverse outcomes in anesthesia practice.[1,11,16,19,20,26-29] A few examples help illustrate this point. The Anesthesia Study Commission, which investigated anesthesia-related fatalities in metropolitan Philadelphia between 1935 and 1944, identified respiratory factors such as airway obstruction, hypoxia, and aspiration as the probable cause of death in approximately 19% of cases.[27] A large, multicenter study by Beecher and Todd, conducted about a decade later when curare and other muscle relaxants were first entering clinical practice, led to the recognition of excess mortality associated with perioperative respiratory depression.[1] In the 1970s, Utting and

colleagues analyzed a 7-year series of anesthesia accidents reported to the Medical Defence Union of the United Kingdom.[29] Of 227 cases resulting in death or brain damage, 36% involved adverse respiratory events such as esophageal intubation, ventilator misuse, and aspiration.

Critical-incident studies have offered a similar picture. A landmark study of the late 1970s by Cooper and colleagues revealed that 29% of reported incidents were related to respiratory events such as airway mismanagement or failure and misuse of ventilators and breathing circuits.[11] More recently, the Australian Incident Monitoring Study has provided a detailed analysis of the first 2000 cases that have been voluntarily submitted since the late 1980s.[26] In this collection of critical incidents, problems with ventilation accounted for 16% of reports from anesthesiologists in Australia and New Zealand.

II. THE CLOSED CLAIMS PERSPECTIVE

Closed medical malpractice claims represent an important resource for the study of professional liability associated

The opinions expressed herein are those of the authors and do not represent the policy of the American Society of Anesthesiologists.

with airway management. To better appreciate this resource, it is helpful to describe some basic features of claims data.

A medical malpractice claim is a demand for financial compensation by an individual who has sustained injury in connection with medical care. Resolution of a claim usually occurs by either an out-of-court process or litigation. Once a claim is resolved, its file is *closed*. A closed claim file typically contains a broad assortment of documents related to the adverse outcome. These documents may include medical records, narrative statements of the involved health care personnel, expert and peer reviews, deposition summaries, outcome and follow-up reports, and the cost of settlement or jury award.

Claims represent only a small fraction of all adverse outcomes arising from medical care. The Harvard Medical Practice Study of patients in New York State in 1984 reported that approximately 4% of patients sustained an iatrogenic injury during hospitalization.[3] Malpractice claims, however, were filed by only one eighth of all injured patients. Similar findings were described 10 years earlier by the Medical Insurance Feasibility Study in California.[18] These small fractions make it unlikely that claims can be regarded as a representative cross section of all adverse outcomes.

Although claims may not serve as a representative sample of the entire population of adverse outcomes, these cases have a direct and important implication for the study of professional liability: the cost of claims plays an important role in determining the cost of medical malpractice premiums. By studying a large collection of claims, it may be possible to identify types of adverse events that consistently make a large contribution to insurance costs. This information helps focus research and risk management strategies on areas of clinical practice associated with the greatest losses. Successfully reducing losses may lead to lower premiums, with accompanying savings for physicians, patients, and associated third-party participants. Because many types of adverse outcomes are relatively rare, claims files also represent an enriched environment for collecting information about infrequent but catastrophic events. Examining a large set of rare or unusual adverse outcomes with a common theme provides an opportunity to generate hypotheses of causation and remedy that may not be evident to anesthesiologists who experience such cases as isolated events.

Since 1985, the Committee on Professional Liability of the American Society of Anesthesiologists (ASA) has engaged in a structured analysis of closed anesthesia claims in the United States. This undertaking is designated as the ASA Closed Claims Project. Cases involving adverse anesthetic outcomes are retrieved from the closed claims files of 35 U.S. medical-liability insurance carriers who voluntarily participate in this project. Claims for dental injury are not included in this project. In aggregate, the 35 participating carriers provide coverage for approximately 50% of U.S. anesthesiologists. Because several years often elapse between the occurrence of an adverse event and the closure of its associated claim, the majority of cases span an interval from the late 1970s to the mid-1990s. The database now contains more than 6000 cases.

A detailed description of data collection procedures for the Closed Claims Project has been reported previously.[5,9] In brief, each claim file is reviewed by a practicing anesthesiologist, and a standardized form is used to record detailed information on characteristics of patients, surgical procedures, anesthetic agents and techniques, involved personnel, sequence of events, standard of care, critical incidents, clinical manifestations, types of error, responsibility, and outcome. Standard of care is rated on the basis of reasonable and prudent practices at the time of the event. Practice patterns that may have evolved at a later date are not retrospectively applied when the standard of care is rated. An adverse outcome is deemed preventable with better monitoring if the reviewer finds that the use—or better use—of any monitor would probably have prevented the outcome, whether or not such a monitor was available at the time of the event. An acceptable level of interrater reliability has been established for reviewer judgments on the standard of care and preventability of adverse outcomes with better monitoring.[24]

A. PRINCIPAL FEATURES OF ADVERSE RESPIRATORY OUTCOMES AND HIGH-FREQUENCY ADVERSE RESPIRATORY EVENTS

1. Basic Features

Adverse respiratory events constitute the single largest source of injury in the closed claims project (Table 53-1). A detailed analysis of these events was initiated when the database reached a total of 1541 claims.[4] The contrast between adverse respiratory events and other claims was particularly unfavorable. In particular, respiratory-related claims were characterized by a high frequency of devastating outcomes and costly payments (Table 53-2).

Just three mechanisms of injury accounted for nearly two thirds of all claims for adverse respiratory events (Table 53-3). These mechanisms were inadequate ventilation (24% of cases), esophageal intubation (14%), and difficult intubation (DI) (24%). In the 1990s, after the adoption of pulse oximetry and end-tidal CO_2 as monitoring standards, DI (31%) and inadequate ventilation (16%) remained the most common adverse respiratory events, but esophageal intubation (6%) decreased greatly compared with earlier decades (see Table 53-3). The remaining adverse respiratory events were produced by a variety of low-frequency mechanisms including aspiration, airway obstruction, bronchospasm, premature and unintentional extubation, endobronchial intubation, inadequate inspired oxygen delivery, and equipment failure. Special features of low-frequency events are discussed later in this chapter.

Table 53-1 **Most Common Damaging Events**

	Total $n = 6448$	1970s $n = 669$	1980s $n = 2949$	1990s $n = 2718$
Respiratory events	23%	35%	27%	15%
Block related events	15%	10%	12%	20%
Cardiovascular events	12%	11%	11%	12%
Equipment problems	10%	9%	10%	10%
Wrong drug or dose	3%	3%	3%	3%

$N = 6448$.
From ASA Closed Claims Database, 2004.

A detailed display of outcome and payment data for the three most common types of adverse respiratory events is shown in Table 53-4. Death and permanent brain damage were more frequent in claims for inadequate ventilation and esophageal intubation (greater than 90%) than in claims for difficult endotracheal intubation (54%; $P < .05$). Overall, payment for respiratory-related claims ranged from $500 to $11 million (in 1999 dollars). Most claims (69%) resulted in payment. Median payment was highest for inadequate ventilation ($521,000) and lowest for difficult endotracheal intubation ($203,000). Claims for adverse respiratory events generally involved healthy adults undergoing nonemergency surgery with general anesthesia (Table 53-5).

The reviewers judged that better monitoring would have prevented the adverse outcome in 50% of the 1474 claims for adverse respiratory events (Fig. 53-1). This differs from nonrespiratory claims, in which only 9% of cases were judged preventable with better monitoring ($P < .05$). Almost all claims (more than 80%) for inadequate ventilation and esophageal intubation were considered preventable with better monitoring, as opposed to 19% of claims for difficult endotracheal intubation. For the claims considered preventable with better monitoring, the reviewers chose pulse oximetry, capnometry, or both of these devices in most cases. Data on the role of better monitoring in the prevention of adverse outcomes must be interpreted with particular care, as the reviewers were not asked to consider confounding factors such as equipment malfunction, diversion of attention, misinterpretation and misuse of data, or the impact of false-positive and false-negative results. Thus, the reviewers' judgments should be regarded as a near-maximum (and probably unattainable) estimate of the efficacy of better monitoring. It should also be noted that this analysis is based on claims for events that occurred prior to the adoption of pulse oximetry and end-tidal CO_2 as ASA standards.

2. Inadequate Ventilation

The largest class of adverse respiratory events was inadequate ventilation. The distinguishing feature in this group of claims was the reviewer's inability to identify a specific mechanism of injury. In part, the inability to assign a mechanism of injury may reflect uncertainty on the part of the original health care providers. Because most adverse events occurred before the widespread use of pulse oximetry and capnometry, the uncertainty may be due to the limitations of traditional clinical signs such as chest excursion, reservoir bag motion, and breath sounds. With increasing use of quantitative measures

Table 53-2 **Comparison of Respiratory and Nonrespiratory Events**

	Total		1970s		1980s		1990s	
	Respiratory $n = 1474$	All Others $n = 4974$	Respiratory $n = 231$	All Others $n = 438$	Respiratory $n = 810$	All Others $n = 2139$	Respiratory $n = 413$	All Others $n = 2305$
Incidence	23%	77%	35%	65%	27%	73%	15%	85%
Death or brain damage	78%	29%	90%	39%	80%	31%	67%	26%
Preventable	50%	9%	71%	19%	59%	12%	20%	5%
Substandard care	64%	28%	73%	33%	67%	31%	53%	24%
Payment frequency	69%	48%	79%	57%	71%	52%	59%	42%
Median payment (1999 dollars)	$384,000	$110,250	$529,713	$171,750	$409,150	$100,750	$262,040	$108,406

$N = 6448$.
From ASA Closed Claims Database, 2004.

Table 53-3 **Most Common Adverse Respiratory Events as Proportion of All Respiratory Events in Decade**

	Total *n* = 1474	1970s *n* = 231	1980s *n* = 810	1990s *n* = 413
Inadequate ventilation/oxygenation	24%	37%	24%	16%
Difficult intubation	24%	15%	24%	31%
Esophageal intubation	14%	15%	18%	6%
Aspiration	9%	7%	7%	15%
Airway obstruction	8%	6%	9%	8%
Premature extubation	7%	4%	6%	13%
Bronchospasm	4%	7%	5%	3%

Other adverse respiratory events (inadvertent extubation, inadequate fraction of inspired oxygen, endobronchial intubation) exhibited an overall incidence of less than 5% of all respiratory events. *N* = 6448.
From ASA Closed Claims Database, 2004.

of ventilation, fewer cases have been assigned to the category of inadequate ventilation. These events have declined in occurrence from 37% of all respiratory events in the 1970s to 16% in the 1990s (see Table 53-3). It is also possible that a delayed rather than contemporaneous approach to the investigation of adverse outcomes is not powerful enough to provide an understanding of many events.

3. Esophageal Intubation

Prompt detection of esophageal intubation is a primary concern in anesthesia practice. Claims for esophageal intubation decreased considerably in the 1990s (6%) compared with prior decades (see Table 53-3). An in-depth analysis[4] of claims for esophageal intubation found that the detection of esophageal intubation required 5 or more minutes in the majority of cases (97%).

Incompetence and negligence (e.g., intubation performed by a legally blind anesthesiologist or minimal attention to the patient during the first half hour of the case) provide straightforward explanations for delayed detection. However, we found only eight claims (9%) in which this type of obviously inadequate behavior played a primary role.

Why, then, was delayed recognition such a prominent feature in these claims for esophageal intubation? We speculate that reliance on indirect tests of ventilation may have been an important factor contributing to delay. For example, cyanosis is an indirect test of ventilation that might be used as a clue of esophageal intubation. This approach, however, is limited by the insensitivity of the human eye to the changes in skin color that occur during arterial desaturation.[10,12] Furthermore, effective preoxygenation before intubation may extend the time before significant arterial desaturation develops.[17] In this

Table 53-4 **Outcome, Payment, and Frequency for the Most Common Adverse Respiratory Events**

	Inadequate Ventilation *n* = 355	Esophageal Intubation *n* = 208	Difficult Intubation *n* = 359	All Nonrespiratory Events *n* = 4974
Outcome				
Death	67%*	79%*	43%*	20%
Permanent brain damage	27%*	17%*	11%	8%
Payment in 1999 dollars				
Range	$2745-$10,980,000	$16,775-$9,962,000	$573-$8,540,000	$34-$35,960,000
Median	$521,125*	$460,246*	$203,100*	$110,250
Payment frequency	74%*	79%*	62%*	48%

*$P < .05$ compared with nonrespiratory events; *N* = 6448.
From ASA Closed Claims Database, 2004.

Table 53-5   **Basic Clinical Features of Cases Involving Adverse Respiratory Events**

	Respiratory Events $n = 1474$	All Others $n = 4974$
Age in years (mean ± SD)	40.40 ± 21.10	42.89 ± 19.25
ASA 1-2	43%	46%
Emergency	25%	16%
Gender		
Female	55%	60%
Male	44%	40%
Primary anesthetic		
General	88%	60%
Regional	4%	32%
Monitored anesthesia care	3%	3%
Other*	5%	5%

*Includes combined regional and general techniques, anesthesia standby, and nonoperative events involving an anesthetist. $N = 6448$.
ASA, American Society of Anesthesiologists.
From ASA Closed Claims Database, 2004.

Table 53-6   **Major Hemodynamic Derangements Accompanying Esophageal Intubation Claims**

Hemodynamic Derangement	% of Claims $(n = 94)$
Bradycardia	57
Asystole	55
Hypotension	49
Unspecified dysrhythmia	10
Tachycardia	5
Ventricular fibrillation	1

Percentages sum to more than 100 because of multiple derangements. $N = 1541$. From ASA Closed Claims Database, 1990.
Adapted from Caplan RA, Posner KL, Cheney FW, et al: Adverse respiratory events in anesthesia: A closed claims analysis. Anesthesiology 72:828, 1990.

context, it is not surprising that cyanosis preceded the recognition of esophageal intubation in only 34% of cases.

One might also expect cardiovascular clues to accompany hypoxemia or hypercarbia. Indeed, one or more major hemodynamic derangements were recorded in 79 of the 94 claims (84%) for esophageal intubation.

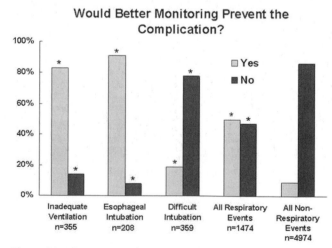

Would Better Monitoring Prevent the Complication?

Figure 53-1 Percentage of adverse respiratory events considered preventable or not preventable by better monitoring. Yes/No bars do not sum to 100% because of claims in which an assessment of preventability could not be made. *$P = .05$ compared with nonrespiratory claims; $N = 6448$. (From ASA Closed Claims Database, 2004.)

In order of frequency, these derangements included bradycardia, asystole, hypotension, unspecified dysrhythmia, tachycardia, and ventricular fibrillation (Table 53-6). It is particularly noteworthy that hemodynamic derangements preceded the recognition of esophageal intubation in 60 claims (65%). One can readily appreciate that the life-threatening nature of such derangements could have drawn effort away from detection of the underlying problem. The severity of the hemodynamic changes also suggests that the respiratory and metabolic consequences of esophageal intubation were so far advanced that some degree of irreversible damage had already occurred. Thus, from the standpoint of timely detection and intervention, skin color and routine hemodynamic measurements do not seem to provide useful clues of esophageal intubation.

Auscultation of breath sounds is another widely used test of ventilation. In this series of claims, breath sound auscultation was documented in 62 of the 94 claims for esophageal intubation (63%). In three of these cases (5%), breath sound auscultation led to a correct diagnosis of esophageal intubation. In 30 cases (48%), auscultation led to the erroneous conclusion that the endotracheal tube (ET) was located in the trachea when it was actually in the esophagus. This result was termed a *misdiagnosis of endotracheal intubation*. The diagnostic error in such cases was recognized in a variety of ways, including later reexamination with direct laryngoscopy, absence of any object in the trachea at the time of an emergency tracheostomy (despite ongoing "ventilation" through an ET), resolution of cyanosis following reintubation (often by a second participant), and discovery of esophageal intubation at autopsy. In 29 of the 62 claims (47%) in which auscultation was documented, the records did not contain sufficient information to determine how the auscultatory findings were interpreted.

The preceding paragraph presents the grim finding that breath sound auscultation was associated with a misdiagnosis of endotracheal intubation in nearly half of cases (48%). Let us try to place these data in a more favorable context by devising an analysis based upon a best-case scenario in which we assume that auscultation led to a correct diagnosis in (1) the 3 cases in which it actually did so, (2) the 29 cases in which the role of auscultation was unclear, and (3) the 32 cases in which there was no information about the use of auscultation. With this approach, the results are still unsettling: misdiagnosis occurred at a rate of 32% (30 out of 94 cases).

Although the limitations of auscultation have been well described previously,[2] this set of claims provided the first evidence for a recurring pattern of risk: *if esophageal intubation has occurred, the use of auscultation to distinguish between endotracheal and esophageal location may delay the restoration of effective ventilation by producing a false impression of correct endotracheal placement.* We do not wish to imply that the risk of auscultation is related primarily to the mechanical act of listening to breath sounds (which is innocuous by itself) or the simple existence of false-positive and false-negative results (which can occur with any test). We speculate that the risk develops when auscultatory findings are obtained in a clinical environment that promotes misinterpretation. The risk of misinterpretation may be greatest when quantitative data from capnometry and oximetry are unavailable and other indirect clues of esophageal intubation (e.g., gastric distention, cyanosis, hemodynamic changes) are not readily evident or not yet manifest.

The most likely setting for misinterpretation of breath sounds is probably the first few minutes following esophageal intubation in the patient who has been adequately preoxygenated during an otherwise uncomplicated induction of general anesthesia. In the context of this transiently benign-appearing state, there may be a tendency to interpret equivocal or ambiguous auscultatory findings as normal. The reasoning process leading to this error might take a course similar to the following: "The breath sounds are somewhat distant, but everything else seems fine. Therefore, the abnormal quality of breath sounds is more likely due to obesity (or has some other underlying condition that can hamper auscultation), rather than esophageal intubation." Because quantitative data from capnometry and oximetry are also subject to misinterpretation, these monitors cannot be regarded as definitive remedies. The fundamental problem is the potential for error that arises from the interaction between preconceived notions of likelihood, reflex clinical behaviors, conflicting environmental data, the potential for a rapid and poorly reversible cascade of critical events, and the inherent limitations of all diagnostic tests (see Chapter 8). The theoretical background for exploring this type of interaction and developing more effective clinical algorithms has been reviewed by Gaba and colleagues.[14,15]

4. Difficult Intubation

Claims for DI were distinguished by a relatively small percentage of cases in which care was considered less than appropriate (46% versus more than 80% for inadequate ventilation and esophageal intubation) and a similarly small percentage of cases in which better monitoring would have prevented the complication (19% versus more than 80% for inadequate ventilation and esophageal intubation). Although these findings seem outwardly favorable, the comparisons are not so attractive from the perspective of risk reduction. If the majority of cases of DI cannot be linked to obvious inadequacies in care or deficiencies in monitoring, it is unlikely that claims analysis alone can point to effective or broad-based remedies. Simulators, algorithms, and drill routines have generated considerable interest in recent years. These newer educational tools and management strategies may provide an important opportunity for clinicians to gain concentrated exposure to relatively infrequent events. An evidence-based guideline for management of the difficult airway (DA) has been developed by the ASA.[25] Key features of this guideline are discussed in Chapter 9.

B. LOW-FREQUENCY ADVERSE RESPIRATORY EVENTS

1. Basic Features

The foregoing discussion has focused on the most common mechanisms of respiratory injury in the closed claims database. A formal study of low-frequency adverse respiratory events was conducted in 1991 when the closed claims database had reached 2046 cases.[8] Although these events are much less common—each category representing no more than 5% of the overall database—sufficient claims have been collected to permit the identification of recurrent themes that may contribute to liability. Five categories of events have been studied in depth, each category containing at least 40 claims and together encompassing 300 claims, or about 15% of the overall database. These categories are airway trauma, pneumothorax, airway obstruction, aspiration, and bronchospasm. Death or brain damage occurred in nearly half (47%) of these cases, and the median payment was $60,000 (Table 53-7). Airway trauma was reanalyzed in detail in 1999.[13]

2. Airway Trauma

Airway trauma was the most common type of low-frequency airway event, accounting for 266 of 4460 claims or 6% of the overall database.[13] DI was associated with 103 of these claims (39%). The most frequent sites of injury were the larynx, pharynx, and esophagus (Table 53-8), together accounting for 70% of injuries associated with airway trauma claims. Esophageal and tracheal injuries were more likely to be associated with DI than other airway trauma claims. In contrast, laryngeal and temporomandibular joint injuries were rarely

Table 53-7 **Low-Frequency Adverse Respiratory Events**

Type of claim	n (% of total)	Death (%)	Brain Damage (%)	Payment Frequency (%)	Median Payment ($)
Airway trauma	97 (4.7)	12	0	60	22,000
Pneumothorax	67 (3.3)	24	10	63	19,000
Airway obstruction	56 (2.7)	64	23	63	300,000
Aspiration	56 (2.7)	45	5	66	60,000
Bronchospasm	40 (1.9)	70	18	53	218,000
All infrequent respiratory*	300 (14.6)	37[†‡]	10[†]	60[†‡]	60,000[†]
Other respiratory	462 (22.6)	70	23	75	233,000
All nonrespiratory	1284 (63.7)	22	9	59	40,000

*Because more than one adverse respiratory event occurred in 16 claims, the total number of claims for 316 events is 300. $P \leq .01$ compared with other respiratory claims ([†]) or nonrespiratory claims ([‡]). N = 2046. From ASA Closed Claims Database, 1991.
Adapted from Cheney FW, Posner KL, Caplan RA, et al: Adverse respiratory events infrequently leading to malpractice suits. A closed claims analysis. Anesthesiology 75:932, 1991.

associated with DI. Pharyngeal and esophageal injuries most commonly consisted of lacerations or perforations leading to mediastinitis or mediastinal abscess. The most common laryngeal injuries included vocal cord paralysis (30 cases), granuloma (15 cases) and arytenoid dislocation (7 cases). None of the 27 temporomandibular joint injuries were associated with DI.

These claims provide several useful insights. Circumstances surrounding DI clearly put the tissues of the pharynx and esophagus at risk. The clinical implication is that patients in whom endotracheal intubation has been difficult should be observed for, or told to watch for, the

development of signs and symptoms of pharyngeal abscess or mediastinitis. Because soft tissue infections may develop slowly over a period of days, an apparent lack of complications in the first few hours after surgery should not be regarded as a definitive outcome in patients who have experienced DI. This is especially important to remember in the ambulatory surgery setting.

Although it is easy to understand how DI may lead to trauma of the larynx, it is less apparent why laryngeal injuries appeared so infrequently associated with DI. The reason for vocal cord paralysis, granuloma, and arytenoid dislocation with routine intubation was not apparent from the data available in the claim file. Similarly, it is curious that temporomandibular joint injury was present only with routine intubation. One might expect that temporomandibular joint injury would be more commonly associated with DI, in which forces applied to the jaw during airway manipulation and laryngoscopy might be more intense or prolonged than those encountered during routine intubation. These observations suggest that many injuries to the larynx and temporomandibular joint may be related to predisposing factors or underlying characteristics of patients that we do not yet understand. A similar phenomenon has been observed in the review of closed claims for peripheral nerve injuries.[7,21]

Table 53-8 **Sites of Airway Trauma**

Location of Injury	Total (% of 266)	Difficult Intubation n (% of site)
Larynx	87 (33%)	17 (20%)*
Pharynx	51 (19%)	26 (51%)
Esophagus	48 (18%)	30 (62%)*
Trachea	39 (15%)	25 (64%)*
Temporomandibular joint	27 (10%)	0 (0%)*
Nasopharynx, nose	13 (5%)	4 (31%)

Distribution of airway trauma sites and presence of concomitant difficult intubation.
*$P \leq .05$ versus other sites combined. N = 4460. From ASA Closed Claims Database, 1999.
Adapted from Domino KB, Posner KL, Caplan RA, et al: Airway injury during anesthesia: A closed claims analysis. Anesthesiology 91:1703, 1999.

3. Pneumothorax

Pneumothorax was the second most common type of low-frequency airway event.[8] Clinical activities that were not directly or clearly related to airway management were associated with 43 of the 67 claims for pneumothorax (64%; Table 53-9). In particular, five types of nerve

Table 53-9 **Clinical Factors Associated with Pneumothorax Claims**

Clinical Factor	Claims	% of Total
Airway related		
Airway instrumentation	13	19
Barotrauma	11	16
Non–airway related		
Regional block	27	40
Central line	5	7
Spontaneous/unknown	5	7
Other	6	9
Total	67	100

N = 2046. From ASA Closed Claims Database, 1991.
Adapted from Cheney FW, Posner KL, Caplan RA, et al: Adverse respiratory events infrequently leading to malpractice suits. A closed claims analysis. Anesthesiology 75:932, 1991.

blocks (supraclavicular, intercostal, stellate ganglion, interscalene, and suprascapular) were responsible for 40% of pneumothorax claims. Airway instrumentation was associated with pneumothorax in 19% of cases. The actual mechanism of pneumothorax was not anatomically proved in most cases but was usually attributed to laryngoscopy, ET placement, or bronchoscopy on the basis of clinical events and reviewer judgments. Barotrauma was the cause of pneumothorax in 11 claims (16%), mostly arising from obstruction of the expiratory limb of a mechanical ventilator or the use of excessive tidal volumes (seven cases).

A notable feature of pneumothorax claims was the marked disparity in outcome between events associated with airway instrumentation and events arising from nerve blocks and central-line placement. In the subset of 24 claims involving airway instrumentation, the outcome in 16 cases (67%) was death or permanent brain damage. In contrast, there were no instances of death or brain damage in the 16 cases of pneumothorax that arose after nerve blocks or central-line placement. We speculate that this difference may be due at least in part to the more rapid compromise of respiratory and circulatory function that occurs under conditions of mechanical ventilation and positive-pressure gas delivery. Not surprisingly, the median payment for pneumothorax associated with nerve block or central-line placement was only $6000 whereas the median payment for cases associated with airway instrumentation was $75,000.

4. Airway Obstruction

Airway obstruction accounted for 56 claims or approximately 3% of the database.[8] Most cases (89%) occurred during general anesthesia. Obstruction was attributed to an upper airway site in 39 claims (70%), although an exact cause or site was identifiable in only half of these claims. Laryngospasm was the most common cause of upper airway obstruction, accounting for 11 (28%) of 39 cases. Other causes of upper airway obstruction included foreign body (four cases), laryngeal polyps (two cases), laryngeal edema (one case), and pharyngeal hematoma (one case). In 10 cases of upper airway obstruction, emergency tracheostomy was performed. Causes of lower airway obstruction (21% of claims) included blood clots or mucous plugs in the tracheal lumen or external compression related to mediastinal tumor masses or blood. ET obstruction accounted for 9% of cases and was attributed to blood clots in the lumen of the ET or kinking of the tube itself. Other factors associated with claims for airway obstruction included concurrent DI (17 cases, 30%), operation on the airway (13 cases, 23%), and pediatric age group (10 cases, 18%). The outcome in almost all claims for airway obstruction (87%) was death or brain damage.

5. Aspiration

Claims for aspiration accounted for 3% of the database (56 cases).[8] Almost all cases (95%) occurred in patients who received general anesthesia. The aspirated material was gastric contents in 88% of cases; other cases involved aspiration of blood, pus, or teeth. Approximately one third (34%) of aspirations took place during anesthetic induction just prior to endotracheal intubation (34%). In six of these cases, aspiration occurred during a rapid sequence induction; in another six, the aspiration occurred under circumstances in which the reviewer believed that a rapid sequence induction was indicated but not used. Another one third of aspiration cases (36%) took place during the maintenance phase of mask general anesthetic. Of note, only two cases occurred (4%) during the maintenance phase of general endotracheal anesthesia. Aspiration occurred in one of these cases when the ET was removed to facilitate the passage of a nasogastric tube. In the other case, aspiration occurred while an ET with a leaking cuff was being replaced with a new tube. The remaining cases took place during emergence from anesthesia (18%).

Two clinical factors—pregnancy and emergency surgical status—were particularly prevalent in claims for aspiration. Obstetric patients account for 12% of the overall database but represent 29% of all aspiration claims (P = .05). Emergency surgery patients account for 19% of the database but represent 45% of all aspiration claims (P = .01). It is also noteworthy that 23% of aspiration claims involved a problem with airway management such as DI (nine cases) or esophageal intubation (four cases). This relationship was previously reported by Olsson and colleagues.[22]

Overall, aspiration accounted for only 3% of claims in the database. In terms of contemporary experience, this is consistent with the observation by Warner and colleagues[30] that the incidence of aspiration in more than 200,000 patients who underwent elective and emergency surgery between 1985 and 1991 was very low (1 in 3216). These observations suggest that current strategies to prevent aspiration in the United States are generally successful. It is interesting to contrast this picture with the findings of Tiret and colleagues' prospective survey[28] of anesthesia complications in France between 1972 and 1982. This large study identified 163 complications that were totally attributable to anesthesia. Among these, aspiration accounted for 17% of all complications and 30% of complications that were specifically related to respiratory events. Moreover, almost 50% of cases in the Tiret series occurred in the postanesthetic period. This high incidence of aspiration in the Tiret study has been attributed to a lack of postanesthetic care units in French hospitals during the years encompassed by the study.[28]

6. Bronchospasm

Adverse outcomes arising from bronchospasm accounted for 40 claims or almost 2% of the database.[8] Most of these claims (80%) occurred during the administration of general anesthesia as the primary anesthetic technique. Nearly half (48%) of the patients had a medical history that included at least one of the following: asthma, chronic obstructive pulmonary disease, or smoking. In cases involving the administration of general anesthesia, the first occurrence of bronchospasm was more often at the time of intubation (69%) than during maintenance (25%) or emergence (6%).

Twenty percent of claims for bronchospasm were associated with the conduct of regional anesthesia (RA). In most of these cases, bronchospasm occurred during cesarean section when endotracheal intubation was required for management of a failed block or a high block in a patient with a history of asthma. These cases illustrate the concept that RA does not in itself obviate the risk associated with intraoperative management of reactive airway disease. In particular, the risk of bronchospasm may be especially pronounced in this setting because relatively modest doses of intravenous agents are often employed in an effort to minimize anesthetic effects on the fetus.

Bronchospasm claims were also notable in cases that involved a difficult differential diagnosis. The claims files indicated that clinicians had difficulty distinguishing between bronchospasm and the presence of esophageal intubation (six cases) or pneumothorax (four cases). End-tidal carbon dioxide concentration was not used in any of the six cases in which the failure to make a correct and timely differential diagnosis between esophageal intubation and bronchospasm led to an adverse outcome. Because end-tidal carbon dioxide is now an ASA standard for verification of ET placement, it is possible that this pathway of injury will become less common. However, it is important to recognize that failure to differentiate between bronchospasm and esophageal intubation may still occur in cases in which bronchospasm is so severe that ventilation is impossible and carbon dioxide cannot reach the detector in clinically useful amounts. In this circumstance, fiberoptic bronchoscopy might prove helpful.

C. EMERGING TRENDS FROM THE ASA CLOSED CLAIMS PROJECT

The database of the closed claims project is now sufficiently large that it can be studied for evidence of changing trends in the overall distribution of adverse events and outcomes. In doing so, two key limitations must be emphasized. First, these data cannot be used to generate any general estimates of risk. This limitation arises from a lack of denominator data, a probable bias toward severe outcomes, and partial reliance on the observations of direct participants. Second, the resolution of a claim is a lengthy process. Typically, this leads to a delay of about 5 years between the occurrence of a claim and its entry into the database. Thus, the most recent trends (which are usually of greatest interest) must be viewed as especially tentative because they may show considerable change as additional claims are resolved and processed.

In 1999, an examination of trends was conducted.[5] At that point the database consisted of more than 4000 claims drawn from 35 U.S. insurance organizations. Two major trends were evident. The first trend involved the severity of injury. This showed a general decrease and was specifically characterized by a declining incidence of claims for death and brain damage. Between 1970 and 1979, for example, 56% of claims involved death or brain damage. In contrast, death and brain damage accounted for only 31% of claims that occurred in 1990 to 1994. Second, the contribution of adverse respiratory events to death and brain damage was declining. During the earliest interval between 1970 and 1979, 56% of claims for death and brain damage arose from respiratory system events. This percentage decreased to 49% between 1980 and 1989 and further decreased to 38% in the group of claims occurring from 1990 onward.

Some tentative associations in this trend can be postulated. In the 1990s, there were several changes in monitoring and clinical practice that may have had an impact on adverse respiratory events. Pulse oximetry and end-tidal capnometry have been widely available since the mid-1980s. Moreover, the ASA Standards for Basic Intra-Operative Monitoring specify the use of pulse oximetry for basic intraoperative monitoring (as of January 1, 1990) and end-tidal CO_2 for verification of endotracheal intubation (as of January 1, 1991).

Is the presence of these monitors reflected in the pattern of liability for closed claims? This question was explored in 2002 when the overall database contained 5480 cases.[6] Claims for death and brain damage in the

1980s and 1990s were compared ($n = 1870$). Respiratory events declined from 48% to 23% of death and brain damage claims. A focused examination of the three most common adverse respiratory events (inadequate ventilation, esophageal intubation, and DI) revealed an important pattern. In aggregate, these outcomes constituted 34% of the 1980s death and brain damage claims. In the 1990s, death and brain damage associated with inadequate ventilation and esophageal intubation declined from 25% to 9%. This decline was seen in claims in which end-tidal CO_2 or oxygen saturation or both were monitored.

As mentioned previously, evidence-based guidelines for management of the DA have been developed by the ASA.[25] The impact of this set of guidelines on claims involving DA management has been studied in the closed claims project. DA problems were encountered during all phases of anesthesia management, including preinduction, induction, maintenance, emergence, postanesthetic care unit (PACU) care, and intensive care unit settings.[23] Death and brain damage were more common in DA claims arising from non-operating room/PACU locations as well as in the setting of difficult mask ventilation, "cannot intubate, cannot ventilate" emergencies, and persistent intubation attempts.[23]

Clinicians often worry that the proliferation of practice guidelines will lead to a general increase in liability. It is important to remember that modern, evidence-based guidelines have a relatively flexible place in medical practice that differs from that of standards. Standards are typically used for straightforward aspects of care that command high levels of agreement and acceptance. Noncompliance implies an action that is outside a clearly recognized norm; in some instances, such actions may be accompanied by sanctions. Guidelines are employed for more complex aspects of care that cannot be precisely codified and accepted in a near-uniform fashion. Thus guidelines are intended as *recommendations* that can assist the anesthesiologist and the patient in making decisions about health care. Guidelines may be accepted, modified, or even rejected according to specific clinical needs and constraints. This means that not following a guideline, under some clinical conditions, can still be a decision that is consistent with reasonable and prudent practice. In DA malpractice claims, the ASA guideline for management of the DA was rarely an issue in litigation. In the few claims in which the guideline was a factor, it was used for the defense more often than the plaintiff.[23]

III. CONCLUSION

The database of the ASA Closed Claims Project indicates that adverse events involving the respiratory system continue to constitute an important source of liability in anesthetic practice. These events represent a particularly urgent target for research and preventive strategies because they are characterized by a high frequency of severe outcomes and costly payments.

Inadequate ventilation and DI account for nearly half of all adverse respiratory events. The occurrence of injuries related to inadequate ventilation has been decreasing, but DI remains a recurring problem. The use of capnography to confirm ET placement seems to have reduced the severity of outcomes associated with delayed recognition of esophageal intubation.

The in-depth analysis of low-frequency respiratory events also provides valuable lessons. Complications associated with airway trauma may not manifest in the immediate postoperative period. This suggests that explicit follow-up plans and communication are particularly important for outpatients who have experienced airway management difficulties. Severe bronchospasm is not a common cause of claims in the overall database, but the desire to minimize fetal exposure to anesthetic agents may be a factor leading to a relatively high incidence of bronchospasm claims in obstetric patients receiving general anesthesia for cesarean section.

Overall, reviewers have found that most claims involving adverse respiratory events might have been prevented by the use of pulse oximetry and capnography (either alone or in combination). Because most claims took place before the widespread use of these two monitors, it is difficult to know whether this perception is accurate in its own right or a reflection of wishful hindsight and unrealistic expectations. Tentative support for a preventive role comes from the observation that adverse respiratory events constitute a decreasing proportion of database claims, particularly for claims occurring in the 1990s.

ACKNOWLEDGMENTS

The Closed Claims Project is supported by funds from the American Society of Anesthesiologists. The project committee gratefully acknowledges the contributions of insurance companies who have granted access to closed claims files and the members of the American Society of Anesthesiologists who have served as reviewers of closed claims and participants in studies of peer review.

REFERENCES

1. Beecher HK, Todd DP: A study of the deaths associated with anesthesia and surgery based on a study of 599,548 anesthesias in ten institutions, 1948-1952, inclusive. Ann Surg 140:2, 1954.

2. Birmingham PK, Cheney FW, Ward RJ: Esophageal intubation: A review of detection techniques. Anesth Analg 65:886, 1986.

3. Brennan TA, Leape LL, Laird NM, et al: Incidence of adverse events and negligence in hospitalized patients: Results of the Harvard Medical Practice Study I. N Engl J Med 324:370, 1991.

4. Caplan RA, Posner KL, Ward RJ, et al: Adverse respiratory events in anesthesia: A closed claims analysis. Anesthesiology 72:828, 1990.

5. Cheney FW: The American Society of Anesthesiologists Closed Claims Project. What have we learned, how has it affected practice, and how will it affect practice in the future? Anesthesiology 91:552, 1999.

6. Cheney FW: Changing trends in anesthesia-related death and permanent brain damage. Am Soc Anesthesiol Newslett 66(6):6, 2002.

7. Cheney FW, Domino KB, Caplan RA, et al.: Nerve injury associated with anesthesia: A closed claims analysis. Anesthesiology 90:1062, 1999.

8. Cheney FW, Posner KL, Caplan RA: Adverse respiratory events infrequently leading to malpractice suits: A closed claims analysis. Anesthesiology 75:932, 1991.

9. Cheney FW, Posner K, Caplan RA, et al: Standard of care and anesthesia liability. JAMA 261:1599, 1989.

10. Comroe JH Jr, Botelho S: The unreliability of cyanosis in the recognition of arterial anoxemia. Am J Med Sci 214:1, 1947.

11. Cooper JB, Newbower RS, Long CH, et al: Preventable anesthetic mishaps: A study of human factors. Anesthesiology 49:399, 1978.

12. Coté CJ, Goldstein EA, Coté MA, et al: A single-blind study of pulse oximetry in children. Anesthesiology 68:184, 1988.

13. Domino KB, Posner KL, Caplan RA, et al.: Airway injury during anesthesia: A closed claims analysis. Anesthesiology 91:1703, 1999.

14. Gaba DM: Human error in anesthetic mishaps. Int Anesthesiol Clin 27:137, 1989.

15. Gaba DM, Maxwell M, DeAnda A: Anesthetic mishaps: Breaking the chain of accident evolution. Anesthesiology 66:670, 1987.

16. Harrison GC: Death attributable to anaesthesia: A ten-year survey, 1967-1976. Br J Anaesth 50:1041, 1978.

17. Heller ML, Watson TR Jr: Polarographic study of arterial oxygenation during apnea in man. N Engl J Med 264:326, 1961.

18. Hiatt HH, Barnes BA, Brennan TA, et al: A study of medical injury and medical malpractice: An overview. N Engl J Med 321:480, 1989.

19. Holland R: Anaesthesia-related mortality in Australia. Int Anesthesiol Clin 22:61, 1984.

20. Keenan RL, Boyan CP: Cardiac arrest due to anesthesia: A study of incidence and causes. JAMA 253:2373, 1985.

21. Kroll DA, Caplan RA, Posner K, et al: Nerve injury associated with anesthesia. Anesthesiology 73:202, 1990.

22. Olsson GL, Hallen B, Hambraeus-Jonzon K: Aspiration during anaesthesia: A computer-aided study of 185,358 anaesthetics. Acta Anaesthesiol Scand 30:84, 1986.

23. Peterson GN, Damino KB, Caplan RA, et al: Management of the difficult airway. A closed claims analysis. Anesthesiology 103:33, 2005.

24. Posner KL, Sampson PD, Caplan RA, et al: Measuring interrater reliability among multiple raters: An example of methods for nominal data. Stat Med 9:1103, 1990.

25. Practice guidelines for management of the difficult airway: An updated report by the American Society of Anesthesiologists Task Force on Management of the Difficult Airway. Anesthesiology 98:1269, 2003.

26. Russell WJ, Webb RK, Van Der Walt JH, et al: Problems with ventilation: An analysis of 2000 incident reports. Anaesth Intensive Care 21:617, 1993.

27. Ruth HS, Haugen FP, Grove DD: Anesthesia Study Commission: Findings of eleven years' activity. JAMA 135:881, 1947.

28. Tiret L, Desmonts JM, Hatton F, et al: Complications associated with anaesthesia: A prospective survey in France. Can Anaesth Soc J 33:336, 1986.

29. Utting JE, Gray TC, Shelly FC: Human misadventure in anaesthesia. Can Anaesth Soc J 26:472, 1979.

30. Warner MA, Warner ME, Weber JG: Clinical significance of pulmonary aspiration during the perioperative period. Anesthesiology 78:56, 1993.

INDEX

Note: Page numbers followed by f refer to figures; those followed by t refer to tables; and those followed by b refer to boxed material.

G